Umphred's
NEUROLOGICAL REHABILITATION

Seventh Edition

Umphred's NEUROLOGICAL REHABILITATION

Rolando T. Lazaro, PT, PhD, DPT
Associate Professor
Department of Physical Therapy
College of Health and Human Services
California State University, Sacramento
Sacramento, California

Sandra G. Reina-Guerra, PT, DPT, MS
Board Certified Pediatric Clinical Specialist
Physical and Occupational Therapy
Shriners Hospital for Children—Northern California
Sacramento, California

Myla U. Quiben, PT, PhD, DPT, MS
Board Certified Neurologic Clinical Specialist
Board Certified Geriatric Clinical Specialist
Associate Professor and Interim Chair
Department of Physical Therapy
University of North Texas Health Science Center
Fort Worth, Texas

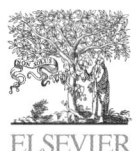

ELSEVIER

Elsevier
3251 Riverport Lane
St. Louis, Missouri 63043

UMPHRED'S NEUROLOGICAL REHABILITATION, SEVENTH EDITION   ISBN: 978-0-323-61117-6

Previous editions copyrighted 2013, 2007, 2001, 1995, 1990, 1985.

Library of Congress Control Number: 2019939395

Senior Content Strategist: Lauren Willis
Content Development Specialist: Lisa Barnes
Publishing Services Manager: Catherine Jacksom
Senior Project Manager: Sharon Corell
Design Direction: Patrick Ferguson

Printed in Canada

Last digit is the print number: 9   8   7   6   5   4   3   2   1

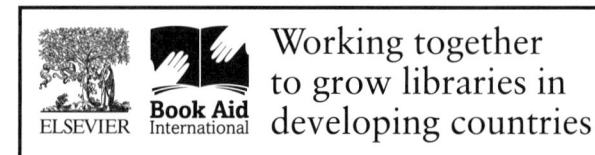

We dedicate this book to Dr. Darcy Umphred, who has inspired generations of physical and occupational therapists to ask brave questions, to trust in the wisdom of patients, and to value acts of kindness both large and small. The work completed for this seventh edition is an expression of the gratitude we feel for Darcy's devotion to the rehabilitation professions. The host of esteemed colleagues who have contributed their knowledge to this edition is a testimony to Darcy's legacy in the neurologic rehabilitation community.

RTL, SRG, MQ

Personally, to me this book has signified love, dedication, commitment, perseverance, resilience, grit, kindness, and understanding—all of which I have learned from my mother. I dedicate this book and all that it stands for to her.

RTL

I would like to dedicate the work on this book to my husband, Mario, and to our children young and old. The gratitude I have for your love and support was the purest motivation, from beginning to end. To Davis Reina-Guerra, when you went away to college, you gave up your bedroom for my office and shared with me your passion for neuroscience—sparking my own, again. Thank you for lending me your keen student's eye and perspective during the editing process.

SRG

To Diana and Eric, for all the times you've both supported me to pursue my passions of learning and for joining me in all my adventures. To Mom and Dad, for instilling a love for reading, grit, and kindness. This is for you. For all my students and UNTHSC colleagues who continue to push me to be a better teacher, leader, and human being: I'm up for the challenge.

MQ

CONTRIBUTORS

Paula M. Ackerman, MS, OTR/L
Program Manager
SCI Post-Acute
Shepherd Center
Atlanta, Georgia

Diane D. Allen, PT, PhD
Professor
Graduate Program in Physical Therapy
University of California San Francisco/San Francisco State University
San Francisco, California

Leslie K. Allison, PhD, PT
Retired [Associate Professor]
Department of Physical Therapy
Winston-Salem State University
Winston-Salem, North Carolina

Myrtice B. Atrice, PT, DPT, CLT
Clinical Manager
Spinal Cord Injury
Shepherd Center, Inc.
Atlanta, Georgia

Joyce Ann, OTR/L
Occupational Therapist
Guild Certified Feldenkrais Practitioner (GCFP)
Highland Park, Illinois

Ronald Barredo, PT, DPT, EdD, FAPTA
Board-Certified Clinical Specialist in Geriatric Physical Therapy
Dean and Professor
College of Health Sciences
Tennessee State University
Nashville, Tennessee

Mark David Basco, PT, DPT
Board-Certified Clinical Specialist in Geriatric Physical Therapy
Certified Exercise Expert for Aging Adults
Director of Physical Therapy
Muenster Memorial Hospital
Muenster, Texas
Lecturer
College of Allied Medical Professions
University of the Philippines Manila
Manila, Philippines

Amy J. Bastian, PhD, PT
Chief Science Officer
Director
Motion Analysis Laboratory Kennedy Krieger Institute
Baltimore, Maryland

Joanna C. Beachy, MD, PhD
Pediatrics, Neonatology
Cohen Children's Medical Center
New Hyde Park, New York
Professor of Pediatrics
Donald and Barbara Zucjer School of Medicine at Hofstra-Northwell
Hempstead, New York

Janet R. Bezner, PT, DPT, PhD, FAPTA
National Board Certified Health and Wellness Coach
Associate Professor
Department of Physical Therapy and Athletic Training
Texas State University
Round Rock, Texas

Elissa C. Held Bradford, PT, PhD
Board Certified Neurologic Clinical Specialist
Board Certified in Multiple Sclerosis
Assistant Professor
Physical Therapist
Doisy College of Health Sciences
Department of Physical Therapy and Athletic Training
Saint Louis University
Saint Louis, Missouri

Annie Burke-Doe, PT, MPT, PhD
Dean/Program Director
Department of Physical Therapy
West Coast University
Los Angeles, California

Nancy N. Byl, PT, MPH, PhD, FAPTA
Professor Emeritus
University of California, San Francisco
School of Medicine
Department of Physical Therapy and Rehabilitation Science
San Francisco, California

Heather Campbell, PT, DPT, MA, OCS (Emerita)
Affiliate Faculty
School of Physical Therapy
Rueckert-Hartman College for Health Professions
Regis University
Denver, Colorado

Laurie Ruth Chaikin, OD, OTR/L, FCOVD
Optometrist and Occupational Therapist
Private Practice
Walnut Creek, California

Doris Chong, BScPT, MSc, DScPT
Freelance Physiotherapist and Lecturer
Hong Kong, Hong Kong

Alain Claudel, PT, DPT
Clinical Electrophysiologic Certified Specialist
Rehabilitation Services
Community Hospital of the Monterey Peninsula
Monterey, California

Elizabeth (Lisa) D'Angelo, PhD, CCC-SLP
Assistant Professor
Communication Sciences and Disorders
College of Health and Human Services
California State University, Sacramento
Licensed Speech-Language Pathologist
Mercy General Hospital
Sacramento, California
Licensed Speech-Language Pathologist
Davis Joint Unified School District
Davis, California

Judith A. Dewane, MHS, DSc
Board Certified Neurologic Clinical Specialist
Associate Professor
Doctor of Physical Therapy
Department of Orthopedics and Rehab Medicine
University of Wisconsin—Madison School of Medicine and Public
    Health
Madison, Wisconsin

Deborah S. Diaz, PT, MA, PhD
Associate Professor
Doctor of Physical Therapy Program
Mary Baldwin University
Fishersville, Virginia

Susan V. Duff, PT, EdD, MPT, OT/L
Certified Hand Therapist
Associate Professor
Department of Physical Therapy
Crean College of Health and Behavioral Science
Chapman University
Irvine, California

Domenique Hendershot Embrey, OTD, MS, OTR/L
Assistant Professor
Department of Occupational Therapy
Samuel Merritt University
Oakland, California

Kenda Fuller, BS Physical Therapy
Co-owner
South Valley Physical Therapy, PC
Private Practice
Denver, Colorado

Mary Lou Anne Galantino, PT, MS, PhD, FNAP, FAPTA
Distinguished Professor of Physical Therapy
Program in Physical Therapy
Stockton University
Galloway, New Jersey
Adjunct Research Scholar
School of Medicine
University of Pennsylvania
Philadelphia, Pennsylvania
Visiting Professor
School of Health Sciences
University of Witwatersrand
Johannesburg, Gauteng, South Africa

Miguel Garcia, MSPT, DPT
Assistant Professor
University of St. Augustine for Health Sciences, Miami Campus
Miami, Florida

William J. Garcia, PT, DPT, OCS, FAAOMPT
Board Certified Orthopedic Clinical Specialist
Assitant Professor
Department of Physical Therapy
College of Health and Human Services
California State University, Sacramento
Sacramento, California

Ellen M. Godwin, PT, PhD, PCS
Adjunct Associate Professor
Department of Physical Therapy
Long Island University
Director
Human Performance Laboratory
State University of New York Downstate Medical Center
Research Physical Therapist
New York Harbor Health Care System
New York City Veterans Administration Medical Center
Brooklyn, New York

Edward James Gorgon, MPhysio, BSPT
Associate Professor
Department of Physical Therapy
University of the Philippines Manila
Manila, Philippines

Lenin C. Grajo, PhD, OTR/L
Director
Post-Professional Doctor of Occupational Therapy Program
Assistant Professor
Programs in Occupational Therapy
Department of Rehabilitation and Regenerative Medicine
Vagelos College of Physicians and Surgeons
Columbia University
New York, New York

Teresa Gutierrez, PT, MS
Pediatric Physical Therapy
Lakewood, Washington

Julia M. Guzman, OTD/OTR/L
Faculty Specialist
Department of Occupational Therapy
University of Scranton
Springfield, New Jersey

Rebecca Hammad, MHS, OTR/L, CLT
Therapy Manager
Post Acute Spinal Cord Injury Program
Shepherd Center
Atlanta, Georgia

John D. Heick, PT, PhD, DPT, OCS, NCS, SCS
Associate Professor
Department of Physical Therapy and Athletic Training
Northern Arizona University
Flagstaff, Arizona

Janet A. Hiley, MS, OTR/L, MBSR
Faculty Emerita
Cabrillo College Stroke Center
Cabrillo College
Aptos, California

Kristin Horn, PT, DPT, NCS
Physical Therapist
Rancho Los Amigos National Rehabilitation Center
Downey, California

Lauren F. Hurt, PT, DPT
Board Certified Neurologic Clinical Specialist
Energy Rehab
Pleasant Gap, Pennsylvania

Kristen Ikeda, PT, DPT, NCS
Board Certified Neurologic Clinical Specialist
Walnut Creek, California

Jennifer L. Keller, MS, PT
Senior Physical Therapist
Center for Movement Studies
Kennedy Krieger Institute
Baltimore, Maryland

Sheri Kiami, DPT, MS
Board Certified Neurologic Clinical Specialist
Associate Clinical Professor
Physical Therapy, Movement, and Rehabilitation Sciences
Northeastern University
Boston, Massachusettes

David M. Kietrys, PT, PhD, OCS, FCPP
Associate Professor and Assistant Vice-Chair
Rehabilitation and Movement Sciences
Blackwood Campus (DPT Program—South)
Rutgers Doctor of Physical Therapy Program—South
Blackwood, New Jersey

Laurie A. King, PhD, PT
Associate Professor
Neurology
Oregon Health & Science University
Portland, Oregon

Rolando T. Lazaro, PT, PhD, DPT
Associate Professor
Department of Physical Therapy
College of Health and Human Services
California State University, Sacramento
Sacramento, California

Sophie Lefmann, PhD, PT
Board Certified Neurologic Clinical Specialist
Lecturer in Physiotherapy (Paediatrics)
School of Health Sciences
University of South Australia
Adelaide, Australia

Rachel M. Lopez, PT, MPT, NCS
Physical Therapy Specialist
Barrow Neurological Institute
St. Joseph's Hospital
Phoenix, Arizona

Marilyn MacKay-Lyons, PT, PhD
Professor
School of Physiotherapy
Dalhousie University
Affiliated Scientist
Physical Medicine
QEII Health Sciences Centre
Halifax, Nova Scotia,Canada

Martina Mancini, PhD
Assistant professor
Neurology
Oregon Health & Science University
Portland, Oregon

Rossniel Marinas, PT, DPT, c/NDT
Board Certified Pediatric Clinical Specialist
Neuro-Developmental Treatment Clinician
Special Olympics (FUNfitness) Clinical Director
Assistant Professor—Doctor of Physical Therapy Program
University of St. Augustine For Health Sciences-Miami Campus
Miami, Florida

Rachel McAhren, BS, DPT
Physical Therapist
Pediatric Physical Therapy—Kids on the Move
Gainesville, Florida

Rochelle Mclaughlin, MS, OTR/L, MBSR
Adjunct faculty
Department of Occupational Therapy
San Jose State University
San Jose, California

Marsha Melnick, PT, PhD
Retired

Nicole Miranda, PT, DPT
Affiliate Faculty
School of Physical Therapy
Rueckert-Hartman College for Health Professions
Regis University
Denver, Colorado
Adjunct Faculty
School of Physical Therapy
South College
Knoxville, Tennessee

Brian M. Moore, PT, DPT
Board Certified Neurologic Clinical Specialist
Assistant Professor
Department of Physical Therapy
College of Health and Human Services
California State University, Sacramento
Sacramento, California

Susanne M. Morton, PT, PhD
Associate Professor
Department of Physical Therapy
University of Delaware
Newark, Delaware

Preeti Nair, PT, PhD
Associate Professor
Department of Physical Therapy
Samuel Merritt University
Oakland, California

Emily Nguyen, BSc, MScPT
School of Physiotherapy
Dalhousie University
Halifax, Nova Scotia, Canada

Preeti Deshpande Oza, PT, PhD, NCS
Board Certified Neurologic Clinical Specialist
Associate Professor
Department of Physical Therapy
Thomas J. Long School of Pharmacy and Health Sciences
University of the Pacific
Stockton, California

Elizabeth Pharo, PT, BSPT
Board Certified Neurologic Clinical Specialist
SCI Therapy Education Coordinator and CCCE
Spinal Cord Injury
Shepherd Center
Atlanta, Georgia

Darbi Breath Philibert, LOTR, OT
Occupational Therapist
New Orleans, Louisiana

Myla U. Quiben, PT, PhD, DPT, MS
Board Certified Neurologic Clinical Specialist
Board Certified Geriatric Clinical Specialist
Associate Professor and Interim Chair
Department of Physical Therapy
University of North Texas Health Science Center
Fort Worth, Texas

Sandra G. Reina-Guerra, PT, DPT, MS
Board Certified Pediatric Clinical Specialist
Physical and Occupational Therapy
Shriners Hospital for Children—Northern California
Sacramento, California

Margaret L. Roller, PT, MS, DPT
Professor
Department of Physical Therapy
California State University, Northridge
Northridge, California

Angela Rusher, PT, DPT
Board Certified Neurologic Clinical Specialist
Instructor/Assistant Director of Clinical Education
Department of Physical Therapy
Samuel Merritt University
Oakland, California

Susan D. Ryerson, PT, DSc
Making Progress: Neurologic Physical Therapy
Falls Church, Virginia
Research Scientist
Medstar National Rehabilitation Hospital
Washington, District of Columbia

Yasser Salem, PT, PhD, NCS, PCS
Board Certified Neurologic Clinical Specialist
Board Certified Pediatric Clinical Specialist
Professor
Department of Physical Therapy
University of North Texas Health Science Center
Fort Worth, Texas
Lecturer
Faculty of Physiotherapy
Cairo University
Cairo, Egypt

Elizabeth Sasso-Lance, PT, DPT
Board Certified Neurologic Clinical Specialist
Clinical Research Physical Therapist
Crawford Research Institute
Shepherd Center
Atlanta, Georgia

Dale Scalise-Smith, PT, DPT, PhD
Professor, Emeritus
Department of Physical Therapy
Utica College
Utica, New York

Osa Jackson Schulte, PT, PhD
Guild Certified Feldenkrais Practitioner/Assistant Trainer (GCFP/AT)
Executive Director and Continuity Assistant Trainer
Feldenkrais Professional Training Program
Movement and Healing Center
Clarkson, Michigan

Claudia R. Senesac, PT, MHS, PhD, PCS
Board Certified Pediatric Clinical Specialist
Clinical Professor
Universiity of Florida
Gainesville, Florida

Eunice Yu Chiu Shen, PT, PhD, DPT
Board Certified Pediatric Clinical Specialist (PCS)
Physical Therapy Consultant
Physical Therapy Services and Volunteer Coordinator
Rainwater Foundation
Monterey Park, California
Physical Therapy Education Coordinator
Medical Therapy Program
Department of Public Health
Children's Medical Services, County of Los Angeles
El Monte, California

Timothy J. Smith, RPh, PhD
Professor Emeritus
University of the Pacific
Thomas J. Long School of Pharmacy and Health Sciences
Stockton, California

Kerri Sowers, PT, DPT, PhD, NCS
Board Certified Neurologic Clinical Specialist
Assistant Professor of Health Science
School of Health Sciences
Stockton University
Galloway, New Jersey

Corrie J. Stayner, MS, PT
Physical Therapist
Barrow Neurological Institute
Phoenix, Arizona
Adjunct Faculty
Physical Therapy Program
Arizona School of Health Sciences
AT Still University
Mesa, Arizona

James Stephens, PT, PhD
Guild Certified Feldenkrais Practitioner (GCFP)
Movement Learning and Rehab
Havertown, Pennsylvania

Bradley W. Stockert, PT, PhD
Professor
Department of Physical Therapy
College of Health and Human Services
Califorinia State University, Sacramento
Sacramento, California

Jane K. Sweeney, PT, MS, PhD, FAPTA
Board Certified Pediatric Clinical Specialist
Professor and Program Director
Pediatric Science
Rocky Mountain University of Health Professions
Provo, Utah
President
Pediatric Rehab Northwest, LLC
Gig Harbor, Washington

Stacey E. Szklut, MS, OLTR/L
Executive Director
South Shore Therapies
Weymouth/Pembroke/Norwood, Massachusetts

Marcia Hall Thompson, PT, DPT, DSc
Assistant Professor
Department of Physical Therapy
Alvernia University
Reading, Pennsylvania

Heidi Truman, CPO
Orthotist
Orthopedic Surgery
University of California, San Francisco
San Francisco, California

Karla M. Tuzzolino, PT, DPT
Board Certified Neurologic Clinical Specialist
Physical Therapist
Mercy Gilbert Medical Center
Gilbert, Arizona
Adjunct Faculty
Physical Therapy Program
Arizona School of Health Sciences
AT Still University
Mesa, Arizona

Darcy A. Umphred, PT, PhD, FAPTA
Emeritus Professor and Retired Chair
Department of Physical Therapy
Thomas J. Long School of Pharmacy and Health Science
University of the Pacific
Stockton, California

Jeric Uy, PhD, PT
School of Health Science
Lecturer in Physiotherapy (Rehabilitation)
University of South Australia
Adelaide, South Australia

Erin Vestal, PT, DPT, MPH, PhD (c)
Board Certified Geriatric Clinical Specialist
Certified Dementia Practitioner
Academic Coordinator of Clinical Education
Assistant Professor
University of St. Augustine for Health Sciences
Miami, Florida

Arvie Vitente, PT, DPT, MPH, PhD (c)
Board-Certified Geriatric Clinical Specialist
Graduate, Education Leadership Institute Fellowship, APTA
Credentialed Clinical Instructor, APTA
Certified Dementia Practitioner
Academic Coordinator of Clinical Education
Assistant Professor
DPT Program
University of St. Augustine for Health Sciences
Miami, Florida

Kristen Webber, MOT, OTR/L, BCPR, ATP
Inpatient Therapy Manager
Spinal Cord Injury
Shepherd Center
Atlanta, Georgia

Gail L. Widener, PT, PhD
Professor
Department of Physical Therapy
Samuel Merritt University
Oakland, California

Over the last 60 years, tremendous changes have occurred in the educational level and research within the professions of physical and occupational therapy. This book has evolved over my lifetime as a physical therapist and movement specialist. In the early 1970's colleagues followed approaches and philosophies developed by master clinicians for treating patients with movement disorders caused by central nervous system (CNS) pathology. Those approaches evolved because master clinicians were experts in analyzing movement and how patients responded to those interventions. Those colleagues analyzed abnormal patterns while their patients tried to perform functional movements. With their understanding of normal movement, they identified what components needed to be corrected and identified ways for those individuals to learn or relearn those functional movements. None of those master clinicians developed those approaches based on neuroscience but instead on movement analysis.

In the 1970's I started developing a model that integrated all the techniques. That model was based on a huge number of types of movement problems presented, such as instability of the scapula, poor postural tone or co-activation of the trunk, lack of neck stability, abnormal extensor or flexor tone in the leg, lack of adequate range or power problems, and others. Also, I tried to analyze how those movements changed in various spatial and functional positions. That model was based on the integration of three very different conceptual frameworks. One was based on the science or current research on the brain, which is and will always be constantly changing but continues to explain why specific movement problems develop given the trauma to specific areas of the brain. The second focused on how and why human movement develops from birth and over the life span. It isn't the position a child uses to develop motor control but how and why the brain uses those patterns to advance motor control and learning to gain upright posture or to regain that function if lost. The third aspect had to do with both the individual patient's internal and external environment as well as that of the clinicians. How the variance in both clinician and patient affected the learning environment and the motivation of the patient to participate is critical.

Empowering colleagues to become critical visual observers of patient movements and behavior in spite of any medical diagnosis seems to be the role of therapists if we are truly movement specialists and are the best professionals to create an environment of learning that empowers the patient to take control over their own motor system and thus their quality of life.

The first edition of the book was published in 1985. Each edition thereafter has always taken a problem-solving approach to movement dysfunction based on observations following neurological problems. From my experience in the last 60 years, I knew there was something special about the brain's ability to learn in spite of trauma. In the 90's, the term neuroplasticity became common. We all learned that in spite of disease or trauma, individuals can learn to move again. This textbook never has been a cookbook for the treatment of any movement problem associated with brain dysfunction but always has tried to identify environments or potential maps for both the clinician and the patient to analyze the movement dysfunctions presented. Although the available science or research of the time, no matter the edition, has always been integrated into the discussion, that research can only provide recommendations of types of evaluations to use for specific movement problems and various treatment approaches or ideas that have the potential of improving function. The analysis needs to be done by the movement specialist.

Science, research, and clinical strategies today should always be used to help colleagues select best tools and treatment approaches, but we must remember that science is always evolving and will never give us only one answer to a clinical problem. The answer to the clinical problem is within the patient and not the research. We need to continue to develop a movement-based conceptual framework that classifies and identifies variance in normal movement across the lifespan and then analyze what components are missing or substituting in abnormal movements. We need to stop relating our research to specific disease and pathology of the brain and analyze the dysfunction in relation to the area of the brain from which that movement problem arises. We have always been hands-on clinicians. If we ever give up (1) using our hands to feel the problems, (2) analyzing the functional movement problem with our eyes, and (3) interacting with the patient as a whole person and what motivates them, we certainly won't truly be movement specialists. We have the potential to truly become those specialists if we can move away from a medical model of disease/pathology and into a movement classification model that embraces all movement dysfunctions no matter the age or medical diagnosis of the patient.

Darcy A. Umphred

OVERVIEW OF THE SEVENTH EDITION

The seventh edition of the *Umphred's Neurological Rehabilitation* textbook contains several significant changes, but the overlying foundational principle remains the same—that clinicians must have a thorough understanding of the patient/client as a total human being to provide the best care that optimizes the person's health and well-being. We continue to use and expand the clinical problem-solving, diagnosis-prognosis approach that this book has taken since its inception. This book orients the student and clinician to the roles that multiple systems within and outside the human body play in the causation, progression, and recovery process of a variety of common neurological problems. Another objective is to orient the reader to a theoretical framework that uses strategies for **enhancing functional movement, enlarging the individual's repertoire for movement alternatives, and creating an environment that empowers the person to achieve the highest levels of activity, participation, and quality of life.**

Methods of examination, evaluation, prognosis, and intervention must incorporate all aspects of the client's nervous system and consider the influences of the external environment on those individuals. In the clinical management of persons with neurological dysfunctions, it is important to highlight the importance of a team approach in the physical rehabilitation of these individuals.

As to be expected, the foundations for contemporary clinical practice in neurological rehabilitation continue to be in a constant state of evolution, and this book has clearly articulated that evolution throughout its seven editions. This book emphasizes evidence-based clinical practice and guides clinicians to generate new hypotheses when there is an absence of clear evidence to guide practice. It is for that reason that this edition has retained information of conventional approaches that remain commonly used by therapists in the world today.

This book is divided into three sections. Section I provides the foundational knowledge necessary to understand and implement a problem-solving approach to for clinical care across the span of human life. The basic knowledge of the function of the human body in disease and repair is constantly expanding and often is changing in content, theory, and clinical focus. This section reflects that change in both philosophy and scientific research. This section has been designed to weave together the issues and concepts related to evaluation and intervention with components of central nervous system (CNS) function to consider a holistic approach to each patient/client's needs. This section delineates the conceptual areas that permit the reader to synthesize all aspects of the problem-solving process in the care of a client.

Section II is composed of chapters that deal with specific clinical problems, beginning with pediatric conditions, progressing through neurological problems common in adults, and ending with aging with chronic impairments. In Section II, each author follows the same problem-solving format to enable the reader either to focus more easily on one specific neurological problem or to address the problem from a broader perspective that includes life impact. The multiple authors of this book use various cognitive strategies and methods of addressing specific neurological deficits. The seventh edition of the text now contains separate and expanded chapters on Balance Dysfunctions and Vestibular Dysfunctions. This edition also contains a new chapter on Concussion Management in response to the emerging body of knowledge related to the examination and physical rehabilitation management of this condition.

A range of strategies for examining clinical problems is presented to facilitate the reader's ability to identify variations in problem-solving methods. Many of the strategies used by one author may apply to situations presented by other authors. Just as clinicians tend to adapt learning methods to solve specific problems for their patients/clients, readers are encouraged to use flexibility in selecting treatment interventions with which they feel comfortable and to be creative when implementing any therapeutic plan. Chapters in Section II also include methods of examination and evaluation for various neurological clinical problems using reliable and valid outcome measures. The identification of impairments in body structures and functions, activity-based functional limitations, factors that create restrictions in participation and affect health quality of life, significant outcome measurement tools in neurologic examination, and patient empowerment are critical aspects of each clinical chapter's diagnostic process.

Section III of the text focuses on clinical topics that can be applied to any one of the clinical problems discussed in Section II, such as pharmacology and cardiopulmonary management in neurorehabilitation. Chapters have been updated to reflect changes in the focus of therapy as it continues to evolve as an emerging flexible paradigm within a multiple systems approach. Two additional chapters that were added in the sixth edition were further enhanced in this edition: (1) the chapter on current technology in rehabilitation that discusses the current technology being used to inform the physical rehabilitation management of individuals with neurologic dysfunctions, and (2) the chapter on the use of medical imaging in neurorehabilitation.

We conclude the overview of this text by recognizing the immense contribution of Dr. Darcy Umphred and her significant influence in shaping the foundations for practice in neurological rehabilitation. A majority of the authors in the sixth edition have agreed to update their chapters for this new edition "one last time for Darcy," with many bringing with them new co-authors with the intent of passing on the torch for the succeeding editions. Taking over a textbook that has been exceptionally successful and transformative for the past several decades is an absolutely a daunting task, and the one main reason for this edition's editors and authors in continuing the book is to keep Darcy's voice, vision, and perspective alive for the next generations of students and clinicians. Those of us who have had the honor and privilege of knowing Darcy will forever have the "Darcy" in us—always seeing the patient as a whole person, recognizing the immense effect of the limbic system in movement, constantly striving to give the best care for each patient, and empowering them to take ownership for their health and well-being. We encourage the reader to learn from the concepts presented in the text and more importantly, to understand Darcy's clinical pearls that have been incorporated in each of the chapters.

Rolando T. Lazaro
Sandra G. Reina-Guerra
Myla U. Quiben

CONTENTS

Umphred's
NEUROLOGICAL REHABILITATION

1

Foundations of Clinical Practice

Rolando T. Lazaro, Myla U. Quiben, and Sandra G. Reina-Guerra

OBJECTIVES

After reading this chapter the student or therapist will be able to:
1. Analyze the concepts of a systems model and discuss how cognitive, affective, sensory, and motor subsystems influence normal and abnormal function of the nervous system.
2. Use an efficient and effective physical therapy diagnostic process that is centered on the patient/client management model.
3. Apply the International Classification of Functioning, Disability and Health (ICF) to the clinical management of patients/clients with neuromuscular dysfunction.
4. Discuss the evolution of enablement, health classification models, neurological therapeutic approaches, and health care environments in the United States and worldwide.
5. Discuss the interactions and importance of the patient, therapist, and environment in the clinical triad and the generation of movement.
6. Consider how varying aspects of the clinical therapeutic environment can affect learning, motivation, practice, and ultimate outcomes for patient/client.
7. Define, discuss, and give examples of a holistic model of health care.
8. Describe the relevance of the movement system to the practice of physical therapy.

KEY TERMS

clinical problem solving
empowerment
International Classification of Functioning, Disability and Health (ICF)

learning environment
movement system
patient/client management model

WHAT ARE THE FOUNDATIONS OF CLINICAL PRACTICE IN NEUROLOGICAL REHABILITATION?

The foundations of physical[1] (PT) and occupational[2] (OT) therapy practice are continuously being retooled. Even at the writing of this edition, professional leaders are still working to refine the *identity* of their respective professions to clarify the core knowledge and skills a therapist should possess. This clarification is necessary to justify consumer access to therapy services, to improve entry-level professional education, and to convey to society the professions' commitment to improve health, function, and quality of life for all. Both professions face the challenges of the current health care climate, which demands therapeutic care models that are efficient, cost-effective, and result in measurable outcomes.[3] In the particular branch of neurological rehabilitation, practitioners must be skilled not only in the choice and application of system-specific interventions but also in their understanding of the patient's/client's function in all aspects, including the central nervous system (CNS) as a movement control center. In this chapter, five foundational elements will be discussed: the complexity of the CNS; professional

roles in rehabilitation for the patient with neurological conditions; the movement system and the PT's identity; models and constructs for the different elements of the patient care management cycle and the practitioner-patient partnership.

COMPLEXITY OF THE NERVOUS SYSTEM AS A CONTROL CENTER

The concept of the CNS as a control center is based on a therapist's observations and understanding of the sensory-motor performance patterns that are reflective of that system. This understanding requires an in-depth background in neuroanatomy, neurophysiology, motor control, motor learning, and neuroplasticity, and gives the therapist the basis for clinical application and treatment. Understanding the intricacies and complex relationships of these neuromechanisms provides therapists with direction as to when, why, and in what order to use clinical interventions. Motor behaviors emerge based on maturation, potential, and degeneration of the CNS. Each movement behavior observed, sequenced, and integrated as part of the intervention strategies should be interpreted according to neurophysiological and neuroanatomical principles, as well as the principles of learning and neuroplasticity. As science moves toward a greater understanding of the neuromechanisms by which behaviors occur, therapists will be in a better position to establish efficacy of intervention. Unfortunately, our observation of behavior is ahead of our understanding of the intricate mechanisms of the CNS that create it. Thus the future will continue to expand the reliability and validity of therapeutic interventions designed to modify functional movement patterns as we better understand the neuromechanisms responsible for the change. First, therapists need to determine what interventions are effective within a clinical environment. Then the efficacy of specific treatment variables can be studied and more clearly identified. The rationale for the use of certain treatment techniques will likely change over time as we better understand the CNS.

PROFESSIONAL ROLES IN NEUROLOGICAL REHABILITATION

Identity, Efficacy, and Advocacy

The rich history of neurological rehabilitation was built upon the foundation of master clinicians who developed unique models of therapeutic interventions through well-honed observations of human movement and how impairments in the neuromusculoskeletal system alter motor behavior and functional mobility. These approaches include those developed by Ayers (sensory integration), Bobaths (Neuro Developmental Treatment [NDT]), Brunnstrom (movement therapy approach), Feldenkrais (Functional Integration and Awareness Through Movement), Knott and Voss (Proprioceptive Neuromuscular Facilitation [PNF]), and Rood (Rood's sensorimotor approach), among others. These were the first behaviorally based models introduced within the health care delivery system, and they have been used by practitioners within the professions of physical and OT since the middle of the 20th century. These individuals, as master clinicians, tried to explain what they were doing and why their respective approaches worked using the available science of the time. From their teachings, various philosophical models evolved. These isolated models of therapeutic intervention were based on successful treatment procedures as identified through observation and described and demonstrated by the teachers of those approaches. In the decades that followed, content related to these techniques has been taught as individual units; many continuing education courses still teach these specific techniques individually. The general model of health care delivery under which these approaches were used was the allopathic model, which began with physician-diagnosed disease and pathology. Various models of health care delivery will be discussed in later sections of this chapter.

In a broader sense, the roles of PTs and OTs in neurological rehabilitation have moved beyond impairment-based interventions. Because a specific treatment has a potential effect on multiple body systems and interactions with the unique characteristics of each patient/ patient clinical problem, establishing efficacy for interventions is extremely difficult. The rationale often used to explain the effectiveness of interventions was based on an understanding of the nervous system as described in the 1940s, 1950s, and 1960s. That understanding has dramatically changed; although this does not negate the potential usefulness of any treatment intervention, it does create a dilemma regarding efficacy of practice.

Efficacy has been defined as the "ability of an intervention to produce the desired beneficial effect in expert hands and under ideal circumstances."[4] When any model of health care delivery is considered, the question the therapist must ask is "Which model will provide the most

efficacious care?" Therapists are not responsible for the diagnosis of a pathological disease, but they are in a position of responsibility to examine body systems for existing impairments, to analyze movement, and to determine appropriate interventions for activity-based functional problems. Some differences in this responsibility may exist between practice settings. In selecting the most appropriate examination tools, the therapist must consider several issues independently or in combination: existing levels of evidence, applicability to the setting and population, practicality, availability of norms, and a test's clinimetric properties.

Within some hospital-based systems, therapists may be expected to use specific tools that are considered a standard of care for that facility, regardless of the applicability and evidence. In some hospitals and rehabilitation settings, a clinical pathway may be used that defines the roles and responsibilities of each person on a multidisciplinary team of medical professionals that may limit the decision making process. The therapist is strongly encouraged to use existing evidence, to consider all the issues related to selecting the most appropriate tests and measures, and to reflect on their own professional values during the decision making process.

Regardless of which clinical setting or role the therapist plays, it is always the responsibility of the therapist to be sure that the plan of care meets the needs of the patient/client, challenges the patient/client to progress appropriately, and renders successful outcomes. If the needs of the particular patient/client do not match the progression of the pathway, it is the therapist's responsibility to recommend a change in the patient's/client's plan of care. Efficacy does not come because one is *taught* that an examination tool or intervention procedure is efficacious; it comes from the judicious use of tools to establish impairments, activity limitations, and participation restrictions, to identify movement diagnoses, to create functional improvements, and to improve quality of life in individuals who come to us for therapy. When a holistic view of the patient/client is the foundation in therapy, it is apparent that outcome tools are not yet available to simultaneously measure the interactions of all body systems, making it difficult to apply models that purport to balance quality and cost of care. We must guard against the tendency to default to a narrow bank of "efficacious" interventions and measurement tools, and to the exclusion of techniques that have clinical effectiveness.

Evidence-based practice is basic to the care process.[5-7] Therapists should always be able to defend their choice and use of intervention approaches; this becomes even more relevant as the cost of health care rises. Clinicians need to identify which of their therapeutic interventions have demonstrated positive outcomes for particular clinical problems or patient populations and which have not.[8] Those that remain in question may still be judged as useful. The basis for that judgment may be a patient satisfaction, an outcome that has become a critical variable for many areas in health care delivery[9,10] with a growing body of supportive evidence.[11-15] A discussion of patient satisfaction will be expanded in following section on the patient-practitioner relationship.

The potential for OTs and PTs to become primary providers of health care in the 21st century is becoming a greater reality (e.g., within the military system as well as in some large health maintenance organizations [HMOs]).[16-21] The role a therapist in the future will play as that primary provider will depend on that clinician's ability to screen for disease and pathological conditions and to examine and evaluate clinical signs that will lead to diagnoses and prognoses that fall inside and outside of the scope of practice. These clinicians must also select appropriate interventions that will lead to the most efficacious, cost-effective treatment.

The foundation of neurological clinical practice is expanding for both the professions of OT and PT. In recent years, OTs are advocating for practice and policy changes to address the negative effects of fragmented health care[22] on patients/clients. Examples of these issues as identified in professional OT literature are (1) inconsistent patient/client access to care based on region of the country and type of insurance, (2) poor information hand-off between practitioners and clinician-patient, and (3) lack of transition services to bridge patient/client needs between home and work environment. In response, a key action of the OT profession is to advocate for practitioners in their discipline to seek credentialing as Certified Care Managers (CCMs). As described by Robinson and colleagues (2016) "occupational therapists have the training and skills to understand the complexity of medical issues and care, and the ways complex conditions disrupt everyday functioning."[22]

Relevant to both OTs and PTs in neurological rehabilitation settings is clear *communication* in multidisciplinary teams, which is paramount to patient safety and service delivery efficacy. Improvements in patient safety have been closely tied to interprofessional practice and clinician education.

To conclude this section's highlights on professional identity, efficacy, and advocacy, the reader should refer to the sections in this chapter on *the movement system* and *movement system diagnosis*—two rapidly evolving topics in the profession that will most assuredly shape the future of the doctoring profession in the United States.

THE PRESENT AND OUR FUTURE: THE MOVEMENT SYSTEM AND THE PHYSICAL THERAPIST'S IDENTITY

Movement has long been implied as the core of PT practice for more than 40 years; however, the concept of movement as a physiological system surfaced more recently. Many leaders in the profession have alluded to a professional identity with a component of movement as central the profession.

In 1975, Helen Hislop, PT, PhD, FAPTA, one of the founding leaders in PT, called attention to the profession's identity crisis and proposed pathokinesiology as defining science of PT during the profession's 1975 prestigious lectureship, the Mary McMillan lecture.[23] Florence Kendall, PT, FAPTA, in the 1980 McMillan lecture,[24] pointed out the distinction of PTs beyond procedures or modalities. She associated many medical specialties with specific body systems and proposed the musculoskeletal system, being the linked most to movement, as the PT's focus.[24] The American Physical Therapy Association (APTA) House of Delegates in 1983 adopted a definition of PT that identified the diagnosis and treatment of human movement dysfunction as the primary focus of PT patient management. In 1990, with input from Kendall and another leader in the profession, Scott Irwin, the movement system was defined in Steadman's Medical Dictionary as a physiological system that functions to produce motion as a whole or of its body parts.[25,26] Years later, Shirley Sahrmann, PT, PHD, FAPTA, in her 1998 McMillan lecture,[25] challenged the profession in defining its identity and to further develop the concept of movement as a physiological system.[25] Only at a later time did the concept gain ground again when Dr. Cynthia Coffin-Zadai, in the John Maley Lecture in 2004, discussed the human movement system, the complexity of the diagnostic process related to movement, and called for advancing diagnostic classification categories.[27] Two years later, the Diagnosis Dialog, a series of conferences to discuss diagnosis in PT, was convened by Barbara Norton, PT, PhD, FAPTA, and continued for the next 10 years.[28]

Clearly, evolving discussions on movement as the profession's focus have been occurring for many years, and attempts to organize and get consensus on the body of knowledge has been challenging. Agreement on defining, describing, organizing, and labeling concepts of movement as the profession's "system" has proven to be daunting. Consider

that PTs—clinicians, educators, and researchers—come from multiple philosophies in examination and intervention approaches, in addition to varied frameworks of clinical decision making and practice. The lack of professional consensus on the language and definitions related to movement, and the complexity of the diagnostic process on labeling movement dysfunction, have limited the profession from establishing a unique and singular statement on who and what PTs do. The lack of professional identity has been a dialogue extending many years, even if there seems to be unanimous agreement across many PTs that we are "movement experts."

Finally, after many years of discussion and debate on movement, in 2013 the House of Delegates of the APTA adopted a vision that highlighted and asserted that movement is an integral part of the PT profession. The vision states, "The physical therapy profession will transform society by optimizing movement to improve health and participation in life."[29] With this vision came guiding principles to communicate how the profession and society will look when the vision is achieved. The first principle, on Identity,[29] articulates that the movement system will be the core of PT practice, education, and research.

One of the first steps undertaken to meet this vision was the development of a definition of the movement system to standardize the framework and language. In 2015 the APTA released its definition along with a description of the relationship of the movement system to PT practice.[30] The movement system is defined as a "collection of systems (cardiovascular, pulmonary, endocrine, integumentary, nervous, and musculoskeletal) that interact to move the body or its body parts."[30] (Fig. 1.1).

The Identity statement reiterates the long-standing discussion on the PT identity associated with the movement system. The new vision and Identity statement linked the profession to a system of the body, a feature that has long been associated with established professions but has been missing in PT. Discussions that began more than 40 years ago are currently coming into fruition with defining the PT's role in health care as experts in the movement system.

Shortly then, the House of Delegates adopted the position, the Management of the Movement System, in which APTA endorses the development of diagnostic labels and/or classification systems that

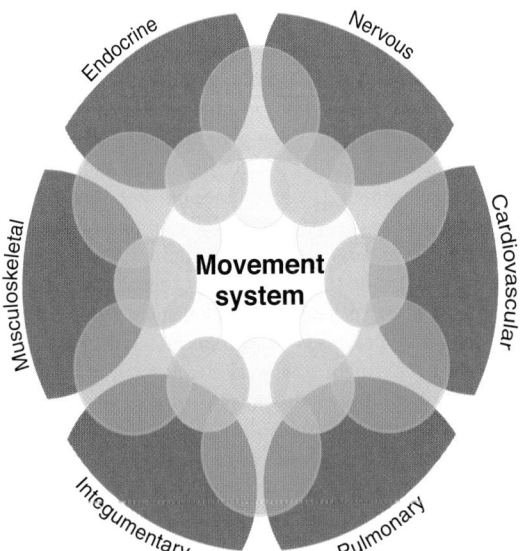

Fig. 1.1 The American Physical Therapy Association Movement System. (Reprinted from http://www.apta.org, with permission of the American Physical Therapy Association.© 2019 American Physical Therapy Association. All rights reserved.)

reflect and contribute to the PT's ability to properly and effectively manage disorders of the movement system.[30] The formation of the APTA Movement System Task Force, along with the position statement, iterates commitment to moving the profession towards the movement system as the profession's core and identity.

In 2016, APTA held the Movement System Summit, with more than 100 PT clinicians, educators, researchers, and leaders, with the goals of describing the implications of using movement system diagnostic labels and developing an action plan to integrate movement system concepts into practice, education, and research.[31] Participants' tasks included identifying activities or tasks that are essential to a movement system examination and criteria for diagnostic labels specific to the movement system. Recommendations from the Summit and the APTA Task Force were forwarded to the APTA Board of Directors for review and action.

In 2018 the APTA Movement System Task Force assembled two work groups to move forward with an action plan item from the Summit to "promote the development, implementation and dissemination of diagnostic classification systems/labels that adhere to the established and validated criteria."[32] As of spring of 2019, templates developed from the two work groups, the Movement System Diagnosis Work Group and the Task Analysis Work Group, are currently under review of the APTA Board of Directors for consideration. Over the next several years, the integration of the movement system is expected to continue as the profession debates and discusses strategies to infuse the movement system into practice, education, and research.

With many systems interacting to produce movement, so must the PT consider all of the systems contributing to movement. An individual moves the way they do because of many contributing factors—it is the therapists' task to determine which system contributes most to movement dysfunction and eventually prioritize which impairments need to be addressed. Therapists who focus on the movement system must consider the effects of all the components involved rather than examining a specific part of the anatomical system affected by a lesion.

The Guide to Physical Therapist Practice[33] *(The Guide)* describes examination as a comprehensive screening and specific testing process comprised by the patient history, systems review, and tests and measures of body structure and function, activities, and participation. It is during the examination leading to the evaluation that the therapist develops a hypothesis of the possible impairments that cause movement dysfunction based on the information from the history, results of the systems review and standardized tests, and movement analysis. However, the movement observation as envisioned to assist the choice of outcome measures and the diagnosis specific to the movement system is not explicitly identified in *The Guide* as a component of the patient/client management (PCM) model, nor is it a standard component clearly documented as part of clinical examination.

The Academy of Neurologic Physical Therapy (ANPT) Movement System Task Force posits that movement observation and analysis is central to the process of assigning a movement system diagnosis.[34] While the diagnostic process is a common in clinical practice, a clear, straight-forward movement observation and analysis of tasks or activities are not typically included in practice[34] or in documentation. The ANPT Task Force further acknowledged the absence of validated tools that accurately identify movement system dysfunction and recommend the development of a systematic process of observation and analysis. To date, the recommendation is to have the patient/client perform key tasks methodically and to observe performance that will provide insight on potential impairments that contribute to movement dysfunction. The core tasks recommended for movement observation include sitting, standing, sit-to-stand and stand-to-sit, step up and down, and reach, grasp, and manipulation. Hedman et al, 2018.[34]

These tasks are likely to change or to be added onto with further discussions regarding what activities/tasks at the minimum should be observed to provide the most insight on movement dysfunction, impairments that contribute to it, and lead to a diagnosis. Currently, there are no standardized methods on the performance of recommended tasks across patient populations. The ANPT Task Force has formed two subgroups, one that specifically is developing diagnostic labels for individuals with postural control dysfunction and the other is developing methods for task analysis that will lead to standardized movement observation. Over time, these diagnostic labels and movement observation procedures will be validated and refined for clinical use.

Movement System Diagnosis: What Is This?

The PCM model identifies a PT diagnosis determined after the evaluation process. A movement system diagnosis is determined after a consideration of all possible sources of movement dysfunction (Fig. 1.2), along with pertinent information from the patient history, systems review, and results of tests and outcome measures from the examination. Prior PT-related diagnostic labels were typically based on pathoanatomical models in which the diagnosis process focused on identification of pathology or anatomical causes that produced movement dysfunction.[35,36] In contrast to medical diagnoses or pathoanatomical-based diagnosis, movement system diagnostic labels are envisioned to be based on clear description of clusters or patterns of movement observations and associated examination findings that have a greater potential drive interventions.[34,35] Movement system diagnoses are envisioned to help identify targeted interventions that address specific movement patterns or impairments that limit the ability to function or participate in the environment. Examples of diagnostic labels specific to the movement system have been published[37,38]; however, these have not been validated through rigorous research nor are they universally used in clinical practice.

The ANPT Task Force recommended characteristics for the development of clinically meaningful movement system diagnosis. These include: a theoretical framework grounded on movement science, an emphasis on movement observation and analysis of core standardized tasks central to the examination, a cluster of movement observation and examination findings across tasks and health conditions, and non-ambiguous labels that are descriptive, unique, and applicable across health conditions.[34]

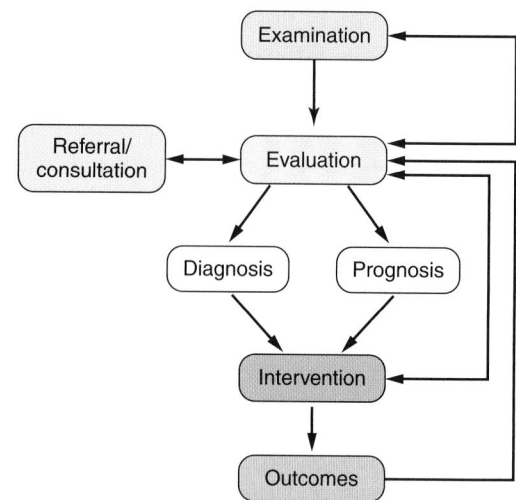

Fig. 1.2 The Process of Physical Therapist Patient and Client Management. (Reprinted from http://www.apta.org, with permission of the American Physical Therapy Association.© 2019 American Physical Therapy Association. All rights reserved.)

To date, activities are occurring across the profession at the APTA and its component levels to promote and develop the transition to the movement system throughout the profession. There is much work to do to integrate the movement system across practice, education, and research. Initial steps include the development of standardized movement observation and analysis that will inform therapists' clinical decision making leading to diagnostic labels. Movement system diagnoses, once developed, will need to be validated and examined for clinical utility. Academic curricula based on the movement system and movement system diagnosis will need to permeate entry-level education and diffuse to both academic and clinical faculty. Similarly, research on the clinical utility, validity, and predictability of diagnostic labels will be necessary as PTs characterize diagnoses of the movement system and associate these diagnoses first and foremost with PT. The transition will likely be lengthy and challenging, and universal professional acceptance will be dependent on the entire profession embracing the concepts of the movement system and claiming it as the profession's identity.

MODELS AND CONSTRUCTS FOR THE DIFFERENT ELEMENTS OF THE PATIENT CARE MANAGEMENT CYCLE

Therapeutic Models of Neurological Rehabilitation: What Are "Models" of Intervention? How Are They Useful?

In the development of a prescriptive therapy plan, the therapist's clinical decision making is informed by knowledge of the patient's health condition, the function of all the body systems, and the relationship to activity limitations and/or inability or difficulty in participating in functional tasks and activities. Therapists are also responsible for analyzing the interactions of all other systems and how they compensate for or are affected by the original medical problem. To accomplish these tasks, therapists use a variety of *models* in the patient/client care management cycle. Models of practice serve as road maps for foundation for clinical outcomes. They are also used to create a common language for health professionals. Practice models that focus on disablement—what the patient/client cannot do—were used by clinicians early on. As the practices evolved, clinicians realized the power of recognizing what the patient can do enhances their ability to improve their activity and participation.

To understand how and why disablement, enablement, and health classification models have become the accepted models used by PTs and OTs, it is important for the reader to review the evolution of health care within our culture. The dominant model of health care in Western society began with the allopathic model, and even nowadays it forms the conceptual basis for health care in industrialized countries.[39] The allopathic model assumes that illness has an organic base that can be traced to discrete molecular elements. The origin of disease is found at the molecular level of the individual's tissue. The first step toward alleviating the disease is to identify the pathogen that has invaded the tissue and, after proper identification, apply appropriate treatment techniques including surgery, drugs, and other proven methods.

It is implicit in the allopathic model that licensed physicians have the sole responsibility for the identification of the cause of the illness and for the judgment as to what constitutes appropriate treatment. PTs and OTs have never been responsible for the medical diagnosis or treatment of diseases or pathological conditions but rather are responsible for providing therapeutic interventions to help patients achieve their desired quality of life. Improvements in movement function and task participation can be achieved, even when the patient/client disease

or pathology is chronic and unchanged; thus the evolution to more holistic models of diagnosis and health classifications.

A holistic model (*holos,* from the Greek, meaning "whole"), also known as the biopsychosocial model of health care, seeks[40] to involve the patient/client in the process and take the mystery out of health care for the consumer. It acknowledges that multiple factors are operating in disease, trauma, and aging and that there are many interactions among those factors. An expanded biopsychosocial model includes emotional, environmental, political, economic, psychological, and cultural factors as influences on the individual's potential to maintain health, to regain health after insult, or to maintain a quality of health in spite of existing disease or illness. Measures of success in health care delivery have shifted from the traditional standard of whether the person lives or dies to the assessment of the extent of the person's quality of life and ability to participate in life after some neurological insult. Moreover, "quality of life" or living implies more than physical health. It implies that the individual is mentally and emotionally healthy as well. It takes all dimensions of a person's being into consideration regarding health. From the beginning, even Hippocrates emphasized treatment of the person as a whole, and the influence of society and of the environment on health.

An approach that takes this holistic perspective centers its philosophy on the patient/client as an individual.[41] The individual with this orientation is less likely to have the physician look only for the chemical basis of his or her difficulty and ignore the psychological factors that may be present. Similarly, the importance of focusing on an individual's strengths while helping to eliminate impairments, and activity limitations in spite of existing disease or pathological conditions, plays a critical role in this model. This influences the roles PTs and OTs will play in the future of health care delivery and will continue to inspire expanded practice in these professions.[42]

Since 2001, when 191 members states of the World Health Organization adopted the International Classification of Functioning, Disability and Health (WHO-ICF), the degree and quality human function has been the focus and framework for population health research and health policy actions. Application of this model is reshaping PT and OT professional education and clinical practice, including diagnosis, prognosis, outcomes measurement, and multidisciplinary patient management. The ICF model evolved from a linear disablement model to a progressive model that encompasses more than disease, impairments, and disablement. It includes personal and environmental factors that contribute to the health condition and overall well-being of individuals. The ICF model is considered an enablement model as it not only considers dysfunctions, but helps practitioners and researchers to understand and use an individual's abilities in the clinical presentation. The ICF recognizes disability not only as a medical or biological dysfunction but as a result of multiple overlapping factors including the impact of the environment on the functioning of individuals and populations. The ICF model is presented in Fig. 1.3.

It is easy to integrate the ICF model into behavioral models for the examination, evaluation, diagnosis, prognosis, and intervention of individuals with neurological system pathologies (Fig. 1.4). Whether an individual's activity limitations, impairments, and strengths lead to a restriction in the ability to participate in life activities, the perception of poor health or restriction in the ability to adapt and adjust to the new health condition will determine the eventual quality of life of the person and the amount of empowerment or control he or she will have over daily life. The importance of the unique qualities of each person and the influence of the inherent environment helped to drive changes in world health models. The ICF is widely accepted and used by therapists throughout the world.[5]

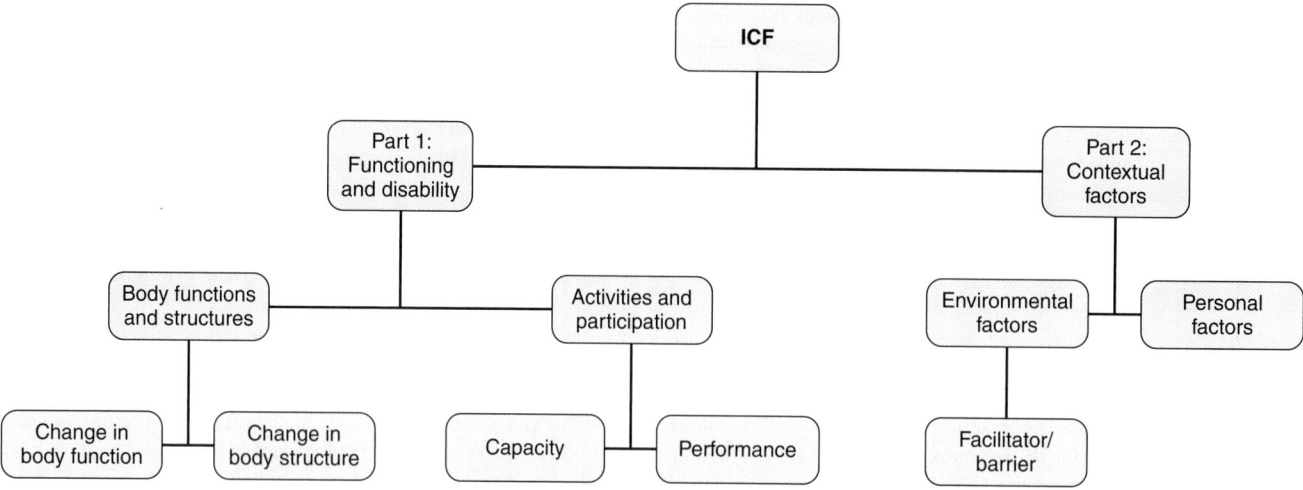

Fig. 1.3 Structure of the International Classification of Functioning, Disability and Health *(ICF)* Model of Functioning and Disability. (Reprinted from http://www.apta.org, with permission of the American Physical Therapy Association © 2019 American Physical Therapy Association. All rights reserved.)

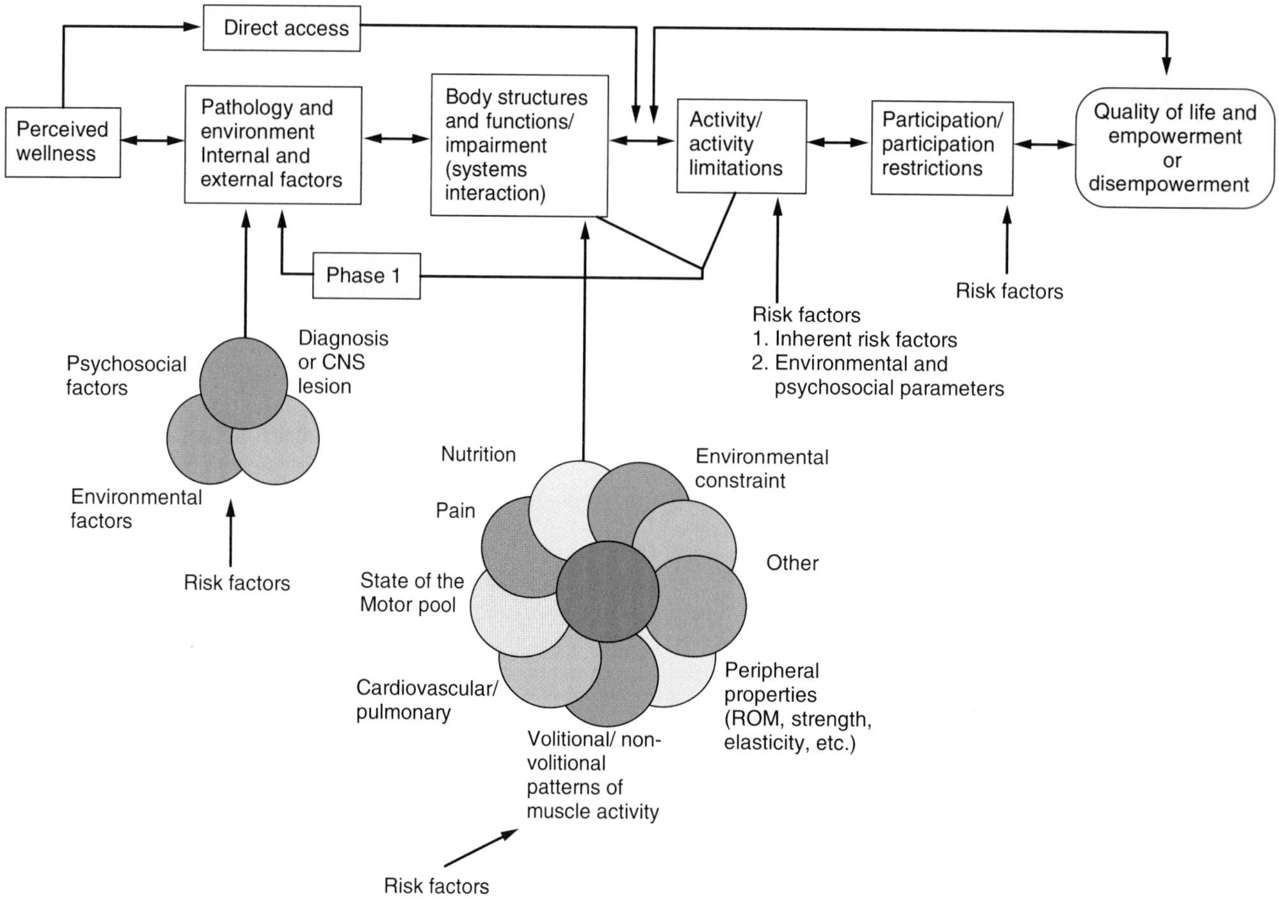

Fig. 1.4 Behavioral model for evaluation and treatment based on the International Classification of Functioning, Disability and Health *(ICF)* enablement schema. *CNS,* Central nervous system; *ROM,* range of motion.

Conceptual Frameworks for Patient/ Client Care Management: Who Needs to Use a Framework?

A patient/client care management framework is useful to convey the timing and relevance of each step and process that takes place between the patient/client and clinician. The structure of a framework provides an account of each task and responsibility a therapist fulfills in the course of a documented episode of care. A framework model can provide a sequential, developmental pathway, by which students can develop problem-solving strategies. Thus frameworks are beneficial for both the seasoned practitioner, new program graduate, and student. An example of a widely used framework in PT is the PCM model, as described in *The Guide*.[33] The PCM model[5] identifies the process used in PT to manage the patient and make clinical decisions. The six distinct elements are critical in clinical reasoning and decision making in neurology PT: examination, evaluation, diagnosis, prognosis, intervention, and outcomes. The PCM model is presented in Fig. 1.2.

PATIENT-CLIENT MANAGEMENT: EXAMINATION

The examination, the required first step for all patients/clients, is a comprehensive screening and specific testing process. Three components comprise the examination: patient/client history, systems review, and tests and measures of body structure and function, activities, and participation. During this initial step, the therapist develops a hypothesis of the possible impairments that cause movement dysfunction. The information from the history, results of the systems review, and tests provide the foundation to hypothesize the underlying cause/s of impairments that contribute to activity limitations and participation restrictions.

Medical Screening by the Therapist

Therapists must be able to screen patients/clients for signs of disease and pathological conditions.[19] This screening process is used to determine whether the individual shows signs and symptoms that are outside a therapist's scope of practice and therefore should be referred to another practitioner such as a physician. If the signs and symptoms both fall within the clinician's scope of practice and overlap with that of other disciplines, the therapist must refer and decide (1) to treat to prevent problems until the other practitioner's treatment can be performed, (2) to manage the limitations in activity and participation in spite of the pathological process, or (3) to manage functional loss and impairments that may correct the pathological cause. In some cases, the overlap with other disciplines may not necessitate an immediate referral, but interactions among the professionals managing the patient/client care must be made when needed to ensure the best outcome from intervention. However, when the information obtained by the therapist indicates a possible immediate and life-threatening condition, the therapist must act accordingly by referring the patient/client to a physician or medical emergency responders.

Examination With a Movement System Framework

Critical to the examination with a movement system framework is identifying the movements that are atypical. This observation of movement includes identification of the individual's movement abilities and limitations during performance of activities or tasks. Several strategies to observe and analyze movement exists along with their own definitions; explicit examination of movement dysfunction occurs variably across settings and among clinicians. Although many clinicians examine movement to some degree, no standardized approach to movement observation and analysis currently exists and consistent terminology to describe movement dysfunction is lacking.

As researchers continue to unravel the mysteries of brain function and learning, their understanding of how children and adults initially learn or relearn after neurological insult is often explained with new and possibly conflicting theories. Behavioral responses observed as functional patterns of movement, whether performed by a child, adolescent, young adult, or older person, are still visually identified by a therapist, family member, or innocent observer as either normal or abnormal.

Human beings exhibit certain movement patterns that may vary in tonal characteristics, amplitude, aspects of the specific movement sequences, and even the sequential nature of development. The range of acceptable behavior does have limitations, and variations beyond those boundaries are recognizable by most people. A 5-year-old child may ask why another child walks on his or her toes with the legs stuck together. If questioned, that same 5-year-old child may have the ability to break down the specific aspects of the movement that seem unacceptable even from a child's lens. From birth, a sighted individual observes human movement and after numerous observations over time will begin to see patterns that may be perceived as normal. Although variability in human movement exists, most everyday human movement patterns have a range of "normal," and therefore many elements are predictable, such as appearance of developmental milestones in children, and the variety of ways a person performs a sit-to-stand. This concept does provide flexibility in analysis of normal movement and its development. Some children choose creeping as a primary mode of horizontal movement, whereas others may scoot. Both forms of movement are normal for a young child. In both cases, each child would have had to develop normal postural function in the head and trunk to carry out the activity in a normal fashion. Thus, for the child to develop the specific functional motor behavior, the various components or systems involved in the integrated execution of the act would require modulation in a plan of action. Because the action must be carried out in a variety of environmental contexts, the child would need the opportunity to practice in those contexts, identify errors, self-correct to regulate existing plans, and refine for skill development. Thus each movement has a variety of complex systems interactions, which when summated are expressed by means of the motor neuron pool to striated muscle tissue function. The specifics of that function, whether fine or gross motor control, or full-body or limb-specific movement, still reflect the totality of the interaction of those systems. No matter the age of the individual, the motor response still reflects that interaction, and the behavior can be identified as normal and functional; functional but limited in adaptability; or dysfunctional and abnormal. Therapists must be able to (1) organize observational skills for any movement pattern, (2) identify components of the movement, (3) identify missing or abnormal movement patterns, and (4) select and administer interventions to incorporate the missing strategies or normalize the missing components.

The concept of the CNS as a control center is based on a therapist's observations and understanding of the sensory-motor performance patterns that are reflective of that system. This understanding requires an in-depth background in neuroanatomy, neurophysiology, motor control, motor learning, and neuroplasticity and gives the therapist the basis for clinical application and treatment. Understanding the intricacies and complex relationships of these neuromechanisms provides therapists with direction as to when, why, and in what order to use clinical treatment techniques. Motor behaviors emerge based on maturation, potential, and degeneration of the CNS. Each movement behavior observed, sequenced, and integrated as part of the intervention strategies should be interpreted according to neurophysiological and neuroanatomical principles, as well as the principles of learning and neuroplasticity. As science moves toward a greater understanding of the neuromechanisms by which behaviors occur, therapists will be in a better position to establish efficacy of intervention. The rationale for the use of certain treatment techniques will likely change over time as we better understand the CNS.

One can be confident that no infant will be born, jump out of the womb, walk over to the physician, and shake hands or say "hi" to mom and dad before learning to roll or control posture of the trunk and head. Instead, typical motor development requires new motor plans that lead to the infant's ability to achieve functional movement through motor learning. These new motor programs will be modified and reintegrated along with other programs to develop normal motor control in more complex patterns and environments because of neuroplasticity. Each pattern and the advancement from one pattern to another require time and repetition for mastery.

Two important aspects of the clinical problem-solving process emerge when observing movement. First, the examination of motor function is based on the interaction of all components of the movement system and the cognitive and affective influences, as stated previously. Second, as part of the diagnostic process, the therapist needs to recognize which aspects of the movement are deficient, absent, inaccurate, or inappropriate when cross-referenced with the desired movement outcome. Some patients/clients may not have had the opportunity to experience the desired skill because of a congenitally defective nervous system, whereas others may have lost the skill as a result of changes within the CNS or disuse. In either case the normal accepted patterns and variability remain the same.

Specific activity limitations and the impairments within the body systems that affect the individual's ability to control quiet postures or dynamic movement in any activity become a focus in the diagnostic process. The functional loss itself may or may not reflect specific diseases or pathological conditions within the CNS but does reflect specific impairments within that person's body.

Following the examination, a therapist must draw conclusions regarding those examination results and their interactions. That interpretation leads to a PT diagnosis. The interpretation of the examination results and their interaction with the therapist's and patient's/client's desired outcomes within a defined time period, the available resources, and the individual's potential lead to the prognosis. Selection of the best and most efficient resources to achieve the desired outcome will lead to establishment of the treatment intervention plan.

PATIENT-CLIENT MANAGEMENT: EVALUATION AND DIAGNOSIS

The evaluation refers to the synthesis of the findings from the examination components with the goal of establishing a diagnosis and prognosis. The interpretation of results and resulting clinical judgments guide the plan of care and interventions.

Diagnosis is a conclusion drawn regarding specific diseases and pathological processes within the human body; when made by a physician it is considered a medical diagnosis. Diagnosis made by a PT is a conclusion drawn regarding the status of body systems, activity and participation, and their interactions considering the patient's/client's personal factors and the environment. In consideration of each of these elements of examination subcomponents, the relative contribution to an overall movement disorder is determined. PTs use recognized movement problems to establish problem lists and intervention sequences. Using functional behavioral models such as the ICF model, clinicians are becoming comfortable with the *identification of body system problems (impairments), activity limitations (functional limitations), and participation restrictions*, and the conceptual understanding that a diagnosis[28] of a *movement system* dysfunction is very different from that made by a physician.

Differential Diagnosis Within a Therapist's Scope of Practice

Once a clinician determines that the patient's/client's need for service falls within his or her respective scope of practice, then the examination

continues and results in the development of a PT diagnosis, prognosis, and plan of care. The use of the ICF model will help the therapist to best capture the patient's/client's abilities, impairments, activity limitations, and participation restrictions, and the personal and environmental (contextual) factors that may influence progress. The information can then be used to determine the patient's/client's goals, address the individual's needs, and optimize function and quality of life. The patient's/client's functional goals and expectations may include activities of daily living, job skills, recreation and leisure activities, or the skills required for performance of typical societal roles. Each of these goals are associated with examination tools that can result in realistic, objective, measurable outcomes.

Two important clinical components affect the accuracy of the PT diagnosis and prognosis. First, the clinician must establish accurate, nonbiased results. This fact seems obvious, but with the pressures of third-party payers, family members, and other care providers and the desire to have the patient improve, it is easy to submit to drawing a conclusion based on *desired* outcomes rather than facing what is truly present and realistic. The second factor deals with the honesty of the interaction between the therapist and the patient/client. This "bonding" is critical for obtaining accurate examination results. Safety, trust, and acceptance of the patient as a human being play key roles in therapeutic outcomes and thus in efficacy of practice.[43–46]

The specific cognitive process used by therapists before formulation of a PT diagnosis might be conceptualized as a nine-step process. As the therapist enters into the clinical environment of the patient/client, he or she starts collecting data that might be relevant to the analysis of the clinical problem (step 1). This includes information obtained through observation, history taking, chart review, and interviews. The therapist must take that array of divergent information and determine what data are relevant to the case while disregarding what may be irrelevant information (step 2). This body of knowledge is then differentiated into various body systems that might be affected by the identified problems. If a specific system does not seem to be affected, then it can be eliminated, at least temporarily, from the diagnostic process (step 3). In general, administration of self-report measures and performance-based testing will provide an overview of the strengths and limitations of the individual in terms of function (step 4). After performing examination procedures and observing patterns of movement and specific normal and abnormal responses, the therapist once again diverges his or her thought processes back to separate large body systems to classify problems in the appropriate system (step 5). The therapist further subdivides these large systems into their components to assess specific subsystem deficits and strengths (step 6). This will allow the therapist to categorize objective measurements of impairments that are recognized as deficits within subsystems. Clusters of specific signs and symptoms will emerge that will help to direct the clinicians to a therapy diagnosis. Once the therapist has obtained these clusters of symptoms within specific subsystems, two additional convergent steps need to be completed. First, the presence and lack of impairments and how those impairments interact to cause dysfunction in a major body system are determined (step 7). Second, how those impairments affect the interaction of the major system with other major body systems is determined (step 8). These first eight steps tell the therapist exactly why the individual has difficulty performing specific functional activities. The problem list that incorporates the severity of impairments that have interacted to cause loss of function gives the clinician the therapy diagnosis. The number and extent of impairments along with an understanding of the cause of loss of function will lead the therapist to establishment of various prognoses and identification of optimal intervention strategies.

The last step (step 9) requires the therapist to diverge his or her thought processes back to the patient's/client's total environment to determine the accuracy of the diagnosis, prognosis, and selected treatment interventions as they interact with the individual as a whole. This is the "putting them all together" step where the clinician synthesizes all the information and makes sure that the individual is front and center in the process. Although some completion of this diagnostic process may occur within minutes after a patient/client and therapist begin their interactions, the process is continual, and at any time a therapist may need to go back to previous steps to obtain and analyze new and relevant information.

PATIENT/CLIENT MANAGEMENT: PROGNOSIS

The Guide[33] defines prognosis as the determined, predicted outcome of improved movement function. Intermediate levels of improvement and the optimal level of function are included in the prediction. Documentation of prognosis also requires prediction of the amount of time to reach each level within a course of PT.

How Long Will It Take to Get From Point A to Point B?

If a patient/client has a variety of impairments, activity limitations, and participation restrictions, then a variety of appropriate prognoses may be formulated. These prognoses could be used to speculate the amount of time or number of treatments it will take to get from the existing activity limitations and participation restrictions (point A) to the desired outcomes (point B). The intended outcomes provide information on whether the intervention will (1) improve activity through changes, adaptations, and learning within the patient as an organism or (2) improve function through compensation and modification of the external environment. Once the PT diagnosis has been established, a clinician must consider many factors when making a prognosis. Some factors are related to the internal environment of the patient/client, such as number and extent of impairments, level of physical conditioning or deconditioning, the ability and motivation to learn, participate, and change, and the neurological disease or condition that led to the existing problems. The patient's/client's support systems have a dramatic impact on prognosis. Cultural and ethnic pressures, financial support to promote independence, availability of appropriate skilled professional services, prescribed medications, and the interaction of all of these factors need to be considered. Specific environmental factors such as belief in health care and agreement about who has the responsibility for healing can create tremendous conflict among current health care delivery systems, the patient/client, the family, and the clinician.[44,47,48] In the ICF model, all of these variables influence the prognosis and must be considered in the patient/client management model.

Once a prognosis has been established, the therapist's next step is to identify the intervention strategies that will guide the patient/client to the desired outcome within the time period identified.

PATIENT/CLIENT MANAGEMENT: INTERVENTIONS

The Guide[33] defines interventions as any purposeful interaction to produce changes in a patient's/client's condition. Interventions should be consistent with the patient's diagnosis and prognosis and may also include interactions with others directly involved in the individual's care. Therefore, within this definition, an intervention includes direct, hands-on movement guidance, verbal instructions, and family education. Chapter 8 of this text describes interventions for patient's with neurological movement disorders. Foundationally, however, therapeutic interventions are based on knowledge of the movement system and the interactions of the patient-provider relationship.

Most treatment interventions used for patients/clients with CNS pathology incorporate principles of neuroplasticity, adaptation, motor control, and motor learning in various environmental contexts. Thus the consideration of the basic science of central and peripheral nervous system function and a behavioral analysis of movement must be included in any conceptual model used as a foundation for the entire diagnostic process.

The established plan of care determines the interventions and the method toward the achievement of the agreed-on outcome goals. The therapist, in collaboration with the patient/client, can choose from restrictive and nonrestrictive treatment environments and interventions to best achieve identified goals. The recognition and value of a holistic approach to illness are receiving increasing attention in society. Interventions designed to improve both the emotional and physical needs of patients/clients during illness has been recognized and advocated as a way to help individuals regain some control over their lives. Currently, the task of PTs and OTs is to empower the patient/client to be more responsible for their own health, in addition to the health and well-being of the community. This means that the consumer must play a critical role in the decision making process within the entire health care delivery system, including optimizing adherence to prescribed interventions.[49] The current increasing limitations placed on the delivery of medical care forces the patient/client to be more responsible for their health. Levin[50] points out that there is a lot that patients can do for themselves. Most people can assume responsibility to care for minor health problems. The opioid epidemic has forced our medical system to look at other options for managing pain. The use of nonpharmaceutical methods (e.g., hypnosis, biofeedback, meditation, and acupuncture) to control pain is becoming common practice.

The available choices of interventions will depend on the therapist's skill, the level of function and ability of the individual to control his or her own neuromuscular system, and treatment tools and strategies that are available in the clinic. Yet, freedom within that established environment must exist if learning by the patient/client is to occur.

PATIENT/CLIENT MANAGEMENT: OUTCOMES

Although patient/client satisfaction is a critical variable within the ICF model, there are always problems with satisfaction and outcomes versus identification of specific measurable variables within the CNS that are affecting outcomes. One reason for the problem of integrating patient satisfaction with PT and OT services within a neurorehabilitation environment is the large discrepancy between the variables we can measure and the variables within the environment that are affecting performance. For example, a neurosurgeon once asked the question to one of the editors, "Do you know how to prove the theories of intervention you are teaching?" The answer was, "Yes, all I need are two dynamic PET units that can be worn on both the patient's and the therapist's heads while performing therapeutic interventions. I also need a computer that will simultaneously correlate all synaptic interactions between the therapist and the patient to prove the therapeutic effect." The physician said, "We don't have those tools!" The response was, "You did not ask me if the research tools were available, only if I know how to obtain an efficacious result." Thus the creativity of the therapist will always bring the professions to new visions of reality. That reality, when proven to be efficacious, assists in validating the accepted interventions used by the professional. Therapists have a responsibility to provide evidence-based informed practice to the scientific community, but more important, also to the patient/client. Therapeutic discovery usually precedes validation through scientific research. This discovery leads the way to, first, effective interventions, followed by efficacious care. If research and efficacious care always have to come before the application of therapeutic procedures, nothing new will evolve because discovery of care is most often, if not always, found in the clinic during interaction with a patient. Thus the range of therapeutic applications will become severely limited and the evolution of neurological care stopped if that discovery is ignored because there is no efficacy as defined by current research models. However, performing interventions because the approaches "have been typically done in the past" could be wasteful and irresponsible.

A therapist, through professional education, efficacy of preexisting clinical pathways, and clinical experience, can generally identify the most effective interventions and the most expedient way to guide a patient/client toward the desired outcome. However, the patient/client response to intervention is not always immediate or complete and may not lead the individual in the most direct path to the desired outcome. For example, if a therapist and patient/client are working on coming to standing patterns and the patient/client begins to fall, the therapist would need to guide the patient/client back into the desired movement patterns and not allow the fall. In that way the patient/client is working on the identified outcome. Falling as a functional activity should be taught as a different intervention and would be considered part of a different clinical map. The degree to which the therapist needs to control the response of the patient/client will determine the extent to which the intervention would be considered contrived. Contrived interventions can, in time, lead to functional independence of the patient, but as long as the therapist needs to control the environment, functional independence has not been achieved.

Patient and Provider Relationship Is a Determinant of Outcomes

There are many ways to get to a desired outcome. Involving the patient/client in the goal setting and intervention planning process will lead to the best results. These interactions require the patient/client to trust the therapist as a guide and teacher. The patient/client-provider relationship includes concepts of the learning environment.

Learning Environment

The learning environment may be the critical factor in the success or failure of therapeutic interventions. The therapist, patient/client, and the environment formulate and maintain this environment. To comprehend the dynamics of the learning environment and function with optimal success, the clinician must do the following:

- Develop the learning process and provide an environment that promotes learning.
- Investigate the use of sensory input and motor output systems, feedforward and feedback mechanisms, and cognitive processing as means for higher-order learning.
- Use the principles and theories of motor control, motor learning, and neuroplasticity to facilitate learning and carryover of treatment into real-life environments.
- Obtain knowledge of both the patient's and the provider's learning styles. If these learning styles are not compatible, then the clinician is obligated to teach using the patient's preferred style.
- Attend to the sensory-motor, cognitive, and affective aspects of each patient/client, regardless of the clinical emphasis at any given time.

There are four distinct and interactive components of the learning environment: the internal and external environments of the patient, and the internal and external environments of the clinician (Fig. 1.5).

Patient's/Client's Internal Environment

A critical component of the ability to learn is the patient's/client's *internal environment.* When a lesion occurs within a body system, it directly and indirectly affects the entire internal environment. If the lesion occurs before initial learning, then habilitation must take place. These individuals may possess a genetic predisposition for a specific learning style, even though one has not yet been established. The therapist should test the inexperienced CNS by creating experiences in various contexts that require a variety of types of higher-order processing to discover optimal methods of learning that best suit the CNS of the individual. Then the therapist can use those methods in treatment. If previous learning has occurred, then the therapist needs to know what those are and whether they have been affected by the neurological insult so that proper rehabilitation can be instituted.[51]

One way to determine preferential learning styles is by taking a thorough history. Leisure activities and job choices often give clues to learning styles. For example, a patient/client who loved to take car engines apart or build model ships demonstrates a preference for the visual-kinesthetic learning style, whereas a patient/client whose preference for pure enjoyment was sitting in a chair and reading a book demonstrates a probable preference toward verbal learning. Again, this does not mean that the patients/clients in the examples mentioned could not selectively use all methods, but it does illustrate the issue of preference. Both the position of the lesion and the preferential learning style can play key roles in matching the learner with a particular treatment environment and identifying potential for recovery of function. For example, if a patient/client has had a massive insult to the left temporal lobe and before the trauma showed poor ability in using the right parieto-occipital lobe, then spatial or verbal strategies may be ineffective in the relearning process. However, an individual with the same lesion who had high-level right parieto-occipital function before the insult will probably learn at a much faster rate if visual-kinesthetic strategies are used to promote learning.

Patient's/Client's External Environment

The patient's/client's *external environment* is the second critical component.[52] All external stimuli—noise, lighting, temperature, touch, humidity, and smell—can modulate the individual's responses. External inputs can invoke either negative or positive influences on internal mechanisms and alter the patient's/client's ability to manipulate the world. Therefore a therapist should make every effort to be aware of

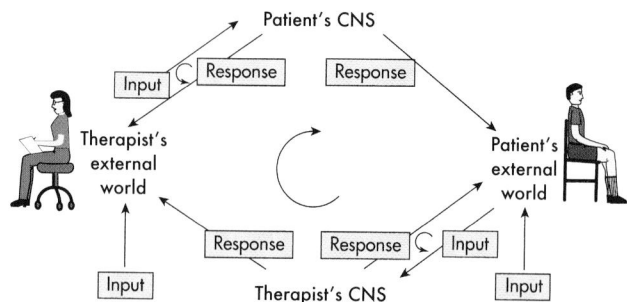

Fig. 1.5 Clinical Learning Environment. *CNS,* Central nervous system.

what externally is influencing the patient/client.[53–56] Any behavioral change displayed by the patient/client, such as a change in mood or attitude, or a change in muscle tone could serve as an indicator to the therapist that an environmental effect may have occurred.

Clinician's Internal Environment

The third critical component is the *internal environment of the clinician.*[57] The clinician should be aware of personal internal factors that can influence patient responses. Everyone has preferential styles of teaching and learning, yet many of us may be unaware of what they are and how they affect our outlook on life and interactions with other people.

Clinician's External Environment

The fourth component of the learning environment is the *clinician's external environment.* It is generally expected that personal life should never affect professional work. However, to accept this assumption may be to deny that emotions affect behavioral patterns. Response patterns can vary without cognitive awareness when an individual is emotionally upset or under stress. Each individual is unique. Therefore it is difficult to analyze the specifics related to each individual's learning environment. However, six basic learning principles have been established that are relevant to both the patient and the clinician in any learning environment.[58–60] Box 1.1 presents the six principles of the learning experience.

Although all six learning principles seem simple, their application within the clinical setting is not always as obvious. *Principles 1 and 2* are intricately linked with the appropriateness and difficulty of tasks presented to patients/clients. If a patient/client is asked to perform a task that requires a sequence of movements be performed (e.g., moving from supine to sitting, dressing, or maneuvering a wheelchair), to succeed, the patient must be able to plan the entire task and modulate all motor control during the sequence of the entire activity. If steps are not mastered, if sequencing is inappropriate or absent, or if motor control systems are not modulated accurately, dependence on the clinician to solve the problem is reinforced. Clinicians must differentiate missing components (impairments) from functioning systems and create an environment that encourages and allows the CNS to adapt and learn ways to regain that control. The clinician must also facilitate the patient's/client's ability to intrinsically self-correct during practice. This assumes that the patient is able to recognize the error to make the correction. Errors that lead to learning are encouraged, but errors that that always lead to failure do not help the patient to learn avenues of adaptation.

The level of difficulty or challenge of the task can be intricately linked with success. Changing the level of difficulty of a task is used to tease out specific impairments or as a progression of activity. The greater the task difficulty or complexity, the greater the challenge and consequently the greater the satisfaction if success is achieved. On the other hand, failed performance on a very difficult challenge can be demoralizing for the patient.

There is a subtle interplay among degree of difficulty, challenge, and success. Selecting tasks that are age appropriate, clinically relevant, and goal related is a challenge to the therapist. For the patient/client to be successful, the therapist must be a creative problem-solver and knowledgeable about the patient's needs, abilities, and goals. If the tasks are too simple or if the patient considers them unimportant, boredom will ensue, and progress may not be achieved. If the tasks are too difficult, the patient may feel defeated and may turn away from

> ## BOX 1.1 Six Principles of the Learning Experience
>
> 1. Individuals need to be able to solve problems and practice those solutions as motor programs if independence in daily living is desired. This requires the use of intrinsic feedback systems to modulate feedforward motor plans as well as correct existing plans.
> 2. The possibility of success must exist in all functional tasks, regardless of the level of challenge to the patient.
> 3. An individual will revert to safer or more familiar motor programs or ways to solve problems and succeed at functional tasks when task demands are new, difficult, or unfamiliar.
> 4. The learning effect occurs in multiple areas of the central nervous system (CNS) simultaneously when teaching and learning are focused within one area of the CNS.
> 5. Motivation is necessary to drive the individual to try to experience what would be considered unknown. Simultaneously, success at the activity is critical to keep the individual motivated to continue to practice.
> 6. Clinicians need to be able to analyze an activity as a whole, determine its component parts, and use problem-solving strategies to design effective individualized treatment programs. At the same time, if independence in living skills is an objective, the therapist needs to teach the patient those problem-solving strategies rather than teaching the solution to the problem.

them. In such cases, a child tends to withdraw physically, whereas an adult usually avoids the problem. This avoidance can be manifested in different ways—being late to therapy, having to leave early, or always needing to go to the bathroom are all avoidance behaviors that may be linked to inappropriate tasks.

The *third learning principle* describes a behavior inherent in all people: reversal. When confronted by a problem, individuals revert to patterns that produce feelings of comfort and competence when solving the problem. In Fig. 1.6, a 2-year-old child is confronted with just such a conflict. The bridge he wants to cross is unstable. The main goal is to cross the bridge in a manner that the patient thinks will result in the highest probability of success. Therefore the child reverts to previous movement that has proven to be successful—scooting. As the child gains confidence, he sequences from scooting to four-point bunny hopping, then creeping, on to cruising, and finally to reciprocal walking. Although reverting to more familiar or comfortable ways of solving problems is normal, it becomes problematic if used for a prolonged period of time. For example, if a patient/client with residual hemiplegia has spent a week modifying and controlling a hypertonic upper extremity pattern during a simple task and is now confronted with a more difficult problem, the hypertonia within the limb will most likely return with the added complexity of the task. The pattern or plan for standing is different from that for walking, and the emotional implications of walking are very high. The clinician should anticipate the possibility of the patient/client returning to a more stereotypical pattern. This possibility must also be explained to the patient/client. Anticipating that less efficient patterns will usually return as the tasks demanded increase in complexity, the clinician can attempt to modify the unwanted responses and let the patient/client know that the response is actually normal given the CNS dysfunction, but that movement can be changed and normalized with practice. The key to comprehension of this concept is not the behavior itself; instead, it is the attitude of a therapist toward a new

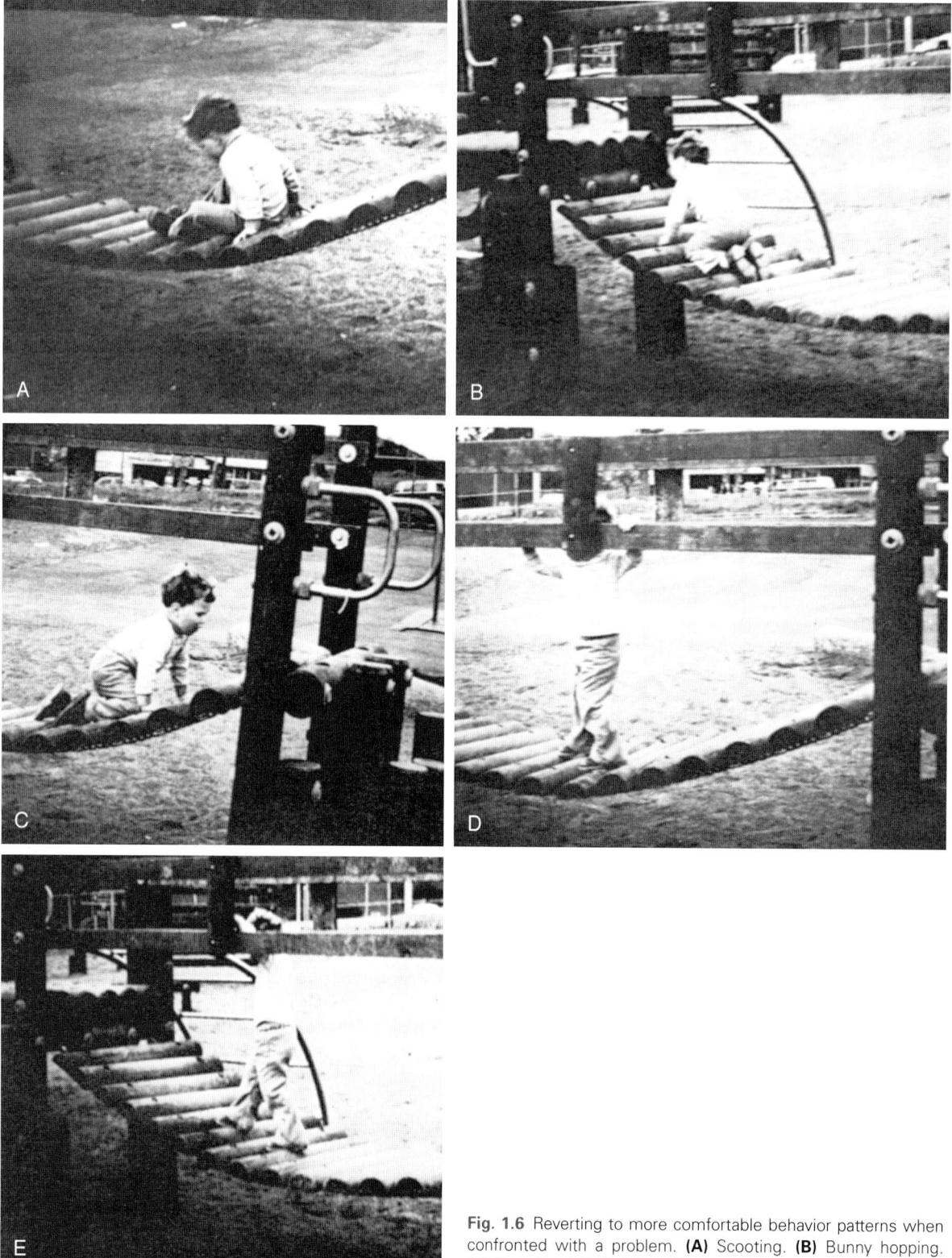

Fig. 1.6 Reverting to more comfortable behavior patterns when confronted with a problem. **(A)** Scooting. **(B)** Bunny hopping. **(C)** Creeping. **(D)** Cruising. **(E)** Walking.

task presented to the patient/client. If the clinician expects the patient to be successful, the patient/client will also expect success. If failure occurs, both parties will be disappointed, and a potentially negative clinical situation will be created; however, if the patient/client succeeds, both will have expected the result and their attitude will be neither excited nor depressed. On the other hand, a clinician who expects the patient/client to revert to an old behavior can prepare the patient/client. If the individual reverts, neither party will be disappointed; but if no reversion occurs, both will be excited, pleased, and encouraged by the higher functional skill. By understanding the concept, the clinician can maintain a very positive clinical environment without the constant negative interference of perceived failure when a patient/client does revert.

The *fourth learning principle* deals with the totality of the patient/client. Whether the area of emphasis is motor performance, emotional balance, or perceptual integration, all areas interact and influence movement. Therefore understanding and respect for all factors are important if optimal patient function is a primary objective. This does not suggest that therapists should address each aspect of personality; however, integration of the patient's/client's physical, mental, and spiritual areas should be a responsibility of the staff. Awareness of possible adverse effects of one learned behavior on other CNS functions can help to avoid potential problems. For example, if working on lower extremity patterns creates extreme upper extremity hypertonicity through associated patterns, the clinician is not dealing with the patient/client as a whole.

The unknown creates fear and curiosity for most individuals, and the *fifth learning principle* points out that for most patients/clients the unknown is all encompassing, whatever the degree of prior learning. For a patient whose only difficulty is a flaccid upper extremity, functional activities such as toileting, dressing, or eating will be troublesome. Motivation is a critical factor for success. Maintaining motivation to try while ensuring a high degree of success is an important teaching strategy that tends to encourage present and future learning.

An additional comment regarding patients/clients who lack motivation should be made. If a patient chooses to be totally dependent and has no need to become independent, then participation with tasks will likely be minimal. For example, Mr. Salas, a 63-year-old bank president with a wife, 4 children, and 10 grandchildren, survives an operable brain tumor with residual right hemiparesis and minimal cognitive-affective deficits. The patient's work history indicates that he was highly success oriented. Unknown to most persons is that for 63 years Mr. Salas desired to be a passive-dependent person, but circumstances never allowed him to manifest those behaviors. With the neurological insult, he is in a position to actualize his needs. Until the patient desires to improve, therapy will probably be ineffective; thus motivating the patient becomes critical. This might be accomplished in a variety of ways. Knowing that Mr. Salas values privacy, especially with respect to hygiene, that he thoroughly enjoys dancing and birdwatching in the forest, and that he ascribes importance to being accepted in social situations, such as cocktail parties, helps the therapist to create a learning environment that motivates this patient toward independence. Being independent in hygiene requires certain combinations of motor actions, including sitting, balance, and transfer skills. Being able to birdwatch deep in an unpopulated forest requires ambulation skills, tolerance of the upright position for extended periods of time, and endurance. Being socially accepted depends to a large extent not only on grooming but on normal movement patterns, especially in the upper extremity and trunk. Creating a therapeutic environment that stresses independence in the three goals identified by the patient will simultaneously create further independence in other areas. Whether the patient decides to return to banking and other activities in conflict with his personality will need to be addressed later. Another way to motivate Mr. Salas is to place him in an environment in which he is not satisfied, such as a nursing home or his own home with an assistant rather than his wife to help him with his needs. Dissatisfaction with the current external environment will generally motivate an individual to change or may trigger depressive symptoms. Obviously, creating a positive environment for change versus a negative one would be the method of choice.

The *sixth learning principle* has been discussed in earlier sections. To be a successful teacher of motor skills and to assist the

patient in recovery of function, the clinician should be able to break more complex motor plans and functional tasks into smaller component parts. These parts can then be taught successfully and then integrated back into the whole activity for optimal learning to occur. The therapist should always strive to allow each patient/client to solve movement problems and develop strategies for reaching the outcome goals, rather than producing the desired outcome for or with the patient.

Many additional learning principles from the fields of education, development, and psychology can be used to explain the behavioral responses seen in our patients/clients. It is not expected that all therapists will intuitively or automatically know how to create an environment conducive to helping the patient achieve optimal potential. Yet all can become better at creating a beneficial learning environment by understanding how people learn. The critical importance of being honest and accurate with prognosis and how that will ultimately affect function outcomes, participation in life, and quality of life cannot be overemphasized.[61]

The principles presented in this chapter deliver a strong message: individuals need to solve problems, and most want to solve the problem given a chance that the solution will be successful. Unless the task fits the individual's current capability, adaptation using whatever is available will become the consensus that drives the motor performance through the CNS. Learning is taking place in all aspects of life, and the patient/client must ultimately take responsibility for the means to solve the problem.[62]

CONCLUSION

The roles of PTs and OTs have evolved over the past several decades to include benefits to the patient for overall health, wellness, and disease/injury prevention. Medical screening and early detection of neurological problems should facilitate early referral of the consumer to a medical practitioner. Similarly, patients/clients may reenter PT or OT after a neurological insult as someone who has a chronic movement dysfunction or degenerative condition that may be getting worse and who needs some instruction to regain motor function.

Neurological rehabilitation will continue to take place in a constantly changing health care environment and ever-evolving delivery system. The balance between visionary and pragmatist must be maintained by the practitioner. By the end of the 21st century, neurological rehabilitation will have evolved into a new shape and form, will take place within a very different health system, and will involve the patient as the center of the dynamic exchange among wellness, disease, function, and empowerment.

We are getting closer to fully defining who we are and our distinct roles and responsibilities in the health care environment. It is also a time of distinct challenges with changes and uncertainties will most likely affect health care delivery. Increased globalization means that these changes and challenges will not be confined to one area but can potentially change the world. The seventh edition of this text also reminds us that regardless of these changes, there are foundations of our neurological rehabilitation practice that remain constant. Although the PCM process is changing, we recognize the importance of a more universal language an process. Such processes should (1) inform data gathering for the purpose of identifying a movement, function, and participation deficit, (2) guide the design of a plan of care, (3) prognosticate the likelihood of success following targeted interventions, and (4) assess outcomes following therapeutic intervention. We recognize that the unique relationship of the therapist and the patient/client in the therapeutic process has evolved into a partnership, with a set of negotiated, collaborated, and shared therapeutic goals. We reiterate the importance of the therapeutic environment to success in therapy. Finally, we highlight the value of learning in the healing and recovery process.

ACKNOWLEDGMENT

All the present authors and editors would like to express their deepest gratitude to Dr. Darcy A. Umphred and Dr. Margaret L. Roller who helped develop this chapter in the previous editions of the text.

REFERENCES

To enhance this text and add value for the reader, all references are included on the companion Evolve site that accompanies this textbook. This online service will, when available, provide a link for the reader to a Medline abstract for the article cited. There are 62 cited references and other general references for this chapter, with the majority of those articles being evidence-based citations.

Movement Analysis Across the Life-Span

Dale Scalise-Smith and Darcy A. Umphred

OBJECTIVES

After reading this chapter the student or therapist will be able to:

1. Comprehend the complexity and interlocking nature of human development over a lifetime.
2. Differentiate traditional theories of development from contemporary theories.
3. Analyze the differences among various subsystems within the human organism.
4. Identify elements of physiological changes over a lifetime.
5. Analyze normal movement strategies and identify subsystems' responsibility for success of a motor task.
6. Identify normal changes in motor strategies over a lifetime and synthesize differences between normal movement patterns and pathological movement problems across the life cycle.

KEY TERMS

abnormal movement strategies
developmental theory
neuroconstructivism
nonlinear dynamics

normal movement strategies
stages of motor development
systems theory

As physical and occupational therapists assume greater roles in primary care of patients/clients, they recognize the importance of a multifactorial approach. To competently evaluate functional movement across the life-span, clinicians must possess knowledge and skills in the development of skilled, refined movement across domains. Only then will therapists be prepared to perform the necessary evaluative and diagnostic testing and effectively develop and implement plans of care aimed at minimizing impairments, maintaining or regaining functional skills, and improving quality of life.

Throughout much of the 20th century, developmental researchers were heavily focused on skill acquisition from infancy through early childhood.[1-3] In the 1970s, as research paradigms directed at motor development and motor learning evolved, it became evident that changes in motor skills were not limited to childhood but occurred throughout the life-span. Consequently, the concept of life-span development came to incorporate the prenatal period through older adulthood.

During infancy (birth to 1 year) and childhood (1 to 10 years) acquisition of motor skills coupled with cognitive and perceptual development are the primary foci of developmental researchers and clinicians. As the young child transitions to adolescence (11 to 19 years) and has the opportunity to experience motor behaviors across different environmental contexts, more complex behaviors emerge. Adulthood (20 to 59 years) signals a period when skills are refined and motor behaviors mature. Only through practice and repetition are skills attained and retained. Individuals who continue to use motor learning strategies into late adulthood (60 years through death) often report more successful aging than those who do not engage in such motor skills.[4-6]

Identifying mechanisms that enable individuals to be successful in acquisition and retention of functional motor behaviors is critical to examining variables that alter or impair these same behaviors in other individuals. Kandel and colleagues[7] suggested that "the task of neural science is to understand the mental processes by which we perceive, act, learn, and remember" (p. 3). This view supports the interactive and collaborative nature of intrinsic and extrinsic systems to accomplish motor learning tasks.

Given the interactive nature of different subsystems, it would seem most effective for clinicians to recognize the need for implementing a multidimensional approach when devising intervention programs. To discuss the interactive nature of these issues, this chapter will (1) briefly provide a historical perspective of theories of motor development, (2) discuss domains (cognition, memory, perception, and so on) associated with life-span motor development from prenatal development through older adulthood, (3) discuss the impact of various body systems on motor skill acquisition, retention, or deterioration, and (4) describe behavioral changes that may positively or negatively influence motor performance across the life course.

With the focus of this book on neurological rehabilitation, it is imperative to incorporate the complex and interactive nature of the physiological, cognitive, and perceptual systems. Although readers can read about movement development across the life-span, it will not integrate into clinical practice until the therapist understands movements of the patient and how those movements reflect the summation of systems interacting to allow that individual to express movement, whether that be as a functional task, a written script, or the use of verbal language. Without that link between identified movement and motor control expressing that movement, often the therapist misses critical clues to the analysis of the central nervous system (CNS) of the patient and how best to provide an environment that provides the opportunity for that individual to improve functional skills and quality of life. For that reason, figures have been inserted to help the reader understand the differences among movement patterns across the life-span.

THEORIES OF DEVELOPMENT

Development is often portrayed as a series of stages through which an infant progresses with a fixed order to the sequence.[8] A developmental theory may be characterized as a systematic statement of principles and generalizations that provides a coherent framework for studying development. Historically, development was thought to be linear, occurring in an invariant sequence and resulting in behavioral changes that are direct reflections of the maturation of anatomical and physiological systems.[9,10] Development is generally examined in terms of quantitative and qualitative change. Although it is universally accepted that acquisition of developmental skills is not reversible, the underlying principles surrounding the emergence of these behaviors has evolved over the past 50 to 75 years.

Early developmental theorists used neuromaturational models of CNS organization as the framework for conceptualizing development.[1,2] These researchers provided elaborate descriptions of posture acquisition and a blueprint delineating skill development. Research focused on the emergence of cognitive and affective behaviors and ignored the processes and mechanisms involved in acquiring motor skills.[11] Several investigators attributed developmental changes to intrinsic variables such as maturation of the CNS, whereas others associated changes with extrinsic variables involving the environment.[1,2,12,13]

During the 1930s and 1940s, Arnold Gesell and Myrtle McGraw led a cadre of avant-garde researchers exploring the field of infant motor development. Gesell[1,14] described the normative time frame for when behaviors emerge, and McGraw[2] examined the underlying mechanisms responsible for the emergence of these behaviors. The underlying premise, the foundation for their elaborate descriptions of motor development, was based on maturational processes in the CNS.

Gesell, a pioneer in developmental research, was a proponent of the theory that nature drives development.[15] He proposed that growth is a process so complicated and so sensitive that intrinsic factors are solely responsible for influencing development. He used the evolutional thinking of Darwin and Coghill to explain changes in motor behaviors. Coghill,[16] in his work with salamander embryos, reported that motor behaviors, like swimming, emerge in an orderly sequence as connections of specific neural structures appear. Coghill concluded from his observations of emergence of behaviors in the salamanders that human infant motor behaviors appear in a predictable sequence and at predictable chronological ages.

With Coghill's research as the foundation for his thinking, Gesell embraced the concept of a hierarchical organization of the CNS. He believed that the emergence of motor behaviors was contingent on maturation in the CNS and concluded that only after the emergence of higher-level neural structures would complex motor behaviors appear. Within this constrained theoretical perspective, extrinsic or environmental stimuli, human or otherwise, were thought to have little impact on the appearance of motor behaviors. Gesell concluded that infant development is preprogrammed foundations and linear, emerging at predetermined stages or periods in time.[15] Perhaps his greatest contribution to

motor development was the conceptualization of milestones as markers to evaluate infant behavior.

Although McGraw was a proponent of ontogenic development as one variable influencing motor development, she did not believe, as Gesell did, that it was the sole determinant.[17] Rather, McGraw attempted to explain the emergence of motor behaviors through environmental influences as well as CNS maturation.[2] She examined the temporal and qualitative aspects of motor skill acquisition through her study of Jimmy and Johnny,[18] a study of twin brothers in which one twin was provided an exercise program, whereas no intervention was afforded the other twin. She found temporal and qualitative differences in the boys' acquisition of motor skills and attributed differences in acquisition of these behaviors to disparities in practice opportunities.

McGraw believed that the acquisition of the movement (process) is as important as when (chronological time frame) the behavior is acquired (the outcome). She further elaborated that, within the constraints imposed by the developing CNS, a rich and challenging environment can and does facilitate temporal efficiency in acquisition of motor behaviors. And finally, she proposed that practicing motor skills influences emergence of the same behavior.

Sufficient evidence exists to support the premise that although some predetermined processes occur at relatively similar points in development, not all motor behaviors emerge at the same biological, chronological, or psychological age in every individual. Although motor milestones provide information regarding outcome, no information can be derived about the process of attaining motor skills from those specific milestones. Perhaps a more realistic explanation may be that emergence of new skills occurs out of a need to solve specific problems within the environment. Working within this context, it is evident that traditional theories of development and maturation fail to adequately encapsulate the innate variability in human development.[11,12]

Within the last few decades, researchers employed more contemporary theories of development when designing studies involving infants and young children.[19–21] These investigators examined the process of skill acquisition rather than using traditional methods that assess outcome as a measure of motor development.[22]

Although early pioneers in developmental research described development as linear, uniform, and sequential, Thelen and Smith[23] depict development as "messy," "fluid," context-sensitive, and nonlinear. Linear and nonlinear dynamics are derived from mathematics. Linear dynamics is described by the proportional relationship of the initial condition to the outcome, whereas no such proportional relationship exists in nonlinear dynamics. Nonlinearity is used to describe complex systems, in this case biological or more specifically human systems.[24] Within these complex systems exists a level of unpredictability, given the interactive and interdependent nature of biological systems.

Thelen and Smith[23] suggested that, although traditional theories of development support the premise that behaviors emerge in accordance with a relatively fixed temporal sequence, an organism may exhibit "precocial" abilities when the context is altered and the behavior emerges earlier than expected. These authors stated that immature systems exhibit behaviors that are variable and easily disrupted. Although development of some organisms in a controlled laboratory environment may reflect more traditional perceptions of development, outside, in a more naturalistic environment, development is more likely to be flexible, fluid, and tentative. Thelen and Smith also found that factors most likely to have an impact on performance are the "immediacy of the situation" and the "task at hand" rather than "rules" of the performance. Given this perspective, Thelen and Smith[23] identified six goals as essential to developmental theory. These goals are as follows:

1. To understand the origins of novelty.
2. To reconcile global regularities with local variability, complexity, and context-specificity.
3. To integrate developmental data at many levels of explanation.
4. To improve a biologically plausible yet nonreductionist account of the development of behavior.
5. To understand how local processes lead to global outcomes.
6. To establish a theoretical basis for generating and interpreting empirical research (p. xviii).[23]

Thelen and Smith urged developmental researchers to devise paradigms that attempt to explain development in terms of diversity, flexibility, asynchrony, and "the ability of even young organisms to reorganize their behavior around context and task" (p. 18).[23]

Contemporary theorists inferred that developmental changes are nonlinear and emergent and may be the result of the interactive effects of intrinsic and extrinsic variables. This divergence from traditional thinking compelled avant-garde scholars to propose new theories.[23,25,26] Investigators described behaviors as complex, interactive, cooperative, and reflects an ability to organize and regroup around task and context, rather than conforming to a rigid structure and rule-driven hierarchy, as many earlier cognitive researchers believed.[23,26] Contemporary theorists exploit technology to derive a model to explain variability and flexibility in developing, mature, and aging populations.[26]

GENERAL SYSTEMS THEORY

Systems theory, first described by von Bertalanffy in 1936, was not discussed in great detail until 1948. In 1954 von Bertalanffy and colleagues from three other professions met to discuss systems movement.[28] Theorists then applied systems theory to a variety of human and nonhuman systems. As theorists became acquainted with systems theory, they became more receptive to alternate theoretical proposals of growth and development in living organisms.

Systems theory may be applied as a transdisciplinary model examining relationships of structures as a whole.[28] "The notion of a system may be seen as simply a more self-conscious and generic term for the dynamic interrelatedness of components"[28]; von Bertalanffy proposed this theory to more adequately describe biological systems, investigate principles common to all complex organisms, and develop models that can be used to describe them.[28]

Principles that embody general systems theory include nonsummative wholeness, self-regulation, equifinality, and self-organization.[28] Contrary to systems theory in disciplines such as traditional physics, in which systems are said to be *closed,* von Bertalanffy suggested that biological systems are open and modifiable and that changes in the system are the result of the dynamic interplay among elements of the system.[28]

Embedded in the general systems theory is nonlinear dynamics, a concept in which behaviors are not described as the sum of their parts. Thus within a nonlinear model, a mathematical model is derived.[26,29] Characterized within this model is the notion that systems may change in a sudden, discontinuous fashion. During development a small increase or decrease in one parameter leads to changes in the behavior. This abrupt change, identified as a bifurcation, causes the system to move out of its previous state and toward a new state of being.

Throughout development, periods of rapid differentiation or change occur when an organism is most easily altered or modified. These periods were identified by Scott[30] as "critical periods." Physiological systems are most vulnerable during these periods and may be seriously affected by both intrinsic and extrinsic factors acting on the system. These periods occur at different times for different body systems. Understanding systems theory and the concept of critical periods is crucial to all aspects of motor development.

As scientists began to revisit theories of motor development, they discarded some of the traditional theories and embraced contemporary concepts of nonlinear dynamics.[26,27,29] Proponents of nonlinear dynamics contend that modifications in motor behaviors are the result of dynamic interactions among the musculoskeletal, peripheral and central neuromuscular, cardiovascular and pulmonary, and cognitive and emotional systems.[28] These interactive, multidimensional elements are vulnerable to changes in organizational and behavioral abilities (system) over time.[30,31] Some theorists propose that as skills are acquired and organizational or behavioral changes occur, the system is driven to identify the most efficient and effective strategy to produce motor behavior(s).[30,31] Yet others purport that variability implies that typical healthy individuals may use a variety of strategies to produce the same behavioral outcome and that variability is an indication of the individuals' flexibility in responding to unpredictable perturbations.[26,32] Implicit in nonlinear dynamics is the concept of critical periods in development.[30–33] Investigators suggested that interventions imposed during a critical period may more easily positively or negatively modify the behavior. Recognizing the crucial role systems theory and critical periods play in development is essential to comprehending how developmental skills emerge. The multifactorial nature of nonlinear dynamics illustrates the complexity of development and the difficulty in identifying the appropriate variables that influence motor skill development.

With use of concepts previously described, it is reasonable to expect that a small change in any subsystem may result in a large change in a motor behavior. This is evident in work by Thelen and colleagues examining stepping in infants 8 weeks of age.[31,34–36] They reported that introducing a small change in one element of the system, identified as a small weight applied to an infant's leg, resulted in the infant being unable to step. The authors deduced that small changes in one subsystem, in this case the musculoskeletal system, may result in a change in the outcome. Additionally, adverse events during vulnerable periods of childhood can negatively impact the immune system leading to inflammatory responses that negatively impact health and risk for chronic disease and cognitive deficits in adulthood.[37] This lends support to the hypothesis that modifying one aspect of a multicomponent system, especially during a critical period, may cause the system to evolve into an entirely new behavior.

Periods of rapid differentiation, although often observed during early life, have also been observed across the life-span. Changes in anthropometric measures, such as weight gain during pregnancy, influence coordination between limbs and cause emergence of a different gait pattern. Changes in one system, in this case the endocrine system, result in increased ligamentous laxity at the pelvis and also contribute to gait alterations.

Menopause may be another critical period. During menopause, decreases in hormone production are thought to lead to osteoporosis and cardiac disease.[38] Examples described previously provide evidence across the life-span that the dynamic interplay within a system and among systems may significantly influence emergence and disappearance of behaviors.

Although research in the beginning of the 20th century was heavily focused on development of the very young, studies during the latter part of the century were directed toward research on aging. Technological advances in medicine have dramatically increased life expectancies. During the 20th century, the number of individuals in the United States older than 65 years old grew from 3 million to 35 million.[39] Perhaps the most significant statistic is that the oldest old grew from 100,000 in 1900 to 4.2 million in 2000.[39] By 2011 the Baby Boomer generation began turning 65 years old, and the number of older individuals will increase sharply between 2010 and 2030.[39] By 2030, Americans over the age of 65 years will represent nearly 20% of the population, and by 2050 the number of individuals over the age of 85 years is predicted to grow to 21 million in the United States and 400 million worldwide.[5,39] Given this incredible demographic transformation and that current policymakers are, in large part, the generation directly affected by these statistics, a significant paradigm shift in funded research has evolved over the past quarter century. "As such, aging and death are inseparable partners to growth and development" (p. 32).[40] Recognizing that a critical mass of Americans are entering older adulthood, terminology that operationally defines and is then applied consistently when referring to the aging population or an individual is imperative.

Biological and Chronological Age

Age can be described in terms of chronological age and biological age.[41] Chronological age is the period of time that a person has been alive, beginning at birth. In infants it is measured in days, weeks, or months, whereas in adults it is expressed in terms of years and at times decades.

Although chronological age is measured in terms of temporal sequencing, biological age is related more to functioning and physiological aging of organ systems.[42] For example, a triathlete may have biologically younger cardiovascular and pulmonary systems than same-age peers who do not perform high-level aerobic activities. Another example might be a child who underwent precocious puberty. Precocious puberty, identified as puberty earlier than 8 years of age in girls and 9.5 years in boys, results in acceleration in a biological system before same-chronological-age peers.[43] Physiological changes include elevated hormonal levels, which would then stimulate development of breast tissue and early menstruation in girls. Changes in the musculoskeletal system include early closure of the epiphyseal plates, resulting in significantly smaller stature. Conversely, these young women's reproductive cycles are significantly skewed. Women would also have menopause and aging issues associated with hormonal changes earlier than other women of the same chronological age. Although no consistent method has been established for measuring biological age, there is general agreement that a wide variability of biological aging exists and that a number of factors contribute to accelerated or decelerated biological aging.

Aging

"Aging refers to the time-sequential deterioration that occurs in most animals including weakness, increased susceptibility to disease and adverse environmental conditions, loss of mobility and agility, and age-related physiological changes" (p. 9).[44] Goldsmith's description of aging is typically viewed as an inevitable fact of life. This perspective evolved as technological advances and new evidence emerged indicating that age-related changes are more medically treatable than previously thought.[41,44,45] Scientists are hesitant to attribute a decline in functional movement in older adults to a decline in physiological systems or to diminished opportunities for practice or conditioning.[4] Rowe and Kahn reported that "with advancing age the relative contribution of genetic factors decreases and [of] the nongenetic factors increases" (p. 446).[4] Age-related factors that are modifiable may be used to identify individuals who may or may not age successfully. For instance, lifestyle choices, including diet, physical activity, and other health habits, and behavioral and social factors have a potent effect and accelerate or decelerate aging. Evidence to support this was initially derived from a 10-year study conducted by Rowe and Kahn.[46] The

authors identified three critical factors that contribute to aging successfully: avoidance and absence of disease, maintaining cognitive and physical functioning, and "sustained engagement in life."[46] Recently researchers suggested that Rowe and Kahn's classification of successful aging is too restrictive and may lead to classifying individuals with relatively minor health problems as unhealthy.[47] McLaughlin and colleagues[48] suggested that a critical variable in defining successful aging is first identifying what the goal is for measuring successful aging. Building on Rowe and Kahn's conceptual model of successful aging, recently researchers suggested shifting the focus from older adulthood to a life course approach.[47,49] The life course approach is a more holistic model focused on "aging well" and promoting healthy lifestyle choices for both physical and mental well-being across the lifespan, well before older adulthood.[49] Aging, a complex and dynamic phenomenon, is impacted by temporal modulation between and within systems/subsystems. Only then can researchers determine how best to define and measure successful aging. Although controversy exists regarding defining successful aging, factors that contribute to successful aging hinge on higher levels of physical activity, increased social interactions, and positive perception of health. Factors thought to negatively impact successful aging include smoking, chronic diseases (arthritis, diabetes), and impaired cognition.[50,51] Consequently, developing a healthy lifestyle early in life may be critical to maintaining good health and may play a significant role in successful aging.[5,6] Moving away from a deficit model, researchers are now conceptualizing aging as a lifelong process influenced by development, lifestyle choices, social relationships, health, and experiences influencing aging from a physical and behavioral perspective.[5,47,49,52,53]

Factors associated with aging are generally identified as either age related or age dependent. Age-dependent changes within organ systems are observed in individuals at a similar age, whereas age-related changes may be accelerated or decelerated in same-age individuals on the basis of intrinsic or extrinsic factors related to lifestyle. Just as variables associated with lifestyle (extrinsic factors) influence aging, genetics (intrinsic factors) also play a significant role. From a genetic perspective, structural and functional changes are generally thought to be a consequence of aging and are therefore predictable and consistent across physiological systems.[6] Variables thought to influence the genetic potential for longevity include environmental factors such as toxins, radiation, and oxygen free radicals. Free radicals are highly reactive molecules produced as cells turn food and oxygen into energy.[52,54] In summary, the use of biological age rather than chronological age may be a more accurate reflection of an individual's true age.

Theories of Aging

Throughout the 20th century, the average life expectancy of individuals living in the United States increased. The second half of the 20th century signaled a shift in the focus of human development research, from infant and child development to older adult development.

Scientists view aging as a progressive accumulation of changes over time that increases the probability of disease and death.[55] Given that portrayal of aging, researchers have proposed myriad hypotheses regarding aging. Aging theories evolved because there is no single factor or mechanism responsible for physiological aging.[41] Biological aging theories, similar to developmental theories, are attributed to complex, underlying mechanisms.[41,44,45,56] Although theorists attempt to classify aging theories, these theories are rarely mutually exclusive. Some theories were formulated around control of physiological functioning, others around cellular changes, and still others around genetic causes.

Neuroendocrine theory is based on the premise that hormones play a significant role in aging.[45,49] Hormones are vital to repairing and regulating bodily functions. Hormone production decreases significantly during aging and limits the body's ability to repair and regulate itself as effectively. Although hormonal decline is one plausible explanation for age-related changes, it does not account for all changes. Harman[57] proposed the free radical theory on the basis of his investigations that examined the effects of radioactive materials on human tissue.[57]

Harman reported that when human tissue is exposed to radiation, a byproduct is formed. He identified the byproduct, an unstable compound, as a free radical. Over time, human tissue with free radicals showed evidence of biological defects consistent with accelerated aging. Harman postulated that accumulation of free radicals in human tissue may also occur as a part of the normal aging process. This became known as the free radical theory of aging.[57–59]

Free radicals are highly reactive molecules that damage proteins, lipids, and deoxyribonucleic acid (DNA). In some instances, free radicals combine with enzymes and turn into water and a harmless form of oxygen that moves harmlessly through the cells.[58] In other instances the oxygen binds with intrinsic or extrinsic sources that influence the aging process.

Scientists have suggested several different ways that free radicals influence aging through intrinsic and extrinsic mechanisms.[58,59] An example of an intrinsic mechanism would be chronic infections that extend phagocytic activity and expose tissues to oxidants, creating cumulative oxidative changes in collagen and elastin. Extrinsic sources of free radicals include environmental toxins—for example, industrial waste and cigarette smoke.

Human exposure to intrinsic and extrinsic free radicals causes large numbers of reactive oxygen molecules to interact with DNA, leading to mutations thought to be the cause of a variety of diseases, including cancer, atherosclerosis, amyloidosis, age-related immune deficiency, senile dementia, and hypertension. Although some scientists suggest that aging has many factors that can accelerate or decelerate the process, other scientists suggest a much simpler, preprogrammed theory, known as the Hayflick limit. [41,58–60]

Hayflick and Moorhead[60,61] proposed that there is a finite number of times that a normal cell is capable of dividing. Current thinking is that cells are capable of dividing up to 50 times. Cell division is recognized as one way in which cells age and, after attaining the maximum number of divisions, finally die.

The factor thought to limit a cell's ability to divide infinitely is the presence of telomeres. Telomeres are minute units at the end of the DNA chain.[60] Each time a cell divides a small amount of the telomere is used in the process. Eventually, when cells have exhausted the supply of telomeres available, the cell is unable to divide and cell death ensues.

Telomerase, a substance that can lengthen telomeres, is available in human cells. Typically, telomerase is switched off in all cells except the reproductive cells. The availability of telomerase in reproductive cells allows for many more divisions than previously observed in the Hayflick limit. In addition to the presence of telomerase in reproductive cells, scientists have also discovered that telomerase remains active in cancer cells. Both reproductive and cancer cells divide well beyond the 50-division limit. Consequently, scientists are now working toward activating telomerase in all cells to slow or stop aging. If scientists are successful in activating telomerase in other cells, it may stimulate skin cell regrowth for burn patients and cure diseases that result from failure of aging cells to divide, as in macular degeneration or Hutchinson-Guilford progeria syndrome.[62,63] The downside of this is that scientists may have a difficult time controlling the telomerase and in fact may see more uncontrolled cell growth—cancer—one of the greatest threats to prolonged existence.

Although many aging theories are directed at mechanisms that negatively influence aging, other theories are focused on factors that have a positive impact on aging processes. One such process is the caloric restriction theory.[57,59,60,64] Liang and colleagues,[64] with use of several genetic mouse models, investigated the impact of dietary control on the life-span. The authors reported that the mice did, in fact, have their life-spans extended when their dietary intake was controlled. Although these findings are potentially significant, given the small sample size and model examined, these data were not generalizable to all species. The researchers suggested that these preliminary data provide a foundation for scientists to examine whether dietary control will extend the life-span in humans as it did in the mouse models.

Sleimen-Malkoun and colleagues proposed a framework that aging is "driven by complexity changes and dedifferentiation within and between the different functional subsystems."[65] Additionally, they suggested that their view diverged from a more traditional perspective and suggested that if we better understand how different subsystems interact and how the interactions change as a consequence of the adaptive processes across the life-span, we might develop a model that promotes healthy, active, and successful aging.

Although a large body of literature exists examining the underlying mechanisms associated with aging, it seems inconceivable that any one mechanism is responsible for age-related changes. More likely is that aging may be attributed to multiple factors, including lifestyle choices, in combination with the physiological and environmental factors.[66]

Belsky and colleagues conducted longitudinal research examining aging of adults in their third and fourth decades of life.[5] They found participants with accelerated aging were less physically able, had cognitive changes, were less healthy, and physically appeared older.

In summary, current research is challenging more traditional perspectives on aging. Rather than focusing on declining motor behaviors in older adults attributable to declining physiological systems, decreased practice or conditioning, or decreased ability to perform skilled behaviors,[67–70] researchers are suggesting that promoting health and well-being across the life-span might mitigate decline in older adults.[5,6,37,47,49] This suggests that physical or occupational therapy intervention may provide adults with strategies to positively impact performance over the life course, with a focus on promoting successful aging and maintaining skills.

The exogenous and endogenous variables across the life course are thought to be interrelated and provide an expansive description of the deleterious changes at the cellular, organ, and system level that accompany both aging and many age-associated diseases. The accumulation of damage is in DNA, proteins, membranes, and organelles, as well as the formation of insoluble protein aggregates. Many organ systems, such as the cardiovascular system, the brain, and the eye, are not programmed for indefinite survival. Consequently, the inability to maintain the integrity of tissues and organs is the end result of the multidimensional aspect of aging.

PHYSIOLOGICAL CHANGES IN BODY SYSTEMS ACROSS THE LIFE-SPAN

Organ systems undergo critical physiological changes across the life-span. These alterations are observed most often during periods of rapid differentiation. Applying concepts of dynamic systems theory to life-span development may help to explain how small changes in biological systems have a significant impact on the individual as a whole.

Examining interactions among variables within different body systems may provide insight into when one system may play a greater or lesser role in acquisition, retention, or deterioration of functional motor behaviors. The next section will examine how different systems develop and their contribution to functional movement.

Musculoskeletal System

Structural and functional adaptations in the musculoskeletal system are evident across the life-span. The musculoskeletal system provides a structural framework for the body to move and serves as protection for the internal organs.

Skeletal muscle tissue first appears during the fifth week of embryonic development and continues to develop into adulthood.[60,71] During this early period of embryonic development, the differentiation of musculoskeletal system is rapid: during the fifth week of embryonic life the limb buds appear, by the seventh week muscle tissue is present in the limbs, and limb movements emerge as early as the eighth week of prenatal life.[42,72,73]

Whereas many of the structural aspects of the musculoskeletal system are formed prenatally, muscle and bone continue to grow into adulthood. Motor skill acquisition involves considerable variability among young children from age 5 months through 3 years. During this time, the rate of growth of muscle tissue is reportedly two times faster than that of bone.[74]

Structural and functional differences in the musculoskeletal system of a child versus an adult are attributed to the presence and predominance of muscle fiber types. For example, infant muscles are composed predominantly of type I (slow-twitch) fibers, whereas adult muscles contain types I and II (fast-twitch) fibers. Behaviorally, infant movements are characterized predominantly by postural movements. The capacity to produce a greater repertoire of movements, including rapid or ballistic movements, emerges later in development.

Distinct differences also exist in temporal differentiation of the muscular systems of males and females of the same chronological age. Through adolescence, boys show evidence of a significantly greater increase in fiber size compared with girls.[75] In addition, differences exist in the age at which the number of muscle fibers dramatically increases. Girls reportedly have a steady increase in the muscle fibers from 3.5 to 10 years of age. In contrast, boys have two periods of rapid differentiation in the number of muscle fibers. The first period occurs from birth until 2 years of age and the second from ages 10 to 16 years.[75] Although the pace slows considerably, muscle fiber development continues in men and women well into middle adulthood.

Age-related changes evident in the musculoskeletal system include decreased fiber size, loss of muscle mass, denervation of muscle fibers, decline of total muscle fiber number, and decreased quantity of fast-twitch fibers.[76–79] Muscle mass peaks in the third decade of life and then begins to decline with approximately 10% lost by the fifth decade and 20% to 40% decrease between the seventh and eighth decades.[80–82] Muscle force production likewise decreases at a rate of about 30% between 60 and 90 years of age. Additional musculoskeletal changes documented in older adults include decreased tensile strength in bone, reduced joint flexibility, and limited speed of movement. Decreased muscle mass in a person older than 60 years may be attributed to decreased size, fewer type II muscle fibers, and an increase in fat infiltration into the muscle tissue.[83,84] Clinically these factors manifest as reduced muscle force production during high-velocity movements.

Currently, scientists are examining the premise that, as an individual ages, muscular changes are more likely attributable to decreased motor activity levels and are age related rather than being solely age dependent.[78,83] Acknowledging that investigators had previously found that muscle power deteriorates more quickly with age, scientists set out to measure training effects in older adults.[69,85] These investigators concluded that with training older adults were capable of improving strength, power, and endurance. Modifying musculoskeletal tissue may take longer in older adults and requires that other body systems are capable of modifying performance levels to adjust to the increased demands of the musculoskeletal system.[86] The skeletal system, similar to the muscular system, experiences periods of growth, stability, and degeneration. The immature skeletal system is composed primarily of preosseous cartilage and physes (growth plates).[87] More simply, bone in infants and young children is flexible, porous (lower mineral count), and strong with a thick periosteum.[87,88] Given these properties of immature bone, a child is less likely to have a fracture because the periosteum is strong and consequently the bones absorb more energy before the break point is reached. In addition, if a fracture does occur, healing is usually quicker because callus is formed faster and in greater amounts in children than in adults.

A primary difference between the child's and the adult's skeletal system is the presence of the growth plate complex in children. Whereas primary ossification occurs prenatally, secondary ossification is not complete until the child reaches skeletal maturity, generally at age 14 years in girls and 16 years in boys.[88,89]

Even after bones have attained their full length, they continue to grow on the surface. This is termed *appositional growth* and continues throughout most of life. During childhood and adolescence, new bone growth exceeds bone resorption and bone density increases. Until age 30 years, bone density increases in most individuals, and bone growth and reabsorption remain stable through middle adulthood. Later in adulthood, resorption exceeds new bone growth and bone density declines.[90]

Women exhibit more loss of bone mass than men do.[91] Decreased bone density in women is generally attributed to differences in the types and levels of hormones present. Although the difference is most significant during menopause, premenopausal women still lose bone density at a higher rate than their male peers do.

Osteopenia is the presence of a less-than-normal amount of bone and, if not treated, may result in osteoporosis. Progressive loss of bone density, observed into older adulthood, is commonly identified as osteoporosis. Osteoporosis is more common in women than in men and is a major cause of fractures and postural changes in both sexes.[92]

Overall, much of the growth in the musculoskeletal system is related to demands placed on the system. Intrinsic and extrinsic forces imposed on the musculoskeletal systems of typically and atypically developing children may lead to structural and functional differences in their respective skeletal structures. Consequently, temporal sequencing, acquisition, and characteristics of motor behaviors emerge differently in typically and atypically developing children. Similarly, age-related changes in older adulthood may be accelerated in direct proportion to decreased levels of activity.[93] Older adults who maintain more active lifestyles and place greater physical demands on their musculoskeletal systems are more likely to have an improved bone density and muscle mass than their peers who are not as active.[94]

Sarcopenia, the age-related loss of muscle mass, and dynapenia, the loss of muscle strength, each contribute to changes in power and function.[76,81,95] Researchers examining sarcopenia in older adults reported that men are affected more by sarcopenia than women.[83,96] In fact, men with sarcopenia manifest four times the rate of activity limitations than do men with a normal muscle mass. Additionally, research suggests that while there is a relationship between changes in muscle mass and strength, they are not necessarily proportional, as many neuromuscular factors contribute to force production.[80,76] Therefore, it is important to differentiate between sarcopenia and dynapenia and to examine the interactive effects, as these might be more sensitive indicators of muscle function than strength or mass alone.[97]

Reid and colleagues suggested that changes in neuromuscular activation changes may precede changes in muscle mass or strength and may be the initial mechanism that influences muscle power loss as a consequence of aging.[98] Investigators noted increased adipose tissue in skeletal muscle of older adults impacting the older adult's muscle power and performance.[98,99] The increase in fat in muscle tissue is now recognized as myosteatosis. JafariNasabian and colleagues[81] proposed a similar term for changes in bone-osteosteatosis described as the process where adipose tissue infiltrates into the bone marrow. Examining bone, muscle, and fat changes across the life course and evaluating how these changes impact functional performance, mobility, and risk for falls and fractures is important to planning and implementing therapeutic interventions in older adults.[81]

While sarcopenia, osteopenia/porosis, and obesity are recognized and exist as unique entities, the presence of the triad is now characterized as osteosarcopenic obesity syndrome.[81] Increased body fat is redistributed to muscle and bone as well as abdominal and visceral organs as a consequence of aging. Osteosarcopenic obesity syndrome is composed of two newly recognized components that might exist independently or as components of the syndrome: osteopenic/osteoporotic obesity and sarcopenic obesity.[81]

Finally, while it may take longer for older individuals to regain strength or flexibility than a young adult or child, musculoskeletal tissue is modifiable throughout life.[95] Modifying the strength and flexibility of an older adult requires that other bodily systems be capable of modifying performance levels to meet the increased needs of the musculoskeletal system. Therapeutic interventions focused on reversing the physiological changes in bone and muscle may improve musculoskeletal health, functional performance, and quality of life in older adults. Recognizing the interconnections between bone, muscle, and fat, therapeutic approaches should focus efforts on all of these tissues to maximize the impact.[99]

Although strength is critical to musculoskeletal function, flexibility is equally as important. Flexibility incorporates joint motion and the extensibility of the tissues that cross the joint. The degree of flexibility changes across the life-span as a direct result of aging and activity level.[12] Changes in flexibility are evident throughout life: limited at birth, increasing until the individual approaches adolescence, and then gradually decreasing. Exceptions may be seen in athletes, dancers, and other individuals involved in activities that incorporate flexibility training. Loss of flexibility as a consequence of age may have a negative impact on functional independence in older adults. Flexibility is thought to be directly proportional to the amount, frequency, and variability of motor activities performed. As activity increases, so does flexibility. Conversely, as individuals exhibit decreased levels of motor activity, often associated with age, flexibility decreases.[90]

By age 70 years, flexibility is thought to have decreased by 25% to 30%.[79] Although this was purported to be age dependent, it may be more likely that it is age related.[78] Regularly performing exercise directed toward improving strength and flexibility can reverse the effects of inactivity for most individuals, even those older than 90 years of age.[76,78,93] As scientists continue to examine functional changes across different systems as a consequence of age, physical and occupational therapists must educate individuals regarding the importance of embracing a physically active lifestyle and methods to enhance quality of life at each stage in an individual's life. Although all systems contribute to an individual's health and wellness across the life-span, the cardiovascular and pulmonary systems play a key role (see Chapter 29).

Cardiovascular and Pulmonary Systems

The cardiovascular system is composed of the heart, lungs, and associated vascular complex. It is responsible for pumping blood through the coronary, pulmonary, cerebral, and systemic circulations, with the goal of perfusing all bodily tissues for the delivery of oxygen and vital nutrients and picking up waste products for elimination. The pulmonary system is responsible for oxygen transport, gas exchange, and removal of airborne pollutants that may enter during respiration (see Chapter 29).

The interdependent nature of the cardiovascular and pulmonary systems is evident in the fact that, each minute, all of the body's blood travels through the lungs before being returned to the left side of the heart for ejection into the systemic circulation.[100] Because of this relationship, changes in heart function can dramatically affect lung function, and vice versa. In addition, these two systems are connected as part of a larger closed pressure-volume loop through the peripheral circulatory structures. Likewise, any alteration in the function of the peripheral vessels will affect both the heart and lungs, and vice versa.

The function and homeostasis of the cardiovascular, pulmonary, and peripheral vascular systems are influenced by both internal and external forces.[100] Internal mechanisms of control are based on the autonomic nervous system, the relative health of the anatomic structures involved, the growth and development of the structures, and the behavioral and emotional adaptations of a particular individual. All those internal mechanisms are subject to changes with growth and development, aging, lifestyle choices, and the unique life experiences of an individual. Growth and development primarily affect the physics of the system by altering volumes, lengths, smooth and myocardial muscular tension, and physiological capacitance within the system to support the growing body. Numerous effects of aging have an impact on the adaptability of the system. Behavioral and emotional responses influence both autonomic and volitional cardiovascular and pulmonary reactions to stress. External forces include movement, environment, and activity level, which alter the gravitational forces on the closed pressure-volume system. An increased activity level causes exercise stress, which requires an altered demand for oxygen and nutrients to the structures providing the work. Finally, emotional stress needs to be considered as an external factor. Behavioral responses to stress can affect functional movement and cause maladaptive coping mechanisms on any or all systems. As with anything, the age, cognitive status, and relative health of an individual will dictate the potential success of these endeavors.

Because oxygen transport and exchange are the primary requirements for sustaining life, efforts toward maximizing the efficiency of the cardiovascular and pulmonary systems represent a fundamental component of therapeutic practice. It is critical that no matter where a patient falls in the life-span, strategies for screening, prevention, and rehabilitation of the cardiovascular and pulmonary systems be incorporated into a comprehensive plan to promote optimal mobility, function, and independence.[101] It is essential for therapists to keep in mind that all interventions have a direct or indirect impact on these systems and that it is their responsibility to monitor and manage those responses to maintain safety.

A detailed understanding of the anatomy of the heart, lungs, and vessels, as well as the physiology and interrelationship of the organs involved, is essential to the practice of both physical and occupational therapy. Refer to Chapter 29 for additional information. For pediatric therapists, the added knowledge of normal growth and development of these structures is critical.

From weeks 3 to 8 of fetal life, the cardiac structures are formed.[71,72,102] All other structures of the cardiovascular system are fully developed and functional shortly after birth. Although the left and right ventricles are of similar size at birth, by 2 months of age the muscle wall of the left ventricle is thicker than that of the right ventricle.[103] This is attributable to the fact that the left ventricle is responsible for pumping blood to the whole body, requiring a higher internal pressure and contractile force, whereas the right ventricle is responsible for pumping blood only to the lungs, a relatively low-pressure function in a healthy individual.

It bears mentioning that the heart's function begets structure. Therefore if function becomes impaired, the structure is likely to adaptively change. For example, if the resistance in the vascular system from the right ventricle to the lungs becomes increased, the right ventricle must pump harder, with a greater volume of blood, to overcome the resistance.[104] Over time, this will increase the size of the ventricular walls because the myocardium is muscular tissue that is as equally capable of hypertrophy as skeletal muscle tissue.

Structurally, the heart doubles in size by year 1, and its size increases fourfold by year 5. Many of the changes associated with size are complete by the time the child has reached maturity. Recall that cardiac output (CO) is equal to stroke volume times heart rate. As the size of the heart increases (increasing the volume capacity for each stroke), the heartbeat decreases and the blood pressure increases.[105] Heart rate in a newborn infant is generally 120 to 200 beats per minute (bpm), 80 bpm by 6 years of age, and 70 bpm by 10 years of age.[103,106] Systolic blood pressure (defined as maximal pressure on the artery during left ventricular contraction or systole) is 40 to 75 mm Hg at birth and increases to 95 mm Hg by 5 years of age.[103] Blood pressure continues to rise into adolescence. The capacity to maintain exercise for longer periods and greater intensities increases through early childhood. Although cardiovascular disease is generally associated with adults, children as young as 5 years of age may show signs of or be at risk for cardiovascular disease if they do not engage in regular aerobic activity.[103,107]

Development of the pulmonary system occurs late in prenatal and early postnatal life.[106] As the lungs increase in size, tripling in weight during year 1, the capacity and efficiency increase while the respiratory rate decreases.[106] Physiological performance of the cardiovascular and pulmonary systems improves in response to growth and development. Although the vital capacity of a 5-year-old child is 20% of an adult's, this is not usually a limiting factor during exercise.[105] Overall, aerobic capacity increases during childhood and is slightly higher in boys than in girls. The overall work capacity of children increases most dramatically from 6 through 12 years of age.[105] Peak oxygen consumption is achieved early in adulthood and changes in direct relation to activity levels. Lungs of an average adult at rest take in about 250 mL of oxygen every minute and excrete about 200 mL of carbon dioxide.[108] As activity levels change across the life course, so do the structural and functional capacities of the cardiovascular and pulmonary systems.

Many of these changes are a result of changes in the elasticity of the tissues, efficiency of the structures, and ability to increase workload. CO decreases approximately 0.7% per year after age 20 years so that by age 75 years the CO is 3.5 L/min, down from 5 L/min at age 20 years.[108] Functional changes include a decrease in the overall maximum heart rate from 200+ bpm through young adulthood to 170 bpm by age 65 years.[103] Older adults typically have less elastic vessels, with increased resistance to the blood volume. Consequently, older adults reach peak CO at lower levels than do younger individuals. These cardiovascular changes may be compounded by inactivity, resulting in decreased capacity to perform activities that raise metabolic demands and increase the requirement for oxygen transport.[109]

Cardiovascular health also plays a significant role in the health of the brain, in particular white matter.[110] As individuals age, cardiovascular health changes leading to hypertension and elevated resting heart rate

are related to white matter health and the associated macro- and micro-structural changes. Pulse pressure, defined as the difference between a person's systolic and diastolic blood pressure, is recognized as a good indicator of cardiovascular and white matter health in older adults. That is, higher systolic and lower diastolic blood pressures may indicate increased arterial stiffness and reduced vessel compliance. Additionally, body mass index (BMI) also impacts cardiovascular and white matter health. As BMI increases, white matter health decreases, suggesting that changes in cardiovascular and white matter health are possible by controlling BMI through lifestyle changes such as nutrition and exercise.[110]

Throughout life, performance of motor activities and activities of daily living (ADLs) is highly dependent on the integrity of an individual's cardiopulmonary and cardiovascular systems. Introduction of aerobic activities during early childhood has implications for improved health and wellness across the life-span.[5] Although aging has a negative impact on performance and efficiency of the cardiovascular and pulmonary systems, aerobic exercise has a positive impact on these systems. Howden and colleagues[111] examined changes in cardiac stiffness and maximum oxygen uptake in healthy sedentary middle-aged adults participating in a 2-year intensive exercise program. They suggested that maintaining a regular exercise training program may reduce cardiac stiffness and improve the overall health of the cardiovascular system. These findings are consistent with the work of other researchers examining the impact of aerobic activity on body systems.[112] Aerobic exercise improves the elasticity of blood vessels, enhances cardiac contractility, and improves the oxygenation to different organs. Changes in the cardiovascular and pulmonary systems have a significant impact on the overall health of other systems and consequently on body functioning. Information from these systems, including blood pressure and oxygen saturation rates, is communicated through the nervous system. The nervous system, in turn, regulates responses of the cardiovascular and pulmonary systems through the autonomic nervous system.

Neurological System

The nervous system encompasses the CNS and the peripheral nervous system (PNS). The CNS includes the brain and spinal cord, and it is responsible for all bodily functions. The PNS includes both the autonomic and the somatic nerves and is responsible for transporting impulses to and from the CNS.[5] The capacity for humans to produce behaviors far beyond those of other animals is directly related to the complex abilities of the CNS and interneuronal communications.

Over the past three decades, technological advances have enabled neuroscientists to dramatically improve their understanding of the molecular changes in the nervous system over time.[113] Development of the CNS is coordinated through intrinsic influences involving the temporal and spatial coordination of synaptic connections with genetic processes, along with extrinsic or environmental factors. Initially, development of the CNS is dependent on precise connections formed between specific types of nerve cells and begins with the recruitment of cells that form the neural plate, which gives rise to the neural tube, and then differentiation of regions of the brain begins.[5,114] Changes in the nervous system are predicated on critical periods, or times when different regions of the brain are sensitive to change, and occur across the life-span.[5,30,115,116]

Each region of the brain is thought to undergo critical or sensitive periods at different ages. One of the most critical periods in development of the CNS occurs from birth through 1 year of age. During this period, when the system is most vulnerable to change, intrinsic and extrinsic variables may influence the nervous system structurally and functionally. In late adulthood, gray matter is thought be vulnerable to the effects of aging, with the frontal and temporal regions most susceptible to age-related changes.[116,117]

Differentiation of cells in the nervous system begins during the embryonic period and continues throughout adulthood.[5,113] Development of the nervous system during embryonic life involves the overproduction of glial cells and neurons that, after they are no longer useful, die. Additional developmental changes noted in the nervous system include increased myelination within the brain and an increase in neuronal size.[71] Much of the growth may be attributed to these changes in the nervous system and may account for the development of the infant's brain, which increases to one half the size of the adult brain during the first year of life. Neural development, particularly in the cerebral cortex, documented early in development, may emerge out of environmental demands and the need to solve problems (tasks). Consequently, experiences can alter neural networks, and more complex experiences lead to increasing complexity of the neural structures.[118] As individuals age, brain weight and volume decreases.[116,119] Brain volume decreases an average of 0.2% to 0.5% per year.[116] Atrophy, noted in both gray and white matter, is not thought to be equally distributed, with upwards of 15% to 20% decrease in white matter.[52,116,119]

Whereas researchers long supported the premise that decline of the nervous system begins generally after age 30 years, more recent studies indicate that adults, even older adults, can form new neural connections and grow new neurons as an outgrowth of learning and training.[113,115,120] Before the work of Eriksson and colleagues, researchers and clinicians believed that structural changes in older adults, such as decreased numbers of corticospinal fibers, intracortical inhibition, and neuronal degradation in centers in the CNS, particularly the cerebellum and basal ganglia, were inevitable.[123] In contrast, more recent research challenged traditional constructs that the only possible changes in the adult human brain were the result of negative changes caused by aging or pathology.[122] Instead these researchers reported that the brain retains a level of neuroplasticity and is capable of changing into late adulthood. Employing strategies that promote neuroplasticity may provide more positive and cost-effective experiences and reduce the rate of cognitive decline in older adults.[115,116] They suggested a direct relationship exists between learning a novel task, juggling, and structural changes in the gray matter.[122] The authors caution that these structural changes were task specific and limited to the training period. Reexamination of magnetic resonance imaging (MRI) scans, after 3 months of no training, demonstrated that subjects no longer displayed the same structural changes as during juggler training.

Loss of neurons in the centers controlling sensory information, long-term memory, abstract reasoning, and coordination of sensorimotor information negatively affects function.[116] For some individuals this may not have significant implications. For others, CNS changes create serious functional losses. Alterations in the CNS, including altered neural control and decreased efficiency in temporal sequencing of muscle synergies, may play a role in postural instability and impaired sensation.[52,77,116] Although the CNS, similar to other bodily systems, may have the capacity to compensate for some age-related changes, the degree of compensation may be modulated by the complexity of the task and continuation of "practice" over time. Although some investigators have reported that neuromuscular systems in older adults may not be as flexible as systems in younger adults, new studies examining changes in mature and aging systems are still in the early stages. Neuromuscular systems in older adults may not be as capable of rapidly reorganizing muscle synergies to produce variable functional responses.[121] The researchers did say that this may be related not solely to the aging neurological system but to other factors including experience, cardiovascular and musculoskeletal fitness, and current

level of functional independence. Other scientists suggested an alternative view that repetition of motor activities may stimulate new growth in dendrites located proximal to neurons previously lost.[52,77] Implicit in performance of many functional activities is cognition. If changes in cognition coexist with changes in other systems, it may be difficult to accurately interpret the underlying causes.

Cognitive System

Cognition may be defined as awareness, perception, reasoning, and judgment.[123] Cognitive development involves processes of perception, action, attention, problem solving, memory, and mental imagery. Action, from the perspective of physical or occupational therapy, may be referred to as *functional movement(s)* and incorporates all the processes described previously to successfully perform a specific task.

Jean Piaget, one of the most recognized scientists in developmental psychology of the 20th century, was particularly intrigued with how biological systems affect what individuals "know."[123,124] He observed interactions among children of different ages and hypothesized that younger children's thought processes were different from those of older children as evidenced through the differences in responses between them to the same questions.

Piaget proposed that cognitive development moved in a linear, stagelike progression, each stage of which involves radically different schemes.[124] He suggested four stages of cognitive development, identified as sensorimotor state (infancy), preoperational (toddler and early childhood), concrete operational (childhood and early adolescence), and formal operational (adolescence and adulthood).[123] He proposed that (1) sensorimotor behaviors stimulate cognitive development and (2) problem solving as a measure of cognition enables infants and young children to identify and modify motor behaviors.

Piaget's theory of cognitive development focused around how humans adapt within the environment and how these adaptations or behaviors are controlled.[124] He postulated that behavioral control is mediated through schemas or plans, generated centrally. These schemas provide a representation of the world in an effort to formulate an action plan. At birth, infants' earliest schemas are organized around reflexive behaviors that are modified as the infant adapts to the affordances and constraints of the environment.

Piaget suggested that adaptations occur through two processes: assimilation and accommodation.[124] He defines *assimilation* as a process of altering the environment around cognitive structures. An example of assimilation is when an infant, initially breast-fed, is transitioned to bottle feeding. *Accommodation* refers to changes of the cognitive structures to meet changing demands of the environment. Accommodation may be involved when an infant transitions from nutritive sucking (breast or bottle) to nonnutritive sucking (pacifier).

Much of Piaget's work was based on descriptive case studies. Although some aspects of his theory were supported by subsequent studies, other aspects of his work have not been shown to have empirical evidence. The inconsistencies of research findings examining Piaget's stages of development may be indicative of the dynamic and nonlinear nature of development and, more specifically, cognition.

Rather than postulating that infants are reflexive beings with little or no volitional movements early on, it may be more appropriate to view infants as competent beings with volitional and complex behaviors present at birth.[125] Brazelton reported that a newborn infant turns toward the mother's voice rather than toward an unfamiliar voice. In addition, research conducted by Meltzoff and Moore[126] provides evidence supporting the complex nature of infant behavior. They found that infants as young as 2 to 3 weeks of age can imitate facial gestures performed by adults. Their work was supported by subsequent studies performed by independent investigators using different procedures and in different environments.[127] These findings, contrary to Piaget's proposal that infants were not capable of imitative behaviors until 1 year of age, provided scientists with a new perspective on infant behavior.

Contemporary researchers approach developmental theory from a dynamic and nonlinear model.[23,114,118,128] Over the past 10 years, advances in technology (e.g., diagnostic imaging, functional magnetic resonance imaging [fMRI], magnetoencephalography [MEG], event-related potentials [ERPs]) have dramatically improved the ability to document change within the developing brain.[114] These technological advances coupled with developmental paradigm shifts and computer modeling have led developmentalists to propose new theoretical frameworks to explain cognitive development. One model, called *neuroconstructivism,* incorporates intrinsic constraints and abilities of the CNS at the most basic cellular level with extrinsic influences involving environmental experiences and interactions.[114,118] Fundamental to the neuroconstructivist theory is the principle of context dependence, in which representations emerge in direct response to the structural changes in the cognitive system. Embedded within neuroconstructivism is the concept of the infant as interactive, in contrast to more traditional developmentalists' perception of the infant as passive. Experiences that individual infants engage in vary through processes involving competition and cooperation. The processes employed during development may result in differing pathways or trajectories of development through which the outcome or behavior is realized. Despite the variability in the individual developmental trajectories, the behavioral outcome is often similar.

This model is purportedly applicable to typical and atypical development as well as mature and aging systems. In contrast, whereas the processes and interactions among multiple interactive constraints (biological and environmental) may be similar in typical and atypically developing systems, the constraints may differ. Hence the outcome or emergent behavior may be different.

Current theories lend support to the concept that the cognitive system integrates multimodal input to process, interpret, store, and retrieve information as a mechanism for information processing and problem solving.[123] Changes in cognition, defined as relatively permanent changes in behavior, cannot be measured directly but rather must be inferred from changes observed across multiple systems.

As the ability of infants to act on the environment develops, their ability to accurately detect and process relevant information becomes more efficient, lending support to the interdependence of the motor, cognitive, and perceptual systems.

Information processing, defined as the ability to understand human thinking, is a critical factor that must be examined within the cognitive system. Initially, infants and young children cannot recognize relevant cues or chunk information for storage. As children's developing systems become more adept at integrating information from multiple systems and more efficient at processing information, they begin to process relevant information more effectively. Consequently, infants and young children may not use or interpret information as efficiently as older children.

The integrative nature of movement, cognition, and perception is evident in developmental psychology literature.[129] Given that these domains are interrelated, one area cannot be examined in isolation of other interrelated systems. Acquisition of motor skills is the primary mechanism for evaluating cognition and perception in prelinguistic children. In addition, as individuals grow older, changes in any system may influence functional movement. Finally, when examining functional movements, therapists must always consider the individual's cognitive and perceptual abilities.

As higher-level cognitive processing skills become apparent, the child can accurately identify relevant cues, filter irrelevant cues, and process information more efficiently. One such higher-level cognitive processing skill is executive functioning. Adolescence signals a period during which executive functioning begins to mature.[130] This period may be characterized as critical in CNS development. During this critical period, production of mature, adult-like decisions requires selective attention and increased integration of information via the prefrontal cortex (PFC). During the maturation process, adolescents may exhibit inconsistent decision making, resulting in less-than-optimal outcomes. By young adulthood, as the individual approaches maturity, optimal executive decision making becomes more consistent.

Human systems are continuously pelted with sensory information through some or all of the sensory modalities. At any one time, more sensory information is available than can possibly be processed. Consequently, the individual must learn to select information relevant to the task and chunk the information for processing.

Another example of the multidimensional processes involved in higher order tasks such as functional movement is found in a study conducted by Hazlett and Woldorff.[131] They proposed that implicit in motor tasks are concepts of cognition including attention, perception, and information processes. This multimethodological approach examined (1) the influence of attention on sensory and perceptual processing, (2) the executive control of attention by higher centers of the brain, and (3) the processes underlying multisensory integration and the mechanisms by which attention interacts with such integration processes.[131] Processing information acquired from different sensory systems may be directly related to changes to the respective sensory system.

Throughout the life-span, physical growth and development of many systems have an impact on the acquisition and performance of motor skills. Changes in one system and the interactive effects on all other systems can lead to deleterious changes in motor performance as a whole.

Changes in cognitive function in older adults are variable. Examining micro- and macro-level changes is critical to understanding the relationship between structural and behavioral changes.

Consequences of aging include slowed information processing and increased time necessary to perform motor skills.[119] Even though learning may take more time in older adults, once a behavior is learned, retention is similar to that of younger individuals. Of significance for older adults is delayed performance of long-standing tasks, such as driving a car, which may have serious consequences for the driver, passengers, or others in the immediate vicinity of the vehicle. Delays in processing and task execution pose risks to the older person or individuals with CNS deficits and may affect the individual's level of independence and quality of life.[132] These changes are directly related to state-imposed mandatory driving tests for older adults.[119]

Researchers have suggested that some individuals with higher cognitive reserve, attributed to higher educational level and socioeconomic status among other factors, have better compensation and neural plasticity in the face of neural insults, and clinicians should employ strategies to maintain cognitive functioning and/or slow cognitive decline.[115,116] With technological advances introduced over the past three decades, clinicians and researchers are better able to measure structural changes influencing aging.[133] Researchers suggested that the brain and nervous system in older adults, similar to young children, may also be vulnerable to even small changes.[116] Consequently, examining structural and functional changes will be important to better differentiate factors influencing changes.[117] The relationship between cognitive function, brain integrity, compensation, and plasticity are central to a better understanding of normal and impaired cognitive processing in older adults.[115]

Evidence is mounting in support of the premise that physical exercise has a positive effect on the rate of cognitive aging and cognitive performance,[134-138] suggesting that the impact of these normal aging responses can be reduced through structured physical activities. Exercise provides benefits to overall functioning with little cost or side effects. Hence future efforts should focus on delineating the most effective types of exercise programs, frequency, and duration that yield the best outcomes. Recently, evidence emerged supporting the positive impact of social and leisure activities on maintaining cognitive performance in mid-life and older adults.[47,138,139]

Physical and occupational therapists have expertise and would serve as key contributors in developing best practices for exercising with older adults. Therapists are well positioned to work with patients in identifying physical activities that they previously or currently enjoy and find ways to modify the activities to the patients' abilities, as a means of encouraging increased levels of physical activity. Finally, group exercises may be a means to integrate social and leisure activities with exercise to improve participation and benefits to patients.

While older adults experience deterioration in the processing and retrieval of information, the extent of the decline is not consistently predictable. Cognitive deficits most frequently observed in older adults include word retrieval, recall, dual-task execution, and activities involving rapid processing or working memory.

Memory

Memory can be broken down to three types: working, declarative, and procedural. Working memory, short-term memory, is the equivalent of the RAM of a computer.[123] This is the mechanism that enables a child who does not appear to be attending to what the parent is saying to repeat what the parent has just said. Given the temporary nature of this memory, no space in the hippocampus or amygdala is required. Working memory may in fact be more of a cortical phenomenon. Declarative memory is what is typically envisioned when we think of intermediate or long-term memory. Declarative memory is the area where long-term information about everything an individual has ever learned or information acquired is stored, including facts, figures, and names.[123] An example of declarative memory is a second-grade teacher recalling the name of a student she had in her class 15 years previously. Declarative memory is analogous to the hard drive in the computer. The third type of memory is procedural memory. Procedural memory involves all motor activities, actions, habits, or skills that are learned through repetition in motor practice.[123] Examples of procedural memory include walking, playing an instrument, and driving a car.

Different structures in the brain are involved in declarative and procedural memory. Declarative memory involves the hippocampus and other medial-temporal lobe structures, and procedural memory involves interconnected brain structures in frontal/basal-ganglia circuits, including frontal premotor and related regions.[140] Declarative memory is able to rapidly acquire new knowledge from a single experience/exposure.[140,141] While new knowledge acquired through declarative memory can be implicit and explicit, long-term explicit knowledge is thought to solely be acquired through declarative memory. A variety of factors are thought to influence declarative memory including age, sex, sleep, and stress.[140]

Rovee-Collier and colleagues[142-144] have conducted numerous studies related to memory retention in prelinguistic children. Evidence exists to support the premise that infants as young as 2 to 3 months of age are capable of identifying relevant cues and chunking this information for later retrieval. One caveat is that retrieval of such information is possible only when the specifics of the behavior are retained. Infant memories are tightly linked to the specific information related to the task, environment, and stimulus. Consequently, a slight change in any of these three components may result in an inability to retrieve information from infant memory. Retention of information is directly proportional to the infant's age. As an infant grows older, the period for which information is retained increases.

While declarative memory continues to develop through childhood into young adulthood, procedural memory matures in childhood and is thought to influence some aspects of language.[145] As children grow older, they develop more effective and efficient strategies to retain information. During adolescence the brain enters a plastic period, particularly in the frontal lobes. Neuronal connections that control sleeping and eating habits; regulate motor behavior; and modulate impulses, decision making, memory, and other high-level cognitive functions change significantly during adolescence. Given the plasticity of the adolescent's brain, it is highly probable that environmental stimuli influence intrinsic changes in the adolescent's CNS.

Across the life-span, some aspects of cognition seem to be impaired or changed before others. One area most susceptible to age-associated changes is the PFC. This particular area of the brain is where information critical to executive function, attention, and working memory is stored.[146] Although memory is one component of cognition that is generally acknowledged to deteriorate as an individual moves toward older adulthood, not all aspects of memory are affected at the same time or in the same way. Additionally, older adults are thought to compensate for changes in memory by keeping lists and writing things down.[119] Using these strategies, performance of older adults may be better than younger adults depending solely on memory.

Episodic memory is reportedly the first to be impaired, then working memory (short-term memory).[146] Episodic memory is thought to begin declining in the fifth decade.[116] Implicit memory and semantic memory remain intact for a much longer period of time. Little information is available about procedural memory, memory of how to perform tasks. Researchers have suggested that an older adult's declarative memory is also affected by normal and neuropathological aging.[45,146] These investigators suggested that although older adults with deterioration in declarative memory are able to perform tasks, the individual is unable to retain information and consequently unable to learn tasks.[45] Many factors negatively or positively influence memory, including the nature of encoding or processing that information, such as the source of the material or time of day material is presented.[146]

Although evidence exists that many aspects of memory decline with age, recent evidence supports the premise that variables other than encoding and retrieving information may have a significant impact on memory and remembering in older adults.[116,147,148] Researchers at the University of Kuopio examined memory in older persons and focused on neuropsychological processes as a method for evaluating memory and other functions of the frontal lobe.[148] The investigators reported that elderly subjects with subsequent degradation of the frontal lobe had memory loss. These researchers suggested that some aspects of memory loss could be staved off through memory-sharpening activities and games, limitation of alcohol consumption, and participation in activities designed to retain details of skills and tasks. Combining physical and cognitive activities in a training program were also found to improve performance in executive functioning (attention and working memory), episodic memory, and processing speed of older adults for at least 1-year following physical-cognitive training.[136]

May and colleagues[147] examined the role of emotion in memory tasks for older adults and found that older adults seem to be motivated to remember information that is emotionally relevant and meaningful. These findings lend support to yet another system, the emotional system, and its impact on an older adult's memory and task performance.

Emotional System

Although current literature examines the emotional development of children, evidence documenting how emotions are mediated, at a neurobiological level, are still emerging.[149] Emotion is modulated through the amygdala and measured through neuroimaging techniques including positron emission technology (PET) and fMRI scans. The amygdala appears to undergo changes throughout infancy and childhood into adolescence, increasing in volume until age 4 in females and age 18 in males.[149] In addition to the amygdala, the PFC plays an important role in emotional regulation, particularly in early childhood, and decreases in adolescence into early adulthood. If the connection between the amygdala and the PFC is weak, the ability to modulate emotional responsivity may be negatively impacted. Parental control appears to be an important factor in emotional regulation. The better input of parental control on emotion during sensitive periods in development, the better the individual's self-regulatory capacity later in life.

Zinck and Newen[150] proposed a classification of emotion that might provide a clearer understanding of responses within and between individuals and factors that affect emotion. The authors characterized emotion into four categories based on when the emotions appear developmentally. Emotion is characterized as a means of communicating state, expectations, and reactions of an individual.[150] Emotions are "interpersonal/interactive" behaviors that enable the individual to communicate to the world. The four categories are pre-emotions, basic emotions, primary cognitive emotions, and secondary cognitive emotions. Pre-emotions and basic emotions function as basic mental representations, whereas primary cognitive and secondary cognitive emotions are categorized as cognitive attitudes.

Pre-emotions are characterized as innate behaviors, present at birth, nonspecific, nonintentional, and used for communication to others about the state of the infant.[150] Pre-emotions are identified as comfort and distress. These responses may be positive or negative responses depending on the situations. Pre-emotions are the most fundamental sensations followed by basic emotions.

Basic emotions and developmental timing of basic emotions include joy at 2 to 3 months, anger at 3 to 4 months, sadness at 3 to 7 months, and fear at 7 to 9 months. These emotions are said to emerge in the absence of conscious processing of stimuli. These responses are shared by other mammals, and do not involve complex cognitive processing. These behaviors lead to faster and more stereotypic responses.[150]

Primary cognitive emotions are characterized as basic emotions with more specificity, in addition to a cognitive component. Primary cognitive emotions are highly dependent on the individual's cognitive development as well as cultural variations and socialization.

Secondary cognitive emotions are depicted as complex constructs that involve social relations, with consideration for expectations of the future. Consequently, secondary cognitive emotions are highly dependent on personal experiences and culture. The authors provide an example of how one situation—high performance in academics—would be perceived by different cultures. Whereas a child from one culture might receive praise for and exhibit pride in high academic performance, a child from another culture could have such performance deemphasized and display shame. In addition to cognition, secondary cognitive emotions incorporate social constructs of family, culture, previous experiences, and environment in formulating complex responses.[151] These responses are cumulative, using previous experiences to render new responses.

Examination of emotion in adults often involves a retrospective analysis of the behavior over a specified period of time. Although the focus of the research may be directed toward emotion, memory cannot be disentangled from the emotion. With regard to aging in older adults, researchers generally have reported that emotions—in particular, negative emotions—diminish later in life. Some researchers have suggested that diminished negative emotions may be attributed to decreased functioning in the amygdala.[152] Still other investigators have suggested that, rather, a decline in the functioning of the amygdala and decreased ability to recall negative experiences may be attributed to the socioemotional selectivity theory (SST).[153] The SST involves prioritization of memories and which temporal boundaries play a role in prioritization. Specifically, older adults do not perceive negative emotions as a priority; hence older adults are more likely to process positive emotions than negative.

Problems in normal emotional development are documented in the literature, focused on childhood and adulthood emotional problems stemming from either pathological conditions or environmental conditions during childhood.[154-159] Within the literature, the reader can find discussions of emotional intelligence in adults and how emotional skills such as empathy or cultural sensitivity might be taught.[160-166] Specific aspects of an emotion or mood change and how that might assist or hinder an individual within a psychosocial environment can be located,[167-170] but the integration of the entire emotional system and its normal changes throughout life require additional study. Future research directed toward aging and emotion has potential to broaden the theoretical perspective by examining emotional experiences in an ecological context.[171,172] In addition, identifying, measuring, and analyzing variables that appear to make a difference in social and professional success will be a central focus of future studies.[173] (See Chapter 4 on the limbic system and its influence on motor control and Chapter 5 on psychosocial adaptation and adjustment for additional information.)

Language

Consistent with all areas of development, acquisition of language, receptive and expressive, is measured quantitatively and qualitatively. Critical to the acquisition of receptive and expressive language is sensory, cognitive, perceptual, and motor development in the infant and child. Researchers have found evidence that language development emerges through nonverbal gestures or "signs"[174-178] and is evident as early as 6 months of age.[177,178] As the number of nonverbal gestures increases, verbal communication reportedly emerges earlier than in infants who do not use nonverbal gestures.[175,177,178] "Gestures thus serve as a signal that a child will soon be ready to begin producing multi-word sentences."[179] Having a large number of gestures at 18 months of age positively affects later language development and is the foundation for later linguistic abilities.[176]

Imitation, such as "mama" or "dada," is often the first form of verbal communication, progressing to spontaneous single-word utterances. Infants produce their first spoken single-word utterances as early as 12 to 15 months of age.[180] During this time the child's brain is undergoing rapid differentiation in Broca's area; at the same time, motoric ability to communicate verbally is emerging. Consequently, it is evident that intrinsic (neurodevelopmental) constraints and extrinsic (environmental) factors affect the emergence of receptive and expressive language. Investigators examining utterances in children and adults reported that utterances produced by children do not approximate those of adults until 14 years of age.[181,182] Recently researchers reported that, consistent with findings of earlier investigators, articulatory movement speed increases from birth to adulthood.[182] Throughout childhood, as language acquisition emerges, children become more sophisticated in communicating and more fully integrate information from intrinsic and extrinsic sources to produce more complex utterances.[180]

Maner and colleagues[181] reported that children exhibited increased variability when a five-word sentence was embedded in longer sentences than when the child spoke only the five-word sentence. These findings led the investigators to infer that a relationship existed between language processing and movement in young children.[183] In addition, adults reportedly modified the five-word sentence when it was embedded in the longer sentence, but 5-year-olds did not modify the utterance. Sadagopan and Smith[184] replicated the work of Maner and colleagues[181] and found that children aged 5 to 16 years exhibited more variability when the five-word sentence was embedded in a more complex sentence compared with when the five-word sentence was spoken in isolation. Young adults (21 to 22 years old) reportedly did not exhibit this same variability. In addition, investigators reported that the duration of the simple and complex utterances differed between children and adults. Unlike the youngest children (5 and 7 years), duration of the utterances decreased in adults. This finding provided evidence for the investigators' theory that adults altered or shortened the complex utterances, given the shorter duration taken to utter the complex sentence. Whereas earlier researchers reported that both adults and children decrease their rate of speech during complex sentences,[185] more recently investigators suggested that adults may increase their rate of speech production. Sadagopan and Smith[184] reported that although both children and adults slow the rate of speech production, children exhibited a much slower rate than adults in producing complex sentences. Hence investigators concluded that whereas adults' rate of speech production did explain some of the difference in utterance duration for the simple and complex sentences, it did not fully explain the differences. This led investigators to suggest that differences in utterance duration may be attributed to both faster rate of speech and altered or shortened complex sentences containing the simple five-word phrase.

Researchers focused on expressive language in adults reported that older adults speech patterns demonstrate more interrupted speech than younger adults and used nonnormative language that might be attributed to increased word-finding difficulties.[186] Speech in adults (65 to 85 years) resembled that of children (<11 years of age).[187] While older adults had more instances of nonnormative word use than younger adults, the words used were often characterized as more optimal than younger adults. Perhaps some of these expressive language changes noted in older adults are related to the high incidence of hearing loss.[187] Older adults experience decreased perception of high-frequency sounds and dynamic range. Researchers used fMRI to document regions activated when examining aspects of expressive language and found that different regions were activated in older adults. Changes in physical and physiological structures as well as decreased motor control in older adults and children may be factors impacting similar language challenges. The dynamic nature of language is grounded in the constructs of dynamical systems theory involving intrinsic and extrinsic mechanisms. These mechanisms evolve over time and are highly sensitive to changes within and between systems.

Perceptual System

As researchers continue to examine the interactive and interdependent roles of body systems, the perceptual system must not be omitted. Perception, yet another process important to performance of functional movements, involves acquisition, interpretation, selection, and organization of sensory information. Perception is the very essence of the interaction between organism and environment. Every movement gives rise to perceptual information and in turn guides the organism to adapt movements accordingly.[12,188]

Initially perception revolves around the infant's visual exploration of people, objects, and environmental activities. Infants are capable, at birth, of visually exploring their environment, people, and objects.[124] Investigators have suggested that infants use information acquired through visual exploration to develop new methods of exploring and discovering cues about the environment such as depth, distance, surface definition, and dimensionality of objects.[189]

A second phase of perceptual exploration emerges as an infant's exploratory behaviors transition to functional movements such as reaching and kicking. Through these exploratory behaviors emerge additional mechanisms for acquiring information about the environment.[6,188] Throughout development, active exploration enhances perceptual information through each new encounter and enables the infant to recognize distinctive features and similar characteristics that allow the infant to differentiate between objects. The information generated from exploration provides new input to many subsystems, in particular the sensory, motor, and cognitive systems that enable the individual to gain new knowledge about the environment and the action.

Development of the infant's perceptual system is dependent on acquiring new information about the affordances of the task that may influence performance of the action. As the infant develops the capacity for independent mobility, the expanse of the environment increases, as do the opportunities to integrate prior knowledge with newly acquired information to discover unchartered surroundings. This again supports the interactive and interdependent nature of systems throughout development. As maturation progresses, infants develop the ability to evaluate information acquired from various systems and to make decisions about the optimal strategy for successfully navigating over or around a surface. With maturation, successful navigation of new environments depends on opportunities for exploration that may involve other processes in addition to motor processes. An example of this may be seen in a person trying to locate a building in an unfamiliar city. Adults typically use maps as a visual representation of the surroundings that allow them to find the location. Infants and young children are most accurate in locating desired targets through active exploration. This allows the child to acquire spatial information critical to locating the destination at a future time.

If perception is the process of integrating and organizing intrinsic and extrinsic input, then changes in sensory systems as a consequence of aging are certain to affect perception.[190] The visual perceptual processing system is most often identified as altered in older adults. Specifically, researchers have reported that although older adults are capable of discriminating between variation in depth perception in a manner similar to that of younger adults, they are less able to discriminate between three-dimensional shapes of objects.[191] Clearly the perceptual system is closely associated with many other body systems, and therefore age-related or age-associated structural and functional changes in associated systems will affect the perceptual system.[192] Older adults secure input from multiple areas/systems to address issues associated with cognitive and perceptual changes. This suggests that increasing visual challenges increases the need for compensatory activity. Age-related changes in the visual acuity necessitate use of assistive devices such as glasses.

In addition, May and colleagues[147] found that older adults placed less emphasis on perceptual aspects of an event than they did on the emotional components when encoding information. They suggested that older adults may find emotional information to be more meaningful than perceptual information and may retain more elaborate, detailed processing of emotional data than perceptual information.

Decreased processing speed is well documented in older adults and directly impacts visual perceptual abilities.[193] Physical activity is one factor that positively impacts age-related perceptual decline. The structural and functional changes associated with physical activity are thought to delay the onset of degenerative changes in the brain. Findings continue to build supporting the premise that older adults participating in physical activities have maintained visuospatial skills and related cognitive functions.[193,194]

MOTOR DEVELOPMENT

Movement is the primary mechanism by which prelinguistic children communicate with their environment. That said, it is no wonder that development of motor skills is greatest during the first 2 years of life. Motor development may be defined as the acquisition, refinement, and integration of biomechanical principles of movement in an effort to achieve a motor behavior that is proficient.[13]

Early developmental researchers referred to infants as *reactive,* inferring that, early on, infants are responsive to stimuli rather than capable of initiating functional movements. Young infants were characterized as "reflexive" beings producing stereotypic primitive and postural responses to stimuli. Emergence of these reflexive motor behaviors was based on traditional models of CNS organization and motor development theories. Traditional theories of human development emerged from animal models and studies involving spontaneously aborted fetuses.[16,195] Traditionally, sucking and stepping behaviors were examples of developmental reflexes. By definition, a reflex is a consistent response to a consistent stimulus. By use of traditional models of CNS organization, developmental reflexes, present at birth, become integrated as higher centers assume control over lower centers and then volitional movements begin to emerge.

Over the past two to three decades, advances in technology have enabled scientists to gain more insight into fetal and infant motor abilities. More recently, research has generated evidence that behaviors emerge out of a need to solve a problem in the environment rather than solely as a result of maturation in the CNS.[196] Given this evidence supporting the premise that newborn infants are capable of producing complex volitional movements, previous views of the infant as passive and "reflexive" are no longer accurate. In addition, continuing to refer to early infant motor behaviors as "reflexes" may also not accurately reflect the behavior. A reflex is defined as a consistent response given in response to a consistent stimulus. Perhaps use of the term *innate motor behaviors* to reflect behaviors that are present at birth may be more appropriate. See Fig. 2.1A–C, for a visual explanation of how the complexity of the stepping reaction of a newborn infant and the learned programming for upright posture and balance, including biomechanical range and force production, will lead to the integration of stepping in standing. Similarly, as an individual ages loss of some of the postural power, effectiveness of balance reactions, and fear can create a potentially dangerous environment for an elderly person (see Fig. 2.1D–E). Likewise, an individual with an abnormal or inefficient stepping pattern (see Fig. 2.1F) should automatically stand out to a therapist analyzing movement dysfunction. If a clinician does not have a clear picture in his or her mind of the movement pattern desired, then easily or quickly identifying the system or subsystem motor impairments seen in a patient's movement dysfunction may be outside a therapist's analytical repertoire.

Contemporary research refutes the assertion that infants are reactive organisms.[114,118] In contrast, contemporary studies purport that infants are competent and capable of producing complex interactive behaviors at birth.[124,197] Additional support for the complex nature of a newborn infant is evident in the infant's ability to discriminate and turn toward his or her mother's voice rather than toward the voice of an adult with whom the infant is unfamiliar.

Evidence from studies examining motor development indicate that motor behaviors do not always emerge in a linear and predictable sequence, nor do all individuals achieve the same skills at the same chronological age.[10,197] Rather, emergence of motor behaviors in an alternate sequence may be attributed to the intrinsic and extrinsic constraints that contribute to motor development in a nonlinear fashion and is not necessarily indicative of atypical development. Fig. 2.2A is an example of a child who had a very large head at birth. His head circumference was in the 99.9th percentile and remained so for the first 3 years of his life. His Apgar score at birth was 10, or normal. He was slow in rolling over and coming to sit and spent much of his time playing with his hands and feet and visually exploring the environment. Fig. 2.2B and C illustrate that his focus was on fine motor development throughout his first year, especially when he was placed in a vertical position. He loved to play catch when placed in a sitting position and accurately propelled the ball toward a partner when playing by age 1 year. His early gross motor development was within the normal range but below the mean. He started independently walking at age 14 months and began running on the same day. Fig. 2.2D–F illustrate that once he gained control over the heavy weight of his head, he quickly caught up in gross motor skill. And, like any child, he has taken full advantage of his environment to play and learn.

Over the past several decades the incidence of obesity in children and adolescents has increased dramatically.[198] The incidence of obesity has increased in all age groups and sexes, and currently 20% of all children are classified as obese, with a prevalence greater among children who are African American or Hispanic. With the increase in overweight and obese children, the Centers for Disease Control and Prevention (CDC) defined the terms overweight (>85% BMI) and obesity class I-III. One of the most striking increases of obesity in an age group was noted in children aged 2 to 5 years. Obesity is said to be one of the greatest threats to public health.[199–201] Several factors are thought to impact the increase in obesity including SES, nutrition, participation in organized sports, access to safe walkable environments, as well as screen device use.[200,201] The use of screen devices include television (TV), smartphones, tablets, computers, and video-gaming systems place children at risk for obesity associated with decreased physical activity, sleep deprivation, and increased intake of sugary drinks and foods.[200] While adolescents are recognized as high-end users of screen devices, it is estimated that up to 50% of 3-year-olds have a tablet. Children with obesity are at increased risk for asthma, sleep apnea, musculoskeletal problems, precocious maturation, polycystic ovarian syndrome, and hepatic steatosis. Children may also have mental health issues directly related to their weight issues, including low self-esteem, depression, decreased quality of life, and bullying. Children with obesity are five times more likely to have obesity as adults than individuals not obese as children. Estimates of previous research indicate that 64% of preadolescent children and 80% of adolescent children with obesity have obesity as adults.[201] Obesity in childhood that continues into adulthood places an individual at higher risk for chronic diseases associated with obesity including hypertension, hyperlipidemia, type II diabetes, and cardiovascular disease.[202] Given the relationship between obesity and physical activity, obesity may play a role in an individual's motor performance.

Motor performance, measured both qualitatively and quantitatively, is highly dependent on the task, the environment, and the individual. Changes in motor performance emerge in accordance with age-dependent changes, within different systems, and with respect to environmental affordances and constraints. As skills emerge in speech, language, and cognition, other previously achieved skills may "regress." In reality, acquisition of a new skill requires more attention than the previously attained skills; consequently, the infant or child's attention is divided between the tasks. Lindenberger and colleagues[203–205] conducted studies investigating life-span changes in resource allocation

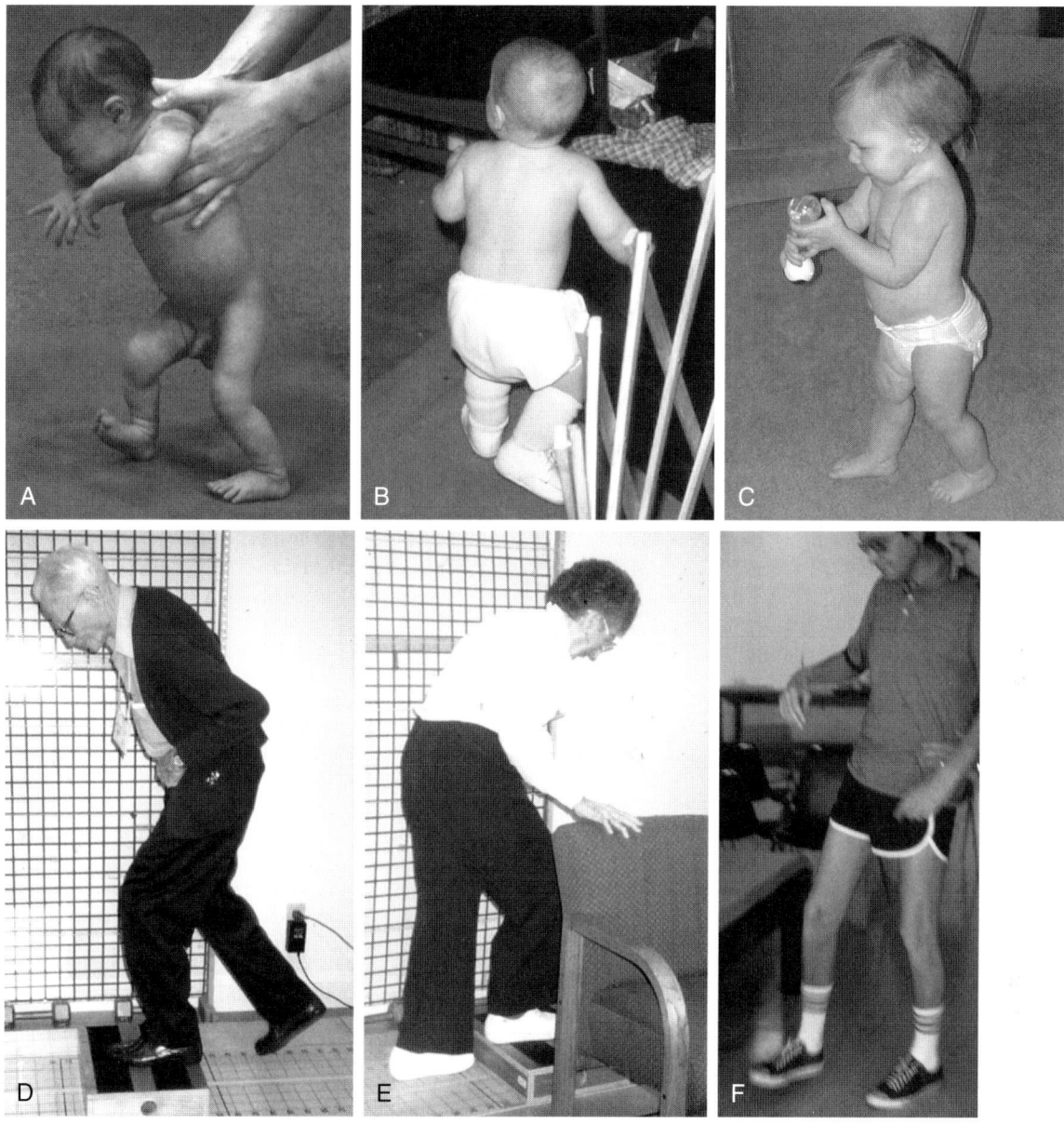

Fig. 2.1 Development and Integration of Stepping, Upright Vertical Posture, and Vertical Balance Reaction. **(A)** Automatic stepping in a newborn infant. **(B)** Early cruising or side-stepping using multiple points of support. **(C)** Early bipedal independent stepping. **(D)** 90-year-old patient stepping. **(E)** 78-year-old patient with falling problems. **(F)** Abnormal stepping after traumatic brain injury.

during multitask activities. The researchers found that for young children certain tasks require more attention and attempting to perform such a task in conjunction with a task requiring less attention causes deterioration in performance of both tasks. Hence deterioration of a previously attained skill is more likely a result of attentional demands of young children performing high-attention tasks rather than a true "regression" of the skill. This progression is illustrated by a child confronted with a new environment, who will seem as if he or she has regressed in motor performance while confronting and solving a task-specific challenge—for example, crossing over a suspension bridge that moves from side to side is compliant to body weight and creates a perceptual challenge from the visual surround. Once the child understands the task, his attention is directed toward developing effective strategies to solve a problem and successfully perform the motor

behavior of crossing the bridge. Stability or consistency in performing a skilled movement is achieved by self-organization through practice and repetition.[23] Performance of skilled movements, such as those observed in athletes, is measured not only on the consistency in performing the task but also on the skilled performance of the task under variable conditions.[23] Conversely, decreased frequency in performing a motor skill as an effect of age may result in a less rich repertoire of normal variability and may be a contributing factor to a decline in motor skills.[32] Just as motor skills emerge from a multifactorial interweaving of maturation and experience, deterioration in motor performance may be attributable to alterations in various systems that occur as part of the aging process. Emergence of motor behaviors is never the same for any two individuals, nor does decline in functional motor behaviors follow the same time line. Fig. 2.3 illustrates how standing

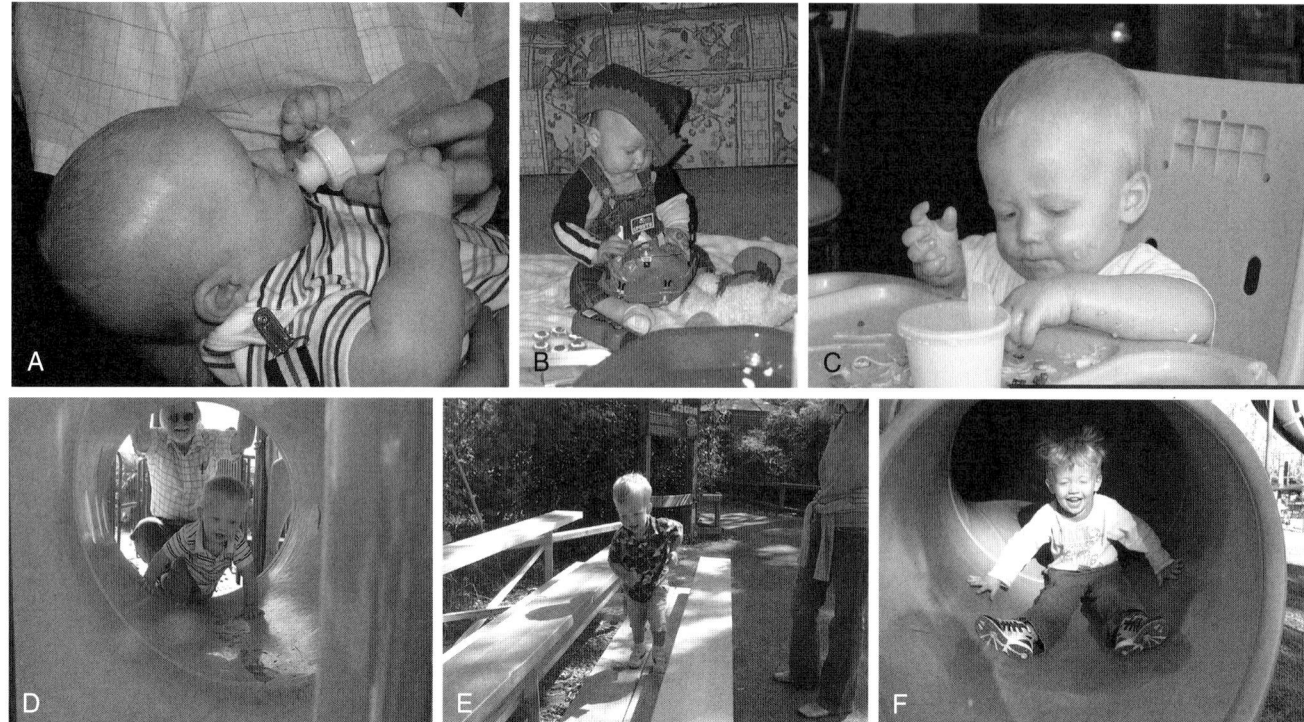

Fig. 2.2 Head size can affect when a child initiates independent movement activities and whether he or she develops gross or fine motor skills. **(A)** A 2-month-old being fed (note large head). **(B)** Child at 5 months old placed in sitting has overcome delayed head control in vertical. **(C)** By 9 months old, the child has gained normal head control as well as fine motor skills. **(D)** Head control in horizontal crawling. **(E)** Child running at 2 years of age. **(F)** Normal head control on slide. By 1 year of age, head size is no longer a variable.

patterns will change with practice, be maintained as long as practice continues, become extremely efficient within a specific environmental context, or become deficient after CNS injury.

Prenatal (0 to 40 Weeks' Gestation) Development

Motor behaviors emerge early in embryonic life. By the tenth week of fetal life the variety of observed movements increases, as does the frequency of the movements. Complex movements are present by gestational age (GA) 12 weeks, and goal-directed movements may be seen as early as GA 13 weeks. Facial movements, including sucking, swallowing, and yawning, are evident in the second and third trimesters. The fetal activity level increases so that by week 14 GA, periods of quiet (no activity) are only 5 to 6 minutes in duration. Investigators have documented 15 fetal movements visible by 15 weeks of age.[206] After initial observation of a motor behavior, it remains part of the fetal repertoire. Pooh and Ogura's[206] research lends support to the premise that before delivery fetuses are in fact capable of producing complex motor behaviors.

The dynamic nature of birth and the associated change from the intrauterine to the extrauterine environment alter the production of movements previously observed in fetal life.[73] As the newborn infant adapts to the forces in the extrauterine environment, motor behaviors emerge. These complex behaviors lend additional evidence to the premise that at birth infants are competent beings.

The extrauterine environment poses many challenges for the newborn infant. Consequently, fetal behaviors observed by ultrasonography may not be evident postnatally until the infant learns to adapt to the new environment by modifying movements to accommodate to the new forces imposed by gravity. Newborn infants must learn to use

new strategies to generate functional motor behaviors, given the different environmental constraints.

Infancy (Birth to 12 Months)

As alluded to earlier, newborn infants possess a rich array of motor behaviors. During the first year of life, motor behaviors are the primary mechanism for learning. Every movement is a new and unique opportunity to gain knowledge about the environment. During each movement, new information is gathered in an effort to solve environmental problems, and as a result this motor planning fosters cognitive development. Similarly, each movement provides feedback that intrinsically enables the infant to modify movements in accordance with changes in the environment, the skill, or growth parameters.[207] This interdependence between perception and motor behaviors allows one domain to facilitate acquisition of skills in the other domain in a reciprocal fashion.

Given the capabilities of a newborn infant, many behaviors previously identified as reflexes are in fact functional motor behaviors that the infant is capable of modifying. Evidence that one such behavior, sucking, is not a reflex was supported by studies examining sucking rates when stimuli were varied.[208,209] Researchers reported that the sucking response varied depending on the level of hunger or environmental stimuli. In addition, when the stimulus is introduced after feeding, after the infant is satiated, the stimulus may produce no response or a diminished response, thus refuting the idea that sucking is reflexive.

Consequently, rather than refer to these behaviors as *developmental reflexes,* it seems more accurate to refer to such motor behaviors, evident at birth, as *innate motor behaviors.* Innate motor behaviors are,

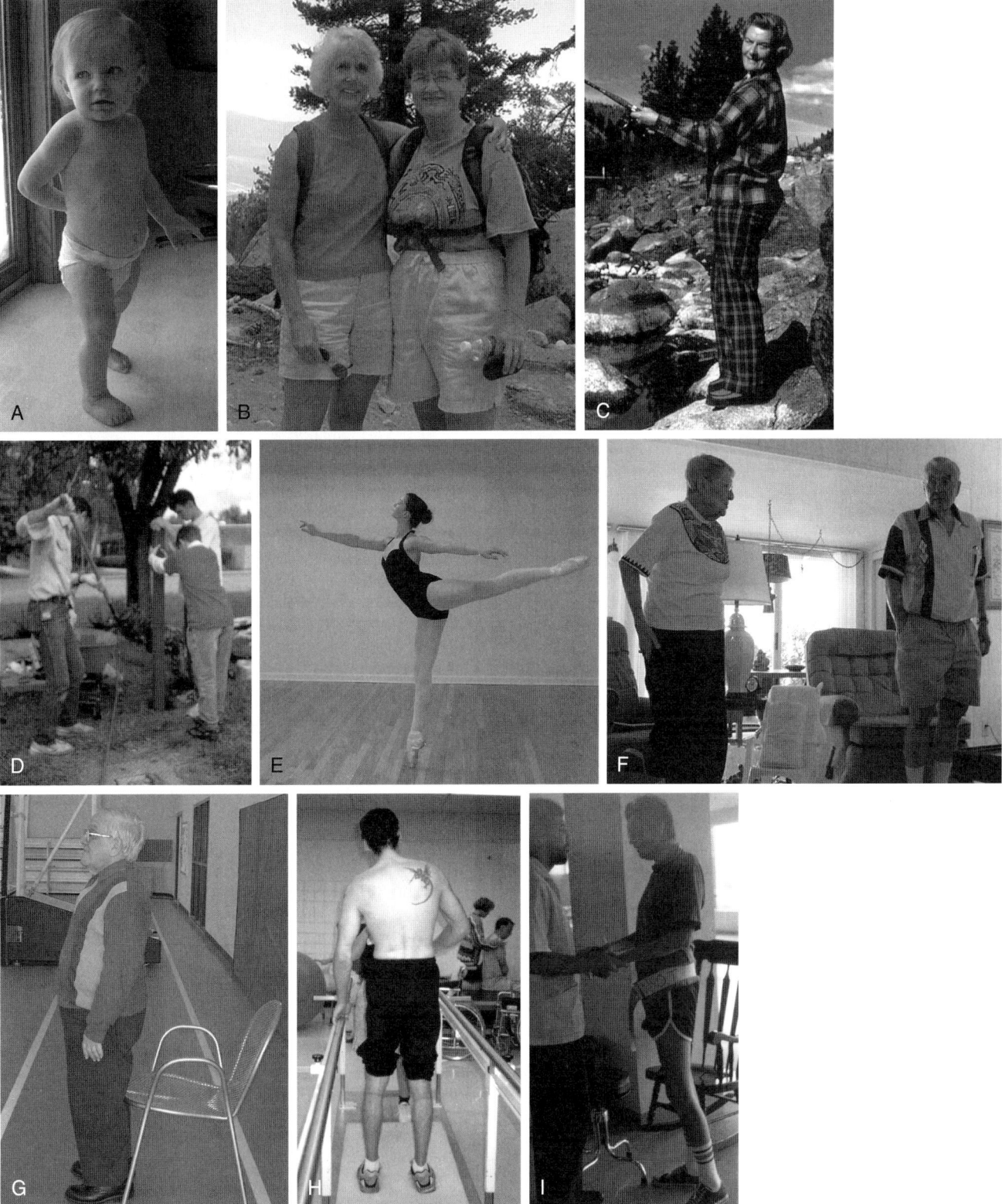

Fig. 2.3 Standing as a functional activity will become procedural with practice and be maintained over a lifetime as long as impairments do not preclude practice or injury to the central nervous system (CNS). **(A)** Early standing. **(B)** Relaxed standing as adults. **(C)** Standing on uneven surfaces. **(D)** Procedural standing during a functional activity. **(E)** Advanced skill in standing as ballet dancer. **(F)** Maintained functional standing in healthy 83-year-old elderly couple. **(G)** Elderly man developing verticality impairment. **(H)** Subtle abnormal standing after head injury. **(I)** Multiple subsystem problems in standing after CNS injury.

in essence, functional behaviors present at birth that are modifiable given alterations in feedback from intrinsic or extrinsic mechanisms.

Additional evidence exists to refute the concept that other motor behaviors are reflexes. Stepping is one such behavior. Thelen and Fisher[20,34,35] conducted a series of experiments examining the stepping reflex in young infants. Early developmentalists hypothesized that stepping reflexes, present at birth, became integrated and then later emerged as a volitionally controlled movement. Thelen and Fisher[20,35] found that when one variable, weight, was altered, infants mimicked "integration" or emergence of the behavior. Young infants who were stepping had weights added to their lower extremities, to simulate weight gain over the first few months. These infants stopped stepping. Similarly, infants who did not step were submersed in chest-deep water, simulating less weight in the lower extremities, and stepping appeared. Obviously, the presence and absence of this behavior was mediated by weight gain in the lower extremities and not by CNS control as early developmental researchers had postulated. Consequently, upright mobility emerges when the infant is able to garner the force production in the lower extremities to modulate stepping. This is just one example of the significance of one system on another and the interdependent nature of body systems. Recognizing the interdependence of systems may provide one explanation for the presence or absence of motor behaviors at any given time. These concepts have been transferred into the therapeutic practice environment when working with individuals who cannot generate enough force to produce the movement given the body size or cannot produce the postural stability to reinforce the stepping pattern or one of a variety of other motor components that support normal upright stepping or walking. (See Chapter 3 for theories of motor control and learning, Chapter 8 for therapeutic approaches to assist a patient with learning or relearning motor control, and Chapter 38, which introduces emerging practices to bridge the gap between normal human movement development and technologies.)

At birth, an infant is capable of turning toward the sound of her or his mother's voice and visually focusing on objects 8 to 12 inches from the face.[124] These behaviors are apparent when the infant's head is supported, given that at birth the newborn infant does not have the neck strength to maintain head control against gravity. Similarly, auditory and visual stimuli continue to bombard the infant and challenge the motor system, fostering the need to attain head control.

Infant motor behaviors during the first 3 months of life are focused on acquisition of head control in all planes of movement. Once the infant has achieved head control in the supine and prone positions, the complexity of the tasks increases exponentially on the basis of the new challenges and stimuli presented to the infant. For example, while in the prone position an infant may reach for an object out of reach and then roll to attain the desired object. Improvements in visual acuity enable an infant to visually track people and objects at greater distances while challenging the infant to seek out the stimuli.

By age 3 to 4 months, as the infant is able to maintain head control in the upright position for longer periods, coordinated eye-hand activities begin to emerge. Acquisition of manipulative skills involves perception and lends support for the coupling of developing cognitive, sensory, and motor systems.[25,188] Bushnell and Boudreau[8] added that if the infant is unable to achieve a motor skill and this skill is coupled with a sensory or cognitive task, that task may not be attained. Bushnell and Boudreau's[8] research focused on the role of motor development in achieving skills in other domains.

Reaching is one such task that the researchers suggest may serve to promote skills in cognitive and sensory domains. Initial reaching activities enable the infant to gain information relevant to depth perception, and coupling this information then allows the infant to modulate parameters associated with reaching. For example, the infant

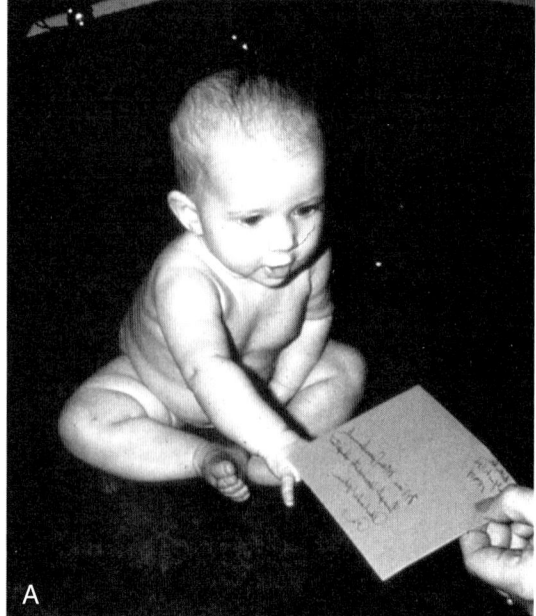

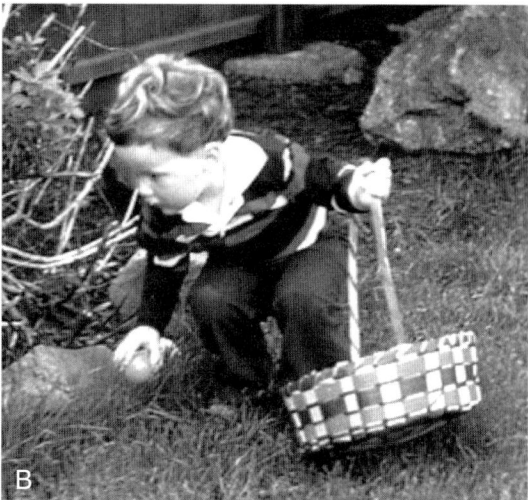

Fig. 2.4 Reaching Activity. (A) Error in reaching leads to learning, and **(B)** reaching becomes accurate during a complex motor task.

must learn to vary the distance moved and force necessary to attain an object given a series of opportunities. Infant grasping and reaching may initially seem inefficient, but with practice under varying situations, efficiency and accuracy improve across multiple domains with varying rates. Fig. 2.4 illustrates both the error that provides feedback and the success during complex movement patterns after practice.

As infants develop an upright sitting posture, they use their upper extremities for support. Sitting, a functional motor behavior, is tightly linked to the performance of most ADLs and occupational and leisure-time activities. Fig. 2.5 depicts development of functional sitting over a lifetime. A delay in attaining independent sitting may directly affect upper extremity control, alter attainment of skills in other domains, and ultimately affect an individual's level of functional independence.

As upright trunk posture is attained and independent sitting emerges, usually by 6 months of age, and infants then begin to explore using their manipulative skills. Manipulative skills are composed of reaching and grasping behaviors. Upper-extremity interlimb coordination bimanual and unimanual tasks include retrieving objects

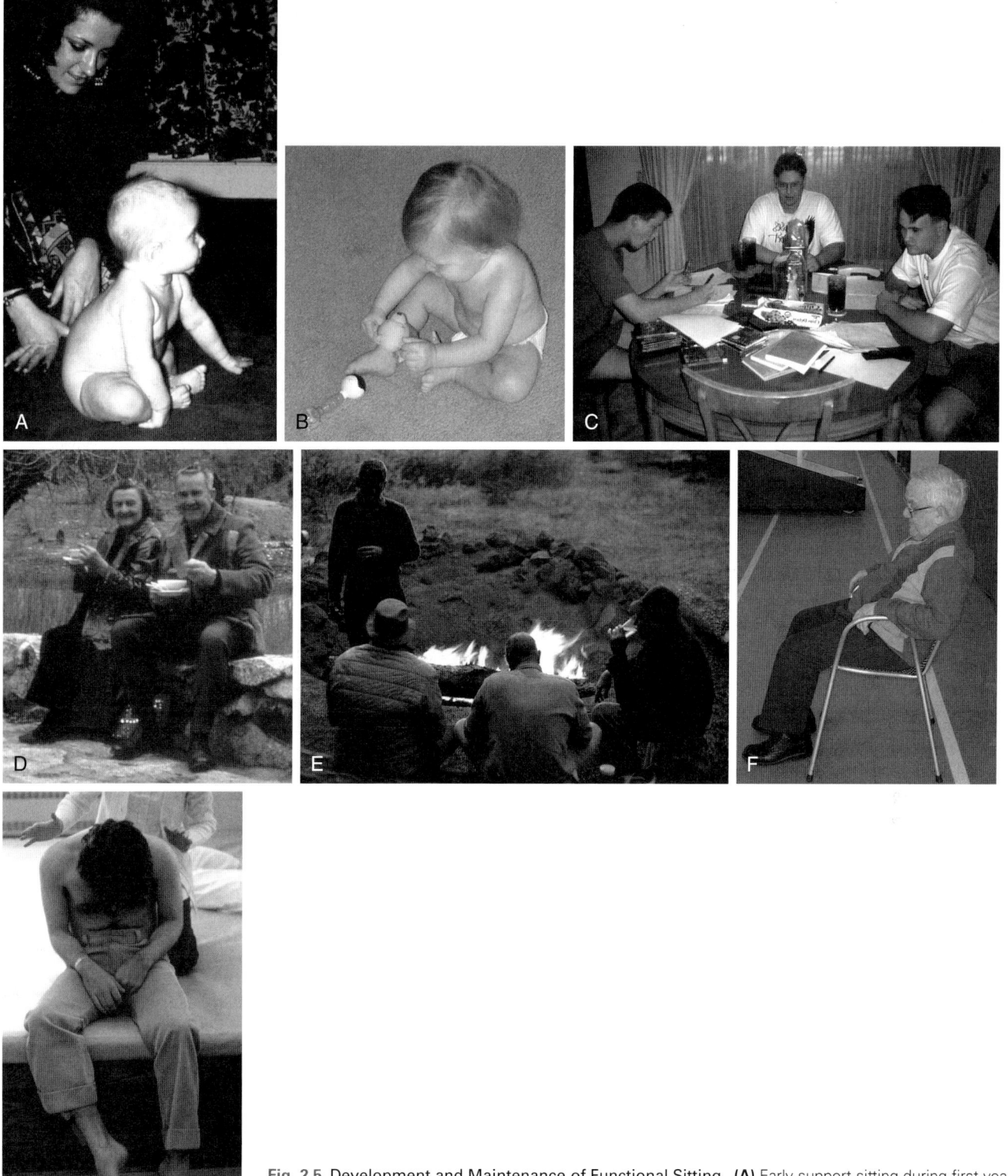

Fig. 2.5 Development and Maintenance of Functional Sitting. **(A)** Early support sitting during first year. **(B)** Independent sitting during play. **(C)** Functional sitting in adolescents while studying. **(D)** Adults sitting without support while eating. **(E)** Sitting as part of a social interaction of an adult group. **(F)** Functional changes in sitting in the elderly. **(G)** Loss of adequate sitting programs after closed head injury.

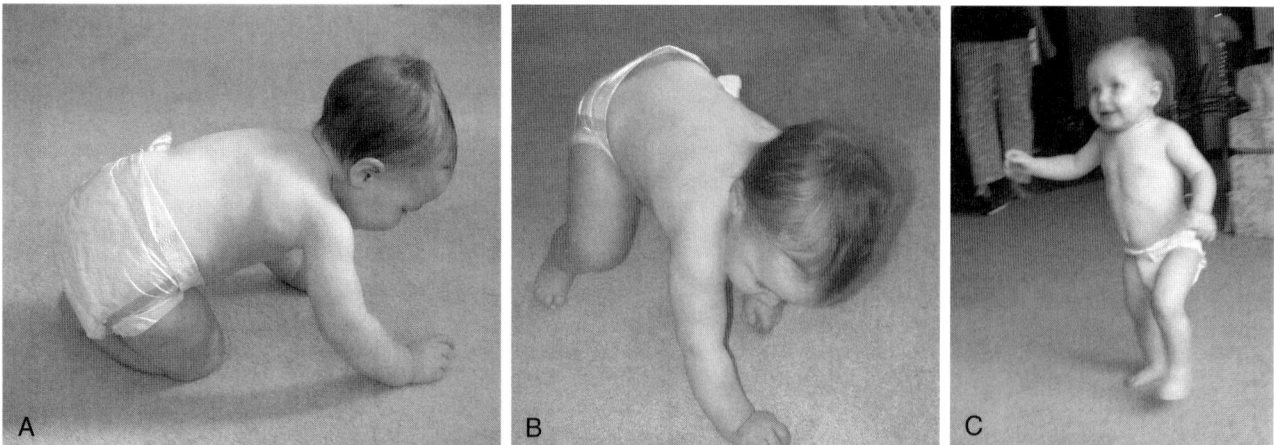

Fig. 2.6 Emergence of Upright Mobility. (A) Quadruped in preparation for quadrupedal creeping. **(B)** Moving from quadruped into standing. **(C)** Moving in vertical.

(placed within reach); holding two objects, one in each hand; using two hands to hold an object (bottle); and holding a toy in one hand while retrieving another object with the free hand.[210]

During the second half of year 1, the infant is focused on mobility, initially prone (rolling, crawling), then creeping on all fours, and then upright (cruising and ambulation). Adolph and Berger[25] reported that as coordination of upper- and lower-extremity movements with trunk control emerges and infants begin upright mobility, they spend up to 50% of their day performing balance- and mobility-based activities, varying the surface, distance, and other parameters each time the task is performed (Fig. 2.6). On the basis of research conducted with infants acquiring independent mobility, Adolph and Berger[25] estimate that an infant walks up to 29 football fields each day.

Acquisition of independent mobility is complicated by new manipulative skills, as discussed by Corbetta and Thelen.[210] They found that while infants are achieving independent mobility, their manipulative skills are highly variable and vacillate between bimanual and unimanual tasks depending on the nature of other tasks with which the infant is involved. Infants may revert to performing bimanual activities, with upper extremities coupled and movements synchronized, during early acquisition of independent mobility, signaling the presence of multiple tasks requiring attention. Unimanual control signals uncoupling of the upper extremities and asynchronous manipulation in young children.

Analyzing the early development of a child is often done at specific times over the first year, such as at birth, 2 months, 6 months, and 9 months. As important as understanding and analyzing a complex phase of development such as 3 months is analyzing the changes in motor control and learning of a specific motor function over a period of time. The development of head control is a good example of how the nervous system adapts and learns given different environmental restraints over a period of time. The complexity and integration of movement patterns involved in a child gaining functional control over the head in all spatial environments can be delineated into many components. Each component can then become a variable in determining how and if a child has or will develop a specific movement pattern such as head control (see Fig. 2.2).

Weight is one factor that plays a role in acquisition of motor skills. Dinkel and colleagues[211] examined sitting development in infants who were normal and overweight. While the authors did not see differences in the temporal aspects of skill acquisition, they noted that overweight in-

fants employed different postural strategies than normal weight infants. Overweight infants demonstrated lower sway amplitude during sitting skills acquisition, and their sway pattern was more confined to mediolateral movement than their normal-weight counterparts. As they became more skilled in performing the behavior, the postural control resembled strategies employed by normal weight infants.

Early Childhood (1 to 5 Years)

Whereas the first year of life is characterized by periods of rapid physical growth and acquisition of motor skills, the second year signals a slower rate of growth, refinement of current skills, and acquisition of new motor skills.[212] Concurrently the toddler experiences rapid differentiation in other domains including cognition, speech, and social-emotional domains.

At the onset of the second year of life, independent ambulation becomes refined as other forms of mobility wane. Dynamic balance in an upright bipedal posture evolves as the infant develops more mature gait characteristics. Modification of parameters indicative of a more mature gait include narrowing of the base of support, decreased cocontraction in the lower extremities, and improved intralimb coordination, as well as learning to modulate displacement and velocity.[25] As gait matures and toddlers have more opportunity to explore their environment, more challenges appear. Attempts to solve these problems and challenges result in the appearance of more complex motor behaviors that include running, climbing, and jumping. Toddlers find particular pleasure in throwing, kicking, and catching balls. In addition, toddlers assert their independence through such activities as propelling themselves with riding toys.

Toddlers continue to explore and assert independence through activities involving bimanual and unimanual tasks. Challenges to fine motor skills of toddlers involve manipulating functional objects (large buttons, eating utensils, crayons, door knobs, and blocks; opening and closing jars to retrieve small objects [cereal, raisins]). Achieving these tasks enables the toddler to perform rudimentary aspects of ADLs such as eating and dressing and adds another degree of independence. Fig. 2.7 illustrates development of ambulatory skill over a lifetime.

Preschool-aged children pedal a tricycle and use a narrow base of support to walk along a balance beam. By age 3 years most children ascend stairs using alternating feet and by 4 years most descend stairs alternately. Fig. 2.8 shows a preschooler descending stairs. The gait pattern matures with reciprocal arm swing and a heel-to-toe gait

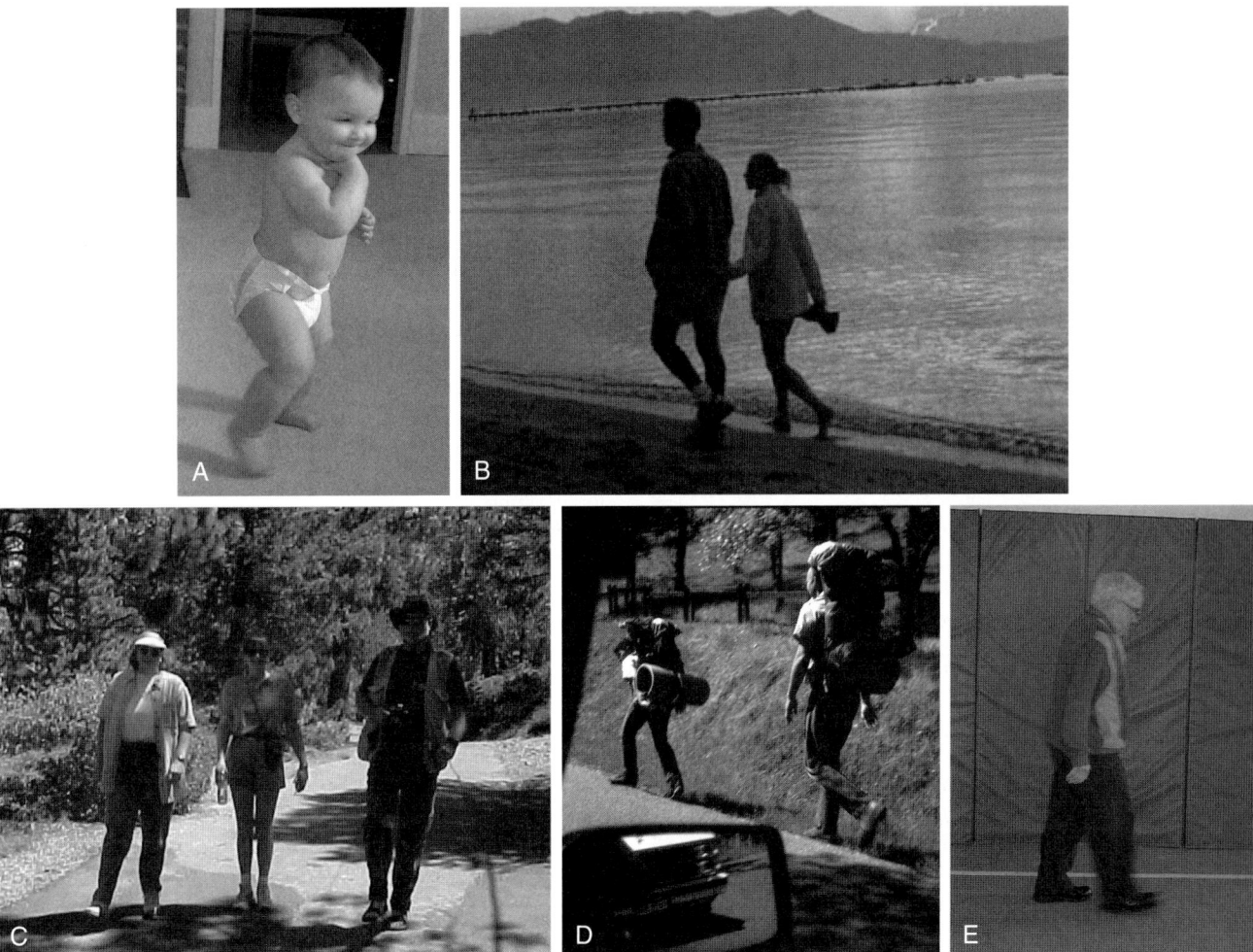

Fig. 2.7 Functional Ambulation Over the Life-Span. (A) Early independent walking. **(B)** Two young adults walking on sand. **(C)** Three adults of different body sizes, each walking independently. **(D)** Hiking with backpacks requires motor adaptations. **(E)** Elderly man walking with visual guidance instead of visual anticipation, creating potential functional impairments.

pattern. Early in the preschool period, children mimic a "true" run and have difficulty efficiently controlling all aspects of the behavior. Finally, receipt and propulsion of balls of all shapes and sizes improve qualitatively.

Fine motor skills expand significantly during the preschool period. The environmental demands of preschool and day care preparation for entering primary grades are the driving force behind acquisition of many manipulative behaviors. Most children begin to cut with scissors, copy circles or crosses, use a crayon to trace a circle, match colors, and often demonstrate hand preference. Although maturity certainly plays a role in skill performance, the efficiency with which skills are performed is also influenced by genetics, affordances and constraints of the environment, practice, and intrinsic motivation.

Use of digital screen devices has changed the way children play or spend leisure time. Lin and colleagues[213] examined fine motor proficiency in preschool children using screen devices as compared to children using blocks and other fine motor manipulatives. The researchers indicated that fine motor skill development was better in preschool children using manipulatives than those using screen devices. Expanding research in this area is critical to fully examining the impact using digital devices on fine motor skill development.

Equally as important is gross motor performance and physical activity in preschool age children. The incidence of obesity in preschool children increased dramatically in children age 2 to 5, with a greater increase in males than females.[198] Efforts to reduce obesity found to be most effective included family behavioral training (FBT) and parent behavioral training (PBT). These training programs provided parents and children with ways to improve nutrition, time spent on digital devices, and physical activity for parents and their children.

Childhood (5 to 10 Years)

Childhood is characterized as a period when children begin their formalized education, usually in a structured environment separate from their families. Consequently, a new set of dynamics comes into play. Children take on new roles with peers and adults outside of the family. During this period of social-emotional change, other systems also undergo changes.

Motor skills that children display during this period include galloping, hopping on one foot for up to 10 hops (hopscotch), jumping rope, kicking a ball with improved control (soccer), and bouncing a large ball (basketball). Often these skills emerge while playing with peers during directed (physical education or community-based team sports)

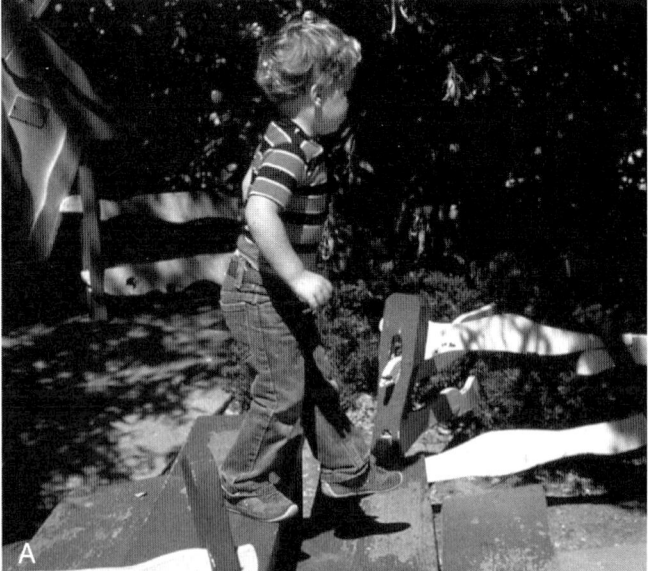

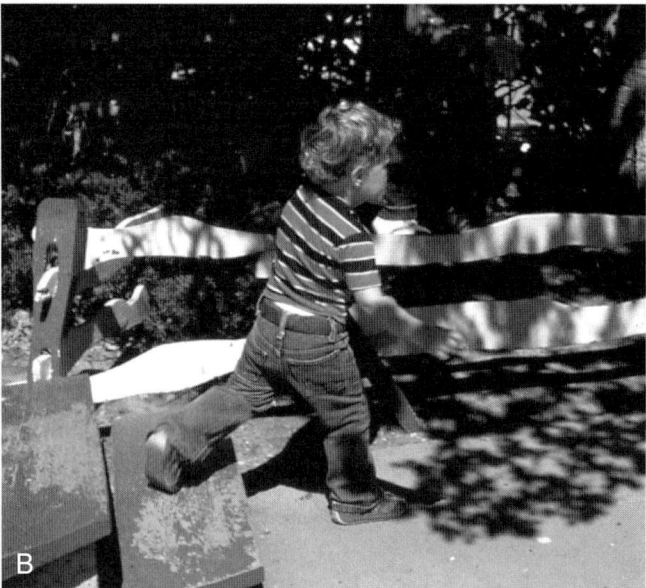

Fig. 2.8 Child Descending Stairs Successfully. (A) Attention on stepping down. **(B)** Success at the task.

and nondirected (recess) periods. Mobility, balance, and fine motor skills improve dramatically. Girls and boys exhibit similar abilities in speed up to age 7 years, but by age 8 years boys begin to outperform girls.[212]

During childhood, manipulative skills increase exponentially. Fig. 2.9A–E shows the amazing skill developed between birth and age 4 years. Manipulative skills assume a predominant role as part of the academic experience, requiring high levels of practice and opportunities for refinement of the skills. Hand preference is confirmed by this age. As components of independence, many of the manipulative skills achieved are directly related to self-care activities. Skills that improve dramatically include dressing, including fastening and unfastening clothing; tying shoes; using an implement for writing (coloring and handwriting); and successfully manipulating utensils not only to eat, but to socially interact while eating. As children approach preadolescence (9 to 12 years of age), manipulative

skills improve dramatically. Children produce cursive handwriting and complex drawings.

Perceptual development often improves significantly, often in direct relationship to the demands of the tasks along with practice, feedback, and motivation.[212] Visual-perceptual systems are nearing maturity and allow children to participate in sophisticated activities such as archery, baseball, dance, and swimming. Fig. 2.10 helps bring to light complex skill development during a lifetime. That skill development may begin with a fun team sport activity and lead to a lifetime of professional accomplishment.

The musculoskeletal system enters a period when muscle growth is rapidly increased, accounting for a large percentage of the weight gained during this period.[212] Constraints and affordances of the musculoskeletal system along with demands of the tasks and environment are highly interactive and influential in skilled activities. Children are generally flexible because muscle and ligamentous structures are not firmly attached to bones. Although this allows for flexibility, it also poses risks for musculoskeletal injury. Care should be taken when participation in high-level athletic activities is a consideration.

Qualitative changes in coordination, balance, speed, and strength improve while existing motor skills become more refined and controlled, more efficient, and more complex.[212] Qualitative improvements of motor skills may be attributed to an asynchronous growth in children's limbs in relation to the trunk. Consequently, better leverage is attained. Motor skills strongly influence social domains as boys and girls begin to perform in organized sports teams in school and the community. Competition within sports becomes a powerful force in motivating children to practice motor skills or directing children away from organized sports. Children with poorly developed motor skills, as a result of either genetics or opportunity, may be excluded from team activities and experience social isolation.[212] Similarly, a child may have the genetic potential to become a master in an area that uses a specific motor task, but if he or she is never introduced to the specific environment, such as playing a piano, and the motor skill is never actualized.

Children identified as obese reportedly have poorer gross and fine motor skills, decreased physical fitness, and often exhibit delayed motor development.[202] Children aged 5 to 6 years who are obese were noted to have poorer fine motor skills, balance, postural control, balance, and agility.[214] Skills identified as less proficient include running, hopping, kicking, sliding, and dribbling. Obesity in childhood often leads to obesity in adulthood/older adulthood, may negatively impact the individual's quality of life, and place the individual at increased risk for chronic diseases in adulthood.

Adolescence (11 to 19 Years)

Early adolescence signifies a period characterized by improved quantitative performance and qualitative changes in skills along with physical growth (size and strength).[13] By age 12 years, reaction times closely resemble those of the mature adult. Although skills involving balance, coordination, and eye-hand coordination also continue to improve with respect to perceptual development and information processing, the rate is not as dramatic. Elite athletes, in contrast, often continue to show steady improvement in qualitative and quantitative skill performance well into adulthood.

During later adolescence, when periods of physical growth have stabilized, motor skills acquired previously continue to develop in speed, distance, accuracy, and power. Many adolescents are involved in competitive sports. However, few exhibit performance levels identified with elite athletes. Those athletes that do reach this high level of skill

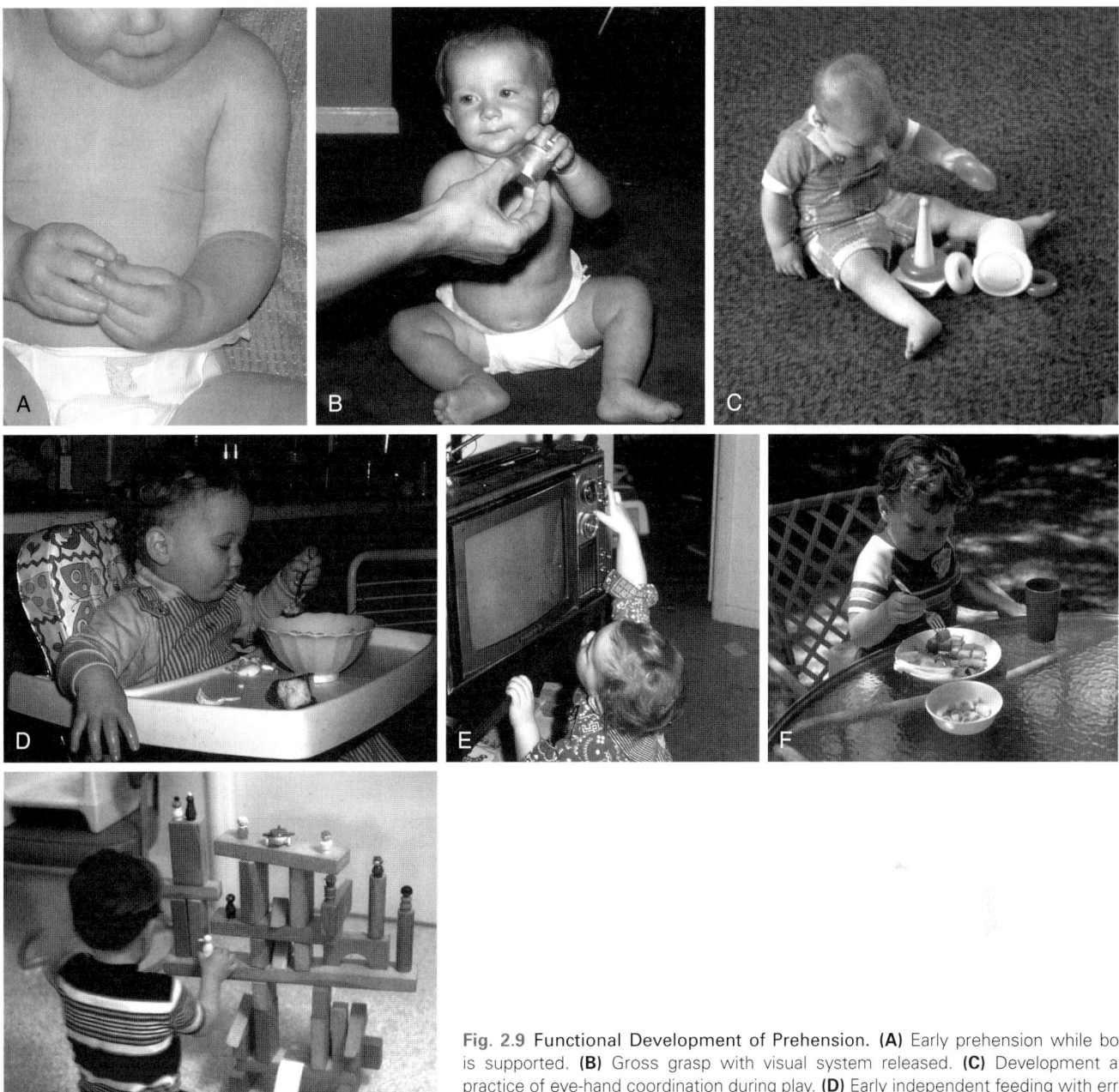

Fig. 2.9 Functional Development of Prehension. (A) Early prehension while body is supported. **(B)** Gross grasp with visual system released. **(C)** Development and practice of eye-hand coordination during play. **(D)** Early independent feeding with error. **(E)** Functional use of individual digit. **(F)** Eating with few errors while using utensils. **(G)** Fine motor prehension while simultaneously using force and direction of the upper extremity with little error during play.

often have a genetic predisposition, environmental affordances, adequate opportunities for high-level practice and performance, and strong motivation. More often, adolescents performing in competitive sports will find this is their avocation rather than their vocation (see Fig. 2.10).

Manipulative skills of adolescents resemble those of adults. Greater dexterity of the fingers for more complex tasks including art, sewing, crafts, knitting, wood carving, and musical performance enables adolescents to perform these motor tasks with greater precision and proficiency.

Upwards of 81% of the 11- to 17-year-old children and youth fail to meet their recommended physical activity levels.[215] TV and digital screens (smartphones, tablets, videogames, computers) usage places adolescents at higher risk for developing obesity. The risk for becoming obese is thought to stem from decreased physical activity, increased intake of sugary drinks/foods, and disrupted sleep. Recently the subgroup with the greatest increase in obesity is 16- to 19-year-old females.[198] Current estimates are that 21% of white adolescent females are classified as obese.[201] Efforts by public health officials to reduce the incidence of obesity in children and adolescents led to a parent challenge to control screen time and intake of sugary beverages and food, as well as increase physical activity and limit the use of digital devices prior to bedtime. Family and parent participation was found to be an effective intervention strategy with parents serving as role

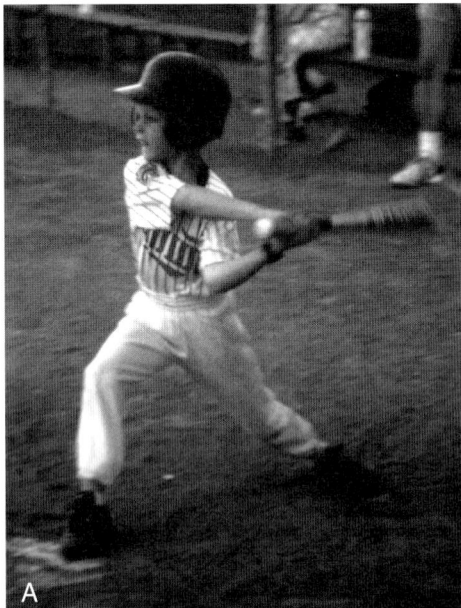

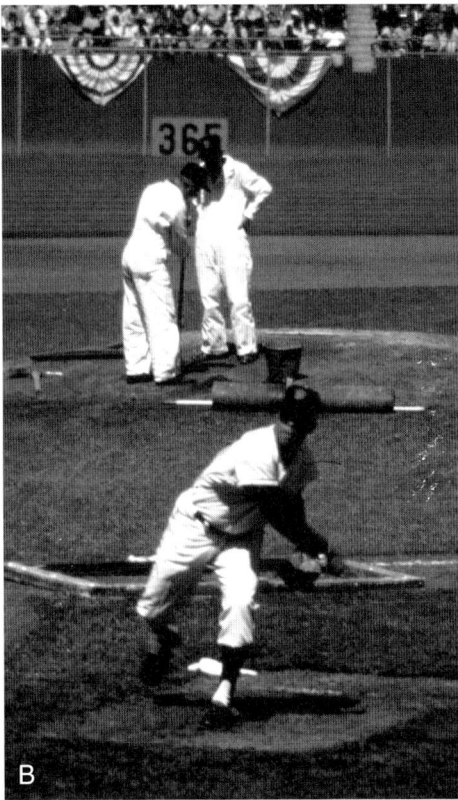

Fig. 2.10 Complex Skill Development. (A) Child participating in a team sport. **(B)** Adult demonstrating advanced skill development as a professional baseball player.

models for improving physical activity and modifying nutritional intake and reducing the likelihood the individual will develop comorbid conditions such as cardiovascular disease, hypertension, type II diabetes, or hyperlipidemia. Additionally, engaging children and adolescents in physical activity is thought to improve motor competence and self-concept of physical abilities among these groups and improve their overall health across the life course.[215]

Adulthood (20 to 39 Years)

Motor performance is relatively consistent in adulthood. Skillful performance of movements may be characterized not only through consistency, but also through the infinite ways in which the skill is performed. Hence change is generally focused on leisure activities or elite athletic competition. Leisure activities of many adults involve exercise of some form. Maintaining a healthy lifestyle through exercise and fitness is one method for staving off effects of aging and degenerative diseases. Although many adults participate in exercise for health and wellness, others who do not routinely exercise are at risk for obesity and associated health problems. Obesity is thought to negatively impact an individual's emotional and physical well-being as well as functional performance.[216] Often some of the physical activity expressed through the motor system is an example of parent-child bonds and creates a fun environment for play. Parent-child interaction through physical activity provides a positive environment that is thought to decrease the incidence of obesity in children and adolescents.[217] When a task-specific activity is selected and challenged by family members, the motivation to perform becomes high. An example of a parent-child activity can be seen in Fig. 2.11A. An observer might think that all three individuals are performing similarly with similar strategies. In reality, single-leg stance increases in difficulty as the base of support decreases and the body size changes. Note that the smallest individual has the smallest foot and the largest base of support in proportion to his body size. The adolescent is not as tall as his father, but his foot size is significantly larger, which (1) increases his base of support, (2) gives him less input proportional to his foot size or representation on the somatosensory cortex, and (3) gives him higher degrees of freedom when shifting his weight, which can either increase or decrease the task difficulty depending on practice. Fig. 2.11B shows the way both taller individuals use strategies to initially assume the upright stance position while the smaller child attained the single leg stance by stepping from a table. Body height, weight, and amount of practice all are variables that will help determine outcome. All three individuals achieve success, although the specific motor patterns and strategies used to succeed may be different. In Fig. 2.11C, a child with severe sensory organization problems would not be able to solve the challenge presented in Fig. 2.11A, because he cannot even begin to stand independently on a large, stable surface. Again, therapists need to be able to match the motor program impairments causing the child with learning disabilities to fail at the task and identify what programs are needed or expressed in the success of all three individuals in Fig. 2.11A.

The peak of muscular strength occurs at 25 to 30 years of age in both men and women. After that period, muscle strength decreases as result of a reduction in the number and size of the muscle fibers.[218] Loss is related to genetic factors, nutritional intake, exercise regimen, and daily activities.

Middle Adulthood (40 to 59 Years)

Changes associated with aging have been identified in the neuromuscular, musculoskeletal, and cardiovascular and pulmonary systems. These age-associated changes can greatly affect motor performance, although the degree is highly variable. Between 30 and 70 years of age, strength loss is moderate, with about 10% to 20% of total strength lost, for most activities—insignificant and undetectable by the individual.[77,219] Participating in regularly scheduled exercise regimens that emphasize aerobic and strengthening activities may reduce effects associated with aging. Furthermore, developing muscle mass and competence in motor skills early in life may have long-term positive effects on adult skills and reduce the risk of disability and frailty later in life.[220]

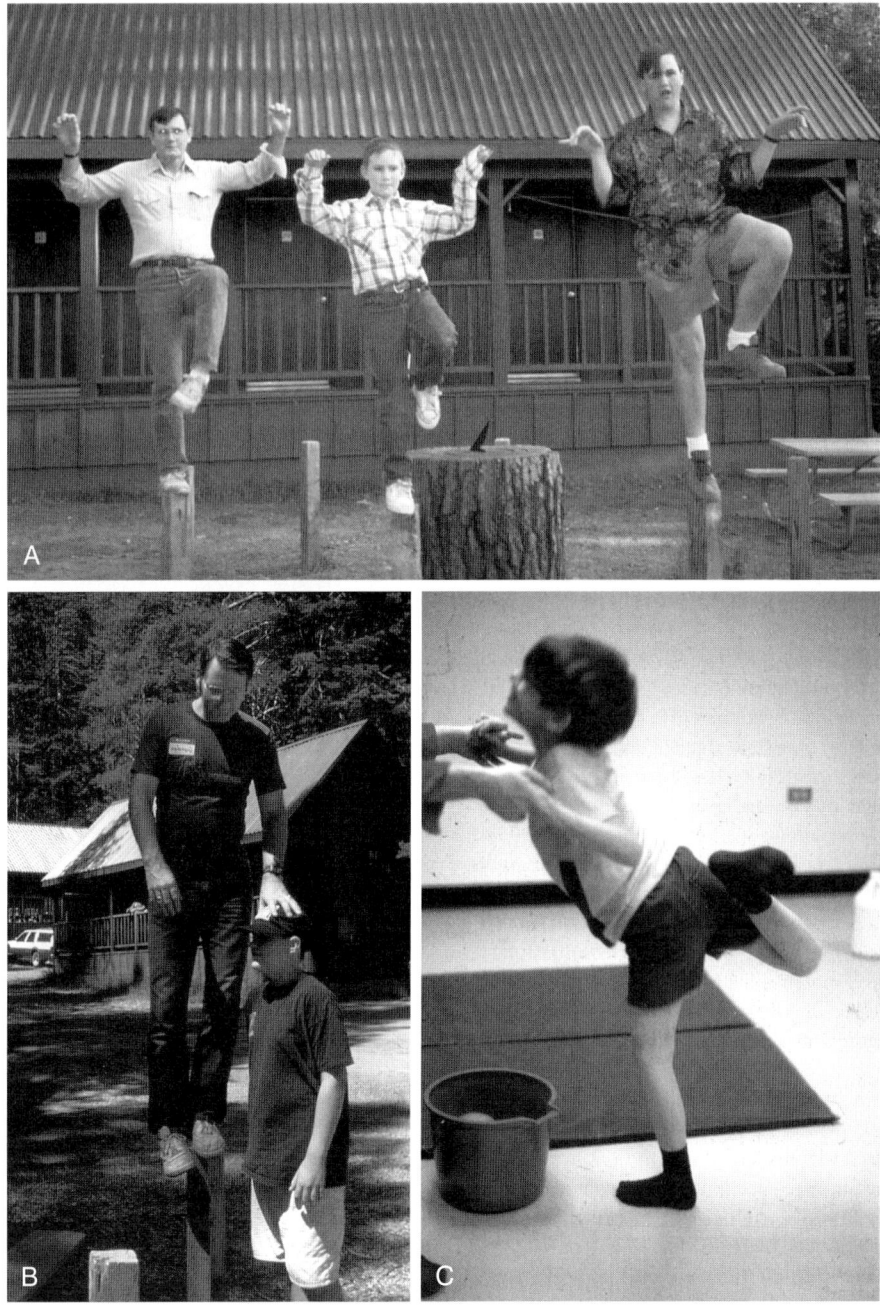

Fig. 2.11 A Complex Task Performed by Individuals With Different Foot Size and Body Composition. (A) Three individuals of differing age, body composition, and experience successfully performing the same task. **(B)** The strategy used by the adolescent and adult to find verticality. **(C)** A child with learning difficulties failing at independent one-legged stance.

Older Adulthood (60+ Years)

Age-related changes may be attributed to alteration in perception, compensations in the neural mechanisms, and changes between and within the different systems involved in motor skill performance.[221] Integrated effects may include slowing in movement production and increased activation of agonist-antagonist muscle groups. An example of agonist-antagonist activation is during dynamic balance activities.[222] After age 70 years, most individuals incur losses in muscle strength of up to 30% over the next 10 years. Overall, the loss of muscle strength through adulthood may be as much as 40% to 50% by the time an individual reaches 80 years of age.[73] The percentage decline

is inversely related to the demand by the individual for repetition of the movements. Continuing to regularly play preferred activities including tennis, running, golf, or skiing may significantly decrease the percentage of loss of strength compared with individuals who do not participate in such activities.

Although some effects are age associated and may be reduced with regular exercise and increased motor activity, not all are modifiable. Willardson[94] reported that older adults who maintain more active lifestyles are more likely to have a more favorable outcome than are peers who were not as active. Fig. 2.12 is an example of an 81-year-old adult who regularly bicycles 8 to 10 miles 3 to 4 times/week. He

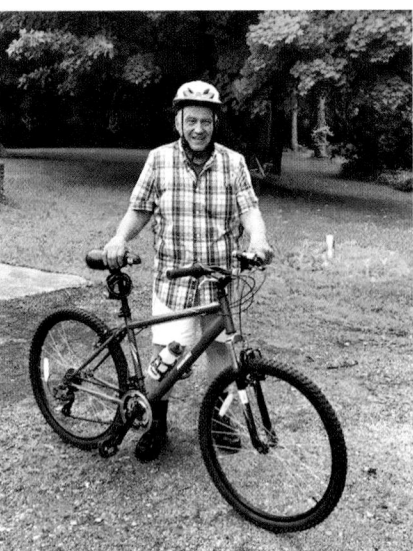

Fig. 2.12 Image is an example of an 81-year-old adult who regularly bicycles 8 to 10 miles 3 to 4 times/week.

attributes his overall health to regular exercise he and his spouse continue to participate. Findings by Hamer and colleagues[223] and Voelcker-Rehage and Willimczik[120] supported the findings of Willardson[94] in regard to older adults and lifestyle. Hamer and colleagues[223] indicated that even when older adults participate in regular exercise later in life, there were still significant health benefits. In addition, Voelcker-Rehage and Willimczik[120] found that older adults aged 60 to 69 years were able to acquire and refine a novel task (juggling) at a level comparable to children 10 to 14 years old and adults 30 to 59 years old. Only young adults aged 15 to 29 years performed at a higher skill level. Furthermore, adults older than age 70 years were found to have limitations in their ability to learn the novel motor skill. Moreover, as individuals age, they generally have a decreased ability to produce force, and they tend to coactivate agonist-antagonist muscles.[224] The researchers suggested that older adults may coactivate agonist-antagonist muscles as a strategy to (1) modulate movement variability and (2) maintain accuracy in movement. The investigators also reported that older adults' coactivation strategy compromised the subjects' ability to rapidly accelerate their limbs in exchange for improved accuracy of control.

One factor contributing to loss of motor performance and/or quality of movements in older adults is being overweight or obese.[202] Maintaining an exercise regime as part of one's life course reduces the incidence of obesity, preserves the white matter, and improves motor control of older adults.

In addition, information processing appears to be slowed in older adults.[221] Motor times have also been found to be delayed in older adults, particularly when a higher-level force is required.

Temporal coupling also appears to be altered in older adults.[221] Perhaps as individuals age, they are less able to modulate timing of muscles during contraction and relaxation phases and are more likely to coactivate agonist-antagonist muscles. The outcome behaviors are typified by poorly coordinated motor activities and increased time to produce adequate muscle force to elicit the behavior.

In addition to reduced efficiency in movement production, variability in performance of motor skills also increases with age. Although small changes in individual systems may not have a significant effect on functional movements, the compounding effects of changes in several systems may have serious implications for older adults and place them at increased risk for falls and injuries.[66] Fig. 2.13A and B are

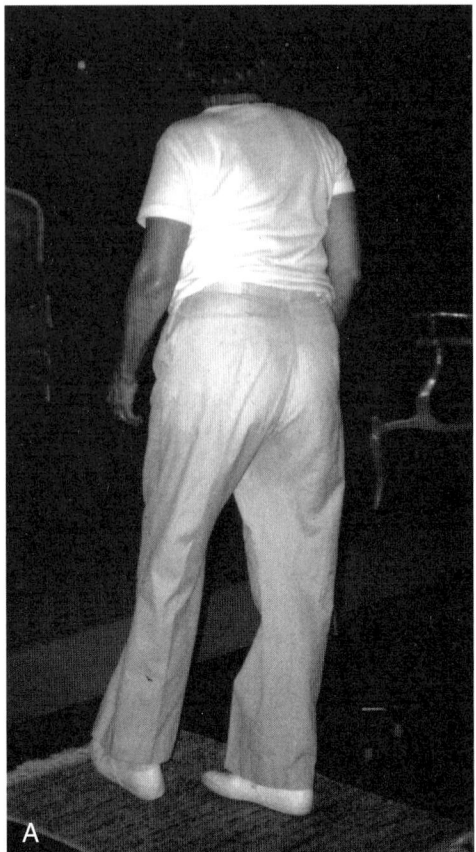

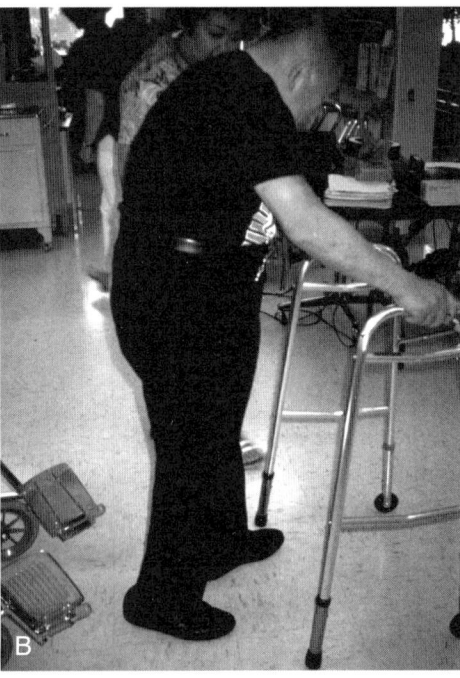

Fig. 2.13 As individuals age, more sedentary lifestyles, preexisting long-term health issues such as chronic obstructive pulmonary disease or chronic back pain, and a decrease in environmental challenges can lead to a higher risk of falls. **(A)** Woman with chronic back problems leading to a fixed trunk. **(B)** Man with chronic obstructive pulmonary disease and a fixed flexed posture resulting from inactivity.

examples of movement dysfunctions seen within an elderly population. These alterations are limiting the individual's ability to respond to a given motor task. As individuals age, there can be a large number of potential alterations in the body systems that limit CNS and musculoskeletal options when the individual tries to accomplish a motor activity. These limitations can place individuals at high risk of failure of any one motor task. The greatest fear within this group is not death; it is falling, and as a result losing independence. Prevention will be more and more important as the world's population of elderly individuals enlarges on a yearly basis.

Thirty percent of all community-dwelling elderly persons fall at least once each year.[219,225] Factors contributing to falls include intrinsic and extrinsic variables.[226–228] Intrinsic alterations in the older adult have implications for performance of motor skills and potential for falls. Risks associated with falls increase with age and when functions of the neuromuscular, musculoskeletal, cardiovascular and pulmonary, and sensory systems deteriorate. This deterioration of covariant factors and not age itself is more closely related to health and wellness and end-of-life age.[229] Another critical variable that is closely associated with motor decline in the aging is the individual's social interactions and participation in life.[230] Research has yet to determine whether a decrease in motor performance results from a decrease in participation in life.

Researchers examined manipulative skills in older adults and reported changes in muscle performance and flexibility.[63,231,232] These changes resulted in decreased hand function associated with impaired performance of ADLs. One thought is that decline in perceptual speed may play a significant role in fine motor abilities of older adults (Fauth et al., 2017).

STRATEGIES FOR FOSTERING ACQUISITION AND RETENTION OF MOTOR BEHAVIORS ACROSS THE LIFE-SPAN

Movements occur out of a need to solve problems in the environment. Solving these problems is not dependent on any one system but rather is a collaborative effort of multiple systems. The clinician is responsible for examining the patient's performance by evaluating the underlying conditions and the strategies that the individual may use to modify a behavior. Fig. 2.14A–F presents an example of individuals standing up from a chair. The first panels (see Fig. 2.14A and B) show a child whose feet are not on the surface because the child's legs are not long enough. No matter the variance of the task, the child was motivated to succeed. The second individual (see Fig. 2.14C and D), an elderly man, has lost the ability to shift his weight forward over his feet and thus is rising posterior on his heels, which will require anterior flexor power to prevent him from falling backward. The third individual (see Fig. 2.14E and F) has residual motor problems after a stroke. She has been taught to come to stand over her less-involved leg versus centering her base of support between her two feet. The specific way an individual learns, maintains, and relearns a specific motor task as a functional activity will vary, but the important principle will be to empower the individual to succeed with fluid, dynamic motor pattern options. Therapists need to visualize movement and place the movement pattern of the individual on top of that image. The specific motor impairments will then become obvious, and treatment options will be generated. Examination is vital to this process, although it often occurs in an environment far removed from the patient's natural surroundings.

Through acquisition of motor skills, individuals of all ages are afforded the opportunity to meet the environmental demands imposed by work, play, family, or personal activities. Refer to Fig. 2.14 as an example of common motor activities used at work, play, and home. Motor skill acquisition, retention, and decline are influenced by constraints or affordances that affect opportunities for practice in an environment that challenges and drives the individual to perform optimally. The patient's investment in achieving a successful outcome can help foster persistence in reaching the desired outcome. Practitioners recognize the importance of patient's goals in motivating him or her to move beyond his or her current functional abilities. Creating an environment that challenges the patient to attempt and complete movements in preparation for successfully completing preferred activity(ies) enables the therapist and patient to work collaboratively and achieve the goals, designing sessions that enable the patient to complete movements that culminate in the preferred activity and working toward his or her stated goal.

Fine motor abilities are implicit in performance of instrumental activities of daily living (IADLs) and should be examined during functional evaluations. Additionally, therapeutic intervention focused on improving ADL-related performance in older adults should consider the role of perceptual speed and variability in the overall approach to intervention.

Practice, the primary method for acquisition and retention of motor tasks, is exciting for very young children because each attempt is a new opportunity to achieve the outcome and reach a new level of independence. In contrast, practice in adolescent and adult populations may not be seen in the same light but rather as tedious and boring. Instead, physical and occupational therapists have the responsibility to challenge the cognitive, affective, motor, perceptual, sensory, and physiological systems through patient-selected activities. Activities directed toward the age and needs of the individual, such as interactive dance mats for adolescent patients or ballroom dancing for the older adult, may provide the motivation necessary to practice the task a sufficient number of times to achieve the desired outcome. Fig. 2.15A–H show age-appropriate challenges to individuals. The activity used with a child may be inappropriate for use with an adult, although a similar motor behavior may be the desired outcome. If the individual identifies the activity, he or she will be more motivated and more likely to practice a desired skill. Carryover from a clinical setting to a home or environmental setting is critical when looking at movement function over a life-span.

Strategies used to achieve desired motor outcomes may include a variety of feedback mechanisms to correct errors and identify more efficient strategies to attain the motor skill. Embracing the concept of enablement rather than disablement may also serve to motivate the patient because individual abilities are acknowledged and promoted while strategies are used for acquisition or relearning of motor skills. The needs of adolescent and adult patients are unique and differ significantly from those of the young child or infant.

Opportunities for exploration that engage the infant or young child are the primary motivation for movement. Although motor activities serve as the primary focus, engaging the infant or child provides stimulation that promotes development across multiple domains (e.g., cognition, social, communication). Environmentally challenging activities place demands on the child that maintain a level of curiosity or motivation and encourage persistence in attaining a motor skill that is successful and efficient. As the child matures, play-based activities shift the focus, depending on the expected outcomes. Overall, play is the primary mechanism that children use to mimic adult-like behaviors. Finally, children and adults use play or leisure activities as a means of promoting skill acquisition and proficiency across all developmental domains.

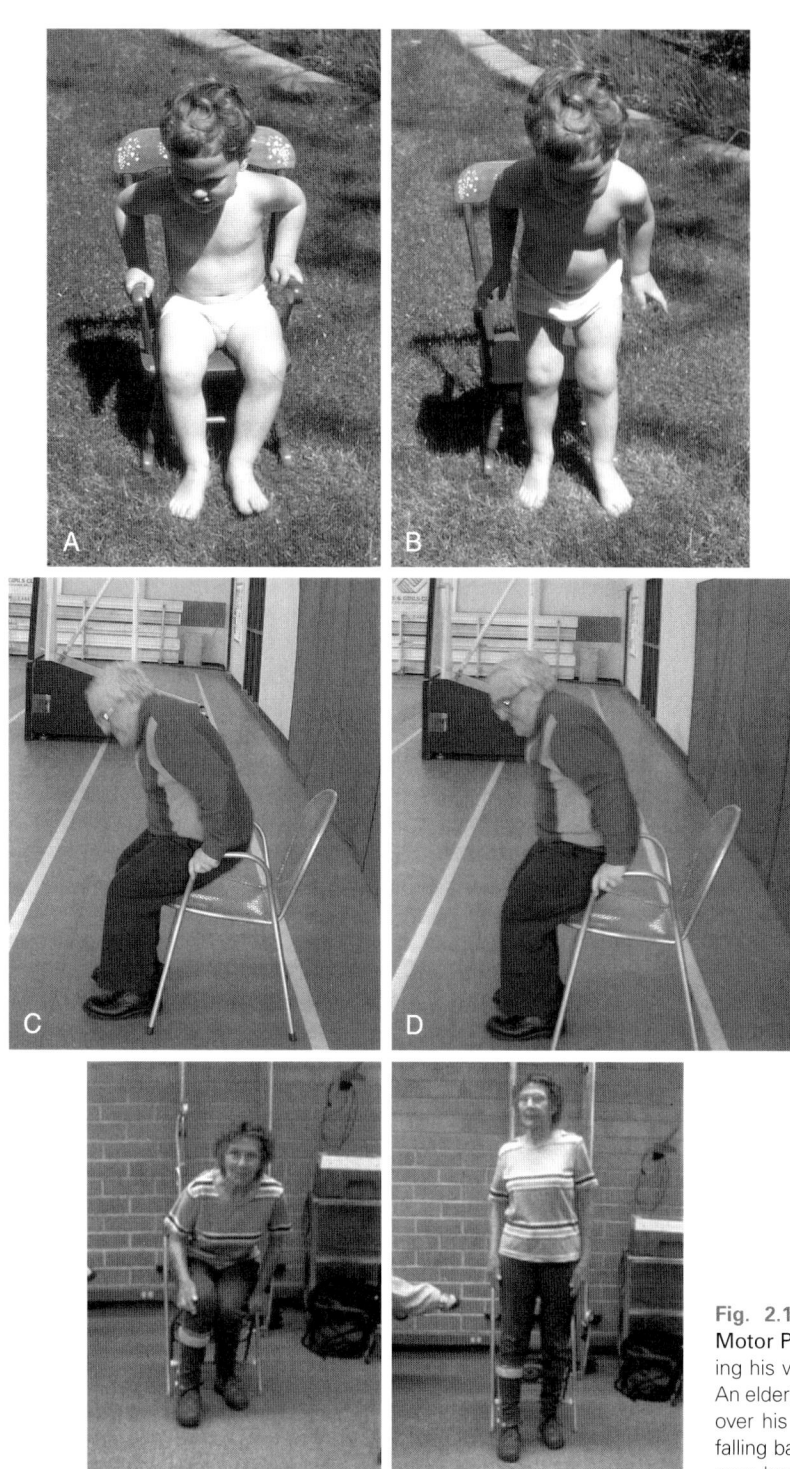

Fig. 2.14 Three Individuals Coming to Stand Using Different Motor Patterns. **(A** and **B)** A child rising to stand from a chair by shifting his weight over his base of support and rising vertically. **(C** and **D)** An elderly man rising to stand without adequate weight shifting forward over his base of support, requiring additional flexor power to prevent falling backward into the chair. **(E** and **F)** A woman after a stroke rising over her less involved leg, thus decreasing her symmetrical weight distribution and ability to step in any direction with either foot as a response to center of gravity shifting outside her base of support.

Development of Head Control as an Example of Movement Development Across the Life-Span and Its Impact on Quality of Life

When analyzing the development of head control by viewing movement of a young child over the first few years, it becomes clear that the motor control of the head in all spatial positions is very complex, requiring the integration of a variety of movement patterns. The infant needs to develop both the flexors that bend the head forward as well as the flexors that tuck the chin. These flexor patterns will be integrated into diagonal movements in order to roll over from supine to prone. A neck-righting program orients the body to the head

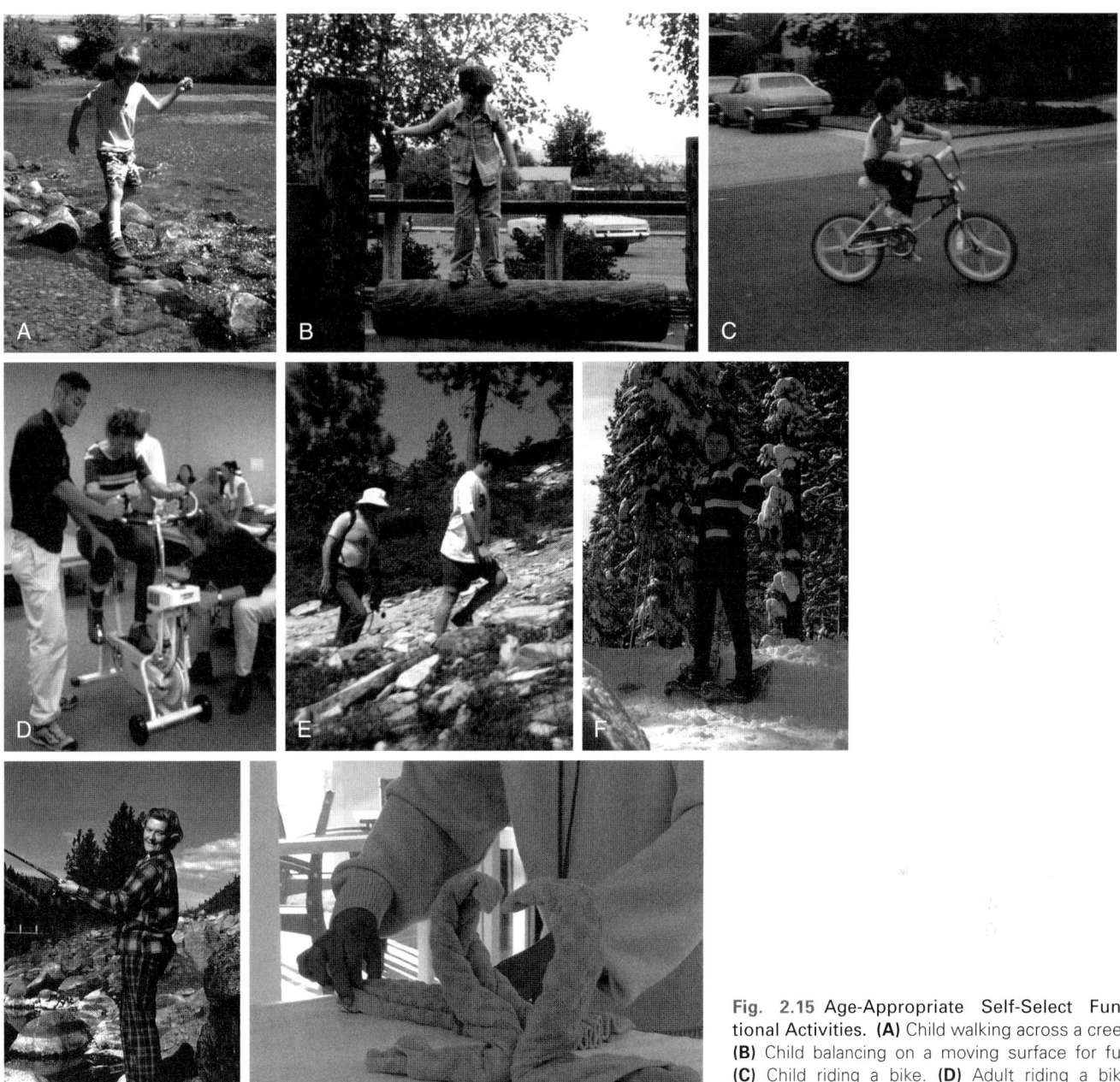

Fig. 2.15 Age-Appropriate Self-Select Functional Activities. (A) Child walking across a creek. **(B)** Child balancing on a moving surface for fun. **(C)** Child riding a bike. **(D)** Adult riding a bike. **(E)** Adult walking up a hill. **(F)** Adult using snowshoes. **(G)** Adult fishing. **(H)** Adults folding towels into figures for fun.

when the head is initially moving. Although the neck-righting program is present at birth, it will take the child a couple of months to gain the power necessary to independently flex and rotate the head against gravity with the body following the head in order to roll over. As the flexor power improves, it will be integrated into patterns of coactivation with postural extensors. The extensor movements of the head include (1) extension from a flexion position through hyperextension and/or rotation of the head in all spatial planes; and (2) postural extension, holding and/or stabilizing each vertebra within the spinal column. These postural programs help coactivate the flexors and postural extensors simultaneously to stabilize the

head in space. There are a variety of motor programs that assist in gaining this control of the head. Head-righting reactions, using the semicircular canals, are programmed to right the head, or bring it to face vertical, no matter where the head is in space. The righting programs need the underlying power to produce the force necessary to right the head. The heavier the head, whether in weight of the cranium or its positioning against gravity, the harder it is to right the head to vertical. Thus it could be hypothesized that if the head were in a vertical position or vertical in reference to gravity, it would be easier to control the head in space. The force production would be nominal compared with the force production needed when bringing the head up from horizontal or just holding it against gravity when horizontal. There are motor programs triggering extensor tone due to the position of the otoliths in the inner ear. The degree of tone will depend upon whether the head is horizontal in supine, vertical, or in between. This response has been labeled the *tonic labyrinthine reaction* (TLR). The TLR is strongest in the supine position because of the optimal pull of the otoliths by gravity. When an individual is supine, the tactile input from pressure to the surface of the skin increases extensor tone. Thus in the supine position the tactile input and the information from the hair cells of the otoliths are activating the motor pool of the extensors and simultaneously decrease the motor pool of the flexors. These systems decrease the ability of the motor control system to generate flexor tone in supine. When the child is placed prone, the skin sensitivity decreases extensor tone.

Flexor Control

Fig. 2.16A–F illustrates the patterns of a healthy 4-week-old when being pulled to sit and returned to the floor. Initially the child has difficulty flexing his head when trying to pull the head into flexion from the supine position because of both the extensor tactile system and the labyrinthine mechanism, which inhibit the flexors while facilitating the extensor muscles. This can be seen in Fig. 2.16A–C. This lack of adequate flexor control would be considered normal for the child's age but also defined as a head lag (see Fig. 2.16A–C). As the child approaches vertical, his weight is shifted down through his buttocks and over his base of support. At that point the head control

kicks in (see Fig. 2.16D and E). This motor control of the head in vertical incorporates both postural extensors and flexors while optimizing the use of optic and labyrinthine righting and stretch to both flexors and extensors muscle groups (see Fig. 2.16D). The child is able to maintain better control of head and neck flexors when lowered back down to supine (see Fig. 2.16E and F). This ability to control the head while transitioning from sitting to supine illustrates the fan swing principle: once the flexor program is elicited in the vertical position, it can maintain head control for a longer period of time and through more degrees of motion as the head movement progresses from vertical to horizontal.

Over the next month the child will develop flexor control in space by using head righting, muscle strength, and facilitation of the nervous system to keep the head and eyes oriented toward an object as the head travels through space. Motor control over flexor patterns becomes more flexible, and the power needed to perform tasks increases. Fig. 2.17A–C demonstrates the pull to sit pattern in a healthy 3-month-old infant. She not only has learned to dampen the influence of the TLR in the supine position and the skin's influence on the extensor motor pool, but also has learned that by flexing most of her body parts (flexion facilitates flexion) she will gain additional flexor control of the head when pulled from supine (see Fig. 2.17A). This flexion continues as the child goes through midrange (see Fig. 2.17B) and continues as the child approaches vertical (see Fig. 2.17C). Unfortunately, the child does not have the integrated motor control over flexion and extension or the balance reactions in sitting to extend the legs as she approaches vertical. This movement is a prerequisite for gaining control of long

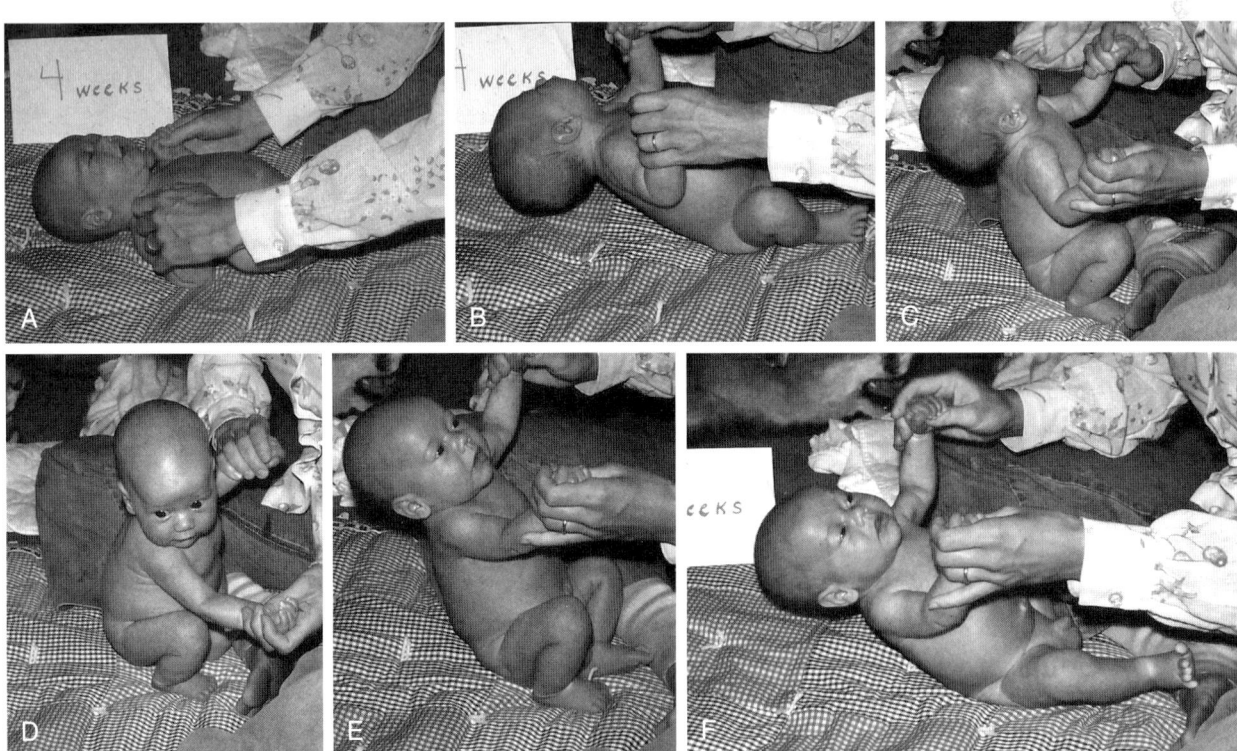

Fig. 2.16 A 1-Month-Old Child Being Pulled to Sit From Supine and Lowered Back Down. (A) Starting position in supine. **(B)** Pulled toward vertical, maximal resistance from gravity, inadequate response to stretch by neck flexors. **(C)** Position of ears and otoliths inhibits flexors; thus inadequate head righting is still seen. **(D)** Child in vertical, weight through hips, quick stretch to head in all directions facilitates head control. **(E)** Child lowered back toward horizontal continues to have adequate head control. **(F)** Maximal stretch from gravity; child still retains adequate neck flexion.

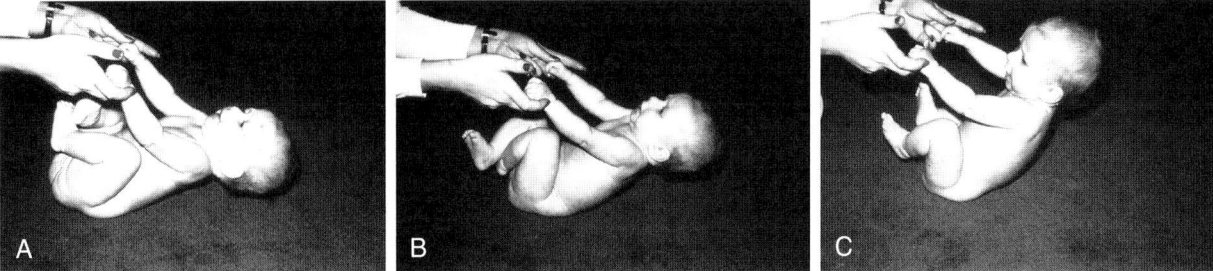

Fig. 2.17 A 3-Month-Old Healthy Child Pulled to Sit. (A) Initial stretch in horizontal pulls in neck flexion along with flexion of the hips and knee. **(B)** Adequate neck flexion persists as child looks at therapist while being pulled to sit: midrange. **(C)** Transitioning to vertical; less stress on neck flexors, yet flexion persists in lower extremities.

sitting in vertical. These new motor movements will become the foundation for balance reactions in vertical sitting.

A month later the child's nervous system integrates the flexor patterns into smooth movement through 90 degrees of motion from supine to sitting (Fig. 2.18A–C). The child also demonstrates a more integrated response to being lowered backward from vertical (see Fig. 2.18D). Yet the child's motor system has not developed the rotatory aspects or control of the diagonal flexor patterns as shown in Fig. 2.18E. These rotatory patterns will develop as the child practices

rotation in rolling and then incorporates that rotation when coming to sit in a partial rotation pattern.

The child will not be able to independently initiate motor control over the adult pattern of coming to a sitting position for at least 3 to 5 years but certainly should gain that control by age 6 (Fig. 2.19). As the child's age increases, the movement patterns become more complex, and additional motor programs are learned and integrated. This aspect of head control will be maintained and integrated in movement patterns as the individual explores the environment.

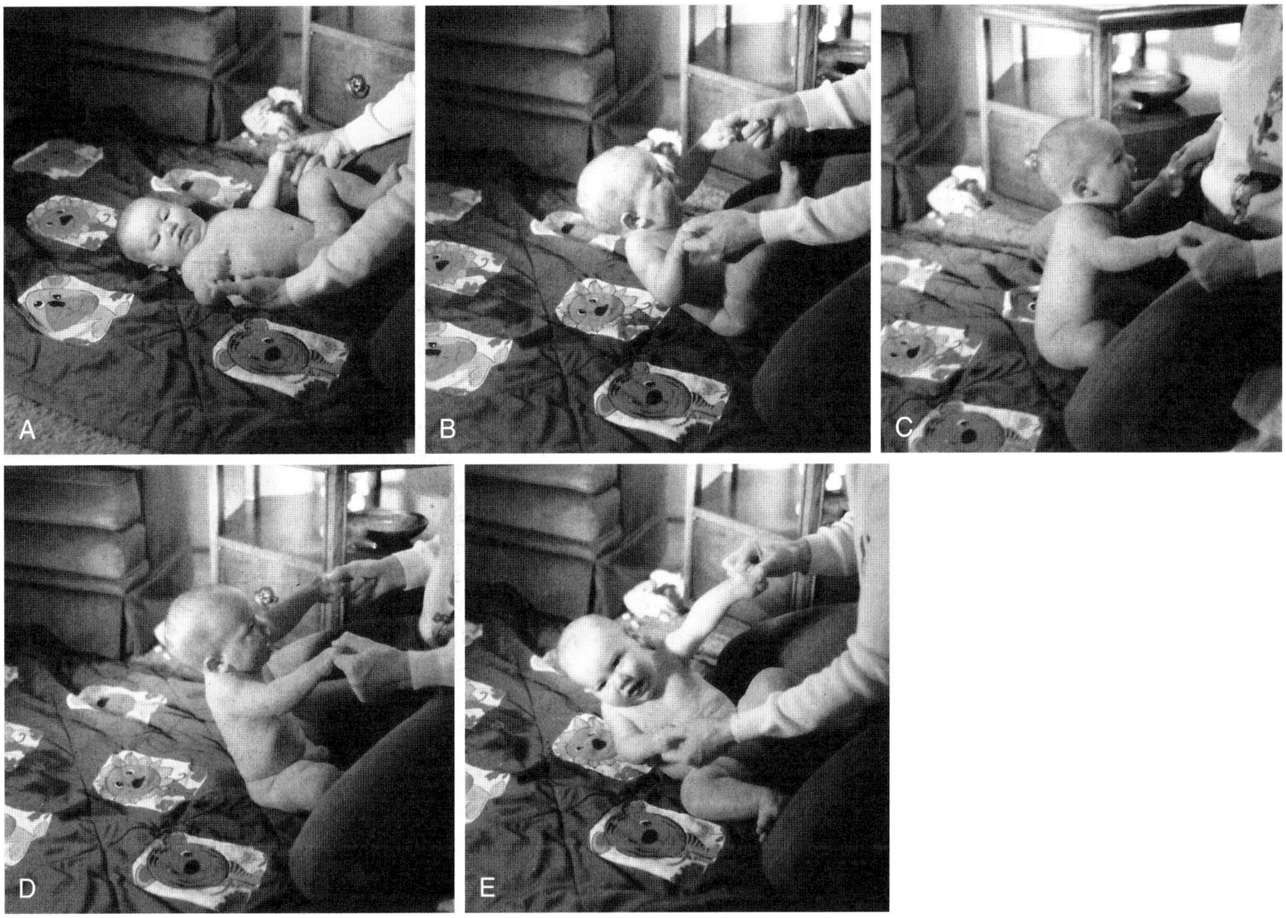

Fig. 2.18 Pull to Sit in 4-Month-Old-Healthy Child. (A) Child looks as therapist places finger to the child's head—recognized tactile stimulus, relaxed supine. **(B)** Child pulled to sit, neck tucked and hips flexed. **(C)** In vertical, child relaxes hip flexors in order to have sitting balance. **(D)** Child lowered toward supine maintains neck and trunk control. **(E)** Rotation added into lowering to supine pattern; neck response is inadequate.

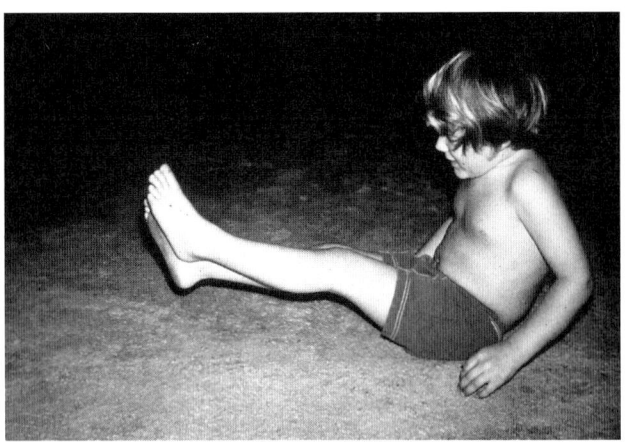

Fig. 2.19 Normal 6-Year-Old Using Adult Independent Coming-to-Sit Pattern.

Extensor Control

As the child develops flexion, the child also needs to develop the extensor control of the head. There are two extensor component patterns used by the CNS to control extension. The first pattern is controlling extension of the head from a totally flexed position (as if an individual were looking down at his shoes) to a hyperextension position (as if an individual in a standing position were looking up at the stars). This pattern has a large range of motion, and the power needed will change depending on the head's position in space, in relation to gravity, as well as the weight of the head itself. The second pattern is considered "postural" and requires the small muscles of the neck and the shoulder and trunk to hold each vertebra in relation to the vertebra above and the vertebrae below. This is the boney support encompassing the spinal cord. Similarly, in the upper cervical region as the flexor and extensor patterns work together in a coactivation pattern, chin tucking occurs. This pattern allows the head to remain stable in space, keeping the eyes and the ears horizontal to the surroundings, a key component for perceptual learning. This movement pattern is often called *optic and labyrinthine righting of the head* because both the eyes and the ears provide stimuli to trigger this motor response.

Assessment of Head Control

Most individuals analyze the development of postural control by evaluating the extensor aspect of head control in the prone position. But the prone position is not the first position in which a child begins to achieve independent head control. Fig. 2.20A–C illustrates a newborn (2 days old) extending both the long extensors (see Fig. 2.20A and B) as well as

moving into the postural extensor pattern component when tucking the chin (see Fig. 2.20C). While prone the newborn child has very little independent control over extension and can just clear the airways (Fig. 2.21). This same limitation is not present when the child is in a supported vertical position. After a week the extensor patterns in the vertical position have already become more functional and demonstrate better motor control and greater power. Fig. 2.22A–C shows the same child at 1 week of age while supported in a vertical position. Fig. 2.22C is a beautiful example of the postural pattern one expects to see consistently later in the child's development. Obviously, he is practicing these movements every time he is vertical and given these limited degrees of freedom. Looking at the same child at 1 month of age (Fig. 2.23), the integration of these postural movements is continuing down his entire spine. This does not mean he can hold this pattern for an extended period of time but does illustrate his ability to move with control into a total postural extension pattern and hold it at least briefly. On the same day and about 15 minutes later, the child (Fig. 2.24) was placed prone on the floor, clearly demonstrating that he has not developed the necessary power to control his head or upper trunk for postural extension in the prone position. Although he is more relaxed prone at 1 month than at birth (see Fig. 2.21) and can lift and turn his head in both directions, it will still be 1 or 2 additional months before he can extend his head and trunk enough to prop on his elbows. It will take more time to roll from prone to supine.

While the cervical and upper thoracic muscles are developing postural power, they need to learn to hold the head in space against gravity for longer periods of time. Postural function

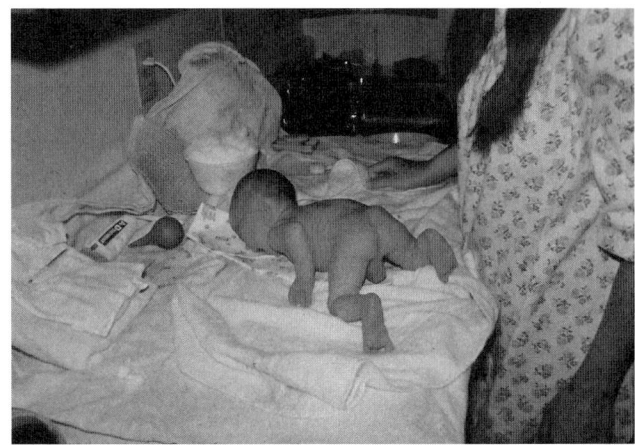

Fig. 2.21 When Placed Prone, the Newborn Has Excessive Flexion.

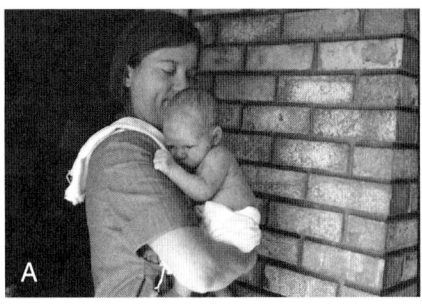
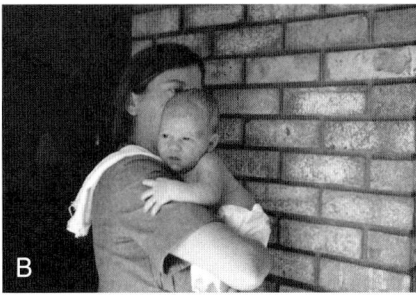
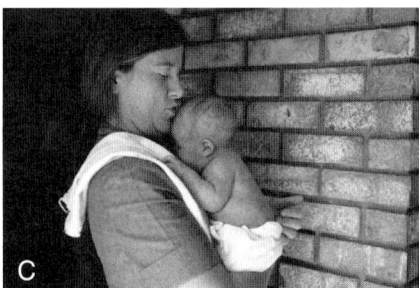

Fig. 2.20 Newborn Neck Extension in Supported Vertical Position. **(A)** Newborn lacks postural extension of trunk and head. **(B)** Newborn initiates neck extension, showing that patterns exist. **(C)** Newborn moves into postural extension of upper cervical region.

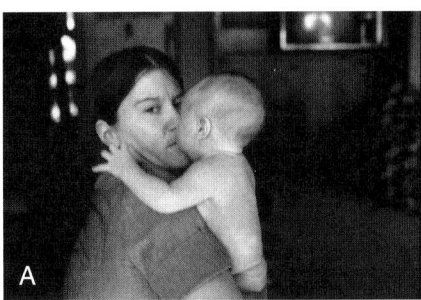 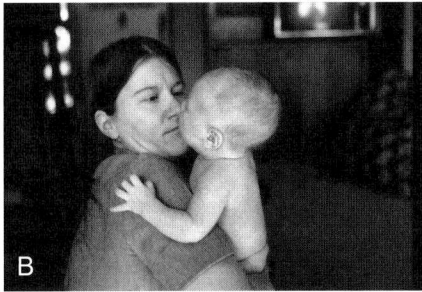 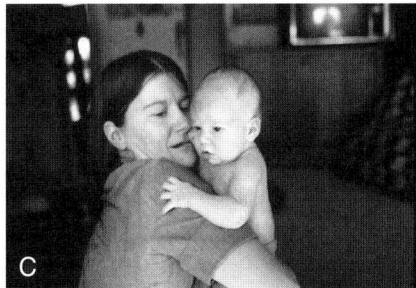

Fig. 2.22 Child 7 Days Old in Vertical Extension. (A) Child eliciting active neck and truck extension in vertical at 7 days. **(B)** Child does not have adequate righting of the head in vertical at 7 days but is responding. **(C)** Child pulls into postural extension of the neck and trunk, allowing for binocular vision at 7 days.

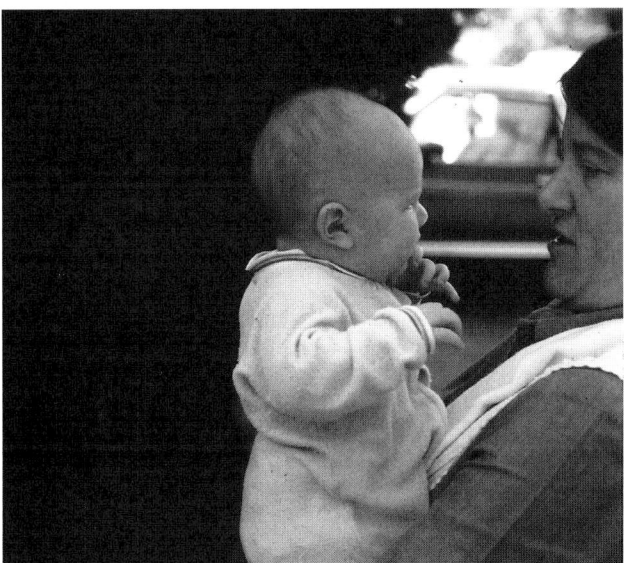

Fig. 2.23 A 1-month-old child, when supported in a vertical position, shows postural extension of the neck and trunk while looking at his mother.

requires coordination and coactivation of the short extensors of the neck and the neck flexors—especially the sternocleidomastoid, hyoid, and scalene muscles—in order to tuck the chin and balance the head in space. These movement patterns play a key role in stabilization of the head in order to move the head in and out of vertical space. The motor control system uses both righting and balance reactions in order to gain full head and neck control of vertical space. The movements become more and more complex, modifying and integrating various additional motor programs in order to have greater flexibility to control and move the head. These patterns give the eyes and ears the visual and auditory orientation needed to process consistent external environmental information. Fig. 2.25 illustrates an individual after head injury who has lost his automatic righting of the head in vertical. He has the ability to bring his head to vertical by hyperextension of the neck but does not do so automatically. This hyperextension pattern dramatically changes the motor patterns of head, neck, and trunk control, which will affect his upright behaviors including balance, gait, feeding, and social interactions.

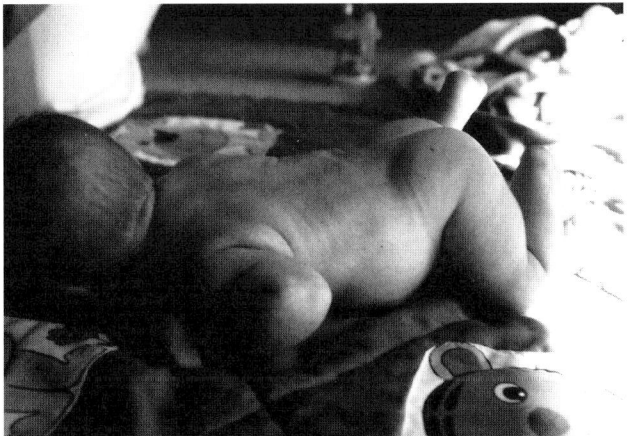

Fig. 2.24 Same child when placed prone, 15 minutes after Fig. 2.23 was taken. This child demonstrates that when prone he still has a flexor bias and has little adequate postural extension in this position.

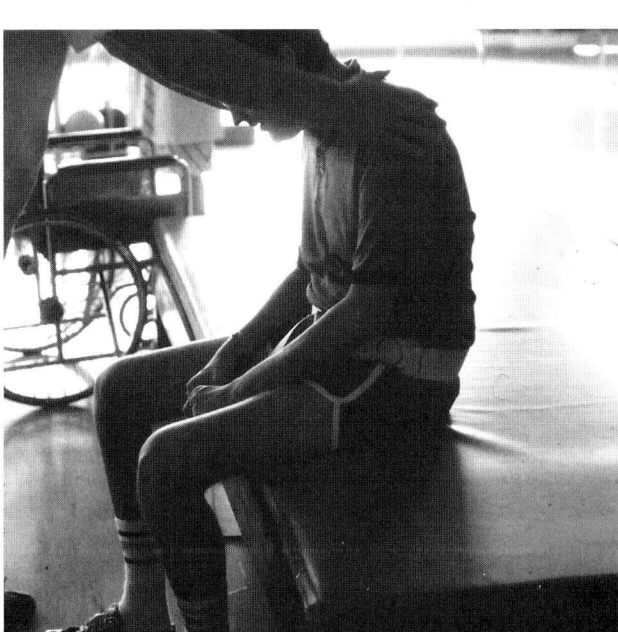

Fig. 2.25 An individual who sustained a closed head injury with residual lack of postural neck extension has poor head control in vertical.

Application of the Development of Head Control to Rehabilitation

The reason the patterns of head extension in vertical have been presented is to illustrate that motor control progresses from vertical to horizontal and then from horizontal to vertical. Therapists think of the prone position as the first position in which the child develops extensor control because it is the first position in which an observer sees independent selection of extensor movement. However, extensor control begins when an individual passively brings a young baby to sitting or standing. The baby learns to control the head with small movements that displace the center of gravity. Understanding this stage of head control may be a critical component of working with a neurologically impaired youngster or an adult.

Analysis Between Normal and Impaired Motor Function

Differentiating normal age-related reactions of any movement impairment is the responsibility of a movement specialist. For example, differentiating the movement of a normal child who has a lag in head control (see Fig. 2.16B and C) from the movement of a child who does not demonstrate any head control (Fig. 2.26A–E) should guide the therapist in a decision about where to begin treatment. It is an unrealistic expectation for the child in Fig. 2.25 to gain flexor head control by starting at supine. After the child has been pulled to sit, flexor power production is beyond the control of the child's motor system. Once the child is vertical, the influence of gravity on the weight of the head has decreased. The vertical position also inhibits any influence of the otoliths when supine. The upright position helps to facilitate the labyrinthine and optic righting of the head. Fig. 2.26D and E demonstrates how the tone within the neck and shoulder girdle changes once the head attains a vertical position. A therapist should not only see a change to more normal tonal patterns but also observe relaxation of the facial muscles—closure of the mouth and a more functional position of the eyes in space for visual processing.

Movement demonstrates the ease or difficulty the motor system is experiencing while trying to complete an activity. The activity analyzed may be a basic pattern such as head control or a complex one as seen in Fig. 2.3E. Differentiating between the movements in Figs. 2.15A and 2.25A should guide the clinician in establishing realistic prognoses. The first child, with practice and CNS maturity, should automatically develop head control, whereas the second child has gone beyond his age-appropriate movement delays and has abnormal responses to the stretch stimuli.

Similar analysis can be made when looking at the extensor component of head control. The vertical position that optimizes extension is kneeling or standing because compression down through the joints and spine facilitates extension. Using kneeling or standing may pull in too much extension, especially if it results in hyperextension. In that case sitting may be appropriate even though it may facilitate flexion. When kneeling or standing, if inadequate extension still exists, then adding additional compression down though the head or shoulder girdle may help. Using an apparatus that takes away some of the weight of the head or trunk reduces the demand on the nervous system and may help the individual regain postural neck, shoulder girdle, and upper trunk control. As the individual begins to demonstrate that control, the therapist can slowly take away the assistance with the expectations that the individual will gain independence in that activity.

As the individual ages, changes in the control of the head can lead to new problems. Fig. 2.13B is an example of a man who has a fixed flexed posture. If the flexed posture is permanent, treatment alternatives must take into consideration the impact this posturing will have on all ADLs. As stated earlier, any patient can exhibit a range of problems in head control. How those movement impairments present themselves and which treatment alternatives a therapist might select

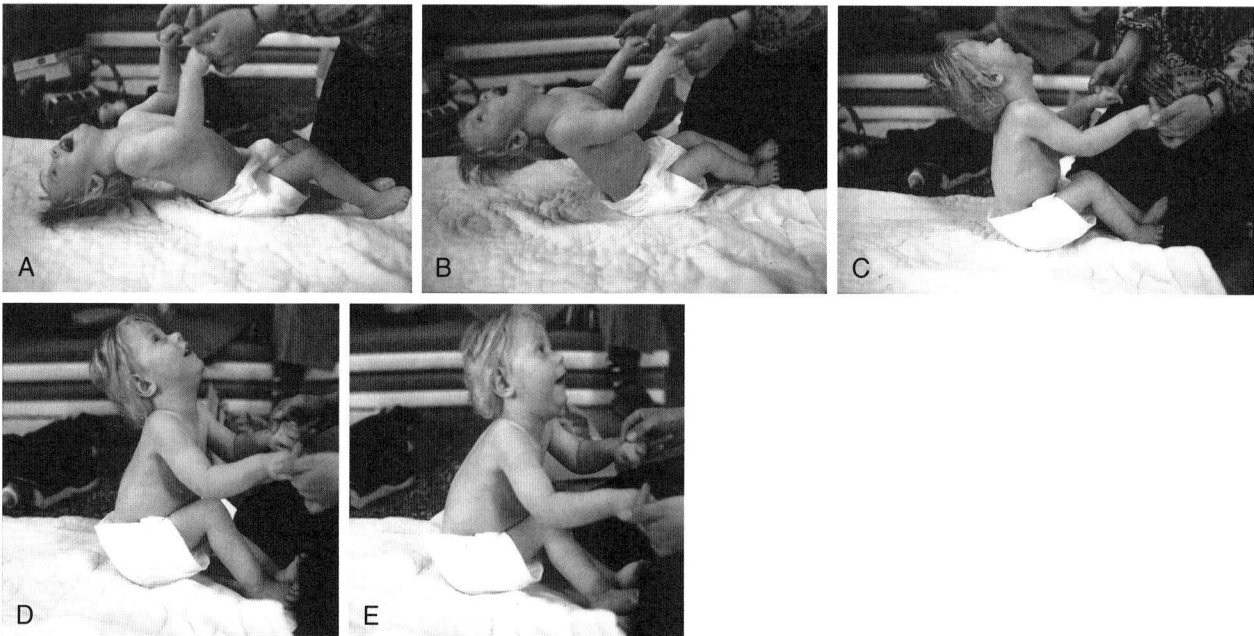

Fig. 2.26 Child 2½ years old with cerebral palsy being pulled to sit, and muscle action facilitated once vertical. **(A)** Initial pull toward sit; no response to stretch of neck flexors. **(B)** Continued pull toward vertical, head at end range of neck extension. **(C)** Trunk in vertical but neck remains in horizontal; no flexor response. **(D)** Child pulled beyond vertical as trunk extensors begin to activate from stretch and mouth closure is beginning. **(E)** Therapist facilitates head into vertical as mouth continues to relax and close and eyes are looking at a target.

will depend on the clinician's ability to analyze normal movement and create an optimal environment for patients to engage and practice those patterns.

Clinical Example

Cervical torticollis in a child is an imbalance in rotation of the neck and muscle groups secondary to position of the fetus in utero. Cervical torticollis in adults is a focal dystonia or an imbalance of excitation and inhibition of the neck muscles. These patients have impaired integrative balance responses. Standard medical intervention is botulinum toxin injections followed by physical therapy focusing on range of motion and strengthening exercise. The emphasis needs to be on restoring and progressing head control from vertical to supine—that is, trying to help the neck muscles to retrain a stable condition in the vertical position by using a collar for support. Compression down through the cervical and thoracic spine can facilitate flexors, extensors, and rotator muscles. Then, as in the infant, with arms fixed on a stable support surface, slowly let the patient move out of vertical toward horizontal, moving only as far as head control is maintained, which may be as limited as 10 to 20 degrees. Repeat this activity many times in order for this activity to become procedural. Patients can hold onto some stable support object at home in order to practice. The challenge for both the therapist and the patient is to retrain head control in order for the individual to be able to participate in life.

Head Control Development Summary

Normal development of head control has been highlighted because so many clinicians become frustrated with patients who do not have adequate head control. The examples of the development of head control serve as a foundation for every movement pattern that people use, whether stationary or in motion. The process used to analyze the development of head control can be used to analyze all movement patterns, whether the movement problem is caused by a bodily system (biomechanical, cardiopulmonary, CNS, or another system problem) or by some environmental factor.

SUMMARY

Clinicians must focus best practice toward successful patient management geared toward promotion of function and prevention of chronic illness or disability for the youngest of the young to the oldest of the old. As practitioners, we must embrace tenets central to the *Healthy People 2020* project.[233] Physical and occupational therapists serve as role models for individuals of all ages and educate diverse groups of individuals about the multifaceted, interactive systems involved in the acquisition, retention, and deterioration of motor behaviors. Recognizing internal and external constraints or affordances that influence motor behaviors enables the clinician to devise a plan of care and the scientist to design a study targeting the needs of the whole person. Analyzing, understanding, and visually recognizing movement patterns that are efficient, fluid, and goal oriented and that vary across the life-span are the first steps or prerequisites to evaluating abnormal movement patterns that do not fall within a normal parameter. Fig. 2.27A–G shows an example of rolling, a basic movement strategy controlled by the child midway through the first year of life that can become an extremely challenging activity after a CNS insult. Differentiating between components of a normal movement and deviations that prohibit normal movement falls into the clinical expertise of occupational and physical therapists Without the knowledge of normal movement, analysis of the causation of abnormal movement would be difficult if not impossible. This chapter has been written to help the reader understand normal movement across the life-span. It is the first step, and in sighted individuals the analysis begins as soon as visual images are recorded in the visual cortex.

Scientists acknowledge that development is characterized as nonlinear, emergent, and dynamic, rather than sequential, predictable, and stage like. Dynamic systems theory, although it does have certain limitations, provides a better explanation for development than do neuromaturational theories. The emphasis or responsibility does not lie with any one system but varies across different systems because of age, genetics, or experience.[127] That said, future studies directed at examining human movement and optimal variability through nonlinear dynamics may provide new perspectives in motor development and control. Although the research may provide valuable insights into how the brain develops and exactly what controls which aspects of movement, the movements themselves and the sequences children use to move from one functional skill to the next may not vary tremendously.

Human behavior is by nature complex. As such, no one system or skill develops in isolation but rather emerges from a complex interaction among multiple systems. Complex behaviors are evident beginning in utero and continuing throughout life. No one theory explains the development of complex motor behaviors, and none encompass the essence of interindividual and intraindividual variability in aging. Aspects of various theories provide evidence that an integrative perspective is a more accurate reflection of aging. As theorized earlier, lifestyle choices and other modifiable behaviors have potent effects on aging. Activities should be promoted that the individual enjoys and strategies employed that encourage the individual to participate in preferred motor activities across his or her life-span, in a safe and supportive environment. After the individual executes the task(s) in a supported environment, the next step is participating in real-life leisure activities with family and peers and providing additional social interactions. Interventions designed to provide older adults with strategies to positively influence successful aging, rather than being sought after a negative outcome of aging is realized, may improve the quality of life. Optimal quality of life is what all individuals hope to obtain, whether learning to reach a cracker, climbing the highest mountain, or playing a game of bridge.

Maintaining that quality before the end of life, no matter the age, is often based on movement function. The patient, whenever possible, should determine identification of the specific function. Identification of the necessary steps to get from existing skill to desired skill is the role of a movement specialist, whether that therapist is dealing with preventive care or postinsult care.

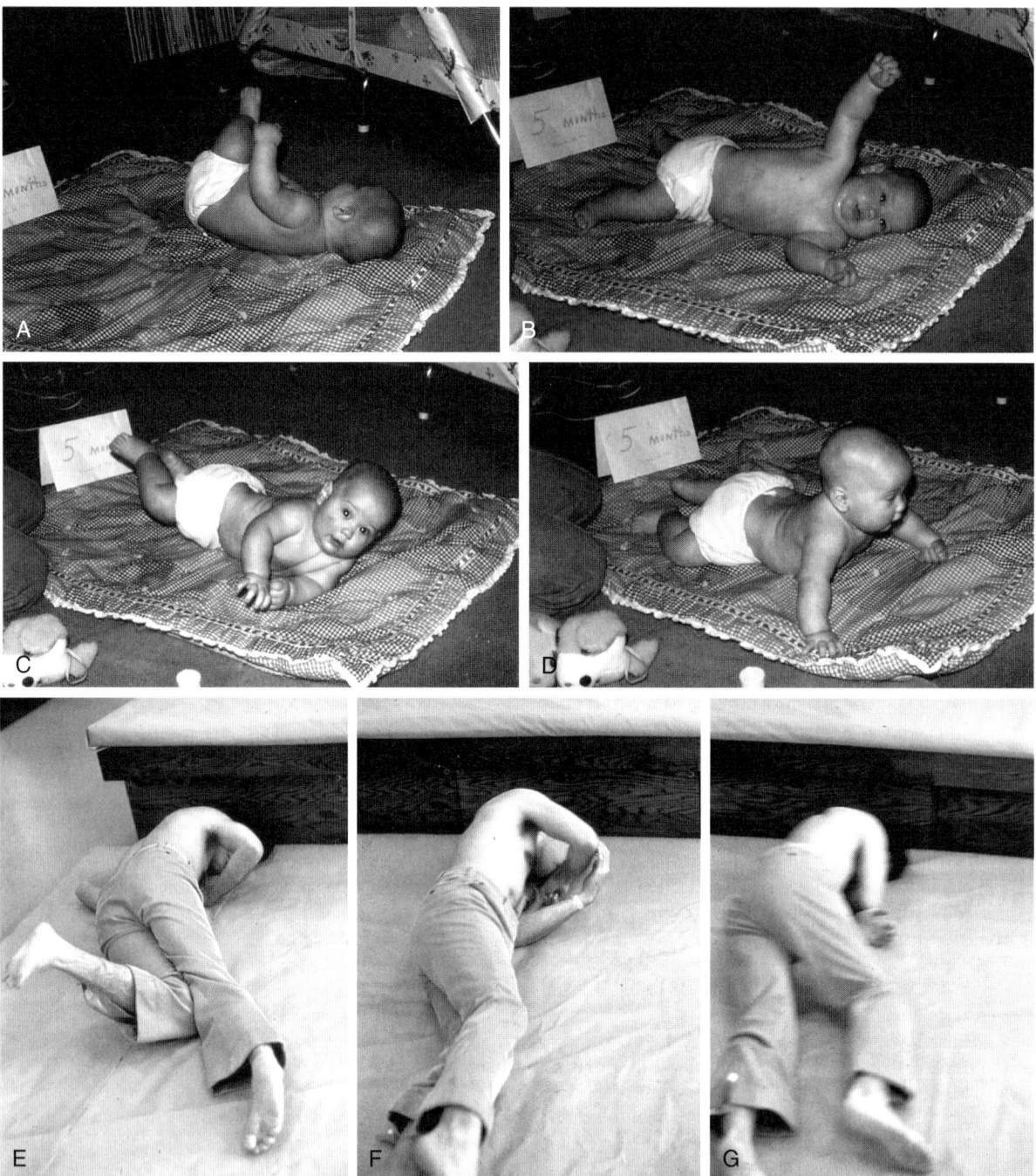

Fig. 2.27 Rolling—An Activity Achieved Within the First Year. (A) Child beginning rolling in supine position. **(B)** Child semiprone with trunk rotation. **(C)** Child brings arm through to become symmetrical while proceeding toward prone position. **(D)** Child prone with postural extension. **(E)** Adult with traumatic brain injury; first try at rolling toward prone position from supine. **(F)** Adult's second try at rolling, changing programming. **(G)** Once prone, he is stuck, unable to extend.

REFERENCES

To enhance this text and add value for the reader, all references are included on the companion Evolve site that accompanies this textbook. This online service will, when available, provide a link for the reader to a Medline abstract for the article cited. There are 233 cited references and other general references for this chapter, with the majority of those articles being evidence-based citations.

3

Contemporary Issues and Theories of Motor Control, Motor Learning, and Neuroplasticity*

Margaret L. Roller, Susan V. Duff, Darcy A. Umphred, and Nancy N. Byl

OBJECTIVES

After reading this chapter the student or therapist will be able to:
1. Identify the evolution of motor control theories and discuss the utility of current theory in clinical practice.
2. Identify body structures and functions that contribute to the control of human posture and movement.
3. Relate the cognitive, associative, and autonomous stages of motor learning to behavior and skill performance.
4. Describe the variety of practice conditions that may be used to enhance motor learning within a practice session.
5. Apply motor learning variables related to person, task, and environment within the therapeutic setting.
6. Discuss neuroplasticity theories that explain how the nervous system adapts to demands placed on learning and performance.
7. Discuss the relationships between motor control, motor learning, and neuroplasticity in the production of functional movement behaviors.

KEY TERMS

motor control theory	motor learning	neuroplasticity

The production and control of human movement is a process that varies from a simple reflex loop to a complex network of neural patterns that communicate throughout the central nervous system (CNS) and peripheral nervous system (PNS). Neural networks and motor pattern generators develop as the fetus develops in utero and are active before birth. These simple patterns become building blocks for more skilled, complex, goal-directed motor patterns as a person develops throughout life. New motor patterns are learned through movement, interactions with rich sensory environments, and challenging experiences that drive a person to solve problems. The personal desires and goals of the individual shape the process of learning new motor skills at all stages of life. If a condition exists or develops or if an event occurs that damages the nervous system and prevents normal transmission, processing, and perception of information in the PNS and CNS, movement control becomes abnormal, slow, labored, uncoordinated, or weak—or movement may not be produced at all. The damaged nervous system is able to repair itself, change, and adapt to some extent by means of nerve regeneration and neuroplasticity. However, when nerve cells die and neural connections are not viable, there are alternative pathways within the nervous system that can take the place of the normal processes and provide some means of meeting the movement goal—whether it is to walk, use an arm to eat, or make a facial expression. This process of change, healing, or motor learning depends on many factors, including inherent elements of the individual such as age, the extent of tissue damage, and other physiological and cognitive processes as well as external factors such as interactions with sensory and motor system challenges and goal-directed practice of meaningful, functional motor skills.

This chapter introduces the reader to basic concepts of motor control, motor learning, and neuroplasticity. Figures and tables are provided to emphasize and summarize concepts. Patient case examples are used to illustrate concepts in this chapter as they apply to the evaluation and management of people with neurological conditions.

MOTOR CONTROL

Motor control is defined as "the systematic transmission of nerve impulses from the motor cortex to motor units, resulting in coordinated contractions of muscles."[1]

This definition describes motor control in the simplest terms—as a top-down direction of action through the nervous system. In reality, the process of controlling movement begins before the plan is executed and ends after the muscles have contracted. The essential details of a movement plan must be determined by the individual before the actual execution of the plan. The nervous system actively adjusts muscle force, timing, and tone before the muscles begin to contract, continues to make adjustments throughout the motor action, and compares movement performance with the goal and neural code (instructions) of the initial motor plan. This extension of the definition takes into account that the body *accesses sensory information* from the environment, *perceives* the situation, and *chooses a movement plan* appropriate to the task that the person wants to complete; this plan is then *coordinated* within the CNS. Finally the plan is *executed* through motor neurons in the brain stem and spinal cord that communicate with muscles in postural and limb synergies as well as muscles in the head and neck that are timed to fire in a specific manner. The movement that is produced supplies *sensory feedback* to the CNS to allow the person to (1) modify the plan during performance, (2) know whether the goal of the task has been achieved, and (3) store the information

---

*Videos for this chapter are available at studentconsult.com.

for future performance of the same task-goal combination. Repeated performance of the same movement plan tends to create a preferred pattern that becomes more automatic in nature and less variable in performance. If this movement pattern is designed and executed well, it means that the person has developed a new skill. If this pattern is incorrect and does not efficiently accomplish the movement goal, it means that the outcome is abnormal.

Theories and Models of Motor Control

A summary and historical perspective of motor control theories is given in Table 3.1. The control of human movement has been described in many different ways. The production of reflexive, automatic, adaptive, and voluntary movements and the performance of efficient, coordinated, goal-directed movement patterns involve multiple body systems (input, output, and central processing) and multiple levels within the nervous system. Each model of motor control that is discussed in this chapter has both merits and disadvantages in its ability to supply a comprehensive picture of motor behavior. These theories serve as a basis for predicting motor responses during patient examination and treatment. They help explain motor skill performance, potential, constraints, limitations, and deficits. They allow the clinician to (1) identify problems in motor performance, (2) develop treatment strategies to help patients remediate performance problems, and (3) evaluate the effectiveness of intervention strategies employed in the clinic. Selecting and using an appropriate model of motor control is important for the analysis and treatment of patients with dysfunctions of posture and movement. As long as the environment and task to be performed necessitates change in the CNS, and the individual has the desire to learn, the adaptable nervous system will continue to learn, modify, and adapt motor plans throughout life.

Motor Programs and Central Pattern Generators

A motor program (MP) is a learned behavioral pattern defined as a neural network that can produce rhythmic output patterns with or without sensory input or central control.[14] MPs are sets of movement commands, or "rules," that define the details of skilled motor actions. An MP defines the specific muscles that are needed; the order of muscle activation; and the force, timing, sequence, and duration of muscle contractions. MPs help to control the degrees of freedom of interacting body structures and the number of ways in which each individual component acts. A generalized motor program (GMP) defines a pattern of movement with a lesser degree of specificity, rather than defining every individual aspect of a movement. GMPs allow for the adjustment, flexibility, and adaptation of movement features according to environmental demands. The existence of MPs and GMPs is a generally accepted concept; however, hard evidence that an MP or a GMP exists has yet to be found. Advancements in brain imaging techniques may substantiate this theory in the future.[14,15]

In contrast to MPs, a central pattern generator (CPG) is a genetically predetermined movement pattern.[16,17] CPGs exist as neural networks within the CNS and have the capability of producing rhythmic, patterned outputs resembling normal movement. These movements have the capability of occurring without sensory feedback inputs or descending motor inputs.[18] Two characteristic signs of CPGs are that they result in the repetition of movements in a rhythmic manner and that the system returns to its starting condition when the process ceases.[19] Both MPs and CPGs contribute to the development, refinement, production, and recovery of motor control throughout life.

The Person, the Task, and the Environment: An Ecological Model for Motor Control

Motor control evolves so that people can cope with their environment. A person must focus on detecting information in the immediate environment (perception) that is determined to be necessary for performance of the task and achievement of the desired outcome goal. The individual is an active observer and explorer of the environment, which enables the development of multiple ways in which to accomplish (choose and execute) any given task. The individual analyzes a particular sensory environment and chooses the most suitable and efficient way to complete the task. The *person* consists of all functional

TABLE 3.1   Theories of Motor Control

Motor Control Theory	Author and Date	Premise
Reflex Theory	Sherrington, 1906[2]	Movement is controlled by stimulus-response. Reflexes are combined into actions that create behavior.
Hierarchical Theory	Jackson, 1932[3]	Higher centers are in control of lower centers.
Motor Program Theory	Adams, 1971[4,5] Schmidt, 1976[6]	Cortical centers control movement in a top-down manner throughout the nervous system. Closed-loop mode: sensory feedback is needed and used to control the movement. Adaptive, flexible motor programs (MPs) and generalized motor programs (GMPs) exist to control actions that have common characteristics. Open-loop mode: movements are preprogrammed, and feedback is used to update the program.
Ecological Theories	Gibson and Pick, 2000[7,8]	The person, the task, and the environment interact to influence motor behavior and learning. The interaction of the person with any given environment provides perceptual information used to control movement. The motivation to solve problems to accomplish a desired movement task goal facilitates learning.
Systems Model	Bernstein, 1967[9] Shumway-Cook, 2017[10]	Movement emerges to control degrees of freedom. Multiple body systems overlap to activate synergies for the production of movements organized around functional goals. Considers interaction of the person with the environment.
Dynamical Systems Theory	Turvey, 1977[11] Kelso and Tuller, 1984[12] Thelen et al., 1987[13]	Patterns of movements self-organize within the characteristics of environmental conditions and the existing body systems of the individual. Functional synergies are developed naturally through practice and experience and help solve the problem of coordinating multiple muscles and joint movements at once.

Cano-de-la-Cuerda R, Molero-Sanchez A, Carratala-Tejada M, et al. Theories and control models and motor learning: clinical applications in neurorehabilitation. *Neurologica*. 2015;30(1):32-41.

and dysfunctional body structures and functions that exist and interact with one another. The *task* is the goal-directed behavior, challenge, or problem to be solved. The *environment* consists of everything outside of the body that exists, or is perceived to exist, in the external world. All three of these motor control constructs (person, task, environment) are dynamic and variable, and they interact with one another during learning and the production of a goal-directed, effective motor plan.[10]

Body Structures and Functions That Contribute to the Control of Human Posture and Movement

Keen observation of the quality of motor output during the performance of functional movement patterns helps the therapist to determine activity limitations and begin to hypothesize impairments within sensory, motor, musculoskeletal, cardiopulmonary, and other body systems.

Table 3.2 shows the body system processes involved in motor control, their actions, and the body structures included. The following chapter sections explain these processes in more detail.

Role of Sensory Information in Motor Control

Sensory receptors from somatosensory (exteroceptors and proprioceptors), visual, and vestibular systems as well as taste, smell, and hearing fire in response to interactions with the external environment and to movement created by the body. Information about these various modalities is transmitted along afferent peripheral nerves to cells in the spinal cord and brain stem of the CNS. All sensory tracts with the exception of smell then synapse in respective sensory nuclei of the thalamus, which acts as a filter and relays this information to the appropriate lobe of the cerebral cortex (e.g., somatosensory to the parietal lobe, visual to the occipital lobe, vestibular, hearing, and taste to the temporal lobe). Sensory information is first received and perceived and then associated with other sensory modalities as well as memory in the association cortex. Once multiple sensory inputs are associated with one another, the person is able to *perceive* the body, its posture and movement, the environment and its challenges, and the interaction and position of the body with objects within the environment. The person uses this perceptual information to create an internal representation of the body (internal model) and to choose a movement program, driven by motivation and desire, to meet a final outcome goal. Although the sensory input and motor output systems operate differently, they are inseparable in function within the healthy nervous system. Agility, dexterity, and the ability to produce movement plans that are adaptable to environmental demands reflect the accuracy, flexibility, and plasticity of the sensorimotor system.

The CNS uses sensory information in a variety of ways to regulate posture and movement. Before movement is initiated, information about the position of the body in space, body parts in relation to one another, and environmental conditions is obtained from multiple sensory systems. Special senses of vision, vestibular inputs that respond to gravity and movement, and visual-vestibular interactions supply additional information necessary for static and dynamic balance and postural control as well as visual tracking. Auditory information is integrated with other sensory inputs and plays an important role in the timing of motor responses with environmental signals, reaction time, response latency, and comprehension of spoken word. This information is integrated and used in the selection and execution of a movement strategy. During movement performance, the cerebellum and other neural centers use feedback to compare the actual motor behavior with the intended motor plan. If the actual and intended motor behaviors do not match, an error signal is produced and alterations in the motor behavior are triggered. In some instances, the control system anticipates and makes corrective changes before the error signal is detected. This anticipatory correction is termed *feedforward control*. Changing one's gait path while walking in a busy shopping mall to avoid a collision is an example of how visual information about the location of people and objects can be used in a feedforward manner.

Another role of sensory information is to revise the reference of correctness (central representation) of the MP before it is executed again. For example, a young child standing on a balance beam with the feet close together falls off of the beam. An error signal occurs because of the mismatch between the intended motor behavior and the actual motor result. If the child knows that his feet were too close together when he fell, then he will space his feet farther apart on the next trial. The child will then use this information about what happened, falling or not falling, in planning movement strategies for balancing on any narrow object such as a balance beam, log, or wall in the future.

Sensory information is necessary during the acquisition phase of learning a new motor skill and is useful for controlling movements during the execution of the motor plan.[10,20,21] However, sensory information is not always necessary when a person is performing

TABLE 3.2   Components of Motor Control: Body System Processes Involved in Motor Control, Their Actions, and the Body Structures Included

Process	Action	Body Structures Involved
Sensation	Acquires sensory information and feedback from exteroceptors and proprioceptors	Peripheral afferent neurons, brain stem, cerebellum, thalamus, sensory receiving areas in the parietal, occipital, and temporal lobes
Perception	Combines, compares, and filters sensory inputs	Brain stem, thalamus, sensory association areas in the parietal, occipital, visual, and temporal lobes
Choice of movement plan	Use of the perceptual map to access the appropriate motor plan	Association areas, frontal lobe, basal ganglia
Coordination	Determines the details of the plan, including force, timing, tone, direction, and extent of the movement of postural and limb synergies and actions	Frontal lobe, basal ganglia, cerebellum, thalamus
Execution	Executes the motor plan	Corticospinal and corticobulbar tract systems, brain stem motor nuclei, and alpha and gamma motor neurons
Adaptation	Compares movement with the motor plan and adjusts the plan during performance	Spinal neural networks, cerebellum

well-learned motor behaviors in a stable and familiar context.[20,21] Rothwell and colleagues[21] studied a man with severe sensory neuropathy in the upper extremity. He could write sentences with his eyes closed and drive a car with a manual transmission without watching the gear shift. He did, however, have difficulty with fine motor tasks such as buttoning his shirt and using a knife and fork to eat when denied visual information. The importance of sensory information must be weighed by the individual, who is unconsciously filtering and choosing appropriate and accurate sensory inputs to use to meet the movement goal.

Sensory experiences and learning alter sensory representations, or cortical "maps," in the primary somatosensory, visual, and auditory areas of the brain. Training, as well as use and disuse of sensory information, has the potential to drive long-term structural changes in the CNS, including the formation, removal, and remodeling of synapses and dendritic connections in the cortex. This process of cortical plasticity is complex and involves multiple cellular and synaptic mechanisms.[22] Plasticity in the nervous system is discussed further in the third section of this chapter.

Choice of Motor Pattern and the Control of Voluntary Movement

A choice of body movement is made based on the person's perception of the environment, his or her relationship to objects within it, and the goal to be met. The person chooses from a collection of plans that have been developed and refined over his or her lifetime. If a movement plan does not exist, a similar plan is chosen and modified to meet the needs of the task. Once the plan has been chosen, it is customized by the CNS with what are determined to be the correct actions to execute, given the perceived situation and goal of the individual.

Coordination

The movement plan is customized by communications between the frontal lobes, basal ganglia, and cerebellum, with functional connections through the brain stem and thalamus. During this process specific details of the plan are determined. Postural tone, coactivation, and timing of trunk muscle firing are set for proximal stability, balance, and postural control. Force, timing, and tone of limb synergies are set to allow for smooth, coordinated movements that are accurate in direction of trajectory, order, and sequence. The balance between agonist and antagonist muscle activity is determined so that fine distal movements are precise and skilled. This process is complicated by the number of possible combinations of musculoskeletal elements. The CNS must solve this "degrees of freedom"[23] problem so that rapid execution of the goal-directed movement can proceed and reliably meet the desired outcome.[9,24] Once these movement details are complete, the motor plan is executed by the primary motor area in the precentral gyrus of the frontal lobe.

Execution of Movement Plans

Pyramidal cells in the corticospinal and corticobulbar tracts *execute* the voluntary motor plan. Neural impulses travel down these central efferent systems and communicate with motor neurons in the brain stem and spinal cord. The corticobulbar tract communicates with brain stem motor nuclei to control muscles of facial expression; mouth and tongue for speaking and eating; larynx and pharynx for voice and swallow; voluntary eye movements for visual tracking, saccades, and vergence; and muscles of the upper trapezius for shoulder girdle elevation. The corticospinal tract communicates with motor neurons in the spinal cord. The ventral corticospinal tract system communicates primarily with proximal muscle groups to provide the appropriate amount of voluntary activation needed to stabilize the trunk and limb girdles, thus allowing for dexterous distal limb movements. The lateral corticospinal tract system communicates primarily with muscles of the arms and legs—firing α motor neurons in coordinated synergy patterns with appropriate activity in agonist and antagonist muscles so that movements are smooth and precise. Other motor nuclei in the brain stem are programmed to fire just before corticospinal tract activity in order to supply postural tone and anticipatory muscle activity. These include lateral and medial vestibular spinal tracts, the reticulospinal tract, and the rubrospinal tract systems. Adequate and balanced muscle tone of flexors and extensors in the trunk and limbs is supplied automatically, without the need for conscious control. These brain stem nuclei have tonic firing rates that are modulated up or down to effectively provide more or less muscle tone in body areas depending on stimulation from gravity, limbic system activity, external perturbations, or other neuronal activity.

Adaptation

Adaptation is the process of using sensory inputs from multiple systems to adapt motor plans, decrease performance errors, and predict or estimate consequences of movement choices. The goal of adaptation is the production of consistently effective and efficient skilled motor actions. When all possible body systems and environmental conditions are considered in the motor control process, it is easy to understand why there is often a mismatch between the movement plan that is chosen and how it is actually executed. Errors in movements occur and cause problems that the nervous system must solve in order to deliver effective, efficient, accurate plans that meet the task goal. To solve this problem, the CNS creates an internal representation of the body and the surrounding world. This acts as a model that can be adapted and changed in the presence of varying environmental demands. It allows for the ability to predict and estimate the differences between similar situations. This ability is learned by practicing various task configurations in real-life environments. Without experience, accurate movement patterns that consistently meet desired task goals are difficult to achieve.[25]

Anticipatory Control

Anticipatory control of posture and postural adjustments stabilizes the body by minimizing displacement of the center of gravity. Anticipatory control involves motor plans that are programmed to act in advance of movement. A comparison between incoming sensory information and knowledge of prior movement successes and failures enables the system to choose the appropriate course of action.[15,26]

Flexibility

A person should have enough flexibility in performance to vary the details of a simple or complex motor plan to meet the challenge presented by any given environmental context. This is a beneficial characteristic of motor control. When considering postural control, for example, a person will typically display a random sway pattern during standing that may ensure continuous, dynamic sensory inputs to multiple sensory systems.[27] The person is constantly adjusting posture and position to meet the demand of standing upright (earth vertical), as well as to seek information from the environment. Rhythmic, oscillating, or stereotypical sway patterns that are unidirectional in nature are not considered flexible and are not as readily adaptable to changes in the environment. Lack of flexibility in postural sway may actually render the person at greater risk for loss of balance and falls.

Role of the Cerebellum

The primary roles of the cerebellum in motor control are to maintain posture and balance during static and dynamic tasks and to coordinate movements before execution and during performance.[28] The cerebellum processes multiple neural signals from (1) motor areas of the cerebral cortex for motor planning, (2) sensory tract systems (dorsal spinal cerebellar tract, ventral spinal cerebellar tract) from muscle and joint receptors for proprioceptive and kinesthetic sense information resulting from movement performance, and (3) the vestibular system for the regulation of upright control and balance at rest and during movements.[29] It compares motor plan signals driven by the cortex with what is received from muscles and joints in the periphery and makes necessary adjustments and adaptations to achieve the intended coordinated movement sequence. "Instructions" for movements that are frequently repeated are stored in the cerebellum as procedural memory traces. This increases the efficiency of its role in coordinating movement. The cerebellum also plays a role in the function of the reticular activating system (RAS).[30] The RAS network exists in the brain stem tegmentum; it is a network of nerve cells that maintain human consciousness and help people focus attention and block out distractions that may affect motor performance. Damage to the cerebellum, its tract systems, or its structure creates problems of movement coordination—not execution or the choice of which program to run. The cerebellum also plays a role in language, attention, and mental imagery functions that are not considered to take place in motor areas of the cerebral cortex (see Table 3.2).

The cerebellum plays the following four important roles in motor control[31]:

1. *Feedforward processing*: The cerebellum receives neural signals, processes them in a sequential order, and sends information out, providing a rapid response to any incoming information. It is not designed to act like the cerebral cortex and does not have the ability to generate self-sustaining neural patterns.
2. *Divergence and convergence*: The cerebellum receives a great number of inputs from multiple body structures. It processes this information extensively through a structured internal network and sends the results out through a limited number of output cells.
3. *Modularity*: The cerebellum is functionally divided into independent modules—hundreds to thousands—all with different inputs and outputs. Each module appears to function independently, although each shares neurons with the inferior olives, Purkinje cells, mossy and parallel fibers, and deep cerebellar nuclei.
4. *Plasticity*: Synapses within the cerebellar system (between parallel fibers and Purkinje cells and synapses between mossy fibers and deep nuclear cells) are susceptible to modification of their output strength. The influence of input on nuclear cells is adjustable, which provides great flexibility in adjusting and fine-tuning the relationship between cerebellar inputs and outputs.

Role of the Basal Ganglia

The basal ganglia are a collection of nuclei located in the forebrain and midbrain and consisting of the globus pallidus, putamen, caudate nucleus, substantia nigra, and subthalamic nuclei. The basal ganglia have primary functions in motor control and motor learning. They play a role in deciding which motor plan or behavior to execute at any given time and have connections to the limbic system; they are therefore believed to be involved in "reward learning." The basal ganglia play a key role in eye movements through midbrain connections with the superior colliculus and help to regulate postural tone as a basis for the control of body positions, preparedness, and central set (i.e., the nervous system's internal model of strategies for reactive balance control).[32] Refer to Chapter 18 for additional information on the basal ganglia.

Information Processing

The processing of information through the sensory input, motor output, and central integrative structures occurs by various methods to produce movement behaviors. These methods allow us to deal with the

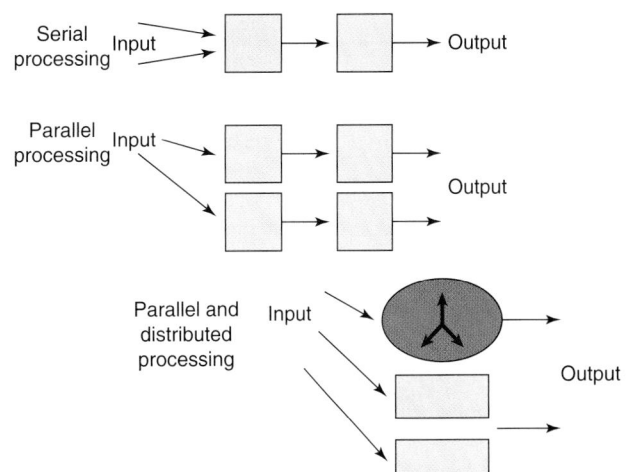

Fig. 3.1 Methods of Information Processing.

temporal and spatial components necessary for coordinated motor output and to anticipate, so that a response pattern may be prepared in advance. *Serial processing* is a specific, sequential order of processing of information (Fig. 3.1) through various centers. Information proceeds in lockstep through each center. *Parallel processing* is processing of information that can be used for more than one activity, and by more than one center simultaneously or nearly simultaneously. A third and more flexible type of processing of information is *parallel-distributed processing*.[33] This type of processing combines the best attributes of serial and parallel processing. When the situation demands serial processing, this type of activity occurs. At other times parallel processing is the mode of choice. For optimal processing of intrinsic and extrinsic sensory information by various regions of the brain, a combination of both serial and parallel processing is the most efficient mode. The type of processing depends on the constraints of the situation. For example, maintaining balance after an unexpected external perturbation requires rapid processing, whereas learning to voluntarily shift the center of gravity to the limits of stability requires a different combination of processing modes.

In summary, information processing reinforces and refines motor patterns. It allows the individual to initiate compensatory strategies if an ineffective motor pattern is selected or if an unexpected perturbation occurs. And, most important, information processing facilitates motor learning.

Movement Patterns Arising From Self-Organizing Subsystems

Coordinated movement patterns are developed and refined via dynamic interaction among body systems and subsystems in response to internal and external constraints. Movement patterns used to accomplish a goal are contextually appropriate and arise as an emergent property of subsystem interaction. Several principles relate to self-organizing systems: reciprocity, distributed function, consensus, and emergent properties.[34]

Reciprocity implies information flow between two or more neural networks. These networks can represent specific brain centers—for example, the cerebellum and basal ganglia (Fig. 3.2). Alternatively, the neural networks can be interacting neuronal clusters located within a single center—for example, the basal ganglia. One model to demonstrate reciprocity is the basal ganglia regulation of motor behavior through direct and indirect pathways to cortical areas. The more direct pathway from the putamen to the globus pallidus internal segment provides net inhibitory effects. The more indirect pathway from the putamen through the globus pallidus external segment and subthalamic

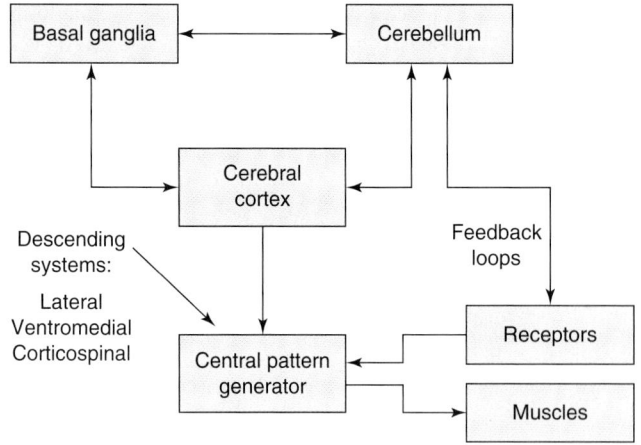

Fig. 3.2 Systems Model of Motor Control.

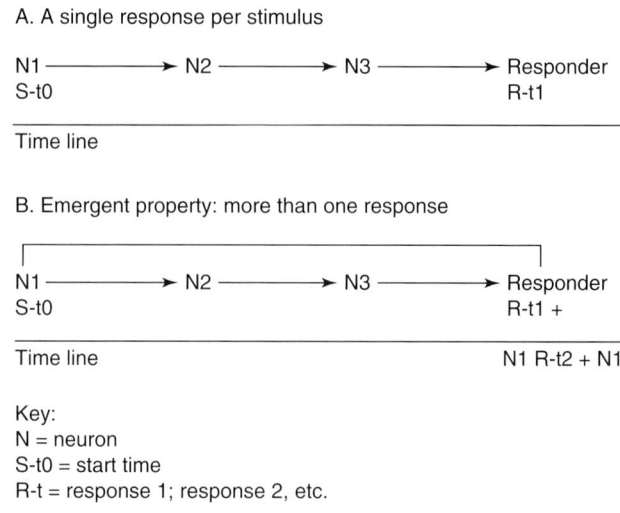

Key:
N = neuron
S-t0 = start time
R-t = response 1; response 2, etc.

Fig. 3.3 Emergent Property.

nucleus provides a net excitatory effect on the globus pallidus internal segment. Alteration of the balance between these pathways is postulated to produce motor dysfunction.[35,36] An abnormally decreased outflow from the basal ganglia is postulated to produce involuntary motor patterns; these produce excessive motion such as chorea, hemiballism, or nonintentional tremor. Alternatively, an abnormally increased outflow from the basal ganglia is postulated to produce a paucity of motions, as seen in the rigidity observed in individuals with Parkinson disease (see Chapter 18).

Distributed function presupposes that a single center or neural network has more than one function. The concept also implies that several centers share the same function. For example, a center may serve as the coordinating unit of an activity in one task and as a pattern generator or oscillator to maintain the activity in another task. An advantage of distributing function among groups of neurons or centers is to provide centers with overlapping or redundant functions. Neuroscientists believe such redundancy is a safety feature. If a neuronal lesion occurs, other centers can assume critical functional roles, thereby producing recovery from CNS dysfunction.[37–42]

Consensus implies that motor behavior occurs when a majority of brain centers or regions reach a critical threshold to produce activation. Also, through consensus, extraneous information or information that does require immediate attention is filtered. If, however, a novel stimulus enters the system, it carries more weight and receives immediate attention. A novel stimulus may be new to the system, may reflect a potentially harmful situation, or may result from the conflict of multiple inputs.

Emergent properties may be understood by the adage "the whole is greater than the sum of its parts." This concept implies that brain *centers,* not a single brain center, work together to produce movement. An example of the emergent properties concept is continuous repetitive activity (oscillation). In Fig. 3.3A, a hierarchy is represented by three neurons arranged in tandem. The last neuron ends on a responder. If a single stimulus activates this network, a single response occurs. What is the response if the neurons are arranged so that the third neuron sends a collateral branch to the first neuron in addition to the ending on the responder? In this case (see Fig. 3.3B), a single stimulus activates neuron No. 1, which in turn activates neurons No. 2 and No. 3, causing a response as well as reactivating neuron No. 1. This neuronal arrangement produces a series of responses rather than a single response. This process is also termed *endogenous activity.*

Another example of an emergent property is the production of motor behavior. Rather than having every MP stored in the brain, an abstract representation of the intended goal is stored. At the time of motor performance, various brain centers use the present sensory information combined with past memory of the task to develop the appropriate motor strategy. This concept negates a hardwired MP concept. If MPs were hardwired and if an MP existed for every movement ever performed, the brain would need a huge storage capacity and would lack the adaptability necessary for complex function.

Controlling the Degrees of Freedom

Combinations of muscle and joint action permit a large number of degrees of freedom that contribute to movement. A system with a large number of degrees of freedom is called a *high-dimensional system.* For a contextually appropriate movement to occur, the number of degrees of freedom must be constrained. Bernstein[9] suggested that the number of degrees of freedom could be reduced by muscles working in synergies—that is, coupling muscles and joints of a limb to produce functional patterns of movement. The functional unit of motor behavior is then a *synergy.* Synergies help to reduce the degrees of freedom, transforming a high-dimensional system into a low-dimensional system. For example, a step is considered to be a functional synergy pattern for the lower extremity. Linking together stepping synergies with the functional synergies of other limbs creates locomotion (interlimb coordination).

Functional synergy implies that muscles are activated in an appropriate sequence and with appropriate force, timing, and directional components. These components can be represented as fixed or "relative" ratios, and the control comes from input given to the cerebellum from higher centers in the brain and the peripheral or spinal system and from prior learning (see Chapter 19).[39,41,43] The relative parameters are also termed *control parameters.* Scaling control parameters leads to a change in motor behavior to accomplish the task. For example, writing your name on the blackboard exemplifies scaling force, timing, and amplitude. Scaling is the proportional increase or decrease of the parameter to produce the intended motor activity.

Coordinated movement is defined as an orderly sequence of muscle activity in a single functional synergy or the orderly sequence of functional synergies with appropriate scaling of activation parameters necessary to produce the intended motor behavior. Uncoordinated movement can occur at the level of the scaling of control parameters in one functional synergy or inappropriate coupling of functional synergies. The control parameter of duration will be used to illustrate scaling. If muscle A is active for 10% of the duration of the motor activity and muscle B is active 50% of the time, the fixed ratio of A/B is

1:5. If the movement is performed slowly, the relative time for the entire movement increases. Fixed ratios also increase proportionally. Writing your name on a blackboard very small or very large yields the same result—your name.

Timing of muscle on/off activation for antagonistic muscles such as biceps and triceps or hamstrings and quadriceps must be accurate for the coordination and control of movement patterns. If one muscle group demonstrates a delayed onset or maintains a longer duration of activity overlapping with triceps "on" time, the movement will appear uncoordinated. Patients with neurological dysfunction often demonstrate alterations in the timing of muscle activity within functional synergies and in coupling functional synergies to produce movement.[44,45] These functional movement synergies are not hardwired but represent emergent properties. They are flexible and adaptable to meet the challenges of the task and the environmental constraints.

Finite Number of Movement Strategies

The concept of *emergent properties* could conceivably imply an unlimited number of movement strategies available to perform a particular task. However, limiting the degrees of freedom decreases the number of strategies available for selection. In addition, constraints imposed by the internal environment (e.g., musculoskeletal system, cardiovascular system, metabolic activity, cognition) and external environment (e.g., support surface, obstacles, lighting) limit the number of movement strategies. Horak and Nashner[32] observed that a finite number of balance strategies were used by individuals in response to externally applied linear perturbations on a force plate system. With use of a lifespan approach, VanSant[46] identified a limited number of movement patterns for the upper limb, head-trunk, and lower limb for the task of rising from supine to standing.

The combination of these strategies produces the necessary variability in motor behavior. Although an individual has a preferred or modal profile, the healthy person with an intact neuromuscular system can combine strategies in various body regions to produce different movement patterns that also accomplish the task.[47,48] Persons with neurological deficits may be unable to produce a successful, efficient movement pattern because of their inability to combine strategies or adapt a strategy for a given environmental change (e.g., differing chair height for sit-to-stand transitions).

Variability of Movements Implies Normalcy

A key to the assessment and treatment of individuals with neurological dysfunction lies in variability of movement and in the notion that variability is a sign of normalcy, and stereotypical behavior is a sign of dysfunction.

Age, activity level, the environment, constraints of a goal, and neuropathological conditions affect the selection of patterns available for use during movement tasks.[49] When change occurs in one or more of the neural subsystems, a new movement pattern emerges. The element that causes change is called a *control parameter*. For example, an increase in the speed of walking occurs until a critical speed and degree of hip extension are reached, thereby switching the movement pattern to a run. When the speed of the run is decreased, there is a shift back to the preferred movement pattern of walking. A control parameter shifts the individual into a different pattern of motor behavior.

This concept underlies theories of development and learning. Development and learning can be viewed as moving the system from a stable state to a more unstable state. When the control variable is removed, the system moves back to the early, more stable state. As the control variable continues to push the system, the individual spends more time in the new state and less time in the earlier state until the individual spends most of the time in the new state. When this occurs,

the new state becomes the preferred state. Moving or shifting to the new, preferred state does not obviate the ability of the individual to use the earlier state of motor behavior. Therefore new movement patterns arise when critical changes occur in the system because of a control parameter, but they do not eliminate older, less-preferred patterns of movement.

Motivation to accomplish a task in spite of functional limitations and neuropathological conditions can also shift the individual's CNS to select different patterns of motor behavior. The musculoskeletal system, by nature of the architecture of the joints and muscle attachments, can be a constraint on the movement pattern. An individual with a functional contracture may be limited in the ability to bend a joint only into a desired range, thereby decreasing the movement repertoire available to him or her. Such a constraint produces adaptive motor behavior. Dorsiflexion of the foot needs to meet a critical degree of toe clearance during gait. If there is a range of motion limitation in dorsiflexion, then biomechanical constraints imposed on the nervous system will produce adaptive motor behaviors (e.g., to achieve toe clearance during gait). Changes in motor patterns during the task of rising from supine to standing are observed when healthy individuals wear orthoses to limit ankle dorsiflexion.[50] The inability to easily open and close the hand with rotation may lead to adaptations that require the shoulder musculature to place the hand in a more functional position. This adaptation uses axial and trunk muscles and will limit the use of that limb in both fine and gross motor performance. Refer to Chapter 19 for more information in this regard.

Preferred, nonobligatory movement patterns that are stable yet flexible enough to meet ever-changing environmental conditions are considered *attractor states*.[10] Individuals can choose from a variety of movement patterns to accomplish a given task. For example, older adults may choose from a variety of fall-prevention movement patterns when faced with the risk of falling. The choice of motor plan may be negatively influenced by age-related declines in the sensory input systems or a fear of falling. For example, when the Multi-Directional Reach Test[51] is being performed, an older adult may choose to reach forward, backward (lean), or laterally without shifting her center of gravity toward the limits of stability. She has the capability of performing a different reaching pattern if asked but prefers a more stable pattern.

Obligatory and stereotypical movement patterns suggest that the individual does not have the capability of adapting to new situations or cannot use different movement patterns to accomplish a given task. This inability may be a result of internal constraints that are functional or pathophysiological. The patient who has had a stroke has CNS constraints that limit the number of different movement patterns that can emerge from the self-organizing system. With recovery, the patient may be able to select and use additional movement strategies. Cognition and the capability to learn may also limit the number of movement patterns available to the individual and the ability of the person to select and use new or different movement patterns.

Obligatory and stereotypical movement patterns also arise from external constraints imposed on the organism. Consider the external constraints placed on a concert violinist. External constraints can include, for example, the length of the bow and the position of the violin. Repetitive movement patterns leading to cumulative trauma disorder in healthy individuals can lead to muscular and neurological changes.[51-55] Over time, changes in dystonic posturing and changes in the somatosensory cortex have been observed. Although one hypothesis considers that the focal dystonia results from sensory integrative problems, the observable result is a stereotypical motor problem.

To review, the nervous system responds to a variety of internal and external constraints to develop and execute motor behavior that is efficient to accomplish a specific task. Efficiency can be examined in terms of metabolic cost to the individual, type of movement pattern used, preferred or habitual movement (habit) used by the individual, and time to complete the task. The term *attractor state* is used in dynamical systems theory to describe the preferred pattern or habitual movement.

Individuals with neurological deficits may have limited repertoires of movement strategies available. Patients experiment with various motor patterns in order to learn the most efficient, energy-conscious motor strategy to accomplish the task. Therapists can plan interventions that help to facilitate refinement of the task to match the patient's capability, allowing the task to be completed using a variety of movement strategies rather than limited stereotypical strategies, leading to improved function.

Errors in Motor Control

When the actual motor behavior does not match the intended motor plan, an error in motor control is detected by the CNS. Common examples of errors in motor control are loss of balance; inappropriate scaling of force, timing, or directional control; and inability to ignore unreliable sensory information, resulting in sensory conflict. Any one or combination of these errors may be the cause of a fall or an error in performance accuracy.

Errors also occur when unexpected factors disrupt the execution of the MP. For example, when the surface is unreliable (unstable, moving), this will force the individual to adapt motor responses to meet the demand of the environment. Switching between closed environments (more stable) and open environments (more unpredictable) will challenge the individual to adapt motor responses. When an individual steps off a moving sidewalk, a disruption in walking occurs. The first few steps are not smooth because the person has to switch his movement strategies from one incorporating a moving support surface to one incorporating a stationary support surface.

Errors occur in the perception of sensory information, in the selection of the appropriate MP, in the selection of the appropriate variable parameters, or in the response execution. Patients with neurological deficits may demonstrate a combination of these errors. Therefore an assessment of motor deficits includes analysis of these types of errors. If a therapist observes a motor control problem, there is no guarantee that the problem has arisen from within the motor system. Somatosensory problems can drive motor dysfunction; cognitive and emotional problems express themselves through motor output. Thus it is up to the movement specialist to differentiate the cause of the problem through valid and reliable examination tools (see Chapter 8). Once the cause of the motor problem has been identified, selection of interventions should lead to positive outcomes.

All individuals, both healthy and those with CNS dysfunction, make errors in motor programming. These errors are assessed by the CNS and are stored in past memory of the experience. Errors in motor programming are extremely useful in learning. Learning can be viewed as decreasing the mismatch between the intended and actual motor behavior. This mismatch is a measure of the error; therefore a decrease in the degree of the error is indicative of learning. Errors, then, are an important part of the rehabilitation process. However, this does not mean that the therapist allows the patient to practice errors over and over. The ability of the patient to detect an error and correct it to produce appropriate and efficient motor behavior is one key to recovery and an important consideration when intervention strategies are developed. This is discussed further in the next section of this chapter.

Motor Control Section Summary

Motor control theories have been developed and have evolved over many years as our understanding of nervous system structure and

function has become more advanced. The control of posture and movement is a complex process that involves many structures and levels within the human body. It requires accurate sensory inputs, coordinated motor outputs, and central integrative processes to produce skillful, goal-directed patterns of movement that achieve desired movement goals. We must integrate and filter multiple sensory inputs from both the internal environment of the body and the external world around us to determine position in space and choose the appropriate motor plan to accomplish a given task. We combine individual biomechanical and muscle segments of the body into complex movement synergies to deal with the infinite "degrees of freedom" available during the production of voluntary movement. Well-learned motor plans are stored and retrieved and modified to allow for flexibility and variety of movement patterns and postures. When the PNS or CNS is damaged and the control of movement is impaired, new, modified, or substitute motor plans can be generated to accomplish goal-directed behaviors, remain adaptable to changing environments, and produce variable movement patterns. The process of learning new motor plans and refining existing behaviors by driving neuroplastic changes in the nervous system is discussed in the next sections of this chapter.

MOTOR LEARNING

Therapeutic interventions that are focused on restoring functional skills to individuals with various forms of neurological problems have been part of the scope of practice of physical therapists (PTs) and occupational therapists (OTs) since the beginning of both professions. These two professions have emerged with a complementary background to examine, evaluate, determine a prognosis, and implement interventions that empower patients to regain functional control of activities of daily living (ADLs) (e.g., getting out of bed, bathing, walking, and eating, as well as working, playing, and interacting socially) and resume active participation in life after neurological insult. These two professions specialize in the analysis of movement and possess knowledge of the scientific background to explain why the movement is occurring, what strengths and limitations exist within body systems to produce that movement, and how different therapeutic interventions can facilitate or enhance functional movement strategies that remediate dysfunction and ultimately carry over into an individual's improved performance of ADLs and participation in life. PTs and OTs are also knowledgeable about diseases affecting body systems (neurological, musculoskeletal, integumentary, cardiopulmonary, and integumentary systems) and how the existence or progression of these pathological states affects motor performance and quality of life. Consideration and training of caregivers and family members to help patients maintain functional skills during transitional disease states is also a component of practice and of treating the patient in a holistic manner.

It is therefore important for clinicians to understand how individuals learn or relearn motor tasks and how the learning of motor skills can best be achieved to optimize outcomes.

Motor learning results in a permanent change in the performance of a skill because of experience or practice.[56] The end result of motor learning is the acquisition of a new movement or the reacquisition and/or modification of movement.[57] The patient must be able to prepare and carry out a particular learned movement[58] in a manner that is efficient (optimal movement with the least amount of time, energy, and effort),[59] consistent (same movement over repeated trials),[60] and transferable (ability to perform the movement under different environments and conditions) to be considered to have learned a skill.

Learning of a particular motor task allows patients to use select motor skills to optimize function. This type of learning is expressed in explicit (declarative) and implicit (procedural) memory. Explicit memory is expressed by conscious recall of facts or knowledge.[61] An example of this could be the patient verbally stating the steps needed when going up the stairs with the use of crutches. Conversely, implicit learning involves movement performed without conscious thought (e.g., riding a bike or walking). The interplay of explicit (cognitive and emotional) and implicit memory affects ultimate learning to influence the time needed to learn or relearn a functional movement and use it in everyday activity.

The learning of a motor skill is measured indirectly by testing the ability of a patient to perform a particular task or activity over time or in different environmental contexts or conditions. The testing must be done over a period of time to determine long-term learning and minimize the temporary effects of practice. In *retention tests,* a patient performs the task under the same conditions in which the task was practiced. This type of test evaluates the patient's ability to learn the task. This is in contrast to *transfer tests,* in which a patient performs the activity under different conditions from those in which the skill was practiced. This evaluates the ability of the patient to use a previously learned motor skill to solve a different motor problem.

Motor skills can be categorized as discrete, continuous, or serial. Discrete motor skills pertain to tasks that have a specific start and finish. Repetitive tasks are classified as *continuous* motor skills. Serial skills involve several discrete tasks connected in a particular sequence that rapidly progress from one part to the next.[59] The category of a particular motor skill is a major factor in making clinical decisions regarding the individual-, task-, and environment-related variables that affect motor learning. This is discussed later in the chapter.

An Illustration of Motor Learning Principles

Motor learning is the product of an intricate balance between the feedforward and feedback sensorimotor systems and the complex central processor—the brain—for the end result of acquiring and refining motor skills. People go through distinct phases when they learn new motor skills.

Observe the sequential activities of the child walking off the park bench in Fig. 3.4A–C. A clear understanding of this relationship of walking and falling is established. In frame *A,* the child is running a feedforward program for walking. The cerebellum is procedurally responsible for modulating appropriate motor control over the activity and will correct or modify the program of walking when necessary to attain the directed goal. Unfortunately a simple correction of walking is not adequate for the environment presented in frame *B.* The cerebellum has no prior knowledge of the feedback presented in this second frame and thus is still running a feedforward program for stance on the left leg and swing on the right leg. The cerebellum and somatosensory cortices are processing a massive amount of mismatched information from the proprioceptive, vestibular, and visual receptors. In addition, the dopamine receptors are activated during the goal-driven behaviors, creating a balance of inhibition and excitation. Once the executive or higher cognitive system recognizes that the body is falling (which has been experienced from falling off a chair or bed), a shift in motor control focus from walking to falling must take place. To prepare for falling, the somatosensory system must generate a sensory plan and then relay that plan to the motor system through the sensorimotor feedback loops. The frontal lobe will tell the basal ganglia and the cerebellum to brace and prepare for impact. The basal ganglia are responsible for initiating the new program, and the cerebellum carries out the procedure, as observed in Fig 3.4C. The child succeeds at the task and receives positive peripheral and central feedback in the process. It is possible that this experience has created a new procedural program that in time will be verbally labeled "jumping." The entire process of the initial motor learning takes 1 to 2 seconds. Because of the child's motivation and interest (see Chapter 4), the program is practiced for the next 30 to 45 minutes. This is the initial acquisition phase and helps the nervous system store the MP to be used for the rest of the child's life. If this program is to become a procedural skill, practice must continue within similar environments and conditions. Ultimately the errors will be reduced and the skill will be refined. Finally, with practice, the program will enter the retention phase as a high-level skill. The skill can be modified in terms of force, timing, sequencing, and speed and is transferrable to different settings. This ongoing modification and improvement are the hallmarks of true procedural learning. Modifications within the program will be a function of the

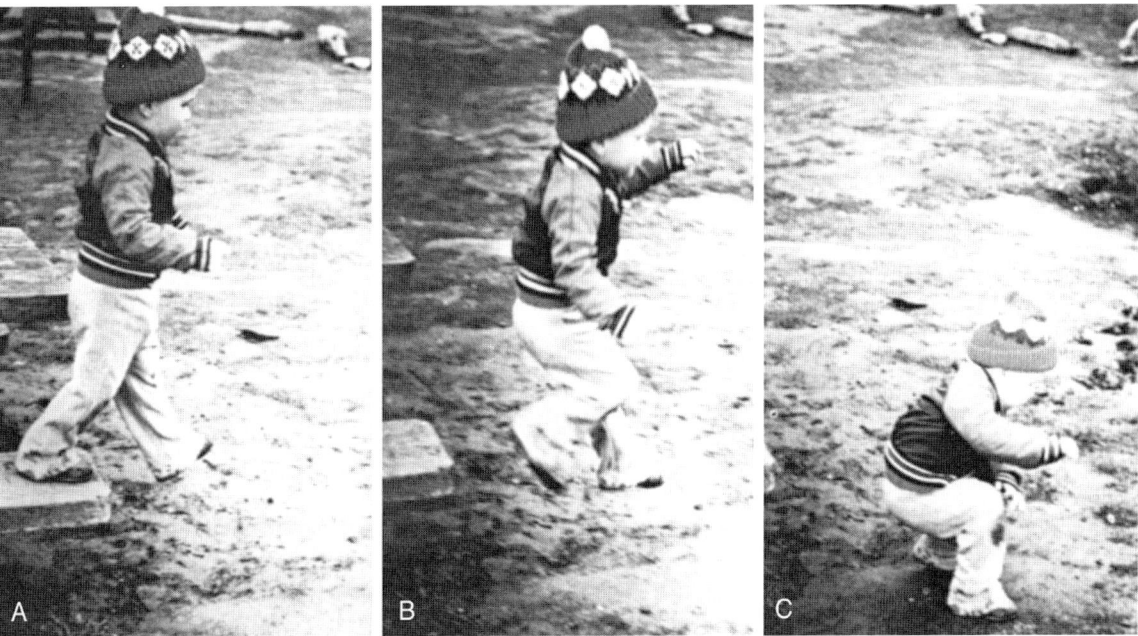

Fig. 3.4 (A) Experiencing the unknown. **(B)** Identifying the problem. **(C)** Solving the problem.

plasticity that occurs within the CNS throughout life as the child ages and changes body size and distribution. Similar plasticity and the ability to change, modify, and reprogram motor plans will be demanded by individuals who age with chronic sensorimotor limitations. Unfortunately, in many of these individuals, the CNS is not capable of producing and accommodating change, which creates new challenges as they age with long-term movement dysfunctions.

Stages of Motor Learning

Several authors have developed models to describe the stages of motor learning. These models are presented in Table 3.3. Regardless of the model, it is widely accepted that the process of learning a motor task occurs in stages. During the initial stages of learning a motor skill, the intent of the learner is to understand the task. To be able to develop this understanding requires a high level of concentration and cognitive processing. In the middle and later stages, the individual learns to refine the movement, improve efficiency and coordination, and perform the skill within different environmental contexts. The later stages are characterized by automaticity and a decreased level of attention needed for successful completion of the task. It is important to emphasize early that because the activities performed by a learner during each stage of learning will be different, the role of the clinician, the types of learning activities, and the clinical environment must also be different.

The learning model described by Fitts and Posner[64] consists of a continuous progression through three stages: cognitive, associative, and autonomous.

A learner functions in the *cognitive stage* at the beginning of the learning process. The person is highly focused on the task, is attentive to all that it demands, and develops an understanding of what is expected and involved in performance of the skill. Many errors are made in performance; questions are asked; cues, instructions, and guidance are given by the clinician; and demonstrations are found to be helpful in this phase of learning. Performance outcomes are variable and inconsistent, but the improvements achieved can be profound.

During the *associative stage* the learner refines movement strategies, detects errors and problem solves independent of therapist feedback, and is becoming more efficient and reliable at achieving the task goal. The length of time spent in this phase tends to be dependent on the complexity of the task. The ability to associate existing environmental inputs with motor plans for improved timing, accuracy, and coordination of activities to accomplish a task goal is improved. Although variability in performance decreases, the patient continues to explore solutions to best solve a movement problem.

Focused practice with repetition over time leads to the automatic performance of motor skills in the *autonomous stage* of learning. The individual is in control of the learned movement plan and is able to use it with little cognitive attention while involved in other activities. Skills are performed with preferred, appropriate, and flexible speed, amplitude, direction, timing, and force. Consistency of performance is a hallmark of this phase, as is the ability to detect and self-correct performance errors. Individuals who do not have the cognitive skill to remember the learning can go through a much longer repetitive practice schedule to learn the motor skill, but there will be very little carryover into other functional movements or activities.[62,65,66]

In summary, the overall process of the stages of motor learning as introduced by Fitts and Posner[64] suggests that first a basic understanding of a task be established, along with a motor pattern. Practice of the task then leads to problem solving and a decrease in the degrees of freedom during performance, resulting in improved coordination and accuracy. As the learner continues to practice and solves the motor task problem in different ways and with different physical and environmental constraints, the movement plan becomes more flexible and adaptable to a wide range of task demands.

Bernstein[9] presented a more biomechanical perspective as he addressed the problem of degrees of freedom during motor learning. He also broke the motor learning process down into three stages: novice, advanced, and expert. He proposed that these three stages are necessary to allow a learner to reduce the large number of degrees of freedom that are inherent in the musculoskeletal system, including structure and function of muscles, tendons, and joints. He proposed that as a person learns a new motor skill, he or she gains coordination and control over the multiple interacting variables that exist in the human body to master the target skill.

The *novice stage* is defined by the coupling of movement parameters—degrees of freedom—into synergies. During this stage some joints and movements may be "frozen" or restrained to allow successful completion of the task. An example of this is posturally holding the head, neck, and trunk rigid while learning to walk on a narrow surface.

The *advanced stage* is achieved by combining body parts to act as a functional unit, further reducing the degrees of freedom while allowing better interaction and consideration for environmental factors. He considers that motor plans must be adapted to the dynamic environmental conditions in which the task must be performed. In this stage the learner explores many movement solutions, reduces some degrees of freedom, develops more variable movement patterns, and learns to select appropriate strategies to accomplish a given task. This stage of motor learning is accomplished through practice and experience in performing a task in various environments. To achieve this stage the learner progressively releases some couplings, allowing more degrees of freedom, greater speed and amplitude of movement, and less constraints on the action. Performance of the task becomes more efficient, is less taxing on the individual, and is executed with decreased cognitive effort. Variability of performance becomes an indicator that a level of independence in the activation of component body parts during a given task has indeed been achieved.

In Bernstein's *expert stage,* degrees of freedom are now released and reorganized to allow the body to react to all of the internal and external mechanisms that may act on it at any given time. At the same time, enhanced coactivation of proximal structures is learned and used to allow for greater force, speed, and dexterity of limb movements.[67]

Gentile presented a two-stage model of motor learning.[68,69] She considered motor learning from the goal of the learner and strongly considered how environmental conditions influence performance and learning.

Stage one requires the patient to problem solve strategies to get the idea of a movement and establish a motor pattern that will successfully meet the demands of the task. As with the models presented previously, this process demands conscious attention to the components of the task and environmental variables to formulate a "map" or framework of the

Motor Learning Model	Stage One	Stage Two	Stage Three
Fitts and Posner (1967)[62]	Cognitive	Associative	Autonomous
Bernstein (1967)[9]	Novice	Advanced	Expert
Gentile (1998)[63]	Get in the ballpark, Acquire the plan	Develop consistency and adaptability	

TABLE 3.3 Stages of Motor Learning—Three Models

movement pattern. Once this framework is established, the patient has a mechanism for performing the task; however, errors and inconsistency in performance accuracy are often present.[70]

During *stage two*, the patient attains improved consistency of performance and the ability to adapt the movement pattern to demands of specific physical and environmental situations. Greater economy of movement is achieved, and less cognitive and physical effort is expended to reach the task goal. Practice in appropriately challenging conditions leads to consistent, efficient, correct execution while maintaining adaptive flexibility within the motor plan, allowing the patient to react quickly to changing conditions of the task.

The three motor learning theories just presented simplify a complex process into simple stages to give a broad picture of the development of skilled movement performance. Each theory can be used to assist the therapist in the process of teaching and facilitating long-term learning or relearning of motor skills before and after insult to the nervous system. The ultimate goal of motor learning is the permanent acquisition of adaptable movement plans that are efficient, require little cognitive effort, and produce consistent and accurate movement outcomes.

Variables That Affect Motor Learning

The ecological model (constraints theory) of motor control and learning states that motor learning involves the individual, the task, and the environment.[63] For a purposeful and functional movement to occur, the *individual* must generate movement to successfully meet the *task* at hand, as well as the demands of the *environment* where the task must be performed. For motor learning to be successful, several variables related to each of these three constructs must be taken into account.

Variables Related to the Individual

The clinician must first differentiate general motor performance factors that are under the control of the individual's cognitive and emotional systems and those that are controlled by the motor system itself. These concepts are presented in Fig. 3.5. There are many cognitive factors—such as arousal, attention, and memory, as well as cortical pathways related to declarative or executive learning—that have specific influences over behaviors observed after neurological insult.[71,72] Other factors—such as limbic connections to cortical pathways affected by motivation, fear and belief, and emotional stability and instability—also dramatically affect motor performance and declarative learning. Some of these factors may also limit activity and participation. Therapists must learn how to discriminate between problems due to motor output, somatosensory input, cortical processing, and limbic emotional state problems and to identify how the last two systems affect motor

output. With that differentiation, clinicians should also be able to separate specific motor system deficits from motor control problems arising from dysfunction within other areas of the CNS. Last, the patient's fitness level; current limitations in strength, endurance, power, and range of motion; or pain level may also influence learning.[57,73–78]

Variables Related to the Task

The two major variables related to the task itself that must be considered when facilitating motor learning include practice of the task and feedback related to task performance.

Practice. Practice is defined as "repeated performance in order to acquire a "skill."[79] As the definition implies, multiple repetitions of the task are usually required to be able to achieve skillful performance of a task. With other variables being constant, more practice results in more learning.[57] To be effective, these repetitions must involve a process of problem solving rather than just repetition of the activity.[80] The therapist can manipulate variables related to practice in order to optimize motor learning in an individual with a pathological movement pattern.

Practice conditions. The term *practice conditions* refers to the manner in which the task or exercise is repeated with respect to rest periods, the amount of exercise, and the sequence in which these tasks or exercises are performed.

According to the apportionment of practice in relation to rest periods, massed tasks or exercises can be classified as *massed practice* or *distributed practice.* Massed practice is when the rest period is much shorter in relation to the amount of time the task or exercise is practiced.[81] This is contrasted against distributed practice, in which the time between practice sets is equal to or greater than the amount of time devoted to practicing a particular task or activity such that the rest period is spread out throughout the practice.[82] In terms of neurological physical therapy practice, it is important to consider the effect of physical and mental fatigue when a person is training. For example, physical fatigue sets in during massed practice of a particular balance exercise activity in standing and may cause a patient to fall. Moreover, individuals who are cognitively impaired may not respond positively to sustained activity that requires considerable concentration and therefore might fail in the performance of the skill. On the other hand, to be functional and useful in daily life, certain activities have to be performed without significant amounts of rest. For example, taking significant rest breaks when one is ambulating for even a short distance limits the person's ability to use walking in a functional manner. Sometimes a patient needs more rest periods in the initial stages of learning a skill to compensate for impairments in muscular endurance or cardiopulmonary function with the intent of decreasing these rest periods to achieve skill performance that reflect how that activity is used in real-life situations. Therefore therapists should consider the skill demands and desired results when they are choosing one practice type versus another.[82]

Complete, functional tasks or activities can usually be divided into smaller subcomponents for practice. The way those subcomponents are practiced relative to the entire task or activity can be manipulated to optimize motor learning. This includes practice of the entire task or parts of the task, whole learning, pure-part learning, progressive-part learning, or whole-part learning methods. Fig. 3.6 summarizes these concepts.

Whole learning suggests that the learner practice the entire movement as one activity. Asking a person to stand up incorporates the entire activity of coming to stand from sitting. Simple movements such as rolling, coming to sit, coming to stand, and walking might best be taught as a whole activity as long as the individual has all the component parts to practice the whole.

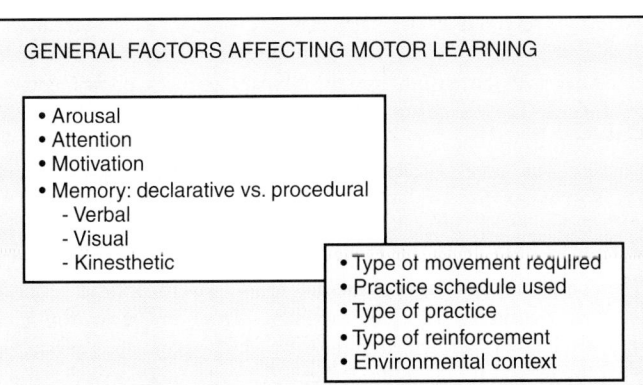

GENERAL FACTORS AFFECTING MOTOR LEARNING

- Arousal
- Attention
- Motivation
- Memory: declarative vs. procedural
  - Verbal
  - Visual
  - Kinesthetic

- Type of movement required
- Practice schedule used
- Type of practice
- Type of reinforcement
- Environmental context

Fig. 3.5 Concepts Affecting Motor Learning.

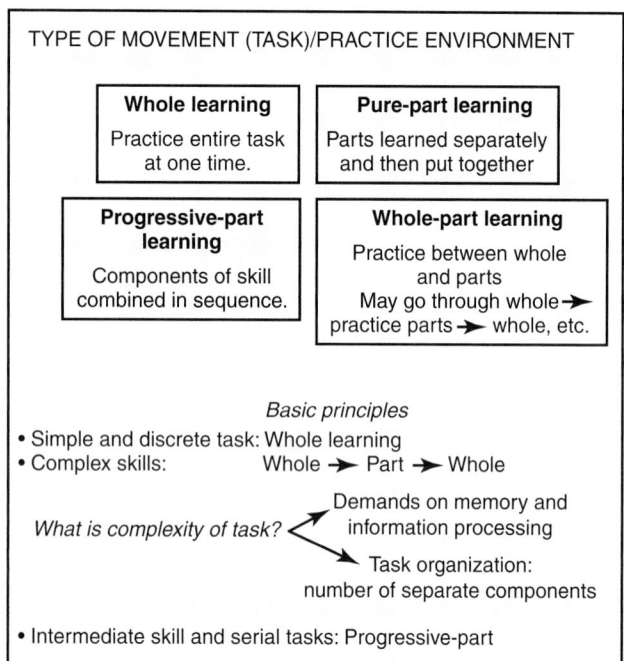

TYPE OF MOVEMENT (TASK)/PRACTICE ENVIRONMENT

Whole learning
Practice entire task at one time.

Pure-part learning
Parts learned separately and then put together

Progressive-part learning
Components of skill combined in sequence.

Whole-part learning
Practice between whole and parts
May go through whole → practice parts → whole, etc.

Basic principles
- Simple and discrete task: Whole learning
- Complex skills: Whole → Part → Whole

What is complexity of task? 〈 Demands on memory and information processing
Task organization: number of separate components

- Intermediate skill and serial tasks: Progressive-part

Fig. 3.6 Type of Movement (Task) and Practice Environment.

In pure-part learning the therapist introduces one part first; then this part is practiced by the learner before another new part is introduced and practiced. Each part is critical to the whole movement, but which one is learned first does not matter. Learning a tennis serve is an excellent example of an activity that can be taught as a pure part. Learning to toss the ball vertically to a specific spot in space is a very different and separate part from swinging the tennis racket as part of the serve. Learning to squeeze the toothpaste onto the brush is a very different movement strategy from brushing the teeth.

Progressive-part learning is used when the sequence of movements and the component parts to be learned need to be programmed in a specific order. Line dancing is an activity taught using progressive part learning. Individuals with sequencing deficits must often be taught using progressive parts, or they will mix up the ordering of parts during an activity. Therapists see this in the clinical arena when an individual stands up from a wheelchair and then tries to pick up the foot pedals and lock the brakes. Given that problem, such a patient must practice progressive-part learning by first locking the brakes, then picking up the foot pedals, and finally standing. If the activity is not practiced using progressive-part learning, the patient will have little consistency in how the parts are put together, thereby placing that him at high risk of failing at the functional task.

Whole-part learning can be used when the skill or activity can be practiced between the whole and the parts. In the clinical environment, a common application of this concept is *whole to part to whole learning*.[83] First the therapist has the patient try the whole activity, such as coming to stand or opening a door. Next, the therapist has the patient practice a component part that is deficient (e.g., gripping the doorknob). Finally the whole activity is practiced as a functional pattern. In this way therapists work on the functional activity and then work on correcting the impairment or limitation, such as power production, range, or balance. Then they go back to the functional activity in order to incorporate the part learning into the whole. An example might be asking a patient to first stand up from a chair. As she tries to stand she generates too much power, holds her breath, and cannot repeat the activity more than once. The therapist decides to practice a component

part by first assisting the patient to a relaxed standing posture, then having her eccentrically begin to sit into a partial squat, and then having her return to standing. As the patient practices, she will increase the range of motion and eventually will sit and return to stand. Once that is accomplished, she will continue to practice sit to stand to sit as a whole activity.

Therapists change the sequence in which component parts of a task are practiced using blocked or random practice. In *blocked practice* the patient first practices a single task over and over before moving to the next task. With *random practice* the component skills are practiced in random order without any particular sequence. The contextual interference effect explains the difference in motor performance found when these two types of practice are compared. Studies have shown that performance may be enhanced by using blocked practice; however, learning is not enhanced by using this type of practice. Random practice has been shown to enhance learning because this type of practice forces the learners to come up with a motor solution each time a task is performed.[84,85]

Feedback. The use of feedback is another important variable related to motor learning. Feedback is defined as the use of sensory information—visual, auditory, or somatosensory—to improve performance, retention, or transfer of a task. Internal feedback pertains to sensory information that the patient receives that can be used to improve performance of that particular task or activity in the future. The therapist provides extrinsic or augmented feedback with the intent of improving learning of the task. In people with neurological dysfunctions, extrinsic feedback is important because the patient's intrinsic feedback system may be impaired or absent.

Extrinsic feedback can further be classified as knowledge of performance (KP) or knowledge of results (KR). KP is given concurrently while the task is being performed and can therefore also be called *concurrent feedback*. Feedback given concurrently, especially during the critical portions of the task, allows the patient to successfully perform the activity.

KR pertains to feedback given at the conclusion of the task (therefore it is also called *terminal feedback*) and provides the patient with information about the success of his or her actions with respect to the activity. KR can be classified as faded, delayed, or summary. In faded feedback the therapist provides more information in the beginning stages of learning of the skill and slowly withdraws that feedback as the patient demonstrates improvement in the performance of the task. With delayed feedback, information is given to the patient when a period of time has elapsed after the task has been completed. The intent of this pause between the termination of a task and feedback is to give the patient some time to process the activity and generate possible solutions to the difficulties encountered in the previous performance of the task. In contrast, summary feedback is provided after the patient has performed several trials of a particular task without receiving feedback. Studies show that subjects who were given more frequent feedback, compared with those who received summary feedback, performed better during the task acquisition stage of learning but worse on retention tests.[86,87]

Additional concepts related to long-term learning are presented in Fig. 3.7.

Variables Related to the Environment

Therapists can alter environmental conditions to optimize motor learning. Gentile[68,69] described the manipulation of the environment in which a task is performed to make an activity more appropriate for what the patient is able to do. Patients with neurological dysfunction may benefit from practicing in a *closed environment* that is stationary and predictable. It allows the skill to be practiced with minimal

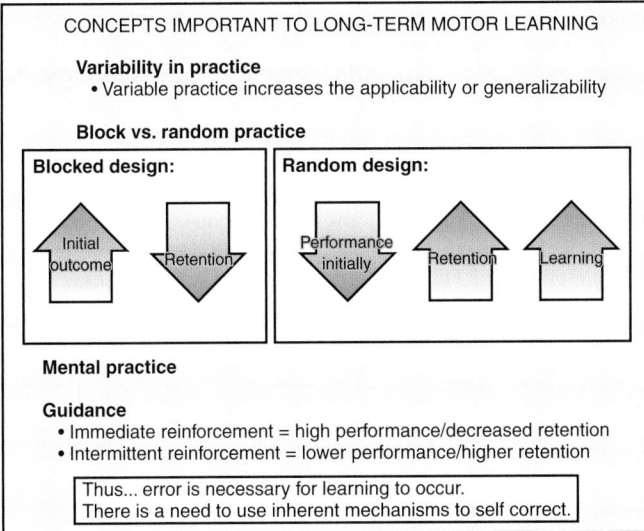

CONCEPTS IMPORTANT TO LONG-TERM MOTOR LEARNING

Variability in practice
• Variable practice increases the applicability or generalizability

Block vs. random practice

Blocked design:	Random design:

Mental practice

Guidance
• Immediate reinforcement = high performance/decreased retention
• Intermittent reinforcement = lower performance/higher retention

Thus... error is necessary for learning to occur.
There is a need to use inherent mechanisms to self correct.

Fig. 3.7 Concepts Important to Long-term Learning.

distractions or challenges from the environment, enabling the patient to plan the movement in advance. An example of this would be performing gait training in a quiet, empty therapy gym. As the patient improves, it is important to practice this activity in an *open environment* that is less predictable, more distracting, or in motion to provide a real-world application of the task. An example of this would be gait training the patient in a busy gym environment, in a crowded cafeteria, on a moving walkway, or in a noisy hallway.

If prior procedural learning has occurred, then creating an environment that allows the program to run in the least restrictive environment should lead to the most efficient outcome in the shortest time.[74,75] If a patient must learn a new program, such as walking with a stereotypical extension pattern, then goal-directed, attended practice with guided feedback will be necessary. It may be easier to bring back an old ambulatory pattern by creating an environment to elicit that program than to teach a patient to use a new inefficient movement program.[76–78]

A therapist must identify what MPs are available and under what conditions. This allows the therapist to (1) determine whether deficits are present, (2) anticipate problems in performance, and (3) match existing programs with functional activity challenges during training. Similarly, knowing available MPs and the component body systems necessary to run those programs aids the therapist in the selection of intervention procedures.

If the patient has permanent damage to either the basal ganglia or the cerebellum, then retaining the memory of new MPs may be difficult and substitution approaches may become necessary. Through evaluation, the clinician must determine whether anatomical disease or a pathological condition is actually causing procedural learning problems and whether identifying and teaching a substitution pattern or teaching the patient to compensate with an old pattern will allow him to succeed at the task. However, therapists should never forget that the plasticity of the CNS can promote significant recovery and adaptation through the performance of attended, goal-directed, repetitive behavior.[88,89]

The provision of an appropriate level of challenge to the learner can optimize motor learning. The clinician must learn to expertly manipulate the environment to best facilitate learning. A task that is too difficult for the patient will result in persistent failure of performance, frustration, and lack of learning; then the only option will be to compensate through available patterns of movement that limit function.

An activity that is too easy and routinely results in 100% success also does not result in learning because the learner becomes bored and no longer attends to the experience. The most beneficial level of challenge for training will create some errors in performance, require the patient to solve problems to meet the demands presented, and allow a level of success that inspires continued motivation to practice and achieve a higher standard of skill.

PRINCIPLES OF NEUROPLASTICITY: IMPLICATIONS FOR NEUROREHABILITATION

Rehabilitation, Research, and Practice

Rehabilitation is the process of maximizing functional learning. The integration of basic neuroscience into clinical practice is critical for guiding the questioning of researchers and maximizing the recovery of patients. Over the past 30 years, researchers have made enormous advances in understanding the adaptability of the CNS. Because of this revolution, clinicians have moved toward a focus on recovery rather than compensation. There is sufficient evidence that the CNS continues to develop and mature from infancy into adolescence. During early and late adulthood, the CNS can recover from serious disease and injury, maintaining sensory, motor, and cognitive competency through spontaneous healing, appropriate medical management, physical exercise and activity, balanced nutrition, and opportunities to learn. Across the life-span, individuals can maximize independence and quality of life by capitalizing on learning from enriched environments, task-specific training, and attentive, progressive, self-generated, goal-oriented, repetitive behaviors. Unfortunately the nervous system can adapt negatively to repetitive and atypical patterns of movement based on neuromuscular deficits, structural anomalies, pain, abnormal biomechanics, or bad habits (see the section on motor learning earlier in this chapter). To promote recovery versus negative adaptation, rehabilitation professionals must be cognizant of a patient's learning potential and be aware of the resources available at the environment, task, and individual level.

The paradigm shift in rehabilitative intervention strategies based on neuroplasticity is ongoing. Researchers in basic and translational science must collaborate with clinicians to determine how research findings can influence recovery.[92–94] Furthermore, clinicians cannot simply provide the same familiar treatment of yesterday because it is comfortable and requires minimal effort. Rehabilitation professionals must be dynamic, enthusiastic, evidence-based, and committed to lifelong learning, ready to accept the challenge and unique opportunity to work with other members of the health care team to translate neuroscience to practice. Failure to translate research findings into clinical practice will significantly impede the potential for patient recovery.

Over the past 50 years, conferences have begun to address key issues in neuroscience and rehabilitation to move the field forward.[95–100] In 1966, the Northwestern University Special Therapeutic Exercise Project (NUSTEP) conference in Chicago brought researchers, basic scientists, educators, and master clinicians together for 6 weeks to identify commonalities in approaches to interventions and to integrate basic science into those commonalities. A huge shift from specific philosophies to a bodily systems model occurred in 1990 in Norman, Oklahoma, the site of the Second Special Therapeutic Exercise Project conference (II STEP). During the next 15 years, motor learning and control concepts began to influence the intervention philosophies of both occupational and physical therapy. Simultaneously, newer approaches such as locomotion training with partial weight support,[101,102] task-specific training,[103,104] constraint-induced movement therapy,[105,106] neuroprotective effect of exercise,[107] mental and physical practice,[108,109] patient-centered therapy,[110–112] and sensorimotor training[113] were frequently found in peer-reviewed literature. The third STEP conference, Summer Institute on Translating Evidence into Practice (III STEP), occurred in July 2005 in Salt Lake City, Utah. At this conference, unique clinical models for intervention were embraced that continue to direct professional education. The IV STEP Conference, with a focus on the 4 P's in rehabilitation (prediction, prevention, plasticity, and participation),[98–100] took place in July 2016 at The Ohio State University in Columbus. The IV STEP conference highlighted the progress made since the III STEP Conference and challenged attendees to push forward as new breakthroughs provide an impetus for ongoing change in personalized rehabilitation. Related conferences included the recent Progress in Clinical Motor Control: Neurorehabilitation at Pennsylvania State University in State College in July 2018. These conferences further challenge the research and rehabilitation community to provide strong evidence for intervention strategies aimed at fostering neural recovery and function. Although the inclusion of new, evidence-based, intervention strategies into clinical practice continues to lag behind research findings, the goal of integration remains.

There are many challenges to implementing effective, neuroscience-based interventions. The first is the patient. Patient-centered therapy is critical for effective therapeutic outcomes. The patient can be both the obstacle to successful recovery[114,115] and the critical link to success.[116,117] To achieve optimum neural adaptation, the patient must be attentive during self-generated goal-directed novel progressive activity. There is no measurable neural adaptation with passive movements or passive stimuli. To achieve a change in neural response, a stimulus must be novel and the individual must attend to it. This adaptive process can be implicit or explicit. For example, if the process is explicit, the individual is aware, makes a decision about what to do, and receives some feedback regarding the appropriateness or accuracy of the outcome.[118] This progressive decision making has to be done repetitively and advance in difficulty over time. Adaptive behaviors may be difficult to achieve when a person is depressed, feels hopeless, lacks motivation or cognition, is emotionally unstable, or neglects of one or more parts of the body.

Another obstacle to bringing scientific evidence into practice is the barrier created by living in a society in which the economics of health care rather than the science or patient benefits drive the delivery of services. When a physician or therapist recommends a new approach to intervention, the third-party payer may deny payment for service because it is "experimental." Furthermore, third-party payers may deny the opportunity to apply findings from animal studies to human subjects. Another constraint from the third-party payer is the timing of intervention. Despite the evidence that the CNS can be modified under conditions of goal-oriented, repetitive, task-relevant behaviors years after stroke, insurance companies deny coverage of service late in the recovery process. The insurance company may interpret "medically necessary services" as the services provided during the first 30 days after injury, the time when the greatest spontaneous recovery occurs. Furthermore, even though neural adaptation research confirms that enriched environmental conditions and sensory inputs can facilitate both greater and continued recovery, the insurance company may claim that the services[119–122] are simply for maintenance. Thus as the science of neuroplasticity continues to develop, it is critical to improve the interface between the scientist, the practitioner, the patient, and the third-party payer. It is vital that clinicians and researchers regularly inform third-party payers about current research evidence.

Integration of Sensory Information in Motor Control

One's understanding of neural adaptation must include attention to sensory as well as motor systems. In virtually all higher-order perceptual processes, the brain must correlate sensory input with motor output to assess the body's interaction with the environment accurately. Thus a problem in the somatic motor system affects the motor output system. Both systems are independently adaptive, but functional neural adaptation involves the interaction of both sensory and motor processing.

The sensory system provides an internal representation of the inner and outer worlds to guide the movements that make up our behavioral repertoire. Movement is controlled by the motor systems of the brain and the spinal cord. Our perceptual skills reflect the capabilities of the sensory systems to detect, analyze, and estimate the significance of physical stimuli. (Augmented therapeutic intervention for each sensory system is discussed in Chapter 8.) Our agility and dexterity reflect the capabilities of the motor systems to plan, coordinate, and execute movements. The task of the motor systems in controlling movement is the reverse of the task of sensory systems in aiding or updating internal representations. Perception is the end product of sensory processing, whereas an internal representation is the beginning of motor processing.

Sensory psychophysics looks at the attributes of a stimulus: its quality, intensity, location, and duration. Motor psychophysics considers the organization of action, intensity of muscle contraction, recruitment of distinct motor neuron populations, coordination and accuracy of movement, and the speed of movement. The complex behaviors in the sensory and motor systems depend on the modalities available. The distinct modalities of pain, temperature, light touch, deep touch, vibration, and stretch are found in the sensory system; whereas the modalities of reflex responses, intra- and interlimb rhythmic patterns, automatic and adaptive responses, and voluntary fine and gross movements are found in the motor system.[123–143] Although all motor movement requires integration of sensory information for motor learning, once motor control has been attained, the system can often run on very little feedback. The relationship of incoming sensory information is particularly complex in voluntary movement, which constantly adapts to environmental variance. For voluntary movements, the motor system requires muscle contraction and relaxation with appropriate timing and sequencing, recruitment of appropriate muscles and their synergies, the distribution of the body mass, and appropriate postural adjustments.

There must be adjustments to compensate for limb inertia and the mechanical arrangement of muscles, bones, and joints before and during movement to ensure and maintain accuracy. The control systems for voluntary movement involve (1) a continuous flow of sensory information about the environment, body/limb orientation, and degree of muscle contraction; (2) the spinal cord; (3) the descending systems of the brain stem; and (4) the motor pathways of the cerebral cortex, cerebellum, and basal ganglia. Each control system is organized hierarchically and in parallel and uses sensory information relevant for the functions it oversees via feedback and feedforward mechanisms. These systems control activation of sensations and movement as well as inhibition (e.g., globus pallidus). Some brain regions are engaged during new learning (e.g., cerebellum) and others during maintenance of learning (e.g., globus pallidus, hippocampus). The hierarchical but interactive organization permits lower levels to generate reflexes without involving higher centers, whereas the parallel system allows the brain to process the flow of specific types of sensory information to produce discrete types of movements.[144,145]

Ultimately the control of graded fine movement involves the muscle spindle, which contains the specialized elements that sense muscle length and the velocity or changes in spindle length. In conjunction with the tendon organ, which senses muscle tension, the muscle spindle provides the CNS with continuous information on the mechanical

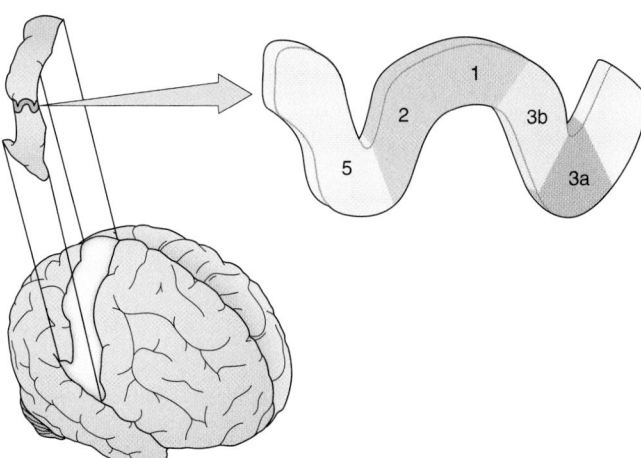

Fig. 3.8 Classification and Anatomical Locations of Cortical Map.

TABLE 3.4 Neuroprotective Motor Enrichment Factors Affecting Outcomes

	Negative Plasticity	Positive Plasticity
Stimulation	Disuse, unskilled	Intensive, skilled
Quality of sensory input	Noisy, nonspecific	Appropriate, specific
Modulation	Not challenging	High stakes, novel, challenging
Outcome	Negative behaviors	Positive behaviors

state of the muscle. Ultimately the firing of the muscle spindles depends on both muscle length and the level of gamma motor activation of the intrafusal fibers. Similarly, joint proprioceptors relay both closed- and open-chain input and mobility (range) information from within the joint structures to the CNS. This illustrates the close, integral relationship between sensory and motor processing.[146]

Foundation for the Study of Neuroplasticity

The principal models for studying cortical plasticity have been based on the representations of the movement and skin of the hand in the New World owl monkey (Aotus) and the squirrel monkey (Saimiri). These primate models have been chosen because their central sulci usually do not extend into the hand representational zone in the anterior parietal (S1) or posterior frontal (M1) cortical fields. In other primates the sulci are deep and interfere with accurate mapping. Even though there are differences in hand use among primates, in all primates the hand has the largest topographical and distinct representation for the actual size of the extremity. Thus the hand has the greatest potential for skilled movement and sensory discrimination. Findings from studies of this cortical region are applicable across the different cortices as well as the other cornerstones of the brain such as the thalamus, basal ganglia, brain stem, and cerebellum.[147,148] See Fig. 3.8 to identify specific anatomical locations and their respective classifications.

To understand neural adaptation and be able to apply the principles to practice, it is essential to measure change objectively. Positive change in neural structure can be measured with a variety of imaging techniques (e.g., magnetic resonance imaging [MRI], functional MRI [fMRI], magnetoencephalography, magnetic source imaging [MSI], and diffusion tensor imaging [DTI]). The types of outcomes that can be expected are summarized in Table 3.4. Electroencephalography (EEG) can be used to examine recovery patterns and dynamic change during select activities.[149,150] The specific type of intervention to address the principles of neuroplasticity may vary, but the outcomes must be clearly documented.

Research has now begun to explore the role of neurotrophic factors and genetics and the potential for neural recovery and adaptation. For example, the protein brain-derived neurotrophic factor (BDNF), which serves to improve the function of neurons, has been found to influence neuroplasticity and motor learning.[151] The release of BDNF is reportedly activity-dependent, with increased levels noted in response to aerobic exercise and skill learning.[152,153] However, there is variability in the release of BDNF in the case of genetic polymorphisms or

variations in DNA. In reference to BDNF, a common single-nucleotide polymorphism has been reported, called val66met, which involves an amino acid substitution from valine to methionine at codon 66. This substitution results in a BDNF val66met polymorphism and a reduction in the activity-dependent release of BDNF.[154] As more information is gained from this line of research, among other contributing factors, we may be better able to predict which individuals will best respond to particular intervention strategies and which will need alternative programming to foster responsiveness.

Principles of Neural Adaptation

To achieve maximal neural adaptation, several basic principles must be kept in mind (Box 3.1). Learning is the key to neural adaptation. Plasticity is the mechanism for encoding, the changing of behaviors, and both implicit and explicit learning. During neural adaptation, the fundamental questions are as follows: As we learn, how does the brain change its representations of inputs and actions? What is the nature of the processes that control the progressive elaboration of performance abilities? In different individuals, what are the sources of variance for the emergence of improved performance? What changes in cortical plasticity facilitate the development of "automatic" motor behaviors? Why are some behaviors hard to change? What limits plasticity processes? What are the critical elements of brain circuitry, genes, synapses, neural chemistry, neuronal networks, and neural connections for the restoration of lost function? What guidelines must be followed to drive the greatest change in brain structure and function? How do spontaneous compensatory behavioral strategies contribute to or interfere with restoring lost neuronal function? How does the less affected side following stroke contribute to or interfere with neuroplastic changes and restoration of function? Does damage to the brain alter the neuronal response to learning (e.g., cascade of cellular activity for healing altered circuitry, new neural connections)?

The most informative studies on neuroplasticity are those specifically directed toward defining the changes induced by learning. One approach has been to document the patterns of distributed neural response representation of specific inputs before and after learning. In particular, neuronal responses have been measured in the primary auditory, somatosensory, and motor cortices in animals. These animal studies have been paired with behavioral studies in humans. Both the animal and human studies provide strong evidence documenting the ability of the brain to functionally self-organize. This capacity for change occurs not only during development but also in adulthood, specifically after learning-based activities. The basic processes for neural adaptation are discussed in the following paragraphs.

1. *Neural circuits must be actively engaged in learning-based activities to prevent degradation and atrophy.*

We know that if infants are deprived of sensory and motor experiences during development, the brain does not develop sufficiently. For example, without exposure to light, there is a reduction in the number of neurons in the visual cortex.[155] Similarly, if infants are

BOX 3.1 Neuroplasticity Principles Translated to Guide Clinical Practice

Basic Principles

The task of translating basic science to clinical practice over time is a challenging one. There is no exact protocol. Learning activities must be adapted and matched to the abilities, goals, and objectives of each individual. Based on research evidence, the following principles can help to guide training:

1. *Use it or lose it*—Stay active and keep challenging learning. Failure to regularly engage specific and general brain functions can lead to functional degradation.
2. *Use it and improve it*—Engaging in training behaviors that drive specific brain functions can lead to enhancement of the function.
3. *Be specific*—The training experience must match the desired outcome; the nature of neural plasticity is dictated by the nature of the training.
4. *Repetition is essential*—Learning requires repetition, progressive in difficulty and spaced over time.
5. *Intensity matters*—Plasticity changes require a sufficient training intensity to ensure the durability of pathways.
6. *Salience is important*—The training must be salient and must match the outcome behavior desired and the goals of the individual.
7. *Age must be addressed*—Training-induced plasticity occurs most readily in a young brain, but neural adaptation continues across the life-span with learning-based training. With aging, greater efforts at variety, integration, and discovery may be needed.
8. *Transference*—Plasticity in response to one training experience can also enhance the acquisition of similar behaviors and adaptations in other experiences and other parts of the body.
9. *Interference*—Plastic changes after one training experience may interfere with the acquisition of changes in similar systems.
10. *Patient expectation*—Patient expectation can facilitate the outcomes of training; patients who expect to get better can enhance their learning.
11. *Reward or feedback*—Feedback enables the modification of training behaviors, correction of errors, and improvement in the accuracy of learning.
12. *Environment*—The environment can be enriched simply by noticing everything in the environment, expanding the environment to include new opportunities, and providing opportunities to interact with others.
13. *Fun*—Learning is greatest when it is associated with discovery and fun.
14. *Helping others*—The fitness of the brain is maintained best when individuals look beyond themselves to help and involve others.

Integrate the Principles of Neural Adaptation Into Neurorehabilitation

In embarking on a rehabilitation program with someone, it is important to match the principles of neuroplasticity to interactions with the patient, the family, the health care team, and the job, emphasizing the importance of the following:

1. Thinking positively about health and recovery; expecting to get better
2. Setting clear goals and objectives for retraining
3. Encouraging the family to be involved in the retraining activities
4. Creating learning activities that are attended-goal directed, repetitive, progressed in difficulty, increased in variety and depth, spaced over time, rewarded, and complemented with feedback on accuracy
5. Linking activities temporally (in time) and spatially but progressively sequenced; making the stimulus strength adequate for detection and appropriate to avoid abnormal behaviors
6. Integrating training behaviors into meaningful functional activities
7. Making training activities age appropriate
8. Integrating training activities across multiple sensory modalities appropriate for desired outputs
9. Performing training activities in different postural orientations and different environments, thus facilitating the best performance
10. Matching training behaviors with progression of healing and recovery as well as development
11. Strengthening positive responses with meaningful rewards

12. Making it difficult to use the unaffected side (e.g., wearing a glove)
13. Avoiding activities that stimulate the repetition of abnormal movements
14. Maintaining high levels of attention and cognitive function within the context of all daily activities; avoiding habitual unattended behaviors
15. Maintaining self-esteem
16. Avoiding an egocentric focus; thinking about how to help and be involved with others
17. Being fit, thinking "tall," and challenging balance by interacting in new unstable environments

Research-Validated Outcomes Following Central Nervous System Training

With thoughtful, attentive, regular physical exercise; integrated learning-based activities; daily learning; and specific practice to improve skills, there is scientific evidence confirming the following positive outcomes:

1. Strengthened and elaborated neuronal interconnections
2. Improved health and vigor of nerve cell populations (including neurotransmitters, nerve brain growth factors, dopamine)
3. Increased physical size of brain centers and a slowing down of shrinkage and atrophy of the brain with aging and disuse
4. Increased accuracy of neuronal processing
5. Improved strength of associative memory processes and the capacity for the brain to remember what is seen, heard, felt, or learned
6. Faster brain processing and more reliable connections to improve sharpness and completeness of how our brain represents and records information
7. Improved coordination of neuronal activities across brain subsystems
8. Improved abilities to broaden and control one's attention, shift attention, and take in more information with better acuity
9. Improved integration in vision, listening, feeling, and awareness of joint and trunk position in space
10. Improved ability to suppress noise and distractions to stay on track
11. Improved security of mobility and more reliable postural reactions to protect from falling in familiar and stable as well as unfamiliar and unstable environments
12. Reactivation of long underpracticed skills that support independent mental and physical actions (e.g., riding a bike, skipping, throwing and catching balls, playing an instrument)
13. Restoration of fluency, self-confidence, liveliness, and happiness
14. Increased longevity
15. Increased blood flow and oxygen to the heart and nervous system
16. Physical exercise combined with attended learning-based exercise in order to decrease the risk for heart disease, cancer, metabolic failure, and Alzheimer disease

Methods of Measuring Neural Adaptation
Neurophysiological and Neuroanatomical Outcomes

Neurophysiological and neuroanatomical changes can be measured in the CNS with learning. Measurements have been made with a variety of techniques (e.g., neurophysiological mapping after craniotomies, electroencephalography [EEG], magnetic source imaging [MSI], functional magnetic resonance imaging [fMRI], electromyography [EMG], cortical response mapping with positron emission tomography, diffusion tensor imaging [DTI], and spectroscopy with the potential for neurochemical analysis of neurotransmitters, growth hormones, inhibitors, corticosteroids). With learning it is possible to measure the following:

1. Achievement of specialized cortical representations of behaviorally important inputs
2. Growth in the number of neuron populations excited with progressively greater specificity in the neuronal representations and stronger temporal coordination
3. Strengthening of neural connections (synapses) following important behavioral inputs

BOX 3.1 Neuroplasticity Principles Translated to Guide Clinical Practice—cont'd

4. Increased oxygenation
5. Decreased atrophy of the brain
6. Shortening of the time between the stimulus and neuronal activation (latency)
7. Modification of the amplitude of neuronal firing
8. Improvement in the ability to turn off neurons once fired
9. Increased ability to inhibit unwanted neuronal firing in response to an input
10. Shortened integration time between the processing of inputs and production of outputs
11. Specialization of representational firing in response to familiar inputs
12. Improved temporal sequencing of firing following familiar inputs
13. Increased myelination
14. Increased complexity of dendrites and change in number and complexity of synapses
15. Increased consistency of response (e.g., density of neuronal responses)
16. Improved selective excitation
17. Increased specificity of neuronal response
18. Increased salience of the response
19. Change in cortical (and noncortical) topography
20. Increased area of representation
21. Smaller receptive fields
22. Increased density of receptive fields
23. Improved precision and order of receptive fields

Clinical Documentation of Outcomes After Learning-Based Training

Basic science and clinical research studies report positive correlations between functional outcomes and neural adaptation. With timely prevention, appropriate management of acute insults to the CNS, spontaneous recovery, and thoughtful attention to activities of daily living (ADLs) and task practice, disabling CNS problems can be minimized. Furthermore, early treatment after CNS injury or onset of disease may prevent more extensive damage to the brain. Learning activities may not only be neuroprotective but also drive more complete recovery of function. Changes in neural adaptation can be measured clinically in terms of improvements in function, including the following:

1. Fine and gross motor coordination
2. Sensory discrimination
3. Balance and postural control
4. Reaction time
5. Accuracy of movements
6. Rhythm and timing of movements
7. Memory storage, organization, and retrieval
8. Alertness and attention
9. Sequencing
10. Logic, complexity, and sophistication of problem solving
11. Language skills (verbal and nonverbal)
12. Interpersonal communication
13. Positive sense of well-being
14. Insight
15. Self-confidence
16. Self-image
17. Signal/noise detection; able to make finer distinctions
18. Ability to "chunk" information for memory and use
19. Learning skills including faster learning
20. Achievement of developmental milestones
21. Appropriate sensitivity of the nervous system (e.g., reduction in hyperactivity and sensory defensiveness)
22. Ability to perform a skill from memory

23. Flexible behaviors; variability in task performance
24. Flexibility for experience-based learning

Practical Suggestions for Maintaining Physical and Brain Health Across the Life-Span[39,135]

Make living a learning experience by creating goal-directed activities that require attention and can be progressed in difficulty or variety over time. Where possible, provide conditions where feedback about performance is received. Try to maintain variability in activities and vary the environments for performing the same and different tasks. Take some risks by changing activities that are familiar and comfortable. Walk around on unstable surfaces as well as familiar surfaces with the eyes closed to challenge balance and postural reactions. Assume different positions to perform common tasks. More specifically,

1. Integrate low- to moderate-intensity physical exercise into the day, balanced with healthy eating, good hydration, and stress management.
2. Stop all negative learning behaviors; minimize or eliminate bad habits.
3. Be actively engaged at the cutting edge of all activities; minimize habitual behaviors.
4. Improve skills; progressively practice to perform each task better and use mistakes to guide practice.
5. Improve language listening skills and expand the words and the language used.
6. Be a lifelong learner; take classes, go to lectures, listen to audio books, and discuss what was learned with others.
7. Engage in conversational listening (review what is remembered about a conversation right after the conversation ends).
8. Keep hobbies alive; mix life with work and play.
9. Consider learning to play a musical instrument (e.g., take lessons, practice, and carefully listen while playing).
10. Sing along with music; sing out loud in the car (loud, clearly, and slowly), and consider joining a choir to share the joy of singing with others.
11. Take time and opportunities to dance; consider taking some lessons.
12. Volunteer in the community to interact with others.
13. Wear a hearing aid if one has been prescribed; wear glasses if they are needed.
14. Improve everyday activities by learning something new or by challenging observation and recall skills: have a puzzle out and add pieces or have challenging crossword puzzles to work on.
15. Play games that require fine motor skills (e.g., shuffling cards, Ping-Pong, bowling, tennis).
16. After walking to the store, reconstruct all of the things that were seen on the way and at the store and what was accomplished.
17. When waiting for scheduled appointments, review the details of the environment; examine what has changed since the last visit.
18. Before going to social gatherings, try to remember the names of the people who are expected to be there; afterward, review who was there by name.
19. When idle or waiting, instead of sitting, walk around and mentally review items in the environment, organize these items, review tasks that need to be done (including steps required), play a game.
20. Find different ways to get to common places; evaluate which way is fastest, easiest, most interesting, most fun.
21. Constantly read and listen to the news, attend lectures, listen to or watch educational programs.
22. When with others, especially with children or grandchildren, play progressive or problem-solving games (e.g., Boggle, chess, card games, checkers).
23. Look beyond the self; think what you can to do make others happy.
24. Avoid stress; instead enjoy life and share joy with others.
25. Take a walk or ride a bike every day.
26. Find something fun to do every day.

Data from Byl N, Merzenich MM, Cheung S, et al. A primate model for studying focal dystonia and repetitive strain injury: effects on the primary somatosensory cortex. *Phys Ther.* 1997;77:269–284; Kleim J, Jones TA. Principles of experience-dependent neural plasticity: implications for rehabilitation after brain damage. *J Speech Lang Hear Res.* 2008;51(1):S225–S239; and Merzenich M. *Soft-Wired: How the New Science of Brain Plasticity Can Change Your Life.* 2nd ed. San Francisco, CA: Parnassus Publishing; 2013.

not exposed to sound, there is a reduction in the neurons in the auditory cortex.[156] Even in adults, when neural circuits are not used over an extended period of time, they begin to degrade, and the unused area of the brain is allocated to serve another part of the body.[157] Similarly, if task performance is practiced, then the topography expands and becomes more detailed, as might occur in someone who is blind and reads Braille.[158] It is also interesting to note that although a person is blind, the visual cortical areas may become active when the individual is reading Braille.[159] Similarly, a person who is deaf may demonstrate activation of the auditory cortex when visual stimuli are presented.

2. *With skill learning, the distributed cortical representations of inputs and brain actions "specialize" in their representations of behaviorally important inputs and actions.*

A minimal level of repetitive practice is needed to acquire a new skill that will be maintained over time. This may lead to specialization or change in the underlying neurophysiological processing.[160–162] Such specialization develops in response to selective cortical neuron responses specific to the demands of sensory, perceptual, cognitive, and motor skill learning.[163–166] This adaptation has been clearly documented in animal studies. For example, if an animal is trained to make progressively finer distinctions about specific sensory stimuli, then cortical neurons come to represent those stimuli in a progressively more specific and "amplified" manner.

3. *Important behavioral conditions are essential to the learning phase of plasticity.*
   a. If behaviorally important stimuli repeatedly excite cortical neuron populations, the neurons will progressively grow in number.
   b. Repetitive, behaviorally important stimuli processed in skill learning lead to progressively greater specificity in the spatial and temporal dimensions.

4. *The growing numbers of selectively responding neurons discharge with progressively stronger temporal coordination (distributed synchronicity).*

Through the course of progressive skill learning, a more refined basis for processing stimuli and generating actions critical to skilled tasks is enabled by the multidimensional changes in cortical responses. Consequently, specific aspects of these changes in distributed neuronal responses are highly correlated with learning-based improvements in perception, motor control, and cognition.[167–170] In these processes the brain is not simply changing to record and store content but is selectively refining its processing capacities to fit each task at hand by adjusting its spatial and temporal filters. Ultimately it establishes its own general processing capabilities. This process of "learning to learn" determines the facility with which specific classes of information can be stored, associated, and manipulated. These powerful self-shaping processes of the forebrain machinery are operating not only on a large scale during development but also during experience-based management of externally and internally generated information in adults. This self-shaping with experience allows the development of organization of perception, cognition, motor, and executive management skills.

5. *The growing numbers of selectively responding neurons discharge with progressively stronger temporal coordination (distributed synchronicity).*

The process of coincidence-based input co-selection leads to changes in cortical representation. Coincident, temporally and spatially related events that fire together are strengthened together. In skill learning, this principle of concurrent input co-selection results from repetitive practice that includes the following:
   a. A progressive amplification of cell numbers engaged by repetitive inputs.[169–171]

b. An increase in the temporal coordination of distributed neuronal discharges evoked by successive events to mark features of behaviorally important inputs is a consequence of a progressive increase in positive coupling between nearly simultaneously engaged neurons within cortical networks.[169,172]
   c. A progressively more specific "selection" of all input features that collectively represent behaviorally important inputs is expressed moment by moment in time.[171,172] Thus skill learning results in mapping temporal neighbors in representational networks at adjacent spatial locations when they regularly occur successively in time.[88,173,174] Changes in activation patterns, dendritic growth, synapses, and neuronal activities may also be observed.

The basis of the functional creation of the detailed, representational cortical maps converting temporal to spatial representations is related to the Hebbian change principle.[175] This principle applies to the development of interconnections between excitatory and inhibitory inputs within the cortical pyramidal neurons and their connections to extrinsic inputs and outputs. On the basis of the Hebbian principle, the operation of coincidence-based synaptic plasticity in cortical networks results in the formation, strengthening, and continuous recruitment of neurons within neuronal "assemblies" that "cooperatively" represent behaviorally important stimuli.

6. *Plasticity is constrained by anatomical sources and convergent-divergent spread of input.* Every cortical field includes the following:
   a. Specific extrinsic and intrinsic input sources
   b. Dimensions of anatomical divergence and convergence of its inputs, limiting dynamic combination Hebbian input co-selection capacities[176,177]

Anatomical input sources and limited projection overlap to enable change by establishing input-selection repertoires and to determine the limits for change. There are relatively strict anatomical constraints at the "lower" system levels, where only spatially limited input, coincidence-based combined outcomes are possible. In the "higher" system hierarchies, anatomical projection topographies are more powerful, with neurons and neuronal assemblies developing that respond to complex combinations of features of real-world objects, events, and actions.

7. *Plasticity is constrained by time constants governing coincident input co-selection and by time structures and potentially achievable coherence of extrinsic and intrinsic cortical input sources.*

To effectively drive representational changes with coincident input-dependent Hebbian mechanisms, temporally coordinated inputs are prerequisite, given the short duration (milliseconds to tens of milliseconds) in the time constants that govern synaptic plasticity in the adaptive cortical machinery.[178] Consistently uncorrelated or low discharge-rate inputs induce negative changes in synaptic effectiveness. In addition, stimuli occurring repetitively simultaneously can also degrade the representation. These negative effects also contribute importantly to the learning-driven "election" of behaviorally important inputs.

8. *Cortical field–specific differences in input sources, distributions, and time-structured inputs create different representational structures.*
   a. There are significant differences in the activity from afferent inputs from the retina, skin, or cochlea generated in a relatively strictly topographically wired V1 (area 17), S1 proper (area 3b), or A1 (area 43) compared with the inferotemporal visual, insular somatosensory, dorsotemporal auditory, or prefrontal cortical areas that receive highly diffuse inputs (see Fig. 3.8). In the former cases, heavy schedules of repetitive, temporally coherent inputs are delivered from powerful, redundant projections in

strictly topographically organized thalamic nuclei and lower-level, associated cortical areas. Yet neighboring neurons can share some response properties, neurons, or clusters of neurons that respond selectively to learned inputs. These neurons are distributed widely across cortical areas and share less information with neighboring neurons. In the "lower" levels, afferent input projections from any given source are greatly dispersed. Highly repetitive inputs are uncommon, inputs from multiple diffuse cortical sources are more common with more varied complex input combinations. These differences in input schedules, spreads, and combinations presumably account for the dramatic differences in the patterns of representation of behaviorally important stimuli at "lower" and "higher" levels.[179]

b. Despite these differences in representational organization across the cortex, it progressively differentiates cortical cells to accomplish specific operational tasks. There is a serial progression of differentiation to allow the development of functional organization, which enables an individual to progressively master more elaborate and differentiated perceptual, cognitive, monitoring, and executive skills.

c. The sources of inputs and their field-specific spreads and boundary limits, the distributions of modulatory inputs differentiated by cortical layers in different cortical regions, the basic elements and interconnections in the cortical processing machine, and crucial aspects of input combination and processing at subcortical levels are inherited (see reference Quinn[180] for review). Although these inherited aspects of sensory, motor, and cortical processing circuits constrain the potential learning-based modification of processing within each cortical area, changes in representation can occur as a result of environmental interaction and purposeful behavioral practice.

9. *Temporal dimensions of behaviorally important inputs also influence representational "specialization."* In at least four ways, the cortex refines its representations of the temporal aspects of behaviorally important inputs during learning.

a. First,

(1) The cortex generates more synchronous representations of sequenced and coincident associative input perturbations or events, not only recording their identities but also marking their occurrences. These changes in representation appear to be primarily achieved through increases in positive coupling strengths between interconnected neurons participating in stimulus- or action-specific neuronal cell assemblies.[165,180a,181–201] The strength of the interconnectedness increases representational salience as a result of downstream neurons being excited in direct relation to the degree of temporal synchronization of their inputs.

(2) Increasing the power of the outputs of a cortical area drives downstream plasticity. Hebbian mechanisms operating within downstream cortical (or other) targets also have relatively short time constants. The greater the synchronicity of inputs, the more powerfully those change mechanisms are engaged. The strength of the interconnections also helps protect against noise. For example, by simple information abstraction and coding, the distributed representation of the "signal" (a temporally coordinated, distributed neuronal response pattern representing the input or action) is converted at the entry levels in the cortex into a form that is not as easily degraded or altered by "noise." The strength of the interconnectedness also confers robustness of complex signal representation for spatially incomplete or degraded inputs.

b. Second,

(1) The cortex can select specific inputs through learning to exaggerate the representation of specific input time structures. Conditioning a monkey or a rat with stimuli that have a consistent, specific temporal modulation rate or interstimulus time, for example, results in a selective exaggeration of the responses of neurons at that rate or time separation. In effect, the cortex "specializes" for expected relatively higher-speed or relatively lower-speed signal event reception.

(2) Both electrophysiological recording studies and theoretical studies suggest that cortical networks richly encode the temporal interval as a simple consequence of cortical network dynamics.[202,203] It is hypothesized that the cortex accomplishes time-interval and duration selectivity in learning by positively changing synaptic connection strengths for input circuits that can respond with recovery times and circuit delays that match behaviorally important modulation frequency periods, intervals, or durations. However, studies on including excessive, rapid, repetitive fine motor movements can sometimes lead to serious degradation in representation if the adjacent digits are driven nearly simultaneous in time. This may be associated with negative learning and a loss of motor control.[204]

c. Third,

(1) The cortex links representations of immediately successive inputs presented in a learning context.

(2) As a result of Hebbian mechanisms, it establishes overlapping and neighboring relationships between immediately successive parts of rapidly changing inputs yet retains its individualized, distinct cortical representation.[88,205]

d. Fourth,

(1) The cortex generates stimulus sequence-specific ("combination-sensitive") responses, with neuronal responses selectively modulated by the prior application of stimuli in the learned sequence of temporally separated events.

(2) These "associative" or "combination-sensitive" responses have been correlated with evidence of strengthened interconnections between cortical cell assemblies representing successive event elements separated by hundreds of milliseconds to seconds in time.[206,207] The mechanisms of origin of these effects have not yet been established.

e. *Temporal dimensions of behaviorally important inputs also influence representational "specialization."* Cortical networks engage both excitatory and inhibitory neurons by strong input perturbations. Within a given processing "channel," cortical pyramidal cells cannot be effectively reexcited by a follow-up perturbation for tens to hundreds of milliseconds. These integration "times" are primarily dictated by the time for recovery from inhibition, which ordinarily dominates poststimulus excitability. This "integration time," "processing time," or "recovery time" is commonly measured by deriving a "modulation transfer function," which defines the ability of cortical neurons to respond to identical successive stimuli within cortical "processing channels." For example, these "integration" times normally range from about 15 to about 200 ms in the primary auditory receiving areas.[208–210] Progressively longer processing times are recorded at higher system levels (e.g., in the auditory cortex, they are approximately a syllable in length, 200 to 500 ms in duration) in the "belt cortex" surrounding the primary auditory cortex.[211]

f. These time constants govern—and limit—the cortex's ability to "chunk" (i.e., separately represent by distributed, coordinated discharge) successive events within its processing channels. Both neurophysiological studies in animals and behavioral training studies in human adults and children have shown that the time constants governing event-by-event complex signal representation are highly plastic. With intensive training in the correct form, cortical "processing times," as reflected by the ability to accurately and separately process events occurring at different input rates, can be dramatically shortened or lengthened.[212–215]

10. *Plasticity processes are competitive.*

a. If two spatially different inputs are consistently delivered non-simultaneously to the cortex, cortical networks generate input-selective cell assemblies for each input and actively segregate them from one another.[172,214,216–218] Boundaries between such inputs grow to be sharp and are substantially intensity independent. Computational models of Hebbian network behaviors indicate that this sharp segregation of nonidentical, temporally separated inputs occurs secondary to a wider distribution of inhibitory versus excitatory responses in the emerging, competing cortical cell assemblies that represent them.

b. This Hebbian cell assembly formation and competition appear to account for how the cortex creates sharply sorted representations of the fingers in the primary somatosensory cortex.[173,219] The Hebbian network probably accounts for how the cortex creates sharply sorted representations of native aural language-specific phonemes in lower-level auditory cortical areas in the auditory and speech processing system of humans. If inputs are delivered in a constant and stereotyped way from a limited region of the skin or cochlea in a learning context, the associated skin surface or cochlear sector is an evident competitive "winner."[169,220] By Hebbian mechanisms, the cortical networks will co-select that specific combination of inputs and represent it within a competitively growing Hebbian cell assembly. The competitive strength of that cooperative cell assembly will grow progressively because more and more neurons are excited by relevant behavioral stimuli with increasingly coordinated discharges. That means that neurons outside of this cooperative group have greater numbers of more coordinated outputs contributing to their later competitive recruitment. Through progressive functional remodeling, the cortex clusters and competitively sorts information across sharp boundaries dictated by the spatiotemporal statistics of its inputs. If it receives information on a heavy schedule that sets up competition for a limited input set, it will sort competitive inputs into a correspondingly small number of largely discontinuous response regions.[221,222]

c. Competitive outcomes are, again, cortical level dependent. The cortex links events that occur in different competitive groups if they are consistently excited synchronously in time. At the same time, competitively formed groups of neurons come to be synchronously linked in their representations of different parts of the complex stimulus and collectively represent successive complex features through the coordinated activities of many groups.

d. Neurons within the two levels of the cortex surrounding A1 (see Fig. 3.8) have greater spatial input convergence and longer integration times that enable their facile combination of information representing different spatiotemporal details. Their information extraction is greatly facilitated by the learning-based

linkages of cooperative groups that deliver behaviorally important inputs in a highly salient, temporally coordinated form to these fields. With their progressively greater space and time constants, still higher-level areas organize competitive cell assemblies that represent even more complex spatial and serial-event combinations. Note that these organizational changes apply over a large cortical scale. In skill learning over a limited period of training, participating neuronal members of such assemblies can easily be increased by many hundredfold, even within a primary sensory area such as S1, area 3b, or A1.[169,172,204,214,223]

e. In extensive training in complex signal recognition, more than 10% of neurons within temporal cortical areas can come to respond highly selectively to a specific, normally rare, complex training stimulus. The distributed cell assemblies representing those specific complex inputs involve tens or hundreds of millions of neurons and are formed by enduring effectiveness changes in many billions of synapses.

11. *Learning is modulated as a function of behavioral state.*

a. At "lower" levels of the cortex, changes are generated only in attended behaviors.[170,171,179,223–225] Trial-by-trial change magnitudes are a function of the importance of the input to the animal as signaled by the level of attention, the cognitive values of behavioral reinforcement, and internal judgments of trial precision, or error based on the relative success or failure of achieving a target goal or expectation. Little or no enduring change is induced when a well-learned "automatic" behavior is performed from memory without attention. Interestingly, at some levels within the cortex, activity changes can be induced even in nonattending subjects under conditions in which "priming" effects of nonattended reception of information can be demonstrated.

b. The modulation of progressive learning is achieved by the activation of powerful reward systems releasing the neurotransmitters norepinephrine and dopamine (among others) through widespread projections to the cerebral cortex. Norepinephrine plays a particularly important role in modulating learning-induced changes in the cortex.[214,225,226]

c. The cortex is a "learning machine." During the learning of a new skill, neurotransmitters are released trial by trial with application of a behaviorally important stimulus or behavioral rewards. If the skill can be mastered and thereafter replayed from memory, its performance can be generated without attention (habituation). Habituation results in a profound attenuation of the modulation signals from these neurotransmitter sources; plasticity is no longer positively enabled in cortical networks.

12. *Top-down influences constrain cortical representational plasticity.*

Attentional control flexibly defines an enabling "window" for change in learning.[212] Progressive learning generates progressively more strongly represented goals, expectations, and feedback[227,228] across all representational systems that are undergoing change and to modulatory control systems weighing performance success and error. Strong intermodal behavioral and representational effects have also been recorded in experiments that might be interpreted as shaping expectations.[229,230] These shaping expectations would be similar to those observed in a human subject using multisensory inputs such as auditory, visual, and somesthetic information to create integrated phonological representations, to create fine motor trajectory patterns that underlie precise hand control, or to make a vocal production.

13. *The scale of plasticity in progressive skill learning is massive.*
    a. Cortical representational plasticity must be viewed as arising from multiple-level systems broadly engaged in learning, perceiving, remembering, thinking, and acting. Any behaviorally important input (or consistent internally generated activity) engages many cortical areas. Repetitive training drives all cortical areas to change.[164,177,231] Different aspects of any acquired skill are contributed from field-specific changes in the multiple cortical areas that are remodeled in its learning.
    b. In this kind of continuously evolving representational machine, perceptual constancy cannot be accounted for by brain representations in constant locations; relational representational principles must be invoked to account for it.[164,232] Moreover, representational changes must obviously be coordinated level to level. It should also be understood that plastic changes are also induced extracortically. Although it is believed that learning at the cortical level is usually predominant, plasticity induced by learning within many extracortical structures significantly contributes to learning-induced changes that are expressed within the cortex.
14. *Enduring cortical plasticity changes appear to be accounted for by local changes in neural anatomy.*

    Changes in synapse turnover, synapse number, synaptic active zones, dendritic spines, and the elaboration of terminal dendrites occur in a behaviorally engaged cortical zone.[177,233–238] Through many changes in local structural detail, the learning brain is continuously physically remodeling its processing machinery, not only across the course of child development but also after behavioral training in an adult with a neural insult.
15. *Cortical plasticity processes in child development represent progressive, multiple-staged skill learning.*
    a. There are two remarkable achievements of brain plasticity in child development. The first is the progressive shaping of the processing to handle the accurate, high-speed reception of the rapidly changing streams of information that flow into the brain. In the cerebral cortex, shaping appears to begin most powerfully within the primary receiving areas of the cortex. With early myelination, the main gateways for information into the cortex are receiving strongly coherent inputs from subcortical nuclei, and they can quickly organize their local networks on the basis of coincident input co-selection (Hebbian) mechanisms. The self-organization of the cortical processing machinery spreads outward from these primary receiving areas over time to ultimately refine the basic processing machinery of all the cortex. The second great achievement, which is strongly dependent on the first, is the efficient storage of massive content collections in richly associated forms.
    b. During development, the brain accomplishes its functional self-organization through a long parallel series of small steps. At each step, the brain masters a series of elementary processing skills and establishes reliable information repertoires that enable the accomplishment of subsequent skills. Second- and higher-order skills can be viewed as elaborations of more basic mastered skills and the creation of new skills dependent on combined second- and higher-order processing. That hierarchical processing is enabled by greater cortical anatomical spreads, by more complexly convergent anatomical sources of inputs, and by longer integration (processing, recovery) times at progressively higher cortical system levels. This integrating process allows for progressively more complex combinations of

information integrated over longer time epochs as one ascends across cortical processing hierarchies.
    c. As the cortical machinery functionally evolves and consequently physically "matures" through childhood developmental stages, information repertories are represented in progressively more salient forms (i.e., with more powerful distributed response coordination). Growing agreement directly controls the power of emerging information repertoires to drive the next level of elaborative and combinatorial changes. It is hypothesized that saliency enables the maturation of the myelination of projection tracts delivering outputs from functionally refined cortical areas. More mature myelination of output projections also contributes to the power of this newly organized activity to drive strong, downstream plastic change through the operation of Hebbian processes.
    d. As each elaboration of skill is practiced, neuromodulatory transmitters enable change in the cortical machinery. The cortex functionally and physically adapts to generate the neurological representations of the skill in progressively more selective, predictable, and statistically reliable forms. Ultimately the performance of the skill concurs with the brain's own accumulated, learning-derived "expectations." The skill can then be performed from memory, without attention. With this consolidation of the remembered skill and information repertoire, the modulatory nuclei enable no further change in the cortical machinery. The learning machine, the cerebral cortex, move on to the next elaboration. Thus the cortex constructs highly specialized processing machinery that can progressively produce great towers of automatically performable behaviors and progressively mature hierarchies of information-processing machinery capable of achieving more powerful complex signal representations, retrievals, and associations. With this machinery in a mature and efficient operating form, there is a remarkable capacity for reception, storage, and analysis of diverse and complexly associated information.
    e. The flexible, self-adjusting capacity for refinement of the processing capabilities of the nervous system confers the ability of our species to represent complex language structures. This self-adjusting capacity also allows humans to develop high-speed reading abilities; remarkably varied complex modern-era motor abilities; and abstract logic structures characteristic of a mathematician, software engineer, or philosopher. This refinement of the nervous system also creates elaborate, idiosyncratic, experience-based behavioral abilities in all of us.

Neuroplasticity and Learning

How are learning sequences controlled? What constrains learning progressions? Perhaps the most important basis of control in learning progressions is representational consolidation. Through specialization, the trained cortex creates progressively more specific and more salient distributed representations of behaviorally important inputs. Growing representational salience increases the power of a cortical area to effectively drive change wherever outputs from this evolving cortical processing machinery are distributed (e.g., in "higher system levels distributed and coordinated [synchronized] responses" more powerfully drive downstream Hebbian-based plasticity changes).

A second powerful basis for sequenced learning is progressive myelination. At the time of birth, only the core "primary" extrinsic information entry zones (A1, S1, V1) in the cortex are heavily myelinated.[239,240] Across childhood, connections to and interconnections between cortical areas are progressively myelinated, proceeding from these core areas out to "higher" system levels. Myelination in the posterior parietal, anterior, and inferior temporal and prefrontal cortical areas is not "mature" in the human forebrain until 8 to 20 years of age. Even in the mature state, it is far less developed at the "highest" processing levels.

Myelination controls the conduction times and therefore the temporal dispersions of input sources to and within cortical areas. Poor myelination at "higher" levels in the young brain is associated with temporally diffuse inputs. They cannot generate reliable representational constructs of an adult quality because they do not effectively engage input-coincidence–based Hebbian plasticity mechanisms. That ensures, in effect, that plasticity is not enabled for complex combinatorial processing until "lower" level input repertoires are consolidated (i.e., become stable, statistically reliable forms).

Although myelination is thought to be genetically programmed, some scientists hypothesize that myelination in the CNS is also controlled by emerging temporal response coherence and is achieved through temporally coordinated signaling from the multiple branches of oligodendrocytes that terminate on different projection axons in central tracts and networks. It has been argued that central myelination is positively and negatively activity dependent and that distributed synchronization may contribute to positive change.[241] If the hypothesis that coherent activity controls myelination proves to be true, then the emerging temporal correlation of distributed representations of behaviorally important stimuli is generated level by level. This is done by changes in coupling in local cortical networks in the developing cortex. It would also directly drive changes in myelination for the outputs of that cortical area. These two events in turn would enable the generation of reliable and salient representational constructs at that higher level. By this kind of progression, skill learning is hypothesized to directly control progressive functional and physical brain development through the course of child development. This is accomplished both by refining ("maturing") local interconnections through response dynamics of information processing machinery at successive cortical levels and by coordinated refinement ("maturing") of the critical transmission pathways that interconnect different processing levels.

Another constraint in the development of neural adaptation may be the development of mature sleeping patterns, especially within the first year of life.[242] Sleep enables the strengthening of learning-based plastic changes and resets the learning machinery by "erasing" temporary unreinforced and unrewarded input produced over the preceding awake period.[243–245] The dramatic shift in the percentage of time spent in rapid-eye-movement sleep is consistent with a strong early bias toward noise removal in an immature, unorganized, and poorly functionally brain. Sleep patterns change dramatically in the older child, in parallel with a strong increase in a daily schedule of closely attended, rewarded, and goal-oriented behavior. This research should be further explored in patients with CNS damage. This population often has poor breathing habits and capabilities that lead to decreased oxygenation and often broken sleep cycles. It has yet to be determined how much impairment, breakdown, and associated interaction diminishes neuroplasticity.

Top-down modulation controlling attentional windows and learned predictions (expectations and behavioral goals) must all be constructed by learning. Delays in goal development could create an important constraint for the progression of early learning. In the very young brain, prediction and error-estimation processes could be weak if stored higher-level information repertoires are ill formed and unreliable. As the brain matures, stored information enables attentional and predictive controls to operate more reliably. This provides a stronger basis for success and error signaling with modulatory control nuclei, enabling syntactic feedback to increase representational reliability.

Attention, reward and punishment, accuracy of goal achievement, and error feedback gate learning through a modulatory control system critical for learning. The modulatory control systems that enables learning is plastic, with their process of maturation providing constraint or facilitation of progressive learning. These subcortical nuclei are signaled by complex information feedback from the cortex itself. The salience and specificity of that feedback information grows over time. The ability to provide accurate judgment of error or goal-achievement signaling must progressively grow. The nucleus basalis, nucleus accumbens, ventral tegmentum, and locus coeruleus must undergo their own functional self-organization based Hebbian plasticity principles to achieve "mature" modulatory selectivity and power. The progressive maturation of the modulatory control system occurs naturally with development or training. This system can provide other important constraints on the progression of skill development involving regulation of postural/balance control and fine motor coordination.

What facilitates the development of permanent "automatic" motor behaviors? The creation and maintenance of cortical representations are functions of the animal's or human's level of attention at a task. Cortical representational plasticity in skill acquisition is self-limiting. Because the behavior becomes more "automatic," it is less closely attended, and representational changes induced in the cortex fade and ultimately disappear or reverse (unlearning effects).[246–248] The element of behavioral performance that enables maintenance of the behavior with minimal involvement of the cortical learning machinery is probably stereotypical movement sequence repetition. As a movement behavior is practiced, an effective, highly statistically predictable movement sequence is adopted that enables the storage of the learned behavior in a permanent form that requires minimal to no attention. If behavioral performance declines or brain conditions change to render a task more difficult, attention to the behavior will need to increase, producing an invigorated cortical response to the new learning challenge.

By this view, the cerebral cortex is clearly a learning machine. William James[249] was the first to point out that the great practical advantage for a self-organizing cortex was the development of what he called "habits." When a skill is overlearned, it will engage pathways that are so reliable that they can be followed without attention.

Why are some habits retained and others lost? Can sensorimotor learning be sustained when the adaptive representations of the learned behavior "fade" in the cerebral cortex? These areas have not been well researched. However, there are several possibilities. Habits could come to be represented in an enduring form extracortically. The cortex could modify processing in the spinal cord, the basal ganglia, the red nucleus, or the cerebellum. For example, the learning of manual skills requires a motor cortex, but overlearned motor skills may not be significantly reduced by the induction of a wide area four lesion.

Another possibility is that behaviorally induced cortical changes endure in a highly efficient representational form that can sustain the representation of its key features on the cortex itself, engaging only limited distributed populations of cortical neurons to represent the behavior with high fidelity. Thus recall of past learning may take less time to restructure than reformatting new learning, whether it be a cognitive or motor task. The fact that a monkey improves its discriminative abilities or movement performance after modifying the cortical neuron response with heavily practiced behaviors supports this alternative. However, many behaviors, such as musical performance, require constant, attended practice at a highly cognitive level to maintain both the representational changes and the performance. It also appears that continued learning with heavily practiced behaviors may be neuroprotective with aging, maintaining function despite loss of cortical neurons as a natural part of aging.

INTEGRATION AND IMPLEMENTATION INTO CLINICAL PRACTICE

Over the years, learning has been linked with critical periods of development, with the assumption that if a particular skill or behavior was not learned during the critical period, the opportunity to acquire that skill was lost. After this critical period of development, aging was associated with inevitable deterioration of brain and neurophysiological function. Yet today there is substantial evidence that the brain is an incredibly specialized representational machine that can adapt to meet the specific inputs that engage it. The beauty of the brain is that it not only self-organizes but also stores the contents of its learning to create a foundation that increases in depth and breadth and makes predictions on even novel inputs to facilitate acute and efficient operations. The earlier the exposure to multisensory stimuli, the easier it is for competitive neuronal processes to adapt and to make extensive connections. With growing neuronal specificity and salience, more powerful predictions continue until there is greater learning and mastery.

Among the important findings of the 20th century was the validation that the brain is a learning machine that operates throughout life. The aging process can restrict the ability to store information and may reduce both the complexity of the information processed and the individual's ability to retrieve it. But if an individual is able to maintain good hydration, balanced nutrition, physical exercise, and regularly goal-directed progressive learning, CNS pathways of representation and prediction can not only be preserved but can continue to adapt. These activities can also slow the aging process. Thus it is possible to drive improvement in function in individuals with abnormalities related to development, disease, injury, or aging. Learning is not necessarily specifically staged but rather represents complex abilities developed mostly from system interaction and integration. Therapists must develop the ability to determine what inputs are reliable and salient to effectively create functional and physical brain maturation, adaptation, and learning. In the face of different types of challenges (structural, emotional, pathological), clinicians must develop more effective strategies that can help facilitate neural adaptation, learning, substitution, and representational changes allowing meaningful maintenance and improvement in function despite anatomical or physiological variances in structure. Although strong behavioral events can be associated with measurable neural adaptability, new, more permanent neural connections and synapses must be strengthened with repetition and increased complexity. Patients with CNS disorders may have sustained damage to certain areas of the brain, which may not recover; however, with learning-based activities it is possible to reorganize the brain, stimulate neurons from adjacent areas, establish new synapses and dendritic pathways,[250] and activate neurons in the contralateral, uninjured parts of the brain.[251-257] Creating the best environment to learn a skill may initially need to be contrived, with limitations controlled externally by the therapist's hands or clinical arena. In time, those limitations must be eliminated and variability within the natural environment reintroduced to achieve true learning and ultimate neuroplasticity.

The elements of neuroscience research on neural adaptation have been summarized into 14 principles to guide rehabilitation programs designed to facilitate experience-dependent plasticity.[123,258,259] These principles, outlined in Box 3.1, are similar to those suggested by Nudo[162] as well as Kleim and Jones[161] and Byl and colleagues.[260] Although these principles are particularly relevant to patients with a head injury or stroke, they are also relevant for aging adults[261-265] and those with neurodegenerative disease. These principles are not meant to be exhaustive or mutually exclusive but to highlight the principles of experience-dependent plasticity. They can also serve as a reference for therapists who are designing creative intervention programs based on the translation of basic science to clinical practice and to help organize the extensive research on neuroplasticity.

These principles can be applied across a broad range of activities and conditions to improve cognition and intellect as well as physical capability. Priming the system before learning can take many forms, including aerobic exercise, cortical stimulation, and skill learning. As reviewed earlier, BNDF, which is necessary for activity-dependent learning, can be increased with aerobic exercise and skill learning.[151] Yet the influence of BDNF polymorphisms in different individuals needs further research. It is clear that the timing of enrichment (e.g., sensory and motor training) is important not only during development but across the life-span. An exercise program initiated too early (e.g., in less than 24 hours after acute neural injury) may be associated with an exaggeration of cellular injury.[266] Yet waiting too long to intervene can limit the efficacy of the learning-based training experience.[267] Learning-based training may also be enhanced with cortical stimulation,[268] repetitive transcranial magnetic stimulation (rTMS),[269] transcranial direct current stimulation (tDCS),[270] bilateral mechanical priming,[271] and mental imagery.[271] It is critical to create a positive foundation to maximize learning (e.g., good hydration to maximize blood flow and oxygenation of tissues, adequate nutrition to energize the body, and aerobic activity to increase endorphins and BDNF, as well as positive expectations of getting better [limbic system]). Rehabilitation specialists must not only translate basic neuroscience into practice but participate in clinical research, serve as advocates for patients, ensure access to appropriate rehabilitative services, and be politically active in health care reform.

To ensure maximum neural adaptation, rehabilitation programs must include strong, carefully outlined home programs. Therapists must educate patients and their families about the principles of neuroplasticity to empower them to create progressive learning activities at home and in the community. Patients should revisit health care team members to facilitate ongoing learning. Patients must become their own best therapists, consistently motivating themselves to learn something new, perform attended behavioral activities, observe and integrate new information from their environment, have fun, stay engaged with family/friends/community, and avoid habitual stereotypical behaviors. Learning should be an excuse to travel to new places and learn new skills. Every day should include a new learning experience. Learning and aerobic exercise may not only be neuroprotective but could be critical for slowing down the natural neurodegenerative aspects of aging. Computer gaming, new technology, and robotics can be integrated to expand daily learning-based activities at home.

The maximum attainment of skilled performance cannot necessarily be determined. The original injury can be used only as an estimate of the damage with some indicators for prognosis and recovery. The rest of the success of rehabilitation and restoration of function will reside with the motivation and commitment of the individual. How that motivation and commitment are initially established and continually reinforced is based on the patient, the therapist's interactive skills and emotional bond, and the family and other support systems surrounding the patient.

CASE STUDY 3.1   The Person With Parkinson Disease

People with Parkinson disease develop an array of deficits in motor control that interfere with multiple ADLs and can eventually degrade quality of life. When motor control deficits are evaluated in this population, the severity of the disease, the activity level of the person, and the medication schedule are important considerations. Following are several motor control deficits that are evident in this disease.

Motor control impairments of rigid tone and bradykinesia create alterations in stride length, speed, and step frequency in the gait pattern of persons with Parkinson disease. The person may demonstrate a gait pattern characterized by decreased amplitude of leg movement, duration of the gait cycle, trunk rotation, and arm swing. Difficulty initiating gait, or "freezing," is an observable motor control problem, and small shuffling steps and a festinating gait pattern are also common. Impaired righting and balance reactions can contribute to gait instability. When the demands on gait velocity and frequency are altered, metabolic cost increases and the ability of the individual to safely complete the functional movement with appropriate coordination of postural and motor control is challenged.

A practical outcome measure that can be used to capture the effect of these motor deficits on functional mobility is the Timed Up-and-Go (TUG) test. This quick test can be used to capture the time it takes for a person to initiate sit-to-stand, transition from sit-to-stand, walk 3 m, turn around, walk back, turn, and sit down. During the performance of these sequential movement patterns the clinician can observe gait deviations, postural abnormalities, movement amplitude, and safety awareness. Episodes and duration of "freezing," or failed initiation, can be accounted for, and the number of steps to turn 180 degrees can be documented.[272] The overall time to complete the test can supply the clinician with objective data related to fall risk.

Overshooting or undershooting the 3-m line before turning may be demonstrated. Although patients with Parkinson disease are able to prepare the motor strategy and use advance information, the primary problem is slow onset of execution of movement; therefore changing motor patterns (e.g., switching from walking to turning) can be quite difficult.

To illustrate the multiple motor control deficits, imagine a patient performing the TUG.[273] The person may have difficulty accelerating to walk and decelerating to turn around and decelerating on approaching the chair and sitting down. Postural instability may be observed during transfers and turning, and a loss of balance in the backward direction without the activation of an automatic stepping response may occur. The motor control deficits exhibited in the patient with Parkinson disease are numerous and intertwined, and their severity is influenced by the progression of the disease. As mentioned earlier, the patient cannot appropriately control the increase and decrease in the rate of force production, which is evident in the acceleration and deceleration phases of the movement. If the rate of force production is altered, the amplitude of force production may also be affected.

The person may have a decreased ability to predict and prepare the motor pattern for turning before the actual turn. There appears to be a slow initiation of the turning task. This phenomenon could be caused by an inability to sequence the motor behavior as a whole. Several researchers have observed that the person completes one movement before starting the next movement in the sequence rather than executing a smooth, continuing movement pattern.[45] Another reason for the decrease in the ability to perform this task smoothly is the patient's dependence on visual feedback. Relying more heavily on visual feedback to accomplish a task slows the movement.

The movement deficits observed may also be a result of the inability to effectively coordinate movements such as those observed between postural and motile components of the task. Postural strategies may be classified on a continuum that includes postural preparations, postural adaptations, and postural reactions.[274] The person with Parkinson disease may not predict and make appropriate postural adjustments before the movement and may have deficits in adaptive and reactive postural responses (e.g., righting and equilibrium reactions, and adapting to environmental demands). In the case of the TUG, movement and balance strategies are assessed when the patient stands up and sits down. If the patient does not use a controlled descent into the chair but rather falls backward, what are the possible causes for the sudden descent? The patient's goal may be to land in the chair, but the preferred pattern may be to fall into the chair. The individual may not be able to predict the time and force needed to activate the muscles for a smooth descent, the individual may be deconditioned and not have the strength or endurance to perform a smooth descent, or the individual may not have the balance strategies required to perform this maneuver.

The patient with Parkinson disease is one example of a patient with a neurological condition that affects motor output and control. Regardless of the diagnosis, all aspects of motor control need to be examined, and activity-based tests must be conducted to determine how the impairments interact to affect the execution of functional tasks. A few key deficits in gross and fine motor control and postural control are examined in this example. It is not within the scope of this chapter to present all the motor and postural control deficits but to highlight the complexity of patients with neurological pathology. Accurate identification of motor control problems in patients assists the therapist and the patient in the development of realistic functional goals and effective intervention programs.

REFERENCES

To enhance this text and add value for the reader, all references are included on the companion Evolve site accompanying this textbook.

This online service will, when available, provide a link for the reader to a Medline abstract for the article cited. There are 274 cited references and other general references for this chapter, with the majority of those articles being evidence-based citations.

4

The Limbic Network: Influence Over Motor Control, Memory, and Learning*

Marcia Hall Thompson and Darcy A. Umphred

OBJECTIVES

After reading this chapter the student or therapist will be able to:

1. Describe the structures of the limbic network.
2. Understand the complexity of the limbic network and the influence of the limbic network on both behavior and function.
3. Describe the behavioral responses directly and indirectly influenced by the limbic network.
4. Identify signs of both positive and negative limbic network influence on observable behavior, motor learning, neuroplasticity, and functional responses.
5. Identify patient populations with the potential for negative limbic network influence over observable behavior, motor learning, and ultimately functional outcome.
6. Differentiate between limbic-driven motor control responses and frontal, cerebellar, and basal ganglia motor regulation of motor responses.
7. Describe the role of the limbic network on both declarative and procedural learning.
8. Describe physical therapy examination procedures or tests and measures that could identify the presence of limbic network involvement requiring intervention and establish a responsive intervention baseline.
9. Describe interventions or program modifications with potential to improve motor learning through integration of limbic network treatment techniques into current intervention models.
10. Understand the influence of the therapist over the limbic network and behavioral and functional responses.

KEY TERMS

amygdala
declarative memory and learning
emotional behavior
F²ARV (*f*ear and *f*rustration, *a*nger, *r*age, *v*iolence/withdrawal) continuum
General Adaptation Syndrome (GAS)
hippocampus
hypothalamus

limbic network
limbic neutral state
motor learning
MOVE (*m*otivation or *m*emory, *o*lfaction, *v*isceral, autonomic nervous system, *e*motional)
procedural memory and learning
therapeutic alliance
therapeutic environment

INTRODUCTION

Our understanding and respect for the limbic network has expanded since the publication of the sixth edition, particularly when analyzing emotions, behavior, learning, and their influence on activities and participation in normal personal and societal roles. At no time has this understanding been more critical, with the prevalence of known mental health challenges faced within our country. In the United States, 18.3%, or 44.7 million adults, experience mental illness (AMI) or a mental, behavioral, or emotional disorder each year.[1] This represents approximately one in five adults, which theoretically could reflect one to two patients of a given therapist's treatment load per day. Beyond those mental health disorders that can be considered functional disorders of the limbic system, the prevalence of key central

nervous system (CNS) disorders, in which the structures of the limbic network are involved, is also high, including patients with acquired brain injury (ABI, such as concussion or traumatic brain injury [TBI]), cerebrovascular accident (CVA), tumors, inflammatory disorders, Alzheimer disease, Parkinson disease, and vestibular disorders. Clearly, the prevalence of coincident limbic system impairment in our patients may therefore be substantial within the practice of any physical therapist.

This chapter has been prominently positioned within this textbook on basic neurological rehabilitation. Traditionally, the limbic system may have only been discussed within a basic science course of neuroanatomy and neurophysiology. In other curricula, the role of the limbic system in declarative memory and emotional responses may be presented as part of a discussion on behavior or cognitive function within a psychology course. Yet today, motivation and attention are stressed and accepted as key factors in neuroplasticity and motor learning.[2-4]

---

*Videos for this chapter are available at studentconsult.com.

Therapists are familiar with the need to prioritize primary body system impairments as they relate to a movement disorder. Moreover, they are familiar with the need to individualize treatment to the primary impairment(s) identified through the evaluation process. However, they are less comfortable with those "other systems" encountered as Doctors of Physical Therapy or Occupational Therapy in their role as functional diagnosticians. The profession's acceptance of the foundational, integrated role of the cardiopulmonary system to the function of all other systems has advanced, and the acceptance of the role of the limbic system(s) needs to be similarly advanced, given the current evidence illuminating the role of the limbic network in motor output, control, and learning. Coincident is the opportunity to identify, develop, and validate requisite screening and examination tools that help physical therapists to determine the state of the limbic network and its implications for diagnosis, prognosis, and treatment planning. This chapter is intended to continue to advance our understanding of and respect for this complex, integrated system, such that its contribution is considered within the evaluation of every patient regardless of setting or diagnosis.

This chapter is designed to address this opportunity regardless of experience, from the student learner to the more seasoned clinician. For the student learner, the first section of the chapter is an overview of the limbic network and a discussion of limbic behavior and how to begin to differentiate true motor responses from those entangled in limbic interactions. For the therapist learner desiring ongoing clinical mastery, the second section delves into the anatomy and physiology of the limbic network and the the biology of learning and memory, neurochemistry, and neuroplasticity. The third section discusses the immediate relevance of this material to both the student and the practicing clinician—how can we apply our understanding of the limbic network to our patient assessments, treatment, environment, and interactions? In other words, how might it change what we do as rehabilitation professionals "come Monday morning"? And finally, in the last section, current advances and future research possibilities in the role of the limbic network and its impact on the professional roles of physical and occupational therapists are explored.

THE LIMBIC NETWORK

Our discussion must begin with a working definition of the limbic network and an overview of its function. It is not easy to find a generally accepted definition of the "limbic network or complex," its boundaries, and the components that should be included. Mesulam[5] likens this to a 5th century BC philosopher's quotation: "the nature of God is like a circle of which the center is everywhere and the circumference is nowhere." Brodal[6] suggests that functional separation of brain regions becomes less clear as we discover their interrelatedness through continuing research. He sees the limbic network reaching out and encompassing the entire brain and all its functional components and sees no purpose in defining subdivisions. Although the anatomical descriptions of the limbic network may vary from author to author, the functional significance of this system is widely acknowledged in defining human behavior and behavioral neurology.[7]

Morgane and colleagues describe the limbic network as both an "anatomical entity as well as a physiological concept." Historically termed a limbic *system*, more current evidence suggests it to Limbic *network* comprises several emotional, behavioral, learning, and memory neuroanatomical subsystems. The term "limbic *cortex*" refers to only an anatomical part of the network and the two C-shaped gyri surrounding the corpus callosum, specifically comprising the cingulate gyrus, the parahippocampal gyrus, and the olfactory lobe.

Brooks[8] divided the brain anatomically and functionally into a limbic brain and a nonlimbic somatomotor brain, Fig. 4.1 with the somatomotor portion involved in both the perception of afferent sensory input and the generation of efferent motor output. Historically, the limbic brain was seen as primitive and essential for survival, sensing the "need" to act.[8] Today, the limbic network is considered in evolutionary terms as an older brain system that provides fundamental support (alertness, motivation, memory, and learning) to enable the phylogenetically newer brain systems to regulate more complex behaviors, movement, and function. Thus the overall purpose of the limbic network is to initiate need-directed motor activity for survival based on experience, through its neuronal connections up to the frontal lobe (intentional responses) or down to the brain stem (automatic responses), thus regulating motor output.

We will discuss the neuroanatomy and neurobiology as they relate to both function and dysfunction of the limbic network later in this chapter, but briefly outline the major interacting systems, structures, and neurotransmitters here. The limbic network can generally be thought to include two system divisions: the prefrontal-limbic "forebrain" system (emotional and behavioral) and the limbic midbrain (motor control and movement). The major structures comprising the network include the limbic cortex (anterior cingulate cortex/gyrus [ACC]), parahippocampal gyrus, and olfactory lobe), the prefrontal cortex, amygdalar complex, limbic thalamus, stria medullaris (epithalamus), hippocampus, nucleus accumbens (NAc), the ventral tegmental area (VTA), and midbrain raphé nuclei of the basal ganglia. These structures are primary components of the network as well as essential neuromodulators upon the network. As one example, the ACC, amygdala, and hippocampus serve to connect the limbic network and the prefrontal cortex, while the network is modulated by the hypothalamus, basal ganglia, and midbrain. Given the broad structural components, the neurotransmitters of the system are also extensive and include serotonin, norepinephrine (NE), dopamine, and acetylcholine. As one major example, dopamine plays a critical role in the motivation to move as well as motor function (Fig. 4.2).[9,10]

This summary does not account for the direct and indirect influences of the limbic network upon other body systems. In the past, review of the literature on the limbic network was limited to

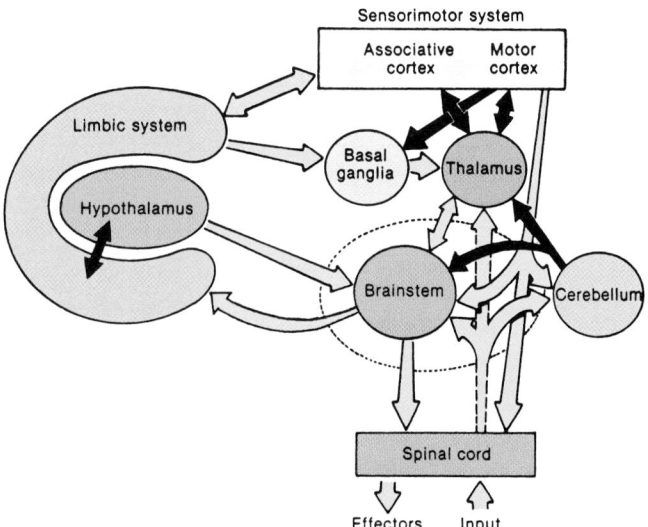

Fig. 4.1 Divisions and interconnections between the limbic and nonlimbic cortices (sensory and motor areas).

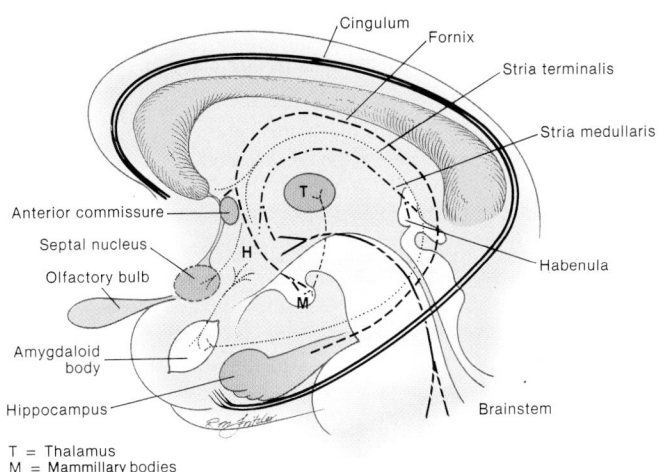

T = Thalamus
M = Mammillary bodies
H = Hypothalamus

Fig. 4.2 Interlinking Neuron Network Within the Limbic Network. (Adapted from Kandel ER, Schwartz JH, Jessell TM. *Principles of Neural Science.* 4th ed. New York: McGraw-Hill; 2000.)

CLINICAL CASE 4.1

A patient example of limbic interactions can be found in a case description of a middle-aged woman admitted to the intensive care unit (ICU) with multiple pelvic fractures and diagnosed with severe internal bleeding, kidney failure, pneumonia, pulmonary emboli, and severe clotting in the lower extremities. The physician took her husband aside to let him know that she was going to die, to which her husband replied, "I understand. Juggling one system problem is easy, juggling two systems takes a little practice, and three-system involvement may challenge the best medical skill. She is presenting four or five body system failures, and you are sure no one can juggle that many problems." The doctor said yes, and the patient's husband then said, "Please keep juggling and don't worry about me, because if you do, I would then be one more ball to juggle." And it did seem that every time the doctors got a handle on a body system problem, another system would fail. She required services from an endocrinologist, infection control specialists, interventional radiologists, a pulmonologist, a hematologist, a vascular surgeon, an internal medicine specialist, a urologist, and a nephrologist. Each specialist shared his or her limited experience with a complex clinical problem like this and that there was nothing in the literature to help his or her respective understanding. After 2{1/2} months in the ICU, the woman survived. The physician who had foretold her death met again with the patient and her family. He stated, "How are you still alive? I know what we did medically, but that was not enough to keep you alive." And he was right. No model within each respective field could account for her recovery. However, the piece not considered within her medical management was the beliefs and spiritual strength of the patient and her family, a positive limbic network influence on the function of each failing body system.

investigating potential interactions of other systems with nuclei within the limbic network. This is no longer the case, as neuroscience research has helped to identify the critical nature of behaviors modulated or influenced by the limbic network. Based on research at a cellular level,[11–13] a consciousness level,[14–17] a bodily systems level,[18–20] and a quantum level[21–23] it is now clear that many systems are affected by the complex limbic network, and most notably, the motor systems.[24–31] A patient example of the complex and critical interactions between the limbic network, body systems, and its influence upon human behavior can be considered in Clinical Case 4.1.

The Limbic Network "MOVEs" Us

Moore[32] eloquently describes the limbic network as the area of the brain that moves us. The word *MOVE* can be used as a mnemonic for the functions of the limbic network that drive movement. As seen in Fig. 4.3 the M (motivation, memory) depicts the drive component of the limbic network; the O (olfaction) refers to the sense of smell and of other sensory inputs that drive motor, emotional, or visceral responses; the V (visceral) outlines the visceral and autonomic responses that serve as an indicator of the limbic network state; and E (emotional), the value or significance of individual feelings, attitudes, and beliefs that possess emotional significance for attention and learning.

Motivation

"The most powerful force in rehabilitation is motivation."[26] Without motivation the individual will not attend to the task and the neurobiology of learning will not occur. Motivation drives our motor system to develop motor programs that will enable us to perform and execute movements with the most efficient patterns available. In addition, motivation drives our ability to integrate the somatosensory map of functional skills[2] (cortical) and attention (limbic) necessary to process both sequential and simultaneous components (parts) of the movement task to be learned (whole).

Moore[32] considers motivation and memory as part of the MOVE system. Esch and Stefano[33] link motivation with reward, illustrating how the limbic network "learns" through repetition and reward. They state that the concept of motivation includes drive and satiation,

goal-directed behavior, and incentive. They recognize that these behaviors maintain homeostasis and ensure the survival of the individual and the species. Motivation mediated by limbic (forebrain) and subcortical structures forms an interlocking neural network with the cognitive representation within the frontal regions and thus plays an important role in movement execution.[26,34]

Memory

The brain stores sensory and motor experiences as memory. Current theory supports a "dual memory system," each utilizing different pathways in the nervous system. Terms such as *verbal* and *nonverbal* and *intrinsic* and *extrinsic* have been given to these two memory systems. For this discussion, two specific categories of learning—*procedural* and *declarative*—will be used, although in today's neuroscience environment, the terms *implicit* and *explicit* memory are used as frequently. The limbic network plays a key role in both declarative and procedural aspects of memory and learning.[35–38] Before the limbic network's impact on learning and memory can be delved into, a clear understanding of what is meant by these functions is needed. Declarative (explicit) memory entails the capability to recall and verbally report experiences. This recall requires deliberate conscious effort, whereas the procedural counterpart is the recall of "rules, skills, and procedures (implicit),"[39] which can be recalled unconsciously. Both categories of learning have been correlated to limbic function.[40–42] These systems do not operate autonomously, and many therapeutic activities seem to combine these memory systems to achieve functional behavior.[39] The limbic amygdala and hippocampal structures and their intricate circuitries play a key role in the declarative aspect of memory.[35–38] The hippocampus may be more concerned with sensory and motor signals relating to the external environment, whereas the amygdala is related

Limbic Network Function – MOVE

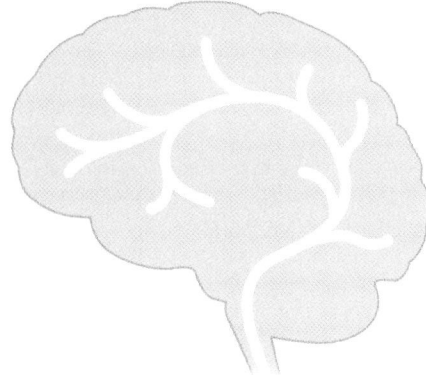

Memory and motivation: drive
- Memory: attention and retrieval, declarative learning
- Motivation: desire to learn, try, or benefit from the external environment

Olfaction
- Only sensory system that does not have to go through the thalamus as a second-order synapse in the sensory pathway before it gets to the cerebral cortex

Visceral (drive: thirst, hunger, and temperature regulation; endocrine functions)
- Sympathetic and parasympathetic reactions
- Hypothalamic regulation over autoimmune system
- Peripheral autonomic nervous system (ANS) responses that reflect limbic function

Emotion: feelings and attitude
- Self-concept and worth
- Emotional body image
- Tonal responses of motor system affected by limbic descending pathways
- Attitude, social skills, opinions

Fig. 4.3 Limbic Network Function—MOVE.

more to those of the internal environment. They both contribute in relation to the significance of external or internal environmental influences.[43,44–49] Procedural learning is vital to the development of sequence-specific learning and motor control. Acquisition and learning (memory) of new motor tasks involves dopaminergic projections from the VTA to the primary motor cortex for motor execution and initiating neuroplastic change, and from the NAc for the reward and reinforcement of that motor learning. The dorsal prefrontal cortex and the ACC are more active in the skill acquisition phase of motor learning than in the execution of pre-learned motor skills, consistent with the need for motivation as a requisite. Consolidation and retention occur as information passes through the limbic network nuclei; it is stored in cortical areas and retention and retrieval occurs without limbic involvement.[10,50–54]

Olfaction

The *O* refers to olfaction, or the incoming sense of smell, which exerts a strong influence on alertness and drive. This is clearly illustrated by the billions of dollars spent annually on perfumes, deodorants, mouthwashes, and soap as well as scents used in stores to increase customers' motivations to purchase. Olfactory input first synapses within the olfactory bulb. Subsequently, afferents travel to and synapse within the cerebral cortex without second-order synapse in the thalamus, as well as with structures within the limbic network. Although collaterals do project to the thalamus, unlike all other sensory afferent information, olfaction does not need to use the thalamus as a relay center to access the cortical structures.[39,55] Olfactory input that enters the limbic network may be used to calm or to arouse the patient, based upon the specific odor selected; for example, the use of aromatherapy to promote muscle relaxation prior to therapeutic massage.[56,57] Thus olfaction indirectly influences motor output via the limbic network's influence on muscle tone through brain stem modulation of the indirect or "emotional" motor pathways. Through brain stem connections to the reticular activating system, olfaction can have a powerful effect upon alertness. The evaluation of this system seems even more critical when a patient's motor control system is locked, with no volitional movement present. Research has shown that retrieval processing and retrieval of memory have a distinctive emotionality when they are linked to odor-evoked memories.[58,59]

Beyond olfaction, input from the other senses may not be reaching the cortical levels, such as in patients with lesions in the internal capsule or thalamus, and the patient may have a sensory-deprived environment. If the sensory input to the patient is deprived, the limbic network may place the patient in a "limbic low" state and the patient may withdraw physically or mentally, lose focus or attention, decrease motivation, and demonstrate a decrease in motor tone and output. Conversely, if the sensory input to the patient is excessive, whether through internal (patient/systems generated) or external (therapist, environment generated) feedback, the limbic network may go into an alert, protective mode, or "limbic high" state. The patient may withdraw physically or mentally, lose focus or attention, decrease motivation, and become frustrated or even angry. The resultant overload on the reticular system may be the reason for the shutdown of the limbic network versus dysfunction of the limbic network itself. Both are part of the same neuroloop circuitry and as such, in either situation, the CNS will not function optimally and learning will diminish. All these behaviors may be expressed within the hypothalamic-autonomic system as motor output, no matter where in the loop the dysfunction occurs. Having a functional understanding of the neuroanatomical sectors and their relationships with each other helps therapists unravel some of the challenging patient presentations after CNS insult.[60,61]

Therapists often try to increase motor activity through sensory input; however, they must cautiously avoid indiscriminately bombarding the sensory systems. The limbic network may demonstrate overload from stimulation at the same time the spinal motor generators reflect inadequate activation. One way that a therapist might assess for potential limbic overload would be to closely monitor the autonomic nervous system (ANS) responses, such as blood pressure, heart rate, internal temperature, and sweating, versus observing or measuring muscle tone.

Visceral or Autonomic

The *V* represents visceral or autonomic drives to movement. At the heart of the limbic network is the hypothalamus, the primary regulator of autonomic and endocrine functions. The hypothalamus controls and balances homeostasis of the internal and peripheral (skin) organ systems through regulation of sympathetic and parasympathetic reactions. Protective drives such as thirst, hunger, temperature regulation, and sexuality are controlled by this system.[39] However, the hypothalamus is also an important modulator of the limbic network, given its direct connections with the limbic midbrain,[39] the amygdala, and hippocampus, as well as close reciprocal interaction with most centers of the cerebral cortex, brain stem, and spinal cord. As such, the fact that autonomic and somatomotor responses controlled by the hypothalamus are closely aligned with the expression of emotions[62–65] and strong emotions and emotionally linked memories can change or support movement has clearly been established.[66]

Of clinical importance is that autonomical responses may reflect the presence of a limbic network imbalance that may go unnoticed by therapists. For example, patients with unstable body temperature regulation may exhibit signs of hypothalamic-pituitary involvement and overactivity.[39] Similarly, severe sweating of the palms or increased oral motor activity may be the first sign that the stress of an activity is becoming overwhelming to a patient. A therapist must continually monitor the patient's response behaviors to ascertain that they reflect true or desired motor output and not limbic influences over the motor system.

Emotional

E relates to emotions: the feelings, attitudes, and beliefs that are unique to that individual. These beliefs include psychosocial attitudes and prejudices, ethnic upbringing, cultural experiences, religious convictions, and concepts of spirituality.[67] When stimuli or tasks are endowed with emotional value or significance, a patient's attention is drawn to those with emotional significance, selecting these for attention and learning. Emotionally charged events will leave a more significant impression and enhance subsequent recall. All these aspects of emotions are strongly linked to the amygdaloid complex of the limbic network, and activity within the frontal lobe.[34,68,69] As a primary emotional center, it regulates not only our self-concept but our attitudes and opinions toward our external environment and the people within it. One aspect of self-concept is the emotional component of body image. A second self-concept deals with the patient's perceived worth or value to society, the world, and their role within it.[70] Both of these attitudes may be changed through enhanced mood or positive experience, enabling emotions to influence what is perceived and learned via the amygdala's reciprocal connections with the cortex.

Preconceived attitudes, social behaviors, and opinions have been learned by filtering the input through the limbic network. If new attitudes and behaviors need to be learned after a neurological insult, the status of the amygdalar pathways seems crucial. Damage to these limbic structures may prevent learning[71]; thus socially maladaptive behavior may persist, making the individual less likely to adapt to the social environment. It is often harder to change learned social behaviors than any other type of learning.[72–75] Because our feelings, attitudes, values, and beliefs drive our behaviors through both attention and motor responses, the emotional aspect of the limbic network has great impact on our learning and motor control. If a patient is not motivated to participate and places little value on a motor output, then low complacency results, and little learning will occur.[76–78] On the other hand, if a therapist places an extremely high value on a motor output as the expression of motor control success without interlocking that with the patient's sense of control, the behavioral response (limbic influence) may lead to inconsistency, lack of compliance/participation, and thus lack of motor learning and carryover.[76] In addition, it can cause the patient significant stress, which can prevent recovery and in some cases, cause disease.[79]

Repeated experience of reinforcement and reward leads to learning, changed expectancy, changed behavior, and maintained performance.[80] Emotional learning through the limbic network is very hard to unlearn once the behavior has been reinforced over and over.[81,82] For that reason, motor behavior that is strongly linked to a negative emotional response might be a very difficult behavior to unlearn. Repetition of motor performance with either the feeling of emotional neutrality or the feeling of success (positive reinforcement) is a critical element in the therapeutic setting. Consistently making the motor task more difficult just when the patient feels a need to succeed may decrease positive reinforcement or reward, lessen the patient's motivation to try or participate, and decrease the probability of true independence once the

patient leaves the clinical setting. When pressure is placed on therapists to produce changes quickly, strategic and meaningful repetition and thus long-term learning are often jeopardized. Rapid progression based solely upon therapist/clinic requirements may impede progress and yield a dramatic effect on the quality of the patient's life and the long-term treatment effects once he or she leaves the medical facility. Motor control theory (see Chapter 3) coincides with limbic research regarding reinforcement. Inherent feedback within a variety of environmental contexts allowing for error with correction leads to greater retention.[83] Repetition or the opportunity to practice a task (motor or cognitive) in which the individual desires to succeed will lead to long-term learning.[84] Without practice or motivation, the chance of successful motor learning is minimized. This continues to highlight the importance of both therapeutic environment and therapeutic alliance, which we will discuss in greater detail.

Multiple nuclei and interlinking circuits of the limbic network play crucial roles in behavioral and emotional changes[85–87] and declarative memory.[9,86–102] The loss of any link can affect the outcome activity of the whole circuit. Thus damage to any area of the brain can potentially cause malfunctions in any or all other areas, and the entire circuit may need reorganization to restore function.

THE NEUROSCIENCE OF THE LIMBIC NETWORK

The limbic network comprises a group of nuclei, tracts, and cortical areas that lie beneath the cortex and surround the thalamic structures. All of the areas of the limbic system are interconnected with each other through both simple and complex reverberating neural pathways. There are extensive connections between the limbic system and the hypothalamus and brain stem structures, these together play a substantial role in the regulation of homeostasis and autonomic control. Similarly, there are extensive connections to the structures of the basal ganglia, thus influencing motivation to move, as well as initiation and modulation of motor output.[103] A limited overview of the anatomy and physiology of the limbic network is presented in the following sections, designed to guide our understanding of the limbic network. The complexities of the network and its complex circuitry can be found upon deeper review of primary and secondary evidence.[7,39,104–108]

Neuroanatomy
Basic Structure and Function

Broca[109] first conceptualized the anatomical regions of the limbic lobe as forming a ring around the brain stem. Today, neuroanatomists do not differentiate an anatomical lobe as limbic, but rather refer to a complex network that encompasses cortical, diencephalon, and brain stem structures.[39] This description is less precise and includes (but is not limited to) the orbitofrontal and prefrontal cortex, hippocampus, parahippocampal gyrus, cingulate gyrus, dentate gyrus, amygdaloid body, septal area, hypothalamus, and some nuclei of the thalamus.[39,110–114] Anatomists stress the importance of looking at the interrelated structures, pathways, and functional loops within the complex limbic region.[85,115]

The limbic network can be best visualized as consisting of both cortical and subcortical structures, with the hypothalamus located at the central position (Figs. 4.4 and 4.5). The hypothalamus is surrounded by a circular alignment of the subcortical limbic structures linked with one another and the hypothalamus. These subcortical structures include the amygdalar complex and the hippocampal formation as the major input structures, and the anterior nuclei of the thalamus (limbic thalamus), as well as the NAc, the fornix, and the septal nuclei areas. The septal area projects to emotion-generating

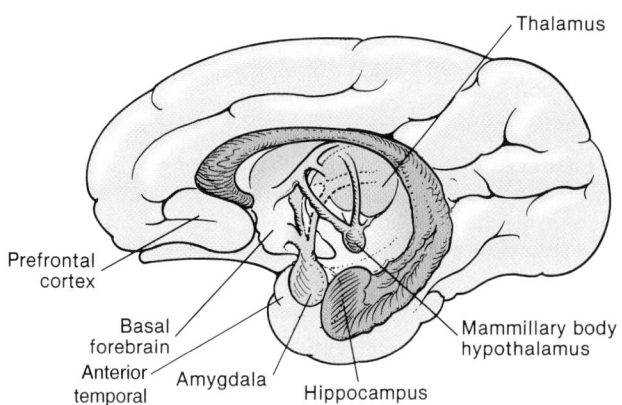

Fig. 4.4 Anatomy of the Limbic Network: Schematic Illustration.

are neuroanatomists who include the olfactory system and the basal forebrain area (cognition and memory) within the network as well (see Fig. 4.5). Olfaction is included as part of a "mesolimbic" system, linking olfaction to the midbrain structures of the NAc and the VTA.

Vitally linked to the limbic network is the excitatory reticular activating system and other brain stem nuclei of the midbrain. Some consider components of the midbrain a very important region for emotional expression.[92] Derryberry and Tucker[92] found that attack behavior aroused by hypothalamic stimulation is blocked when the midbrain is damaged and that midbrain stimulation can be made to elicit "attack behavior" even when the hypothalamus has been surgically disconnected from other brain regions. Recent research has clearly identified the neurochemical precursors to this aggressive behavior.[39,62,118–120] This "septo-hypothalamic-mesencephalic (midbrain)" continuum, connected by the medial forebrain bundle (see Fig. 4.5), is suggested as vital to the integration and expression of emotional behavior.[121] The linking of other brain structures to emotions came initially from the work of Papez,[122] who first identified the hippocampal-fornix circuit. He saw this as a way of combining the "subjective" cortical experiences with the emotional subcortical (hypothalamic) contribution. Earlier, Broca[109] labeled the cingulate gyrus and hippocampus "circle" as "the great limbic lobe." Today, the concept of the limbic network and its interaction with sensory inputs and motor expression has become extremely complex.[123] Mood can change motor output, and motor activity can change mood.[124,125]

Klüver and Bucy[126] linked the anterior half of the temporal lobes and the amygdaloid complex to the limbic network. They showed changes in behavior, with specific loss of the amygdaloid complex and anterior hippocampus input, resulting in (1) restless overresponsiveness, (2) hyperorality, or examining objects by placing them in the mouth, (3) psychic blindness of seeing and not recognizing objects and the possible harm they may entail, (4) sexual hyperactivity, and (5) emotional changes characterized by loss of aggressiveness. These changes have been named the *Klüver-Bucy syndrome*.[127] Myriad connections link the amygdala to the olfactory pathways, the frontal lobe and cingulate gyrus, the thalamus, the hypothalamus, the septum, and

areas and plays an important role in feelings of social connectedness and bonding. The fornix contains major efferent fibers from the hippocampus, as well as carrying some afferent fibers to the hippocampus from structures in the thalamus and basal forebrain.[116] The cingulate fasciculus carries amygdalic and hippocampal projections to and from the prefrontal cortex, linking many basic perceptual strategies, such as body schema, hearing, vision, and smell, to the emotional and learning centers of the limbic network.[117]

The subcortical structures are again similarly surrounded by a ring of cortical structures collectively called the *limbic cortex*, which includes the frontal cortex, the ACC/gyrus, the parahippocampal gyrus, and the uncus. The limbic network circuitry contains parallel and reverberating connections between the subcortical and limbic cortex structures, the anterior nuclei of the thalamus *(limbic thalamus)*, as well as to the limbic forebrain NAc and limbic midbrain structures: VTA and midbrain raphé nuclei of the basal ganglia. There

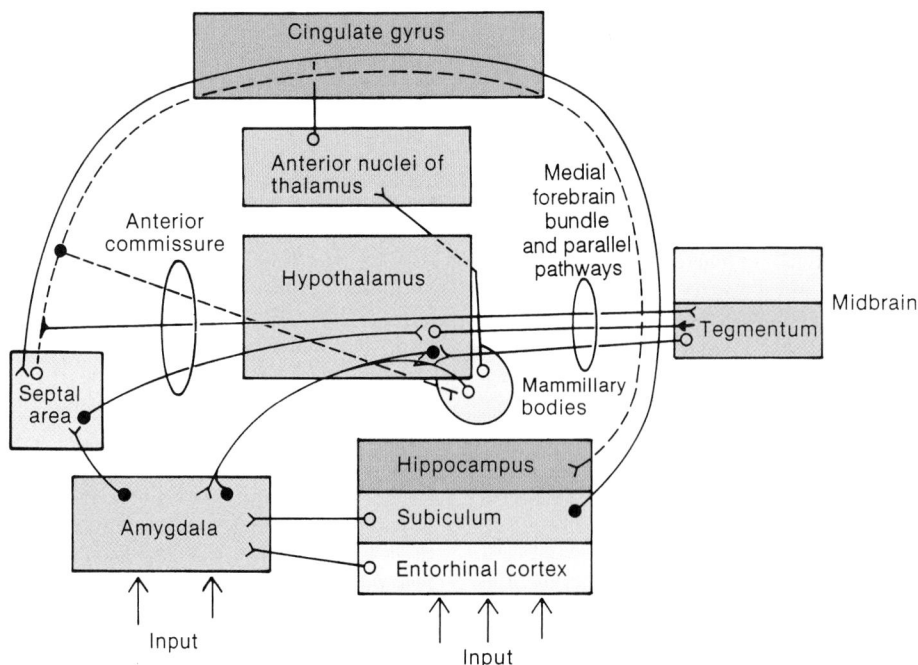

Fig. 4.5 Limbic network circuitry with parallel and reverberating connections and with medial forebrain bundle.

the midbrain structures of the substantia nigra, locus coeruleus, periaqueductal gray matter, and the reticular formation. The amygdala receives feedback from many of these structures it projects to by reciprocal pathways.

At the heart of the limbic network is the hypothalamus. The hypothalamus, in close reciprocal interaction with most centers of the cerebral cortex and the amygdala, hippocampus, pituitary gland, brain stem, and spinal cord, is a primary regulator of autonomic and endocrine functions and controls and balances homeostatic mechanisms. Autonomical and somatomotor responses controlled by the hypothalamus are closely aligned with the expression of emotions.[62–65]

In the temporal lobe, anteromedially is the amygdaloid complex of nuclei, with the hippocampal formation situated posterior to it. Located medial to the amygdala is the basal forebrain nuclei, which receive afferent neurons from the reticular formation, the hypothalamus, and the limbic cortex. From this basal forebrain, efferents project to all areas of the cerebral cortex, the hippocampus, and the amygdaloid body, providing an important connection between the neocortex and the limbic network. These nuclei represent the center of the cholinergic system, which supplies acetylcholine to limbic and cortical structures involved in memory formation.

Interlinking the Components of the System

The limbic network has many reciprocating interlinking circuits among its component structures, which provide for much functional interaction as well as allow for continuing adjustments with continuous feedback (see Fig. 4.2).[39,62] Neuroimaging has helped reduce uncertainty concerning the anatomical pathways, and neurochemistry has widened the possibilities of variations across synaptic connections.[128–130] The largest of the interlinking pathways is the fornix, providing efferent and afferent connections to the hypothalamus and connecting the limbic network structures.[131] The stria terminalis, another of the linking circuitry components, originates in the amygdaloid complex and follows a course close to the fornix to end in the hypothalamus and septal regions. The amygdala is also directly connected to the septal region by a short pathway, the *diagonal band of Broca*. These pathways serve as foundation for emotion memory and bonding. A third pathway, the uncinate fasciculus, connects the amygdala and the orbitofrontal cortex serving as a foundation for decision making.[39,132,133]

The medial forebrain bundle and other parallel circuits (see Fig. 4.5) are vital connections of the limbic network.[134] These pathways course through the lateral hypothalamus to terminate in the cingulate gyrus in its ascending limb and in the reticular formation of the midbrain in its descending part; these pathways have strong interconnections and control over the periaqueductal gray area, and thus influence upon descending modulation of pain signals.[135]

Commissural fibers from the vestibular nuclei run through the lateral medullary reticular formation (parvicellular reticular formation [PCRF]) and connect the vestibular nucleus to the reticular formation. The PCRF and the solitary nucleus receive both vestibular and nonvestibular input from the cortex, cerebellum, and the limbic network and are considered functionally as the "vomiting center." It also receives heavy input from the chemoreceptor region in the floor of the fourth ventricle (area postrema), resulting in vomiting in response to noxious chemicals. The PCRF also projects fibers to the parabrachial nuclei that contain the respiratory centers and to the hypoglossal nucleus to activate and coordinate the protective gag reflex.[136] Visceral autonomic input from multiple sources, including the vestibular nuclei, converges on the parabrachial nucleus. The locus ceruleus and autonomical brain stem nuclei also receive vestibular nuclear input.[137–141] Thus cardiovascular activity and respiration

(brain stem–mediated autonomic activity), as well as vomiting, are highly influenced by the status of the vestibular system and the limbic system. This helps us to understand how cold to the neck or forehead, pressure to the wrist, or taste or olfactory input of ginger depresses autonomic reactions and nausea in response to chronic vestibular or interneuronal connection problems. There are three different types of drugs that neuroanatomically suppress or modulate vestibular input and thus have a dramatic effect on dizziness and nausea.[142] Additionally, functional magnetic resonance imaging (fMRI) confirms that there is increased activity within the inferior frontal cortex when nausea is induced by either vestibular stimulation or ingestion of an emetic.[143] This research supports that there is a strong interconnection among vestibular input, limbic nuclei, and autonomic responses.[144]

There are also connections between the parabrachial nucleus and higher brain centers, including the amygdala, which is known to be critical in the development of conditioned avoidance, such as found in agoraphobia, as an example. Thus vestibular input results in a sensory stimulus that may induce a state of general autonomic discomfort as a trigger of avoidance that precedes the onset of a panic attack.[14,136,138,144] Vestibular firing rates are further modulated and regulated by the dorsal raphe nucleus of the midbrain and rostral pons. The dorsal raphe nucleus is the largest producer of serotonin in the brain, which further explains the significant linkage between vestibular dysfunction and anxiety, and sleep deprivation and anxiety.[145]

Additionally, animal research has shown that bilateral vestibular lesions result in changes in the morphology and function of the hippocampus, specifically associated with hippocampal atrophy. The hippocampus contributes to spatial and gravitational orientation, cognition, learning, and memory (spatial and nonspatial), which are symptoms and functional limitations often identified by individuals with vestibular dysfunction.[146–154]

Central pattern generators found in the caudal brain stem and the spinal cord are understood to generate fixed rhythmic motor output patterns such as biting and swallowing. These motor tracts receive direct and indirect afferent information from the periphery and are part of the interneuronal projection system to motor neurons, contributing to the activity within the motor neuron pool.[155–157] Their output is linked to the proximal (axial) and distal motor control system through the ventromedial and lateral descending motor pathways, modulated by a variety of structures, and regulated by the prefrontal area.[135,158–162] Their output is also strongly linked to the limbic network, resulting in an emotional context linked to the motor output.[158,163] The functional motor implication of these tracts is determined by whether the fibers project as part of the medial or lateral descending system. The medial components of this system originate within the medial portion of the hypothalamus, and the lateral portion originates in the limbic network (lateral hypothalamus, amygdala, and bed nucleus of the stria terminalis). The medial system, through the locus coeruleus, periaqueductal gray matter, and raphe spinal pathways, contributes to the general level of activity of both somatosensory and motor neurons. As such, the limbic network can have an effect on both somatosensory input and motor output. A change in activity in this system can alter the level of excitation at the first order synapse, thus altering the processing or sensitivity to that afferent information as it enters the nervous system. Similarly, it can alter the level of motor activity and thus motor output or expression, which may account for the increase in extensor muscle tone and extension seen with anger and the flexion and decrease muscle tone seen with depression. The lateral system seems to be involved in more specific motor output related to emotional behavior and may explain some of the loss of fine motor skill when one is placed in an emotional situation such as competition. The clinical relevance of this information highlights the need during patient examination to differentiate whether observed postural/muscle tone abnormalities are deficits within the motor system itself, or are a result of limbic system influence on that motor output. The clinician would need to observe and assess the emotional state, as well as how it changes with patient mood or activity, or with modification of the therapeutic environment. If the abnormal state consistently alters with mood shifts of control of emotional variables, then limbic involvement causing motor control disturbances could be identified. Human social behavior requires motor expression, yet that behavior is driven through the limbic circuitry.[164–167]

These links enable the limbic network itself and the non–limbic-associated structures to act as one neural task system. No portion of the brain, whether limbic or nonlimbic, has only one function.[39] Each area acts as an input-output station. At no time is it totally the center of a particular effect, and each site depends on the cooperation and interaction with other regions. The concept of neuroplasticity within the motor system and motor learning is well understood by physical therapists, but less understood is the integration of this emotional system interaction with sensory and motor components of motor performance and learning. Research is identifying that these neurocircuitries are present and interactive, and therefore should be considered.[164]

Neurochemistry

Discussion of the limbic network's intricate regulation of many neurochemical substances is not within the scope of this chapter. Yet therapists need to appreciate how potent this system can be with respect to the influence of neurochemical imbalance or loss on motor control, memory, or motor learning. The amount of research reflecting new understanding of the role of neurochemistry in brain function highlights the importance of frequent review of the literatures.[168–176]

More than 200 neurotransmitters have been identified within the nervous system.[39] The hypothalamus, the physiological center of the limbic network (see Figs. 4.1 and 4.5), is involved in neurochemical production and is essential for the passage of information along specific neurochemical pathways within the network. Squire and colleagues[177] consider it the major motor output pathway of the limbic network, which also communicates with every part of this system.

Neuropeptides

The importance of neuropeptides is being recognized relative to the limbic network's role in the regulation of affective and motivated behaviors.[34,39,135,178–180] Certain nuclei of the hypothalamus produce and release these neuroactive peptides, which have long-acting effectiveness as neuromodulators, controlling the levels of neuronal excitation and effective functioning at the synapses. Through their long-lasting effects, they regulate motivational levels, mood states, and learning. These peptide-producing neurons extend from the hypothalamic nuclei to the ANS and to the nuclei of the limbic network, where they modulate neuroendocrine and autonomic activities. Lesions in the medial hypothalamus affect hormone production and thus alter regulation of many hormonal control systems.[39] For example, head injury may lead to medial hypothalamic lesions general hyperactivity, signs of hostility after minimal provocation, as well as huge weight gain resulting from the increase of insulin in the blood (increasing feeding and converting nutrients into fat) and loss of satiety.

The nuclei of the amygdaloid complex represent the center of the cholinergic system, which supplies *acetylcholine* to limbic and cortical structures involved in memory formation. Depletion of acetylcholine in patients with Alzheimer disease relates to memory loss.[135,181–183,184]

Monoamines

The monoamines play a critical role in many aspects of function and dysfunction within the limbic network. As a quick overview, the noradrenergic system (noradrenaline and adrenaline) plays a significant general role in the body's response to stressors. In the brain, the noradrenergic system is located primarily in the locus coeruleus and plays a significant role in modulating behavioral and cognitive function within the cortex.[185] The adrenal corticosteroids also contribute to modulation of long-term potentiation within the hippocampus.[186] Novelty or reward-seeking and motivational behaviors of the limbic network seem to be dopamine dependent,[187] whereas coordination of circadian body rhythm and sleep (critical for motor performance and learning) is influenced by levels of all of the monoamine neurotransmitters.[188–190]

A functional deficiency in monoamines, especially *serotonin*, is hypothesized to be a primary cause of depression.[191,192] The serotonin systems originate in the rostral and caudal raphe nuclei in the midbrain. Ascending serotonergic tracts start in the midbrain and ascend to the limbic forebrain and hypothalamus; they are concerned with mood and behavior regulation. Damage to the ascending pathways contributes to depression as a mood disorder. In addition, newer evidence has highlighted the important role serotonin plays in motor control.[193]

Descending pathways from the raphe nuclei to the substantia gelatinosa are involved in pain mechanisms. Through a complex sequence of biochemical steps, a reduction in serotonin in the raphe nuclei contributes to the increased sensitization of the presynaptic terminals of the cutaneous sensory neurons. Increased central sensitization of these terminals can lead to a hyperactive withdrawal reflex or hypersensitivity to cutaneous sensory input.[39] This would account for the behavior patterns seen in patients with head trauma, when the therapist sees a flexed posture with a withdrawn or depressed affect associated with an extreme sensitivity to touch or even cutaneous input from clothing, air, etc.

Lesions in the lateral hypothalamus lead to damage of *dopamine*-carrying fibers that begin in the substantia nigra and filter through the hypothalamus to the striatum of the basal ganglia. Lesions, either along this tract or within the lateral hypothalamus, lead to aphagia and hypoarousal, as well as marked passivity with decreased functioning. Decreased sensory awareness contributing to sensory neglect is also present in lateral hypothalamic lesions. Disruptions of the indirect (hypothalamic) and direct (independent of hypothalamus) pathways from the mammillary bodies to the anterior thalamus contribute highly to loss of spatial orientation and memory.[194] Bilateral infarcts within the mammillothalamic tract result in acute Korsakoff syndrome.[195]

Dopamine is critical for motor cortex plasticity and motor skill acquisition and learning.[196] Dopamine released from the VTA in the midbrain projects to the primary motor cortex (M1) and enables motor skill acquisition.[52] Moreover, the dopaminergic VTA neurons projecting to M1 are activated when rewards are obtained during motor skill acquisition, but not during task execution in later associative or autonomous stages of motor learning, or when rewards are not associated with performing a skilled movement. Dopamine released from the VTA to the NAc and the frontal cortex plays an important role in reward processing for motor learning.[51] Furthermore, in animal study, destruction of the VTA dopaminergic neurons prevented improvements in forelimb reaching, but learning recovered on administration of levodopa directly into the M1 of these VTA-lesioned animals. Of note is that lesioning the VTA did not affect performance of an already learned skill, meaning movement execution remained intact.[52]

It is hypothesized that the underlying pathophysiological mechanism of one form of schizophrenia involves an excessive transmission of *dopamine* within the mesolimbic tract system.[39] The dopaminergic cell bodies are located in the VTA and the substantia nigra. Some of these neurons project to the limbic network, specifically to the NAc, the stria terminalis nuclei, parts of the amygdala, and the frontal entorhinal and ACC, serving to modulate the flow of neural activity through the limbic network.[39] The NAc may serve a critical role, acting as a filtering system with respect to affect and certain types of memory through its influence over the hippocampus, frontal lobe, and hypothalamus.[39]

The specific roles of the *noradrenergic* pathway are numerous and affect almost all parts of the CNS. The center for the noradrenergic pathways is located within the caudal midbrain and upper pons. Its nucleus is referred to as the *locus coeruleus*. This nucleus sends at least five tracts rostrally to the diencephalon and telencephalon.[39] Of specific interest for this discussion are the projections to the hippocampus and amygdala, which have an excitatory effect on the regions where they terminate.[39] Thus the activation of this system will heighten the excitation of the two nuclei within the limbic network that are involved in declarative learning and memory. This excitation or hyperactivation may cause "overload" or impair focus of attention and learning.[197] Decreased activity may prevent learning and memory. Attention to task may depend on continuing noradrenergic stimulation. These tracts, travelling rostrally from the midbrain, play a key role in alertness. The correlation of alertness and attention to performance and learning of motor tasks can be demonstrated.[39]

In conclusion, the neurochemistry of the limbic network is intricately linked to the neurochemistry of the brain and the body organs regulated by the hypothalamus. All systems within the limbic circuitry seem to be interdependent, with the summation of all the neurochemistry being the determinants of the specific processing of information. Similarly, the interdependence of the limbic network with almost all other areas of the brain and the activities of those areas at any time reflect the complexity of this system.

Neurobiology of Learning and Behavior

Strub and Black[198] view behavior as occurring on distinct interrelated levels that represent behavioral hierarchies. Starting at level 1, a state of alertness to the internal and external environment must be maintained for motor or mental activity to occur. The brain stem reticular activating system brings about this state of general arousal by relaying in an ascending pathway to the thalamus, the limbic network, and the cerebral cortex. To proceed from a state of general arousal to one of "selective attention" requires the communication of information to and from the cortex, the thalamus, and the limbic network and its modulation over the brain stem and spinal pattern generators.[39,199]

Level 2 of this hierarchy lies in the domain of the hypothalamus and its closely associated limbic structures. This level deals with subconscious drives and innate instincts. The survival-oriented drives of hunger, thirst, temperature regulation, and survival of the species (reproduction) and the steps necessary for drive reduction are processed here, as well as learning and memory. Most of these activities relate to limbic functioning. If an individual or patient is in a perceived survival mode, little long-term learning regarding either cognition or motor programming will occur. Thus making the patient feel safe is initially a critical role for the therapist. This approach may require placing the therapist's hands on the patient initially to take away any possibility of falling. The therapist would first deal with the emotional aspect of the patient's environment and then shift to the motor learning and control component, in which the patient is empowered to practice and self-correct within the program she or he can control.

On level 3 only cerebral cortical areas are activated. This level deals with abstract conceptualization of verbal or quantitative entities. It is

at this level that the somatosensory and frontal motor cortices work together to perceptually and procedurally develop motor programs. The prefrontal areas of the frontal lobe can influence the development of these motor programs, thus again illustrating the limbic influence over the motor system.[200–203]

Level 4 behavior is concerned with the expression of social aspects of behavior, personality, and lifestyle. Again, the limbic network and its relationship to the frontal lobe are vital. The shift to the World Health Organization International Classification of Functioning, Disability and Health (WHO-ICF) model, which reflects patient-centered therapy, has actualized the critical importance of this level of human behavior.[204–208]

The interaction of all four levels leads to the integrative and adaptable behavior seen in the human. Our ability to become alert and protectively react is balanced by our previous learning, whether it is cognitive-perceptive, social, or affective. Adaptability to rapid changes in the physical environment, in lifestyles, and in personal relationships results from the interrelationships or complex neurocircuitry of the human brain. When insult occurs at any one level within these behavioral hierarchies, all levels may be affected.

A fifth level of limbic function may one day be recognized as the link between the hard science of today and unexplained medical mysteries of healing. Meanwhile, how might the function of the limbic system explain certain mysteries, such as why some people heal from terminal illnesses spontaneously, others heal in ways not accepted by traditional medicine,[213,214] and others just die without any known disease or pathological condition?[67,105,215,216] It is proposed that a characteristic of the fifth level of limbic function is the patient's strong, emotional belief[67] that he or she will heal or will not heal. How conscious intent drives hypothalamic autoimmune function is being unraveled scientifically, and clinicians often observe these changes in their patients. Through observation it becomes apparent that patients who believe they will get better, often do, and those who believe they will not, generally do not. Whether belief comes from a religious, spiritual, or hard science paradigm, that belief drives behavior, and that drive has a large limbic component. Intellectual curiosity and human compassion motivates practitioners to explore these mysteries that otherwise might remain unexplained, overlooked, disbelieved, or forgotten.

As Western medicine continues to explore the intricate neurochemistry of the limbic network,[209–212] alternative medicine is establishing effectiveness and efficacy for various interventions, approaches, and philosophies (see Chapter 39). The intersection of evidence and treatment efficacy is this: there is an interlocking dependence among somatosensory mapping of the functional skills[2] (cognitive), attention (limbic) necessary for any type of learning, and the sequential, multiple, and simultaneous programming of functional movement (motor). The limbic amygdala and hippocampal structures and their intricate circuitries play a key role in the declarative aspect of memory and learning.[35–38] The dorsal prefrontal cortex and the ACC were activated more when the subjects learned[53,54] a new sequence than they were when subjects simply paid attention to a pre-learned sequence.[51,52] Once this syntactical, intellectual memory is learned and taken out of short-term memory by passing through limbic nuclei, the information is stored in cortical areas and can be retrieved at a later time without limbic involvement.[50]

Limbic Influence on Memory and Motor Learning

Recovery of function after injury may involve mechanisms that allow reorganizing of the structure and function of cortical, subcortical, and spinal circuits. In very young infants, areas within opposite hemispheres may "take over" function, whereas in more mature brains reorganization of existing parallel and silent pathways within and between hemispheres, as well as synaptogenesis are accepted recovery mechanisms within the expanding knowledge of neuroplasticity.[217–220] For complex behavior, such as in motor functioning requiring many steps, the limbic network, cortex, hypothalamus, basal ganglia, and brain stem work as an integrated unit. As such, damage to one area may cause the whole system to initially malfunction. In addition, a lesion in one area may cause secondary dysfunction of a different area that was not damaged by the primary lesion. Without appropriate task (activity), internal and external environmental challenge designed to promote neuroplasticity, the initial malfunction can become permanent.[221] The optimal rehabilitation timing for neuroplastic change has not yet been firmly established; however, it is accepted that there are key plastic "time windows."[222] The use of drug therapies to alter cellular activity and plasticity within these key windows after CNS damage has become a huge area of pharmaceutical research.[223–229] This line of research is focused on the effect of the sensorimotor representation of movement within the cortex, which is a net effect of the stimulation of multiple pathways. The activation of specific direct, indirect, or modulating pathways engaged during the process of function-induced neuroplasticity, such as those of the limbic network, is less understood.

"Ultimately, to be sure, memory is a series of molecular events. What we chart is the territory within which those events take place."[32] The brain stores sensory and motor experiences as memory. In processing incoming information, most sensory pathways from receptors to cortical areas send vital information to the components of the limbic network. For example, extensions can be found from the visual pathways into the inferior temporal lobe (limbic network).[39,230,231] Visual information is "processed sequentially" at each synapse along its entire pathway, in response to size, shape, color, and texture of objects. In the inferior temporal cortex, the total image of the item viewed is projected. In this way the sensory inputs are converted to become "perceptual experiences." This also applies to other sensory stimuli, such as tactile, proprioceptive, and vestibular. The process of translating the integrated perceptions into memory occurs bilaterally in the limbic network structures of the amygdala and the hippocampus.[39,43,168,232–241]

Before the limbic network's impact on learning and memory can be investigated, a clear understanding of what is meant by these functions is needed. Current theories support a "dual memory system" consisting of different pathways in the nervous system. Terms such as *verbal* and *nonverbal, habit* versus *recognition, intrinsic* and *extrinsic,* and *procedural* and *declarative* have been given to these two memory systems. These systems do not operate autonomously, and many therapeutic activities seem to combine these memory systems to achieve functional behavior.[39] As such, in reality, the complexity of memory is not a two-category system. Verbal and nonverbal memory both interact with declarative function.[242] Even within spatial memory, additional areas of integration and parallel circuitry have been identified.[243,244]

For this discussion, two specific categories of learning—procedural and declarative—will be used, although in today's neuroscience environment, the terms *implicit* and *explicit memory* are used as frequently. Both categories of learning have been correlated to limbic function.[40–42] Declarative (explicit) memory entails the capability to recall and verbally report experiences. This recall requires deliberate conscious effect, whereas the procedural counterpart is the recall of rules, skills, and procedures (implicit),[39] which can be recalled unconsciously.

Procedural learning is vital to the development of motor control. A child first receives sensory input from the various modalities through the thalamus, terminating at the appropriate sensory cortex. That information is processed, a functional somatosensory map is formulated,[2,245] and the information is programmed and relayed to the motor cortex. From there, it is sent to both the basal ganglia and the cerebellum to establish plans for postural adaptations, refinement of motor programs, and coordination of direction, extent, timing, force, and tone necessary throughout the entire sequence of the motor act. Procedural learning and memory do not *require* limbic network involvement as long as an emotional value is not placed on the task. This memory deals with skills, habits, and stereotyped behaviors. Summarizing, the frontal lobe, basal ganglia, and cerebellum are critical nuclei for changing and modulating existing programs.[39] Storage and subsequent retrieval of memory of these semiautomatic motor plans are thought to occur throughout the motor control system.[39] This motor system is involved in developing procedural plans used in moving us from place to place or holding us in a position when we need to stop.[39] The complexity of this process has had an impact on the study of motor control and variables that might affect that control.[246]

Unlike procedural learning and memory, declarative (explicit) learning and memory require the wiring of the limbic network and are closely associated with limbic function. Declarative thought deals with factual, material, semantic, and categorical aspects of higher cognitive and affective processing.[247] A strong emotional and judgmental component is linked with declarative thought. Thus as soon as a motor behavior has value placed on the act, it becomes declarative as well as procedural, and the limbic network may become a key element in the success or failure of that movement.[248,249] Most functional tasks or activities practiced in a clinical setting have value attached to them. That value can be clearly seen by observing the emotional intent placed on the activity by the patient.[250]

Two reciprocal pathways, or circuits, within the limbic network are intimately involved in the process of declarative learning and memory (1) the amygdaloid, dorsomedial thalamic nucleus, and cortical pathways and (2) the hippocampal, fornix, anterior thalamic nucleus, and cortical pathways. Both pathways contribute in relation to the significance of external or internal environmental to learning of a concept or task.[43–49] The amygdala may be more concerned with sensory and motor signals relating to the internal environment, whereas the hippocampus is concerned more with those of the external environment. The hippocampus is rich in stem cells and may be a primary nuclear mass that directs the bodily systems to heal after injury. This is especially true when the external environment is enriched and nurtures the emotional environment for that healing.[251,252]

For initial declarative learning and memory, function of the hippocampus and the amygdala of the limbic network is required.[39] These two structures play an important role within the "cortico-limbo-thalamo-cortical" circuit, which plays a significant role in memory storage.[39] For memory formation to occur in early motor learning (acquisition), there must be a storing of the "neural representation" of the stimuli in the association and the processing areas of the cortex. This "cortico-limbo-thalamo-cortical" circuit serves as the "imprinting mechanism" by which pathway activation by stimulus is reinforced. Limbic involvement in the declarative memory and learning processes creates a chemical bond that allows cortical storage of "stimulus representation" necessary for subsequent recognition and recall of the information.[39,44,233,235,236] Therefore on subsequent stimulation, a stimulus recognition or recall would be elicited. In the associative phases of recall and transfer of learning, stored representations of any interconnected imprints might be evoked simultaneously.[39]

The amygdaloid circuits seem to deal with strongly emotional and judgmental thoughts, whereas the hippocampal circuits are less emotional and more factual. The amygdala may be more involved in emotional arousal and attention, as well as motor regulation, whereas the hippocampus may deal with less emotionally charged learning. It

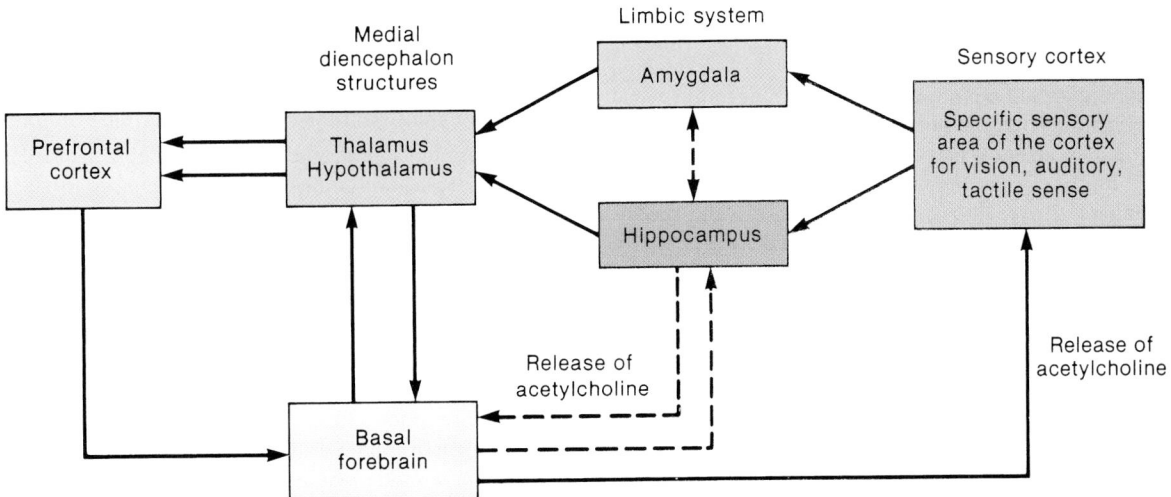

Fig. 4.6 The basal forebrain closes the circuit and causes changes in sensory area neurons, which could lead to correct perception and stored memory. This is neurochemical-dependent.

is postulated that the amygdala is the area of the brain that adds a "positive association," associating a stimulus and reward and placing an emotional value memories or learning. In this way, stimulus and reward are associated by the amygdala, and an emotional value is placed on them.[253,254] These limbic circuits seem crucial in the initial processing of material that leads to learning and memory. Once the thought has been laid down within the cortical structures, retrieval of that specific intermediate and long-term memory does not seem to require the limbic network, although new associations will need to be run through the system.[39,233,235,43]

The hippocampus and amygdala are also linked both structurally and functionally to each other and to specific thalamic nuclei in the medial diencephalon. The medial diencephalon is an important relay station along the pathway that leads from the specific sensory cortical region to the limbic structures in the temporal lobe to the medial diencephalic structures and ends in the ventromedial part of the prefrontal cortex (Fig. 4.6).[39,255,256] A vital processing area for all sensory modalities is located in the region of the anterior temporal lobe. Patients with temporal epileptic seizures and whose temporal lobes have been surgically removed develop global anterograde amnesia—that is, amnesia develops for all senses, and no new memories can be formed. Experimental removal of only the hippocampus does not bring about these changes, although processing is slowed down. When both the hippocampus and the amygdala are removed bilaterally, the amnesia is both retrograde and anterograde. A third component in the memory pathway involves pathways between the amygdala, hippocampus, and the thalamic nuclei in the medial diencephalon. When the medial diencephalic region is damaged by neurological trauma such as strokes, neoplasms, infections, or chronic alcoholism, global amnesias result. Given that the limbic network and the diencephalon cooperate in the memory circuits, the destruction of these pathways causes the same amnesic effect.

As shown in Fig. 4.6, memories may be stored in the sensory cortex area, where the original sensory input was interpreted into "sensory impressions." Today, concepts regarding memory storage suggest that declarative memory is stored in categories similar to a filing system. Those categories or files seem to be stored in several cortical areas bilaterally depending on the context.[257,258] This system allows for easy retrieval from multiple areas. Memory has stages and is continually changing. It was once thought that the hippocampus only dealt with

long-term memory, but it is now accepted that it also supports multi-item working memory.[259] To go from short-term to long-term memory, the brain must physically change its chemical structure (a plastic phenomenon). Memory first begins with a representation of information that has been transformed through processing of perceptual systems. The transferring of this new memory into a long-lasting chemical bond requires the neuronal network of the limbic complex. Owing to the multiple tracts or parallel circuits in and out of the limbic network and throughout neocortical systems, patients, even with extensive lesions, can often learn and store new information.[39,260] This may also explain why damage to the limbic network structures does not destroy existing memory nor make it unavailable because it is actually stored in many places throughout the neocortex. The circular memory circuit illustrated in Fig. 4.6 shows only one system. The reader must remember that many parallel circuits function simultaneously. The circular memory circuit shown reverts to the original sensory area after activation of the limbic structures to cause the necessary neuronal changes that would inscribe the event into retrievable stored memory.[261] This information can be recognized and retrieved by activation of storage sites anywhere along the pathway.[39,262] Patients with brain lesions localized in the limbic network components of the amygdala and hippocampus have the ability to acquire and function with "rule-based" games and skills but have lost the capacity to recall how, when, or where they gained this knowledge or to give a description of the games and skills learned. Relating this to clinical performance, patients may develop the skill in a functional activity but not the problem-solving strategies necessary to associate danger or other potentially harmful aspects of a situation that may develop once out of the purely clinical setting.[119,263–266] Similarly, if a patient needs to learn a procedural task such as walking, transfers, eating, and so on, it may be extremely important to direct the attention off the task while the task is being practiced procedurally.

The last station or system to be added to the circuit is the "basal forebrain cholinergic system," which delivers the neurochemical acetylcholine to the cortical centers and to the limbic network, with which it is linked. Visual recognition memory can be augmented or impaired by administration of drugs that enhance or block the action of acetylcholine.[267–269] The loss of this neurotransmitter is linked to memory malfunctioning in Alzheimer disease and plays a key role in dementia problems in Parkinsonism.[270] Currently, many chemicals are being studied for their influence on brain structures and specially limbic structures.[271,272]

The hippocampus and the amygdala are involved in recognition memory.[273] Hippocampal (indirect) and nonhippocampal (direct and independent) pathways influence the anterior thalamus and thus play an important role in memory, particularly spatial memory and location of objects in space.[194] The the amygdala is necessary for the association of memories derived through the various senses with a specific recognition recall. For example, a whiff of ether might bring to mind a painful surgical experience or the sight of some food may cause a recall of its pleasant smell. Removal of the amygdala brings out the behavior shown in Klüver-Bucy syndrome. For patients with this neurological problem, familiar objects do not bring forth the correct associations of memories experienced by sight, smell, taste, and touch and relate them to objects presented.[274] Association of previously presented stimuli and their responses appear to be lost. Animals without amygdaloid input had different response patterns that ignored previous fears and aversions. Thus the amygdala adds the "emotional weight" to sensory experience. Loss of the amygdala takes away many positive associations and potential rewards, thereby altering the shaping of perceptions that lead to memory storage.

When stimuli are endowed with emotional value or significance, attention is drawn to those possessing emotional significance, selecting these for attention and learning. This would give the amygdala a "gatekeeping" function of selective filtering. The amygdala may enable emotions to influence what is perceived and learned by reciprocal connection with the cortex. Emotionally charged events will leave a more significant impression and subsequent recall. The amygdala alters perception of afferent sensory input and, hence, affects subsequent actions.[36,275,276]

In the human, memory functioning has been associated with the phenomenon of long-term potentiation observed in hippocampal pathways.[39] This potentiation of synaptic transmission, lasting for hours, days, and weeks, occurs after brief trains of high-frequency stimulation of hippocampal excitatory pathways. Whether this long-term potentiation occurs presynaptically, postsynaptically, or both has not yet been established.[39,135,277] The adrenal corticosteroids contribute to modulation of long-term potentiation within the hippocampus.[186] Recent literature has linked a neurotropic factor usually considered for long-term potentiation within the hippocampus as a factor in amygdala-dependent learning, thus reiterating the interaction between these two nuclei and their role in memory and learning.[36]

Learning and memory evoke alterations in behavior that reflect neuroanatomical and neurophysiological changes.[39,210] These alterations include the phenomenon of long-term potentiation as an example of such changes. The hippocampus demonstrates the importance of input of long-term potentiation in associative learning. In this type of learning, two or more stimuli are combined through the "associative" interaction of afferent inputs. As such, tetanizing of more than one pathway needs to occur simultaneously. If only one pathway is tetanized, the effect is decreased synaptic transmission. Thus long-term potentiation serves as one model for understanding the neural mechanism for associative learning. Hormones interact with this neural mechanism, which, if combined with stress, can change the specific circuitry active during the experience.[278] As an example, the amygdala is not only involved in learning related to emotional experiences but is also responsible for changing motor expression or conditioned response generated as part of an autonomic expression, such as with fear.[164,279] Limbic responses to input stimuli need to be differentiated from limbic memory and initiation of a response without the stimuli. Although this is an area of practice not yet fully understood,

clinical implications to patient examination and evaluation will be generally discussed later in this chapter.

Limbic Influence on Emotions and Behaviors: The F²ARV and General Adaptation Syndrome Continua

Noback and co-workers[280] state that the limbic network is involved with many of the expressions that make us human, namely, emotions, behaviors, and feeling states. That humanness is highly individual even in patients with normal functioning limbic networks, and even greater variance with involvement of the primary or modulating limbic network structures or pathways.

As a brief clinical example, a patient with severe brain injury with decreased responsiveness (Ranchos Los Amigos Level of Consciousness II–III) may show increased alertness and an increase in base muscle tone or motor function through effective use of sensory stimuli. Alternatively, although the desired response may be improved alertness or a motor response, a patient may become highly oversensitive to a strong odor or noxious tactile stimuli,[281] and the response may become autonomic or behavioral instead, reflected in an increased heart rate or blood pressure, or even as fear or anger.[57] Overstimulation may move the patient into a "protective state of survival," whereas a pleasant/personally desirable smell, touch, or sound (e.g., melody) will more likely lead to "safety." The former can lead to strong emotions or responses such as anger; the latter often leads to bonding, engagement (attention), and motivation to learn.[16]

Both motivation ("feeling the need to act") and concentration ("ability to focus on the task") are interlinked with the limbic network and are both critical to participation in the motor activities. The amygdaloid complex with its multitude of afferent and efferent interlinkages is specially adapted for recognizing the significance of a stimulus, and it assigns the emotional aspect of feeling the need to act. These neuroanatomical loops have tremendous connections with the reticular system. Hence, some authors call it the reticulolimbic network.[39,74] The interaction of the limbic network and the motor generators of the brain stem and ultimate direct and indirect modulation over the spinal system lead to need-directed and therefore goal-directed motor activity. It also filters out insignificant from significant information through selective processing, storing the significant for memory, learning, and recall. These interconnected neuroloop circuitries reinforce the concept that areas have both specialization and generalization and thus work closely together with other areas of the brain.[81,282]

Some of the earliest understanding of the limbic network was limited to that of a primary protective role in "fight or flight." With normally functioning limbic networks, patients can appropriately recognize the significance of a stimulus, effectively filter out insignificant from significant stimuli or information, and appropriately assign a need to act. However, in the impaired patient, inaccurate stimulus interpretation and therefore action/reaction occur. The therapist needs to be aware that a patient may overrespond to stress, frustration, or fear of failure in both cognitive and motor activities. A small or unfiltered stimulus may generate one of two powerful and predictable limbic motor response programs: the fear and frustration, anger, rage, and violence continuum (F²ARV) and the general adaptation syndrome (GAS). The F²ARV and GAS continua are often interrelated in individuals who have direct or indirect limbic network involvement.

Fear and frustration, anger, rage, and violence or withdrawal continuum. One sequence of behaviors used to describe the emotional circuitry of the limbic network through the amygdala is the F²ARV continuum (Fig. 4.7).[74,283,284] This continuum begins with fear or frustration. This fear can lead to avoidance behavior.[285] If the event inducing the fear or frustration continues to heighten, avoidance behaviors can continue to develop.[285] In a simple example, we recall or

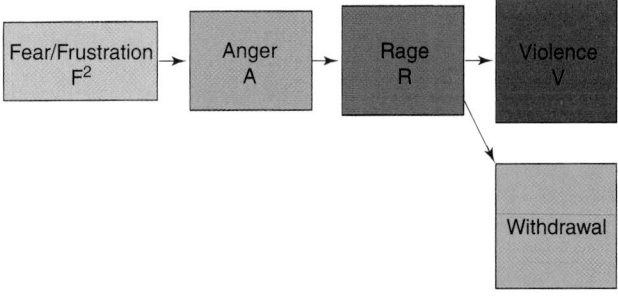

Fig. 4.7 Fear and Frustration, Anger, Rage, and Violence or Withdrawal: F^2ARV Continuum.

have seen these behaviors in our teens and as young adults, when the challenges faced in high school can lead to *avoidance* of activities. Alternately, extreme fear and frustration can also lead to *anger*. Anger is a neurochemical response that is perceived and defined cognitively (at the cortical level) as anger. If the neurochemical response continues to build or is prolonged, the anger displayed by the person may advance to *rage* (internal chaos) and finally into *violence* (strong motor response). A common societal example is in the case of domestic discord and violence. Women who attain the level of rage may become withdrawn and thus become victimized by a partner who is also in rage or inflicting physical or emotional violence.[286] Another current example is posttraumatic stress disorder (PTSD), in which the prolonged stress of deployment and unique challenges of warfare lead to limited adaptive reserves in warriors and returning veterans.

How quickly and completely any individual will progress from fear to violence is dependent on several factors. First, the genetic neurochemical predisposition (initial wiring) will influence behavioral responses.[284] Second, "soft-wired" or conditioned responses resulting from experiences and reinforced patterns will influence output. For example, it is commonly known that abusive parents were usually abused children[283,287]; they learned that anger quickly leads to violence and that the behavior of violence was somehow acceptable. Last, the quality and intensity of the stimulus initiating the continuum will influence the level of response.

The neurochemistry within an individual's CNS, whether inherently active or altered through drugs or injury, will have great influence on the plasticity of the existing wiring.[263,288] Repetitive or prolonged exposure to negative environmental stimuli may also lead to a chronically imbalanced neurochemical state that results in a lowered threshold or tolerance to a given stimulus. Chemistry or wiring can become imbalanced from damage, environmental stress, learning, or other potentially altering situations, changing an individual's control over this continuum.[39,227–229,289,290] When neurochemical imbalance exists, these behaviors will persist, and balance may be restored only through natural neurochemical activity (e.g., sleep, exercise, diet, spirituality) or medication support (chemical replacement).

Therapists need to be acutely aware of this continuum in patients who have diffuse axonal shearing within the limbic complex. Diffuse axonal shearing is most commonly seen and reported in research on individuals with head trauma (see Chapter 23).[291,292] Resulting lesions within the limbic structures may cause an individual to progress down this continuum at a rapid speed. This point cannot be overemphasized. Patients with an accelerated F^2ARV continuum, whether through prior learning or due to the injury, may physically strike out at a clinician or caregiver out of simple frustration during care. Knowing the social history of the patient and the causation of the injury often can help the therapist gain insight into how an individual patient might progress

down this continuum. Not all head-injured patients had prior difficulty with the F^2ARV continuum; however, it is important to note that many individuals received their head injuries in violent confrontational situations or in wartime conflict. Some individuals, primarily females, when confronted with stress, anger, and potential violence from another, will withdraw and become depressed. This behavior, similar to violence, will change the structure of the limbic network.[293] A brief patient example of accelerated limbic-driven responses along the F^2ARV continuum is described in Clinical Case 4.2.

General adaptation syndrome. The autonomic responses to stress also follow a specific sequence of behavioral changes and are referred to as the *general adaptation syndrome*.[294–300] The sequential stages of GAS are a direct result of limbic imbalance and can play a dramatic role in determining patient progress.

Stress can be caused by many internal or external factors, often unique to the individual. Examples include pain, acute or chronic illness or the ramification of illness, confusion, sensory overload, and a large variety of other potential sources. The initial reaction to a stressor is a neurochemical change or "alarm" that triggers a strong sympathetic nervous system reaction. Heart rate, blood pressure, respiration, metabolism, and muscle tonus will increase. It is at this stage that the grandmother lifts the car off the child as in our previous example. If the overstimulation or stress does not diminish, the body will protect itself from self-destruction and trigger a subsequent parasympathetic

---

CLINICAL CASE 4.2

A 40-year-old man presented with moderate physical and severe cognitive functioning deficits resulting from a brain aneurysm, associated with violent episodes of rage. He would escalate very rapidly along the F^2ARV continuum when presented with unpredictable environmental stimuli, such as passing another patient with his wheelchair in the hallway. Although his physical rehabilitation had progressed well and he had made functional gains in mobility, because his assaultive outbursts posed risks to other patients as well as to caregivers, this patient appeared to be heading for placement in a locked facility, a more restrictive environment than he would need considering his level of physical limitation. Although this unfortunate man had no short-term memory function or insight into his behaviors, assessment revealed that he was highly responsive to calming music and was able to access some intact long-term memories that could be used to elicit a relaxation response. A highly positive or neutral limbic state of deep relaxation was therefore facilitated using meaningful, calming music, and simple verbal cues were presented/timed to develop a conditioned response that any staff member could then call forth with the verbal cue alone. The entire rehabilitation team was briefed on the use of this intervention and reported success using this approach during nursing care and rehabilitation interventions when the patient would become resistant or angry in response to clinician instructions. The patient was able to be trained to self-regulate by giving himself the same verbal cue when confronted with challenging situations. This treatment supported the patient's ability to regain emotional controls and allowed him the opportunity to be placed in a less-restrictive community environment. The patient never recalled a previous music therapy treatment session and asked each time to have the purpose of the treatment explained to him. But his body remembered the set of behavioral experiences, and he quickly complied with the relaxation procedure. The success of this approach demonstrates that even in the absence of short-term memory and other cognitive functions usually considered essential for new learning, the skillful engagement of positive limbic states and intact areas of patient functioning (strengths) can support development of new adaptive skills, which can be generalized to new environments.

response. At this time, all clinical symptoms reverse and the patient exhibits a decrease in heart rate, blood pressure, and muscle tonus. The bronchi become constricted, and the patient may hyperventilate and become dizzy, confused, and less alert. As the blood flow returns to the periphery, the face may flush and the skin may become hot. The patient will have no energy to move, will withdraw, and again will exhibit decreased postural tone and increased flexion.

This stress or overstimulation syndrome is characterized by common symptoms as described earlier.[34,301–308] If the acute symptoms are not eliminated, they will become chronic and the behavior patterns much more resistant to change.

GAS is often seen in the elderly, with various precipitating health crises[298] (and also in neonatal high-risk infants), victims of head trauma, and other patients with neurological conditions. The initial alarm can be precipitated by moderate to maximal internal instability with less intensive external stress, or by minimal internal instability with severe external sensory bombardment. For instance, in the elderly, stresses such as change of environment, loss of loved ones, failing health, and fears of financial problems can each cause the patient's system to react as if overloaded.[300] As another example, individuals with head trauma, vestibular dysfunction, inflammatory CNS problems, and brain tumors often possess hypersensitivity to external input such as visual environments, noise, touch, or light. In these individuals, typical clinical environments and therapeutic activities may create a sensory overload and trigger a GAS response.

Stress, no matter what the specific precipitating incident (confusion, fear, anxiety, grief, or pain), has the potential to trigger the first steps in the sequence of this syndrome.[301–306,309] The clinician's sensitivity to the patient's emotional system will be the therapeutic technique that best controls and reverses the acute condition.

Similarly, patients with dizziness and instability, particularly within visually stimulating environments, can develop feelings of panic, which can evolve into full attacks and agoraphobic responses.[310] These individuals avoid participating in activities that put them within visually overstimulating environments in an effort to control the dizziness and prevent the associated autonomic reactions. Similar types of reactions have been documented, such as space-motion discomfort (SMD),[137] postural phobic vertigo,[310] visual vertigo,[311] and dizziness of "psychogenic" origin. Often these individuals are referred first to psychology or psychiatry. However, there is an underlying physiological explanation for these symptoms. In a majority of individuals with SMD, there is a documented increase in vestibular sensitivity (increased vestibulo-ocular reflex [VOR] gain) and an impairment in velocity storage (shorter VOR time constant).[312] In addition, the dorsal raphe nucleus (dorsal reticular nucleus of the midbrain and rostral pons) is the largest serotonin-containing nucleus in the brain and directly modulates the firing activity of the superior and medial vestibular nuclei. It is this interaction between serotonin and vestibular function that helps to explain the link between vestibular and anxiety disorders. It can also help explain how patients with sleep disorders or other serotonin-depleting disorders develop vestibular-like symptoms and anxiety.[145,313] A comprehensive clinical example of the influence of the limbic system in patients with vestibular dysfunction can be found in Clinical Case 4.3.

CLINICAL CASE 4.3

A 25-year-old first-grade teacher with a history of whiplash has been referred by the neurology department 5 months after a motor vehicle accident with complaints of severe dizziness and imbalance. She is unable to recall the accident; however, there was evidence to suggest that she struck her head on the steering wheel and briefly lost consciousness. Results of diagnostic testing (MRI and electroencephalography) are inconclusive. Medical management to date has been limited to central depressant medications (alprazolam [Xanax] and diazepam [Valium]; see Chapter 36). She has received physical therapy since the accident for neck and back pain, which exacerbated her symptoms. She denies specific assessment or treatment of her dizziness or imbalance until this time. Her medical history includes a hospitalization 3 months after the motor vehicle accident with "intractable migraine, postconcussive syndrome." Of note is a previous head injury 2 years before with moderate to severe postconcussive syndrome, including vertigo and migraines. She has been referred for psychological assessment and management and was recently diagnosed with obsessive-compulsive disorder. She is now referred to physical therapy for a full postural control and vestibular assessment. The differential medical diagnosis is postconcussive syndrome, rule out aphysiological performance (psychogenic and secondary gain). The physician believes that a large part of her problem is based within the medical psychiatric domain, but he is willing to widen his paradigm to include other possibilities and obtain additional data to assist in his patient's management. The patient's goal is to eliminate the dizziness and imbalance and return to normal activity and work.

Phase I: Evaluation

Unaware of being observed, a well-groomed young woman walks into physical therapy extremely slowly, holding the wall, watching the ground, and stopping periodically to close her eyes. Her color is pale, her build small and thin, and her clothing loose. Her steps are shortened in length and widened in width, with limited time spent in the swing phase. She walks en bloc (rigidly) without arm swing, with no segmental movement of the head or trunk. She periodically stops and closes her eyes as people move around her. There is visible extraneous eye movement, although no spontaneous nystagmus noted. She is pleasant and cooperative with no overt signs of anxiety in quiet sitting.

System Impairments (Patient Report and Observation)

* Dizziness with severe nausea and vomiting (at least once weekly)
* Dizziness Visual Analog Scale 7.5/10 and Dysequilibrium Visual Analog Scale 7.0/10 (with 10 representing the most severe symptoms imaginable)
* Decreased concentration and memory; forgetfulness
* Diplopia and visual blurring, with headaches
* Photophobia and hyperacusis
* Emotional instability: fight or flight; in both active F2ARV and active GAS (autonomic) states:
  * Rapid change from a state of calm to fits of rage with her family and other support systems.
  * Anger and rage alternated with reports of depression and avoidance.
* Decreasing body mass as observed by loose clothing and supported by reports of severe nausea
* Central depression of vestibular function (treated with medication)

Activity (Patient Report)

* Impaired balance for function, with near falls in dark and eyes-closed environments. Patient reports one true fall in the shower with her eyes closed.
* Impaired balance within visually challenging environments.
* Sleep deprivation and extreme fatigue.
* Long-term stress and sensory intolerance and overstimulation

It is important for a clinician to remember that the long-term *stress* associated with a chronic disability of this nature can result in a decrease in serotonin, which influences the hypothalamus and alters modulation of the vestibular nuclei through the dorsal reticular nucleus. Loss of sleep can alter levels of serotonin and other neurotransmitters. A decrease in serotonin results in further depression and *loss of sleep,* resulting in a physiological *fatigue.* It also can result in an increase in sensitization of presynaptic terminals of the cutaneous sensory nerves, contributing to the *sensory bombardment* and overstimulation.[314]

Participation in Life (Patient Report)

- She attempted to return to work as a first-grade teacher but had a severe exacerbation of all symptoms in the classroom.
- She is unable to drive and requires assistance for shopping.
- She lives alone in an apartment and is independent in function, modified by her symptoms.
- Disability Rating is $\frac{4}{5}$ (recent severe disability and medical leave).[315]
- Dizziness Handicap Inventory (DHI) score is significant for physical and emotional impact of her dizziness, including depression. (Total disability score is $\frac{78}{100}$, functional subscore $\frac{28}{32}$, emotional subscore $\frac{30}{40}$, and physical subscore $\frac{20}{28}$.[316])

Based on the signs and symptoms obtained in the intake phase and subjective reporting, the preliminary physical therapy hypothesis would be the presence of a probable vestibular dysfunction of a mixed central and peripheral etiology, sensory integration dysfunction, and anxiety overlay. The patient clearly has limbic network overload. It will be the therapist's responsibility to differentiate that from physical motor system problems with the assessment and treatment. The examination phase is designed to confirm or refute and redirect this hypothesis. (See Chapter 21 for clarification of specific vestibular tests and measures.)

Oculomotor

Oculomotor examination was performed, with results supportive of the hypothesis of vestibular involvement, although inconclusive for peripheral versus central versus combination origin.

Gaze instability—Clinical dynamic visual acuity test revealed a significant five- to six-line deterioration in dynamic visual acuity when head was moving, with loss of postural control in posterior-left direction and symptom exacerbation during testing.

Balance Stability

- SOT of sensory balance function[317] showed an across-the-board dysfunction pattern,[24] although results were incomplete because the patient was not able to complete all 18 trials of the test protocol as a result of extreme symptoms (nausea, respiratory, and anxiety symptoms, particularly on conditions 2, 3, 5, and 6).
- Total dependence (overreliance) on visual information for postural stability.
- Poor position and control of the center of gravity, shifted significantly leftward and anterior of midline.
- Excessive use of a hip strategy for basic equilibrium (versus ankle), even on stable surfaces or the smallest perturbation.
- Inability to effectively:
  - Use somatosensory or vestibular sensory cues on functional demand (reweight)
  - Organize the sensory inputs to the CNS to facilitate appropriate motor output
  - Dampen ANS/vegetative response, particularly in visual-vestibular mismatch conditions (SOT 3 and 6)
- Aphysiological criteria—Aphysiological responses were evident within the SOT raw data traces (exaggerated sway frequency and lateral sway responses). Motor Control Test (of automatic motor responses) results would have strengthened conclusions made regarding an aphysiological component, but were unavailable to this clinician at the time of the examination.[317]

Function and Gait

Self-selected velocity of 1.82 ft/s (normal preferred gait speeds in a 20- to 30-year-old woman should be closer to 3.47 ft/s).[24] The patient watched the floor for the entire distance with no head or trunk or arm movement. Thus vision was clearly directing each step, and her preferred head position was compensatory

to decrease extraneous visual flow or input. When she was encouraged to focus on a distant object, velocity declined to 1.34 ft/s and the patient veered consistently leftward 100% of the distance. She could be encouraged to walk at 2.86 ft/s (normal encouraged gait speeds should approach 6.43 ft/s), but with an increase in instability and a leftward loss of balance; however, at this low velocity, she could regain her balance without therapist assistance.

The interactions of the patient and therapist (limbic bonding, as referred to previously within this chapter) became a critical element in the examination. The patient had to trust the therapist that if she followed the therapist's direction in examination, she would not fall or incur additional symptoms outside her control. The therapist, during the evaluation, empowered the patient to take responsibility for her functional movement while making sure the patient was successful if willing to take the risk. This aspect of the therapeutic alliance (interaction) is a limbic-neutral technique, and its success or failure will be reflected in the motor responses of the patient.

Confirmatory Tests and Measures

- Intact sensation but extreme hypersensitivity to vibratory input (with strong ANS response)
- Normal strength and range of motion

Multiple rests were required throughout the examination to decrease symptomatology (nausea, increased respiration, sweating) to patient tolerance. Testing reproduced all subjective dizziness, and there was a resultant gross instability with loss of balance in the posterior direction, necessitating assistance. Imbalance, nausea, and anxiety were residual for 10 min after testing.

In the evaluative phase, the working hypothesis after the examination phase was as follows:

- **Diagnoses** as identified by therapist:
- *Medical*—probable mixed central and peripheral vestibular presentation, without confirmatory medical diagnostics or diagnosis. Further medical workup was requested.
- *PT Rehabilitation*[318]—Primary Problem: Practice Pattern 5D: Acquired impairment of the central nervous system; Secondary Problem: Practice Pattern 5A: Primary prevention of falls
- **Characterized** by (1) space-motion discomfort (SMD) with gaze instability resulting from VOR impairment (probable high gain); (2) central processing impairment; (3) postural control impairment with over-reliance on vision; and (4) limbic high state with autonomic response.
- **Prognosis:** Fair for modified community level independence, physiologically complicated by history (repeated concussions) and chronicity. Improvement intra-trial is a positive physiological sign. However, anxiety overlay and history may have psychogenic versus physiological impact on recovery.
- **Red Flags:** Watch for (1) additional central signs, (2) signs of secondary gain, (3) F^2ARV and GAS limbic cascade, or (3) social service issues.

Phase II: Intervention

1. There are three objectives of the treatment phase driven by findings in the clinical assessment:
   a. Monitor and manage limbic symptoms through environment change of input systems (vision, auditory, kinesthetic) with the goal of the limbic network going neutral if possible.
   b. Maximize sensory integration, central processing, compensatory impairments of the vestibulospinal reflex (balance control) and VOR (gaze control).
   c. Integrate gains in balance and gaze control into functional activity with and without emotional overlays.
2. Treatment approach:
   a. Patient-oriented approach.
      Goal: Maximize internal locus of control and trust; quiet the limbic influence (facilitate limbic neutral) to set an environment appropriate for motor learning and functional change.

Continued

CLINICAL CASE 4.3—cont'd

Techniques:
- Awareness and validation of the problem. Provide the patient with objective findings of organic and functional involvement (sensory organization, dynamic visual acuity, and other testing). Many of these patients have been told for years that it is "in their head." The statement is accurate, but the intent is condescending and implies some psychological dysfunction.
- Awareness of and participation in the plan and approach. The treatment plan should have strong emotional meaning to the patient to turn the "limbic key" to maximize involvement and motivation. It should be goal directed intra- and inter-session. Achieving proper motivation and reward maximizes neuroplastic change.[319]
- Therapeutic Alliance: The correct patient-therapist pairing for effective execution of the plan. Safe clinician contact may actually be part of the rehabilitation plan, with gradual reduction based on limbic and functional improvements.
- Therapeutic Environment: The correct environment to effect change. Use appropriate voice (timbre, pitch, and volume), appropriate pacing (onset of sound or other stimuli), sound, light, consistency, and predictability.

b. Balance retraining using sensory reorganization (reweighting).
   Gaze stability (VOR) retraining
   Goal: Appropriate timing and predictability of sensory treatment: "dose" to achieve desired limbic and functional outcomes.
- Expose the patient to the problematic sensory conditions identified during the examination, presenting first the easier conditions and progressing in terms of difficulty and complexity on the basis of patient response. Force the development of sensory integration, compensation, or substitution, as well as the development of new and appropriate movement strategies.
- Provide for selective attention through predictable, short segments of sensory integrative challenge.
- Avoid sensory overload through proper exercise prescription (intensity, duration, repetitions, and frequency) during sensory integrative treatment.
- Provide for maximal motor learning environment by keeping the limbic network quiet while achieving the correct balance between error detection and correction versus demotivation through making mistakes.
- Provide knowledge of performance and knowledge of results frequently. As one example, computerized visual biofeedback provides direct one-on-one feedback of body position in space and motor performance.

c. Functional activity requires complex integration of balance and gaze control.
- Gait training at controlled pacing in stable environments, progressing to changing pace within predictable visual environments, to unstable visual environments and variable surface environment.
- Hippotherapy (term derived from Greek "hippo" meaning "horse,") is a therapeutic riding activity that is meaningful to the patient. Performed in a controlled environment, the rhythmic cadence provided by the animal provides predictable sensory input (somatosensory, vestibular, auditory, and olfactory), controlled rhythmic visual flow, and neutral warmth in a

meaningful, goal-directed activity (as identified by the patient). This can be a very limbic-neutralizing activity when fear is controlled as a factor.

d. If the patient does not progress in a physiologically normal manner or limbic signs remain unchanged (or increase), then psychological management may take precedent over (or be required before) recovery in rehabilitation (motor learning and neuroplasticity within the CNS) can be achieved.
- Successful life outcome is affected by early management. The extent to which a mild dizziness problem becomes chronic is dependent mainly on the psychological reaction to the symptoms.[310]
- There are specific management strategies associated with anxiety-type disorders within psychology, including use of medications. One theory of recovery from psychology problems is referred to as exposure. Although exposure is meant to cause habituation of the patient to the triggering events, in our case exposure actually will lead to forced use of the appropriate sensory system(s) as required in activities of daily living.

Conclusion

What makes this a clinical problem within the domain of the limbic network is that this woman's limbic network was overriding all other systems. At first glance this person was referred to therapy with typical vestibular and balance dysfunction. She was anything but typical and could not be approached with a "standard protocol," or failure for both the therapist and the patient was inevitable. The role of the patient within this setting was to gain an appreciation and integration of how her vestibular, motor, and limbic networks were interacting and when she went into system overload and why. The therapist's role was to (1) help the patient gain this body awareness, (2) empower the patient with regard to her potential for recovery, (3) design interventions that would nurture patient success, (4) collaborate with the patient on needed interventions regarding practice and novelty within the environment along with consistency of practice, and (5) allow the patient to improve at a pace her CNS could manage.

The long-term permanent changes that may or may not have occurred with this patient's vestibular, motor, or limbic networks are not known. The essential role of complete history taking and dedication to reality by the therapist is obvious. The therapist's success within this case was dependent on her ability to listen and watch (visually, auditorily, and emotionally [limbic]) as the patient unfolded the mystery of her CNS problems. The patient was the key to successfully unlocking her complex subsystem problems. In the health care world of stress, limited visits, and expected outcomes after intervention, it is far too easy to blame the patient for our failure as clinicians. It is also easy to quickly identify that the patient has problems in other system areas outside our scope of practice and thus infer that it is those areas that are limiting improvement. The difficulty is that all professions are doing the same thing, and the patient is drowning in the repercussions of the waves. Partnering interventions both with other professionals and with the patient should optimize an environment that nurtures long-term learning and plastic changes within the CNS. The limbic network drives our attention, our motivation, and our willingness to take risks into unknown environments. How you as a clinician accompany those patients throughout the learning experience will depend on your limbic network as much as theirs.

Although there are physiological reasons underlying the vestibular system disorder in a majority of these cases, the symptoms triggered are part of a spectrum of limbic responses to aberrant vestibular, cerebellar, and brain stem interactions. Normal clinic activity or typically appropriate therapeutic activity may trigger an autonomic cascade versus the desired somatomotor response. The rehabilitation of the resultant visual and postural movement dysfunction is typically more complicated in the absence of limbic network management. The clinician's strategic prescription (or "dosing") of therapeutic activities with

careful monitoring of the patient's emotional system and physiological response will be one of the therapeutic techniques that best controls the aberrant responses and allows vestibular adaptation and compensation to occur. This must be done to manage limbic network activity for successful motor learning to occur.

Developing limbic network assessment tools (or repurposing existing tools) for their ability to screen or identify the presence of direct or indirect limbic involvement is of critical value. In addition, the ability to discriminate the type of limbic involvement (decreased responsiveness and withdrawal from increased responsiveness or overresponsiveness) is important to treatment planning. Treatment techniques will be discussed later in the chapter. However, the specific techniques appropriate for treating these syndromes are tools all therapists possess. These tools range from simple variations in approach (e.g., lighting, sound, and smell) to more formal therapeutic techniques, such as the Feldenkrais approach, or the Bonny Method of Guided Imagery and Music.[320] How each clinician uses those tools is a critical link to success or failure in clinical interaction.

Limbic Influence on Motor Performance and Function

Kandel and colleagues[39] state that functional behavior requires three major systems: the sensory, the motor, and the motivational or limbic systems. When a seemingly simple action, such as swinging a golf club, is analyzed, the sensory system is recruited for visual, tactile, and proprioceptive input to guide the motor systems for precise, coordinated muscle recruitment and postural control. The motivational (limbic) system does the following: (1) provides intentional drive for the movement initiation, (2) integrates the total motor input, and (3) modifies motor expression accordingly, influencing both the autonomic and the somatic somatomotor systems. It thereby plays a role in controlling the skeletal muscles through input to the frontal lobe and brain stem and the smooth muscles and glands through the hypothalamus, which lies at the "heart" of the limbic network (Fig. 4.8).

The motivational or limbic component is further understood to be linked to the NAc, which has been described as the "limbic-motor interface." The NAc has been found in animal studies to link motor responses with the value of expected rewards associated with a given motor plan. The expected reward is encoded with a behavioral response within a given neural signal. The spatial and motor components of a given behavioral response are similarly encoded together, including the timing and accuracy components of a movement. It is important to note that within this encoding process, the predictability of the behavior and reward are critical for activation of the

NAc neurons. This supports the concept that predictability within the therapeutic tasks, environment, and alliance are critical to motivation and, as such, to motor output and learning.[321]

Though *MOVE* has been used to delineate specific functions of the limbic network that drive movement, it is important to remember that these functions are highly interactive and individual. Our unique memory storage, our variable responses to different environmental contexts, and our control or lack thereof over our emotional sensitivity to environmental stimuli all play roles in the expression of our motor output, motor performance, and function. As such, an understanding of the influence of the limbic network on an individuals' function helps further define our need to assess the state of this system—and for those findings to factor into our treatment plans.

To appreciate the sensory system's influential interaction with the limbic network directly, the reader might also look at the literature on music and how it interacts with emotions.[322,323] Most people can give examples of instances where music has elicited immediate and compelling emotional responses of various types. Pleasant and unpleasant musical stimuli have been found to increase or decrease limbic network activity and influence both cognitive and motor responses, although the neurological mechanisms are not completely understood.[324–327] Consider the clinical implications. Reflect on the typical treatment environment: frequent and variable noise, loudspeaker announcements, piped-in music, and a cacophony of therapists' voices can quickly overload the CNS of a patient and result in a limbic response versus a desired motor or functional response. These responses can be highly emotional or *limbic high*, resulting in visceral behavior and affecting motor expression. Alternately, the response may be calming or relaxing to a *limbic neutral* state, allowing for full engagement (motivation, attention) in the movement or task at hand. Musical consonance or dissonance (stable versus unstable) of an auditory stimulus is subjectively experienced by the listener as pleasant or unpleasant. Listening to music uniquely affects limbic emotional states, and the influence may direct the hypothalamus in regulation of blood

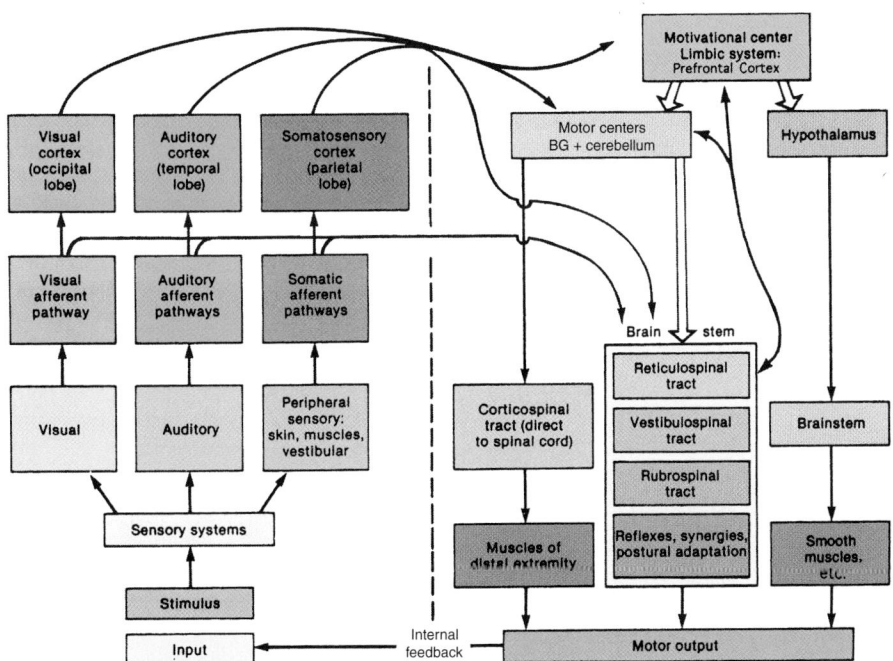

Fig. 4.8 Motivational System's Influence Over the Somatomotor and Autonomic Nervous Systems. (Adapted from Kandel ER, Schwartz JH, Jessell TM. *Principles of Neural Science.* 4th ed. New York: McGraw-Hill; 2000.)

flow within the CNS.[327] With music or sound being just one input system, the therapist must consider that sensory influence from smell, taste, touch, proprioception, and vestibular and organ system dysfunction can lead to potential limbic involvement in all aspects of CNS function and directly affect the emotional stability of the patient.

CLINICAL IMPLICATIONS OF THE LIMBIC STATE

Today the medical profession is rediscovering the importance of how the systems interact with and influence one another.[328,329] Similarly, it is very important for movement specialists to look at movement not only from a biomechanical, muscular, neurological, cardiopulmonary, or integumentary system perspective, but also to accept that interactions between systems highly influences movement. What is less understood, or perhaps considered, by physical therapists are the interactions between the environment and behaviors, learning and movement, including the therapeutic alliance between therapist and patient. Cognitive impairment and limbic network involvement can lead to tremendous errors in motor responses even when the motor system is intact.

Although far from yielding a complete understanding, this research and knowledge are increasing daily and force today's therapist not only to recognize limbic behavior but also to develop an understanding of how involvement of the limbic network will positively and negatively affect the movement of each patient. Therapists can no longer think of motor control and motor learning as controlled exclusively by an anatomically unique motor system, nor can we understand movement using motor control or motor learning principles alone. Therapists must consider how the limbic network strongly influences motor sequencing and control, behaviors that influence function and participation (attention, motivation, and cooperation), as well as beliefs and attitudes. Any of these factors may affect outcomes through influence on engagement or empowerment over treatment planning and/or responsibility for, and compliance with, home programs. Without an understanding of limbic interactions and modulations over motor expression, patient performance and outcomes may show greater variability, even with consistent and accepted interventions. And, given the limitations in today's health care delivery models, stresses, and the growing dependence on home programs, without a keen awareness of the limbic responses of both the patient and the provider, a therapist will have reduced influence over the best functional outcome for their patients.

The complexity of the limbic network and its associated influence over both the motor control system and cortical structures are enormous. A therapist dealing with a patient with motor control or learning problems needs to understand how the limbic network affects behavioral responses and functional performance. This understanding should lead to a greater awareness of the individual factors associated with limbic network involvement, as well as the clinical activities (interventions) and environmental factors that will result in positive neuroplastic change and motor learning. Without this knowledge of how to differentiate limbic from other system dysfunction within the physical therapist evaluation, objective measurements of motor performance or cognitive abilities may be inaccurate, inconsistent, or variable between therapists or sessions without apparent explanation. Similarly, with aberrant limbic activity (high or low), a patient's ability to store and retrieve either declarative or procedural learning may be negatively affected, thus limiting the patient's ability to benefit from traditional interventions or to achieve optimal quality of life.

Examination and Evaluation

Throughout this chapter we have discussed negative limbic influences or states and positive limbic states. Negative limbic states include the overloaded or overactive state, termed *limbic high*, whereas underactive limbic network states can be termed *limbic low* (underactive). The optimal state of any human limbic network is one that is devoid of negative limbic influences, or a *limbic neutral* state. A limbic neutral state provides a strong foundation for procedural learning to occur. We discuss how various disorders are typically associated with negative limbic states in Table 4.1.

Therapists are familiar with the need to prioritize primary body system impairments as they relate to a movement disorder. Moreover, they are familiar with the need to individualize treatment to the primary impairment(s) identified through the evaluation process. Logically, the next consideration for medical and rehabilitative professionals is how we determine or assess the limbic network state of our patients, using qualitative versus quantitative assessment. The master clinician can surmise this intuitively, based upon both observation and experience. But how do we develop this as a requisite skill in our students and colleagues, and can we agree that there is an opportunity to do so? Considering the evidence presented within this chapter, one might challenge that there is a *need* to do so. And if this is true, what existing assessment tools are there to assist us in doing so?

TABLE 4.1	Interactions Among Limbic State, Medical Conditions, and Behaviors	
Limbic State	**Often Associated With**	**Observed Behaviors**
Neutral	Health and wellness	Relaxed state
Low	Depression and stroke	Decreased eye contact and crying Lack of motivation
High	Anxiety and panic disorders Vestibular disorders Mild or traumatic head injury Blast injury, PTSD	Anxiety, anger, fear, increased respiratory rate, higher blood pressure, high muscle tension or tone, and hyperactivity
Overload (F²ARV, GAS)	Traumatic head injury Blast injury, PTSD, frail individual (either young or old), and physiologically unstable individual	Violence, extreme withdrawal, loss of inhibition, and reversal of expected behavior

Many individuals with neurological dysfunction fall into these categories.
GAS, General adaptation syndrome; *F²ARV,* fear and frustration, anger, rage, violence; *PTSD,* posttraumatic stress disorder.

Traditionally, observation was our main assessment tool in the identification of these impairments. Observation of patient presentation and behaviors would provide an astute clinician with insight into the system. It was not included as a standard part of the assessment, but rather a notation of extremes. There are no assessment tools validated to provide insight into the limbic network state. This certainly makes sense given the broad-reaching structural and functional influences of the system as outlined within this chapter. Similarly, beyond strategic management of the environmental stimuli for patients with head injury or clear agitation, there was no clear path from observation to screening to assessment to intervention.

As such, it is recommended that we agree to the importance of elevating the limbic network to a primary body system that has significant, well-established influence over movement. As the movement specialists, it is therefore recommended that we commit to the validation and/or development of screening and assessments of the limbic state. Screening of the system is designed to be binary, ruling individuals either in or out of the limbic impaired group. Just as in the identification of fall risk, high specificity and potential errors in ruling in might be considered. However, despite the absence of such tools, we can propose that observation of limbic-associated presentation and behaviors could trigger a therapist to be alert and to set the therapeutic environment in general. In Table 4.2 we outline the ways in which a therapist might use existing skills and knowledge to quickly screen patients for negative limbic network involvement, with examination of the system if negative influence (*limbic high* or *limbic low* state) is suspected. It might be recommended that all at-risk patients by history, as well as those individuals who have primary or secondary involvement of the limbic structures or have neurochemical risk, undergo examination. The potential population of individuals is described in examples throughout the foundations of this chapter, common disorders summarized at the end of this chapter, and outlined again for the reader here, in the context of the evaluation, in Table 4.2.

Interventions

No single input causes any one or multiple limbic responses, nor does one treatment counteract their progression. Being aware of clinical signs is critical. In a time when therapists are often rushed by the realities of a full schedule or stressed by a third-party or short discharge demands, a clinician may inadvertently miss key signs and opportunities to treat. In addition, he or she may actually create a less optimal environment by physically moving faster than the pace best tolerated by the patient, who may need more time to process stimuli or to practice a target skill. The challenge for both the therapist and the patient is to find harmony within the given environment to allow for optimal outcomes. If a therapist misses these limbic signs that reflect

TABLE 4.2 Patient Evaluation—From Screening Through Examination

	Limbic Low	Limbic High
Observation (behaviors)	*Vision*—decreased eye contact; downward cast eyes *Voice*—low volume and rate and poor articulation *Muscle*—low muscle tone; decreased extensor muscle tone and often increased flexor tone. *Posture*—flexed posture; forward head; and may have flexed extremities, often have poor postural trunk coactivation. *Activity level*—slowed movements/decreased responsiveness or engagement and decreased attention, motivation, and fatigues quickly.	*Vision*—decreased eye contact; darting or scanning eye movement *Voice*—increased rate, variable volume, and poor articulation *Muscle*—high muscle tone; increased extensor muscle tone. *Posture*—extended posture; may have extended extremities. *Sensory*—lower thresholds to stimuli *Activity level*—hyperactive or hypervigilant; "nervous" behaviors (twitching, leg or finger tapping, fidgeting, etc), agitated or irritated engagement; attention deficit.
Systems review	*Skin*—pallor *Respiratory rate/quality*—slowed, shallow or deep; heavy sighs and yawns	*Skin*—can be red, blotchy in color *Sensory*—tactile sensitivity or hypersensitivity; dysesthesias; and Allodynia *Respiratory* rate/quality—rapid and shallow
History	*Psychological*—depression, bipolar depression; grief; substance abuse *Neurological*—left CVA; normal pressure hydrocephalus; acquired cerebral disorders (stroke, tumor, and ventricular disorders); progressive cerebral disorders (PD, MS, ALS, etc) *Cardiopulmonary*—primary cardiac disorders *Chronic disorders/illness*—chronic pain; prolonged hospitalization; multifactorial disequilibrium; and dysequilibrium of aging	*Psychological*—Anxiety? PTSD? Bipolar depression; fear/fear of falling. (Can come from a prior abusive environment) *Neurological*—right CVA; late phase dementia, Parkinson disease; head injury (traumatic of any severity; concussion; blast injury); and vestibular dysfunction *Cardiopulmonary*—primary cardiac disorders; COPD and primary respiratory disorders *Musculoskeletal*—MVA *Social/vocational*—contact sports and military service (with or without blast exposure); domestic violence *Chronic disorders/illness*—chronic pain
Examination (examples, but not limited to)	*Vital signs*—decreased HR, RR, and gait velocity *Tests and measures:* Positive and Negative Affective Scale (PANAS) Depression Anxiety Stress Scales (DASS21) Geriatric Depression Scale (GDS)	*Vital signs*—increased HR, RR, gait velocity *Tests and measures:* Positive and Negative Affective Scale (PANAS) Depression Anxiety Stress Scales (DASS21) Agitated Behavior Scale Ranchos Level of Cognitive Function (RLOCF) Moss Attention Rating Scale

ALS, Amyotrophic lateral sclerosis; *COPD,* chronic obstructive pulmonary disease; *CVA,* cerebrovascular accident; *HR,* heart rate; *MS,* multiple sclerosis; *MVA,* motor vehicle accident; *PD,* Parkinson disease; *PTSD,* post-traumatic stress disorder; *RR,* respiratory rate.

the emotional state of the patient, the patient may perceive that the therapist doesn't truly care about him or her as a person and thus the therapeutic alliance (patient/therapist bond) may be negatively affected.

The positive and negative effects of sensory input or the therapeutic environment on the limbic system, on motor output, and on behaviors are as much a part of the treatment plan as are the therapeutic activities. The *limbic network state* may support or limit consistent responses of the motor systems and thus dampen procedural learning and limit the success of the therapeutic setting. The optimal therapeutic environment for an individual is a positive limbic state where the system is open to learning and not trying to protect or withdraw from the learning environment. This state would be described as *limbic neutral,* or devoid of negative limbic influence, to ensure a strong foundation for both declarative and procedural learning to occur. Carryover of procedural learning into adaptive motor responses needs to be practiced with consistency.[39] If a patient is frustrated or angry and simultaneously has hypertonicity, then a therapist might spend the entire session trying to decrease the abnormal motor response when the causation may be limbic. If the patient could be helped to neutralize the emotional system during the therapy session and achieve a *limbic neutral* state, then the specific problems could be treated effectively and with confidence that whatever motor problems exist are truly motor-driven. Differentiating the limbic network component from the motor control system when establishing treatment protocols has not typically been within the spectrum of a therapist's skills, but is a skill that must be developed and practiced if rehabilitation professionals are to be considered movement specialists.

The critical responsibility of physical therapists is to strategically manage the interaction between sensory inputs of the **therapeutic alliance** and the **therapeutic environment** and thus the activation of the limbic network or *limbic network state.* Successful management of these components, paired with the correct **tasks or therapeutic activities**, serves to set a strong, neutral foundation for effective motor learning to occur. Initially practicing motor skills with a limbic neutral environment will lead to motor learning. The therapist should then slowly introduce limbic stimuli and continue to practice the motor learning. In that way, the motor system learns the control no matter the emotional environment society might introduce.

Therapeutic Alliance: Clinician and Patient

The concept of patient/client-centered therapy has evolved to become an important aspect of health care delivery.[204–206,330–337] The desire to improve or regain function can be self-motivated, but very often is instilled through the clinician to the patient that his or her best interests and unique goals are the focus of the health care team. This belief is based on trust, hope, and attainable steps toward desired and realistic goals, all of which are limbic driven. Patients know when their desires, interests, and needs as unique and valued members of society are considered as part of therapy. They first believe and then recognize that they are persons with specific problems and desired outcomes when the therapist empowers them to link those beliefs to their own therapeutic environment. Although they may have specific medical diagnoses, be placed on clinical pathways, administered drugs, and sent off to the next facility in a couple of days, patients need to feel that they, as individuals, have not lost all individuality and that someone cares. That need is a feeling of security and safety that bonds a patient to a therapist along the journey of learning.[338–340]

Before understanding and becoming compassionate regarding the needs of other people, such as patients with signs and symptoms of neurological problems, therapists need to understand their own limbic network and how it affects others who might interact with

them.[288,341–345] The emotions felt by the therapist learner in pursuit of mastery and the ability to have the intellectual memory of the learning are also limbic functions. These behavioral or limbic responses will play an important role in our own lives, but also may either positively or negatively influence the lives and recovery of our patients/clients, and we will investigate this concept further in this chapter.

Many types of emotions create motivation, such as pleasure, reward processes, emotions associated with addiction, appreciation of financial benefits, amusement, sadness, humor, happiness, and depression.[33,346–350] Some emotions tend to drive learning, whereas others may discourage learning, whether that learning be cognitive or motor. If a person is fearful or apprehensive, motor performance and the ability to learn either a motor skill or intellectual information will be very different[118,293,351–356] from that of an individual who feels safe, is given respect, and becomes part of the decision making process and thus functions inherently with control.[39,209,213,355,357–359]

An individual will naturally have feelings of loss and reservations or fears about the unknown future after injury to any part of the body, but especially the CNS. Yet that individual needs to be willing to experience the unknown to learn and adapt. The willingness, drive, and adaptability of that individual will affect the optimal plasticity of the CNS.[360] The limbic network is a key player that drives and motivates that individual. The lack of awareness of that variable or its effect on patient performance will ultimately lead to questions and doubts about the effectiveness and efficacy of both assessment and intervention results. Similarly, if this system is overwhelmed either internally or externally, it will dramatically affect neuroplasticity and motor learning as well as cognitive, syntactical learning.

At the conclusion of this chapter it is hoped that therapists will comprehend why there is a need to learn to modulate or neutralize the limbic network so that patients can functionally control movement and experience cognitive learning. Then therapists need to strategically reintroduce emotions into the activity and allow the patient to once again experience movement and cognitive success during various levels of emotional demands and environments. This change in the emotional environment will create novelty of the task. This novelty is a critical motivator for learning and will drive neuroplasticity.[361–363]

Yet a therapist deals with the limbic network of patients on a moment-to-moment functional level throughout the day. Fig. 4.9

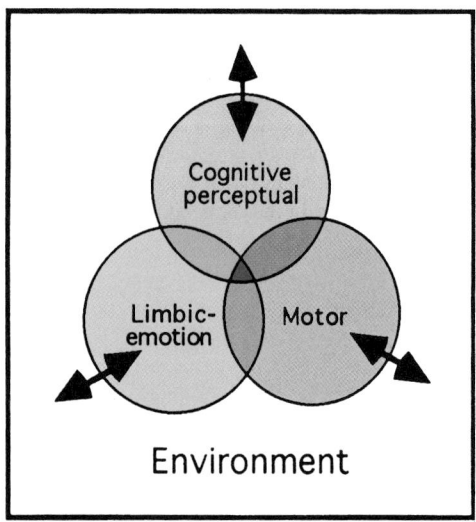

S.S. '94

Fig. 4.9 Interlocking Co-Dependence of All Major Central Nervous System Components.

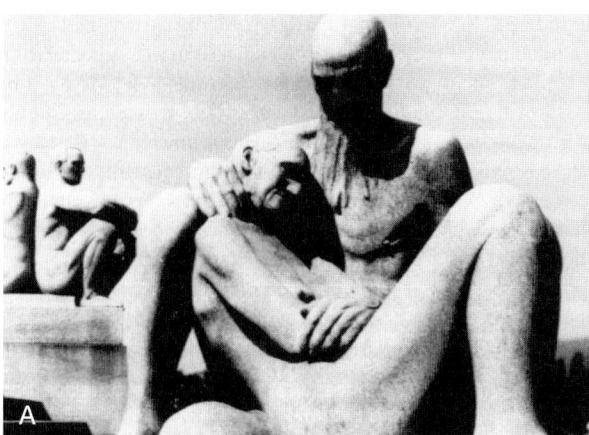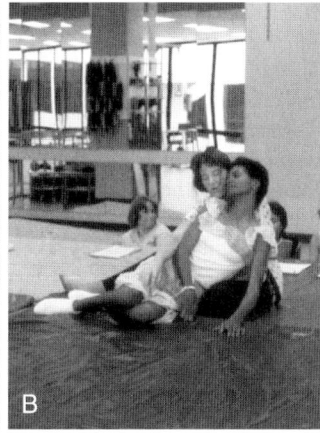

Fig. 4.10 (A) Grief, depression, and compassion responses are seen in the center figures, and rigid, stoic, distancing behaviors are observed in the two left statues. (B) Compassion is easily recognized in the clinic between a therapist and the patient. (A, From Vigelund Sculpture Grounds in the Frogner Park, Oslo, Norway. Adapted from photo by Normann.)

illustrates the interlocking co-dependency of all major CNS components with the environment. At no time does any system stand in isolation. Thus, from a clinical perspective the therapist should always maintain focus on the whole environment and all major interactive components within it, while directing attention to any specific component. How the feedback (internal and external) to the patient's CNS changes the neurochemistry and membrane potential, triggers memory, creates new pathways, or elicits other potential responses is not the responsibility of the clinician or therapist. The responsibility of the clinician is accurate documentation of changes and consistency of those changes toward desired patient outcomes. The professions that focus on movement science are interacting more closely with the neurosciences and other biological sciences and many related professions to unravel many of these mysteries and create better assessment and intervention procedures for future patients.

Because of the potency of the limbic network's connections into the motor system, a therapist's sensitivity to the patient's emotional state would obviously be a key factor in understanding the motor responses observed during therapy. In Fig. 4.10 an entire spectrum of motor responses can be observed in four statues. A patient who feels safe can relax and participate in learning without strong emotional reactions. The woman being held in Fig. 4.10A is safe and relaxed. The man and woman are interacting through touch with deep pressure, warmth, and compassion that are often observed in the patient-therapist interaction of an experienced or master clinician. In Fig. 4.10B, the patient and clinician seem to flow together during the treatment as if they shared one motor system. When looking at the therapist and patient or looking at the man and woman in the statue, it becomes obvious that the two figures seem to flow together. In the statue, those two figures make one piece of art.

With clinical emphasis on patients generating and self-correcting motor programming, it would perhaps seem reasonable for a therapist to conclude that he or she need not, or should not, touch the patient. This conclusion may be accurate when considering the motor system in isolation and assuming that patients can self-correct errors in motor programs. When correction by the therapist is through words rather than touch, external feedback through the auditory system has replaced internal feedback from the somatosensory system. The voice, as well as touch, can be soothing and instill confidence.[364] Yet language in and of itself will not replace the trust and safety felt both physically and emotionally through the deep pressure of touch as illustrated in

Fig. 4.10. Bonding and trust occur much more often through touch than through conversation.[365] Recall, also, that verbal instructions require intact auditory processing and translation from declarative to procedural information, a cognitive ability that the patient may not possess.

Referring again to Fig. 4.10A, the two men in the statue on the left demonstrate a lack of bonding. In fact, if the artist could have brought them closer together, they might just have rejected or repelled each other with greater intensity. If one of the men were the therapist and one the patient, little interaction would be occurring, and thus an assumption that learning is occurring is probably false. The therapist could do nothing to the other person (and vice versa) without that person perceiving the act as invasive, negative, or even disrespectful, with little consideration of the person's individual values. The therapist's responsibility is to open the patient's receptiveness to learning, not to close it.[366,367]

These pictures clearly illustrate two types of therapist-patient interactions, or *therapeutic alliance*. If an artist can clearly depict the tonal characteristics of emotion, certainly the therapist should be able to recognize those behaviors in the patient.[39,368] Achieving a limbic neutral state in the patient through an effective therapeutic alliance is an essential foundation for successful intervention and functional outcome. There are many core tenets and techniques necessary to effectively achieve this neutral state, internal and external therapeutic environment, and optimal performance and learning in the patient. The first component of a successful intervention is self-awareness on the part of the helping professional. "Behavioral activity can often tell us about the inner state of another or ourselves" (p. 19).[369] The willingness to be aware of one's own internal state increases the therapist's ability to perceive subtleties in the patient's responses. Differentiating how a patient learns and emotionally responds to therapy from how the clinician learns and emotionally responds to the patient/therapist bond and to therapeutic environments allows the therapist to create a situation where patient can more easily learn. Subsequently, the therapist must establish predictability for their patient's interventions through *Trust, Responsibility, Flexibility and Openness, and Vulnerability.*

Trust. Trust is a critical component of a successful therapy session.[370] The therapist gains the patient's trust by his or her actions. The therapist may also build trust through sincere acknowledgment that the patient has life-limiting functional problems and that those problems are limiting normal participation. Trust is further developed when the therapist's words can be supported by data. When the therapist can illustrate the presence of functional limitations and generate a treatment plan with the patient using objective data, a bond of trust between the patient and the therapist are created.[371] In today's environment the use of reliable, valid, objective tests and measures allows for this form of communication, which has not existed to the same extent in the past. Honesty and truth lead to trust.[105,372–376]

A trusting relationship is strengthened when an agreement or "contract" can be established that sets the boundaries for discomfort (fatigue, dizziness, nausea, and imbalance) or pain that the patient will experience within a therapeutic session. As one example, telling a person that you will not hurt them is a therapist-patient contract. If the therapist continually ranges a joint beyond a pain-free range, that behavior is dishonest and untruthful and will not lead to trust. Trust can be earned by stopping as soon as the patient verbalizes symptoms or shows pain with a body response such as a grimace. Being sensitive to a patient's pain, no matter the cause, and working with the patient to eliminate that pain often lead to very strong bonding and trust that will lead to compliance and learning. Ignoring the pain may be perceived as insensitivity and lack of caring, which can lead to distrust and often resistance to learning or performance.

As another example, a patient with vestibular dysfunction associated with significant dizziness and nausea will experience symptoms within the course of recovery (adaptation and compensation), but those symptoms must be carefully controlled in intensity and duration. Symptoms poorly controlled can trigger an ANS or GAS cascade and elevate the limbic state, preventing learning and recovery and destroying trust.

Because these symptoms can be overt or covert, the therapist needs to be aware of both the physical and emotional responses of the patient. The use of analog or perceived exertion scales can be a valuable way to make the covert more overt to the therapist. Symptoms are valuable to the therapist as well as the patient to cooperatively create environments for change. The intensity of those stimuli need close monitoring because they can dramatically affect motor responses and ultimately overwhelm the CNS and prevent learning. Compliance to participation is limbic, and the limbic system has tremendous control over intentional movement, no matter the context of the environment.[105]

Once a patient gives his or her trust, a clinician can freely move with the patient and little resistance caused by fear, reservations, or need to protect the self will be felt or observed. When the patient is *limbic neutral* (the limbic network is emotionally neutralized), the tightness or limitations in movement that are present on examination can be considered true impairments within those systems or subsystems. Examination and interventions at this time will more consistently reflect true motor performance. Once limbic neutral has been achieved and examination is complete, it is recommended, for example, that if the pain is a result of peripheral tightness or joint immobility, the therapist does not elicit pain during that session. Deal with those issues in the next session after gaining the trust of the patient. Trust by the therapist or the patient does not mean lack of awareness of potential danger. Trust means acceptance that although the danger is present, the potential for harm, pain, or disaster is very slight and the expected gain is worth the risk (in this case, delay in intervention). In Fig. 4.11, the student's trust that the instructor will not hurt her can be seen by her lack of protective responses and by her calm, relaxed body posture. The student is aware of the potential of the kick but trusts her life to the skills, control, and personal integrity of the teacher. Those same qualities are easily observed in patient-therapist interactions when watching a gifted clinician treat patients. The motor activities in a therapeutic setting may be less complex than in Fig. 4.11, but in no way are they less stressful, less potentially harmful, or less frightening from the patient's point of view.

In addition, therapists must first trust themselves enough to know that they can effect changes in their patients.[17,377] Understanding one's own motor system, how it responds, and how to use one's hands, arms, or entire body to move someone else is based partly on procedural skills, partly on declarative learning, and partly on self-confidence or self-trust. Trusting that one, as a therapist, has the skill to influence the motor response within the patient has a limbic component. If a therapist has self-doubts about therapeutic skills, that doubt will change performance, which will alter input to the patient. This altered input can potentially alter the patient's output and vary the desired responses if the patient's motor system cannot run independently.

Responsibility. Very close to the concept of trust is the idea of responsibility. Accepting responsibility for our own behavior seems obvious and is accepted as part of a professional role.[378] Accepting and

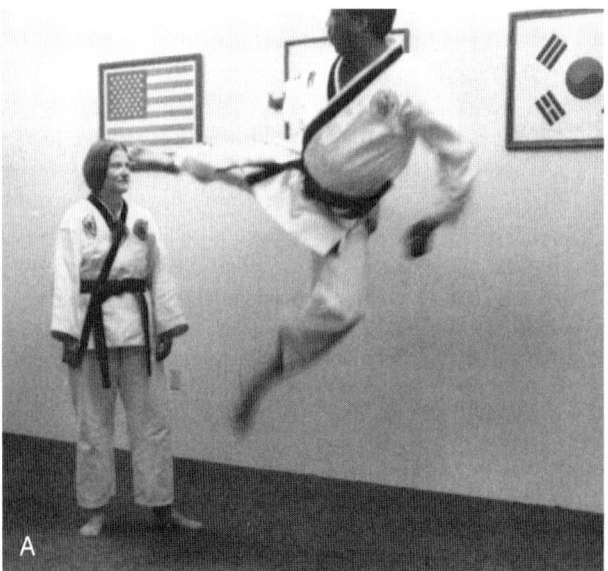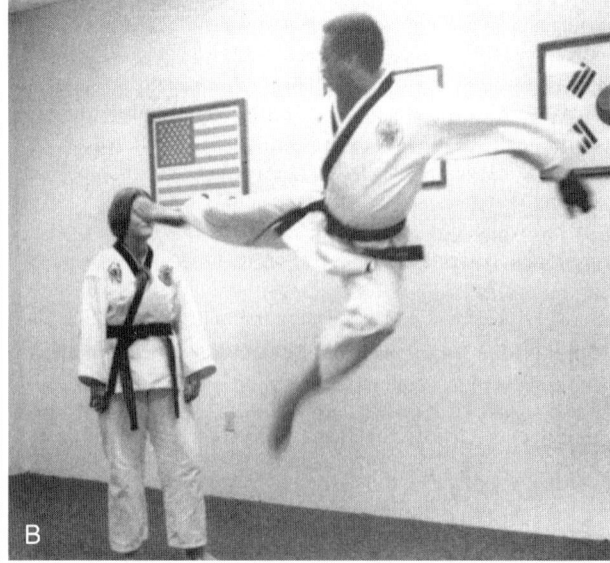

Fig. 4.11 Trust Relaxes the Limbic Network's Need to Protect. **(A)** The skill of the teacher is obvious. **(B)** The student trusts that she is in no danger.

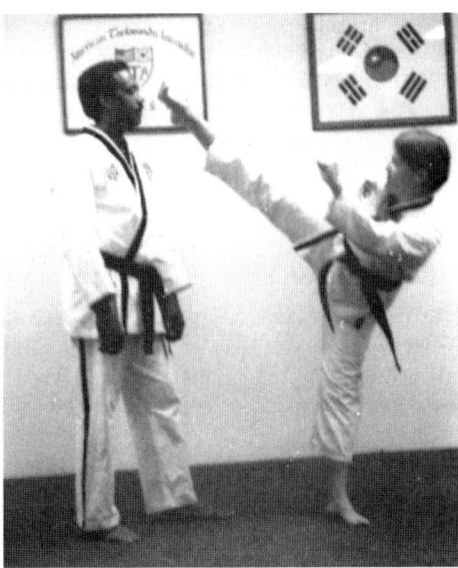

Fig. 4.12 The teacher relinquishes the task to the student, and the student trusts the teacher is right even if self-doubt exists.

allowing the patient the right to accept responsibility for her or his own motor environment are also key elements in creating a successful clinical environment and an independent person.[204–206,318,379,380]

Fig. 4.12 illustrates the concept through the following example: The instructor asked the student to perform a motor act, in this case, to perform a kick to the teacher's head. The kick was to be very strong or forceful and completed. The student was instructed not to hold back or stop the kick in any way, even though the kick was to come within a few inches of the teacher's head. This placed tremendous responsibility on the student. One inch too far might dangerously hurt the instructor, yet one inch too short was not acceptable. The teacher knew the student had the skill, power, and control to perform the task and then passed the responsibility to the student. The student was hesitant to assume the responsibility, for the consequence of failure could have been very traumatic. However, the student trusted that the teacher would not ask for the behavior unless success was fairly guaranteed. That trust reduced anxiety and thus neutralized the neurochemical limbic effect on the motor system of the student, giving her optimal motor control over the act.[381] Once the task was completed successfully, the student gained confidence and could repeat the task with less fear or emotional influence while gaining refinement over the motor skill.

Although the motor activities described in this example are complex and different from functional activities practiced within the clinic by therapists and patients, the dynamics of the environment relate consistently with patient-therapist roles and expectations. A gifted clinician knows that the patient has the potential to succeed. When asked to perform, the patient trusts the therapist and assumes responsibility for the act. The therapist can facilitate the movement or postural pattern through the use of his and her hands and own body movements, thereby ensuring that the patient succeeds. This feeling of success by the patient stimulates motivation for task repetition, which ultimately leads to learning. The incentive to repeat and learn becomes self-motivating and then becomes the responsibility of the patient. As the therapist relinquishes control and empowers the patient to more and more of the function, novelty to the learning is occurring.

Current literature has shown that people are more motivated by novelty and change than by success at mastery or accomplishment of a goal.[96,381,382] The limbic complex and its interwoven network throughout the nervous system play a key role in this behavioral drive.[383] The task itself can be simple, such as a weight shift, or as complex as getting dressed or climbing onto and off of a bus. No matter what the activity, the patient needs to accept responsibility for her or his own behavior before independence in motor functioning can be achieved. Although the motor function itself is not limbic, many variables that lead to success, self-motivation, and feelings of independence are directly related to limbic and prefrontal lobe circuitry. The variance and self-correction within the movement expression also create novelty and motivation to continue to practice.[96,381–384]

As another clinical example of responsibility, in a patient with vestibular dysfunction and dizziness compounded by anxiety, symptoms of dizziness are necessary during treatment to drive CNS change. The therapist has a responsibility to prescribe the appropriate activities, dosage (intensity, timing, and so on), and environment to retrain sensory organization and balance (motor output). The patient can be given the responsibility of monitoring and managing her or his own symptoms within these activities. For instance, empowering the patient to determine the maximal level of dizziness within the therapeutic activity is an example of how the patient and therapist can develop an optimal level of interaction and potential positive therapeutic outcomes. A tool as simple as a verbal or visual analog scale can empower the patient to manage symptoms, dampen the limbic network response, and improve motor output for balance control.

Flexibility and openness. Another component of a successful clinical environment deals with learning and flexibility on the part of the therapist. A master clinician sees and feels what is happening within the motor control output system of the patient. Letting go of preestablished beliefs concerning what will happen is difficult.[385,386] It is important for a clinician to be open to what is present as the motor expression. This openness is critical to actually identifying what is being expressed by the nervous system of the patient. Master clinicians do not get stuck on what they have been taught but use that as a foundation or springboard for additional learning. Learning is constantly correlated to memories and new experiences.

To the therapist, each patient is like a new map, sparsely drawn or sketchy at the beginning, but one that is constantly revised as the terrain (patient's condition) changes. The initial medical diagnosis may link to many paths provided within the map, but the comorbidities can result in great variance among patients.[387] That initial map might be a critical care pathway for the patient, given her or his neurological insult. That pathway is a map, but only a sketchy one, and may not even be a map that a particular patient falls within, in spite of his or her medical diagnosis. It is the therapist's responsibility to evaluate the patient and determine whether that pathway or map will work or is working and when features of that map need to be changed, or altered, further. That is, the therapist must let go of an outdated map or treatment technique and create a new one as the environment and motor control system of the patient change. This transference or letting go of old maps or ideas is true for both the patient and the therapist. If a position, pattern, or technique is not working, then the clinician needs to change the map or directions of treatment and let the patient teach the therapist what will work. The ability to change and select new or alternative treatment techniques is based on the attitude of the therapist toward selecting alternative approaches. Willingness to be flexible and open to learning is based on confidence in oneself, a truly emotional strategy or limbic behavior. Master clinicians have learned that the answers to the patient's puzzle are within the patient, not the textbooks.

Fig. 4.13 depicts two maps, each with a beginning point and a terminal outcome or goal. The parameters of the first map illustrate the boundaries of that therapist's experience and education. The clinician, through training, can identify what would seem to be the most direct

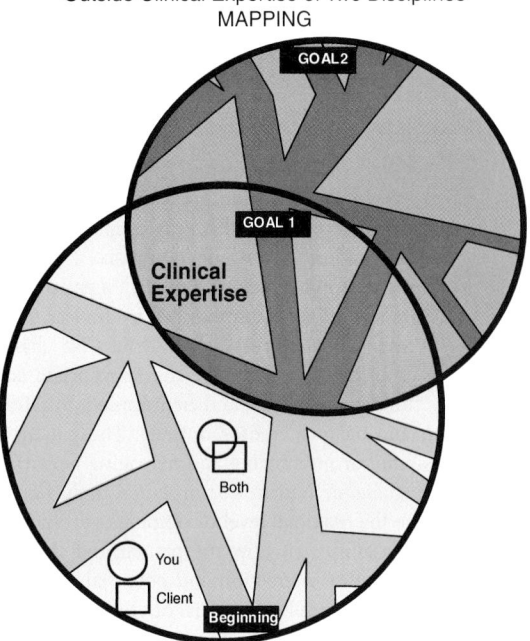

Outside Clinical Expertise of Two Disciplines
MAPPING

Fig. 4.13 Concept of clinical mapping including patient and therapist and the interactions and importance of overlapping professional goals and staying within the professional expertise.

and efficient route toward the mutually identified goal of the therapist and patient. When the patient becomes a participant within the environment or map, what would seem like a direct path toward a goal might not be the easiest or most direct path for the patient. If empowerment of the patient leads to independence, then allowing, even encouraging, the patient to direct therapy may provide greater variability, force the patient to problem-solve, and lead to greater learning. The therapist needs to recognize when the patient is not going in the direction of the goal. For example, the patient is trying to perform a stand-pivot transfer and instead is falling. If it is important to practice transfers, then practicing falling is inappropriate and the environment (either internal or external) needs modification. Falling can be learned and practiced at another time. Once both strategies are learned, the therapist must empower the patient to take ownership of the map. In the examples of transferring, if the therapist asks the patient to practice transfers and if the patient starts to fall, a change in required motor behavior must be made and the opportunity given to the patient to self-correct. In that way the patient is gaining independent control over a variety of environmental contexts and outcomes. Within the same figure (see Fig. 4.13) is a second map. That second map might represent another professional's interaction and goal with the same patient. It is during these overlapping interactions that both professionals can empower the patient to practice, and that practice will help lead to those functional goals established by both practitioners. In some situations, a clinician from one profession may guide a patient toward obtaining the functional skill necessary for a member of the second profession to begin guiding the patient toward the expected outcomes of the second profession. These interlocking dependencies of the patient and the professions are illustrated in Fig. 4.13. If the patient begins therapy striving for the first goal and ends at the functional outcome of the second goal, then additional functional outcomes have been achieved and both professions interacted for the ultimate prognosis for the patient. That interaction requires respect

and openness of both professionals toward each other as well as toward the patient. Those attitudes and ultimate behaviors are limbic-driven.

Matching maps should be a collaborative effort instead of coincidence. These collaborative efforts include interactions with all professions within the rehabilitation setting. Occupational and physical therapists are very familiar with collaboration, and both often approach interventions as a team effort. There are many additional therapists and individuals within that same setting who could also collaborate. Recreational therapists, psychologists, nurses, family members, and music therapists are but a few. Within a profession such as music therapy, the existence of two maps may overlap within a multidimensional environment. When a physical or occupational therapist needs to challenge a patient, the music therapist may be able to calm the system at the same time (overlapping maps). Research on affective responses to consonance and dissonance in music supports the creation of a map within a rehabilitation environment that could overlap with either physical, occupational, or speech therapy. Words such as *relaxed* or *calm* correlated positively with higher levels of consonance in the music, whereas adjectives associated with negative emotions (*unpleasant, tense, irritable, annoying, dissonant,* and *angry*) were found to correlate positively with higher levels of dissonance.[281] Creating a whole environment where potential frustrations within motor learning could be balanced with higher levels of consonance in the music would potentially balance the limbic network emotional response within the overlapping maps and bring balance or stability to the limbic network's influence on motor learning and control. A later study by Peretz and colleagues[327] related the same variables to a happy-sad rating task. Given the research evidence for activity within the limbic network as it relates to music,[323,388] motor learning,[389] and cognitive enhancement,[390] a natural multiple map system would be easy to incorporate within a therapeutic setting. The clinician needs to appreciate the uniqueness of each map while holding onto the concept of the interaction of the two maps.

Vulnerability. To receive input from a patient that is multivariable and simultaneous, a therapist has to be open to that information. If a clinician believes that he or she knows what each patient needs and how to get those behaviors before meeting the patient, then the case falls into a category of a recipe for treating the problem. Using the recipe does not mean the patient cannot learn or gain better perceptual and cognitive, affective, or motor control, but it does mean that the individuality of the person may be lost. A more individualized approach would allow the clinician to identify through behavioral responses the best way for the patient to learn how to sequence the learning, when to make demands of the patient, when to nurture, when to stop, when to continue, when to assist, when to have fun, when to laugh, or when to cry. An analogy might be going to a fast food restaurant versus a restaurant where each aspect of the meal is tailored to one's taste. It does not mean that both restaurants are not selling digestible foods. It does mean that at one eating place the food is mass-produced with some choices, but individuality, with respect to the consumer, is not an aspect of the service. Unfortunately, managed care, limited visits, reduced time for treatment, and therapists' level of frustration all are pushing therapeutic interventions toward a "one size fits all" philosophy that may increase the time needed for learning, not reduce it.

To be open totally to processing the individual differences of the patient, the clinician must be relaxed and nonthreatened, and feel no need to protect himself or herself from the external environment. This environment needs to project beyond the therapist-patient relations and envelop all disciplines interacting with the patient.[391] For these interactions to occur, the clinician's emotional state requires some vulnerability, allowing him or her to be open to new and as-yet-unanalyzed or unprocessed input. This vulnerability implies the role not of an expert who knows the answers beforehand but of an expert investigator. Being open must incorporate being sensitive not only to the variability of motor responses but also to the variability of emotional responses on the part of the patient.[392,393] This vulnerability leads to compassion, understanding, and acceptance of the patient as a unique human being. It can also be exhausting. Therapists need to learn ways to allow openness without taking on the emotional responsibility of each patient.

A clinical example can be used to help identify unique characteristics of the patient that will set the stage for effective learning. A 72-year-old woman has sustained a left CVA. She comes from a low socioeconomic background and was a housekeeper for 40 years for a wealthy family of high social standing. She addresses you (the therapist) with "yes, ma'am" or "no, ma'am" and does just what is asked, no more and no less. It may be very hard to empower this patient to assume responsibility for self-direction within the therapeutic setting. She may not feel she has the right or the power to assume such responsibilities within a setting (a medical facility) that may, from her perception, have high social status. The concept of empowerment may play a crucial role in regaining independent functional skill and control over her environment.[204–206,380,394–396] However, to get optimal outcomes from this patient/clinician interaction, the therapist must find an environment, wherein this person feels worthwhile and empowered to regain functional movement to participate in life activities. This can be very challenging to a therapist but comes automatically to a master clinician. It means that both the patient and the therapist need to be vulnerable and open to the unknown for learning.

Not only does the therapist need to recognize when a patient has not accepted responsibility for motor control or has withdrawn from the therapy environment, but must also notice when the observable motor control is exaggerated by limbic reactions. Newspapers sometimes carry a story that generally reads as follows: "Seventy-nine-year-old, 109-pound arthritic grandmother picks up car by bumper to free trapped 3-year-old grandson." We read these articles and doubt their validity, questioning the sensationalism used by the reporter. But we know that these events are real. That elderly lady picked up the car out of fear of severe injury to her grandchild. Emotions can create tremendously high tonal responses, either in a postural pattern, such as in a temper tantrum, or during a movement strategy, such as picking up a car. Conversely, fear can immobilize a person and make it impossible to create enough tone to run a motor program or actually move. Evaluating muscle power or tone production in relation to emotional state (versus a pure reflection of motor control) is an aspect of evaluation often overlooked.

Therapeutic Environment

The *therapeutic environment* refers to both the internal and external environmental influences upon the individual that may positively or negatively influence a desired therapeutic outcome, and certainly the therapeutic alliance can contribute to that environment. The therapist must establish consistency and predictability within the treatment environment through (1) facilitating or ensuring neutral or stable function of the patient's body systems or milieu; (2) facilitating a limbic-neutral learning environment; and (3) linking reward and other motivational factors to desired motor/task outcomes.

Facilitating the internal environment. First, consider that the structure and function of an individual's body systems influence function of the limbic network and prepare the brain for motor learning. More specifically, the neurobiology must include adequate neurochemicals to enable effective transmission between the key motor learning structures, including the emotional/behavioral prefrontal-limbic "forebrain" system, the cerebellum, and the motor control limbic midbrain and its cortical M1 projections. Similarly, the

environment should avoid oxidative or other stressors that negatively impact effective neurochemical production or transmission.

Nutrition and hydration. The functions of noradrenergic receptors of the locus coeruleus decline in the presence of hyperoxia-induced oxidative stress. The negative effect of hyperoxia and high levels of oxidative stress are blocked by antioxidants, as determined through animal study.[397,398] Foods high in anthocyanin and other antioxidants, or "super foods" such as key legumes, blueberries, cranberries, raspberries, strawberries,[399] etc. have been shown to be neuroprotective during high periods of stress, which can lead to impaired motor learning through "accelerated aging" and cognitive decline. Motor learning and coordination as well as memory are also highly dependent upon calcium. Calcium-dependent plasticity is present in many synapses within the motor output and control loops, and reductions in calcium may result in deficits in long-term potentiation at these various synapses.[400]

Adequate hydration plays a role in behavior (mood, motivation), cognitive (attention), and motor performance. Even small amounts of dehydration (even less than 5%) have been found to impair performance in tasks that require attention, psychomotor, or immediate memory skills.[401]

Sleep and biorhythms. Coordination of circadian body rhythm and sleep are critical for motor performance and learning, and as such, lack of or altered patterns of sleep have a negative effect upon performance and retention.[189,402,403] Sleep influences and is influenced by levels of all of the monoamine neurotransmitters, thus affecting mood, cognition, and learning.[188,189]

Motor learning occurs "off-line" during sleep and is important for memory consolidation that is unrelated to practice. It is likely that procedural memory is consolidated during stage 2 non-rapid eye movement (REM) sleep as well as in REM sleep. Interestingly, sleep of 60 to 90 minutes duration that occurs between practice and retention testing has shown to improve motor task performance when compared with those who stay awake.[189]

Medication compliance and effectiveness. Effectiveness of prescribed medication is a complex issue, extending beyond compliance, with recommended dosing to include evaluation of effectiveness of prescribed dosing. The physical and occupational therapist play an important, supportive evaluative and educational role in both of these areas. Serotonin and dopamine are two key neurotransmitters required for effective motor control, yet endogenous effectiveness can be impaired, and exogenous over- and under-medication can also reduce their effectiveness. In the case of serotonin, in addition to difficulties in determining optimal dosing for effective neuromodulation, up to 50% of individuals with depression are prone to discontinue their prescribed selective serotonin reuptake inhibiting (SSRI) medication.[404] In the case of dopamine, there are two problems; first, the challenges associated with delivery of an effective dose of its precursor, L-dopa; and second, the changing effectiveness of dopamine replacement as the disease progresses in years and severity. Initially, upon starting therapy, the neurons of the substantia nigra are responsive to dopamine replacement, but they lose their sensitivity; the drug's prolonged effectiveness drops after about 10 years of the disease.[405] Within a given day, individuals may experience a sudden improvement of symptoms followed by a rapid decline in symptomatic relief, termed the "On-Off" phenomenon.[406–408] The "On" phase is of longer duration earlier in the disease; efficacy is decreased, and this phase is of very short duration after years of therapeutic dosing. Overmedication can occur.[409] In both cases, evaluation of movement control and/or changes can give the prescribing provider valuable information to assist with achieving optimal dosing.

Achieving an optimal external environment. It is critical that a therapist facilitate a limbic-neutral environment to optimize motor learning. Obtaining a limbic-neutral impact or learning environment is critical before evaluating functional movement to accurately determine true motor system involvement. Highlighting this again as an example, it can be difficult to differentiate hypertonicity resulting from or worsened by stress from true spasticity or clinical hypertonicity. Patient motivation, alertness, and concentration are critical to motor learning because they determine how well we pay attention to the learning and execution of any motor task. These processes of learning and doing are inevitably intertwined: "We learn as we do, and we do only as well as we have learned."[410]

A neutral limbic environment is one that has mitigated all obvious external stressors (extraneous activities or interruptions, visual interference, auditory interference, olfactory interference, etc.) and internal, patient-specific stressors. These patient-specific stressors require observation and intuition on the part of the therapist, and may be triggered by past memories or experiences associated with less obvious individuals or sensory inputs within the environment. The treating professional can also become aware, during assessments or treatments, of environmental sensory input that may trigger stress responses in patients who have limbic network involvement or who may have experienced traumatic physical or emotional injuries. These triggers can be something as simple as the therapist's tone of voice in a sentence to the patient or as complex as the multiple-noise environment of a busy rehabilitation setting. Some patients may need to be scheduled for early morning, during lunchtime, or in the late afternoon to provide a decrease in the auditory environment.

The same awareness can lead a therapist to identify something within the environment that could result in a positive emotional state for learning. Positive emotional states may create a limbic environment in which the therapist can link reward and pleasure associations to new motor sequences. As one example, music or pleasurable sounds can be used to help neutralize or balance the limbic influence on motor expression, as discussed earlier in this chapter and also in Chapter 39. Within the therapeutic environment, it may be advantageous to purposefully facilitate positive or pleasant physical and affective experiences using music before engaging individuals in more challenging therapeutic interventions. Although it may be impractical to provide appropriate music selections on the basis of individual assessment in the therapeutic environment (e.g., physical, occupational, music), other modalities such as heat, massage, or ultrasound treatment may also elicit relaxed, receptive physical states.

Predictability of the environment is also an important consideration. Gentile presents a taxonomy for the acquisition of motor skills. In this taxonomy, Gentile describes a continuum of predictability, from "closed skills" that are highly predictable and self-paced to "open skills" that are less predictable and externally paced.[411] A classic example of closed versus open would be a private room (closed) versus the middle of the gym (open), highlighted above. Closed, predictable activities provide the patient with the greatest control over themselves and their environment.

Decreasing stimulation versus increasing facilitation may lead to attention, calmness, and receptiveness to therapy. When the patient feels that control over her or his life has been returned, or at least the individual is consulted regarding decisions (informed consent as opposed to forced choices), resistance to therapy or movement is often released and stress is reduced. Even patients in a semi-comatose state can participate to some extent. As a clinician begins to move a minimally responsive patient, resistance may be encountered. If slight changes are made in rotation or trajectory of the movement pattern, the resistance is often lessened. If the clinician initially feels the resistance and overpowers it, total control has been taken from the patient. Instead, if the clinician moves the patient in ways her or his body is

willing to be moved, respect has been shown and overstimulation potentially avoided. This highlights the importance of a physical or occupational therapist managing and strategically planning the treatment environment for all patients, not just for those with known head injury or trauma.

Linking motivation and reward. These words are strong and reflect the importance of the limbic network in rehabilitation. Motivated behavior is geared toward reinforcement and reward, which are based on both internal and external feedback systems. Repeated experience of reinforcement and reward leads to learning, changed expectancy, changed behavior, and maintained performance.[80] Emotional learning, which certainly involves the limbic network, is very hard to unlearn once the behavior has been reinforced over and over.[81,82] For that reason, motor behavior that is strongly linked to a negative emotional response might be a very difficult behavior to unlearn. For example, a patient who is willing to stand up and practice transfers just to get the therapist off his back is eliciting a movement sequence that is based on frustration or anger. When that same patient gets home and his spouse asks him to perform the same motor behavior, he may not be able to be successful. The spouse may say, "The therapist said you could." The patient may respond, "I never did like him!" Thus repetition of motor performance with either the feeling of emotional neutrality or the feeling of success (positive reinforcement) is a critical element in the therapeutic setting. Consistently making the motor task more difficult just when the patient feels ready to succeed will tend to decrease positive reinforcement or reward, lessen the patient's motivation to try, and decrease the probability of true independence once the patient leaves the clinical setting. When pressure is placed on therapists to produce changes quickly, repetition and thus long-term learning are often jeopardized, which may have a dramatic effect on the quality of the patient's life and the long-term treatment effects once he or she leaves the medical facility. Motor control theory (see Chapter 3) coincides with limbic research regarding reinforcement. Inherent feedback within a variety of environmental contexts allowing for error with correction leads to greater retention.[83] Repetition or the opportunity to practice a task (motor or cognitive) in which the individual desires to succeed will lead to long-term learning.[84] Without practice or motivation the chance of successful motor learning is minimal to nonexistent.

Goal-directed or need-directed motor actions are the result of the nervous system structures acting as an interactive system. Within this system (see Fig. 4.14), all components share responsibilities. The limbic network and its cortical and subcortical components represent the most important level. In response to stimuli from the internal or external environment, the limbic network initiates motor activity out of the emotional aspect of feeling the need to act. This message is relayed to the sensory areas of the cerebral cortex, which could entail any one or all association areas for visual, auditory, olfactory, gustatory, tactile, or proprioceptive input. These areas are located in the prefrontal, occipital, parietal, and temporal lobes, where they analyze and integrate sensory input into an overall strategy of action or a general plan that meets the requirements of the task. Therefore these cortices recognize, select, and prepare to act as a response to relevant sensory cues when a state of arousal is provided by reticular input. The limbic cortex (uncus, parahippocampal gyrus/isthmus, cingulate gyrus, and septal nucleus) has even greater influence over the somatomotor cortices through the cingulate gyrus, both directly and indirectly through association areas.[412-414] The thalamus, cerebellum, and basal ganglia contribute to the production of the specific motor plans. These messages of the general plan are relayed to the projection system. The limbic structures through the cingulate gyrus also have direct connections with the primary motor cortex. These circuits certainly have the potential to assist in driving fine motor activities through

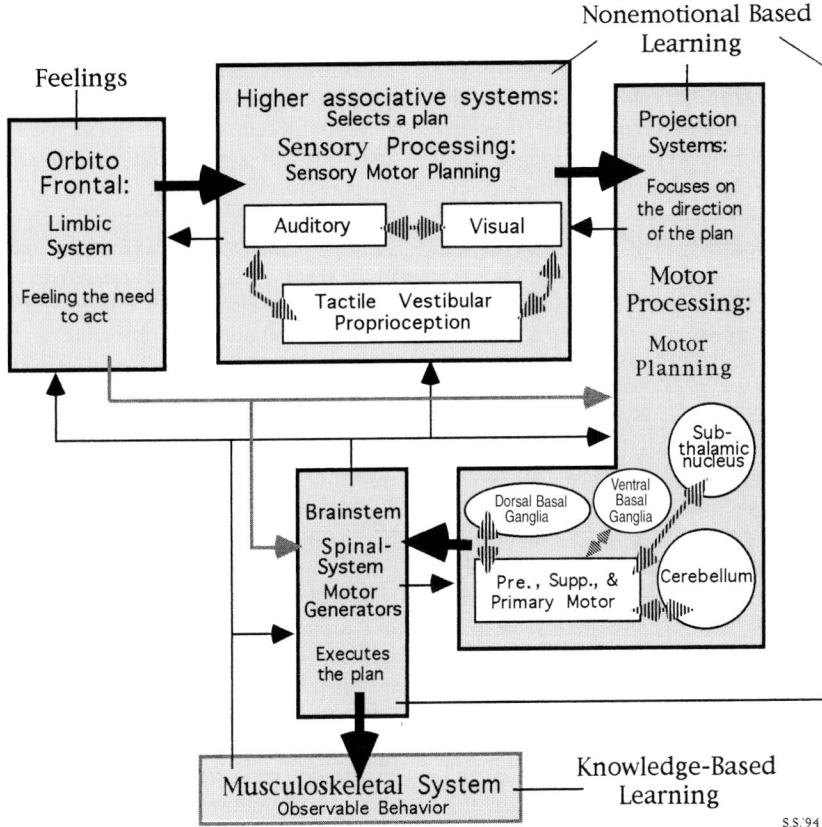

Fig. 4.14 Functional and dynamic hierarchy of systems based on both limbic and motor control interactions. (Adapted from Brooks VB. *The neural basis of motor control*, New York, 1986, Oxford University Press.)

corticobulbar and corticospinal tract interactions. The thalamus, cerebellum, basal ganglia, and motor cortices (premotor, supplementary motor, and primary motor) contribute to the production of the specific motor plans.[39] Messages regarding the sensory component of the general plan are relayed to the projection system, where they are transformed into refined motor programs. These plans are then projected throughout the motor system to modulate motor generators throughout the brain stem and spinal system.[39] Limbic connections with (1) the cerebellum, basal ganglia, and frontal lobe[39,415–419] and (2) the motor generator within the brain stem enable further control of limbic instructions over motor control or expression. If the limbic and the cognitive systems decide not to act, goal-driven motor behavior will cease. An individual's belief (emotional and spiritual) can inhibit even the most basic survival skills, as has been clearly shown in history when individuals with particular religious beliefs were pitted against vicious predators and those people chose not to defend themselves.

Within the projection system and motor planning complexes, the specifics are programmed and the tactics are given a strategy. In general, "what" is turned into "how" and "when." The necessary parameters for coordinated movement are programmed within the motor complex as to intensity, sequencing, and timing to carry out the motor task. These programs, which incorporate upper motor neurons and interneurons, are then sent to the brain stem and spinal motor generators, which in turn, through lower motor neurons, send orders regarding the specific motor tasks to the musculoskeletal system. The actions performed by each subsystem within the entire limbic–motor control complex constantly loop back and communicate to all subsystems to allow for adjustments of intensity and duration and to determine whether the plan remains the best choice of responses to an ever-changing three-dimensional world.[60,416,417]

The limbic network has one more opportunity to modify and control the central pattern generators and control the body and limbs through direct connections to the spinal neuronetwork.[135,199,420–422] That is, the limbic network can alter existing motor plans by modulating those generators up and down or altering specific nuclear clusters and varying the patterns themselves. Therapists as well as the general public see this in sports activities when emotions are high, no matter the emotion itself. Individuals who have excellent motor control over a specific sport may find high-level performance difficult as the stress of competition increases. Having control over emotional variance as well as motor variance with a functional activity is an accurate example of empowerment. Thus for a therapist to get a true picture of a patient's motor system function, the limbic network should be flowing in a neutral or balanced state without strong emotions of any kind. Generally, that balance seems to reflect itself in a state of safety, trust, and compliance. Once the motor control has been achieved, then the therapist must reintroduce various emotional environments during the motor activity to be able to state that the patient is independent.

In summary, the limbic complex generates need-directed motor activity and communicates that intent throughout the motor system.[199,421,423,424] This step is vital to normal motor function and thus patient care. Patients need the opportunity to analyze correctly both their internal environment (their present and feedforward motor plans and their emotional state) and the external world around them requiring action on a task. The integration of all this information should produce the most appropriate strategy available to the patient for the current activity. These instructions must be correct, and the system capable of carrying out the motor activity, for effortless, coordinated movement expression to be observed. If the motor system is deficient, lack of adaptability will be observed in the patient. If the limbic complex is faulty, the same motor deficits might present themselves. The therapist must differentiate what is truly a motor system problem versus a limbic influence over the motor system problem.

Schmidt[425] stresses the significance of "knowledge of results feedback" as being the information from the environment that provides the individual with insights into task requirements. This insight helps the motor system correctly select strategies that will successfully initiate and support the appropriate movement for accomplishing the task. This knowledge of results feedback is required for effective motor learning and for forming the correct motor programs for storage.[426,427]

The reader may better understand the role of the limbic network in motor programming through a nonmedical example. Imagine that you are sitting in your new car. The dealer has filled the tank with necessary fuel. The engine, with all its wires and interlocking components, is totally functional. However, the engine will not perform without a mechanism to initiate its strategies or turn on the system. The basal ganglia or frontal lobe motor mechanism plays this role in the brain. The car has a starter motor. Yet the starter motor will not activate the motor system without the driver's intent and motivation to turn the key and turn on the engine. The limbic complex serves this function in the brain. Once the key has been turned, the car is running and ready for guidance. Whether the driver chooses reverse or drive usually depends on prior learning unless this is a totally new experience. Once the gear has been selected, the motor system will program the car to run according to the driver's desires. It can run fast or slow, but for the plan to change, both a purpose and a recognition that change is necessary are required. The car has the ability to adapt and self-regulate to many environmental variables, such as ruts or slick pavement, to continue running the feedforward program, just as many motor systems within the CNS, especially the cerebellum, perform that function. The limbic network may emotionally choose to drive fast, whereas one's cognitive judgment may choose otherwise. The interactive result will drive the pedal and brake pressure and ultimately regulate the car. The components discussed play a critical role in the total function of the car, just as all the systems within the CNS play a vital role in regulating behavioral responses to the environment.

Brooks[8] distinguishes insightful learning, which is programmed and leads to skills when the performer has gained insight into the requirements, from discontinuous movements, which need to be replaced by continuous ones. This process is hastened when patients understand and can demonstrate their understanding of what "they were expected to do." Improvement of motor skills is possible by using programmed movement in goal-directed behavior. The reader must be cautioned to make sure that the patient's attention is on the goal of the task and not on the components of the movement itself. The motor plan needs programming and practice without constant cognitive overriding. The limbic/frontal system helps drive the motor toward the identified task or abstract representation of a match between the motor planning sequence and the desired outcome. The importance of the goal being self-driven by the patient cannot be overemphasized.[200,204–206,428,429]

Without knowledge of results, feedback, and insight into the requirements for goal-directed activity, the learning is performing by "rote," which merely uses repetition without analysis, and meaningful learning or building of effective motor memory in the form of motor holograms will be minimal. Children with cognitive and limbic deficits can learn basic motor skills through repetition of practice, but the insights and ability to transfer that motor learning into other contexts will not be high.

Schmidt[425] suggests that to elicit the highest level of function within the motor system and to enable insightful learning, therapy programs should be developed around goal-directed activities, which means a

strong emotional context. These activities direct the patient to analyze the environmental requirements (both internal and external) by placing the patient in a situation that forces development of "appropriate strategies." Goal-directed activities should be functional and thus involve motivation, meaningfulness, and selective attention. Functional and somatosensory retraining uses these concepts as part of the intervention. Specific techniques such as proprioceptive neuromuscular facilitation, neurodevelopmental therapy, the Rood method, and the Feldenkrais method can be incorporated into goal-directed activities in the therapy programs, as can any treatment approach, as long as it identifies those aspects of motor control and learning that lead to retention and future performance and allows the patient to self-correct.[425] With insights into the learned skills, patients will be better able to adjust these to meet the specific requirements of different environments and needs, using knowledge of response feedback to guide them. The message then is to design exercise activities or programs that are meaningful and need-directed, to motivate patients into insightful goal-directed learning. Thus understanding the specific goals of the patient, patient-centered learning, is critical and will be obtained only by interaction with that patient as a person with needs, desires, and anticipated outcomes.[430,431] A therapist cannot assume that "someone wants to do something." The goal of running a bank may seem very different from that of birdwatching in the mountains, yet both may require ambulatory skills. If a patient does not wish to return to work, then a friendly smile and the statement, "Hi, I'm your therapist, and I'm going to get you up and walking so you can get back to work," may lead to resistance and decreased motivation. In contrast, a therapist who knows the goal of the patient may help him or her become highly motivated to ambulate; that patient may be present in the clinic every day to meet the goal of birdwatching in the mountains, although never wishing to walk back into the office again.

Therapeutic Activities

Strategic exercise prescription has a significant effect upon limbic activity and motor learning. First, exercise has a positive effect on high and low limbic network states, such as seen in chronic stress, anxiety (high), or in depression (low), for example. A recent Cochrane Collaboration Review investigated the effect of exercise upon depression through meta-analysis.[432] Though there were methodological errors, the authors were able to conclude that exercise is moderately more effective than a control intervention for reducing symptoms of depression, but not more effective than psychological or pharmacological interventions alone. Individuals with depression can be considered to exhibit a low limbic state, which has been discussed as impairing motor learning. No similar systematic review has been published through the Cochrane Collaboration for anxiety. No Clinical Practice Guidelines could be identified to guide exercise prescription for the depression or anxiety populations, which would be reflective of limbic network involvement.

Exercise similarly establishes an internal environment favorable for neuroplasticity and for neuroprotection. Specifically, high-intensity aerobic exercise facilitates an exercise-induced response of peripheral brain-derived neurotrophic factor (BDNF), which improves the ability to achieve neuroplastic change and motor learning.[433] For a discussion of neuroplasticity and the positive effects of exercise on neuroplastic change and motor learning in the cortex, the reader is referred to Chapter 3. What is less discussed is the effect of exercise on interaction between motor and limbic networks for effective motor learning.[434] High intensity exercise also improves neurotransmission of dopamine and glutamate in the basal ganglia, both of which play important roles in the initiation and control of movement.[435,436] As such, a positive neuroprotective effect can decrease the rate of degeneration of the dopaminergic cells within the basal ganglia; this can reduce the amount of medication required by an individual to control their symptoms and improve learning and carry-over to function.

Patient education concerning all aspects of limbic network influence on motor performance and learning can provide insight, enabling patients to achieve acceptance and engagement. In particular, education in those aspects of their internal and external environment within their control (sensory inputs, sleep, pharmacological management, etc.) may help maximize patients' participation in interventions, activities, and in societal roles.

Emerging Interventions

Advances in surgical neuromodulation of the limbic circuitry underlying these disorders offer hope for individuals suffering from addiction, PTSD, or memory disorders. Emerging evidence shows that deep brain stimulation (DBS) to specific nuclei within the limbic system may be at least as successful as traditional pharmacological therapies to improve dynamic memory and learning processes.[437] In a single patient case investigation, Freund and colleagues reported that treatment with DBS of the nucleus basalis in the basal forebrain enhanced the synthesis of nerve growth factor, resulting in markedly improved cognitive function, specifically attention, concentration, alertness, and drive.[438] The critical importance of these cognitive functions to motor learning has been stated frequently throughout the evidence presented within this chapter.

Advancements in genetic profiling and genetic modification bear close attention, with meaningful influence upon all aspects of brain function. As one example, it is understood that adequate dopamine must be present for brain plasticity, motor skill acquisition, and motor learning, given projections from the midbrain VTA to the M1 primary motor cortex.[52] Electrical stimulation of the VTA resulted in improved function of the dopaminergic pathway and improved expression of the gene c-fos in M1 by more than 142%, which has been shown to improve the function of the primary motor cortex. Five genetic polymorphisms have been identified as having effect upon dopaminergic neurotransmission. Specifically the DRD2/ANKK1 genotype has been significantly associated with motor learning and its modulation through medication management of dopamine precursors (L-dopa).[439] These genetic variations help to explain the individual differences in patient response to medications designed to improve motor performance (in Parkinson disease [PD]); insight into pharmacological management can be based upon these biological subgroups. The knowledge of genetic variation and specific polymorphisms that negatively impact motor learning can direct future efforts in genetic modification. The knowledge of genetic advancements may assist physical and occupational therapists to help their patients understand their unique positive, neutral, or negative responses to interventions or pharmacological management.

COMMON DISORDERS WITH LIMBIC NETWORK PROBLEMS

Throughout the existence of humankind, emotions have been identified in all cultures. A child knows when a parent is angry without a word being spoken. A stranger can recognize a person who is sad or depressed. People walk to the other side of the road to avoid being close to someone who seems enraged. Emotions are easily recognizable as they are expressed through motor output of the face and body. Emotions similarly have an impact on functional motor control. The effect and intensity of emotions and limbic influence on motor control are an important part of the therapy evaluation. Many lesions or neurochemical imbalances within the limbic network drastically affect the success or failure of physical, occupational, and other therapy programs. This chapter does not discuss in detail specific problems and their treatment, but instead it is hoped that identification of limbic involvement may help the reader develop a better understanding of its role in specific medical disorders or neurological conditions. Table 4.1 helps differentiate the level of limbic activity with observed behavioral states cross-referenced with various medical conditions.

Grief, Depression, and Anxiety

Notably, 6.7% or 162 million people had at least one major depressive episode in the past year.[440] Depressive disorders are the sixth-most-costly health condition and the most costly among mental health and substance abuse disorders, with $71 billion spent in 2013.[441]

Dysregulation within the structures of the cortico-limbic network play a role in clinical depression and the major depressive disorders (MDD).[442–444]

Individuals with MDD demonstrate changes in volume within key limbic structures, specifically lower cingulate (cognitive division) volume and higher amygdala volumes. Individuals with clinical depression also demonstrate changes in neurochemistry, primarily associated with a reduction of *serotonin* production.[192] Ascending serotonergic tracts start in the raphe nuclei of the midbrain and ascend to the limbic forebrain and hypothalamus; they are concerned with mood and behavior regulation.

Emotions such as depression or grief can be expressed by the motor system, typically classified within a limbic low state.[39,445] Thus the observed or behavioral responses are usually withdrawal, decreased postural extension with increased flexion, and reported feelings of fatigue and/or exhaustion (see Fig. 4.15A and B). Sensory overload, especially in the elderly, can create low muscle tone and excessive flexion. Again, because of the strong emotional factor, these motor responses are considered to be the result of the limbic network's influence over motor control.[199] These individuals can develop an associated sense of learned helplessness, which therapists should identify in an effort to mitigate it.[277] When patients are encouraged or allowed to become dependent, their chances of benefiting from services and regaining motor function are drastically reduced.[446,447]

Fear

Fear is an emotional response and thus is initiated and controlled by the limbic network, specifically the reticulolimbic network.[39,74] The amygdala recognizes the significance of stimuli, adds the "emotional weight" to sensory experiences or memory, and assigns it with a feeling associated with the need to act. That ascribed "need" to act can be either appropriate, exaggerated, or accelerated. The resultant response or action can either be commensurate with the need (realistic), or can generate an inappropriate response, such as a GAS or F²ARV response. Fear typically is associated with a limbic high state, but can, over prolonged periods of the stress associated with fear, result in a general adaptation avoidance or limbic low state.

Fig. 4.16A illustrates two people riding a rollercoaster, which may or may not generate emotions of fear. The boy looks scared and obviously exhibits fear. However, the woman's expression could be one of either joy or fear, based upon her motor responses. Her facial expression with fixed eyes could represent a limbic motor reaction, which could be a semiautomatic fear response. The amygdala nuclei also play a critical role in regulation of facial responses to fear, pain, or other incoming stimuli.[448] In Fig. 4.16B, the rollercoaster has stopped, and she still has the same expression. In fact, it took over a minute before she was able to relax her face and regain the feeling that she had some control over her emotional reaction. This was followed by crying and observable frustration at her inability to control her initial response.

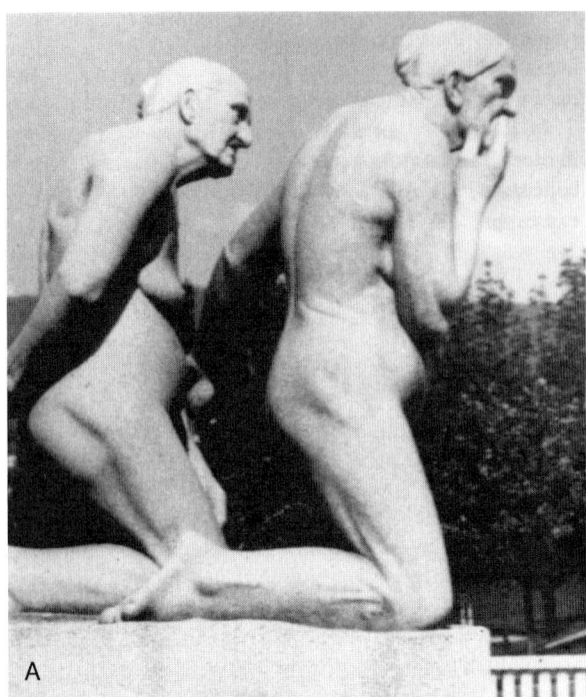
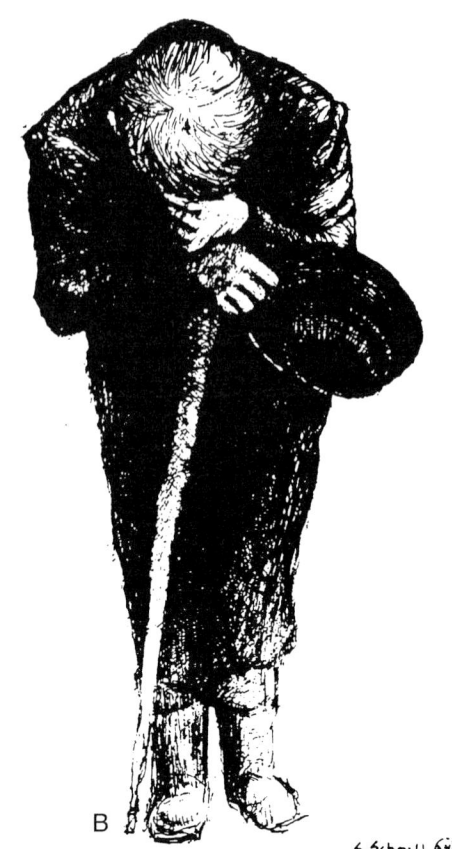

Fig. 4.15 **(A)** Behavior responses elicited by concern, pain, and grief. **(B)** Pain or grief elicits flexion and can modify postural extension. (**A,** From Viegelund Sculpture Grounds in the Frogner Park, Oslo, Norway. Adapted from photo by Normann.)

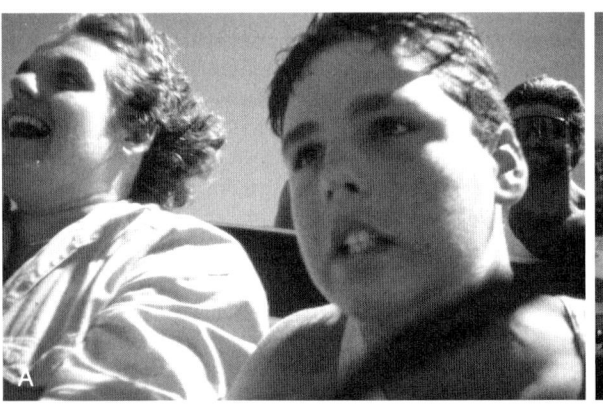
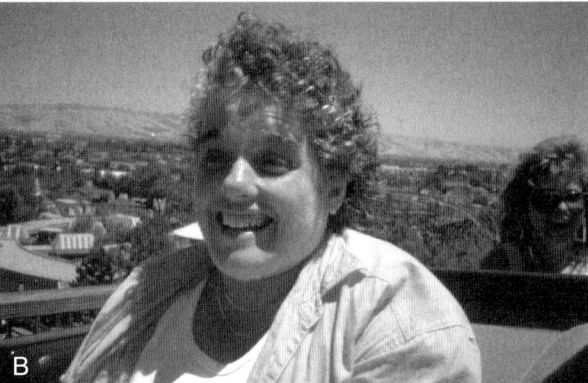

Fig. 4.16 **(A)** Two individuals riding a roller coaster. Individual on right looks scared; this facial expression represents fear. The facial expression of the individual on the left could represent enjoyment, with eyes open and a smile, or extreme fear, with hyperextension of her head causing her mouth to open. **(B)** Individual's facial expression after the roller coaster stopped. She was unable to relax her facial muscles for more than 2 minutes because she had been so scared or demonstrated extreme fear.

These responses are often observed in healthy normal individuals such as those seen in Fig. 4.6, but similarly can be seen in patients who are extremely fearful, no matter the cause.

Fear of falling is a common problem in the elderly, especially in those individuals who have functional limitations resulting from a neurological disorder.[449,450] Therapists working with individuals who have a fear of falling need to first acknowledge that the fear is normal and then must establish a strong therapeutic alliance. That therapeutic alliance must establish trust of the clinician and predictability for the patient and provide the patient with maximal opportunity for control over their mobility and safety during interventions. The specifics of the therapeutic alliance were previously discussed in this chapter.

Fear of pain is another emotional response housed within the limbic network that drives many individuals' motor responses. Whether individuals have fear of movement after a musculoskeletal injury,[448] fear of going to the dentist after a dental procedure,[451] fear of pain intensity after a chronic pain problem,[452] or fear of falling,[453] fear will drive motor responses, and that fear will often lead to a lower quality of life.[449] For that reason alone, therapists need to differentiate the limbic system's and the motor system's summated responses when observing the movement patterns of the individual in therapy.

Anxiety and Posttraumatic Stress Disorder

Individuals with anxiety disorders display excessive anxiety and behavioral disturbances that can interfere with daily activities. An estimated 19.1% of US adults had any anxiety disorder in the past year; 31.1% experience anxiety at some point in their lifetime.[454] These individuals can be classified between a limbic neutral and a limbic high state at baseline.

PTSD is considered an anxiety disorder that specifically develops following a traumatic event, typically one that is life-threatening. It includes perceptual, cognitive, affective, physiological, and psychological components, and is characterized by emotional dysregulation, a hyperarousal state, vivid and intrusive memories of the event(s), and exaggerated fear-avoidance behaviors.[455] An estimated 3.6% adults were diagnosed with PTSD in the past year, with a lifetime prevalence of 6.8%. Of those, 30.2% of cases are categorized as "mild" and as such, represent highly functional individuals.[456] However, even the most "mildly" affected of these individuals can most typically be classified within a limbic high state at baseline.

PTSD as a disorder can be a sequelae of many types of trauma associated with emotion, including mild head injury or concussion from accident or domestic abuse, or a frightful experience such as a near-drowning. This problem is especially apparent when treating soldiers injured on the battlefield who have returned home; it is considered a signature injury of war-related activities.[457] The presence of lower density in the limbic and para-limbic cortices was found to be associated with a diagnosis of PTSD, the degree of trauma, and psychotherapy treatment outcome from eye movement desensitization and reprocessing (EMDR).[458]

A therapist always needs to understand the environment within which the injury occurred, as well as being aware of preexisting complications. In an injury sustained in a violent confrontation or in a frightful experience, the emotional system was at a high level of metabolic activity at the time of the insult. With knowledge of that information, a therapist should assess the state of the limbic network for high (anxiety, fear) or low (depression, avoidance) influence.

Both environmental noise and "background" music, such as present in many clinics, may present in auditory triggers that elicit limbic network and ANS activity, with the potential for eliciting the F²ARV continuum. In treating more than 200 patients following trauma, Körlin[459] found that certain kinds of musical elements often triggered intrusive and traumatic re-experiences of the event. (For a theoretical discussion of this phenomenon, see Goldberg.[460]) The phenomenon of auditory triggering has implications for the rehabilitation setting, where patients may be recovering from traumas related to accident, injury, or difficult medical procedures.

Suicide and domestic violence have become a more common occurrence between deployments, necessitating a dramatic shift in mental health policy in the last 5 years.[461–464]

Anger

Anger itself creates muscle tone through the amygdala's influence over the basal ganglia and the sensory and motor cortices and their influence over the motor control system. This is clearly exhibited in a child throwing a temper tantrum (see Fig. 4.17) or an adult putting his fist through a wall. How far a patient or a friend will progress through the F²ARV continuum (discussed earlier within this chapter) depends on a large number of variables. When a patient loses control, the therapist must first determine whether the intervention forced the patient beyond her or his ability to control. If so, changes within the therapeutic environment need to be made to allow the patient opportunities to develop control and modulation over that continuum.

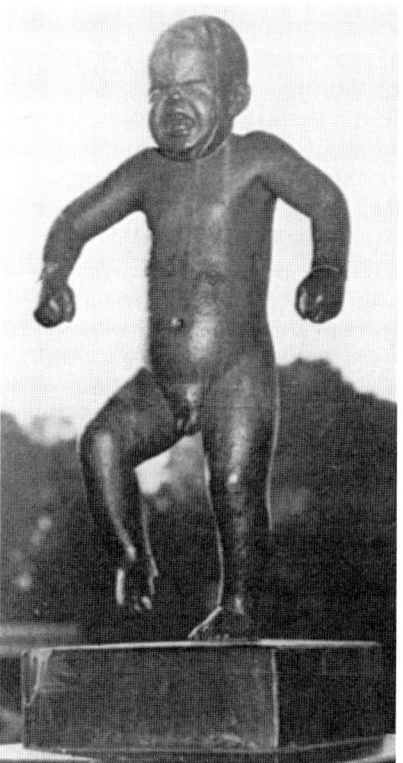

Fig. 4.17 Extensor behavior responses caused by anger. (*Angry Boy*, Vigelund Sculpture Grounds in the Frogner Park, Oslo, Norway.)

Creating opportunities to confront frustration and fear or even anger in real situations while the patient practices modulation will lead to independence or self-empowerment. The patient simultaneously needs to practice self-directed motor programming without these emotional overlays. Thus true motor learning can result. In time, practicing the same motor control over functional programs when confronted with a large variety of emotional situations should lead to independence in life activities and thus meet a therapeutic goal.

Similarly, being unaware of a patient's anger may lead the therapist to the false assumption that that individual has adequate inherent postural tone to perform activities such as independent transfers. If the patient is angry with the therapist and performs the transfer only to get the therapist "off my case," when the patient is sent home she or he may be unable to create enough postural extension to perform the transfer. Thus this transfer skill was never functionally independent because the test measurements were based on limbic or frontal influence over the extensor component of the motor system. The patient needs to learn how to do the activity without the emotional overlay. When a therapist is unwilling, unaware, or unable to attend to these variables, the reliability or accuracy of functional test results becomes questionable.

Substance Abuse and Dependence

The National Institutes of Health National Institute on Drug Abuse (NIDA) has estimated the annual cost related to substance use disorders, crime, lost work productivity, and health care to the United States at more than $740 billion annually.[465]

The NIDA Division of Neuroscience and Behavior (DNB) advances the science of substance abuse and addiction through basic and clinical research. Whether medical, illicit, or recreational (such as in alcohol consumption), drugs and alcohol can have dramatic effects on the CNS and often are associated with limbic behavior.[466] A large body of animal and human evidence over the last several decades has shown that the mesocorticolimbic reward pathway plays a critical role in the process of addiction. The NAc is a critical structure within that neural circuitry that contributes to reward processing, goal-directed behavior and motivation.[437] Recent research has investigated the effect of bilateral stereotactic ablation of the NAc in humans to block the mesocorticolimbic dopamine circuit, resulting in the reduction of drug-seeking behaviors in individuals addicted to opioids. Although full remission has not yet been achieved, decreased symptoms of withdrawal were experienced making it a viable future treatment option.[467]

Korsakoff's syndrome is perhaps the most well-known of the disorders resulting from chronic alcoholism and its related nutritional deficiencies. This syndrome is identified by the structural involvement of the diencephalon, specifically the mammillary bodies and the dorsal medial and anterior nucleus (AN) of the thalamus[39] (see the anatomy section and Fig. 4.4). The most dramatic sign observed in a patient with Korsakoff syndrome is severe memory deficits.[447,468–470] These deficits involve declarative memory and learning losses, but the most predominant problem is short-term memory loss.[471] As the disease progresses, patients generally become totally unaware of their memory loss and are unconcerned. Initially, confabulation may be observed,[472] but in time most patients with a chronic condition become apathetic and somewhat withdrawn and are in a profound amnesic state. They are trapped in time, unable to learn from new experiences because they cannot retain memories for more than a few minutes and are unable to maintain their independence[447,468–470,473]; many may become social isolates and homeless. Beyond the notable implications to motor learning through rehabilitation processes, the severe memory limitations paired with the lack of insight into those losses should be considered within the management plan from a safety and a behavioral point of view.

The use of alcohol affects not only adults but also children and adolescents. Still another population of children affected by alcohol abuse has surfaced as a specific clinical problem. These children are infants who have the effects of fetal alcohol syndrome. A variety of researchers have investigated the effects of alcohol and other toxic drugs on neuromotor and cognitive development.[474–479]

The use of systemic drugs such as cocaine and alcohol can lower the threshold for seizures. Cocaine reduces seizure threshold in patients with underlying epilepsy (direct toxic effect) or indirectly by contributes to poor compliance with antiepileptic medications, poor diet, or poor sleep habits.[480] The anterior temporal lobe and its connections with the hippocampus and amygdala have a lower threshold for epileptic seizures than do other cortical structures.[39] These seizures are often accompanied by sensory auras and alterations in behavior, with specific focus on mood shifts and cognitive dysfunction.[481] Similarly, the AN of the thalamus is an integral part of the limbic system that plays a role in modulating alertness and is involved in learning/memory, but is also associated with intractable seizures. DBS of the AN has been shown not only to reduce seizure activity, but also to improve learning.[482]

Obviously, the precise association between behavior and emotions or temporolimbic and frontolimbic activity is not understood, yet the associations and thus their impact on a therapeutic setting cannot be ignored.[294,483]

Disorders of Cognition and Memory

The most challenging of the disorders of cognition and memory is Alzheimer disease. The reader is referred to Chapter 27 for a detailed description and discussion. But relative to the limbic network, the hippocampus and nucleus basalis are the most severely involved structures, with associated neurofibrillar degeneration of the anterotemporal, parietal, and frontal lobes.[181–183,447,484] The initial symptoms fall into emotional, social, and cognitive categories. Depression and

anxiety often are seen during the early phases because of the neuronal degeneration within the prefrontal lobes and limbic network.[183,485–487] During the second stage, the emotional, social, and intellectual changes become more marked. Patients have difficulty with demands, business affairs, and personal management. Their memory and cognitive processing continue to deteriorate, whereas their awareness of the problem is often still insightful, causing additional anxiety and depression. During this phase patients may be unable to recognize familiar objects and become fearful because they are losing control of the environment both internally and externally. Thus the patient may become combative out of a defensive autonomic "fight-or-flight" response. For that reason, therapists need to make sure the patient feels safe during therapy to optimize learning and compliance.

The third phase of advancing Alzheimer disease manifests itself with moderate to severe aphasia, apraxia, and object agnosia, or the failure to recognize objects. Distractibility and inattentiveness are also common during this third stage. In the final stage, the individual becomes uncommunicative, with little meaningful social interaction, and often takes on the features of the Klüver-Bucy syndrome. Thus they exhibit emotional outbursts, inappropriate sexual behaviors, severe memory loss, constant mouth movements, and often a flexor-type postural pattern. In this latter phase, the patient is virtually decorticate and clinically indistinguishable from persons with other dementias. The prognosis of Alzheimer disease was only a few years ago totally bleak, but today there are hopes that in the future, pharmacological interventions may slow and even reverse the damage inflicted by this disease.[488–491]

The continual degeneration of the limbic network through each phase is a key distinguishing factor in Alzheimer disease and constantly affects the behavioral patterns of the individual.[492–498] The neurochemical state within the limbic network can be influenced by the drugs often used to prevent or slow the progression of Alzheimer disease (see Chapter 36).[499–503] Similarly, gene therapy may prove to have great therapeutic value given the genetic predisposition identified in some patients with Alzheimer disease.[39,504–507] Because music is able to activate many different brain areas, music therapy can be particularly valuable in the treatment of persons at all stages of Alzheimer disease.[508] Long after declarative memory is lost, individuals can sing entire songs (procedural memory), dance with a loved one they no longer recognize (procedural memory), or be soothed and calmed by hearing someone who cares about them singing familiar favorite songs or lullabies (limbic response). In earlier phases of the disease, individuals who have lost words can recall words such as song lyrics through the linking with melody. When melody is lost, individuals still retain rhythmic responses. In the final, palliative stage of Alzheimer disease care, agitated patients are observed to calm to simple music such as familiar lullabies. Thus Alzheimer disease patients are able to continue to respond to music through the progression of the disease, and the response to rhythm may represent overlearned motor responses that are tied to positive limbic states. For example, nonambulatory individuals, when presented with familiar and preferred music, may stand and move with the rhythm of the sound. Their bodies may remember how to dance with the spouse whose name they no longer know.[509] A physical or occupational therapist can instruct a caregiver to use music as part of everyday activities. The therapeutic effects of music to engage and maintain attention, activate long-term memory, and modulate emotion states are well suited to the needs of both the person with Alzheimer disease and his or her caregivers.[509]

Hippocampal and anterior cingulate volumes have been correlated with both gait and executive function. Hippocampal, anterior cingulate, and NAc volumes have been correlated with stride length. Older adults with mild cognitive impairment demonstrated significantly slower gait speed and shorter stride length when asked to walk quickly.[510]

Head Injury

A detailed understanding of nontraumatic and traumatic head injury can be found in Chapters 22 and 23. The behavioral sequelae after any head injury reflect many signs of limbic involvement. In studies of both the pediatric and adult populations,[117,511–516] behaviors of impulsiveness, restlessness, overactivity, destructiveness, aggression, increased tantrums, and socially uninhibited behaviors (lack of social skills) are frequently reported. These behaviors all reflect a strong emotional or limbic component. Given Moore's concept of a limbic network that MOVEs us and the F²ARV continuum regarding emotional control over noxious or negative input, it is no wonder so many patients have difficulty with personal and emotional control over their reactions to the therapeutic world. If the imbalance were within the patient, then the external environment would be one possible way to help center the patient emotionally.[517,518] This centering requires that the therapist be sensitive to the emotional level of the patient. As the patient begins to regain control, an increase in external environmental demands would challenge the limbic network. If the demand is excessive, the patient's emotional reaction as expressed by motor behavior should alert the therapist to downgrade the activity level.

Head injuries affect many areas of the CNS, however, no matter the commonalities of the site or extent of the lesions. Each patient is different because of prior learning, conditioning of the limbic network, and their respective perception of quality of life.[519] The overall limbic state (low, neutral, or high) and response of two patients to the same clinical learning environment may have great variance and should be carefully observed, evaluated, and documented by the clinician. The therapist should provide undivided attention to the patient at all times and be willing to make moment-to-moment adjustments within the external environment to achieve a neutral limbic state and help the patient maintain focus on the desired learning. A patient with spasticity, rigidity, or ataxia may exhibit an increase in motor responses when in a limbic high state, when the limbic network becomes stressed. The therapist must differentiate a true motor output and control problem from limbic over- or under-activity that negatively influences the motor control systems. Therapists should be able to identify the true underlying cause of the motor control problem and plan their respective treatments accordingly.[520]

Traumatic Injury

Diffuse axonal injury sustained within a traumatic closed head injury can result in severe limbic network instability.[291,292,511–513,521] The long associative bundles or fibers that transverse the cortex on a curved route can be sheared by an impact or a blow to the head, or sustain microtrauma through stretch, particularly one with torsion in the mechanism of injury. One of these long associative bundles is the cingulate fasciculus, which carries the amygdala and hippocampal projections to and from the prefrontal cortex. Many basic perceptual strategies, such as body schema, hearing, vision, and smell, are linked into the emotional and learning centers of the limbic network through the cingulate fasciculus.[117] Thus declarative learning through sensory and cognitive processing can become impossible. If the pathways to and from the hippocampus and amygdala are sheared bilaterally, total and permanent global anterograde amnesia will be present.[522,523] If destruction of both tracts on one side occurs, but the contralateral side is left intact, the individual can compensate, but learning will be slower or the rate of processing delayed.[74] If only one tract on one side is damaged, such as the tract to and from the hippocampus, the amygdaloid system on the same side will compensate but be slower than without the lesion.[74] Thus the

specific degree of involvement will vary and depend on the extent of shearing. Those with total shearing on both sides will usually be in a deep coma and will not survive the injury.[524] Those with less severe insult will show signs ranging from total amnesia to minor delays in declarative learning.[525] The emotional problems of traumatic head injury can often be associated with other limbic problems such as posttraumatic stress syndrome. This problem is especially apparent when treating soldiers injured on the battlefield who have returned home.[457]

Cerebral contusions (bruises) have long been a primary sign of traumatic head injury.[526] Regardless of area of impact, the contusions are generally found in the frontal and temporal regions. There are long-term neuropsychological ramifications after mild traumatic brain injury even when there is no loss of consciousness.[514] The regions most frequently involved are orbitofrontal, frontopolar, anterotemporal, and lateral temporal surfaces. The limbic network's connection to these areas would suggest the potential for direct and indirect limbic involvement. The greater the contusion, the greater the likelihood that the limbic structures might simultaneously be involved. Impulsiveness, lack of inhibition, and hyperactivity are a few of the clinical signs associated with orbitofrontal or limbic involvement.[527] The dorsomedial frontal region, involved in the hippocampal-fornix circuit (once referred to as the *Papez circuit*),[122] when damaged seems to induce a pseudo-depressed state, including slowness, lack of initiation, and perseveration.

Nontraumatic Head Injuries

Nontraumatic head injuries include anoxic or hypoxic brain injury. Lack of oxygen to the brain, regardless of the cause, seems not only to have a dramatic effect throughout the cortex but also results in selective damage to the hippocampal regions.[528] The loss of hippocampal declarative memory systems bilaterally would certainly provide one reason for the slowness in processing so commonly observed in head injury.[529] A hypothesis could also be made regarding the limbic network's interrelation with other cortical and brain stem structures. In cases of hypoxia, many structures interconnecting in the limbic network are potentially affected, so information sent to the limbic network may be distorted. These distortions could cause tremendous imbalances within the limbic processing system, with not only attention and learning problems but also the hypothalamic irregularity often seen in head trauma. Individuals who demonstrate obstructive sleep apnea, another cause of hypoxia, have been shown to have an imbalance in the hippocampal area.[530] This imbalance may lead to severe cognitive dysfunction.[531] This preexisting hypoxic environment certainly can have a long-term effect on any patient who has CNS damage at any age.

A therapist always needs to understand the environment within which the injury occurred as well as being aware of preexisting complications. If the event was anoxic, then those areas with the highest oxygen need or at the highest metabolic state might be the most affected or damaged after the event. Knowing that information, a therapist's analytical problem-solving strategies should guide her or him toward limbic assessment.

Vestibular Disorders

The vestibular system has extensive neuronal connections and commissural influences on the limbic network and structures; conversely, the limbic network has significant influence on the vestibular nuclei. Details of the neuroanatomical connections have been described previously in this chapter, and a detailed discussion of vestibular disorders can be found in Chapter 21.

It is generally accepted that vestibular dysfunction results in erroneous input to the CNS. This erroneous sensory information creates a mismatch between the external (afferent) cues and the internal conceptual model for movement contained by the cerebellum. This mismatch creates an imbalance in vestibular and cerebellar signals to the CNS, flooding the central limbic structures and resulting in symptoms such as vertigo, motion sickness, nausea, or decreased postural control. Detection of this mismatch results in an attempt by the cerebellum to compensate for the imbalance, which becomes a core tenet of recovery.[136] Alternately, this neural stimulation may create an internal stressor and trigger an adverse limbic response, such as a GAS response.

Newer evidence from animal research has demonstrated that vestibular lesions result in dramatic changes in the morphology and function of the hippocampus. Of note is that bilateral vestibular lesions have been associated with hippocampal atrophy. The hippocampus makes unique contributions to memory, both spatial and nonspatial. Thus vestibular lesions impair learning and memory, particularly those tasks that require spatial processing. In addition to the more well-known deficits in spatial and gravitational orientation for balance control, vestibular lesions can also result in impaired cognition, learning, and memory through damage to this connection. Decreased concentration, thought processes, and memory are among the most common complaints in patients with vestibular disorders. In the past these complaints were often attributed to competitive resources, suggesting that cognitive resources were being devoted to the basic tasks of staying balanced during function. It is now clear that there is a true physiological explanation for these secondary symptoms, which are quite limiting to activity and participation in normal daily activities, particularly working. It has also been suggested that treatment activities that stimulate the function of the vestibular system also stimulate activity within the hippocampus and can improve memory, which has important implications for treatment.[146–154]

Thus vestibular dysfunction can influence the therapeutic environment both in the assessment and the treatment of this system. However, the vestibular system is not a primary consideration of most physicians and therapists during evaluation. On the basis of benchmarking data from within specialized balance centers, the average patient with a vestibular disorder (dizziness or imbalance) travels within the medical system an average of 52 months before finding a solution. During this time, he or she has seen on average four physicians. There is also at least one visit to the emergency department in crisis and one visit to a psychiatrist. Typically, there has been no rehabilitation referral or intervention during this time.[532]

The patient with a chronic vestibular disorder can have myriad symptoms, including vegetative, autonomic, motoric, cognitive, psychological, and behavioral symptoms that are often misdiagnosed during this search for an outcome as other, more serious medical diagnoses. As an example, of those patients diagnosed with dizziness or imbalance of a psychological origin, evidence has determined that more than 70% of these patients have underlying vestibular dysfunction on key vestibular function tests (electronystagmography and calorics, rotary chair, computerized dynamic posturography, auditory brain stem response, and acoustic reflexes).[310,311,316,533,534] Conversely, of those patients with chronic dizziness and imbalance, only 16% were found to have dizziness of a true psychogenic origin.[535] Acknowledgment of a patient's symptoms, use of data, and explanation (in understandable detail) that there is a physiological explanation for his or her complaints builds the patient-therapist relationship and begins to neutralize the patient's abnormal limbic state (anxiety versus depression). It can lower the GAS or autonomic cascade, maximizing the **treatment** time before the onset of limiting symptoms (i.e., raising the **symptom** threshold).

Even patients with motion sickness have documentable physiological and functional changes. Some of the best current evidence is in our military personnel with symptoms of motion sickness. On examination, these soldiers have physiological changes identifiable by results of rotary chair (60% with abnormally long-time constants) and computerized dynamic posturography (70% with abnormal Sensory Organization Test [SOT] condition 5 and 6).[536]

Patients who have sustained a mild head injury, postconcussive syndrome, blast exposure or injury (positive or negative pressure event), or whiplash often have concomitant involvement of the vestibular apparatus or nuclei. This often goes undetected within the initial medical workup and management plan excepting in specialty vestibular practices.[536–540] When the disorder is undetected and left unchecked, the patients do not respond to standard treatment interventions. They also complain of atypical symptoms or responses to these typical treatments. When the patient does not respond in predictable ways to standard treatment, the label "aphysiological" is applied, particularly in situations where disability or secondary gain is a factor. Fortunately there are well-established performance criteria that can effectively differentiate true balance or vestibular impairment from embellishment for secondary gain.[541] (Refer to Chapters 20 and 21.)

In treatment, recovery is based on long-term compensation mediated by the cerebellum, and symptoms must be reproduced for recovery to occur. However, stimulation of the vestibular system must be controlled, with every effort made to maintain a limbic (emotional) neutral state. Some patients have true vestibular dysfunction that affects only motor responses, whereas other patients have true limbic psychiatric problems that do not manifest themselves with vestibular symptoms. These two behaviors are located at the polar ends of the curve between limbic motor and vestibular motor dysfunction. Before prescribing appropriate intervention strategies, the clinician must be clear regarding the degree of limbic overlay on the vestibular dysfunction, and the question "What are the best vestibular and limbic interactive environments that will challenge and drive neuroplastic change?" must be answered. Although researchers[310,316] have identified tools that differentiate the two extremes, today researchers are trying to clarify the midrange of patients who clearly have symptoms on the basis of the interaction of both systems.[541,542] Development of tools that can further discriminate whether the behaviors are first driven by vestibular and followed by limbic responses, or vice versa, is a key to treatment planning. The reader is again referred to Clinical Case 4.3, outlining the complex interactions between the vestibular system and limbic network.

Parkinson Disease

The motor impairments seen in individuals with PD are widely accepted, understood, and treated by physical and occupational therapists and are discussed in detail within Chapter 18 and throughout this chapter. An important consideration not commonly factored in by physical and occupational therapists is that individuals diagnosed with PD often have limbic involvement in addition to their motor involvement. In addition to primary and secondary depression discussed below, dopamine plays a direct role in both the motivation to move and motor function.[10] From a motor perspective, recall that dopamine is released from the VTA in the midbrain and projects to the primary motor cortex (M1), effecting motor output and enabling motor skill acquisition.[52] Dopaminergic VTA projection neurons are activated when rewards are obtained during motor skill acquisition, but not during task execution in later stages of motor learning. In addition, reward-seeking and motivational behaviors of the limbic network's connection to the NAc and frontal cortex are dopamine-dependent.[51,187]

As one unique example of linked limbic and motor output, a masked expression is widely accepted as a cardinal motor sign of this disease and is linked directly to the rigidity expressed within the motor system. Yet, a masked expression is also associated with fear as an emotion (see Fig. 4.6). Similarly, the ability to extinguish this fear response or masked expression is also based on the infralimbic prefrontal lobe and the number of dopamine receptors.[543] These areas may not be directly damaged by PD, but the amount of available dopamine is dramatically reduced. Given this interaction, patients with PD may have difficulty facially expressing what they are feeling. Thus when a therapist sees a patient with a fixed facial expression, that therapist cannot draw a conclusion from that facial expression.

Similarly, depression is commonly seen in individual with degenerative disease.[544,545] Although thought first to be reactive to the disease state, depression also results from a neuroanatomical perspective through involvement of the limbic system and its associated motor responses. Depression from a motor response perspective causes lower postural tone with increased flexion in the neck (see Fig. 4.17B). This flexed pattern within the trunk is also considered the postural pattern of individuals with PD. The question thus arises, "Is the tone generated from the motor system alone, from the limbic influence on the motor system alone, or from a combination of the two?"

Procedural learning impairments are not early symptoms of PD, but emerge with progression of the disease, independently of cognitive dysfunction or dopaminergic medication.[546] As the disease progresses, motor learning studies have shown that persons with PD have difficulty in initiating and maintaining movement without external cues. It is thought that these external cues reroute movement initiation from the automatic basal ganglia pathway through nonautomatic pathways.[547] Effective external cues typically include musical rhythms or marches, rhythmic tones, tactile directional cues, or visual cues.[548] However, extrinsic or declarative verbal cues that help to provide motor sequencing may provide cognitive interference to learning in individuals with PD. Extrinsic verbal cues designed to focus attention to missing components, for example, step length or arm swing, have been shown to improve performance.[547]

Cerebrovascular Accidents

The reader is referred to Chapter 22, which offers a detailed discussion of stroke. The most common insult in CVA results in occlusions in the distributions of the middle cerebral artery.[39] When this occlusion is in the right cerebral hemisphere, studies have shown that patients are often confused and exhibit metabolic imbalance.[549] A primary problem associated with this confused state is inattention and impulsivity. After brain scans, it has been shown that focal lesions existed within both the reticulocortical and limbic cortical tracts, suggesting direct limbic involvement in many middle cerebral artery problems.[5] Conversely, individuals with left MCA distribution involvement present with an increase in attention to deficits, frustration with functional limitations, and cautious engagement in rehabilitation interventions. In each of these presentations, the patient may show emotional components out of sync with their actual neurophysiological deficit; the patient with right CVA may present as limbic low to neutral, whereas the patient with left CVA may present with higher frustration or fear, in a limbic high state.

With the use of MRI, specific lesion deficits after CVA can help physicians and therapists identify specific motor and limbic behavioral problems that would limit quality of life of the patients.[457,550,551] Many patients who have had a CVA do not have direct limbic involvement, yet the stresses placed on the patient,[552,553] whether external or internal, are often reflected in the limbic network's influence over cognition and the motor control systems.[554] Personal (emotional), performance, or physical stresses experienced within the rehabilitation process increase activity within the limbic network and overflow into the motor system via the reticulospinal pathways. Increased activation of the

reticulospinal pathways results in increased hypertonicity within the muscles of the involved extremities due to the lack of cortical inhibition. The patient is usually unaware of this buildup of hypertonicity but can release it once attention is drawn to it. Neuromuscular rehabilitation interventions serve to introduce therapeutic handling or sensorimotor techniques that serve to reduce extraneous stress and limbic input upon the reticular system and its outputs, thus decreasing overall tonus. This reduction in the overall limbic network activity enables the therapist to facilitate more normal task-specific engagement of motor output.

Similar to individuals with other neurological disorders, there are two types of depression to consider. The first is the reaction to the CVA and losses itself, and the next is the depression resulting from involvement of the limbic network structures and their connections to the primary motor cortex. Differentiating the contribution of the two can be quite challenging. The first step would be to insure appropriate medication focused on a possible reactive depression component, followed by interventions focused on increasing the activity of a depressed limbic network through therapeutic alliance and maximized engagement.

Often mistaken for depression is a post-stroke phenomenon called pseudobulbar affect (PBA). Also known as "emotional lability" or "emotional incontinence," PBA is a disinhibition syndrome characterized by uncontrollable outbursts of crying or emotion that can happen at any time, even in inappropriate social situations; it is typically disproportionate to the emotions actually being experienced. Prevalence estimates range from 9.4% to 37.5%, resulting in an estimated 1.8 to 7.1 million affected individuals in the United States across several neurological disorders, including amyotrophic lateral sclerosis (ALS), multiple sclerosis (MS), Alzheimer disease, stroke, PD, and traumatic brain injury.

In PBA, the corticolimbic pathways modulated by serotonin and the widespread pathways modulated by glutamate are disrupted. Although the neuroanatomical processes are still being investigated, one component of the disorder appears linked to a reduction of the inhibitory input from the frontal lobe that results in disinhibition of the limbic responses.[555,556] About 30% to 35% of individuals with PBA suffer from associated depression and anxiety and have poor social functioning. Current treatment has typically been focused on tricyclic antidepressants and SSRIs designed to increase availability of serotonin at the synapses in corticolimbic and cerebellar modulation pathways.[555] Physical and occupational therapy interventions have been heavily focused on patient and family education surrounding the behavioral versus the neurological basis of the disorder. With the introduction of newer pharmacological agents, such as dextromethorphan the therapist's role expands to assist in the evaluation of medication efficacy and maximized, positive behavioral outcomes.

Tumor

Brain tumors are discussed in detail in Chapter 25. Any brain tumor, regardless of whether it directly affects the limbic structures, will certainly arouse the limbic network because of the stress, anxiety, and emotional overlay associated with the diagnosis. The degree of emotional involvement will obviously affect the declarative learning of the patient as well as the limbic network's influence over motor response.

Tumors specifically arising within limbic structures[557,558] can cause dramatic changes in the patient's emotional behavior and level of alertness, especially with hypothalamic tumors.[559] The behaviors reported include aggressiveness, hyperphagia, paranoia, sloppiness, manic symptoms, and eventual confusion.[39] Tumors within the hypothalamus cause not only behavioral abnormalities but also autonomic endocrine imbalances, including body temperature changes, menstrual abnormalities, and diabetes insipidus.[198]

When the tumor is located within the frontal and temporal lobes, associated with limbic structures, psychiatric problems may manifest, ranging from depression to anorexia to psychosis.[198,560] Obsessive-compulsive disorder resulting from limbic tumor has been used as a tumor marker for relapse.[561] Amnesia has been reported in patients with dorsomedial thalamus, fornix, midbrain, and reticulolimbic pathway lesions. This again reinforces the importance of the limbic network's role in storage.[124,198,562]

The neurochemistry within the limbic network is very complex and will be discussed within the next large section, but even without a keen understanding of the specific chemistry, therapists need to recognize behavior and mood changes within the patient. These changes often signal neurochemical problems affecting the individual's motor system. If medical intervention includes medicine, pharmacists should be able to explain how those behaviors are being regulated by pharmacological intervention. Literature is now reporting that what were once thought to be idiopathic seizures are now believed to be neurochemical imbalances within the limbic structure and may someday be controlled with medications that directly affect the immune system.[563]

Ventricular Swelling

Ventricular swelling resulting from trauma to or inflammation in the CNS or following spinal defects in utero are discussed throughout a variety of chapters in greater detail. Although the effects of ventricular swelling after trauma, inflammation, and in utero cerebrospinal malformations are not discussed in great detail in the literature with respect to limbic involvement, the proximity of the lateral and third ventricle to limbic structures cannot be ignored. It is common knowledge that most people exposed to hot, humid weather begin to swell; become more irritable, less tolerant, and moody; and may complain of headaches. Some people become aggressive, others lethargic. All these behaviors are linked to some extent with limbic function. Thus ventricular swelling causing hydrocephalus, whether caused by trauma, inflammation, or obstruction, would potentially affect the limbic structures. Reported behavioral changes such as seizures, memory and learning problems, personality alterations, alertness, dementia, and amnesia can be tied to direct or indirect limbic activity.[39]

Chronic Pain

Although not considered a mental health disorder, chronic pain sequelae manifest in behavioral and emotional change. According to the U.S. Department of Public Health, in 2016 approximately 20 percent of adults living in the U.S. were living with chronic pain.[564]

Pain is a complex phenomenon, and the more it is understood, the more complex it becomes⁻ (see Chapter 30).[565–570] Hippocampal volume has been identified as a variable in pain ratings in the elderly.[571] Similarly, the amygdala plays an important role in regulation of and the emotional reaction to both chronic and acute pain.[572,573] Whether the pain is peripherally induced or centrally induced because of trauma or emotional overload, often the same motor responses will exist. A withdrawn flexor pattern from pain makes postural activities exhausting because of the work it takes to override the existing central pattern generators. Thus daily living activities, which constantly require postural extension against gravity, may be perceived as overwhelming and just not worth the effort. The therapist needs to learn to differentiate between peripheral physical pain and central or emotional pain and between mixed peripheral and central induced pain. To the patient, "pain is pain!"[569,574–580] With the current opioid epidemic, primary care physicians as well as physical therapists have recognized that pain, especially chronic pain, is a common, complex, and challenging condition, having a biological component as well as being associated with the limbic system.[581,582] Thus when dealing with both

chronic and acute pain patients, the importance of the patient's emotional acceptance of the plan of care co-established by the therapist and the individual receiving care cannot be overemphasized.[583]

Summary of Clinical Problems Affected by Limbic Involvement

It is easy to identify limbic problems when behaviors deviate drastically from normal responses. It is much more difficult to determine subtle behavior shifts in patients. The therapist should be sensitive to these minor mood shifts because they may represent early signs of future problems. Similarly, noting that a particular patient is always irritable and has difficulty learning on hot days should help direct the therapist toward establishing a treatment session that regulates humidity and temperature to optimize the learning environment. The limbic network is not just a neurochemical bundle of nuclei and axons found within the brain. It is a pulsating center that links perception of the world and the way an individual responds to that perception. Quality of life is a value, and that value has a strong limbic component. If functional outcomes leading to maintaining or improving the quality of life of our patients is the goal of both physical and occupational therapy,[318,584,585] then the limbic network is no less important during examination, evaluation, prognosis, and intervention than the motor system itself.

THE "MIND, BODY, SPIRIT" PARADIGM: INSIGHTS ON THE LIMBIC SYSTEM FROM A MASTER CLINICIAN

By DARCY UMPHRED

As neuroscientists, safe and deep within a Western allopathic model of linear research, establishing efficacy and evidence-based practice for what is taught to new learners is critically important.[318,379,586] Yet there are too many unexplainable behavioral unknowns occurring daily in the clinical environment that cannot be researched using standard Western research tools common to physical or occupational therapists. Identifying with treatment approaches that base their philosophy on energy fields, flow patterns of those fields through the body, rhythms that do not seem to be proven as existing, or planes of consciousness and belief seems to contradict that comfortable groundedness of basic science. (Refer to Chapter 39 on Complementary and Integrative Therapies.) Thus for many health care practitioners, denial of all those potential parameters that might affect evaluation and intervention outcomes is an easy way to feel safe and linked to what is believed to be efficacy- or evidence-based practice within respective professions. Most allopathic medical physicians within the clinical environment are the first to reject what seem like irrational claims or ideas regarding philosophical approaches. Therapists are not far behind those physicians with their attitudes and verbal expressions toward both patients and colleagues who bring in ideas regarding potential approaches that seem to be outside of our reductionist, linear research models used to establish efficacy. In the clinical arena, clinicians are realizing that effectiveness of practice with objective outcome measures is another way to establish evidence. Similarly, effectiveness can be subdivided into variables that pose questions. Researchers might be able to select variables that can be researched to establish efficacy of treatment approaches used within a clinical environment. Western medicine has taught both medical practitioners and therapists to strongly question anything that reflects concepts of energy, healing, or spiritual beliefs with regard to outcomes of therapy. Yet electromagnetic tools have been embraced by physicians and neuroscience researchers in the form of computed tomography, MRI, PET, and fMRI to diagnose and study neurological damage and neuroplasticity. These evaluation and research tools create their own electromagnetic field while the human body is placed within that field.[587,588] Practitioners can still deny that there is a natural energy field and that this field has anything to do with health, but it is getting harder and harder to deny the presence of such a force. All of us have received an electric shock between our body and a metal surface. That shock is called an *electromagnetic charge*, and the voltage depends on the inherent voltage of that individual. Where did this voltage come from? What is meant by *inherent voltage of an individual?* We all have learned that there is a static electromagnetic field around us, but it is very hard to identify how that charge might affect our body systems. As long as practitioners do not inquire about the physics of these energy fields and the bioelectric or biochemical reactions of our human cells to these fields, the idea that the electromagnetic and electrochemical fields have nothing to do with neuroplasticity and changes with patients after neurological insults unfortunately can remain a myth. Over a decade ago, some allopathic physicians stepped out of their established model and developed a subspecialty in psychoneuroimmunology. Checking PubMed for articles from 2018, a reader can find over 2400 published articles under the term *psychoneuroimmunology*. This subspecialty incorporates the relationships among emotion, the endocrine and immune systems, and the CNS and peripheral nervous system.[328,207,208,589] As the limbic neuronetwork intricately links various nuclei that deal with emotion, endocrine production, and autoimmunity, there is little doubt that this system is involved with belief in healing, emotions, and spirituality.[590,591] "Despite such conceptual progress, the biological, psychological, social and spiritual components of illness are seldom managed as an integrated whole in conventional medical practice."[329]

Fortunately or unfortunately, there are scientists and therapists who are "myth busters" and who challenge the rigid paradigm of linear research, stating that there are many more variables and systems involved in neurorecovery or neuroplasticity than have yet been identified. Physicians and neuroscientists studying the effects of disease and neuroplasticity after trauma[587] or application of drugs[592–594] are trying to unravel a complex maze of chemical and electrical reactions at the level of the cell membrane.[104] Quantum physicists are studying the universe and the electromagnetic pull of suns on planets and solar systems on one another.[595–597]

Science is a long way from unraveling the mysteries explored by cellular biologists and quantum physicists and how they might relate to each other. But many scientists trust that there is a relationship. As humans, we are made up of billions of these cells; each cell has a membrane potential and the ability to adapt and change; and they play an important role in the existence of our species. Similarly, the universe is made up of billions of masses; each has some relationship to energy pull, whether that be one solar system in relation to another, one planet in relationship to a sun, one moon in relationship to a planet's oceans, one person in relationship to the gravity on a planet, or one person in relationship to another person. If those cells are what make a person human, and if what holds the person together is electromagnetic energy, then it is hard to ignore the possibility that one person might affect another person just by being present.[593]

Therapists want to study the interaction of brain responses between a practitioner and the patient during a therapeutic treatment session.[598] It is obvious that this interaction cannot be explained by one variable within linear space, nor that it is one variable alone that is causing all change over a linear set in time. Establishing efficacy on what seems to be a multidimensional construct using a basic science research model is not realistic. Thus efficacy research on the totality of the mind, the physical body, and the human spirit eludes basic scientist researchers in a manner similar to the way that researching the effectiveness of intuition eludes psychiatric researchers.

As research practitioners we use various tools to manipulate both the internal and external environments within which our patients function to measure effectiveness of specific or generalized outcomes. Each person is so complex and unique that finding the best combination of tools and environments has a very person-specific answer.[594,599] Thus what we as researchers are trying to do is find evidence that shows that one treatment paradigm has a better chance of creating change than another, without placing rigid restrictions that say all persons will optimally benefit from any one particular approach.[600–607] MRI, PET, and fMRI tools are certainly capable of identifying changes in the CNS after interventions. Even when researchers or clinicians try to control as many variables as possible, many additional external and internal input possibilities exist.

This brings us full circle to the question regarding additional variables that might affect health, well-being, and recovery outcomes from therapeutic interventions.[608–618]

After 40 years of clinical practice and hearing Western physicians say, "Physical therapy and occupational therapy just make the patients *feel* better," it is obvious, first, that many physicians do not understand the depth and breadth of our professions or what is provided to the patients. Second, those physicians do not understand the limbic interconnections to "feel better" and how that might drive the neuroplasticity of the CNS and the autoimmune system's response to disease or pathology.[14,615,619–624] Similarly, after many patients have been observed over the last 40 years regaining consciousness, whether the vegetative state lasted 6 months, 9 months, a year, or 4 years, the fact remains that each individual shifted from what might be considered a level 2, 3, or 4 on the Rancho Levels of Cognitive Functioning to a 6, 7, or 8 on the same scale after 5 to 20 minutes. This reality made me ask the question from the beginning of my professional career, "What are the variables that cause changes in these patients?" The answers are not yet fully understood, although the behavioral outcomes keep presenting themselves. Every time a patient comes out of this vegetative state, I (DAU) feel wondrous, emotional, and humbled. Something happens that is far beyond our scientific understanding, something simple but extremely complex, cellular, and universal, all at the same time. Similarly, the bond between that therapist and that patient is very strong and deeply spiritual. The memory of those patients stays forever embedded in the mind of the therapist even if the clinical environment existed for only 30 minutes. All the words used to explain such clinical experiences link closely to the limbic network and its role in creating change, both within the therapist and the patient; certainly at this time, these experiences fall outside the paradigm of Western medical science. According to a report on the BBC, the use of appropriate fMRIs shows that many individuals in a vegetative state are awake but still have little to no awareness because of the severe brain injury.[625] This explains the fact that a therapist "feels" that a patient is aware but does not explain how the therapist-patient interaction brings that patient to a conscious state of attention.

Medical schools and health science programs are becoming increasingly aware of the need to train the practitioners of the future to enter into a healing relationship with the whole patient,[626,627] a relationship that empowers the patient to engage endogenous healing capacities, even while we work to better understand these mechanisms through both basic and applied research. Master clinicians have long appreciated this dynamic healing relationship, which affects both the therapist and patient. Thus even when our patients can verbally communicate with the therapist, it is still important to listen directly to the body and, on a deeper level, to more subtle input that we do not yet have the ability to describe and quantify with scientific method. It has been demonstrated that even for persons in very low awareness and response states, appropriately selected music can provide time-organized and emotionally meaningful stimuli to gently activate intact neural networks, and to communicate with the person still alive inside the disabled body.[628] The sounds we make and the way we touch communicate to the deeper levels of being and do not require words to convey caring, instill hope, and motivate the will to keep trying to get better.

The success or failure of many forms of alternative medical practice, and for that matter Western allopathic medicine and therapeutic practices, may depend on the limbic network.[597,613,629] At times research can prove unequivocally that certain variables do not show a healing effect, after double blind studies.[630] If a patient "believes" an intervention will work, even if it is a placebo, the chances of success far exceed those when the patient does not think it will work.[631–634] If it is a placebo and the body heals, then logic dictates that the body and the mind did the healing. Similarly, when the drug itself aided in neuroplasticity and change, is it the drug itself or the individual's belief that the drug will work that creates the change or both? How these changes occur is yet to be totally understood, but research substantiates that both neurochemical and neuroelectrical changes occur within an individual's physical body when the individual believes that change is possible.[67,105,610,619,630,633]

When I was a novice therapist, a nurse once said, "I am very glad you are not a nurse because you are so idealistic. You believe these patients in comas are going to wake up and walk out of here. And what is even worse is that most of them do!" That moment should have told me that I would be clashing with allopathic doctrine throughout my professional career, but instead I was confused about the nurse's use of the term *idealistic*. If the patients awoke and walked back into life with function and quality, then should that not be considered a *realistic* expectation? In that same job situation, my boss asked me to treat all the patients who were considered vegetative; once they were awake, my colleagues would treat them from there. My response was, "Emotionally for both the patient and myself, I could not do that. Once I bonded with a person, gained his or her trust, and found the patient was willing and capable of regaining consciousness, I could not just abandon the patient and go on to another person." The significance of that statement took many years to understand, and it was not until I began my study of the limbic network that I truly comprehended the accuracy of that perception, once considered naïve.[610,621,629,635,636] It was not until the writing of the 6th edition of this chapter that I could shrug off comments such as "This has nothing to do with physical therapy."[13,213,328,329,637]

After 45 years of practice and often treating individuals in front of colleagues in workshop situations, I cannot deny that something more than just "feeling good" occurs during physical or occupational therapy interventions although that feeling good is certainly a limbic response. When working with patients, I find myself feeling very open and bonding in some way that is neither "physical" nor "mental"—and thus the only option left is a definition of "spiritual." If, when treating a patient in a vegetative state, that bond tells me that the patient is lost within another plane of consciousness and wants to regain consciousness as defined by healthy people, and the physical body of the patient seems capable, then the treatment is goal directed, the direction of the intervention is identified, and thus the outcome is selected by the patient. The map has been established, and together the patient and the therapist proceed. As with all therapists, the intervention will be guided by the motor responses and control of the patient and the window within which the patient can run those programs independently. At times, when treating patients in a vegetative state, I feel unable to locate the "spirit"; at other times it feels as if that person has not decided whether to venture to an awake state, but more often I sense a frightened, confused individual who just wants to find her or his way back to what we call "life or reality." Those patients often gain

consciousness during therapy. It is not a miracle, nor can I ever say, "I healed something."[252] The term *healing* refers to a concept of "whole." The only person who can regain the structure of the whole is the patient.[638]

As a therapist, I am a teacher or a guide, helping others relearn and regain control over their respective lives. If after a 30-minute treatment session a person regains feeling and control of an extremity 18 years after a CVA or regains functional use of a hand 6 years after incomplete spinal cord injury, there is more to the intervention than merely following a clinical pathway or a treatment regimen geared to all individuals at a specific stage of a disease process or a specific motor impairment.

One variable that always seems to be present when patients achieve dramatic recovery is strong motivation by the patient to retain the control and an appreciation for the instruction on how to do that. A strong bond or compassionate appreciation for each other always seems to be present as another interlocking variable. Thus the clinical question "What is spirituality?" presented itself to me more than 40 years ago. It is a variable that is very difficult to define. That variable, when researched, has been shown to affect health and healing in individuals with health problems. *Spirituality* and *healing* are both words that each individual defines according to her or his own beliefs, cultural experiences, and use of verbal language.[106,107,639–646] The literature is available for those who wish to pursue this topic.[524,274,647–654]

Over the last 7 years since the sixth edition of this text was published, thousands of articles dealing with health, healing, spirituality, energy fields, quality of life, energy medicine, and emotional balance have been published in a large variety of types of journals.[655,656] The reader is encouraged to survey internet resources not only for evidence published in mainstream medical journals but also to understand that patients will glean information about complementary therapy from many other sources, such as blogs, advertisements, and online chat rooms. Refer to Chapter 39 for discussion of these topics as well as related literature. Within this chapter a system that affects all areas of the CNS and peripheral function has been discussed. How this system is affected by or affects one's spirituality is open for many lifetimes of future study.[657,658] Yet if spirituality affects healing and an individual believes that this potential is available, then this variable may play a critical role in patient compliance, neuroplasticity, and the limbic interface with other treatment procedures. Ignoring this variable is no different from ignoring cognitive perceptual deficits when dealing with abnormal motor behavior. Owing to the strong emotional foundation for an individual's spirituality, one could easily assume that the limbic network plays a strong role in establishing and storing memories that reflect these beliefs.

Until we can measure simultaneous synaptic activity of all interactions within the therapist's and the patient's CNS, we will not, from a grounded neuroscience efficacy base, be able to demonstrate exactly what occupational, speech, music, cognitive, or physical therapists do, even though we know they play a role.[659] Until then, outcomes need to be measured objectively. Even if interactions seem unmeasurable and subjective, clinicians still need to record the event change in the patient record and not bury that outcome deep somewhere in the subconscious level of the therapist's mind. The mind, the body, and the spirit are connected as a whole. If therapists treat only one part, it may help the whole, but if the whole is treated simultaneously, the outcome is more likely to change the whole.[660,661] The concept is no different from focusing on strengthening an isolated muscle and hoping it will lead to functional use versus strengthening that muscle in functional patterns and in relation to other muscles that also work together within that movement sequence.

After years of clinical experience and thousands of patients responding positively to various interventions, the question arises regarding clinical decision making and choice of interventions. There is not a "variable" that has been identified that guides that decision. It has been shown that humans bring to consciousness about 10% of all incoming information. Yet the human brain is making decisions using 100% of the input information. Given that relationship, quite a bit of human decision making may be based on nonconscious information regarding the external and internal world.[105,662,663] Thus the word all neuroscientists shudder over—*intuition*—may to a large extent be the unraveling of that nonconsciously received data.[664,665] I have effectively taught colleagues how to feel blood pressure and heartbeats of clinical partners by just barely touching the top of the hand, which might be explained by the high level of sensitivity of Meissner corpuscles within our skin.[661] If a clinician can sense an autonomic response such as heart rate when touching a patient's skin, then knowing how the limbic network is interacting within a motor response can also be deduced. This would allow the clinician to modulate the rate used to move the patient during an activity such as bed mobility, while maintaining a consistent state of the motor generators. That steady state should decrease any need for limbic fear by the patient. Fear has been shown to be very detrimental to motor performance.[666-668] Therapists may interpret these tactile responses as intuitive, but they are not. When one clinician seems to know how fast to move the patient and another clinician has no idea how to determine that decision or control that variable, we say it is the *art* of therapy and not the *science*. Yet it is the science of therapy. Similarly, helping someone shift consciousness levels seems similar to hypnosis. The exact identification of these variables is very hard, let alone finding reliable and valid research tools. This may just be a case of one clinician being open to receiving information and processing it. The other therapist, for some reason, is either not receiving or not processing the available information. This is not an example of "intuition."

Intuition has been a source of fascination over centuries. Recently, with consumer dissatisfaction with health care and the upsurge in alternative medical practices, intuition has again sparked the interest of scholars and the public. To many it reflects mystery, magic, and even voodoo. Individuals with a strong ethnic, cultural, and even religious bias may find it hard to scientifically analyze this human strategy. For more than 43 years my husband has answered questions I have posed in my mind. It took at least the first decade of our marriage for my left brain to actually accept that I was not subvocalizing the thought or that he could not have extrapolated the thought from an environmental stimulus. Yet he consistently has told me that I did vocalize the thought because he hears me ask the question or state a fact in my voice patterns. Obviously, my thoughts have traveled to the primary and associative receiving areas of his left temporal lobe and he "hears" the thought in my voice. The dilemma that confronted me as a scientist is, if the information did not come in through his eighth cranial nerve, then how did it enter into his system and get to his temporal lobe? The answer would seem to be intuition. A definition might be knowing something without entering the data through traditional input systems. The next question is, "What is intuition?"

Unfortunately, after 40 years of study, I cannot answer that question. I do acknowledge that it is something, it can be learned, and master clinicians use it as a part of their clinical decision making, even if they choose not to verbalize it to their colleagues or even acknowledge it within their conscious mind. Much research and literature are available regarding intuition.[105,669-692] Yet the answer to that simple question "What is intuition?" is unavailable and does not seem so simple. No answer exists that has shown to be definitively efficacious and reliable, although research over the last 15 years has begun to identify components of intuition.[665,669-688,693]

It may be that intuition is more than one variable and can be accessed in more than one way. In fact, after studying various alternative medical practices, all using very different interventions based on different philosophies and belief systems, it seems as if all approaches may be tapping into the same human system, just opening to that system through different paradigms.

In the late 1960s, I (DAU) was beginning to present an integrated approach to neurological disabilities. I was integrating various treatment philosophies using the behavioral responses of patients and known science to guide intervention. I was told at that time that integrating approaches could not be done and that I would potentially injure patients by using approaches from different philosophical techniques. Today, of course, with our understanding of motor control, motor learning, and neuroplasticity, an integrated approach from the 1960s based on a systems model is a tool available to all therapists. However, researchers think that those tools were based on the science of the time, and thus they reject many of those techniques because they think they were based on inaccurate understanding of science. The master clinicians of the time based their techniques on movement responses of the patient and how those patients regained normal control over those movements. Today, I now present a similar model based on today's science of the brain, movement analysis across the life-span, and the external and internal environments of both the therapist and patient. This incorporates complementary approaches to intervention and the concept of intuition.

There are a number of variables that seem to open one's intuition: bonding, being dedicated to the patient, having openness in listening to the patient, letting preconceived knowledge be a springboard from which to expand that knowledge, having not only a willingness to learn but an insatiable appetite to continue learning, and possessing the ability to let go of one's importance and just be another person within the environment. These variables may be the best place for a learner to begin learning how to develop this skill. It would seem as if intuition is like an aptitude. Some individuals come into this life already with a high level of potential, others are nurtured to develop that potential, and still others never have an opportunity or an environment in which to develop those strategies. Some individuals have had strong intuitive senses from childhood but share those experiences with few, if any, other people.

Experiencing intuition is an all-knowing experience. One knows something first, then one can become emotional regarding that knowledge. It is a knowledge that has a "wholeness" component and that can develop a strong emotional base on the limbic system. For example, I *knew* I was going to lose a parent. Which parent, I did not know, but I moved home for a year to make sure there wasn't anything I should have said to either parent before I went on with my life. A year later I was married and home for a holiday. When my husband and I left my parents' home, I cried all the way back to our dwelling across the country because I knew I would never see my father again. I was right; he passed two weeks before I was to return home six months later. My father had been a very healthy man with no health issues that would indicate any life-threatening health problems. I had known what was going to happen as a whole (intuition) and then had had a very strong emotional response to that intuition. Also, when my brother called to say that our father was critically ill, I had already adjusted to the probability of his loss and was the one individual within the family who could make cognitive decisions or answer press questions by phone. If I were to hazard a guess, the intuitive center is probably in the right anterior temporal lobe, owing to the "whole" understanding and its strong emotional connection. If that proves true, it will solidify the limbic network's connection to intuition. Experiences often create the first questions that lead to hypotheses and later to research that establishes efficacy.

During the first 10 years of my professional life, I (DAU) hid from most people that aspect of my person because I was becoming a neuroscientist and wanted to be grounded in scientific efficacy like all my colleagues. Unfortunately, my clinical experiences did not allow me to hide that intuitive aspect of my clinical decision making from my family or close colleagues or those colleagues who recognized that something had happened during a treatment that made no sense whatsoever. Those individuals recognized changes within the patient that, although very positive, should not have happened or were very far from our basic scientific understanding.

In 1980 I treated a woman who had a severe head injury and who after 6 months was at a Rancho level III. After 30 minutes of intervention the woman volitionally moved all of her limbs and trunk without cognitive confusion. That motor function and cognition might be partially explained by recent research using fMRI.[625] But something that goes far beyond today's fMRI followed the intervention. I innocently stepped out of the safety of scientific understanding. I shared with my colleagues this woman's medical and social history. That information was critical to their understanding the course of progression of this woman through the rehabilitation process and the future plan of care. I discussed the patient's social background, her education, her family, her children, and her husband, who had shot her in the head. This all made perfect sense, until the head of the department asked me how I knew that information. I said, "I read it in the chart." The director informed me that I had not seen the chart. I said, "You told me?" The director responded with, "We did not discuss the case!" I asked if I had been wrong, and the director said "no." In fact, she was amazed at how accurate I had been and just wondered how I had known that about the patient.

At that moment, my life was changed. I could no longer hide whatever this "intuition" was, nor could I truthfully tell colleagues what I had done during interventions without bringing up this topic. Also, I could only tell them ways to develop intuition but had no understanding of the basic neuroscience behind its function. I could not tell anyone exactly what it was because I did not have any verbal knowledge of how and where the information is processed, so I could not translate that knowledge into verbal language to explain it to colleagues. That unknown is still present, although some of the variables may have been identified. The future will unravel those answers. What I have found since that day is that "masters," whether they are physicians, therapists, or teachers, often use this additional source of information gathering to help them in their clinical reasoning. I do not make this statement lightly nor without tremendous professional risk. I will leave you with an interaction that solidified my belief that this direction of scientific study needs to be pursued. Two decades ago, I was a keynote speaker at an international neurosurgical conference on brain tumors. I was the token "other," and the only speaker who was not a neurosurgeon. I presented the topic "The Limbic System's Influence on Motor Output." With this audience of 500 neurosurgeons and 50 token others, I, of course, used charts and pictures and based every sentence on efficacy-based scientific research. At dinner that night when all the speakers were together, the master neurosurgeon whom everyone acknowledged asked if he could sit next to me. I was aghast—a little nervous but honored nonetheless. He opened by saying, "I think many physical and occupational therapists are intuitive." With that, I knew him, his life, his experiences, and so on. Of course, I needed to let my left brain validate my intuition, and I said, "Yes, it is like walking into a room, looking at a patient, knowing where and what type of tumor the patient has, and using instruments such as positron emission tomography (PET) scan to validate what you already know." He responded with a smile and said, "Yes, it is exactly like that!" I do not need to continue to discuss the fascinating interactions of that night but leave the reader

with the thought that even the master of the masters in neurosurgery uses intuition as a variable in clinical decision making. It gave this man one additional bit of information that his colleagues could not use in clinical reasoning. No physician or therapist uses intuition as the only variable; intuition just gives additional information that helps in the process of clinical reasoning. It would seem as though intuition is highly integrated into the limbic network and often gives direction to a therapist as to the selection of specific examination tools to validate that assumption, and then gives insight as to which intervention tools would best match the person's needs.

As said previously, intuition is knowing something. As a result one can experience great emotion: "*I know, thus I fear.*" If the sequence of events begins with an emotion or fear and leads to what is perceived as knowledge or truth, one might question whether intuition was the driving force behind the belief. When emotions become elevated an individual may progress with "*I fear, thus I think I know.*" Research that looks at intuition assumes that when the limbic network is involved, the experience is highly emotional, and one might argue that an individual can be highly emotionally charged and still be neutral as far as a balance in emotions. Fear is not what drives intuition; instead it is emotional balance. Emotional balance or centering is not a state of being without emotion but rather a heightened state of emotional awareness without emotion, all at the same time. To become truly intuitive, one needs to become emotionally centered. In our everyday world where each of us is overstimulated as a day-to-day experience, this emotional balance is extremely difficult to achieve. It is even harder to find that balance in a clinical arena where patients are arriving with more acute diseases along with chronic secondary problems, often patients' schedules overlap with other patients' time, and therapists not only are limited in time for intervention but also find that the number of allowed visits falls well short for optimal opportunity for learning by the patient. That reality does not mean that the therapist's responsibility has changed. It is always up to the therapist to find those avenues by which better care may be provided within the existing environment. This reality just says that the challenges and questions are enormous. Finding emotional balance within that environment is very hard. Yet intuition seems to be a variable that gives some colleagues additional information that is then used as part of the clinical reasoning process.

Intuition, as a variable, needs to be identified, studied, researched, and taught once it is clearly understood. It is up to all of us to find the answers to these questions and the solutions to today's clinical problems and develop evidence-based practice to progress into the 21st century.[694,695]

The concept of integration of mind, body, and spirit as a critical element in maintaining or regaining quality of life between birth and death is not new.[696-699] Western society has tried to separate this concept into three distinct categories. The mind is made up of perception, cognition, and emotion. The body is made up of all systems external to the nervous system such as peripheral organs, muscles, bones, and skin. Both the peripheral and central motor systems, which control the body, are also included in the concept of body. The last component, the spirit, is a transcendental concept and is thought to depend on individuals' beliefs. Some individuals believe that spirit means belonging to a religious order. Others define spirit or spirituality as beyond religion—the essence that links the person to a greater energy force. For decades this last category has been considered outside the domain of responsibilities of Western allopathic health care delivery and was comfortably relegated to religious leaders or spiritual guides.

Today, everything is changing. Some scientists refer to energy fields around cells; others talk about energy fields around solar systems. Complementary practitioners talk about energy fields around the living organisms. Physicians are being taught cultural sensitivity training while in medical school to be more empathetic to the populations of people they will service. Physical therapy curricula are responsible for creating culturally sensitive professionals.[700–703]

Occupational therapy programs are responsible for including spirituality as one of the competencies a graduate is to have met.[704,705]

None of these professions have identified how these competencies relate to evaluation and intervention outcomes after treatment, but even the accrediting bodies believe they are important. Thus even at the entry level, for student therapists, emphasis is placed on making sure not only that the therapists' limbic systems have become sensitive to spirituality, but also that they be able to identify its significance in their patients' lives. Where does the interaction of the mind, body, and spirit play a critical role in quality-of-life issues and empowerment of the patient? The answers to that question cannot be found within this text or any other text in print today. Individuals with strong beliefs in a specific paradigm that includes spirituality can project the answer to this question, but establishing efficacy is an entirely different issue. Our professions are tethered to research, science, behavioral observations, and current knowledge. We as clinicians can stretch that tether. Much of our early treatments developed from behavioral observations that included individuals' beliefs, which clearly required the limbic network for processing, storage, and direct effect on bodily system reactions. If a patient lacks motivation, a therapist knows part of the job is to motivate the person. If the person believes his "God" will heal him, the therapist should never undermine that belief because everyone knows it cannot hurt and often creates a positive change.[706] How that interaction occurs is unknown today, but clinical observation would reinforce that it does help. Because spirituality uses belief and hope, memory of those feelings must be processed and later stored with the help of the limbic network.

These dilemmas exist with every professional dealing with health and wellness and quality-of-life issues. I (DAU) will leave you with one additional example. I spent over 2 months in the ICU a few years ago after a severe fall that caused two fractures to the pelvis, followed by severe internal hemorrhages. To summarize the medical problems, I had 18 initial arterial ruptures treated with radiological interventional surgery, followed by four more ruptures 1 week later leading to more surgery. I also had bilateral kidney failure, a large pulmonary embolism on the right side, pulmonary collapse in the left inferior lobe, massive internal infections, infusion of 12 units of blood, thrombophlebitis, fevers of over 105°F, very low blood pressure, and low oxygen absorption, along with external bleeds through most external orifices. In addition, the two bleeds destroyed my adrenal glands bilaterally, throwing me into another life-threatening imbalance of chemistry within my body. The doctor kept telling my husband with confidence that I would die. As my husband had been told this many times before, he kept telling the doctor he would wait for 3 days after I had been declared dead before he would accept that conclusion. Two weeks after the initial hospitalization, the doctor came into the room. He shut the door, sat down in a chair, addressed both of us and asked, "I know what medical problems you have had, I know that we did everything medically that we could, but it was not enough, so *how come you are still alive*?" I responded with, "There is a lot more to healing than what we understand, and that is what is fun about being a health professional." Life has taught me the lesson, whether as an intuitive, as a neuroscientist, or as a therapist, that there will be unknowns or mysteries along one's life journey. Sometimes one can solve the problems or answer the questions, but more often than not, one just has to file them in memory with the hope that one will sometime find an answer. The unknowns are always present even as answers are discovered. Having those unknowns creates an exciting challenge and adventure for every clinician who has or will have the opportunity to interact with individuals who have been brought into the health care delivery system because of a CNS problem. Those individuals want to be considered as a whole human being even if part of their physical body is dysfunctional. A circle has been drawn, and this chapter needs to end with a question. What is that whole? Refer to Case Study 4.1 as a clinical example.

REFERENCES

To enhance this text and add value for the reader, all references are included on the companion Evolve site that accompanies this textbook. This online service will, when available, provide a link for the reader to a Medline abstract for the article cited. There are 706 cited references and other general references for this chapter, with the majority of those articles being evidence-based citations.

5

Psychosocial Aspects of Adaptation and Adjustment During Various Phases of Neurological Disability*

Rochelle Mclaughlin and Janet A. Hiley

OBJECTIVES

After reading this chapter the student or therapist will be able to:

1. Describe adaptation and adjustment as parts of a flexible, flowing, and dynamic human process of meaning-making, not as static disembodied, stages.
2. Describe elements of the grief process that foster greater clarity and literacy around dominant cultural narratives around grief and the importance of mourning throughout the life-span and especially during times of significant life changes.
3. Integrate elements of mindfulness, resilience, coping, emotion-focused problem solving, and learning styles into the treatment process.
4. Integrate the family, community, and our human need for belonging with the patient's styles of coping and capacity for resilience into therapeutic treatment strategies.
5. Expanding our network of inner and outer resources of support available to us as a way to be strengthened as essential elements for coping and healing ourselves.
6. Accept the role of patient advocate, knowing state law as part of state licensure requirements, and the responsibility to report any abuse.

KEY TERMS

acceptance
adaptation
adjustment and coping
bonding
emotion-focused problem solving
family network, belonging, and community

inner and outer support systems
loss, grief, and suffering
meaning-making
mindfulness
resilience and stress hardiness

It is a part of the human condition to have intense life experiences that can range from relatively benign to absolutely catastrophic, and there are incredibly complex ways in which we might respond and adjust to these kinds of life experiences. Adjusting to a disability is an ongoing process, just as adjusting to all other aspects of life is for everyone. This process of moving forward is a lifelong one. To move forward with a disability, it is important to turn toward and acknowledge and be present to and acknowledge the situation at hand, thereby opening oneself up to the potential hidden within the situation. If we turn away from and deny the situation, we are at risk of never fully coming to terms with and adjusting to the experience.

Adjusting to a disability is not unilateral. It is layered and deep. The family and support system must be involved in this process. Therapists may be tempted to treat the impairment in isolation and not be involved in the adjustment process for the individual or their support system. This would be a major mistake. Technicians address the mechanical (technical) aspects of treatment, but clinical professionals must treat the whole person and must be involved in the process of adjustment at all times. It

is a fatal flaw to reduce the individual to just the impairment and not see or try to understand the bigger picture with regard to what is really being called for during treatment intervention. A technician may obtain good physical results, but if the individual has not begun the process of adapting to the life-altering event, the physical results may never be maximized. If an individual's support system has not been adjusting to the impairment, he or she may hold the patient back from optimal functioning or put unnecessary pressure simply out of a lack of knowing how to respond to the situation. Proper training and practice can foster the empowerment of the patient and the support system. In this chapter, we will pursue topics that cover important aspects of the adjustment process for the individual with a disability and his or her support system.

PSYCHOLOGICAL ADJUSTMENT

In clinical practice, theoretical foundations for adjustment to disability appear to be elusive because they represent a fluid process: all people are constantly changing. This is especially true for people who have recently become physically disabled. They do not reach a certain state of adjustment and stay there but progress through a series of adaptations. Therapists see patients in a crisis state[1-6] and therefore identify

---

*Videos for this chapter are available at studentconsult.com.

their adjustment patterns from this frame of reference. How well the individual adjusts to the crisis, however, does not necessarily indicate how well he or she will adjust to all aspects of the disability or the rate of progress from one point of adaptation to another.[6–15] Disabilities are an unimaginable insult to an individual's self-perception and identity.[16–19] A month or even a year after the injury may not be long enough to put the disability into perspective.[10,16,17,19–22]

For most people, progressing from the shock of injury to the acceptance of and later adaptation to disability is a process filled with psychological ups and downs and may not be linear. The process may even be considered like a spiral rather than a linear progression, and the word "progress" is used loosely here.

Several authors have discussed the possible stages of adjustment and grieving.[10,14] The research of Kübler-Ross[23] into death and dying has application to this topic of adjustment to disability. She discussed the concept of loss and grief in relation to life; loss of function may result in just as profound a reaction. The practice of mindfulness may be important in disengaging individuals from automatic thoughts, habits, and unhealthy behavior patterns, and thus could play a key role in fostering informed and self-endorsed behavioral regulation and adjustment to catastrophic life events.[24] Peretz[25] and others[26–28] discuss the grieving process in relation to the loss of role function as well as loss of body function. These losses must be grieved for before the patient can fully benefit from therapy or adjust to a changed body and lifestyle. Therapists must be aware that the patient can and must deal with the death of certain functional abilities. At the same time our dominant North American culture does not foster the skills of grieving over the course of one's life-span. Death is largely swept under the rug, and grief and sadness are not given much space in our fast-paced lifestyles. So we all are developmentally challenged to know what appropriate grief looks or feels like, and most of us might even be inclined to say, "Enough already, it's time to move on now, get on with it, move on . . . etc.," even if we may not say this out loud. You are encouraged to notice when this might arise in yourself without condemning yourself but acknowledging this as powerful cultural messages we swallow being raised in this dominant North American narrative. So how do we proceed if we as practitioners lack the skills to wrestle with our own suffering? If you are like most of us, you learn to numb yourself from your suffering or the suffering of others. And today's society offers us a smorgasbord of options to numb out now more than ever before. What can we do then? We can learn to grieve, to engage with and acknowledge our own suffering, and to "adapt" right alongside our patients. At the same time, the development of mindfulness in our own lives is essential to ground us within our own embodied experiences of the present moment so that we are not so easily swept up by other people's suffering. We must begin to build a strong sense of rootedness within oneself to enhance our therapeutic use of self.

Some authors have questioned the concept of stages of adjustment[1,29] and call for more empirical research into adaptation and adjustment; this has been started.[30] One alternative concept that has been developed is cognitive adaptation theory.[31] This concept examines self-esteem, optimism, and control. In this theory, if the individual feels good about himself or herself and has an optimistic view of life and a sense of control over life, the individual will adapt to the functional limitations and will participate in life. Cognitive adaptation theory does not consider the organic changes that may take place when brain damage has occurred, but the basic goals are very much worth taking into consideration. These should be examined in relation to the limbic system (see Chapter 4) because limbic involvement is crucial to reaching all goals and plays a key role in establishment of motivation.

The components of successful psychological adjustment to a physical disability (activity limitations) are varied and complex. To bring a patient to a level of function that is of the highest quality possible for that individual, therapists must look holistically at the psychosocial aspects and at the adjustment processes involved, evaluate each component, and integrate the processes into the therapeutic milieu to promote growth in all areas. There is much more to evaluation and treatment than just the physical component; the mind and body have intricately interrelated influences, and both must be considered, evaluated, and treated individually and as a whole.

WE UNDERSTAND MORE ABOUT SUFFERING THAN WE THINK

Clinical professionals have a wellspring of knowledge to draw from beyond their extensive traditional education. We are all human beings, and being human comes with a great deal of innate suffering. If we bring awareness to the fact that we have all suffered in our lives, we may not feel so separate from our patients. We may realize that we have more to offer our patients than just the knowledge we have gained about their disability and how we might help them gain function. The more we allow ourselves to slow down and be present with suffering— our own or that of another—the more we will be able to be open to the mystery and joy of our lives just as they are without requiring them to be any different.[32] It may be our lifetime's journey to be servants of the healing arts; this is our job, and it also takes enormous skill and bravery to bear witness to the full catastrophe of the human condition.[32] One of the benefits of our profession is the stimulus to examine our lives through the experiences of others. This can improve our function and help us grow as professionals and individuals, but if we are not open to the patients' experiences, we may not find a reason to examine and grow from our own experiences.

If we haven't endured great suffering personally, we have borne witness to it—"9/11" is a perfect example of this. If we acknowledge this fact, then maybe we can acknowledge that we are more connected to our patients than we once thought and that we have more to offer our patients in terms of their ability to adjust to their disability than we may have imagined. It is within the wrestling with suffering where meaning-making arises. Honoring, acknowledging, and appreciating human suffering (our own and that of others) is the cornerstone of adaptation. When we are mindful of this grappling with life's challenges, we can't help but be transformed, and a new normal ushers its way into place over and over again. Within the pains blossoms wisdom and insight, a deeper capacity to feel life deeply, maybe even to have our heart's broken on schedule, maybe even a capacity to wonder at it all and to act accordingly and with discernment.

Frank Ostaseski, after years of working in hospice and training hospice workers, in his book *The Five Invitations* offers these suggestions rooted in mindfulness practice, which are helpful pointers for therapists:
1. Don't Wait.
2. Welcome Everything, Push Away Nothing.
3. Bring Your Whole Self to the Experience.
4. Find a Place of Rest in the Middle of Things.
5. Cultivate Don't Know Mind.[33]

AWARENESS OF PSYCHOLOGICAL ADJUSTMENT IN THE CLINIC, SOCIETY, AND CULTURE

Working with individuals with functional limitations requires that we cultivate a holistic and all-encompassing perspective: to visualize how they might best participate within their own homes and communities and in the context of their society and a given time. This is a dynamic and constantly evolving process. The clinician must develop an intervention that will appropriately stimulate the individual and all their potential caregivers to maximize the potential for the highest-quality life possible. The skilled clinician initially evaluates the individual's physical and cognitive capabilities, depending on the type of functional limitations. The more subtle psychological aspects of the patient's ability to function need to be assessed at some level. These include the individual's support system and/or family network and the ability to adjust to the imminent changes in lifestyle. It would be a tragic situation for a clinician to ignore the individual's psychological adjustment or consider it to be less important in any way.[19,34-37]

Livneh and Antonak[38] have introduced a consolidated way to look at adaptation as a primer for counselors, which should be examined by therapists. They use some of the same basic concepts, such as stress, crisis, loss and grief, body image, self-concept, stigma, uncertainty or unpredictability, and quality of life, to frame their approach. They also consider the concepts of shock, anxiety, denial, depression, anger and hostility, and adjustment in a format that is usable by the therapist.

Livneh and Antonak[38] mention that one of the aspects that the therapist must watch out for is a form of coping called *disengagement.* This style of coping may be demonstrated through denial or avoidance behaviors that can take many forms. It can result in substance abuse, blame, or just refusal to interact. Research regarding people with head injuries has demonstrated that if a premorbid coping style for a person was to use alcohol or other drugs, the patient may revert to these same styles of coping, which can result in poor physical and emotional rehabilitation.[39] It is important to help the individual out of this quagmire. The skills of a therapist are likely not enough to do this in the short time that the patient is in treatment, so a referral to social work, psychology, or psychiatry is recommended to help support the long-term process. It is still the therapist's job to understand the process of adjustment, the indications regarding how an individual is adjusting, as well as key concepts for how to engage with an individual who is adjusting. It is also essential for the clinician to build skills for how to set personal boundaries without numbing out, to build skills of caring for oneself deeply and on many levels, and to build a practice of extending self-compassion to oneself, so that the clinician is less likely to be overwhelmed by the process of adjustment and disability and has greater capacity to stay centered in the face of human suffering, adjustment, and growth.

In light of all this, it is still the primary job of the therapist to help promote and maximize the engagement in functional activities. These activities are behaviors that are goal oriented (patient, family, and therapist driven), demonstrating problem solving and information seeking and involving completion of steps to positively move forward into life with the disability and maximize independence (promoting function).

The rest of this section introduces the reader to some of the psychological change components that may be assessed and acknowledged. The last section will attempt to demonstrate possible ways that these components can be taken into account as an aspect of therapy.

Growth and Adaptation

The clinician must keep in mind the context from which the patient is coming. Just days or even hours ago the individual may have been going about daily life without difficulty. The trauma may be multifaceted: (1) physical trauma, (2) emotional trauma occurring to the individual's support system, and (3) trauma of each of these systems interacting (the support system trying to protect the individual, and the patient trying to protect the support system). The interaction of these multifaceted components of the trauma may lead to posttraumatic stress. Posttraumatic stress can happen anytime after the life-changing or traumatic event. The level of distress can become disabling in and of itself, and our medical system will label the response a "syndrome" if the level of distress becomes paralyzing. The posttraumatic stress

"syndrome" may be observed more often in women,[40] but because of cultural barriers it can be hidden in men. It happens more often when there has been a near-death situation.[41,42] The patient may blame others, try to protect others, or be so self-absorbed that little else in the world may be seen or heard. It may be helpful to get psychological help for the individual early in therapy, even without the label of a "syndrome," if the level of distress is preventing optimal outcomes or creating obstacles in therapy.[4,15,43-46] Keeping in mind that even the concepts of "optimal outcomes" and "obstacles in therapy" can dehumanize our patients and can become blocks in our own capacity as clinicians to bring our own humanity to the patient-therapist relationship. These are moral and ethical concerns that skilled clinicians need to remain vigilant of throughout our career working in our culture's industrialized systems of health care that seek a bottom line that can often be a financial one with fierce productivity standards.

One of the most important jobs the therapist does is to develop a trusting relationship with the patient. Through this relationship the individual can be guided to focus on the goals of therapy and work on a positive perspective about the future. One of the errors of the medical system is that of focusing on the disease outcomes and pathology and not on the person and their capabilities and helping boost the integrity and personal sovereignty of the individual as a whole person.[19] If we focus solely on the loss, we may cause the individual to see only the injury, disease, or condition and nothing else. In a Veterans Administration hospital, spouses of people with spinal cord injuries formed a group in which the group's focus was on why the partners got married in the first place; the group never looked at the physical limitations as disabling. After a little while, people came to the conclusion that they did not marry their spouses for their legs and the fact that the legs no longer worked was not a major issue after all. This started the decentering from the medical disability model, and the focus started to be placed on the people and the families' future. If we can help patients focus on their functions and interests and not their dysfunctions, the effect of therapy after treatment will be much better. More work needs to be done to help patients see the potential they will have in the future to live their lives with the highest quality possible.[35,47-51] The World Health Organization developed a model that differentiates the disease pathology model of medicine and focuses on individuals' activities in life and the ability to participate in those interactions. The therapy world has enthusiastically accepted this model, the International Classification of Functioning, Disability, and Health (ICF), and the professions of both occupational and physical therapy use it as a reference model for practice.

Focusing on how to participate, move, and function in the world is one of the keys to helping the patient and the family work toward its future.[34,50,52-55] The therapist needs to help the patient focus on the direction of treatment objectives and demonstrate how therapy translates into meeting the patient's goals.[19,56] To discover the patient's true goals, the therapist must gain the trust of the patient and establish sound lines of communication. Distrust from health professionals may obstruct the adjustment process and lead to negative consequences.[57] Whenever possible, the patient's support system should be enlisted to help establish realistic support for the patient and the goals of both the patient and the family. It has been found that if the patient trusts the health professional, the patient will be more adherent and will seek assistance when it is needed.[58,59]

A New Normal

When we experience a decline in our ability to carry out our everyday routine tasks, regardless of the cause of our "disability," we may experience incredible degrees of despair. Many societies emphasize a very specific idea of what it means to be normal. At least in our modern,

North American model, there doesn't appear to be a great deal of flexibility in what this standard of normal is, regardless of one's cultural background. When an individual fails to live up to or no longer fits this norm, there can exist a tremendous amount of mental and emotional suffering. Because our bodies and minds are so intricately interconnected, our physical being is adversely affected by the mental and emotional anguish. On top of what the individual may already be experiencing physically, suddenly there is another layer of mental-physical anguish that is far too easily ignored, unappreciated, and unattended to by clinical professionals. However, once we are aware of the multifaceted potential for human suffering with regard to adjusting to a disability, we may be empowered to assist the individual with a non-linear, multifaceted approach. Researchers and theorists from various psychotherapy traditions have begun to explore the potential value of the therapeutic relationship by making direct references to different levels of validation as a means of demonstrating warmth, genuineness, empathy, and acceptance and reiterate how important it is for therapists to reflect back to the patient that their feelings, thoughts, and actions make sense in the context of their current experience and the cultural norms at large. In addition, the therapist articulates an expectation that the treatment collaboration will be effective in an attempt to convey hope and confidence in their ability to work together.[60]

We can guide our patients in identifying a new normal for themselves, all the while allowing them and their support system to grieve the "loss" of the old normal. As the Harvard psychologist Ellen Langer described in her book *Mindfulness*, "if we are offered a new use for a door or a new view of old age [or disability], we can erase the old mindsets without difficulty."[61] We can offer our patients a new view of themselves by showing them what they are capable of as they rebuild their lives. We can also help them honor and acknowledge what is present in this moment for them, we can help reflect back to them what they are capable of, and to appreciate their humanity and their wholeness as they are, without needing them to be any other way.

People who choose to go into this line of work and to be a part of the helping rehabilitation profession tend to be compassionate people. This is of course a wonderful quality to bring to our patients. At the same time, however, we need to be vigilant of the desire we may bring into our work with the underlying goal to take away another person's suffering. This kind of attitude to our work can bring about burnout and compassion fatigue. If we notice this underlying desire, it is helpful to just notice it as it is, maybe inquire about where we may have picked up this narrative, identify if it is useful to the situation, and letting it go. Let's consider this a bit more.

A woman who has lived with multiple sclerosis for over 30 years describes how the relief of suffering does not require restoring physical function to some perceived level of normality. Nor is she saying that our job is to relieve suffering. She states, "Suffering is relieved to the extent that patients can learn to integrate bodily disorder and physical incapacity into their lives, to accommodate to a different way of being" (p. 591).[62] It may be that we can bring healing to ourselves, our patients, and our culture to appreciate the potential for a new narrative around our customary approach to suffering, which is implies that in general we want relief from suffering and sometimes at significant costs. Maybe the new narrative we could foster is one where suffering does not need to be "relieved." We may wonder about who we are as people and health care practitioners, often bringing a narrative of "us" as clinicians, being the ones to take away or "relieve" someone else's suffering. Is this necessary or even helpful? What if we learned to approach our own suffering, our patient's suffering, and the suffering of the world with a view that it is to be honored and appreciated as a profoundly meaningful human experience, not to be disregarded or something to "get rid of"? There is potential within our suffering to

bring profound meaning to our lives. More recent research is demonstrating that when we wrestle with life's challenges or when we give ourselves the space to suffer during challenges and changes, these experiences can help us make meaning of our lives. The process of grappling with these difficulties and intensities, while holding ourselves and others with compassion and clarity, can bring new narratives we so desperately need in these times. So let us wonder together about the implications of this. Feelings of sadness, anger, despair, longing, and fear can all be appropriate responses to change. How might we hold space for and honor these human experiences? There are almost no role models for this way of being in the midst of most of our dominant systems of our industrialized existence, including our health care institutions, but we can always learn, and practicing mindfulness can foster this capacity in meaningful ways.

According to research by De Souza and Frank,[62] their subjects with chronic back pain expressed regret at the loss of capabilities and distress at the functional consequences of those losses. They found that facilitating adjustment to "loss" was more helpful than implying the potential for a life free of pain as a result of therapeutic interventions. The word "loss" is in quotations here to recognize that the language we use to imply a certain kind of meaning on someone else's experience needs to be considered thoughtfully and held in awareness. Language is powerful, and it is important to recognize that it is possible for people to not experience their situation necessarily as a "loss" but consider the experience as a gift or both. Or we could say experiencing that loss comes with a gift.

There is a broad continuum of experience a human being may ascribe to their situation, and we need to be alert to our own biases about a person's potential experience and honor that and not need to impose our own biases and views upon their experience. How do we know what they may be experiencing? Well, we could ask them, with an open, curious awareness, "How is it for you now? What is this experience like for you?" So often in our modern North American culture we are taught to not show our pain and suffering, to numb and subjugate our experience. Through our own personal practice, integrating a mindful holding and honoring of our own human experiences, the griefs, the sadness, the fears, the joys, and the wonder, we become more capable of holding another's full human experience and not needing them to be different from what "it" is.

We can sense this capacity in each other. Consider this: you may know people in your life you feel safe sharing your deepest truth and feelings with and others you can sense are not fully capable of holding your pains and difficulties or your joys for that matter. As clinicians, we can develop and build our capacity to hold another person's experience as meaningful for them without needing them to sugarcoat or subjugate it for our sake to make us feel better.

Guiding the individual through practice and repetition of basic functional activities will allow the patient to identify for himself or herself how to live successfully in this world again and cultivate this "different way of being" in action, while participating in daily life. At the same time we can encourage our patients to mindfully plan for and visualize their future (see the practice section later) during specific times of their day so that their minds are not in constant worry mode or rehearsing, which can cause a great deal of anxiety about the future. We can assist our patients in using emotion-focused and problem-focused problem-solving strategies as they plan for their future, in the present moment, especially in a medical environment where shorter rehabilitation stays are the norm. And we can do all of this without needing their suffering or pain to go away and without needing them "to get on with it already" and "to adapt."

Without any need to apologize for their situation, just simply being with them in the moment in a nonjudgmental way and allowing them to

BOX 5.1   Practice: Mindful Planning and Visualization of Future

- Find a time when you are alone; you need only a few minutes every day for this practice.
- Allow this time to be specifically for future planning and visualization, not worrying.
- If you find yourself worrying about the future at other times during the day, acknowledge that there will be a specific time devoted to planning and visualizing. Worrying throughout the day will bring a great deal of mental anguish during times when you need to focus attention on an important task or rehabilitation intervention.
- Use a journal to record thoughts and ideas on paper so that the thoughts do not have to stay in the mind and be rehearsed. Write down concerns, your emotions, and feelings, as well as your desires and plans.
- Try to let go of planning during daily activities and tasks until the next scheduled mindful planning session, or, if necessary, allow this moment to be the next planning session but be sure to stop whatever else you are doing and be fully present in the planning process.

grieve (and honoring our own grief) can be a powerful tool for healing. Acknowledging the loss, pain, and the suffering may help patients move forward with their lives in a new way. "Acceptance [of what is] doesn't, by any stretch of the imagination, mean passive resignation. Quite the opposite. It takes a huge amount of fortitude and motivation to accept what is—especially when we don't like it—and then work wisely and effectively as best we possibly can with the circumstances we find ourselves in and with the resources at our disposal, both inner and outer, to mitigate, heal, redirect, and change what can be changed" (Box 5.1).[63]

Societal and Cultural Influences

Culture, subcultures, and the culture and beliefs of the given family are all aspects of the patient that the therapist must be aware of.[22,53,64–70] This concept gets into the beliefs about the world and maybe a belief about the cause of the disability or at least how the patient is viewing the disability. Asking "Do you notice any beliefs about why this happened?" can lead to an insightful experience. "Causes" may range from "things like this just happen," "sometimes bad things happen to good people," to "God is punishing me," "I deserved it," or even "life is against me."

From an early age, people in our society are exposed to misconceptions regarding the disabled.[71–74] If in the therapeutic environment, however, the patient and family have their misconceptions challenged constantly, they may start reformulating their concept of the role of the disabled person. As this process progresses, therapists and other staff can help make the expectations of the disabled person more realistic. Therapists can schedule their patients at times when they will be exposed to people adjusting to their disabilities. For example, use of individuals who have been successfully rehabilitated as staff members (role models) can help to dispel misconceptions that people with disabilities are not employable.[75–77]

This process of adaptation to a new disability can be considered as a cultural change from a majority status (able bodied) to a minority status (disabled). Part of the adaptation process can be considered as an acculturation process, and the therapist can help facilitate this process.[16,73,78,79]

The cultural background of the individual also contributes to the perception of disability and to the acceptance of the disabled person. Trombly and Radomski[80] state that perception and expression of pain, physical attractiveness, valuing of body parts, and acceptability of types of disabilities can be culturally influenced. One's ethnic background can also affect intensity of feelings toward specific handicaps, trust of staff,[80] and acceptance of therapeutic modalities.[81–85]

The successful therapist will be sensitive to the cultural values of the patient and will attempt to present therapy to the patient in the most acceptable way. For example, in the Mexican culture it is not polite to just start to work with a patient; rapport must first be established. Sharing of food may provide the vehicle to accomplish rapport. Thus the therapist might schedule the first visit with a Mexican patient during a coffee break. The therapist must remember that the patient may be the one who may have difficulty adjusting to the therapist and that the therapist may need to adjust to the patient, especially in the early stages of therapy.

Gaining trust is one of the crucial links in any meaningful therapeutic situation.[59,86,87] Trust will create an environment that facilitates communication, productive learning, and exchange of information.[76,87] Trust is important in all cultures and will be fostered by the therapist who is sensitive to the needs of the patient. This sensitivity is necessary with every patient but will be manifested in many different ways, depending on the background and needs of the individual in a therapy. A patient of one culture may feel that looking another person in the eyes is offensive, whereas in another culture refusal to look into someone's eyes is a sign of weakness or lack of honesty (shifty eyed).[88] Thus, although it is impossible to know every culture or subculture with which the therapist may come into contact, the therapist must attempt to be sensitive to the background and needs of the patient. Even if the therapist knows the cultural norms, not every person follows the cultural patterns. Thus every patient needs to be treated as an individual in the therapeutic relationship with respect, dignity, and sovereignty. It should be the therapist's job to be sensitive to the subtle nonverbal and verbal cues that indicate the level of trust in the relationship. The therapist will obtain this information by being open to the patient and their context, not open to a textbook. The patient is the owner of this information and will share it with everyone he or she trusts and those who care to ask. It is OK if we mess up sometimes; this is inevitable. Being human and working in diverse health care settings is dynamic and complex. Holding ourselves in compassion when this happens, learning from the situation, and (if it is called for) apologizing are essential.

Trust is often established in the therapeutic relationship through the therapeutic process of doing physical activities. For example, the act of working with a patient in transferring from the chair to the bed can either build trust or destroy the potential relationship. If the patient trusts the therapist just enough to follow instructions to transfer but then falls in the process, it may take quite some time to reestablish the same level of trust, assuming that it can ever be reestablished. This trusting relationship is so complex and involves such a variety of levels that the therapist should be as aware of attending to the patient's security in the relationship as to the physical safety of the patient in the clinic.[59,86] If the patient believes that the therapist is not trustworthy in the relationship, then it may follow that the therapist is not to be trusted when it comes to teaching and learning to participate in newly difficult activities of daily living (ADLs). If the patient does not know how to safely go about their daily activities and thus has not yet built trust in their body or their skill to navigate their ADLs, then lacking trust in the therapist will only compound the stress of the situation.[59,86,89]

The patient's culture may be unfamiliar to the therapist, even though both the clinician and patient may be from the same geographical region. A patient's problems of poverty, unemployment, and a lack of educational opportunities[77,87,90,91] can all result in the therapist and patient feeling that therapy will be unsuccessful, even before the first session has begun. Such preconceived concepts held by both parties may not be warranted and must be examined. These preconceived concepts can be more reflective of failure of rehabilitation than any physical limitation of the patient.

Cultural and religious values may also result in the patient feeling that he or she must pay for past sins by being disabled and that the disability will be overcome after atonement for these sins. Such a patient may not be inclined to participate in or enjoy therapy. The successful therapist does not assault the patient's basic cultural or religious values but may recognize them in the therapy sessions. If the therapist feels that the culturally defined problems are impeding the therapeutic process, the therapist may offer the patient opportunities to reexamine these cultural "truths" in a nonjudgmental way and may help the patient redefine the way the physical limitations and therapy are seen.[92] Religious counseling could be recommended by the therapist, and follow-up support in the clinic may be given to the patient to view therapy not as undoing what "God has done" but as a way of proving religious strength. Reworking a person's cultural and religious (cognitive) structure is a sensitive area, and it should be handled with care and respect and with the use of other professionals (social workers and religious and psychological counselors) as appropriate.

The hospital staff can be encouraged to establish groups in which commonly held values of patients can be examined and possibly reframed or incorporated.[16,92–98] Such groups can lead the patient to a better understanding of priorities and may help the person see the relevance of therapy and the need to continue the adjustment process. This can also prepare the patient to better accept the need for support groups after discharge. The therapist may be able to use information from such group sessions to adjust the way therapy sessions are presented and structured to make therapy more relevant to the patient's values and needs. Value groups or exercises[99] can be another means used by the therapist for evaluation and understanding of the patient.

Beliefs and values of cultures and families can play a profound role in the course of treatment. Such things as physical difficulties, which can be seen, are usually better accepted than problems that cannot be seen, such as brain damage that changed an individual's cognitive abilities or personality.[100] A person with a back injury may be seen as lazy, whereas a person with a double amputation will be perceived as needing help. At the same time, in some cultures a person who has lost a body part may be seen as "not all there" and should be avoided socially. Therefore being attuned to the culture and beliefs of the patient is imperative in therapy. The reader is encouraged to refer to texts on cultural issues in health care such as *Culture in Clinical Care* by Bonder, Martin, and Miracle[101]; *Cultural Competence in Health Care: A Practical Guide* by Rundle, Carvalho, and Robinson[102]; and *Caring for Patients from Different Cultures* by Galanti[103] for more detailed discussions on how culture and beliefs affect health care.

Attachment and Evolving Sense of Self: Foundations of Adjustment

The persons we serve in rehab are fellow travelers on a human, developmental, and evolving journey through life—with its experiences, losses and gains, encounters, and opportunities and obstacles. Any treatment we provide is in the context of that journey as a "self" with its ongoing times of crisis, disequilibrium and chaos, reorganization, and integration and change. The therapist seeks to support the person in their current crisis or condition as well as accompany in service of that evolving meaning-making self. And it is helpful to understand where they are in their evolution as a self, not as an evaluation of their stage but as an understanding of their meaning-making.

As humans we are intrinsically, neurobiologically social. From the time of infancy attachment and development, a growing sense of self and other and of efficacy is gradually formed in the container of relationship with a primary caregiver. Burgeoning research on this primary biological, neurological social core process has shown how sense of other and self, relational constructs are developed and then

continually grown. We are evolved "in relation." It is the medium in which we learn and know self, other, and the world and adapt, grow, and evolve. Research has identified basic "good enough" caregiver qualities crucial to a healthy sense of self, and these core qualities in primary relations become internalized as part of growth and development. They can also be thought of as the qualities of a good container for growth and healing. Family, school, friendships, and groups may hold these qualities to greater or lesser degrees, and we need to consider their capacity to be containers.

The following are some basic qualities ideally present for an infant:[104]
- Physical presence, eye contact, physical contact, consistency, reliability, and interest
- Protection
- Attunement
- Soothing and reassurance
- Expressed delight
- Unconditional support and encouragement
- Felt sense of safety
- Felt sense of comfort
- As the child develops, encouragement and support for inner and outer exploration

Diane Fosha[105] identifies these similar qualities as therapeutic holding:
- Empathic attunement
- Recognition, affirmation, validation, and valuing of patient's experience
- Expressed care, compassion, and concern
- Authenticity and encouragement
- Expressed delight

These all help undo the sense of being alone. It can be said that in general these are attributes from without and internalized within that help promote healing, integration, resilience, and growth. These are also functions of community that can be of primary support for patients, families, and caregivers.

Parents who have experienced obstacles in bonding with an infant born with severe illness or disability can access help and support in this area and also take hope that these are potentially areas of continued growth and healing. Health providers must all give primary support for bonding and the primary relationships. Promising research also shows that deficiencies in attachment can be healed and repaired throughout life with attention and support. No one has perfect experiences (see, among others, D. J. Brown, Elliott *Treating Attachment Disorders in Adults*).

The holding environment and secure-base experience are themselves corrective emotional experiences for patient in large part because they reduce or "undo" the patient's sense of being alone with her or his painful experience.[106]

Persons undergoing new injury, insult, or conditions are often experiencing huge changes in perception, processing, and sense of self. They need support as they undergo an often long and slow process of reorientation, recalibration, and reintegration of a changing sense of self. In this regard, the therapist must be attuned to the present state as well as the long and wide view.

Respect for the current stage and state must be maintained while cultivating openings, opportunities, and seeds for adaptation and integration. Digestion of trauma and change cannot be forced. Healing and growth are a spiraling process with seeming backslides as well as gains. Mindfulness practice, where possible for patients, caregivers, and family, can offer experientially gained insight that promotes greater flexibility, acceptance, and perspective on change, identity, and sense of self over time. When experiencing crisis, the notion of a fixed identity dependent on good health, job and family roles, certain physical, mental, or other capacities can be shattered or injured. Much support, holding, and mirroring are needed to both grieve real losses and validate the patient's experience and value. Many disciplines as well as community and personal networks have a potential role to play over time in supporting the person and their network of caring others who are experiencing their own losses and changes. As time goes on, support groups, consumer groups, community programs, chaplains, counselors, mindfulness groups, or individual support might eventually be incorporated. The trajectory of when a person or family is interested or willing to pursue some of these may vary greatly.

The Evolving Sense of Self: Growth Over the Life-Span

Background to circumstances of health, illness, and changes in abilities and circumstances is the great life project, what Robert Kegan calls the evolution of meaning,[107] the person's capacity to make sense of life in an adaptive manner, to "make whole." The spirit is always engaged in a progressive motion, in giving itself new form an endeavor that requires courage and involves losses and eventual gains. This constructive-developmental approach pays attention to the developmental ongoing activity of meaning-making constructing.

> *Meaning is in its origins, a physical activity, a social activity, a survival activity (in doing it we live). This evolving is the "primary human motion."*
>
> *Processes of internalization are intrinsically related to the movement of adaptation.*
>
> **—Kegan**

Growth is a matter of both differentiation and reintegrating into new connection in a spiraling process, what Piaget calls "decentration," the loss of an old center, and what Kegan calls "recentration," the recovery of a new center.[108] We undergo a series of transformations and imbalances and rebalances, "hatching out" of one self and reforming a larger self and larger relationship with the world, with life, finding new states of equilibrium in the world, "between the progressively individuated self and the bigger life field." And this ongoing conversation with life "is marked by periods of dynamic stability or balance followed by instability and qualitatively new balance."[109] In each new stage, we are defending, surrendering, and reconstructing a center.[110]

Understanding this adaptive conversation forms a background of our understanding how to better serve patients in pain and transition. As humans, we have this process in common. We are fellow travelers in an evolving life project. We are engaged in growing a point of view. Kegan says, "This activity is about knowing and being, about theory-making and investments and commitments of the self. The same ongoing tension between self-preservation and self-transformation is descriptive of the very activity of hope itself."[111]

Undoing Aloneness: The Need for Community, Friendship, Belonging.

From infancy on, it is essential to know that we exist in the heart and mind of another. This is our core relational need—to be recognized, seen, and known and to matter to one another. There are two powerful and profound yearnings in human existence and experience. One is unity: to be included, to be part of, close to, joined with, to be held, admitted, and accompanied. The other is a desire for agency and differentiation: to be independent, to have a unique and separate integrity, and to choose one's own direction.[112] There is an ongoing dynamic tension between these yearnings, and as we grow in development, we spiral through different balances leaning toward one or the other. We are increasing our understanding and differentiation as well as expanding our integration of the world and life. This very much models the experiences of mindfulness practice: that one is knowing, becoming more familiar increasing perception and specificity of

understanding self and experience, and simultaneously expanding the sense of an "I" to include more of life. A sense of safety is essential to this life enterprise of evolving stages of self and other and our construct of the world.

The good-enough "holding environment," described by Winnicott in infancy, is something that accompanies us throughout life. We live in a series of holding environments, in our history of embeddedness. They are the mediums that hold us and include us, and from which we differentiate. As Kegan says, "Your buoyancy or lack of it, your own sense of wholeness or lack of it, is in large part a function of how your own current embeddedness culture is holding you."[113,114]

"Good enough" holding environments—as in infancy and beyond—are containers and mirrors to the self we are and a bridge to the self we are becoming, and a stable presence for the transition in between when one self with its evolutionary truce is gone and the organization of new meaning-making is in transition. Cultures of embeddedness are often inadequate in our society and modern way of life, especially in times of crisis and change. We need to really consider how to create or connect to these ongoing supports of continuity through change.

Mitigating a sense of aloneness and isolation aids healing and recovery. We share a common humanity, and we all take on different roles in life at different times. As social beings, we need to be connected. Humans can bear hardship with the feeling of being accompanied by others. Healing and living fully happen in relation to others. Illness, crisis, disability, and stress can easily lead to isolation and a negative spiral of effects. We need positive mirroring and authentic affirmation of strengths and value. We need to be included and belong, as well as be valued for our uniqueness and agency. We need to know we positively affect others. Some of the most effective community programs have started as tiny grassroots initiatives and have simply grown out an unmet need, which include the Cabrillo College Stroke Center (https://www.cabrillo.edu/academics/strokecenter) and the Shurig Center for Brain Injury Recovery (https://www.schurigcenter.org). Because there was such a big need, they often grew into established vibrant and funded programs over time. Having regular times to meet and share with others provides an important buffer for individuals, caregivers, and families.

In speaking to our need to live in the context of community, Kegan says, "among its most important benefits is its capacity to recognize a person, a marriage, a family, over time and to help the developing system recognize itself amid the losses and recoveries of normal growth." Healing communities can provide a safe support and serve to affirm and recognize individuals, acknowledge losses and growth, and value people. A crisis or illness with loss often includes a loss of how one creates meaning.[115]

The patient's loss and grief brought on by disability or injury can be experienced as the "dying of a way to know the world which no longer works, a loss of an old coherence with no new coherence immediately to take its place. And yet a new balance again and again does emerge . . . Still, it is a new life not a return or recovery. We will never restore the (old) balance—but there is a new balance that can be achieved. We are not going back, but we are coming through- to a new integration, a new direction."[116]

As therapists, we are accompanying and collaborating with the person in their meaning-making process when their process has been threatened. Fosha, et al, reminds therapists, "We are wired to heal, to right ourselves, to grow and transform. It is what neuroplasticity is about."[117] Furthermore, "People have a fundamental need for transformation. We are wired for growth and healing. And we are wired for self-righting and resuming impeded growth. We have a need for the expansion and liberation of the self, the letting down of defensive barriers and the dismantling of the false self. We are shaped by a deep desire to be known, seen, and recognized, as we strive to come into contact with parts of ourselves that are frozen."[118]

We want to take note of the state of the person's vitality and life-force and notice areas of aliveness and obstacles to that life force. Areas of aliveness and wellness needed to be seen and felt, along with more difficult emotions. As Hildegaard de Bingen noticed, the tendency of a living thing is to return to its essence after being wounded, and promoting aliveness and healing involve a lot of time to see who a person is.[119] The long-range view of healing and resources for patients beyond our own contact is of primary importance. We want to encourage healthy social connectedness and hope to expand those possibilities.

Building Resilience: Felt Sense as an Underpinning for Positive Strengths and Neural Integration

Felt sense, a most basic way that we know our experience, is actually a skill that can be cultivated and used to support our more accurate and fully owned bodily perception, emotional knowing and regulation, and neural integration. Increasing capacity for felt sense—bringing attention in present time to the sensory sensations of the body—provides a way to anchor in the body and breath, self-regulate, and increase self-knowledge. Wellness can be described as a byproduct of our ability to tolerate our internal experience.[120] Having a stable caring environment along with mindful felt sense (an internalized holding) increases that capacity to be with our experience. Hendel and others refer to the the body as the place of deep emotional knowing.[121] It is an important stepping stone, increasing capacity for meta-cognition, a sense of insightful "knowing that you know" important to healing and growth. Felt sense is an important part of bringing attention and anchoring positive states in the body and thus wiring them into the brain.

As the qualities of the good enough caregiver (including how we care mentally and emotionally for ourselves) are the food for optimal brain development, in the same way the capacity to feel and sense and drink in positive states and experiences supports positive neuroplasticity in the service of adjustment and healing.[122,123]

Bringing attention to one's experience and amplifying the positive felt experience make them more "known." Gergely's research on marked expressivity, marked affectivity is mirrored with exaggerated content and tone so that the experience is "marked" as having happened, as important, and as belonging to the self.[124,125] In other words, it is known, owned, and wired in the brain more effectively and with greater efficiency, a way that neuroplasticity is utilized for healing. This capacity is increasing the ability to receive positivity, making the most of it, and in the process building up strengths and capacities so the process becomes a self-enhancing loop.

The development of the capacity for felt sense and safety, is the doorway to digest emotions associated with suffering and release subconscious, adaptive action tendencies.[126] Fosha describes in her Accelerated Experiential Dynamic Psychotherapy model that all affective states, in an adequate holding environment, are seeds for deeply transformative experience and development. Understanding this important insight can orient us to highlight this holding environment and build it into the way we structure and enact therapeutic environments and experiences as a foundational support. Presence, being with, cultivating sensing, and mindfulness all affect the quality of the healing capacity.[127] Mindfulness and positive relational experiences of safety, being seen and known, heard, and acknowledged, grow areas of interconnectedness in the corpus callosum, hippocampus, and prefrontal cortex. These relational experiences can happen in ongoing groups and cultures of belonging. Another resource of patients with capacity to develop attention and for caregivers is classes in mindfulness, which in addition to other benefits mentioned, is protective against depression and depression relapse. A secondary condition resulting from brain injury or other neurological events can be clinical depression, which must be addressed by the care team.

Establishment of Self-Worth and Healthy Body Image

The true value of a human being is determined primarily by the measure and the sense in which he has attained liberation from the self.

—Albert Einstein

Self-worth is composed of many aspects, such as body image, sexuality, and the ability to help others and affect the environment. The body image of a patient is a composite of past and present experiences, familial and cultural influences, and the individual's perception of those experiences. Because body image is based on experience, it is a constantly changing construct. An adult's body image is substantially different from the body image of a child and will no doubt change again as the aging process continues. A newly disabled person is suddenly exposed to a radically new body, and it is that individual's job to assess the body's capabilities and develop a new body image. Because the therapist is at least partially responsible for creating the environmental experiences from which the patient learns about this new body, the therapist must be aware of the concept. In the case of an acute injury, the patient has a new body from which to learn and experience. The therapist can promote positive feelings as the therapist instructs the patient how to use this new body and to accept its changes.[1,16,20,27,128,129]

Because in "normal" life we slowly observe changes in our bodies, such as finding one gray hair today and watching it take years for our hair to turn totally white, we have the luxury of slowly adapting to the "new us." Change usually does not happen quite so slowly and "naturally" when trauma or a disease affects the nervous system. This sudden loss of function can create a void that only new experiences and new role models can fill.

The loss of use of body parts can cause a person to perceive the body as an "enemy" that needs to be forced to work or to compensate for its disability. In all cases the body is the reason for the disability and the cause of all problems. The need for appliances and adaptive equipment can create a sense of alienation and lack of perceived "lovability" resulting from the "hardness of the hardware." People tend to avoid hugging someone who is in a wheelchair or who has braces around the body because of the physical barrier and because of the person's perceived fragility; a person with physical limitations is certainly not perceived as soft and cuddly.[20,27,53,103,128] Both the perception that these individuals are not lovable and their labored movements can sap the energy of the disabled and discourage social interaction or life participation. To accept the appliances and the dysfunctional body in a way that also allows the disabled person to feel loved can be a significant challenge.

In the case of a person who will be disabled for the long term, such as the person with cerebral palsy or Parkinson disease, the therapist is attempting to teach the patient how to change the previously accepted body image to one that would allow and encourage more normal function. In short, the therapist has two roles. One role is to help lessen the disabled body image. The second is to teach a functional disabled body image to a newly disabled person. The techniques may be the same, but in both cases the patient will have to undergo a great amount of change. The person with a neurological disorder or neurologically based disability may assume that he or she will not be capable of accomplishing many things with his or her life. The therapist is in a unique position to encourage development of and maximize the patient's level of functional ability. The individual may then expect more of himself or herself. The newly disabled person must change the expectations; however, he or she has little concept of what is realistic to expect of this new body. At this point, role models can be used to help shape the patient's expectations. If the patient is unable to adjust to the new body and accept the body image and self-expectations, life may be impoverished for that individual. Pedretti[130] states that the patient with low self-esteem often devalues his or her whole life in all respects, not just in the area of physical dysfunction.[1,16,20,27,128,130]

One way the patient can start exploring this new body is by exploring its sensations and performance. Dr. Jon Kabat-Zinn developed a guided "body scan" meditation that can help individuals learn how to become more connected and in tune with the sensations of the body.[63] This kind of practice is about learning to pay attention to the body in a new way and can be very helpful in developing an accurate body image and improve self-awareness. For example, the patient with a spinal cord injury may also use the sensation of touch to "map out" the body to see how it responds.[131] Including the whole body, encompassing the felt experience as part of sensory awareness, even though that may include unfamiliar sensations, numbness, and lack of sensation, is helpful in this regard. They may ask themselves the following questions: Is there a way to get the legs to move using reflexes? Can positioning the legs in a certain way aid in rolling the wheelchair or make spasms decrease? Such exploration will start the patient on the road to a self-informed and personally empowered evaluation of his or her abilities.

The therapist's role is to maximize the patient's perceptions of realistic body functioning. Exercises can be developed that encourage exploration of the body by the individual and, if appropriate, the significant partner. Functioning and building an appropriate body image will be more difficult if intimate knowledge of the new body is not as complete as before injury.[9] The successes the patient experience in the clinical setting, coupled with the patient's familiarity with his or her new body, will result in a more accurate body image and contribute to the patient's feelings of self-worth.

The last aspect of self-worth is often overlooked in the health fields. This aspect is the need that people have to help others.[132] People often discover that they are valuable through the act of giving. Seeing others enjoy and benefit from the individual's presence or offering increase self-worth. Situations in which others can appreciate the patient's worth may be needed. Unless the patient can contribute to others, the patient is in a relatively dependent role, with everyone else giving to him or her without the opportunity of giving back. Achieving independence, understanding common interdependence, and then reaching out to others, with therapeutic assistance if necessary, facilitate the individual's more rapid reintegration into society. The therapist should take every opportunity to allow the patient to express self-worth to others through helping and giving back to their family and community.

The ability to expand one's definition and experience of oneself is a key factor in adjusting to a disability. Expanding the experience of oneself in terms of all the roles and responsibilities one has or gently holding an experience of oneself that is so much greater than just the physical realm can help the individual comprehend the enormity of who he or she is. As humans, we have the capacity to understand how we are so much greater than just the job we once performed and so much greater than the role we once played. This practice can cultivate understanding of how complex our species is, it can humble us by acknowledging the vastness of our place within the universe and on this planet, and how much we have to offer the world (God knows the world certainly needs us), differently abled or not (see the journal activity in Box 5.1).

Sense of Control

Oh, I've had my moments, and if I had to do it over again, I'd have more of them. In fact, I'd try to have nothing else. Just moments, one after another, instead of living so many years ahead of each day.
        —*Nadine Stair, 85 years old, Louisville, Kentucky*

In her poignant quote, Nadine Stair speaks to an understanding that we all have the capacity to choose how we will experience every given moment of our lives. There is so little in life that we actually have

control over and our dominant culture doesn't teach what we do have control over, which is how we relate to every moment of our lives. We can intentionally choose to be present, and once we know this is so, we have control over our quality of attention, our level of attention, and our intention. So as humans we can develop these capacities and in doing so we build a greater and greater sense of self-control over our lives. While this sounds simple, it can be profoundly life changing and empowering on many levels. All the while we are exercising our choice to be intentionally present in a specific way and we are building neuroplasticity to choose every single time so that we will more likely be present when the going gets tough.

As Drs. Roizen and Oz stated in their book *You: The Owner's Manual*, we can control our health destiny.[133] Although we can't always control what happens to us (no matter how fit we are), there are some things we can control: our attitude, our determination, and our willingness to take our own health into our own hands.[133]

Adjusting to a disability can make patients feel as though they have very little control over their lives; they may feel helpless, as though their health is in everyone else's hands but their own. This feeling can cause incredible suffering and emotional anguish on top of their physical or cognitive disability. If we focus solely on treating the disability and ignore what may be going on for our patients mentally and emotionally, we may be creating even more suffering for them. Clinical professionals have the opportunity to guide their patients toward a new way of relating to their disability by focusing on what they do have control over as well as identifying ways in which they may relate differently to those situations over which they do not have control.

Dr. Jill Bolte-Taylor says this eloquently in a passage from her book:

I've often wondered, if it's a choice, then why would anyone choose anything other than happiness? I can only speculate, but my guess is that many of us don't exercise our ability to choose. Before my stroke, I thought I was a product of my brain and had no idea that I had some say about how I responded to the emotions surging through me. On an intellectual level, I realized that I could monitor and shift my cognitive thoughts, but it never dawned on me that I had some say in how I perceived my emotions . . . What an enormous difference this awareness has made in how I live my life.[134]

"I had some say in how I perceived my emotions." Let's wonder out loud about this statement. As Dr. Bolte-Taylor describes, all of us have the choice to be in relation to the present moment fully, or we can allow our thoughts and emotions to "take us for a ride" as though we were on automatic pilot.[109] If we allow our minds and emotions to take over our experience of the present moment without any awareness or personal choice, we can feel powerlessness and be dragged along into rehashing our past events that led up to the disability, which can create more suffering and emotional anguish. We also may be rehearsing what our lives will be like without allowing the dust to settle, without waiting until we have a clearer picture of what implications the disability may have for us. An unacknowledged rehashing and rehearsing can create an incredible sense of lack of control over one's life, which can lead to anxiety and depression.

Approximately 70% of our thoughts in any particular waking state can be considered to be daydreams, and they can often be unconstructive.[135] In an experience sampling method, Klinger and his colleagues found that "active, focused problem-solving thought"[136] made up only 6% of the waking state. According to Baruss, "it would make more sense to say that our subjective life consists of irrational thinking with occasional patches of reason"[135] while we are participating in our daily activities. Especially when one is participating in menial, basic self-care activities, our mind is most often in another place. For the most part, our modern North American culture does not teach the skills of mindful, present moment awareness or emotional intelligence.

If an individual is frequently disconnected from the present moment, tending to unconsciously ruminate over negative past or future events, he or she may experience significant negative effects from this perpetual distraction. Unacknowledged rumination, absorption in the past, rehashing, or fantasies and anxieties about the future can pull one away from what is taking place in the present moment. Awareness or attention can be divided without conscious choice, such as when people occupy themselves with multiple tasks at one time or preoccupy themselves with concerns that detract from the quality of engagement with what is focally present, and this can increase a sense of disempowerment, anxiety, and depression.[137] Anxiety and depression can be signs of underlying problems that are unacknowledged. Anxiety and depression are not the problem in and of themselves.

Being sad and feeling depressed or anxious, for example, are completely appropriate responses to so many situations that ail us culturally, socially, ecologically, economically, politically, and personally. So we must be careful in our "diagnosis" of what ourselves or others may be experiencing and feeling and not necessarily labeling "the ailments," the suffering, the strong emotional experiences as dysfunctional when the responses to those events or situations may be completely appropriate to the situation and may actually help bring meaning to one's life, motivation, and emotion-focused problem solving, discernment, and skillful action.

On the other hand, according to Drs. Roizen and Oz,[133] emotions can cause high blood pressure, as well as disrupting the body's normal repair mechanisms. Low-level, perpetual, and unacknowledged states of stress can also constrict our blood vessels, making it even harder for enough blood to work its way through the body. At the same time, stress is also shown to encourage bonding responses that actually work to bring people together in community (https://www.ted.com/talks/kelly_mcgonigal_how_to_make_stress_your_friend). Also called the "tend and befriend reflex," stress can be our friend if we can change our relationship to stress, acknowledge it, honor it for the message it may be sending, and hold it gently in awareness. Learning relaxation techniques such as yoga and meditation can help us build the skills of awareness, clarity, and self-compassion to honor these strong emotions and feelings of stress in our bodies. Learning to allow and honor our human experience, learning how to relate to our feelings and emotions with clarity, discernment, and care is an essential process of learning how to be in skillful relationship to our feelings. Numbing and subjugating our feelings, as our modern North American culture often teaches, is not the answer.

However, we know now that all mind states affect our bodies profoundly whether we are feeling joy, wonder, and awe or jealousy, rage, and hopelessness—for example, a feeling of helplessness appears to weaken the immune system, yet joy and wonder release hormones associated with well-being.[133] We can teach ourselves and our patients to be mindful of and pay attention to our mind states, feelings, and thoughts during therapeutic intervention. In this way and with the skills of mindful awareness, we can encourage a greater sense of personal control and facilitate greater mental and emotional equilibrium and adjustment to the individual's disability. According to a 2008 article by Ludwig and Kabat-Zinn in *JAMA,* "the goal of mindfulness is to maintain awareness moment by moment, disengaging oneself from strong attachment to beliefs, thoughts, or emotions, thereby developing a greater sense of emotional control, balance, and well-being."[138]

The key here is in the practice of loosening attachments or clinging to any specific mind state so that as we begin to notice mental phenomena, we can choose how we wish to respond. We can let go of the thought and focus our attention on the present moment at hand, or we

can hold the thoughts, emotions, and feelings in awareness. We can honor and appreciate our experience as it is without needing it to be any other way, or we can choose another thought or feeling or emotion altogether. Of course this sounds easy, but this takes practice and attitude of kindness, patience, compassion, and a specific kind of intention. One intention is to develop the capacity to build greater and greater degrees of awareness of the sensations of our bodies and to recognize and appreciate the messages of our bodies. Anat Baniel, in her book *Move into Life,* describes how research shows that the moment we bring attention and awareness to our body's movements moment by moment, the brain resumes growing new connections and creating new pathways and possibilities for us.[139]

According to a research study by Dr. Jon Kabat-Zinn[140] of the Stress Reduction Program at the Center for Mindfulness in Medicine, Health Care, and Society, the practice of mindfulness meditation used by chronic pain patients over a 10-week period showed a 65% reduction on a pain rating index. Large and significant reductions in mood disturbance and psychiatric symptoms accompanied these changes and were stable on follow-up. Another study looked at brain imaging and immune function after an 8-week training program in mindfulness meditation.[141] The study demonstrated that this short program in mindfulness meditation produced demonstrable effects on brain and immune function. The results of a clinical intervention study by Brown and Ryan[137] showed that higher levels of mindfulness were related to lower levels of both mood disturbance and stress before and after the Mindfulness-Based Stress Reduction (MBSR) intervention. Increases in mindfulness over the course of the intervention predicted decreases in these two indicators of psychological disturbance. Evidence has indicated that those faced with a life-threatening illness often reconsider the ways in which they have been living their lives, and many choose to refocus their priorities on existential issues such as personal growth and mindful living.[142]

These findings suggest that meditation may change brain function and immune function in positive ways. "Meditation," as it is taught in this 8-week program, is simply an awareness and attention training: a way of learning how to pay attention in the present moment to our bodies, thoughts, and emotions, and coming to understand how our thoughts and emotions affect our bodies. It may sound simple but actually can be incredibly challenging due to our cultural conditionings. However, an instant stress reliever can be bringing awareness to the breath. Deep breathing can act as a mini-meditation, and from a longevity standpoint, it is an important stress reliever.[133] Shifting to slower breathing in times of tension can help calm us and allow us to perform, whether mentally or physically, at higher levels.[133]

Another study, focused on Coping Effectiveness Training (CET), consisted of weekly 60-minute psychoeducational group intervention sessions focused on six topic areas and was adapted from the protocol Coping Effectively with Spinal Cord Injury.[143] The treatment protocol was structured to provide education and skill building in areas of awareness of reactions to stress; situation appraisal; coping strategy choice; interaction among thoughts, emotions, and behaviors; relaxation; problem solving; communication; and social support.[144] There was a significantly positive correlation between the learned coping strategies and the disabled individual's ability to adjust in a healthy way.

Hope, Grief, and Spiritual Aspects to Adjustment for the Patient and Therapist

To feel the consequence of your absence is what awakens in you the ability to feel absence. Seeing the end of something precious to you gives you the chance of loving it well. Loving and grieving are joined at the hip, for all the beauty, soul, and travail that brings. Grief is a way of loving what has slipped from view. Love is a way of grieving that which has not yet done so. We would do well to say this aloud for many days, to help get it learned: Grief is a way of loving, love is a way of grieving. They need each other in order to be themselves. You can learn how to be a faithful witness, to be wrecked on schedule, to put your grief in your carry-on bag together with your other treasured things.

Grief has to be learned, which means it has to be taught. Which means it is possible not to learn it. When we keep insisting on grief being a feeling, or a process that needs management and closure, we are talking about grief as an affliction, the same way we talk about dying. But something changes when we start seeing grief as a skill that needs learning, which is what it is. As a culture we are grief-impaired not because we don't have what we need to feel bad, but because we are grief-illiterate. We aren't taught to grieve; we are taught to handle grief, to resolve grief, to get on the other side of it.

—*Stephen Jenkinson, from* **Die Wise: A Manifesto for Sanity and Soul** *(2015)*[145]

Through the process of grappling with great suffering, we have the potential to grow deeper levels of understanding of life, meaning, and purpose, and from this process and practice of navigating and wrestling with life's challenges, we come into contact with our own and shared humanity, the heartbreak that seems to be a perpetual part of being human in these times of personal, global, economical, political, cultural, and ecological crisis. Our capacity and willingness to show up for the heartbreak change how we are in relationship to ourselves, to our bodies, and to life itself. As clinical professionals we need to be more than just aware of this capacity, we need to be practitioners of it and model it in our lives and work. This is a process of developing a self-evident knowing and embodied experience of how our greatest sufferings can act as potential windows to great depth of meaning in the process of living with fresh eyes as we relate to ourselves and behave and act in the world differently and with a chosen narrative rather than a default one.

Experiences of transcendence can be considered a potential problem for developing these capacities, as we are often taught in this culture that numbing and subjugating one's experience is a sought after way of relating to difficulties, and we are provided with a plethora of opportunities and numbing devices to choose from, such as excessive busyness, sugar, industrialized food products, media, pornography, gambling, drugs, alcohol, and gaming, just to name a few. So it is possible that we could use spiritual practices as a way to numb ourselves when life becomes uncomfortable. However, with a strong mindfulness practice in development, practices of transcendence can provide a process that can help us create a new normal for ourselves, as transcendence can alter our culturally pervasive narratives and stories about how we are meant to relate to our lives, and we can get glimpses of other-than-human perspectives and broader, more encompassing meaning of our lives. Our North American culture narrative perpetuates a view of "the living" as able-bodied, with full-time-plus work that brings in an income so that we can be "independent" consumers and play the worshipful part on the stage of an epic global economy. Our physical body, our relationship to the physical-linear realm, and a clinging to all of "the stuff" are of utmost importance in this cultural narrative. Youthful health and appearance and the endless acquisition of more stuff are presented endlessly in our media culture. A great rupture in this narrative can happen when we sustain a fissure in our capacity to fulfill this pervasive narrative, which can cause us to suffer greatly.

As described by Dr. E. Cassel in the *New England Journal of Medicine*, "Transcendence is probably the most powerful way in which one is restored to wholeness after an injury of personhood. When experienced, transcendence locates a person in a far larger landscape. The sufferer is not isolated by pain but is brought closer to a transpersonal source of meaning and to the human community that shares those meanings. Such an experience need not involve religion in any formal sense; however, in its transpersonal dimension, it is deeply spiritual."[146] Parker Palmer, a writer and teacher, describes it this way: "Treacherous terrain, bad weather, taking a fall, getting lost—challenges of that sort, largely beyond our control, can strip the ego of the illusion that it is in charge and make space for true self to emerge."[147] Eckhart Tolle describes how unnecessary suffering ensues when we are so completely identified with and hang our identities purely on form—physical form, thought form, and emotional form.[148] The more we are identified with and grasping to the physical realm of our human existence, without any recognition or acknowledgement of a realm beyond the human one, the more we suffer when our attachment to stuff or "form" becomes torn through disability or even death of all kinds. In Stephen Jenkenson's book *Die Wise*, he describes how our modern, North American, death-phobic culture is in part a product of this kind of obsession with the living and how we go to great lengths even to die, not dying.[145]

So, it seems a paradox of sorts and a particular challenge to develop the capacity to both release our attachments to unconscious, hand-me-down narratives that can play out in our lives and in our beliefs about our lives and at the same time to open to our humanity as it relates to our capacity to wrestle with life-changing circumstances as well as (and maybe most importantly to) the simple, mundane acts of engaging with our daily lives with openness and curiosity. "For all of us, our willingness to explore our fears and to live inside helplessness, confusion, and uncertainty is a powerful ally. Acknowledging our repeated exposure to human suffering—our own and others'—and the seductive draw of numbness and melancholy that provides temporary escape is necessary if we are to be renewed."[32] Dr. Santorelli goes on to say that "there is no way out of one's inner life, so one had better get into it."[32] "On the inward and downward spiritual journey, the only way out is in and through."[147]

Practice: Developing Attitudes of Willingness to Hold It All in Awareness

1. Become aware of the moments when "resistance to what is" or "clinging to what is" is or "not wanting this . . ." or "not wanting that . . ." is noticed. This may manifest itself as anxiety, sadness, fear, depression, powerlessness, or anger. All valid feelings to be noticed, honored, and acknowledged for the potential messages they bring. Feel the embodied experience of these feelings and emotions without needing them to be any other way keeping in mind that grief is not resistance; it's a valid response to real loss that may also have longing, yearning, as well as resistance/clinging associated with it. Sit quietly and be with the feeling holding in awareness with attitudes of curiosity, self-compassion, and gentleness.
2. As soon as anger arises (for example), notice how it manifests itself physically in the body. It may be tension in the muscles, a quickened or palpitating heartbeat, or sweating. See if you can just allow it space to be experiences, acknowledged, and honored.
3. Note what the sensation feels like in the body without trying to make the moment different than it is. Acknowledge whatever is present in the moment. Note that we are not the anger, we are the awareness of it.
4. Focus awareness on the sensation of the breath as you hold the intense emotion in awareness. Sensing into the breath.
5. Note what the awareness does. Note what they emotion or feeling does. What challenges arose? How did you work with them? What did you learn about yourself? Journal any thoughts or feelings about the practice.

Dr. Jon Kabat-Zinn, in his book *Coming to Our Senses*, states, "It seems as if awareness itself, holding the sensations without judging them or reacting to them, is healing our view of the body and allowing it to come to terms, at least to some degree, with conditions as they are in the present moment in ways that no longer overwhelmingly erode our quality of life, even in the face of pain or disease."[63]

Mystery surrounds every deep experience of the human heart: the deeper we go into the heart's darkness or its light, the closer we get to the ultimate mystery of God [the Universe].[147]

Religious and spiritual beliefs can be assistive in the process of adjusting to a disability. Johnstone, Glass, and Oliver highlight that religion and spirituality are important coping strategies for people with disabilities.[68] According to Dr. Jill Bolte-Taylor in her book *My Stroke of Insight: A Brain Scientist's Personal Journey*, "Enlightenment is not a process of learning but a process of unlearning."[134] Western society rewards the skills of the "doing" left brain much more than the "being" right brain, which can significantly hinder our process of spiritual deepening. The focus of our lives becomes more about obtaining positions, roles, and "stuff." We begin to identify ourselves with all of this when in reality the positions, roles, and things can be taken from us at any moment. "When we are obsessed with productivity, with efficiency of time and motion, and with projecting reasonable goals and making a beeline toward them, it seems unlikely that our work will ever bear fruit, unlikely that we will ever know the fullness of spring in our lives."[147]

There is a much deeper definition of ourselves that goes beyond all of the material possessions and the roles that we may ever play. According to Eckhart Tolle,[148] when forms that we identify with, that give us a sense of self, such as our physical bodies, collapse or are taken away, it can lead to a collapse of the ego, because ego is identification with "form." When there is nothing to identify with anymore, who are we? When forms around us die, or death approaches, Spirit is released from its imprisonment in matter. We can finally understand that our essential identity is formless, spiritual.[148] Cultivating greater understanding of these concepts, developing an embodied experience of them ourselves, and delving more into the experience of spirit can provide a great deal of relief for all of us who are suffering.

There is a wonderful quote by former Secretary-General of the United Nations U Thant, as he describes how he envisions the spiritual:

Spirituality is a state of connectedness to life.
It is an experience of being, belonging and caring.
It is sensitivity and compassion, joy and hope.
It is harmony between the innermost life and the outer life or the life of the world and the life of the universe.
It is the supreme comprehension of life in time and space, tuning of the inner person with the great mysteries and secrets that are around us.
It is the belief in the goodness of life and the possibility for each human person to contribute goodness to it.
It is the belief in life as part of the eternal stream of time, that each of us came from somewhere and is destined to somewhere, that without such belief there could be no prayer, no meditation, no peace, and no happiness.[149]

Spirituality is something that provides hope, connection with others, and reason or meaning of existence for many (if not most) people. It is amazing that the medical community has been slow to accept the power of spirituality because this is an area that gives meaning to so many people's lives. Spirituality has been linked to health perception, a sense of connection with others, and well-being.[67,68,150–156]

The Western medical system was based on diagnosis of pathology and how best to cure disease, but there has been a slow but fruitful shift toward including a more holistic view of the healing process and prevention. The National Institutes of Health now has a National Center for Complementary and Alternative Medicine (http://nccam.nih.gov). Almost every major hospital and university in the country now has an integrative health center (e.g., https://stanfordhealthcare.org/medical-clinics/integrative-medicine-center.html and https://oshercenter.org). Although this small but steady shift in the focus of medicine has gained momentum, one of the dangers of the medical system is still the entrapment in pathology to the point where the patient may not see anything but his or her pathology. Spirituality can help the patient and the family to see that there is more to life than pathology, stimulate interaction with others, put the functional limitations in perspective, give meaning to life (and the disability), and give the person hope and a sense of well-being.[67,68,150,152,153,157,158] This is what we all want for the patient and the family.

Adjustment Using the Stage Concept

Each person has his or her own coping style, and each should be allowed to be unique. Kerr[159] describes five possible stages of adjustment, but please hold these stages lightly as we can oversimplify human experiences and want to rush people along the stages if we feel like it's not quick enough for us, especially considering our dominant cultural view that we need to "move on" or "get on with it already," and if we are not progressing through these kinds of stages, we might even get slapped with a diagnosis of depression or anxiety disorder etc.:

Shock: "This really isn't happening to me."
Expectancy for recovery: "I will be well soon."
Mourning: "There is no hope."
Defense: "I will live with this obstacle and beat it." "I am adjusted, but you fail to see it."
Adjustment: "It is part of me now, but it is not necessarily a bad thing."

In light of current research, it is important for the therapist to realize that these are not lockstep stages and are to be thought of as concepts to help with the understanding of common reactions of some individuals.[160,161] Some individuals may settle in one stage for quite some time or may even skip stages altogether, whereas others may move through the stages quickly. This is an incredibly individual process.

Shock

The individual in shock does not recognize that anything is actually wrong. The patient may totally refuse to accept the diagnosis. The patient may even laugh at the concern expressed by others. This stage is altered when the person has an opportunity to test reality and finds that the physical or cognitive condition is actually limiting the ability to participate in functional activities.

Expectancy for Recovery

There is a dignity to acknowledging and grieving for what is lost. The patient in the stage of expectancy for recovery is aware that he or she is disabled but also believes that recovery will be quick and complete. The person may look for a "miracle cure" and may make future plans that require total return of function. Total recovery is the only goal, even if it takes a great deal of time and effort to achieve. Key signs of this stage are resentment of loss of function and the feeling that the whole body or mind is necessary to do anything worthwhile. The patient's ability and capability to take on reality of situation is going to be very individual in capacity and timing. Great sensitivity must be used in being authentic and also mindful of the state and condition of the patient. It cannot be overstressed that hope needs to be encouraged. Hope is qualitatively different than having a wish or expectation. One can hope that life will have goodness and continue to enfold while having a disability. While one seeks healing and improvement and wishes for outcomes that specifically may not be either reachable or guaranteed.

This can all be a very gradual process on everyone's part, and often there are some great unknowns. Humans have natural protections, and sometimes systems under great stress cannot process too much too soon. Holding environments acknowledge where the person is while believing and promoting the next growth is of essence. In the case of an individual who has experienced a stroke or a brain injury, we know now that the brain is capable of repairing itself throughout a lifetime—though we need to be clear that we do not know how much recovery will occur, if any. This all depends on the severity of the damage and the lifestyle of the patient—for example, smoking, stress, and/or lack of participation in meaningful activity, all of which impede progress.

Mourning

During the stage of mourning the individual feels that all is lost, that he or she will never achieve anything in life. Suicide is often considered. The individual may feel that characteristics of the personality (such as courage or will) have also been lost and must be mourned as well. Thus motivation to continue therapy or the will to improve may be impeded. The prospect of total recovery may no longer be held, but at the same time there appears to be no other acceptable alternative. This feeling of despair may be expressed as hostility, and as a result therapists may view the individual as a "problem patient." It is possible for a patient to remain at this stage with feelings of inadequacy, dependence, and hostility. However, it is also possible for therapeutic intervention to facilitate movement to the next stage by creating situations in which the patient may feel that "normal" aspirations and goals can be achieved. In this circumstance, normal would not include such "low-level" activities as dressing or walking; these are all activities that were taken for granted before the injury. Normal, though, would include performing the job the patient was trained to do. Such activities would also include playing with or caring for a child or family. This would be seen as self-actualization by Maslow.[162]

Defense

The defense stage has two components. The first represents a healthy attitude in which the patient actually starts coping with the disability. The individual takes pride in his or her accomplishments and works to improve independence and become as "normal" as possible. The person is still very much aware that barriers to normal functioning exist and is bothered by this fact but also realizes that some of the barriers can be circumvented. This healthy stage can be undermined and possibly destroyed by well-meaning family, friends, and therapists who encourage the individual to see only the positive aspects and who do not allow the patient to examine feelings about the restrictions and barriers of the condition. Conditions that lead to the final stage of adjustment are the realization that the prior or "whole" body or mind is not needed to actualize his or her life goals and that needs can be actualized in other ways. A therapist should watch for opportunities to facilitate this transition. There is a fine line between hopelessness and hope of regaining function. Taking away any hope of regaining quality of life leads to helplessness and may take away the motivation for neuroplasticity within the patient's central nervous system. Thus helping the patient be realistic and reality oriented while not taking away hope is a skill all therapists need to cultivate.

The negative alternative during the defensive stage is the neurotic defensive reaction. The patient refusing to recognize that even a partial barrier exists to meeting normal goals typifies this. The patient may try to convince everyone that he or she has adjusted.

Adjustment

In the final stage, adjustment, the person sees the disability as neither an asset nor a liability but as an aspect of the person, much like a large nose or big feet. He or she is accepting what is to the degree they are able, not resisting what is. Functional limitation or inability to participate in any life activity is not something to be overcome, apologized for, or defended. Kerr[159] refers to two aspects or goals of this stage. The first goal is for the person to feel at peace with his or her god or greater power: the patient does not feel that he or she is being punished or tested. The second goal is for the patient to feel that he or she is an adequate person, not a second-class citizen. Kerr[163] believes that "[i]t is essential that the paths to those more 'abstract goals' be structured if the person is to make a genuine adjustment." She also believes that it is the health care professional's job to offer that structure.

Acceptance or adjustment is at least as hard to achieve and maintain in life for the disabled person as happiness and harmony are for all people.[164] Adjustment connotes putting the disability into perspective, seeing it as one of the many characteristics of that person. It does not mean negating the existence of or focusing on the condition. Successful adjustment may be defined as a continuing process in which the person adapts to the environment in a satisfying and efficient manner. This is true for all human beings, able-bodied or disabled. There are always obstacles to overcome in attempting the goal of a happy and successful life.[16,93,164,165]

People and circumstances change. Maintaining a balanced state of adjustment is not easy, especially for the person with limitations. I recall a woman who had achieved a relatively stable state of acceptance of her quadriplegic condition. One day she called in a panic because, as she saw it, she "wasn't adjusted anymore." She had moved into a college dormitory and wanted to go out for a friendly game of football with her new friends but suddenly saw how physically limited she was. She had come to terms with her disability in a hospital and had never had to face this situation. After discussing this, she was able to put things into perspective and was able to talk over her feelings of isolation with her friends, who, without hesitation, altered the game to include her. Keeping a balanced perspective is a challenge in a world that changes constantly.

White[166] stated that without some participation, there can be no affecting the environment and thus no sense of self-satisfaction. Fine[167] and King[168] point out that without satisfaction from affecting the environment, reinforcement is insufficient to carry on the behavior, and the behavior will be extinguished. Thus satisfaction and performance must be linked. If the patient has not adjusted to his or her new body, however, little satisfaction can be gained from such everyday activities as walking, eating, or rolling over in bed.[169] To define adjustment on a purely performance basis is to run the risk of creating a "mechanical person" who might be physically rehabilitated but, once discharged, may find that he or she lacks satisfaction, incentive, and purpose. The psychological state of adjustment is what makes self-satisfaction possible.

Body Image

Self-care is never a selfish act—it is simply good stewardship of one of the greatest gifts I have been given, the gift I was put on this earth to offer to others. Anytime we can listen to true self and give it the care it requires, we do so not only for ourselves but for the many others whose lives we touch.[147]

Self-care and body image are inextricably connected, and when we build the skills of caring for ourselves (and modeling this behavior for our patients), we affect how we relate to our bodies and we can heal our relationship to our bodies, and this affects how we think about our bodies. Body image is an all-encompassing concept that considers how the person, and to some extent, the support systems view the person and roles that are expected to be assumed. Taleporos and McCabe[20] found that patients had negative feelings about their bodies and general negative psychological experiences after injury. Even when patients do not have disfigurements that are readily observable, they often still report changes in body image and negative feelings of self-worth.

Self-care is an important practice for our health, sense of self-worth, and well-being particularly when we are going through intense life experiences, and caring for ourselves on many levels can build a strong and resilient body image. Our culture often neglects self-care as an important part of building resilience and stress-hardiness, yet caring for oneself can significantly enhance our view of ourselves, especially when that view may be tested. Self-care can include eating food that is life-enhancing, getting adequate sleep, not saying yes to every activity or opportunity, participating in support groups and counseling services, getting a massage, spending time with friends and family who nourish us, and listening to our favorite music. As clinicians we can support our patients by encouraging them to establish self-care routines that support their resilience, health, and well-being.

Questions about any physical performance are within the domain of therapy. If the patient is asking for information regarding sex (e.g., positioning options), it is a subject that needs to be addressed in a respectful manner. If the questions are regarding fertility, capability, and the like, then these should be referred to an appropriate medical person. None of these questions should be discouraged or neglected, because this area is important for your patients' motivation and sexual health.[170,171] It is important for the therapist to know that in spinal cord injury, fertility will generally not be impaired for a woman, but issues of lubrication before sex should be addressed by the appropriate person. Men may have erection problems and ejaculation issues, but these too can be addressed by the appropriate medical practitioner. It is now known that fertility in spinal cord–injured men may be possible and should not be ruled out.[172,173–176]

Support System

Earlier literature hinted that partner relationships may be negatively affected by a member being disabled. Within the last few years, this concept has been questioned in regard to some disabilities such as adult-onset spinal cord injuries,[177] whereas pediatric spinal cord injury and other disabilities may result in relationship problems.[178,179] It has been shown that adjustment and quality of life can be adversely affected by the physical environment being inadequate, thus making the person more dependent. The result of the dependence appears to be poor relationships.[180–182] This can also be seen with the families in which a member has had a brain injury.[183,184] In studies on muscular dystrophy, it was found that physical dependence is not the only variable that needs to be considered. Psychological issues need to be identified and considered as part of intervention.[185,186] Recent literature has identified a number of elements that the patient and the family may need help to work on, such as "to assist them to develop new views of vulnerability and strength, make changes in relationships, and facilitate philosophical, physical, and spiritual growth."[185] Turner and Cox[185] also felt that the medical staff could facilitate "recognizing the worth of each individual, helping them to envision a future that is full of promise and potential, actively involving each person in their own care trajectory, and celebrating changes to each person's sense of self."[185] Man[186] observed that each family copes differently in relation to a brain-injured family member and that the family's structure should be explored to develop intervention guidelines. It has also been noted that health care professionals should view the situation from the family's perspective to approach and support the family's adaptation.[187] This

should be done to help the patient and the family accept the disability but at the same time help them keep the negative views of society in perspective.[71] In general, it has also been found that family support is a significant factor in the patient's subjective functioning[188,189] and that social engagement is productive.[90,190] According to Franzén-Dahlin and colleagues,[191] enhancing psychological health and preventing medical problems in the caregiver are essential considerations to enable individuals with disabilities to continue to live at home. Their research found that evaluating the situation for spouses of stroke patients was an important component when planning for the future care of the patient.

When working with children, it is important to realize that they often feel responsible for almost anything that happens in life, such as divorce, siblings getting hurt, or general arguments between parents. It is important that the therapist help the patient and the siblings realize that they are not responsible for the patient's condition. Part of this magical thinking that often appears is the concept that "bad things happen to bad people." Thus the child may consider themselves as bad because a bad thing has happened, or the adult is bad just because the disease or trauma has occurred. It is important to be sensitive to this ideation and help dispel this maladaptive thought pattern because it is not true or productive for the patient, the siblings, parents, or spouses within a family and may cause further adjustment problems later in treatment. Siblings of the patient should be encouraged to see their roles as good siblings and should not be placed in the role of caretakers of a sibling with special needs. In this way, all children can grow naturally without any one of the children being overly focused on. At the same time, it is a fact of life that the disabled child will probably need physical assistance, therapy, increased medical care, and thus and more time devoted to him or her, and this is just a fact of life.

It should always be noted by the medical establishment that having a disability is expensive in ways that we are often not aware of. There are obvious medical costs of therapy, surgery, drugs, wheelchairs, or orthoses, but there are other costs such as the possibility of extra cost of transportation, catheters for urination, wheelchair maintenance, adaptive clothing, and the like that are continuing costs not covered by most insurance plans. These costs add up and contribute to the emotional costs and demands on the family. The significant others may feel the need to work more to have the money to cover such expenses, but then that person is not around to help out. This is but one of the many dilemmas that must be acknowledged for the support system of the disabled person. The family may be encouraged to contact groups such as the Family Caregiver Support Network (www.caregiversupportnetwork.org) to get information and assistance on such diverse topics as being a caregiver, legal and financial aid, and communications (this group tends to focus on the adult but still may be a wonderful aid). Such groups will give information to all who need it and help to empower the family. This takes the focus off of the medical condition and may help the family to gain a better, more balanced perspective on the condition.

Loss and the Family

In this chapter, the patient's support system is referred to as the *family.* The family may be composed of spouses, parents, children, lovers (especially in gay and lesbian relationships), friends, employers, or interested others such as church groups, civic organizations, or individuals. The people in the support system may go through the same stages of reaction and adjustment to loss that the patient does.[1,9,167,192–194]

Family Needs

The family will, at least temporarily, experience the loss of a loved family member from the normal routine. During the acute stage, the family may not have concrete answers to basic questions regarding the extent of injury, the length of time before the injured person will be back in the family unit, or possibly whether the person will live.

During this phase, the family network will be in a state of crisis.[9] New roles will have to be assumed by the family members, and the "experts" will not even tell them for how long these roles must be endured. If children are involved, they will probably demand more attention to reassure themselves that they will remain loved. Depending on the child's age, the child will have differing capabilities in understanding the loss (see the section on examination of loss). Each member of the family may react differently to bereavement, and each may be at a different stage of adjustment to the disability (see the section on adjustment). One member may be in shock and deny the disability, whereas another member may be in mourning and may verbalize a lack of hope. The family crisis that is caused by a severe injury cannot be overstated.[99,193-196]

Role changes in the family may be dramatic.[65,75,93,197-199] Members who have never driven may need to learn that motor skill; one who has never balanced a checkbook may now be responsible for managing the family budget; and those who have never been assertive may have to deal forcefully with insurance companies and the medical establishment.[9,58,200,201]

The family may feel resentment toward the injured member. This attitude may seem justified to them because they see the person lying in bed all day while the family members must take over new responsibilities in addition to their old ones. In a study by Lobato, Kao, and Plante,[202] Latino siblings of children with chronic disabilities were at risk for internalizing psychological problems. The medical staff may not always understand the stress that family members are under and may react to the resentment expressed either verbally or nonverbally with a protective stance toward the patient. Siding with the "hurt" patient may alienate the family from the medical staff and may also drive a permanent wedge between family members. This long-term situation may undermine the compliance of family members' involvement in home programs and, ultimately, the successful outcome of long-term intervention.

As clinicians, it may be at times that the only way we may be of service in certain situations is to be a compassionate witness to all that is unfolding in our own or in another person's life. Holding the enormity of the situation in our awareness while staying grounded in our own embodied experience of the present moment is essential. It may be that all we can do is to be a nonjudgmental, engaged, curious listener and life-learner, allowing ourselves to be touched by the other person's (or even our own) suffering. It may be that we are all starving for someone to just be present enough and grounded enough within themselves that they can bear witness to all that is unfolding on personal, communal, and global levels. This kind of listening is learned, and it is not taught in our dominant culture, so clinicians who wish to have this skill will have their work cut out for them to seek out this kind of learning experience. San Jose State University's Mindfulness-Based Occupational Therapy Advanced Certificate program (open to all health care practitioners) and the Center for Mindfulness at the University of Massachusetts Medical School are both such places for this kind of specialized training. These authentic teachings are essential to this kind of way of being and relating to our lives and our work, and they can help us bring healing to an otherwise disembodied, disconnected, dysfunctional system of hierarchy and institutionalization.

Parental Bonding and the Disabled Child

The parental bonding process is complicated and is still being studied.[48] The process may start well before the child is even conceived. The parents often think about having a child and plan and fantasize about future interactions with the child; after conception the planning and fantasizing increase. During the pregnancy the parents accept the fetus as an individual, and after the birth of the child the attachment process is greatly intensified. The "sensitive period" is the first few minutes to hours after the birth. During this time the parents should have close physical contact with the child to strongly establish the attachment that will later grow deeper.[203,204] There is an almost symbiotic relationship between mother and child at this time: infant and mother behaviors complement each other (e.g., nursing stimulates uterine contraction, breast milk production, and oxytocin release). In the early stages of bonding, seeing, touching, caring for, and interacting with the child allow for the bonding process. When this process is disturbed for any reason, such as congenital malformations or hospital procedures for high-risk infants, problems may occur then and later.

When the parents are told that their child is going to be malformed or disabled, it is a profound shock if they were not informed in advance of the baby's birth. The dream of a "normal" child is given up, and the parents must go through the loss or "death" of the child they expected before they can accept the new child. Parents often feel guilty. Shellabarger and Thompson[205] state that parents often feel the deformed child was their failure.[1] The disabled child will always have a strong impact on the family, sometimes a catastrophic one.[1,8,9,205,206] A study by Ha and colleagues[207] found that compared with parents of nondisabled children, parents of disabled children experienced significantly higher levels of negative affect, poorer psychological well-being, and significantly more somatic symptoms. Older parents were significantly less likely to experience the negative effect of having a disabled child than younger parents.

In a study by Arnaud and colleagues,[208] greater severity of impairment was found to not always be associated with poorer quality of life; in the moods and emotions, self-perception, social acceptance, and school environment domains, less severely impaired children appeared to be more likely to have poor quality of life. Pain was associated with poor quality of life in the physical and psychological well-being and self-perception domains. Parents with higher levels of stress were more likely to report poor quality of life in all domains, which suggests that factors other than the severity of the child's impairment may influence the way in which parents report quality of life.

Parents must be encouraged to express their feelings and emotions, and they must be taught how to deal with the issues at hand. Techniques for accomplishing these goals are discussed in later sections.[48,204,206]

The Child Dealing With Loss

If a parent is injured, the young child may experience an overwhelming sense of loss. Child care may be a problem, especially if the primary caregiver is injured. The child might feel deserted by the injured parent and may long for the attention of the remaining parent. This will increase the strain on all family members.[65]

If the child is the patient, his or her life will have undergone a radical change: every aspect of the child's world will have been altered. Loved ones, loved objects, and a sense of safe place will help restore the child's feeling of security. It is of major importance to explain to the child in very simple terms what is going on and to allow the child the opportunity to express feelings both verbally and nonverbally. It is important to use play and art as the medium of communication for children.

The hospital setting is threatening to all people, but children are especially susceptible to loss of autonomy, feelings of isolation, and loss of independence. Senesac has stated that the severity of the disability is not as important a variable in the emotional development of the child as are the attitudes of parents and family.[2,8] Parents must attempt to be aware of the child's inability to understand the permanence (or transience) of the loss of function.[8] They will also need to help the child feel secure by bringing in familiar and cherished objects. A schedule should be established and kept to promote consistency. Play and art should be encouraged, especially types that allow the child to vent feelings and deal with the newness of the experience and the environment. Any procedures or therapies should be presented in a relaxed and playful way so that the child has time to think and to feel as comfortable as possible about the change. The parents may often need to be reminded to pay attention to the children in the family without disabilities during this acute stage.

The Adolescent Dealing With Loss

The adolescent is subject to all of the feelings and fears that other patients express. Adolescents are in a struggle to achieve autonomy, initiation, and independence, and they often are ambivalent about their feelings. When an adolescent is suddenly injured and has to cope with being disabled, it can be a massive assault on the individual's development.[165,209] According to research conducted by Kinavey,[51] findings imply that youth born with spina bifida face biological, psychological, and social challenges that interfere with developmental tasks of adolescence, including identity formation. Therapists are urged to direct intervention toward humanizing and emancipating the physical and social environment for youth with physical disabilities to maximize developmental opportunities and potential while fostering positive identity and initiation into adolescence and young adulthood. Our culture lacks structures in place that can help initiate a child through these monumental growth periods. Programs are recently being developed to provide a container for these kinds of rite of passage experiences to initiate our children into adulthood and beyond including programs for children experiencing catastrophic life difficulties, and most of them accept applications for scholarships for low-income families. As clinicians we can provide resources and encouragement related to the significance of experiences of initiations for youth, especially youth who may be experiencing crisis.

Kingsnorth and colleagues[50] stated that with advances in health care, an increasing number of youth with physical disabilities are surviving into adulthood. For youth to reach their full potential, a number of critical life skills must be learned. Specific learning opportunities are important, as youth with physical disabilities may be limited in the life experiences necessary to acquire these skills. Therapists are in the unique position of fostering these kinds of environments to encourage adolescents to engage in critical life skills such as emotion-focused and problem-focused problem solving, decision making, values-based intentional goal setting, critical thinking, mindfulness-based communication skills, assertiveness and self-advocacy, the establishment of healthy personal-boundaries, self-awareness, self-compassion, being/becoming a life-learner, and developing skills for resilience and stress hardiness. Life skills differ from instrumental daily living skill, though it is best to work on developing life skills in the midst of our daily lives so that our daily living skills (the activities required to function independently in the community including skills such as financial management, meal preparation, and navigating community) become catalysts for our personal growth and development.

Family Maturation

The family also has a maturational aspect. If the injured person is a child and if the family is young with dependent children at home, the adjustment may not be the problem that it would be for a family whose children are older. In the latter case, parents have begun to experience freedom and independence, and they may find adjusting to a restricted lifestyle difficult or even intolerable. They may have the feeling that they have already "put in their time" and "should now be free." If the disability interrupts the child's developmental process, future conflict may arise because the parents may eventually expect retirement, relaxation, and freedom as our dominant North American culture teaches. Parents may feel guilty and try to repress this response.

The reverse may also be true. The parents may be feeling that the children have left them ("empty nest syndrome"), and they may be too willing to welcome a "dependent" family member back into the home. This may lead to excessive dependence or anger toward the parents on the part of the patient. All these factors need to be taken into consideration by the therapist when therapy is presented to the patient and family.

The therapist can develop a greater understanding of the patient and family by being aware of common human developmental patterns. These patterns identify some of the major processes of adjustment that need to be considered during the therapeutic process, but we need to understand that every person and family will have their own unique way of processing the circumstances, and we need to honor, acknowledge, and appreciate, and if we are fortunate enough to be open-minded enough to learn from, perspectives and ways of being and relating to life's challenges that may not be of our dominant North American culture.

Coping With Transition

Learning to suffer, wrestle with tragedy, and grapple with catastrophe is a skill set that we are not taught to any degree in our modern North American culture. In fact, we are systematically taught how to numb and subjugate challenging circumstances, and we are given ample opportunities to do so; this cultural training begins at an early age. Media, refined and processed highly addictive food products, excessive busyness and consumption, gambling, alcohol, drugs, pharmaceuticals, and others all constitute an epic part of our cultural experience across the life-span. We all participate in and perpetuate this system to some degree. The benefit, if there is such a thing, is that we can all tap into the experience of it ourselves, because we have our own embodied experience of how this feels and what this looks like in our daily lives.

We call it "Coping with Transition," with the subtle, undercurrent of meaning that "we need to just get over it already"—whatever *that* is. "Just cope, please, for all our sakes, so we don't have to be with the messiness of too much grieving, too much anger, or too much despair." The subtle message is, "It's just too uncomfortable for me, and I wasn't taught how to be in wise relationship to suffering, so please just get on with it so we can get on to meeting your goals so I can get paid for being a "good therapist" who helps their patients meet goals." Witnessing suffering, our own and that of others (including the planet-in the case of the 6th wave of extinctions; Kolbert, 2014),[210] makes us all uncomfortable because we were born into and trained to be suffering-phobic, strong-emotion phobic, and death-phobic. So it is likely you will notice this in yourself. We all need to learn, on the job, with training in mindfulness under our belts, to develop a new relationship to suffering, where we can become engaged, compassionate witnesses to what is unfolding.

Without this skill development, we may be more likely to have our own present-moment experience co-opted by another's to the degree that we dissociate and fall back on the standard cultural narratives we've learned since childhood. With the developing skills of learning how to be in relationship to the messiness of life's human (and otherwise) tragedies, we can learn to stay grounded and rooted in our being, all the while being present to and in some level of acceptance of what needs to be seen and heard and witnessed without needing to numb or subjugate our experience. Begin a process of learning how to be a compassionate witness to your own suffering, your own emotions, and your own embodied experiences. This is the only way that you will be able to support someone through the trauma of catastrophic, life-changing circumstances. If you haven't already, engage in mindfulness training as soon as possible and begin.

With all of this in mind, in the acute stages of a family member's injury, we can support the family in grappling with the crisis at hand by bearing witness to their experience without needing to change it in any way and just noticing what comes up for you personally as you notice and listen to all that is unfolding. During this phase (that can take any length of time), the family must first be allowed the space to cope, in their own way, with the emotional impact of what is happening with a loved one. When we force our views that our patient's grief or anger or any other strong emotion must be overcome, we may be engaged in perpetuating dysfunctional North American cultural conditioning or what Dr. Robert Masters calls *spiritual bypassing.*

> *Spiritual bypassing, a term first coined by psychologist John Welwood in 1984, is the use of spiritual practices and beliefs to avoid dealing with our painful feelings, unresolved wounds, and developmental needs. It is much more common than we might think and, in fact, is so pervasive as to go largely unnoticed, except in its more obvious extremes.*[211]

In a previous version of this chapter, you will see a standard narrative of the stages of coping listed. It helps to know the literature that is out there around these kinds of stages, but they may be more useful if we hold them lightly and in perspective of the larger cultural narrative around coping that we are all complicit in perpetuating. For example, Brammer and Abrego[212] have developed a list of basic coping skills that they have broken into five levels. In the first level, the person becomes aware of and mobilizes skills in perceiving and responding to transition and attempts to handle the situation. In the second level, the person mobilizes the skills for assessing, developing, and using external support systems. In level three, the person can possess, develop, and use internal support systems (develop positive self-regard and use the situation to grow). The person in level four must find ways to reduce emotional and physiological distress (relaxation, control stimulation, and verbal expression of feelings). In level five, the person must plan and implement changes (analyze discrepancies, plan new options, and successfully implement the plan). Using this model, the therapist and family can evaluate the coping skill level of the family. The therapist and staff are often prompted to promote movement toward the next level of coping with the transition. The stages listed are not the problem in and of themselves. The problems arise when we begin forcing or manipulating our patients, however good our intentions, "to move on already," and we might even work to try to move them on to the next stage, as previously described. This is a pervasive problem we have all been privy to; it is applauded as an integral part of the health care system and way of doing things, and so it helps to hold this reality and realization with gentleness and self-compassion.

Another complex challenge we face as clinicians is encouraging a balanced perspective about disability. One consequence of hospitalization in managing the care of a newly disabled person is that the hospital staff can often focus on the disability rather than on the individual's strengths.[77,193,213] Centering on the disability can lead to a situation in which patient, family, and staff see only the functional limitations and not the potential ability of the patient.

Decentering from the loss of function and holding the whole person of view are important and will be examined further in this chapter. If the family relationship was positive before the disability and if the patient is cognitively intact, then the focus can be directed toward the relationship's strengths as well as toward the patient's and family's individual cognitive and emotional strengths.[92] In the initial acute stage of adjustment, crisis intervention may help the family use its strengths and at the same time deal with the situation at hand.

To adequately grapple with the crisis at hand, in the context of shortened hospital stays, the therapist can encourage the family to do the following:

1. Be encouraged to focus on (rather than deny) the crisis caused by the disability; acknowledge and explore the situation to stimulate emotion-focused and problem-focused problem solving; identify and work through doubts of adequacy, guilt, and self-blame; identify and honor the grief process; gently notice and hold in awareness any anticipatory worry; be offered instruction in mindfulness skills to assist in building skills of stress-hardiness, resilience, and self-compassion and basic information and education regarding the crisis situation; and be helped to create a bridge to resources in the hospital and in the community for support and to see their own family and community as potential resources.[49,214–217]
2. Be helped to remember how they have dealt successfully with crises in the past and to implement some of the same strategies in the present situation.

Work with the family as a unit during crisis to help strengthen the family and facilitate more positive attitudes toward the patient. These attitudes by the family will improve the patient's attitudes or feelings toward the injury and hospitalization.[93,199,218–221] Encouraging family-unit functioning in this situation can decrease the amount of regression displayed by the patient. If the family is encouraged to function without the patient, however, more damage than good may be done.[1,165]

TREATMENT VARIABLES IN RELATION TO THERAPY

Skilled therapy intervention focuses on maximizing participation in functional activities, participation in life, and behavioral change. Livneh and Antonak[160] promote the following activities for the health professional:

1. Assisting patients to explore the personal meaning of the disability. "Training patients to attain a sense of mastery over their emotional experiences." A way of doing this would be to help the patient look at his or her thoughts, emotions, and mental formations with clarity and discernment and to put them into perspective. Mindfulness training can be particularly helpful with this skill.
2. Providing patients with relevant medical information. "These strategies emphasize imparting accurate information to patients on their medical condition, including its present status, prognosis, anticipated future functional limitations, and when applicable, vocational implications." This may be done by helping the patient and family access resources such as PubMed (www.ncbi.nlm.nih.gov/pubmed) online or find medical references in the library. Education about the condition of disability for patient, family, friends, teachers, and others can be essential for assisting communication, understanding, supportive behaviors, and realistic expectations. For example understanding specifics of communication deficits common to aphasia, cognitive processing, perception, stimulation tolerance, attention, distractibility, or social pragmatics can ease the way for successful communication, relations, and tasks. In some cases, the patient may be able to be the one to take charge of educating others about a condition and needs; in other cases an advocate will fill that role. Some neurological conditions may increase lability, impulsivity, volatility, distractibility, etc., and both the patient and supportive others can learn to work with this as possible. Familiarity and knowledge are a form of empowerment. Interdisciplinary referral, consultation and collaboration among speech, counseling, social work, educators, occupational and physical therapies, and involved support systems are called for. The more effective the teamwork and collaboration, the more successful is the reinforcement of interventions and strategies

for recovery. Caregiver education and support is another important focus.

3. Providing patients with supportive family and group experiences. "These strategies permit patients (usually with similar disabilities or common life experiences) and, if applicable, their family members or significant others, to share common fears, concerns, needs, and wishes." This can be done in rather unobtrusive ways such as scheduling patients with the same disability at the same time so that they meet in the waiting room or while doing group mat activities. Another option is hiring individuals with limitations who are health care professionals and can discuss and role model positive behaviors and answer relevant questions from the patient's perspective. Remember that patients are all potential teachers for you as well as other patients.

4. Teaching patients adaptive coping skills for successful community functioning. "These skills include assertiveness, interpersonal relations, decision making, emotion-focused and problem-focused problem solving, suffering-literacy, emotion-literacy, creating values-based narratives to live by, discernment when it comes to dysfunctional cultural messages perpetuated by the dominant North American narratives, stigma management, and time management skills." This would entail role-playing disturbing situations that may occur in the community, such as an able-bodied person asking why the patient is in a wheelchair; preaching to the wheelchair user because he or she must have offended God in some way—otherwise the person would not be in a wheelchair; or telling a woman that it is such a shame that she is disabled because she is so good looking and could have found a man if it were not for the disability.

ROLE OF THE THERAPEUTIC ENVIRONMENT

Whenever possible in therapy the functional activity should be presented and structured to promote empowerment, problem solving, and adjustment. Adjustment and adaptation to life form a dynamic process that allows for the person to interact with life in a way that encourages the person to find meaning and purpose in life (Fig. 5.1).[17,81,222–225] This section examines issues the therapist and staff should know to create a therapeutic environment that will facilitate psychological adjustment

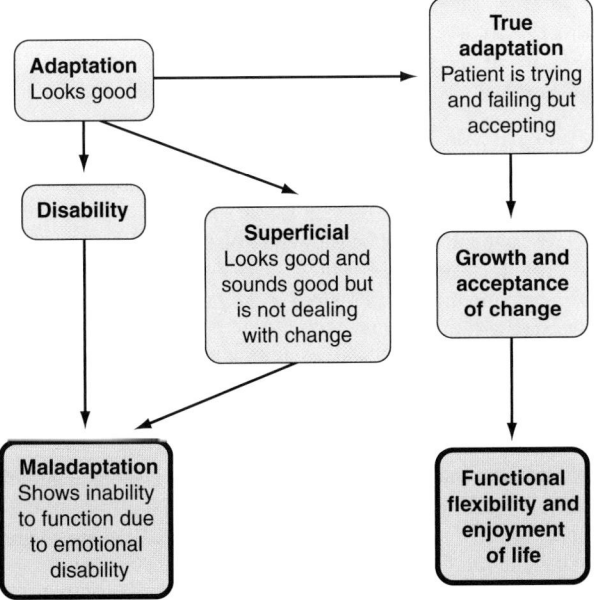

Fig. 5.1 Possible Directions of the Adaptive Process.

and independence of the patient with activity limitations. We all know there is increasing pressure to meet goals quickly due to shorter hospital stays, so keeping this in mind will help us maintain a human perspective as we navigate these institutionalized structures that we do not have much say over. With this in mind, the physical and the attitudinal environment of the treatment facility plays a major role in the way the patient views the services that are rendered and their desire to build rapport with the treatment team.

Recall a time before you became a member of the medical community. Think about how you experienced doctors wearing their white coat uniforms, keep in mind how you experienced the unfamiliar smells of the hospital, how busy it all seemed, and how puzzling the secret medical language and the medical technology and devices were. It all seemed overwhelming then, and it still is to newcomers, especially newly admitted patients and their families. The hospital usually appears impersonal,[226] sterile, monotonous, and confusing, and all personal status accumulated outside the hospital means little on the inside.

The therapist needs to take the setting into account when engaging with patients. The environment can be altered in a variety of ways. Therapy staff could wear street clothes, decorate the department or hospital with posters and lively colors, and allow patients to bring some personal items into the hospital.

The nature of the therapy process can often lead the therapist to see only the disability and not the person—as occurs, for example, when a patient is referred to by his or her disability rather than by name. This stereotyping of those with disabilities can lead the therapist to concentrate on the lack of abilities rather than on the strengths of the patients, and it reduces the patient to the disease. The real danger is that the patient and family will also start to focus on the functional limitations of the patient and feel that their family relationship is now permanently altered. The accuracy of this perception may have to be evaluated as part of the adjustment process. The wife of a man with paraplegia said with a sudden burst of insight, "I didn't marry him for his legs—this doesn't change the relationship." Often so much attention is directed toward the disability that tunnel vision develops. One way to try to get a better perspective is to look at the bigger picture. A variety of questions can be asked that may help the therapist gain greater insight into the patient as a person (Box 5.2).

After the therapist is aware of the strengths of the patient, these strengths may be capitalized on therapy to help the patient realize them and build confidence. Patients often reported that they were not complimented in therapy and especially that they never received feedback that their bodies were desirable[227] or that they were doing things correctly.[11,77,228] A logical thought by the patient is, "If the therapist cannot see anything desirable about me, and the therapist deals with the individuals with similar problems all the time, then there must not be anything good about me." Positive, sincere comments to the patient and family can add a motivational factor to treatment that may have been missing.[77,220]

Providing opportunities to be outdoors can help patients cultivate a sense of connection with something that is larger than themselves. At the most basic level there is more oxygen outside, and in general the air is fresher than indoors. "And looking at a faraway horizon or sky can help us gain needed perspective on our small world, bounded by our bodies and our lives."[229]

The last and possibly the most important aspect in creating an environment that will foster growth and adjustment in the patient is a staff whose members are well adjusted and aware of their own personal needs. Just as coping skills are necessary for the patient, the staff, too, must actively engage in skills that build stress hardiness and resilience as well as self-compassion and mindfulness. The therapist must also engage with his or her own personal reactions to the sometimes devastating situations others are experiencing.[77,220,230] For example, exposure to such situations, without having built the skills and know-how to acknowledge

---

The following questions can be considered by therapist:

What would this person be doing if he or she did not have this condition?

What is stopping the person from reaching these goals now?

What are his or her positive traits?

What has this person been doing for a living, how has he/she been in the world, how has this person contributed to life?

What will this person do for a living?

What has this person done for enjoyment, and what might this person do in future?

How will this person bring others enjoyment?

What would this person be doing if there was no disability?

How is the disability stopping the person from actualizing their goals? (These are the goals that can be worked on.)

Similar questions can be asked of the patient to explore ways of helping the patient have a meaningful life, and the therapist could choose from among these questions to orient a discussion:

What skills are you needing/wanting to address now?

What are you needing/wanting to address in therapy now?

What important things would you be doing now if there were no barriers?

What activities or forms of productivity were you involved in before, and which were important to you?

Which of these things do you still do?

What if anything is preventing you from doing these things now?

What adjustments might enable you to participate in these activities?

What kind of balance do you want in your life among self-care, work, recreation, family time, time with others, rest, spiritual life?

How does this condition currently affect your being a lover of life, family, significant other, and so on?

Consider an important life goal or meaningful activity, and what a new approach might be.

How much different would your life look if it were not for this condition?

Are any of the above changed or prevented by your condition, and if so how?

---

one's own emotional landscape, the capacity to honor and stay grounded within one's own experience, and to identify when one needs somatic-integrated psychotherapy. Staff needs to care for their own mental and emotional well-being to be able to be in skillful relationship as workers on the front lines of incredible human suffering. This emotional energy needs to be engaged skillfully so that the energy does not turn into dysfunction within the staff interaction or become a destructive force for the patient.

To decrease the possibly destructive nature of unacknowledged or unappreciated emotions and feelings, the staff should be made aware of their own coping styles, and they should be allowed to express their reactions in a positive, supportive group. Group meetings can be useful in providing a container for the community of practitioners to express, honor, and acknowledge challenges that may arise. This is not a psychotherapy session (although psychotherapy may be warranted in some situations) but rather an opportunity to problem solving, express feelings, and to be heard and acknowledged as a community. These sessions can make use of the four elements of crisis intervention mentioned in the previous section as well as information from others.[220] The staff can use these sessions to better understand their various reactions and responses to stress and explore their coping styles.[198,220,231,232] Ideally, this knowledge of coping styles and stress reduction will decrease staff burnout and aid the staff to help patients and their families engage with stress more skillfully.[165,228–232] MBSR developed out of the University of

Massachusetts Medical School's Center for Mindfulness is a course series that is recommended for health care practitioners wanting to build their own skills for stress hardiness, resilience, and emotional intelligence. MBSR courses held in most hospitals, universities, and communities can be found online at www.umassmed.edu/cfm/mbsr.

The need to have a staff that is supportive is of paramount importance because the attitude of rehabilitation personnel has emerged as one of the chief motivating factors in rehabilitation.[1,93,163] In fact, the use of humor has been found to be assistive in the process of adjustment. In a study by Solomon,[233] aging well was related to aspects of humor. It seemed to affect aging well through its relationship with perceived control. Physical health, satisfaction with housing, and relationships with family and friends were also positively influenced by humor.

We have already explored the complex circumstances that we live in a suffering-phobic culture and that learning to be in skillful relationship to our own and another's suffering, grief, and despair is essential for the work we do as therapists, but what about the value of distracting oneself when we just need to do so? Of course, in fact, one suggestion by McCreaddie and Wiggins[234] is that stress can be coped with through distraction, which lessens the negative physical effects of stress. Humor is also known to have a number of potential benefits in relation to interpersonal skills or social support.[235] Specific aspects such as empathy, intimacy, and interpersonal trust have all been positively correlated with a sense of humor and subsequently with interpersonal relationships. According to McCreaddie and Wiggins,[234] a degree of rapport with the patient is necessary before humor should be used, and humor should be used only after a level of empathy, caring, and competence has been clearly demonstrated. This interaction of therapy and societal interactions explain why the World Health Organization model went from a disability or handicap model to a model of functional ability and participation in life. Although the International Classification of Diseases (ICD-9 or ICD-10) deals with physicians and disease categories, therapy clearly separates itself into a clear model that stresses the strength of an individual and his or her potential to participate in and have quality of life (https://www.who.int/classifications/icf).

Rogers and Figone[169] developed the following suggestions that could benefit the therapist when trying to create a supportive environment:

1. It is helpful to use the same staff member to develop the relationship and provide continuity of care.
2. Concerned silence is most appreciated, although pushing is sometimes necessary.
3. Staff members should anticipate the need to repeat information graciously.
4. Cumbersome, hard-to-repair adaptive equipment should not be used after discharge.
5. Give patients responsibility so that they feel they have some control over therapy.
   a. The patient should be allowed to pick his or her own advocate from the team.
   b. The patient should be given a choice of activities (e.g., which exercise comes first).
   c. Health care professionals should avoid placing the patient in an inferior status.
6. Personal matters are better discussed with staff members with whom the patient has developed a relationship.[2,215]
7. Willingness to allow the patient to try and fail is more helpful than controlling the patient.

Bolte-Taylor[134] developed "forty things I needed the most" during her rehabilitation for her stroke. Here are a few:

1. I am not stupid, I am wounded. Please respect me.
2. Come close, speak clearly, repeat yourself if necessary, and enunciate.

3. Approach me with an open heart, slow your energy down, and take your time.
4. Be aware of what your body language and facial expressions are communicating to me.
5. Make eye contact with me, encourage me.
6. Honor the healing power of sleep.
7. Protect my energy. No talk radio, TV, or nervous visitors! Keep my visitations brief.
8. Speak to me directly, not about me to others.
9. Clarify for me what the next step or level is so I know what I am working toward.
10. Celebrate all of my little successes. They inspire me.

CONCEPTUALIZATION OF ASSESSMENT AND TREATMENT

Assessment

The one component that weaves through all of Rogers and Figone's[169] seven points is the need for the therapist to be involved with the patient in a therapeutic relationship—that is to develop a sense of where the patient is coming from. To know where the patient is coming from is to be aware of and sensitive to the person's total psychosocial frame of reference.[2,215]

The therapist who knows his or her own beliefs, reference points, and prejudices can evaluate whether an assessment result or treatment sequence reflects the patient's needs and values or those of the therapist. In the first half of this chapter, some assessments were discussed that could be summarized into the following three major components:

1. Preinjury
   a. Values and prejudices (value systems, culture, and prejudgments) of the patient and family members before the injury
   b. Developmental stage of the patient and family members
   c. Cognitive level of the patient and family members
   d. Ability of the patient and family members to handle crisis
2. Components to be evaluated leading to adjustment
   a. Loss and grief process for the patient and family members
   b. Adjustment process for the patient and family members
   c. Transitional stages for the patient and family members
   d. Role changes for the patient and family members
   e. Age or cognitive level of patient and family members[9,165,215,236]
   f. Sexual adjustment for the patient and spouse
3. Techniques used to elicit adjustment and independence
   a. Crisis intervention strategies
   b. Letting the patient and family take control
   c. Expression of emotion, both verbally and nonverbally
   d. Emotion-focused and problem-focused problem solving
   e. Role playing
   f. Praise
   g. Education
   h. Support groups

Once an assessment has been made of the patient and family members' stages of psychological adjustment, the patient's occupational history and roles, and their preinjury attitudes and beliefs, a treatment protocol can be established. This protocol will need to incorporate steps toward stage change and possibly attitudinal change. Because these changes require learning on the part of the patient and family, an environment that optimally facilitates these changes need to be established.[9,76,93,99,182,197,237–239]

Therapy can be seen as a form of education in which the patient and the patient's family are taught how the patient could care for and optimally function with his or her body. However, the education process is not limited to the physical aspects of therapy. The patient is also encouraged to experience, view, and wonder about their body and the experience of disability and to begin to articulate their needs and be given the opportunity to make decisions for themselves whenever possible. If the staff is nonverbally telling the patient and the family that the patient is not capable of making decisions and is not capable of being independent, it follows that the patient may indeed feel dependent and incapable of making decisions. Giles[198] and others[194,198,237,240,241] stated that there was an inverse relationship between independence and distress. Distress causes further anxiety and decreases the learning potential of the patient. Thankfully, there are many ways for the therapist to encourage resilience, stress-hardiness, adaptation, and independence on the part of the patient and his family.

Specific Therapeutic Interventions

"Engagement in leisure-like activities may not only help people feel better in the immediate context of coping with rehabilitation treatments, but may help sustain coping efforts as individuals learn to live with ongoing functional limitations."[242]

Problem-Solving Process

The family unit, including the patient, should be encouraged to take active control over as much of the patient's care and decision making as possible.[19,22,53,195,198,236–238,240,241,243–245] This can be done in every phase of the rehabilitation process. A family conference with the rehabilitation staff should actively involve the patient and family in all stages of planning and treatment, up to and including discharge. The family (including the patient) should be briefed ahead of time to prepare questions that they want answered or problems that need to be addressed. Rogers and Figone[169] report that conferences with family members that excluded the patient engendered suspicion[2,198]; therefore if the patient is capable, the patient may educate the family in regard to what is happening in the hospital and in rehabilitation. Conversely, family involvement facilitates and shortens the rehabilitation process and encourages reintegration into the community.[8,194,237,241] The family can also be educated regarding the side effects and interactions of medication with publications such as the *Physicians' Desk Reference.*[246] Later in the rehabilitation process, the patient and family can be encouraged to arrange transportation services, find and evaluate housing, and supervise attendant care. All these activities allow the patient and the family to be more in control of the environment and thus feel independent.

In the context of one-on-one therapy, giving choices can foster patient responsibility and independence. Making a decision about the order of treatment activities (such as on which side of the bed to transfer out of or which direction to roll one's wheelchair first) can give the individual a sense of self-worth that can continue to grow. This can cultivate a belief by the patient and family that they are strong, with basic needs that can be respected and met. Moving out of the role of the victim, the patient begins to exercise responsibility and to take action, such as applying for extended health benefits or getting a second consultation when an important medical decision needs to be made. If the patient and family start to realize that they do not have to be a casualty of the medical establishment and if they find ways to control what they can within the medical establishment,[93,222,247] they are better able to discard the role of victim.

The steps of crisis intervention, which were mentioned in the previous section, can be used to help the family understand and analyze their needs in the crisis situation. Once the family has discerned that they may be discovered that they are in crisis, they will then be able to draw upon strategies and skills that they can use to overcome present and future problems.

Our dominant cultural way of coping with difficulty primarily deploys problem-based problem-solving strategies, yet emotion-focused problem solving is a skill that can be developed and can be an important element in the process of adjusting to a disability, and the therapist can use these techniques to help the patient and family gain intentional, values-based planning to enhance independence and a sense of control over the situation.[19,53,194,198,237,238,240,241,243,244]

Rather than having the patient learn how to accomplish each specific activity, the patient or family can be encouraged to think through the process from the problem to the solution and to accomplishment of the task. To achieve this activity analysis, the patient would have to know the basic principles behind the activity[169] and may then be responsible for educating the family. An example of this would be a transfer from the wheelchair to the toilet. If the therapist simply has the patient memorize the steps in the task, the patient or family members will not necessarily be able to generalize this procedure to a transfer to the car. If the patient learns the principles of proper body mechanics, work simplification, and movement, the patient or family member may be more able to generalize this information to almost any situation and solve problems later when the therapist is unavailable.[240] Rogers and Figone[169] have noted that although the patient and family may fail at times during these trials, the therapist should let them be as independent and responsible as possible: let them try it their way, even if they are not successful the first time.

Pictures or slides of a restaurant, movie theater, or public building can be used to facilitate discussion and problem solving by the family unit when analyzing potential architectural barriers in the environment. Thus in the future when the family is presented with a problem or a barrier, they will have the resources to overcome it rather than be devastated by it.

Role playing in combination with support groups can also be used to defuse potentially painful situations and operate independently. While the patient is still in the safe environment of the rehabilitation setting, simulations of incidents can be created for them to practice problem solving with supervision to help anticipate potential situations. They can be asked what they would do when a stranger (possibly a child) approaches the patient and asks why he or she is in a wheelchair or is disabled, or what they would do when a waiter asks the family member to order for the disabled patient. All of these situations are potentially devastating for all involved; however, if role playing and support groups are used in advance to help all members of the family (patient included) to satisfactorily handle and feel in control of the situation, the family will not be as likely to be traumatized by a similar occurrence. The result is that the family will not be as inclined to be overwhelmed by social situations and will be able to socialize in a much freer, more gratifying way.[78,80,248,249]

Cognitive-behavioral therapy has been used for patients and spouses with success.[94-96] Psychosocial support groups have been called for throughout the literature.[92,214,217,224,237,250-252] Throughout the therapeutic process, the patient and the family need to be praised frequently, and credit needs to be given for the gains made by the patient and family members. Granted, the therapist may have engineered the gains, but the family and patient are the ones who need the reinforcement. As Bolte-Taylor[134] suggested, celebrate all of the little successes—they can help inspire the patient and their family. Through gratifying experiences the family will unite to overcome the disability. They need to know that they can survive in the world without having the medical staff constantly there to solve the family's problems. In short, they need the strategies and resources that will allow them to be independent outside the medical model.

Yet another way to encourage independence can be applied to working with parents of disabled children.[13] The parents should be educated about normal and abnormal growth and development, including physical, cognitive, and emotional growth, so that the family can maintain some perspective and objectivity about their child's various levels.[8,92,224]

The parents can then better understand the needs of those children with disabilities and those without in the family. Armed with this knowledge, the parents and children will be less likely to be frustrated with unreal expectations or unreal demands. Education for the parents could take place at local colleges, online, at the hospital, or even in a parent's group.

Support Systems

Groups are often used to increase motivation, provide support, increase social skills, instill hope, model our humanity, and help the patient and family realize that they are not the only ones who have a disabled family member. This will help the patient and family establish a more accurate set of perceptions about the disabled individual and allow for greater independence of the patient and family.[1,9,93,161,249,253] Problem solving can be encouraged, and value systems can be clarified and bolstered. Patient or family support groups, including healthy peer groups, can be used to relieve pressure that might otherwise be vented in therapy. Lawrie Williams, a mother of two daughters who experienced serious medical challenges, is the author of a series of articles about parental roles in family-centered care. One article in particular highlights the role parents can play in helping other families through parent-to-parent support programs. Williams first experienced the support of another parent when one of her daughters was young, and later realized she could use her own experiences professionally. For the past 6 years, Williams has been the coordinator of the Parent Support Program at the Center for Children with Special Needs, Children's Hospital and Regional Medical Center in Seattle, Washington.[254]

Livneh and Antonak[160] found that in a chronic-care ward family involvement helped the patient and the family improve their status. Schwartzberg[237] and Schulz[154] and others[1,99,132,236,255-257] have reported great success in the use of support groups with individuals who had brain damage. Support groups can also be used to educate the patient about the patient's disability to increase independence.[1,194,236,241,258,259]

Kreuter and colleagues[259] and Taanila and colleagues[13,258] found that independent physical functioning and knowledge about one's condition were exceedingly important in moving through the phases of the rehabilitation process.[76,222,253,260] A guide to facilitating support groups has been published by Boreing and Adler,[261] and it has been found to be useful, especially by laypeople establishing such groups.[76,93,99,194,237,258-262]

The Adult Patient With Brain Damage

The adult patient with brain damage and the needs of the family will be specifically, yet briefly, explored here. Brain damage can affect the cognitive, perceptual, emotional, social, and neurological systems of the individual and can be incredibly disruptive and catastrophic to the patient's and family's lives. When a person sustains a brain injury and is hospitalized, emotional support for the family (patient included) is the primary need to be met initially. The therapist should attempt to convey warmth and a caring attitude, especially during the family's initial contacts.[263] Typical complaints about the acute period involve impersonal hospital routines and lack of definite information about the patient's status.[13,93,217,264] Unfortunately, definitive information is usually not available at the earliest stages.

Later the family must deal with the physical changes in the patient's body; what may be even more injurious to the family are the psychological, cognitive, and social changes in the patient.[1,8,9,16,18,19,250] People with cerebrovascular accidents have been found to be more clinically depressed than orthopedic patients are. The libido[251] and the emotional systems are also affected.[76,214] It has further been shown that persons who survive a cerebrovascular accident or other impairment and who have a full return of function do not return to normal life because of a lack of social and emotional skills.[1,9,93,161,249,253] Families of cerebrovascular accident victims have also reported that social reintegration is the most difficult phase of rehabilitation.[265] Lack of socially appropriate behaviors has been one of the most troublesome complaints of people who deal with the person with a traumatic brain injury. Therapists may be able to help alter this difficulty by encouraging appropriate behavior and by structuring therapy situations to provide opportunities for the patient to practice appropriate behavioral and social interaction skills. A technique called *dialectical behavioral therapy* has been used with people with mental health disorders, and it appears to be a promising approach. One study by Miller and colleagues[266] found significant reductions in suicidal symptoms; the most highly rated skills included distress tolerance and mindfulness skills. The goals of a dialectical behavioral therapy program designed for individuals with mild traumatic brain injury include decreasing the individual's self-defeating behaviors and cognitions, cultivating understanding of the individual's abilities and impairments, and increasing behavioral and cognitive skills that will lead to a greater sense of self and feelings of self-esteem. The program is designed to improve each patient's ability to accept his or her life as it is and function independently.[267]

Better follow-up care needs to be implemented when dealing with the adult with brain damage.[1,99,132,236,255–257] In some areas there are outpatient, privately funded programs that can help support the brain-injured individual and his or her family on discharge from hospital settings. These resources must be recommended for follow-up care as needed.

It may not be possible for the patient and family to constantly come to the clinic for support and follow-up, but Skype or Zoom conversations can be scheduled on a periodic basis, or the exchange of text messages and emails can also be used. With the increased availability of online video conferencing capabilities, follow-up may be performed online by patients living in rural areas. In-person or online conferencing support groups are being used increasingly to facilitate patient and family adjustment and accommodation to disability, as well as reentry into the community.[1,16,93,220,227,236,258,268]

CONCLUSION

The practice area of neurological rehabilitation and the implications of our work in fostering and supporting our patients and patients in the process of learning how to be in relationship to disability is an extraordinarily complex and encompassing practice. We all have, as a part of our own humanity, experiences of adaptation and adjustment through our life-spans to draw from and as therapists. We are given unlimited opportunities to bring our own humanity to bear in this dynamic and humbling work. It may be that beyond the intensifying productivity standards and potential for cynicism and burnout that is increasingly becoming a reality of our work. There is a well of insight, wisdom, and compassion we can draw from to cultivate and develop as clinicians. Our practice, with the support of community, is in seeking out opportunities to build our own inner and outer resources of support, strengthening our capacity to remain centered, modeling qualities of reciprocity, connection, and self-care to the best of our abilities in the therapeutic relationship, all the while sustaining the course even in the midst of challenging circumstances.

Acknowledgment

The present authors and editors would like to thank Gordon U. Burton PhD, OTR/L for his significant contribution on this chapter in the previous edition of the text.

CASE STUDY 5.1 Putting Evaluations and Techniques Into Practice

Diane, a divorced 42-year-old woman with a college-age daughter, was happily employed as a junior high art teacher when she had a left hemorrhagic CVA resulting in right spastic hemiplegia and motor speech impairment. She had right-handed dominance prior to the stroke. She is in grief over the losses of her job as a teacher and her accomplished art skills that relied on her dominant hand. She is devastated and angry about these losses and the difficulties ahead. She is experiencing fear and stress about how she will manage financially and practically. Connecting with other patients in similar circumstances is very important to her. The value and authenticity of this sharing is acknowledged by members of the team. A very independent person, Diane still wants to work. She hopes to learn to drive an adapted car in the future, pending thorough evaluation and training. She wants to live as independently as possible and be able to participate in all those activities that brought meaning, purpose, and joy to her life. Diane's friends, colleagues, and siblings have been supportive. Her daughter took a semester off from college and will be returning to school in a few months.

Treatment

What is key here is the manner of proceeding in collaboration, with therapists looking for opportunities within the therapy experience to listen and reflect what is being discovered and for gains to acknowledge. Diane has been participating in occupational therapy and physical therapy treatments working to treat spasticity, learning methods to decrease tone, and using splinting. Mindful sensing and breathing are incorporated into the treatment as well as reporting nuances of awareness of felt experience: familiarizing, being aware of, and owning the experience of the body as it is in the moment. All kinds of feelings of grief, strangeness, and frustration may arise throughout treatment sessions. Her goal in PT is to progress to walk independently with walker and quad cane and to transfer safely. She is working with the speech therapist on motor speech and swallowing techniques. Currently her speech is labored but understandable. Diane is working with OT on dressing using nondominant L side assistive devices, and she is learning one-handed kitchen skills with assistive methods and devices. Spasticity, pain, and therapy appointments are all physically, mentally, and emotionally fatiguing.

Initially Diane will participate in peer-support groups to foster mental and emotional processing of her situation, to work with processes of acceptance, adjustment, and coping, and to provide an atmosphere to cultivate relationships, bonding, a sense of belonging, build resources for resilience, and enhance inner and outer resources such as emotion-focused problem solving, mindfulness, and building a sense of community and connectedness.

The current treatment plan is to collaborate with Diane to plan and implement energy conservation strategies and break down very sizable goals into workable steps. She has high hopes, and it will be important to keep steps incrementally achievable, to recognize small gains, and to honor the challenge and work involved so that the healing and rebuilding processes are not overwhelming. This can be an opportunity to explore mutuality, interdependence, and independence in the context of community.

The treatment team is collaborating with Diane to explore interests, strengths, and needs to address potential job or job-training possibilities. While there are new restraints, there are also deepening capacities growing out of these challenging circumstances. The OT and Diane will work together to problem solve what adaptations, support, and stamina issues need to be considered. While Diane has great grief over losing her dominant hand for art work, OT will invite alternative approaches with her nondominant hand, offering participation in art activities. This exploration will need to be sensitive to Diane's capabilities and perhaps allow a new approach, one following her lead, permission to experiment in a new medium with no agenda other than doing something new,

Continued

CASE STUDY 5.1   Putting Evaluations and Techniques Into Practice—cont'd

and engage in a creative process using her nondominant hand and thus different brain engagement.

The medical social worker, in communication with the rehab team, will be working with Diane and support persons to assess finances, services, and access to resources for her goals. She will also be referred to vocational rehab counseling once she feels more stabilized in her daily functioning and has a realistic picture of her activity tolerance and fatigue. The rehab team contributes to vocational rehab assessment. There is discussion of exploring the future possibility of canine companions, which Diane has heard about and is very interested in.

REFERENCES

To enhance this text and add value for the reader, all references are included on the companion Evolve site that accompanies this textbook. This online service will, when available, provide a link for the reader to a Medline abstract for the article cited. There are 268 cited references and other general references for this chapter, with the majority of those articles being evidence-based citations.

6

Differential Diagnosis of the Patient With a Neurological Condition

John D. Heick and Rolando T. Lazaro

OBJECTIVES

After reading this chapter the student or therapist will be able to:

1. Identify the difference between differential diagnosis for medical screening, and differential diagnosis for diagnosis of impairments, activity limitations, and participation restrictions.
2. Analyze the concept of body system and subsystem screening to be used with patients with unknown or known preexisting neurological dysfunction.
3. Develop a mechanism for body system screening to be used with patients with preexisting neurological dysfunction.
4. Analyze the significance and importance of performing a medical screening for all patients who interact in a therapeutic environment with clinicians.

KEY TERMS

causational systems interaction
medical screening

patient referral
review of systems

INTRODUCTION

The term *differential diagnosis* means different things to different clinicians. In this text the term will be used to answer the question that all therapists should ask themselves when they are performing the initial evaluation of a patient: Does the patient present a condition that is within the scope of physical or occupational therapy practice that the clinician can treat? If the answer is no, then the clinician has two choices. The first is to continue to manage the patient to work on those issues that can be improved with physical or occupational therapy intervention AND refer the patient to another health care provider that can help identify and treat the other condition the patient may have. The other option is to refer the patient out to another health care practitioner who is capable of diagnosing and managing the presenting condition.

This initial process of differential diagnosis is performed by the clinician while doing a thorough history and neurological examination to rule out serious neurological conditions and rule in the patient's condition. In this case, the patient likely presented with multiple "red flags," which are signs and symptoms that act as warnings to alert the therapist to investigate further. In the case that a patient does have a serious neurological condition, therapists need to appreciate that clusters of tests or clusters of red flag signs and symptoms are most useful to identify serious neurological conditions and that the reliance on only one test or positive red flag sign or symptom is not as conclusive to the decision making process for the clinician.

Evidence has suggested that identifying clusters of several red flags improves the sensitivity or specificity of a condition. For example, Raison and colleagues[1] found that combining asking a patient about bowel and bladder disorders and asking the patient about saddle paresthesia and identifying two positive answers to these red flags improved the specificity to 0.92 in those patients whose magnetic resonance imaging (MRI) confirmed spinal cord compression. Kollensperger and colleagues[2] found that clustering red flags for confirming multiple system atrophy, a condition that mimics Parkinson disease, resulted in a specificity increase to 98.5%, sensitivity to 84.2%, positive predictive value to 96%, and negative predictive value of 92.7% when clustering 2 out of 6 red flag categories.

In the neurological examination, one sign or symptom that appears as a red flag does not mean that the examination is stopped and does not mean that there is complete certainty of predicting the cause; it just increases the probability of that condition. For example, an upgoing plantar response to the Babinski test as the one positive test is considered to be a reliable marker for upper motor neuron lesion. If the clinician identifies the red flag and stops the neurological examination on the patient at that point in time, the clinician might miss the other potential positive tests or signs and symptoms that would help to clarify the patient's diagnosis. Simply stated, red flags are used as warning signs to alert the therapist to investigate further and consider the complete examination. Red flags may occur through multiple approaches that are specific to the setting. Red flags may come from questioning the patient. Yet Premkumar and colleagues[3] recently reported that individual red flag questions were not as effective as clusters of red flag questions, albeit in patients with low back pain. Red flags may also come as objective findings or positive neurological tests. Evidence continues to build on the compilation of red flag questions and red flag objective findings and the use of clinical decision rules to assist therapists in differentiating one condition compared to another.

Evidence suggests that clustering of red flag questions and tests improves the probability of the specific condition, but this has not been explored as well with neurological conditions as it has with orthopedic conditions. After the physical examination, the next step is to evaluate the results of the examination. This systematic approach helps the therapist to identify clusters of positives and thus form clinical patterns that are consistent with specific diagnoses.

The neurological examination should be performed systematically every time. When considering a direct access primary care clinic where physical therapists work, there may be an increased probability of patients coming in with serious conditions that warrant immediate referral to another health care provider. These could be potentially life threatening and include conditions such as stroke or a patient with progressive neurological system decline such as in transverse myelitis. Transverse myelitis may initially present with low back pain and paresthesias, and rapidly progress to weakness in the extremities and bowel and bladder incontinence. In many situations like this example, this may involve additional tests and measures that the patient has to undergo to rule out conditions and ultimately identify the condition. In the multiple practice settings where occupational and physical therapists work, therapists may have a variety of resources to assist in identifying conditions, such as referral sources to assist in ordering blood work or imaging for therapists who work in the hospital, emergency department, or settings that are in close proximity to a physician, nurse practitioner, or physician's assistant. On the other side of the spectrum, many therapists have little to no resources available to them to assist in identifying conditions, such as in school settings.

In those settings that have a variety of resources, such as the ability to quickly receive blood work or imaging, therapists must form relationships across disciplines to understand how to facilitate this process and advocate for their patients. Understanding neuroanatomy and how neurological conditions present is pivotal to improving clinical decision making and facilitating the right test for the patient with a neurological condition. For example, a patient with a suspected stroke that presents at a direct access clinic may present with a specific clinical pattern that helps the therapist conclude the location of the deficit. Anterior circulation deficits may be anterior cerebral or middle cerebral artery presentations. Anterior cerebral artery strokes in a patient may present with lower extremity weakness more than upper extremity weakness, whereas middle cerebral artery strokes present with contralateral hemiparesis and speech deficits. Posterior circulatory deficits could likely be seen in a patient presenting with vertigo, dizziness, altered mental status, or visual field deficits. By knowing this, therapists can assist with imaging requests that correspond to the patient's clinical presentation. For example, anterior circulatory strokes are easier to catch by head computed tomography (CT).[4] Middle cerebral artery strokes are best identified with noncontrast head CT with angiography. Head CT with angiography can be used to identify diffuse atherosclerosis and has an odds ratio of 23.6 for ischemic stroke identification. CT angiography with the addition of noncontrast head CT increases the specificity to 88% and sensitivity to greater than 70%.[4] Small lesions such as transient ischemic attacks are hard to identify on CT, with a sensitivity of only 12%. Posterior circulatory lesions require MRI to identify (sensitivity 80%, specificity 95%).[4]

In all settings, the therapist starts with the initial examination which includes taking a thorough history, including an investigation of the patient's medical history, presenting complaints, and a systems review (Box 6.1). In terms of differentially diagnosing the patient in the outpatient setting, a review of systems (Box 6.2) is done by ensuring that a questionnaire that asks about body systems is completed by the patient, and the therapist reviews these questions with the patient to make sure the patient understands. Fig. 6.1 is an example of an intake

---

BOX 6.1 Systems Review Checklist

SYSTEMS REVIEW (note if subjective or objective information: note as impaired or not impaired)

Cardiovascular and Pulmonary ☐ Not impaired ☐ Impaired
☐ Blood Pressure: _____
☐ Edema
☐ Heart Rate _____
☐ Respiratory Rate _____
Integumentary ☐ Not impaired ☐ Impaired
☐ Integrity
☐ Scars
Musculoskeletal ☐ Not impaired ☐ Impaired
☐ Gross ROM WNL
☐ Gross Strength WNL
☐ Gross Symmetry: Symmetrical
Height: _____
Weight: _____
Neuromuscular ☐ Not impaired ☐ Impaired
☐ Gross Balance
☐ Gross Gait
☐ Gross Locomotion
☐ Gross Transfers
☐ Gross Transitions
☐ Motor Function (control, learning)
Communication, Affect, Cognition, Learning ☐ Not impaired ☐ Impaired
☐ Age-appropriate Communication
☐ Orientation × 4
☐ Emotional/behavioral responses
Language:
☐ Preferred Language: _____
☐ English verbal comprehension
    ☐ Fluent
    ☐ Limited
    ☐ Interpreter needed
☐ Reading comprehension
    ☐ Fluent
    ☐ Limited

Adapted from Intake Form, California State University Sacramento Neurologic Probono Clinic. Courtesy D Michael Mckeough, Department Chair.

---

form/medical history questionnaire that includes items for systems review and review of systems. In the inpatient setting, by contrast, a systems review and review of systems is initiated by performing a chart review to investigate the patient's medical history followed by a physical examination of the patient. For example, in a patient with a chief complaint of inability to walk secondary to a middle cerebral artery stroke, it would be important to take their vital signs, scan their integumentary system for signs and symptoms of arterial and venous compromise, as well as to perform a complete neurological examination. A review of systems is also necessary to determine which other body systems may be pathological—whether related or not to the primary diagnosis. This history and the findings of the physical examination will lead to a diagnosis that may necessitate additional tests and measures, which may include laboratory tests or imaging that the patient needs a referral to receive. Especially in the care of the patient with a neurological condition, the therapist needs to be certain of the decision of treat, treat and refer, or refer. The identification of a condition that implicates the central nervous system after the examination of the patient, when the patient is sent to the therapist with a different

BOX 6.2   Review of Systems

When conducting a general review of systems, ask the patient about the presence of any other problems anywhere else in the body. Depending on the patient's answer you may want to prompt him or her about any of the following common signs and symptoms* associated with each system:

General Questions
___Fever, chills, sweating (constitutional symptoms)
___Appetite loss, nausea, vomiting (constitutional symptoms)
___Fatigue, malaise, weakness (constitutional symptoms)
___Excessive, unexplained weight gain or loss
___Vital signs: blood pressure, temperature, pulse, respirations, pain, walking speed
___Insomnia
___Irritability
___Hoarseness or change in voice, frequent or prolonged sore throat
___Dizziness, falls

Integumentary (Include Skin, Hair, and Nails)
___Recent rashes, nodules, or other skin changes
___Unusual hair loss or breakage
___Increased hair growth (hirsutism)
___Change in nail beds
___Itching (pruritus)

Musculoskeletal/Neurological
___Joint pain, redness, warmth, swelling, stiffness, deformity
___Frequent or severe headache
___Change in vision or hearing
___Vertigo
___Paresthesias (numbness, tingling, "pins and needles" sensation)
___Change in muscle tone
___Weakness; atrophy
___Abnormal deep tendon (or other) reflexes
___Problems with coordination or balance; falling
___Involuntary movements; tremors
___Radicular pain
___Seizure or loss of consciousness
___Memory loss
___Paralysis
___Mood swings; hallucinations

Rheumatological
___Presence/location of joint swelling
___Muscle pain, weakness
___Skin rashes
___Reaction to sunlight
___Raynaud phenomenon
___Change in nail beds

Cardiovascular
___Chest pain or sense of heaviness or discomfort
___Palpitations
___Limb pain during activity (claudication; cramps, limping)
___Discolored or painful feet; swelling of hands and feet
   Pulsating or throbbing pain anywhere, but especially in the back or abdomen
___Peripheral edema; nocturia
___Sudden weight gain; unable to fasten waistband or belt, unable to wear regular shoes
___Persistent cough
___Fatigue, dyspnea, orthopnea, syncope

___High or low blood pressure, unusual pulses
___Differences in blood pressure from side to side with position change (10 mm Hg or more; increase or decrease/diastolic or systolic; associated symptoms: dizziness, headache, nausea, vomiting, diaphoresis, heart palpitations, increased primary pain or symptoms)
___Positive findings during auscultation

Pulmonary
___Cough, hoarseness
___Sputum, hemoptysis
___Shortness of breath (dyspnea, orthopnea); altered breathing (e.g., wheezing, pursed-lip breathing)
___Night sweats; sweats anytime
___Pleural pain
___Cyanosis, clubbing
___Positive findings during auscultation (e.g., friction rub, unexpected breath sounds)

Psychological
___Sleep disturbance
___Stress levels
___Fatigue, psychomotor agitation
___Change in personal habits, appetite
___Depression, confusion, anxiety
___Irritability, mood changes

Gastrointestinal
___Abdominal pain
___Indigestion; heartburn
___Difficulty in swallowing
___Nausea/vomiting; loss of appetite
___Diarrhea or constipation
___Change in stools; change in bowel habits
___Fecal incontinence
___Rectal bleeding; blood in stool; blood in vomit
___Skin rash followed by joint pain (Crohn disease)

Hepatic/Biliary
___Change in taste/smell
___Anorexia
___Feeling of abdominal fullness, ascites
___Asterixis (muscle tremors)
___Change in urine color (dark, cola-colored)
___Light-colored stools
___Change in skin color (yellow, green)
___Skin changes (rash, itching, purpura, spider angiomas, palmar erythema)

Hematological
___Change in skin color or nail beds
___Bleeding: nose, gums, easy bruising, melena
___Hemarthrosis, muscle hemorrhage, hematoma
___Fatigue, dyspnea, weakness
___Rapid pulse, palpitations
___Confusion, irritability
___Headache

Genitourinary
___Reduced stream, decreased output
___Burning or bleeding during urination; change in urine color
___Urinary incontinence, dribbling

Continued

BOX 6.2 **Review of Systems—cont'd**

___Impotence, pain with intercourse
___Hesitation, urgency
___Nocturia, frequency
___Dysuria (painful or difficult urination)
___Testicular pain or swelling
___Genital lesions
___Penile or vaginal discharge
___Impotence (males) or other sexual difficulty (males or females)
___Infertility (males or females)
___Flank pain

Gynecological
___Irregular menses, amenorrhea, menopause
___Pain with menses or intercourse
___Vaginal discharge, vaginal itching
___Surgical procedures
___Pregnancy, birth, miscarriage, and abortion histories
___Spotting, bleeding, especially for the postmenopausal woman 12 months after last period (without hormone replacement therapy)

Endocrine
___Change in hair and nails
___Change in appetite, unexplained weight change
___Fruity breath odor
___Temperature intolerance, hot flashes, diaphoresis (unexplained perspiration)
___Heart palpitations, tachycardia
___Headaches
___Low urine output, absence of perspiration
___Cramps
___Edema, polyuria, polydipsia, polyphagia
___Unexplained weakness, fatigue, paresthesia

___Carpal/tarsal tunnel syndrome
___Periarthritis, adhesive capsulitis
___Joint or muscle pain (arthralgia, myalgia), trigger points
___Prolonged deep tendon reflexes
___Sleep disturbance

Cancer
___Constant, intense pain, especially bone pain at night
___Unexplained weight loss (10% of body weight in 10–14 days); most patients in pain are inactive and gain weight
___Loss of appetite
___Excessive fatigue
___Unusual lump(s), thickening, change in a lump or mole, sore that does not heal; other unusual skin lesion or rash
___Unusual or prolonged bleeding or discharge anywhere
___Change in bowel or bladder habits
___Chronic cough or hoarseness, change in voice
___Rapid onset of digital clubbing (10–14 days)
___Proximal muscle weakness, especially when accompanied by change in one or more deep tendon reflexes

Immunological
___Change in skin or nail beds
___Fever or other constitutional symptoms (especially recurrent or cyclical symptoms)
___Lymph node changes (tenderness, enlargement)
___Anaphylactic reaction
___Symptoms of muscle or joint involvement (pain, swelling, stiffness, weakness)
___Sleep disturbance

*Cluster of three to four or more lasting longer than 1 month.
Reprinted from Goodman, Heick and Lazaro. *Differential Diagnosis for Physical Therapists*. 6th ed. St. Louis, MO: Elsevier; 2018.

---

referring diagnosis, is important to verify as soon as possible. This will aid in recognition of a specific diagnosis and lead to a more accurate prognosis. One way to think about a systems review is that it directs the therapist on whether to investigate that system. For example, in the patient that presents with a middle cerebral artery stroke and left neglect, the therapist needs to be concerned about the integumentary system, especially of the left upper extremity if the patient has a lesion of the dorsal column medial lemniscus tract.

The therapist organizes the history and physical examination (including tests and measures) findings into clusters, syndromes, or categories. In the neurological examination, therapists identify clusters of findings that suggest the presence of disease or an adverse drug event and warrant communication with a physician. The therapist then considers using the World Health Organization (WHO) International Classification of Functioning, Disability and Health (ICF) model[5] to examine the influences of both internal and external factors to the patient's health. The ICF framework classifies the health components of function and disability. The ICF framework focuses on the three perspectives that influence the patient: body, individual, and society. By reflecting on these influences, therapists can then pair outcome measures that correctly identify how these three perspectives influence the individual with a neurological condition.

DIFFERENTIAL DIAGNOSIS: MEDICAL SCREENING

The *Guide to Physical Therapy Practice*[6] clearly describes the therapist's responsibility to refer patients with health concerns to other practitioners (Fig. 6.2). In the practice of treating patients with neurological conditions, many times the therapist needs to refer the patient back to the physician. This usually occurs due to the patient's sudden changes in mental and/or physical status. This may also be associated with a recent exacerbation of symptoms such as pain, weakness, numbness, dizziness, falls, or confusion. Therapists may also detect signs or symptoms not related to the patient's primary neurological condition but instead related to a comorbidity or a medication side effect. The systems review and review of systems may reveal a need to refer the patient for a dermatological, cardiovascular, or other system involvement not related to their primary neurological condition that requires attention by a physician (Fig. 6.3).

As a health care professional and especially in a direct access clinic, it is the therapist's duty to screen the patient within their scope of practice. In screening the patient the therapist may (1) identify signs and symptoms consistent with existing medical conditions, (2) identify signs and symptoms suggesting that an existing medical condition may be worsening, (3) identify neurological

Family/Personal History

Date: _____

Patient's name: _____   DOB: _____   Age: _____

Race/ethnicity: ☐ American Indian/Alaska Native   ☐ Asian
                 ☐ Black/African American   ☐ Caucasian/white
                 ☐ Hispanic/Latino   ☐ Native Hawaiian/Pacific Islander
                 ☐ Multiracial   ☐ Other/unknown

Language: ☐ English understood   ☐ Interpreter needed   ☐ Primary language:

Medical diagnosis: _____   Date of onset: _____

Physician: _____   Date of surgery (if any): _____   Therapist: _____

Past Medical History
Have you or any immediate family member (parent, sibling, child) ever been told you have:

(Do **NOT** complete) **For the therapist:**

Circle one:

			Relation to patient	Date of onset	Current status
• Allergies	Yes	No			
• Angina or chest pain	Yes	No			
• Anxiety/panic attacks	Yes	No			
• Arthritis	Yes	No			
• Asthma, hay fever, or other breathing problems	Yes	No			
• Cancer	Yes	No			
• Chemical dependency (alcohol/drugs)	Yes	No	**Therapists:** Use this space to record baseline information. This is important in case something changes in the patient's status. You are advised to record the date and sign or initial this form for documentation and liability purposes, indicating that you have reviewed this form with the patient. You may want to have the patient sign and date it as well.		
• Cirrhosis/liver disease	Yes	No			
• Depression	Yes	No			
• Diabetes	Yes	No			
• Eating disorder (bulimia, anorexia)	Yes	No			
• Headaches	Yes	No			
• Heart attack	Yes	No			
• Hemophilia/slow healing	Yes	No			
• High cholesterol	Yes	No			
• Hypertension or high blood pressure	Yes	No			
• Kidney disease/stones	Yes	No			
• Multiple sclerosis	Yes	No			
• Osteoporosis	Yes	No			
• Stroke	Yes	No			
• Tuberculosis	Yes	No			
• Other (please describe)	Yes	No			

Fig. 6.1 Example of an Intake Form/Medical History Questionnaire. From Goodman C, Heick J and Lazaro R. *Differential Diagnosis for Physical Therapists*, 6th ed. St. Louis, MO: Elsevier; 2018. Reprinted with permission

Continued

Personal History

Have you ever had:

• Anemia	Yes	No	• Chronic bronchitis	Yes	No
• Epilepsy/seizures	Yes	No	• Emphysema	Yes	No
• Fibromyalgia/myofascial			• GERD	Yes	No
pain syndrome	Yes	No	• Gout	Yes	No
• Hepatitis/jaundice	Yes	No	• Guillain-Barré syndrome	Yes	No
• Joint replacement	Yes	No	• Hypoglycemia	Yes	No
• Parkinson's disease	Yes	No	• Peripheral vascular disease	Yes	No
• Polio/postpolio	Yes	No	• Pneumonia	Yes	No
• Shortness of breath	Yes	No	• Prostate problems	Yes	No
• Skin problems	Yes	No	• Rheumatic/scarlet fever	Yes	No
• Urinary incontinence			• Thyroid problems	Yes	No
(dribbling, leaking)	Yes	No	• Ulcer/stomach problems	Yes	No
• Urinary tract infection	Yes	No	• Varicose veins	Yes	No

For Women:

History of endometriosis	Yes	No
History of pelvic inflammatory disease	Yes	No
Are you/could you be pregnant?	Yes	No
Any trouble with leaking or dribbling urine?	Yes	No

Number of pregnancies _____   Number of live births _____

Have you ever had a miscarriage/abortion? Yes   No

General Health

1. I would rate my health as (circle one):   Excellent   Good   Fair   Poor
2. Are you taking any prescription or over-the-counter medications? If yes, please list: _____ Yes   No
   _____
3. Are you taking any nutritional supplements (any kind, including vitamins)   Yes   No
4. Have you had any illnesses within the last 3 weeks (e.g., colds, influenza, bladder or kidney infection)?   Yes   No
   If yes, have you had this before in the last 3 months?   Yes   No
5. Have you noticed any lumps or thickening of skin or muscle anywhere on your body?   Yes   No
6. Do you have any sores that have not healed or any changes in size, shape, or color of a wart or mole?   Yes   No
7. Have you had any unexplained weight gain or loss in the last month?   Yes   No
8. Do you smoke or chew tobacco?   Yes   No
   If yes, how many packs/pipes/pouches/sticks a day? _____ How many months or years? _____
9. I used to smoke/chew but I quit.   Yes   No
   If yes: pack or amount/day _____ Year quit _____
10. I would like to quit smoking/using tobacco.   Yes   No
11. How much alcohol do you drink in the course of a week? (One drink is equal to 1 beer, 1 glass of wine,
    or 1 shot of hard liquor) _____
12. Do you use recreational or street drugs (marijuana, cocaine, crack, meth, amphetamines, or others)?   Yes   No
    If yes, what, how much, how often? _____
13. How much caffeine do you consume daily (including soft drinks, coffee, tea, or chocolate)? _____
    _____
14. Are you on any special diet?   Yes   No

Fig. 6.1, cont'd

15. Do you have (or have you recently had) any of these problems:
- ☐ Blood in urine, stool, vomit, mucus
- ☐ Dizziness, fainting, blackouts
- ☐ Fever, chills, sweats (day or night)
- ☐ Nausea, vomiting, loss of appetite
- ☐ Changes in bowel or bladder
- ☐ Throbbing sensation/pain in belly or anywhere else
- ☐ Skin rash or other skin changes

- ☐ Cough, dyspnea
- ☐ Dribbling or leaking urine
- ☐ Heart palpitations or fluttering
- ☐ Numbness or tingling
- ☐ Swelling or lumps anywhere
- ☐ Problems seeing or hearing
- ☐ Unusual fatigue, drowsiness

- ☐ Difficulty swallowing/speaking
- ☐ Memory loss
- ☐ Confusion
- ☐ Sudden weakness
- ☐ Trouble sleeping
- ☐ Other: _____
- ☐ None of these

Medical/Surgical History

1. Have you ever been treated with chemotherapy, radiation therapy, biotherapy, or brachytherapy (radiation implants)?   Yes   No
   If yes, please describe: _____
2. Have you had any x-rays, sonograms, computed tomography (CT) scans, or magnetic resonance imaging (MRI) or other imaging done recently?   Yes   No
   If yes, what?_____ When? _____ Results? _____
3. Have you had any laboratory work done recently (urinalysis or blood tests)?   Yes   No
   If yes, what?_____ When? _____ Results (if known)? _____
4. Any other clinical tests?   Yes   No
   Please describe: _____
5. Please list any operations that you have ever had and the date(s):
   Operation_____ Date _____
6. Do you have a pacemaker, transplanted organ, joint replacement, breast implants, or any other implants?   Yes   No
   If yes, please describe:_____

Work/Living Environment

1. What is your job or occupation?_____
2. Military service: (When and where): _____
3. Does your work involve:
   - ☐ Prolonged sitting (e.g., desk, computer, driving)
   - ☐ Prolonged standing (e.g., equipment operator, sales clerk)
   - ☐ Prolonged walking (e.g., mill worker, delivery service)
   - ☐ Use of large or small equipment (e.g., telephone, forklift, computer, drill press, cash register)
   - ☐ Lifting, bending, twisting, climbing, turning
   - ☐ Exposure to chemicals, pesticides, toxins, or gases
   - ☐ Other: please describe
   - ☐ Not applicable; none of these
4. Do you use any special supports:
   - ☐ Back cushion, neck cushion
   - ☐ Back brace, corset
   - ☐ Other kind of brace or support for any body part
   - ☐ None; not applicable

History of falls:
- ☐ In the past year, I have had no falls
- ☐ I have just started to lose my balance/fall
- ☐ I fall occasionally
- ☐ I fall frequently (more than two times during the past 6 months)
- ☐ Certain factors make me cautious (e.g., curbs, ice, stairs, getting in and out of the tub)

I live:
- ☐ Alone ☐ With family, spouse, partner
- ☐ Nursing home ☐ Assisted living ☐ Other_____

For the physical therapist:
Exercise history: determine level of activity, exercise, fitness (type, frequency, intensity, duration)
Vital signs (also complete Pain Assessment Record Form, Appendix C-7 on ⓔ)
Resting pulse rate: _____ Body temperature: _____ Respirations: _____ Oxygen saturation: _____
Blood pressure: 1st reading _____ 2nd reading _____
   Position: Sitting   Standing   Extremity: Right   Left

Fig. 6.1, cont'd

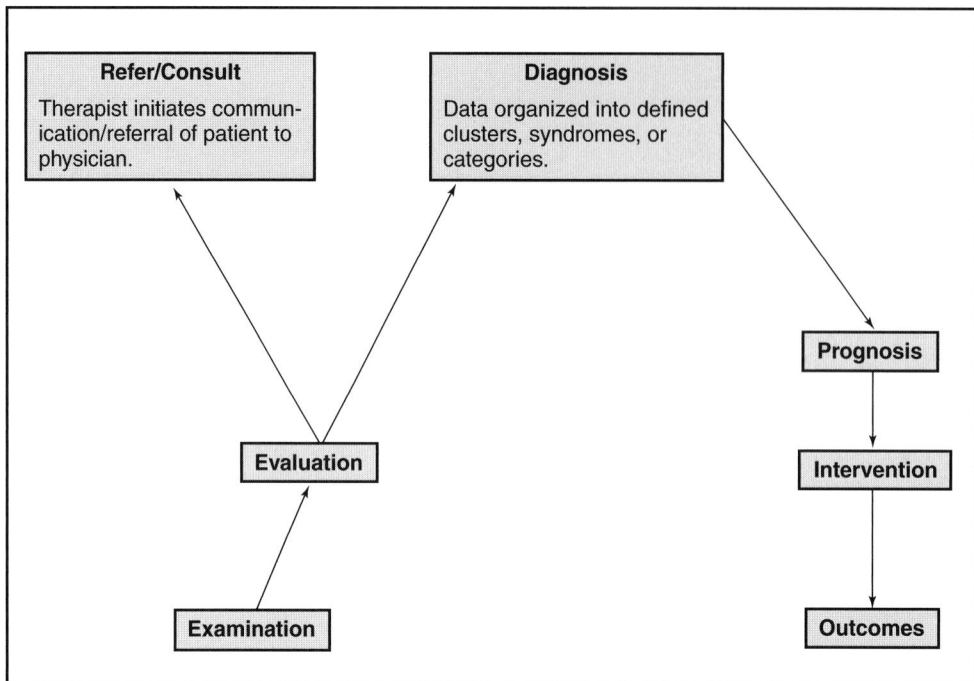

Fig. 6.2 Patient/Client Management Process Showing Therapist Referring the Patient Back to the Physician. (Modified from Umphred DA [Chair]: Diagnostic Task Force, State of California, 1996–2000., California Chapter of the American Physical Therapy Association.)

manifestations that suggest an acute or life-threatening crisis, and (4) identify signs and symptoms suggestive of the presence of an occult disorder or medication side effect. This medical screening has always taken place within the clinical framework of physical therapist (PT) practice, but as direct access practitioners, this screening must become more comprehensive, requiring outcome measures and documented evaluation results. Fig. 6.4 is an example of an examination scheme that leads into a clinical decision to treat the patient, to treat *and* refer the patient, or to refer the patient. This figure suggests referring the patient may also include the decision to refer the patient to another practitioner (e.g., dietician, social worker, clinical psychologist) for services such as wellness clinics that encourage participation in movement activities to maintain gains experienced in therapy or once the patient has reached a plateau in rehabilitation. The following material focuses on the components of this scheme most directly related to the medical screening process leading to a patient referral.

Identifying Patients' Health Risk Factors and Previous Conditions

Owing to the considerable overlap in symptomatic presentation of impairment-related conditions and those requiring physician examination, identifying existing health risk factors for occult diseases is important. Numerous factors have an effect on the patient's risk for compromised health status, including age, sex, race, occupation, leisure activities, preexisting medical conditions, family medical history, medication usage (over-the-counter and prescription drugs), tobacco use, and substance abuse or the interaction of some of these conditions.

Of these, a personal history of a current or recent medical condition, current medication use, and a positive family history (e.g., mother and aunt with a history of breast cancer, father diagnosed with prostate cancer at the age of 58 years) are the most relevant risk factors for the potential presence of an occult condition. For example, the history of a previous episode of depression significantly increases the risk of a second episode compared with the risk that someone who has never had an episode of depression will have his or her first such episode.[7] The greater the number of existing risk factors, the more vigilant the therapist should be for the presence of warning signs suggestive of disease and the more extensive the other medical screening components will need to be. Those increased risk factors, whether within one system or multiple systems, can lead to clinical behaviors that are the summation of the systems problems and their interactions that affect movement. Physicians should be able to depend on the therapist to recognize these interactive symptoms and refer the patient back to either the referring physician or to another specialist.

There are different methods to collect this medical history and patient profile information, including a review of the medical record and use of a self-administered questionnaire, depending on the practice setting and patient population. Fig. 6.1 is an example of a self-administered questionnaire that could be completed by the adult patient, a family member, or a caregiver. A quick review of this information should occur, if possible, before the patient interview is begun. The therapist will have a head start in organizing the history and physical examination, knowing what to prioritize and at least initially what parts of the examination can be deemphasized.

Affirmative answers to previous or current illness questions should direct the therapist to consider what the potential impact may

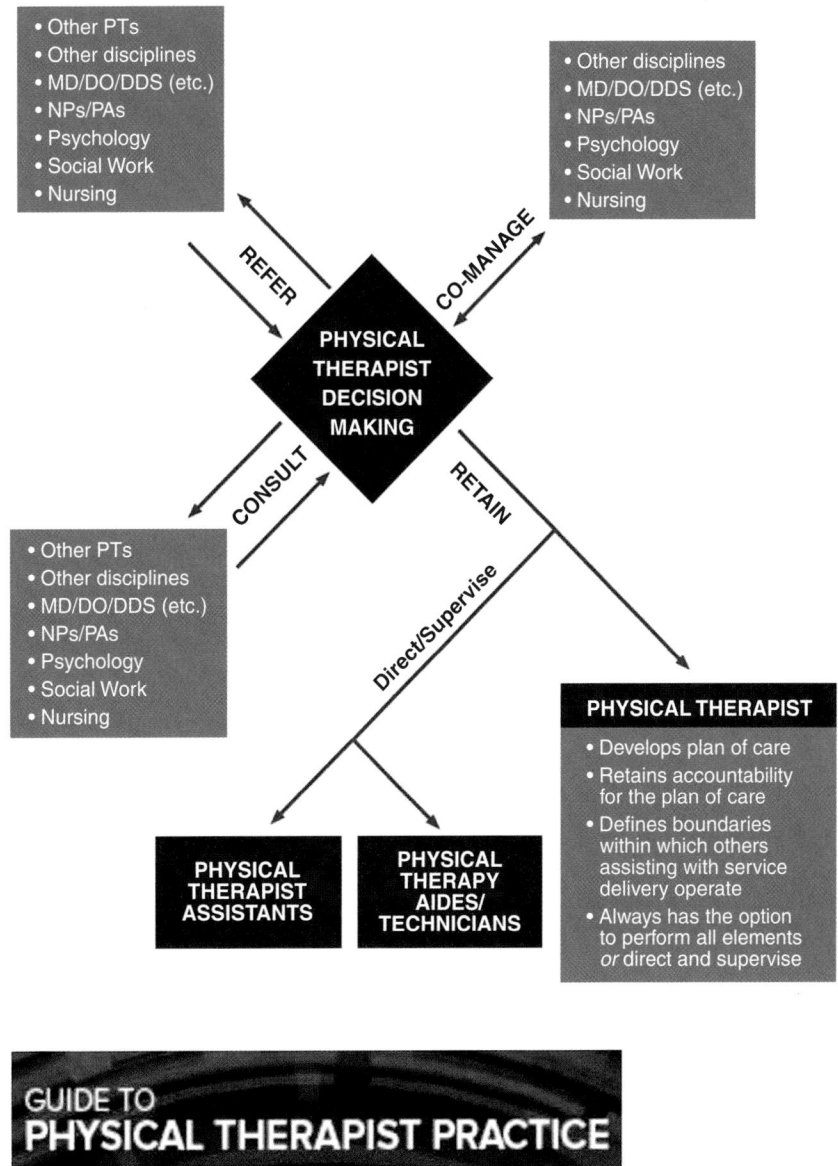

Other PTs
- Other disciplines
- MD/DO/DDS (etc.)
- NPs/PAs
- Psychology
- Social Work
- Nursing

- Other disciplines
- MD/DO/DDS (etc.)
- NPs/PAs
- Psychology
- Social Work
- Nursing

REFER   CO-MANAGE

PHYSICAL THERAPIST DECISION MAKING

CONSULT   RETAIN

- Other PTs
- Other disciplines
- MD/DO/DDS (etc.)
- NPs/PAs
- Psychology
- Social Work
- Nursing

Direct/Supervise

PHYSICAL THERAPIST ASSISTANTS

PHYSICAL THERAPY AIDES/ TECHNICIANS

PHYSICAL THERAPIST
- Develops plan of care
- Retains accountability for the plan of care
- Defines boundaries within which others assisting with service delivery operate
- Always has the option to perform all elements *or* direct and supervise

GUIDE TO
PHYSICAL THERAPIST PRACTICE

2014 by American Physical Therapy Association

Fig. 6.3 The Physical Therapist Decision Making Process. (Reprinted from http://ww.apta.org, with permission of the American Physical Therapy Association. © 2019 American Physical Therapy Association. All rights reserved.)

be on the patient's symptoms, choice of examination and interventions, rehabilitation potential, and risk for additional illness. For example, the presence of existing chronic kidney disease (e.g., renal failure) should alert the therapist to numerous potential complications including patient fatigue, weakness, and impaired concentration, all of which could interfere with rehabilitation efforts. Chronic renal failure is also marked by paresthesia and muscle weakness, which could mistakenly be associated with other neurological conditions. Renal osteodystrophy is yet another complication associated with chronic renal failure. The concern for compromised bone density should direct the therapist to use techniques that carry a reduced risk of skeletal injury. A series of follow-up questions for the affirmative answers will assist the therapist in determining the relevance

(if any) of each item (see Fig. 6.5 for examples of follow-up questions for selected information categories).

Symptomatic Investigation of Functional Restriction

The chief presenting symptoms or limitation in activity typically provides the reason for therapy services being sought and can provide the initial warning sign(s) of potential medical issues needing to be addressed. Despite pain not typically being the chief complaint of many patients with primary neurological conditions, a relatively mild pain is often the initial complaint associated with a serious pathological condition; a dull diffuse ache is often the initial presenting complaint associated with tumors of the musculoskeletal system.[8] This relatively minor complaint may easily be overlooked by therapists working with

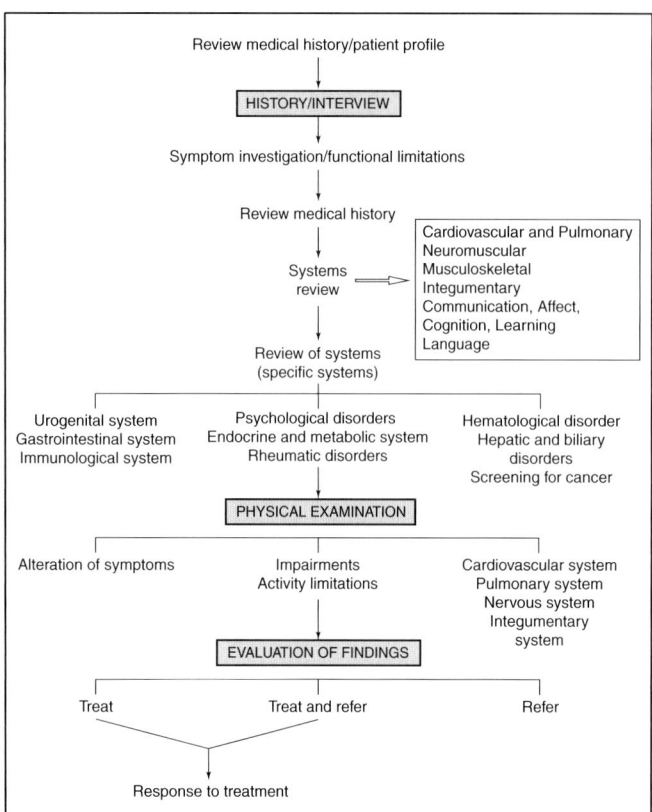

Fig. 6.4 Examination scheme that leads into a clinical decision to treat the patient, to treat *and* refer the patient, or to refer the patient. (Modified from notes from course by W.G. Boissonault, 1998 as published in Umphred DA, Lazaro RT, Roller ML, Burton GU. *Umphred's Neurological Rehabilitation.* 6th ed. St. Louis, MO: Elsevier; 2013.)

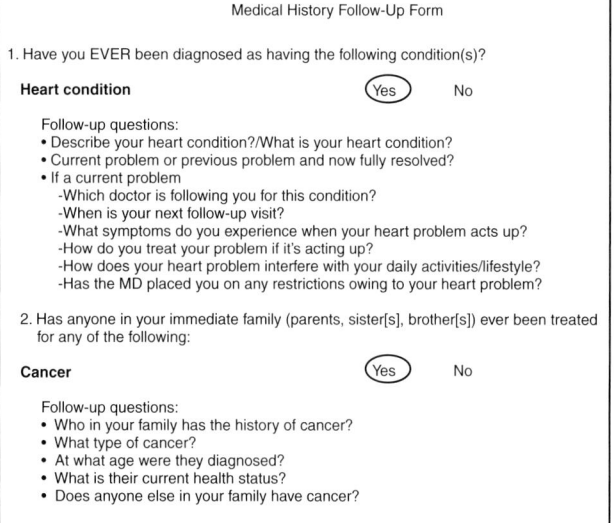

Fig. 6.5 Potential follow-up questions for affirmative answers on the self-administered questionnaire. (From W.G. Boissonault course notes, 1998 as published in Umphred, Lazaro, Roller, et al. *Umphred's Neurological Rehabilitation.* 6th ed. St. Louis, MO: Elsevier; 2013.)

patients who have neurological involvement and signs and symptoms (e.g., weakness, numbness) that are much more debilitating and cause more functional limitations than the pain complaints. Although investigating pain complaints may not be the initial priority for therapists, at a later visit such questioning is very important, especially if the pain continues, increases in intensity, shifts, or enlarges its region with no causation. Effective medical screening involves the interpretation of a patient's description of symptoms, functional limitations, and the corresponding physical examination findings. Descriptions of symptoms associated with neuromusculoskeletal impairments (loss or abnormality of physiological, psychological, or anatomical structure or function) generally reveal a fairly consistent and predictable pattern of onset and change over a defined period of time. In addition, the neurological and musculoskeletal impairments noted during the physical examination should match with the functional limitations described by the patient or the caregiver. If these expectations are not met, it does not necessarily mean the patient has cancer or an infection, but doubt should be raised on the therapist's part whether therapy is indicated.

Patients many times are not aware that presenting signs and symptoms suggest a condition better addressed by a physician as opposed to a PT or an occupational therapist (OT). For example, a 67-year-old male patient had a cerebrovascular accident 6 months ago with resultant mild residual left hemiplegia. At the time of discharge from rehabilitation services, he was independent in all activities of daily living, but residual left upper extremity weakness remained. When visiting his internist for a routine checkup, he complained that over the prior 3 weeks he had lost some functional skills and was having difficulty with self-care. The physician then referred the patient to the therapy clinic for evaluation and treatment. The patient states he has been less active and just needs some help regaining his motor function. During the patient interview he states that he is experiencing a deep, dull, aching sensation in the lower lumbar spine and right buttock. He assumes it has developed as a result of his inactivity and thus saw no reason to bother the physician with this problem. As the patient continues to describe his difficulties, he also notes a constant deep ache in the right shoulder that he relates to increased use of his right arm to compensate for the left arm weakness. The physical examination of the low back, pelvis, and right shoulder reveals that the existing symptoms do not vary with active or passive range of motion, resisted testing, or postural holding. In addition, quantity of motion is normal for these regions and motor programming appears intact. At this point the therapist cannot explain the symptoms from an impairment standpoint; therefore depending on other examination findings, including the patient profile and medical history, communication with the internist may be warranted.

Symptom Pattern

Aspects of the patient's chief complaint other than symptom location are very relevant to the process of differential diagnosis, in particular a description of how and when the symptoms changed over a defined period of time. Complaints of pain, paresthesia, and numbness associated with primary musculoskeletal conditions typically change in a consistent manner over a 24-hour period. The patient will report that the symptom intensity increases with the assumption of specific postures such as left side lying or sitting or with specific activities such as walking, driving, or 2 hours of computer work. Conversely, patients typically can relate paresthesia or pain relief with avoiding certain postures or activities, the assumption of certain postures, wearing an arm sling, and so on. Night pain investigation also falls under this subcategory of patient data. Pain that wakes an individual from sleep and for which changing positions in bed does not provide relief is more concerning than if the pain is positionally related. If the pattern of symptom aggravation and alleviation is that there is no consistent pattern, such as pain that comes and goes independently of the patient's posture, activities, or time of day; night pain is the patient's most intense pain; or paresthesia or pain moves from one body region to another inconsistently with common pain referral patterns or identified medical conditions, then the therapist should consider if the patient is a candidate for physical or occupational therapy

In general, when symptoms such as weakness or numbness associated with primary neurological conditions are investigated, the 24-hour reference point to assess symptom change is not realistic. Except for an acute onset or exacerbation, these symptoms tend not to fluctuate that quickly with change in posture or position. Understanding the pathogenesis of primary neurological disorders will allow for detection of symptom change unusual for the patient. This will lead to follow-up questions to determine whether this change may represent a medically serious condition. Similarly, a change in the biomechanical alignment of a joint (e.g., the shoulder) may immediately alter the patient's pain response, indicating a direct relationship between musculoskeletal imbalance in joint stabilization and gravitational pull, for which therapy would be appropriate.

History of Symptoms

The therapist must also scrutinize the patient's report of the onset of the symptoms. Pain and paresthesia or numbness associated with neuromusculoskeletal impairments typically can be related to trauma, either on a macro or a micro level, or to a medical event such as a cerebrovascular accident. More often than not it is repetitive overuse or cumulative trauma that leads to tissue breakdown and inflammation. Patients with neurological impairments resulting in postural abnormalities and abnormal movement patterns are at risk for such conditions. If a patient's symptoms are truly insidious, meaning not related to macro or micro trauma, or there has not been a significant change in activity level that reasonably accounts for the complaints, the therapist should again be concerned about the source of the symptoms. A worsening of symptoms such as numbness, weakness, spasticity, or swelling associated with an existing medical condition should be investigated by the therapist with the same scrutiny. The therapist always needs to ask, "Is there a reasonable explanation for the worsening?" An increase in the intensity of the complaints or the involvement of additional body regions could signal a progression of the disease.

Review of Systems

By design, *review of systems* screening allows the therapist to detect symptoms secondary (and potentially unrelated) to the reason therapy has been initiated.[9] The review of systems allows for a general screening of body systems for symptoms suggesting the presence of an adverse drug reaction, occult disease, or worsening of an existing medical condition. Suspicions of any of these scenarios would warrant communication with a physician. A set of sample checklists of symptoms and signs for each body system that can be used by the PT during the patient interview can be found in Box 6.2. To keep the checklists manageable in length, the therapist should investigate presenting complaints and symptoms and the patient's medical history before the review of systems. For example, on review of the cardiovascular and peripheral vascular systems associated with heart conditions, important items appear to be omitted, such as chest pain, claudication, a history of heart problems, hypertension, high cholesterol levels, and circulatory problems. If symptoms have already been investigated by use of a body diagram, the therapist would already know whether the patient has chest pain. If symptom change (aggravation or alleviation) over a 24-hour period has already been investigated, the therapist would know whether claudication is an issue. Finally, if the patient's medical history has already been discussed, the therapist would know whether heart problems, hypertension, or circulatory problems existed.[10]

All of the checklists in Box 6.2 need not be used for every patient. The location of symptoms will direct the therapist in deciding which checklists should be included in the initial examination. Fig. 6.6 and Table 6.1 can be used to link pain location with visceral systems that could be the source of the complaints. Table 6.2 provides a summary of potential pain locations and diseases of the pulmonary, cardiovascular, gastrointestinal, and urogenital systems. Other symptom characteristics can also alert the therapist to the possible involvement of the endocrine, nervous, and psychological systems. Symptoms, including pain and paresthesias that come and go irrespective of posture, activity, or time of day and that appear to move among the various body regions, can be associated with these systems as well as the visceral systems. In addition to the identification of the location and characteristics of symptoms, a patient's medical history will also help the therapist decide which systems to screen. A positive medical history, such as a heart problem, would direct the therapist to investigate the patient's condition, including possible use of the cardiovascular and peripheral vascular checklist as well as the questions listed in Box 6.2. The therapist also needs to be aware of the medications taken by the patient to medically manage these pathological conditions. Similarly, therapists need to be able to analyze how the drugs potentially affect functional movements and functional loss. Often, that means a therapist must have a working professional relationship with a clinical pharmacist. Use of a general health checklist (see Box 6.2) can assist the therapist in prioritizing the inclusion of the checklists in the systems review checklists box during the initial visit. The symptoms noted in this checklist can be associated with disease of most of the body's systems, as well as with systemic disease and adverse drug events.

If the patient or caregiver (on the patient's behalf) replies "yes" to any *review of systems* question, the therapist must determine whether there is a reasonable explanation for the complaint, whether the physician is aware of the complaint, and, if so, whether the complaint has worsened since the patient last saw the physician. When the given explanation is not satisfactory, the physician is unaware of the

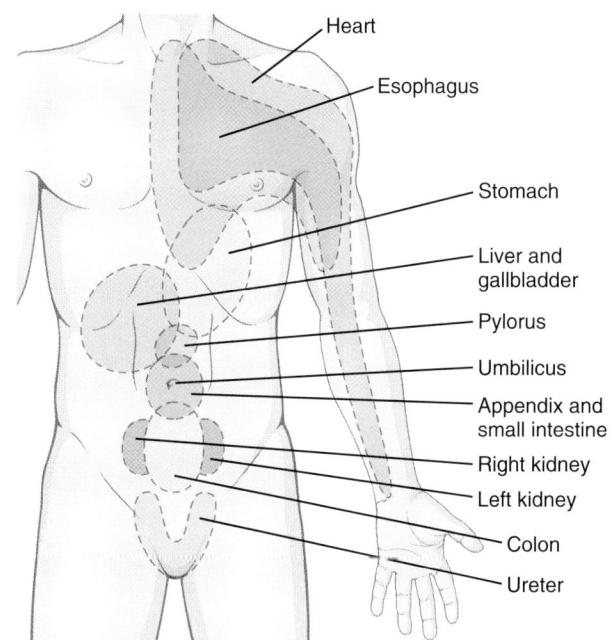

Fig. 6.6 Areas of Referred Pain From Different Visceral Organs. (From Hall J. *Guyton and Hall Textbook of Medical Physiology.* Elsevier; Philadelphia 2016.)

TABLE 6.1   Visceral Pain Patterns

Structure	Segmental Innervation	Possible Areas of Pain Referral
Pelvic Organs		
Uterus including uterine ligaments	T10–L1, S2–S4	Lumbosacral junction Sacral Thoracolumbar
Ovaries	T10–T11	Lower abdominal Sacral
Testes	T10–T11	Lower abdominal Sacral
Retroperitoneal Region		
Kidney	T10–L1	Lumbar spine (ipsilateral) Lower abdominal Upper abdominal
Ureter	T11–L2, S2–S4	Groin Upper abdominal Suprapubic Medial, proximal thigh Thoracolumbar
Urinary bladder	T11–L2, S2–S4	Sacral apex Suprapubic Thoracolumbar
Prostate gland	T11–L1, S2–S4	Sacral Testes Thoracolumbar
Digestive System Organs		
Esophagus	T6–T10	Substernal and upper abdominal
Stomach	T6–T10	Upper abdominal Middle and lower thoracic spine
Small intestine	T7–T10	Middle thoracic spine
Pancreas	T6–T10	Upper abdominal Lower thoracic spine Upper lumbar spine
Gallbladder	T7–T9	Right upper abdominal Right middle and lower thoracic spine, including caudal aspect scapula
Liver	T7–T9	Right middle and lower thoracic spine
Common bile duct	T6–T10	Upper abdominal Middle thoracic spine
Large intestine	T11–T12	Lower abdominal Middle lumbar spine
Sigmoid colon	T11–T12	Upper sacral Suprapubic Left lower quadrant of abdomen
Cardiopulmonary System		
Heart	T1–T5	Cervical anterior Upper thorax Left upper extremity
Lungs and bronchi	T5–T6	Ipsilateral thoracic spine Cervical (diaphragm involved)
Diaphragm (central portion)	C3–C5	Cervical spine

Modified from Boissonnault WG, Bass C. Pathological origins of trunk and neck pain, I. Pelvic and abdominal visceral disorders. *J Orthop Sports Phys Ther.* 1990;12:192–207, with permission of the Orthopaedic and Sports Sections of the American Physical Therapy Association.

TABLE 6.2   Linking Pain Patterns and Visceral Systems

Pain Location	Visceral Systems
Right shoulder (including shoulder girdle)	Pulmonary Cardiovascular Gastrointestinal
Left shoulder (including shoulder girdle)	Cardiovascular Pulmonary
Upper thoracic or midthoracic spine	Cardiovascular Pulmonary Gastrointestinal
Lower thoracic and upper lumbar or midlumbar spine	Peripheral vascular Pulmonary Gastrointestinal Urogenital
Lumbopelvic region	Gastrointestinal Urogenital Peripheral vascular

complaint, or the symptom is worsening, communication with the physician is warranted. Similarly, most physicians look at direct causation: complaint to disease. Therapists need to look at system causation because we see the end result of the combinations of the problems: disease, maturation, environmental factors, and other nondisease causations. All the checklists do not need to be covered during the initial visit. If the patient says "no" for each of the general health items, the patient's health history is uneventful, and the therapist is comfortable with the description of the chief complaints (including pattern and onset), then the therapist can proceed with the evaluation of specific impairments and functional limitations with some confidence that therapy interventions are very likely appropriate. The review of systems then takes a lower priority. The result is that the therapist could decide to delay the use of the appropriate systems review checklists until the patient's second or third visit. If the patient answers "yes" to general health items and has an inconsistent pain pattern, the appropriate review of systems then takes a higher priority and should be covered during the initial visit.

Musculoskeletal System

Box 6.3 provides the checklist for the musculoskeletal system. The general health checklist also provides a level of screening for conditions of the musculoskeletal system, as with all other body systems. Infections, metastatic cancers, and rheumatic disorders (e.g., rheumatoid arthritis) are problems associated with this system. Identifying patient risk factors for these conditions is a key for recognizing when to be suspicious. For example, those at highest risk for musculoskeletal

BOX 6.3   Musculoskeletal System Screening

Insidious onset of symptoms
Atypical pain pattern (aggravating or alleviating factors)
Night pain (progressive and/or nonpositional)
Early morning stiffness lasting longer than 30 to 60 min
Inadequate relief of symptoms with rest or rehabilitation
Inability to alter symptoms during the physical examination
Lack of impairments that match patient's functional limitations
Atypical physical examination findings (e.g., masses, unexplained atrophy, or weakness)

cancers are those (1) over the age of 50 years and under 20 years, (2) having a previous history of cancer (e.g., breast, lung, prostate, thyroid, and kidney—the most common cancers to metastasize to the axial skeleton), (3) having a positive family history of cancer, and (4) having had exposure to environmental toxins. Those individuals at highest risk for musculoskeletal infections report or demonstrate (1) current or recent infection (e.g., urinary tract, tooth abscess, skin infection), (2) history of diabetes with use of large doses of steroids or immunosuppressive drugs, (3) elderly age, and (4) spinal cord injury (SCI) with complete motor and sensory loss.[11] Last, the primary risk factors for rheumatoid arthritis include (1) female sex, (2) age (peak) 30 to 40 years, and (3) positive family history.[12]

The other category of musculoskeletal conditions for which therapists need to be vigilant is fractures. The pain and deformity associated with most sudden-impact, traumatic fractures make for an obvious presentation. However, trauma sufficient to cause a fracture may not be so obvious in a patient with decreased bone density. Lifting a gallon of milk, experiencing a mild slip or bump, or trying to open a window that is stuck may be sufficient to cause a fracture in a patient with a history of chronic renal failure, multiple sclerosis, rheumatoid arthritis, hyperparathyroidism, gastrointestinal malabsorption syndrome, and long-term corticosteroid, heparin, anticonvulsant, and cytotoxic medication use. The most common locations for such fractures include vertebral bodies, the neck of the femur, and the radius. Observation of posture and body position may provide a clue that something may have changed structurally. For example, with vertebral compression fractures the thoracic kyphotic curve may be accentuated, accompanied by a very pronounced apex of the curve that was not present before. With femoral neck fracture the lower extremity is often positioned in external rotation and appears shortened compared with its counterpart.[13]

Causing potential confusion for the clinician are diseases (especially in the early stages) of the musculoskeletal system, which may mimic mechanical musculoskeletal conditions. The patient may report a specific event or time of onset of symptoms, and a pain pattern of increasing pain with weight bearing on the involved extremity over time and lessening relief of pain with assumption of non-weight-bearing positions—all typical findings with impairment-driven symptoms. The therapist may also be able to provoke symptoms during the physical examination as the involved bony area is mechanically loaded. When the history and physical examination findings are evaluated, an unusual finding or pattern will emerge, or the patient will not respond to treatment as expected, making the therapist step back and consider alternative hypotheses regarding the origin of patient symptoms, especially if the risk factors listed earlier are present.

Integumentary System

Screening of the integumentary system is not typically based on the presence or absence of pain, paresthesia, or numbness. As with the nervous system, some degree of screening of the integumentary system occurs with every patient regardless of the presenting diagnosis. Skin cancer has the highest incidence of all the cancers,[14] and therapists generally see a number of exposed body areas during the postural

---

BOX 6.4 Skin Lesion Screening—Pathological Characteristics

Multivariant color
Black or blue-black color
Irregular borders
Nondistinct ("fuzzy") borders
Size: 6 mm or larger in diameter
Asymmetrical shape
Friable tissue
Ulcerations
Evolving (changing size, shape, color)

---

assessment and regional examination that make up the physical examination. In fact, as noted in Fig. 6.4, screening the skin begins during the patient interview. During the interview the therapist can be looking at areas of exposed skin such as the face, neck, arms, and feet. As with screening of the other body systems, the therapist's goal is not to identify a melanoma or differentiate squamous cell and basal cell carcinoma but simply to identify skin lesions with atypical presentations. Once the patient has been referred to the physician, disease will be ruled out or diagnosed. Box 6.4 can be used to assess any mole or other skin marking. The items noted are atypical for a benign lesion, more suggestive of a pathological condition.[15] Selected items from Box 6.4 have been highlighted, resulting in an acronym—A (asymmetry), B (borders), C (color), D (diameter), and E (evolving)—that has been used to educate the public for self-screening.[16] If the therapist notes any of these findings and the patient reports a recent change in the size, color, or shape of the lesion, and that a physician has not looked at the lesion, a referral would be warranted.

Besides skin lesions, abnormal general skin color can be a manifestation of a number of conditions. Table 6.3 summarizes abnormal skin color changes. Occasionally, some of the most obvious abnormalities are the most difficult to note when one is so focused on items more directly related to therapeutic intervention.

Nervous System

As with the integumentary system, the nervous system is screened to a degree for all patients. The systems review provides a very gross, general screening of the nervous system. The therapist should be vigilant for the presence of any of these items in all patients during the initial and subsequent visits. For patients with preexisting findings from this checklist, the therapist must be vigilant for a worsening of the observed abnormalities. Covering the items in the nervous system checklist should add little time to the therapist's initial examination. Assessing for facial asymmetries and tremors can take place during the interview. Observation of balance, movement patterns, and muscle atrophy can occur while watching the patient ambulate into the examination area, during the interview, and as the patient changes positions during the physical examination. Last, impaired mentation may become apparent during the interview or the physical examination as the patient struggles to appropriately answer questions or follow directions. Case Studies 6.1 and 6.2 illustrate the importance of this general screening.

CASE STUDY 6.1

A 55-year-old elementary school teacher was referred with a diagnosis of C5 to C6 and C6 to C7 degenerative disk disease. Her chief complaint was pain in the posterior cervical region and reports of neck weakness. Functionally, the patient's primary concern was her increasingly difficult time making it through her workday. She taught first-grade students, so much of her workday was spent with her neck and trunk in a forward flexed position. The patient believed that this persistent flexion posturing was a significant factor for the worsening of her symptoms as her workday progressed. As the patient interview continued, the physical therapist observed tremor of the patient's right hand and forearm. When questioned about the observed tremor, the patient stated it started about 4 months ago. When further questioned, she admitted the tremor appeared to be getting worse, but since it did not interfere with her

Continued

CASE STUDY 6.1—cont'd

activities, she did not mention it to her physician. No other significant neurological findings were noted. After the initial examination was completed, the therapist collaborated with the patient to develop goals and a plan of care related to the complaints of neck pain and weakness. The therapist also discussed his concern about the tremor and requested permission from the patient to call the patient's primary care physician (who is also the referring physician) so he can communicate his finding of resting tremor. The physician facilitated a referral of the patient to a neurologist who diagnosed the patient with Parkinson disease. In this example, differential diagnosis revealed the presence of a new symptom (tremor of the right hand) that was not consistent with the medical diagnosis of degenerative disk disease. This symptom triggered the decision by the therapist to continue with physical therapy management and refer the patient back to the physician for that specific clinical sign, which led to the additional diagnosis of Parkinson disease. The patient was medically managed with medications for Parkinson disease, and she was also referred to physical therapy for further examination and management of impairments, activity limitations, and participation restrictions related to Parkinson disease.

CASE STUDY 6.2   Written by Brian Moore, PT, DPT, NCS

The patient was a 57-year-old Hispanic male who was referred to physical therapy for an episode of low back pain that occurred two weeks ago. He worked as an auto body technician but had not returned to work at the time of initial evaluation. Past medical history included recurrent episodes of low back pain and controlled hypertension and hypercholesterolemia. During the initial interview the patient reported two falls that occurred in the last 3 months due to tripping, once while walking across a parking lot and the other during a walk with his wife. He reported weakness in the right lower extremity and muscle twitching in the right lower extremity.

Pertinent physical therapy examination findings included the following:
Normal strength and range of motion in the upper extremities
Pain on palpation in the paraspinal muscles
Deep tendon reflexes were present and symmetrical except for the Achilles tendon reflexes, which were exaggerated and symmetrical

The therapist concluded that the clinical findings were consistent for a symptom modulation rehabilitation approach to address recurrent back pain with the patient presenting with a directional preference into extension. Following 8 weeks of treatment to improve movement control and optimize function, the patient's report of low back pain had resolved. However, the patient reported worsening weakness in the right leg, with weakness in the left lower extremity in addition to symptom complaints of cramps and stiffness in bilateral lower extremities. Due to the worsening in functional status, the patient was referred back to the patient's primary care physician. The patient was then referred to a neurologist due to the clear neurological signs of bilateral lower extremity weakness.

The patient presented to the neurologist 2 months following the end of the episode of care with the physical therapist. He was no longer able to rise from a chair to stand without assistance and required assistance from his wife to maintain his balance while walking. The patient was diagnosed with amyotrophic lateral sclerosis (ALS), given the presence of upper motor neuron (UMN) and lower motor neuron (LMN) signs found on physical examination and electrodiagnostic testing. Results of the neurological examination, laboratory, and imaging findings were important to exclude other motor neuron disorders that mimic the presentation of ALS, including progressive demyelinating disorders of the peripheral nervous system (chronic inflammatory demyelinating polyneuropathy) and central nervous system (multiple sclerosis) in addition to paraneoplastic syndrome, cervical myelopathy, Lyme disease, human immunodeficiency virus, and syringomyelia. Individuals with neuromuscular disorders may go years living with a progressive disorder in a pre-symptomatic phase prior to symptoms emerging such as tripping while walking or slurring of speech (i.e., dysarthria). Following the emergence of initial symptoms there is a worsening of the presentation that may manifest as weakness in the lower extremities or slurred speech. Such symptoms progress over the course of months to years. Depending on the speed of the progression and presence of clear neurological signs, individuals may go 4 to 16 months before referral to a neurologist.[17] In this case the physical therapist decided to continue treatment then referred the patient to a physician because of worsening symptoms that do not seem to be consistent with the initial diagnosis of low back pain.

TABLE 6.3   Abnormal Color Changes of the Skin

Color Change	Physiological Change	Common Causes
White, pale (pallor)	Absence of pigment or pigment changes Blood abnormality Temporary interruption or diversion of blood flow Internal disease	Albinism, lack of sunlight Anemia, lead poisoning Vasospasm, syncope, stress, internal bleeding Chronic gastrointestinal disease, cancer, parasitic disease, tuberculosis
Blue (cyanosis)	Decreased oxygen in blood (deoxyhemoglobin)	Methemoglobinemia (oxidation of hemoglobin), high blood iron level, cold exposure, vasomotor instability, cerebrospinal disease
Yellow	Jaundice, excess bilirubin in blood, excess bile High levels of carotene in blood (carotenemia)	Liver disease, gallstone blockage of bile duct, hepatitis pigment (conjunctivae are also yellow) Ingestion of food high in carotene and vitamin A
Gray	High level of metals in body	Increased iron, bronze-gray; increased silver, blue-gray
Brown (hyperpigmentation)	Disturbances of adrenocortical hormones	Adrenal pituitary Addison disease

From Shapiro C, Skopit S. Screening for skin disorders. In: Boissonnault WG, ed. *Examination in Physical Therapy Practice—Screening for Medical Disease.* 2nd ed. New York: Churchill Livingstone; 1995.

BOX 6.5 Depression Screen

Depressed or irritable mood
Psychomotor agitation or retardation
Apathy
Sleep disturbance
Weight gain or loss
Fatigue
Feelings of worthlessness
Impaired concentration
Suicidal ideation (recurrent)
Recent loss of family member

Depression. Depression is a commonly encountered mental health disorder.[7,18-20] The systems review checklists in Box 6.5 contain items the therapist can use to help make the decision to refer a patient for consultation. For the first eight items on the depression checklist, concern should be raised when the therapist detects four or five of the items present daily for a minimum of 2 weeks and resulting in the patient having difficulty functioning at home, work, or school, socially, or in rehabilitation. Of the four or five items, one of them should be depressed or irritable affect or apathy. An exception to the 2-week time frame is during periods of bereavement. When people are faced with a significant loss, it is not uncommon for them to experience a number of the checklist items as they work through the grieving process.[7] It is reasonable for these people to experience these symptoms for up to 2 months. A neurological event such as a cerebrovascular accident could easily trigger a major clinical depressive disorder, and the depression could significantly impede rehabilitation progress. The therapist may be in a position to facilitate a psychological consultation.

Clinicians must screen the general adult population for depression. The two-item (PHQ-2) and nine-item Patient Health Questionnaires (PHQ-9) are validated tools for depression screening. According to recommendations by the US Preventive Services Task Force (USPSTF) and American Academy of Family Physicians, the PHQ-9 or a clinical interview must be performed if PHQ-2 was found to be positive for depression.[21]

Suicide. Considering that approximately 15% of people with true major clinical depression commit suicide,[7] therapists need to be vigilant for warning signs that the patient may be considering this action. See the suicide screening shown in Box 6.6 for a list of warning signs. Once the patient acknowledges suicidal ideation, follow-up questions would be appropriate to investigate the patient's plan and how readily available the resources are regarding the reported method of attempt. This is all-important information to be reported when the therapist contacts the physician. Therapists should be very familiar with their facility's "suicide protocol or procedure" in terms of what information should be collected from the patient and who should be contacted.

BOX 6.6 Suicide Warning Signs

History of major clinical depression, chemical dependency, schizophrenia, or previous suicide attempt
Expressions of hopelessness
The sense that the patient is "giving up"
An abrupt improvement in patient mood

PHYSICAL EXAMINATION

In addition to this discussion of observation screening for the integumentary and nervous systems, other screening principles are associated with the physical examination. The therapist should have expectations of physical examination findings based on the existing medical diagnosis and data from the history. There should be a correlation between the described activity limitations and the noted impairments. A patient's complaint of right shoulder pain would be expected to increase or decrease in intensity with palpation, movement assessment, or special tests. The inability to alter a patient's complaints and the lack of neuromusculoskeletal impairments one would expect with a particular medical diagnosis should raise concern about the source of the symptoms.

The *Guide to Physical Therapy Practice* describes the systems review, in part, as a brief or limited examination of the anatomical and physiological status of the cardiovascular and pulmonary, integumentary, musculoskeletal, and neuromuscular systems, as well as the assessment of communication, learning, and affect. For the purposes of this chapter the discussion will focus on assessment of height and weight and assessing heart rate and blood pressure. Being overweight or obese can significantly increase the risk of development of a number of serious conditions. Using patient height and weight to calculate body mass index (BMI) can be a valuable measure to identify patients who may need a dietary consultation to prevent disease states or minimize morbidity associated with current illnesses.

Resting blood pressure and pulse rate and rhythm are also important values to be routinely measured. A 30-second monitoring period after a 2- to 5-minute rest period is recommended to obtain baseline rate values.[22] Resting blood pressure values can also provide important screening information. As with assessing pulse rate, resting blood pressure should be assessed after a 5-minute rest period. Variations from the normative values may lead therapists to additional assessment of the vascular system and the central autonomic nervous system and then to a patient referral.

Examination Summary

For many patients a single red flag finding does not warrant a referral, but a cluster of history and physical examination findings does increase disease probability to the point where a referral is indicated. Two examples that are germane to a number of individuals with neurological conditions are deep vein thrombosis (DVT) and pulmonary embolus (PE). DVT affects approximately 2 million individuals in the United States annually, making it the third most common cardiovascular disease.[12,23] Approximately 50% of those with a DVT are asymptomatic in early stages. Clinicians are challenged to identify patients at greater risk for this condition who do not have the obvious signs and symptoms of calf pain, swelling, and redness. The revised Wells Clinical Decision Rule (CRD) determines whether the patient is "likely" or "not likely" have DVT, and is recommended in outpatient settings (Table 6.4). It should be noted that there is an increased risk of DVT in the population of patients with SCI because of hypercoagulability, changes in the epithelial structure of the blood vessels, and decreased blood circulation.[24]

Similarly for PE, a clinical decision rule exists for screening (Table 6.5). PE is associated with high morbidity and mortality, highlighting the critical nature of timely detection. Hull describes PE as one of the "great masqueraders" of medicine because of the often nonspecific presenting symptoms and signs.[25] Wells and colleagues estimate that 50% of PEs go undiagnosed.[26]

Clinician concern regarding the possibility of a DVT and/or a PE being present would warrant urgent communication with the patient's physician.

TABLE 6.4 Revised Wells Clinical Decision Rule for Deep Vein Thrombosis

Clinical Presentation	Score
Previously diagnosed DVT	1
Active cancer (within 6 months of diagnosis or receiving palliative care)	1
Paralysis, paresis, or recent immobilization of lower extremity	1
Bedridden for >3 days or major surgery within the previous 12 weeks	1
Localized tenderness in the center of the posterior calf, the popliteal space, or along the femoral vein in the anterior thigh/groin	1
Entire lower extremity swelling	1
Unilateral calf swelling (>3 cm larger than uninvolved side)	1
Unilateral pitting edema	1
Collateral superficial veins (nonvaricose)	1
An alternative diagnosis is as likely (or more likely) than DVT (e.g., cellulitis, postoperative swelling, calf strain)	−2
Total points	

Key: ≥2: DVT likely; <2: DVT unlikely.
Medical consultation is advised in the presence of low probability and medical consultation is required with moderate or high score

DVT, Deep vein thrombosis.
From Le Gal G, Carrier M, Rodger M. Clinical decision rules in venous thromboembolism. *Best Pract Res Clin Haematol.* 2012;25:303–317.

TABLE 6.5 Simplified Wells Criteria for the Clinical Assessment of Pulmonary Embolism

Clinical Presentation	Score
Clinical symptoms of DVT (leg swelling, pain with palpation)	1.0
Other diagnosis less likely than pulmonary embolism	1.0
Heart rate >100 bpm	1.0
Immobilization for 3 or more days or surgery in the past 4 weeks	1.0
Previous history of DVT/PE	1.0
Hemoptysis	1.0
Malignancy	1.0
Screening clinical probability assessment	
PE likely; medical consult advised	Total score: 2 or more
PE unlikely; review all other factors then document findings	Total score: 0 or 1

DVT, Deep vein thrombosis; *PE*, pulmonary embolism
Data from Douma RA. Validity and clinical utility of the simplified Wells' rule for assessing clinical probability for the exclusion of pulmonary embolism. *Throm Haemost.* 2009;101(1):197–200 and Gibson NS. Further validation and simplification of the Wells' clinical decision rule in pulmonary embolism. *Thromb Haemost.* 2008;99:229–234.

RESPONSE TO TREATMENT

Frequently the therapist will decide referral of the patient to a physician is not warranted and will proceed to determine whether physical therapy is warranted or no intervention recommended. As treatment is initiated and progresses, the therapist must remain vigilant for the appearance of symptoms and signs discussed throughout this chapter. In addition, correlating subjective and objective changes as treatment progresses will help the therapist decide whether further intervention is warranted or whether referral back to the physician or other health care practitioner is appropriate. For example, if a patient reports a significant improvement or worsening, one would expect the therapist to note a corresponding change in posture, movement ability, palpatory findings, or neurological status. If the expected correlation between patient report and physical examination findings is not found, the therapist should begin considering that therapy may not be warranted. A careful review of systems and symptom investigation is necessary.

CONCLUSION

If all diseases manifested with a high fever, coughing up blood, and blood in the urine, the medical screening process would be a simple one. Unfortunately, many diseases initially manifest with subtle complaints, intermittent symptoms or mild pain, stiffness, subtle weakness or paresthesias, or acute dementia. If these complaints are brought to a physician's attention by the patient, they often are not severe enough to warrant extensive diagnostic testing. Many patients or family members simply ignore symptoms or physiological changes, rationalizing that everything is okay, the family member is just old, or he or she simply does not like to see physicians or is too busy. All of the scenarios can account for patients with occult disease seeing therapists. The fact that PTs and OTs tend to spend a moderate amount of time with patients over a period of weeks or months can facilitate the detection of subtle manifestations. In addition, as therapists develop rapport with patients and family members, information may be shared that they were uncomfortable disclosing initially. Always remember that acute dementia is never normal and is reflective of an acute problem rather than simply of aging.

The responsibilities of the PT and OT related to screening for symptoms and signs that indicate the involvement of another health care practitioner are clearly stated in the *Guide to Physical Therapy Practice.* The process associated with differential diagnosis allows for the appropriate medical screening yet keeps therapists within their scope of practice. The therapist simply communicates to the physician the list of clinical findings. The physician will determine whether new or additional medical tests are needed to rule out or diagnose specific diseases. Facilitating the timely referral of patients to physicians is an important role for therapists working within a collaborative medical model. It is this model that best serves the needs of our patients. For additional information related to the medical screening process, the readers are directed to the *Goodman's Differential Diagnosis* 6th edition textbook (Elsevier) and several other texts available in the market.

With changes in health care delivery and physicians also being asked to see more patients in less time, it is critical that all health care practitioners include an adequate medical screening component to their examinations. If quality-of-life issues are truly an important component of health care delivery, then medical screening will continue to be a professional expectation and responsibility placed on each PT and OT. Because consumers are accessing therapeutic services through more direct means, that responsibility will remain and grow in importance as part of both professions' education and practice. Over the next few years the roles of PTs and OTs will continue to evolve in the arena of primary care. Medical screening performed by the therapist will guide patients to a physician and could become a key component of maintaining the health and quality of life of that consumer.

In the future another choice will have to be considered as part of the role of a movement specialist. The results of differential diagnosis assessments may determine that neither a medical referral nor therapeutic intervention itself is appropriate. In this situation, the patient might benefit from community activities but would not need a movement specialist, especially if the physician also has determined that medical intervention is not necessary.

ACKNOWLEDGMENT

The chapter authors would like to thank Dr. William Boissannault and Dr. Darcy Umphred for their excellent work in developing this chapter in the fifth and sixth editions of the text. Their work was particularly important at that time, when physical therapists were defining their roles related to diagnosis by a physical therapist, differential diagnosis and screening for possible medical conditions.

REFERENCES

To enhance this text and add value for the reader, all references are included on the companion Evolve site that accompanies this textbook. This online service will, when available, provide a link for the reader to a Medline abstract for the article cited. There are 26 cited references and other general references for this chapter, with the majority of those articles being evidence-based citations.

7

Examination and Evaluation of Functional Movement Activities, Body Functions and Structures, and Participation*

Deborah S. Diaz

OBJECTIVES

After reading this chapter the student or therapist will be able to:
1. Differentiate the medical diagnosis made by the physician from the diagnosis made by a movement specialist.
2. Identify the differences among activity limitations, participation restrictions, and impairments in specific body structure and function.
3. Choose appropriate examination tool(s) from each category of the International Classification of Functioning, Disability and Health model.
4. Identify resources used to analyze the usefulness and psychometric properties of outcome measures
5. Evaluate the results of the examination to establish a physical therapy diagnosis that drives intervention planning.

KEY TERMS

activity limitations
evaluation
examination

impairments
participation restrictions

INTRODUCTION

People who experience neurological disease or dysfunction are often cared for by therapists (physical therapists [PTs] and occupational therapists [OTs]) who are experts in the assessment of and treatment of movement disorders. Movement therapists' (PT and OT) role in working with patients with neurological dysfunction is to address the impact of the condition on the patient's functional status and ability to engage in society. The neurological examination is a process used by therapists to determine the implications of a neurological condition on patients' ability to perform important functional activities. The results gleaned from a neurological examination inform therapists about the movement diagnosis, prognosis, long-term and short-term goals, and plan of care. The neurological exam is performed in part or whole throughout the episode of care to document patient progress and stimulate changes in the plan of care.

Whether the neurological condition is recent/acute or long-standing/chronic, movement therapists must first screen their patients on two levels. First, a medical screening exam is important to answer the question, "is my patient sufficiently medically stable that it is safe to proceed with the examination?" If the therapist notes "red flags," meaning the patient's medical condition is unstable and requires immediate and, in some cases, emergent care, treatment from a physician or other health care provider is warranted. When the patient is deemed medically stable, movement therapists must determine appropriateness for therapy and ask, "Am I the appropriate professional to address this patient's limitations in light of his/her goals and preferences?" If the answer to this question is "no," the movement therapists must refer the patient to the appropriate professional for the most suitable care.[1]

When the patient is deemed both medically stable and appropriate for therapy, the neurological examination commences. Ideally, the neurological examination begins with a review of the medical record, which can inform the therapist about the following: (1) onset and cause of the condition, (2) comorbid conditions, (3) social context (meaning family and work responsibilities), (4) home environment, (5) avocations, and (6) patient age. This information should help the therapist to formulate questions for the subsequent patient interview and plan the objective evaluation.

A framework for clinical decision making regarding comprehensive examination in the movement therapies is the International Classification of Function developed by the World Health Organization (see Chapter 1). There are numerous tools available to measure the impact of neurological conditions at each of the levels of the International Classification of Functioning, Disability and Health (ICF), Body Function and Structure Impairments, Activity Limitations and Participation Restrictions. All tests and measures of each of these levels must be rigorously tested for their psychometric or clinometric properties (validity, reliability, sensitivity, specificity, etc.). Throughout the neurological examination, movement therapists should frame the data they plan to gather and the results they find into the levels of the ICF.

Therapists can use several tools to assess patient status after neurological damage. Multiple body function and structure impairments may contribute to an impaired ability to perform functional activities. Therapists select measurement tools that address specific sensory, motor, or cognitive systems which contribute to activity performance.

Activity measures specifically assess patient functional performance of activities of daily living objectively. These tools typically rate

---

*Videos for this chapter are available at studentconsult.com.

performance on an ordinal or interval scale, which provides the opportunity to measure progress or decline. Although the change in score on a performance measure is objective and reflects decline or improvement in function, it is not possible, simply from the score, to know the cause of this change. The clinician must hypothesize the most likely cause at the body function and structure level and specifically examine the impairment to confirm or deny the hypothesis. In many cases a combination of body function and structure impairments contribute to scores on activity performance measures.

A third category of assessment addresses participation outcome measures (OMs) that are designed to assess a client's involvement or restriction in domestic, community, social, and civic life situations. Most often these measures address the client's perspectives regarding the impact of the neurological condition upon quality of life, interpersonal interactions, and quality of involvement in domestic, community, social, and civic life situations.

To evaluate the results of the neurological examination at the body function and structure, activity and participation levels must be synthesized by the therapist to proceed to the meaningful next steps. Therapists must critically evaluate the results to establish the client's diagnosis, prognosis, and plan of care while considering the individuals' goals and preferences.[2] In addition, the neurological examination is an ongoing, repetitive process throughout the episode of care. The therapist must constantly assess the patients' health status to identify evidence of recovery or decline. As the patient recovers the ability to perform more complex movement activities, therapists must consider further assessment at the body function and structure level, as well as the activity level. It may be that changes at the body function and structure level contribute to improved function and interventions should change to reflect this improvement.

In addition, improvement in activities may require a different measurement tool because the patient's recovery goes beyond the capability of the measure to document change. In other words, the assessment tool may have a ceiling effect to which the patient outperforms. In all cases, the rigor and intensity of therapy interventions must morph to require continual and significant effort on the patient's part.

History and Systems Review

The first encounter with a patient begins with a history of the present illness in which the patient reports the experience surrounding the onset and sequelae of the condition. During the interview, the therapist gathers information including the patient's perspective on the onset and course of the current condition, comorbid conditions, social context, meaning family and occupation responsibilities, home environment, avocations, and age. The therapist attends to information that is different from or in addition to the medical record. It is imperative that the therapist fully understands as a result of this subjective assessment, the patient's primary concerns, goals, and priorities for this episode of care.[2-4]

During the interview, while the therapist listens attentively, she or he also observes how the patient moves and interacts. Important physical details to note include, eye contact, facial symmetry, posture, and movement of the extremities and trunk. In addition, to screen for impairments in cognition, speech production, perception, and aphasia, the therapist should attend to the patient's clarity and coherence of speech and whether the patient attends to all parts of the environment.

Upon concluding the history and review of systems, the therapist notes the important objective tests and measures to gather next. The therapist should, based on the patient's stated goals and priorities, identify both functional activities to assess and the body function and structure impairments that likely contribute to movement dysfunction. The therapist should have a plan for completing this part of the neurological examination in the most efficient yet thorough manner.

Tests and Measures

Ideally, this phase of the examination begins with the observation of functional activity that reflects the patient's stated goals. During movement analysis of these functional activities, the therapist notes the qualities of movement that vary from neurotypical movement without neurological pathology. Although visual observation is important, it is vital that the examiner use assessment tools that are objectified and quantifiable to track change over time. Please refer to the section on "Choosing the best appropriate examination tool," found later in this chapter, for several lists of relevant tests and measures used in physical therapy practices.

TESTS OF ACTIVITY AND FUNCTIONAL PERFORMANCE

Measures at the activity level quantify patient functional status ranging from balance skills to walking ability and other tasks important to everyday function. Tests of skills at the activity level may range from a single item that documents a narrow set of skills to multidimensional tests used to discern the elements of an activity that are most problematic and require skilled therapeutic interventions. Those activity measures that include a single or small set of skills may be used to assess client ability generally. These tests are quick and easy to perform and can screen out those who do not require in-depth study and screen in those with more significant involvement. At the other end of the Activity assessment spectrum are multiple item tests. These multiple item tests are more time consuming but test more skills that might be overlooked when using shorter assessments. One way to consider these is that a short tool can screen for general problems, whereas the multiple-item tests provide information in more detail and can be used as a follow-up to the short, single-item tests. For example, the Timed Up and Go (TUG) test is an excellent measure that predicts risk for falls in many populations. People who score below a "cutscore" on the TUG test are at higher risk for falling. But which dimension(s) of balance should a therapist devote time and attention to minimize the fall risk? One might consider follow-up testing using a multidimensional balance assessment like the Berg Balance Scale, the Fullerton Advanced Balance Scale, or the Mini-Best Test. From these multi-item tests, a clinician can deduce which elements of balance that the client needs to work on the most.

Outcome scales for functional tests may be found in ordinal format (e.g., Functional Independence Measure [FIM], Barthel Index, Katz Index of Independence in Activities of Daily Living). Each has its unique point value and range, varying from a two- to three-point scale (e.g., Tinetti Performance-Oriented Mobility Assessment [POMA]) to a seven-point scale (e.g., FIM). A few tools supply ratio scale data (e.g., the TUG test, Functional Reach Test, and measures of gait velocity). Test data presented in ratio scale format will more clearly show incremental changes, thereby facilitating the comparison of pretherapy to posttherapy performance.

TESTS OF BODY FUNCTIONS AND STRUCTURES

After identifying problems with the performance of functional activities, the clinician then focuses on body functions and structures that likely contribute to difficulty in daily activities. Consistent with the ICF model, the intent is to identify which body systems or subsystems are intact and functioning normally and those systems that could be optimized as the patient works to maximize functional tasks and participate in life. Identifying which body systems and subsystems that are not normal may lead the clinician to surmise the likely cause of the functional loss.

Impairment is defined as the loss or abnormality of physiological, psychological, or anatomical structure or function at the organ system level.[5] The clinician must distinguish between primary impairments and secondary impairments. Primary impairments are a direct consequence of the client's specific disease or pathological condition. Secondary impairments are changes in the structure and function of body systems that could have many causes. Secondary impairments may result from unaddressed primary impairments after the onset of the neurological condition, modified movement patterns after onset resulting in stress or compromise to a body structure or function, normal aging, disuse, repetitive strain, lifestyle, and many more. Secondary impairments may be premorbid. In this case an impairment that did not interfere with activities and skills prior to onset may now interfere with moving adaptively after onset. For instance, someone with a C6 spinal cord injury must have full elbow extension and significant shoulder external rotation to passively lock the elbows for transfers and prop sitting. Prior to the injury, a slight elbow flexion contracture may go undetected, but afterward, the consequences are dire, prohibiting the individual from transferring independently.

Moreover, the clinician must remember that, although functional limitations are usually caused by a combination of specific impairments, it is possible that impairments may not contribute to specific functional problems for some clients. If this is the case, the clinician should decide whether these impairments, if left uncorrected, will result in the development of activity limitations or other complications later. Simultaneously, the patient must be a part of this discussion to prioritize which impairments to address given the patient's goals.

The ultimate goal of any therapeutic intervention program is to maximize the client's health and wellness. Measuring progress toward these goals is critical.

Clinicians are challenged with selecting and administering examination tools that reflect the patient's health, wellness, and response to therapeutic interventions. Examination tools that assess activity limitations typically require a lot of change to be clinically significant. Clinicians should document baseline performance of the functional activity and repeat the performance assessment at regular intervals. However, during rehabilitation programs, therapists address patients' activity limitations and impairments of body systems that contribute to functional problems. It is reasonable to expect short-term improvement in impairments prior to small change in functional tasks and activities.

Box 7.1 illustrates impairments that may be seen in patients/clients with movement disorders caused by neurological dysfunctions. These impairments are further classified as those that are within the central nervous system and those that are outside the central nervous system and result from interaction with the environment. These impairments are further discussed in detail in various sections of this book.

Range-of-motion (ROM) testing is one example of a common neuromusculoskeletal system examination procedure. Clinicians depend heavily on ROM measurements as an essential component of their examination and consequent evaluation process. It is imperative that the data obtained from this procedure be reliable. It has been suggested that the main source of variation in the performance of ROM testing is the method used. Standardizing methods and procedures will improve the reliability of the data gathered.[6]

An impairment in ROM can be the result of other body system impairments. ROM measurements may be used to determine the effect of tone, balance, movement synergies, pain, and so forth on the neuromuscular system and ultimately on behavior. Most important, the clinician needs to remember that the ROM needed to perform a functional activity is more critical than "normal," anatomical, biomechanical ROM values and must be considered when labeling and

---

BOX 7.1 Identification and Classification of Impairments

Impairments Within the Central Nervous System
1. Tone and reflexes
2. Synergies (volitional or reflexive)
3. Sensory integration and organization
4. Balance and postural control
5. Speed of movement
6. Timing
7. Reciprocal movement
8. Directional control, trajectory, or pattern of movement
9. Accuracy
10. Emotional influences
11. Perception
12. Cognition, memory, and ability to learn
13. Levels of consciousness

Impairments Outside of the Central Nervous System and Interaction With the Environment
1. Range of motion
2. Muscle strength or power production
3. Endurance
4. Cardiac function
5. Circulatory function
6. Respiratory function
7. Other organ system interactions
8. Hormonal and nutritional factors
9. Psychosocial factors

---

measuring impairments. For example, full ROM in the shoulder is seldom needed unless activities of daily living, work, or leisure activities require it, such as performing a tennis serve or reaching overhead to paint a ceiling. When needed for specific tasks, goniometric measurements of ROM are appropriate, but at other times a functional range measurement may be sufficient.

Muscle strength testing is another commonly used examination procedure. Clinicians use various methods of quantifying strength including "traditional" manual muscle testing (MMT) and the use of a dynamometer. As with ROM, strength should be correlated with the patient's functional performance. Again, the clinician may find a client to have $\frac{3}{5}$ strength in the shoulder flexor muscle groups or find grip strength to be 35 kg, but the more important question should be "What does this mean in terms of the client's ability to perform activities of daily living, and/or can he use that power in a functional activity?" The clinician is also advised to make the distinction between muscle strength and muscular endurance as it relates to function. A client may have sufficient lower-extremity strength and power to get up from the seated position; however, this does not necessarily mean that the client has muscular endurance to perform the task repeatedly during the day as part of normal everyday activities.

The status of the cardiac, respiratory, and circulatory systems significantly affects a client's functional performance. Blood pressure, heart rate, and respiration give the clinician signs of the patient's medical stability and the ability to tolerate exercise. The clinician may also obtain the results of pulmonary function tests for ventilation, pulmonary mechanics, lung diffusion capacity, or blood gas analysis after determining that the client's pulmonary system is a major factor affecting medical stability and functional progress. Various exercise tolerance tests also attempt to quantify functional work capacity and serve as a guide for the clinician performing cardiac and pulmonary rehabilitation.

A client who has difficulty performing activities of daily living and who has neurological impairments in the central motor, sensory, perceptual, or integrative systems needs to undergo examination procedures to establish the level of impairment of each involved system and to determine if and how that system is contributing to the deficit motor behaviors. Functional evaluation tools used may include the FIM, the Barthel Index, the Tinetti POMA, or the TUG test. The results of these tests will help to steer the clinician toward the most useful impairment tools to use to evaluate limitations in the various body systems. Impairment tools may include the Modified Ashworth Scale for spasticity, the Upright Motor Control Test for lower-extremity motor control, the Clinical Test of Sensory Interaction on Balance (CTSIB), or the Sensory Organization Test (SOT) for balance and sensory integrative problems, or computerized tests of limits of stability on the SMART EquiTest, among others.

The clinician is also advised to investigate the interaction of other organs and systems as they relate to the patient's functional limitations. For example, electrolyte imbalance, hormonal disorders, or adverse drug reactions may explain impairments and activity limitations noted in other interacting systems.

TESTS FOR PARTICIPATION AND SELF-EFFICACY

In ICF terminology, *participation* is defined as an individual's involvement in a life situation. Domestic life, interpersonal interactions and relationships, and community, social, and civic life are some examples of aspects of participation that can be examined for each individual. *Participation restriction* is the term used to denote problems that individuals may experience in involvement in life situations. When considering participation, it is important to obtain the individual's perception of how the medical condition, impairments, and activity limitations affect his or her involvement in life and community. Therefore many of the tests for participation and self-efficacy are in self-report format. The Activities-specific Balance Confidence (ABC) Scale, Short Form 36 (SF-36), and Dizziness Handicap Inventory (DHI) are examples of tests that can be used to gather information under this domain. These tests allow an individual to assess his or her health quality of life after an incident that affected activity and participation.

CHOOSING THE APPROPRIATE EXAMINATION TOOL

Selecting appropriate OMs is key in clinical decision making, documenting patient change over time and in response to interventions, justifying payment for skilled therapy, and communicating with the health care team, including the patient. Deciding which OMs to use can be a daunting task. One repository of OMs in rehabilitation is the Rehabilitation Measures Database found at the Shirley Ryan Ability Lab (https://www.sralab.org/rehabilitation-measures). A brief search of this database using the term "neurologic physical therapy outcome measures" returned more than 400 assessments. This large amount is clearly overwhelming for clinicians looking for assessments for their patients. Some mechanism for organizing outcomes must be used to make wise selections. One useful organizing tool is the aforementioned ICF model in which the clinician can choose measures based on whether they assess limitations in Body Structure and Function, Activity, or Participation. However, categorizing more than 400 measures into these categories is still daunting. In 2006 the American Physical Therapy Association (APTA) in partnership with the Research Section of the APTA formed the Evaluation Database to Guide Effectiveness (EDGE) Task Force in an attempt to standardize OMs and distill them to a core set.[7]

The Academy of Neurologic Physical Therapy (ANPT) formed multiple diagnosis-specific EDGE Task Forces that provided recommendations for measures by level of the ICF, patient, practice setting, utility in research, and entry-level physical therapy education. There are currently six EDGE documents available on the ANPT website (www.neuropt.org) that include StrokEDGE,[8] MS EDGE,[9] Traumatic Brain Injury EDGE,[10] Spinal Cord Injury EDGE,[11] Parkinson Disease,[12] and Vestibular Disorders.[13] The EDGE Task Forces' recommendations for PT education are divided into OMs that "students should learn to administer" and those "students should be exposed to." Combining the recommendations from each EDGE Task Force and eliminating redundancy, graduates of PT education programs should know how to administer 52 different OMs and be exposed to an additional 55 OMs, making 107 OMs in neurological patient/client management courses alone. The specific EDGE Task Force recommendations are included in Appendix 7.A.

In July of 2018, the Journal of Neurologic Physical Therapy and ANPT identified a core set of OMs for neurological rehabilitation.[7] The authors used the Consensus-based Standards for the selection of health Measurement Instruments (COSMIN) checklist to examine the literature related to OMs in neurological rehabilitation. Their criteria were that each measure could be applied to patients at different levels of acuity, with varied neurological conditions and in different practice settings. Nine action statements were addressed with the first six addressing specific activities necessary for function on a daily basis. The seventh addressed documentation, whereas eight and nine made recommendations for using the core set of OMs and their results. The Action Statements and the associated OMs are included in Appendix 7.B.

Another way to approach assessment tools is to categorize them by the type of information that the clinician and patient seek. Those heavily involved with clinical practice may find this type of organization most valuable for their particular circumstances as they could easily identify possible tests and measure to use based on a particular patient problem or presentation that they would like to closely monitor for progress. Please refer to Appendix 7.C.

Moreover, there are OMs that are specifically valuable for the pediatric population. A list of the more common OMs can be found in Appendix 7.D.

For all measures, the reader is referred to the Rehabilitation Measures Database (search "Rehabilitation Measures Database") for the most recent data and literature for each measure.

The ability to choose the appropriate examination tool(s) for a particular client will depend on several factors:

1. The client's current functional status (ambulatory vs. nonambulatory)
2. The client's current cognitive status (intact vs. confused or disoriented)
3. The clinical setting in which the person is being evaluated for treatment (acute hospital, rehabilitation, outpatient, skilled care, or home care)
4. The client's primary complaints (pain vs. weakness vs. impaired balance)
5. The client's goals and realistic expectation for recovery, maintenance, or prevention of functional loss (acute injury, chronic problem, or progressive disease process)
6. The type of information desired from the test (e.g., if the test is discriminative or predictive). The reader is encouraged to read the two articles on "outcome measures in neurological physical therapy practice"[20,21] published in the *Journal of Neurologic Physical Therapy* for a detailed discussion on this subject.
7. The psychometric properties of the test on the specific patient population/diagnosis
8. The ability of the test to detect significant change over time

The evaluator should select examination tools that address three objectives: first, to measure the client's primary problems (activity limitations, impairments, and participation restrictions); second, supply outcome values necessary for setting realistic treatment goals in collaboration with the client and family; and third, to plan efficient and effective intervention strategies.

Many of the examination tools that measure a client's ability to perform functional activities have been accepted as valid, reliable, and useful for the justification of payment for services rendered. The number of activity limitations and the extent of the client's participation limitation are often reasons why an individual either has access to therapy services directly or is referred by a medical practitioner. For this reason, the third-party payers expect to receive reports concerning positive changes in the client's functional status to justify therapeutic services. The initial list of functional or activity limitations or participation restrictions helps the therapist to determine the extent of, expectations for, and direction of intervention, but it does not determine why those limitations exist. The answer to this question is critical in the evaluation process. Examination tests and procedures that identify specific system and subsystem impairments help the therapist to determine causes for existing participation and activity limitations. These tools must be objective, reliable, and sufficiently sensitive to provide needed communication to third-party payers to explain the subsystem's baseline progress during and after the intervention. These tools should also supply explanations for residual difficulties in the event that the functional problems themselves do not demonstrate significant objective change or show progress within the time frame estimated.

Examination Process in Practice

The following case scenario synthesizes the clinical examination and evaluation process used by PTs and OTs.

Assume that a clinician has been called in to examine a client who has sustained an anoxic brain injury during heart surgery. The client's cognitive ability is within normal limits, and he is highly motivated to get back to his normal activities. He is retired; he loves to walk in the park with his wife and to go on birdwatching experiences in the mountains with their group of friends. The clinician must select which functional tests to use to obtain an objective initial status and target the client's problems. Currently the client requires assistance with all gross mobility skills and is demonstrating difficulty balancing in various postures and performing activities of daily living. Results of functional testing reveal that the client demonstrates significant limitations, requiring moderate assistance in the activities of coming to sit, sitting, coming to stand, standing, walking, dressing, and grooming. Assume that the client also displays impairment limitations in flexion ROM at the hip joints caused by both muscle and fascia tightness and hypertonicity within the extensor muscle groups. He has compensated to some degree and is able to perform bed mobility independently. Upper extremity motor control is within normal limits, and thus the client is capable of performing many activities of daily living as long as his lower trunk and hips are placed in a supportive position and hip flexion beyond 90 degrees is not required. The client has general weakness from inactivity, and power production problems in his abdominals and hip flexor muscles owing to the dominance of extensor muscle tonicity. Once he is helped to stand, the extensor patterns of hip and knee extension, internal rotation, slight adduction, and plantarflexion are present. He can actively extend both legs after being placed in flexion, but he is limited in the production of specific fine and gross motor patterns. Thus a resulting balance impairment is present owing to the inability to adequately access appropriate balance strategies caused by the presence of tone, limb synergy production,

and weakness in the antagonists to the trunk and hip extensors. Through the use of augmented intervention, the client is noted to possess intact postural and procedural balance programming; however, both functions are being masked by existing impairments. The decision is made to perform impairment measures, including assessments of ROM at the hip, knee, and ankle joints; the ability to produce strength in both the abdominal and hip flexor muscle groups; and volitional and nonvolitional synergic programming, balance, and posture, and volitional control over muscle tone. The demand on ROM, power production, and specific synergic programming will vary according to the requirements of the functional activities performed.

Using a clinical decision-making process, the clinician will conclude that the impairments that are being targeted to measure will vary from one functional activity to the next. For instance, if this client is demonstrating difficulty rising from a chair, the target impairment may be quantified with a ROM measurement. This same ROM impairment may also contribute to problems with moving about the base of support in functional sitting. The clinician makes the determination as to the extent to which the impairment interferes with each functional problem for that particular client.

These objective measurements help the clinician to explain which outcomes would be expected to be achieved first and why. These measurements are recorded as part of intervention charting and help to objectively demonstrate that the client is improving toward functional independence. They also give an indication of what the client still needs to reach the desired outcome, the rate of learning that is taking place, and an estimation of recovery time that is still required. These objective measurements give to the clinician and the client a better avenue to discuss expectations with family members, other medical practitioners, and third-party payers. In this example, assume that, after intervention, functional ROM in the hip was achieved. However, this improvement did not result in an improvement in the activity problems because synergic programming prevented adequate hip flexion during one or more functional activities. Understanding and measuring the difference between lack of ROM as a result of muscle or fascia tightness versus lack of range from abnormal synergic patterning helps the clinician to communicate why a client is successful in one activity and may still need assistance in another.

Scores obtained from tests of activity, participation, and impairments supply statistically important measurements that can then be used to discuss the limitations placed on the therapeutic environment by fiscal intermediaries. Therapists must be clear when documenting the initial status and the target status for clients so that the recommended intervention and length of stay may be justified.

When making a determination of the potential impact of an intervention on improving a client's problems, clinicians must remember that a key factor in this process of examination and evaluation is the acceptance of the movement dysfunction or impairment by the client. A mobility problem or impairment may be clearly identified by a functional test or impairment test; however, the client may deny that the problem even exists. Acceptance of the problems by the client and a willingness to change are critical to the client's adherence to the intervention strategy.

As mentioned earlier, the identification of potential impairments was done after functional testing to streamline the examination process. After performing the functional examination, the therapist postulated that the client might have impaired motor control, muscle weakness, sensory deficits, pain, and decreased endurance that may have been causing the functional limitations. MMT revealed lower-extremity strength of $1/5$ in both ankle motions, $2/5$ in both knees, and $3-/5$ in both hips. Upper extremities tested as $1/5$ finger flexors (incomplete grip), ²⁄₅ wrist motions, and 3+/5 in both elbow motions. Shoulder and trunk strength were within functional limits for all motions. Sensory testing indicated absent touch and proprioceptive sensations from the foot to the knee of both lower extremities, with impaired sensation from the thighs to the hips. Both hands and wrists tested absent to touch and proprioception, with the elbows and shoulders testing intact. The client's endurance was limited to short bouts of activity (3 to 5 minutes), with rapid muscular and cardiovascular fatigue. The presence of these impairments helped to explain the resultant functional limitations tested earlier.

In terms of standardized functional tests, the multidisciplinary FIM could give insight into this patient's ability to function in multiple domains and categories. Baseline scores on the Berg Balance Scale could be collected because this client is expected to regain further function in balance and postural control as recovery from the condition occurs. As the client regains strength and peripheral sensory ability, he may be able to perform the TUG test and the 10-Meter Walk Test. These functional assessments paint a better picture of what the client can and cannot do, as well as provide a way to measure functional progress in various activities throughout rehabilitation.

Because the patient's prior status included enjoying walks in the park with his wife and birdwatching experiences in the mountains with friends, it is important to keep in mind that the patient likely desires to return to these activities that relate to his role as husband and friend. The clinician is encouraged to add measures of satisfaction with life and to link the outcome assessment results to goals to return to walks in the park and bird watching in some format.

ACKNOWLEDGMENTS

The author recognizes Drs. Peggy Roller, Rolando Lazaro, and Darcy Umphred, who authored this chapter in the sixth edition of the text.

REFERENCES

To enhance this text and add value for the reader, all references are included on the companion Evolve site that accompanies this textbook. This online service will, when available, provide a link for the reader to a PubMed abstract for the article cited. There are 21 cited references and other general references for this chapter, with the majority of those articles being evidence-based citations.

CASE STUDY 7.1[a]

The patient is a 30-year-old man who was referred to outpatient physical therapy after a 1-week stay in an acute care facility following an exacerbation of relapsing-remitting multiple sclerosis (MS). His height was 2.05 m (6 feet 9 inches), and his weight was 133.81 kg (295 pounds). The patient was first diagnosed with MS 4 years ago. He developed optic neuritis during the exacerbation and was treated with corticosteroid pulse therapy. The patient's past medical history included depression, gastroesophageal reflux disease, migraine headaches, and hyperlipidemia. After being diagnosed with MS, the patient had to stop working. Before the most recent hospitalization, the patient lived with his sister in a single-story home with five stairs to enter with a railing. At that time he was able to ambulate independently without an assistive device and to complete all activities of daily living without any assistance.

An outpatient physical therapy initial examination was conducted 1 week after the patient was discharged from the hospital. He reported that he was using a wheelchair to get to and from appointments, and inside his home. He was alert and oriented to person, place, and time, although responses were delayed and speech was slightly slurred. There were no complaints of pain, and the patient stated that fatigue and temperature had not affected him.

Several tests of functional movement activities were performed first. The patient was able to roll to the right and left with minimal assistance, with rolling to the right being less difficult for the patient. He needed supervision to move from supine to sitting.

The patient required moderate assistance to perform a sit-to-stand transfer. He was able to ambulate five steps with a front-wheeled walker (FWW) and moderate assistance of one person.

After examination of the patient's functional movement activities, several tests of body function and structures were then administered. Passive range of motion for all joints in both upper and lower extremities was within normal limits. The patient presented with ³⁄₅ (fair) strength of the right upper and lower extremities and good (⁴⁄₅) strength of the left upper and lower extremities during MMT. Light touch and superficial pain sensations tested intact from C4 to S2 dermatomes bilaterally.

Sitting balance was scored as ¾ (good) because the patient was able to accept moderate challenges. Standing static balance was 10+/4 (poor plus); the patient was able to maintain balance with handheld support and occasional minimal assistance.

Observational gait analysis was performed, and impairments in gait included the following: decreased step length bilaterally, wide base of support, decreased weight bearing through the right lower extremity, and lack of toe-off. It was also noted that ataxic type movements were present with ambulation.

The Gait Abnormality Rating Scale (GARS) was performed, and the patient scored a ³²⁄₄₈, indicating increased fall risk. The Tinetti Performance-Oriented Mobility Assessment (POMA) was also administered. The patient scored ⁸⁄₂₈, indicating a high risk for falls. Several tests were performed using the Natus Balance Master. The sit-to-stand test showed that the patient had difficulty maintaining balance immediately after rising and had more weight on his left lower extremity. The results were abnormal, based on the norms for the patient's gender and age. Next, the weight-bearing squat test was done. During this test the patient was not able to maintain equal weight through bilateral lower extremities, with the patient bearing weight more on the left side. The patient then performed the limits of stability test, which revealed an inability to lean his center of gravity (COG) over his right lower extremity, or forward onto his toes. The patient then performed the rhythmic weight-shift test; he was not able to complete the forward-backward component of the rhythmic weight-shift test without falling, and he also had difficulty with directional control and velocity during lateral weight shifting.

Last, tests for participation and self-efficacy were administered. The Activities-specific Balance Confidence (ABC) Scale questionnaire was given to the patient to assess the patient's balance self-efficacy. The patient had a score of 20%, indicating a low level of physical functioning. He scored 10% on being able to bend down, pick a slipper up off the floor, and reach for a can on a shelf at eye level with the use of an FWW.

The data collected at initial examination revealed limitations in functional performance resulting from impairments in balance, gait, strength, and motor control, giving the therapist the various movement diagnoses that reflected problems. Intervention frequency and duration was set at three times per week for 8 weeks. The prognosis that the patient would be able to ambulate independently in the community with an assistive device in 8 weeks was good, given the patient's willingness to participate in physical therapy, positive outlook, family support, and positive response to medical interventions. The plan of care that was developed focused on improving activity limitations such as transfers and gait and impairments such as weakness and imbalance. The expected outcomes were set to be achieved in 8 weeks, and anticipated goals were set to be achieved in 4 weeks.

[a]Case study modified from Larsen-Merrill J, Lazaro R: Use of the NeuroCom balance master training protocols to improve functional performance in a person with multiple sclerosis. *J Stud Phys Ther Res* 21:1–16, 2009.

Summary of Recommendations From the Evaluation Database to Guide Effectiveness (EDGE)

1. StrokEDGE[14]

OUTCOME MEASURE	ICF CATEGORY			ENTRY-LEVEL EDUCATION	
	Body Structure/ Function	Activity	Participation	Students Should Learn to Administer	Students Should Be Exposed
6-Minute Walk	X	X		X	
10-Meter Walk		X		X	
Berg Balance Test		X		X	
Dynamic Gait Index		X		X	
Fugl-Meyer	X			X	
Functional Reach	X	X		X	
Orpington Prognostic Scale		X		X	
Postural Assessment Scale for Stroke	X			X	
Stroke Impact Scale			X	X	
Tardieu Spasticity Scale	X			X	
Timed "Up and Go" test		X		X	
5 Times Sit-to-Stand	X	X			X
Action Research Arm Test	X	X			X
Activities-specific Balance Confidence Scale		X	X		X
Ashworth Spasticity Scale	X				X
Assessment of Life Habits			X		X
Chedoke-McMaster Stroke assessment	X				X
Dynamometry	X				X
EuroQOL			X		X
Functional Independence Measure		X			X
Fugl-Meyer (Sensory)	X				X
Hi-Level Mobility Assessment Tool (HiMAT)		X			X
Modified Rankin Scale		X			X
Motricity Index	X				X
Nottingham Assessment of Somatosensation	X				X

Stroke Adapted Sickness Impact Scale-30			X		X
Short Form 36 (SF-36)			X		X
Stroke Rehabilitation Assessment of Movement		X			X
Vo₂max	X				X
Wolf Motor Function Test		X			X
2. Spinal Cord Injury EDGE[15]					
6-Minute Walk	X	X		X	
10-Meter Walk		X		X	
ASIA Impairment Scale				X	
Berg Balance Test		X		X	
Functional Independence Measure		X		X	
Handheld Myometry				X	
Manual Muscle Test				X	
Numeric Pain Rating Scale				X	
Timed "Up and Go" test		X		X	
Modified Ashworth Spasticity Scale	X				X
Capabilities of Upper Extremity Functioning Instrument		X			X
Craig Handicap Reporting and Assessment Technique		X	X		X
Dynamic Gait Index		X			X
Functional Gait Assessment		X			X
Multidimensional Pain Inventory, SCI Version	X				X
Penn Spasm Frequency Scale	X				X
Reintegration to Normal Living Index			X		X
Satisfaction with Life Scale			X		X
Medical Council SF-36			X		X
Sickness Impact Profile			X		X
Spinal Cord Injury Independence Measure		X			X
Walking Index for Spinal Cor Injury II		X			X
World Health Organization Quality of Life—BREF			X		X
3. Multiple Sclerosis EDGE[16]					
12-item MS Walking Scale		X		X	
2-Minute Walk Test		X		X	
6-Minute Walk		X		X	
9-Hole Peg Test		X		X	
Activities-specific Balance Confidence Scale		X	X	X	
Berg Balance Test		X		X	
Dizziness Handicap Inventory	X	X	X	X	
Dynamic Gait Index		X		X	
Fatigue Scale for Motor and Cognitive Functions	X			X	
Functional Independence Measure	X	X	X	X	
MS Quality of Live (MSQOL-54)		X	X	X	
Rivermead Mobility Index		X		X	
Static Standing Balance Test	X			X	
Timed 25-Foot Walk		X		X	
Timed "Up & Go" Test with Cognitive/Manual Tasks		X		X	

Continued

Trunk Impairment Scale	x	x		x	
Visual Analog Scale (for fatigue)	x			x	
Functional Reach		x		x	
12-Minute Walk/Run		x			x
Box and Blocks Test	x				x
Disease Steps	x				x
4-Square Step Test		x			x
Functional Assessment of MS	x	x	x		x
Maximal Inspiratory/Expiratory Pressure	x				x
Oxygen Uptake (max and peak)	x				x
MS Functional Composite	x	x			x
MS Impact Scale			x		x
Modified Fatigue Impact Scale	x				x
SF-36			x		x

4. Traumatic Brain Injury EDGE[17]

6-Minute Walk	x	x		x	
10-Meter Walk		x		x	
Action Research Arm Test		x		x	
Agitated Behavior Scale	x	x		x	
Berg Balance Test		x		x	
Coma Recovery Scale-Revised	x			x	
Community Balance and Mobility Scale	x	x		x	
Community Integration Questionnaire			x	x	
Dizziness Handicap Inventory	x	x	x	x	
Functional Independence Measure	x	x	x	x	
High-Level Mobility Assessment		x		x	
Modified Ashworth Scale	x			x	
Moss Attention Rating Scale	x			x	
Rancho Levels of Cognitive Functioning	x			x	
Balance Error Scoring System		x			x
Disability Rating Scale	x	x	x		x
Functional Assessment Measure	x	x	x		x
Patient Health Questionnaire	x				x
Quality of Life after Brain Injury			x		x
Sydney Psychosocial Reintegration Scale			x		x

5. Parkinson EDGE Task Force Recommendations[18]

Mini-BEST Test	x	x		x	
Montreal Cognitive Assessment	x			x	
5 Times Sit-to-Stand	x	x		x	
6-Minute Walk	x	x	x	x	
10-Meter Walk		x	x	x	
Functional Gait Assessment		x	x	x	
9-Hole Peg Test		x	x	x	
PDQ-8 or PDQ 39					x
Activities-specific Balance Confidence Scale			x		x

MDS-UPDRS revision-Part 1 & 3	x				x
Timed "Up and Go" Cognitive	x	x	x		x
MDS-UPDRS revision—Part 2		x	x		x
Freezing of Gait Questionnaire		x	x		x
Parkinson Fatigue Scale		x	x		x
6. Vestibular EDGE Task Force Recommendations[19]					
4-Square Step Test		x		x	
Berg Balance Test		x		x	
Functional Reach		x		x	
Modified Functional Reach		x		x	
CTSIB	x			x	
mCTSIB (no dome)	x			x	
Romberg	x			x	
Unipedal Stance	x	x		x	
Activities-specific Balance Confidence Scale		x	x	x	
Dizziness Handicap Inventory	x	x	x	x	
Dynamic Gait Index		x		x	
Functional Gait Assessment		x	x	x	
Timed "Up and Go"	x	x	x	x	
Timed "Up and Go" Cognitive	x	x	x	x	
5 Times Sit-to-Stand	x	x		x	
Gait Velocity				x	
30-s Chair Stand Test	x	x		x	
Dix-Halpike	x			x	
Roll Test	x			x	
Sidelying Test	x			x	
Head Impulse Test/Head Thrust Test	x			x	
Balance Error Scoring System (BESS)	x				x
BEST Test	x	x			x
NeuroCom Sensory Organization Test	x				x
Vertigo Handicap Questionnaire		x	x		x
Vestibular Disorders Activities of Daily Living Scale		x	x		x
Vestibular Rehabilitation Benefit Questionnaire		x	x		x
UCLA Dizziness Questionnaire		x	x		x
Disability Rating Scale		x	x		x
Fukuda Stepping Test		x			x
Head Shaking Nystagmus Test	x				x

EDGE, evaluation database to guide effectiveness.
Tables are organized according to the international classification of functioning, disability and health (ICF) category and recommendations regarding inclusion of specific content in entry-level education.

Core Set of Outcome Measures for Adults With Neurological Conditions Undergoing Rehabilitation: A Clinical Practice Guideline

Outcome Statement Number	Area of Assessment	Relevant Outcome Measures
Action Statement 1	Static and dynamic sitting and standing balance assessment	Berg Balance Scale (BBS)
Action Statement 2	Walking balance assessment	Functional Gait Assessment (FGA)
Action Statement 3	Balance confidence assessment	Activities-specific Balance Confidence (ABC) Scale
Action Statement 4	Walking speed assessment	10-Meter Walk Test (10mWT)
Action Statement 5	Walking distance assessment	6-Minute Walk Test (6MWT)
Action Statement 6	Transfer assessment	5 Times Sit-to-Stand (5TSTS)
Action Statement 7	Documentation of patient goals	Goal Attainment Scale (GAS)
Action Statement 8	Use of the core set of outcome measures	
Action Statement 9	Discuss outcome measure results and use collaborative/share decision making with patients	

Adapted from Moore JL, Potter K, Blankshain K, et al. A core set of outcome measures for adults with neurologic conditions undergoing rehabilitation: a clinical practice guideline. *J Neurol Phys Ther*. 2018;42(3):174–220.

Relevant Outcome Measures to use for Selected Impairment, Activity Limitations, or Participation/Quality of Life Restrictions

What Do You Want to Test?	Outcome Measures
Cognition, mental status	Mini-Mental State Examination (MMSE) Montreal Cognitive Assessment (MoCA)
Depression	Geriatric Depression Scale (GDS) Beck Depression Scale Zung Depression Scale
Level of consciousness	Rancho Los Amigos Levels of Cognitive Functioning (TBI) Coma/Near Coma Scale Glasgow Coma Scale (GCS) Glasgow Outcome Scale (GOS)
Shortness of breath/ Level of perceived exertion/level of aerobic fitness	Borg Scale of Dyspnea Borg Rate of Perceived Exertion Scale (RPE) VO_{2ma}
Joint range of motion	Goniometry Inclinometry
Sensation	Rivermead Assessment of Somatosensory Performance Nottingham Assessment of Somatosensation Semmes-Weinstein Monofilament Test (superficial touch/light pressure only) Fugl-Meyer Assessment (FMA) Sensory Exam
Use of sensory systems for balance and postural control	Sensory Organization Test (SOT) on computer force plate systems such as NeuroCom or Bertec Modified Clinical Test of Sensory Interaction on Balance (mCTSIB) on foam or computer force plate system
Strength (force production)	Dynamometry Upright Motor Control Test (UMC) Stroke LE
Power	5 Times Sit-to-Stand (5TSTS) Medical Research Council (MRC) Grading System (0–5 Scale)
Spasticity/ muscle spasms	Ashworth Scale, Modified Ashworth Scale (MAS) Tardieu Scale, Modified Tardieu Scale Penn Spasm Frequency Scale (SCI)
Motor performance (synergy, selective voluntary motor control)	Fugl-Meyer Assessment (FMA) Motor for UE and LE Stroke Rehabilitation Assessment of Movement (STREAM) (also includes mobility) NIH Stroke Scale (includes sensory, consciousness) Rivermead Motor Assessment Limits of Stability (LOS)
Endurance	6-Minute Walk Test (6MWT) 2-Minute Walk Test (2MWT) 3-Minute Walk Test (3MWT) 12-Minute Walk Test (12MWT)

Continued

What Do You Want to Test?	Outcome Measures
Upper extremity (UE) fine motor control UE function	9-Hole Peg Test (9-HPT) Box and Block Test (BBT)
UE synergy vs. selective control	Action Research Arm Test (ARAT) Arm Motor Ability Test (AMAT) Wolf Motor Function Test (WMFT) Jebsen Taylor Arm Function Test Chedoke Arm-Hand Inventory Motor Activity Log (MAL) (P) STREAM—UE subscale Fugl-Meyer Assessment (FMA) Motor—UE Frenchay Activities Index (FAI) (IADLs)
Trunk control	Trunk Control Test Trunk Impairment Scale Segmental Assessment of Trunk Control (SATCo)—peds
Pain perception	Visual Analog Scale (VAS) Pain Faces Pain Scale (FPS) Numeric Pain Rating Scale (NPRS)
Gait speed Gait ability	10-Meter Walk Test (10MWT) 25-Foot Walk Test Dynamic Gait Index (DGI) Functional Gait Assessment (FGA) (high level, stairs) Tinetti Gait Subscale (gait deviations) Modified Gait Assessment Rating Scale (mGARS) Functional Ambulation Category (FAC) Walking Index for SCI (WISCI-II) SCI Functional Ambulation Inventory (SCI-FAI)
Wheelchair mobility assessment	Wheelchair Assessment Tool (WAT) Functional Evaluation in Wheelchair (FEW)
Balance fall risk	Berg Balance Scale (BBS) 7-Item Short Form Berg Balance Scale (7-Item BBS) Timed Up-and-Go (TUG) Test Balance Evaluation Systems Test (BEST Test) Mini BEST Test Brief BEST Test Functional Reach Test (FR) Dynamic Gait Index (DGI) Functional Gait Assessment (FGA) 5 Times Sit-to-Stand (5TSTS) Tinetti Performance-Oriented Mobility Assessment (POMA) Fullerton Advanced Balance Test (FAB) (high level skills) Brunel Balance Test Activities-specific Balance Confidence (ABC) Scale Sensory Organization Test (SOT) Composite Score Romberg Sharpened Romberg Single Leg Stance Test (SLS)
Balance perception	ABC Scale Falls Efficacy Scale (FES)—Tinetti FES: Swedish Version (higher level skills)
Dizziness perception	VAS Dizziness

What Do You Want to Test?	Outcome Measures
Oculomotor testing (reflexive and voluntary)	Dynamic Visual Acuity Test (DVA) Gaze Stabilization Test (GST) computerized Head Impulse Test (HIT) [AKA Head Thrust Test (HTT)] Video Head Impulse Test (VHIT) Spontaneous Nystagmus Gaze Evoked Nystagmus Head Shaking Nystagmus Vibration Induced Nystagmus Test VOR Cancellation Smooth Pursuit/Tracking Saccades/2-target Test
Motion sensitivity (positional Nystagmus)	Dix-Hallpike Test Motion Sensitivity Quotient (MSQ)
Functional mobility	Walky-Talky Test Physical Performance Battery 4-Square Step Test (FSST) Hi MAT (TBI population)
Ataxia	Fregly Graybiel Ataxia Test Battery
Burden of care Level of functional independence Handicap	Functional Independence Measure (FIM) Modified Rankin Scale (MRS) stroke Craig Handicap Assessment and Reporting Technique (CHART, CHART-19) Disability Rating Scale (DRS)—Rappaport
Self-care and activities of daily living (ADLs) status	Barthel Index (BI) Katz Index Vestibular ADL Scale (VADL)
Quality of life outcome measures (QOL)—general and specific	Short Form 36 or 12 (SF-36, SF-12) European Quality of Life Measure (Euro QOL) Multiple Sclerosis QOL 54 Scale (MSQOL-54) Modified Fatigue Impact Scale (MS population) Fatigue Severity Scale Parkinson Disease Questionnaire (PDQ) Stroke–Adapted Sickness Impact Scale (SA-SIP30) Stroke-Specific QOL Scale (SS-QOL) Stroke Impact Scale (SIS, SIS-16) Dizziness Handicap Inventory (DHI) Satisfaction with Life Scale (SWL)
Effect of degenerative disease on motor control, ADLs, and/or function	United Parkinson Disease Rating Scale (UPDRS) United Huntington Disease Rating Scale (UHDRS) Kurtzke Expanded Disability Status Scale (MS) ALS Functional Rating Scale
Stage or classification of disease, disorder, or diagnosis	Hoehn and Yahr Scale (H&Y) (PD) American Spinal Injury Association (ASIA) (SCI) Rancho Los Amigos Levels of Cognitive Functioning (TBI) NIH Stroke Scale (Stroke severity)
Wearable and instrumented technology for balance and gait testing	iTUG (instrumented TUG test) iCTSIB (use of sensory systems for postural control) iSWAY (postural stability) iSAW (instrumented stand and walk test) iWALK (gait) GAITRite (gait) Zeno Walkway (gait) APDM Wearable Sensors (mobility)
Severity of stroke and prognosis	Orpington Prognostic Scale STREAM (DC destination)

Continued

What Do You Want to Test?	Outcome Measures
Level of functional mobility post-stroke	Postural Assessment Scale for Stroke Patients (PASS)
	Modified Rankin Scale (MRS)
	STREAM (Mobility Subscale)
	Chedoke-McMaster Stroke Assessment
Pediatric gross motor function	Gross Motor Function Measure (GMFM)
	Gross Motor Function Classification Scale (GMFCS)

Adapted from instructional materials developed by Peggy Roller PT, DPT, MS.

Selected Pediatric Assessment Tools by International Classification of Functioning, Disability and Health Categories

ICF CATEGORY: BODY STRUCTURE/FUNCTION	
What Do You Want to Test?	**Assessment Tools**
Anthropometrics	Body Composition (BMI) Height/Weight Leg Length
Cardiopulmonary	Blood Pressure Heart Rate Oxygen Saturation, Respiratory Pattern and Rate Skin Color Skin Turgor
Coordination	Clinical Observation of Motor and Postural Skills (COMPS) Florida Apraxia Screening Test Gross Motor Performance Measure (GMPM) Selective Control Assessment of the Lower Extremity Test of Ideational Praxis
Endurance/energy expenditure	Early Activity Scale for Endurance (EASE) Energy Expenditure Index 6-Minute Walk Test 30-s Walk Test
Fitness	Fitness Gram Presidential Physical Fitness Test
Pain	Children's Hospital of Eastern Ontario Pain Scale (CHEOPS) CRIES Scale (Cries, Require Oxygen, Increased Vital Signs, Expression, Sleep) Faces Pain Scale FLACC (Faces, Legs, Activity, Crying, Consolability Behavioral Pain Scale) Individualized Numeric Pain Scale (INRS) Numeric Scale Oucher Scale Visual Analogue Scale
Posture/balance	Early Clinical Assessment of Balance (ECAB) Movement Assessment of Infants (MAI) Pediatric Balance Scale (PBS) Pediatric Clinical Test of Sensory Interaction for Balance (P-CTSIB) Pediatric Reach Test (Pediatric Functional Reach Test) Timed Up and Down Stairs Test

Continued

Posture/structural integrity	Adam Forward Bend Test Anterior/Posterior Drawer Test Apley Test Arch Index Beighton Scale of Hypermobility Craig Test Galeazzi Sign Heel Bisector Angle Lachman Test Navicular Drop Test McMurray Test Ryder Test Talar Tilt Transmalleolar Axis
Range of motion/muscle length	Ely Test Hamstring Length Test Modified Ober Test Popliteal Angle Prone Hip Extension Test Spinal Alignment and Range of Motion Measure (SAROMM) Straight Leg Test Thomas Test
Reflexes	Movement Assessment of Infants (MAI)
Sensory processing	Infant/Toddler Sensory Profile Sensory Integration and Praxis Test Sensory Profile
Spasticity	Modified Ashworth Scale (MAS)5 · Modified Tardieu Test
Strength/muscle power	Manual Muscle Testing Dynamometer Measurement Muscle Power Selective Control Assessment of the Lower Extremity (SCALE)
Visual motor/perception	Developmental Test of Visual Motor Integration Test of Visual Motor Skills-3 (TVMS-3)

ICF CATEGORY: ACTIVITY

What Do You Want to Test?	Assessment Tools
Gait/walking	Dynamic Gait Index Functional Mobility Assessment Observational Gait Scale (OGS) Standardized Walking Obstacle Course Timed Obstacle Ambulation Test Timed Up and Down Stairs test Timed "Up and Go" (TUG)
Gross Motor	Alberta Infant Motor Scales (AIMS) Bruininks-Oseretsky Test of Motor Proficiency (BOTP-2) Gross Motor Function Measure (GMFM) Gross Motor Performance Measure High Level Mobility Assessment Tool (HIMAT) Motor Function Measure Peabody Developmental Motor Scales Second Edition (PDMS-2) Test of Gross Motor Development, 2nd Edition (TGMD-2) Test of Infant Motor Performance (TIMP)

Fine motor	Bruininks-Oseretsky Test of Motor Proficiency (BOTP-2) Jebsen Taylor Test of Hand Function 9-Hole Peg Test Peabody Developmental Motor Scales Second Edition (PDMS-2) Assisting Hand Assessment Shriner Upper Extremity Assessment Melbourne Unilateral Upper Limb Function (MUUL)
Play	Preschool Play Scale Test of Playfulness (ToP)
Developmental screening	Ages & Stages Questionnaires (ASQ-3) Assessment, Evaluation, and Programming System for Infants and Children (AEPS)–Second Edition Bayley Infant Neurodevelopmental Screener (BINS) Carolina Curriculum for Infants and Toddlers with Special Needs, Third Edition Carolina Curriculum for Preschoolers with Special Needs FirstSTEp: Screening Test for Evaluating Preschoolers Motor Skills Acquisition in the First Year and Checklist

ICF CATEGORY: PARTICIPATION AND QUALITY OF LIFE

What Do You Want to Test?	Assessment Tools
Multidomain	Assessment of Life Habits (LIFE-H) Canadian Occupational Performance Measure (COPM) Children's Assessment of Participation and Enjoyment (CAPE) Participation and Environment Measure-Children and Youth (PEM-CY) Preferences for Activities of Children (PAC) School Function Assessment (SFA) Vineland Adaptive
Quality of life	Child Health Index of Life with Disabilities Kidscreen · Pediatric Quality of Life Inventory (PEDS QL) Pediatric Outcomes Data Collection Instrument (PODCI) Quality of Well-Being Scale (QWB)
Health status	Child Health and Illness Profile Adolescent Edition (CHIP-E) Child Health Questionnaire (CHQ) Child Health Assessment Questionnaire (CHAQ) Health Utilities Index-Mark 3

From Section on Pediatrics, Fact Sheet. List of Pediatric Assessment Tools Categorized by ICF Model. Available at: https://pediatricapta.org/includes/fact-sheets/pdfs/13%20Assessment&screening%20tools.pdf.

8

Interventions for Individuals With Movement Limitations

Rolando T. Lazaro, Myla U. Quiben, and Sandra G. Reina-Guerra

OBJECTIVES

After reading this chapter the student or therapist will be able to:

1. Appreciate the complexity of motor responses and discuss methods used to influence body.
2. Analyze the similarities and differences among interventions that address impairments in specific body systems, and functional training.
3. Identify the role of augmented feedback in neurological interventions.
4. Select appropriate intervention strategies to optimize desired outcomes.

5. Analyze variables that may both positively and negatively affect complex motor responses and a patient's ability to perform functional activities and participate in the community.
6. Discuss interventions in neurorehabilitation with regards to current evidence, clinical implications, and considerations for utility.
7. Consider the contribution of the patient/client, available support systems, research evidence, neurophysiology, and the best practice standards available to optimize outcomes.

KEY TERMS

augmented intervention
evidence-based practice

functional training
intervention for impairments

Before discussing therapeutic interventions, the therapist must identify the learning environment within which the patient/client will perform tasks/activities. That environment is made up of the therapist and the patient/client, all internal body control mechanisms of the patient/client, and the external restraints and demands of the environment. Although this text focuses on relearning functional movement, the reader must always consider many factors that influence the patient/client management, including how other organs or body systems will be affected by or will affect the therapeutic outcome, both during and after rehabilitation, in relation to long-term quality of life. An examination and evaluation are performed before intervention to establish movement diagnoses. A physical therapy diagnosis must link impairments at the body structure and function level to activity limitations and participation restrictions, as well as provide a prognosis of the patient's/client's potential for functional improvement. Personal factors, such as motivation, family support, financial support, patient values, and cultural biases, must be considered as part of the prognosis.[1-3] Therefore the physical therapy diagnosis and prognosis guide the selection of intervention strategies. This text addresses interventions for patients/clients with movement system dysfunction associated with nervous system impairments. Prognostic accuracy and appropriate goal setting require clinical reasoning to distinguish if a specific activity limitation is due to an acute event or if the limitation has developed over a lifetime as a result of small traumas and adjustments to life.

Both the American Occupational Therapy Association (AOTA) and the American Physical Therapy Association (APTA) have developed standards of professional practice to guide therapists in the patient/client management process.[2,3] "The body of online tools to support

evidence-based practice is growing, including diagnosis-specific interventions. Some tools are open access such as the Physiotherapy Evidence Database (PEDro)[4] while others require professional membership."[5,6] Through the use of current evidence-based practice of sensorimotor processing, motor control, motor learning, and neuroplasticity theories and body systems models, the therapist must determine the inherent motor control and learning flexibility the patient demonstrates while executing functional activities and participating in life. This chapter and text cannot establish for the reader the exact treatment sequence that should be used for every patient but presents an example of a decision making pathway in Box 8.1. Functional goals must be established that lead to the patient's/client's ability to participate within his or her environment and whenever possible lead to or maintain the quality of life desired by the patient/client. Before beginning any intervention, the therapist must determine the treatment strategies that will be used to help the patient/client attain the desired functional outcomes. The specific environment used by the therapist to optimize patient performance will depend on the functional level and amount of motor control exhibited by the patient. In some cases the therapist may be constrained to use the existing environment and will need to modify it to meet the intent of the therapeutic session. The following classifications can be used to document the specific role of the therapist within the intervention session:

Functional training: Practice of a functional skill that is meaningful, goal directed, and task oriented. Patients will experience errors and self-correct as the program becomes more automatic and integrated. An example would be gait training on a tile surface, rugs, inclined surfaces, compliant surfaces such as grass, and so on, to practice ambulation.

BOX 8.1 Treatment Strategy Categories

Compensation Training

Use of an assistive device or orthotic to compensate for a permanent impairment or lost body system function.

Substitution Training

Teaching the patient to use a different sensory system or muscle(s) group to substitute for lost function of another system. An example of sensory substitution might be teaching the patient to use vision to substitute for an impaired vestibular system or somatosensory system for balance function. Substitution within the motor system might be teaching hip hiking to substitute for lack of dorsiflexion of the ankle during swing phase of gait.

Habituation Training

Activity-based provocation of symptoms with the goal of symptom reduction with repetitive practice. An example would be teaching head movement to a patient who has a chronic labyrinthitis and severe nausea with any head movement.

Neural Adaptation

Driving changes in structure and function of the central or peripheral nervous system with repetitive, attended practice. This category would be considered neural plasticity. This category of treatment strategy takes the greatest repetition of practice and requires a strong desire by the individual to gain the functional ability and realize the potential of the central nervous system to change.

Intervention for impairments: Treatment focus is on correcting an impairment in the body system with interventions such as muscle strengthening, stretching, sensory training, endurance training.

Whether the intervention approach is via functional training or intervention for impairments, the clinician may use *augmented feedback* strategies to optimize the patient's response to the intervention strategy. The external feedback received by the patient (auditory, visual, kinesthetic, tactile, etc.) will limit the response patterns (e.g., reducing degrees of freedom, reduction or enhancement of tone) for successful performance of the desired movement. Examples of these are provided in the later portion of this chapter.

Patients/clients with central nervous system (CNS) damage often benefit from a combination of interventions from the above categories. An example of this might be the early phase of partial body weight supported treadmill training (BWSTT), where a therapist or assistant guides the patient's/client's leg during swing and stance phases while the body harness supports a proportion of the patient's/client's total weight (augmented feedback) to maintain balance and decrease the power needed to generate a more typical gait pattern. This augmented intervention is done in a functional pattern within an environment that perturbs the patient's/client's base of support. This perturbation moves each foot reciprocally backwards and the body forward, triggering a stepping reaction. In the case of an individual after a cerebrovascular accident (CVA), one leg will still respond normally, thus helping to trigger a between-limb reciprocal stepping action of the involved leg. In the case of bilateral involvement, both legs may need placement, requiring more external assistance. The intent of the intervention is to correct an impairment, leading to functional training to trigger normal motor programs necessary for gait. Simultaneously, augmented training done by a therapist includes manual assistance in the direction and rate of stepping, and placement of the involved leg throughout the gait cycle. In

this previous example, therapists need to make sure they are aware of the patient's center of gravity and do not move the foot before it should be at "push off" during the gait cycle. When selecting from a variety of treatment interventions, it is important for the therapist to consider that each intervention comes with different strategies and rationales that contribute to the expected outcome. All interventions should address the needs of the patient and must consider any emotional and cognitive restraints. Because these intervention strategies can be used simultaneously and in various combinations, it is important for the clinician to determine how and why the outcomes were influenced by the intervention. Without understanding the interactions of intervention methods and the outcome, treatment effectiveness and future clinical decision making remain unpredictable, and unique practice patterns and pathways are hard to identify with consistency.[7] A conscientious clinician knows how and why the decisions are made along the intervention pathway, communicates this rationale clearly, and leaves a legacy of effective patient/client care. The reader must remember that intervention encompasses multiple interactive environments where intervention decisions are often made moment by moment during any treatment period. The challenge to the clinician is to determine what is being done, why it is working, how to continue its effectiveness, and how to assess/measure the progress of the successful intervention. The clinician must also determine how to empower the patient/client (emotionally, cognitively, and motorically) to participate in the intervention with inherent, automatic mechanisms that lead to fluid, flexible, and functional outcomes that are independent of the therapist and not purely exclusive to the environment within which the activity is occurring. The efficacy of a specific treatment is often yet unestablished in the laboratory and research literature; therefore the patient's/clinician's thoughtful choice of interventions and outcome measures is the first step in determining treatment effectiveness. Once efficacy has been established through larger controlled studies within the clinical environment, researchers can begin to tease out separate variables and establish efficacy as part of evidence to justify clinical decision making.

HISTORY OF DEVELOPMENT OF INTERVENTIONS FOR NEUROLOGICAL DISABILITIES

In the mid-1900s the interventions by physical therapists (PTs) and occupational therapists (OTs) were separate. In general, PTs worked on gross motor activities, with specific emphasis on the lower extremities and the trunk, whereas OTs worked on the upper extremities and fine motor activities. Both professions focused on daily living skills, with those involving the arms falling within the domain of the OT and those involving the legs falling within the domain of the PT. Activities that required gross motor skills such as sitting, coming to stand, walking, walking with assistive devices, and running fell within the purview of the PT, whereas grooming, hygiene, and eating were the responsibility of the OT. Currently, this approach is not as commonly practiced owing to the understanding of motor learning, neuroplasticity, and motor programming and control. In the past, it was also accepted that the PT worked on specific system problems such as weakness, inflexibility, lack of coordination, and voluntary control, whereas the OT worked on functional activities integrated within the environment (such as dressing) and the patient's emotional needs and desires (occupational expectations). According to the terminology of the mid- to late 20th century, PTs were trained to identify and correct impairments that caused functional limitations, whereas OTs were trained in activity analysis and treatment that identified and optimized the functional activities that resulted from the impairments. Few clinicians seemed to focus on the sequential or interactive aspect of lack of function with specific impairments. Thus, after the onset of a stroke, the PT would strengthen and evaluate range of motion (ROM) of the leg and trunk, whereas the OT would encourage the patient to try to functionally use the arm. Both therapists hoped the patient would accept responsibility for continued improvement through practice. What both professions discovered was that the patient generally did not regain normal motor control. The patient may be able to walk and move the shoulder, but the movement strategies were generally stereotypical, were abnormal in patterns, and took tremendous effort by and energy from the patient to perform. Over time, patients lost the motivation to even try, and thus what had been gained through therapy may have been lost from lack of practice once they got home. There was also minimal recovery of functional hand use, often because of the tremendous effort a patient had to use to move the shoulder to place the hand somewhere. Once that effort had been used, the tightness and increased tone in the hand prevented functional use. Although measurable, functional, independent skills as were achieved, typical movement patterns and motor control were rarely restored, and quality of life was clearly affected for the patient and family.

During the decade or two before the 1960s, clinicians began to question the traditional therapeutic intervention strategies. Several renowned clinicians[8–32] in neurological rehabilitation pioneered the development of new concepts that allowed basic science to infiltrate the clinical arena. The intervention strategies of Jean Ayers, Berta Bobath, Signe Brunnstrom, Margaret Johnstone, Susanne Klein-Vogelbach, Margaret Knott, Dorothy Voss, and Margaret Rood, among others, became popular. Colleagues observed these master clinicians and could easily see that the "new" interventions were much more effective and provided better outcomes than previous interventions. Each approach focused on multisensory inputs introduced to the patient in controlled and identified sequences. These sequences were based on the inherent nature of synergistic patterns[8,24,33,34] and motor patterns observed in humans[8,10,35] and lower-order animals[36] or a combination of the two.[22,24] Each method focused on the individual patient, the specific clinical problems, and the availability of alternative treatment approaches within an established framework. Some of these approaches focused on specific neurological medical diagnoses. The treatment emphasis was then on specific patients and their related movement disorders. Children with cerebral palsy and head injuries[10,26,31] and adults with hemiplegia[11,12,24,35] were the three most frequently identified medical diagnoses associated with these approaches.

The timeline and evolution of clinical practice and research in the therapy professions can be derived in great part by understanding the products of a series of conferences, currently known as the STEP Conferences.[37] A summary of the four STEP conferences follows in this section to give the reader contextual perspective of present day intervention strategies for prevention of primary and secondary impairments, the choice and application of predictive measures, strategies to enhance patient participation, and ongoing research to examine exercise-induced brain plasticity.

Beginning in 1968 at Northwestern University with NUSTEP, and most recently in 2016 at the University of Ohio for IV Step, master clinicians and academics along with research scientists of the day have come together to try to (1) identify the commonalities and differences between therapeutic approaches, (2) integrate and use the neuroscience of the day to explain why these approaches worked,[38] and (3) promote the translation of new knowledge into clinical practice. Parallel to the STEP conferences, most dogmatism no longer persists with respect to territorial boundaries between PTs' and OTs' perceived ownership of a certain body systems or treatment approaches; this as result of the adoption of a systems model when looking at impairments, activity limitations, and participation in life interactions.[39]

Since the 1970s, substantial clinical attention has also been paid to children with learning and language difficulties.[8,16,40] Now these concepts and treatment procedures have been applied across the age spectrum for all types of medically diagnosed neurological problems seen in the clinical setting (refer to section Intervention Strategies of this text). This expansion of the use of any of the methods for any pathological condition manifested by insults from disease, injury, or degeneration of the brain seems to be a natural evolution given the structure and function of the CNS and commonalities in system problems and activity limitations that take the individual away from participating in life.

Since the II Step Conference in 1990, the boundaries for interventions began blurring. Intervention approaches such as proprioceptive neuromuscular facilitation (PNF) were then integrated into the care of patient's with orthopedic problems and patients with neurological impairments. Currently, few universities within the United States teach separate sections or units on specific approaches but rather teach students to identify impairments, when and how these interfere with functional activities, and what body systems may contribute to activity limitations or participation restriction.

For example, assume that a patient/client with hemiplegia exhibited signs of a hypertonic upper-extremity pattern of shoulder adduction, internal rotation, elbow flexion, and forearm pronation with wrist and finger flexion. Brunnstrom[11] would have identified that pattern as the stronger of her two upper-extremity synergies. Michels,[24] although using an explanation similar to Brunnstrom's to describe the pattern, would have elaborated and described additional upper-extremity synergy patterns. Bobath would have asserted that the patient/client was stuck in a mass-movement pattern resulting from abnormal postural reflex activity.[33] Although the conceptualization of the problem certainly determined treatment protocols, the pattern all three clinicians would have worked toward was shoulder abduction, external rotation, elbow extension, forearm supination, and wrist and finger extension. The rationale for the use of this pattern within an intervention period would vary according to the philosophical approach. One clinician might describe the pattern as a reflex-inhibiting position (Bobath).[34] Another would describe the pattern as the weakest component of the various synergies (Brunnstrom),[11] whereas still another might identify the pattern as producing an extreme stretch and rotational element that inhibited the spastic pattern (Rood).[28] How those master clinicians sequenced treatment from the original hypertonic pattern to the opposite pattern and then to the goal-directed functional pattern would vary. Some would facilitate push-pull patterns in the supine and side-lying positions and rolling. Others would look at propping patterns in sitting or at weight-bearing patterns of patients in the prone position, over a ball or bolster, or in partial kneeling. All have the potential of improving the functional pattern of the upper extremity and modifying the hypertonic pattern. One method may have been better than the others given a particular patient, but in truth, improved patient performance may have stemmed not from the method itself but rather from the preferential CNS biases of the patient and the variability of application skills among the clinicians themselves. That is, when a therapist intentionally uses specific augmented feedback to modulate the motor system's response to an environment but does not identify the other external feedback present within that environment (e.g., lighting, sound, touch, environmental constraints), therapeutic results will vary. Because of variance, efficacy of intervention is often questionable, although the effectiveness of that therapist may be easily recognized.

Because of the overlap of intervention strategies and the infiltration of therapeutic management into all avenues of neurological dysfunction, various multisensory models were developed during the early 1980s.[16,41–44] These have continued to evolve into acceptable methods in the current clinical arena. Although these models attempted to integrate existing techniques, in reality they have created a new set of holistic treatment approaches. In July 2005, the III STEP conference[45] was held in Utah to again bring current theories and evidence-based practice into the current clinical environment. The history of the three STEP conferences demonstrates the evolution of evidence-based practice from the first conference, where basic science was the only evidence to justify treatment, to the second conference, where evidence in motor learning and motor control began to bring efficacy to intervention. By the time the third conference was held, the research in neuro/movement science regarding true efficacy within practice and the reliability and validity of our examination tools set the stage for standards in practice.[46] No proceedings from that third conference were published, but over the preceding years, articles covering most of the presentations had been published in *Physical Therapy*. The ultimate goal would be to develop one all-encompassing methodology that allows the clinician the freedom to use any method that is appropriate for the needs and individual learning styles of the patient as well as to tap the unique individual differences of the clinician. Although intervention currently is based on an integrated model, the influence of third-party payers, the need for efficacy of practice, and time constraints often factor into the therapist's choice of intervention. Visionary and entrepreneurial practice ideas that have the potential to be effective will always be a challenge to future therapists. Those ideas generally originate within the clinical environment and not the research laboratory. For that reason, clinicians need to communicate ideas to the researcher, and then those researchers can develop research studies that test the established efficacy or refute that effectiveness. Few researchers are master clinicians, and few clinicians are master researchers; thus collaboration is needed as the professions move forward in establishing evidence-based practice.

Today's therapists have replaced many of the existing philosophical approaches with patient-centered therapeutic interventions. Patient performance, values and preferences, available evidence, and the expertise of the clinician often play key roles in the clinical decision making process. Control of the combination of movement responses and modulation over specific central pattern generators or learned behavior programs will allow the patient opportunities to experience functional movement that is task oriented and environmentally specific. With goal-directed practice of the functional activity, neuroplastic changes, motor learning, and carryover can be achieved.[47] With a better scientific basis for understanding the function of the human nervous system, how the motor system learns and is controlled, and how other body systems, both internal and external to the CNS, modulate response patterns, today's clinicians have many additional options for selection of intervention strategies.[48–57] Whether a patient would initially benefit best from neuromuscular retraining, functional retraining, or a more traditional augmented or contrived treatment environment is based on the specific needs identified during the examination and evaluation process.

No matter what treatment method is selected by a clinician, all intervention should focus on the active learning process of the patient. The patient should never be a passive participant nor should the patient be asked to perform an activity when the system problems only create distortion or demonstrate total lack of control of the desired movement. With all interventions requiring an active motor response, whether to change a body system impairment such as by increasing or reducing the rate of a motor response, modulate the tonal state of the central pattern generators and learned motor behaviors, or influence a functional response during an activity, the patient's CNS is being asked to process and respond to the external world. That response needs to become procedural and controlled by the patient without any augmentation to be measured as functionally independent. In time, the ultimate goal is for the patient to self-regulate and orchestrate modulation over this adaptable and dynamic integrated sensorimotor system in all functional activities and in all external environments.

A problem-oriented approach to the treatment of any impairment or activity limitation implies that flexibility and neural adaptation are key elements in recovery. However, adaptation should not be random, disjointed, or non–goal oriented. It should be based on methods that provide the best combination of available treatment alternatives to meet the specific needs of the individual. Development of a clinical knowledge bank enables the therapist to match treatment alternatives with the patient's impairments, activity limitations, objectives for improved function, and desired quality of life. A therapist no longer bases treatment on identified approaches, although specific aspects of those approaches may be treatment tools that will meet the patient's needs and assist him or her in regaining functional control of movement. Intervention is based on an interaction among basic science, applied science, the therapist's skills, and the patient's desired outcomes.[52–55,58–60] In most cases, multiple intervention strategies must be included, but the therapist needs to be able to identify why those selected treatments will lead to system improvement, as well as documenting those findings using reliable standardized and acceptable clinical methods and terminology. These intervention strategies must be dynamic yet also understandable and repeatable. As new scientific theories are discovered, new information must be integrated to continue to modify treatment approaches.

INTERVENTION STRATEGIES

Functional Training

Functional training is a method of retraining the motor system using repetitive practice of functional tasks in an attempt to reestablish the patient's/client's ability to perform activities of daily living (ADLs) and participate in specific life activities. This method of training is a common and popular intervention strategy used by clinicians owing to the fact that it is a relatively simple and straightforward approach to improving deficits in function. A system problem such as weakness in the quadriceps muscle of the leg can be treated by muscle strengthening in a functional pattern that can be easily measured. Because of its inherent simplicity, functional training is sometimes misused or abused by clinicians. Most patients with neurological deficits have multiple subsystem problems within multiple areas, which forces the CNS to use alternative movement patterns to try to accomplish the functional task presented. If the therapist accesses a motor plan such as transfers but allows the patient to use programs that are inefficient, inappropriate, or stereotypical, then the activity itself is often beyond the patient's ability. The patient may learn something, but it will not be the normal program for transfers. This activity often leads to additional problems for the patient.

The intricate relationship of body system problems, impairments, and functional limitations that decrease participation in the rehabilitation process are discussed. Functional training can be implemented once the clinician has identified the patient's activity limitations. The clinician must first answer the questions: "What can the individual do?" "What limitations does the patient have when engaging in functional activities in his or her daily environments?" "Are there motor programs that are being used to substitute for typical motor function?" and "Can the therapist use functional training to improve body system problems within the context of the functional skill?" Once the therapist develops an understanding of the potential reasons for activity limitations and can alleviate the substitution and compensation for the deficit, functional tasks should be identified and practiced.

Effect of Functional Training on Task Performance and Participation

The main focus of functional training is the correction of activity limitations that prevent an individual from participating in life. However, through repetitive practice of functional tasks and gross motor patterns, many of the patient's impairments can also be affected. For example, if a therapist practices sit-to-stand transfers with a patient in a variety of environments and performs multiple repetitions of each type of transfer, not only can learning be reinforced, but the patient can also gain strength in the synergistic patterns of the lower extremities that work against gravity to concentrically lift the patient off of the support surface and eccentrically lower him or her down. Weight bearing through the feet in a variety of degrees of ankle dorsiflexion during transfer training will effectively place the ankles in functional positions. The act of standing also helps the trunk and neck extensors to engage in postural control. Varying the speed of the activity during the treatment can stimulate cerebellar adaptation to the movement task. Moving from one position to another with the head in a variety of positions stimulates the vestibular apparatus and may assist in habituating a hypersensitive vestibular system, allowing the patient to change body positions without symptoms of dizziness, resulting in a higher quality of life. Repetitive practice also affects the vasomotor system and may assist in habituating postural hypotensive responses.

Functional training should access the patient's highest level of independent and uncompensated movement—this is often challenging. For example, early gait training for patient's with acute stroke may take place in artificial environments, such as within parallel bars. If the therapist providing the training is not cognizant of the quality and goal of the patient's postural control and body movement, the patient/ may use a dysfunctional, inefficient motor program. An example outcome of prolonged, ineffective gait training within the parallel bars can be seen in a patient with CVA who relies heavily on the nonparetic upper extremity for support on one bar, resulting in the next compensation of forward trunk lean, then hip retraction and knee hyperextension on the hemiparetic limb during single limb stance phase. If this misuse of functional training is not recognized, the patient may have long-lasting dysfunctional use of both the upper and lower extremity.

Instead, the astute therapist will use strategies to help the patient to safely and gradually explore appropriate movement strategies, provide the patient with a variable practice environment for walking (e.g., out of the parallel bars), and ultimately improve the plasticity of the patient's nervous system during recovery. Functional training is the best method of intervention when the patient has some motor abilities with limitations such as limited ROM or inadequate muscle power from disuse. Functional training will use existing abilities until fatigue sets in, which may be after only one or two repetitions. Increasing the repetitions and/or the power necessary to complete the tasks will lead to functional improvement. An intervention approach in the early 1990s that evolved as an offshoot of functional training was labeled *clinical pathways.* These pathways were established by health care institutions to improve consistency of management of patients who met specific medical diagnostic criteria. It has been proven that the implementation of these pathways reduces variability in clinical practice and improves patient outcomes.[61] Health care practitioners also became aware that some individuals do not fall into these pathways and need to be treated according to the specific clinical problems that the patients were presenting.

Selection of Functional Training Strategies

What is the "ideal" procedure for effectively and efficiently using functional training as a treatment intervention? First, it is suggested that the clinician identify and select procedures that will use the patient's strengths to regain lost function and correct system limitations—"What can the individual do?" The clinician is also advised to avoid activities that may be too difficult and elicit compensatory strategies that may result in the development of abnormal, stereotypical movement and potentially create additional impairments. An example of this is using transfer training when the patient is unable to perform the task with some element of success. Once in a situation where the patient fails to perform the task, the patient uses approaches to prevent from falling, not activities that allow the patient to safely transfer. The therapist's decision regarding what functional patterns or activities to practice, and in what order, will depend on several factors. The therapist must choose functional activities that are necessary for the patient to perform independently or manage with less help before being discharged home. For PTs, safe transfers and ambulation are generally the focus of functional training. For OTs, independent bathing, dressing, and feeding are major foci. Yet both PTs and OTs also need to be sensitive to the activities that the patient or the patient's family want to improve to enhance the quality of life for everyone involved in the person's case. The ability to get in and out of a car might be the most important activity due to frequent trips to the physician's office and the primary caregiver's limited abilities to physically assist.

It is suggested that the clinician modify or "shrink" the environment to allow normal motor programs to run. An example of this might be to limit the ROM an individual is allowed while performing a rolling pattern. The therapist may opt to start this movement with the patient in a side-lying position. The amount of patient movement may be even further limited by the therapist stabilizing the patient's hips by using the therapist's one leg in kneeling position against the patient's posterior pelvis and the therapist's other leg in half-kneeling position with the top leg of the patient over the therapist's half-kneeling leg. In this way, the individual's body can be totally controlled by the therapist; the patient can be encouraged to roll the upper part of his trunk both backward with the arm reaching back and then forward with the arm coming across the body toward a weight-bearing pattern on the hand. The therapist can change the rate of movement and also use his or her knees to control the range that the patient is allowed. The environment can be progressively "enlarged" to allow the patient/client to perform the activity in a functional context. Although this narrowing of the functional environment would be considered a contrived environment and must not be recorded as functional as defined in a functional or activities-based examination, it may allow the nervous system the opportunity to control and modify the motor programs within the limitations of its plasticity at the moment. This therapeutic technique could be used within a functional training environment or may fall into an augmented treatment approach category, given an individual who has neurological problems that prevent normal movement.

The goal of therapy is to move toward functional training as quickly as the patient's motor system can control the movement. As learning and repetition assist the CNS in widening the response pattern during a functional activity, the patient's ability to respond to variance within the environment will enlarge and assist in gaining greater independence. An example of this application of functional training might be asking a patient/client to perform a stand-to-sit transfer. The patient is first guided down to sitting onto a large gym ball, a high-low table, or a stool that allows the patient to sit only one-fourth to one-half of the way down before returning to stand. As the patient develops increased strength and balance and improved control over abnormal limb synergies and tone in this pattern, then a smaller gym ball or a lower point on a high-low table can be used. Finally, the patient is asked to sit down onto a ball/mat or chair that results in sitting with the hips and knees at 90 degrees. Once the patient can sit down and return to a vertical position, the next task will be to sit down, relax, and then stand up. When this task is done easily, the patient will be functionally able move from standing to sitting and to reverse the movement pattern to sitting to standing.

Although many clinicians understand the importance of running motor tasks within an appropriate biomechanical, musculoskeletal, and sensorimotor window in which the patient has the ability to perform procedures functionally, it may be argued that in many cases this particular type of treatment strategy is simply not possible in a real-world situation. For example, given the current health care environment, if the patient is given a limited number of visits to achieve the desired outcome, the clinician may conclude that there is no choice but to "allow as many degrees of freedom as possible" or, in other words, to "force the window open" no matter the abnormal movement patterns used or the limitations in independent functional control that they may produce.

In summary, the clinician should first identify and emphasize the patient's strengths and use those strengths to efficiently and effectively achieve functional change. Next, the clinician must prioritize activities that need to be addressed; the choice of what activities to emphasize during therapeutic training always poses a dilemma to therapists. One should keep in mind that, although several skills may be learned by training them simultaneously, it may make more sense to concentrate on the safe performance of one or two necessary functional tasks rather than having the patient end up being able to perform multiple tasks that require considerable outside assistance for safety. The need to work functionally on additional activities may also be an opportunity for the clinician to request additional therapy visits for the patient/client, arguing that there is a reasonable expectation that more intervention would result in a greater increase in function and a greater decrease in the risk for potential injury than if the intervention were not continued. The use of valid and reliable functional outcome measures becomes critically important in case management. These tools objectively measure the effect of the intervention, help to predict the potential risks if the therapy is not continued, and ultimately aid in the justification to continue therapeutic intervention.

One important variable that has clearly been identified with respect to functional training is "task specificity."[50,62–70] Although it is important that a patient be independent in as many ADLs as possible, often the therapist, the patient, and the family need to prioritize which activities are most important to the quality of life of the patient. If walking into the mountains to do "birdwatching" is one important goal to the patient, then creating an environment that would closely resemble the environment of that activity is crucial. Similarly, practice within that environment is a key to successful carryover. If the patient wants to walk into the mountains and the family expects the patient to walk into his or her old job, a therapist must accept that motivation will drive behavior and task specificity will drive learning. Carryover into any other functional activity such as walking into the office building to go back to work may not be the motivating factor that will guide that individual's desire to perform that motor task. Whether the patient ever goes back to work is not the variable that should be used as part of the motivational environment for task-specific gait training geared to walking in the mountains and is not a decision for which the therapist is responsible. Therapists need to elicit the most important activities for the patient and use the specificity of that task to optimize motor learning and functional recovery.

CASE STUDY 8.1   Functional Training: Ambulation

Teaching a patient to ambulate can be approached in many ways. Assume that the objective for a particular session is ambulation. First, the patient may be asked to ambulate in the parallel bars using the upper extremities to assist in forward progression of the movement to decrease fear and to assist in maintaining balance. Once the patient can perform this ambulatory activity, the therapist might decide to progress the patient's ambulation by introducing a walker, which has four points of support. Ambulating with the walker will again increase power production in the legs and create an environment of safety for the patient. Once walking with the walker can be performed at various speeds and distances, the therapist may advance the activity to using two canes, then one cane depending on the patient's balance, coordination, and need. While the patient is practicing ambulating with cane(s), he may also be walking supported on a treadmill to increase endurance, velocity of gait, and power. Once the patient can ambulate safely with a cane, the therapist may decide to transition to walking without any assistive devices. Again, the patient may first be asked to walk on a treadmill while holding on with his arms until he feels safe walking and no longer needs an assistive device. The therapist could transition to ramps, obstacles, uneven ground, and so on. All these activities would require the individual to begin with functional control. All the activities are focused on regaining independence in the functional activity of walking, using repetitive practice. Training can continue with or without an assistive device, with consideration that a device itself will usually limit the environments within which a patient can ambulate independently.

Intervention for Impairments

The therapeutic examination results in the identification of activity limitations and possible body system and subsystem impairments that are causing the functional movement disorders. Directly addressing these system impairments is another intervention strategy that involves the intervention for impairments with the expectation that improving these will result in a corresponding improvement in function. For example, when a patient has the inability to stand up without assistance (activity limitation) and the clinician determines the cause to be lower-extremity weakness, an appropriate approach may be to strengthen the lower extremities. Numerous studies have shown the effectiveness of addressing impairments directly in improving the functional performance of individuals with neurological conditions such as cerebral palsy,[71,72] stroke,[73–81] multiple sclerosis,[82–87] Parkinson disease,[88–92] and other neuromuscular diagnoses.[93–104] Considering the previous case, the strengthening interventions should reflect the task and the environment within which the impairment was identified. The clinician should attempt to create a training situation so that the patient may be able to run the necessary motor programs with all the required subsystems in place. For example, training sit-to-stand with weakness in the hip and knee extensors is much less likely to automatically result in the improvement of sit-to-stand function if the therapist begins the activity in sitting, where generation of extension is most difficult, than if the strengthening training was performed with repetition of practice starting in standing and going to sit and back again to stand. By decreasing the degrees of freedom of the eccentric control of the hips and knees when going from stand to sit, the functional training activity has turned into specific impairment training. The therapist can ask the patient to eccentrically lengthen the extensors only in a limited range and then concentrically contract back to standing. As the power increases, the degrees of freedom can also be enlarged until the patient is able to complete the task of stand to sit while simultaneously regaining the sit to stand pattern.

In pure impairment training, a patient might also be asked to straighten the knee when sitting or to extend the hip when prone. These three exercises have the potential of training impaired strength, but only the first example forces the training within a functional pattern. Similarly, the therapist could train the sit-to-stand pattern using various seat heights that encompass many of the components that force the use of normal movement synergies and postural control, using the environment in which that activity is typically performed, versus performance of strengthening exercises against resistance in an open chain exercise program.

The decision to treat the impairments causing the activity limitations or to correct the functional problems themselves is influenced by many factors. One critical factor is the therapists' ability to isolate the cause of the atypical movement pattern. Different impairments may potentially contribute to atypical movement; thorough movement analysis and testing should elicit the impairments that at contribute most to movement dysfunction and that should be targeted during interventions. It would appear that for certain tasks to be completed the patient must possess the "threshold amount" of basic movement components required for the task. Task specificity within this limited environment will result in more meaningful changes in function.

Augmented Therapeutic Intervention

Some treatment alternatives require little if any hands-on therapeutic manipulation of the patient during the activity. For example, the patient practices transfers on and off many support surfaces with standby guarding only. The patient self-corrects or uses inherent feedback mechanisms to self-correct error to refine the motor skill. This ultimate empowerment allows each individual to adapt and succeed at self-identified and self-motivated objectives first with augmented intervention and finally without any assistance. Often, allowing the patient to attempt movement without assistance enables the therapist to evaluate what components of the task the patient can control and what components are not within the patient's current capabilities, especially if normal, fluid, efficient, and effortless movement is the desired outcome. In some cases, the therapist may use hands-on skills or augmented aids such as BWSTT, which would substitute for many aspects of the environment and allow the patient to succeed at the task—*but* the control and feedback during the activity would be considered augmented feedback and fall into that classification.

Augmented techniques make up a large component of the therapist's specific interventions tool box. Augmented training may be done as part of a functional, task-specific activity but could also be administered in nonfunctional positions, depending on therapeutic goals. In augmented training the therapist may use a piece of equipment to be part of the patient's external environment for the patient to succeed at the task. For example, in BWSTT a harness is used to take away the demand of gravity on the limbs during gait and the demand of the postural trunk and hip muscles for stability. Before the therapist or the patient can consider the movement as independent, those aspects must be removed from the environment. In the previous example, the individual needs to transition from maximal body weight support during ambulation to not needing any external support during ambulation. The patient must assume *total ownership* of the functional responses. Then and only then has independence been achieved. At that time, functional retraining can be used with the intent of enlarging the environmental parameters to allow for maximal independence. Augmented techniques are often the early choices for treatment of patients who have neurological insults. It cannot be emphasized enough that once the patient has the ability to perform without augmented

methods and does so in functional, efficient ways, those augmented techniques need to be selectively eliminated.

Once a clinician has chosen to augment the clinical environment, the patient needs to learn efficient motor behaviors within the limitations of that environment. The patient influences the therapist's decision making strategies by selecting inefficient or ineffective motor responses to a given task demand. If the response is effortless, efficient, and noninjurious to any part of the body and meets the patient's expectations and goals, then the therapist knows the strategies selected were effective even if the therapist augmented the intervention. If the movement itself is available to the patient, then there is a high probability that the patient will be able to regain that movement control, regardless of the need for early augmentation to achieve the skill. If the response does not meet the desired goal for any reason, then the therapist must determine why. Often, it is because the therapist did not identify the correct body system impairments. Which solution is best may be more patient than approach dependent. Fig. 8.1 summarizes the use of these intervention approaches as a roadmap for neurological rehabilitation.

The clinician has little basis for decision making without a comprehensive understanding of the neurophysiological mechanisms of (1) the various techniques introduced to modify input, (2) where that information will be processed and how that might affect motor output, (3) prior learning and the ability for new learning, and (4) the patient's willingness and motivation to adapt.

The number of available augmented feedback techniques is almost infinite. This section presents an overview of a classification system that can be used to help the reader develop a greater understanding of why certain responses occur and why the selection of certain techniques is appropriate and should positively affect the desired motor responses. This section focuses on intervention strategies that have been accepted, have been used within the traditional Western health care model, and are efficacious. There are other classification systems a clinician might use when analyzing movement problems seen in patients with neurological dysfunction. For example, a therapist may see in a patient a problem primarily with tone, such as hypertonicity, hypotonicity, rigidity, dystonia, flaccidity, intentional and nonintentional tremors, ataxia, and combinations of or fluctuations in the total movement strategies. Given this specific classification schema, one still uses the available treatment strategies or uses an input modality that may modify the specific tone problem that was causing the movement dysfunction.

The primary goal of this section is to help the reader develop a classification system based on the primary input modality used when introducing an augmented treatment technique to facilitate a sensory system and provide feedback to the CNS to help a patient learn or relearn motor control.

When the primary input system for a technique is identified, at no time do we suggest that it is the only input system affected. For example, when a proprioceptive technique is introduced, tactile cutaneous receptors are also simultaneously firing. If there is a "noise" component (such as with vibration or tapping with the fingers), then auditory input has been triggered as well. There is evidence that a given sensory modality may "cross over" or fuse with a completely different modality, helping in the synthesis of motor responses. In addition, there is evidence that the principles of neuroplasticity are applicable across modalities (e.g., auditory, visual, vestibular, somatosensory). Sometimes responses occur in a modality that does not appear to be related. For example, olfaction may improve tactile sensitivity of the hand. This concept is called *cross-modal training* or *stimulation*.[105,106] Yet, a classification schema based on a primary modality promotes

Patient/client enters clinical environment

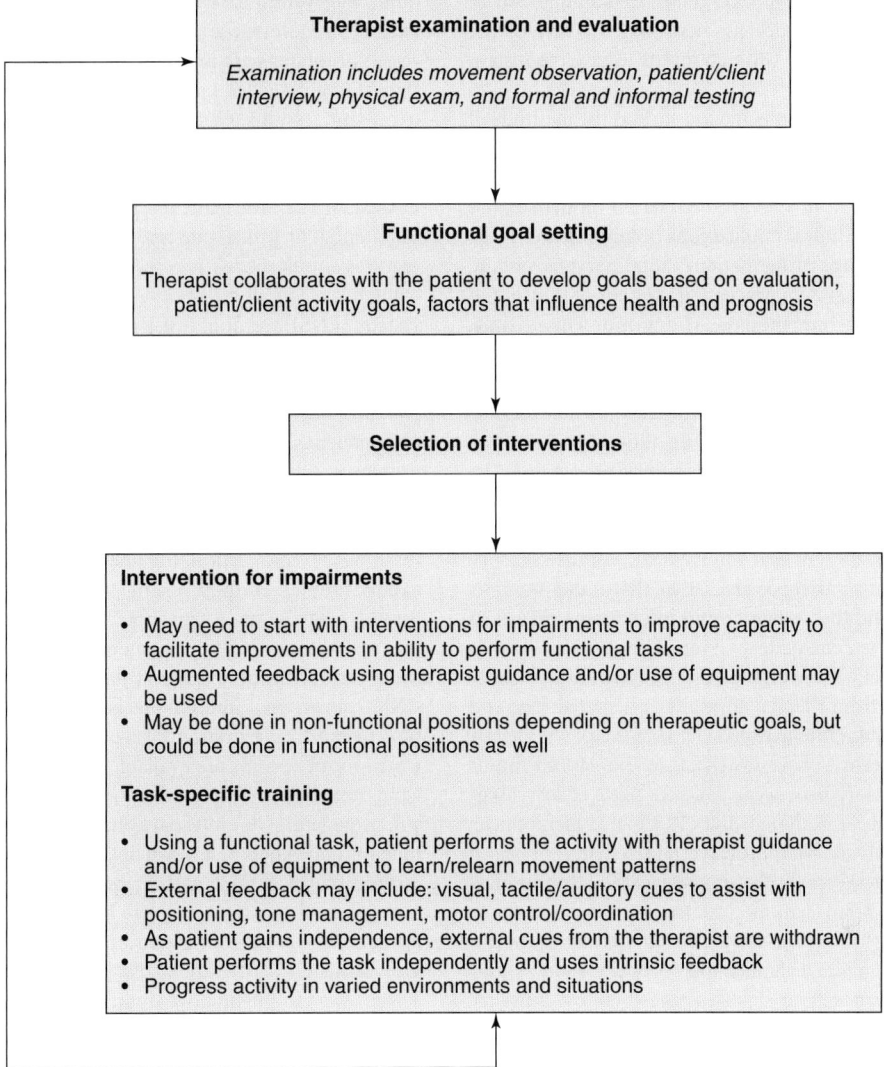

Fig. 8.1 Roadmap for Neurological Rehabilitation. (Modified from the original work of Jan Davis, OTR, San Jose State University.)

logical problem solving because the therapist can select from available treatment procedures that theoretically provide similar information to the CNS and help in the organization of appropriate motor responses. The motor system and its various motor programmers adapt to the environment to achieve functional motor output toward a goal. Both external and internal feedback are critical for adaptation and change. External feedback in this chapter is considered a mechanism to help the patient's CNS optimally learn and adapt. Obviously, as the patient learns, internal feedback will allow the person to run feedforward motor programs without the need for external feedback for control. External feedback will, it is hoped, be used only when the outside surrounding needs the feedforward program to change to adapt to a new environment (refer to the Chapter 3 section on motor learning). Therapists must realize that even if the primary goal may be to facilitate or dampen a motor system response, diverging pathways may also connect with endocrine, immune, and autonomic systems. According to motor control theory, the clinical picture is a consensus of all interacting body systems (see Chapter 3). Research tools are not yet available

to measure those systems interacting simultaneously, although functional magnetic resonance imaging (fMRI) studies are beginning to help researchers and clinicians identify what happens to the nervous system with input from the environment and how that information is processed. Efficacy using reliable and valid measurement tools must then be based on outcomes, with an understanding of the best available scientific knowledge as a rationale for why the outcome is present.

This classification system is based on identified input, observed responses, current research on the function of the CNS, and the various systems involved in the control and modification of responses. An understanding of normal processing of input and its effect on the motor systems helps the clinician to evaluate and use the intact systems as part of treatment. Research with fMRI is currently allowing greater insight into specific brain regions that are being used during various cognitive and motor activities.[107–122] Yet the specific interactive nature of multisensory input, memory, motivation, and motor function is still unknown. When the response to certain stimuli does not help the patient select or adapt a desired motor response, then the classification schema for augmented input provides the clinician with flexibility to select additional options. This can be done by spatially summating input, such as using stretch, vibration, and resistance simultaneously, or temporally summating input, such as increasing the rate of the quick stretch or increasing the time between inputs to give the system ample time to respond.

Many factors can influence motor behavior, such as the methods of instruction, the resting condition of the nervous system, synaptic connections, cerebellar or basal ganglia or cortical processing, retrieval from past learning, motor output systems, or internal influences and neuroendocrine balance. Its clinical implications become clearer if the therapist retains a visual image of the patient's total nervous system, including afferent input, intersystem processing, efferent response, and the multiple interactions on one another. At any moment in time, multiple stimuli are admitted into a patient's input system. Before that information reaches a level of primary processing, it will cross at least one if not many synaptic junctions. At that time the information may be inhibited, excited, changed or distorted, or allowed to continue without modification. If the information is at the first synapse, the patient will have no sensation. If it is inhibited at the thalamus, again the patient will not perceive sensation, but that does not mean other areas of the brain will not be sent that information, because sensory information is also sent to a variety of areas after that initial synapse. Research studies have found that sensory input information may even affect gait and other movement patterns even if the patient has no perception of the input.[123,124] If the input is changed, then the processing of the input will vary from the one normally anticipated. The end product after multiple system interactions will be close to, will be farther away from, or will seem to have no effect on the desired motor pattern. Furthermore, sensory processing can take place at many segments of the nervous system. Although the CNS is not hierarchical, with one level in total control over another, certain systems are biased to affect various motor responses. At the spinal level the response may be phasic and synergistic. Brain stem mechanisms may evoke flexor or extensor biases, depending on various motor systems and their modulation. Cerebellar, basal ganglia, thalamic, and cortical responses may be more adaptive and purposeful.[124–127] Thus the therapist must try to discern where the input or the feedback is being affective or short circuited.

Remembering input as a possible option for intervention will always allow the therapist to differentiate the same five alternatives—no response, facilitating (heightening), inhibiting (dampening), distorting, or normal processing. These alternatives can occur anywhere in the system at synaptic junctions. Finally, motor output is programmed and a response is observed. If the response is considered normal, the clinician assumes that the system is intact with regard to the use and processing of the inputs. If the response is distorted or absent, little is known other than there is a lack of the normal processing somewhere in the CNS or an insufficient amount of input was used. One way to differentiate motor problems from problems with other systems is to use other functional activities that have programs similar to the body system program identified as impaired. If a program, such as posture, demonstrates deficiencies in one functional pattern, then the therapist must determine if it is also deficient in other patterns. If the postural motor problem affects all motor performance, then the therapist had determined that a motor program deficit exists and will have to determine how to correct that problem. If, on the other hand, the program runs smoothly and effortlessly when certain demands are taken away, such as resistance from gravity, position in space, need for quick responses, and so forth, then it may be that the problem is within another subsystem such as cognition, perception, the biomechanical system, or the cardiopulmonary system or is a power-production problem that can be corrected by slowly increasing the demand on the postural system through repetitive practice using various additional input interventions. Differentially screening motor impairments as pure CNS motor problems (muscle recruitment, firing rate, balance) versus problems with another system (perception of vertical) becomes critical in a managed-care system that funds only a certain number of treatment sessions. Once normal processing has been identified, understanding of deficit systems and potential problems can be analyzed more easily. To reiterate, this requires awareness of the totality of the individual (i.e., the patient's personal preference of stimuli and the uniqueness of processing and internal influences). A systems model requires simultaneous processing of multiple areas, with interactions being relayed in all directions. A patient's CNS and peripheral nervous system (PNS) are doing just that, and the therapist must develop a sensitivity toward the patient as a whole while interacting with specific components. With input from the patient and family, it is the therapist's responsibility to select methods most efficacious and effective for each patient's needs in relation to that person's specific neurological problems. This viewpoint, based on a variety of questions, leads to a problem-oriented approach to intervention. Because the output or response pattern is based on α motor neuron discharge and thus extrafusal muscle contraction, the *first question* is posed: what can be done to alter the state of the alpha motor neuron pool or motor generators? *Second*, what input systems are available, either directly or indirectly, that will alter the state of the motor pool? *Third*, which techniques use these various input systems as their primary modes of entry into the CNS? *Fourth*, what internal mechanisms need modification or adaptation to produce a desired behavior response from the patient? *Fifth*, which input systems are available to alter the internal mechanism and what outcomes are expected? *Sixth*, what combination of input stimuli will provide the best internal homeostatic environment for the patient to learn and rehearse a more optimal response pattern? For example, assume that a patient with a residual hemiplegia resulting from an anterior cerebral artery problem has a hypertonic lower extremity that produces the pattern of extension, adduction, internal rotation of the hip, extension of the knee, and plantarflexion inversion of the foot. The answers to the first two questions are based on the knowledge that the proprioceptive and exteroceptive systems can drastically affect spinal central pattern generators and that these input systems are intact at spinal, brain stem, cerebellum, and thalamic levels and may even project to the cortex.

Appropriate selection of specific techniques will provide viable treatment alternatives. Awareness that a patient's/client's response pattern is an inherent synergistic pattern leads to a better understanding of the clinical problem. Knowing that the patient/client is unable to combine the alternative patterns, such as hip flexion with knee extension needed for the late stage of swing phase through the early aspects of stance phase during gait, the therapist can use the other inherent processes to elicit these and other patterns. BWSTT is an example of an augmented treatment intervention in which the clinician assists the patient to place the leg and foot with each step while the apparatus controls balance and posture to provide an experience of normal gait while requiring the patient to have only the strength to manage partial body weight.[128–133] Finally, techniques such as combining standing and walking with the application of quick stretch, vibration, or rotation, or having the patient reach for a target or follow a visual stimulus while walking, provide a variety of combinations of therapeutic procedures to help the patient learn or relearn normal response patterns. Furthermore, combining techniques gives the clinician a choice of various procedures and promotes a learning environment that is flexible, changing, and interesting. The therapist must, again, make the transition from applying contrived therapeutic procedures during functional tasks to allowing the patient to practice the task without the therapist interceding and without external feedback.[134] In that way the patient uses inherent feedback to self-correct feedforward motor programming and then to continue running the appropriate movement strategies.

Proprioceptive System Integration of Stretch, Joint, and Tendon Receptors

Proprioceptive training is proposed to benefit somatosensory and sensorimotor function through cortical reorganization that occurs in response to repetitive active or passive movement. Proprioception[135] as an input system has a direct effect on program generators at the spinal level.[136] However, because of its importance in motor learning and motor adaptation to new or changing environments, proprioception also has significant connections to the cortical and cerebellar neural networks. Its divergent pathways have synapses within the brain stem, diencephalon, and spinal system. Proprioceptive input can potentially influence multiple levels of CNS function, and all those levels can potentially modulate the intensity or importance of that information through many different mechanisms.[136,137] Proprioceptors are found in three peripheral anatomical locations: the stretch receptors, the tendon, and the joint. The afferent receptors responsible for relaying sensory information through those sites are discussed in the following subsections.

Muscle stretch receptors

Stretch. Stretch, quick stretch, and maintained stretch are all sensory input systems that use the stretch receptors in the muscles and heighten the motor pool.[138–140] Stretch simultaneously heightens both the muscle response to stretch and potentially heightens the sensitivity of the agonistic synergy. It will also lower the excitation of the antagonistic muscle and those muscles that are part of the antagonistic synergy. Stretch information will be sent to higher centers for sensory integration and perception. The cerebellum uses this incoming feedback to maintain and/or regulate motor nuclei in the brain stem that will influence the state of the α and γ motor neurons. This allows for cerebellar feedforward regulation (refer to Chapter 19). There are many ways to apply stretch to the muscles. The therapist can use (1) the hands and their respective muscle power to apply a stretch, (2) a manual weight system of some sort that maintains the stretch through the range, (3) a suspension system such as used in Pilates exercises, (4) the patient's own body weight against gravity, (5) a complex robotic system that computerizes the amount of stretch depending on the individual's specific data, or many other creative ways to apply stretch to muscle fibers within the belly of the muscle tissue. As stated previously, stretch can also be applied to the antagonist muscle or muscle synergy to dampen agonist function. Thus stretch can be used to enhance tone in the agonist or to decrease tone of the agonist through the antagonist. The therapist should always remember that even though a response may not look obvious, as long as the peripheral nerves and motor neurons within the spinal system are intact, these approaches will change the state of the motor pool.

Table 8.1 lists a variety of treatment procedures believed to use proprioceptive input from the muscles as a primary mode of sensory stimulation. The varying intensity, amount of tension, or rate of the stimuli, in addition to the original length of the muscle before application of the stimulus, will determine its firing. Remember, afferent information is projecting to many areas above the spinal system, and the result will be regulation or modulation, ultimately affecting activity.[136]

Resistance and strengthening. Resistance is often used to facilitate intrafusal and extrafusal muscle contraction. Resistance can be applied manually, mechanically, and by the use of gravity. Resistance recruits more motor units in the target muscles. Although muscles can contract both in an isometric and an isotonic fashion, most

TABLE 8.1 Treatment Suggestions Using Proprioceptive Input from the Muscles

1. Resistance
2. Quick stretch to agonist
3. Tapping: tendon and/or muscle belly
4. Reverse tapping: gravity stretches; tapping agonist into shortened range
5. Positioning (range)
6. Electrical stimulation
7. Pressure or sustained stretch
8. Stretch pressure
9. Stretch release
10. Vibration: facilitatory frequency for small vibrator, relaxation for total-body vibration
11. Gravity as a prolonged stretch
12. Active motion

contractions consist of a mixture of the two. Certain muscle groups, such as the flexors, benefit from isometric exercise, as well as isotonic exercise in both eccentric and concentric modes. Under normal circumstances, the flexors are used for repetitive or rhythmical activities. The extensors, on the other hand, usually remain contracted in an effort to act against the forces of gravity. Therefore the extensor groups benefit best from isometric and eccentric resistance.[141]

When resistance is applied to a voluntary muscle, spindle afferent fibers and tendon organs fire in proportion to the magnitude of the resistance. Resistance is more facilitative to an isometrically contracted muscle than in an isotonic contraction.[40] As isometric resistance is increased or continued, more motor units are recruited, thereby increasing the strength of extrafusal contraction.[29] Eccentric isotonic contraction refers to the lengthening of muscle fibers with resistance added to the distal segment, as in lowering the arms while holding a heavy weight. Eccentric contraction uses less metabolic output and promotes strength gains in less time.[29] Resistance is an important clinical treatment and has been used and will continue to be used by clinicians within multiple treatment philosophies over the next millennium.[11,22,28,32,71,142–148] The complexity of neural adaptation after resistive exercises may lead to a different training environment depending on age, athletic status, and specific body system deficits.[149] Combining resistive training with guided imagery or other types of adjunct interactions has conflicting results.[149–151] Yet there are still questions regarding optimal resistive training, in particular, the parameters of load and work frequency,[152,153] and whether one resistive technique is better than another.[154,155] Research certainly has shown that resistance training does enhance functional abilities across age groups,[145,156,157] but[158] again the specific resistive training techniques are often not identified. The terms *resistive training*, *weight training*, and *strength training* are often used synonymously, and thus specifics are yet to be identified in the research. How all these uses of resistive exercises will play out in the future is up to future researchers in the field of movement science. Very costly high-technology tools have been added to aid in resistive training.[159,160] Given the needs of individuals after neurological insults, cost becomes a major factor, and finding creative and cost-efficient ways to apply resistance may become a common research question in the future.

Tapping. Three types of tapping techniques are commonly used by therapists. Tapping of the tendon is a fairly nondiscriminatory stimulus. Physicians use this technique to determine the degree of stretch sensitivity of a muscle. A normal response would be a brisk muscle contraction. Because of the magnitude of the stimulus and the direct effect on the α motor neuron, this technique is not highly effective in teaching a patient to control or grade muscle contraction.[161] Instead, tapping of the muscle belly, a lower-intensity stimulus, is more satisfactory. Reverse tapping is a less frequently described technique, but it can be used. The extremity is positioned so gravity promotes the stretch, instead of the therapist manually tapping or actively inducing muscle stretch. Once the muscle responds, the therapist taps or passively moves the extremity to help the muscle obtain a shortened range. An example of reverse tapping would be tapping the triceps muscle when the patient is bearing weight on the extended elbow and actively trying to achieve full elbow extension. Timing of this technique is important. Gravity quickly stretches the triceps. If the timing follows the quick stretch to the extensor, then the flexors will be dampened and active extension more likely a motor response. If the therapist taps the elbow toward extension when the flexors' motor neurons are sensitive, then those flexor muscles may respond to the stretch and contract, taking the arm farther into flexion.

Positioning (range). The concept of submaximal and maximal range of muscles is highly significant to clinical application. Bessou and colleagues[162] monitored the neuronal firing of muscle spindles at different ranges of motion. Upper motor neuron lesions can alter the sensitivity of the spindle afferent reflex arc fibers by not using presynaptic inhibition to normally dampen incoming afferent activity.[163] Therefore ROM should be carefully assessed on an individual basis, particularly in a patient with an upper motor neuron lesion, to determine the maximal or submaximal range for an individual. Therapists always need to determine whether the difference between optimal range and functional ROM is different. If a patient will never need to use full ROM, then spending long periods of time trying to stretch a shoulder or hip to end-range of tissue mobility may not be the best decision with regard to intervention. Therapists also need to carefully evaluate excessive range resulting from hypermobility and hypotonicity. In those situations, external support of the affected joint or limb needs to be considered in all functional positions in order to prevent complications such as pain.[164–166]

Stretch pressure. The muscle belly is the stimulus focus of stretch pressure. The therapist slowly applies pressure to the muscle belly. It is used to decrease or release tone in the target muscle, allowing for the (temporary) recovery of voluntary movement.[105,167] Generally this type of stimulus is applied and maintained for a period of time (e.g., 5 to 10 seconds). It is not a quick stimulus and may be using the tendon organ to dampen tone. This type of pressure technique is also used in a variety of complementary approaches (see Chapter 39).

Stretch release. This technique is performed by placing the fingertips over the belly of larger muscles and spreading the fingers in an effort to stretch the skin and the underlying muscle. The stretch is done firmly enough to temporarily deform the soft tissue so the cutaneous receptors and Ia afferent fibers may produce facilitation of the target muscle. It is easy to determine quickly whether the response is efficacious by just feeling and looking at the response of the patient.

Manual pressure. Manual pressure can be facilitatory when it is applied as a brisk stretch or friction-like massage over muscle bellies. The speed and duration at which the manual pressure is applied determine the extent of recruitment from receptors. Paired with volitional efforts, manual pressure can lead to motor function and, with repetition, motor learning.

Vibration. There are two types of vibratory methods used therapeutically. The first deals with the use of a handheld vibrator to facilitate Ia receptors to enhance agonist muscle contraction in hypotonic muscles or to facilitate Ia receptors of antagonistic muscle fibers to inhibit hypertonic agonists. Currently the use of vibration to facilitate Ia responses within specific muscle function has been used to show how proprioception can be used to alter upright standing.[168,169] The second type of vibratory method is a total-body vibration to facilitate postural tone and balance and is applied through the feet in a standing position.[170–173]

Bishop[174,175] wrote an excellent series of articles on the neurophysiology and therapeutic application of vibration in the 1970s. High-frequency vibration (100 to 300 Hz or cycles per second) applied to the muscle or tendon elicits a reflex response referred to as the *tonic vibratory response*. Tension within the muscle will increase slowly and progressively for 30 to 60 seconds and then plateau for the duration of the stimulus.[176] Some researchers found that at cessation of the input the contractibility of the muscle was enhanced for approximately 3 minutes.[176,177] The discrepancy in the research may reflect the way the individual is using the input, both from a direct effect on the motor generator and from supraspinal modulation over the importance of the input, which may affect the overall learning and plasticity of the CNS. To facilitate hypotonic muscle, the muscle belly is first put on stretch, and then vibratory stimuli are applied.[178] To inhibit a hypertonic muscle, the antagonistic muscle could be vibrated.[174,178] The use of vibration can be enhanced by combining it with additional modalities such as resistance, position, and visually directed movement. Vibration also stimulates cutaneous receptors, specifically the pacinian corpuscles, and thus can also be classified as an exteroceptive modality.[179] Because of its ability to decrease hypersensitive tactile receptors through supraspinal regulation, local vibration is considered an inhibitory technique (it is also discussed later in the section on exteroceptor-maintained stimulus).

Amplitude or amount of displacement must also be considered when vibration is analyzed as a modality. It has been reported that high amplitude causes adverse effects, especially in patient's with cerebellar dysfunction.[175] Vibration is not recommended for infants because the nervous system is not yet fully myelinated and the vibration might cause too much stimulation. The reader is also cautioned about using vibration over areas that have been immobilized because of the underlying vascular tissue potential for clotting. Vibration on or near these blood vessels could dislodge a clot, causing an embolism. Vibration also needs to be used cautiously over skin that has lost its elasticity and is thin (e.g., that in older persons) because the friction itself from the vibration can cause tearing. The therapist must always keep in mind the environment and the functionality of an intervention procedure. The use of vibration may assist the patient in contractions and somatosensory awareness, but it is an unnatural way to facilitate either system and thus needs to be removed as part of an intervention as soon as the patient demonstrates some sensory awareness and/or volitional control over a movement component.

Within the past decade, the use of vibration of specific muscle groups of the neck has been studied to determine its effect on upright standing and the interaction with and without eyes open.[168,169] These studies showed that by vibrating specific muscle groups, those muscles would actively contract and change the position of the head in space but that with eyes open the effect was minimized in relation to global postural control. A similar study examined the effect of vibration on various muscles within the lower extremities and how that affected various postural responses.[180,181] These researchers found that different frequencies affected different muscle groups. The one consistent thing all studies have shown is that vibration does facilitate Ia muscle fibers, which in turn affect muscle contraction of the agonist receiving the vibration. Other sensory systems can assist or override the effect of vibration, but that is because of superspinal influence over motor generators.

Total-body vibration is currently being used to determine if it affects motor performance. Studies have shown that whole-body vibration can enhance motor performance in high-level athletes performing sprints and jumps,[170,171] as well as improve trunk stability, muscle tone, and postural control in individuals after stroke while in geriatric rehabilitation.[173] Its application for individuals with neurological dysfunction is inconclusive.[182,183] Studies specifically directed toward the elderly again show promise, but further research is needed for specificity.[184–186] Future research will need to determine the effect of total-body vibration when introduced to all populations of individuals with neurological dysfunction.[187] At that time, both amplitude and magnitude will need to be identified to replicate studies. Total-body vibration certainly falls under primarily proprioception but also could be classified under combined proprioceptive techniques or multisensory classification techniques because the input affects the muscle spindles, the joints, the vestibular system, and possibly the auditory system with the low frequency noise. And every time vibration is applied, the skin receptors will initially fire although most will adapt quickly to prolonged use of any stimuli.

The tendon. The tendon receptors are specialized receptors located in both the proximal and the distal musculotendinous insertions. In conjunction with the stretch receptors, the tendon plays an important role in the mediation of proprioception.[136,137,188–193]

The principal role of the tendon is to monitor muscle tension exerted by the contraction of the muscles or by tension applied to the muscle itself. Research has demonstrated that the tendon is highly sensitive to tension and acts conjointly with the stretch receptors to inform higher centers of continuing environmental demands to modulate or change existing plans; these higher centers in turn regulate tonicity and the state of the motor pool.[46,136] The tendon (Ib) signals not only tension but also the rate of change of tension and provides the sensation of force as the muscle is working.[188] A fundamental difference between the tendon organ and the stretch receptors is that the stretch receptors detect length, whereas the tendon monitors tension and force. The stretch receptors regulate reciprocal inhibition, whereas the tendon modulates autogenic inhibition. Table 8.2 lists a variety of treatment approaches using the tendon to inform higher centers regarding needed changes and regulation over spinal generators.

Maintained stretch to the tendon organ. Maintained stretch to a muscle has the potential for triggering the tendon organ if tension is great enough. Once the maintained stretch fires the tendon organ, autogenic inhibition of the same muscle occurs. A therapist will feel a release of the agonist muscle, allowing for elongation of the contractile components. Simultaneously, the tendon organ's sensory neurons will facilitate motor neurons to the antagonist muscle, thus heightening its sensitivity and potential for activity. This is the technique used when a joint has developed range restriction. The clinician always needs to differentiate whether the tightness found within the joint is caused by compensatory muscles considered *movers* protecting injured postural muscles beneath or by tightness just from positioning, disuse, or fear.

Inhibitory pressure. Pressure has been used therapeutically to alter motor responses. Mechanical pressure (force), such as from cones, pads, or the orthokinetic cuff developed by Blashy and Fuchs,[194]

TABLE 8.2 Treatment Suggestions Using Proprioceptive Input From the Tendon

1. Extreme stretch
2. Deep pressure to tendon
3. Passive positioning in extreme lengthened range
4. Extreme resistance: more effective in lengthened and shortened range
5. Deep pressure to muscle belly to put stretch on tendon
6. Small repeated contractions with gravity eliminated

provided continuously is inhibitory. That pressure seems most effective on tendinous insertions. It is hypothesized that this deep, maintained pressure activates pacinian corpuscles, which are rapidly adapting receptors. A variety of researchers have studied these receptors and their relationship to regulating vasomotor reflexes,[195] modulating pain,[196–200] and dampening other sensory system influence on the CNS.[177,199]

This inhibitory pressure technique also works when pressure is applied across the longitudinal axis of a tendon. The pressure is applied across the tendon with increasing pressure until the muscle relaxes. Constant pressure applied over the tendons of the wrist flexors may dampen flexor hypertonicity and elongate the tight fascia over the tendinous insertion.

Pressure over bony prominences has modulatory effects. A common example is pressure on the medial aspect of the calcaneus, which dampens plantarflexors and allows contraction of the lateral dorsiflexor muscles. Pressure over the lateral aspect of the calcaneus also dampens calf muscles to allow for contraction of the medial dorsiflexor muscles.[28] Localized finger pressure applied bilaterally to acupuncture points has been shown to relieve pain and reduce muscle tone.[200–204] This technique has also been found to be particularly effective when used in a low-stimulus environment and when combined with deep breathing. This combination of pressure (manually applied), environmental demands (low), and parasympathetic activity (slow, relaxed breathing) illustrates various systems interacting together to create the best motor response. The real world requires the patient to respond to many environmental conditions while relaxed or under stress. Thus once a patient begins to demonstrate normal adaptable motor responses, the therapist needs to change the conditions and the stress level to allow the patient to practice variability. As described, this practice should incorporate motor error, especially error or distortions in the plan, yet still achieve the desired goal. As the patient self-corrects, greater demand and variability should be introduced.[205]

Joint receptor approximation. Approximation of the joint mimics weight bearing and facilitates the postural extensor system, and thus use of the treatment technique is thought to improve balance.[206] Gravity creates approximation and its greatest force is produced down through the body in vertical postures. Approximation should help to stabilize any joint that is in a load-bearing situation by eliciting coactivation of the muscles around the joint in question. In standing, gravity creates approximation down through the entire spine, hips, knees, and ankles. When in a prone position on elbows, the load goes down again through the upper spine while simultaneous going down through the shoulder girdles of both arms. If a therapist increases that load by adding pressure down through the joints in question, then an augmented intervention has been added to the therapeutic environment. Using weight belts around the waist or a weighted vest on the trunk can facilitate the postural coactivation needed during standing or walking.[207–209] At times, approximation can be used to heighten normal postural tone while simultaneously dampening excessive tone in the other leg. For example, patients/clients who have CNS insult often have an imbalance in function within the two lower extremities. This can be very frustrating for the therapist because bringing the patient to standing to assist in regaining normal postural extension of one leg triggers the other into a strong extensor pattern, causing plantarflexion and inversion of that foot. One way to use approximation in treating both legs simultaneously might be to first bring the patient from sitting onto a high-low mat. Then the therapist can raise the mat high enough that the patient can be lowered into standing on the normal-functioning leg. At the same time the patient's other leg can be bent at the knee, and that knee placed on a stool or chair. This allows approximation down through the entire leg that is in standing position while approximating the trunk, hip, and knee of the other leg in the kneeling position. The therapist can work on standing and weight shifting in one leg while dampening abnormal tone in the kneeling leg. As the kneeling leg starts to regain postural coactivation in its hip, postural function will often be felt in the knee and ankle.

Traction and distraction. One or more joints are distracted by a force that causes it or them to separate or pull apart, similar to the swing phase of the leg during ambulation or the arms in a reciprocal pattern to each leg. This distraction of the joint receptors also puts stretch on the muscles, which combines to facilitate the pattern into which the limb is moving. Simultaneously, distraction dampens the antagonistic movement pattern, which allows the agonist movement to continue. A therapist will often use manual traction to get relaxation of hyperactive extensor muscles or for limited mobility.[210] Often therapists do not think of the traction when applying resistance to a limb. For example, a mistake made is placing ankle weights to facilitate limbs that are ataxic. Ataxia is an imbalance in coactivation and smooth movement of both agonist and antagonist muscle groups.[211] The weight itself slows down the excessive movement by the resistance. However, weight on the ankle creates traction that will facilitate only the flexor group and often creates an additional imbalance in the ataxic leg.[212] When the weights are removed, the patient often is more ataxic. Table 8.3 lists a variety of treatment approaches using the joints to facilitate or inhibit motor output.

Combined proprioceptive input techniques. Many techniques succeed because of the combined effects of multiple inputs to the proprioceptive system of stretch, joint, and tendon receptors. Some of these combined techniques described in this section include ballistic movements; total-body positioning; PNF patterns; postexcitatory inhibition (PEI) with stretch, range, rotation, and shaking; heavy work patterns; Feldenkrais (see Chapter 39)[213–215]; and manual therapy.[23,198,216]

Ballistic movement.   Ballistic movements are characterized by muscle contractions that occur in very high velocities over a short period of time. They are effective because of their combined proprioceptive interaction. The patient/client is asked to quickly initiate a movement, such as shoulder flexion while prone over a table with the arm hanging over the side. This component is volitional, but the patient then maintains a passive role. As the patient relaxes, the movement patterns become automatic. The physiology behind the automatic movement is easy to understand. As the muscle approaches the shortened range, the amount of ongoing γ afferent activity decreases. Thus both the agonist α motor neuron bias and the inhibition of Ia and II receptors of the antagonistic α motor neurons decrease. Simultaneously, the antagonistic muscle is being placed on more and more stretch. This stretch, as well as the lack of inhibition on the

antagonistic α motor neurons, will encourage the antagonistic muscle to begin contraction and reverse the movement pattern. The tendon organs also play a key role in ongoing inhibition. As the muscle approaches the shortened range and tension on the tendon becomes intense, the tendon organ increases its firing, thus inhibiting the agonistic muscle in the shortened range while facilitating the antagonistic muscle. This technique is highly movement oriented, and the traction applied by gravity to the shoulder joint while swinging the arm further facilitates the movement. These ballistic movements are part of the program generators within the spinal system that facilitate reciprocal movements of the limb. As the patient performs the movement, there is little need for conscious attention to drive the movement; it will run automatically. The role of the Ib fibers during this open chain or movement pattern is definitely different from its role in a closed chain or weight-bearing environment.[189] Supraspinal influence over programmed activity also plays a role in the effectiveness of this treatment.[217] The specific rationale for why ballistic movements have functional carryover may be explained by recent research into cerebellar function and the importance of mechanical afferent input in regulation of movement (see Chapter 19).

The clinician using this technique must exercise caution. ROM can easily be obtained through ballistic movement. Consequently, the clinician must always determine before therapy the reasons for specific clinical signs and whether the total problem will be corrected through an activity such as a ballistic movement. This is the diagnostic responsibility of the professional. If one component of the problem is alleviated, such as limitation of range, while other components are ignored, this can be a dangerous technique. If the lack of range is a result of muscle splinting because there is lack of postural tone or joint stability, then ballistic movement has the possibly increasing the problem. For example, assume that the rotator cuff muscles are slightly torn and the movers of the shoulder are superficially splinting to prevent further tearing. Ballistic movement that causes relaxation of more superficial muscles will place more responsibility for shoulder stabilization on the rotator cuff muscles and may increase the tear on the rotator cuff muscles causing increased pain.

Total-body positioning.   Total-body positioning implies the use of positioning and gravity to dampen afferent activity on the α motor neurons and thus cause a decrease in tone, or relaxation.[218] Currently, the rationale for why relaxation of striated muscle occurs after this treatment implies that the effect of the flexor reflex afferents is being dampened by a combination of input and interneuronal activity. These changes in the state of the muscle tone will not be permanent and will revert to the original posturing unless motor learning and adaptation within the central programmer occur simultaneously. Thus, for this treatment to effect permanent change, a large number of systems need modification. This modification can be augmented by techniques that facilitate autogenic inhibition, reciprocal innervation, labyrinthine and somatosensory influences, and cerebellar regulation over tone.[219] Changing the degree of flexion of the head also alters vestibular input and the state of the motor pool. But again, the patient's CNS needs to be an active participant and will ultimately determine whether permanent learning and change are programmed.

Proprioceptive neuromuscular facilitation.   To analyze and learn the principles, techniques, and patterns that constitute PNF, a total approach to treatment, refer to the texts by Adler and colleagues,[220] Voss,[221] and Sullivan and colleagues.[32] This approach is used extensively for patients with musculoskeletal and neuromuscular problems, with research on this method encompassing more populations with lower motor neuron and musculoskeletal problems than upper motor neuron lesions.[149,216,222–230] When proprioceptive techniques are packaged in specific movement patterns, it may be referred to as PNF. When individual

---

TABLE 8.3   Treatment Suggestions Using Proprioceptive Input From the Joints

1. Manual traction (distraction) to joint surfaces to facilitate joint motion
2. Manual approximation (compression) to joint surfaces to facilitate cocontraction or postural holding
3. Positioning: gravity used to approximate or apply traction
4. Weight belts, shoulder harnesses, and helmets to increase approximation
5. Wrist and ankle cuffs to increase traction
6. Wall pulleys, weights, manual resistance
7. Manual therapy[23]
8. Elastic tubing to provide compression during movement

proprioceptive techniques are discussed alone, the specific sensory function is being acknowledged, and these techniques can be integrated into many rehabilitation intervention strategies.

Postexcitatory inhibition with stretch, range, rotation, and shaking. The concept of PEI is based on the action potential or electrical response pattern of a neuron at the time of stimulation and on the entire phase response until the neuron returns to normal. At the time of stimulation, the action potential will build and go through an excitatory phase. The neuron then enters an inhibitory phase or refractory period during which further stimulation is not possible. This is referred to as the *PEI phase* or *postsynaptic afferent depolarization.*[105] These phase changes are extremely short and, in normal muscle, asynchronous with respect to multiple neuronal firing. In a hypertonic muscle, more simultaneous firing occurs. When the muscle is lengthened, and thus tension is created, more fibers will be discharged. It is hypothesized that if the hypertonic muscle is placed at the end of its spastic range and a quick stretch is applied and held, then total facilitation followed by total inhibition will occur because of PEI. As the inhibition phase is felt, the therapist can passively lengthen the spastic muscle until the facilitatory phase sets in repolarization. At that time the clinician holds the lengthened position. Increased tone will ensue, followed by inhibition and continued lengthening. Holding the range (not allowing concentric contraction during the excitatory phase) is critical. If the muscle is held as the tone increases, the resistance and stretch are then maximal and probably further facilitate the inhibitory phase.

Rood's heavy work patterns. Rood's concepts of cocontraction in weight-bearing positions such as on elbows, on extended elbows, kneeling, and standing blend with current concepts of motor learning. Concepts explain the rationale why postural holding in shortened range for periods of time are valid interventions. Rood stressed the need for patients to work in and out of those shortened ranges to gain postural control and to practice directing the limbs during both closed and open chain activities.

Feldenkrais. The Feldenkrais concepts[213,214] of sensory awareness through movement place emphasis relaxation of muscles on a stretch, including distracting and compressing joints for sensory awareness. Both techniques reflect combined proprioceptive techniques. Taking muscles off the stretch slows general afferent firing and thus overload to the CNS. Compression and distraction of joints enhance specific input from a body part while simultaneously facilitating input of a lesser intensity from other body segments. This combined proprioceptive approach enhances body schema awareness in a relaxed environment. It also integrates empowerment of the patient by use of visualization and asking for volitional control. (See Chapters 27 and 39 for additional information.)

Exteroceptive or Cutaneous Sensory System

Differentiation of receptor site as augmented intervention. Humans have many different types of tactile receptors. Some are superficial, and others are deep within the layers of the skin. These receptors have been identified within the chapter on motor learning. Their use as augmented intervention strategies is discussed in the following section.

A list of treatment techniques using the exteroceptive (tactile) input system as their primary mode of entry can be found in Table 8.4. Interventions that use cutaneous stimuli include neutral warmth, light touch, and maintained pressure, among others. Specific stimuli for the varied receptors and the expected responses to cutaneous stimuli are presented in the table.

Treatment alternatives using the exteroceptive system. The function of the exteroceptive system is to inform the nervous system

TABLE 8.4 **Suggested Treatment Procedures Using Cutaneous Stimuli**

Quick Phasic Withdrawal
1. Stimulus
   a. Pain
   b. Cold: one-sweep with ice cubes, Rood quick ice
   c. Light touch: brush (quick stroking), finger, feather
2. Response
   a. Stimulus applied to an extensor surface: elicits a flexor withdrawal*
   b. Stimulus applied to flexor surface: may elicit flexor withdrawal or withdrawal from stimulus into extension

Prolonged Icing (Repetitive Icing Should Be Used With Caution Because of Rebound Effect)
1. Stimulus
   a. Ice cube
   b. Ice chips and wet towel
   c. Bucket of ice water
   d. Ice pack
   e. Immersion of body part or total body
2. Response: inhibition of muscles below skin areas iced

Neutral Warmth
1. Stimulus
   a. Air bag splints
   b. Wrapping entire body or individual body part with towel
   c. Tight clothing such as tights, fitted turtleneck jerseys, Lycra clothing
   d. Tepid water or shower
2. Response: inhibition of area under which neutral warmth was applied

Light Touch, Rapid Stroking
1. Stimulus
   a. Light intermittent tactile stimulus to an identified dermatome-myotome interaction area
2. Response: facilitation of muscle(s) related to the stimulus area

Maintained Pressure or Slow, Continuous Stroking With Pressure
1. Stimulus
   a. Slowly rubbing the target area with a towel
   b. Wearing Lycra or spandex clothing
2. Response: sensory receptor adaptation and decrease in afferent firing

*Response: adaptation of many cutaneous receptors to stimulus, thus decreasing exteroceptive input, decreasing reticular activity, and decreasing facilitation of muscles underlying stimulated skin.

about the surrounding world. The CNS will adapt behavior to coexist and survive within this environment. Although many protective responses are patterned within the motor system, these patterned responses can be changed or modulated according to momentary inherent chemistry, attitude, motivation, alertness, and so on. Different from some of the other treatment approaches, the function of the exteroceptive input system is not reflexive but rather informative and adaptable.

Quick phasic withdrawal. The human organism reacts to painful or noxious stimuli at both conscious and unconscious levels. If the stimulus is brief and of noxious quality, it will elicit a protective reaction of short duration with use of the long-chain spinal reflex loops. Simultaneously, afferent impulses ascend to higher centers to evoke prolonged emotional-behavioral responses. Stimuli such as pain, extremes in temperature, rapid movement, light touch, and hair displacement are the most likely to cause this reaction by activating free nerve endings. These stimuli are perceived as potentially dangerous and communicate directly with the reticular-activating system and nonspecific thalamic nuclei. These structures have diffuse interconnections with all regions of the cerebral cortex, autonomic nervous system (ANS), limbic system, cerebellum, and motor centers in the brain stem. Research has shown that children who exhibit hyperactive withdrawal reactions also develop negative emotional reactivity and show significantly more avoidance behavior and in time show right frontal asymmetry.[231] These alerting stimuli have been linked to motor seizures in critically ill patients.[232] As indicated by these research studies, therapists need to be aware of these potential responses, especially in patients with severe neurological insult that has resulted in a lower level of consciousness. These low-functioning patients cannot express their feelings nor how their nervous system is reacting to the input. Thus therapists need to be very aware of any motor response a patient may express and try to avoid using stimuli that might trigger these avoidance behaviors.

From observance of the behavior of patient's with chronic neuropathic pain, withdrawal responses seem to become habitual and may be associated with somatosensory (S1) remapping[233]; thus some individuals may have difficulty with discriminating benign stimuli from potentially injurious stimuli. When any movement or touch is perceived as painful, the challenge to both therapist and patient is to agree on the therapeutic dose of a certain intervention and particular session. Therapists need to gain trust, and one way is to not elicit a lot of pain during treatment. Patient responses to pain induced during treatment such as exercise and manual therapy range can from increased patient resistance to joint and overall body movement to a complete loss of trust in the practitioner. Alami and colleagues completed a small study of patients/clients who experienced pain induced by exercise and mobilization (PIEM) during physical therapy and found that patient's desire preintervention education about pain, their particular pain response, and how a physical therapy plan of care can be adapted according to their pain intensity.[233a]

There are some real therapeutic limitations to using stimuli that "load" the spinothalamic system. A painful stimulus will be excitatory to the nervous system and produce a prolonged reaction after discharge.

Because light touch has both a protective and a discriminatory function, techniques such as brushing or stroking the skin with a soft brush have the potential of informing the CNS about (1) texture, object specificity, and error in fine motor responses or (2) danger (eliciting a protective response). If a protective response is triggered, the specific withdrawal pattern will depend on a variety of circumstances. If the stimulus is applied to an extensor surface, then a flexor withdrawal will be facilitated. If the stimulus is placed on a flexor surface, one of two responses occurs. First, the patient might withdraw from the stimulus, thus going into an extensor pattern. Second, the stimulus may elicit a flexor withdrawal and cause the patient to go into a flexor pattern. Which pattern occurs depends on preexisting motor programming bias as a result of positioning and the predisposition of the patient's CNS. Both responses would be considered normal. The condition or emotional state of the nervous system and whether the stimulus is considered threatening also determine the sensitivity of the response, again reinforcing the systems' interdependence. These responses are protective and do not lead to repetition of movement or motor learning. For that reason, along with the emotional and autonomic reactions, a phasic withdrawal to facilitate flexion or extension is not recommended as a treatment approach unless all other possibilities have been eliminated.

Short duration, high-intensity icing. Cold is another stimulus that the nervous system perceives as potentially dangerous. The use

of ice as a stimulus to elicit desired motor patterns is an early technique developed by Rood and was referred to as *repetitive icing*. An ice cube is rubbed with pressure for 3 to 5 seconds or used in a quick-sweep motion over the muscle bellies to be facilitated. This method activates both exteroceptors and proprioceptors and causes a brief arousal of the cortex. This method can produce unpredictable results. Although initially a phasic withdrawal pattern generator response will be activated immediately after the reflex has taken place, the "rebound" phenomenon deactivates the muscle that has been stimulated and lowers the resting potential of the antagonistic muscle.[234] Therefore a second stimulus to the same dermatome-myotome neural network may not elicit a second response. However, because of reciprocal innervation, the antagonistic muscle may effect a rebound movement in the opposite direction. Icing may also cause prolonged reaction after discharge because of the connections to the reticular system, limbic system, and ANS. Thus the ANS would be shifted toward the sympathetic end. Too much sympathetic tone causes a desynchronization of the cortex.[235] Although the resting state of the spinal generator may be altered briefly, if the heightened state persists, the cause is most likely fear or sympathetic overflow (see Chapter 4). This state is destabilizing to the system and most likely will not lead to any motor learning. Because of unpredictable response patterns to Rood's repetitive icing, this technique is seldom used.

The therapist is cautioned not to use short-duration, high-intensity icing to the facial region above the level of the lips, to the forehead, or to the midline of the trunk. These areas have a high concentration of pain fibers and a strong connection to the reticular system.[13,236]

Ice should not be used behind the ear because it may produce a sudden lowering of blood pressure.[237] The therapist should also avoid using ice in the left shoulder region in patients with a history of heart disease because referred pain from angina pectoris manifests itself in the left shoulder area, indicating that the cold stimulus might cause a reflexive constriction of the coronary arteries.[238] In addition, the primary rami located along the midline of the dorsum of the trunk have sympathetic connections to internal organs. The cold stimulus may alter organ activity and perhaps produce vasoconstriction, causing increased blood pressure and reduced blood supply to the viscera.[239,240]

Brief administration of ice can have beneficial effects if the nervous system's inhibitory mechanisms are in place. For instance, in children with learning disabilities or adults with sensorimotor delays, the application of ice to the palmar surface of the hands will cause arousal at the cortical level because of the increased activity of the reticular activating system. This arousal response presumably produces increased adrenal medullary secretions, resulting in various metabolic changes. Therefore icing should be used selectively. If the patient has an unstable ANS, icing should be eliminated as a potential sensory modality.[241]

Prolonged use of ice. Physicians have used therapeutic cold for the treatment of individuals with high fever and/or intracranial pressure with the intent of reducing the body temperature or brain swelling to prevent brain damage.[242] This procedure is done with cooling pans or blankets. Whole-body cryotherapy has been used to reduce inflammation and pain and overcome symptoms that prevent normal movement. This type of therapy consists of the use of very cold air maintained for 2 minutes in cryochambers. A recent study looked at this type of therapy for injured athletes. It was found that the procedure did not cause harm to the individual.[243] This approach does not seem realistic for use in occupational or physical therapy clinics.

A variety of approaches that incorporate prolonged icing techniques have been used in therapy clinics for decades. The PNF approach may be the most common.[22] Inhibition of hypertonicity or[244] pain is the goal for the use of any of these methods. With prolonged cold, the neurotransmission of impulses, both afferent and efferent, is reduced. Simultaneously the metabolic rate within the cooled tissue is reduced (see Chapter 30). Caution must be exercised with regard to the use of this modality. However, for effective treatment results, the patient (1) should be receptive to the modality, (2) should be able to monitor the cold stimulus (sensory deficits should not be present), and (3) should have a stable autonomic system to prevent unnecessary adverse effects of hypothermia. Research of the past decade has consistently shown that cryotherapy is an effective tool for reducing pain and has helped individuals regain integration of axial musculature after neurological insults.[245–248] Individuals of all ages seem to respond similarly, which allows therapists to use this therapeutic tool across generations.[249]

Ice immersion of the contralateral limb was used decades ago to get a reflexive decrease in temperature in the affected limb. It was believed that this intralimb reflex was an effective way of treating pain without directly treating the limb, and recent research has validated that belief.[250]

Ice massage is another form of prolonged icing and is often used to treat somatic pain problems.[251] It is also used over high-toned muscles to dampen striated muscle contractions. Caution must be used when eliminating pain without correcting the problem causing pain. For example, if instability causes muscle tone and pain, then icing might decrease pain while causing additional joint instability and potential damage. The end result would be an increase, not a decrease, in pain and motor dysfunction.

Maintained stimulus or pressure. Because of the rapid adaptation of many cutaneous receptors, a maintained stimulus will effectively cause inhibition by preventing further stimuli from entering the system. This technique is applied to hypersensitive areas to normalize skin responses. Vibration used alternately with maintained pressure can be highly effective. It should be remembered that these combined inputs use different neurophysiological mechanisms. It is often observed that low frequency–maintained vibration is especially effective with learning-disabled children who have hypersensitive tactile systems that prevent them from comfortable exploration of their environment. When children themselves use vibration on the extremities, their hypersensitive systems seem to normalize and they become receptive to exploring objects. If that exploration is accompanied by additional prolonged pressure, such as digging in a sandbox, the technique seems to be more effective because of the adaptive responses of the nervous system.

Maintained pressure approaches using elastic stockings, tight form-fitting clothing (e.g., wet suits, expanded polytetrafluoroethylene [Gore-Tex] biking clothing), air splints, and other techniques can be incorporated into a patient's daily activity without altering lifestyle. The use of TheraTogs in children with various hyperactivity conditions has become an accepted therapeutic tool. They add some resistance, some support, and maintained pressure.[252] TheraTogs have also been shown to be effective in assisting individuals with hemiplegia to regain abductor control.[253]

In this way, patients can self-regulate their systems, allowing greater variability in adapting to the environment. Owing to the multisensory and multineuronal pathways used when peripheral input is augmented, traditional linear, allopathic research on human subjects is extremely difficult to design or measure with control, but outcome studies demonstrating efficacy are possible. Initially, efficacy confirmed by observation was acceptable. Concrete evidence is still scarce; repeat studies with use objective measures are needed.

Light discriminatory touch. Once an individual can discriminate light touch both for protection and for discriminatory learning, a lot of therapeutic tools become available to the therapist. Using boxes with an opening so the individual can insert a hand and arm but

cannot see what is inside, a patient can work on discriminating textures, objects, letter, numbers, and so on while working on higher-order processing. Once this touch has been integrated, the patient can also use light touch to determine balance, position in space, and various other types of perceptual tasks.[254]

Vestibular System

Vestibular treatment techniques. The vestibular system is a unique sensory system, critical for multisensory functioning, making it a viable and powerful input modality for therapeutic intervention. Any static position and any movement pattern will facilitate the labyrinthine system; therefore vestibular function and dysfunction play a role in all therapeutic activities. To conceptualize vestibular stimulation as spinning or angular acceleration minimizes its therapeutic potential and also negates an entire progression of vestibular treatment techniques.[15,44,255–257] Linear movements in horizontal and vertical postures and forward-backward directions occur early in development and should be considered one viable treatment modality. These movements seem to precede side-to-side and diagonal movements, which are followed by linear acceleration and end with rotational movements. All these movements can be done with assistance or independently by the patient in all functional activities. It is important to remember that the rate of vestibular stimulation determines the effects. A constant, slow, repetitive rocking pattern, irrespective of plan or direction, generally causes inhibition of total-body responses via the α motor neuron but not the spindles,[258] whereas a fast spin or fast linear movement tends to heighten both alertness and the motor responses. Again, the vestibular mechanism is only one of many that influence the motor system. Thus the system interaction must be constantly reassessed.

As already indicated, constant, slow, repetitive rocking patterns, irrespective of plane or direction, generally cause inhibition of the total-body responses. Yet any stimulus has the potential of causing undesired responses, such as increased or decreased tone. When this occurs, the procedure should be stopped and reanalyzed to determine the reason for the observed or palpated response. For example, assume that a patient, whether a child with cerebral palsy, an adolescent with head trauma, or an adult with anoxia, exhibits signs of severe generalized extensor hypertonicity in the supine position. To dampen the general motor response, the therapist decides to use a slow, gentle rocking procedure in supine position and discovers that the hypertonicity has increased. Obviously, the procedure did not elicit the desired response and alternative treatment is selected, but the reason for the increased hypertonicity needs to be addressed.

It is possible that the static positioning of the vestibular system is causing the release of the original tone and that through increasing of the vestibular input the tone also increases. It may also be that the facilitatory input did indeed cause inhibition but the movement itself caused fear and anxiety, thus increasing preexisting tone and overriding the inhibitory technique. Instead of selecting an entirely new treatment approach, a therapist could use the same procedure in a different spatial plane, such as a side-lying, prone, or sitting position. Each position affects the static position of the vestibular system differently and may differentially affect the excessive extensor tone observed in the patient. The vertical sitting position adds flexion to the system, which has the potential of further dampening extensor tone. This additional inhibition may be necessary to determine whether the slow rocking pattern will be effective with this patient. It would seem obvious that if a vestibular procedure was ineffective in modifying the preexisting extensor tone, then use of a powerful procedure, such as spinning, would be inappropriate. Selection of treatment techniques should be determined according to patient needs and disability. Patients either with an acoustic tumor that perforates into the brain stem or with generalized inflammatory disorders may be hypersensitive to vestibular stimulation, whereas other patient's, such as a child with a learning disability, may be in need of massive input through this system. Heiniger and Randolph[44] and Farber[15,105] present in-depth analyses of various specific vestibular treatment procedures commonly used in the clinic. The literature clearly establishes the causation of one vestibular imbalance, dizziness, for all age groups.[259–262] Certainly individuals can have vestibular problems and will present themselves as being dizzy or hypersensitive to movement of the head.

General body responses leading to relaxation. Any technique performed in a slow, continuous, even pattern will cause a generalized dampening of the motor output.[263] During handling techniques, these procedures can be performed with the patient in bed, on a mat while horizontal, sitting at bedside or in a chair, or standing. The movement can be done passively by the therapist or actively by the patient. Carryover into motor learning will best be accomplished when the patient performs the movement actively, without therapeutic assistance. In a clinical or school setting, a patient who is extremely anxious, hyperactive, and hypertonic may initiate slow rocking to decrease tone or feel less anxious or hyperactive. The reduction of clinical signs allows the patient to sit with less effort and to be more attentive to the environment, thus promoting the ability to learn and adapt.

It is the type of movement, not the technique, which is critical. The concept of slow, continuous patterns is used in Brunnstrom's rocking patterns[11] in early sitting, in PNF mat programs, and in therapeutic ball exercise programs; the use of these patterns can be observed in every clinic. Although the therapist may be unaware of why Mr. Smith gets so relaxed when slowly rocked from side to side in sitting, this procedure elicits an appropriate response. The nurse taking Mr. Smith for a slow wheelchair ride around the hospital grounds may do the same thing. Once the relaxation or inhibition has occurred, the groundwork for a therapeutic environment has been created to promote further learning, such as learning of ADL skills. The technique in and of itself will relax the individual but not create change or learning.

Pelvic mobilization techniques in sitting use relaxation from slow rocking to release the fixed pelvis. This release allows for joint mobility and thus creates the potential for pelvic movement performed passively by the therapist, with the assistance of the therapist, or actively by the patient. This technique often combines vestibular with proprioceptive techniques, such as rotation and elongation of muscle groups, which physiologically modify existing fixed tonal response through motor mechanisms or systems interactions. Simultaneously, slow, rhythmic rocking, especially on diagonals, is used to incorporate all planes of motion and thus all vestibular receptor sites to get maximal dampening effect, whether directly through the vestibulospinal system or indirectly through the cerebellum and reticular spinal motor system. The same pelvic mobility can be achieved by placing the patient (child or adult) over a large ball. The ball must be large enough for the patient to be semiprone while arms are abducted and externally rotated, and the legs relaxed (either draped over the ball or in the therapist's arms). Again, this position allows for maintained or prolonged stretch to tight muscles both in the extremities and in the trunk while doing slow, rhythmical rocking over the ball. The pelvis often releases, and the patient can be rolled off the large ball to stand on a relaxed pelvis preliminary to gait activities. A word of caution must be given regarding use of a large ball for relaxation. It is much easier to control the ball when someone is assisting that control from the opposite direction (in front of the patient). If slow rocking is done and the therapist is keeping his or her voice monotonous for further relaxation, the individual assisting will also relax. One author has had family members fall asleep and slowly or quickly fall to the floor.

Techniques to heighten postural extensors. Any technique that uses rapid anteroposterior or angular acceleration of the head and body while the patient is prone will facilitate a postural extensor response. Scooter boards down inclines, rapid acceleration forward over a ball or bolster, going down slides prone, and using a platform or mesh net to propel someone will all facilitate a similar vestibular response of righting of the head with postural overflow down into the shoulder girdle, trunk, hips, and lower extremities. Rapid movements while on elbows, on extended elbows, and in a crawling position can also facilitate a similar response. Depending on the intensity of the stimulus, the response will vary. In addition, the patient's emotional level during introduction to various types of stimuli may cause differences in tonal patterns. Clinical experience has shown that facilitatory vestibular stimulation promotes verbal responses and affects oral-motor mechanisms. Children with speech delays will speak out spontaneously and respond verbally.

Because facilitatory vestibular stimulation biases the sympathetic branch of the ANS, drooling diminishes and a generalized arousal response occurs at the cortical level. Therefore the appropriate time to teach adaptive rehabilitative techniques is after vestibular stimulation.[264]

Facilitatory techniques influencing whole-body responses. Tactile, vestibular, and proprioceptive inputs also assist in the regulation of the body's responses to movement.[40,105] As stated previously, the vestibular system, when facilitated with fast, irregular, or angular movement, such as spinning, not only induces tonal responses but also causes massive reticular activity and overflow into higher centers. Thus increased attention and alertness are often the outcome. The tracts going from the spinal cord, brain stem, and higher subcortical structures must be sufficiently intact to permit the desired responses from this type of input. If a lesion in the brain stem blocks higher-center communication with the vestibular apparatus, then massive input may cause a large increase in abnormal tone. The therapist needs to closely monitor any distress or ANS anomalies.[265]

Autonomic Nervous System

The ability to differentiate tone created by emotional responses versus tone resulting from CNS damage is a critical aspect of the evaluation process. Emotional tone can be reduced when stress, anxiety, and fear of the unknown have been reduced. This is true for all individuals. The patient with brain damage is no exception. Six treatment modalities[266] that normally produce a parasympathetic or decreased sympathetic (flight or fight) response are as follows:

1. Slow, continuous stroking for 3 to 5 minutes over the paravertebral area of the spine
2. Inversion, eliciting carotid sinus reflex along with other somatosensory receptors (refer to the discussion of vestibular system earlier in the chapter)
3. Slow, smooth, passive and active assistive movement within a pain-free range (refer to Maitland grade II movements)[23]
4. Deep breathing exercises
5. Progressive muscle relaxation
6. Cranial sacral manipulation (see Chapter 39)

When pressure is applied to both the anterior and posterior surfaces of the body, measurable reductions may be recorded in pulse rate, metabolic activity, oxygen consumption, and muscle tone.[237,267] These pressure techniques are identified as an intricate part of the many intervention approaches such as therapeutic touch,[27,238] Feldenkrais,[213–215,268] Maitland,[23] massage,[269,270] and myofascial release.[9,202,271–273] Although not verbally identified, other techniques (e.g., neurodevelopmental treatment [NDT],[34,35] Rood,[32,44,105] Brunnstrom,[11] and PNF[32]) also place an important emphasis on the response of the patient to the therapist's touch.

Treatment Alternatives Using the Autonomic Nervous System

Slow stroking. Slow stroking over the paravertebral areas along the spine from the cervical through lumbar components will cause inhibition or a dampening of the sympathetic nervous system. The technique is performed while the patient is in the prone position. The therapist begins by stroking the cervical paravertebral region in the direction of the thoracic area, using a slow, continuous motion with one hand. Usually a lubricant is applied to the skin, and the index and middle fingers are used to stroke both sides of the spinal column simultaneously. Once the first hand is approaching the end of the lumbar section, the second hand should begin a downward stroking at the cervical region. This maintains at least one point of contact with the patient's skin at all times during the procedure. The technique is applied for 3 to 5 minutes—and no longer—because of the potential for massive inhibition or rebound of the autonomic responses.[40,263] It is also recommended that at the end of the range of the last stroking pattern, the therapist maintain pressure for a few seconds to alert both the somatic and visceral systems that the procedure has concluded. Eastern medicine recognizes the importance of the ANS in total-body regulation to a greater extent than Western medicine does. The concepts of meridians and acupressure and acupuncture points are all intricately intertwined with the ANS (see Chapter 39). For that reason, a technique such as slow stroking would potentially interact with meridians and does extend over the row of acupuncture points referred to as *shu points* and relates to visceral reflexes connecting smooth muscle and specific organ systems. It is believed that this continuous, slow, downward pressure modulates the sympathetic outflow, causing a shift to a parasympathetic reaction or relaxation. Whether a result of the pressure on the sympathetic chain, some energy pressure over meridian points, a pleasant sensation, or something unknown, slow stroking does elicit relaxation and calming.[44,105] Patients/clients with large amounts of body hair or hair whorls are poor candidates for this procedure because of the irritating effect of stroking against the growth patterns and the sensitivity of hair follicles.

Slow, smooth, passive movement within pain-free range. Increasing ROM in painful joints is a dilemma frequently encountered by therapists caring for a patient with neurological damage. Having the patient communicate the first perception of pain and then moving the limb in a slow, smooth motion toward the pain range may elicit a variety of behaviors. In patients with fear and guarding, one strategy is for the therapist to stop the motion at the patient's stated point of pain, then retreat back into a pain-free area, or "safety range," then approach again, possibly with a slight variation in rotation or direction: often the patient will relinquish the safety range with improved comfort. The second finding is that if the motion toward the pain range is slow, smooth, and continuous, then frequently much of the range that was initially painful becomes pain free. The hypothesis is that slow, continuous motion is critical feedback for the ANS to handle imminent discomfort. The slow pattern provides the ANS time to release endorphins, thus modifying the perception of pain and allowing for increased motion. If the therapist stabilizes the painful joint and prevents the possibility of that joint going into the pain range, rapid, oscillating movements can often be obtained within the pain-free range. This maintains joint mobility and often, as an end result, increases the pain-free range. This technique is not unique to the treatment of individuals with neurological problems; it is often used as a manual therapy procedure.[202,274,275] Furthermore, one can move slowly into a range that actually shortens muscles. If held for 30 seconds, the muscle that is too short can relax, promoting greater motion in the opposite direction. This can be called *strain-counterstrain*—inhibiting firing by maintaining a position of active insufficiency, making the muscle too short.

Manual therapy[23,143,276–279] can be used to describe the pain and joint changes occurring at the joint level. As the fields of orthopedics and neurology merge into one system,[216] with the brain acting as an organ controlling the entire system and its components, the question of whether the pain reduction is centrally or peripherally triggered may be an important one. The answer is probably both. For example, thumb pain can increase the sensation of the nervous system to the point that even cutaneous and proprioceptive receptors act as nociceptors.

Maintained pressure. As discussed earlier, pressure has been a common technique in neurological rehabilitation. Farber[15] discusses a variety of techniques that facilitate a reduction of tone or hyperactivity. Pressure to the palm of the hand or sole of the foot, to the tip of the upper lip, and to the abdomen all seem to produce this effect. The pressure need not be forceful, but it should be firm and maintained.[280] This same technique is defined as inhibitory casting when applied through the use of an orthosis (see Chapter 32).

Progressive muscle relaxation. Progressive muscle relaxation is practiced during both meditation and treatment approaches such as Feldenkrais.[268,280,281] These methods of relaxation tend to trigger parasympathetic reactions, which in turn slow down heart rate and blood pressure and trigger slow, deep breathing (see Chapters 16 and 39). The Alexander technique has also been shown to cause relaxation while simultaneously increasing postural tone.[282]

Treatment considerations using olfactory, gustatory, auditory, and visual systems. Boxes 8.2 to 8.5 present a summary of treatment considerations using the olfactory, gustatory, auditory and visual,

Combined multisensory approaches. Although all techniques have the potential to be multisensory, the specific mode of entry may focus on one sensory system, as already described, or it may target two or more input modalities along with automatic motor programming.

BOX 8.2   Treatment Considerations Using the Olfactory Sense

Smell evokes different responses by means of the limbic system's control over behavior. Pleasant odors, such as vanilla or perfume, can evoke strong moods. Unpleasant odors can facilitate primitive protective reflexes, such as sneezing and choking. Sharp-smelling substances such as ammonia can elicit a reflex interruption of breathing.[283,284]

- Odors such as vanilla and banana have been used to facilitate sucking and licking motions.[285,286]
- Ammonia and vinegar have been used clinically to elicit withdrawal patterns and increase arousal in semicomatose patients.[287]
- When odors are used as a stimulant, the therapist must be aware of all behavior changes occurring within the patient. Arousal, level of consciousness, tonal patterns, reflex behavior, and emotional levels all can be affected by odor.
- Odors such as body odor, perfumes, hairspray, and urine can affect the patient's behavior although the smell was not intended as a therapeutic procedure. Some patient's, especially those with head traumas and inflammatory disorders of the central nervous system, often seem to be hypersensitive to smell. In these cases the therapist needs to be aware of the external olfactory environment surrounding the patient and to make sure those odors that are present facilitate or at least do not hinder desired response patterns.[288]
- There may be a cultural sensitivity to various smells that would suggest a cultural learning linked with emotional responses to smell.[289–291] Therefore if a therapist is going to use smell as part of therapy, identification of the individual's prior likes and dislikes is very important. Family members and close friends will be the best people to consult in order to get this information.
- Because of limited research in this area, caution must be exercised to avoid indiscriminate use of the olfactory system.

BOX 8.3 Treatment Considerations Using the Gustatory Sense

- Gustatory input is generally used as part of feeding and prefeeding activities. The oral region is sensitive not only to taste but also to pressure, texture, and temperature. For that reason, feeding would be classified as a multisensory technique that uses gustatory input as one of its entry modalities.
- Specific input modalities are based on the combined taste, texture, temperature, and affective response pattern (i.e., both a banana and an apple may be sweet, yet the textures vary greatly). When mashed, both fruits may have a pudding-like texture, yet the patient's emotional response may differ. Disliking the taste of banana but enjoying apple may cause startling differences in the patient's response during a feeding session.

BOX 8.4 Treatment Considerations Using the Auditory System

- Because of the complexity of the auditory system, a potentially large number of types of input modalities exists. Although some of them might not be considered traditional therapeutic tools, they are nonetheless techniques that affect the central nervous system (CNS). Some treatment alternatives focus on the following:
  - Quality of voice (pitch and tone)[292]
  - Quantity of voice (level and intensity)[293]
  - Affect of voice (emotional overtones)[294,295]
  - Spatial and temporal sound (how fast a stimulus occurs, and how frequently)[296–300]
  - Extraneous noise (sound)[301]
  - Auditory biofeedback[302–308]
  - Language[309]
  - Volume, level, and affect of voice[310–312]
  - Auditory perception[313–315]
- The therapist's voice can be considered one of the most powerful therapeutic tools. The emotional inflections used by the clinician certainly have the potential to alter patient response.[294,295] Knowing which emotional tone best coincides with a patient's need at a particular moment may come with experience or sensitivity to others' unique needs.
- The varying level of sound or extraneous noise in a clinical setting can at times be overwhelming. Timer alarms, messages over loudspeakers, conversations, computers, printers, or a child crying all are encountered in the clinical environment, and all could be occurring simultaneously. patients with CNS damage may not have the ability to filter sensitivity to all these intermittent noise sensations.[307]
- Decreasing auditory distracters or sudden noises can drastically improve the patient's ability to attend to a task or to succeed at a desired movement.[316,317]
- Music is used for encouraging not only motor function but also memory[318,319] and socialization.[320–322] Rhythmic sound perceived as an enjoyable sensation certainly has the effect of creating motor patterns in response to that rhythm.
- Auditory biofeedback is generally thought of as a procedure in which sound is used to inform the patient of specific muscle activity.[306,308] The level or pitch may change in relation to strength of muscle contraction or specific muscle group activity.

BOX 8.5 Treatment Considerations Using the Visual System

- Any light, no matter the degree of complexity, has the potential to affect a patient's central nervous system (CNS). That input not only reaches the optic cortex for sight recognition and processing but also projects to the brain stem and to the cerebellum through the tectocerebellar tract. Simultaneously, these afferents activate the reticular-activating and limbic spinal generators through the tectospinal tract.[263,323]
- The five categories of visual-system treatment alternatives should not be considered fixed, all-inclusive, or without overlap. The first three categories (color, lighting, and visual complexity) are common everyday visual stimuli. Combined, they make up the visual world.
  - Colors. Cool colors, a darkened room, and monotone color schemes all seem to have an inhibitory effect. In contrast, intermittent visual stimuli, bright colors, bright lights, and a random color scheme seem to alert the CNS and have a generalized facilitatory effect.[324–326]
  - Lighting. patients may find that the high-frequency flutter of fluorescent lamps to be irritating and causes distraction. The types of visual stimuli that may cause seizures and are seen by patients within rehabilitation settings include computers, video games, television, and venetian blinds.[327] For that reason, any change in lighting should alert the clinicians to watch for changes in their patients' behavior.
  - Visual Complexity. The visual system is the primary spatial sense for monitoring moving and stationary objects in space.[328,329] When brain damage occurs, the ability to identify objects, localize them in space, pick them out from other things, and adapt to their presence may be drastically diminished.[239] Because of the distractibility of many patient's, reducing the visual stimuli within their external space can help them to cope with the stimuli to which they are trying to pay attention. Using rooms that have been stripped of such stimuli as furniture and pictures can reduce not only distractibility but also hyperactivity and emotional tone.

TABLE 8.5 Examples of Treatment Modalities/Techniques Using Combined Sensory Input Systems

Sweep tapping[330]

Brunnstrom rolling (hand)[43]

Raimiste sign[43]

Stretch pressure[330]

Digging in sand, and so on

Gentle shaking[330]

Prone activities over ball[54,330,331]

Sitting activities on ball[54]

Mat activities

Resistive exercises: resistive rolling; resistive patterns: PNF[332–334]; resistive gait[335]; isokinetics[336,337]; wall pulleys; rowing[43]

Feeding[54,93,330]: maintained pressure: walking to back of tongue; resistive sucking (straw, Popsicle); use of textures (peanut butter, applesauce); maintained pressure to top lip

Inverted TLR[330,338]

Touch bombardment[330]: tactile discrimination in sand, etc.; pool therapy

Joint compression more than body weight[339,340]

Throwing and catching: balloon; heavy ball

Variance in movement: quick action directed by vision; postural activities in front of mirror; therapist using voice command to assist patient with movement

High-level movements: walking on a balance beam; trampoline activities (running, jumping, skipping)

PNF, Proprioceptive neuromuscular facilitation; *TLR,* tonic labyrinthine reflex.

As stated before, Table 8.5 categorizes a variety of treatment techniques that are clearly multisensory. The therapist, analyzing how the summated effect of the combined input and automatic responses influences patient performance, gains direction in anticipating treatment outcomes in terms of the problem-solving process. Because the potential combinations of multisensory input classification are enormous, only a few examples of combinations are included in the text to illustrate the process a clinician might use when classifying a new technique or a new approach to intervention. When clinicians select augmented treatment interventions to help a patient as part of somatosensory retraining or functional retraining or to establish a procedural program, the basic science understanding behind the clinical decision helps to develop questions for future research, determine a prognosis regarding outcomes, and rationally explain why or why not an intervention was effective. Prioritization of which techniques to continue using must be based on understanding and integration of neurophysiological mechanisms, learning environments, concepts of motor learning and control, and what motor impairment or body system problems are affecting functional performance and on the patient's and family's needs, motivations, and goals. A simple rule a therapist might follow would be to take away the least natural technique first. That technique would be the most artificial or contrived. An example using only one sensory system might help to clarify this point. For example, a therapist might assist a patient with elbow flexion during a feeding pattern by (1) vibrating the biceps, (2) quickly tapping the biceps, or (3) quickly stretching the biceps a little beyond midrange by using gravity. The first option would be the least natural and obviously the least socially acceptable. The third option is the most natural and closest to what might occur in the real environment in which the patient will need to function. Remember, these contrived techniques are used to assist patients who cannot control or perform the motor programs or functional activities without assistance or who need assistance in learning to modulate motor control for greater functional adaptability. If the therapist added verbal feedback or music, as well as asking the patient to visually look at the target, the example would become multisensory.

Within the following section are examples of combined multisensory approaches that might be used to augment sensory feedback to obtain a better environment for regaining functional control.

Sweep tapping. Sweep tapping is usually used to open a hypertonic flexor-biased hand. Many isolated techniques, such as sweep tapping[105] or rolling,[11] would be considered primarily proprioceptive-tactile in sensory origin. During sweep tapping, the clinician first uses a light-touch sweep pattern over the back of the fingers of one of the hands. This stimulus is applied quickly over the dermatome area that relates to muscles the patient is being asked to contract. Second, the therapist applies some quick tapping over the muscle belly of the hypotonic muscle. The first technique is tactile and believed to stimulate the reflex mechanism within the cord to heighten motor generators and increase the potential for muscle contraction of the hypotonic muscle or to dampen the hypertonic flexors. The second aspect, tapping, is a proprioceptive stimulus used to facilitate afferent activity within the muscle spindle of the extensors, thus further enhancing the patient's potential for muscle contraction. At the same time the patient will be asked to voluntarily activate the extensor motor system, which then automatically augments tactile, proprioceptive, and auditory input with functional control.

Taping. Taping procedures normally used in peripheral orthopedic muscle imbalances and pain have the same potential for patients with neurological problems. This adaptation would be a modification of both splinting and slings. Research has been done to demonstrate efficacy of taping to offset peripheral instability in individuals with neurological system impairments.[253,341-345] The concepts and ideas remain that taping has implications when treating individuals with neurological problems. Taping hypotonic muscle groups into a shortened range should effectively reduce the mechanical pull of gravity on both the muscle groups and joints and prevent the CNS from developing the need for compensatory stabilization or hypertonicity. If hypertonicity is the result of peripheral instability, then taping a hypertonic muscle into its shortened range should stabilize the peripheral system and eliminate the need for the CNS to create the hypertonic pattern. On the other hand, taping can also be used to heighten information about proprioception and joint position, providing feedback to avoid hyperextension or hypermobility of a joint. This is especially true when there is an imbalance of intrinsics and extrinsics in the hand.

Oral-motor interventions. There are more research articles available on specific oral-motor dysfunctions in patients with neurological problems[346-351] than on interventions. These are studies using fMRI of the CNS during oral-motor activity, but the transition to intervention again is limited.[352,353] Systematic reviews of potential oral-motor interventions are even fewer.[354]

When dealing with oral-motor intervention, the complexity of combined proprioceptive-tactile input becomes enhanced by adding another sensory input, such as taste. Implementation of one of a variety of feeding techniques clearly identifies the complexity of the total input system. When taste is used, smell cannot be eliminated as a potential input, nor can vision if the patient visually addresses the food. The following explanation of feeding techniques is included to encourage the reader to analyze the sensory input, processing, and motor response patterns necessary to accomplish this ADL task. The complexity of the interaction of all the various systems within the CNS is mind boggling, but if the motor response is functional, effortless, and acceptable to the patient and the environment, then the adaptation should be facilitated after attended repetitive behaviors.

Several feeding techniques have been developed in the past by master clinicians such as Mueller,[355] Farber,[105] Rood,[28] and Huss.[263] These techniques were not easily mastered or understood through reading alone. Competence in feeding techniques is best achieved through empirical experience under the guidance of a skilled instructor. Currently, some evidence base for implementation of feeding techniques or related motor activities can be found in the literature.[55,356,357]

The facial and oral region plays an important role in survival. Facial stimulation can elicit the rooting reaction. Oral stimulation facilitates reflexive behaviors, such as sucking and swallowing. Deeper stimulation to the midline of the tongue elicits a gag reflex. These reactions and reflexes are normal patterns for the neonate. When these reactions and reflexes are depressed or hyperactive, therapeutic intervention is a necessity. Oral facilitation is an important treatment modality for infants and children with CNS dysfunction. Therapeutic intervention during the early stages of myelination can be crucial to the development of more normalized feeding and speech patterns.

Similarly, adults with neurological impairment often have difficulty with oral-motor integration. Problems with swallowing, tongue control, and hypersensitive and desensitized areas within the oral cavity and also with mouth closure or chewing are frequently observed in adults with CNS damage.[346,347]

Before basic feeding techniques are implemented, clinicians need to understand how the CNS and PNS work collaboratively with the musculoskeletal system to control and perform these complex oral-motor functional movements.[136,358,359] Feeding therapy is preceded by observation and examination. With a pediatric patient, the therapist should observe breathing patterns while the patient is feeding, to determine whether the child can breathe through the nose while sucking on a nipple. In addition, the child's lips should form a tight seal around the nipple. Formal assessments should include functional assessments, developmental milestones, and behavioral manifestations. Medical charts and results from neurological examinations should be consulted for baseline data.

Postural mechanisms can influence feeding and speech patterns in patient's with neurological dysfunction.[31,357,360] A patient with a strong extensor pattern may have to be placed in the side-lying, flexed position to inhibit the forces of the extensor pattern. The ideal pattern for feeding is the flexed position, which promotes sucking and oral activity. Basic reflexes such as rooting, sucking, swallowing, and bite and gag reactions should be elicited and graded in children and evaluated in adults. The head needs to be in slight ventriflexion to pull in the postural stabilization of the neck and tongue. This is necessary to effectively facilitate programs that provide functional swallowing and control of foods by the tongue.

The facial region and the mouth have an extraordinary arrangement of sensory innervation. Therefore oral techniques must be used with utmost care. Anyone who has visited the dentist can attest to the feeling of invasiveness when foreign objects are placed in the mouth. With this in mind, the therapist should begin each treatment session by moving the autonomic continuum toward the parasympathetic end. Activation of the parasympathetic system should lower blood pressure, decrease heart rate, and, more important, increase the activity of the gastrointestinal system. Neutral warmth, the inverted position, and slow vestibular stimulation should help to promote parasympathetic "loading." Another approach that is applicable to feeding techniques is the application of sustained and firm pressure to the upper lip. An effective inhibitory device is a pacifier with a plastic shield that applies firm pressure on the lips. Perhaps this is why a pacifier is a "pacifier." Adults can acquire resistive sucking patterns with a straw and plastic shield and achieve the same results.

Sometimes children or adults are not cooperative and will not open their mouths.[361,362] Rather than the mouth being pried open, the jaw is pushed closed and held firmly for a few seconds. On release of the pressure, the jaw reflexively relaxes. The receptors in the temporomandibular joint and tooth sockets may be involved in the production of this response.

A common problem seen in neurologically impaired infants and adults with head trauma is the "hyperactive tongue," which is often accompanied by a hyperactive gag reflex. To alleviate this problem, the receptors have to be systematically desensitized. The technique called *tongue walking* has met with clinical success.[15,44] It entails using an instrument such as a swizzle stick or tongue depressor to apply firm pressure to the midline of the tongue. The pressure is first applied near the tip of the tongue and progressively "walked back" in small steps. As the instrument reaches the back of the tongue, the stimulus sets off an automatic swallow response. The instrument is withdrawn the instant the swallow is triggered. This technique is repeated anywhere from 5 to 30 times a session, depending on individual responses.

Another technique, which might be called *deep stroking*, is used to either elicit or desensitize the gag reflex. Again, an instrument such as a swizzle stick is used to apply a light stroking stimulus to the posterior arc of the mouth. The instrument should lightly stretch the lateral walls of the palatoglossal arch of the uvula. Normally, the palatoglossal muscle elevates the tongue and narrows the fauces (the opening between the mouth and the oropharynx). Just behind the palatoglossal arch lies another arch, called the *palatopharyngeal arch.* Normally, this structure elevates the pharynx, closes off the nasopharynx, and aids in swallowing. Touch pressure to either arc incites the gag reflex. This touch pressure should be carefully calibrated. A hyperactive gag reflex may be best diminished by prolonged pressure to the arcs, whereas light, continuous stroking may be more facilitatory in activating a hypoactive gag reflex. A child or adult who has been fed by tube for extended periods of time will often have both hypersensitive reactions in various parts of the oral cavity and hyposensitive areas in other locations. This problem needs to be assessed to formulate a complete picture of the patient's difficulties.

The use of vibration over the muscles of mastication appears to be physiologically valid. Muscle spindles have been identified in the temporal and masseter muscles.[42] Selected use of vibration on the muscles of mastication enhances jaw stability and retraction. For protraction to be facilitated, the mandible is manually pushed in.[105]

To promote swallowing, some therapists use manual finger oscillations in downward strokes along the laryngopharyngeal muscles and follow up with stretch pressure. Ice is beneficial as a quick stimulus to the ventral portion of the neck or the sternal notch. In addition, chewing ice chips provides a thermal stimulus to the oral cavity and a proprioceptive stimulus to the jaw and teeth; it also increases salivation for swallowing.

It is recommended that a therapist work closely with a colleague who has experience working with functional feeding before independently beginning to work with patient's. The possible complications that might develop with individuals aspirating food cannot be overemphasized.[363]

The therapist can quickly realize that feeding as a proprioceptive, tactile, and gustatory input modality is extremely complex and often incorporates other sensory systems. Breaking down the specific approaches into finite techniques helps the clinician to categorize each component and then reassemble them into a whole. The job of dividing and reassembling the parts becomes more and more difficult as the number of input systems enlarges.[238]

Head and body movements in space. Proprioceptive and vestibular input is one of the most frequent combination techniques used by therapists. In fact, patient success in almost all therapeutic tasks depends on the coordinated input of these two sensory modalities.

If the head is moving in space and gravity has not been eliminated from the environment, vestibular and proprioceptive receptors will be firing to inform the CNS whether it should continue its feedforward pattern or adapt the plan because the environment no longer matches the programmed movement. Depending on the direction of the head motion and the way gravity is affecting joints, tendons, and muscles, the specific body response will vary according to the degree of flexibility within the motor system. Bed mobility, transfers, mat activities, and gait all incorporate these two modalities. Although all these functional movements can be performed without these feedback mechanisms, the CNS cannot adapt effectively to changing environments without input from these systems. For that reason alone, a thorough examination of the integrity of both systems and the effect of their combined input seems critical if any ADL is to be used as a treatment goal.

The use of a large ball or a gymnastic exercise ball can be classified under the category of proprioceptive-vestibular input. Many activities can be initiated over a ball. When a child or adult is prone on a ball, righting of the head can often be elicited by quickly projecting the child forward while the therapist exerts control through the feet, knees, or hips. If the weight of the head is greater than the available power, then a more vertical and less gravitationally demanding position can be used. As the head begins to come up, approximation of the neck can be added. Vibration of the paravertebral muscles might also assist. Rocking forward or bouncing the patient who is weight bearing on elbows or extended elbows will facilitate postural weight-bearing patterns through the two identified sensory input systems. Having a patient sitting on a therapy ball doing almost any exercise will require vestibular and proprioceptive feedback for appropriate adaptive responses to be made. The combination seems to play a delicate role in the maintenance of normal righting and the equilibrium response so important in functional independence.

A trampoline, balance board, or similar apparatus has the potential to channel a large amount of vestibular-proprioceptive input into the patient's CNS. In fact, a trampoline is so powerful it can often overstimulate the patient and cause excitation or arousal in the CNS.

The trampoline and balance board are generally used to increase balance reactions, orient the patient to position in space and to verticality, and increase postural tone. A patient with poor balance, poor postural tone, or inadequate position in space and verticality perception may be justifiably fearful of these apparatuses because of the rate, intensity, and skill necessary to accomplish the task. Because fear creates tone and that tone may be in conflict with the motor response from the patient, caution must be exercised with either modality. (See Chapter 21 for further discussion of the interactions of sensory systems and balance.)

Gentle shaking. A specific technique of gentle shaking can be listed under a combined vestibular, muscle spindle, and tendon category. This technique is performed while the patient is in a supine position and the head ventriflexed in midline. The head is flexed 35 to 40 degrees to reduce the influence of the otoliths and unnecessary extensor tone through the lateral vestibulospinal tract. This flexed position should be maintained throughout the procedure. The therapist places one hand under the patient's occiput and the other on the forehead. Light compression is applied to the cervical vertebrae. This technique activates the deep-joint receptors (C1 to C3) and muscle spindles in the neck along with the vestibular mechanism, which in turn connects with the cerebellum and motor nuclei with the brain stem. If the technique is performed slowly and continuously in a rhythmical motion, total-body inhibition will occur. If the pattern is irregular and fast, facilitation of the spinal motor generators will be observed.

Any one of these techniques can be implemented as a viable treatment approach in considering vestibular-proprioceptive stimuli. The selection of an approach or a method will depend on patient preference, patient response, the clinician's application skills, and the need for therapeutic assistance.

Innate Central Nervous System Programming

The responses of the PNS and CNS to various external stimuli determine the individuality of an organism and its survival potential within the environment. As organisms become more and more complex, the types of external stimuli and the internal mechanisms designed to deal with that input also increase in complexity. As the CNS develops structurally and functionally, inherent control over responses to certain common environmental stimuli seems to be manifested. Different areas of the motor system play different roles in the regulation of motor output. No area is dominant over another. Each area is interdependent on both the input from the environment and the intrinsic mechanisms and function of the nervous system.

As mentioned earlier, the PNS is intricately linked to the CNS and vice versa. Damage to one could potentially alter the neuropathways, their function, and ultimately behavior anywhere along the dynamic loops. Nevertheless, although researchers currently emphasize the dynamic interactions of all components,[364–371] clinicians have observed for decades different motor problems when different areas of the brain are damaged. Thus when individuals with neurological damage are discussed, it seems paramount to identify inherent synergy patterns available to humans, especially if those patterns become stereotypical and limit the patient's ability to adapt to a changing environment.

The authors do not recommend or discredit the use of any stereotypical or patterned response as a treatment procedure. Acknowledging the presence and stressing the importance of knowing how these motor programs affect patients' functional skills are important. Without this knowledge, therapists working with either children or adults with CNS dysfunction limit their understanding of the normal CNS, the normal motor control mechanism and its components, and the interactive effect of all systems on the end product: a motor response to a behavioral goal.

To conceptualize a systems model, the reader must replace the hypothesis of a stimulus response–based concept of reflexes[267] with a theory of neuronetworks that may be more or less receptive to environmental influences.[372] That sensitivity is modulated by a large number of interconnecting systems throughout the CNS and by the internal molecular sensitivity of the neurons themselves. Specific motor patterns seem to be organized or programmed at various levels or areas within the CNS. These synergies or patterned responses are thought to limit the degrees of freedom available to programming centers such as the basal ganglia and cerebellum[14,219] and to enable more control over the entire body. Having soft-wired, preprogrammed, patterned responses allows organizing systems to activate entire sequences of plans and modify any components within the total plan. Modification and adaptation then become the goal or function of the motor system in response to both internal and external goal-directed activities. The specific location of soft-wired programs is open to controversy, as is the complexity of programming at any level within the CNS. Recognizing that these neuronetworks exist with or without external environmental influences would suggest that patterns can and will present themselves without an identified stimulus. In the past, when an external influence was not correlated with an identifiable stereotypical motor pattern, it was referred to as a *synergy*. When a stimulus was identifiable, the entire loop was called a *reflex*. Reflexes and preprogrammed, soft-wired neuronetworks such as walking are interactive or superimposed on one another to form the background combinations for more complex program interactions. This superimposed network may encompass spinal and supraspinal coactivity, which makes it difficult to specify a level of processing. The exact control mechanisms that regulate the specific pattern may again be a shared responsibility throughout the nervous system, thus providing the plasticity observed when disease, trauma, or environmental circumstances force adaptation of existing plans, as discussed in the neuroplasticity section.

When specific patterned responses are observed, the reader must always hold simultaneously the interaction of all other motor programming options. In this way the therapist can easily conceptualize the variations within one response and the reason why, under different environmental and internal constraints, the motor response pattern may show great variations within the same general plan. Similarly, the expected motor response may not be observable, although it would seem appropriate and anticipated. The clinician must remember that the more complex the action (e.g., rolling compared with dressing compared with playing hockey), the greater the need for integration and coordination over pattern generators. Similarly, the more complex the desired action (especially in new learning), the greater the potential for needed perceptual-cognitive and affective interactions and the greater the potential for gratification and also for failure.

Certain patterned responses or neuronetworks might be considered more simplistic or protective in function. These patterns were once thought to be hard-wired spinal reflexes. It is now known that these reflexes, as well as complex pattern generators, exist at the spinal level and that their responses affect brain stem, cerebellar, and cortical actions. These centers simultaneously affect the specifics of the spinal neuronetwork responses.[123,124,373] With patients/clients who have low functional control over the spinal or brain stem motor networks, identifying existing patterns, optional patterns as a response to environmental demands, and obligatory patterns not within the control of the patient's intentional repertoire of patterns becomes a critical evaluative component before prognosing or identifying the most appropriate interventions.

Recognizing specific patterns and how those patterns and others might affect functional movement or positional patterns has clinical significance. For instance, a child with spastic cerebral palsy shows extension and "scissoring" when the pads of the feet are stimulated. Sometimes the extension pattern is so strong that the child will arch backward. Sustained positions that oppose pathological patterns are believed to elicit autogenic inhibition. Contraction-relaxation techniques also work on the autogenic inhibition principle.[22]

Just as afferent input can be used to alter tone and elicit movement, it can also become an obstacle when the therapist tries to coordinate complex movement patterns. The human palmar and plantar grasp patterns are often thought of as reflexive patterns, as seen in a newborn.[374-376] A persistent grasp pattern is a common occurrence in children and adults with a CNS insult. This dominant grasp is often reinforced by the patient's own fingers and frequently prevents functional use of the hand. If a withdrawal pattern is elicited every time a patient is touched, the patient not only will be unable to explore the environment through the tactile-proprioceptive systems but also will experience arousal by the influence of the cutaneous system over the reticular activating system. Severe agitation could likely be a behavioral outcome from such a persistent reflex.

As with any treatment procedure, a clinician should determine whether the technique will help the patient to obtain a higher level of function. The clinician must learn to recognize not only specific patterns but also what combinations of responses of pattern generators would look like. If the reader overlaid the map of the pattern generators for any combination of programs, a complex neuronetwork would result. To some it would verify chaos theory, and to others it would verify the end result of multiple systems interacting. The neuronetwork complexity of multiple input can be overwhelming. Thus a therapist must always be observant of the specific behavioral response and the moment-to-moment changes in behavior during a treatment session, even if the specific neuronetwork is not understood.

The clinician needs to observe whether the specific patterned response is (1) triggered by afferent input, (2) triggered by volitional intent, or (3) activated without environmental input including position in space or cortical intent. In the third case, the entire motor system needs to be evaluated to determine which portion might be modulating the observable behavior. Differentiating these motor components will help in selecting appropriate examination tools, making the movement diagnosis, prognosing, and selecting interventions.

Holistic Treatment Techniques Based on Multisensory Input

As already mentioned, a variety of accepted treatment methods exist. Each approach focuses on multisensory input introduced to the patient in controlled and identified sequences. These sequences are based on the inherent nature of synergistic patterns,[8,33] the patterns observed in humans[8,10,377] and lower-order animals,[36] or a combination of the two.[22,31] Each method focuses on the total patient, the specific clinical problems, and alternative treatment approaches available within each established framework. Certain methods have traditionally emphasized specific neurological disabilities. Cerebral palsy in children[10,26,31,378-380] and hemiplegia in adults[11,12,24,34,381,382] are the two most frequently identified. In the past two decades, substantial clinical attention has been paid to children with learning difficulties.[15,40,383-385] Yet the concepts and treatment procedures specific to all the techniques have been applied to almost every neurological disability seen in the clinical setting. This expansion of the use of each method seems to be a natural evolution because of the structure and function of the

CNS and commonalities in clinical signs manifested by brain insult. Literature in occupational and physical therapy management of individuals with various other neurological problems has also enriched therapists' identification of efficacious interventions, as well as those that should be removed from the toolbox.[386-391]

Additional Augmented Interventions: Current Focus

Four augmented therapeutic intervention approaches that have become accepted over the past decade are (1) body weight supported treadmill training (BWSTT), (2) constraint-induced movement therapy (CIMT), (3) imagery (discussed in the section on the visual system) and virtual reality, and (4) robotic training. Each is discussed as a separate intervention philosophy, but the reader must remember that these are *augmented intervention* programs. Before an individual would be considered functionally independent, the patient must be able to perform the functional activity in a natural environment, such as ambulation within a home setting or eating using the more involved extremity without having the unaffected extremity restrained. A fourth augmented intervention approach, robotics, will also be presented briefly within this chapter to illustrate how therapists and patients have the capabilities to interface with new and sophisticated technology. The reader is also referred to Chapter 38 for more in-depth detail. One additional augmented approach, the Accelerated Skill Acquisition Program (ASAP), has been described here. This approach is currently undergoing, and research is still needed to establish efficacy. This approach is impairment oriented, emphasizes bimanual activities, and focuses on active, patient-centered collaboration reinforced with self-management and self-efficacy.[392-395] This approach emphasizes attended, repetitive task practice progressing in difficult situations and meets the principles for neuroplasticity.

Body weight–supported treadmill training. Over the past decade, BWSTT has been accepted within the therapeutic community as an alternative approach to teaching gait training for individuals with CNS damage and residual motor dysfunction. Students are introduced to the treatment procedures and potential sequences from total dependence to independence of the patient. Colleagues take continuing education courses to learn to position and drive the various motor components of the gait program while using BWSTT. Both a vertical support (harness) or air-distributed positive pressure to unweight the body and a treadmill are combined for BWSTT. The treadmill perturbs the feet backward or shifts the center of gravity forward, and the ground reaction forces are reduced by the support. The clinical environment unloads the CNS's need to (1) provide protection from falling; (2) trigger and control an effective and efficient postural system reaction; (3) reflexively drive the power stepping reaction necessary to perform upright ambulation; (4) control the balance strategy of stepping to prevent falling; (5) facilitate rhythmic, symmetrical, bilateral stepping; and (6) have a cognitive interface with the various motor programs necessary to run this functional activity. The treadmill perturbation of the lower limb into extension facilitates the transfer of weight to the forefoot. This forward translation forces the feet backward and optimizes the stepping reaction forward. If the moving treadmill is not a sufficient stimulus to trigger a step, this component can be controlled by one or two therapists, depending on whether it is a unilateral or bilateral problem. If the patient does not step, has a delayed stepping response, or steps effectively with only one foot, the therapist(s) can help to initiate the desired response at the patient's feet. The rate of movement or speed of the treadmill can also be controlled, as well as the length of time spent on the affected leg. This treadmill strategy may encourage more symmetrical and faster gait speed in patients after stroke[396] and with Parkinson disease[397-399] compared with standard physical therapy. This control by the therapist helps to facilitate a patient's response even if it is slow or inadequate for normal over-ground ambulation. The question remains whether this type of augmented therapeutic intervention does create the best environment to empower the patient to learn or relearn normal locomotion after a neurological insult.

The literature is mixed with regard to this question. The literature supports BWSTT for individuals with incomplete spinal injury,[390] older adults with Parkinson disease,[391] and some individuals after stroke,[132,392] but other literature suggests that BWSTT is equivalent to or maybe less effective than over-ground gait training with a PT,[400,401] and still other researchers report that there is no difference among different forms of ambulation training.[401] With the literature so inconsistent, the clinician could be confused as to the effectiveness of BWSTT and whether this type of augmented intervention should even be considered. One primary problem with the research literature is the great variance in training and the identified variables selected by researchers within their respective studies.[130,402,403–405] The following are examples of potential variables:

- Walking speeds
- Amount of body weight supported
- Frequency of training
- Length of training
- Aerobic levels of training
- Type of unweighting
- Type and severity of the patient's neurological dysfunction
- Presence of hypertonicity
- Age of patient
- Time since injury
- Level of independence
- Assistance needed during ambulation

There have been some excellent systematic reviews of BWSTT in the literature that help to identify many of the reasons the literature seems so inconsistent.[130,406] The research indicates that the two populations of individuals who most often benefit from use of BWSTT are people with incomplete spinal cord injuries and individuals post stroke. Another problem in BWSTT research is that the harness systems can be uncomfortable at 20% to 30% unweighting.[407] Thus, as stated, the huge number of possible variables and functional ways to measure outcomes using BWSTT or other types of training along with BWSTT has led to confusion in the literature.[401,402,405,408,409] Even with all the confusion regarding these variables, this form of augmented intervention seems to show promise as a protocol for gait training. Future research studies will still need to determine which patients, their degree of motor involvement, the optimal dosage, the time after insult, the best combination of other interactive interventions (e.g., pharmacological, robotic), the specific type of gait impairments, and where within the gait cycle the patient's would most likely benefit from this type of augmented intervention. It is important to continue to obtain evidence to more precisely define the practice guidelines for BWSTT. As has been shown in the past, new treatment ideas gain popularity and become standards of practice without the rigor of establishing an evidence-based practice.[40,45,410,411]

Constraint-induced movement therapy. CIMT (or CI therapy) is a type of intervention for individuals with motor system limitations with the aim of reducing the impact of upper limb functional limitations after a stroke. Major components of CIMT include the restraint of the less impaired limb, behavioral strategies, and supervised practice of functional tasks.

The restraint or immobilization of the less impaired limb and resultant forced use of the affected limb for prolonged periods varies from 6 hours to more than 10 hours per day across the literature. Patients typically participate in 6 to 7 hours of therapy a day; in addition, this training is reinforced in home activities and ADLs.[412–415] A hand mitt or sling is used to constrain the use of the unaffected upper limb while the affected limb is engaged in a forced-use, mass practice of meaningful motor tasks.

Supervised practice of functional tasks is structured to challenge the capacities of the patients. The therapist-patient ratio is typically 1:1, with the therapist present to give tactile and verbal feedback and instruction, along with assistance for the desired skill training. Daily practice lengths vary across literature; early studies implemented 6 hours of practice per day, with more recent studies describing 1 to 2 hours per day using a modified CIMT program.

The focus of CIMT is on shaping behavior to improve functional use of the impaired upper limb.[416,417] Behavioral strategies, such as shaping and adherence logs, are used to promote transfer of training to daily activities. Patients typically keep a daily treatment diary to document the amount and intensity of therapeutic intervention and the amount of time spent wearing the mitt or sling each day for the duration of the intervention.[414]

CIMT and the learned nonuse theory are based on deafferentation experiments in monkeys done by Dr. Edward Taub.[418,419] Taub and colleagues proposed that the inability to move and use the paretic upper limb may arise, in part, from "learned nonuse".[420] Early primate studies demonstrated that if the upper limb was surgically impaired by dorsal rhizotomy to disrupt afferent input to the sensory cortex, the animal stopped using the limb for function. Active mobility was restored by immobilizing the intact upper limb for several days while training the animal to use the affected limb.[420] The results indicated that the inability to use the impaired limb may be a learned behavioral response.

CIMT is based on the theory that impairment in hand and arm function in patients after a stroke is compounded by learned nonuse of that affected upper extremity, which leads to a physical change in the cortical representation of the upper limb in the primary sensory cortex.[421] Learned nonuse develops in the early stages after a stroke in humans as the patient compensates for difficulty using the impaired limb by increasing reliance on the intact limb. This compensation has been shown to hinder recovery of function in the impaired limb.[412] The first report of CIMT for hemiparesis in humans was by Ostendorf and Wolf in 1981.[422] Since then, investigations have demonstrated the effectiveness of CIMT with individuals who have residual upper-extremity weakness as the result of an upper motor neuron lesion.[422–432] CIMT has been shown to be an effective therapy in persons with chronic stroke who have sufficient residual motor control to benefit from the exercises,[423–425,430,433–437] in brain-injured patients,[438,439] in children with hemiplegic cerebral palsy,[414,416,440–443,444] and in patients with Parkinson disease.[445] The CI therapy approach has also been used successfully for the lower-limb rehabilitation of patients with stroke hemiparesis, incomplete spinal cord injury, and fractured hip.[426] Other diverse chronic disabling conditions, including nonmotor disorders such as phantom limb pain and aphasia, may also benefit from CIMT.[426]

The criteria for the inclusion of subjects in most CIMT research studies have focused on voluntary movement ability in the involved upper extremity.[412,416–419,421–433,437] These criteria included the ability to start from a resting position of forearm pronation and wrist flexion and actively extend each metacarpal-phalangeal and interphalangeal joint at least 10 degrees and extend the wrist at least 20 degrees through a ROM.[434] It is estimated that approximately 20% to 25% of the population of patients with chronic stroke with residual motor deficit meet this motor criterion.[415]

Not all patients with hemiparesis have been found to benefit from CIMT. It has not been shown to be beneficial for patient's with severe chronic upper-extremity hemiplegia after a stroke.[446] Attempts to include individuals who did not meet the minimal motor criteria (at least 10 degrees of finger extension and 20 degrees of wrist extension) have failed to demonstrate significant or lasting functional improvements in the involved upper extremity after CIMT.[426,446]

The criteria associated with successful therapeutic components of CIMT therapy are (1) restraint of the unaffected arm with a mitt, sling, or glove for 90% of waking hours for a 2- to 3-week period; and (2) therapeutic sessions with physical and occupational therapy in which patients concentrate on intense, repetitive task training of the more affected upper extremity for 8 hours a day.[a] These same criteria have been identified as challenges to CIMT. Wearing a mitt or sling for 90% of waking hours is very restrictive. Similarly, therapy sessions of 6 hours per day for 2 weeks very intensive and is burdensome for the patient and caregivers. The application of CIMT to real-life clinical environments presents challenges, including the time and physical demands on therapists, the cost to the patient, and the resources required during rehabilitation. This limits its cost-effectiveness and overall effect.[412] Many patients in the acute rehabilitation setting do not qualify for CIMT on the basis of limited motor function.[412] CIMT, by its nature, can prove to be difficult, frustrating, and intense, and progress can be slow. It will create beneficial effects only if all participants put in the time and effort to make it successful.[414] Many subjects who have been presented with the opportunity to participate in CIMT programs and studies have refused because of the intense practice schedule and the necessity of the restrictive device.[447] Therapists have also voiced concerns about patient adherence and safety.[447] Although it has been shown to be effective in laboratory research, CIMT may have limited practicality in some clinical environments.[447] Techniques were modified to address these concerns resulting in modified CIMT (mCIMT); the restriction on the less affected limb was limited to 5 hours per day (Page et al., 2013).[448]

Subjects with chronic stroke hemiparesis who have participated in CIMT rehabilitation programs have demonstrated significant gains in functional use of the stroke-affected upper extremity as measured by the Motor Activity Log,[415] significant reductions in motor impairment on the upper-extremity motor component of the Fugl-Meyer Test,[446] and more efficient task performance as measured by the Wolf Motor Function Test.[449-453] Fine motor improvements have also been measured with use of the Grooved Pegboard Test and other dexterity tests.[412,421] These improvements in impairment and function have been shown to persist at follow-up evaluations up to 2 years after training.[421,432,444,452] Individuals participating in CIMT studies have demonstrated improvements in the amount of use and quality of movement in the more involved upper extremity and carryover of skills from the clinic to real-world activities.[414,422-424] This functional improvement may be significant even if the patient has previously participated in a conventional rehabilitation program.[454] Recent systematic reviews and meta-analyses identified a multitude of outcome measures from those initially mentioned that primarily looked at upper extremity function. Outcome measures identified in the recent systematic reviews on CIMT include the Functional Independence Measure (FIM),[455,456,457,459] Barthel Index (BI),[455,456,459] Action Research Arm Test (ARAT),[455,456,457] Motor Assessment Scale (MAS),[455] Stroke Impact Scale (SIS) participation,[459] quality of life (QoL),[458] and ADLs.[458]

The question of when to begin CIMT after a stroke has not yet been definitively answered. CIMT has been applied to patients with subacute strokes. This early use of CIMT is based on the hypothesis that earlier intervention may prevent learned nonuse and may have a greater impact on overall function. Investigators have found no adverse effects of CIMT in the subacute phase and only slightly greater improvement in motor function of the affected upper extremity.[460] There is some evidence from animal studies to suggest that if CIMT is introduced too early (e.g., 24 hours post stroke), it may be detrimental and potentially harmful to humans. It may cause an increase in the size of the cortical lesion. This is based on studies of "forced overuse" in animals.[461-464] Kozlowski and colleagues[464] found that early forced overuse of the affected limb within the first 7 days after a sensorimotor cortex lesion impeded motor recovery of the affected limb and enlarged lesion volume. Bland and co-workers[461] also forced overuse of the affected forelimb immediately after a focal cortical middle cerebral artery stroke, which increased the lesion size and impaired motor recovery. The relative risks and benefits of "acute" CIMT and its optimal timing remain to be determined.[412]

The neurophysiological mechanisms that are believed to underlie the treatment benefit of CIMT include overcoming learned nonuse and plastic brain reorganization.[454,465] Studies have confirmed that CIMT produces use-dependent cortical reorganization in humans with stroke-related paresis of an upper limb.[424,432,465,466] However, there is some question as to whether the improvements in upper-extremity motor function after CIMT are a result of the reduction of learned nonuse or of overcoming a sense of increased effort during movement.[421] Thus task-specific, goal-oriented training with the affected limb might be similarly beneficial, even without the constraint of the less affected side.

Neuroimaging studies such as transcranial magnetic stimulation (TMS), fMRI, and electroencephalography[325,421] have been used to provide cortical evidence of neuroplasticity and cortical changes after CIMT.[414,427,432,467] These studies have validated that massed practice of CIMT produces a massive use-dependent cortical reorganization. This change increases the area in which the cortex is involved during voluntary movements of an affected limb, even in patients with chronic stroke.[412,468]

The utility of CIMT depends on several factors including economic considerations, limitations of the practice setting, and the cognitive and physical status of the patient. Less intense practice schedule models[467,469,470] and combining CIMT with pharmacological interventions or robotic assistance may help to increase its effectiveness and decrease costs without sacrificing the benefits.[412,471] Studies are underway to determine if massed task-specific practice without constraint can be equally beneficial.[472,473] Systematic reviews and meta-analysis[455-459] demonstrate improvements in upper-extremity movements during functional activities. Interestingly, evidence is limited on the improvements in quality of life and independence in ADL from intense CIMT. mCIMT, developed to address concerns on burden of such an intensive therapy, has demonstrated significant improvements in upper limb movements and independence in ADLs.[459] Despite improvements noted with CIMT and mCIMT, further research is needed to understand the mechanisms that lead to improvements and the most effective functional activities. The evidence on CIMT, along with evidence on task-related training, posit that task-related training of functional activities with behavioral strategies is an effective, feasible approach to the rehabilitation of the upper limb after stroke.

Robotics, gaming, and virtual reality (see Chapter 38). The most recent augmented intervention procedures involve the use of technology to regain control over functional movement. The use of robotics,[474-477] virtual reality,[478-481] and gaming[482-485] in the clinical environment continues to gain popularity as technology for gaming and virtual reality continue to be more affordable, and their applications are becoming more widespread. A thorough discussion of these technologies can be found in Chapter 38.

With the improvements and expansion of computational approaches and faster and more powerful computers, different types of robotic technologies have been tested in neurorehabilitation.[486] Advantages identified to robotic devices in rehabilitation include the ability to provide consistent practice for patients to help decreases variability; decrease therapist burden with decreased hands-in clinical time and provide practice outside of the therapy sessions; and present another mechanism for quantitative examination and tracking of outcomes. The ability to deliver high-dosage and high-intensity training.[487] has been noted to be the most important advantage of robotic technology in rehabilitation. Robot-assisted training aims to provide intensive practice of repetitive, stereotyped, and functional movements with reduced therapist burden.

Systematic reviews and meta-analyses on robot-assisted training have shown mixed results. In a randomized controlled trial (RCT) that incorporated robotic therapy in an intensive task-specific practice of the upper limb,[488] the group that completed an 8-week robotic training performed better than the comparison group on the Fugl-Meyer Assessment (FGA). The improvements were small and of weak significance, which bring into question the clinical relevance. Furthermore, improvements were not retained in follow-up assessments at 16 and 34 weeks. Participants in the conventional therapy group continued to improve during the follow-up sessions, suggesting that functional training may be of better value. A review of 12 RCTs in multiple stages of stroke[489] showed that robotic therapy is not more effective than conventional therapy for upper limb recovery, but when added to conventional therapy, significant improvements were seen in motor recovery of the of the upper extremity. With the costs in human training and robotic device and its limited efficacy, robotic devices are more an adjunct to therapy rather than the primary method of intervention.

The evidence on robotic therapy is variable and difficult to generalize given the heterogeneity of the robotic devices, the participants' characteristics, and the variety of the study designs in the literature. At this time, the role of robot-assisted training for stroke rehabilitation is more of an adjunct to therapy versus replacement to conventional therapy. Further developments on robotic technology may improve the efficacy and costs associated with robotic devices. For this approach to be an essential part of neurorehabilitation and a standard therapeutic modality, further studies with larger populations that demonstrate superior efficacy in motor recovery, that provide functional benefits above and with conventional therapy, and that offer realistic economic feasibility are substantially needed.

Summary of augmented intervention strategies. As with many interventions, the therapist may need to start with augmented approaches to reduce impairments and/or gain functional movement in a controlled environment. As the patient demonstrates improvement in this narrow window of movement or function, the clinician could then increase the challenge with the goal of optimizing functional performance and improving quality of life. A summary of the augmented intervention strategies that facilitate neuroplasticity can be found in Box 8.6.

BOX 8.6 Summary of Intervention Strategies to Facilitate Neuroplasticity

There are many different intervention strategies to use when working with patients with neurological problems. These interventions need to be matched to the needs of the individual patient and be consistent with the patient's goals and objectives. All the intervention strategies should be goal directed and repeated with attention to both the input mechanisms (motivation, sensory) and the output mechanisms (movement). The input and output mechanisms are multifactorial, and they also involve all components of the sensory, emotional, sensorimotor, and motor systems. Although evidence is increasing about the benefit of learning-based activities, research is still needed to help define more precisely when intervention should occur, how intense the intervention should be, how much repetition is needed, how long the learning-based activities need to be continued and spaced, how specific the training needs to be, how quickly behaviors can be progressed and the magnitude of gradation needed, how to keep patients interested, motivated, and compliant in learning, and the magnitude of interference in learning relative to depression, stress, and loss of self-esteem. The intervention strategies can be broadly classified as follows:

1. General body responses leading to quieting of the nervous system[11,263]
   a. Slow rocking in a rocking chair or hammock.
   b. Slow anterior-posterior, horizontal, or vertical movements (chair, hassock, mesh net, swing, ball bolster, riding in a carriage, glider chair).
   c. Rotating equipment such as a bed, chair, stool, hammock, or therapeutic or gymnastic ball (e.g., rhythmical bouncing).
   d. Slow linear, undulating movements, such as in a carriage, stroller, wheelchair, or wagon.
   e. Wrapping up tightly before rocking (e.g., roll self in sheet; put both arms inside tight tee shirt).
   f. Listening to quiet music or natural environmental sounds (e.g., waves).
   g. Repeating activities listed above first with eyes open and then closed.
2. Techniques to heighten postural righting reactions[136]
   a. Rapid or unexpected anterior-posterior or angular acceleration.
      i. Scooter board: pulled or projected down inclines.
      ii. Prone over ball: rapid acceleration forward.

   iii. Platform or mesh net: prone.
   iv. Slides.
   v. Any proprioceptive input that heightens postural extensors (e.g., quick stretch, tapping, resistance, vibration, joint compression). Remember to use the most natural first, such as quick stretch versus vibration.
   b. Rapid anterior-posterior motion in prone position, weight-bearing patterns such as on elbows or extended elbows while rocking and crawling.
   c. Weight-shifting in kneeling, half-kneel, or standing positions (first in vertical and then off vertical within limits of stability by an activity itself [reaching]).
   d. Do activities with eyes closed.
   e. Create dual-task activities such as walking and talking, stepping over obstacles while on unstable surfaces, reading while maintaining balance in a confusing environment.
   f. Challenge balance in distracting environments (e.g., moving surround, multisensory stimuli in visual surround).
3. Facilitatory techniques to influence whole-body responses[33,105,265]
   a. Movement patterns in specific sequences.
      i. Rolling patterns.
      ii. Prop on elbows (prone and side-lying positions) and extend and flex elbows as well as crawling (e.g., side by side, or linear and angular motion).
      iii. Coming to sit (side-lying to sit [using upper trunk and head rotation], prone to four-point position to sit [four-point position to lower trunk rotation to side sit to sit], adult sit [full flexion leading with head]).
      iv. Coming to stand (squat to stand, half-kneel to stand, standing from a chair or stool).
   b. Spinning.
      i. Mesh net.
      ii. Sit and spin toy.
      iii. Office chair on universal joint.

Continued

BOX 8.6 Summary of Intervention Strategies to Facilitate Neuroplasticity—cont'd

c. Any activity that uses acceleration and deceleration of head.
  i. Sitting and reaching.
  ii. Walking.
  iii. Running.
  iv. Moving from sit to stand.
  v. Doing activities with eyes closed, head still, and then eyes closed, head turning.
d. Performing activities that require attention, memory, and cognitive processing at the same time.
4. Combined facilitatory and inhibitory technique: inverted tonic labyrinthine activities
  a. Inverted tonic labyrinthine activities.
    i. Semiinverted in-sitting (head between the legs).
    ii. Squatting to stand (head below heart).
    iii. Thirty degrees to total inverted vertical position beginning in supine.
  b. Somatosensory and sensorimotor stimulation (refer to earlier in this chapter).
    i. Proprioceptive stimulation.
      (a) Vibration over joints.
      (b) Vibration in opposite direction of movement.
      (c) Wear weights around ankles or on belt.

  (d) Position the limbs and the trunk to match a position visually presented.
  (e) Move slowly to the count of a metronome and then change speeds.
  (f) Look at pictures and position the body to match the pictures.
  c. Auditory discrimination (localization).
5. Techniques to facilitate specific task performance
  a. Forced use.
    i. Create training activities in which patients must use the affected extremity.
    ii. Minimize the need to use the unaffected side.
    iii. Use bilateral activities in which both hands and upper extremities are required.
  b. Constraint-induced movement therapy (CIMT) (forced use)[423–425,468,490,491]
  c. Mass task practice
  d. Mental imagery.
  e. Mental practice.
  f. Body weight–supported treadmill training (BWSTT).[394–397,492]
  g. Integration of robotics and technology (see Chapter 38).
  h. Use of gaming (Wii Fit, Brain Fit).[479,482–485]

CONCLUSION

The CNS is in a constant state of change throughout life. The brain is unique to each individual. Each brain has idiosyncrasies but also has an enormous number of predictable responses. These factors affect the success or failure of the patient/client-therapist interaction. In Box 8.7 the reader will find guidelines that may assist in determining the type of interventions (functional, impairment, augmented, or somatosensory training) that will best match the patient's functional movement capability. In answering the questions presented, the therapist will gain a better idea of which examination tools will best help to objectively measure the progress of the patient toward that patient's specific goals. From that thorough examination process, the therapist must decide which treatment is appropriate and the most efficient course of intervention on the basis of the goals of the patient and family, the movement system deficit, the prognosis, the resources available, and the skills of the therapist. Once a decision is made regarding whether the interventions should be based on compensation, substitution, habituation, neural adaptation, or a combination of the four, the team must select the best options available given all the resources. The options include functional retraining, impairment training, augmented and contrived interventions, and somatosensory reintegration. No matter the specifics of the intervention selection, the therapist must cognitively organize intervention options in a sequential process, be willing to change direction or options as the patient changes, and develop greater clinical repertoire of intervention strategies.

When specific augmented interventions are needed, the therapist must select specific interventions according to the needs of the patient, the time available for therapy, the level and extent of the functional involvement, the motivation of the patient and family, the creativity of the therapist, and, of course, the existing pathology, whether it be stable or an active disease process. A therapist must choose whether somatosensory retraining, functional training, impairment training, augmented treatment interventions, or any combination of these four will provide the patient with the most environmentally effective, cost-efficient, and quickest map to functional independence or maximal quality of life. How each therapist combines the interventions with the patient's specific needs will vary according to education, belief, skill, and openness to learning from the total environment itself. Learning should lead to further learning. Answers to unknowns will be found, with new unknowns coming to consciousness. The brain is still more mystery than not, so for most OTs and PTs beginning or ending their practice, the adventure has just begun. *Enjoy the experience.*

BOX 8.7 Conceptual Guidelines for Clinical Decision Making: How to Select Treatment Options for Patients With Neurological Impairments

After performing examination procedures in which you identify problems with activities and participation, you will then be able to classify these into clusters or syndromes (i.e., the physical therapy diagnosis). You then need to formulate a prognosis and determine the intervention options.

To determine the *best* treatment options for a patient with a neurological condition with movement problems, you must simultaneously consider non–physical therapy–based as well as non–neurological system–based limitations along with the specific neurological impairments.

Assume the *best-case scenario* (which never exists) in which there are no limitations in health benefits, from cultural beliefs or family, caused by conflict with other care providers, or in systems other than motor such as cognitive, emotional, vascular, integumentary, pulmonary, cardiac, and so on.

First, what does the patient want to do compared with what his or her motor system can do? Can you work on improvement of impairments and function within activities the patient is motivated to do? *If so, do it!*

BOX 8.7 Conceptual Guidelines for Clinical Decision Making: How to Select Treatment Options for Patients With Neurological Impairments—cont'd

Second, without altering the patient's normal feedback (intrinsic) mechanisms, can he or she perform the functional activity without causing program adaptations that are so stereotypical that those programs may limit future movement functions and carryover?

For example: can you create an activity that will do the following without contriving the environment and while still running flexible, malleable motor programs?
1. Improve range of motion (ROM) or
2. Improve power or
3. Improve coordination or
4. Improve balance or
5. Improve endurance or
6. Any or all of the above
7. Have any similar effect
   If so, do it!

If not, you will need to contrive the environment to create functional change through treatment intervention.

Ask Yourself

1. Where in the activity can you optimize biomechanics, and where are biomechanics deoptimized? If the body was placed at a better biomechanical advantage:
   a. Would the patient be able to run and power the program?
   b. Would the motor program run more fluidly and procedurally?
   c. Would there be greater endurance?
   If your answer is *yes,* then proceed with the activity initially and then increase the range and challenge all components of the program.
2. Throughout the activity, where would the least and greatest power be needed? Does the program run differently at different points throughout the activity depending on power production? Optimize what power you have, while maintaining fluid, relaxed program generators. Hypertonicity will often be observed if you ask for more power than the generators can create in a normal fashion.
3. Look at the program itself.
   a. What CNS components are missing (impairments or functional problems)? These are usually your neurological diagnoses (physical therapy diagnoses).
   b. Can you elicit through treatment intervention corrections of the impairments in any aspect of the program? *If so, how?*
      • Caused by biomechanical advantage
      • Caused by musculoskeletal advantage
      • Caused by the program advantage itself

Optimize:
   • Synergistic advantage
   • Balance synergies
   • Sensory processing
   • And so on

These treatment answers will lay the foundations for your specific intervention strategies.
      c. Can you elicit those components in any other movement programs? If so, these are treatment alternatives, although they will not be task specific and have less immediate carryover.
4. Select movement activities that use existing components procedurally and facilitate or elicit function from impairment component of subsystems.
5. Prioritize functional activities by identifying daily living needs of the patient, goals of the patient, and functional skill of the patient. Determine which impairments affect the greatest number of functional activities. Similarly determine which impairments can be quickly changed to gain functional skill. Decide within the limits of the environment which activities to focus on first.

   For example: assume the patient has poor balance in sitting and standing. He plans to sit in the lounge chair most of the day but walk to the toilet when necessary. Although range, power, and postural control would need to be considered, you might decide to work on standing balance and balance during walking before sitting balance owing to task specificity and functional need. This is not stating that sitting balance is not important; it is prioritizing the activities according to need. Power, range, posture, and so on may determine the specific intervention strategies used to work on standing and walking balance.
6. If normal programming cannot be elicited, look at adaptations and determine alternative interventions such as the following:
   a. Adaptive equipment: biofeedback, orthotics, canes, and so on
   b. Adaptive environments: ramps, rails, lights, changing walkways, changing surfaces (e.g., removing shag carpets)
   c. Encouraging stereotypical and inflexible programs
   d. Combination of a, b, or c

   Make sure that when selection of alternative approaches or adaptations is made, consideration is given to what will be given up by adapting the environment and central nervous system. Consider whether that decision is truly cost efficient and the best alternative to meet the needs and goals of the patient, his or her family, and the physical and cultural environment within which he or she will function.

Case Examples:

CASE STUDY 8.2 Patient With Lack of Head Control

Impaired head control is a common clinical problem in developmentally delayed children or in individuals who have sustained a severe injury to the central nervous system (CNS). Virtually all functional activities are affected by this impairment.
The patient is Timothy, a 16-year-old adolescent male with a closed-head injury sustained 3 months ago. He currently demonstrates the following attributes regarding head control:
• Mild extensor hypertonicity is present in the supine position, and Timothy is unable to rotate his neck or lift his head off the mat.
• In prone position, extensor hypertonicity is absent and hypotonicity prevails. The patient is able to briefly bob his head off the mat in a cervical hyperextension pattern. Mild tonal shifts occur in his trunk and lower extremities when his head is passively turned to either side or when his neck is flexed or extended.
• Timothy is unable to roll or perform any functional activity in the horizontal plane.

• When placed in a long sitting position, he is unable to hold the position and his head remains in total flexion with his chin on his chest. Extensor tone dominates the lower extremities.
• When placed in a short sitting position on a mat table, he is unable to hold the position. General hypotonicity prevails, and his neck remains flexed with chin nearly to chest and his trunk is slightly flexed. When asked to pick up his head, he initiates a partial movement with cervical hyperextension. A position of cervical extension increases his trunk extensor tone. Extensor tone of lower extremities is diminished compared with long sitting.
• When placed upright with the head vertical, he is unable to hold this head position.
• Timothy does not mind being touched and responds well to handling techniques.

Continued

CASE STUDY 8.2   Patient With Lack of Head Control—cont'd

From the analysis of these clinical signs, the following clinical interpretations are presented:

1. In the horizontal position, Timothy has persistence of a motor program that is enhanced by the spatial position and its influence on the vestibular system. The result might be considered persistence of a tonic labyrinthine reflex (TLR). In this patient the dominant synergic pattern is extension. While he is supine, extension prevails. While he is prone, extension is inhibited, although flexion tone is not dominant. Because of the persistence of hyperactivity among the extensor motor generators, the ability to initiate rolling using a neck-righting pattern is prevented. The presence of a mild, asymmetrical tonic neck reflex to both sides and a symmetrical tonic neck reflex has been noted. Because of his instability and low tone, Timothy seems to be using these stereotypical patterns volitionally to assist in gaining some control over his motor patterns. In prone position, Timothy has the ability to move into a neck extension or optic and labyrinthine righting (OLR) pattern but is unable to hold it. Movement and range are present but postural holding is missing.

2. As a result of ventriflexion of the head in sitting, the vestibular apparatus is placed in a position similar to that when prone. In a like manner, the total patterns remain fairly consistent. The decrease in extensor tone in trunk and extremities in short sitting may result from the positioning of hip and knee flexion and kyphosis of the back. The inability to flex the hips with knee extension suggests that total tonal patterns or synergies are dominant. The patient is unable to break out of those dominant patterns. Dominant OLR is not present.

3. When asked, Timothy carries out the command to the best of his motor ability. This suggests the presence of some intact verbal processing, which is translated into appropriate motor acts. Similarly, when asked to pick up his head, he does just that, suggesting some perceptual integrity of body image, body schema, and position in space. Knowing where his head is in space and where to reposition it also suggests that some proprioceptive-vestibular input and processing are occurring.

4. Timothy's enjoyment of being moved in space as related to handling techniques suggests proprioceptive-vestibular integrity. Similarly, his tactile systems seem to be functioning in a discriminatory manner and modifying negative responses of withdrawal and arousal. However, specific tactile perception would need a great deal of further testing. Thus he demonstrates functional strengths in cognition and perception, in limbic motivation, in some areas of sensory integrity, and in control over available but limited motor programming. Yet performance on any functional test would result in identification of an individual whose functional limitations prevent him from independence in any activity. Prognosis must be guarded until the therapist has had an opportunity to augment the environment to determine how quickly he will regain control and retain the learning. The initial plan of care is assumed to focus on development of head control as a preliminary and necessary motor program for all functional daily living activity. The estimated time it will take to regain this function will not be identified until after the first intervention session.

Evaluation of Movement Deficits

The patient is unable to functionally control his head in any position in space, which limits independence in all functional activities. Lack of postural coactivation and adequate control over the motor generators has led to imbalances in the tonal characteristics of flexor and extensor patterns with the compensatory development of stereotypical patterns of movement.

Goal of Intervention Program

The goal is development of independent head control, initially in a vertical midline posture with the intent of enlarging that biomechanical window to include all positions in space.

Now that the clinical problem has been analyzed and the goal of development of head control set, an intervention sequence or protocol must be established. Timothy lacks head control in all planes and in all patterns of movement. Thus flexors and extensors must be facilitated to develop a dynamic coactivation or postural holding pattern of the neck. The categorization scheme can now be of some assistance. The therapist can ask, "Are there any inherent mechanisms that enhance flexors or extensors in a holding pattern?" The OLR reaction should elicit the desired response. Similarly, the clinician can ask, "Are there any inherent motor programs that would prevent righting of the head to face vertical OLR?" The TLR would block or modify the facilitation of OLR. Knowing that the TLR is most dominant in horizontal and least dominant (if at all affected) in vertical is of clinical significance. It is also important to know that the OLR is most frequently tested in a vertical position and seems most active in that position. Awareness that the patient is sensitive to total patterns (e.g., flexion facilitates flexion or extension facilitates extension) gives additional treatment clues.

After all this information has been assimilated, the following treatment could be established.

For enhancement of neck flexors, the patient will be placed in a totally flexed position in vertical, with the head positioned in neutral. The patient will be rocked backward toward supine, allowing gravity to quick stretch the flexors (Fig. 8.2A). As soon as the neck flexors are stretched, the head should be tapped forward and then back to vertical but not beyond. This avoids hyperextension, extreme stretch to the proprioceptors, and the horizontal supine position of the labyrinths, all of which dampen the flexors and facilitate the extensors. The quick stretch and position should optimally facilitate OLR, which should activate the neck flexors. The total flexion of the body similarly facilitates the neck flexors. Once the neck flexors respond, Timothy can be rocked farther and farther backward while maintaining the head in vertical or ventriflexion (see Fig. 8.2B). Once Timothy can be rocked from vertical to horizontal and back to vertical while maintaining good flexor neck control, his CNS has demonstrated inherent control and modification over the stereotypical patterns, such as the TLR in supine with respect to its influence over the neck musculature. This rocking maneuver can be done on diagonals to practice flexion and rotation (see Fig. 8.2C), the key to eliciting a neck-righting, rolling pattern from supine to prone. The total flexed pattern can also be altered by adding more and more extension of the extremities. This decreases the external facilitation to the flexors and demands that Timothy's CNS takes more and more control (internal regulation). Additional treatment procedures can be extracted from a variety of sensory categories. To add additional proprioceptive input, any one of those listed techniques might be used. The rotation and speed of the rocking pattern affect the vestibular mechanism. Auditory and visual stimuli can be used effectively. If the therapist takes a position slightly below the patient's horizontal eye level, the patient (to look at the therapist) will need to look down and flex his head, thus encouraging the desired pattern. Any type of visual or auditory stimulus that directs the patient into the desired pattern would be appropriate. The therapist must remember that neck flexion is one of the identified goals. Rotation was added to incorporate and set the stage for inherent programming that will lead to rolling, coming to sit, and reaching while sitting. Because the postural extensor component still needs integration, total head control has not been attained. To facilitate neck extension, a procedure similar to the one for flexion can be established. A vertical position, thus eliminating the influence of the TLR, would again be the starting position of choice.

With extension facilitating extension, the patient should be placed in as much extension as possible without eliciting excessive extensor tone. An inverted labyrinthine position, a kneeling position, or a standing position would be viable spatial patterns to facilitate OLR of the head and coactivation of postural extensors. The vestibular system sensory category can be checked to identify the treatment procedure for use with an inverted labyrinthine position. The kneeling or standing position places the patient in a vertical position with hip and trunk extension. Kneeling rather than standing is used first because of the influence of the positive supporting reaction in standing and the massive facilitation of total extension. Kneeling avoids total extension while maintaining a predominant extensor pattern. As a result of the gravitational pull of body weight through the joints, approximation to facilitate postural extension is constantly maintained. The upper extremities can be placed in shoulder abduction and external rotation, which tends to inhibit abnormal upper-extremity flexor tone and facilitate postural tone into the shoulder. This extensor tone has the potential through associated spinal reactions to facilitate neck and trunk extension. The arms can be placed in this position over a bolster or ball or by the therapist handling the patient from the rear (Fig. 8.3A). The head should begin again in a neutral position. The patient is rocked forward (see Fig. 8.3B) to facilitate OLR of the head and to elicit a quick stretch to the postural extensors. If the head begins to fall forward, the therapist can tap the patient's forehead immediately after the quick stretch. This tapping action is the reverse tap procedure described under the proprioceptive stretch receptors category. The tapping is done to passively move the head back to vertical.

A variety of additional procedures can easily be combined to summate facilitation to the postural extensors. Tapping, vibration, and approximation through the head to the shoulders are only a few of the proprioceptive modalities; all would be facilitatory. A variety of auditory and visual stimuli could be used to orient the patient to a position in space and thus righting of the head. Techniques listed under the exteroceptive and vestibular systems could also be part of the treatment protocol. The therapist would want to sequence the patient toward prone while the head remained in a vertical postural holding pattern. As the therapist rocks the patient toward prone again, a rotational component should be added (see Fig. 8.3C). The patient will extend and rotate to counterbalance the movement, thus incorporating the neck-righting pattern of extension and rotation necessary when rolling from prone to supine. Resistance to neck extension with or without rotation is an important element in regaining normal functional control. The patient is alert and has some functional use of the arms and legs. This rocking pattern in kneeling can be done as a functional activity. The therapist asks the patient to assist in reaching toward an object with one upper extremity. The therapist can guide the patient in the

reaching pattern in a forward, sideward, or cross-midline direction. While reaching, the patient can be rocked forward to elicit right and equilibrium reactions. In incorporating an activity into the treatment of head control, the patient not only is entertained but also attends to the task rather than cognitively trying to keep his head up. In this way, automatic head control is facilitated, and often postural patterns follow. In a partial kneeling pattern the patient can be sequenced to on-elbow over a bolster or ball or on a chair. These activities should be sequenced from vertical to prone to ensure both total postural programming in prone and optimal integration of OLR, as well as to let the patient experience control of various motor strategies in many different environmental contexts.

Once the patient can maintain good flexor, extensor, and rotational components of head control, the activity should, if possible, be practiced with the patient's eyes closed. If the patient can still maintain head control, labyrinthine righting would be adequate for any functional activity. If the patient loses head control, then additional labyrinthine facilitation would be indicated. If a patient uses only vision to right the head, then any time vision is needed to lead or direct another activity, head control might be lost. Because symmetrical vestibular stimulation plays a key role in activating the neck muscles to hold the head in vertical, it also is a key element leading to the perception of vertical and all the directional activities sequencing out of the concept of verticality. The postural extensor programming for head control needs to be practiced in a standing position and a sitting position. The patient needs to be able to stand quietly without excessive extension to run both postural and balance programs. Similarly, he needs to be able to sit with hip flexion while coactivating postural extension in the trunk and neck.

Head control is a complex motor response. A therapist can facilitate inherent mechanisms to assist a patient in regaining function. Simultaneously, multitudinous external input techniques classified under the various sensory modalities and combined modalities can be used to give the patient additional information. Awareness of one technique and the ability to categorize it appropriately allow easy identification and implementation of many additional approaches. The therapist always needs to remember that the patient must practice the behavior (head control) in a variety of spatial positions during various functional activities. This practice must be functional and no longer contrived.

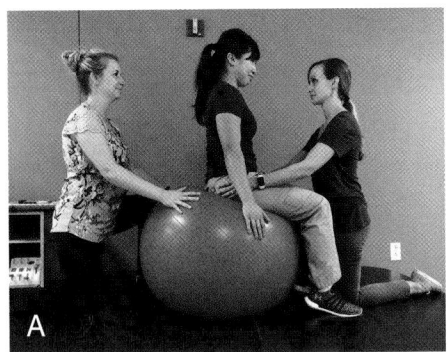 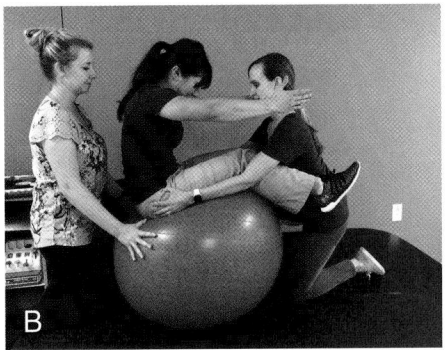 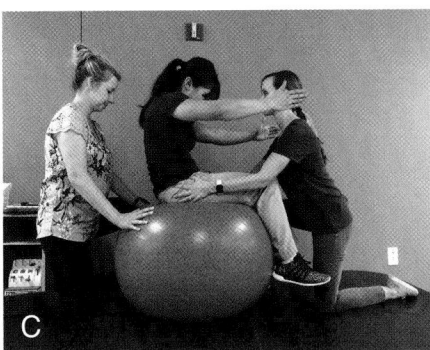

Fig. 8.2 Development of Flexor Aspect of Head Control. (A) Vertical position: head at midline and midrange (total-body flexion) to optimally facilitate neck flexors. **(B)** Facilitating symmetrical neck flexion, using position, gravity, and flexor positions **(C)** Facilitating flexion and rotation to develop pattern necessary for neck-righting pattern.

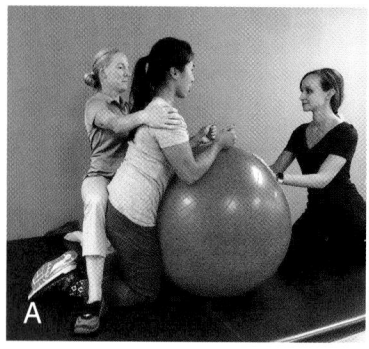 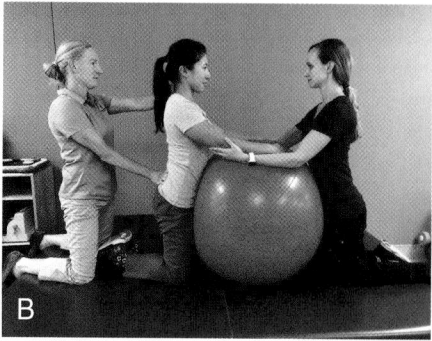 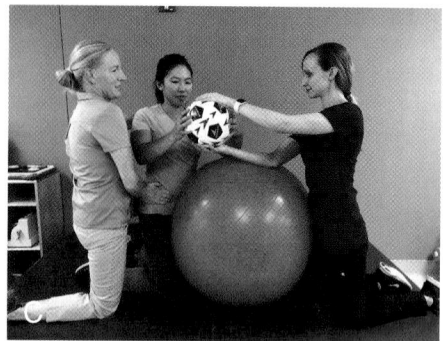

Fig. 8.3 Development of Extensor Aspect of Head Control. (A) Vertical position: head midline with long extensor in midrange and postural extensors in shortened range; body in postural weight-bearing pattern. **(B)** Facilitating symmetrical extension of head, trunk, and hips while inhibiting abnormal upper-extremity tone. **(C)** Facilitating head and trunk extension and rotation to encourage neck righting pattern; patient reaches for an object, which is then placed on the opposite side.

CASE STUDY 8.3 Initial Augmented Intervention Transitioning to Independence in Bed Mobility

Teaching the patient to roll in bed can be approached in a variety of ways to accomplish the goal. The entire rolling pattern may be practiced with enough assistance for the patient to be able to accomplish the goal but also limiting help so that the patient must use the maximum amount of power and range of motion (ROM) available within the key movement pattern.

Rolling

The patient is a 73-year-old man, status post–ischemic infarct in the frontoparietal cortex with resultant left hemiplegia, hemisensory deficit, and left homonymous hemianopia. The patient demonstrates visual-spatial inattention to the left environment. The patient must learn to roll independently in bed for comfort and function. An example of a treatment session aimed at reaching the goal of independent rolling to the right and left may include the following sequence of

activities: (1) begin in side-lying on one side; (2) ask patient to tip back a few degrees and then return to the side-lying position (impairment training within limited ROM); and (3) progressively increase the degree the patient must roll backward, assisting (augmenting) him as needed. By the end of several repetitions, the patient may be rolling from supine to side lying and the movement is functional because he is performing independently. The patient will need to practice many times to relearn the activity before that activity would be considered functional training within the environment practiced. Rolling on a therapeutic mat table is not the same as rolling on a soft mattress at home. There may or may not be carryover. That needs to be identified by the therapist and appropriate steps taken to ensure that independence in all environments is obtained.

Refer to the online video for a demonstration of handling while working on rolling for bed mobility.

ACKNOWLEDGMENT

All the present authors and editors would like to express their deepest gratitude to Dr. Darcy A. Umphred, Dr. Nancy N. Byl, and Dr. Margaret L. Roller who helped develop this chapter in the previous editions of the text.

REFERENCES

To enhance this text and add value for the reader, all references are included on the companion Evolve site that accompanies this textbook. This online service will, when available, provide a link for the reader to a Medline abstract for the article cited. There are 492 references and other general references for this chapter, with the majority of those articles being evidence-based citations.

9

Medical and Developmental Challenges of Infants in Neonatal Intensive Care: Management and Follow-Up Considerations

Jane K. Sweeney, Teresa Gutierrez, and Joanna C. Beachy

OBJECTIVES

After reading this chapter the student or therapist will be able to:

1. Discuss current theoretical frameworks guiding neonatal therapy services in the neonatal intensive care unit.
2. Identify the physiological and structural vulnerabilities of preterm infants that predispose them to stress during neonatal therapy procedures.
3. Outline mentored clinical training components and acute pediatric care experiences to prepare for entry into neonatal intensive care unit practice.
4. Describe how the grief, fear, and emotional trauma may affect behavior and caregiving performance of parents of neonates in the intensive care unit.

5. Differentiate the developmental course and neuromotor risk signs in infants with emerging neuromotor impairment from the characteristics of infants with typical variations in motor behaviors.
6. Identify instruments for neuromotor examination of infants in neonatal intensive care units and in follow-up clinics and compare psychometric features of the tests.
7. Describe program plans and follow-up for neonates and infants in neonatal intensive care unit and home settings.

KEY TERMS

high-risk clinical signs
medical complications of prematurity
neonatal intensive care unit environment
neuromotor assessment

neuromotor intervention
parent instruction
physiological and musculoskeletal risks
subspecialty training

Premature birth continues to be associated with an increased prevalence of major and minor neurodevelopmental disability despite ongoing advancement in newborn resuscitation and neonatal intensive care procedures.[1-3] The risk of neurodevelopmental disability in infants born preterm remains high, with increasing prevalence of mild neurological impairment reported in infants with a late preterm birth (34 to 36 weeks of gestation).[4,5]

Neurodevelopmental and movement assessments combined with brain imaging provide moderate to high prediction of neurodevelopmental outcome.[6,7] Serial clinical examinations and careful monitoring of neurodevelopmental status are critical during the neonatal period, at discharge from the neonatal intensive care unit (NICU), and

sequentially in the outpatient follow-up phase of care. Pediatric therapists with mentored, subspecialty training in neonatology, infant examination, and infant therapy approaches can serve these increasing numbers of surviving neonates at neurodevelopmental risk by

- collaborating with neonatal care teams in NICU rounds and family conferences,
- providing diagnostic data through neurological, developmental, and behavioral examinations
- participating in developmental, feeding, and environmental interventions adapted to each infant's physiological, motor, and behavioral needs

- facilitating parent teaching on developmental and feeding strategies
- reinforcing preventive aspects of health care through early intervention and long-term developmental monitoring

The focus of this chapter is clinical management during the NICU and outpatient follow-up phases for neonates at neurodevelopmental risk and their parents. A theoretical framework for neonatal practice is presented, and an overview of neonatal complications associated with adverse outcomes is provided. In-depth discussion in the neonatal section includes neurodevelopmental examination and pain assessment, intervention plans, and therapy strategies in the NICU. The section on outpatient follow-up addresses critical time periods for neuromotor and musculoskeletal reexamination, assessment tools, and clinical cases.

THEORETICAL FRAMEWORK

Concepts of dynamic systems, neuronal group selection theory (NGST), and parental hope-empowerment provide a theoretical framework for neonatal therapy practice. In this section, three models provide a theoretical structure for practitioners designing and implementing neuromotor and neurobehavioral programs for neonates and their parents.

Dynamic Systems

Dynamic systems theory applied to infants in the NICU refers to multiple interacting structural and physiological systems within the infant as well as to dynamic interactions between the infant and the environment. The synactive model of infant behavioral organization is an example of a neonatal dynamic systems model for establishing physiological stability as the foundation for organization of motor, behavioral state, and attention or interactive behaviors in infants. Als and colleagues[7,8] described a "synactive" process of four subsystems interacting as the neonate responds to the stresses of the extrauterine environment. They theorized that the basic subsystem of physiological organization must first be stabilized for the other subsystems to emerge and allow the infant to maintain behavioral state control and then interact positively with the environment (Figs. 9.1 and 9.2).

To evaluate infant behavior within the subsystems of function addressed in the synactive model, Als and associates[9] developed the Assessment of Preterm Infants' Behavior (APIB). With the development of this assessment instrument, self-regulation, a fifth subsystem of behavioral organization, was added to the synactive model. The self-regulation subsystem consists of physiological, motor, and behavioral state strategies used by the neonate to maintain balance within and between the subsystems (see Fig. 9.2). For example, many infants born preterm appear to regulate overstimulating environmental conditions with a behavioral state strategy of withdrawing into a drowsy or light sleep, thereby shutting out sensory input. The withdrawal strategy is used more frequently than crying because it requires less energy and causes less physiological drain on immature, inefficient organ systems. Neonatal therapists may find a dynamic systems framework useful in conceptualizing and assessing changes in infants' multiple subsystems during and after therapy procedures. In Fig. 9.1 neonatal movement and postural control are targeted as a core focus in neonatal therapy, with overlapping and interacting influences from the cardiopulmonary, behavioral, neuromuscular, musculoskeletal, and integumentary systems. A change or intervention affecting one system may diminish or enhance stability in the other dynamic systems within the infant. Similarly, a change in the infant's environment may impair or improve the infant's functional performance.

This theory guides the neonatal practitioner to consider the many potential physiological and anatomical influences (dynamic systems

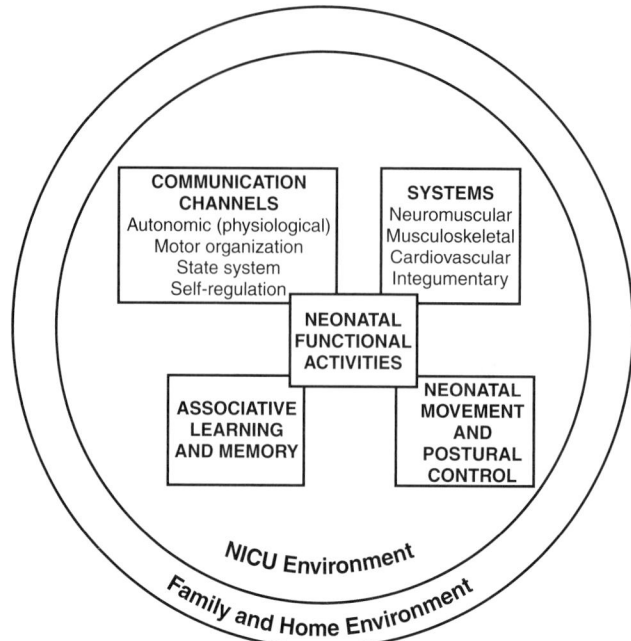

Fig. 9.1 Dynamic systems within neonates and interacting external influences on functional performance. *NICU,* Neonatal intensive care unit. (From Sweeney JK, Heriza CB, Blanchard Y, et al. Neonatal physical therapy. Part II: practice frameworks and evidence-based practice guidelines. *Pediatr Phys Ther.* 2010;22:3.)

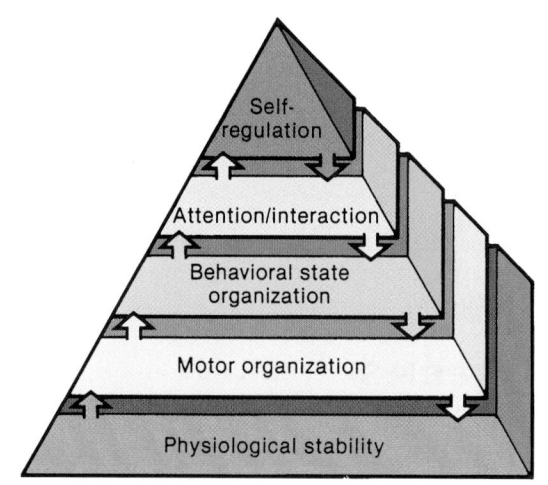

Fig. 9.2 Pyramid of synactive theory of infant behavioral organization with physiological stability at the foundation.

within the infant) that make preterm infants vulnerable to stress during caregiving procedures, including neonatal therapy. In dynamic systems theory, emphasis is placed on the contributions of the interacting environments of the NICU, home, and community in constraining or facilitating the functional performance of the infant.[10]

Neuronal Group Selection Theory

This theoretical framework was developed by Edelman[11,12] on the hypothesis that specific behaviors are the product of neuronal groups, which are dynamically organized to be selected by development. Edelman described three tenets:
- Tenet 1: Development of primary repertoires
  Millions of neurons are interconnected to form functional units known as neuronal groups.

Neuronal groups come together to form primary neuronal repertoires capable of adaptation and accommodation. Formation of primary repertoires does not rely on experience and are endogenously generated.

- Tenet 2: Development of secondary repertoires

  Preexisting primary repertoires are modified by environmental and individual experiences.

  The experience of movement strengthens or weakens repertoires based on value, repetition, or availability of other repertoires. Secondary repertoires develop as a result of this selection.

- Tenet 3: Development of neural maps

  The selection process gives way to neural maps. Neuronal groups are distributed throughout the nervous system. These maps are organized in such a way that distinct and distant areas of perception, cognition, emotion, movement, and posture can be activated simultaneously for one task.

The NGST has been further explored in recent literature as one of the leading theories explaining the dynamic nature of infant development, with variability as one of the main properties of normal movement.[13,14] The continuity of neural functions from prenatal to postnatal life has been well documented over the years. Prechtl[15,16] documented the timing of prenatal, endogenously generated behaviors such as swallowing, sucking, yawning, hand-to-mouth movements, and general body movements.

Preterm infants are born with an innate repertoire of spontaneous movement with specific qualitative characteristics. Variability and complexity of movement are key indicators of central nervous system integrity. Changes in the quality of spontaneous movement with decreased variability may indicate neuromotor dysfunction.[17,18]

Hope-Empowerment Model

A major component of the intervention process in neonatal therapy is developing a therapeutic relationship with the family and supporting family-centered care practices in neonatal care units. A hope-empowerment framework (Fig. 9.3) may guide neonatal practitioners in building the therapeutic partnership with parents; facilitating adaptive coping; and empowering them to participate in caregiving, problem solving, and advocacy. The birth of an infant at risk for a disability, or the diagnosis of such a disability, may create both developmental and situational crises for the parents and the family system.

The developmental crisis involves adapting to changing roles in the transition to parenthood and in expanding the family system. Although not occurring unexpectedly, this developmental transition for the parents brings lifestyle changes that may be stressful and cause conflict.[19] Because parents are experiencing (mourning) loss of the "wished for" baby they have been visualizing in the past 6 months, they may struggle with developing a bond with their "real" baby in the NICU.[20]

A situational crisis occurs from unexpected external events presenting a sudden, overwhelming threat or loss for which previous coping strategies are not applicable or are immobilized.[21] The unfamiliar, high-technology, often chaotic NICU environment creates many situational stresses that challenge parenting efforts and destabilize the family system.[22] The language of the nursery is unfamiliar and intimidating. The sight of fragile, sick infants surrounded by medical equipment and the sound of monitor alarms are frightening. The high frequency of seemingly uncomfortable, but required, medical procedures for the infant are of financial and humanistic concern to parents. No previous experiences in everyday life have prepared parents for this unnatural, emergency-oriented environment. This emotional trauma of unexpected financial and ongoing psychological stresses during parenting and caregiving efforts in the NICU contributes to potential

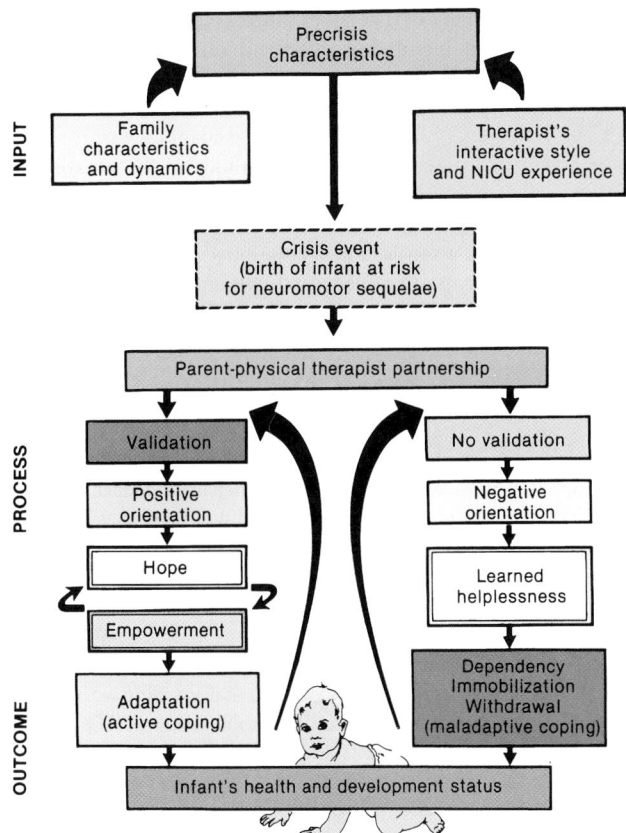

Fig. 9.3 Hope-empowerment *(left)* versus learned helplessness *(right)* processes of the therapeutic partnership between parents and the neonatal therapist. *NICU,* Neonatal intensive care unit.

posttraumatic stress disorder in parents of infants requiring intensive care.[23–26]

The quality and orientation of the helping relationship in neonatal therapy affect the coping style of parents as they try to adapt to developmental and situational crises (see Fig. 9.3). Although parents and neonatal therapists enter the partnership with established interactive styles and varying life and professional experiences, the initial contacts during assessment and program planning set the stage for either a positive or negative orientation to the relationship.

Despite many uncertainties about the clinical course, prognosis, and quality of social support, a positive orientation can be developed by acknowledging and validating parents' feelings and experiences. Validation then becomes a catalyst to a hope-empowerment process in which many crisis events, negative feelings, and insecurities are acknowledged in a positive, supportive, nonjudgmental context in which decision making power is shared.[27] In contrast, a negative orientation may be inadvertently facilitated by information overloading without exploring and validating parents' feelings, experiences, and learning styles. Uncertainty, fear, and powerlessness may be experienced by parents attempting to participate in neonatal therapy activities.

In a hope-empowerment framework, parent participation in neuromotor and feeding intervention allows sharing of power and responsibility and can promote continuous, mutual setting and revision of goals with reality grounding. Adaptive power can be generated by helping parents stabilize and focus energy and plans and by encouraging active participation in intervention and advocacy activities.[27] Exploring external power sources (e.g., online groups supporting parents of infants born preterm) early in the therapeutic relationship may help parents focus and mobilize.[28–30]

Hope and empowerment are interactive processes. They are influenced by existential philosophy: the hope to adapt to what is and the hope to later find peace of mind and meaning for the situation, regardless of the infant's outcome. In describing the effect of an infant born prematurely on the parenting process, Mercer[31] stated that "hope seems to be a motivational, emotional component that gives parents energy to cope, to continue to work, and to strive for the best outcome for a child." She viewed the destruction of hope as contributing to the physical and emotional withdrawal frequently observed in parents who attempt to protect themselves from additional pain and disappointment and then have difficulty reattaching to the infant.

Hope contributes to the resilience parents need to get through the arduous NICU hospitalization period and then begin to face the future in their home and community with an infant at neurodevelopmental risk. Groopman[32] proposed that hope provides the courage to confront obstacles and the capacity to surmount them. He described the process of creating a *middle ground* where truth (of the circumstances) and hope reside together as one of the most important and complex aspects in the art of caregiving.

In a hope-empowerment context, parental teaching activities are carefully selected to contribute to pleasurable, reciprocal interaction between infant and parent. Gradual participation in infant care activities and therapeutic handling in the NICU provides experience and builds confidence for continuation in the home environment.[33]

Conversely, if the parents' learning styles, goals, priorities, values, time constraints, energy levels, and emotional availability are not considered in the design of the developmental program, parents may experience failure, low self-esteem, powerlessness, immobilization, or dependency. The neonatal therapist may recognize signs of learned helplessness in parents when they show nonattendance, noncompliance, negative interactions with infant and staff, or a hopeless, overwhelmed outlook during bedside teaching sessions.

New events in the infant's health or developmental status may create new crises and destabilize the coping processes. In long-term neurodevelopmental follow-up, many opportunities occur within the partnership to validate new fears and chronic uncertainties within a hopeful, positively oriented, therapeutic relationship. This model provides a framework for understanding the processes of hope and empowerment for mediating emotional trauma of parents during the unexpected experience of parenting their baby in a NICU.

NEONATAL COMPLICATIONS ASSOCIATED WITH ADVERSE OUTCOMES

Improvements in neonatal intensive care over the last 30 years have led to increased survival of preterm and term infants. Specific obstetric advances include earlier identification of high-risk pregnancies, improvement in prenatal diagnosis using ultrasound and noninvasive prenatal screening, establishment of specialized tertiary care centers for high-risk pregnancies, and medications such as progesterone to assist in prolonging pregnancy and betamethasone to enhance fetal pulmonary development. Availability of commercial surfactant, advances in ventilator design, and improvement in the management of neonatal respiratory distress have resulted in significantly decreased pulmonary damage after preterm birth (refer to Table 9.6 for a description of ventilators and other specialized equipment in the NICU).

For infants born at 23 weeks gestation, survival has increased from approximately 0% to more than 50%, and for infants born at 26 weeks gestation, survival has increased from 25% to 85% over the past 20 years.[34] Importantly, the incidence of severe neurological injury has decreased over time; however, an increased number of preterm infants will exhibit long-term neurological impairment owing to increased survival.

Preterm Birth

Preterm birth is defined as any infant born alive under 37 weeks gestation. Late preterm infants (born between 34 and 36/7 weeks gestation) comprise more than 70% of all preterm births. These infants are at risk for respiratory compromise, apnea, feeding problems, jaundice, and temperature instability.[35] In addition, they are at increased risk for neurodevelopment delay because a significant amount of brain growth, development, and maturation occurs during the last 6 weeks of gestation.[36]

For infants born less than 34 weeks gestation, mortality and neurodevelopmental impairment increase with decreasing gestational age. Very preterm infants are born between 28 and 32 weeks gestation, and extremely preterm infants are born less than 28 weeks gestation; however, the exact gestational age of the preterm infant is frequently unknown, and infants are frequently categorized by birth weight groups to predict survival and the risk of short and long-term outcomes. Low birth weight (LBW) infants weigh less than 2500 g at birth and are usually under 37 weeks gestation. Very low birth weight (VLBW) infants weigh less than 1500 g and extremely low birth weight (ELBW) infants weigh less than 1000 g at birth regardless of gestational age. The most frequent reasons for an infant to have a birth weight less than expected for their gestational age (i.e., small for gestational age or growth restricted infants) are twin and higher order multiple pregnancy, maternal disease such as pregnancy-induced hypertension, maternal smoking, placental dysfunction, and/or chromosomal abnormalities.

Survival of extremely preterm infants has dramatically increased over time, resulting in increasing numbers of infants with neurodevelopmental delay. The neurodevelopmental outcome of extremely preterm infants assessed at 18 to 30 months of age is reported widely.[37–40] Developmental outcome of Swedish infants born at less than 27 weeks gestation between 2004 and 2007 indicated that 56% had no cognitive, language, or motor impairment, and 20% had moderate to severe impairment.[39] Moderate to severe language delay (16%) or motor impairment (15%) were more prevalent than cognitive disability (11%). Cerebral palsy (CP) was present in 7% of this extremely preterm cohort.

In France, in 2011, 49% of infants born at less than 27 weeks gestation survived to 2 years without detection of neurodevelopmental impairment. CP was present in 7% of this sample. Infants born between 27 and 31 weeks gestation had increased survival without impairment (90%) compared to very preterm infants born at less than 27 weeks gestation. Infants born at full term gestation rarely had neurodevelopmental impairment (2%).[38]

In a study conducted from 2011 to 2015 in the United States, 19% of infants born at less than 27 weeks demonstrated neurodevelopmental delay. Ten percent had significant cognitive delay and 13% had motor impairment. Predictors of developing CP included decreasing gestational age, intraventricular hemorrhage (IVH), and chronic lung disease (CLD), with the incidence of CP decreasing over time.[37] More than 50% of ELBW infants in a US sample had receptive language delay at 30 months, and 23% were severely delayed. Forty eight percent of the infants had some expressive language delay, and 30% were severely delayed. Infants requiring assistance with feeding were at higher risk of expressive language delay (2.3-fold increase). The need for feeding assistance and decreased cognition was significantly associated with receptive language delay.[41]

At 6 to 7 years of age, only 36% of infants born at less than 27 weeks gestation in Sweden had a normal IQ. One-third of these very preterm infants had moderate to severely decreased IQ compared to 2.2% of term infants. The average IQ of preterm infants was 17 points lower than the IQ of term infants. Thirty percent of preterm infants had moderate to severe cognitive delay, specifically in verbal comprehension, working memory, reasoning, and processing speed. Overall, 36.2% of these preterm infants demonstrated no neurodevelopmental delay and 33.6% had moderate to severe delay.[42]

Does cognitive and motor ability at 2 years of age predict outcomes at school age? A cohort of very preterm infants born in Sweden at less than 27 weeks gestation were tested at 2 and 6 years of age. Sixty six percent of infants had no or only mild delays at 6 years. Overall, 21% of infants exhibited improved outcome, 32% had worse outcome, and the remainder were stable. The percentage of infants with moderate to severe disability increased over time from 27% to 34% showing that disability level was inversely related to gestational age. At 6 years of age, decrease in cognitive ability was likely due to decreased executive functioning, a cognitive area not tested at the younger age;[39,42] thus neurodevelopmental testing at 2 years of age identifies most infants at risk for developmental delay and allows them access to needed therapy and educational assistance.

The fetal brain undergoes tremendous growth, development, and maturation during the second and third trimester. The preterm brain is especially vulnerable to injury from hypoxia, medications, stress, and pain. The long-term impact of adverse conditions depends on the gestational age of the infant as well as timing, frequency, nature, and duration of the insult. Expanded description of brain development can be accessed in Volpe's Neurology of the Neonate,[43] a comprehensive resource for health professionals.

Brain development and maturation are categorized into five primary phases (proliferation, migration, organization, synaptogenesis and apoptosis, and myelination). All neurons and glial (support) cells are generated in the germinal matrix, an area adjacent to the ventricle. Neuronal proliferation is nearly complete by 5 months of gestation, well before preterm delivery. Neuronal migration starts at 3 months of gestation and continues for 3 more months, with developing neurons guided by glial cells to form neuronal columns. The organization phase lasts from 5 months gestation through several years after birth. In this phase, neurons are oriented, neuronal projections (axons and dendrites) are elaborated, and interconnections between neurons are generated. Synaptic formation (neuronal interconnections) and elimination (programmed cell death—apoptosis) are present in the third trimester but are most active after birth. Synaptogenesis and apoptosis are experience-dependent and confer plasticity to the preterm brain, ensuring individuality. The final phase of brain maturation involves glial maturation of astrocytes and oligodendrocytes. Astrocytes help maintain the blood-brain barrier, provide nutrient support, regulate neurotransmitter and potassium concentration, and assist in neuronal repair after injury. Oligodendrocytes produce the myelin sheath that covers neurons and facilitates nerve transmission. Myelination starts in the second trimester and continues through adulthood. The oligodendrocytes are especially sensitive to hypoxia and other insults. Disruption of normal myelination results in white matter hypoplasia and periventricular leukomalacia (PVL) (see later discussion) leading to impaired motor function.[43]

Specific insults to the fetal and neonatal brain are associated with impaired neurological functioning and long-term developmental

TABLE 9.1   Conditions Associated With Impaired Neurodevelopment

Condition	Population
IVH PHVD	<28 weeks gestation
PVL	<32 weeks gestation
Cerebellar hemorrhage	Preterm infants
HIE	Term and near term infants
BDP/CLD	All infants
Sepsis	All infants
NEC	Preterm infants
In utero drug exposure	All infants

BPD, Bronchopulmonary dysplasia; *CLD,* chronic lung disease; *HIE,* hypoxic-ischemic encephalopathy; *IVH,* intraventricular hemorrhage; *NEC,* necrotizing enterocolitis; *PHVD,* posthemorrhagic ventricular dilatation; *PVL,* periventricular leukomalacia.

delay. The next section focuses on specific diseases and conditions: IVH, PVL, hypoxic-ischemic (H/I) encephalopathy (HIE), CLD, sepsis, necrotizing enterocolitis (NEC), and in utero drug exposure (Table 9.1).

Intraventricular Hemorrhage

IVH is the most common brain injury in preterm infants born at less than 32 weeks gestation and is a significant risk factor for neurodevelopmental impairment. The incidence of IVH varies inversely with gestational age. The incidence of severe IVH has decreased over time and is currently less than 15% for infants born at under 27 weeks gestation.[44]

The origin of IVH is in the microcirculation/capillary network of the germinal matrix. The germinal matrix is a highly vascularized area due to the high metabolic demand from rapidly proliferating neuronal stem cells. The vessels in the germinal matrix have thin walls and are fragile, predisposing them to rupture and hemorrhage. Preterm infants have impaired cerebral vascular autoregulation. During labor, delivery, and the immediate postpartum transition period, decrease in blood pressure can lead to cerebral hypoperfusion and ischemia and, conversely, increased blood pressure can lead to hyperperfusion and blood vessel rupture. Risk factors for IVH include asphyxia, alterations in serum carbon dioxide, rapid infusion of fluids (especially hypertonic solutions), platelet and coagulation disturbances, anemia, and pain.[45] In infants with gestational age greater than 28 weeks, IVH is rarely seen owing to the developmental involution of vessels in the germinal matrix.

IVH is diagnosed by cranial ultrasound and graded in severity from 1 to 4. The IVH Grade 1 is considered mild, with the hemorrhage confined to the germinal matrix. In IVH Grade 2, the hemorrhage extends into the ventricle (Fig. 9.4). Grade 3 hemorrhage occurs when more than 50% of the ventricle is filled and causes ventricular distention. The evolution of IVH Grade 3 over 10 days is shown in Fig. 9.5. Grade 4 IVH, or periventricular hemorrhagic infarct (PVHI) illustrated in Fig. 9.6, is not caused by germinal blood vessel rupture but, instead, is derived from venous congestion of the terminal veins that border the lateral ventricles, resulting in white matter necrosis and the development of a porencephalic cyst.[46] The usual distribution of PVHI as seen on cranial

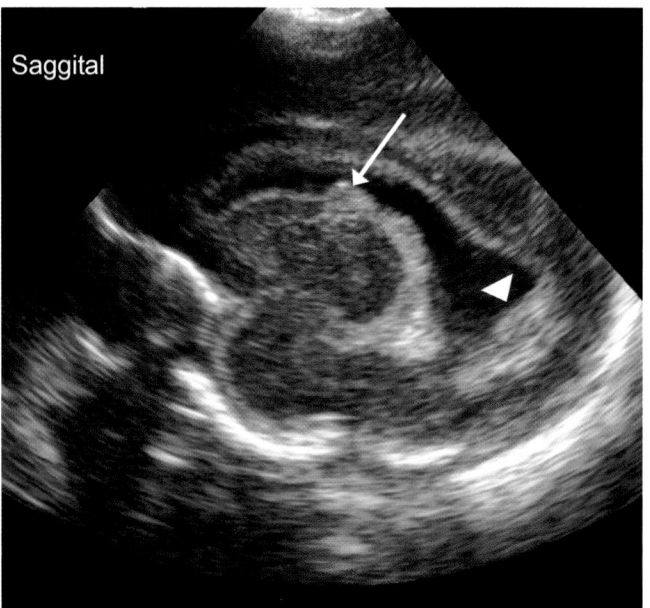

Fig. 9.4 Grade 2 intraventricular hemorrhage, sagittal view on cranial ultrasound. Arrow points to area of germinal matrix bleed in the cardio-thalamic notch. Arrowhead points to blood layering out in the posterior aspect of the lateral ventricle.

ultrasound is initially fan-shaped in the periventricular location. The PVHI lesion is usually unilateral (~70%) and approximately ¾ are associated with severe IVH.[44]

IVH may not be apparent on ultrasound in the first few days after birth, but 90% of IVH can be detected by 4 days of age. Grades 1 and 2 IVH are not associated with a significant increase in neurodevelopmental impairment. Infants with severe IVH (Grade 3 and/or 4) have increased mortality and are at markedly increased risk for developmental disabilities, specifically spastic hemiplegia and diplegia because the motor tracts innervating the lower extremities are in close proximity to the germinal matrix[47] (refer to Fig. 9.7 for schematic diagram of corticospinal [motor] tracks). Infants with small unilateral PVHI have no increased risk of developmental delay compared to infants with Grade 3 IVH. If the PVHI is bilateral or if large or multiple porencephalic cysts are present, the risk for severe motor impairment is significantly increased. The full extent of the hemorrhage may not be appreciated for several days after the initial diagnosis of IVH is made. The extent and impact of cerebral damage from IVH may not be evident on cranial ultrasound at term gestation, and magnetic resonance imaging (MRI) may give more information on the extent of injury. Owing to plasticity of the preterm brain, undamaged portions may assume tasks lost to damage, potentially leading to less impact on neurodevelopmental outcome than anticipated.

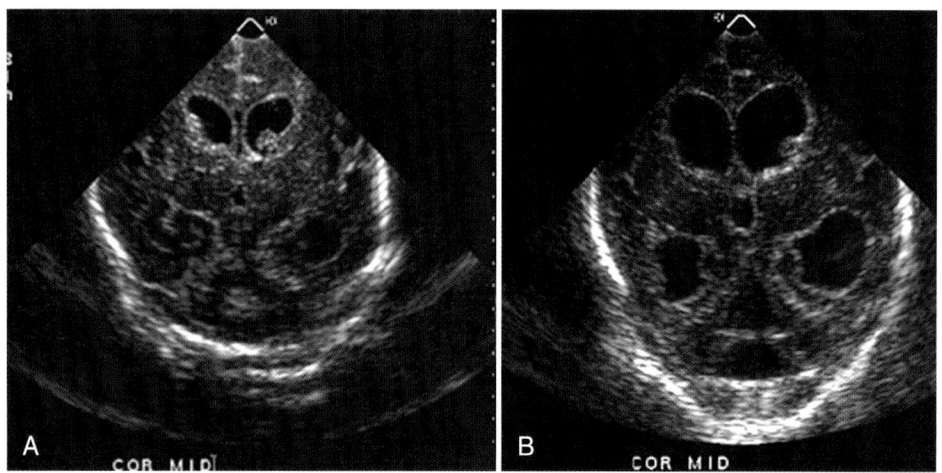

Fig. 9.5 Change in Grade 3 intraventricular hemorrhage in coronal plane on cranial ultrasound. Figure **A** is on day 3 and Figure **B** is 1 week later.

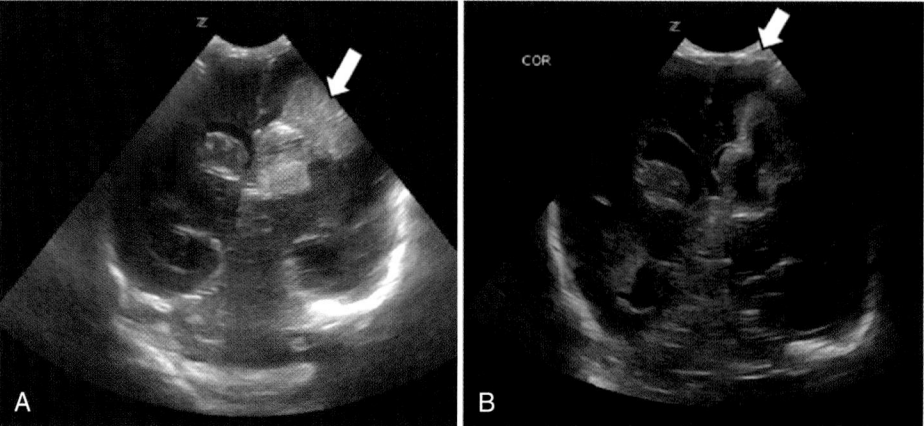

Fig. 9.6 **(A)** Left Grade 4 intraventricular hemorrhage on day of life 3 and **(B)** day of life 9 with initial hyperechoic area and subsequent dissolution of brain matter *(arrow)* as imaged with cranial ultrasound, coronal view.

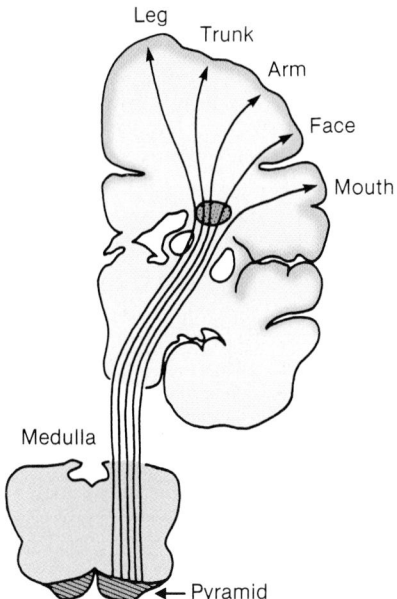

Fig. 9.7 Schematic diagram of corticospinal tract fibers that extend from the motor cortex through the periventricular region into the pyramid of the medulla. The lower motor neurons affected by intraventricular hemorrhage and periventricular hemorrhagic infarct are located in close proximity to the ventricle. Bulbar and upper motor neuron tracts are affected in term infants with hypoxic-ischemic encephalopathy and are parasylvian in location. (From Volpe JJ. Hypoxic ischemic encephalopathy: neuropathology and pathogenesis. In: Volpe JJ, ed. *Neurology of the Neonate*. Philadelphia: WB Saunders; 1995.)

TABLE 9.2 Outcome of Extremely Low Birth Weight Infants With Grade 3 or 4 Intraventricular Hemorrhage With or Without Ventriculoperitoneal Shunt

	No VP Shunt	VP Shunt	
MDI < 70	326/719 (45.3%)	146/214 (68.2%)	<0.001
MDI = 49	130/719 (18.1%)	87/214 (40.7%)	<0.001
PDI < 70	263/711 (37%)	163/214 (76.2%)	<0.001
PDI = 49	146/711 (21%)	113/214 (52.8%)	<0.001
CP	217/767 (28.3%)	128/227 (69.6%)	<0.001

CP, Cerebral palsy; *MDI*, mental developmental index; *PDI*, psychomotor development index; *VP*, ventriculoperitoneal.
From Modified from Adams-Chapman I, Hansen NI, Stoll BJ, et al. Neurodevelopmental outcome of extremely low birth weight infants with posthemorrhagic hydrocephalus requiring shunt insertion. *Pediatrics*. 2008;121:1167–1177.

POSTHEMORRHAGIC VENTRICULAR DILATATION

Approximately 50% of infants with severe IVH (Grade 3 or 4) will develop posthemorrhagic ventricular dilatation (PHVD) caused by either blockage of the normal flow of cerebrospinal fluid (CSF) or decreased absorption of CSF. Approximately 50% to 75% of these infants will develop progressive PHVD resulting in the need for treatment. The severity of ventricular dilatation can be measured on serial cranial ultrasounds.[48,49] Severe ventricular dilatation is usually evident by 2 to 3 weeks after birth while pathological increase in head circumference does not occur until 1 to 2 weeks later. PHVD is treated with serial removal of CSF by spinal tap, subgaleal shunt, or placement of Ommaya reservoir. Removal of CSF has been shown to decrease intracranial pressure and improve cerebral perfusion[50] and increase cortical gray and white matter.[51] In addition, there is indirect evidence that ventricular distention itself may cause secondary brain injury through axonal stretching and disruption, gliosis, and loss of oligodendrocytes (cells that make the myelin sheath).

No consensus has been reached on the optimal management of PHVD.[52,53] Infants with PHVD that does not resolve with serial removal of CSF require ventriculoperitoneal (VP) shunt placement. Significant complications of VP shunt include sepsis, specifically ventriculitis, or shunt malfunction, such as blockage or leaking, necessitating a shunt revision. These complications further impact the neurodevelopmental outcome of infants with VP shunts. The National Institute of Child Health and Development, a consortium of 17 tertiary NICUs, reported results on the neurodevelopmental outcome at 2 years in ELBW infants with Grade 3 and 4 IVH, born between 1993 and 2002.[54] Infants who required shunt placement had significantly worse outcome when compared to infants with Grade 3 or 4 as assessed by the Bayley Scale of infant Development (Table 9.2). A score of less than 70 denotes an infant who is severely delayed. Moreover, the number of infants who were untestable (score = 49) owing to severe neurodevelopmental handicap and the incidence of CP were significantly increased in infants who received a VP shunt compared to infants with only Grade 3 or 4 IVH.[54]

Retrospective studies from the Netherlands indicated that earlier intervention when the ventricles were only moderately dilated significantly decreased the need for VP shunt from 62% to 16% and tended to improve long-term developmental outcome with a decreased incidence of moderate to severe handicap.[48,55] Halting the progression of PHVD and decreasing the need for VP shunt are likely to improve long-term outcome in these infants. With the possibility of spontaneous resolution of PVHD without intervention, identification of factors for accurate prediction is needed to determine which infants will develop persistent PHVD and subsequently require VP shunt placement.

PERIVENTRICULAR LEUKOMALACIA

PVL is the most common ischemic injury to the preterm infant's brain. This injury involves nonhemorrhagic (ischemic) cellular necrosis of periventricular white matter in the arterial watershed area caused by the lack of cerebral autoregulation. Like IVH, PVL is inversely related to gestational age and is present in less than 10% of preterm infants. The PVL lesion can either be cystic or global and may be difficult to identify on radiological images. Cystic PVL (Fig. 9.8) results from the focal dissolution of cellular tissue approximately 3 to 4 weeks after the asphyxial insult and can be identified on ultrasound if greater than 0.5 cm in diameter;[44] however, cysts visualized by cranial ultrasound may disappear over time owing to fibrosis and gliosis; thus the incidence of cystic PVL is considered to be underestimated by cranial ultrasounds. Global PVL results from diffuse white matter injury and myelin loss. This finding can be subtle with moderate ventricular dilatation and/or a mild increase in extraaxial fluid on cranial imaging. Infants with severe PVL have marked ventricular dilatation, increased extraaxial fluid, and decreased head growth.

Brain imaging by MRI obtained at term may be more sensitive in identifying white matter injury from PVL and can be predictive of subsequent neurosensory impairment and cognitive delay present in up to 50% of extremely preterm infants.[56] Newer techniques, such as diffusion tensor imaging (DTI), functional connectivity MRI (fcMRI),

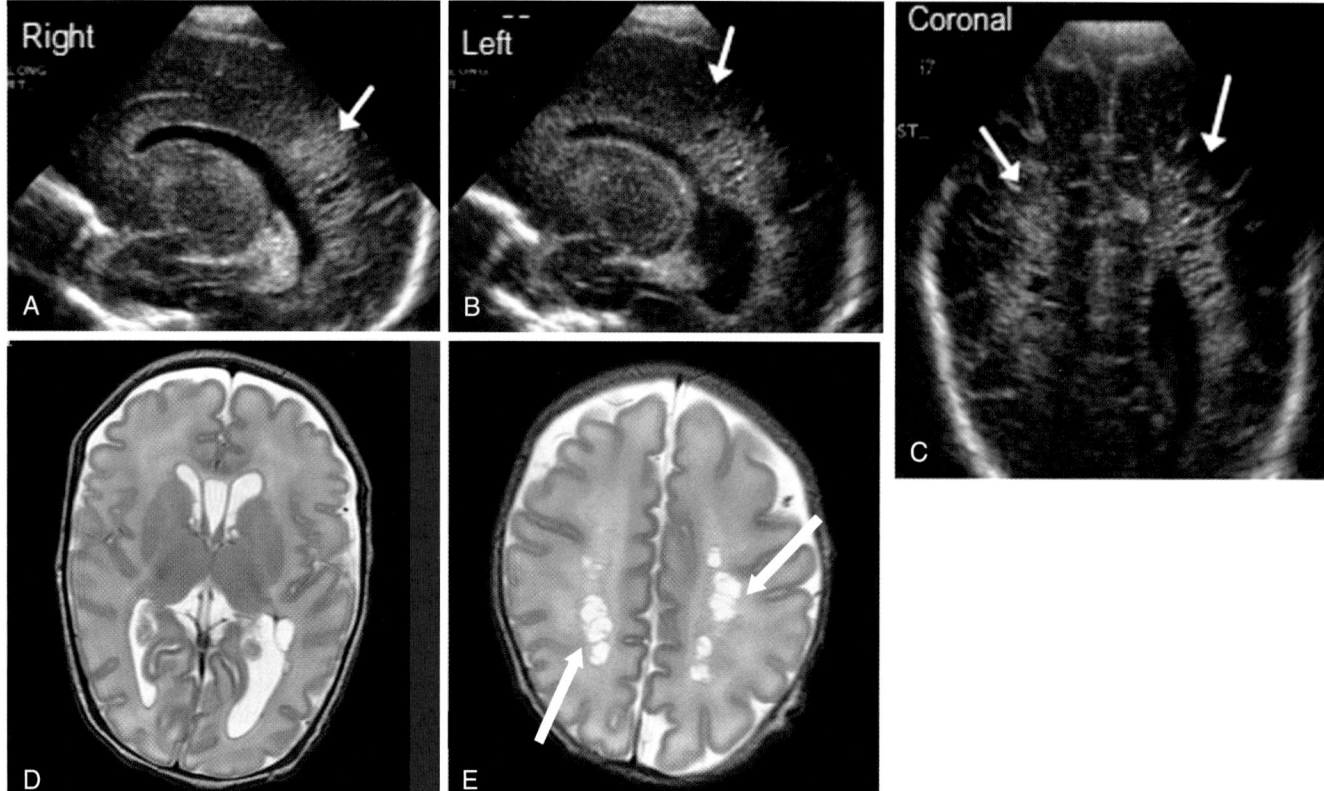

Fig. 9.8 Cystic periventricular leukomalacia is present on cranial ultrasound in sagittal view on the right **(A)** and left **(B)** side of the brain as marked by *arrows*. **(C)** Coronal view. Cysts are evident using magnetic resonance imaging **(D** and **E)**.

and morphometry for analysis of cortical folding, are being investigated as early markers of impaired neurodevelopmental outcome. With DTI, the restriction of water diffusion in the myelin sheath surrounding axons is measured and yields information at the microstructure level about axon caliber change and aberrations in myelination. In addition, DTI allows for visualization of brain fiber tracks and neuronal connectivity. The interaction between areas of the brain at rest and during tasks using changes in blood flow is examined with fcMRI, currently a research tool. Morphometric analysis of sequential MRI scans has been used to create maps of cortical folding with quantification of surface area and degree of gyral formation. White matter injury results in delayed myelination and altered cortical folding.[56]

CEREBELLAR INJURY

The cerebellum is essential for gross and fine motor control, coordination, motor sequencing, and also plays an important role in attention and language.[54] Although the hallmark of damage to the cerebellum is ataxia, recent advances in fcMRI have demonstrated interactions between the cerebellum and nonmotor brain areas involved in language, attention, and mental imagery. Cerebellar injury can also be noted by cranial ultrasound on specific mastoid views. The incidence of cerebellar injury may be as high as 20% in ELBW infants.[57] While the mechanism for damage is unknown, IVH is present in more than 75% of infants with cerebellar injury, implicating similar risk factors. The majority of cerebellar lesions (70%) are unilateral.

Cerebellar lesions are usually clinically silent at birth, and the full impact of the damage is noted over time. As a result of the intricate interconnections between the cerebellum and cerebrum, damage in one area can greatly impact development in other areas of the brain,

thereby amplifying the damage. Preterm infants with isolated cerebellar hemorrhage had significant neurological impairments: hypotonia (100%), abnormal gait (40%), ophthalmological abnormalities (~40%), and microcephaly (17%).[58] Overall, preterm infants with cerebellar hemorrhage had visual deficits and performed significantly lower on tests of gross and fine motor and expressive and receptive language. Infants with both cerebellar injury and IVH had greater motor impairment than infants with isolated cerebellar hemorrhage. Socially, infants with isolated cerebellar hemorrhage exhibited lower communication skills, more withdrawn behavior, and decreased attention skills. Cerebellar injury therefore increases the risk for poor neurodevelopment outcome in cognition, learning, and behavior in preterm infants.[59]

BRONCHOPULMONARY DYSPLASIA

Bronchopulmonary dysplasia (BPD) or CLD is the result of mechanical ventilation and supplemental oxygen delivered to preterm infants to treat their immature lungs that lack surfactant. It was originally defined as an oxygen requirement at 28 days of life in conjunction with classic x-ray findings of atelectasis (areas of collapsed lung) and multiple cysts. The presence of BDP leads to the need for continued respiratory support owing to insufficient air exchange and, frequently, the placement of a tracheostomy tube. With recent treatment advancements such as maternal betamethasone to promote fetal lung maturity, exogenous surfactant, gentler, refined ventilation strategies, and careful supplemental oxygen administration, BPD is now defined as oxygen requirement at 36 weeks corrected gestational age. The level of BPD can be either moderate (requires supplemental oxygen) or severe (requires tracheostomy and ventilator support). The incidence of BPD in infants born at less than 27 weeks gestation or birth weight 500 to 750 g is 60%.[60] The incidence of BPD for infants with birth weight 751 to 1000 g, 1001 to 1250 g, and 1251 to 1500 g is 33%, 14%, and 6%, respectively.[61]

Infants with BPD can have altered pulmonary function, reactive airway disease, asthma, and delayed neurodevelopment. They may have decreased pulmonary reserve and frequent hospitalizations related to bacterial or viral pneumonia.[60] Owing to the need for prolonged ventilation, infants with BPD may develop oral aversion resulting in difficulty with oral feeding and delayed expressive language.[41] Dexamethasone has been used to decrease the dependence on mechanical ventilation but alters brain development, thereby negatively affecting neurodevelopmental outcome.[62,63] Hydrocortisone used instead of dexamethasone may result in lowering the incidence of BPD and appears to have decreased impact on neurodevelopmental outcome at 2 years of age.[61]

SEPSIS

Preterm infants are at high risk of developing sepsis owing to immature immune responses and decreased concentration of acquired maternal antibodies through the placenta. Approximately 2% of infants will be born septic, and 21% will develop sepsis during their NICU stay, with a mortality of 10% to 30% depending on infant age and other confounding factors. Cytokines are released from cells of the immune system in response to bacterial infection and can damage organs (e.g., lungs, kidneys, and brain). Infants with sepsis require increased time on mechanical ventilation and supplemental oxygen and have an increased incidence of BPD with its associated morbidities. Hypotension often accompanies sepsis leading to malperfusion of the brain and impaired development of oligodendrocytes. A two- to threefold increase in the risk for CP and neurodevelopmental impairment is reported in infants with sepsis.[64] For infants with acquired sepsis, an increase in white matter injury is seen on MRI, especially if repeated episodes of sepsis occur.[65]

Central line–associated blood stream infections (CLABSI) are hospital-acquired infections in conjunction with the presence of a central line. Much effort has been focused on decreasing CLABSI such as requiring stringent hand hygiene practices, minimizing central line use, decreasing number of central line interruptions, improving skin care, and enforcing strict infection control monitoring.

NECROTIZING ENTEROCOLITIS

NEC is the most common neonatal intestinal disease with an incidence of 10% in extremely preterm infants. An early presentation occurs within the first month of life, and NEC is frequently associated with intestinal perforation. Surgery is necessary for 50% of infants with NEC when medical management is insufficient or persistent intestinal perforation is present. Surgery is associated with an increased risk of mortality (20% to 40%) compared to infants treated medically. The etiology of NEC is not established, but risk factors include prematurity, umbilical artery catheterization, asphyxia, congenital heart disease, blood transfusion, and enteral feedings. Several viruses (adenovirus, enterovirus, and rotavirus) and bacteria have been implicated as causative agents for NEC. Infants with NEC are usually bacteremic either at the time of presentation of NEC or secondary to intestinal perforation.[66]

Complications of NEC include sepsis, wound infection, and stricture formation that occurs in 10% to 35% of infants and requires additional surgeries to remove the stricture. If removal of intestines is required, wound infection and short gut condition are further

complications. Growth of infants with NEC can be impaired owing to feeding intolerance, prolonged parenteral nutrition, removal of a significant amount of intestine, and repeated surgeries and infections. Persistence of weight at under 10% for age is correlated with decreased neuromotor and neurodevelopmental outcome. Failure to achieve normalization of head growth is associated with abnormal performance at 1 year and probably reflects significant white matter injury. Infants with surgically managed NEC have significantly increased incidence of CP (24% vs 15%), deafness (4.1% vs 1.5%), and blindness (4.1% vs 1%), compared to infants with medically treated NEC.[66,67] A meta-analysis of 7 studies investigating the impact of NEC on neurodevelopmental outcome showed that infants with surgically treated NEC have a statistically significant increase in cognitive, psychomotor, and neurodevelopmental impairment compared to preterm infants without NEC.[67] Impaired neurodevelopmental outcome in infants with NEC is further exacerbated by sepsis with the release of inflammatory cytokines and mediators leading to white matter injury as noted above.[34]

HYPOXIC-ISCHEMIC ENCEPHALOPATHY IN TERM AND NEAR TERM NEONATES

Perinatal asphyxia affects approximately 3 to 5 per 1000 infants annually and can lead to HIE in 0.5 to1/1000 live births. Approximately 15% to 20% of infants with HIE will die, and 25% of the surviving infants will exhibit permanent neurological sequelae. Clinical findings will vary depending on the timing and duration of the H/I insult, preconditioning, fetal adaptive mechanisms, comorbidities, and resuscitative efforts. Impaired oxygen delivery to the fetus leading to asphyxia can result from maternal hypotension, abruption placenta, placental insufficiency, cord prolapse, prolonged labor, and fetal-maternal transfusion. Frequently, infants who develop HIE have associated factors such as abnormal maternal thyroid status, chorioamnionitis, and intrauterine growth retardation.[68]

It is important to note that the injury from a H/I insult is an evolving and progressive process that begins at the time of the insult and continues through the recovery period, allowing the opportunity to decrease the damage from the asphyxial event. The H/I insult leads to decreased oxygen and glucose delivery to the brain causing a shift from aerobic to anaerobic metabolism. This shift causes a decrease in high-energy compounds such as adenosine triphosphate (ATP) production leading to failure of the energy-dependent membrane sodium potassium pump. Sodium enters the neuronal cell causing depolarization and release of excitatory neurotransmitters. This initial phase can last several hours and is marked by significant acidosis, depletion of high-energy compounds, cellular swelling caused by entry of sodium and water, and cellular necrosis causing spillage of intracellular contents into the extracellular space and activation of microglia. The degree of neuronal necrosis is directly related to the duration and severity of the H/I insult. During the reperfusion phase, an increase in free radical production and activation of microglia occur with release of inflammatory mediators caused by improved oxygen delivery. The second phase of energy failure ensues with calcium entering the mitochondria to activate the apoptotic pathway (programmed cell death). During this second phase of energy failure, seizures are often present. Activation of the apoptotic pathway accounts for the majority of cellular death and inactivation of this apoptotic pathway is the target for treatment.[47]

The damage from HIE in term infants is located in the deep structures of the brain (basal ganglia, thalamus, and posterior limb of the internal capsule) as well as in the subcortical and parasagittal white

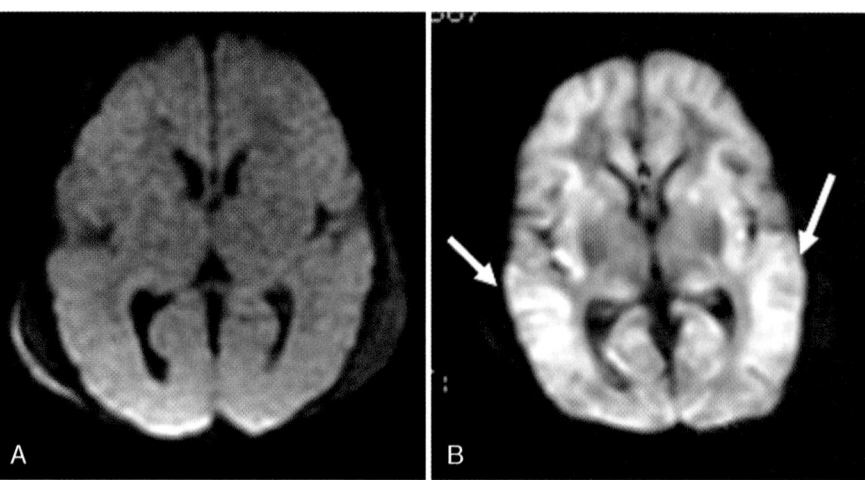

Fig. 9.9 Magnetic Resonance Imaging (MRI) Diffusion Weighted Imaging. **(A)** MRI of normal infants with no areas of increased signal. **(B)** An infant with severe hypoxic-ischemic encephalopathy with arrows pointing to increased signal in the subcortical areas.

matter. Diffusion-weighted imaging MRI (DWI) is an early and sensitive technique to identify damage after the H/I insult. As shown in Fig. 9.9, a marked increase in signal is found in the subcortical and parasagittal white matter as well as in the deep nuclear structures. MRI spectroscopy, usually in the area of the basal ganglia, yields information about the degree of secondary energy failure by analyzing the depletion of the high-energy compound N-acetylaspartate and the presence of lactate. The degree of secondary energy failure is predictive of death and poor neurodevelopmental outcome at 1 and 4 years of age.[69]

The Sarnat score (Table 9.3) classifies the severity of HIE based on clinical signs.[70] Approximately 20% of infants with stage 1 HIE will have long-term sequelae.[71] Infants with Grade 2 or moderate HIE have abnormal tone and reflexes and decreased spontaneous activity. Seizures are a common finding in infants with moderate HIE, and approximately 10% of these infants will die and up to 30% will have neurodevelopmental delay. Infants with severe HIE (Grade 3) have minimal or no spontaneous activity or reflexes, and approximately 50% of these infants will die and, of the survivors, more than 60% to 80% are profoundly impaired. Seizures are present in up to 40% of infants with HIE and are identified either clinically or by EEG or amplitude integrated EEG. Long-term consequences of HIE include bulbar palsies with difficulties in sucking, swallowing, and facial movement.[72] Upper extremity involvement is more prominent than lower extremity deficits. The development of epilepsy occurs in approximately 30% of infants with HIE. Owing to the fact that approximately 50% of infants with moderate or severe HIE treated with hypothermia will exhibit normal neurodevelopmental outcomes, other modalities such as Xenon gas, topiramate, melatonin, tetrahydrocannabis, and erythropoietin are being investigated to enhance the efficacy of hypothermia.

Mild hypothermia (33.5°C) is becoming the standard of care for infants under 36 weeks gestation who present with moderate or severe HIE. Hypothermia has been shown to decrease metabolic demand and therefore help preserve high-energy compounds, delay membrane depolarization, and decrease neuronal excitotoxicity. Free radical production and microglial activation are also decreased. Most

TABLE 9.3   Sarnat Scoring Scale for Encephalopathy

Stage Encephalopathy	Normal	Stage 1 (Mild)	Stage 2 (Moderate)	Stage 3 (Severe)
1. Level of consciousness	Alert, responsive	Hyper-alert, responds to minimal stimulation	Lethargic	Stupor/coma
2. Spontaneous activity	Changes position	Normal or ↓	Decreased	None
3. Posture	Flexed when quiet	Mild flexion distal	Distal flexion, full extension	Decerebrate
4. Tone	Strong flexor tone	Normal or slightly ↑	Hypo- or hyper-	Flaccid or rigid
5. Reflex:				
Suck	Strong	Weak or incomplete	Weak	Absent
Moro	Complete	Intact	Incomplete	Absent
6. Autonomic:				
Pupils	Normal	Mydriasis	Myosis	Variable
HR	100-160	Tachycardia	Bradycardia	Variable
Respirations	Regular	Hyperventilation	Periodic breathing	Apnea, assisted

Modified from Sarnat HB, & Sarnat MS. Neonatal encephalopathy following fetal distress: A clinical and electroencephalographic study. *Arch Neurol.* 1976; 33: 696-705.

TABLE 9.4   Effect of Moderate Hypothermia on Neurological Outcomes at 18 Months Compared With Controls

	Risk Ratio (95% Confidence Interval [CI])	Risk Difference (95% CI)	Number Needed to Treat (95% CI)	P Value
Death or severe disability[a]	0.81 (0.71–0.93)	−0.11 (−0.18−−0.04)	9 (5–25)	.002
Survival with normal outcome[b]	1.53 (1.22–1.93)	0.12 (0.06–0.18)	8 (5–17)	<.001
Mortality	0.78 (0.66–0.93)	−0.07 (−0.12−−0.02)	14 (8–47)	.005
Severe disability in survivors[a]	0.71 (0.56–0.91)	−0.11 (−0.20−−0.03)	9 (5–30)	.006
Cerebral palsy in survivors	0.69 (0.54–0.89)	−0.12 (−0.20−−0.04)	8 (5–24)	.004
Severe neuromotor delay in survivors[c]	0.73 (0.56–0.95)	−0.10 (−0.18−−0.02)	10 (6–71)	.02
Severe neurodevelopmental delay in survivors[d]	0.71 (0.54–0.92)	−0.11 (−0.19−−0.03)	9 (5–39)	.01
Blindness in survivors	0.57 (0.33–0.96)	−0.06 (−0.11–0.00)	17 (9–232)	.03
Deafness in survivors	0.76 (0.36–1.62)	−0.01 (−0.05–0.03)	NA	.47

[a]Severe disability was defined in the CoolCap and TOBY trials as the presence of at least one of the following impairments: Mental Development Index score of less than 70 (2 standard deviations below the standardized mean of 100) on the Bayley Scales of Infant Development; gross motor function classification system level 3 to 5 (where the scale is from 1 to 5, with 1 being the mildest impairment); or bilateral cortical visual impairment with no useful vision. The NICHD trial defined disability as a Mental Developmental Index score of 70 to 84 plus one or more of the following impairments: gross motor function classification system level 2; hearing impairment with no amplification; or a persistent seizure disorder.
[b]Survival with normal outcome was defined as survival without cerebral palsy and with a Mental Developmental Index score of more than 84, a Psychomotor Developmental Index score of more than 84, and normal vision and hearing.
[c]Severe neuromotor delay was determined on the basis of a Psychomotor Developmental Index score of less than 70 in survivors.
[d]Severe neurodevelopmental delay was determined on the basis of a Mental Developmental Index score of less than 70 in survivors.
From Edwards AD, Brocklehurst P, Gunn AJ, et al. Neurological outcomes at 18 months of age after moderate hypothermia for perinatal hypoxic ischaemic encephalopathy: synthesis and meta-analysis of trial data. *BMJ.* 2010;340:c363.

importantly, the activation of the apoptotic pathway is diminished. Transient side effects of hypothermia, such as bradycardia, mild hypotension, thrombocytopenia, and persistent pulmonary hypertension, can be treated medically and are usually not significant. A meta-analysis of published randomized studies comparing infants with moderate and severe HIE treated with either hypothermia or normothermia showed that hypothermic treatment significantly decreased mortality and morbidity (Table 9.4).[73] It is known that hypothermia is most effective when administered prior to the onset of the second phase of energy failure. As the timing of the H/I insult can occur prior to delivery, hypothermia should be initiated as quickly as possible after delivery to increase the likelihood that it will diminish the neuronal damage and improve neurodevelopmental outcome.[47]

MATERNAL MEDICATION

The impact of maternal medications on the developing fetal brain depends on the specific drug or combinations of drugs, as well as on the timing and duration of the drug exposure. Whereas the insults discussed previously cause predominantly cellular necrosis and apoptosis, medications given to the fetus and preterm infant can also cause alterations in the structure and function of genetic material. The hypothesis that factors acting early in life have a long-lasting impact on development is called the Barker hypothesis or the fetal origins of adult disease.[74,75] It is proposed that the biological value of this reprogramming is to prepare the fetus for maximal adaptation through methylation and deacetylation of histones, thereby determining the quantity of specific proteins that are produced. This section will focus on maternal use of opioids, cocaine, cannabis, and selective serotonin reuptake inhibitors (SSRIs) during pregnancy.

Opioids

In the past decade, increasing concern has emerged over the marked use of opioids, both by prescription for pain relief and illicit use, leading to an increase in deaths owing to overdose. Most commonly used are naturally occurring opioids (morphine and codeine) and synthetic opioids (heroin, methadone, buprenorphine, and, recently, fentanyl). Opioids act on receptors present in both the central nervous system and gastrointestinal tract leading to euphoria and constipation, respectively. Continued use of opioids leads to tolerance resulting in a need to increase the drug's dose for the same effect. Physical dependence is manifested by withdrawal symptoms when the drug is discontinued. Addiction is a complex issue including tolerance, dependence, and psychological compulsion to use the drug.

Use of pain relievers, specifically opioids, during pregnancy has increased fivefold during the past decade.[76] These drugs are highly addictive to the mother and can readily cross the placenta and affect the fetus. Methadone and buprenorphine are commonly used in pregnant females to decrease the need for illicit drug use and stabilize maternal narcotic dependence. Opioid use during pregnancy has been associated with premature rupture of membranes, uterine irritability, preterm labor, preeclampsia, and growth-retarded infants.

Neonatal abstinence syndrome (NAS) is a constellation of symptoms in infants exposed prenatally to opioids and, after delivery, are subject to cessation of opioids leading to withdrawal symptomatology. Infants will demonstrate neurological hyperexcitability with high-pitched crying, increased muscle tone, irritability, decreased sleep, hyperalert state, and tremors at rest. Gastrointestinal symptoms can also be present such as vomiting and diarrhea. Impaired oral feeding and an increased need to suck on a pacifier are common. Autonomic signs include sweating, mottling of the skin, increased temperature, and nasal stuffiness. Occasionally, seizures are present. In Ohio, hospital admissions for infants with NAS increased from 1.4 to 5.6 per 1000 live births.[76]

Withdrawal from narcotics occurs 2 to 5 days after delivery depending on the opioid. Withdrawal from heroin and morphine usually starts by 24 hours after delivery. Neonatal withdrawal from maternal methadone or buprenorphine use is delayed up to 5 days after delivery owing to the long half-life on these medications. Severity of neonatal withdrawal symptoms is not exclusively related to the dose of maternal medications, but is influenced by polysubstance drug exposure, cigarette use, and genetics differences. Two commonly used scoring methods for determining the severity of NAS and the need for treatment are scales by Lipsitz[77] and Finnegan and colleagues.[78] The Lipsitz scale has 11 components scored from 0 to 3, with any score over 4 necessitating treatment. The Finnegan scale is a comprehensive assessment with more than 30 elements. A modified Finnegan assessment tool has been validated and is most frequently used.[79]

Nonpharmacological supportive care consists of minimizing environmental stimuli by decreasing light and noise and decreasing irritability with swaddling, holding, pacifier use, and on-demand feeding. Maternal rooming-in and breastfeeding have beneficial effects on decreasing symptoms of withdrawal. This supportive care should be implemented even if the infant is on medications because they continue to demonstrate hyperexcitable behavior and have decreased tolerance to stimulation. Approximately 30% to 80% of in utero opioid-exposed infants will require medical treatment for NAS with either morphine or methadone. Phenobarbital and/or clonidine have been used as adjunctive treatment if symptoms continue. The goal of treatment is to decrease irritability, improve nippling efforts and weight gain, and decrease vomiting and diarrhea. The incidence of apnea and sudden infant death syndrome (SIDS) is increased in opioid-exposed infants. Long-term effects of in utero exposure to opioids include tremulousness, hypertonicity, irritability, and increased crying episodes. In addition, they are less able to interact with people, demonstrate decreased age-appropriate free play, and have delayed fine motor coordination. An appropriate and nurturing home environment is essential after discharge from the hospital to maximize neurodevelopmental outcome.

Cocaine

It is difficult to ascertain the exact frequency of cocaine use during pregnancy because its use is frequently associated with other illicit drugs. Cocaine is extracted from the leaves of the coca plant and induces an intense and immediate euphoric state through inhibiting uptake of neurotransmitters, specially serotonin and dopamine. Dependence can occur, and cocaine is highly addictive with severe and intense cravings lasting for several months with potential recurrence years after cessation of cocaine use.

Cocaine can cause vasoconstriction leading to placental abruption, preterm labor, uterine irritability, and premature rupture of membranes. In the fetus, there is an increased risk for H/I injury and middle cerebral artery stroke. Cocaine also negatively affects fetal neuronal proliferation, migration, growth, and connectivity, which distort neuronal cortical architecture; however, the effects of intrauterine exposure to cocaine are difficult to determine because cocaine use is frequently associated with the abuse of other illicit drugs, cigarettes, and alcohol. Other confounding variables increasing the risk for negative fetal outcomes include inadequate maternal nutrition and limited prenatal care. In a large prospective blinded study, more infants exposed to cocaine in utero were delivered prematurely and exhibited decreased weight, length, and head circumference compared

with matched controls.[80] Neonates with prenatal cocaine exposure demonstrate tremors, hypertonia, irritability, poor feeding ability, and abnormal sleep patterns and are at a threefold to sevenfold increased risk of SIDS.[81] In addition, in utero cocaine exposure has been linked to increased incidence of behavioral problems and special education referrals in school-aged children with abnormalities in executive functioning.

Cannabis

As a result of the legalization of marijuana (cannabis) in many states, an increasing number of pregnant females are using cannabis during pregnancy to treat nausea and vomiting in addition to recreational use. Marijuana use is increased in mothers who are younger (18 to 25 years), habitually smoke, use illicit drugs, have completed high school, are unemployed, and are enrolled in federal subsidy programs (e.g., women, infants, and children nutrition program).[82] Mixed reports about the impact of marijuana on the brain of the developing fetus are a result, in part, of concomitant exposure to cigarette smoking and other confounding drugs (cocaine, opioids, etc). Marijuana readily crosses the blood-brain barrier and modulates the release of specific neurotransmitters from glial and neuronal cells that are important for the normal maturation of the brain in utero. Marijuana use has been implicated in an increased incidence of stillbirths and preterm labor, increased risk of infection, and increased neurological morbidity (specifically IVH and PVL). Infants tend to have decreased birth weight and an increased risk of admission to the NICU. Long-term in utero exposure to maternal marijuana appears to impact attention span and short-term memory, with increased risk of impulsivity and hyperactivity in school-aged children.[83] The American Academy of Pediatrics (AAP) discourages the use of marijuana during pregnancy owing to concerns for the long-term impact on the developing brain. The AAP also discourages the use of marijuana during breastfeeding because the active compound is present in breast milk.[84]

Selective Serotonin Reuptake Inhibitors

Depression during pregnancy can cause serious side effects in both the mother and the developing fetus. At least 600,000 infants are born yearly to mothers who have a major depressive disorder during their pregnancy. It is reported that at least 6% of pregnant woman use SSRIs during pregnancy, and almost 40% of depressed women have been reported to use antidepressants at some time during pregnancy.[85] The most common SSRI medications used to treat anxiety and depression during pregnancy are fluoxetine (Prozac, Fontex, Seromex, and Seronil), sertraline (Zoloft, Lustral, Serlain, and Asenta), paroxetine (Paxil, Seroxat, Sereupin, and Paroxat), fluvoxamine (Luvox and Favoxil), escitalopram (Lexapro, Cipralex, and Esertia), and citalopram (Celexa, Sceropram, Citox, and Cital).[86] A meta-analysis found that maternal depression was significantly associated with an increased incidence of preterm labor and neonatal birth weight less than 2500 g but not intrauterine growth retardation of the fetus.[87] Unfortunately, this study was unable to evaluate the effect of only SSRI therapy on these outcomes.

The SSRI drugs readily cross the placenta and inhibit serotonin reuptake in neuronal cells. The serotonergic system is present early in gestation and is important in fetal brain development. Perturbations in this system are associated with alterations in somatosensory processing and emotional responses. Infants exposed to SSRIs in the third trimester have symptoms similar to withdrawal from opioid exposure (irritability, tremors, jitteriness, agitation, and difficulty sleeping). These symptoms are transient, appearing 2 to 4 days after birth and disappearing by the second week of life.[88] Neonatal feeding difficulties are quite common in infants exposed to SSRIs. Seizures and abnormal posturing are occasionally noted. In addition, infants exposed to SSRIs *in utero* have a twofold increased risk of developing pulmonary hypertension.[89] It is difficult to identify any specific adverse neurodevelopmental outcomes in infants exposed prenatally to SSRIs from published studies because of the variability in the specific SSRI taken, the duration and timing of SSRI use, and the confounding factors of maternal depression and the use of multiple medications.

CLINICAL MANAGEMENT: NEONATAL PERIOD

Pediatric therapists with mentored subspecialty training in neonatology and infant therapy approaches can expand neonatal services by creating clinical protocols and pathways designed to optimize the development and interaction of neonates and parents. The therapeutic partnership between parents and neonatal therapists during developmental intervention in the NICU sets the stage for parental support and competency in caregiving and compliance with follow-up in the outpatient period. General aims of NICU clinical management of infants at risk for neurological dysfunction, developmental delay, or musculoskeletal complications are to

- promote posture and movement appropriate to gestational age and medical stability
- support symmetry and biomechanical alignment of extremities, neck, and trunk while multiple infusion lines and respiratory equipment are required
- decrease potential skull and extremity musculoskeletal deformities and acquired joint-muscle contractures
- foster infant-parent attachment and interaction
- modulate sensory stimulation in the infant's NICU environment to promote behavioral organization and physiological stability
- provide consultation or direct intervention for neonatal feeding dysfunction and oral-motor deficits
- enhance parents' caregiving skills (feeding, dressing, bathing, positioning of infant for sleep, interaction and play, and transportation)
- prepare for hospital discharge and integration into home and community environments

Educational Requirements for Therapists

Examination and intervention for neonates are advanced-level, not entry-level, clinical competencies. Neonatology is a recognized subspecialty within the specialty areas of pediatric physical therapy[10,90,91] and pediatric occupational therapy.[92] No amount of literature review, self-study, or experience with other pediatric populations can substitute for competency-based clinical training with a mentor in a NICU. The potential for causing harm to medically fragile infants during well-intentioned intervention is enormous.[93,94] The ongoing clinical decisions made by neonatal therapists in evaluating and managing physiological and musculoskeletal risks while handling small (2 or 3 lb), potentially unstable infants in the NICU should not be a trial-and-error experience at the infant's expense. Therapists with adult-oriented training and even those with general pediatric clinical training (excluding neonatal) are not qualified for neonatal practice without a supervised clinical practicum (2 to 6 months). The NICU is not an appropriate practice area for physical therapy assistants, occupational therapy assistants, or student therapists on affiliations for reasons outlined by Sweeney and colleagues[10]: "handling of vulnerable infants in the NICU requires ongoing examination, interpretation, and multiple adjustments of procedures, interventions, and sequences to minimize risk for infants who are physiologically, behaviorally, and motorically unstable or potentially unstable." The physical or occupational therapy assistant and student therapist are not prepared, even with supervision, to "provide moment-to-moment examination and evaluation of

> **BOX 9.1   Neonatal Intensive Care Unit Observational Experiences for Entry-Level Students**
>
> - Reviewing neonatal literature and neonatal therapy clinical practice guidelines before site visit to neonatal intensive care unit (NICU)
> - "Shadowing" neonatal nurses to observe:
>   - Neonatal equipment (refer to Table 9.6)
>   - Caregiving routines
>   - Teaching styles with parents and grandparents
>   - Feeding procedures and equipment
>   - Unique culture of the NICU compared with adult intensive care units
>   - Skin-to-skin holding by parent
>   - Environmental adaptations (light, sound, and clustered handling)
> - "Shadowing" neonatal therapist to observe:
>   - Chart reviews
>   - Interdisciplinary rounds
>   - Discharge planning conferences
>   - Behavioral and physiological baseline examinations
>   - Examination and intervention procedures adapted for medically stable infants at varying gestational ages, acuity levels, and behavioral organization
>   - Parental teaching
>   - Collaboration with neonatal nurses for positioning, feeding, and parent instruction
> - Observing and participating with neonatal therapist in NICU follow-up clinic

From Rapport MJ, Sweeney JK, Dannemiller L, et al. Student experiences in the neonatal intensive care unit: addendum to neonatal physical therapy competencies and clinical training models. *Pediatr Phys Ther.* 2010;22:439–440.

the infant and have the ability to modify or stop preplanned interventions when the infant's behavior, motor, or physiological organization begins to move outside the limits of stability with handling or feeding."[10] Appropriate nonhandling, observational experiences for physical therapist or occupational therapist students in the NICU are delineated by Rapport and colleagues,[95] with a wide range of observational learning experiences with a preceptor recommended in this specialized practice environment (refer to Box 9.1 for appropriate nonhandling, observational experiences for entry-level students during hospital clinical affiliations).

Delineation of advanced-level roles, competencies, and knowledge for the physical therapist,[10,91] occupational therapist,[99] and speech pathologist[96-98] in the NICU setting have been described separately by national task forces from the respective national professional organizations. These practice guidelines provide a structure for assessing competence of individual therapists working in NICU settings and offer an ethicolegal practice framework for designing clinical paths and an evidence base for specific neonatal therapy services.

A gradual, sequential entry to neonatal practice is advised by building clinical experience with infants born at term gestation as well as with physiologically fragile older infants and children and their parents. The experience may include managing caseloads of hospitalized children on physiological monitoring equipment, external feeding lines, and supplemental oxygen or ventilators. Participating in discharge planning and in outpatient follow-up of high-risk neonates are other options for providing exposure to examination, intervention, and family issues when the infants and parents are more stable. This clinical experience and a competency-based, precepted practicum in the NICU offer the best preparation for appropriate, accountable, and ethical practice in neonatal therapy.[10,99] In-depth study of perinatal and neonatal medicine and related obstetrical, neonatal nursing, high-risk parenting, and neonatal therapy literature is recommended before pediatric therapy clinicians begin to participate on the intensive care nursery team.

Neonatal Pain and Neurological Assessment

Multiple neonatal neurological and neurobehavioral examinations have been developed to assess the integrity and maturation of the nervous system and to describe newborn behavior. Most of these tests offer information on the quality of motor performance, attention, and interaction and because these assessments are based on gestational age, an accurate calculation of gestational age is necessary at the time of the testing.

Pain Assessment

Despite immature myelinization, premature infants *definitely* perceive pain and retain the memory of painful experiences. Skin receptors are developed by 14 to 16 weeks of gestation. In addition, the density of pain receptors in the skin of neonates at 28 weeks of gestation is considered similar to, and even exceeds, adult density during maturation from birth to 2 years of age.[100,101] Blackburn[102] explained that although pain transmission in neonates occurs mainly through the slower, unmyelinated C fibers, the shorter distance in neonates that impulses travel to reach the brain compensates for the slower rate of transmission and creates substantial pain reception. Early pain experiences may create later increased sensitivity to pain and vulnerability to stress disorders.[103–105] If neonatal therapy assessment or intervention procedures immediately follow a noxious procedure in the NICU, handling techniques may need to be modified or therapy session rescheduled to avoid contributing to a cascade of aversive experiences for the infant. Parents showing distress and concern about infant pain may benefit from training in comfort care techniques of swaddling, pacifier use, touch, soft conversation, and holding.

Psychometric data and clinical use of the pain tools are described for infants as early as 28 weeks of gestation.[106] Many elements in the pain assessments have been identified by Als[9] as signs of excessive stimulation and stress in the preterm infant. Specific extremity movements, such as hand-to-face, elevated leg extension, salute, lateral extension of arms, finger splay, and fisting, have been proposed by Holsti and Grunau[107] as indicators of stress and/or pain.

In addition to practice guidelines on pain assessment developed primarily by neonatal nurses, numerous instruments are available to assess pain in infants. Pain scale data are integrated into NICU nursing assessments and can be a valuable adjunct to the neonatal therapist's baseline and post-therapy observations. Indicators of pain are detailed in the instruments outlined below. These pain assessments provide documentation for pain or distress signs in the following three categories: (1) physiological (heart rate, oxygen saturation, and breathing pattern), (2) behavioral (eye squeeze, brow bulge, facial grimace, and behavioral state, including crying and sleeplessness), and (3) motor (tone and movement in extremities).

- The Premature Infant Pain Profile (PIPP[108]) assigns points for changes in three facial expressions (brow bulge, eye squeeze, and nasolabial fold), heart rate, and oxygen saturation. Gestational age and preprocedural behavioral state are included in the assessment. The maximal PIPP score is 21; the higher the score, the greater the pain. A score of 0 to 6 points indicates minimal or no pain, whereas a score of 12 or more indicates moderate to severe pain.
- The Face, Legs, Activity, Cry, and Consolability Behavioral tool (FLACC) uses grades of 0 to 2 for facial expression, leg activity, general activity, cry nature, and ability to be consoled and has been used in pediatric and adult settings. This test is capable of assessing

pain in normal as well as cognitively impaired children, thereby giving it a high degree of versatility and usefulness.[109] Change in FLACC score has been used to demonstrate that the use of sucrose and a pacifier during venipuncture is more effective in consoling infants younger than 3 months of age compared to infants older than 3 months of age.[110]

- The Neonatal Pain, Agitation, and Sedation Scale (N-PASS) uses five indicators: (1) crying and irritability, (2) behavioral state, (3) facial expression, (4) extremity movement and tone, and (5) vital signs. As with the PIPP scale, additional points are added for decreasing gestational age.[111] Good correlation was established between the N-PASS and the PIPP assessments during routine heelstick in infants younger than 1 month old born at 23 to 42 weeks' gestation.[112]
- The Neonatal Infant Pain Scale (NIPS) has six indicators for pain or distress and can be used with both preterm and full term infants. On a 7-point scale, pain behavior is assessed by facial expression, cry nature, breathing pattern, arm and leg posture, and arousal state.[113]

Neonatal Behavioral Assessment Scale

To document individual behavioral and motor differences in infants at term gestation to 2 months of age, Brazelton and Nugent[114] developed a neonatal behavior scale to assess neuromotor responses within a behavioral state context. The 30- to 45-minute examination consists of observing, eliciting, and scoring 28 biobehavioral items on a 9-point scale and 18 reflex items on a 4-point scale. This interactive test assesses the infant's ability to respond to stimuli and return to an alert state. The reflex items are derived from the neurological examination protocol of Prechtl and Beintema.[115]

The scale was designed to assess newborn behavior in healthy 3-day-old term (40 weeks of gestation) Caucasian infants whose mothers had minimal sedative medication during an uncomplicated labor and delivery. Use of this examination with infants born preterm requires modification of the examination procedure to the environmental constraints of an intensive care nursery and interpretation of findings relative to the gestational age and medical condition of the infant. For preterm infants approaching term gestation (minimum of 36 weeks of gestation), nine supplementary behavioral items are offered. Many of these items were developed by Als[9] for use with preterm and physiologically stressed infants (see discussion of the APIB, later). In the manual,[114] methods of adapting the Neonatal Behavioral Assessment Scale (NBAS) for preterm neonates with accompanying case scenarios are described to illustrate use of the findings to enhance parent-infant interaction and guide developmental interventions.

Six behavioral state categories are outlined in the NBAS: deep sleep, light sleep, drowsiness or semi-dozing, quiet alert, active alert, and crying. Behavioral state prerequisites are provided for each biobehavioral and reflex item to reduce the state-related variables in testing. During the assessment the examiner systematically maneuvers the infant from the sleep states to crying and back to the alert states to evaluate physiological, organizational, motor, and interactive capabilities during stimulation and physical handling. The scoring is based on the infant's best performance, with flexibility allowed in the order of testing, repetition of items encouraged, and scheduling of the assessment midway between feedings to give the infant every advantage to demonstrate the best possible responses.

Four dimensions of newborn behavior are analyzed in the NBAS: interactive ability, motor behavior, behavioral state organization, and physiological organization. *Interactive ability* describes the infant's response to visual and auditory stimuli, consolability from the crying state with intervention by the examiner, and ability to maintain alertness and respond to social or environmental stimuli.

Motor behavior refers to the ability to modulate muscle tone and motor control for the performance of integrated motor skills, such as the hand-to-mouth maneuver, pull-to-sit maneuver, and defensive reaction (e.g., removal of cloth from face). In the assessment of *behavioral state organization,* the infant's ability to organize behavioral states when stimulated and to shut out irritating environmental stimuli when sleeping are analyzed. *Physiological organization* is evaluated by observing the infant's ability to manage physiological stress (changes of skin color, frequency of tremulous movement in the chin and extremities, number of startle reactions during the assessment). For analysis, the information is divided into seven clusters: habituation, orientation, motor, range of state, regulation of state, autonomic stability, and reflexes. The cluster systems are highly useful for clinical interpretation and for data analysis in clinical research. Performance profiles of worrisome or deficient interactive-motor and organizational behavior are identified by clusters of behavior associated with potential developmental risk.[114]

Definite strengths of the NBAS are the well-defined indicators of autonomic stress, analysis of coping abilities of high-risk infants experiencing external stimuli and handling, and quality of infant-examiner interaction. These features generate specific findings to assist therapists in grading the intensity of assessment and treatment within each infant's physiological and behavioral tolerance and in guiding the development of parental teaching strategies to address the individual behavioral styles of infants. The NBAS has proved to be more sensitive to the detection of mild neurological dysfunction in the newborn period compared to classic neurological examinations that omit the behavioral dimensions. This assessment is not predictive but gives a good analysis of the infant's strengths and weaknesses. Improved performance from repeat examinations over time is a better predictor of the infant's ability and potential.

Participation of the parent in the newborn assessment may yield long-term positive effects on infant-parent interaction and later on cognitive and fine motor development. Widmayer and Field[116] reported significantly better face-to-face interaction and fine motor-adaptive skills at 4 months of age and higher mental development scores at 12 months of age when teenage mothers of preterm infants (mean gestational age at birth, 35.1 weeks) were given demonstrations of the NBAS. These demonstrations were scheduled when the premature infants had reached an age equivalence of 37 weeks of gestation.

A four-step examiner training involving self-study, skill test, practice, and certification phases is coordinated through the Brazelton Institute/Touch Points Center, Children's Hospital, Boston, Massachusetts.[117] For clinicians beginning to develop competence in examining at-risk infants, the NBAS provides a system for developing basic handling skills with healthy, term infants without concerns of stressing medically fragile preterm infants during the training period. Learning the NBAS in term infants before entering NICU practice provides familiarity with similar testing and scoring procedures for preterm infants.

Newborn Behavioral Observations System

The Newborn Behavioral Observations (NBO) system, developed from the pioneering work and philosophy of Brazelton, is an interactive, observational tool for use with infants and parents in hospital, clinic, and home settings.[118] The focus is on prematurely born infants and at-risk infants, with emphasis on cultural competence, family-centered care, and infant development. The NBO system helps determine the behavioral profile of the infant and allows the practitioner to

provide parents with individualized and unique information about their infant. This behavioral information promotes positive parent-infant interaction and also a positive partnership between parents and practitioners.

Certification in administering, interpreting, and scoring the 18-item NBO assessment is arranged through the Brazelton Institute/Touch Points Center, Boston, MA, in a 2-consecutive-day format. The training encompasses the following observation categories: (1) habituation to external light and sound; (2) muscle tone and motor activity level; (3) behavioral self-regulation (crying and consolability); and (4) visual, auditory, and social-interactive abilities.[119]

Neurological Assessment of the Preterm and Full-Term Newborn Infant

The Neurological Assessment of the Preterm and Full-Term Newborn Infant is a streamlined neurological and neurobehavioral assessment designed by Dubowitz and colleagues[120] to provide both a systematic, quickly administered newborn examination applicable to infants born preterm or at term gestation and a longer infant examination for children to 24 months of age. A distinct advantage of this tool is the minimal training or experience required by the examiner and the ease of adapting it to the infant and the environment. The adaptability of the test and use of the scoring form with stick figure diagrams have made it useful for implementation in developing countries where English is not widely spoken.

The test includes the six behavioral state categories of the NBAS and seven orientation and behavior items scored on a 5-point grading scale and sequenced according to the intensity of response. The orientation and behavior items consist of the following categories: (1) auditory and visual orientation responses; (2) quality and duration of alertness; (3) irritability (the frequency of crying to aversive stimuli during reflex testing and handling throughout the examination); (4) consolability (the ability after crying to reach a calm state independently or with intervention by the examiner); (5) cry (quality and pitch variations); and (6) eye appearance (absent, transient, or persistent appearance of sunset sign, strabismus, nystagmus, or roving eye movements).

The 15 items that assess movement and tone and the six reflex items evolved from clinical trials on 50 term infants using the clinical assessment of gestational age by Dubowitz and colleagues,[121] the neurological examination of the newborn by Parmelee and Michaelis,[122] and the neurological examination of the full-term newborn infant by Prechtl.[123] The examination format was then used during a 2-year period on more than 500 infants of varying gestational ages. After 15 years the authors revised the assessment in the second edition by eliminating seven items, expanding the tone pattern section, and developing an optimality score. Reliability data are not reported, but modification of examination procedures occurred during the pilot phase that promoted objectivity in scoring and a high interrater reliability among examiners, regardless of experience level.

The examination protocol is available in two formats: (1) Hammersmith Short Neonatal Neurological Examination and (2) Hammersmith Infant Neurological Examination (HINE; age range, 2 to 24 months) (see later in this chapter). The examination forms are illustrated with stick figures and can accommodate both baseline and repeat assessments. For neonatal therapy examinations the forms can be effectively combined with a narrative impression, treatment goals, and plan of care. A numerical score for each item and a summary score are provided in the revised edition of the test. The authors advised that the scoring system was primarily intended for the purpose of research and for numerical charting of progress with sequential examinations. Because of the continued clinical emphasis on patterns of responses, selected parts of the protocol (without summary scoring) are appropriate for examining premature or acutely ill infants on ventilators, in incubators, or attached to monitoring or infusion equipment. Scheduling of examinations is recommended two-thirds of the way between infant feeding sessions.

Evolution of neurological patterns in infants with IVH, PVL, and HIE is described in the test manual and correlated with brain imaging. Abnormal neonatal clinical signs associated with long-term neurological sequelae were persistent asymmetry, decreased lower-extremity movement, and increased tone. Infants with IVH had significantly higher incidence of abnormally tight popliteal angles, reduced mobility, decreased visual fixing and following, and roving eye movements. The authors cautioned that early signs of motor asymmetry in neonates with cerebral infarction may be associated with normal outcome, but normal neonatal neurological examinations after cerebral infarction do not exclude the possibility of later hemiplegia.[124]

Long-term follow-up data beyond 1 year have not been reported with this examination. Dubowitz and colleagues[125] reassessed 116 infants (27 to 34 weeks of gestation) at 1 year of age. Of 62 infants assessed as neurologically normal in the newborn period, 91% were also normal at 1 year of age. Of 39 infants assessed as neurologically abnormal in the newborn period, 35% were found to be normal at 1 year of age. The predictive value of a negative test result with this instrument was 92%, and the predictive value of a positive test result was 64%.

Assessment of Preterm Infant Behavior

Als[9] designed the APIB to structure a comprehensive observation of a preterm infant's autonomic, adaptive, and interactive responses to graded handling and environmental stimuli. It involves six maneuvers with increasing challenging and complex interactions with a highly structured format. As previously described in the theoretical framework section of this chapter, this assessment is derived from synactive theory and is focused on assessing the organization and balance of the infant's physiological, motor, behavioral state, attention and interaction, and self-regulation subsystems. The APIB has testing sequences and a scoring format similar to those used in Brazelton's NBAS, with increased complexity and expansion for premature infants.

Administration and scoring of the APIB may require 2 to 3 hours per infant and often two or more sessions with the infant depending on examiner experience and infant stability. Although the APIB may be an instrument of choice for the clinical researcher, it is not usually practical (time efficient) for many neonatal clinicians with heavy caseloads in managed-care environments. Extensive training and reliability certification are required to safely administer and accurately score and interpret the test for clinical practice or research.

Neonatal Individualized Developmental Care and Assessment Program

Als and colleagues[126] developed Neonatal Individualized Developmental Care and Assessment Program (NIDCAP) to document the effects of the caregiving environment on the neurobehavioral stability of neonates. This naturalistic observation protocol includes continuous observation and documentation at 2-minute intervals of an infant's behavioral state and autonomic, motor, and attention signals, with simultaneous recording of vital signs and oxygen saturation. Documentation occurs before, during, and after routine caregiving procedures. The infant's strengths, weaknesses, and coping skills are identified. A narrative description of the infant's responses to the stress of handling by the primary nurse and to auditory and visual stimuli in the NICU environment is provided to assist caregivers and parents in identifying the infant's behavioral cues and providing appropriate in-

teraction. Options are described in the care plans for reducing aversive environmental stimuli and modifying physical handling procedures. This clinical tool allows neonatal therapists to determine the infant's readiness for assessment and intervention by observing the baseline tolerance of the infant to routine nursing care before superimposing neonatal therapy procedures.[127] Sequential documented observations occur weekly or biweekly. Parental involvement is strongly encouraged and instrumental in facilitating a smooth transition from hospital to home. Examiner training in the NIDCAP may be coordinated through the NIDCAP Federation International[128] where priority is given to NICU teams, rather than to individuals.

NICU Network Neurobehavioral Scale

Lester and Tronick[129] designed a tool for preterm and drug-exposed infants from 30 weeks of gestation to 6 weeks postterm. The test includes items from the NBAS, APIB, Finnegan abstinence scale, and other neurological assessments and consists of 115 items in general categories of neurological and neuromotor integrity (tone, reflexes, and posture), behavioral state and interaction (self-regulatory competence), and physiological stress abstinence signs (drug-exposed infants). This test is state dependent and gives a comprehensive and integrated picture of the infant. More than half of the test items are infant observations, and 45 items require physical handling of the infant. Test-retest reliability of preterm infants indicated correlations of 0.30 to 0.44 at 34, 40, and 44 weeks of gestation. This test is useful for the management of drug-exposed infants but may have limited predictive value. Training and certification in administration and scoring of the test are coordinated through Brookes Publishing Company and available in the United States and internationally with use of videoconferencing for lectures and demonstrations.

Test of Infant Motor Performance

Developed by Campbell and colleagues,[130,131] the 42-item Test of Infant Motor Performance (TIMP) is focused on evaluating postural control, spontaneous movement, and head control for neonates at 34 to 35 weeks of gestation to 16 weeks postterm. Functional motor performance is assessed through observation of infant movement and through responses to various body positions and to visual or auditory stimuli. Because the elicited reflex and tone items on the TIMP may contribute to physiological and behavioral stress for infants born preterm, a shorter form of the test is available, the Test of Infant Motor Performance Screening Items (TIMPSI).[132] The elicited tone and reflex items in the screening test still require judicious use with the tone and reflex items and careful monitoring with hospitalized late preterm infants.

Psychometric components of the TIMP have been developed. These components include (1) construct validity[131] and ecological validity,[133] (2) concurrent validity at 3 months of age with the Alberta Infant Motor Scale (AIMS),[134] and (3) predictive validity at 5 to 6 years of age with the Bruininks-Oseretsky Test of Motor Proficiency[135] and at 4 to 5 years of age with the Peabody Developmental Motor Scales and Home Observation for Measurement of the Environment: Early Childhood.[136] Training on test procedures is available through 2-day workshops or through a self-guided training method with a CD-ROM from the test developer.[137]

Neurobehavioral Assessment of the Preterm Infant

The Neurobehavioral Assessment of the Preterm Infant (NAPI) was developed by Korner as a developmental test to assess medically stable infants from 32 weeks to term gestation using a sequence of specific movements. This test focuses on tone, reflexes, movement, response to visual and auditory stimulation, and observation of cry and state. This tool does not require a specific preassessment state as is required by the previously mentioned tests, but starts with the infant asleep. It does not take as long to administer (<½ hour) than the previously described tests and is easy to analyze. The data are categorized into seven clusters and compared with standardized scores. With repeated examinations over time, persistent deviations from the normative scores indicate that the infant is at risk for developmental delays and is in need of close follow-up. In addition, the NAPI has been shown to be predictive of short-term and long-term neurodevelopmental outcomes.[138]

General Movement Assessment

The assessment tools reviewed so far in this chapter require direct handling of the infant. Infants born preterm are particularly vulnerable to developing physiological stress during the maneuvers required by most tools available for infant assessment. Instead, noninvasive, repeated observation and assessment are needed to accommodate the concurrent motor variability, immature nervous system, and physiological vulnerability of the preterm infant.[139] Based on the pioneering work of Prechtl examining the continuity of prenatal to postnatal fetal movement,[140] this criterion-referenced test focuses on evaluating the quality of spontaneously generated movements in preterm, term, and young infants until 16 weeks postterm. A wide repertoire of spontaneous motility in the fetus including isolated limb movements, stretches, hiccups, yawning, and breathing movements can be identified as early as 9 weeks.[139–142]

General movements (GMs) are spontaneously generated, complex movements involving the trunk, limbs, and neck in varied speed and intensity. These movements are among the number of movement patterns emerging during fetal life and continuing until approximately 16 weeks postterm, when goal-oriented movements appear. The quality of movement is assessed through observation and scoring of videotaped spontaneous movement of an infant in supine position without stimulation or handling.[143] A distinct difference occurs between the GMs in the preterm infant and those in the term and postterm infant. GMs in the term infant, and for the first 8 weeks, change in amplitude and speed, taking on a writhing quality. The writhing movements gradually give way to the fidgety movements, which are present in awake infants between 9 and 16 to 20 weeks postterm. Fidgety movements are small, circular movements of small amplitude and varying speed involving the neck, trunk, and extremities.[139]

This neonatal and young infant assessment instrument has gained substantial attention in the past 20 years for its high reliability, sensitivity, and predictive validity. In a comprehensive review of the psychometric qualities of neuromotor assessments for infants, the GM assessment was rated among the tools with the highest reliability, averaging interrater and intrarater correlation coefficient, or *k,* greater than 0.85.[144] Multiple studies have corroborated the predictive validity and sensitivity of this method. The sensitivity for identifying abnormal movement is lower during the preterm period and writhing movement stage, but improved during the fidgety movement period of the older infant. Sensitivity as high as 95% has been reported.[145]

Hadders-Algra[146] created a scoring system for infant general movements based on the original work of Prechtl. Many similarities are described between the two approaches in the observation of complexity and variation in general movements of neonates.[147] Hadders-Algra has expanded the general movement assessment by profiling preterm infants with mild neurological impairment[148] and by extending the observational movement assessment from 3 to 18 months of age in a new assessment, The Infant Motor Profile.[149,150]

Testing Variables

Neuromuscular and behavioral findings in the newborn period may be influenced by several variables. Increased reliability in examination

results and in clinical impressions may occur when these variables are recognized. Medication may produce side effects of low muscle tone, drowsiness, and lethargy. Such medications include anticonvulsants, sedatives for diagnostic procedures (computed tomography [CT] scan, electroencephalography, and electromyography), and medication for postsurgical pain management. Intermittent subtle seizures may produce changes in muscle tension and in the level of responsiveness. Mild, ongoing seizures may occur in the neonate as lip smacking or sucking, staring or horizontal gaze, apnea, and bradycardia. Stiffening of the extremities occurs in neonatal seizures more frequently than clonic movement. Fatigue from medical and nursing procedures can result in decreased tolerance to handling, decreased interaction, and magnified muscle tone abnormalities. Fatigue may also result when neurodevelopmental assessment is scheduled immediately after laboratory (hematologic) procedures, suctioning, ultrasonography, or respiratory therapy. Tremulous movement in the extremities may be linked to conditions of metabolic imbalance (hypomagnesemia, hypocalcemia, and hypoglycemia), and low muscle tone may be associated with hyperbilirubinemia, hypoglycemia, hypoxemia, and hypothermia.[151]

Summary

Practitioners must be aware of the normative and validation data and of the predictive characteristics of the test(s) administered to allow appropriate interpretation of the results. Specific clinical training with a preceptor is essential to administer, score, and interpret neonatal assessment instruments accurately; to establish interrater reliability; and to plan treatment based on the evaluative findings. Even low-risk, healthy preterm infants are vulnerable to becoming physiologically and behaviorally destabilized during neurological assessment procedures.[94] This risk is reduced with precepted, competency-based clinical training in the NICU.

Intervention Planning

Level of Stimulation

The issue of safe and therapeutic levels of sensory and neuromotor intervention is a high priority in the design of developmental intervention programs for infants who have been medically unstable. The concept of "infant stimulation," introduced by early childhood educators in the 1980s to describe general developmental stimulation programs for healthy infants, is highly inappropriate in an approach based on concepts of dynamic systems, infant behavioral organization, and individualized developmental care.

For intervention to be therapeutic in a NICU setting, the amount and type of touch and kinesthetic stimulation must be customized to each infant's physiological tolerance, movement patterns, unique temperament, and level of responsiveness. Rather than needing more stimulation, many preterm or acutely ill term infants have difficulty adapting to the routine levels of noise, light, position changes, and handling in the nursery environment. General, nonindividualized stimulation can quickly magnify abnormal postural tone and movement, increase behavioral state lability and irritability, and stress fragile physiological homeostasis in preterm or chronically ill infants. Implementation of careful physiological monitoring and graded handling techniques are essential to prevent compromise in patient safety and to facilitate development. Infant modulation, rather than stimulation, is the aim of intervention. Techniques of sensory and neuromotor facilitation and inhibition developed for healthy infants and children are inappropriate for the developmental needs and expectations of an infant with physiological fragility or premature birth history (<37 weeks of gestation).

Timing

The timing of neurodevelopmental examination and intervention for infants in the NICU is based on the medical stability of the infant and, in some centers, gestational age. All therapy activities must be synchronized with the schedules of the neonatal nurses and intensive care unit routines.

Neonatal therapists should not interrupt infants in a quiet, deep sleep state but instead wait approximately 15 minutes until the infant cycles into a light, active sleep or semi-awake state. Higher peripheral oxygen saturation has been correlated with quiet rather than with active sleep in neonates. Preterm infants reportedly have a higher percentage of active sleep periods in contrast to the higher percentage of quiet sleep observed in term infants.[169] Allowing the preterm infant to maintain a deep, quiet sleep by not interrupting is a therapeutic strategy for enhancing physiological stability.

Timing of parental teaching sessions is most effective when they express readiness to participate in the care of the infant. Some parents need time and support to work through the acute grief process related to the birth of a fragile, potentially impaired child before they can begin to participate in developmental activities. Other parents find the neonatal therapy program to be a way of contributing to the care of their infant that also helps them cope with often overwhelming fears, stresses, and grief.

Physiological and Musculoskeletal Risk Management

Many maturation-related anatomical and physiological factors predispose preterm infants to respiratory dysfunction (Table 9.5). For this reason many preterm neonates require the use of a wide range of respiratory equipment and physiological monitors (Table 9.6). Pediatric therapists preparing to work in the NICU and those involved with designing risk management plans are referred to the neonatal nursing literature for evidence and perspectives on assessing and managing neonatal stressors during interventions in the NICU.[152–154] Owing to the fact that infants born prematurely or experiencing critical illness communicate through subtle behavioral cues, their understated language is "not easily interpreted unless caregivers understand how infants' ability to respond to stress reflects their maturation and neurodevelopment."[155] Their behavioral cues are considered more subtle and more likely to be disregarded than those of infants born at term gestation.

In this subspecialty area of pediatric therapy practice, neonatal therapists are responsible for preventing physiological jeopardy in LBW infants while providing developmental services in the NICU. Before examination, discussions with the supervising neonatologist and clinical nurse are advised regarding specific precautions and the safe range of vital signs for each infant. Medical update and identification of new precautions before each intervention session are recommended because new events in the last few hours may not have been recorded or fully analyzed at the time therapy is scheduled. The nurse should be invited to maintain ongoing surveillance of the infant's medical stability and provide assistance in interpreting physiological and behavioral cues during neonatal therapy activities in case physiological complications occur. Physiological and behavioral baseline before intervention and physiological and behavioral recovery documentation are fundamental expectations. If medical complications develop during or after therapy, immediate, comprehensive co-documentation of the incident with the clinical nurse and discussion with the neonatology staff are essential to analyze the events, outline related clinical teaching issues, and minimize legal jeopardy.

Numerous potential musculoskeletal and physiological risk concerns are prevalent during neonatal therapy activities. These risk areas include

- fracture, dislocation, or joint effusion during the management of limited joint motion
- skin breakdown or vascular compromise during splinting or taping to reduce deformity
- apnea or bradycardia during therapeutic neuromotor handling with potential deterioration to respiratory arrest

---

TABLE 9.5 **Factors Contributing to Decreased Tolerance to Evaluative and Therapeutic Handling in Preterm Infants**

System

Pulmonary
- Surfactant deficiency prior to 35 weeks
- Initial noncomplaint lungs owing to retained fetal fluid and surfactant deficiency
- Rib cage more complaint than lungs leading to retractions and pectus, stabilized by prone position
- Diaphragm fatigue leading to decreased respiratory stability
- Central (prematurity) and obstructive apnea
- Decreased gag reflux with concern for aspiration

Neurological
- Increased risk of intraventricular hemorrhage (IVH) owing to persistence of vascular germinal matrix through 32 weeks
- Decreased tolerance of stimulation

Cardiac
- Patent Ductus Arteriosus (PDA) causes either:
  - Persistence of increased pulmonary vascular resistance leading to right-to-left shunting
  - Decreased pulmonary vascular resistance leading to excess blood flow to the lungs

Hypothermia
- Caused by decreased brown fat stores
- Head-to-body ratio increased leading to heat loss if not covered
- Immaturity of skin leading to fluid loss and heat loss
- Causes increased oxygen consumption

TABLE 9.6   Equipment Commonly Encountered in the Neonatal Intensive Care Unit

Equipment	Description
Thermoregulation	
Radiant Warmer	Unit composed of mattress, adjustable side panels, and radiant heat source controlled either manually or by servo-control.
	Advantage: ready access to infant
	Disadvantage: increases convective heat loss, insensible heat loss, and encourages excessive stimulation
Double Walled Incubator	Enclosed unit providing heat and humidity controlled either by environmental or servo control. Access to infant is through port holes or opening up incubator
	Advantage: barrier to tactile stimulation, decrease heat loss
	Disadvantage: difficult to gain access to infant and no decreased ambient noise
Respiratory Assistance	
Oxyhood	Clear hood that fits over infant's head to provide heated and humidified supplemental oxygen
Nasal Cannula (NC)	Delivers specific concentration of oxygen via soft nasal cannula, usually <2 L/min
Humidified High Flow NC	Delivers specific concentration of heated and humidified oxygen via slightly larger soft nasal cannula, usually <6 L/min with some distending pressure to assist in lung inflation.
Continuous Positive Airway Pressure	Nasal prongs or mask provides constant pressure and heated and controlled oxygen delivery provided by bubble or ventilator.
Conventional Ventilator	Delivers positive pressure ventilation with positive end expiratory pressure and either a specific delivered pressure or volume.
High Frequency Ventilator Oscillator	Delivers shorts bursts of supplemental oxygen at high rate (240–720 breaths/min) with active inhalation and exhalation.
Jet	Delivers shorts bursts of supplemental oxygen at high rate (240–480 breaths/min) with active inhalation and passive exhalation, is noisy, and requires conventional ventilator.
Monitors	
Cardiorespiratory	Displays heart rate, respiratory rate, and blood pressure with high and low limits.
Oxygen (O_2) Saturation	Measures arterial oxygen saturation and uses a light sensor.
Transcutaneous carbon dioxide (CO_2)	Measures partial pressure of O_2 and CO_2 noninvasively using a heated sensor.
Near Infrared Spectroscopy (NIRS)	Noninvasive method to measure tissue (brain, renal, intestinal) oxygen saturation to ensure adequate oxygen delivery.
Amplitude Integrated Electro-encephalogram (aEEG)	Continuous recording of cerebral electrical activity to evaluate presence of seizures and maturation of the brain.

- oxygen desaturation or regurgitation with aspiration during feeding assessment or oral-motor therapy
- hypothermia from prolonged handling of the infant away from the neutral thermal environment of the incubator or overhead radiant warmer
- propagation of infection from inadequate compliance with infection control procedures in the nursery

Signs of overstimulation may include labored breathing with chest retractions, grunting, nostril flaring, color changes (skin mottling, paleness, and gray-blue cyanotic appearance), frequent startles, irritability or drowsiness, sneezing, gaze aversion, bowel movement, and hiccups. Signals of overstimulation expressed through infants' motor systems are finger splay (extension and abduction posturing), arm salute (shoulder flexion with elbow extension), and trunk arching away from stimulation.[9] Harrison and colleagues[153] found that motor activity cues of preterm infants were correlated with low oxygen saturation and should be carefully monitored during caregiving procedures to minimize physiological instability.

Even a baseline neurological examination, usually presumed to be a benign clinical procedure, may be destabilizing to the newborn infant's cardiovascular and behavioral organization systems. The physiological and behavioral tolerance of low-risk preterm and term neonates to evaluative handling by an experienced neonatal physical therapist was studied in 72 newborn subjects.[94] During and after administration of the Neurological Assessment of the Preterm and Full-Term Newborn Infant, preterm subjects (30 to 35 weeks of gestation) had significantly higher heart rates; greater increases in blood pressure; decreased peripheral oxygenation inferred from mottled skin color; and higher frequencies of finger splay, arm salute, hiccups, and yawns than term subjects. Neonatal practitioners must examine the safety of even a routine neurological examination and weigh the risks and anticipated benefit of the procedure given the expected physiological and behavioral changes in low-risk, medically stable neonates.[94]

High-Risk Profiles

Four high-risk profiles are observed from a dynamic systems perspective. In these profiles movement abnormalities, related temperament or behavioral characteristics, and interactional styles associated with motor status are identified.

Irritable, hypertonic infant. The first high-risk profile involves the *irritable, hypertonic infant.* These infants classically have a low tolerance level to handling and may frequently reach a state of overstimulation from routine nursing care, laboratory procedures, and the presence of respiratory and infusion equipment. They may express discomfort when given quick changes in body position by caregivers and when placed in any position for a prolonged time. Predominant extension patterns of posture and movement are associated with this category of infants. Quality of movement may appear tremulous or disorganized, with poor midline orientation and limited antigravity movement into flexion as a result of the imbalance of increased proximal extensor tone. Visual tracking and feeding may be difficult because of extension posturing or the presence of distracting, disorganized upper-extremity movement. In addition, increased tone with related decreased mobility in oral musculature may complicate feeding behavior. Hypertonic infants frequently demonstrate poor self-quieting abilities and may require consistent intervention by caregivers to tolerate movement and position changes. These temperament characteristics and the signs of neurological impairment previously discussed may place infants at considerable risk for child abuse or neglect as the stress and fatigue levels of parents rise and as coping strategies wear thin during the demanding care required by irritable, hypertonic infants.[156] Hypertonic, irritable infants constituted large percentages of neonatal therapy caseloads in the 1970s through the 1990s, but advances in neonatal pulmonary management have now decreased the numbers of infants with pulmonary conditions matching this neurobehavioral profile. Instead, infants with intermittent hypertonic postures and behavioral agitation now consistently present in NICUs have NAS and are experiencing a withdrawal process from prenatal drug exposure.

Lethargic, hypotonic infant. Conversely, the *lethargic, hypotonic infant* excessively accommodates to the stimulation of the nursery environment and can be difficult to arouse to the awake states, even for feeding. The crying state is reached infrequently, even with vigorous stimulation. The cry is characteristically weak, with low volume and short duration, and related to hypotonic trunk, intercostal, and neck accessory musculature and decreased respiratory capacity. These infants are exceedingly comfortable in any position, and when held they easily mold themselves to the arms of the caregiver. Depression of normal neonatal movement patterns is common. To compensate for low muscle tone when in the supine position, some preterm infants appear to push into extension against the surface of the mattress in search of stability. Although potentially successful in generating a temporary increase in neck and trunk tone, the extension posturing from stabilizing against a surface in supine lying interferes with midline and antigravity movement of the extremities. Such infants dramatically respond to containment positioning in side-lying and prone positions. Drowsy behavior limits these infants' spontaneous approach to the environment and decreases their accessibility to selected interaction by caregivers. Feeding behavior is marked by fatigue, difficulty remaining awake, weak sucking, and incoordination or inadequate rhythm in the suck-swallow process, with the need for supplementation of caloric intake by gavage (oral or nasogastric tube) feeding. The risk for sensory deprivation and failure to thrive is high for hypotonic infants because they infrequently seek interaction, place few if any demands on caregivers, and remain somnolent. Representing this profile in the NICU are infants of diabetic mothers who are large for gestational age and difficult to arouse for feeding in the NICU. A similar behavioral profile of drowsy behavior and slow progression with oral feeding proficiency is common in infants with intrauterine growth restriction.

Disorganized infant with fluctuating tone and movement. The third high-risk profile is the *disorganized infant with fluctuating tone and movement* who is easily overstimulated with routine handling but remains relatively passive when left alone. Disorganized infants usually respond well to swaddling or containment when handled. When calm, these infants frequently demonstrate high-quality social interaction and efficient feeding with coordinated suck-swallow sequence. When distracted and overstimulated, however, these infants appear hypertonic and irritable. Caregiving for intermittently hypertonic, disorganized, and irritable infants can be frustrating for parents unskilled in reading the infant's cues, in implementing consolation and containment strategies, and in using pacing techniques during

feeding. This profile of infant motor and behavioral disorganization represents a large proportion of infants in a typical neonatal therapy caseload.

Neonatal brachial plexus injury (NNBPI). A fourth high-risk profile is the term infant with *neonatal brachial plexus palsy.*

Neonatal brachial plexus injury (NNBPI), also known as obstetric brachial plexus palsy (OBPP), occurs in 1 out of 1000 live births. An uncommon, unpreventable, and unpredictable complication of child birth, NNBPI is the result of a stretch to the brachial plexus when pulling the infant's head away from the shoulder at the time of delivery.[157–159] Recent reports have questioned early assumptions on the cause of the injury, citing multiple factors including prenatal causes such as increased intrauterine mechanical forces and maladaptation.[160] Regardless of the cause, the end result is varied injury to the nerve with resulting muscle weakness or paralysis. The extent of the resulting paralysis depends on the extent of the nerve injury, ranging from a neuropraxic injury (mildest) to complete avulsion (most severe). The initial presentation depends on the level of the injury. For example, an infant with NNBPI at the level of C-5-C-6+/-C7, also known as Erb's palsy, presents with shoulder adduction, internal rotation, elbow extension, forearm pronation, and wrist flexion.[161] The prognosis depends on the severity of the injury.

Two classification systems guide early management and ongoing follow-up of infants with NNBPI.[162] The first system identifies four groups with differing clinical presentations depending on the injury location. Infants in Group I with injury to the nerve roots C5 to C6 are characterized by weakness of the deltoid and biceps with active elbow flexion and wrist/hand function. The rate of full, spontaneous recovery for these infants is reported to be 90%. In group II, infants with injury to C5, C6, and C7 nerve roots present with absent or weak wrist extension in addition to deltoid and biceps paresis and have a recovery rate of approximately 65%. In group III, the rate of recovery drops to 50% for an infant with injury to nerve roots from C5 to T1, which is manifested by paralysis or paresis of the entire arm. Finally, infants in group IV with proximal injury to nerve roots from C5 to T1 and Horner syndrome present with a flail upper extremity and ptosis of the ipsilateral eye. The rate of recovery for infants in group IV drops to 0%.

The second classification system is based on the type and extent of injury to the nerve roots. A transient nerve injury resulting from compression, ischemia, or stretching of the axonal structure is known as neurapraxia. A transient or permanent nerve injury known as axonotmesis results from rupture of the axonal fibers with preservation of all other structures (endoneurium, perineurium, and epineurium). A likely permanent injury may occur from damage to the axon and supporting structures, the endoneurium and perineurium. Finally, a complete transection of the entire nerve will result in a permanent injury.[162]

Regardless of the etiology or the classification scheme, the clinical presentation of NNBPI will guide early management and follow-up from a pediatric therapist's perspective. General agreement exists that early multidisciplinary management optimizes recovery for infants who fail to regain function within the first few weeks of life.[163–166]

Individualized early handling and NNBPI positioning while hospitalized. Early physical therapy evaluation while the infant is still in the hospital can play an important role in establishing a baseline. This examination includes pain assessment and overall neurodevelopmental evaluation to rule out other asymmetries or atypical patterns of posture, movement, and tone. Musculoskeletal examination of passive and active range of motion for neck rotation are also recommended to rule out congenital muscular torticollis, a common comorbidity.[162,166,167]

After the severity of weakness or paralysis is established, a management plan with emphasis on overall comfort, pain management, and protection of the injured arm are implemented as follows:

- Providing support to affected upper extremity to prevent injury to the shoulder joint is recommended for infants when the affected arm is flaccid. Not allowing the upper extremity to dangle during feeding, holding, and carrying the infant will minimize the risk for shoulder subluxation during the acute phase.[166] Using a sling or pinning the clothing can be useful for short-term management of Erb's palsy where the shoulder is the most involved joint. Additional care must be taken when more global paralysis is present, and the infant has a flail wrist. In that case, a soft splint may be used in addition to sling or pinning to prevent wrist deformity. Infants may experience pain and discomfort during the first 2 weeks of life; this possibility must be taken into consideration to guide decisions regarding the use of short-term immobilization of the upper extremity. The presence of clavicular or humeral fractures will make it necessary to immobilize the upper extremity for at least 2 weeks.
- Positioning in supine or side lying on the nonaffected side is recommended to prevent twisting or additional compression of the affected arm. Frequent changes in head position are recommended to prevent development of plagiocephaly and/or torticollis. Infants with NNBPI are at higher risk of developing asymmetrical head position caused by sensory loss and neglect of the affected upper extremity.
- Gentle passive range of motion can be initiated particularly in the elbow, wrist, and hand. The presence of physiological flexion and normal joint mobility in the neonate are considered when implementing PROM, especially in the shoulder. Many infants born at term gestation do not have passive range of shoulder flexion beyond 90 to 100 degrees in the first 1 to 2 weeks, and care must be taken not to exceed what would be considered normal compared to the uninvolved upper extremity. It is recommended that passive movement of the shoulder be performed within the normal range for a newborn and within the limits of pain.[162,166,167]
- Early somatosensory awareness of the involved hand is important to minimize neglect especially if sensory loss is suspected. Promoting hand-to-mouth movement on the affected side and providing sensory input can be effective and recommended unless the infant's response to touch suggests possible hypersensitivity and nerve pain, which can be present early after the birth injury.[162,163,166] Pain assessment and documentation are an integral part of early management.[162,166,167]

NNBPI discharge planning and parent teaching. Strong consensus exists on the importance of parent education as an essential component for the early and ongoing management of infants with NNBPI. Most infants with NNBPI are term infants who are otherwise healthy. Unless a medical complication keeps them in the hospital, the infants are likely discharged within the first 2 days of life. It therefore may fall on the parents to implement the early management strategies at home without immediate support. Parental anxiety and comfort with management of the infant's arm need to be assessed and considered when deciding how early and how frequently to arrange follow-up in the outpatient clinic or in the home. Parents are often afraid of harming the affected upper extremity or inflicting pain on their infant and must be reassured, empowered, and educated early on. Activities and positioning practices that can be implemented within the routine of daily care are the most effective to build confidence and ensure compliance.[162,163,166]

- If indicated and initiated in the hospital, parent teaching occurs on how to support the infant's upper extremity to maintain comfort,

prevent twisting or possible subluxation of a flaccid shoulder caused by lack of joint stability and support. Parents are taught to support the arm when feeding the infant, carrying or holding him or her to prevent the upper extremity from dangling or getting caught under infant's body.[162,166]
- Positioning in supine or side lying over the nonaffected side to keep the affected arm free from compression and prevent possible twisting of the shoulder. Parent education must include monitoring head position and frequent repositioning to prevent plagiocephaly and/or torticollis.
- Promoting somatosensory awareness by encouraging the infant to bring the affected hand to the mouth, gentle massage to the upper extremity if tolerated by infant, and early visual orientation to the affected hand.[162,163,166]
- Teaching dressing and undressing of the affected arm is imperative to prevent twisting or undue pulling on the affected arm. Parents are taught how to dress with upper body garments by gently sliding the sleeve over the affected arm first for dressing and removing the sleeve from the affected arm last for undressing.[162,163]
- Gentle passive range of motion of the elbow, wrist, and hand while protecting the affected shoulder from movement. If shoulder pain is not an issue, parents can be taught how to gently move the shoulder within the infant's normal range of movement and within the level of comfort.[162,163,167,168]
- Follow-up appointment within 1 week to 10 days from discharge is recommended.

NNBPI ongoing follow-up. Consistent and frequent follow-up with a pediatric physical therapist with specialization in infant therapy procedures is essential. The infant therapy goals are created to (1) prevent muscle contractures and maintain full range of motion in all joints, (2) individualize and progress parent education, (3) continuously monitor functional recovery, (4) address all developmental needs of the infant, and (5) ensure access to multidisciplinary team when paralysis persists.[162,163,167,168] It is generally accepted that infants with NNBPI benefit from a multidisciplinary approach (including physical and occupational therapy) to address the full range of developmental needs. A persistent paralysis of the upper extremity will have an impact on trunk control, transitions, symmetry, and play. The management of these infants requires a holistic, developmental approach considering the impact that the lack of upper extremity functional use has on development as a whole.[162,163,165,167]

While physical and occupational therapy are essential for the ongoing management of infants with NNBPI, when paralysis persists it will be necessary for the infant to have access to subspecialized neurosurgical consultation. The consensus, according to current literature, is that if by 3 months of age the infant has not gained function of the biceps muscle, referral for a multidisciplinary brachial plexus clinic should be considered for evaluation for early exploratory surgery option and potential nerve graft procedure.[159,161,162,168]

These four high-risk profiles identify infants with varied motor and behavioral challenges and suggest a need for identifying different tolerance levels of handling and interaction even though long-term developmental goals may be similar. Outpatient surveillance of neonates is advised to monitor the course of even mildly abnormal motor and interactive behaviors and also to support the caregiving stresses of parents. Infants with brachial plexus injuries require specialized, continuous follow-up and particular surveillance of the bicep muscle to determine early need for neurosurgical consultation.

Intervention Strategies

This section addresses components of intervention for enhancing movement, minimizing contractures and deformity, promoting

TABLE 9.7 Evidence-Based Recommendations for Neonatal Physical Therapy

Type	Recommendations	Level of Evidence	References
Prevention	Collaborate with caregivers to reduce risk of skull deformity, torticollis, and extremity malalignment through diligent positioning for symmetry and neutral alignment	Level II Level II Level II	Van Vlimmeren et al., 2007[170] Vaivre-Douret et al., 2004[171] Monterosso et al., 2003[172]
Examination	Conduct baseline observation to determine physiological and behavioral stability (readiness) for evaluative handling	Level II	Sweeney and Blackburn, 2013[94]
	Provide continuous physiological and behavioral monitoring during and after evaluative handling to determine adaptation to evaluative handling and to signal the need for modification of pace and sequence, given expected physiological changes, particularly during neuromotor test procedures	Level II	Sweeney and Blackburn, 2013[94]
Intervention	Collaborate with caregivers to create a developmentally supportive environment with modulated stimulation from light, noise, and handling	Level I Level II Level I	Symington and Pinelli, 2006[175] Westrup et al., 2004[176] Peters et al., 2009[177]
	Support body position and extremity movement—(1) supine: semiflexed, midline alignment using blanket for swaddling containment or "nest" of positioning rolls; (2) prone: vertical roll under thorax; horizontal roll under hips	Level II Level II Level II Level II	Vaivre-Douret et al., 2004[171] Monterosso et al., 2003[172] Short et al., 1996[178] Ferrari et al., 2007[179]
	In selected neonates with movement impairment or disorganization consider therapeutic handling carefully graded in intensity and paced to facilitate head and trunk control, antigravity movement, and midline orientation	Level II	Girolami and Campbell, 1994[180]
	Consider gradual exposure to multimodal stimuli for stable neonates approaching hospital discharge	Level I	Symington and Pinelli, 2006[175]
	Provide opportunities for independent oral exploration through positioning with hands to face, and for nonnutritive sucking to improve state organization and readiness to feed	Level I	Pinelli and Symington, 2005[181]
	Determine readiness for and advancement of oral feeding trials using infant behavioral cues	Level II Level II	Kirk, Alder, and King, 2007[182] McGrath and Medoff-Cooper, 2002[183]
	Encourage parental involvement with feeding while providing interventions for physiological stability (pacing and slowed flow rate)	Level III Level II	Law-Morstatt et al., 2003[184] Chang et al., 2007[185]
	Consider hydrotherapy before feeding for stable infants with movement impairment	Level IV	Sweeney, 2003[186]
Education	Educate parents on behavioral cues and developmental status to mitigate parental stress and improve parental mental health outcomes	Level II Level I Level II	Kaaresen et al., 2006[187] Melnyk et al., 2006[188] Byrne et al., 2019[189]
	Implement multiple methods of instruction for parents and caregivers (demonstration, discussion, video, and written materials)	Level IV	Dusing, Murray, and Stern, 2008[190]

From Sweeney JK, Heriza CB, Blanchard Y, et al. Neonatal physical therapy. Part II: practice frameworks and evidence-based practice guidelines. *Ped Phys Ther.* 2010;22:2–16.

feeding behaviors appropriate to corrected age, developing social interaction behaviors, and fostering attachment to primary caregivers. Management approaches are presented for body positioning, extremity taping, sensory and neuromotor intervention, neonatal hydrotherapy, and oral motor therapy. Parent support and education processes are described. Evidence-based practice recommendations for neonatal therapy are outlined in Table 9.7 and Box 9.2.

Many complexities exist in the management of a neonatal therapy caseload in an intensive care unit. A high degree of adaptability and creativity is demanded from the neonatal therapist in response to many ongoing, simultaneous challenges: (1) constant physiological and behavioral monitoring; (2) frequent modification of techniques to adapt to the constraints of medical equipment, tubes, and lines; (3) flexible scheduling of interventions to coincide with visits of the parents and peak responsiveness of the infants; and (4) ongoing coordination and reevaluation of goals, plans, and follow-up recommendations with NICU team members. Willingness to change an established assessment plan, treatment strategy, or therapy schedule to meet the

BOX 9.2 Hierarchy of Evidence

Level I
Randomized controlled trials (RCTs) or systematic reviews of RCTs

Level II
Small RCTs, cohort studies, or systematic reviews of cohort studies

Level III
Case-control studies or systematic reviews of case-control studies

Level IV
Case series (no control group)

Level V
Opinion of experts or authorities

Data from Oxford Centre for Evidence-Based Medicine, www.cebm. net, adapted with permission from Sweeney JK, Heriza CB, Blanchard Y, et al. Neonatal physical therapy. Part II: practice frameworks and evidence-based guidelines. *Pediatr Phys Ther.* 2010;22:13.

immediate needs of the infant, parents, or NICU staff is paramount. For infants with prolonged periods of only borderline stability during minimal handling by nurses, neonatal therapy services may be limited to consultation on body positioning and assistance to parents in creating and maintaining a calm, developmentally supportive bedside environment. Despite an active referral in place, best practice involves deferring evaluative handling by the neonatal therapist until infant stability and responsiveness are evident. Productivity standards of billable hours used for other caseloads of stable pediatric or adult patients in the hospital are not appropriate for the NICU setting and necessitate negotiation and reinterpretation with rehabilitation or therapy department managers to protect both the infant and the neonatal therapist. Tolley[191] reported an expected mean productivity of 5.0 billable hours (range 4 to 6.5 hours) for hospital-based pediatric physical therapists among hospitals surveyed across 32 states and the District of Columbia. Productivity expectations for neonatal therapy services have not been reported.

Positioning

A diligently administered positioning program can greatly assist infants in incubators, on mechanical ventilators, or on respiratory support through mask or nasal prongs, to simulate the flexed, midline postures of term gestation newborns swaddled in an open crib. Preterm infants characteristically demonstrate low postural tone, with the amount of maturation-related hypotonia varying with gestational age. Infants born prematurely do not have the neurological maturity or the prolonged positional advantage of the intrauterine environment supporting the development of flexion. They are instead placed unexpectedly against gravity and presented with a dual challenge of compensating for maturation-related hypotonia and adapting to ventilatory and infusion equipment that frequently reinforces extension of the neck, trunk, and extremities.

Imbalance of excessive extension may occur in preterm infants with prolonged mechanical ventilation who appear to gain postural stability in the nonfluid extrauterine environment by leaning into or stabilizing against a firm mattress while in the supine position. De Groot[192] explained the postural behavior of preterm infants as an imbalance between low passive muscle tone and active muscle power. She theorized that because preterm neonates may have prolonged periods of immobility, exaggerated active muscle power can be observed in the

BOX 9.3 Potential Components of Hypertonic Postural Profile

Hyperextended neck
Elevated shoulders with adducted scapulae
Decreased midline arm movement (hand to mouth)
Excessively extended trunk
Immobile pelvis (anterior tilt)
Infrequent antigravity movement of legs
Weight bearing on toes in supported standing

extensor musculature, particularly in the trunk and hips. This imbalance of extension is viewed as nonoptimal muscle power regulation that may negatively influence postural stability, coordinated movement, and, later, hand and perceptual skills.[192]

Some neonates, especially those born at less than 30 weeks of gestation, may attempt to posturally stabilize by hyperextending the neck in supine or side-lying positions to compensate for maturation-related hypotonia.[193] Neck hyperextension posturing, without a balance of movement into flexion, may trigger later development of a host of related abnormal postural and mobility patterns to compensate for inadequate proximal stability.[192] In some infants, excessive postural stabilizing into neck hyperextension may contribute to sequential "blocking" or limiting mobility in the shoulder, pelvis, and hip regions. The potential components of this high-risk, hypertonic postural profile appear in Box 9.3.

Shaping of the musculoskeletal system occurs during each body position experienced by neonates in the NICU. A variety of positional deformities in the extremities and skull can result from inattention to alignment. In Table 9.8, common neonatal positional deformities, musculoskeletal consequences, and functional limitations are outlined. Supporting the skeletal integrity of infants born prematurely is challenging in the midst of numerous equipment obstacles, restricted physical handling because of physiological instability, and limited spontaneous movement. Infants with gastroesophageal reflux are frequently positioned on elevated surfaces or wedges that make symmetrical, midline postures difficult to maintain. Skull flattening may continue to evolve after NICU discharge from overuse

TABLE 9.8 Musculoskeletal Malalignment and Functional Limitations in Neonates

Positional Deformity	Consequences	Functional Limitations
Plagiocephaly	Unilateral, flat occipital region; head turn preference; high risk for torticollis	Limited visual orientation from asymmetrical head position; delayed midline head control
Scaphocephaly	Bilateral, flat parietal and temporal regions	Difficulty developing active midline head control in supine position from narrowing of occipital region
Hyperextended neck and retracted shoulders	Shortened neck extensor muscles; overstretched neck flexor muscles; excessive cervical lordosis; shortened scapular adductor muscles	Interferes with head centering and midline arm movement in supine position; interferes with head control in prone and sitting positions; limits downward visual gaze
"Frog" legs	Shortened hip abductor muscles and iliotibial bands; increased external tibial torsion	Interferes with movement transitions into and out of sitting and prone positions; interferes with hip stability in four-point crawling; prolonged wide-based gait with excessive out-toeing
Everted feet	Overstretched ankle invertor muscles; altered foot alignment from muscle imbalance	Pronated foot position on standing; retained, immature foot-flat gait with potential delay in development of heel-to-toe gait pattern from excessive pronation

From Sweeney JK, Gutierrez T. The dynamic continuum of motor and musculoskeletal development: implications for neonatal care and discharge teaching. In: Kenner C, McGrath JM, eds. *Developmental Care of Newborns and Infants.* 2nd ed. Glenview, IL: National Association of Neonatal Nurses; 2010.

of infant seats, reflux wedges, and limited prone play experiences. Plagiocephaly (asymmetrical occipital flattening) and a secondary torticollis may emerge when a strong head turn preference remains, and parents do not vary the direction of head turn for sleeping and infant seat use.

Thirty years ago an abnormal postural profile in preterm infants was linked to body positioning in the NICU and identified when the infants returned for High Risk Infant Follow-up. Retracted shoulder posture (scapular adduction with shoulder elevation and external rotation) was often present. These postures were found to interfere with later reaching, shoulder stability in the prone position, and rolling during the first 18 months of life.[194,195] Excessive tibial torsion and out-toeing gait were reported in preterm infants at 3 to 8 years of age and traced to prolonged "frog leg" (excessive abduction and external rotation with foot eversion) in the NICU.[196,197]

Diligent NICU positioning programs have greatly reduced these postural malalignment outcomes due to collaborative efforts by nurses, parents, and neonatal therapists. Goals of neonatal positioning procedures guiding musculoskeletal and developmental positioning practices include the following:
- Optimize alignment toward neutral neck-trunk position, semi-flexed, midline extremity posture, and neutral foot position
- Support posture and alignment within "containment boundaries" of rolls, swaddling blanket, or other positioning aids; avoid creating a barrier to spontaneous movement, and allow space for partial movement of extremities
- Create positions that promote alert states for enhanced short-duration interaction and sleep states to promote comfort and physiological stability
- Offer positions that allow controlled, individualized exposure to proprioceptive, tactile, visual, or auditory stimuli while monitoring signs of behavioral and physiological stress from potential overstimulation

The use of blanket or cloth diaper rolls or varied commercial neonatal positioning aids may modify increasing imbalance of extension in selected preterm or chronically ill infants and promote movement and postural stability from positions of flexion. After the infant is facilitated into a flexed posture in the side-lying position, posterior rolls behind the head, trunk, and thighs provide a surface against which the infant can posturally stabilize while a flexed midline posture is maintained. An additional anterior roll between the extremities and the use of a pacifier may promote further midline stabilization in flexion (Fig. 9.10). Small neonates can be maintained in a flexed,

symmetrical posture in a circular nest with cloth body straps and foot support against the walls of the nest (see Fig. 9.11). Increased frequency of extremity movements across midline and reduced spine hyperextension were reported in neonates positioned in a circular nest compared to the supine position without a nest.[179,198] Postural asymmetry was reduced when infants were positioned in the nest with an elastic swaddling blanket.[199]

Individualized application of a swaddling blanket can strategically support body alignment while allowing extremity movement in prone, supine, and side positions. Creating space inside swaddling containment for spontaneous kicking is critical for reducing risk of hip dysplasia from excessive hip adduction and extension position.[200] Improved neuromuscular development and motor organization, less physiological distress, longer sleep duration, and improved behavioral self-regulation were documented in swaddled infants.[201] During routine nursing care procedures of bathing,[202,203] heel sticks,[204] and weighing,[205] swaddling was found to modulate physiological and behavioral stress in neonates.

Endotracheal tube placement may contribute to the neck hyperextension posture in infants requiring mechanical ventilation. This iatrogenic component can be avoided by repositioning ventilator hoses to allow enough mobility for slightly tucked chin and partially flexed trunk posture. For neurologically impaired infants with severe pulmonary disease necessitating prolonged ventilatory support, inattention to the alignment of the neck and shoulders may lead to the development of a contracture in the neck extensor muscles (Fig. 9.12).

During the hospital stay, infants on ventilators (Fig. 9.12) are routinely positioned to enhance extremity and trunk flexion in the prone position, improve oxygenation, and decrease irritability.[206–209] Monterosso and colleagues[172] reported that using a small vertical roll along the torso (sternum to pubis) improved hip flexion and scapular alignment (decreased scapular adduction) in the prone position. Vaivre-Douret and associates[171] found that repositioning neonates at 3 to 4 hour intervals in alternating positions (prone, supine, side) in a semicontoured nest contributed to semiflexed body position at hospital discharge compared to extensor postures of infants placed only in prone with a roll under hips (Fig. 9.13). They observed spontaneous head and extremity movements in supine and side positions more than in prone.

A wide range of detailed positioning techniques are reported for application in NICU settings.[210,211] A positioning competency assessment

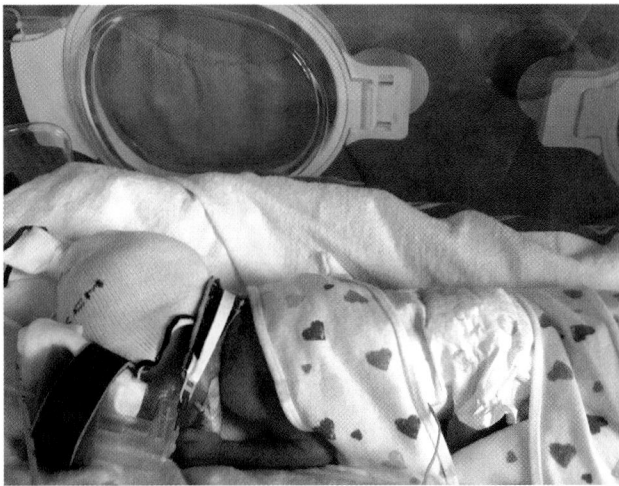

Fig. 9.10 Infant positioned on side with diaper rolls to reduce extension postures.

Fig. 9.11 Preterm infant positioned prone in nest with rolls to promote extremity flexion and hand toward mouth.

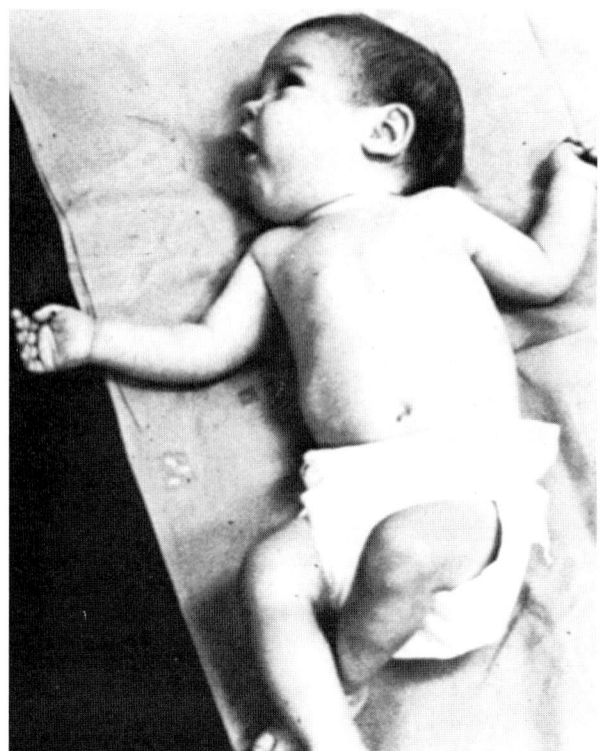

Fig. 9.12 Clinical presentation of contracture in neck extensor muscles related to hyperextension posture during prolonged mechanical ventilation.

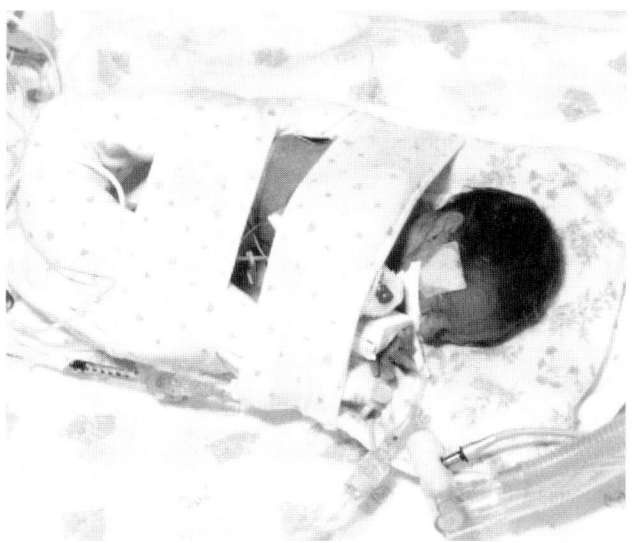

Fig. 9.13 Infant with endotracheal tube and ventilator positioned prone in nest with straps. (Reprinted from Hunter JG. Neonatal intensive care unit. In: Case-Smith J, O'Brien JC, eds. *Occupational Therapy for Children.* 6th ed. St Louis: Mosby; 2010.)

tool to support positioning consistency with positioning interventions by NICU care givers was developed by Coughlin and associates.[212] The Infant Positioning Assessment Tool (IPAT) has been used as an education tool with a 2-point scoring system for body posture at six areas: head, neck, shoulders, hands, hips, and lower leg (knees, ankles, and feet). Repositioning is indicated with an IPAT score of 8 or lower to adjust alignment and provide improved positioning support materials.

After infants are moved from an incubator to an open crib in the NICU, a transition to a standard mattress without positioning aids is recommended to allow time for adaptation to the type of mattress and bed environment to be used at home. Infants are also transitioned to the supine sleeping position at least a week before hospital discharge to model sleep safety for the home environment to reduce the risk of sudden infant death associated with the prone sleeping position and other factors.[213]

The neonatal therapist provides consultation on body alignment of infants in car seats when the LBW infant has not passed the peripheral oxygen saturation test for 90 minutes in the car seat conducted by the neonatal nurse before discharge. Some infants require the use of a car bed with body harness when they are unable to tolerate the upright position of a car seat without oxygen desaturation. Other infants may require a smaller car seat designed for infants at weights of 4 pounds.

Extremity Taping

The presence of perinatal elasticity encourages early management of congenital musculoskeletal deformities in the neonatal period (birth to 28 days of age). A temporary ligamentous laxity is presumed to be present in the neonate related to transplacental transfer of relaxin and estrogen from the mother. In addition to the influence of maternal hormones, the rapid growth of the neonate can foster correction of malalignment if the deforming forces are expeditiously managed. This peak period of hyperelasticity offers pediatric physical therapists with advanced orthopedic expertise many opportunities to manage congenital joint deformities.[214]

Intermittent taping of foot deformities (Fig. 9.14) is highly adaptable to the nursery setting than either casts or splints and is more effective in achieving mobility than range-of-motion exercises. Access to the heel for drawing blood, inspection of skin, determination of vascular status, and placement of intravenous lines can be accomplished with the tape in place or by temporary removal of the tape as needed. Therapists without a sound knowledge of arthrokinematic principles and techniques should not attempt the taping procedure, which involves articulation of the joint(s) into a corrected position before taping. Other components of the taping process include application of an external skin protection solution under the tape, application of an adhesive removal solution when removing the tape, observance of skin condition and vascular tolerance, development of a taping schedule beginning with 1 hour and increasing by 1-hour intervals as tolerated, and clinical teaching with selected neonatal nurses for continuation of the taping if needed on night shifts and weekends. The goal of inpatient taping for infants with congenital foot deformities is preparation for outpatient orthopedist management and likely shorter periods of casting in the outpatient period with parents informed and skilled with foot and ankle mobility techniques. Taping is not appropriate for medically fragile infants on minimal handling protocols or for infants younger than approximately 33 weeks of gestation because of potential epidermal stripping from tape removal or vascular compromise from inadvertent, excessive compression by either the tape or the underwrap layer.

The availability of thin, self-adherent foam material now allows taping on an underwrap (bandage) layer rather than on the infant's skin (Fig. 9.16, A and B). Although this method creates a definite advantage in skin protection, it may cover the calcaneal region for blood drawing. Compromise in alignment may occur if the underwrap layer is applied loosely; conversely, restriction in circulation may be observed by edema or purple-blue color changes in the toes if the underwrap is excessively tight around the foot or ankle. An alternative approach for infants with mild equinovarus deformity is using a neonatal intravenous infusion board on the lateral surface of the foot secured

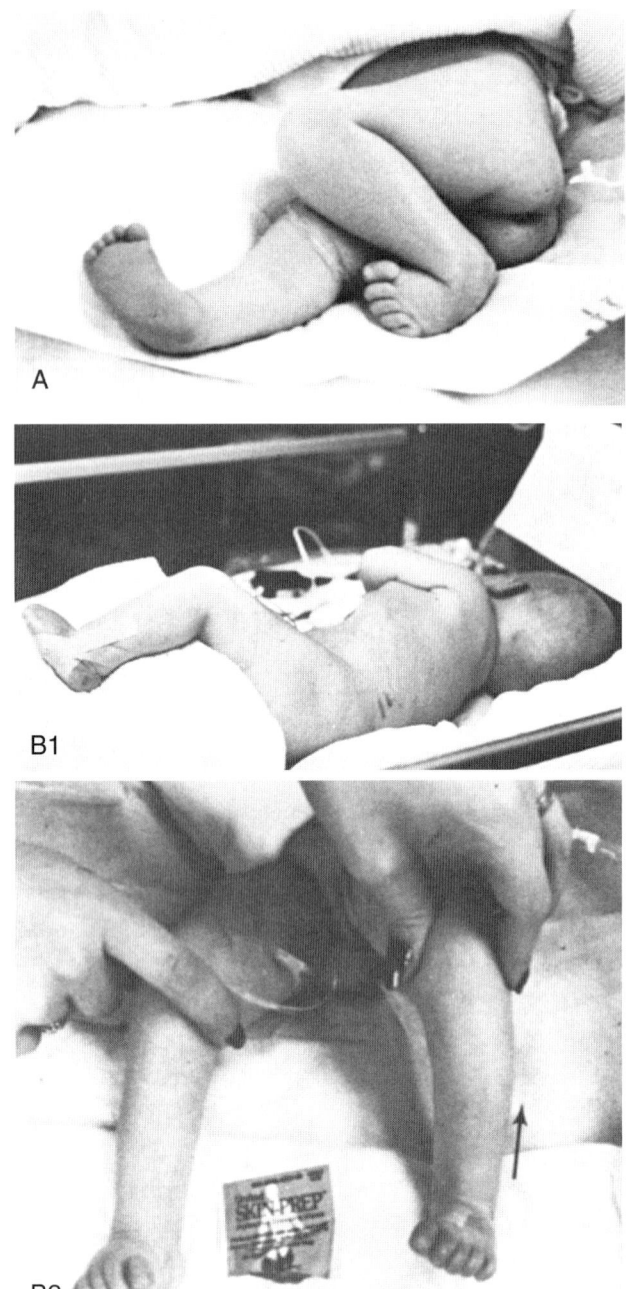

Fig. 9.14 (A) Infant with lumbar meningomyelocele demonstrating marked varus foot deformities before taping. (B1 and B2) Significant correction in alignment of varus foot deformities in neonate with a lumbar meningomyelocele. **B1,** Lateral stirrup with open heel taping procedure. **B2,** Moderate correction.

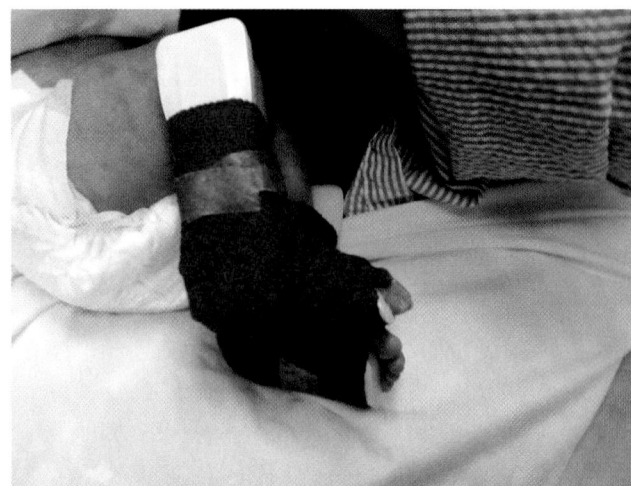

Fig. 9.15 Mild equinovarus foot deformity is held in corrected position with padded, flexible intravenous (IV) board and elastic wrap.

with elastic bandage (Fig. 9.15). Regardless of the taping or soft splinting technique used, specific bedside guidelines for wearing time and removal are needed. Tape or splint removal by the bedside nurse should occur with observation of color changes in toes, capillary refill greater than 2 seconds, skin rash, edema, or prolonged fussy behavior.

Infants with wrist drop from radial nerve compression related to intravenous line infiltration also benefit from the use of taping (Fig. 9.17). The wrist is supported in a functional position of slight extension. As muscle function returns, the taping is used intermittently to reduce fatigue and overstretching of the emerging, but still weak, wrist extensor musculature.

Instead of using rigid, thermoplastic materials or taping, soft foam straps with Velcro closures provide an alternative method of support for wrist drop or hand-wrist malalignment (Fig. 9.18). The splinting material is illustrated in Fig. 9.19 with a small notch for the thumb on the longer strap placed across the palm and the shorter strap for the wrist band (longer strap attaches to posterior wrist band by Velcro). The wearing time is increased by 1-hour intervals to a 3-hour total wearing time and is often synchronized with nurse caregiving schedules (approximately 3-hour intervals) for alternate on-off application. Collaboration with neonatal nurses on wearing schedule, skin and vascular tolerance, alignment, and parental teaching is critical for successful integration of soft splints into the care plan.

Therapeutic Handling

Use of tactile, vestibular, proprioceptive, visual, and auditory stimuli to facilitate infant development has been reported and reviewed by many authors.[215–219] Selection and application of the sensory or neuromotor treatment options in neonatal therapy must occur with judicious attention to the prevention of sensory overload and related physiological consequences. Decision making on the type, intensity, duration, frequency, and sequencing of intervention within the context of infant physiological and behavioral stability can be learned only in a mentored clinical practicum in the NICU setting. The current general guidance on intervention is more observation, less handling, protection from bright lights and loud conversation, and readiness for handling determined on the basis of behavioral and physiological cues of the infant.

Primary aims of therapeutic handling include assisting the newborn to achieve maximal interaction with parents and caregivers and facilitating the experience of postural and movement patterns appropriate to the infant's adjusted gestational age. Helping infants reach and maintain the quiet, alert behavioral state and age-appropriate postural tone appears to enhance opportunities for visual and auditory interaction and for antigravity movement experiences. The typical early movement experiences include hand-to-mouth movement, scapular abduction and adduction, anterior and posterior pelvic tilt, free movement of the extremities against gravity, and momentary holding of the head in midline.[220]

Behavioral state and some movement abnormalities can be modified by creative swaddling and gentle weight shifts and nesting in the

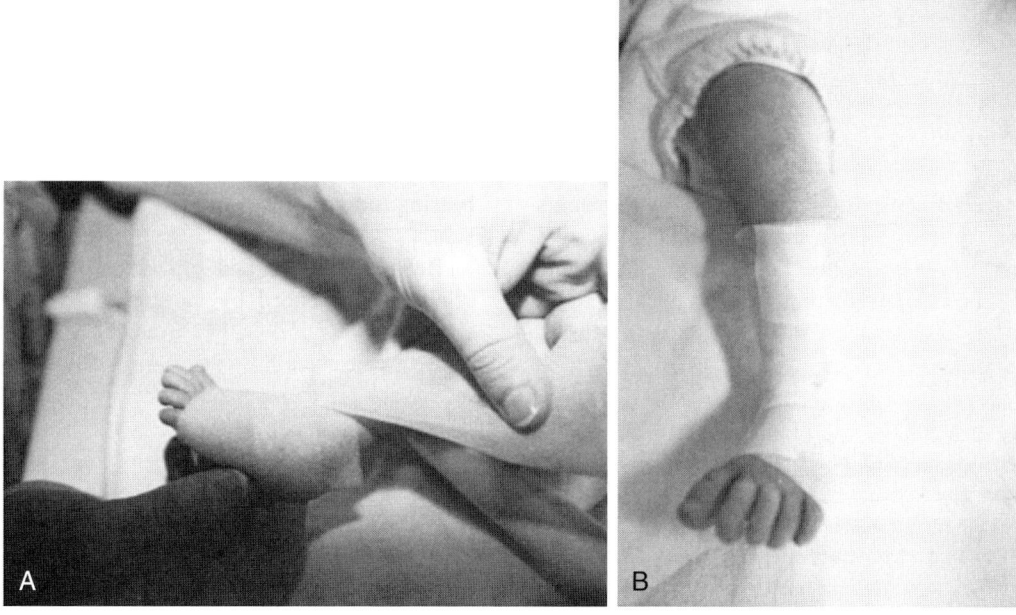

Fig. 9.16 Taping of Varus Foot Deformity. **(A)** Thin foam layer. **(B)** Silk tape in lateral stirrup over foam layer.

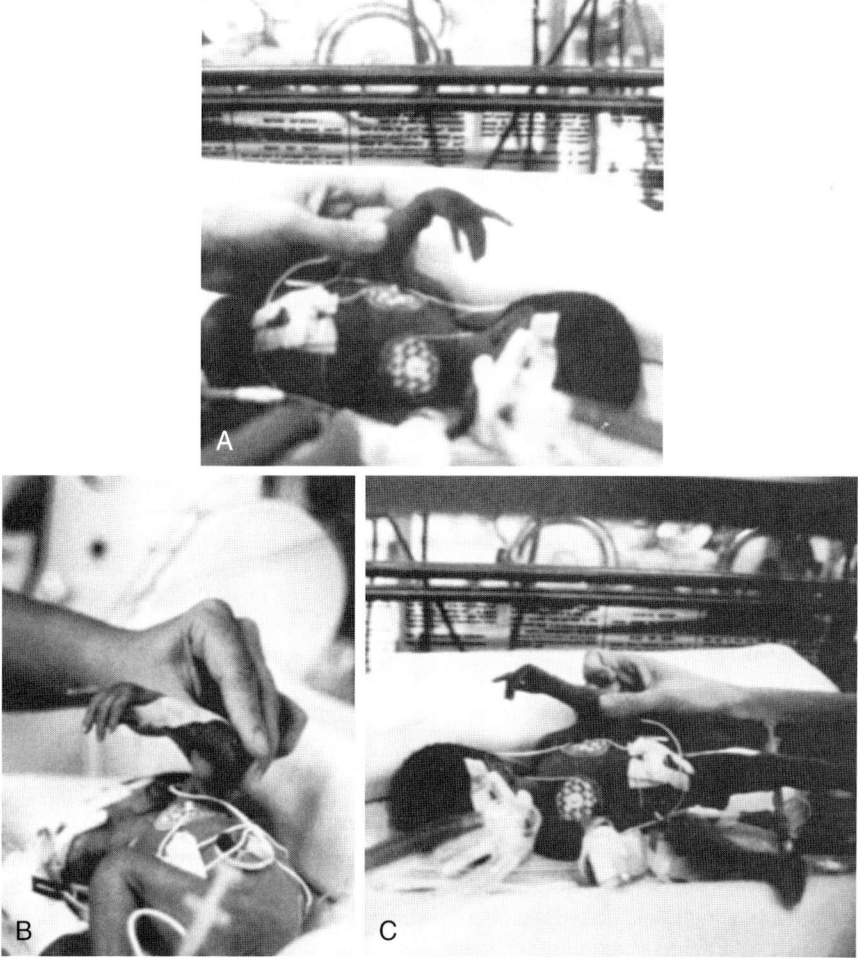

Fig. 9.17 Management of Wrist Drop in Medically Fragile Neonate. **(A)** Wrist drop before taping. **(B)** Taping procedure. **(C)** One week after taping.

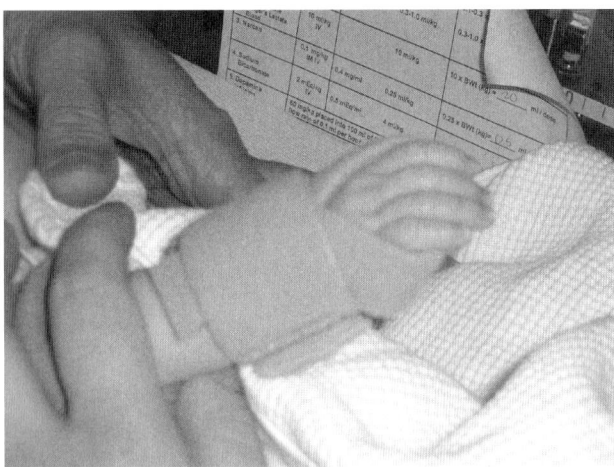

Fig. 9.18 Soft Wrist Extension Splint.

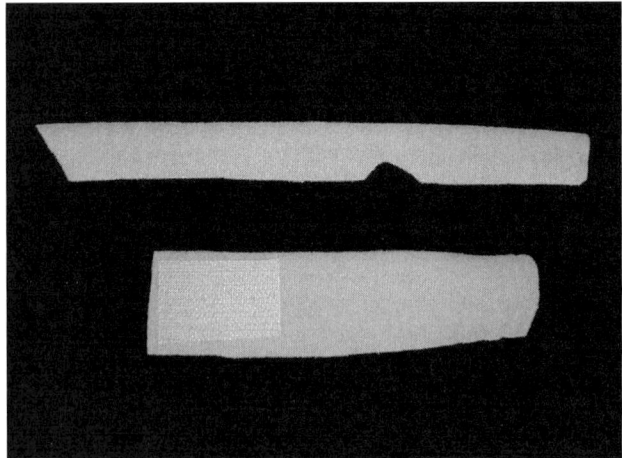

Fig. 9.19 Soft Splint Materials. The long strap is used across the palm with the notch for the thumb. The short strap wraps around the wrist to stabilize the long strap on the dorsum of the hand.

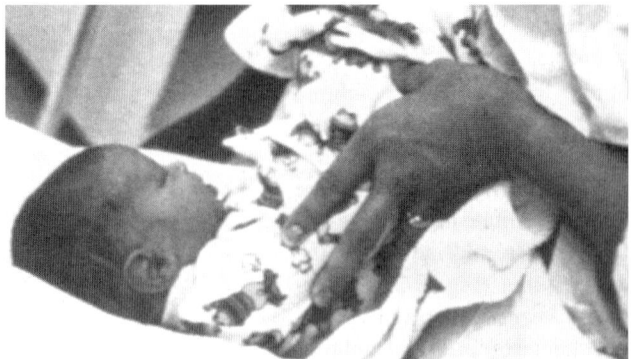

Fig. 9.20 Potential respiratory compromise to the infant from neck extensor muscle elongation in excessively flexed position while supine.

tently unreliable because of motion artifacts from either the infant's spontaneous movement or the therapist's handling of the infant, reliable readings of oxygen saturation may be taken approximately 1 minute after the infant's body is not moved.

Easily overstimulated preterm infants may not tolerate multimodal sensory stimulation but may instead respond to a single sensory stimulus.[216] Implementation of any components of a neonatal therapy or developmental procedure can be instituted only in collaboration with the shifts of bedside nurses in charge of the infant's 24-hour day in the NICU. Collaboration with nurses is a major component of precepted neonatal therapy training and requires integration into and valuing of the unique culture of the NICU. Part of the NICU culture is the unique ecology of environmental light and sound modifications, medical procedures, equipment, and caregiving patterns. Observing and analyzing the effects of the environment on an infant's behavior, physiological stability, postural control, and feeding function are critical elements for establishing a prehandling baseline status before each neonatal therapy contact as well as guiding parent teaching on infant strengths and vulnerabilities. Research on the risks and benefits of neonatal therapy and developmental procedures is critically needed to guide future directions of neonatal developmental practice.

Neonatal Hydrotherapy

Modified for use in an intensive care nursery setting, the traditional physical therapy modality of hydrotherapy has been adapted and implemented into neonatal therapy programs in some NICUs. Neonatal hydrotherapy was conceptualized in 1980 at Madigan Army Medical Center in Tacoma, Washington, and results of a pilot study of physiological effects were first reported in 1983.[223]

Indications for referral of medically stable infants to the hydrotherapy component of the neonatal therapy program include (1) muscle tone abnormalities (hypertonus or hypotonus) affecting the quality and quantity of spontaneous movement and contributing to the imbalance of extension in posture and movement; (2) limitation of motion in the extremities related to muscular or connective tissue factors; and (3) behavioral state abnormalities of marked irritability during graded neuromotor handling or, conversely, excessive drowsiness during handling that limits social interaction with caregivers and lethargy that contributes to feeding dysfunction.

Infants are considered medically stable for aquatic intervention when ventilatory equipment and intravenous lines are discontinued and when temperature instability and apnea or bradycardia are resolved. A standard plastic bassinet serves as the hydrotherapy tub, and the water temperature is prepared at 37.8°C to 38.3°C (100°F to 101°F). An overhead radiant heater is used to reduce temperature loss

caregiver's lap. Swaddling the infant in a blanket with flexed, midline extremity position appears to promote flexor tone, increase hand-to-mouth awareness, inhibit jittery or disorganized movement, and elicit quiet, alert behavior. These effects can also be accomplished in skin-to-skin holding of infants against the parent's chest, implemented routinely with stable infants.[221,222] Application of neonatal therapy techniques must be contingent on both the infant's readiness for interaction and the need for a recovery break in interaction related to sensory overload. Teaching parents and caregivers to read and respond to the infant's motor cues for interaction, feeding, change of body position, and rest breaks is a critical quality-of-life component of the infant's NICU therapy program.

A semiinverted supine flexion position (Fig. 9.20) with preterm neonates should be used with caution, even for diaper changes. This position may be used in therapy procedures with older infants (6 months old) to facilitate elongation of neck extensor muscles and decrease the neck hyperextension posture, but with neonates the position may compromise breathing from positional compression of the chest and from potential airway occlusion associated with maximal flexion of the neck. The use of cardiorespiratory and oxygen saturation monitors during therapeutic handling activities is recommended for objective measurement of physiological tolerance. Although the peripheral oxygen saturation values from monitors may be intermit-

and enhance thermoregulation in the undressed infant. Agitation of the water is not included in the hydrotherapy protocol in the NICU.

After medical clearance and individualized criteria for the maximum acceptable limits of heart rate, blood pressure, and color changes during hydrotherapy have been received from the neonatal staff, the baseline heart rate and blood pressure values are recorded and pretreatment posture and behavioral states are observed. The undressed infant is swaddled and moved into a semiflexed, supine position. The blood pressure cuff is placed around the distal tibial region to continuously measure heart rate and blood pressure at 2-minute intervals during the 10-minute water immersion period. After being lifted into the water, the swaddled infant is given a short period of quiet holding in the water without body movement or auditory stimulation to allow behavioral adaptation to the fluid environment (Fig. 9.21). A second caregiver (e.g., nurse or parent) is recruited to stabilize the infant's head and shoulder girdle region while the neonatal therapist provides support at the pelvis (Fig. 9.22).

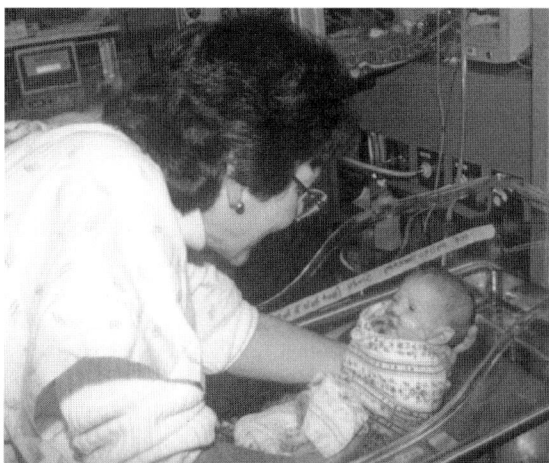

Fig. 9.21 Adjustment to water immersion before introduction of guided movement during neonatal hydrotherapy.

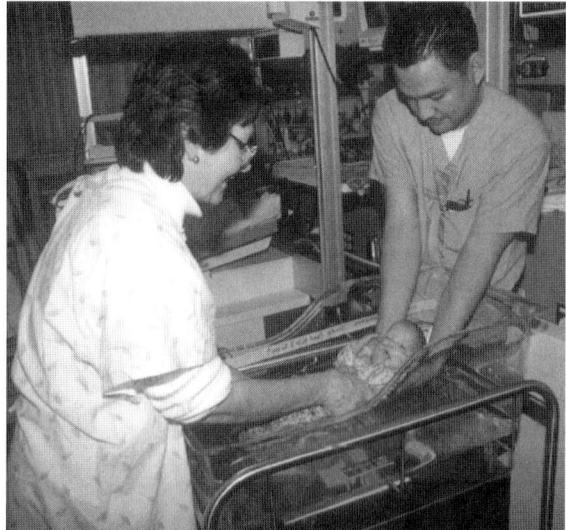

Fig. 9.22 Swaddled infant is supported in neonatal hydrotherapy tub by neonatal physical therapist and neonatal nurse. The blanket is gradually loosened to encourage spontaneous, midrange movement of the extremities.

Within the loosened boundaries of the swaddling blanket, the movement techniques involve midline positioning of the head and slow, graded movement incorporating slight flexion and rotation of the trunk, followed (if tolerated) by progression distally to the pelvic girdle region and finally to the shoulder girdle region. After guided trunk extensor flexion with partially dissociated movement at the shoulder or pelvic girdle, most infants will demonstrate active extremity movement in the water and the swaddling blanket is adjusted (or removed) to allow more movement or more stability depending on the response of the infant. The improved range and smoothness of spontaneous extremity movement is facilitated by the buoyancy and surface tension of the water. Movement experiences in the supine, side-lying, and prone positions are offered as tolerated. If the movement therapy becomes stressful, with agitation or crying by the infant, body movement is stopped immediately, and the infant is either consoled or removed from the water and held with warmed towels. Compromise in hemodynamic stability (increased heart rate, increased blood pressure, decreased respiratory rate) and decrease in arterial oxygen tension during crying have been well documented in neonates.[224] Careful monitoring of behavioral tolerance to hydrotherapy (with avoidance of crying) is considered critical for reducing physiological risk with hydrotherapy.

Multiple therapeutic benefits have been observed from the selective use of 10-minute aquatic intervention sessions. Improved postural tone with semiflexed posture is obtained with less time and effort by the therapist and with higher behavioral tolerance by the infant than when a similar therapeutic handling approach is used without the medium of water. Postural tone changes are frequently maintained for 2 to 3 hours when aquatic intervention is followed by flexed, midline body positioning in the side-lying or prone position supported by positioning rolls, swaddling blanket, and containment nest. Mild flexion contractures of knees and elbows and dynamic hip adduction contractures can be safely and quickly reduced by gentle muscle elongation techniques in warm water. Enhancement of visual and auditory orientation responses (e.g., visual fixing and tracking, auditory alerting, and localization to human voices), prolonged high-quality alertness, and longer periods of social interaction with caregivers are clinically observed during and after hydrotherapy sessions.

Improved sleep quality and behavioral organization were documented in 12 preterm infants (less than 36 weeks of gestation) after a 10-minute hydrotherapy session in a NICU in Brazil.[225] In this study the infants were used as their own controls, and responses were measured by a Neonatal Facial Coding System scale and by sleep-wake cycles from an adapted NBAS.

A later study of neonatal hydrotherapy effects on stress reduction was conducted in Brazil with 15 neonates at a mean adjusted age of 34.2 weeks at the time of testing. Salivary cortisol levels and cardiopulmonary measures indicated short-term, significant decreases in stress after a 10-minute hydrotherapy session with gentle, facilitated movements in a plastic bucket in the NICU. No changes were found in pain responses before and after hydrotherapy using the Neonatal Infant Pain Scale.[226]

Feeding performance may improve when hydrotherapy is scheduled 30 minutes before feeding to prepare the infant for arousal to the quiet, alert state and for flexed, midline postural changes for optimal feeding. A sample of 31 preterm infants received both a 10-minute hydrotherapy session and a 10-minute rest period control condition (crossover design) before bottle feeding by a nurse blinded to the order of the treatment phase. Mean duration of feeding was significantly decreased ($P < .004$) after hydrotherapy compared with the rest condition. Mean daily weight gain after hydrotherapy was significantly higher ($P < .026$) than after the rest condition. All infants consumed

100% of the required feeding volume after the 10-minute hydrotherapy session, indicating that potential overstimulation or fatigue did not occur. On a short-term basis, weight gain was enhanced.[186]

Therapeutic bathing techniques are incorporated into the parental teaching program to foster early parental participation in child care and in specific neonatal therapy activities during the inpatient period to prepare for carryover into the home environment. This early pleasurable involvement of parent and child in hydrotherapy and therapeutic bathing may provide a strong base for future participation in aquatics as a family leisure sports activity and, if needed, as an adjunct to an outpatient therapy program.

When oriented to treatment goals and trained in specific hydrotherapy techniques for individual infants, the nursing staff can effectively carry on the hydrotherapy program established by the neonatal therapist. This release of the neonatal therapist's role to nurses allows additional use of hydrotherapy on evening and night shifts and continued teaching and supervision of parents during evening and weekend visits (Fig. 9.23).

An additional advantage of neonatal hydrotherapy is cost-effectiveness, with the use of equipment readily available in the newborn nursery and the short time (10 minutes) required for therapeutic swaddled bathing. Hydrotherapy becomes labor efficient for the neonatal therapist when it is incorporated into nursing care plans and conducted by nurses and parents, with the therapist assuming a supervisory role.

Although many clinical benefits may be obtained by judicious use of hydrotherapy in the newborn nursery, pilot study data obtained on physiological changes in high-risk infants during hydrotherapy clearly indicate a physiological risk.[223] This risk (7% increase in blood pressure and heart rate in the pilot sample) must be carefully evaluated relative to each infant's general medical stability and baseline heart rate and blood pressure status before hydrotherapy can be included safely in a neonatal therapy program. In collaboration with the neonatology and nursing staff, the therapist must use established criteria for general medical stability and the maximal limits during hydrotherapy for blood pressure, heart rate, and acceptable color changes; this step is essential for risk management. Physiological monitoring of mean blood pressure and heart rate with a neonatal vital signs monitor during aquatic intervention is recommended. The blood pressure cuff is a pneumatically driven device that is not electronically connected to the infant and can be safely immersed in water. Hypothermia is a

recognized risk with both infant bathing and neonatal hydrotherapy. Body temperature should be measured routinely before and after the hydrotherapy session with a thermometer with a digital display. A risk-benefit analysis of the potential physiological risk to each infant and the expected therapeutic benefits is strongly advised before hydrotherapy techniques are incorporated into a neonatal therapy program.

Oral-Motor and Feeding Therapy

Feeding difficulties in preterm neonates may be related to neurological immaturity, depressed oral reflexes, prolonged use of an endotracheal tube for mechanical ventilation with subsequent oral tactile hypersensitivity, insufficient postural tone, or drowsy behavior. Because behavioral state affects the quality of feeding behavior, feeding performance may be significantly improved by specific arousal or calming procedures before feeding and synchronizing feeding according to behavioral readiness cues.[227] Other variables influencing feeding may include decreased tongue mobility, decreased latch and lip seal on nipple, tactile hypersensitivity in the mouth, inefficient and uncoordinated respiratory patterns, reflux or regurgitation insufficient proximal stability from hypotonic neck and trunk musculature, or posturing of the neck and trunk in extension.[228]

Three instruments for assessing oral-motor and feeding behaviors in the nursery are the Neonatal Oral-Motor Assessment Scale (NOMAS),[229] the Early Feeding Skills (EFS) Assessment for preterm infants, and the Supporting Oral Feeding in Fragile Infants, (SOFFI) method.[230–232] The NOMAS is used to evaluate the following oral-motor components during sucking: rate, rhythmicity, jaw excursion, tongue configuration, and tongue movement (timing, direction, and range). Tongue and jaw components are analyzed during nutritive and nonnutritive sucking activity. Cutoff scores were derived from a pilot study with the instrument: a combined score of 43 to 47 indicated "some oral-motor disorganization"; a score of 42 or less indicated oral-motor dysfunction.[229] The absence of a category to evaluate breathing pattern, work of breathing or respiratory exertion, and physiological variables during feeding limits the use of this instrument to low-risk, healthy neonates.

The EFS Assessment is a 36-item observational measure of oral feeding readiness, feeding skill, and feeding recovery.[230] The assessment tool includes examination of physiological and behavioral stability, behavioral feeding readiness cues, oral-motor coordination and endurance, coordination of breathing and swallowing, and post-feeding alertness, energy level, and physiological state. Preliminary content validity and intrarater and interrater reliability procedures were described as "stable and acceptable" (correlation data not reported) with predictive, concurrent, and construct validity testing recently reported.[231] This tool is specifically designed for feeding examinations in the NICU environment and with emerging psychometric testing will be a relevant instrument in managing neonates with feeding impairment.

The SOFFI method provides a decision making algorithm for bottle feeding to guide neonatal practitioners and parents in observing infant behavior to guide pacing (pausing, restarting, and stopping) of the feeding rather than focusing on volume consumed. The individualized starting and stopping of feedings is determined by the infant's physiological and behavioral responses.[232] Feeding outcomes of the SOFFI Method, compared to typical NICU feeding methods, showed significantly less trunk arching, gagging and discomfort, spitting and vomiting with meals, as well as fewer feeding therapy referrals in preterm and term infants at 3 to 5 months corrected age.[233]

General strategies during feeding may include semiflexed, swaddled alignment in an elevated sidelying position.[234] Techniques such as use of a pacifier during gavage feedings,[181] light manual support to the

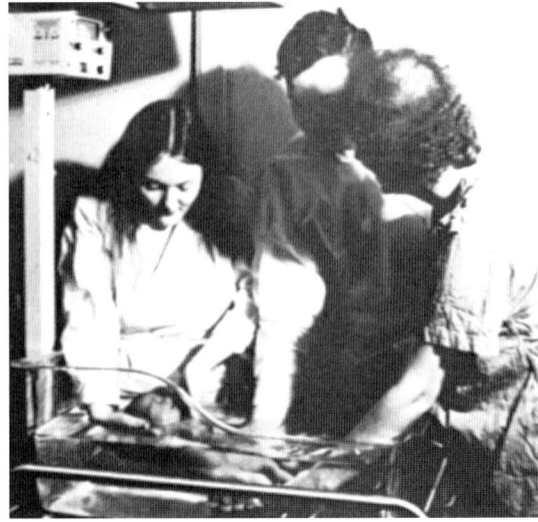

Fig. 9.23 Parents being trained in hydrotherapy techniques for later therapeutic bathing at home.

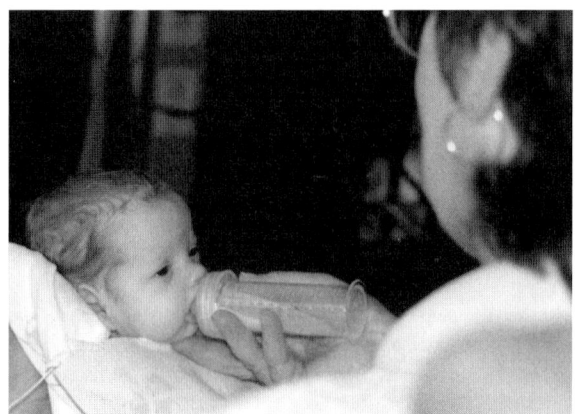

Fig. 9.24 Swaddled preterm infant fed in semiupright position with light support under chin.

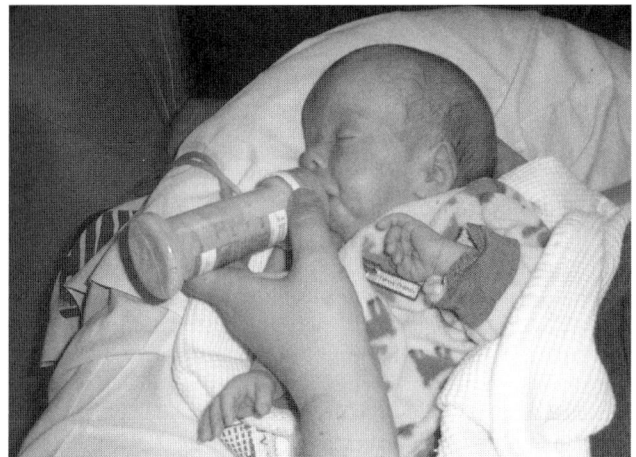

Fig. 9.25 Preterm infant fed in elevated, side-lying position to control milk flow rate and enhance swallow—respiratory coordination.

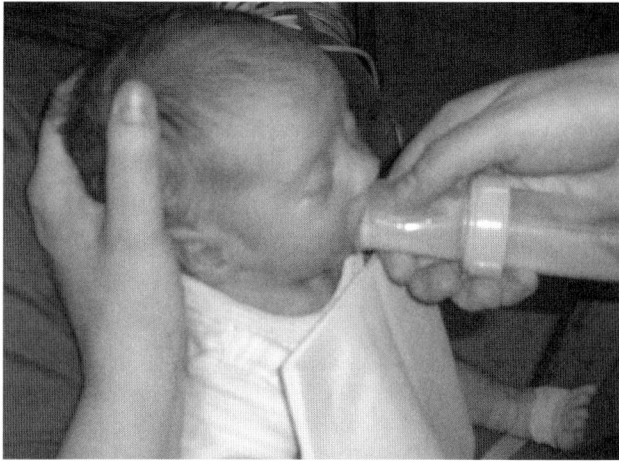

Fig. 9.26 Term infant with cleft palate fed with specialized nipple (Haberman Feeding System) in upright sitting to minimize regurgitation and milk backflow into middle ear.

jaw, and use of specialized feeding equipment are frequent components of oral-motor therapy programs (Fig. 9.24). Scheduling of feeding based on the infant's readiness (behavioral cues of physiological stability, hunger, and alertness) is shown to be effective in helping infants advance the frequency of oral feedings.[235,236]

For some infants, oral intake by bottle may be improved by individualizing nipple selection according to contour, length, hole size, texture, and compression resistance. Wolf and Glass[228] advised evaluation of the flow rate of liquid from various types of nipples and analysis of the effects of nipple size, shape, and consistency on an infant's sucking proficiency. Feeding infants in the side-lying position may decrease flow rate and improve tongue position, particularly if tongue retraction is present (Fig. 9.25). The timing of movement therapy or neonatal hydrotherapy 30 minutes before feeding may improve performance by preparing postural tone, facilitating oral musculature, and enhancing alertness.

Infants with orofacial anomalies (e.g., cleft palate and hypoplastic mandible) often respond to bottle feeding with a Haberman feeding system (Medela, McHenry, Illinois), which allows control of the flow rate through a valve in the bottle and manual compression of the nipple. The Haberman feeder is an ideal option for infants with large bilateral cleft lip and palate because of the long, flexible nipple, which allows formula to be released from manual compression of the nipple by caregivers instead of requiring negative pressure for suction by the baby (Fig. 9.26). Placement of the nipple on the middle of the tongue is advised regardless of the location of the palate or lip defect. Another bottle system for infants with cleft palate also uses a valve to prevent backflow of milk from the nipple, but the infant is able to functionally compress the nipple to express milk without manual assist from caregivers. This features allows self-pacing of sucking rhythm by the infant (Infant Specialty Feeder, Dr. Brown's Medical, St. Louis, MO).

Specialized feeding support and teaching for breast feeding is optimally managed by lactation consultants (nurses; educators) in the NICU. Breast feeding aids allow supplementation of oral intake during breastfeeding through a small tube that goes to the mouth from a sterilized bag containing infant formula or breast milk (e.g., Lact-Aid, JJ Avery, Denver, Colorado). A plastic covering to assist infants in securing a latch on the nipple is used frequently (nipple shield, Medela, McHenry, IL).

Monitoring the infant's physiological tolerance, breathing pattern, and work of breathing is critical during oral-motor examination, intervention, and feeding trials. Heart rate values may be monitored from either the cardiorespirograph or with peripheral oxygen saturation from a pulse oximeter. Color changes, diminished tone in facial muscles, and behavioral stress cues (e.g., restlessness and trunk arching) must be carefully monitored to allow appropriate response to early signs of fatigue, overexertion, and potential airway difficulty. Regurgitation with aspiration of milk or formula into the lungs may occur during feeding trials, with complications of pneumonia, cardiopulmonary arrest, and associated asphyxia. Because of these risks, feeding trials should not be attempted by neonatal therapists untrained in current preterm infant feeding approaches and in managing the respiratory and general physiological monitoring components of neonatal feeding.

Success during feeding activities enhances parent-infant interaction and perceived competency in parenting. Building parent confidence in infant breast or bottle feeding can start early by learning body positioning, pacing, interpreting the infant's behavioral cues, and selecting feeding equipment.

Parental Support
Grief Process

Strong, continuous support is essential to help parents through perhaps the most frightening crisis in their adult lives—the potential death or disability of their infant.[237] Although touching and holding infants contribute to infant-parent attachment,[238] parents may initially establish emotional and physical distance from the infant as they cope with the knowledge that the baby may die. During this time of anticipatory grief, peer group support from other parents of prematurely born children can be of immeasurable value. Actively listening to the parents' feelings and concerns and providing support without judgment through their episodes of detachment and anger are critical. Although long-range plans include participation of parents in all aspects of the developmental program, the timing and amount of initial teaching must be individualized to the levels of stress and acute grief present.

When an infant dies, the neonatal therapist begins the important work of closure. This work includes attending memorial or funeral services to support the family, writing a note expressing sympathy to the family, and initiating a personal closure process. Neonatal therapists are advised to find a senior nurse mentor to guide them through the closure process of identifying and dealing with feelings of loss regarding the infant and family. Finding meaning and value in the process of caregiving rather than solely in functional outcomes is an important task in the work of closure and in preventing professional burnout.

Parent/Caregiver Teaching

Collaboration with family members is a keystone in neonatal therapy. Components of the parental/caregiver teaching process may include (1) discussion of the program goals and services in the NICU; (2) orientation to the interdisciplinary follow-up plan after discharge; (3) guidelines for recognizing and understanding the infant's temperament, stress, and stability cues; (4) methods of creating a calm environment with protection from aversive light and sound; and (5) specific instructions on body positioning, oral feeding techniques and equipment, corrected age–appropriate developmental activities, or therapeutic handling techniques. When used in conjunction with verbal instructions and demonstrations, a packet of written guidelines and pictures individualized to the infant's needs may improve parents' overall skills and understanding of the program. Parents benefit from multiple methods of neonatal therapy instruction. While direct demonstration and video instruction were equally effective, the written-pictorial instruction alone was not as effective for parent teaching of motor tasks in the NICU.[189,190]

Teaching strategies are most effective when they are adapted to the learning style of the parents. This adaptation may involve more demonstrations and an increased opportunity for supervised practice for some parents, particularly those with reading or language difficulties that limit use of a written instructional packet. Cultural caregiving practices of the family may necessitate elimination of common procedures such as the use of pacifiers for nonnutritive sucking or hand-to-mouth engagement.

With consultation and collaboration with neonatal therapists, neonatal nurses can incorporate recommendations to support skeletal and motor development into their routine discharge teaching activities. General considerations for discharge teaching may include the following[239]:

- Varying the direction of head turn for sleeping in the supine position to prevent plagiocephaly
- Placing the head in midline with lateral rolls extending along the side of the head and trunk for car seats and swings
- Limiting the use of infant seats and encouraging the use of prone play on the floor with a roll under the arms and upper chest to assist in head lifting and weight bearing on the arms

- Highlighting the importance of the prone play position for strengthening the neck, trunk, and arm musculature to prepare for sitting and rolling
- Reinforcing the value of interdisciplinary follow-up for musculoskeletal and neurodevelopmental monitoring
- Recommending expedient follow-up if parents notice signs of head flattening, persistent lateral head tilt, strong asymmetrical head turn preference, or asymmetrical arm use

In the neonatal period, the quality of infant-parent attachment and comfort level and proficiency in routine caregiving and therapeutic handling set the stage for later-parenting styles. Helping parents find and appreciate a positive aspect of the neonate's motor or other developmental behaviors gives them a spark of hope from which emotional energy can be generated to help them through the marathon of the NICU experience. Empowering parents early in their parenting experience with the infant is crucial. In the life of the child, the effects of parent empowerment will last far longer than neonatal movement therapy and positioning strategies.

CLINICAL MANAGEMENT: OUTPATIENT FOLLOW-UP PERIOD

Purpose of Outpatient Follow-up for the at-Risk Infant

Systematic follow-up of the at-risk infant after discharge from the NICU is an essential component of the clinical management of high-risk infants. The purpose of this follow-up is threefold: (1) monitor and manage ongoing medical issues, such as respiratory problems and feeding difficulties; (2) provide support and guidance to parents and caregivers in care and nurturing of at-risk infants; and (3) assess the developmental progress of infants to ensure that neuromotor impairments and delays in motor development can be identified and intervention initiated as early as possible. Issues of assessment, intervention, and developmental profiles of the high-risk infant after discharge from the NICU are discussed in this section.

Medical Management

The routine medical care of preterm infants after discharge may be provided by a pediatrician or primary care provider. Infants at neurodevelopmental risk are frequently followed by a number of additional professionals, including neurologists, ophthalmologists, cardiac or pulmonary specialists, nutritionists, orthopedists, pediatric social workers, physical and occupational therapists, and infant educators. Communication among these specialists is often minimal, especially when they are located at different facilities, and access to providers may be restricted by policies of varied hospital or managed-care systems. The parent is often confronted with conflicting opinions, demands, and expectations. The follow-up clinic can play a valuable role in this situation by providing case management to assist caregivers in coordinating services, verifying that all needs of the infant are being met, and helping parents set realistic goals and priorities for themselves and their child.

Family Support

The stress that a vulnerable, premature, or at-risk infant brings to a family is well documented. Grief, anger, and depression are common reactions to the trauma and anxiety of an unanticipated premature birth.[240–242] The caregivers of high-risk infants are required to become knowledgeable about complex medical terminology and equipment. At discharge, they often become responsible for the administration of multiple medications of varying dosages, cardiopulmonary resuscitation procedures and equipment, and complicated feeding schedules requiring daily measurement and recording of nutritional intake and output. In addition, families are often faced with an unexpected, large financial obligation to the hospital and the confusion of dealing with different billing agencies and funding sources.

These stresses and demands are even more overwhelming for parents who are young, are single, or do not speak English. In contrast to the 1980s, a greater proportion of at-risk infants now seen in follow-up clinics are living with caregivers other than their biological mothers. These caregivers may include other relatives, such as single fathers, grandparents, aunts and uncles, foster care providers, or preadoptive parents. At the same time the changing demographics of American society are reflected in the increasing ethnic diversity of preterm infants. Whether they are recent immigrants to the United States, seasonal workers, or residents of an ethnic neighborhood, parents from minority ethnic groups are frequently overwhelmed by the complexities and procedures of a large medical institution. To serve this population adequately, a follow-up clinic team should have access to interpreters and include social workers who are knowledgeable about community resources outside the predominant culture. Cultural competence, defined as performing "one's professional work in a way that is congruent with the behavior and expectations that members of a distinctive culture recognize as appropriate among themselves," is an essential prerequisite for professionals working in a high-risk infant follow-up clinic.[243] For the pediatric therapist conducting an evaluation, cultural competence includes familiarity with differing cultural norms regarding personal interaction, child-rearing practices, and family dynamics.

Preterm or at-risk infants may be irritable, hypersensitive to stimulation, less responsive to the social engagement efforts of adults, and more irregular in sleeping and feeding schedules compared with the term infant.[244] The demands such an infant place on caregivers can be extremely stressful, especially when combined with financial concerns and sleep deprivation. Although these stresses may resolve as the infant's schedule and temperament become more stable, some studies raise concerns about their long-term impact on the parent-infant relationship and the infant's social and affective development.[245,246]

The pediatric therapist in the follow-up clinic must be sensitive to these parent or caregiver stresses and concerns, and because social work and nursing services may not be routinely available, the therapist, within the context of the examination, needs to be alert to cues in the behavior of the infant or caregiver that may indicate problems in the home. Thoughtful questions regarding daily routines, feeding patterns, the sleep schedule of the caregiver as well as the infant, the caregiver's impression of the infant's temperament, and the availability of supportive resources can prompt a discussion of concerns that may not be readily communicated to a pediatrician or other professionals involved in the child's care.

Follow-up Clinic Examination and Evaluation Processes

It is widely recognized that preterm infants are at risk for neurodevelopmental and musculoskeletal impairments that may lead to functional limitations.[247,248] Early assessment plays an important role for discharge teaching, follow-up planning, and identifying infants at the highest risk for developmental impairments so they can be appropriately referred for early intervention. As consultants to the multidisciplinary team, pediatric therapists are in a unique position to become involved in the process of identification of infants at risk, care coordination, and follow-up planning. Critical examination periods and signs of neuromotor or musculoskeletal abnormality indicating a need for comprehensive examination by a pediatric physical therapist are described in the next sections.

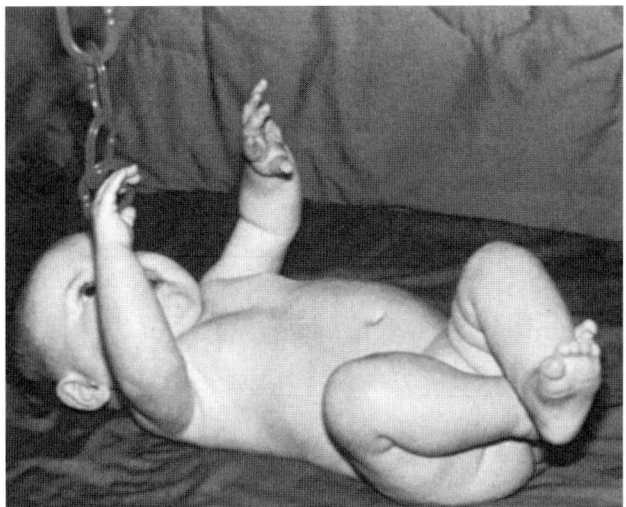

Fig. 9.27 Goal-directed reaching and symmetrical lower-extremity alignment in 4-month-old born at term gestation.

Months 2 to 4

Important changes in postural control, movement, and behavioral organization occur at 2 to 4 months. Head control and balance reactions are emerging, and functional skills are present with orientation around the midline.[249] This is also the time when the transition from GMs to goal-directed movement begins to take place (Fig. 9.27).[18] The pediatric therapist can perform an early developmental follow-up evaluation to provide parent education and monitor changes in infant posture and movement, head control, midline orientation, and visual skills. A marked increase in the prevalence of positional plagiocephaly[170,250] has occurred after positioning practices for sleeping were changed to supine only. In 2016, The American Academy of Pediatrics released a position paper with updated recommendations including supine positioning for sleeping to minimize risk of SIDS.[213] Two to 4 months postterm is a critical window of time for identifying positional preferences in infants and providing parental education to prevent plagiocephaly.

Months 6 to 8

For most LBW infants, medical concerns have resolved at this age and caregivers are raising questions about developmental expectations. This period has great variability in the development of goal-directed behaviors and attainment of motor milestones that are dependent on postural control. General agreement exists that most typically developing infants achieve independent sitting in this time frame.[249] Definitive predictions on long-term prognosis are difficult for a preterm infant at this age. Tools measuring specific milestones have low clinical value owing to variability in the acquisition of motor skills and postural control.[18] A developmental assessment with emphasis on postural control at 6 to 8 months' adjusted age (e.g., Alberta Infant Motor Scale) can document an infant's current level of performance and provide a baseline for subsequent evaluations.

Months 10 to 14

During the first year of life, infants gain increasing levels of postural control and express neurological integrity and capabilities through movement and exploration. Lack of variability and variety in movement strategies may be an early indicator of atypical development. Learning to transition out of supine position and crawling are typically achieved at 10 to 12 months, and by 12 to 14 months most infants have achieved the ability to walk independently.[18,249] By 12 months corrected or chronological age, infants demonstrate a wide repertoire of behaviors in other domains including cognitive and language intertwined with motor development. Multidisciplinary evaluation at 12 months is recommended for infants at risk to create a more comprehensive developmental profile.[251]

Months 18 to 24

With the foundation for gross motor skills well established by 18 months, identifying deficits in the fine motor, cognitive, social adaptive, and language domains that might interfere with school performance becomes the main focus of assessment during this period. High prevalence of positive screening for autism in infants born preterm has been described in the recent literature.[252] These data suggest that while the focus of most follow-up programs for high-risk infants is on motor and cognitive abilities, evidence now supports the inclusion of screening tools to identify early signs of social and behavioral dysfunction. Recent evidence also points to a high prevalence of cerebellar damage or dysgenesis in preterm infants. Cerebellar hemorrhage represents a high risk for cognitive and motor delays in these infants.[252] D'Amore and colleagues reported findings that assessment at 2 years of age can reliably identify developmental impairments.[253]

Comprehensive assessment at 24 months is recommended, including language, fine motor, adaptive, and cognitive skills. Most multidisciplinary follow-up programs stop at this time owing to cost and high rate of attrition.[251] Growing evidence is reported of higher rates of educational and behavioral challenges becoming apparent at school age among children with ELBW; thus ongoing follow-up beyond 24 months is desirable.[253]

Age Correction

Premature infants are scheduled for evaluations in the follow-up clinic according to their corrected age (age adjusted for weeks of prematurity). The issue of whether to adjust for prematurity when assessing cognitive or motor development is an ongoing question. Several researchers have demonstrated that if chronological or unadjusted age is used for standardized testing, the premature infant who is developing appropriately will have a low developmental quotient and test scores indicative of motor delay.[254–257] If age is adjusted for prematurity, the performance of the premature infants is comparable to that of term infants at 1 year. Although some investigators caution that adjustment for prematurity tends to result in overcorrection, particularly for infants born at less than 33 weeks' gestation,[258] the general consensus is that infants born prematurely should be evaluated according to their corrected age.[259]

Neuromotor Assessment Tools for At-Risk Infants

A range of instruments has been designed specifically for examination and evaluation of infants after discharge from the NICU. The choice of instrument for a particular clinical setting depends on the emphasis and purpose of the clinic as well as on the professional disciplines represented in the follow-up team. Evaluation of the at-risk infant with a quantitative, standard assessment tool serves two major purposes in a follow-up clinic:

1. Documentation of the infant's motor status relative to developmental norms or relative to the infant's performance on previous examinations. The information is used to determine the child's developmental progress, rate of change, or extent of motor delay. Achievement of this objective is determined by the scope and focus of the assessment tools used in the evaluation.

2. Identification of a neuromotor impairment to initiate appropriate intervention services. Early identification is not simply a task of detecting signs of neuromotor deviation. The challenge is to identify those infants who are most likely to have an abnormal neurodevelopmental outcome.

A brief review of the infant assessment tools commonly used in follow-up clinics is presented in the following sections.

Bayley Scales of Infant Development

The Bayley Scales of Infant Development (BSID) were first published in 1969 in a format used extensively in clinical and research settings throughout the United States. The BSID-II,[260] a revised version of the BSID, was published in 1993. The goals of the revision process included updating the normative data, extending the upper age level of the test from 30 to 42 months, and adding more relevant test items and materials. The revised test was standardized on 1700 young children representing a distribution of race, gender, geographical region, and level of parental education as an indicator of socioeconomic status. In addition, approximately 370 children with various clinical diagnoses, including autism, Down syndrome, developmental delay, preterm birth, and prenatal exposure to drugs, were tested with the BSID-II. Test scores from these children were not included in the normative data and are intended to provide a baseline of performance for children with these diagnostic conditions.[260]

The expanded age range and updated normative data offered by the BSID-II enhanced its overall use as an assessment tool; however, several areas of weakness were identified in using the BSID-II, particularly with preterm infants.[261] Unlike the protocol of the original test, the administration of items and the scoring procedures for the BSID-II are based on item sets. The appropriate item set for an individual child is usually determined according to the child's chronological age, but the examiner is told to "select the item set that you feel is closest to the child's current level of functioning based on other information you might have."[260] The option to begin testing at different item sets, which can yield different raw scores for the same infant, introduces a level of variability in administration procedures and test results that is inconsistent with the purpose of a standardized test.[261] This problem is magnified for preterm infants because it places even greater importance on the decision of whether to test the infant according to chronological or corrected age.[260]

The third edition of the BSID (BSID-III), published in 2006, is the most recent update.[262] The goals for developing the current edition included updating the normative data, fulfilling the requirements set by the Individuals with Disabilities Education Improvement Act of 2004, strengthening psychometric measures, updating testing materials, simplifying test administration, and improving the test's clinical utility. The BSID-III is a comprehensive assessment for children aged 1 to 42 months to be administered by experienced and trained professionals. This edition comprises five different subscales—cognitive; expressive, and receptive communication; gross and fine motor development; and parental report scales to assess social-emotional development and adaptive behaviors.

The cognitive scale of the BSID-III assesses sensorimotor development, object manipulation and relatedness, concept formation, memory, and simple problem solving. The expressive and receptive language subscales examine verbal comprehension, vocabulary, babbling, utterances, and gesturing. The fine motor subscale examines grasping, motor planning, speed, and visual motor activities, and the gross motor subscale includes sitting, locomotion, standing, and balance. Social-emotional and adaptive behaviors are tested using the parental report scales. Administration times vary depending on the age of the child but can range from approximately 50 minutes for children aged 12 months or younger to 90 minutes for children aged 13 months and older. The child's chronological age (adjusted for prematurity as needed) gives the examiner a starting point. The rules for establishing basal and ceiling levels are the same for the cognitive, language, and motor scales. The child must pass three consecutive items to establish a ceiling, and the test is discontinued after the child fails five consecutive items. The BSID-III has expanded basal and ceiling levels with standardized scores ranging from 40 to 160. The mean for the standardized composite score for the cognitive, language, and motor skills is 100 with standard deviation of 15. The language and motor skills also yield scaled scores with a mean of 10 and standard deviation of 3. In addition, percentile rank, age equivalents, and growth scores can be derived.[262,263]

The BSID-III was standardized on a normative sample of 1700 children from the ages of 16 days to 43 months 15 days living in the United States in 2004. Stratification was based on age, gender, parental education level, ethnic background, and geographical area. Norms for the social-emotional and adaptive behavior scales were derived from smaller groups (456 and 1350 children, respectively), but the same stratification pattern was followed.[262] There are a total of 91 items in the new cognitive scale, including 72 items from the BSID-II. Many items from the former cognitive scale were removed, modified, or moved to other subscales such as language and fine motor scales. The fine and gross motor scales contain a total of 66 items, including 18 new items. The parental report scales are a new addition to assess social-emotional and adaptive behaviors.[262,264]

The psychometric attributes of the BSID-III are as strong as those of the earlier editions and are thoroughly described in the technical manual.[262,263] Reliability coefficients for the subscales and composite scores range from 0.86 to 0.93, with similar or higher coefficients obtained when the reliability was examined testing special groups. Test-retest reliability was examined in a sample of 197 children tested on two separate occasions with an average interval of 6 days. Reliability coefficients ranged from .67 to .94, with an average correlation score of .80. The technical manual describes in great detail the convergent and divergent validity, illustrating the correlation between the BSID-III and other relevant testing tools.[262,264]

Many questions remain on the potential limitations and clinical application of the BSID-III. Administration of the full test is a lengthy procedure, and the composite scores are reported to be higher than those of the BSID-II.[265] Anderson and colleagues[266] examined the ability of the BSID-III to detect developmental delay in 2-year-old extremely preterm children and those born at term with normal birth weights. The study participants were former preterm infants born at less than 28 weeks or weighing less than 1000 g ($n = 221$). Two hundred and twenty healthy full-term infants with normal birth weight were randomly selected as a control group. Developmental assessment was conducted at 2 years (age corrected for prematurity) using the cognitive, language, and motor scales of the BSID-III. The social-emotional and adaptive behavior scales were not used. The authors observed a serious overestimation in the developmental progress of this sample. Questions were raised regarding the sensitivity of this test to detect developmental delay in children. More research is needed to examine this test's sensitivity and the interpretation of test results, especially for high-risk or premature infants. Continued use of the BSID-III should be conducted with caution in the absence of more data to establish the sensitivity of this tool.[264]

Alberta Infant Motor Scale

The AIMS[267] was designed to evaluate gross motor function in infants from birth to independent walking, or birth through 18 months. The stated purposes of the AIMS are (1) to identify infants who are delayed

or deviant in motor development and (2) to evaluate motor maturation over time. The AIMS is described as an "observational assessment" that requires minimal handling of the infant by the examiner. The test includes 58 items, organized by the infant's position, designed to evaluate three aspects of motor performance: weight bearing, posture, and antigravity movements. The normative sample consisted of 2200 infants born in Alberta, Canada.

Raw scores obtained on the AIMS can be converted to percentile ranks for comparison with motor performance of the normative sample. Test-retest and interrater reliabilities, established on normally developing infants, ranged from 0.95 to 0.98 depending on the age of the child. The AIMS reportedly had high agreement with the Motor Scale of the BSID and the Gross Motor Scale of the Peabody Developmental Motor Scales (PDGMS) ($r = 0.93$ and $r = 0.98$, respectively). An evaluation of concurrent validity between the AIMS and the Movement Assessment of Infants (MAI) at 4 and 8 months demonstrated acceptable agreement ($r = 0.70$ and $r = 0.84$, respectively).[268]

Hammersmith Infant Neurological Examination

The HINE is a brief, infant assessment reported to be easily accessible to clinicians in the area of high-risk infant follow-up. The format for the assessment was adapted from the work of Dubowitz and Dubowitz,[120] and the intended age range is 2 to 24 months. The authors divided the examination into two sections with a combination of age-dependent and non age–dependent items. Selected behavioral assessment items were adapted from the Bayley Scales.[262,263] It is considered to be a reliable tool, easily learned, and feasible to administrate in high-risk infant follow-up clinics.[269]

Movement Assessment of Children

The Movement Assessment of Children (MAC) assesses functional gross motor and fine motor skills of children from age 2 months to 24 months.[270] The motor assessment is composed of three sections including head control, upper extremities and hands, and pelvis and lower extremities. In addition, four assessment sections (general observations, special senses, primitive reactions, and muscle tone) contribute to the interpretation of MAC findings for any one child. These four sections assist therapists in making a therapy diagnosis, thereby focusing on the therapist's selection of treatment modalities. The MAC, on average, has five functional test items per month over 23 months of development. It is anticipated that this number of items will allow for accuracy in evaluative and discriminative measures, leading to effective clinical judgments. The MAC can be completed in less than 30 minutes (20 minutes for some children), and it takes 5 minutes to update during reevaluation.

Four hundred and seven assessments were completed on typically developing children aged 2 to 24 months in the greater Denver, Colorado, area. The gestational ages of the children at birth were 37 to 42 weeks, and the majority were Caucasian (77%).

Construct validity of the MAC was established using Rasch analysis with the 407 assessments. In brief, 34 of the 37 super items fit the model based on fit statistics (infit and outfit mean square error values of 0.5 to 1.7). Unidimensionality of the MAC was also achieved: Rasch principal component analysis showed that the model explained 90.4% of the variance. The Rasch analysis also indicated that the MAC has excellent person and item reliabilities. The person reliability index was .98, indicating that the person ability ordering would be stable if these children were assessed on another evaluation tool with the same construct as "the motor super items" of the MAC. Cronbach's α was .97, implying that the MAC super items were internally consistent with little redundancy. The item reliability index was 1.00, indicating that the difficulty hierarchy of these motor super items would be stable if another group of children with the same traits and sample size were tested. (Min-Mei Shih. Personal communication).[271]

The validity, reliability, and sensitivity of the MAC were recently studied in a group of typically developing infants and toddlers from 2 months to 2 years of age. In this study, the construct validity was established and the inter-rater reliability ranged from 0.83 to 0.99. Percent agreement for explanatory items ranged from 0.72 to 0.96. Finally, the stability within age grouping was reported to be consistent.[272]

High-Risk Clinical Signs

Longitudinal studies of LBW infants have been used to identify specific clinical signs or conditions that are most predictive of abnormal neurodevelopmental outcome, such as CP. The conclusions among studies are inconsistent because of the lack of standard criteria for the risk variables, demographic and clinical variation in the study samples, and use of different outcome measures. High-risk motor signs for surveillance by practitioners during high-risk infant follow-up are summarized in Table 9.9.

TABLE 9.9   Motor Impairment "Red Flags" During Neonatal Intensive Care Unit Follow-Up

2 months[a]	Persistent asymmetrical head position; risk for plagiocephaly and torticollis
	Absent midline orientation even when visual stimulation is present
	Jerky or stiff movements of extremities
	Excessive neck or trunk hyperextension in supine position
4 months[a]	Poor midline head control in supine position
	Difficulty engaging hands at midline and in reaching for dangling toy
	Persistent fisting of hands
	Difficulty lifting head and supporting weight on arms in prone position
	Trunk hypertonicity or hypotonicity
	Resistance to passive movement in extremities
	Persistent, dominant asymmetrical tonic neck reflex ("fencing" position of arms)
	Stiffly extended or "scissored" legs with weight bearing on toes in supported standing
8 months[a]	Inability to sit and roll independently
	Inability to transfer objects between hands
	Persistent asymmetry of extremities with differences in muscle tone and motor skill
	Hypertonicity of trunk or extremities
12 months[a]	Inability to pull to stand, four-point crawl, walk around furniture
	Movement between basic positions
	Persistent asymmetry of control in extremities

[a]Ages corrected for prematurity.
Reprinted with permission from Sweeney JK, Gutierrez T. The dynamic continuum of motor and musculoskeletal development: implications for neonatal care and discharge teaching. In: Kenner C, McGrath JM, eds. *Developmental Care of Newborns and Infants.* 2nd ed. Glenview, IL: National Association of Neonatal Nurses; 2010.

Neonatal Period

During the neonatal period through 1 to 2 months after term (40 weeks of gestation), clinical signs suggestive of neuromotor abnormality include stiff, jerky movements or a paucity of movement. Abnormal general movements have reduced complexity and variation. They lack fluency and frequently have an abrupt onset with all parts of the body moving synchronously.[115] Persistence of these movements is considered to be predictive of CP or cognitive impairment.[273]

Infancy

At 4 months of age, hypertonicity of the trunk or extremities is recognized as a high-risk clinical sign.[274] This finding correlates with neck hyperextension and shoulder retraction associated with the tonic labyrinthine reflex in the supine position, which has been identified in other studies as a high-risk sign.[275]

The predictive value of primitive reflexes has been extensively debated. Reflexes and neurological signs, such as the asymmetrical tonic neck reflex (ATNR) and tremulousness, have been correlated with CP in some studies[276] but not in others.[275] The positive support reflex, characterized by stiff extension of the lower extremities when the infant is held in supported standing, is frequently cited as a high-risk sign, but this posture is seen in both term and LBW infants and has not been consistently associated with adverse sequelae.[275] Persistent primitive reflex activity and asymmetry have been identified as early signs of athetoid CP, more common in infants born at term.[277] In Fig. 9.28 a dominant ATNR posture is demonstrated by a 4-month-old infant with athetoid CP. Immature automatic reactions of balance and equilibrium at 4 months, including head righting and the Landau reaction, have been found to be a significant predictor of abnormal neurological outcome.[275]

Comparing an infant's spontaneous, active movements with reflex or passive responses is important in determining risk for neurodevelopmental disability. Systematic observation of kicking activity in LBW infants indicated that infants with neurological impairment demonstrated less alternate kicking movement compared with typically developing LBW infants.[278] Abnormal patterns of kicking, including simultaneous flexion and extension of the hips and knees, were associated with subsequent CP.[279] Abnormalities of kicking described by Prechtl as "cramped-synchronized," that is, limited in variety and characterized by "rigid movement with all limbs and the trunk contracting and relaxing almost simultaneously," were observed in 3-month-old infants who were subsequently diagnosed with CP.[280]

In addition to qualitative differences in motor function, delayed acquisition of motor milestones is an important indicator of neuromotor impairment. In particular, delay in achieving upright, gross motor milestones, such as sitting without support, creeping on hands

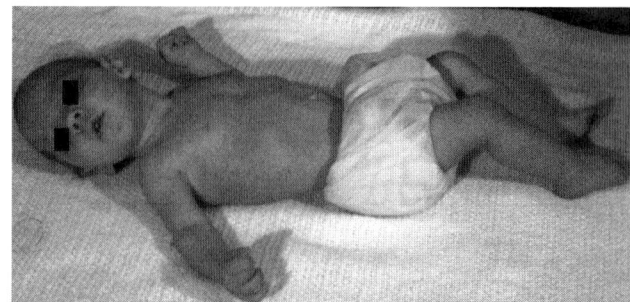

Fig. 9.28 Dominant asymmetrical tonic neck reflex in 4-month-old infant with athetoid cerebral palsy.

to knees, and pulling to stand, was found to be useful in identifying infants with neuromotor impairment.[281]

Challenges to Prediction of Neurodevelopmental Outcome

Accurate prediction of neurodevelopmental outcome of LBW infants on the basis of standard neuromotor tests is particularly challenging because of several complicating factors.

Impact of Medical Status on Test Performance

Infants with LBW often exhibit motor delay or neuromotor deviations because of health or medical status, not because of neurological impairment. Two primary examples are residual influences from habitual positioning in the NICU and chronic medical conditions.

Variations in posture and movement caused by residual influences from time in the neonatal intensive care unit. Although current NICU positioning and handling procedures are increasingly sensitive to the developmental needs of the neonate, the application of life-sustaining interventions (e.g., mechanical ventilation) assumes priority in clinical management. On follow-up evaluation, these infants may show delays in reaching skills and in achieving antigravity postures.

Infants born preterm may exhibit asymmetry related to intrauterine position or prolonged positioning in the NICU necessitated by surgical or medical intervention. On outpatient follow-up examinations, this asymmetry may appear as visual orientation to one side of the body, more mature upper-extremity skill on the same side, and asymmetry of primitive reflex activity. Physical deviations, such as tightness of neck musculature on the preferred side and relative weakness of the opposing muscles, or skull deformities (plagiocephaly) may also be present. Asymmetrical motor function resulting from intrauterine or NICU positioning can usually be distinguished from early spastic hemiplegia or other hemisyndromes by clinical examination and by review of the infant's medical history.[255] Positional asymmetry is generally not associated with differences in muscle tone between the two sides of the body or with neuromotor abnormalities, such as fisting of the hand on the less-active side. Caregivers are advised to promote symmetrical posture through movement and positioning of the infant including strategic placement of the infant in relation to toys, social activity in the room, and use of cushions or rolls to maintain midline positioning for the infant's head and proximal musculature.

Prolonged motor delay from chronic medical conditions. Infants with CLD typically exhibit low muscle tone, delayed gross motor function, and immature balance reactions. Motor skills are often delayed as long as the infant's pulmonary capacity is compromised, but the rate of developmental progress typically accelerates when the respiratory condition resolves.[282] Intervention for infants with persistent respiratory disease includes providing reassurance and support to the caregivers who are dealing with the demands and stresses of parenting a medically fragile child. Caregivers are advised to avoid aggressive physical activity and excessive sensory stimulation that could cause fatigue or tax the infant's limited respiratory capacity. At the same time, the child should be given opportunities to develop skills in nonmotor tasks. Adaptive positioning techniques reduce energy expenditure and fatigue while enabling the infant to be supported in age-appropriate postures (e.g., prone or upright sitting) for developing hand function, vestibular responses, and social skills.

Differences Between Preterm and Term Infant Neuromotor Function

Even when not compromised by chronic illness or neurological impairment, the motor development of preterm LBW infants differs

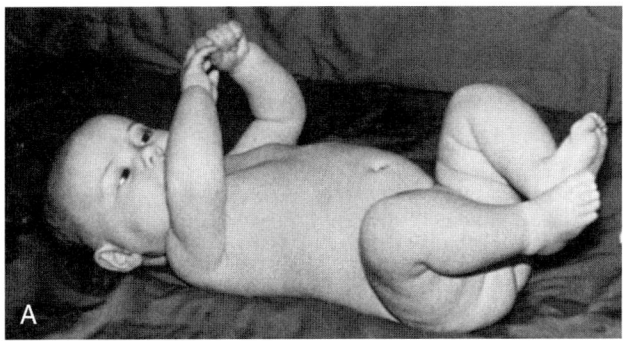

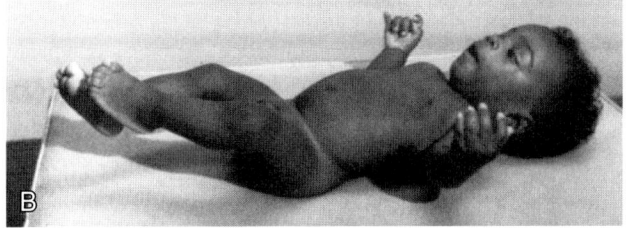

Fig. 9.29 **(A)** Typically developing term infant at 4 months of age demonstrating ability to bring hands to midline and elevate legs with flexion and abduction of hips and dorsiflexion of ankles. **(B)** Infant diagnosed with cerebral palsy at 5 months of age; note inability to bring hands to midline because of shoulder retraction, extension and adduction of hips with limited movement into flexion, and plantarflexion of ankles.

from that of typical term infants. Compared with term infants, healthy preterm infants demonstrate variations in passive and active muscle tone and initially have greater joint mobility, such as increased popliteal angles and low muscle tone in the trunk.[192,193] In the older infant, increased extremity tone is often present, particularly in the hips and ankles. Preterm infants tend to exhibit more neck hyperextension and scapular adduction and fewer antigravity movements in the supine position (Fig. 9.29).

Primitive reflexes such as the ATNR, Moro reflex, and positive support reflex persist longer in preterm infants, even when assessed at corrected age.[192] Gross and fine motor skills are frequently delayed in preterm infants, especially activities requiring active flexion, such as (1) bringing hands to midline and feet to hands; (2) trunk stability required for head control and upright sitting; and (3) trunk rotation for rolling and transitional movements.

Preterm infants exhibit more asymmetry in active movement compared with infants born at term gestation, but asymmetry is usually not observed in passive tone or reflex activity. The asymmetry may be a typical feature of postterm development of relatively healthy preterm infants.[255] For most premature infants, these early variations in movement and posture eventually resolve; however, in the first months of life neuromotor deviations may influence the infant's performance on a standard assessment of motor function or neurological status.

NEUROMOTOR INTERVENTION

Levels of Intervention

Therapeutic intervention for the high-risk infant in the outpatient phase after discharge from the NICU occurs at multiple levels. Type and intensity of intervention depend on (1) the needs of the infant and family; (2) the structure and organization of the follow-up clinic; and (3) the availability of resources in a particular clinical and geographical setting.

Assessment as Intervention

The clinical assessment of an infant is a unique opportunity for intervention on behalf of the infant and family. For the full potential of this interaction to be realized, parents or caregivers must be informed and involved participants in the assessment process, not passive observers. The focus of intervention in this context is on parent or caregiver support with two primary components: education and positive reinforcement for parenting skills.

Education

The educational component of intervention includes enabling the parents of an at-risk infant to recognize their child's unique capabilities and strengths and ability to respond to and influence the surrounding environment. Caregivers learn about their infant's individual responses to stimuli—for example, what causes their child to focus on a stimulus and what elicits stress reactions. Education of parents includes describing typical characteristics and common developmental patterns of the LBW or medically fragile infant that may differ from expectations based on observations of healthy, full-term infants. Parents of at-risk infants are informed about the appropriate sequence and pace of development for their child so they will be realistic in their expectations and interpretation of the child's progress. This anticipatory guidance enables parents to prepare for and maximize learning opportunities.

Reinforcement for Parenting Skills

During the follow-up examination, opportunities to provide positive reinforcement to caregivers need to be emphasized. They should be reassured that they are providing appropriate and beneficial parenting and reminded that the infant's behavioral responses reflect neurobehavioral immaturity or instability rather than an unpleasant personality or negative affective feelings toward the caregiver.

Instruction in Home Management

A critical component of intervention is instruction in specific activities and handling techniques for home management. The recommendations are made on the basis of the therapist's knowledge of the infant's medical and neurological history, current health status, and findings from the neurodevelopmental assessment. The overall purpose may be to maximize a healthy child's growth potential or to promote developmental progress in an infant who demonstrates delay or neuromotor abnormality. In either case, the parent or caregiver must have a clear understanding of the purpose of the activity, what motor behavior will be facilitated or counteracted, the underlying neurodevelopmental process that the activity will support, and the desired response from the infant. Parents can be encouraged to participate creatively in the process of therapy by adapting and modifying the recommendations according to the infant's responses and progress at home.

Although neuromotor handling recommendations are specific to the individual child, some intervention activities are applicable to many preterm infants.

Activities to Counteract Shoulder Retraction

Preterm infants may demonstrate scapular adduction or shoulder retraction postures. This posture may inhibit the infant's ability to bring hands to midline and often results in delayed achievement of upper-extremity skills and rolling. To overcome shoulder retraction, play activities and carrying techniques that bring shoulders forward and hands to midline are encouraged.

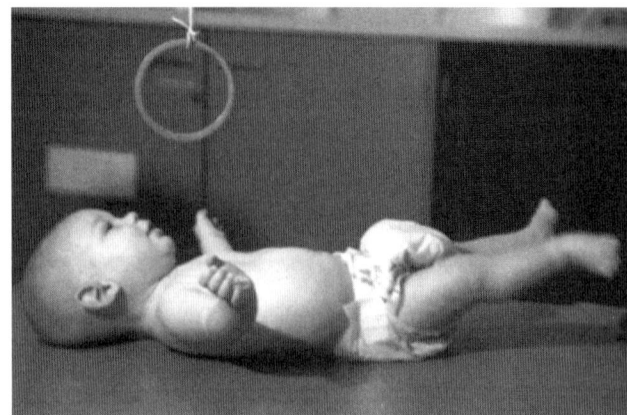

Fig. 9.30 Healthy preterm infant at 4 months of corrected age demonstrating neck hyperextension, scapular adduction and shoulder retraction, and limited antigravity movement into flexion.

Reaching

Most premature infants are immature in reaching skills, reducing their ability to interact with the environment (Fig. 9.30). Activities to counteract shoulder retraction will promote reaching, but the infants should also be provided with other opportunities to practice this skill. Infants who are ready to initiate reaching at 3 to 4 months of age often have only a visually stimulating mobile suspended beyond their reach in the crib. Caregivers are advised to hang toys *within the child's reach* in the crib, playpen, infant seat, or other suitable places. Objects that are suspended, rather than handed to or placed in front of the infant, are preferred to promote the development of directed reach and grasp as well as shoulder stability (Fig. 9.31). Commercially available, relatively inexpensive activity gyms that stand upright on the floor are highly recommended for infants at neurodevelopmental risk.

Head Centering and Symmetrical Orientation

Midline positioning of the head with symmetrical alignment of the trunk and extremities is encouraged to counteract the residual effects of asymmetrical positioning in utero or during hospitalization. Midline orientation will reduce the influence of the ATNR and

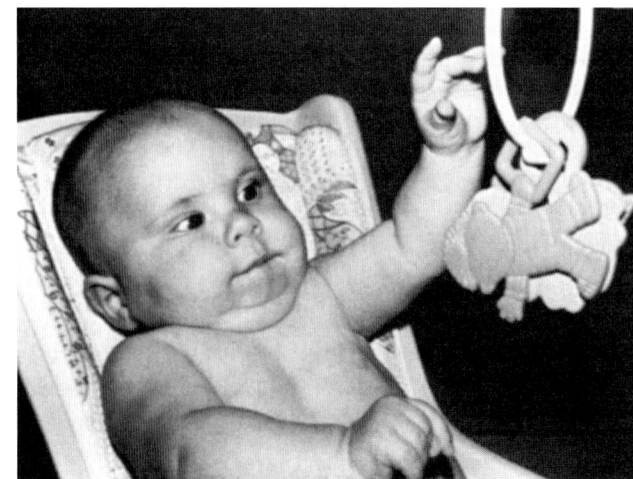

Fig. 9.31 Toys suspended directly in front of infant to encourage symmetrical reaching and midline orientation of head.

promote symmetrical function of the right and left sides of the body. Asymmetry that is not caused by neurological dysfunction tends to resolve when positioning and environmental influences are modified.

Prone Positioning

Active playtime in the prone position with weight bearing on the arms is beneficial for the development of neck and trunk postural and shoulder girdle stability. The prone position also counteracts extension posturing tendencies because the influence of the tonic labyrinthine reflex in the prone position contributes to extremity flexion; however, parents of vulnerable premature infants are often hesitant to place their infants in the prone position for play. Many preterm infants demonstrate a low tolerance for prone positioning, particularly if they have relatively large heads and are visually attentive. Duration of the prone play position can be gradually increased. Visually stimulating objects, including mirrors, musical toys, and the faces of siblings or caregivers, can be arranged in front of the infant to encourage acceptance of the prone position. A roll or wedge positioned under the infant's axillae and upper chest will facilitate the ability to push up in prone, particularly for the infant with low muscle tone. An infant who is apprehensive or stressed when placed on the stomach may tolerate prone lying on the caregiver's chest, where reassuring eye contact can be maintained.

Head Balance

Balance activities to develop active head control are frequently recommended for preterm infants. Tilting responses are usually achieved most effectively with the infant in the parent's lap. Instruction to the caregivers often includes demonstration and practice using a doll before attempts with the infant. Emphasis is placed on the importance of (1) adequate trunk support; (2) movement through small ranges; (3) slow, graded motion; (4) desired head-righting response; and (5) sensitivity to indications of stress or fatigue.

Limited Use of Infant Jumper or Baby Walker

For infants with increased lower-extremity tone or a tendency for toe-standing, the use of baby walkers and jumpers is discouraged because of potential increased stiffness and extension posturing of the legs.[283] Mobile baby walkers are associated with a high risk of injury, including serious trauma such as burns, drowning, and severe head injuries resulting from falls down stairs[284-286]; however, baby walkers are usually enjoyable for infants and may provide caregivers with some needed moments of respite in stressed households. When recommending that time in a baby walker or jumper be restricted, the therapist should help the caregivers find alternative methods of positioning and amusement for the infant. Parents are often reluctant to discard a baby walker, believing that it promotes early ambulation and is beneficial for infants. Informing caregivers of the hazards of infant walkers and research findings indicating walker use may delay the acquisition of gross and fine motor skills enhances the likelihood of their cooperation to eliminate walkers and jumpers.[287,288] The lower-extremity tone and movement effects of semisitting activity centers that allow supported standing and some lateral steps have not been documented.

█ SUMMARY

This chapter on the NICU management and follow-up of at-risk neonates and infants has presented three theoretical models for NICU practice, reviewed neonatal neuropathological conditions related to movement disorders, and described expanded professional services for at-risk neonates and infants in the subspecialty of neonatal therapy. Pediatric therapists participating in intensive care nursery and follow-up teams in the care of high-risk neonates and their parents are involved in an advanced-level practice area that requires heightened responsibility for accountability and for precepted clinical training (beyond general pediatric specialization) in neonatology and infant therapy techniques. Practice guidelines for the NICU from national task forces representing the American Physical Therapy Association, American Occupational Therapy Association, and American Speech-Language, Hearing Association delineated subspecialist roles, proficiencies, and knowledge for neonatal therapy. All three professional organizations concur that the NICU is a restricted and inappropriate practice area for therapy assistants, aides, entry-level students on affiliation, and new graduates.

Inherent to this subspecialty practice is the challenge to design comprehensive neonatal therapy protocols and clinical paths that include standardized examination instruments, comprehensive risk-management plans, long-term follow-up strategies, and systematic documentation of outcome. Ongoing analyses of the physiological risk–therapeutic benefit relationship of neuromotor and neurobehavioral treatment for chronically ill and preterm infants must guide the NICU intervention process. The quality of collaboration between therapists and neonatal nurses largely determines the success of neonatal therapy implementation in the 24-hour care environment of the nursery.

Pediatric therapists working in neonatal units are encouraged to participate in follow-up clinics for NICU graduates to identify and analyze the development of movement dysfunction and behavioral sequelae that may, in the future, be minimized or prevented with creative neonatal treatment approaches. The important preventive aspect of neonatal treatment must be guided by careful analyses of neurodevelopmental and functional outcomes in the first year of life and by the priorities and values of the family.

CASE STUDY 9.1   High-Risk Infant A

Infant A was born prematurely at 29 weeks of gestation with a birth weight of 940 grams. Her neonatal course was complicated by idiopathic respiratory distress syndrome, which was treated with surfactant.

She was first evaluated in the high-risk infant follow-up clinic at 4 months' corrected age (6 months' chronological age). Her mother stated that the infant had several respiratory illnesses after discharge from the NICU. She reported that her infant felt "tense" compared with her older child born at term and seemed to be "a little behind" in overall development. Performance on the Bayley Scales of Infant Development II (BSID-II) generated a Mental Development Index (MDI) of 94 and a Psychomotor Development Index (PDI) of 82. On the Movement Assessment of Infants (MAI) she demonstrated mildly increased lower-extremity muscle tone evident in mild resistance to passive range of motion of her hips and ankles. Persistent primitive reflexes, including the Asymmetric Tonic Neck Reflex (ATNR), Moro reflex, and tonic labyrinthine reflex influence, were present in the supine position. Head balance was immature, but emerging righting reactions were noted. When the infant was observed in the supine position, her posture was extended, but she was beginning to bring her hands to midline. In prone, she had started to push up on elbows, but posture was immature and unstable. Her parents were given recommendations for handling to include holding and carrying positions with shoulders forward to inhibit retraction, frequent play in the prone position, and increased opportunities for reaching in the supine position.

When the infant returned at 8 months' corrected age, her mother reported that progress had been made in the areas of rolling, talking, and sitting. She indicated that the body "stiffness" was less evident, but the infant still did not like to play on her "tummy" and instead preferred to use the baby walker. BSID-II scores at this time were MDI of 101 and PDI of 81. Increased muscle tone observed previously was less evident, and she had full hip mobility but some resistance to passive ankle movement. Muscle tone of the trunk was mildly hypotonic, but age-appropriate antigravity movements were demonstrated in all positions. Primitive reflexes were no longer evident except for the positive

support reflex, characterized by toe-standing tendency during weight bearing. Balance reactions were present but immature in some areas, including head righting into flexion and protective extension reactions. In volitional skills, the infant was now sitting independently for up to 30 seconds, could roll from supine to prone, and could pivot sideways in the prone position. She could pick up a block with either hand and transfer objects. Immaturity was observed in sitting balance, inability to move out of sitting, and failure to move forward on the floor (i.e., low two-point crawl). She attempted to pick up a pellet but was unable to do so. Her parents were advised to discontinue using the baby walker and to maximize playtime on the floor. The infant reportedly enjoyed watching her 4-year-old sibling, so the therapist recommended that he play on the floor beside her. Her mother was also advised to provide the infant with tiny bits of food (e.g., Cheerios) to practice fine motor dexterity.

When seen at 12 months' corrected age, the infant had an MDI of 108 and a PDI of 88. Although not yet walking independently, she was cruising with good weight shift and balance. She was able to creep reciprocally on hands and knees and pulled to stand. She picked up a pellet with an inferior pincer grasp. No deviations of muscle tone or reflex development were observed during examination by the developmental pediatrician. The infant was developing normally and will return for follow-up at 2 years of age. Her parents were advised to call if she was not walking within 2 months or if they had any concerns regarding her pattern of independent walking.

In the management of this child who demonstrated abnormal signs, the primary responsibilities of the pediatric therapist were ongoing assessment and parental guidance and teaching. Although initial concerns about this infant's muscle tone and reflex deviations were present, diagnosing her with a particular condition would have been inappropriate. When followed up over time, the abnormalities resolved and proved to be transient. This child should continue to be followed up in the high-risk infant clinic because she remains at risk for other neurodevelopmental problems that may not become evident until school age.

CASE STUDY 9.2   High-Risk Infant B

Infant B was born prematurely at 29 weeks of gestation with a birth weight of 1200 grams. The neonatal course was complicated by idiopathic respiratory distress syndrome and persistent apnea and bradycardia. Cranial ultrasonography revealed a left subependymal hemorrhage with ventriculomegaly and left-sided periventricular leukomalacia.

She was first seen in the high-risk infant follow-up clinic at 4 months' corrected age (6 months and 17 days' chronological age). The parents stated they had no specific concerns regarding their daughter's development. On the BSID-II the infant received an MDI of 96 and a PDI of 87. On the MAI, muscle tone was normal at rest but increased when she was active or agitated. Tone in the lower extremities was mildly increased with restricted passive movement in the hip adductor and gastrosoleus muscles bilaterally. In the supine position she was frequently in an extended posture and brought her hands to midline only once during the examination. In the prone position she was able to push up and elevate her head while kicking actively. In the prone suspended position, she showed good postural elevation, but movements were stiff. Persistent primitive reflexes included the tonic labyrinthine reflex in supine, ATNR, neonatal positive support reflex, and bilateral ankle clonus. Plantar grasp with toe curling was observed on the right. Righting and equilibrium reactions were emerging. She showed a mature Landau reflex with full extension in prone suspension, which is atypical for her age. In volitional movement, mild asymmetry was evident because she had difficulty bringing her right arm forward when prone and brought her left arm to midline more frequently. Her kicking pattern when supine was low (close to the surface), and she did not elevate her hips. On the right side, hip extension was

accompanied by knee extension and plantarflexion of the ankle. She was not yet reaching for objects, and her hands were frequently fisted, particularly on the right. Her parents were assisted with handling skills to reduce shoulder retraction and extension posturing and to facilitate symmetry in movements and posture.

When the family returned for a follow-up visit at 6 months, they reported that their daughter was making good progress, but she continued to prefer use of her left hand in spite of their efforts to encourage using the right hand. At this evaluation, Bayley Scale scores were an MDI of 94 and a PDI of 83. The infant had made the following developmental progress: (1) rolling from supine to prone (over the right side only); (2) beginning sitting balance; and (3) reaching and grasping objects. She showed a preference for, and greater skill and dexterity with, the left hand. Occasional fisting was still observed on the right hand. She transferred objects only from right to left. Muscle tone continued to be increased in the lower extremities, with restricted passive mobility of the gastrosoleus muscles bilaterally. Toe clawing was observed on the right with minimal spontaneous dorsiflexion observed on this side. Primitive reflexes were integrated except for persistent neonatal positive support and ATNR to the right. Automatic reactions were improved, but balance responses were asymmetrical, with equilibrium reactions and protective extension reactions delayed on the right. Although the developmental progress was encouraging, the persistent asymmetry remained a major concern. The infant was referred to a developmental intervention program with the recommendation that she receive consistent pediatric therapy in her home at least once a week.

The infant was seen in the follow-up clinic at 12 months' corrected age (14 months' chronological age). On the BSID the MDI was 95 and the PDI

CASE STUDY 9.2   *High-Risk Infant B—cont'd*

was 82. She now was creeping reciprocally on hands and knees. When she pulled to stand, she consistently brought the left foot up first. She cruised holding onto furniture with a tendency to stand on her toes on the right. She picked up cubes with either hand but showed partial palmar grasp on the right. She picked up a pellet with an inferior pincer grasp on the left but scooped it into the palm of the right hand. Muscle tone continued to be mildly increased in the lower extremities with Achilles tendon tightness, particularly on the right. She sat independently with a mildly flexed thoracic spine. When moving into and out of sitting, she lacked full trunk rotation, and weight was predominately over the left hip. Language development was considered appropriate for her age. The infant was diagnosed with mild right hemiplegic cerebral palsy. It was recommended that she continue in

the intervention therapy program and return for reevaluation at 2 years of age.

In the management of this child, the role of the pediatric therapist was assessment of neurodevelopmental status and referral to therapy when it became evident that the abnormalities of muscle tone were persisting and interfering with developmental progress. Of note, this child's MDI scores were in the normal range at both the 4- and 8-month examinations. Because the BSID-II does not require infants to perform tasks with both hands, a normal score can be obtained by using just one side of the body. This child should continue to be followed in the high-risk infant clinic after 2 years of age to provide periodic reassessment and guidance to the family as they confront questions of school placement and program planning for their child.

ACKNOWLEDGMENT

We appreciate significant contributions to the case studies by Marcia Williams, PT, MPH, PhD.

REFERENCES

To enhance this text and add value for the reader, all references are included on the companion Evolve site that accompanies this textbook. This online service will, when available, provide a link for the reader to a Medline abstract for the article cited. There are 288 cited references and other general references for this chapter, with the majority of those articles being evidence-based citations.

10

Management of Clinical Problems of Children With Cerebral Palsy*

Claudia R. Senesac and Rachel McAhren

OBJECTIVES

After reading this chapter the student or therapist will be able to:

1. Identify the parameters of the diagnosis of cerebral palsy including motor, family, and psychosocial components.
2. Analyze the multifaceted aspects of the clinical problem and appreciate a multifaceted approach to evaluation and treatment.
3. Analyze treatment strategies and their application to clinical problems.

4. Identify and critique current research for the pediatric patient with cerebral palsy.
5. Identify the therapist's role in the treatment of the child with cerebral palsy, with family involvement, in different settings, and with other health professionals.

KEY TERMS

cerebral palsy
direct intervention
family
indirect intervention

postural and movement compensation
research
spasticity
treatment strategies

OVERVIEW

Perspective

Cerebral palsy (CP) is a misnomer at best. Little[1] suggested the name in the mid-1800s, but there is still no established direct relationship between the identifiable state of the brain and the distortions in posture and movement control that we are able to observe in the individual.[2,3] The condition is not always evident at birth, although the work of Prechtl[4] statistically supports the possibility of a link between the quality of spontaneous movements in the first months of life and later difficulties in coordinated movement expression. Recently in a systematic review of spontaneous infant movement as a predictor of later CP, 47 studies were scrutinized. The authors found that Prechtl's General Movement Assessment had the strongest sensitivity for predictive validity for a later diagnosis of CP.[5] They caution practitioners in the use of this tool in isolation due to a high level of false positive results. In only a small number of children has a specific lesion been identified that corresponds to the observed motor responses of the child, and this elite group includes children with porencephaly and other early developmental malformations of the brain. Whether there is a biochemical element in the brain of a child that distorts the actual motor learning process has not been established. There is a shocking variability in the age at which intervention is initiated for individual children with CP. The continuation of a "wait and see" philosophy in many cases postpones the delivery of services and resultant early intervention. Programs that provide early screening for infants under the Individuals with Disabilities Educational Act (IDEA) utilize a team

of professionals trained in early childhood and typical development to identify children at risk.[6,7] These programs vary from state to state but through Federal and State funding provide services for children 0 to 3 years of age for early intervention. Understanding the process of movement and postural distortion that characterizes children who carry the label of "cerebral palsy" is a critical piece in the delivery of services to this population.

Historically, the evolution of diagnosis and treatment intervention or management is clear and relates to the recognition of the special needs of this minority of society. The British physician, Little, identified the condition on the basis of observable characteristics of movement and posture, or—in other words—the external features of the condition, so the initial efforts at remediation fell to physiatrists and orthopedists such as Deaver and Phelps.[1-3, 8,9] In an article by Kottke and Knapp in 1988 physiatrist Dr. George Deaver was considered the "Grandfather" of physical medicine and rehabilitation, treating individuals with cerebral palsy when others would not consider it. Deaver placed importance on external bracing that was periodically reduced in the hope that the child would take over control of increasing parts of his or her own body.[8] Phelps, an orthopedist, used bracing and surgery and was a significant force in obtaining schooling for these children in the United States.[10,11] He pointed out that these children did not belong in academic classes with children diagnosed as retarded or mentally handicapped, and that children with CP should be exposed to a traditional academic curriculum. In his Children's Rehabilitation Institute in Reisterstown, Maryland, he also advocated restriction of a more functional limb to encourage the use of the one less used, particularly in work with the upper extremities, which was an early introduction of constraint-induced movement therapy (CIMT) known to us today.

---

*Videos for this chapter are available at studentconsult.com.

In the 1950s and 1960s new theories simultaneously emerged of neuromotor behavior that redefined the clinical characteristics of CP and permitted clinicians to orient their intervention strategies to the principles of motor development and motor learning. Kabat, in conjunction with Knott, introduced proprioceptive neuromuscular facilitation (PNF), which was applied to children with movement disorders and to adults with a history of trauma. In 1952 Dorthoy Voss joined Kabat and Knott and expanded on the techniques.[12] The use of diagonal patterns of movement in this approach changed the customary postures of the child and introduced more functional movement patterns in logical learning sequences. Physical and occupational therapist Margaret Rood added the more specific sensory components of ice and light, quick brushing of the skin surface to guide the desired motor response.[13] She spoke of the need to focus attention on both "heavy work" and "light work" during the early development of movement skills. These terms referred to the central body moving over a limb that has been fixed or bearing weight and extremity movement with central stability. Bobath was working in London at this same time and observed the need to have a dynamic distribution between stability and mobility, after finding that inhibition of the reflexive movements was not sufficient to change the functional outcome of the child with CP.[14] Both Rood and Bobath pointed out that the areas of the child's body that appeared to be spastic changed when the body was placed in a different relationship to gravity. This observation held up for reexamination of the prevailing view of the time, namely, that spasticity existed in a tendon or muscle, a specific structure. CP was identified in the mid-1900s as an incident that occurred shortly before, during, or shortly after the birth of the infant. Early intervention was recommended. This timeline was extended to cover the first 2 years of life, which included early cases of meningitis, encephalitis, drowning accidents, and so forth. These factors are true today; however, multiple causes of CP have been documented.[15–17] A systematic review and meta-analysis on the prevalence of CP in 2013 revealed that infants with a gestational age less than 28 weeks and birth weights of 1000 g to 1499 g were at highest risk for CP.[18]

Interestingly, the overall prevalence of CP was found to be 2.11 per 1000 live births, which has remained consistent despite an increased survival rate and improved neonatal care. The Centers for Disease Control and Prevention report a slightly higher incidence of 1.5 to 4 per 1000 births.[19]

Although early clinicians defined CP as a "disorder of posture and movement control," many of the children also had learning problems and inadequate general brain development affecting cognitive skills, reasoning, and judgment. There was a general agreement on categories according to movement characteristics that included spasticity, athetosis, flaccidity, ataxia, and rigidity. Categorization according to the part of the body affected was added to identify hemiplegia, quadriplegia, diplegia, and even monoplegia (affecting one limb), and triplegia (affecting three limbs). It was noted that some children "appeared" to move from one category to another as their body changed with growth and hormonal expression. Therapists began to be aware that a child with high tone could have varying degrees of low tone and muscle weakness underneath when spasticity was inhibited. Fluctuating tone could be confused with ataxia, and the precise intervention strategy might be elusive.

The birth process is complex at many different levels. Sequential hormonal changes alert both the fetus and the mother that it is time for a separation. The infant moves into position for exiting the uterus through the birth canal while the mother's body prepares to participate in the work (labor) of the expulsion. When all goes smoothly, the head of the infant is molded by the passage through the birth canal, and the fibrous sutures of the cranial plates return to their balanced alignment and functional motion. When the birth process is prolonged for any of many reasons, the physiological timing of these changes is interrupted. In the majority of healthy infants born at term, spontaneous movements seem to assist in the activation of the central body (trunk) and the limbs to permit a typical expression of developmental movement responses after birth. Body movement and respiration are coordinated with the infant's physiological rhythms in this initial adaptation to the world of gravity. With complications of the pregnancy or the birth process, these spontaneous movements that are so easily made by the healthy infant become laborious and sometimes impossible, affecting motor actions, postural mechanisms, and the basic physiological rhythms. CP is a heterogeneous collection of clinical syndromes, not a disease, or pathological, or etiological entity.[15–17,19,20] Little described CP as "a persistent disorder of movement and posture appearing early in life and due to a developmental nonprogressive disorder of the brain."[1–3] Current definitions have reiterated that atypical execution of movement and interference with postural mechanisms are the key characteristics of this nonprogressive disorder affecting the developing brain, with wide-ranging presentations.[15,17,19–21]

CP affects the total development of the child. The primary disorder is of motor execution, but common associated dysfunctions include sensory deficits (hearing or vision); epilepsy; learning disabilities; cognitive deficits; emotional, social, and behavioral problems; and speech and language disorders. The degree of severity varies greatly from mild to moderate to severe, and may be combined with multiple comorbidities.[20–23]

Diagnostic Categorization of the Characteristics of Cerebral Palsy

In general, a diagnosis of CP suggests that the individual has a lesion within in the brain affecting the motor control system with a residual disorder of posture and movement control. Varying degrees of associated components are seen with this disorder that further defines the category that a child may fall into: severity of motor abnormalities, anatomical and magnetic resonance imaging (MRI) findings, extent of associated impairments, and the timing of the neurological injury. Further, the severity and type of CP depend on the extent and damage to associated area(s) in the brain affecting the motor cortex. The labeling process helps to identify the parts of the body that are primarily involved. Diplegia, hemiplegia, and quadriplegia indicate that the lower extremities, one side of the body, or all four extremities, respectively, are affected. This can be misleading to the therapist who is working with infants because these children often change their clinical presentation and their respective disabilities. The disorder is not progressive, but the presentation of involvement of body segments may manifest itself differently with hormonal influences as the child grows and his or her structure and tonal distribution changes against gravity. Structure and function are closely related as the child grows and the body matures.

The clinician must be aware that the categorization of CP is based on descriptions of observable characteristics; thus it is a symptomatic description. The *hypertonus* of spasticity prevents a smooth exchange between mobility and stability of the body and interferes with reciprocal innervation. Constriction of respiratory adaptability occurs with poor trunk control. Incrimination of postural tone occurs with an increase in the speed of even passive movement, and clonus may occur in response to sudden passive movement. Although diagnostic terms reflect the distribution of excessive postural tone, the entire body must be considered to be involved. Spasticity, by nature, involves reduced quantity and quality of movement, which makes its distribution easier to identify. Recruitment of the corticomotor neuron pool is affected in the presence of spasticity, and therefore timing issues result in the poor grading of agonists and antagonists.[24] There is also a risk of reduction in the range of limb movements over time when therapy does not include active adaptation in end ranges and organization of postural transitions.[25] Category (spasticity) has the highest occurrence of cases of CP.[17,19] There are several spastic types of CP that require clarification. Fig. 10.1 Spastic diplegia implies that the lower extremities are more involved than the upper extremities but could manifest with varying degrees of arm and hand function, and often the involvement is asymmetrical.[22,23] Hemiplegia displays involvement of one side of the body and can manifest itself with the arm involved more than the leg or the leg involved as much as or more than the arm.[20,22,23] This group of individuals is at risk of developing seizures as they go through puberty; however, a seizure disorder can occur in any of the types of CP as a comorbidity. Quadriplegia, as the term implies, involves the entire body.[20,22,23]

Dyskinetic syndromes, which include athetosis and dystonic types of CP, are characterized by involuntary movements. This type of CP is a result of damage to the basal ganglia, which is responsible for regulating voluntary movements. This area of the brain also is important in regulating emotions, mood, and behavior in general.[26] The term *dyskinetic* is commonly used with children who lack posture, axial, and trunk coactivation. The excessive peripheral movement of the limbs occurs without central coactivation to stabilize the trunk. Dystonic types of CP are dominated by tension and can result in repetitive, sustained movements, or awkward postures.[26] Movement behavior is slow or fast with little control over the movements and may be associated with pain. Athetosis usually has a hypotonic base or underlying tone with slow writhing movements seen at rest, which get more pronounced with increased movement attempts. The child with athetosis can become floppy or be quite spastic within a moment's notice. Muscle tone can fluctuate in both types of dyskinetic CP from hypotonia to hypertonia, making their movements unpredictable. These changes in tone are spontaneous and often related to varied stimuli, which are often specific to each child including—but not limited to—mood, hormones, and environmental influences. Dyskinetic

syndromes may occur with greater involvement in particular extremities, although the condition most often interferes with postural stability as a whole. When pathological or primitive reflexes are used to accomplish movement, there is difficulty with midline orientation and symmetry.

Tonic neck reflexes are observed in this population with the asymmetrical tonic neck reflex (ATNR) the most common although others may also be present. Dyskinetic distribution of postural tone is changeable in force and velocity, particularly during attempted movement by the individual. Midrange control is limited—if present at all—and frequently end ranges of motion are used to accomplish a motor task.[20,22,23] For these reasons, these children have a reduced risk for contractures over time. However, as with any habitual pattern of movement, muscular and joint tightness may occur. Fine motor skills, discrete movements, and skills that require slow control are difficult for these children. Expressive language also may be affected due to changes in muscle tone distribution influencing every muscle in the body, including those that support respiration and speech.

Hypotonicity is another category of CP, but it may also mask undiagnosed degenerative conditions (see Chapter 10). Recent reports suggest that "pure hypotonia" is not an attribute of CP, and further testing to rule out other causation may be indicated.[19,25] Hypotonia in a young infant also may be a precursor of a dyskinetic syndrome. Often, athetoid movements or spasticity are not noticed until the infant is attempting antigravity postures, although there may be some disorganization of movement patterns apparent to the careful observer. Generalized hypotonia may disguise some specific areas of deep muscle tightness with accompanying local immobility in an effort to gain stability for function. Careful examination will assist the therapist in the interpretation of the child's movement strategies.

True *ataxia* is a cerebellar disorder that is seen more frequently as a sequela of tumor removal (see Chapters 20 and 22) than as a problem occurring from birth. Ataxic syndromes are more commonly found in term infants. This type of CP is a diagnosis of exclusion. In a small

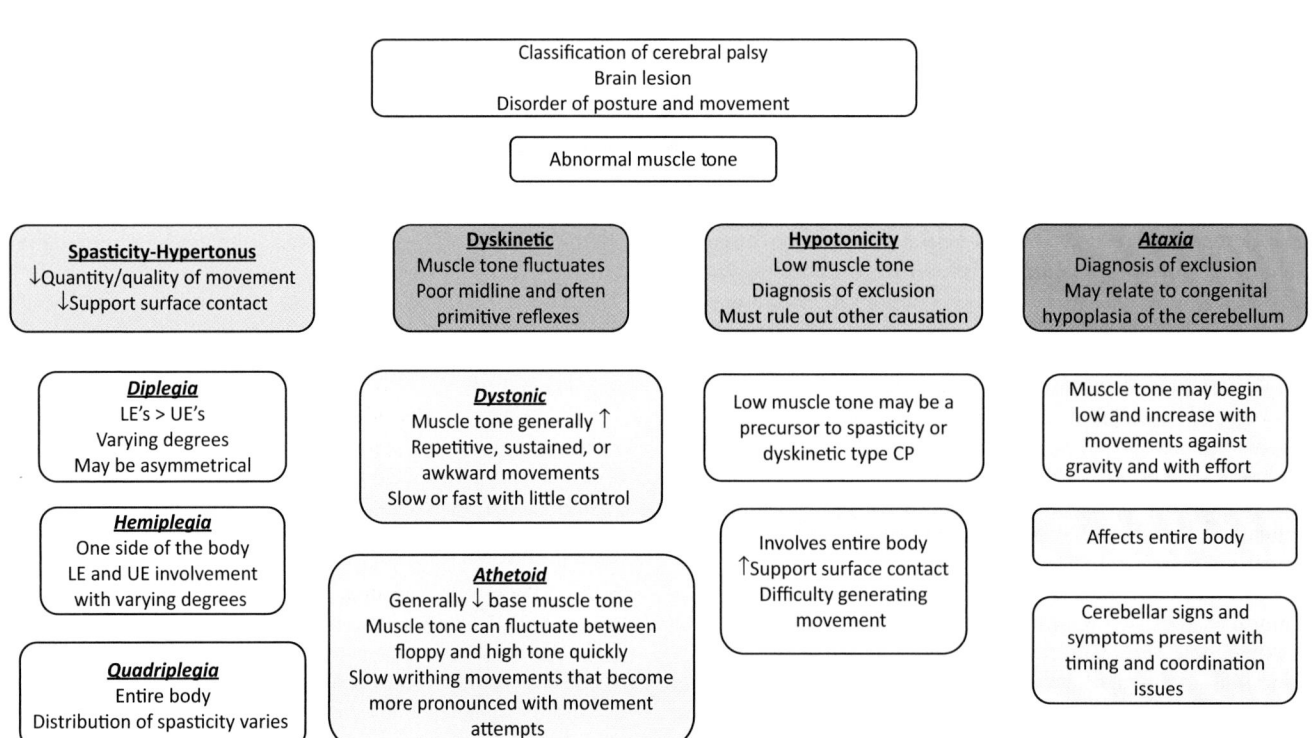

Fig. 10.1 Classification of Cerebral Palsy. *CP,* Cerebral palsy. *LE's,* Lower extremities; *UE's,* upper extremities. (Developed by Claudia Senesac © 2018.)

number of patients there is congenital hypoplasia of the cerebellum. Most of these children are hypotonic at birth and display delays in motor acquisition and language skills.[20] Recruitment and timing issues remain problems in this population. Trajectory of the limbs, speed, distance, power, and precision are frequently documented as problems in this category. Midline is often achieved, but control of midrange movements of the extremities and control of trunk postural reactions are affected. These classifications, even when accurately applied, give the therapist only a *general idea* of the treatment problem and must be supplemented by a specific analysis of posture and movement control during task performance, an interview for home care information, and assessment of treatment responses (see Chapters 6 and 7). The therapist is then ready to establish treatment priorities for the individual child. Refer to Fig. 10.1 for an overview of the classification for types of CP.

Many of the characteristics described in the preceding paragraphs also apply to children who have had closed head traumas or brain infections. Further information can be obtained in Chapters 22 and 26. Some of the treatment suggestions that follow may also be applied in such cases. As with CP, early positioning and handling after trauma may deter later problems.

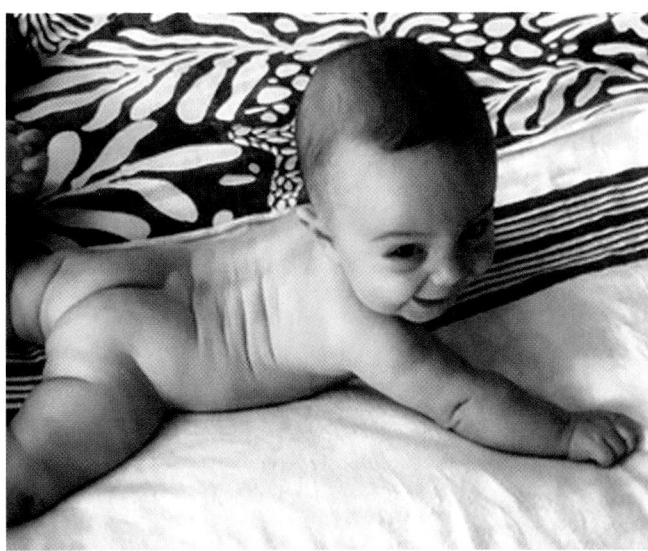

Fig. 10.2 Typical infants accumulate a multitude of experiences as they move smoothly and spontaneously in their environments.

EVALUATIVE ANALYSIS OF THE INDIVIDUAL CHILD

Initial Observations and Assessment

Examination of the individual child begins with careful observation of the interaction between parents and the child, including parental handling of the child that occurs spontaneously. Some additional insight can be gained about the relationship between parent and child by observing how the child is handled both physically and emotionally. Does the child receive and respond to verbal reassurance from the parent in the therapy situation? Are immediate bribes offered to the child? Does parent eye contact increase the child's confidence in responding? Does family communication convey the idea of negativity in the therapy situation or a difficult experience that will soon come to an end? The family orientation will affect the response of the child while working with the therapist. Making connections with the child and family is a critical component to a successful relationship that forms with ongoing treatment.

The therapist working as part of a team may have the advantage of a social worker or psychologist who will relate to the problems and motivations of the parents. Parental responses toward the disabled child arise from the parents' uncertainty, fear, concern for the future, disappointment, distress, and other typical reactions to this unforeseeable life experience. A period of grief is to be expected as their child is often unable to accomplish the milestones and dreams the parents had envisioned for them. Providing clear information for the family in the form of education and interpretation of medical information will assist parents discover how to help their child move forward in all domains. They may be further assisted by opportunities to interact with well-adjusted parents of older children with a diagnosis of CP. Assisting families to make connections with other families and children in the community provides them a supportive network of people who share similar experiences.

A problem-based approach to the assessment and management of the child with CP includes the family as key members of the team.[27] While observing the child, the experienced therapist will want to periodically elicit from the parents their view of the problem and their goals for their child. By listening carefully, the therapist also will be able to discern the emotional impressions that have surrounded previous experiences with professionals. Sometimes what is not said is more

important than what is verbally offered immediately. Listening carefully and clarifying facts are more important than overwhelming the parents with excessive information and suppositions during early contacts. Observation of the family response to information will keep the therapist on track in developing a positive relationship with parents that deepens over time. The therapist's role is often as interpreter of medical information as parents attempt to make some sense of their child's diagnosis.

The next general step is to observe, in as much detail as possible, the spontaneous movement of the child when separated from the parent (Fig. 10.2). Is the child very passive? How does he or she react to the supporting surface (Fig. 10.3)? Are there atypical patterns of movement to reach a toy? Are clearly typical responses occurring with specific interference by pathological synergies or total patterns of movement? Does the child rely heavily on visual communication? Do the eyes focus on a presented object, or does the postural abnormality increase with an effort to focus the eyes? Does the child lead or follow hand activity? Does an effort to move result only in an increase of postural tone with abnormal distribution? Does respiration adapt to new postural adaptations (Fig. 10.4)? Is the child able to speak as well while standing as while sitting? Fig. 10.5 provides key questions to keep in mind during the assessment.

This type of observation is valuable because movement patterns directly reflect the state of the central nervous system (CNS) and can generally be seen while the parent is still handling the child.[28] Once the child is on the mat or treatment table, outer clothing can be removed to observe interactions of limbs and trunk. Observation of the musculoskeletal system without the restriction of clothing allows the therapist to collect information about the initiation of movement, asymmetries, dynamic joint movement, reflexive behavior, support surface contact, and changes that occur with transitions that are difficult to visualize with clothing left on. Movement responses of the child can gradually be influenced directly by the therapist. Many children associate immediate undressing in a new environment with a doctor's office, and the chance to establish rapport is lost. In some instances, it is preferable to have the parent gently remove some of the child's clothing or even to leave the child dressed during the first

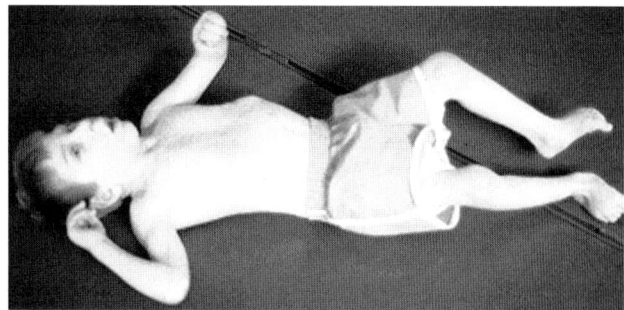

Fig. 10.3 Lack of support surface contact demonstrates difficulty conforming to and activating off of the supporting surface.

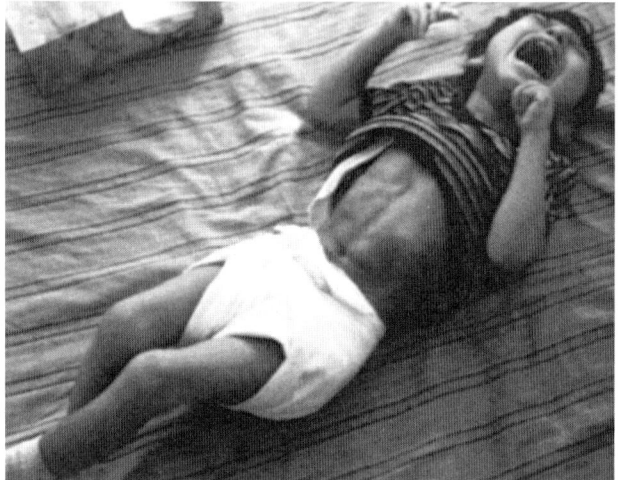

Fig. 10.4 Emotional reactions are also translated into stronger spastic reactions influencing respiratory adaptation.

therapy session. Gaining the trust of the child and parent is crucial during the first few sessions.

The International Classification of Functioning, Disability and Health (ICF)[29,30] is well known in the field of health care and allows one to see the overall interaction of the person with his or her environment, activities, and participation in the presence of the health condition.[29] Fig. 10.6 depicts this health care model with examples of behaviors and information of which the therapist should be cognizant while collecting data for later integration into a treatment plan.

Examination of the child's status is more likely to be adequate if the therapist follows the child's lead when possible. Photos or video recording are beneficial in capturing the interactions and movement patterns of the child; however, parents must be consented prior to using these forms of documentation. Sánchez and colleagues reinforces this idea of video recording as a way to further assess segmental posture of the head and trunk.[31] In addition, the Segmental Assessment of Trunk Control (SATCo) has been found to have excellent reliability and good absolute agreement in children with CP, and offers another objective estimate of sitting trunk control.[32]

Often notes can be organized later to conform to a specific format. It is possible to jot down essential information while observing the child moving spontaneously or while the parent is holding the child. Reactions to the supporting surface will differ in these circumstances. After the session, the therapist will need to record the salient information either electronically, or by hand as part of the evaluation, sending a copy to the primary care physician. Attention should be given to the

typical movements of the child and to those postures that the child spontaneously attempts to control. Building a treatment plan will be based on the strengths of the child noted in these first encounters and will serve as a foundation to build the plan of care (POC). Eye alignment is important; the correspondence between visual and postural activity relates directly to quality of movement control. It is important to note the interaction between the two sides of the body. In noting atypical reactions and compensatory movement patterns, the therapist must also indicate the position of the body with respect to the supporting surface. There is a tendency to compile more pertinent data by learning to cluster observations and relating one to the other. Figs. 10.7 and 10.8 provide examples of how to group data collected during observation and handling of the child. Children are vibrant beings. Their choices of position tell us something about their movement behaviors and how comfortable they are in particular situations. Although it is important to see the child in every position, making smooth transitions from one to another will ensure that the child is secure and give the therapist a more accurate assessment of the child's abilities. Noting the "preferred" position or movement strategy can provide information about the ability to conform to a support surface, the initiation of movement from the surface they are weight bearing on, muscle tightness, muscle tone distribution, and movement variety in the child's repertoire.

Standardized assessments are often used by facilities to document the developmental level of the functioning of a child with disability and to justify treatment. The Gross Motor Function Measure (GMFM) was developed to assess children with CP and has good reliability and validity for children aged 5 months to 16 years.[33–35] This assessment is well studied in the literature and often used to document a baseline and progress, but can also serve to help develop a POC. The Gross Motor Function Classification System (GMFCS), developed in 1997, is often used in conjunction with the GMFM.[36,37] The GMFCS has five levels of classification for gross motor function, emphasizing movement initiation related to sitting, walking, and mode of mobility. Descriptors of motor function span an age range of 2 to 18 years, reflecting environmental and personal factors. Both of these tools have also been used in research studies as a measure to meet inclusion criteria and as outcome measures. The GMFM continues to be investigated for use in different populations and those with visual impairment.[38]

The Pediatric Evaluation and Disability Inventory (PEDI) assesses children aged 6 months to 7.5 years in three domains: social, self-care, and mobility.[39] A computer based version of this instrument, Pediatric Evaluation of Disability Inventory-Computer Adaptive Test (PEDI-CAT), has demonstrated strong construct validity and reliability in children with CP.[40] Both versions of this tool have been used to track outcomes over time. The Functional Independence Measure for Children was developed as a test of disability in children aged 6 months to 12 years. This assessment covers self-care, sphincter control, mobility, locomotion, communication, and social cognition.[36–43] Often the decision to use an instrument to assess development will be left up to the clinician or facility. To date, there is no single tool that will cover all the categories necessary to document change in a child with CP, so the clinician will need to rely on observational skills to describe quality of movement and response to changes in position in space and handling. Each child will differ in the ability to separate from her or his parents. Spontaneity of movement, interest in toys, general activity level, and communication skills will also vary from child to child. Responding to the specific needs of the child enables the therapist to set priorities more effectively. If fatigue is likely to be a factor, it is important first to evaluate those reactions that present themselves spontaneously, followed by direct handling to determine the child's response and

Questions to Guide Therapist-Reminders

Child's name:_____ Caregiver/Parent_____

Date of Birth:_____ Date of Visit_____ Dx_____

1. Does the child make eye contact and interact with caregivers and environment?

2. Does the child adapt to the supporting surface and use the supporting surface contact for movement initiation?

3. Are there *"atypical"* patterns of movement to reach a toy or during movement of any kind?

4. Are *"typical"* responses occurring with specific interference by pathological synergies/reflexive behavior or total patterns of movement?

5. Does the child rely heavily on visual communication? Note the child's ability to communicate.

6. Do the eyes focus on a presented object, or does atypical postural response(s) increase with an effort to focus the eyes?

7. Is the child able to dissociate the eyes from the head and the head from the eyes?

8. Does the child lead or follow hand activity?

9. Does an effort to move result only in an increase of postural tone with abnormal distribution?

10. Does respiration adapt to new postural adaptations?

11. Is the child able to speak while standing as well as sitting?

12. What is the child's response to changes in position?

13. Does the child tolerate transitions of movement when made by the therapist?

14. Does the movement of a limb demonstrate smooth controlled movement without unwanted associated reactions in other parts of the body?

Fig. 10.5 Questions to guide the therapist during the collection of data while assessing the child with cerebral palsy. (Developed by Claudia Senesac © 2018.)

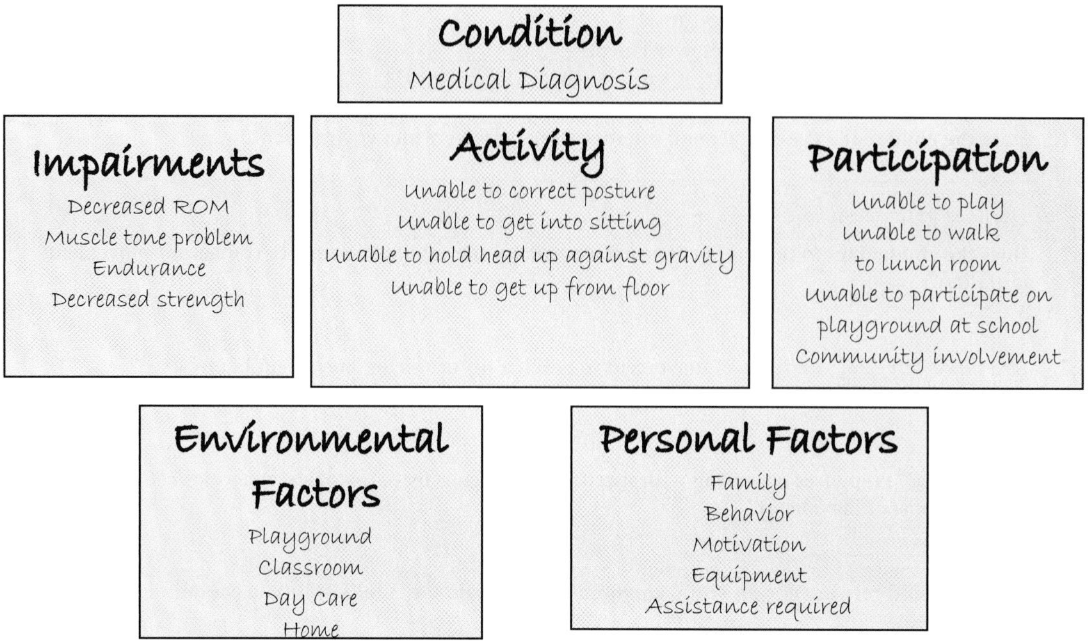

Condition
Medical Diagnosis

Impairments
Decreased ROM
Muscle tone problem
Endurance
Decreased strength

Activity
Unable to correct posture
Unable to get into sitting
Unable to hold head up against gravity
Unable to get up from floor

Participation
Unable to play
Unable to walk
to lunch room
Unable to participate on
playground at school
Community involvement

Environmental Factors
Playground
Classroom
Day Care
Home

Personal Factors
Family
Behavior
Motivation
Equipment
Assistance required

Fig. 10.6 World Health Organization Disablement Model. This table provides all areas of classification in the World Health Organization-International Classification of Functioning, Disability and Health model *(ICF)*. Examples of each category are given as a reference point for collection of data for your assessment. (Adapted from the International Classification Model of Functioning, Disability and Health (ICF) Model–World Health Organization http://www.who.int/classifications/icf/icfbeginnersguide.pdf. Developed by C Senesac ©2018.)

Child's Name: _____   Date: _____   Facility _____

Date of Visit _____   Date of Birth _____   Therapist _____

Position Body Segment Movement Transition	Body Structure Function **Impairments**	Activity **Limitations**	Participation **Restrictions**	**Environmental** Factors	**Personal** Factors

Fig. 10.7 World Health Organizational format for assessment. (Using the WHO terminology to help organize and record data while assessing a patient. Adapted from the International Classification of Functioning, Disability and Health model of the World Health Organization. Developed by Claudia Senesac © 2018.)

Organizational Form by Categories
Assessment Form

Child's name:_____   Date of Visit:_____

Diagnosis:_____   Date of Birth:_____

Category	Response
Standardized Assessments Used	
Specialized Tests/Timed Tests Used	
Skeletal Alignment / ROM	
Muscle Tone	
Primitive Reflexes	
Functional Skills	
Transitional Movements	
Balance	
Muscle Strength	
Family/Participation	
Equipment/Other	
Concerns	
Quality of Movement Postural alignment Patterns of WB Postural stability and control Use and variety of movement patterns Use of compensatory strategies Symmetry versus asymmetry Grading and control of movement Sequencing and planning of motor activities Sensory processing skills	
Other	

Fig. 10.8 Assessment form organized by categories. Organizing and recording data for patient assessment. *WB,* Weight bearing; *ROM,* range of motion. (Developed by Claudia Senesac © 2018.)

potential for more typical movements. Movements or abilities for which there is a major interference from spasticity, primitive reflexive responses, or poor balance reactions (righting, equilibrium, and protective reactions) may be better checked at the termination of the assessment so that the child remains in a cooperative mood as long as possible. Information regarding favorite sleeping positions, self-care independence, and any equipment used at home can be requested as the session comes to a close.

Clinical reasoning involves taking information from the assessment, including observations, results from standardized tools, family input, and the therapist's handling of the child to formulate a treatment plan. Placing this information into a framework that makes sense to the therapist, the physician, other health professionals, and the family will assist in goal writing. Refer to Figs. 10.9 and 10.10 as examples of evaluation formats that are easily incorporated.

Reactions to Placement in a Position

If the child totally avoids certain postures during spontaneous activity, these are likely to be the more important positions for the therapist to evaluate. Observing how the child conforms to the support surface and

Text continued on page 258

Child's Name _____
Date of Visit _____

Facility _____
Therapist _____

Postures - Movement - Compensations - Alignment -	PRONE 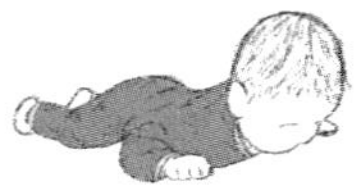 https://babysmilestones.com/first-big-milestone-head-control/	SUPINE 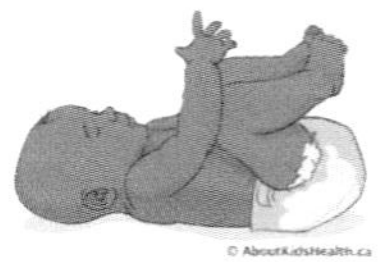 https://www.aboutkidshealth.ca/	SITTING 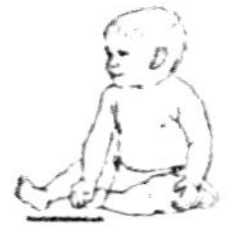 https://clipartxtras.com/download/577eacf80e0766a2a0b3ae28e31e9403e800bc47.html	CRAWLING MOBILITY 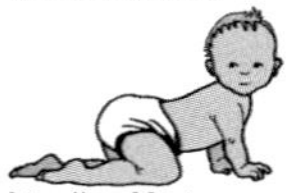 http://worldartsme.com/crawling-babys-cartoons-clipart.html#gal_post_72424_crawling-babys-cartoons-clipart-1.jpg
Initiation of Movement - How Quality				
Body Segments: Head				
Trunk				
Shoulder Girdle				
Pelvis				
UE's				
LE's				
Skeletal Alignment /ROM Muscle Tone				
Primitive Reflexes				
Balance (R,E,PE)				
Muscle Strength				
Other				

Fig. 10.9 Posture Picture Reference evaluation tool for recording and organizing data. *PE*, Physical education; *ACA*, Adjusted chronological age; *CA*, chronological age; *E*, equilibrium reactions; *GM* level, gross motor level; *LE's*, lower extremities; *PE*, protective extension; *R*, righting reactions; *ROM*, range of motion; *UE's*, upper extremities. (Developed by Claudia Senesac © 2018.)

Child's Name _____ Date of Birth _____
Facility _____
Therapist _____

Postures - Movement - Compensations - Alignment -	KNEELING ½ KNEEL http://kip23.narod.ru/vstaem.html	STANDING https://babysmilestones.com/how-can-i-help-baby-learning-to-walk/	WALKING https://babysmilestones.com/how-can-i-help-baby-learning-to-walk/	TRANSITIONS - OBSERVATIONS
Initiation of Movement - How				
Quality				
Body Segments: Head				
Trunk				
Shoulder Girdle				
Pelvis				
UE's				
LE's				
Limitations				
Strengths				
Skeletal Alignment / ROM				
Muscle Tone				
Primitive Reflexes				
Balance (R,E,PE)				
Muscle Strength				
Other				

Fig. 10.9, cont'd

Continued

Child's Name _____   Facility _____
Date of Visit _____   Therapist _____

SUMMARY   CA _____   ACA _____   GM Skill Level _____

Family/Participation	
Equipment/Other	
Concerns	
Recommendations	
Goals	*Short Term* _____ *Long Term* _____
Plan/Frequency	
Additional Comments	

Therapist Signature _____   Date _____

Fig. 10.9, cont'd

Name of Facility
Name of Report i.e. Initial Evaluation/Continuing Stay of Care
From: Therapist   Provider #
        Address   Ph #   Fax #

Patient		DOB:	DOV:
Medicaid #		Dx	ICD 10
Physician		Authorization period	

<u>**Current Functional Status:**</u>

<u>**PMH:**</u>
Other medical conditions:
Medications:
Feeding: **breast fed/formula/finger foods/solids/utensils/cup/**
OM control: **Chewing/tongue lateralization/drooling/teething**

<u>**ROM:**</u>

<u>**Muscle Tone:**</u>   **UE's vs. LE's/proximal vs. distal/ left vs. right/ trunk tone**

<u>**Reflexes:**</u>   **(primitive) appropriate for age/obligatory/non-obligatory**
<u>**Reactions:**</u>   **righting/equilibrium/protective extension**

<u>**Gross Motor Skills/Function:**</u> **GM Skill level_____   CA_____   ACA_____**

<u>**Strength:**</u>

<u>**Fine Motor Skills:**</u>
Speech: expressive/receptive

<u>**Sensation:**</u>   **response to stimulus/hyper vs. hypo**
<u>**Pain:**</u>   **Scale of 1-10/FACES**

<u>**Equipment:**</u>
<u>**Orthotics:**</u>
_____
<u>**Summary of exam:**</u>   **strengths and weaknesses**

<u>**Recommendations/Concerns:**</u>

<u>**Plan of Care:**</u>
        <u>**Goals:**</u>
                STG: (time period)
                LTG: (time period)

<u>**Family Education-HEP:**</u>

<u>**Frequency: therapist will see** *"child"*_____/week/month/other RTC_____</u>

_____   _____
Physician Signature   **DATE**   **Therapist**   **DATE**

By signing as the PCP and/or other authorized provider, I hereby certify that if I am prescribing treatment, I have reviewed each element of the therapy plan of care, that the goals are reasonable and appropriate for this patient, and that if this prescription is for a continuing plan, I have reviewed the patient's progress and adjusted the plan of care goals if necessary.

The prescriber affirms that the services meet the definition of **"medical necessity"** outlined in the Medicaid Therapy Services Coverage and Limitations Handbook.

Fig. 10.10 Evaluation Form Standard Format. *ACA*, Adjusted chronological age; *CA*, chronological age; *DOB*, date of birth; *DOV*, date of visit; *GM*, gross motor; *HEP*, home exercise program; *ICD*, International Classification of Diseases; *LTG*, long-term goal; *OM*, oral motor; *PCP*, primary care physician; *PMH*, past medical history; *RTC*, return to clinic; *STG*, short term goal. (Developed by Claudia Senesac © 2018.)

how much contact there is with the surface will provide information about the ability to initiate movement from the surface. Support surface contact is essential for weight bearing and weight shifting to occur; both are critical for movement. Placement of the child in the previously avoided position will permit the therapist to feel the resistance that prevents successful control by the child.[44] As mentioned previously, this may be held for the end of the assessment. The parent should play an active role in the assessment whenever possible. Continued dialog with the parents reveals factors such as the frequency of a poor sitting alignment at home or a habitual aversion to the prone position. Gathering general information about the child's habits in her or his environment can further enhance the therapists' understanding of how well the child is integrating the visual-motor system, perception, and motor systems; that is, tilting the head when looking at books or watching TV may indicate neck tightness and/or difficulty with functional vision skills.[45] These contributions by the parents establish the importance of good observation and the need for parents and the therapist to work cooperatively as a team. Therapists of different specialties need to initiate continued communication to coordinate therapy objectives. According to the guide for typical development, infants should be able to maintain the posture in which they are placed before they acquire the ability to move into that position alone.[46–47]

The problems presented by CP occur to some extent as a reaction to the field of gravity in which the child moves.[46] Visual perceptions of spatial relationships motivate and determine movement patterns while the child must react at a somatic level to the support surface. It is helpful therefore to attempt placement of the infant or child into developmentally or functionally appropriate postures that are not assumed spontaneously (Fig. 10.11). Resistance to placement indicates an increase in tone, a structural problem, or an inability to adapt to the constellation of sensory inputs for that alignment. A movement that resists control by the therapist will be even less possible for the child. What appears to be a passive posture may hide rapid increases in hypertonicity when movement is initiated or instability of a proximal joint when weight bearing is initiated. A child may have learned to avoid excitation of the unwanted reactions and may fix the body position to avoid the alignment that cannot be controlled. Another child may enjoy the sensory experience of accelerated changes in postural tone and deliberately set them off as a means of receiving the resulting stimulation to his or her system. These movement behaviors provide the therapist with valuable information for treatment planning.

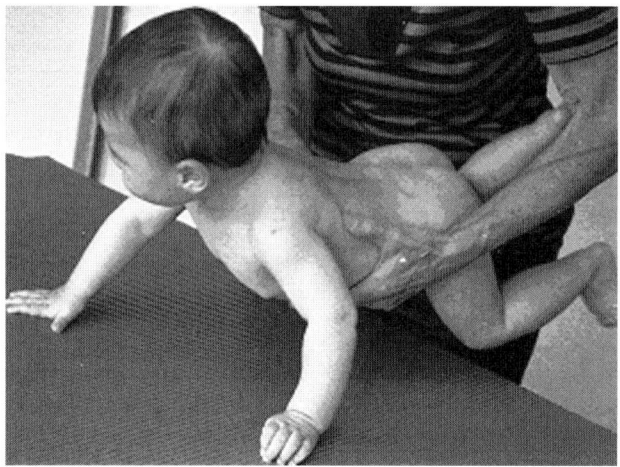

Fig. 10.11 Baby treatment must be dynamic and precisely oriented to individual needs.

VISUAL-MOTOR ASSESSMENT

The visual-motor aspect of performance function is the primary driver of movement in children 0 to 3 years of age. Vision provides motivation, spatial judgment, and orientation to self-body awareness with the external environment needed to control movement of the body in an upright alignment. The child with CP most often demonstrates significant neuromotor delay in the developmental process, which often results in an inadequate establishment of matching of inputs from the postural and visual systems. Visual-motor learning experiences are filled with compensatory responses from both systems. Vision plays an important role in early motor development for learning about, manipulating, and exploring the environment. Therefore vision requires attention during the assessment of motor abilities. (Refer to Chapter 28.)

The visual system in its development has many parallels with the postural system.[48,49] Binocular control and freedom of movement is necessary for the system to function properly. Ambient visual processing must be integrated with central visual processing to take in information that relates to position in space and to focus on a particular target. A simple screening examination may check acuity at 20 feet on the E chart and declare vision to be normal. An ophthalmological examination is needed to determine the health of the eye structures, particularly in the case of infants born preterm. Equally important is a functional vision examination given by a behavioral or developmental optometrist to reveal the level of efficiency that the two eyes have achieved in working together and whether the ability to focus in far and near ranges is well established. Strabismus dysfunctions commonly coexist with CP and may cause the child to receive a double image of environmental objects. Judgments about space are related to a three-dimensional perception of the surrounding environment, which requires coordinated use of the two eyes. Conservative management of eye alignment problems is done with the use of lenses and prisms by the experienced optometrist, which permits the therapist to work for basic head control by the child before compensatory changes are made to the eye muscles. Eye movement differentiates from head movement in much the same way that the hand differentiates from general arm movement, corresponding to general maturation of the central system.

Because the visual system is first a motor system, children with CP most often have difficulty separating eye movement from head movement (referred to as dissociation) and controlled convergence for focal changes. When their posture is supported, eye movement can proceed to evolve in accuracy and complexity. With inadequate alignment of the head in relation to the base of support, the visual system accumulates distortions and inconsistent input, which leads to the formation of an inadequate perceptual base for later motor learning (see Chapters 3 and 28). Even after improvement in the control of posture and movement, the visual system may continue to adapt to the previous faulty visual-motor learning, resulting in perceptual confusion and inefficient organization of body movement in space. The therapist who is working for improved motor control may notice that such a child reacts with adequate postural adaptations when facing the therapist or a support (closed environment—more predictable) and that the movement quality seems to disintegrate when the child faces an open environment or space that is unpredictable.

This immediately jeopardizes the ability of the child to use her or his new responses after leaving the therapy environment. Visual orientation to the environment will dictate alignment against gravity, and the reverse is also true; poor alignment against gravity will affect visual orientation to the environment. An example of this would be the child that is unable to attain and maintain a midline orientation with the head spontaneously. Over time the visual system will adapt to this faulty position and demonstrate great difficulty adjusting to the horizon while the head is in midline. There may be a drive to resort back to a head tilt that is perceived to be the "normal" alignment of the head and neck for visual orientation. Movement, postural stability, and muscle activation are all closely related to vision.[50,51]

By incorporating an understanding of visual observations into intervention strategies, physical and occupational therapists are able to note compensatory adaptations by the complementary systems and to use them to their advantage in effective treatment intervention. Simple interventions may include visual tracking, dissociation of eye movement from the head maintained in midline, dissociation of the head with eyes focused on a fixed target, and visual location of targets in the environment as examples of exercises that could be integrated into a therapy session. The therapist should consider starting these exercises in a gravity eliminated position first to ensure success and then increase the difficult by providing support against gravity. Progressing in difficulty as the child gains success. Understanding the nature of the continuing dynamic interaction between vision, perception, and motor systems and how to incorporate strategies in intervention to address those deficits improves the successful evolution of patients with CP.

POSTURE AND MOVEMENT COMPENSATIONS

Compensatory patterns of movement arise from the motivation of the child to move in spite of various restrictions on the expression of that movement. Components in the developmental process that drive a person to right the head with the horizon and the body upright against gravity are met with interference from the CNS. Visual impressions of the environment motivate movement, and the infant attempts to influence nearby objects or confirm visual impressions by reaching into the environment and touching. As visual awareness enlarges to include more distant targets, the infant is motivated to move toward the object or person seen. With poor balance between flexion and extension and poor grading of agonist with antagonist, the resultant movements are influenced. When the child's body does not respond in a smooth way, the child begins to learn and perfect these uncoordinated attempts. Repetition of inadequate ranges of movement and limited variability of movement patterns begin to establish the atypical appearance of posture in the child with CP.

The characteristics of a body posture or position in space determines the quality of the movement that is expressed. Lack of head control, poor midline organization, and deficient trunk strength begin the process of compensation. From a distorted starting position, the movement initiated is one that is restricted (Fig. 10.12). The lack of "core" stability (trunk control) and the presence of abnormal muscle tone in the body restricts the full available joint range of a limb in attempts to move. This limitation over time is further restricted with developing fascial and muscular stiffness affecting smooth coordinated muscle action. The child continues to learn the atypical responses because the movement patterns tend to be reinforced by repetition as the child accomplishes some movement success during exploration. Compensatory movement patterns evolve out of necessity rather than any feedback as to efficiency or functional smoothness. A child that is motivated to move will do so in any way possible to reach their goal; therefore the development of atypical patterns of movement emerge.

Habitual movement patterns are established on the basis of frequency of use, so the child with CP tends to repeat the atypical responses that have been learned with few variations. In the therapy situation the child has the opportunity to learn new combinations of input to create the basis for more stable postural control. Careful

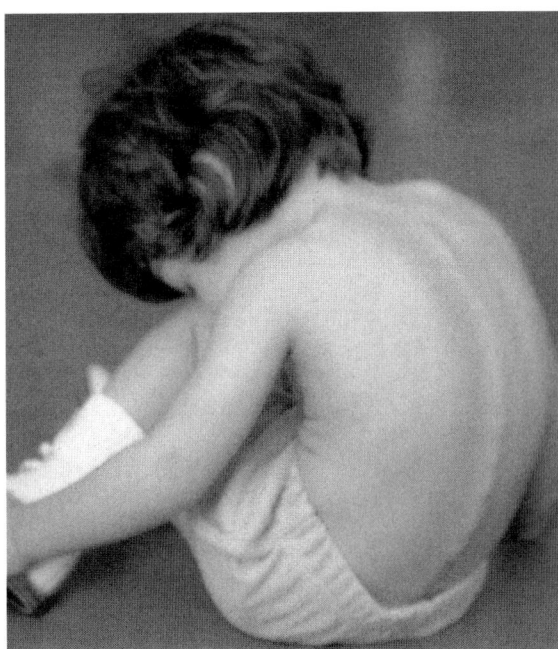
Fig. 10.12 Compensatory postures restrict movement initiation.

analysis of the postural adjustments and movement patterns of the child with CP is crucial to initiate effective intervention strategies.[52] Keep in mind that patterns of movement are additionally influenced by positioning against gravity, head, neck, and trunk position, and the presence of primitive reflexes. Considering the classification of CP and other factors a therapist might be prioritizing when delivering intervention will influence the treatment options that will be most effective. Ultimately, providing more variability and increasing the number of choices a child has for movement also requires repetition for motor learning to occur. The availability of these new movements retrieved from long-term memory to working memory opens up "other" possibilities for the child when enough practice has been provided. There are many factors to be considered in the context of the continuing developmental changes in the child, which makes a simple solution impossible in the treatment of the child with CP. No two children with CP are alike, and each require an individual treatment plan and strategies that are tailored to that child.

Active therapy intervention allows the sensorimotor learning of the child to be modified so that some parts of the compensatory response may become unnecessary and the movement becomes more efficient (Fig. 10.13). This relative approximation of what is expected in a typical response may occur in the area of initiation, timing, strength, or ability to sustain an antigravity alignment. As movement expression and postural stability are better established, the compensatory patterns are used less often, and new movement strategies may begin to be an option for functional tasks. Compensatory processes have their positive aspects.[52] The independence finally achieved by the older child reflects her or his intelligence and motivation, and the family's attitude toward the child and the disability. Developing a positive self-image is a critical part to moving forward and is dependent in part on those that surround and support the child. Compensatory movement patterns may permit greater independence, if and when they do not limit or block the active learning of new motor strategies. Movement is influenced by multiple factors, which include motivation, family, environment, opportunities to practice, comorbidities, muscle stiffness, joint range of motion, medications, and emotional support to mention a few. The therapist will need to keep an open mind and a

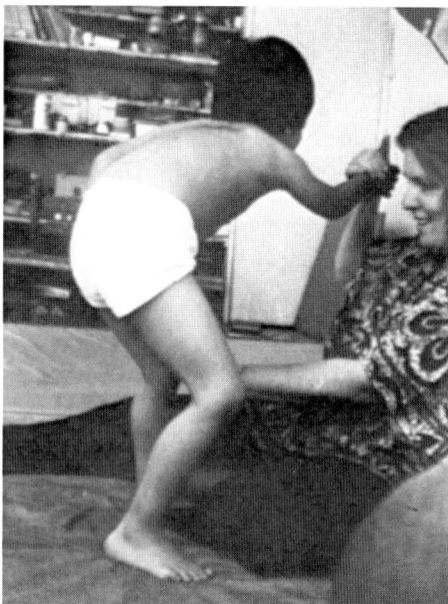

Fig. 10.13 The experience of coming to stand over the more affected side activates diagonal patterns of postural adjustment.

keen awareness of the elements that can affect a child's response to treatment intervention.

OTHER ASSESSMENT CONSIDERATIONS

Nutritional Aspects of Neuromotor Function

Nutrition is viewed as providing an important biochemical base and foundation for enhanced human performance. It is not uncommon for children with CP to have feeding difficulties resulting in poor nutrition. Children with neurodevelopmental problems may present with difficulty managing food and liquids in their mouth, swallowing, and digestive issues. The more severely involved the child the higher the prevalence of feeding issues.[53–55]

Poor nutrition effects energy levels, behavior, and physical and cognitive functioning. In the first 2 years of life patterns for sucking, managing food in the mouth, and control of the related structures (including head control) are developing.[53,56] As the child grows and matures it is critical that they receive the essential nutrients. This can be problematic in someone that has difficulty isolating motor control over large and small muscles throughout their body. Gastroesophageal reflux is also common in infants and older children with developmental problems.[57]

In some infants, reflux decreases or subsides as the muscular stress is reduced in the tissues of the neck, upper thoracic, and cervical region. Furthermore, allergies may also play a role in inadequate caloric intake. To supplement nutritional intake in the child with CP, the individual child must be considered with regard to age, size, activity level, and growth factors.[58,59] The rehabilitative process places increased demands on the entire system and requires fuel to set the stage for improved muscle function.

Protein, carbohydrates, and adequate hydration are sources that build muscle and provide fuel, which provides a foundation for strengthening and the advancement of motor skills in populations without disability.[55,58,60,61] A well-balanced diet will provide the requisite energy for exercise. Little research has been done specifically on children with CP; therefore appropriate levels of protein needed during exercise in this population of children are yet to be determined.

Studies investigating feeding issues in neurodevelopmental disabilities are beginning to emerge in the literature. These studies are exploring assessment tools to better evaluate the problems and potential interventions providing a better understanding for clinicians and families.[58] Therefore it is crucial to discuss these issues with the family using caution in treatment unless specifically trained to do so. A nutritional consultation is warranted when concerns arise in this area.

Consideration of Supplemental Oxygen

Oxygenation of the blood is responsible for the delivery of oxygen to muscle tissue. It is generally accepted that respiratory support increases incrementally to permit faster or stronger movement patterns in a typical individual. Therapists often note that children with CP resist moving into new ranges of movement and that respiratory adaptation does not occur automatically. Supporting the child in the novel posture until a respiratory adaptation is noted results in acceptance of the new experience. Oxygen needs increase in children during growth spurts or when mastering more vertical postural alignments. Increased oxygen is also required for sustained activity such as continuous walking. Incorporating breathing exercises into therapy interventions can help support the child's movement strategies. Children with developmental disabilities have few opportunities to exercise at an intensity level high enough to raise their heart rate. Monitoring oxygen saturation, heart rate, and blood pressure are easily done in a therapy session and can be tracked over time to document progress and to help guide the therapy intervention.

In 2016, Garcia and colleagues performed a careful study of 215 children with CP who were identified by chart review with signs and symptoms of obstructive sleep apnea (OSA) and surveyed with the Pediatric Sleep Questionnaire, for inclusion in the study. They found that children with CP were at a higher risk of OSA with increased severity of their condition, and the risk increased in the presence of seizure activity.[62]

Decreased oxygen levels have been associated with impaired cognitive and physical performance in the literature.[63] In the presence of inadequate peripheral oxygen saturation, low levels of oxygen can be administered during the night. This practice has been used with selected low tone and athetoid children for improved energy during the day during growth changes, but formal study is needed on a larger group of children with CP. Better oxygenation of the tissues can also result in increased nutritional intake and consequently improved energy levels. The therapist should work closely with the primary care physician or pulmonary specialist if there are concerns in this area. It may be suggested that a child have a sleep study to determine oxygen saturation at night while sleeping.

ROLES OF THE THERAPIST

Role of the Therapist in Direct Intervention

The primary role of the therapist is in direct treatment or physical handling of the child in situations that offer opportunities for new motor learning. This should precede and accompany the making of recommendations to parents, teachers, and others handling the child. Positioning for home, general handling, and exercise recommendations should always be tried first by the therapist during a treatment session to ensure that the chosen techniques are successful. As noted for the initial assessment, many interventions will cause a reaction unique to the particular youngster.[23,64] It is the role of the therapist to analyze the nature of the response that is accompanied by adaptation inadequacies, to analyze the movement problems, and to choose the most effective intervention (Fig. 10.14). It will then be possible for other

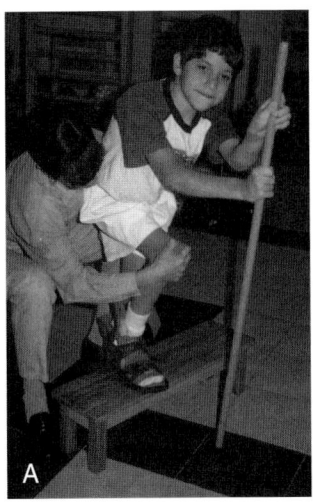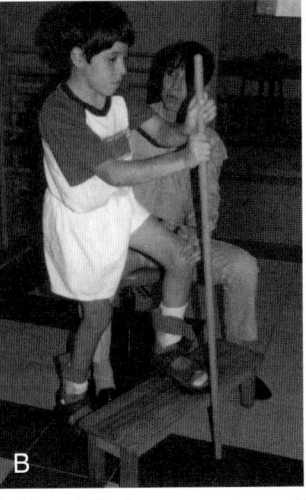

Fig. 10.14 The two sides of the body (**A** and **B**) often respond very differently to the same task, and therapy must be adapted accordingly.

persons to manage play activities and to supervise independent functioning that reinforce treatment goals.

The therapist working with these children becomes an important and trusted resource to the family. At times the therapist who has had the more consistent contact with the child becomes the facilitator of better communication between the parents and medical or health care professionals. The child who starts early and continues with the same therapist may make this person a confidant and share concerns that are difficult or uncomfortable for the child to explain to parents or others. It is a challenge for the therapist who follows the same child for an extended time to come up with appropriate goals and new activities to continue positive change. The therapist should always consider quality of life for each individual in their care. Part of direct intervention is to recognize when the amount of therapy can be reduced and replaced with recreational activities with peers or community involvement. In 2014, Gannotti and colleagues provided a framework for dosing in pediatric rehabilitation for children with CP. This model is strongly based on the ICF model of the World Health Organization and serves as a path to evaluate multiple parameters affecting dosing interventions.[65] This path-based model can serve as a guide for the therapist in decision making related to dosing. There remain many unanswered questions about dosing in children with CP and brain damage. Two papers published in 2014, including Giannotti's study, suggest that a "systematic and in-depth analysis of dosing questions" combined with an "interdisciplinary approach" is critical in advancing research in this area.[65,66]

Case Management and Direct Intervention

Simple documentation of observed changes in a child over a series of regular clinic visits is still too common for many children with CP. Regular appointments, with periodic assignment of a new piece of equipment, do not constitute active treatment. Physical intervention in the form of direct handling of the child is considered a conservative treatment by most physicians. Therapists need to demonstrate their unique preparation and describe their interventions in ordinary language so that families as well as other health care professionals understand the importance of specific treatment versus general programs of early stimulation, which are designed for neurologically intact infants. Demonstrating a clear understanding of the foundational theories that your treatments are based on is essential for justification of your interventions.

The prognosis for change in CP is too often based on records of case management rather than on the effect of direct and dynamic treatment by a well-prepared therapist. Bobath,[67] back in 1965, accurately documented the developmental sequence expected in the presence of spasticity or athetosis. Her book consolidates some observations of older patients that help professionals understand the uninterrupted effects of the CP condition. In any institution, one can observe the tightly adducted and internally rotated legs, the shoulder retraction with flexion of the arms, and the chronic shortening of the neck so commonly seen as the long-term effects of CP. The long-term influence of fluctuating muscle tone results in compensatory stiffness or limited movement patterns to create a semblance of the missing postural stability, while a limited number of movement patterns with limited degrees of freedom are used to function (Fig. 10.15).

Within the clinical community there is increasing evidence that soft tissue restrictions further limit spontaneous movement in children with CP. The fact that these restrictions are often found in infants suggests that they originate early rather than as a gradual result of limited ranges in movement. Because of the tendency of soft tissue to change in response to any physical trauma or strong biochemical change, some of these characteristics might be influenced by the position in utero or originating with traumatic birth experiences, and they could be exacerbated by daily use of limited patterns of movement. Tissue restrictions can also occur with immobilization or general infectious processes.[68] Soft tissue responds to the application of gentle sustained pressure simply from the weight and heat of one's hand with careful consideration by the therapist of techniques used to manipulate the tissue and joints. A therapist must be prepared to defend his or her approach with a solid foundation, theory, and objective outcomes.

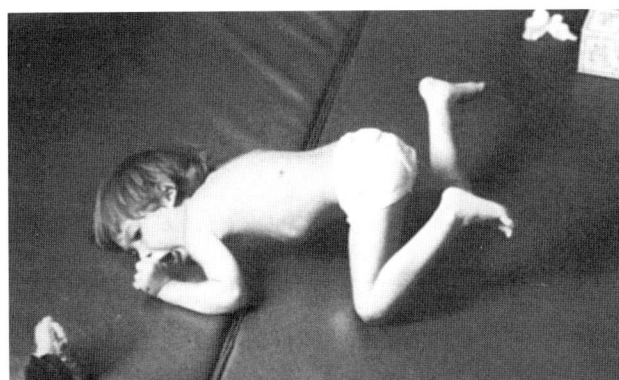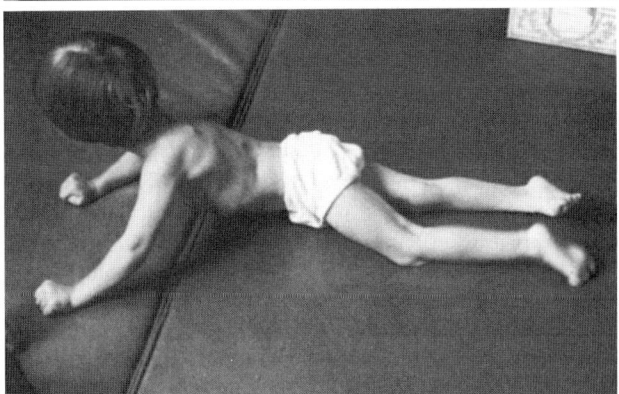

Fig. 10.15 Attempted movement activates atypical patterns and restrictions; restrictions are revealed with limited degrees of freedom available for function.

Objective documentation is important when dealing with any population but is essential for demonstrating therapeutic change.

Applying specific soft tissue treatment techniques to improve mobility and to decrease tonus for any person with a neuromotor disorder creates the need for immediate follow-up with practice of new functional skills using this improved available range of motion. The stretching of muscles in CP has been shown to change muscle tone and to improve range of motion, which can open a window of opportunity to practice functional skills.[69–71] Caution should be exercised to avoid creating excessive tissue mobility in a given area of the body, which can destroy the delicate patterns of coordination that permit synergic function in the person with CP.

Functional activation of the body after each specific mobilization or stretching technique is strongly recommended to integrate the tissue change. Well documented in the literature on current motor control and motor learning is the need to practice, practice, practice.[72] Practice time is related to skill performance; the amount and type of practice are determined by the stage of learning that an individual is in and the type of task to be learned (see Chapter 3 on motor control and learning).[72–76] Interestingly, most of what we know about motor control and motor learning is based on individuals who are "typical," and it is yet to be determined whether the same principles that are considered important in healthy individuals apply to people with disability. However, it makes sense that practice would influence the use of any new or relearned skill.

An occupational therapist, Josephine Moore, emphasized some important points for therapists regarding the concept of increasing functional demands on the central system and the importance of the neck structures in developmental movement sequences. Children with spasticity often have a lack of developmental elongation of the neck, whereas children with athetoid or dystonic movement lack neck stability and consistent postural activation. Tone changes often originate with changes in the delicate postural interrelationship between head/neck and body or with ambient visual processing. An alert therapist will observe these changes and be able to relate them to the initiation of movement and adapt the therapy session to facilitate or inhibit their influence.

Restak,[77] in his book *The New Brain,* confirms the continual reorganization of the brain in response to new input. Several animal and human studies on neuroplasticity have confirmed that the brain reorganizes after an injury and that this reorganization is shaped by rehabilitation and motor skill learning.[78–80]

Our understanding of how the brain works and the mechanisms for neuroplasticity are ever changing. Hartwigsen suggested that having a better understanding of compensatory mechanisms in the brain would increase our understanding of how the brain reorganizes.[81] In 2018, Gaberova and colleagues undertook a systematic review of the literature on task-related functional MRI in children with hemiplegia. The review included sensory, motor, and speech studies. They reported that the sensory system was the most rigid to reorganize and the speech system the most flexible. This appraisal of the literature concluded that reorganization is variable, and dependent on the severity and timing of injury, and the development of each of these individual systems.[82]

In the child with CP, the therapist looks for subtle changes in the child's response to determine newly integrated sensorimotor learning. For example, excessive emphasis on extensor responses in the prone posture for the older child can jeopardize the quality of neck elongation in sitting, so it is essential to work on the components necessary for control of the new posture desired and in reaching for a balance of function versus quality of movement when possible.

Therapy intervention is far from innocuous when it is responsibly applied. A truly eclectic treatment approach comes with clinical experience and personal consideration of observations of the functional problems presented by the complex issue of CP at different ages. Priorities in intervention strategies have a practical aspect, and new developments in our knowledge lead us forward in clinical applications. Continued research and understanding of the intricacies of typical development offer many new clues for new effective interventions. With high-quality treatment intervention, the need for direct therapy service as a crucial aspect of case management for these children is confirmed. Clinical findings in individual case studies need to become part of the professional literature to strengthen the efficacy of intervention in this population.

Special Needs of Infants

The direct treatment of infants deserves special mention because there are significant differences in intervention strategies for the infant and the older child. Aside from the delicate situation of the new parents, the infant is less likely to have a diagnosis and often presents a mixture of typical and atypical characteristics. It is essential that the clinician have a strong foundation in the nuances of typical developmental movement and early postural control.[4,46]

Direct intervention can be offered as a means of enhancing development and overcoming the effects of a difficult or preterm birth. However, it will be important to pursue a diagnosis for the infant who reaches 8 or 9 months of age and continues to need therapy because most third-party payers often require a diagnosis beyond that of developmental delay or prematurity.

Infants with early restrictions in motor control should be followed until they are walking independently, even if they no longer need weekly regular therapy. Infant responses can change rapidly as the therapist organizes the components that contribute to movement control. When present, soft tissue restrictions should be treated initially to have more success with facilitated movement responses. Careful observation is essential because all but the severely involved infant will change considerably between visits. The therapist should invest some time in training the parents to become skilled observers while appreciating the small gains made by their infant and reenforcing the positive changes with the family while remaining realistic and hopeful for the future of their child. It is better to not predict the future motor competency of a child in the early infant stages because the infant will change dramatically over the first year of life. Predictions often limit the therapist in their treatment approach when perceived expectations or limitations are placed on the patient. If one predicts that a child will not stand and walk, the therapist has little impetus to work on those skills. Physiotherapist Mary Quinton,[83] who developed a treatment regime for infants in 2002, wrote specific intervention strategies for babies (Fig. 10.16). In addition, infant massage can be an important adjunct to improve the bonding of mother and child and to improve physiological measures such as abdominal gas, restlessness, and general stiffness.[85,85] Referral to other health care professionals is essential in the presence of possible allergies, new neurological signs, visual or auditory alterations, and persistent reflux or nutritional issues. There is always the possibility of seizures when some brain dysfunction is present, and neurological evaluation should be recommended if this is a concern.

ORIENTATION TO TREATMENT STRATEGIES

The child whose movement is bound within the limitations of hypertonicity suffers first of all from a paucity of movement experience. Because early attempts to move have resulted in the expression of limited typical synergistic postural patterns, the child often experiences the body as heavy or awkward and loses incentive to attempt

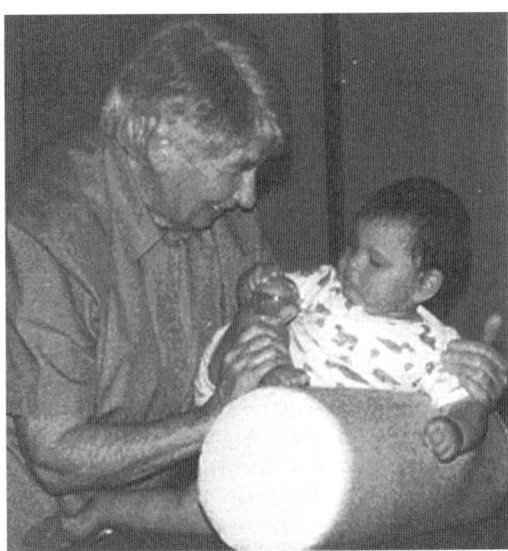

Fig. 10.16 Mary Quinton, British physiotherapist, is widely recognized as the originator of effective infant intervention.

Inhibiting or stopping the movement of one part or even one limb must be done in a way that permits the child to activate the body in a functional way. The child who lies in the supine position with extreme pushing back against the surface is rarely seen when alternative positions, emphasis on head control, and sometimes behavioral management have been implemented early on. The therapist initially may eliminate the supine position entirely but would incorporate into the treatment plan the activation of balanced flexion and extension in sitting with the ability to vary pelvic tilt for functional play and reaching (Fig. 10.17A–C). The child might later be reintroduced to a supine position with postural transitions that support balanced control of the body with more differentiated movement.

One of the primary considerations for the child with spasticity is adequate respiratory support for movement. Mobility of the thoracic cage and the mid-trunk must be combined with trunk rotation during basic postural transitions (Fig. 10.18). Consideration of age-appropriate movement velocity will guide the therapist in choosing activities that challenge better respiratory adaptability and prepare for speech breathing to support vocalization. The therapist will find it helpful to hum or sing or even make silly sounds that encourage sound production by the child during therapy. Movement of the child's body changes respiratory demands and frequently results in spontaneous sound production during therapy. Assessing the ability to sustain a breath to speak is easily done during a therapy session by reciting the letters in the alphabet that can be said with one breath. This should be done with the child supine and in an upright position because trunk control required while sustaining a breath changes with the posture attained against gravity. Consulting with the child's speech and language therapist can provide more ideas for encouraging language and breathing support during therapy sessions. Describing the chest shape and movement of the thorax observed can serve to assist the therapist in problem solving and prioritizing the treatment plan.

movement. The therapist will want to focus on the child's ability to sustain postural control in the trunk in all positions. Central "core" stability to support directed arm movement or weight shifts for stepping may not have developed, so they need to be addressed during therapy intervention. Improved upper extremity control opens the possibility for new learning of more coordinated tasks. Specific work on hand preparation for reach and grasp follows use of the arm for directed movement and often results in improved balance in standing. Any freedom gained in upper body control results in more efficient balance in the upright posture.

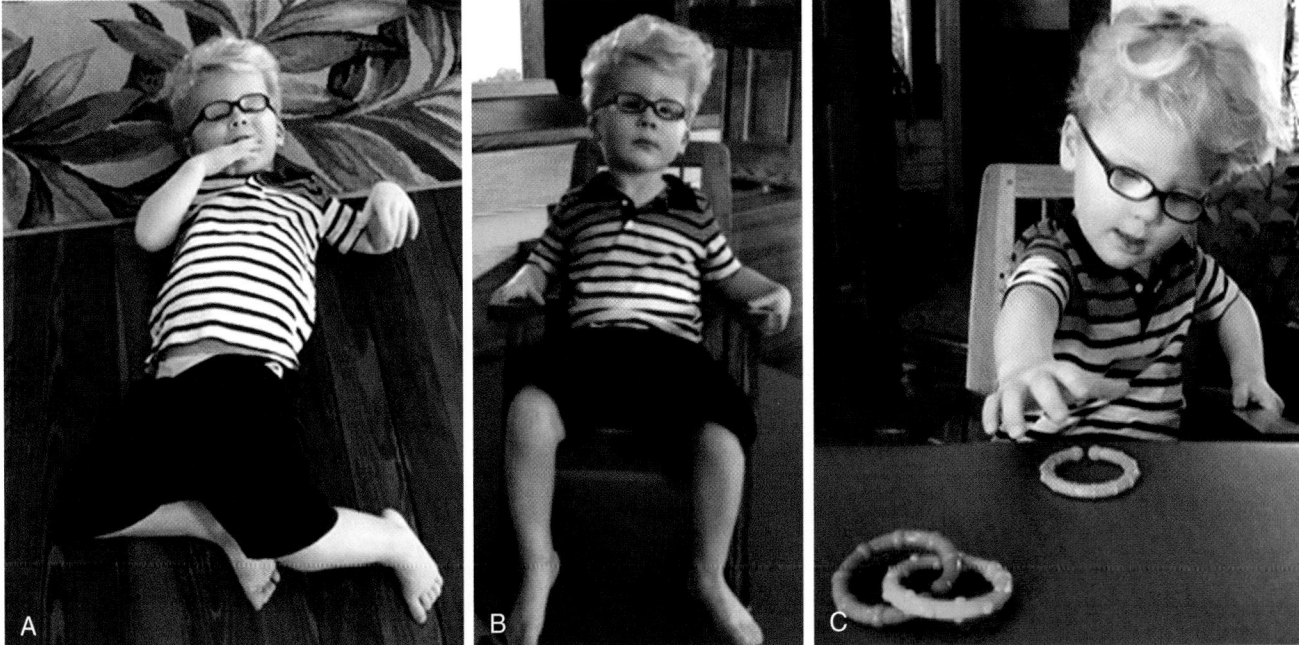

Fig. 10.17 Development of hand use first focuses on bilateral arm activity while keeping the affected hand well within the functional visual field. (A) Asymmetry, atypical tone, and disorganized movements in the supine position. (B) Simple seating can inhibit strong asymmetry and help to organize posture. (C) In a seated position with a work surface in front allows for reaching and play.

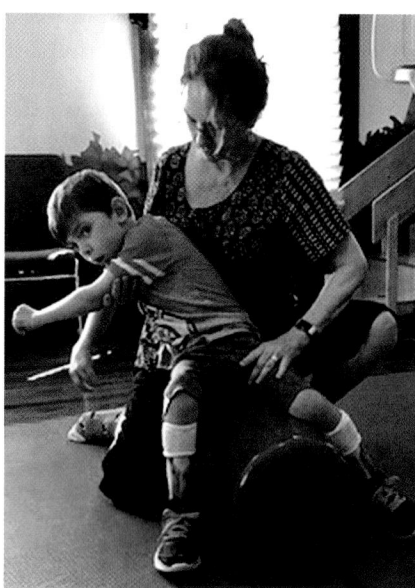

Fig. 10.18 Rotational patterns combined with transitional movements can be used to mobilize the thoracic cage and decrease muscle stiffness.

In some children, respiratory patterns remain immature and superficial, which may be related to the causative factors of the impairment. A lack of postural control limits even the physiological shaping of the rib cage itself because the ribs do not have an opportunity to change their angle at the spine. The therapist must give careful support to sustain the transitional posture of the older child during transient respiratory change. An active respiratory adaptation will increase the variability of postural adaptation. Improved respiratory adaptation will improve trunk muscle tone, just as dynamic trunk alignment facilitates better respiration. Trunk control influences the alignment of the thorax, resulting in the respiratory support and effort a child has to make to sustain adequate oxygenation. These components are closely related. Anytime a child is moved or their position is changed, it is likely to result in respiratory change. Always monitor auditorily (listening carefully to changes in breath sounds), visually, and through palpation as you are treating to pick up the subtle changes that occur.

Weight bearing changes postural tone. The trunk can be helped to experience weight bearing in a variety of alignments by using inflated balls or rolls that offer a contoured surface. The threshold of the original response is gradually altered so that the child begins to learn the new sensations and can follow guided postural transitions. When there are distinct differences between the two sides of the body, attention must be given to lateral weight shifts in sitting and standing. Changes near the vertical midline of the body seem to represent the more difficult input for the compromised system to integrate. It may be necessary to assist sustained weight over one side and then the other to initiate the change. It is important to assist the shoulders to align with the hips and that the visual orientation of the individual brings the head to a correct alignment with regard to the horizon. Young children need special help with segmental rotation of the trunk in the vertical alignment so that the weight-bearing side is relatively forward with dynamic balance of flexion and extension influences (see Fig. 10.13).

Children and adolescents with CP often require a more intense or prolonged sensory cue for a desired movement response to be obtained. Range of movement may require preparation beyond the essential range for the functional goal. In addition, weight bearing against the surface may need to be sustained for a prolonged period of

time in order to facilitate active initiation of movement from the support surface. The therapist is addressing a system that is deficient in its ability to receive, perceive, and use the available input. This makes careful analysis and functional orientation of the sensory input essential. If the microcosm of experience given the child during a therapy session is no more intense than an equal amount of time in her or his living environment, the therapist has failed to use this unique opportunity to deliver a meaningful message to encourage the learning of new motor behavior by striving to improve the child's endurance and tolerance to new movement experiences. During a treatment session, although therapists cannot provide every experience necessary for all movement scenarios, they should provide the component parts necessary for motor skills to be transferred or generalized to other activities in other environments. Recent literature has indicated that the complexity of the task that is practiced and the type of practice may very well enrich generalization. In 2018, Willey and Liu reported that varied practice appeared to influence generalization but not to all conditions, and the transfer effect was not maintained at a 2-week posttest.[86] Wang and Song[87] investigated impaired visuomotor generalization with attentional distraction. This study compared the generalization of two conditions by switching the practice from that of a dual task to a single task. They reported that attention and memory are critical components and should be incorporated into the intervention period to enhance generalization to other untrained tasks regardless of complexity. Kantak and colleagues demonstrated in a small study that training complex activities improved generalization to uncomplicated tasks.[88] Therapists will need to stay abreast of new research in this area to more fully understand the context for motor learning or relearning of new skills.

The therapist working with the child with CP constantly monitors the quality of the child's motor response. These continuing observations guide the manipulation of the environment and the assistance given the child to move toward a functional goal. Is the body tolerating the position? Does the child adapt to the supporting surface and use the supporting surface contact for movement initiation (Fig. 10.19)? Does the movement of a limb demonstrate smooth controlled movement without unwanted associated reactions in other parts of the body? By analyzing the answers to such questions, the therapist is guided to an appropriate sequence of the therapy session and is enabled to set functional treatment goals and to realistically change prognoses.

The therapist makes constant judgments as to the child's responses during therapy, challenging the child's system while ensuring success and moving toward improved control. By using specific intervention strategies, the therapist works to introduce new somatosensory and motor learning. The therapist may introduce a slight modification of the child's response, such as an elongation of a limb as it is being moved. At other times the therapist augments sensory information

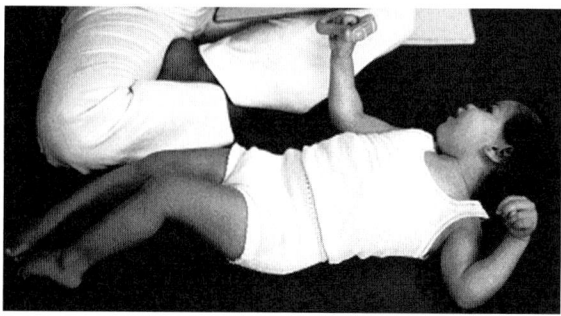

Fig. 10.19 This child has little contact with the supporting surface, resulting in poor movement initiation.

that helps direct a movement. Weight bearing over the feet may be simulated with the young child's foot against the therapist's hand and pressure given through the knee. Visual-motor experiences may be altered with the child's use of prism lenses, prescribed by an optometrist for use during therapy if appropriate.

To be meaningful, sensory input must be contextual and meaningful to the individual who is receiving it. Multiple sensory systems are simultaneously activated by most therapeutic input, and a variety of sights and sounds may be available in the immediate environment. Memory, previous learning, and cognition are activated during the therapy interaction. The therapist makes a continuous reassessment of the child's experiential needs compared with the current input provided. When the therapist works with the child in a more upright alignment during at least part of the session, the CNS is alert and more receptive to the incoming information.

The developmental meaning attached to the sensation of typical movement is complex and starts with the ability to process contrasting stimuli. While several parts of the body are stable, another is moving. Stability of the proximal body permits a limb to extend forcefully or to be maintained in space. Each new level of developmental dissociation of movement increases the complexity of CNS processing. The process of self-feeding illustrates how internal and external stimuli impinge simultaneously on the CNS. The process of guiding a full spoon toward the mouth initially engages the child's attention. The arm is lifted at the shoulder to bring the fragrant food odor to the level of the mouth before elbow flexion takes the spoon to the face (Fig. 10.20). Between 2 and 6 years of age the self-feeding pattern is modified and the elbow moves down beside the body. Now the motor aspect of the task has become procedural and more efficient, permitting the child to participate in social exchanges with the family at the same time that she or he manages independent self-feeding. The complexity of the task increases with the secondary task of social exchange.

A solid understanding of typical developmental sequences is essential for the clinician providing direct treatment intervention.[28,46] Early responses of the typical infant change from a self-orientation to an environmental orientation as new developmental competence emerges. More sophisticated balance in independent sitting occurs

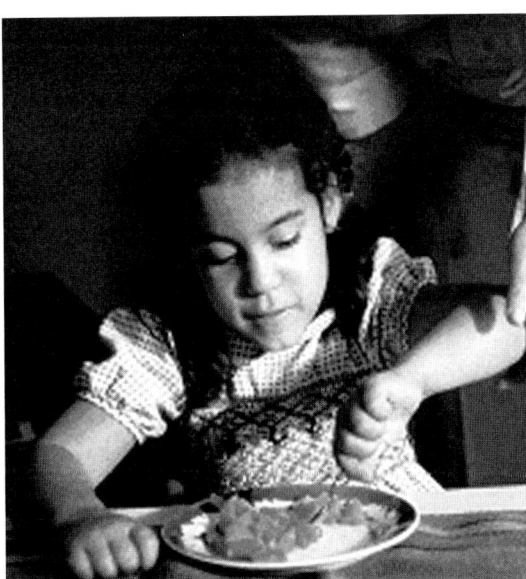

Fig. 10.20 Maintaining the child's elbow in this high position initially permits forearm pronation and activates the shoulder in the typical developmental pattern for improved motor learning.

simultaneously as the ability to pull to standing at a support begins to develop. Such knowledge of developmental details and interplay between developing skills across domains supports the therapist in introducing postural activities at a higher developmental level to integrate more basic abilities. The assisted self-dressing process is an effective way to introduce and integrate new movement and sensorimotor learning while using established movement skills. To sit well, the child needs practice moving over the base of support and coming in and out of sitting, and control of coming to stand from sitting. To walk well, the child may need to practice running to allow practice in changing rate, direction, range, and balance. Sitting is made more dynamic by using a gymnastic ball as a seat. Transitional adaptations of posture may be elaborated during therapy sessions to include more complex alignments. Specific techniques are reviewed in Chapter 8.

With the child dominated by athetoid movement, the therapist's role relates primarily to the organization and grading of seemingly erratic movement responses and establishing function around midline. These children have the ability to balance, but their balance reactions are often extreme in range and velocity often resulting in an ineffective attempt to regain balance. Their movements are rarely in the midline, asymmetrical, and frequently dominated by primitive reflexes, with poor midrange control of the trunk and extremities. Cognitively they are eager to participate and usually are responsive to working on specific goals that relate to functional success. By working to improve central control, the therapist gradually introduces the taking of body weight over the limbs, with assistance, to grade the postural control of the central body. With knowledge of the development of the visual system the therapist can use visual input to improve the child's balance reactions. In these children the therapist may note that disruption of eye alignment or focusing results in a momentary disorganization of postural control (see Chapter 28).

Movement control must become procedural so that it is not interrupted by every environmental distraction. This is more likely to happen when balanced activity of the visual, vestibular, and proprioceptive systems has been achieved. Independent ambulation becomes a spontaneous learned skill when the individual is able to think of something else at the same time or perform a secondary task while ambulating. The therapist begins this process by carrying on a conversation with the child to engage the cognitive attention so that the motor behavior becomes more automatic. The concept of graded stress is discussed in Chapters 4 and 5.

Direct intervention for the hemiplegic child takes into account the obvious difference in postural tone between one side of the body and the other. Treatment for children that addresses itself only to the more affected side of the body will not prove to be effective. The critical therapeutic experience seems to be that of integration of the two sides of the body and the establishment of the midline (see Fig. 10.13). The child with hemiplegia differs from the adult stroke patient in that the adult had a clearly established midline and integration of both sides of the body by learning to cross the midline before the stroke episode. The child with hemiplegia has not had that experience and will need emphasis on this during intervention. The integration of both sides of the body begins early for the typical infant, with lateral weight shifts in a variety of developmental patterns, and leads to postural organization that permits later reaching for a toy while the body weight is supported with the opposite side of the body. The child with a contrast in the sensorimotor function of the two sides of the body needs to experience developmental patterns that include rotation within the longitudinal body axis and lateral flexion of the trunk, with the more affected side forward. The therapist will need to emphasize the experience of supporting the body on the affected side and the experience of initiating movement with this side.

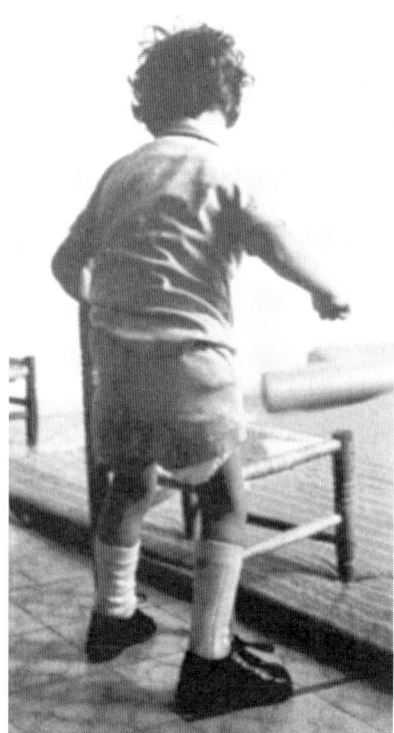

Fig. 10.21 This boy with hemiplegia tries to move a chair by orienting only his more active side to the task and bearing weight only briefly on the more affected side.

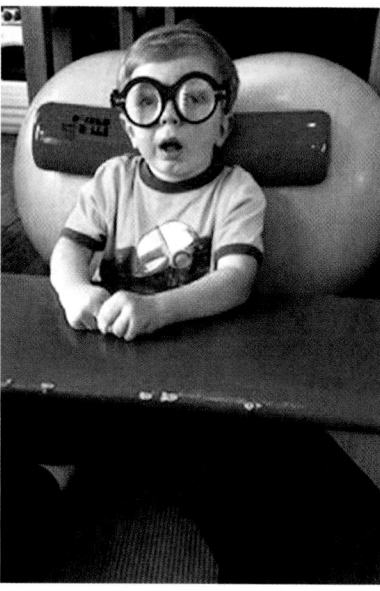

Fig. 10.22 The use of prism lens helps inhibit an upward eye gaze and neck hyperextension in this young boy while maintaining an upright position of his head. He is now ready to interact with toys that might be presented and with his environment.

Development of hand use first focuses on bilateral arm activity while keeping the affected hand well within the functional visual field (Fig. 10.22). The infant or young child works primarily in sitting until dynamic trunk flexion is activated. Pelvic mobility is essential to activate the necessary trunk responses. The therapist may find that dynamic lateral flexion of the more affected side of the body is fully as

difficult for some children as the initial active elongation of that side. There tends to be a high incidence of soft tissue restrictions along the shoulder and neck of the affected side. Children with hemiplegia have difficulty in sustaining a balanced posture against the influence of gravity, and some begin to struggle to do everything with the less affected side (Fig. 10.21). This characteristic contrast in function may contribute to the development of seemingly hyperactive behavior related to the inability of the CNS to resolve contrasting incoming information. Hyperkinetic responses in one side of the body may compensate for relative inactivity in the opposite side. Leg length discrepancy, scoliosis, pelvic obliquity, and shortening between the ribs and pelvis may develop. One goal of treatment is to bring these divergent response levels closer together so that the child can experience more comfortable postural change and can adapt to later school demands. The limbs of the hemiplegic child will change in postural tone as the trunk reactions are brought under active control and lateral weight shifts more clearly to the more affected side. The two hands need the experience of sustaining the body weight simultaneously, as do the two feet. Although the more affected hand may not develop sensation adequate for skilled activity, an important treatment goal is sufficient shoulder mobility to move the arm across the body midline and to assume a relaxed alignment during ambulation. Early treatment increases the possibility that the more affected hand will be used as an assisting or helping hand. There are some children who have such severe sensory loss that active use is minimal, although considerable relaxation can be achieved.

The greater the discrepancy between the sensorimotor experience of one side of the body and the other, the more tendency the system seems to have to reject one of the messages. This can lead to distortions in verticality and is a major interference in bilateral integration. Functional vision evaluation is important to avoid the midline shift problem, which will distort postural control. As body weight is shifted to the more intact side, flexor withdrawal patterns of the limbs increase in frequency and strength in some children. These postural reactions are often associated with lack of full weight bearing on the more affected side. The presence of a lateral visual midline shift or some visual field loss may increase the avoidance of bearing weight on the more affected side. One important therapy goal is the achievement of controlled weight shift through the pelvis during ambulation (Fig. 10.23).

Treatment strategies must incorporate a wide variety of more basic developmental alignments in which pelvic weight shift is a factor. The choice of prone, transitioning from sitting to four-point support, or a simple weight shift while sitting on a bench for reaching will depend on the movement characteristics observed by the therapist during the evaluative session. Diagonal adaptations are useful in the redistribution of tone for upright function. Careful attention must be given to pelvic alignment and mobility because the pelvis has a tendency to be rotated posteriorly on the more affected side in children who have not had adequate early therapy interventions. This can cause increased hip flexion and incomplete hip extension at terminal stance later if the child begins to walk with the more affected side held posteriorly, a characteristic that may be observed during analysis of leg position in gait. Dynamic foot support will facilitate an improved alignment of the base of support and help to facilitate a more functional weight shift when the child is not in the treatment session. The goal of functional movement is best reached through a wide variety of weight-bearing postures, from the obvious developmental alignments to horizontal protective responses, or reaching above the shoulders in sitting and standing to incorporate practical and commonly used adaptations.

The child with low muscle tone is perhaps the greatest challenge for both therapist and parent. Adequate developmental stimulation is difficult unless positioning can be varied. Placing the child in a more

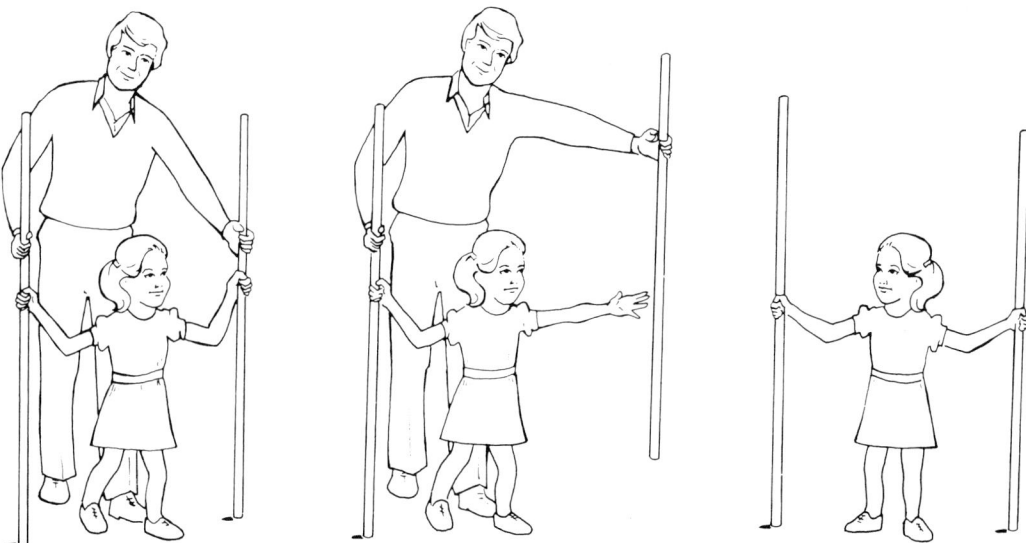

Fig. 10.23 The use of poles was introduced by the Bobaths as a way to achieve graded weight shift for increasingly complex postural adjustments in standing and walking.

upright alignment, although it is achieved with complete support initially, seems to aid the incremental development of postural control. To prepare the low-tone body for function, it is helpful to assess any possible soft tissue restrictions. However, equally important is not to take away muscle tightness that is providing a form of stability for the child without the ability to give him or her another form of stability for functional use. The neck and shoulder girdle are particularly vulnerable when low tone and instability are an issue. Strong proprioceptive input while providing accurate postural alignment is a important part of the treatment session. Strong proprioceptive input, such as axial compression, while accurate postural alignment is ensured as an important part of the treatment session. Gentle traction alternated with approximation as originally described by Bobath in 1975[89] also assists in maintaining antigravity positions and creates postural variance in the practice of antigravity postural reactions. Positioning at home may include a high table that supports the arms, allows for increased trunk extension in good alignment, and permits voluntary horizontal arm motion with the ability to weight bear through the upper extremities. The therapist must be cautious of the tendency of the child to "lock down joints" in the extremities and along the vertebral column for stability in response to trunk instability and initial hypotonicity. This appears as a stiffening response, which can be distributed in the deeper musculature, and contributes to limited adaptability rather than differentiated postural control. It is difficult to ramp up the corticomotor neuron pool even though the child's motor output may remain limited; changes in positioning and opportunities for the child to have other sensory and visual experiences will often serve to motivate the child and contribute to motor learning.

Home handling needs to include a variety of positions during each day for seating and play. Adapting toys and positioning devices will be necessary, and working closely with the family to provide this will afford the child more opportunities to explore visually and motorically. Consistency in these practices is essential for the child with low tone to progress.

The process of undressing and dressing can be a dynamic part of the treatment program for any child and a functional skill that can easily be practiced in a home exercise program. (Fig. 10.24). Diagonal patterns of movement that are incorporated into the removal of socks and shoes assist in the organization of midline orientation. Weight shifts and changes in stability–mobility distribution occur throughout

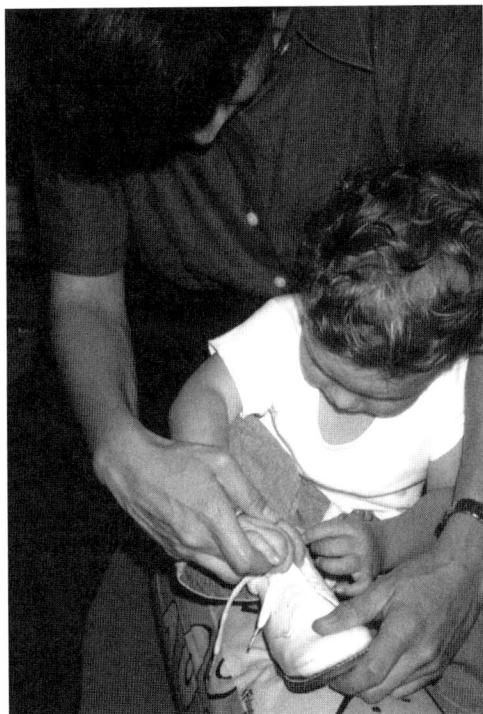

Fig. 10.24 With assistance, this boy with right hemiplegia is helped to improve his self-esteem by exploring dressing.

the dressing process. Concepts of direction and spatial orientation are applied to the relationship of body parts and clothing. Directional vocabulary terms and names of clothing and body parts are learned with this experience. A bench is useful because it permits the adult to sit behind the child who is just beginning to participate actively. The older child with difficult balance reactions can use the bench in a straddle–sit alignment (Fig. 10.25). Aside from the physical and perceptual benefits, this achievement of dressing independently is one that offers the child a feeling of pride and independence. It is also a very practical preparation for the future when it is introduced in keeping with individual developmental and emotional needs (Fig. 10.26).

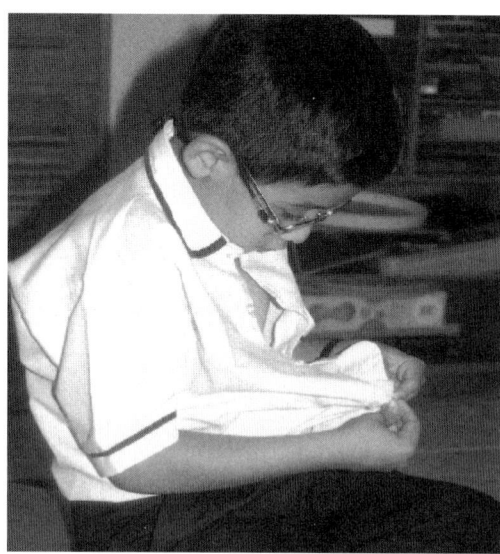

Fig. 10.25 Straddle-sitting on a bench gives this diplegic boy postural stability while he concentrates on the buttoning process.

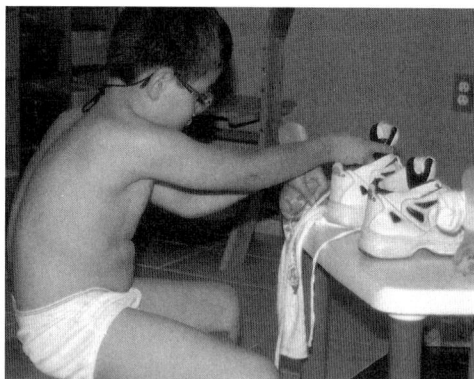

Fig. 10.26 Organization of clothing within reach is essential for success in independent dressing.

Each treatment session regardless of age, severity, or type of CP may begin as a story begins with an introduction analogous to preparation of the body to move. The middle part of the session is the meat of the story providing assistance and facilitation as needed, but challenging the child with new movement experiences. Learning the rules of new movement strategies and making mistakes to form a reference of correctness for future attempts at new skills are all key components in treatment. Near the end of the treatment as in the story, everyone loves a happy ending by performing activities that are achievable and leave the child and family with a feeling of success and a desire to return for more exciting skills. Instruction for a home exercise program is essential to learning new skills. This program should include activities that can easily be incorporated into a daily routine to ensure practice, which is so critical for motor learning.

RESEARCH

Pediatric clinicians are faced with selecting treatments that are efficacious for children with CP. Increasing pressure on clinicians to establish that treatments are effective in improving functional abilities is often dictated by third-party payers. In the past there was little research on pediatric treatment approaches and protocols that withstood the rigors of scientific investigation. Today, several methods that warrant mentioning are undergoing systematic investigation. CIMT

was developed from basic science experiments on deafferented monkeys to overcome learned nonuse of the upper extremity.[90,91] This forced use approach was adapted for adult patients after a stroke; the affected upper extremity is forced to participate in activities and the less involved upper extremity is constrained. Practice is intense, with 6 hours of mass practice for a 2-week period.[92–94] This protocol has been quite successful, with significant improvement in upper extremity movement and use of the affected limb. CIMT is very popular and is now available in some clinical settings in modified dosing. The pediatric patient has also demonstrated a favorable response to this treatment protocol in several single-case studies.

In a clinical randomized trial by Taub and colleagues,[95] children with hemiplegia or brain injury receiving CIMT for 21 consecutive days, 6 hours a day, demonstrated significant improvement in the amount of use, quality of movement, and spontaneous use of the affected upper extremity. These results were sustained at 6-month follow-up. Several studies from around the world are beginning to appear in the literature with varied methods. Most of these studies are promising; however, further investigation is necessary to establish the critical threshold, adequate dosage, and selection process for subjects who will benefit the most.[96–101] Clinicians have been adapting these studies to their therapeutic settings and modify the protocols for clinical use and reimbursement potential as needed. In 2018, Gillick and colleagues investigated combining transcranial direct current stimulation (tDCS) with CIMT in a blinded randomized clinical trial.[102] Twenty participants with a diagnosis of unilateral CP were randomly assigned to a group receiving a sham plus CIMT or tDCS plus CIMT. The results suggested that there were differences between the control group and the experimental group and that tDCS was feasible and safe to use in children.[102] In 2018 Carlson and colleagues investigated the use of MRI and MRS to investigate potential biomarkers in children with perinatal stroke. They demonstrated that MRS may be a promising outcome measure to document the neurophysiology of developmental plasticity in children post perinatal stroke.[103]

Another study by Eliasson and colleagues set out to determine whether CIMT would be beneficial for young children less than 12 months of age with signs and symptoms of hemiplegia.[104] Thirty-seven infants were randomized to one of two groups: CIMT or infant massage. Results indicated that CIMT was more effective than baby massage.[104] Studies are becoming more sophisticated in their design and are looking more closely at mechanisms to explain plasticity. MRI revealed a change in the levels of metabolites serving as biomarkers after CIMT. These results may be indicative of a mechanism for plasticity of the primary motor cortex.[103] Multiple studies have been undertaken in an effort to demonstrate the benefits of this type of therapy for children with hemiplegia. Many of these investigations have reached the level of randomized clinical trials with more stringent outcome measures. The majority of these studies support the use of CIMT.[96–99]

Dosing, delivery, frequency, and method of restraint are all variables that can be manipulated to provide this treatment. Continued study of this therapeutic approach will be ongoing to determine the best combination of modalities to use to maximize the benefits of this intervention. Bilateral training is also a popular approach to improving function in the upper extremities.[105,106]

Treadmill training also has been used in children with CP. The treadmill has been instrumental in rehabilitation for many years with a variety of purposes. This treatment began with animal studies on spinalized cats and rats and their responses to training on a treadmill in the recovery of a walking pattern. Today this treatment is used in many populations, including those with spinal cord injury, traumatic brain injury, Parkinson disease, stroke, and CP. The use of the treadmill in children with CP has shown promising results: improvement in gait pattern, increased walking speed, decreased coactivation in lower extremity musculature, overall gross motor skill improvement, and improved and stabilized energy expenditure. Treadmill training interventions have taken on many different faces, including use of a regular treadmill, commercial equipment, and high-tech body-weight support systems (Figs. 10.27–10.29). Commercial equipment is now available to assist with supporting the body weight of individuals who otherwise would not be candidates for such a treatment. Clinical adaptations also have been incorporated to accommodate smaller bodies on a treadmill, which allows the therapist to assist from behind or from the side. Setting goals for this treatment must be precise, with an understanding of the purpose intended for its use: improving endurance, changing the parameters of the gait pattern, strengthening, and gait training. Each goal must be based on a sound theoretical foundation, which should be referenced to recent research. Researchers currently are investigating the use of several different delivery models, including—but not limited to—virtual reality to improve gait in children with CP,[107] the use of the AlterG anti-gravity treadmill system, and the effects on a variety of outcome measures,[108–110] feasibility of home-based body weight supported treadmill training,[111] and robotic resistance training on the treadmill. Future studies will need to focus on optimal dosing, frequency, ideal walking speed, percentage body weight support for improved gait efficiency, and generalization of improved outcomes. As with any intervention the practice schedule should include variability during the intervention with consideration for increasing the speed, changing the incline, changing of body weight support, walking sideways and backwards, practicing starting and stopping strategies to improve generalization, and introducing a secondary task as in stepping over obstacles presented on the treadmill. Video 1.1 is an example of treadmill training with body weight support and facilitation of a reciprocal pattern using roller skates to improve dissociate of the lower extremities in a young boy with spastic CP. Strength training was never

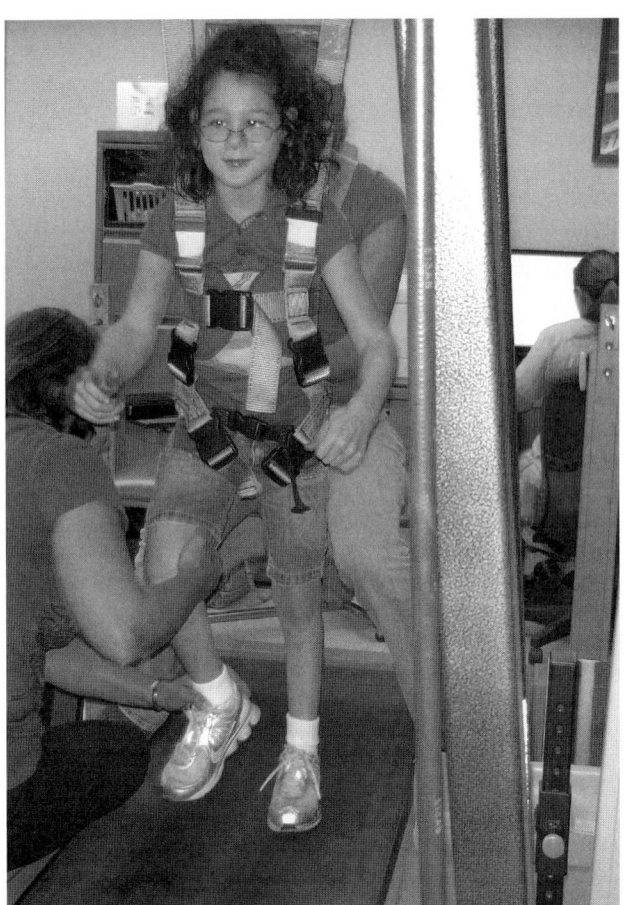

Fig. 10.28 This young girl, who is an independent ambulator with a rollator walker, is participating in partial body weight–supported locomotor training to improve her gait pattern.

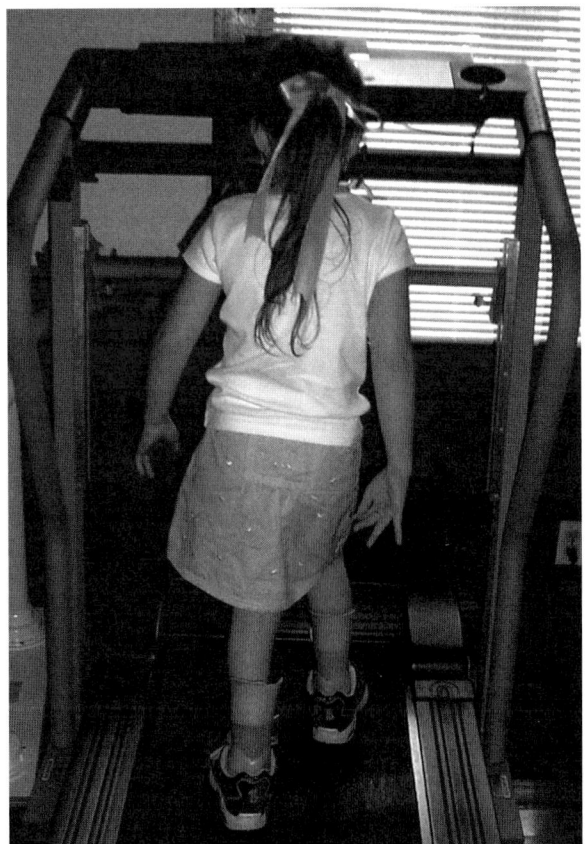

Fig. 10.27 This young girl who has a diagnosis of spastic diplegia is practicing walking on the treadmill without holding on, and incorporating arm swing to improve her stride length.

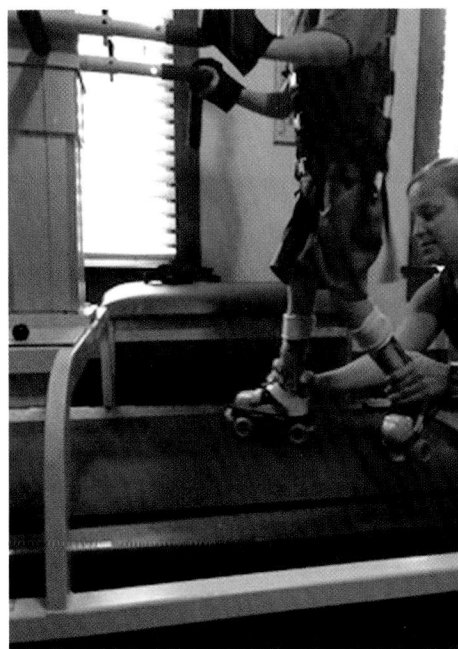

Fig. 10.29 This young boy with spastic quadriplegia is walking on the treadmill with the use of roller skates to provide lower extremity dissociation and reciprocal movement of the legs to decrease muscle stiffness.

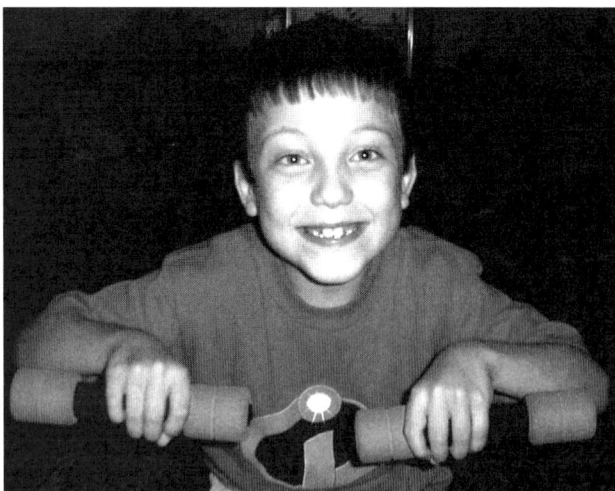

Fig. 10.30 Using free weights to strengthen the upper extremities while stabilizing the trunk while seated on an incline bolster.

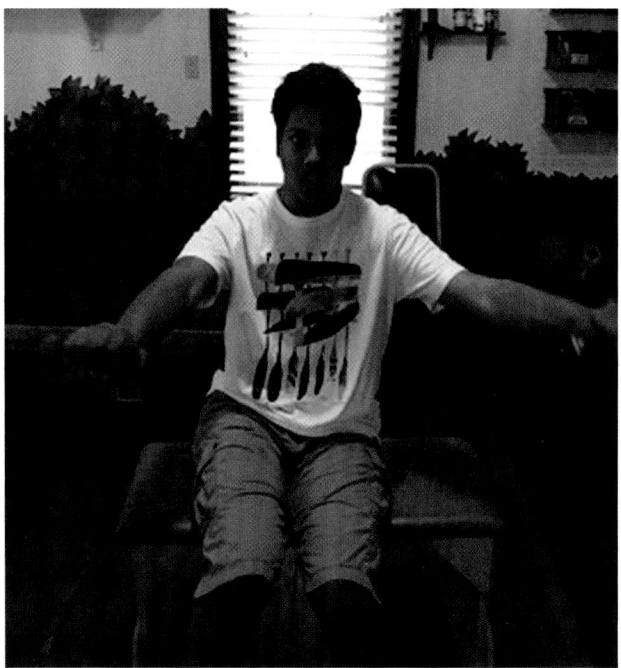

Fig. 10.31 This young adult with athetoid type cerebral palsy is doing exercises to strengthen his rotator cuff muscles with his arms in scapular plane.

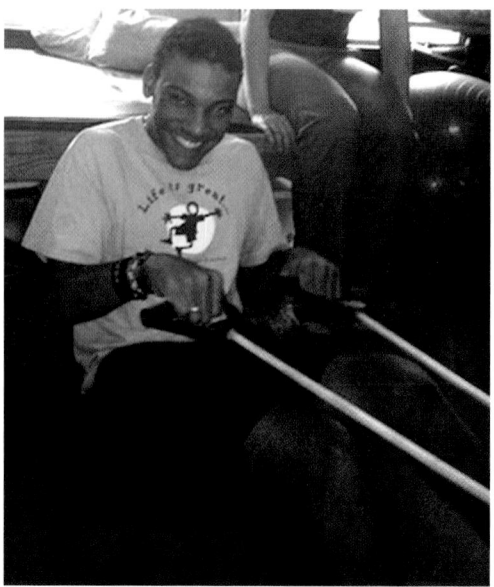

Fig. 10.32 This young man is using stretch cords to work on strengthening his shoulder girdle.

thought possible in the presence of spasticity in children with cerebral palsy. Several studies have now shown that strength can improve in children with spastic cerebral palsy.[112,113] Functional power training was used for a group of 22 children with cerebral pasly for 14 weeks, three times a week for 1 hour of loaded functional exercises including walking, running, and climbing stairs at high movement velocity, resulting in improved strength and walking capacity.[113] Strength was maintained in this group of individuals at a 14-week follow-up posttest. Strength training in the presence of spasticity is also documented in adults as beneficial not only for activity participation, improved range of motion, strength, and physical function but in some cases reduction of spasticity. Strength training in children and adolescents with cerebral palsy has continued with investigations into the intensity, type of contractions to practice, and dosage.[114] In a study by Aviram et al 2017, they looked at the effects of a group progressive resistance circuit program compared to treadmill training.[115] They found that in 95 children who

were adolescents, both groups demonstrated improved motor function as measured by the 10-meter walk test and the 6-minute walk test compared to baseline, end of intervention, and 6 months post. Interestingly, a systematic review of common physical therapy interventions in school-aged children found that strength training demonstrated significant improvements in selected muscle groups but no meaningful change in function. This may indicate that the function assessed was not targeted toward the muscles strengthened in this study. Martin and colleagues[116] and Moreau and colleagues[117] studied muscle architecture as a predictor of maximum strength and its relationship to activity levels in cerebral palsy.[117] They found that ultrasound measures of the vastus lateralis muscle thickness adjusted for age and the GMFCS level were correlated and predictive of maximum torque in children with and without cerebral palsy. A variety of methods for strength training can be incorporated into a clinical treatment setting or home exercise program with anticipated improvement in muscle strength, which may also result in improved functional status for a child with cerebral palsy. Strength training encompasses free weights, aerobic workouts, stretch bands or tubing, and machines that address resistive exercise (Figs. 10.27 to 10.34).[115,118–122] Note strengthening exercises in the "Cage" allowing for lower extremity isolation in Fig. 10.35. This type of therapy is often available with the Thera- suit™ intensive programs detailed in the section on alternative therapies.

Many adjunctive therapies that are popular in combination with other treatments are available to individuals with CP. Electrical stimulation (ES) has been used in a variety of ways with children with CP. In several case reports by Carmick,[123–125] neuromuscular ES (NMES) used in conjunction with task-oriented practice was found to improve sensory awareness, strength, gait parameters, and passive and active range of motion. In a study by Mudge and colleagues, ES was used in conjunction with Botulinum toxin A (BtxA) to improve hamstring extensibility. Six children participated in the study, and no improvement was noted in passive hamstring extensibility as measured by the popliteal angle at 4 weeks compared to BtxA alone.[126] No conclusions can be drawn from the studies mentioned above nor generalized to the population of children with CP due to the small number of subjects and limited current investigations. NMES was used as an adjunct therapy with upper and lower extremity practice protocols.[123–127] NMES has been used in conjunction with 4×/week for 4 weeks of neurodevelopmental therapy (NDT) to improve sitting posture and

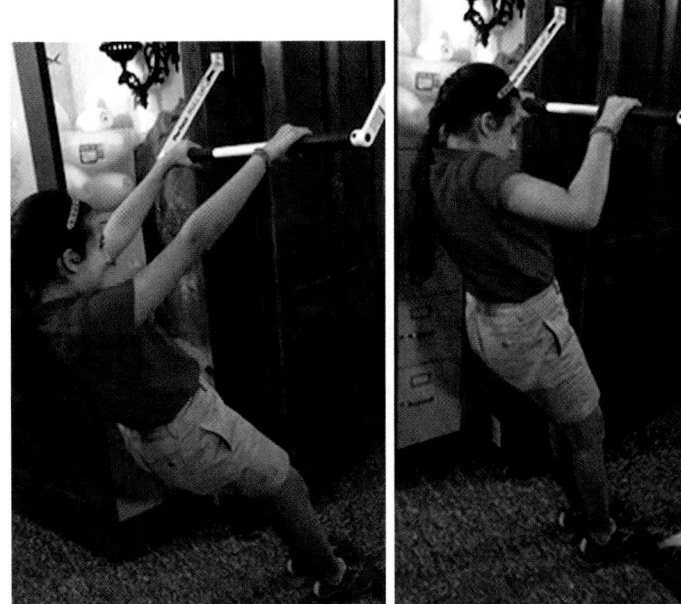

Figs. 10.33 and 10.34 This young girl with mild cerebral palsy is strengthening her shoulder girdle using the pull up bar with her trunk inclined to increase resistance by using her own body weight. This type of exercise targets scapular stabilizers.

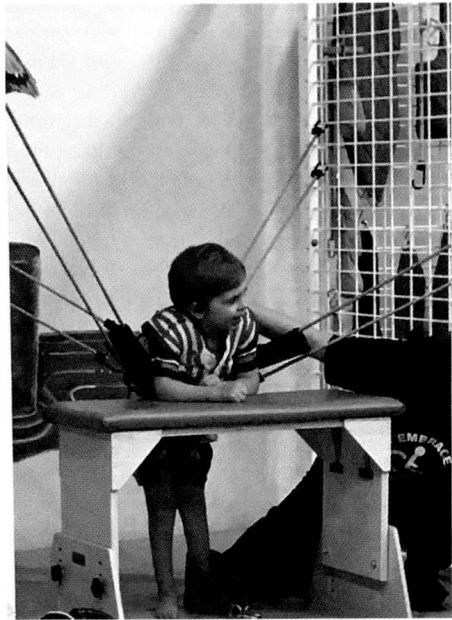

Fig. 10.35 This young patient receives intensive suit therapy. The suit provides varying degrees of compression and support. He is seen here standing with the suit on in the "Cage" using bungee cords to provide additional stability.

balance for 75 children with spastic CP. Significant changes were found in the sitting subset of the GMFM and kyphosis levels of the children with NMES and NDT compared to a control group.[116] NMES was used successfully in combination with gait during an 8-week, daily training program to improve muscle strength and muscle volume of the ankle dorsiflexors in 32 children with unilateral spastic CP.[117] However, although there were significant results found at the end of the 8-week program, only lateral gastrocnemius muscle volume stayed significant at a 14-week follow-up.

A recent study by Qi and co-workers found improved GMFM scores, decreased Comprehensive Spasticity Scale scores, and improved walking speed when NMES was combined with strength training

compared to NMES alone in 100 children with CP.[128] ES has been in the therapy arena for many years, and its selective use with children who have CP may supplement regular therapy sessions with enhanced results. (Therapeutic subthreshold ES at meridian points is discussed in the section on electroacupuncture treatments and in Chapter 39.) ES has had mixed reviews in the literature as a stand-alone therapy and in combination with other modalities. Therapists should be aware of the inconclusive data on ES using good judgment and caution with its use while evaluating its benefits carefully.[117,126]

BtxA, a neurotoxin, has been used to assist in decreasing spasticity because it provides a permissive condition that improves and increases range of motion and practice of new motor patterns and achieves developmental milestones without interference from increased muscle tone. Other positive outcomes from the use of BtxA are decreasing pain, orthotic management, as well as the possible delay in the need for orthopedic surgery until achieving maximal ambulatory ability.[25] Gait, range of motion, and decreased spasticity were noted to be improved in 60 subjects with CP after one local injection of BtxA.[129]

However, BtxA effectiveness is affected by the patient's age, type of CP, and degree of impairment.[129] BtxA has a temporary effect, so the critical element is its combination with other treatment modalities. Dursun and colleagues demonstrated improved range of motion and decreased spasticity in ambulatory children with CP when BtxA was used in combination with serial casting compared to the use of BtxA alone.[130] BtxA injections when used in conjunction with a 2-week physiotherapy program demonstrated significant gross motor function scores in 46 ambulatory children with CP with improvements lasting up to 52 weeks.[131] It has also been used as an alternative to control the progression of hip dislocation, hip pain, and prevention of foot deformities in children with CP.[132–134]

Several studies have initiated comparisons of different products all containing BtxA to assess effectiveness, health costs, and safety as alternatives. All of these have been found to be safe for use in children with CP with reduced economic burden.[132,135] Further studies are ongoing assessing the many uses of BtxA, alternatives, and combinations of therapies for best outcomes. Joint and trunk taping or strapping, and special garments, have been used to provide sensory input and alignment for posture, balance, and strengthening. To date, there is mixed evidence that these adjunctive treatments actually provide the benefits mentioned above. Further objective investigation will be necessary to address the issues presented by these additives to therapy. These alternative adjuncts are considered noninvasive with few side effects other than those associated with adhesive allergy to tape and autonomic nervous system responses such as sweating and overheating. Several different types of tape (athletic, Leukotape P Patella Tape [Notoden, The Netherlands]; Kinesio Tape [Kinesio USA Corporation]) and strapping materials such as Fabrifoam, lycra garments, and compression garments are available commercially. In 2018, Elbasan and colleagues assigned 45 children with CP to one of three therapeutic groups for 6 weeks: (1) NDT; (2) NDT with NMES; and (3) NDT, NMES, plus Kinesio-taping. They found that all groups made significant improvements in postural control and sitting balance; however, group 3 made greater improvements than the other groups.[136] In 2016, Karabay and colleagues reported similar results for postural control and sitting when comparing Kinesio tape, NMES, and NDT conditions.[116] Dos Santos and colleagues[137] investigated the use of Kinesio-taping on sit-to-stand tasks with three conditions in six children with hemiplegic type CP. There were three conditions: (1) Kinesio-tape, (2) no Kinesio tape, and (3) placebo. They reported that children in group 1 increased rectus femoris activity by electromyographic (EMG) monitoring; decreased peak flexion of the trunk, knee, hip, and ankle; and increased trunk extension in the end of sit-to-stand by kinematic measures. The time to complete the sit-to-stand maneuver was not changed. These studies provide the groundwork for further investigation into the use of Kinesio tape as part of a therapeutic intervention.[116,136–138]

Soft tissue mobilization is a method of stretching tight structures that have become restricted from overuse, spasticity, deformities, muscle shortening, surgeries, trauma, and poor nutrition. Inclusive to this group of tissues are fascia, tendons, muscle, ligaments, fat, nerves, vessels, lymphatics, and synovial membranes. This type of stretching has strong roots in osteopathic medicine but is not limited to that area of expertise. Over decades, research investigating the cellular and tissue changes that occur with immobilization has revealed some interesting and shocking alterations in the muscle and collagen fibers. With immobilization, slow muscle fibers show greater atrophy than do fast fibers. There is atrophy, a decrease in peak torque, an increase in fatigue resistance, loss of strength, and reduced central activation when the plantar flexors of the ankle are immobilized.[139,140] In a study of children with severe spasticity, muscle biopsies were performed on the vastus lateralis to determine collagen accumulation in the spastic muscle. An increased accumulation of collagen I fibers in the endomysium of the muscle was noted, with thickening and decreased muscle fiber content in the more severe cases.[141] This study, in combination with what we understand about healthy muscle, reinforces the need to keep the muscles flexible and active to help prevent this accumulation of collagen. Current literature suggests that there is a "redistribution of active nNOS molecules from sarcolemma to sarcoplasm," which serves to initiate other biochemical responses and stimulate the mechanism of muscle atrophy.[142] A small study looked at eight patients who were immobilized for 4 weeks due to fifth metatarsal or fibular fractures. Yoshiko and colleagues found that intramuscular adipose tissue and intermuscular adipose tissue increased; however, this was not statistically significant. Although both intermuscular and intramuscular adipose tissue changed after the period of immobilization, this finding had little effect on muscle atrophy. These changes were studied via cross sectional area using MRI.[143]

Soft tissue mobilization and deep tissue stretching are methods that may improve the ability of the tissue to lengthen and fold, allowing for a more efficient activation of the muscle fibers, thus optimizing the formation of typical synergies during practice of motor skills. It is important for the therapist to realize that these changes in flexibility and muscle stiffness may be only temporary due to multiple factors related to CP.

As mentioned earlier, children with CP often have visual difficulties that are not acuity problems and are not correctable with a standard lens. Vision therapy has demonstrated good results when emphasis is placed on ocular motility and accommodation.[144] When children were given intense visual-oculomotor training, improvement was noted in vision-oculomotor control.[145] Improvement in the child's ability to execute smooth pursuit precision and maximum velocity, improvement of saccadic movement precision and stability, and shortening of the saccadic reaction time were significant after training.[145] In a recent study, Kurz and colleagues began to quantify the temporal intricacies of the α and β cortical oscillations in children with CP.[146] They compared this data with children without neurological deficits. The study demonstrated that children with CP had "uncharacteristic alpha and beta oscillations" within the visuomotor networks of the brain accounting for abnormal motor performance.[146] The accommodative process in children with CP was also found to be slower with a larger error margin potentially interfering in participation in everyday life and classroom learning.[147] Although many clinicians are not experts in the area of vision, vision is an important part of every therapy session. Incorporating vision as an integral part of a therapy session will not only improve the child's orientation in space but will address his or her ability to scan the environment while learning to move through space. Consultation with an expert in this area is warranted when functional vision interferes with movement and cognitive learning abilities.

Many therapies become popular by purporting to be a "fix" for a particular problem associated with CP. The clinician accepts responsibility for making sound judgments concerning treatment and outcomes for children with CP. Not all the treatments used in therapy will be investigated rigorously in a scientific manner. However, when a treatment approach is presented as advantageous for many diagnoses and conditions, with claims of success beyond what is reasonable for those conditions, it is your duty to proceed with caution. Always stop and think what theory and frame of reference the "new" approach is grounded in. Does this "new" therapy make sense with the knowledge you have of anatomy, physiology, neurology, and motor learning? As clinicians we will always be tempted to try new approaches before the scientific community has investigated them thoroughly. Clinicians, because they are creative and innovative, have advanced our professions. It is essential to advance patient care with treatments that are safe and do no harm. Every environment affords research opportunities that contribute to the treatment of children with CP. Single-case reports and single-case studies are the beginning of this process and, although descriptive in nature and with limited generalization, they provide evidence for new therapeutic approaches and further systematic investigation.

MEDICAL INFLUENCES ON TREATMENT

Because the problems of CP are so varied, the condition lends itself to diverse interventions, some of which have a longer life than others. Management of spasticity has always been an area of great concern and interest, and over the years several treatments have been offered to control this positive sign. Various medications have been used to control spasticity and are commonly used together in combination; however, careful monitoring for proper dosage is necessary. Baclofen, benzodiazepines, and dantrolene remain the three most commonly used pharmacological agents in the treatment of spastic hypertonia.[25] (See Chapter 36 for additional information.) The use of the baclofen pump in children with excessive spasticity has gradually increased over the past 20 years. This pump is implanted in the lower abdomen with a catheter leading to the intrathecal space for the administration of the drug. This treatment for spasticity has been effective in children with CP, but it can lead to complications in some patients, such as in standing and gait impairment in ambulatory children, which is due to excessive reduction of muscle tone in the lower extremities. Other adverse events have included headache, nausea, voiding difficulties, and dysarthria.[148] Only a small number of studies have found intrathecal baclofen to be an effective treatment for spasticity for the short term. Further studies are needed to see the true effectiveness of this intervention for children with CP and its long-term effects on spasticity.[149]

Other spasticity management programs are often considered. In 1968 a posterior rhizotomy surgical intervention was developed, with some success reported in reducing spasticity.[150,151] It remained for Peacock and Arens[152] to apply the procedure more selectively and functionally, and to bring it to the United States from South Africa. On the basis of their experience, Peacock and Arens insisted on daily neurodevelopmental (Bobath) treatment for at least 1 year after the surgical intervention. EMG testing before and during the surgery is used to determine which posterior nerve rootlets are creating the spasticity in the lower extremities.[153] The foundations for success are accurate selection of the child, an experienced surgeon, and careful analysis of therapy goals.

An improvement in the surgical technique of the selective dorsal rhizotomy (SDR) procedure was developed by Lazareff and colleagues.[154] They preferred to enter a limited number of levels of the spinal column and work more closely to the cauda equina based on results from a longitudinal study by Fasano and colleagues.[155] Several studies have documented an improvement in function, a reduction of spasticity outcomes, and a significantly less functional decline lasting into adulthood. Research has found that those children who benefit best from SDR have diplegic rather than quadriplegic CP, are younger than 10 years of age, and are those with a GMFCS grade II to III.[156] In a more recent retrospective study by D'Aquino and co-workers,[157] it was found that SDR was safe and effective in reducing spasticity of both the upper and lower extremities without major complications. When combined with physical therapy and careful selection of candidates for the procedure, the functional outcomes over a period of 2 years were lasting.[157] Another study by Oudenhoven and colleagues following 36 children with spastic diplegia for 5 years post-SDR reported that baseline gait quality and GMFCS levels were the greatest positive predictors for good outcomes.[158] In 2018, a study by Park and co-workers found that simultaneous baclofen pump removal and SDR led to improved ambulation and reduced spasticity in a group of 13 children with CP.[159] Although the changes with the modified lower limb Ashworth scores in this study were not found to be significant, all patients had resolution of clonus at the ankles and lower limb hyperreflexia indicating a clear spasticity reduction.[159]

Careful selection of the appropriate candidate for this surgery followed by intense therapy intervention is essential for the success of the procedure and for optimizing motor outcomes. The use of BtxA has gained popularity in this population of children with CP. It has been used locally to affect a change in the individual muscle or motor point injected.[160–167] Both orthopedists and neurologists have taken an interest in the use of BtxA to block selected muscle responses for a temporary period. BtxA has been reported to have fewer side effects than the phenol blocks and is now considered a drug of choice for this type of procedure.[168] These conservative interventions serve to evaluate an individual prior to surgery or to delay surgery until the child is more capable of responding to postsurgical therapy programs.

BtxA is rarely used as the only therapy option and is commonly prescribed in combination with other interventions. Variable results have been found on the true impact of using BtxA in conjunction with rehabilitation interventions. In 2018, Becher and colleagues found no clinically significant changes in muscle strength, walking speed, kinematic gait parameters, and PROM when comparing a group of children with CP who received BtxA prior to a comprehensive physical

therapy program (12 weeks of 3×/week therapy) to a group who received only the comprehensive program.[169] However, another study found significant improvements in the Tardieu Scale, GMFCS, and Visual Analogue Scale for enhanced ambulatory capacity when BtxA and a rehabilitation protocol were combined, compared to those who followed the protocol alone.[170]

BtxA injection combined with serial casting has been shown to improve range of motion, muscle tone, and dynamic spasticity in ambulatory children with CP.[171] Dursun and colleagues looked into the effectiveness of serial casting combined with BtxA and physical therapy for spastic equinus foot in children with CP. They too found improvements in spasticity, passive range of motion, as well as gait function with the Modified Ashworth Scale and the Observational Gait Scale.[130] Therapists should be involved in the decision making process of determining interventions for reduction of spasticity because often they are the most familiar with the child's movement strategies and the postural changes that occur in muscle tone as the child moves against gravity.

Orthopedic surgical intervention continues to be effective in CP to address long-term complications of hypertonia and spasticity such as musculotendinous lengthening, transferring tendons to correct deformities, osteotomies, and joint fusions. Most often a child with CP will have multiple procedures to correct deformities as part of a single event multiple level surgery (SEMLS) to allow for the least amount of hospitalizations and rehabilitation.[25] In any surgery, the outcome is much improved by close coordination between therapist and surgeon, with a functional orientation toward goal setting for the child. A recent systematic review looked into predictors for positive outcomes after SEMLS for children with CP. When assessing the outcome measures of GMFCS, the preoperative Gait Profile Scale (GPS), and the age at surgery, it was found that lower levels of GMFCS and GPS were associated with greater gains in parent-reported satisfaction and gait kinematics.[172] A study by Õunpuu and co-workers found both short- and long-term benefits for children with CP who received a SEMLS that included rectus femoris transfers, as well as gastrocnemius and hamstring lengthening. Significant changes in gait kinematics were found at 1-year postsurgery, as well as sustained improvements in ankle dorsiflexion and knee extension during initial contact found at 11 years postsurgery.[173] Bony surgeries that offer better joint stability are usually planned for the termination of growth. Bracing of the trunk, which is sometimes warranted for scoliosis or kyphosis, is prescribed by the orthopedist. Surgical intervention for spinal deformities is determined by the physician, with consideration of the child's age, condition, and health, and the degree of curvature.

Children with CP differ in their ability to relax completely during sleep, and a small number of these children can benefit from night splints. Consultation with an orthopedist and/or orthotist about the style of night splint to use is suggested. When range of motion is limited, serial casting is often utilized to improve range of motion, to reduce tone, and to decrease excitability of the passive and dynamic stretch reflex at the foot and ankle.[174] These short leg casts are usually applied for a week at a time over the course of 3 to 6 weeks, depending on the progress and response to wearing. New casting materials make it easier to tolerate wearing the casts 24/7; they are lightweight and allow the incorporation of weight-bearing activities while trying to improve range of motion. In addition, there is a variety of lower extremity bracing available, and its selection is dependent on the lower limb segment targeted for control and the outcomes sought in positioning that segment. Bracing also has been shown to improve some gait parameters including walking speed, stride length, and heel-toe gait during ambulation (Fig. 10.36).[175]

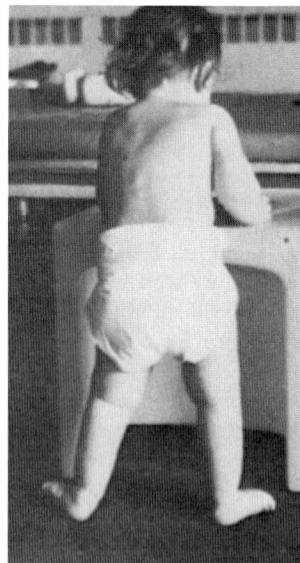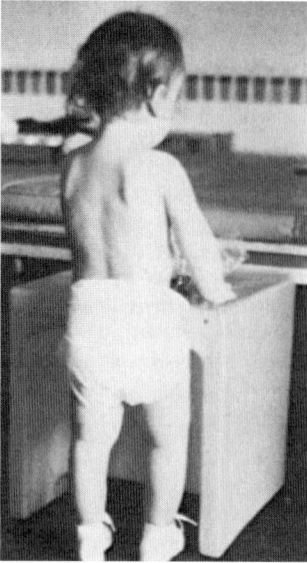

Fig. 10.36 A supportive shoe with inserts provides a more stable base of support for this low-tone child, facilitating more typical trunk reactions and permitting use of the hands for play.

EQUIPMENT

Equipment recommendations must take into account the physical space in the home and the amount of direct treatment available to the child (see Fig. 10.29). Young children in particular can often use normal seating with slight adaptations. This is not only more socially and financially acceptable, but also permits changes as required by the child's developmental progress. The portability of supportive seats or standers encourages the family to take the apparatus along for weekend outings or visits to relatives Fig. 10.37. Chair designs should place children at an age-appropriate level in their environments Fig. 10.38. This permits a better quality of visual exploration and facilitates social exchange with siblings and visiting peers. When planning the amount of physical support needed by the child, the therapist considers varying the structural control in relation to activity (Fig. 10.38). The child who is merely watching the play of others or a television presentation may successfully control trunk and head balance independently with minimal support. However, concentration on hand skills or self-feeding may necessitate trunk control assistance via a chair insert to avoid the child's use of compensatory reactions. As postural reactions become more integrated and hence more automatic, support should be diminished. There are now several options available to the consumer on the internet. Families and therapists alike can search online for commercially available products and alternatives. Some communities may have a lending closet that recycles equipment of children that have outgrown it.

For the more severely disabled child, equipment should be easily and completely washable. Mothers should be able to place special seating inserts into wheelchairs or travel chairs with one hand while holding the child. Wheelchairs should be ordered with consideration for family needs and the child's environment. The most expensive does not always offer the best solution. Control straps and seating should be adaptable and allow for future change on the basis of growth and improved function. The severely limited child needs seating changes at least once every hour during the day to prevent pressure and to provide environment changes as in typical development. Pleasing color, good-quality upholstery, and professional finishing are important not

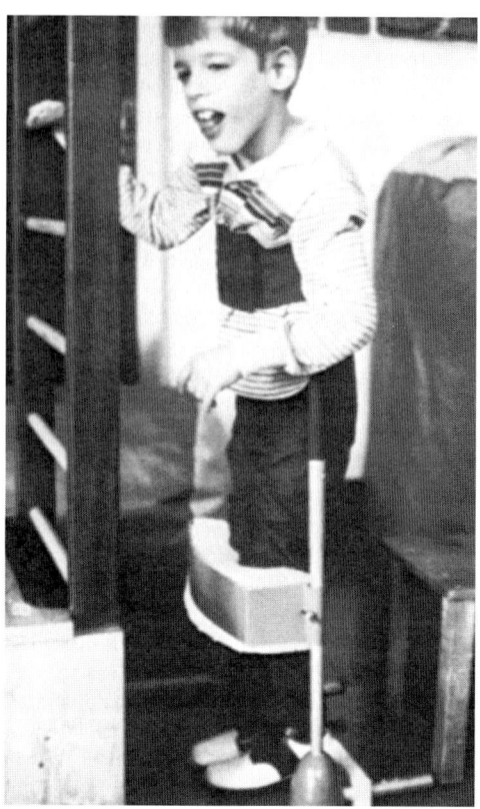

Fig. 10.37 An upright stander is easily incorporated into the home environment, providing the child with an upright position, stimulation, and an opportunity to participate in activities.

only for the child but also for the family members, who are accepting the equipment as part of their personal living environment. Electric wheelchairs provide for independence in the community and can be equipped with a number of different options for driving when there are physical limitations that prevent use of the upper extremities. Careful evaluation of which part of the body will access the switch to drive the chair should be done prior to installation of the device (refer to Video 10.2). Working closely with the vendor, the family, and the individual ensures success. Consulting with a therapist that specializes in wheelchair equipment or attending a wheelchair clinic is highly recommended since this durable medical equipment is always changing and requires justification of medical necessity. Third-party payers require specific documentation to process a claim for a wheelchair. It is essential that the therapist be fully informed about the requirements necessary for billing any durable medical equipment through all third-party payers. In addition, most large items covered through insurance or Medicaid are limited to a 5-year period; that is, wheelchair purchases are only covered every 5 years.

As prices rise and the applicability of insurance changes, the therapist must consider cost effectiveness more carefully. A recent study provided a self-report survey for families on equipment needs and out-of-pocket expenditures and found that most families of children with CP purchased up to 25 items in areas of positioning, mobility, transport, modifications to the home, communication devices, orthoses, self-care, medical, caregivers, and adapted toys. This survey demonstrated the highest number of items were for positioning followed by mobility and then adapted toys.[176] Parents are often desperate to do everything possible for the child and tend to be very susceptible to high-powered advertising and reassuring sales personnel. By providing

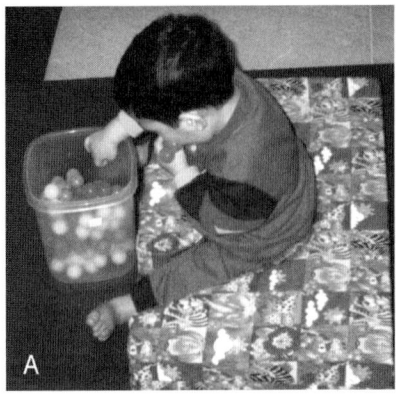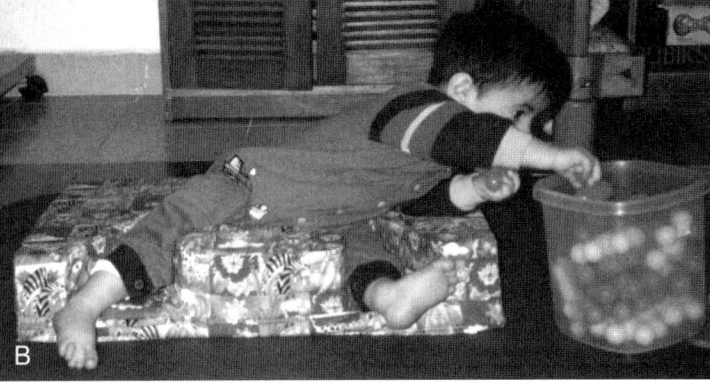

Fig. 10.38 **(A, B)** Use of a simple cut-out space in 3-inch foam gives this 1-year-old child security while requiring more active trunk adaptation during play.

a list of essential equipment features, the therapist will aid the parents in becoming informed consumers. Perusal of several catalogs online or in hard copy permits some comparison of quality and prices. Adaptive equipment fairs are often open to parents and therapists and are great opportunities to actually try the equipment without the burden of the cost. These are usually annual or semiannual events and can be found online or through your equipment vendor. Therapists can forge a relationship with a representative of a medical supply company and then access equipment on loan to try with their patients for short periods of time. Once the appropriate equipment has been purchased, periodic review of equipment used by the child can serve to encourage the family to pass along to someone else equipment items that are no longer needed. Investment in expensive equipment also has the hidden effect of influencing both parent and therapist to continue its use well beyond its effectiveness as a dynamic supplement to treatment. For this reason, more than any other, large investments must be thoroughly researched with regard to their long-term applicability for the child. Many pieces of equipment will be able to grow with the child, and this aspect should always be considered. When anticipating and considering the cost of adaptive equipment needs, it is important for the therapist and family to remember that some of the highest out-of-pocket expenditures come from home modifications and transportation vehicles, as well as the indirect cost of needing specialized care for their child. This typically falls to the mother or father who foregoes paid work to provide for their child.[176]

Adaptive equipment is not the only type of equipment that the therapist must consider for patients. Conditioning and strengthening, now recognized as beneficial to children and adults with CP, open the door for equipment that lends itself to these parameters.[177,178] (Refer to the section on research for evidence of the benefits.) Exercise bikes, treadmills (see Fig. 10.22), light weights (Fig. 10.30), and balance equipment (Fig. 10.39) are all valuable adjuncts to a home exercise program and should be considered, when appropriate, for a particular individual. Many of the commercially available items found at a sporting goods store can be well adapted to fit the needs of the higher functioning person with CP. With more emphasis on working out, sports equipment can even be found in discount stores. Offering to adapt equipment for your patients can encourage and increase compliance with exercises given for home exercise programs.

ALTERNATIVE THERAPIES

Hyperbaric oxygen treatment has gained popularity as a treatment for CP in children. Clinics are beginning to spring up worldwide for this

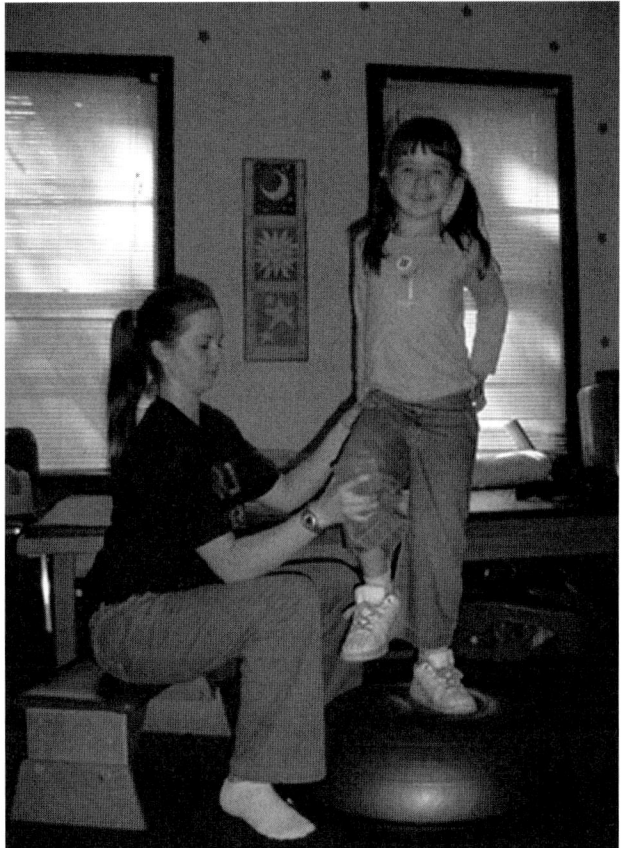

Fig. 10.39 Balance equipment allows for increased complexity in the therapy program with the refinement of balance reactions.

type of therapy. Research on this treatment has been inconclusive, and scientific evidence for its efficacy is lacking.[179,180] Clinicians should keep abreast of the latest developments in the treatment of CP and inform families about the pros and cons of designer treatments. Essentially the Undersea and Hyperbaric Medicine Society (UHM) statement remains unchanged from 2003; that there is not enough evidence to recommend the use of hyperbaric oxygen therapy for CP.[181,182] A systematic review by McDonagh and colleagues[183] found that there was no significant difference between pressurized air and room air pressure, and that the subjects in both groups made gains. In a recent report by Chantre and colleagues the types of conditions for the use of hyperbaric medicine were discussed: acute or long-term chronic pathologies. Continued caution is advised when using this little-known discipline of hyperbaric therapy.[184,185] This topic remains controversial even within the UHM. Several articles and editorials have been written with the overwhelming conclusion that randomized clinical trials should be carried out to determine the effectiveness of this treatment.[179-185]

The Adeli or Therasuit are compression garments with bungee cord–like elastic cords attached to the suit along the trunk and extremities Fig. 10-40. This suit, once referred to as the *therapeutic space suit* or *treatment-loading suit,* was developed for Russian cosmonauts to counteract the adverse effect of long-term zero gravity on the skeletal muscles and bone composition.[186] There remain few studies that suggest that there are benefits for children with CP when they receive therapy in the suit. Ko and colleagues reported in a single case report, that strengthening exercises and gait training in the Adeli suit led to significantly improved spatial-temporal gait parameters, 10-m walking speed, GMFM, and Pediatric Balance Scale from baseline.[187] Although this report demonstrates positive outcomes in this single subject design, it cannot be extrapolated to a larger population of children with CP.[187] The suit allows for controlled practice of activities with resistance, and assistance when necessary; the cords are attached in a variety of ways to give different types of practice repetitions, as well as allowing for the most optimal joint and limb alignment and to dissuade abnormal muscle patterns.[186] Utilizing the suit-orthosis during seated reaching exercises or daily activities may allow for improved postural control and more organized anticipatory postural adjustments, and may assist with arm control.[188] As is prescribed by the proponents of this approach, intense practice is warranted to reap the benefits. This therapy is expensive, and the suit, if bought to use at home, is also very expensive. Rosenbaum[181] has suggested that the benefits of this therapy vary with the type and severity of the involvement, the child's ability to participate in controlled movement, and the tolerance to wearing the suit for extended periods of time. Active participation, initiation, and motivation are known to enhance the long-term learning of motor skills and should be taken into account when determining which patients may benefit from this approach.[74] As clinicians, it is important for us to stay abreast of the latest developments and to provide families with reasonable alternatives. Although intense practice is well known in the literature as being beneficial for motor learning, the addition of the suit brings in a component that "appears" to provide "an extra set of hands," stability, and graded control during practice (Fig. 10.35). In Fig. 10.40 demonstrates the use of bungee cords in the "Cage," which is utilized to accomplish isolated strengthening. In Fig. 10.41 notice how the therapist is utilizing a game to assist with functional skills as part of this intense therapy approach. Caution when describing this approach to families is warranted because some evidence suggests that it may not be appropriate for every child with CP. The long-term effects and measurable outcomes after the use of the Adeli suit are not well documented in the literature.[181,186]

The following questions must be asked: What happens to the motor abilities of the child when the suit is removed? Has the suit actually prevented the development of postural antigravity coactivation of the trunk and proximal axial joints? Are there measurable goals met after intensive suit therapy?

In the mid-1980s Pape[189] published a case series involving five children with CP receiving therapeutic (subthreshold) ES. This case series reported that overnight use of low-intensity ES in combination with standard therapy demonstrated significant improvement in gross motor, balance, and locomotor skills as measured by the Peabody Developmental Motor Scales in children with mild CP.[189] The results

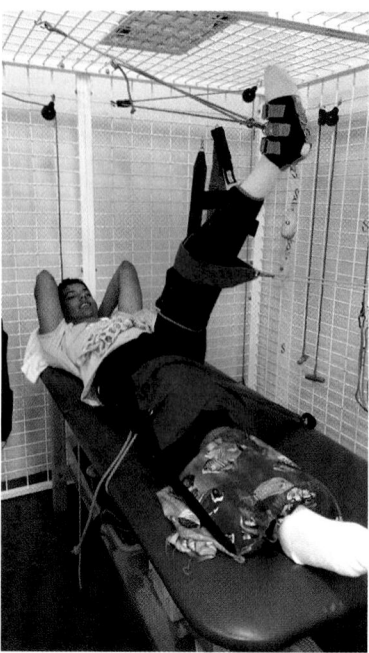

Fig. 10.40 This patient participates in isolated strengthening of lower extremity muscles in the Cage with the use of bungee cords to provide active assistive exercise.

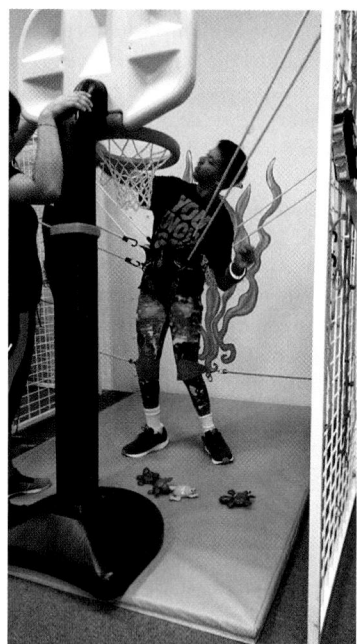

Fig. 10.41 The therapist has followed up with a fun game to bring therapy back to functional skills.

reported were based on observations by individuals who were not blinded to the purpose of the study, and therefore the research design was biased. In a follow-up study, Steinbok and colleagues[190] followed children who had undergone selected dorsal rhizotomy and received therapeutic ES for 1 year. Although this study reported improvement in gross motor function, no other measures were changed: range of motion, spasticity, or strength. Two well-controlled clinical trials investigating this method of threshold electrical stimulation (TES) delivery concluded that no objective effects on motor or ambulatory function or clinical benefit for children and youths with CP were detected.[191,192] In two separate randomized placebo-controlled clinical trials using TES, the results indicated that no significant clinical benefit was observed when compared with NMES.[191,193] (Refer to Chapter 8 for additional discussion.) Parents often report changes with this therapy, but the objective measures do not demonstrate significant results. Clinicians in the field have reported that overnight use of subthreshold ES builds muscle bulk, but unless combined with active participation of the musculature, overall improvement in movement may not be seen. This therapy, for children with CP, requires a special stimulation unit that is subthreshold and capable of being used at night, and which has a shutoff setting that is activated if the electrodes become disconnected from the child. The unit is costly and further requires a clinician who is specially trained in its use to evaluate and periodically update the treatment protocol. Significant benefits for this type of ES have not been documented. In a randomized clinical trial comparing NMES and TES the results demonstrated no statistical difference between the 60 children with CP assigned to either of the NMES, TES, or strengthening groups.[193] This study suggested that children with diplegia may benefit from ES when regular strengthening exercises are difficult to carry out. Another study carried out in 2002 demonstrated similar results and found no clinical benefits during the study.[191] Another form of ES, functional electrical stimulation (FES), is an intervention used during ambulation to support the necessary muscle groups in gait. FES is direct ES to a motor nerve, commonly the peroneal nerve, to produce a functionally useful contraction to prevent drop foot during swing phase by activating the dorsiflexors. It is hoped that FES can improve walking patterns and correct deviations by increasing muscle strength and decreasing muscle spasticity during movement.[194] A literature review on FES as an alternative to orthotic use in patients with a diagnosis of CP found 15 studies that demonstrated a positive orthotic effect and improved dorsiflexion during swing phase. The studies presented here have limitations in their ability to support FES. Only one randomized controlled trial was found in this group, and inclusion criteria for subjects required available dorsiflexion ROM.[194] A systematic review on FES of the ankle dorsiflexors by Moll and colleagues also found evidence for a potential use of FES as an orthotic alternative; however, there lacked support for any functional or therapeutic gains on the child's overall activity and participation.[195] These studies suggest that FES may be a possible and more appealing intervention, with minimal adverse events, for children who are not compliant with brace wear; however, further research needs to be done on its efficacy and long-term effects.

The Peto method or "conductive education" (CE), developed by Andres Peto in Budapest, Hungary, after World War II, has been used in children with disabilities.[196] This approach is an educational versus medical model, as the name implies, and the focus is on the many aspects of child development. It is based on practice and repetition combined with verbal guidance of a trainer (conductor) and self-verbalization by the child as he or she performs the task or activity.[181] Most of the claims that promote its value have come from the Peto Institute in Budapest. The institute has been very selective in choosing candidates for this approach on the basis of the child's potential for independent mobility and function with a good overall prognosis.[181,196] Research into this method of delivery of services to children with CP has been sparse outside the Peto Institute's studies. This approach advocates intense practice of all skills, motor and educational, with an emphasis on self-doing regardless of whether a compensatory pattern is used. Various pieces of equipment are used to facilitate independent skills: wooden slatted beds to allow the child to pull and maneuver, and wooden ladders mounted on the wall to assist

with dressing and transitions. The literature on CE does stress the concept of intense practice for motor learning. Similarly, promoting practice in the CE environment must transfer to home and community for carryover to everyday life situations.[74] A study looking at the attainment of gross motor behaviors in children with CP over an 11-month period 5 days a week reported that children achieved 83% and 89% of their gross motor behaviors in the fall and spring terms, respectively. The evaluators found that all practiced tasks, especially stability and transfer tasks, were attained; however, unpracticed motor behaviors were not achieved.[197] In two recent randomized clinical trials the investigators found no significant long-term effects of CE.[198,199] The authors were careful to point out that larger trials need to be carried out to more fully investigate this approach. In addition, to fully optimize the outcomes of CE, a commitment from the family is essential, as is the case in most therapeutic approaches. It is well understood that for motor learning to be beneficial, skills need to transfer to other environments outside of the treatment arena.[74,197]

The Feldenkrais method was developed by an Israeli engineer, Moshe Feldenkrais, while looking for a solution to his own knee problem. (Refer to Chapter 39 for additional discussion.) He started analyzing body alignment for more efficient movement.[200,201] This form of body work has been used to help dancers, gymnasts, and other skilled persons improve their performance. Some therapists have undertaken the long training necessary to understand typical movement in more detail and to improve the movement coordination of their patients with neuromotor challenges. There remains no published research on this method, but several books and training courses exist that promote its use. Anat Baniel adapted the Feldenkrais method for children, particularly children with disabilities in 2012.[202]

Ida Rolf was trained in physics and had a son with some postural disorganization.[203] She developed a structural approach, called the Rolfing technique, to improve body alignment; the technique uses specific release of deep soft tissue to restore effortless postural control against gravity.[204] She was able to make positive changes in the movement patterns of many children with CP, but she never claimed to treat the disorder itself. The Rolfing technique requires special training, which is a type of deep tissue massage.[205] There are no published research articles on the use of either the Feldenkrais method or the Rolfing technique with children with disabilities.

Dr. William Sutherland,[206] an osteopathic physician, developed direct treatment of the cranium, which is referred to commercially as *cranial therapy* or *cranial sacral treatment.* (Refer to Chapter 39 for additional information.) This type of therapy is purported to have wide application to many disabilities and conditions.[207–209] Today, there are persons trained at many different levels of expertise, so the family of a child with CP seeking this treatment will need to be certain that the practitioner is a professional and that she or he has experience with small children. Cranial treatment has claimed to restore the physiological motion of the craniosacral system, improving circulation of fluids to the brain as well as respiratory function, to which it is believed to be closely linked. In 2011, Wyatt and colleagues investigated the use of cranial osteopathy in 142 children with CP. These children were between 5 and 12 years of age with each receiving 6 sessions of cranial osteopathy. This randomized clinical trial found no significant evidence in improved motor function, sleep patterns, report of pain, or quality of life.[208] Research has been encouraged in this area to substantiate the claims of this approach; however, there remain few rigorous reported studies in the literature.

Equine-assisted therapy (hippotherapy) is a new and popular treatment option for children with CP; it provides motor and sensory input through the movement and gait of the horse. Hippotherapy is thought to affect multiple organ systems including the musculoskeletal, limbic, vestibular, sensory, and ocular systems, allowing likely improvements in posture, mobility, and balance. This therapy approach is fun and provides an opportunity for kids to participate in a more social and community activity. The American Hippotherapy Association (AHA) was founded in 1992 and created an international protocol for use in therapy. Certification standards to become a Hippotherapy Clinical Specialist (HPSC) were established in 1999 with a three-step program and a 3-year training period. Many studies have found hippotherapy to be beneficially effective for coordination, muscle tone, flexibility, endurance, movement patterns, and postural control.[210] A study by Park and colleagues looked at 34 children with CP who received hippotherapy 2×/week for 8 weeks compared to a control group. Improved balance, postural control, and functional performance were found with significantly improved GMFM scores and Pediatric Functional Skill Scale (PEDI-FSS) in the experimental group from baseline.[211] Another randomized controlled trial looked at the effect of hippotherapy on muscle spasticity found decreased scores on the Modified Ashworth Scale for hip adductors after 12 weeks. Decreased spasticity of the hip adductors is purported to allow for improved pelvic kinematics and to lead to improved postural control and balance.[212] When assessing the short-term and long-term effects of riding on motor function for children with CP, it was found that long-term riders (~1 to 4 years of routine practice) demonstrated significant improvements in walking, running, and jumping. The long-term repetition of the horse's pelvic movements is suggested to help reorganize the child's CNS and lead to improved movement patterns during daily and functional activities.[213]

It is important for families to look into the certification of therapists offering hippotherapy, as well as being aware that there are limited number of centers in the United States that provide these services. General health insurance coverage may not cover hippotherapy. Therefore this treatment option can be costly and may not be viable for some families of children with CP.[210] Some communities offer support through grants or through school programs for this type of therapy.

Another alternative treatment used for children with CP is acupuncture, which involves insertion of needles into specific target locations in the skin. Preliminary studies have stated that acupuncture may increase blood flow and oxygenation to surrounding blood vessels, and may play a role in regenerating and repairing injured areas of the brain in children with CP. Acupuncture is an adjunctive therapy for children with CP, and although health insurance may not cover this, it is relatively inexpensive, without serious adverse events, and is considered a simple office procedure. A recent meta-analysis on the effects of acupuncture for CP found that acupuncture in conjunction with rehabilitation training led to improvements in both gross motor function and activities of daily living, as well as reducing muscle spasms.[214] Due to the limited number of studies and sample size in each study, more research is needed to see the true efficacy of acupuncture and the long-term benefits. However, the apparent short-term benefits are encouraging and provide another treatment option or an adjunct to contemporary therapy that the child is already involved in.

Aquatic therapy is an alternative for children with CP diagnosed with all levels of motor impairment. Performing treatment interventions in water may be easier and more beneficial for children with CP due to water's thermal and mechanical properties, including decreased spasticity, improved soft tissue elasticity, and buoyancy, which decrease the effects of gravity and improve joint alignment.[215,216] A recent study looking at aquatic therapy's effect on both motor function and enjoyment in children with CP found aquatic therapy to improve self-reported physical activity enjoyment and gross motor function.[215] Aquatic therapy with an aerobic exercise focus has also demonstrated preliminary results with meaningful changes in gross motor function

and walking endurance in ambulatory children with CP. This 14-week study utilized functional activities including running, jumping, stair climbing, deep water walking, and hopping at a moderate-to-vigorous exercise intensity.[217] For children with higher gross motor abilities, this alternative therapy may be the way to get more participation and motivation for increasing strength and endurance. Aquatic therapy is feasible, fun, more enjoyable, and inexpensive therapy option to land-based therapy with minimal adverse events. More research is needed to understand the dosing and effectiveness for different ages and gross motor levels. Children with varying levels of cognition, interests, spasticity, strength, flexibility, and motor control will react and adjust to aquatic interventions differently. These multiple aspects should be considered when contemplating the best therapy option for each child.[216]

Stem cell therapy is a novel option for children with CP with an increased prevalence in both clinical trials and literature reviews over the past 5 years. Interest in this treatment option has grown in leaps and bounds due to the lack of restorative options for CP. The current belief is that stem cell and other cell-based therapies might be effective for children with CP through its ability to repair and replace damaged brain cells, promote cell survival, and provide immune modulation. Early clinical trials have shown stem cell therapy to be safe and well tolerated with short-term improvements on gross motor outcomes. Many different types of stem cells are being researched, including embryonic stem cells, human amnion epithelial cells, mesenchymal stem cells (umbilical cord blood, placenta, bone marrow, adipose tissue), neural stems cells, etc., with the primary goals of restoring circuitry and normalizing CNS activity.[218] Chahine and colleagues reported a significant improvement of ~1.3 levels on the GMFCS in 11 of 15 children with CP, as well as significant cognitive improvements in 6 of 15, when treated with intrathecal bone marrow mononuclear cells.[219] Although stem cell research appears to be a positive and effective therapy, extensive research is needed to document the efficacy and longitudinal gains of this approach. Establishing the effective dosing, the critical time period for administration of this treatment, the most effective delivery mode, and the criteria for patient selection is prudent before therapists should be advocating for this option with patients' families. Staying up to date on the research for stem cell therapy is in every therapist's best interest due to the possible controversial and ethical conflicts and the widespread interest and discussion in the media.

Whole body vibration (WBV) in oscillation therapy has become increasingly popular in the general population. It is commonly found in local gyms and fitness centers due to its known health benefits of improved flexibility and muscle strength. WBV/oscillation therapy exposes a person's whole body to repetitious low frequency, low amplitude mechanical stimuli while standing on a platform. The belief is that the vibration stimulates muscle spindles to initiate increased and improved muscle contractions through a tonic vibration reflex. Studies that have been performed on children with CP have found WBV improved mobility, posture, gait, leg strength, and decreased spasticity of the knee extensors. WBV is a noninvasive, easy to apply, and relatively safe alternative or adjunct treatment for children with CP.[220]

Cheng and colleagues found that WBV significantly improves ambulatory function with the TUG and 6MWT, as well as decreases spasticity of the lower extremities after an 8-week session with results lasting up to 3 days posttreatment. WBV appears to assist in controlling spasticity and walking function and can be used as a routine treatment or as a spasticity-reducing agent prior to a typical rehabilitation session.[220] In 2015, Saquetto and colleagues reported a meta-analysis reviewing 6 randomized controlled trials with 176 subjects overall and found that WBV may improve gait speed and standing function in children with CP.[221] Utilizing a continuous oscillating platform may also assist with improving both reactive and anticipatory postural control mechanisms that could enhance functional performance in children with CP.[222] Therapists must assess the use of WBV/oscillation therapy on a case-by-case basis for safety and effectiveness. Further research is needed for proper protocols and long-term effects with this population.

DEVELOPING A PERSONAL PHILOSOPHY OF TREATMENT

The practicing therapist continues to learn much about the nuances of typical human development (see Chapter 2).[223] The dynamic interaction of developmental movement components becomes more significant as the therapist acquires greater clinical experience and recognizes developmental change as a reflection of CNS maturation. Increasing knowledge of the functional nature of sensory systems and CNS processing will influence the choice of treatment techniques. Direct intervention will have more depth and specificity to improve the child's control of posture and movement while the therapist appreciates the complex interaction of developmental factors in CP. On the basis of individual experience, each therapist develops a personal philosophy of treatment that incorporates new research findings and evolving perceptions of the problem of CNS dysfunction. Without a philosophical or theoretical orientation for decision making, the therapist may succumb to following each promising treatment idea that is learned without having a clear image of the potential benefits for the specific patient. "Commercial" programs may benefit the child whose needs match the program objectives. An "individualized" program adapts to the needs of the particular child and is shaped by the response of that child during therapy. Without an internalized treatment goal toward which independent techniques are applied, the result may remain ineffective and unconvincing. The therapist in a direct treatment situation must develop a concise visualization of what is to be achieved in each session with the individual child based on a sound foundation. The repetition and practice that are so critical for learning must often be carried out at home, and the therapist becomes responsible for family instruction. Home exercise programs must be tailored for both the child and the family situation, and must be in alignment with the goals and expectations of the family. These programs need to be practical, fun ideas for practice that can be incorporated into the child's home life with reasonable assurance that the activities can and will be carried out regularly. Utilizing the World Health Organization's design of the International Classification of Functioning framework[29,30] allows for a program that improves the child's activities and impairments; however, it also increases their social participation within the family and community. Studies have found participation to be the parents' predominant goal or need.[224] Creative therapeutic ideas for playtime, dressing, grooming, mealtime, and relaxation time are best addressed in the home exercise program because these are everyday tasks that every family encounters, and the family is likely to be compliant. It is important that the family be involved in the development of goals and POC. Most improvements in abilities and skills are accomplished when everyone is working toward common agreed-upon goals. The time spent in therapy throughout the week cannot substitute for all the hours spent at home and at school.

Specialized therapy, like typical development, is potentially a preparation for functional performance. Training in specific coordination skills may be necessary for the older child or adolescent and must begin with a thorough analysis of the whole person who happens to demonstrate the effects of CP. Some children have learned self-care along with brothers and sisters. Others have needed therapy guidance for each achievement. Intelligent children with strong motivation may

only need some assistance in avoiding the use of atypical reactions, whereas others have poor spatial orientation and minimal motivation to achieve independence. The therapist most often needs to create a dialog with the individual who has the problem because parents are often fatigued and without energy to solve the issue of adolescent life skills. Perseverance is key to success with these individuals.

INVOLVING THE FAMILY

To be successful, therapy for the child with CP includes active family participation. Variability of practice in different environments tends to promote more effective motor learning, and parents who learn to help their child early begin to understand the importance of their participation as well as the nature of their child's disability. Parents are in the process of healing their own self-image, which was so injured when they learned of their child's disability. They should not be expected to become therapists per se, but should learn to observe small gains in treatment sessions that offer insight into the child's current strengths and weaknesses.[27] Therapy services have gradually transitioned to this more family-centered approach to allow for family strengths, increased respect between all family members and the therapist, as well as to promote sharing of information to guarantee fully invested care for the child while also empowering the parents. This family-centered care has been associated with progress in both the health and development of the child with CP, as well as improved psychosocial functioning and adjustment in their daily activities.[224]

Parents need to adapt their expectations in keeping with the child's continuing change and emotional maturity. Parenting a child with CP is no easy task, and the therapist will do well to develop respect for this demanding role. No one provides more for the child with CP than the nurturing parent who guides the child to self-acceptance of limitations without destroying personal initiative. This is the child who most often becomes an independent working adult (Figs. 10.42 and 10.43). View Video 10.3 of a young man with athetoid CP negotiating traffic and city streets on his way to the city bus stop to get to job training at the public library. A recent questionnaire completed by 303 caregivers of children with CP demonstrated that a majority of caregivers may not know or understand the GMFCS level assigned to their child, or understand how their child's gross motor development compares to other children. Caregivers preferred having picture references to better understand their child's diagnosis and GMFCS, and reported that it would be helpful to revisit this information routinely to monitor their child's development.[225] It is important that the therapist regularly

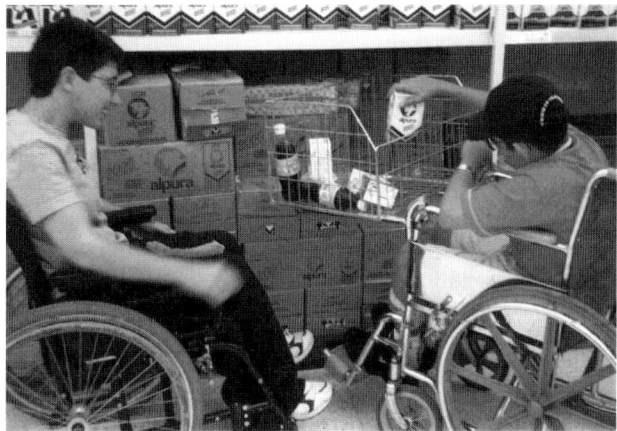

Fig. 10.42 Therapy goals must incorporate functional activities that lead to personal independence if they are to be pertinent for the older child and adolescent.

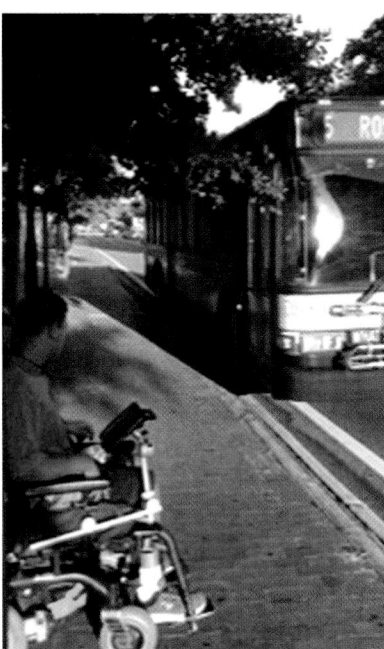
Fig. 10.43 This young man is waiting for public transportation on his way to work at the library.

check in with caregivers and families of children with CP to allow them the opportunity to ask questions and to be fully informed on the child's current status. Families may feel most comfortable discussing and asking motor development questions of the therapist rather than other health care providers due to the amount of time and rapport they have built with the family.

The therapist must give serious thought to priorities in home recommendations. Therapists must consider the size of the family and whether there are siblings, the outside employment of the mother and father, the physical capabilities of the child, the general health status of the child, and the psychological acceptance of the problem within the family. The emotional needs of some parents demand a period of less, rather than more, direct involvement with the child. Other parents must be cautioned that repetition of an activity more times than recommended will not result in faster improvement. This impression is sometimes gained from wide advertising of commercial programs that offer the same activity sequence for every child and demand a large number of daily repetitions. Both parent and therapist must appreciate the need for the CNS to have some time to integrate new sensorimotor experiences and to perfect emerging control of postural adjustments. Excessive control of movement patterns and overprotection by an adult tends to reduce the child's initiation of postural change and decrease active sensorimotor learning. Health needs for good nutrition and adequate rest also must be considered by parents and professionals. The attitude of teachers in the first years is extremely important for the child with CP. Advocating for a positive environment across the settings is advantageous for the child's achievement.

ROLE OF THE THERAPIST IN INDIRECT INTERVENTION

For many children with CP, active treatment is not available. Geographical isolation, socioeconomic factors, poor or lack of insurance coverage, and lack of qualified therapists may interfere with the delivery of direct service. The therapist must then assume the role of

teacher, counselor, or consultant. More often the new role emerges as one in which the therapist tries to meet a combination of needs and is frequently frustrated by lack of time, energy, and community resources. The therapist may be a member of a community team that includes a psychologist, a social worker, and a public health nurse. This sometimes creates more of a behavioral than a traditional medical orientation. Therapists also can be primarily responsible to the public school systems, introducing therapeutic positioning to classroom teachers. For these types of situations, the clinician will find video recordings or photographs a valuable adjunct to direct instruction. The individual child may be filmed with equipment, adequate positions, or therapeutic procedures. Useful topic-oriented video recordings are also available for professionals and families through educational resources and media. Instruction of key personnel in these settings is critical to the success of the therapist's recommendations.

When children have no access to direct treatment, positioning is of paramount importance. The selected support is used to avoid contractures, scoliosis, and permanent limitations in range of movement. Even the most severely limited child should have a minimum of three positions that can be alternated during the day. In addition, the position selected should be as functional as possible for the individual child to allow access to the child's environment. In some cases, this may mean encouraging eye contact. For another child, hand use becomes a possibility with proper trunk support. Each program should be individualized to maximize potential for the child in that environment.

Communication for the nonverbal patient with CP must be an integral part of the therapy or school program.[226] A simple start may be made with pictures to permit choices in food, clothing, and therapy activities. The parents need encouragement to begin the process of letting the child make some simple choices in food, clothing, or preferred activities. Although computers have their place, the child should have the communication device with him or her at all times. Language development in the young child is enhanced by having this type of alternative communication device available while articulation is still difficult. The use of head movement is a powerful influence on muscle tone changes that may cause negative regression in postural or visual control.[227] Care and consideration should be taken when evaluating the body part to access the device. Postural and visual control is essential toward the goal of better function and communication.[228] A solution that was successful with one 9-year-old athetoid girl was moving the elbow back to a switch mounted on the vertical bar of the wheelchair backrest to access her communication device. Any activity that is repeated on a daily basis should be examined in light of possible interference by atypical patterns.

Affordable electronic systems with voice recording, portability, and growth features are available.[229] Communication, which can be achieved by coordinating efforts with the speech pathologist/language therapist, can make the difference between passivity and active participation in the environment. View Video 10.4 of this young boy with dystonic CP using his communication system with eye gaze. His speed and accuracy are remarkable. Play can be encouraged with the use of switch toys and touch-screen computers. New programs have been developed for computers, electronic interactive books, and technology; also, the availability of Bluetooth on multiple devices opens an array of possibilities when an individual is accessing media and their home/office/school environments.

THERAPY IN THE COMMUNITY

Therapists are often concerned with body functions and structure, and neglect to address participation in real-life activities such as school attendance, sports, employment, and involvement in the community.[230,231] Children with mild dysfunction as a result of CP may be successfully incorporated into physical education (PE) classes if the teacher is prepared to make some small adaptations. Teachers generally appreciate the opportunity to discuss with the therapist the specific limitations of the child and those movements that should be encouraged. Taking the opportunity to meet with the PE coach to establish adaptations and modifications or appropriate participation in activities is time well spent for the child's integration into the class. PE class is often rewarding for the child and is important in establishing peer relationships. For better success the child with functional limitations can be incorporated into a class that follows the British form of movement education, which places much less emphasis on intragroup competition and encourages each child to progress at her or his own rate. The therapist and the PE coach can also utilize the Framework for Sustained Participation for strategies to facilitate more frequency and continuous attendance for physical activity. This framework assists in choosing the right activity, encouraging them to want to succeed, providing a sense of belonging, providing the right coach or coaching style, as well as encouraging continuity, passion, and support for the child.[232]

Many communities are now offering after-school programs in adaptive sports, for example, soccer, baseball, and wheelchair sports, to name a few. These programs rely on volunteers in the community to work as "buddies" on the field or on the court to assist as needed for participation by the child with CP. Become familiar with your community to offer suggestions to your patients.

Classroom teachers who lack experience with children who have special needs are understandably reluctant to incorporate a child with movement limitations into the classroom until they know the child. A meeting with the therapist might be used to help the child demonstrate his or her strengths, physical independence, and ability to participate in classroom activities. The child may often play an active role in the problem-solving process necessary for a successful classroom experience. Children often have developed their own ways of managing the water fountain, the locker door, or personal care needs. Demonstrating these abilities reinforces strengths rather than limitations and empowers the child to receive positive responses from curious peers.

As programs that hire therapists move into the fields of prevention and early intervention, the therapist is dealing directly with a population that is not familiar with therapy per se nor aware of the need for this intervention. The therapist may discover a need to reorient previously accepted concepts of general rehabilitation. Clarification of one's own ideas is essential to establish effective communication with others. In some instances, active intervention to help the child will precede the labeling or diagnostic process, and referral to other specialists becomes part of the therapist's responsibility. Philosophically, early therapy becomes an enhancement of typical development rather than a remedial process, and it is advocated in the natural environment by federal funding agencies for children 0 to 3 years of age. Part C of the IDEA provides services for children 0 to 3 years of age, which is family focused and delivered in natural environments.[7] This implies introducing new concepts of quality in early child development to the public. Day care, church, preschool, and Head Start programs are all examples of early childhood settings that incorporate children with impairments.

It is important to keep direct, active treatment available for older children, adolescents, and adults who are motivated to change. Now that more effective procedures are available for changing some of the basic neurophysiological movement characteristics observed in children with CP, it is possible to achieve change with direct treatment of the older patient. The adolescent often responds best to short-term, goal-oriented therapy programs that are patient centered. Motor learning concepts are better understood by both the therapist and the patient, and can be incorporated into activities after mobilizing tissues that have been unused for so many years (see Chapters 3 and 8). With current program directions, many older patients may not have had the opportunity for direct treatment over time by a qualified therapist. For the minimally involved teenager, young adult, and adult with CP the local gym offers an alternative to direct therapy. Muscle weakness is a common impairment all children and adults with CP deal with that affects their ability to perform their activities of daily living. General conditioning is very popular in community programs, including weight training, endurance training, water exercises, yoga, and walking programs. Studies looking into the effect of strengthening interventions for people with CP have found a large effect on strength and physical performance when assessing outcomes of gross motor function, spasticity, kinematic parameters of gait, and range of motion.[114] Although further research needs to be completed to determine which interventions are associated with the greatest improvements in strength and performance, a systematic review assessing the impact of strength training on skeletal morphology in children with spastic CP associates strength training with an increased muscle size, as well as increased strength.[112] Van Vulpen and colleagues found that power training—described as functional high-velocity resistance training—had a significant and effective impact on muscle strength and walking capacity in children with CP. These functional activities were performed at maximal effort for three sets of 608 repetitions.[113] A therapist can be consulted to establish an appropriate program for the individual who wants to work out at the gym on equipment whether typical strength training or power training, attend special classes that are offered, or work out in the pool. When asked, it is the therapist's area of expertise to help identify and make recommendations regarding functional movement and activity participation for adults with developmental disabilities such as CP. (See the section in Chapter 35 on adults with developmental disabilities.)

The movement toward a health orientation as opposed to crisis intervention for illness will also affect services for children and adults with CP. This population does not have an illness or an active disease process, and they strive to lead as normal a life as possible. Many adults with neuromotor disabilities express their preference to participate in the decisions that are made for them regarding their ultimate lifestyle and participation in the community. The therapist who works with this population should familiarize himself or herself with the patient's living situation—family home, group home, or independent living—as well as the support system and work environment if applicable. These factors should be considered when establishing a viable program. Many opportunities for employment and volunteerism exist in communities for individuals with disabilities. This may require that the therapist venture into the workplace to assess accessibility and modifications that can be done in that environment to make for successful integration of the individual into the community. Optimal health for the adult with CP has yet to be described, and much more data must be collected. However, it is an exciting time as our society moves forward in its views and acknowledgment of disability (see Chapter 35).

PSYCHOSOCIAL FACTORS IN CEREBRAL PALSY

We have defined CP as a condition existing from the time of birth or infancy. The developing child has no memory of life in a different body. Movement limitations circumscribe the horizon of the child's world unless the family is able to provide enriching experiences. The development of both intelligence and personality relies heavily on developmental experiences and the opportunity for self-expression.

Participation in fun and exciting family and recreational activities is a way for a child with CP to not only learn new skills, but also to play, to make new bonds with family or friends, and to improve their self-confidence and sense of belonging in their community. The frequency of a child's participation in an activity and their measured enjoyment of participation has been found to be associated with their communication level, gross motor function, and manual ability.[233]

The child with spastic diplegia or spastic quadriplegia may be hesitant in making decisions or reaching out for a new opportunity because the world may seem overwhelming and threatening. The child may find it easier to withdraw toward social isolation. Parents and professionals can help children, adolescents, and adults with CP to avoid these reactions by encouraging independence in thought and in physical tasks. Early choices can be made by the child regarding which clothes to wear or which task to do first. Understanding the child's limitations helps build successes rather than failures. To function in spite of the constraints of spasticity or other movement problems demands considerable effort on the part of the child.

Athetoid children, in contrast, have adapted to failures as a transient part of life. However disorganized their movements, they repeatedly attempt tasks and eventually succeed. Their social interactions reflect this life experience. Most people will sooner or later succumb to the positive smiling approach without analyzing the deeper communication offered by the child. These children are difficult for parents to discipline and structure during their early years. Early treatment with concomitant guidance for young parents ameliorates some of the problems by making the developmental expectations for the child more appropriate. The words of professionals who are in contact with the parents at the time of the diagnosis echo through time to influence future decision making for the child.

Intelligent children with low tone demand that the world be brought to them. Cognitively challenged children may fail to receive sufficient stimulation for optimal development at their functional levels. Many of these children need visual or auditory evaluations and intervention, and some of them need a special educational approach. Whatever the learning potential of the child with CP, it is not always evident early in the child's life. Parents find it difficult to know how to guide a child when they are not certain that an assigned task or calm explanation is understood by the child.

Parental guidance of the child with functional limitations is also influenced by the adults' adaptation to their offspring's problem. Parents need to resolve, in their own way, the emotional impact of the child's disability. Parents need time to grieve the loss of dreams they had for their child, and each person will approach this in his or her own way and time. Each major milestone anticipated in a typical child's life may bring on the grieving process again. Most parents feel inadequate, ignorant, and relatively helpless at being unable to remedy the situation for their child. They need help in feeling good about themselves before they can effectively guide the child toward self-acceptance as an adequate human being. Parents need guidance to provide themselves with opportunities to rest and renew their energies. Therapists can be instrumental during this process by remaining nonjudgmental. (Refer to Chapter 5 for additional information.)

The therapist plays an important role in the psychosocial development of children who receive regular treatment. The child may perceive the therapist as a confidant, disciplinarian, counselor, or friend at various stages of development. Some children accept the therapist as a member of their extended family. This is natural, considering the extent to which therapists influence patients' own self-awareness through changes in their physical bodies. However, it also places a personal responsibility on the therapist to be aware of the continuing interaction and its effect on the maturational process of the child. Long-term relationships with patients and their families must remain professional for the therapist to be effective.

Any evaluation of personality characteristics in a disabled child must take into account the unnatural lifestyle that is imposed by the need for therapy, medical appointments, limited environmental exploration, and hospitalization. The child is expected to separate from parents earlier than the average child and usually confronts many more novel situations. There is little time or physical opportunity for free play. Continuous demands are placed on children to prove their intellectual potential in evaluations of various types. Adults most often monitor their social interaction while they assume a dependent role. Nonetheless, these children's social acceptance frequently rests on their skill in interacting with persons in their environments. It is not fair to the child to evaluate the evolution of personality without considering these experiential factors.[234,235]

DOCUMENTATION

Developing a POC with objective measurable goals is required for documentation of progress in intervention and reimbursement from third-party payers. Carefully extracting a child's strengths and weaknesses from the assessment should drive the POC. Using timed measures, distance, number of repetitions, standardized tools, and other measurable outcomes provides a source of encouragement for families and objective justification for continued intervention.

Data collection is an important task in the treatment of CP. Change occurs at variable rates, but it is important to document the cause and effect of change whenever possible. Photos or video recordings are useful in providing functional comparisons over time. Digital video now allows a specific analysis of movement sequences. Fancy equipment is not necessary to document movement for comparison later. A cell phone provides video and slow motion, which allows you to collect a sample of movement strategies that can be analyzed frame by frame once downloaded. Placing the subject against a spaced grid in varying postures allows for measurement and assessment of alignment. This "basic" method also can be used while filming to assess movement. These ideas may be applied to documentation of treatment effectiveness or be analyzed for an understanding of similar movement problems in other patients. When attempting to document using photographs or filming, consistency in the environment is critical to the outcome and analysis with repeated use. Reliable comparisons made between one time point and another requires the same testing environment, time of day, and conditions. Parental consent is required to use these forms of media.

Methods of intervention or treatment are measurable for research and applicable to the functional problems presented by a diagnosis of CP. Once a specific research question has been formulated, systematic recordings of appropriate data can be gathered over time to accumulate data for a viable study. There is value in longitudinal reporting of a single case or a small group of individuals who have some characteristics in common because this aids our understanding of what we need to inhibit and/or facilitate in the young child to permit optimal function later. Research strengthens our understanding of this condition and further helps to justify our treatments. Clinicians have a difficult time putting into words exactly what takes place during intervention, which further complicates research investigation into the efficacy of treatment. Descriptive analysis of treatment is essential to document and to begin to understand what a therapist does during a therapy session. Understanding what takes place in therapy will help identify questions that could be investigated more closely.

The way in which therapists learn to view a problem determines, to a large extent, the potential range of solutions available to them. CP is a complex of motor and movement inabilities that cluster about the inadequacy of CNS control, visual and soft tissue restrictions, and the amazing ability of the human body to compensate. Therapists need to look critically at developmental processes, qualities of movement, postural adjustments, timing and limitations of movements, and the range of dynamic functional movement. The further development and understanding of motor learning theories offer the researcher novel approaches to the challenge of CP and the resultant disorder of posture control and movement learning. Environmental factors may have as much influence as specific CNS limitations. Early intervention should be analytical, specific, and based on a theoretical foundation. Posture and movement control begin to change with direct treatment. Analysis of the postural components and movement characteristics of children with CP will lead to meaningful research more quickly than will professional reliance on the traditional definitions of the medical condition. Thorough documentation of therapy progress using objective

measures is critical for the development of more effective intervention strategies in the future. In addition, third-party payers including private insurance, Medicaid, and public early intervention programs for children 0 to 3 years of age require either standardized tests and/or other objective measures that are reproducible and reliable.[236]

CASE STUDIES

To understand the problems of children with CP, it is essential to follow some children over time to capture the evolution of family problems. Functional treatment must change according to the developmental level, chronological age, and neuromotor responses of the child. Intervention must be specific to the presenting problem of the moment while the missing aspects of complete motor development are considered. The case studies presented below provide a case description.

CASE STUDY 10.1

AR was a full-term baby born by emergency cesarean section when during labor she developed prolonged bradycardia due to compression of the umbilical cord. Her APGAR scores were 3 at 1 min, 5 at 5 min, and again 5 at 10 min. Her vital signs were depressed with poor recovery at 10 min, and she was transferred to the neonatal intensive care unit (NICU). Her NICU course was unremarkable; however, she spent 4 weeks in the unit. This was the first baby born to this family, and as is common they were unfamiliar with the typical milestones that should occur in development. The Pediatrician was concerned with her initial hypotonia and later development of muscle stiffness, delayed acquisition of speech and language, and motor skills. The Pediatrician referred AR and her family to a neurologist. A diagnosis was subsequently made at 18 months of age of ataxic CP. A magnetic resonance imaging revealed generalized atrophy of the cerebellum also referred to as congenital cerebellum dysplasia. Therapy had been initiated prior to the diagnosis due to developmental delay, and a program was well established. The parents had support of family in the area and were compliant with home exercise recommendations. Mom worked full time, and Dad traveled on his job 2 days/week.

Today AR is 16 years old and walks independently short distances with a reverse rollator walker. She demonstrates timing issues with over- and under-targeting, difficulty with muscle grading interfering with smooth motor execution, and muscle stiffness in all extremities with the right side more involved than the left. AR requires extended processing time, which also influences her

motor planning skills. She remains at high risk for falling. Mom is still working full time, and Dad travels 2 days a week for his job spending 1 night a week out of town during those days. It has been difficult to keep her therapy at 1 day a week, so recently her therapy was reduced to every other week.

Refer to Videos 10.5A–C. Take note in these videos of AR's general movement strategies during gait, transitions, and targeting. Begin to list her strengths and weaknesses related to her impairments and limitations. Use Fig. 10.7 to record your data as you observe AR's movement.

Prioritize your findings. What did you identify as her strong foundation on which to develop your plan of care and to base your goals? Does AR have righting, equilibrium, and/or protective extension reactions? Does AR have midrange control, eccentric control, end range control? What skills does she demonstrate independently? What are the impairments that limit her activities? With her age in mind, what are the issues you see for her in the area of participation in her community?

View Video 10.5D. Note in the video an example of treatment ideas for this child that emphasizes balance, weight shift, reaching outside her base of support, targeting, and problem solving—making this a complex task. How could this activity transfer to something in her own environment? Due to her age and the limited "free time" of the family, home exercises are rarely able to be carried out. What would you suggest to this family that would be beneficial for AR outside of therapy?

CASE STUDY 10.2

WT was born full term with heart complications leading to the need for open heart surgery at 6 days old, placement on the Berlin Heart at 2 months old, and a heart transplant at 9 months old. While on the Berlin Heart, WT had a blood clot travel to his brain causing a cerebral infarction, which resulted in a later diagnosis of spastic left hemiplegic cerebral palsy.

At 9 years of age, WT is now status post left Achilles tendon release and serial casting to promote improved left ankle range of motion. He presents with posturing of the left lower extremity in plantarflexion, mild knee flexion, hip internal rotation, as well as right weight shift with left hip hike and maintenance of left hand in a fisted position. This is clearly demonstrated in the first picture of him standing on the half-BOSU in Fig. 10.44. What impairment should be addressed first? Is the plantar flexed left foot and left hip hike due to the right weight shift or the other way around? Do you feel weakness or lack of proprioception/sensation of the left foot or extremity is more of a factor in his posturing and positioning during standing?

During a recent treatment session, WT participated in an intervention where he alternated between playing the goalie and the soccer kicker. Refer to Videos 10-6A and B for video clips on this patient. Bilateral 0.5-lb ankle weights were donned throughout the task, and he was asked to only dribble and kick with his left leg. Would the ankle weights worn in this task be more beneficial for strengthening or for body awareness? Although using only the left leg for kicking and dribbling encourages a right weight shift, which is already his preference, what are the benefits for performing this task?

See the final two pictures for after-session stance on both a solid surface and the unstable surface performed at the beginning of the session (Figs. 10.45 and 10.46). What are the differences noted? Was the intervention successful? Which aspects of the task impacted WT's impairments the most?

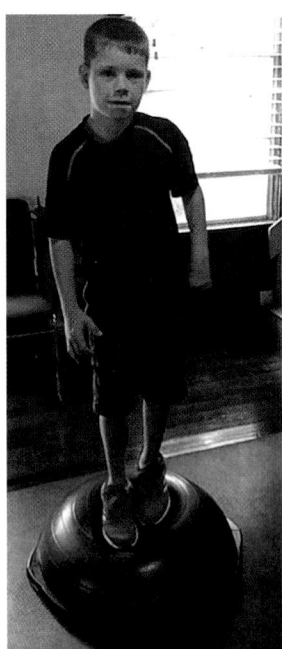

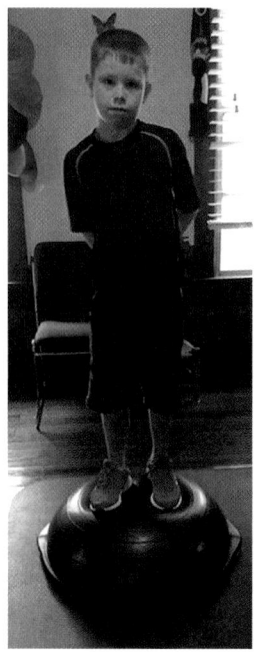

Fig. 10.44 WT (Case Study 10.2) prior to therapy intervention. Note the asymmetry as he stands on an unstable surface (BOSU) and posturing of his left arm. His weight is shifted toward his stronger side. *BOSU,* Both sides up.

Fig. 10.46 WT (Case Study 10.2) after intervention on the unstable surface of the BOSU. Although his weight is more equally distributed over both lower extremities, there is a slight lateral lean to the right. In spite of this he takes more weight through the left leg compared to preintervention. *BOSU,* Both sides up.

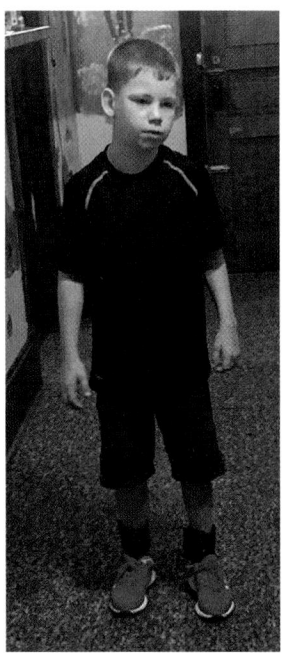

REFERENCES

To enhance this text and add value for the reader, all references are included on the companion Evolve site that accompanies this textbook. This online service will, when available, provide a link for the reader to a Medline abstract for the article cited. There are 236 cited references and other general references for this chapter, with the majority of those articles being evidence-based citations.

DEDICATION

This chapter is dedicated to Christine Nelson—master clinician, true friend, and mentor. Her gifts as a clinician and artistic eclectic approach to the treatment of children were unmatched and often seemed beyond what one could comprehend. She has forever changed those she touched and enlightened all those she taught. Christine will be forever missed, and yet her gift of touch will be everlasting and live on in her patients, students, and friends.

Fig. 10.45 WT (Case Study 10.2) after therapy intervention on a level stable surface. Note a more symmetrical distribution of his weight over both lower extremities.

11

Genetic Disorders: A Pediatric Perspective

Sandra G. Reina-Guerra and Eunice Yu Chiu Shen

OBJECTIVES

After reading this chapter the student or therapist will be able to:

1. Describe the main types of genetic disorders and give an example of each type.
2. Differentiate between genetic disorders diagnosed with clinical versus laboratory methods.
3. Describe three modes of inheritance for single-gene disorders.
4. Recognize key impairments common to many genetic conditions in pediatric patients.
5. Explain the physical or occupational therapist's role in the recognition, referral, and multidisciplinary management of genetic conditions in pediatric patients.
6. Identify resources and strategies for use in clinical decision making, accessing information, and increasing knowledge about genetic disorders.
7. Explain why it is important to include family members in the planning and development of therapy programs for children with genetic disorders.
8. Describe and give examples of three types of assessment tools and state the intended purpose of each.
9. Describe the importance of developing therapy programs for children that are outcome-focused and emphasize functional skills in natural environments.

KEY TERMS

evaluation	genetic disorders	occupational therapist
functional skills	natural environments	physical therapist

The era of genomic medicine has arrived; however, its impact on health care delivery for pediatric patients has not yet been fully realized. Personalized medicine, now expanding to the concept of personalized physical and occupational therapy, is a challenging and exciting undertaking that incorporates evidence from population studies regarding the needs of the unique individual.[1] The Human Genome Project, completed in 2003, quantified an important measure of human "uniqueness": of our approximately 20,500 genes, we are *at least* 99.5% genetically identical to one another.[2] With so little dissimilarity, one may question the hype about a personalized health care approach. The emerging fields of epigenetics and epigenomics offer a partial explanation; though the construction of a single gene may be complex, its work can still be influenced by the chemical compounds attached to it. But does the pediatric therapist have a role in the future of personalized medicine? Professional[3,4] programs are tasked to prepare graduates to participate in translational medicine, and signs are clear that the profession is answering the call. For example, consider the research of physical therapists into mechanotransduction.[5,6] Although the task of achieving clinical competence with genetics and genomics may seem daunting, the need to do so is imperative for the practitioner. After all, the need for personalized health care is as old a concept as "nature versus nurture," and now scientific research is feeding our professional curiosity by facilitating the study of the gene-environment interactions behind many multifactorial genetic conditions.[7]

As in the past several editions of this textbook, this chapter focuses on genetic disorders in children that result in a wide variety of health conditions and associated movement limitations. The impact of such conditions on the child may be evident before or immediately after birth, whereas other conditions may not be diagnosed until later in life, when problems manifest. This chapter provides an overview of common neurological disorders of known genetic origin that pediatric physical and occupational therapists are likely to encounter. Tools such as vocabulary, illustrations, and internet-accessible resources are provided to help clinicians recall basic principles of genetic inheritance and genomics. Case studies are given to provide examples of clinical decision making, including diagnosis, therapy assessment, and prognosis. Last, this chapter includes highlights of advancements in genetics research ranging from the completion of the 2003 Human Genome Project[2] through the present day. See Box 11.1 for a time line of milestones in genetics and genomic research, including gene therapy.

GENOMIC CONSIDERATIONS FOR PEDIATRIC THERAPISTS

An accurate diagnosis of a specific genetic condition is necessary to inform prognosis, as a basis for genetic counseling for the child's family, and often to establish eligibility for therapy and education services.[8]

BOX 11.1   Modern Advancements in Genomics

Human Genome Project, 1990–2003
The 3 million base pairs in human DNA were sequenced; that is, all genes of the human genome were identified and mapped.

1990: Gene Therapy Clinical Trials
The first clinical trial of gene therapy in the United States was approved for the treatment of inherited retinal dystrophy, a single-gene disease.

1995: Genetic Disabilities
The Americans with Disabilities Act (ADA) was extended to ban discrimination in the workplace based on genetic information.

2004: American Physical Therapy Association–Normative Model of Physical Therapist Professional Education
This model states that graduates of physical therapy programs are expected to use their knowledge of genetics to develop prognoses following physical therapy interventions

2002–09: HapMap Project
A catalog of 1 million single-nucleotide polymorphisms (SNPs) was produced to describe patterns of human genetic variation, including risk factors for the development of disease.

2007–08: Next-Generation Genetic Sequencing
NGS increased the output of gene sequences to 70 times faster than prior methods.

2008–15: 1000 Genomes Project
Whole-genome sequencing to catalog the genetic diversity of 2500 humans from 26 global populations. Its open resource database continues to grow and is maintained by the International Genome Sample Resource (IGSR).

2012: The ENCODE Study Publishes 30 Papers, Confirming That the Human Genome Contains Over 20,000 Protein-Coding Genes
2017: US Gene Therapy
December 2016: The US Food and Drug Administration (FDA) approves Spinraza to treat spinal muscular atrophy.
August 2017: The FDA approves the first gene therapy product to treat acute lymphoblastic leukemia in patients up to 25 years of age.
December 2017: The FDA approves the first gene therapy product to treat inherited retinal dystrophy, a single-gene disease.

2017: 48th Annual Mary McMillan Lecture by Dr. Richard K. Shields
"Turning Over the Hourglass": Precision physical therapy and the relationship between movement interventions, human gene regulation, and recovery is described.

2018: National Institutes of Health ALL OF US Research Program–Genomics Working Group
Goal to recruit 1 million US research subjects from diverse backgrounds in order to compile longitudinal health data and promote advancements in precision medicine.

The diagnostic process for genetic disorders includes a combination of clinical assessments by the physician, who collects the child's medical history, and a clinical geneticist, who may construct a family history or "pedigree" to recognize disorders with familiar inheritance patterns. Physical therapists are ideally trained and positioned to contribute to the diagnosis of genetic movement disorders. They are professionally trained to observe, quantify, and interpret human movement across the life-span.[9] Furthermore, pediatric therapists such as those in early intervention (EI) practice have the rare opportunity to spend extended time in the observation and therapeutic handling of involved infants and young children as they develop. Pediatric therapists' evaluations include a comprehensive subjective evaluation, including family history, time line and course of the movement difficulty, a summary of body systems screening, quantified and qualified descriptions of the movements based on expected developmental performance, and measurements of the functional severity of the movement problem(s). Therapists cluster signs and symptoms of medical conditions and diseases and integrate those findings with observed movement to inform the next steps of medical diagnosis, which in many cases may lead to genetic testing.[10]

Genetic tests of varying complexity will be used to confirm a clinical diagnosis, differentiate between diagnoses with similar clinical presentations, and identify the genetic causes of disorders. Pediatric therapists should be prepared to use their knowledge of genetics to contribute clinical evidence that will assist the diagnostic process and choose targeted therapeutic interventions consistent with precision health care.[6,7,11–20] Some genetic disorders are not easily identified, resulting in delayed diagnosis.[21–23] Laboratory testing can be expensive, prolonged, and often inconclusive; therefore pediatricians may refer children to occupational and physical therapy before the nature of their condition is fully known.[8,11–13] Patients are sometimes far removed from hospitals and specialized centers that perform genetic testing and diagnosis; therefore the pediatric therapist is often the first resource to whom families turn for help. Furthermore, many genetic diseases and syndromes are increasingly survivable into adulthood; thus it is vital that physical and occupational therapists incorporate knowledge of the genetic mechanisms that influence disease states and achieve competence in genetics and genomics to deliver care throughout the patient's life-span.[6,11–16]

AN OVERVIEW: CLINICAL DIAGNOSIS AND TYPES OF GENETIC DISORDERS WITH REPRESENTATIVE CLINICAL EXAMPLES

Genetic disorders are typically divided into four categories: chromosomal disorders, single-gene (monogenetic) disorders, multifactorial inheritance disorders, and mitochondrial disorders. **Chromosomal disorders** arise when there is an alteration in either the number or structure of an autosomal or sex (X, Y) chromosome.[21] Numerical or large structural chromosomal abnormalities can be seen through a microscope; therefore a sample of the patient's peripheral blood can be used to detect disorders such as Down syndrome (Fig. 11.1). When there is a suspicion of a clinical spectrum associated with some of the known chromosomal microdeletions, translocations, or inversions, direct deoxyribonucleic acid (DNA) analysis techniques such as fluorescence in situ hybridization (FISH) and microarrays can identify the defective genes and gene products.[21]

Monogenetic disorders are defects of one of the approximately 20,000 protein-coding genes[2,24]; a single gene may be responsible for approximately 6000 known genetic traits.[23] Approximately 4000 of these known traits are diseases or disorders.[22] Indirect DNA analysis techniques such as linkage analysis can be performed to confirm single-gene disorders when the gene or genomic region

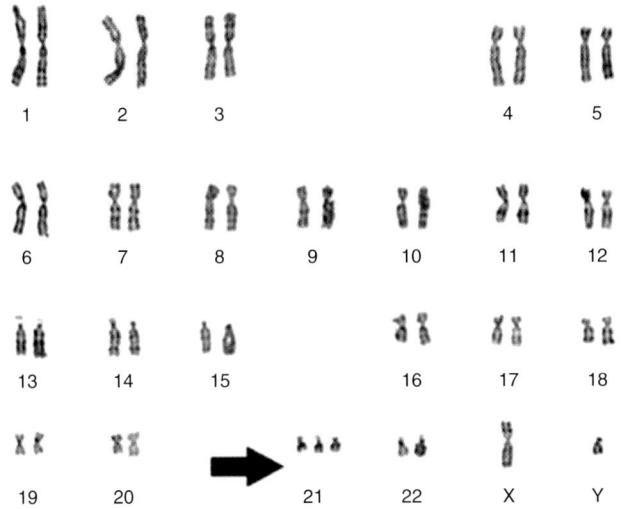

Fig. 11.1 Chromosomes of a child with Down syndrome, (From https://openi.nlm.nih.gov/detailedresult?img=PMC3232533_IPC-4-3-g004&req=4.)

associated with the disorder is unknown.[16] Single-gene disorders may be transmitted through three different patterns: autosomal dominant, autosomal recessive, and sex-linked. *Dominant* refers to the case in which a mutated gene from one parent is sufficient to produce the disorder in offspring. *Recessive* refers to the case in which the disorder will not be expressed unless the offspring inherits a mutated copy of that gene from both parents. It is incorrect to say that a *gene* is recessive or dominant; rather the *trait* or disorder is dominant or recessive.[21]

Inheritance is usually a term reserved for the transmission of a previously recognized family trait to subsequent offspring. However, many genetic disorders arise from new, spontaneous mutations in a *gamete,* the single egg cell from the mother or a sperm cell from the father. The remainder of the gametes of either parent is most likely normal. In the case of a germline mutation, the offspring will be the first in the family to display the *sporadic* or de novo disorder, and the faulty gene can then be passed onto subsequent generations. A disorder that results from a single copy of a mutated gene is referred to as a *dominant* disorder even if it is acquired by a spontaneous mutation. Not all literature sources will include spontaneous mutations in the description of *inherited* disorders.

It is important to understand how a disorder was acquired because the relative risks to other offspring for the disorder vary according to the mode of transmission. For example, the risk of having another child with the same genetic disorder that occurred as a result of a spontaneous mutation is low. However, when one parent is affected by an inherited dominant mutation, the risk of passing that faulty gene onto each child is 50%.[21]

Multifactorial Inheritance Disorders

Most congenital malformations and many serious diseases that have an onset in childhood or adulthood are not caused by single genes or chromosomal defects but rather by a combination of small inherited gene variants acting together with environmental factors.[21,22]

Mitochondrial disorders are caused by alterations in genes that control mitochondrial function (i.e., converting food into energy). Mitochondrial DNA (mtDNA) codes for about 37 genes; mutations are transmitted by maternal inheritance. Mutations in nuclear DNA may follow an autosomal dominant, recessive, or X-linked pattern of inheritance. The clinical manifestations of mitochondrial genetic disorders are extremely variable in severity and timing of presentation. Organs having high energy demand—such as the heart, brain, and skeletal muscle—are more commonly affected than others. The incidence is reportedly 1 in 6000 live births and 1 in 5000 adults.[25] Nongenetic testing includes tests of urine, blood, and spinal fluid as well as muscle biopsy, magnetic resonance imaging (MRI) of the brain and spine, and whole-exome sequencing. Next-generation gene sequencing has led to the discovery of new nuclear genes linked to these disorders. Hence, it was found that disorders arising in children are more often due to mutations in nuclear DNA than mitochondrial DNA; the opposite appears to be true in cases of adult-onset disease.

Currently genetic testing is available for more than 2000 conditions in 500 US laboratories, including samples obtained directly from health care consumers.[26] Specific DNA testing may soon be able to identify nearly all human genetic disorders. This not only allows for accurate and more complete diagnosis but also paves the way for the development of mechanisms for the treatment, cure, and prevention of certain genetic conditions.[26] Table 11.1 lists examples of specific disorders in categories of the most common pattern of inheritance by which each occurs.

Chromosomal Disorders

Cytogenics is the study of chromosomal abnormalities. A karyotype is prepared that displays the 46 chromosomes—22 pairs of autosomes arranged according to length and then the two sex chromosomes, which determine the sex. Modern methods of staining karyotypes enable analysis of the various numerical and structural abnormalities that can occur. Most chromosomal abnormalities appear as numerical abnormalities (aneuploidy) such as one missing chromosome (monosomy) or an additional chromosome, as in trisomy 21 (Down syndrome).[16] Structural abnormalities occur in many forms. They include a missing or "extra portion" of a chromosome or a translocation error, which is an interchange of genetic material between nonhomologous chromosomes. The incidence of chromosomal abnormalities among spontaneously aborted fetuses may be as high as 60%.[27] About one in 150 live-born infants has a detectable chromosomal abnormality; and in about half of these cases, the chromosomal abnormality is accompanied by congenital anomalies, intellectual disability, or phenotypical changes that manifest later in life.[27] Of the fetuses with abnormal chromosomes that survive to term, about half have sex chromosome abnormalities and the other half have autosomal trisomies.[16]

The following section provides a brief overview of common genetic disorders seen by physical and occupational therapists working with children.

Autosomal Trisomies

Trisomy is the condition of a single extranuclear chromosome. Trisomies occur frequently among live births, usually as a result of failure of the parental chromosomes to disjoin normally during meiosis. Trisomy can occur in autosomal or sex cells. Trisomies 21, 18, and 13 are the most frequently occurring; however, few children with trisomies 18 and 13 survive beyond 1 year of age.[27]

TABLE 11.1 Partial Listing of Pediatric Genetic Conditions

Syndrome or Disease	Approximate Incidence (United States)
Chromosomal Abnormalities	
Autosomal Trisomy	
Trisomy 21	1:740
Trisomy 18	1:5000
Trisomy 13	1:16,000
Sex Chromosome Aneuploidy	
Turner syndrome	1:2500 females
Klinefelter syndrome	1:500–1000 males
Partial Deletion	
Prader-Willi syndrome	1:10,000–30,000
Angelman syndrome	1:12,000–20,000
Cri-du-chat syndrome	1:20,000–50,000
Single-Gene Abnormalities	
Autosomal Dominant	
Neurofibromatosis type 1	1:3500
Tuberous sclerosis	1:5800
Osteogenesis imperfecta	6–7:100,000
Autosomal Recessive	
Cystic fibrosis	1:2500–3500 Caucasians (highest ethnic incidence)
Spinal muscle atrophy	1:6000–10,000
Phenylketonuria	1:10,000–15,000
Hurler syndrome	1:100,000
Sex-Linked	
Duchenne muscular dystrophy	1:3500
Fragile X syndrome	1:4000 males, 1:8000 females
Hemophilia A	1:4000–5000 males
Rett syndrome	1:10,000–22,000 females
Multifactorial Abnormalities	
Cleft lip with or without cleft palate	1:1000
Clubfoot (talipes equinovarus)	1:1000
Spina bifida	7:10,000
Mitochondrial Abnormalities	
Mitochondrial myopathy	Rare
Kearns-Sayre disease	Rare

Trisomy 21 (Down syndrome). Trisomy 21 occurs in approximately 1 in every 700 live births,[28] and its incidence is distributed equally between the sexes.[28] The pathophysiological features of Down syndrome are caused by an overexpression of genes on human chromosome 21. Ninety-five percent of individuals have an extra copy in all of their body's cells. The remaining 5% have the mosaic and translocation forms. In the United States, the incidence of Down syndrome increases with advanced maternal age.[28] Detection of Down syndrome is possible with various prenatal tests, and the diagnosis is confirmed by the presence of characteristic physical features present in the infant at birth.[29] Down syndrome is the most common chromosomal cause of moderate to severe intellectual disability.[29] The typical phenotypical features observable from birth are hypotonia, epicanthic folds, flat nasal bridge, upward-slanting palpebral fissures, small mouth, excessive skin at the nape of the neck, and a single transverse palmar crease (Fig. 11.2).

Information compiled by the Centers for Disease Control and Prevention during 1968-2007 indicates that the median survival age of individuals with Down syndrome is 47 years, compared with 1 year in 1968. Improvements in the median survival age were less in races other than white, although the reasons for this remain unclear.[28] Half of all children with Down syndrome have congenital heart defects.[28,29] Congenital heart problems, respiratory infection, and leukemia are the most common factors associated with morbidity and mortality in childhood, whereas a possible increased tendency for premature cellular aging and Alzheimer disease may account for higher mortality rates later in life.[30]

Impairments of visual and sensory systems are also common in individuals with Down syndrome. As many as 77% of children with Down syndrome have a refractive error (myopia or hyperopia), astigmatism, or problems in accommodation.[31] Hearing losses that interfere with language development are reportedly present in 80% of children with Down syndrome. In most cases the hearing loss is conductive; in up to 20% of cases the loss is sensorineural or mixed.[32,33] Obstructive sleep apnea has been reported to exist frequently in young children[32] and adults with Down syndrome.[34] Craniofacial impairments such as a shortened palate and midface hypoplasia—along with oral hypotonia, tongue thrusting, and poor lip closure—frequently result in feeding difficulties at birth.[35] Bell and colleagues studied the prevalence of obesity in adults with Down syndrome and reported it in 70% of male subjects and 95% of female subjects.[36] Children with Down syndrome also appear to have a higher risk of being overweight or obese,[33,37,38] which may be partly a result of the retarded growth and endocrine and metabolic disorders associated with trisomy 21.[33] In a small population study of children with Down syndrome, Dyken and co-workers[39] reported that there was a high prevalence of obstructive sleep apnea associated with a higher body mass index.

Children with Down syndrome may have musculoskeletal anomalies such as metatarsus primus varus, pes planus, thoracolumbar scoliosis, and patellar instability and have an increased risk for atlantoaxial dislocation,[40–42] which has been observed through radiography in up to 10% to 30% of individuals with this syndrome,[40,41] with and without neurological compromise.[43] There is some controversy in the medical community regarding the necessity and efficacy of radiographic screening for the instability.[41,42] Proponents of radiographic screening argue that neurological symptoms of atlantoaxial instability may often go undetected in this population because symptoms are masked by the wide-based gait and motor dysfunction already associated with the disorder. If the child is unable to verbalize complaints or is uncooperative with physical and neurological examinations, symptoms may be missed. There is particular concern about cervical instability if these children undergo surgical procedures requiring general anesthesia[42] and participate in recreational sports such as the Special Olympics.[41] Symptomatic instability can result in spinal cord compression, leading to myelopathy with leg weakness, decreased walking ability,[43] spasticity, or incontinence. Although reportedly rare,

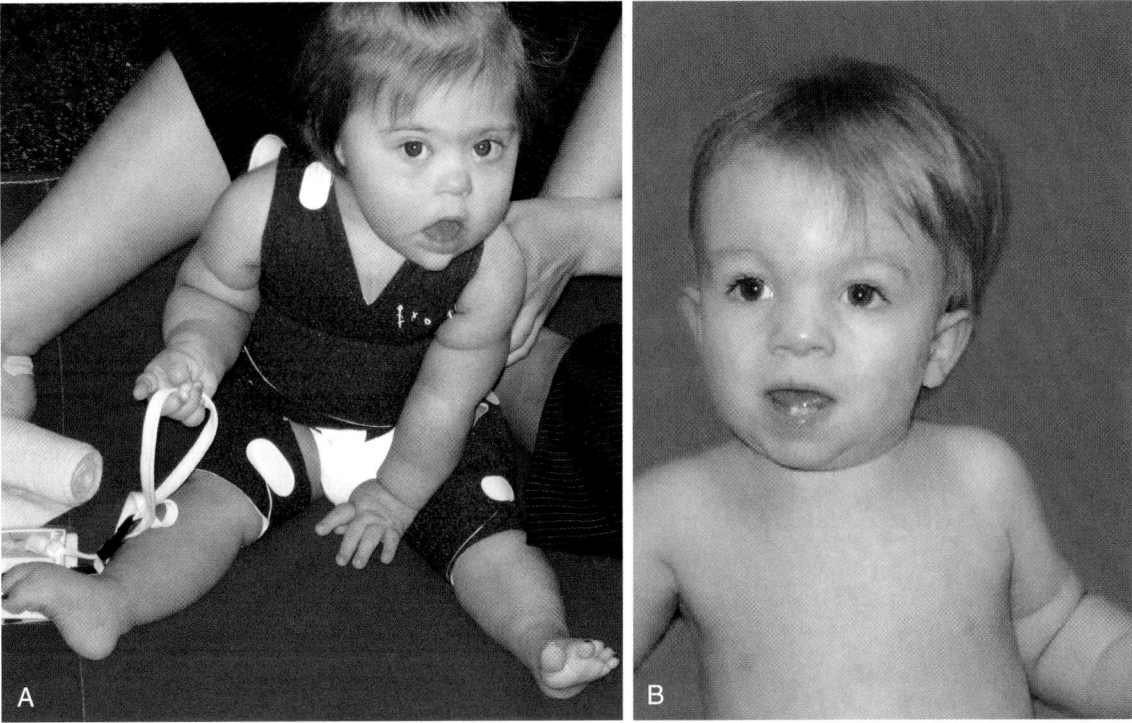

Fig. 11.2 (A) A 10-month-old girl with Down syndrome. **(B)** A 21–month-old boy with the mosaic form of trisomy 18. (Reprinted with permission of Tucker ME, Garringer HJ, Weaver DD. Phenotypic spectrum of mosaic trisomy 18: two new patients, a literature review, and counseling issues. *Am J Med Genet A.* 2007;143:505–517.)

there have been cases where atlantoaxial dislocation has resulted in quadriplegia.[40]

Several researchers have explored the neuropathology associated with Down syndrome. Changes in brain shape, size, weight, and function occur during the prenatal and infant development of babies with Down syndrome, with important differences apparent by 6 months of age.[44] The relatively small size of the cerebellum and brain stem was reported by Crome and Stern in the 1970s.[45] Marin-Padilla[46] studied the neuronal organization of the motor cortex of a 19-month-old child with Down syndrome and found various structural abnormalities in the dendritic spines of the pyramidal neurons of the motor cortex. He suggested that these structural differences may underlie the motor incoordination and intellectual disability characteristic of individuals with Down syndrome. Loesch-Mdzewska[47] also found neurological abnormalities of the corticospinal system (in addition to reduced brain weight) in his neuropathological study of 123 individuals with Down syndrome aged 3 to 62 years. Crome[48] reported lesser brain weight in comparison with normal persons. Finally, Benda[49] noted a lack of myelinization of the nerve fibers in the precentral area, frontal lobe, and cerebellum of infants with Down syndrome. According to McGraw,[50] the amount of myelin in the brain reflects the stage of developmental maturation. The delayed myelinization characteristic of neonates and infants with Down syndrome is thought to be a contributing factor to the generalized hypotonicity and persistence of primitive reflexes characteristic of this syndrome.

Trisomy 18. Trisomy 18, or Edwards syndrome, is the second most common of the trisomic syndromes to occur in term deliveries, although it is far less prevalent than Down syndrome. It occurs in one in 5000 newborns, and approximately 80% of affected infants are female.[51] As with Down syndrome, advanced maternal age is positively correlated with trisomy 18. Most cases of Edwards syndrome occur as random events during the formation of reproductive cells; fewer cases occur as errors in cell division during early fetal development; and inherited, translocation forms rarely occur.[51] Only 10% of infants born with trisomy 18 survive past the first year of life; female and non-Caucasian children survive the longest.[52] The survival of girls averages 7 months, and the survival of boys averages 2 months.[52] Individuals surviving past infancy most often have the mosaic form, and there is high variance in phenotype (see Fig. 11.2).[53]

Individuals with trisomy 18 generally have far more serious organic malformations than seen in those with Down syndrome.[54] Typical malformations affect the cardiovascular, gastrointestinal, urogenital, and skeletal systems. Infants with trisomy 18 have low birth weight and small stature, with a long narrow skull, low-set ears, flexion deformities of the fingers, and rocker-bottom feet. Muscle tone is initially hypotonic, but it becomes hypertonic in children with longer than the typical life-span.[54] The period of hypertonicity in the early years may change to low tone and joint hyperextensibility by preschool and school age. Microcephaly, abnormal gyri, cerebellar anomalies, myelomeningocele, hydrocephaly, and corpus callosum defects have been reported in individuals with trisomy 18.[55]

Common skeletal malformations that may warrant attention from the developmental physical or occupational therapist include scoliosis,[55] limited hip abduction, flexion contractures of the fingers, rocker-bottom feet, and talipes equinovarus.[54] Infants with trisomy 18 may also have feeding difficulties as a result of a poor suck.[56] Profound intellectual disability is another clinical factor that will affect the developmental therapy programs for children with trisomy 18.[55,56]

Trisomy 13. Trisomy 13, also commonly called *Patau syndrome,* is the least common of the three major autosomal trisomies, with an incidence of one in 10,000 to 20,000 live births [21,51] As in the other trisomic syndromes, advanced maternal age is correlated with the incidence of trisomy 13.[57] Fewer than 10% of individuals with trisomy 13 survive past the first year of life[51,52]; girls and non-Caucasian infants appear to survive longer.[51,52] Individuals surviving past infancy most often have the mosaic form, and there is high variance in phenotype.[52] As with Edwards syndrome, most cases of Patau syndrome occur as random events during the formation of eggs and sperm, such as nondisjunction errors during cell division.[57]

Trisomy 13 is characterized by microcephaly, deafness, anophthalmia or microphthalmia, coloboma, and cleft lip and palate.[57] As in trisomy 18, infants with trisomy 13 frequently have serious cardiovascular and urogenital malformations and typically have severe to profound intellectual disability.[58] Skeletal deformities and anomalies include flexion contractures of the fingers and polydactyly of the hands and feet.[7] Rocker-bottom feet have also been reported, although less frequently than in individuals with trisomy 18. Reported central nervous system (CNS) malformations include arhinencephalia, cerebellar anomalies, defects of the corpus callosum, and hydrocephaly.[59]

Sex Chromosome Aneuploidy

The human X chromosome is large, containing approximately 5% of a human's nuclear DNA. The Y chromosome, much smaller, contains few known genes.[21] Females, with genotype XX, are mosaic for the X chromosome, meaning that one copy of their X chromosome is inactive in a given cell; some cell types will have a paternally derived active chromosome and others a maternally derived X chromosome. Males, with genotype XY, have only one copy of the X chromosome; therefore diseases caused by genes on the X chromosome, called *X-linked diseases* (see section on sex-linked disorders), can have a devastating impact in males and less severe in females.[21] In the presence of abnormal numbers of sex chromosomes, neither male nor female individuals will be phenotypically normal.[21] Two of the most prevalent sex chromosome anomalies are Turner and Klinefelter syndromes.

Turner syndrome. Turner syndrome affects females with monosomy of the X chromosome. The syndrome, also known as *gonadal dysgenesis,* occurs in one in 2500 live female births.[60,61] Turner syndrome is the most common chromosomal anomaly among spontaneous abortions.[62,63] Most infants who survive to term have the mosaic form of this syndrome, with a mix of cell karyotypes, 45,X and 46,XX. The *SHOX* gene, found on both the X and Y chromosomes, codes for proteins essential to skeletal development. Deficiency of the *SHOX* gene in females accounts for most of the characteristic abnormalities of this disorder.[61-64] Three characteristic impairments of the syndrome are sexual infantilism, a congenital webbed neck, and cubitus valgus.[65] Other clinical characteristics noted at birth include dorsal edema of hands and feet, hypertelorism, epicanthal folds, ptosis of the upper eyelids, elongated ears, and shortening of all the hand bones.[60,66] Growth retardation is particularly noticeable after the age of 5 or 6 years, and sexual infantilism—characterized by primary amenorrhea, lack of breast development, and scanty pubic and axillary hair—is apparent during the pubertal years. Ovarian development is severely deficient, as is estrogen production.[67] Congenital heart disease is present in 20% to 30% of individuals with Turner syndrome,[66] with a smaller number of cardiovascular malformations in individuals with the mosaic form[68]; 33% to 60% of individuals with Turner syndrome have kidney malformations.[60] Hypertension is common even in the absence of cardiac or renal malformations.[66-69]

There are numerous types of skeletal anomalies, some of which may be significant enough to require the attention of a pediatric therapist. Included among these are hip dislocation, pes planus and pes equinovarus, dislocated patella,[60] deformity of the medial tibial condyles,[55] idiopathic scoliosis,[66] and deformities resulting from osteoporosis.[66]

Sensory impairments include decrease in gustatory and olfactory sensitivity[70,71] and deficits in spatial perception and orientation,[70] and up to 90% of adult females have moderate sensorineural hearing loss. Recurrent ear infections are common and may result in future conductive hearing loss.[69] Although the average intellect of individuals with Turner syndrome is within normal limits, the incidence of intellectual disability is higher than in the general population.[54] Noonan syndrome, once thought to be a variant of Turner syndrome, has several common clinical characteristics; however, advancements in genetics research have shown that the syndromes have different genetic causes.[72,73]

Klinefelter syndrome. Klinefelter syndrome, which occurs in males, is an example of aneuploidy with an excessive number of chromosomes. The most common type, 47,XXY, is usually not clinically apparent until puberty, when the testes fail to enlarge and gynecomastia occurs.[74] Nearly 90% of males with Klinefelter syndrome possess a karyotype of 47,XXY, and the other 10% have variants.[75] The incidence of Klinefelter syndrome (XXY) is about one in 500 to 1000 males, and an estimated half of 47,XXY conceptions are spontaneously aborted.[16] The extra X chromosome(s) can be derived from either the mother or the father, with nearly equal occurrence.[76] Advanced maternal age is widely accepted as a causal factor.[21,75] FISH analysis of spermatozoa from fathers of boys with Klinefelter syndrome suggests that advanced paternal age increases the frequency of aneuploid offspring.[77-79]

Most individuals with karyotype XXY have normal intelligence, a somewhat passive personality, and a reduced libido. Eighty-five percent of individuals with nonmosaic karyotype are sterile. Individuals with karyotypes 48,XXXY and 49,XXXXY tend to display a more severe clinical picture. Individuals with 48,XXXY karyotype usually have severe intellectual disability, along with multiple congenital anomalies, including microcephaly, hypertelorism, strabismus, and cleft palate.[74] Skeletal anomalies include radioulnar synostosis, genu valgum, malformed cervical vertebrae, and pes planus. According to a 2010 systematic review of the literature,[80] the neurocognitive outcomes of people with Klinefelter syndrome include problems of delayed walking in children, persistent deficits in fine and gross motor development, and problems in motor planning.[80,81] Giedd and co-workers published the results of a case-control study examining brain magnetic resonance imaging (MRI) scans of 42 males with Klinefelter syndrome in which they found cortical thinning in areas of the motor strip associated with impaired control of the upper trunk, shoulders, and muscles involved in speech production.[82]

Partial Deletion Disorders

Deletions are examples of mutations that cause changes in the sequence of DNA in human cells. A sequence change that affects a gene's function can cause the final protein product to be altered or not produced at all.

Cri-du-chat syndrome. Cri-du-chat syndrome, also referred to as *cat-cry syndrome* and *5p minus syndrome,* results from a partial deletion of the short arm of chromosome 5. Example nomenclature for a female with this syndrome is (46,XX,del[5p]). The incidence of the syndrome is estimated to be one case per 20,000 to 50,000 live births.[83] Although approximately 70% of individuals with cri-du-chat syndrome are female, there is an unexplained higher prevalence of older males with this disorder.[84] Advanced parental age is not a causal factor. A study completed in 1978 indicated that life expectancy was 1 year for 90% of infants born with this disorder, but now life expectancy is nearly normal with routine medical care.

Primary identifying characteristics at birth include a definitive high-pitched catlike cry, microcephaly, evidence of intrauterine growth retardation, and subsequent low birth weight.[85] Abnormal laryngeal development accounts for the characteristic cry, which is present in most individuals and disappears in the first few years of life. Other features of individuals with this syndrome include hypertelorism, strabismus, "moon facies," and low-set ears.[85] Associated musculoskeletal deformities include scoliosis, hip dislocations, club feet, and hyperextensibility of the fingers and toes. Muscular hypotonicity is associated with this syndrome, although cases with hypertonicity have also been noted.[86] Also, severe respiratory and feeding problems have been reported. Postnatal growth retardation has been documented, with the median near the fifth percentile of the normal growth curve.[87]

Although intellectual disability and physical deformities are more severe with larger deletions,[83] there is evidence that, with early developmental intervention, these children can develop language, functional ambulation, and self-care skills.[88,89]

Prader-Willi syndrome and Angelman syndrome. Prader-Willi syndrome (PWS) and Angelman syndrome (AS) are discussed together because they result from a structural or functional loss of the PWS and AS region of chromosome 15 (15q11-13), which can occur by one of several genetic mechanisms.[90,91] PWS has an incidence of 1 in 15,000 to 30,000,[90] and AS has an incidence of 1 in 12,000 to 20,000.[90,91] These two syndromes illustrate the effect of *genomic imprinting,* which is the differential activation of genes of the same chromosome and location, depending on the sex of the parent of origin (Fig. 11.3).[16]

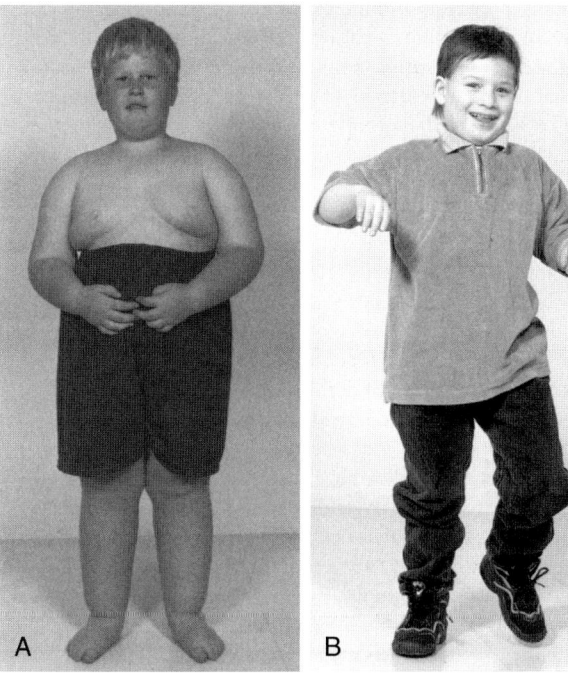

Fig. 11.3 The Effect of imprinting on chromosome 15 deletions. (A) Inheritance of the deletion from the father produces Prader-Willi syndrome. **(B)** Inheritance of the deletion from the mother produces Angelman syndrome. (From Jorde L, Carey J, Bamshad M, et al. *Medical Genetics.* 3rd ed. St. Louis: Mosby; 2005.)

PWS results from a failure of expression of paternally inherited genes in the PWS region of chromosome 15.[90] Conversely, AS results when the maternal contribution in the 15q11.2-q13 region is lost.[91] *OCA2* is a gene located within the PWS and AS region of chromosome 15 that codes for the protein involved in melanin production. With loss of one copy of this gene, individuals with PWS or AS will have light hair and fair skin. In the rare case that both copies of the gene are lost, these individuals may have a condition called *oculocutaneous albinism* type 2, which causes severe vision problems.[91]

Characteristics of PWS in infancy include hypotonia, poor feeding, lethargy, and hypogonadism.[92,93] Developmental milestones in the first 2 years of life are not acquired until approximately twice the normal age.[94,95] Between 1 and 4 years of age, hyperphagia is apparent; if uncontrolled, it will lead to morbid obesity and its associated health complications.[93–96] Most individuals with PWS have mild to moderate intellectual disability, although some have IQ scores within normal limits.[97] Maladaptive behaviors such as temper tantrums, aggression, self-abuse, and emotional lability have been reported.[98] As a result of extreme obesity, many individuals with PWS have impaired breathing, which can produce sleepiness, cyanosis, cor pulmonale, and heart failure.[98] Scoliosis is common but does not appear to be related to obesity.[99]

Clinical diagnosis is confirmed by laboratory genetic testing techniques, including DNA-based methylation testing, FISH probe, and pyrosequencing assays.[93,100] Most cases of PWS are caused by random mutations in parental reproductive cells[94]; others may result from translocation errors.[93,101] Parental studies are important in translocation cases because 20% of those cited in the literature involved familial rearrangements, which may significantly increase the risk of recurrence.[102]

Angelman syndrome, named after Harry Angelman, who first described children with AS in 1965, is characterized by developmental delay or intellectual disability, seizures, ataxia, progressive microcephaly, and severe speech impairments. Tongue thrusting, drooling, and sucking and swallowing disorders occur in 20% to 80% of these children. Individuals often display spontaneous bouts of laughter accompanied by hand-flapping movements and a characteristic walking posture of arms overhead and flexed elbows.[16,91,103] Infants with AS appear normal at birth, but severe developmental delay becomes apparent by 6 to 12 months of age. More unique features of the disorder do not appear until after 1 year of age. Children with AS typically have structurally normal brains on MRI and computed tomography (CT) scans, but electroencephalogram (EEG) findings are often abnormal, showing a characteristic pattern that may assist with diagnosis before other clinical symptoms emerge[91,104]; molecular studies can also confirm the disorder before all of the clinical criteria for this diagnosis are met.[91]

Most cases of AS occur as a result of mutations involving deletion or deficient function of the maternally inherited *UBE3A* gene. This gene codes for ubiquitin protein ligase, an enzyme involved in the normal process of removing damaged or unnecessary proteins from healthy cells. In most of the body's tissues except the brain, both copies (maternal and paternal) of the *UBE3A* gene are active. Only the maternal copy of the gene is normally active in the brain, so if this copy is absent or deficient, the normal cellular housekeeping process breaks down.[91] The risk of having another child with AS can vary from 1% to 50% depending on which of the six known genetic mechanisms is responsible for the disorder.

Translocation Disorders

Translocation errors have been identified in many childhood hematological cancers and sarcomas.[105,106] Such errors are also commonly seen in couples with infertility.[107] Translocation abnormalities occur when genetic material is exchanged and rearranged between two nonhomologous chromosomes (those not in the same numbered pair). The structural abnormality can result in the loss or gain of chromosomal material (an unbalanced arrangement) or no loss or gain of material (a balanced arrangement). Unbalanced arrangements can produce serious disease or deformity in individuals or their offspring. Carriers of balanced arrangements—estimated at one in 500 individuals—often have a normal phenotype, but their offspring may have an abnormal one.[16] There are two basic types of translocations: reciprocal and robertsonian. Reciprocal translocations occur when two different chromosomes break, and the genetic material is mutually exchanged. A robertsonian translocation occurs when there is a break in a portion of two different chromosomes, with the longest remaining portions of both chromosomes forming a single chromosome. The shorter portions that break usually do not contain vital genetic information; therefore the individual may be phenotypically normal.[16] An example notation of a reciprocal translocation is 46,XY,t(7;9)(q36;q34). This individual is male with a normal number of chromosomes but a translocation of genetic material on chromosomes 7 and 9; "q" refers to the short arm of these chromosomes, and the numbers "36" and "34" refer to the location.

Translocations occur in children seen in therapy settings, including about 3% to 5% of children with Down syndrome, and they are found in 40% of all cases of acute lymphoblastic leukemia (ALL).[108]

Acute lymphoblastic leukemia. ALL accounts for one-fourth of all childhood cancers, and it is the most common type of childhood cancer.[109–111] ALL occurs when the DNA of immature lymphoblasts is altered and they reproduce in abnormal numbers, crowding out the formation of normal cells in the bone marrow.[109,112] Sixty percent of cases of ALL occur in children, with the peak incidence in the first 5 years of life. A rise in the incidence of ALL has been reported during major periods of industrialization worldwide[112,113] and is hypothesized to be associated with exposure to radiation[114] and other environmental teratogens[115,116] in the preconception, gestational, and postpregnancy periods.[110,113]

With advancements in medical treatment protocols for pediatric patients, 5-year survival rates have improved to 80%.[111] Children aged 1 to 9 years at diagnosis have a better prognosis than infants, adolescents, or adults diagnosed with ALL.[110] Survival rate statistics since the approval of the gene therapy drug *tisagenlecleucel* for children and adults up to age of 25 years with B-cell ALL are expected to change from previously reported survival rates. Numerous forms[117] of translocation mutations are associated with ALL. Some translocation forms of ALL do not respond well to combination chemotherapy treatment; an example is the translocation that occurs between chromosomes 9 and 22, known as the Philadelphia chromosome.[111,118] Other translocations that result in hyperdiploidy (more than 50 chromosomes)—in particular within chromosomes 4, 10, and 17—may confer a more favorable outcome.[119]

Frequent diagnosis is made when a physician relates the child's history of a persistent viral respiratory infection with other characteristic clinical signs and symptoms consistent with hematopoietic leukemia. The key symptoms of ALL are pallor, poor appetite, lethargy, easy fatigue and bruising, fever, mucosal bleeding, and bone pain.[106] A complete blood count will show a shortage of all types of blood cells, including red, white, and platelets. Diagnosis is confirmed by the presence of lymphoblasts in bone marrow. Radiographs may be necessary to determine metastases, and cerebrospinal fluid will be examined as early involvement of the CNS has important prognostic implications.[113] Cytogenetic studies will be performed to aid in the selection of treatment protocols and determination of prognosis.[111]

Referral to physical and occupational therapists is made for other common problems such as muscle cramps, muscle weakness, impaired gross and fine motor performance, decreased energy expenditure, osteopenia, and osteoporosis.[120]

Monogenetic Disorders

The previous section described genetic disorders that occur because of chromosomal abnormalities involving more than one specific gene. Other genetic disorders commonly seen among children in a therapy setting include those that result from specific gene defects, also known as single-gene disorders. The inheritance patterns of single-gene traits were described by Gregor Mendel in the 19th century. These patterns—autosomal dominant, autosomal recessive, and sex-linked—are discussed separately, and specific examples of syndromes or disorders associated with each type are presented.

Autosomal Dominant Disorders

Mutations on one of the 22 numbered pairs of autosomes may result in isolated anomalies that occur in otherwise normal individuals, such as extra digits or short fingers. Each child of a parent with an autosomal dominant trait has a 50:50 chance of inheriting that trait.[21] Other autosomal dominant disorders include syndromes characterized by profound musculoskeletal and neurological impairments that may require intervention from a physical or an occupational therapist. Three examples of autosomal dominant disorders are osteogenesis imperfecta (OI), tuberous sclerosis, and neurofibromatosis (NFM).

Osteogenesis imperfecta. OI is a spectrum of diseases that result from deficits in collagen synthesis associated with single-gene defects, most commonly of *COL1A1* and *COL1A2,* which are located on chromosomes 17 and 7, respectively.[121] OI is characterized by brittle bones resulting from impaired quality, quantity, and geometry of bone material and hyperextensible ligaments.[122,123] Deafness, resulting from otosclerosis, is found in 35% of individuals by the third decade of life.[54] New knowledge about this disease from molecular genetic studies and bone histomorphometry has expanded the classification subtypes of OI into types I through VIII.[121,124] These classifications are helpful in determining prognosis and management, although there is a continuum of severity of clinical features and much overlap in the features among the different classifications.[124] Types I, IV, V, and VI occur in the autosomal dominant pattern, whereas type VII occurs as a recessive trait and types II and III can occur as either dominant or recessive traits.[121] OI types V and VI account for only 5% of cases, and type VII has been found only in Native Canadian population to date.[124] In 2007, an autosomal recessive OI, designated type VIII, was characterized by white sclerae, severe growth deficiency, extreme skeletal undermineralization, and bulbous metaphyses.[23] This section compares and contrasts only types I through IV.

The overall incidence of OI is one in 10,000 live births in the United States, with types I and IV accounting for almost 95% of all patients with OI.[121] Ninety percent of dominant forms of OI can be confirmed by DNA analysis.[124] Type I is the least severe form, followed by types IV and III, with type II being the most severe.

Type I is characterized by blue sclerae, mild to moderate bone fragility, joint hyperextensibility, and hearing loss in young adulthood.[124] There are no significant deformities; individuals with this type may not sustain fracture until they are ambulatory, and the incidence of fractures decreases with age.[124] Type IV OI is characterized by more severe bone fragility and joint hyperextensibility than in type I. Bowing of long bones, scoliosis, dentinogenesis imperfecta, and short stature are common.[122,124,125]

Children with type IV OI are often ambulatory but may require splinting or crutches.[122]

Children with type III OI have severe bone fragility and osteoporosis; often there are fractures in utero. Type III occurs primarily in autosomal dominant inheritance in North Americans and Europeans.[124] The less frequent autosomal recessive form of OI, type III, is characterized by progressive skeletal deformity, scoliosis, triangular facies, large skull, normal cognitive ability, short stature, and limited ambulatory ability.[122,124,126] The long bones of the lower extremities are most susceptible to fractures, particularly between the ages 2 to 3 years and 10 to 15 years,[54] after which the frequency of fractures diminishes. Intramedullary rods inserted in the tibia or femur may minimize recurrent fractures.[33]

Type II, the most severe form, is most often lethal before or shortly after birth, although there are a few cases of children living up to 3 years.[124,126] Infants with type II OI have multiple fractures, often in utero, and underdeveloped lungs and thorax; therefore many die from respiratory complications soon after birth. Most type II cases are the result of spontaneous mutations. As only one copy of the gene is sufficient to cause the disorder, it is still commonly classified as an autosomal dominant condition. There are fewer cases of autosomal recessive inheritance.[16]

Prevention of fractures is an important goal in working with individuals with OI, but fear of handling and overprotection by caregivers may limit a child's optimal functional independence. Caregiver education in careful handling and positioning should begin in the patient's early infancy, and training in the use of protective orthoses and assistive devices is appropriate from the period of crawling through ambulation.[123,124127], Aquatic therapy can be a valuable treatment strategy for children with OI.[124,127]

Tuberous sclerosis complex. Tuberous sclerosis complex (TSC) is characterized by a triad of impairments: seizures, intellectual disability, and sebaceous adenomas; however, there is a wide variability in expression, with some individuals displaying skin lesions only.[128] Infants are frequently normal in appearance at birth, but 70% of those who go on to show the complete triad of symptoms display seizures during the first year of life. Although tuberous sclerosis is inherited as an autosomal dominant trait, 86% of cases occur as spontaneous mutations, with older paternal age being a contributing factor. TSC affects both sexes equally, with a frequency of one in 5800 births.[129] Mutations in the *TSCI* and *TSC2* genes are known to cause tuberous sclerosis. The normal function of these genes is to regulate cell growth; if they are defective, cellular overgrowth and noncancerous tumor formation can occur.[129] Tumor formation in the CNS is responsible for most of the morbidity and mortality due to TSC,[129] followed by renal disease associated with the formation of benign angiomyolipomas.[128] Diagnostic criteria for TSC have been established, and the determination can be made clinically; results of genetic testing are currently viewed as corroborative.[128] Hypopigmented macules are often the initial finding. These lesions vary in number and are small and ovoid. Larger lesions, known as *leaf spots,* may have jagged edges.[129] Sebaceous adenomas first appear at the age of 4 to 5 years, with early individual brown, yellow, or red lesions of firm consistency in the nose and upper lip. These isolated lesions may later coalesce to form a characteristic butterfly pattern on the cheeks. Also known as hamartomas (tumor-like nodules of superfluous tissue), the skin lesions are present in 83% of individuals with tuberous sclerosis.[47]

Delayed development is another characteristic during infancy,[130] particularly in the achievement of motor and speech milestones. Cerebral cortical tubers are present in over 80% of patients and account for cognitive disability, including autism.[128] Ultimately 93% of individuals who are severely affected will have seizures, usually of the myoclonic type, in early life, progressing in later life to grand mal seizures. Seizure development is the result of formation of nodular lesions in the cerebral cortex and white matter.[47] Tumors are also found in the walls of the ventricles. Neurocytological examination reveals a decreased number of neurons and an increased number of glial cells and enlarged nerve cells with abnormally shaped cell bodies. Surgical excision of seizure-producing tumors has been successful in some cases.[128]

Other associated impairments include retinal tumors and hemorrhages, glaucoma, and corneal opacities.[129] Cyst formation in the long bones and in the bones of the fingers and toes contributes to osteoporosis. Cardiac and lung tissues are also affected by TSC, and these effects are included in the major diagnostic criteria.[128]

Neurofibromatosis. Three genetically distinct disorders that cause tumors to grow in the nervous system compose the neurofibromatosis group. There are three recognized forms of NFM: neurofibromatosis 1 (NFM1), neurofibromatosis 2 (NFM2), and schwannomatosis.[131–133] This section focuses on NFM1 and NFM 2. Neurofibromas[134] or connective tissue tumors of the nerve fiber fasciculus impede the development and growth of neural cell tissues[132,133] and are the hallmark feature of NFM1. Neurofibromas are noncancerous, and malignant changes are rare in children,[135] but an increased risk of malignancy has been observed in adult patients with NFM1, and this is a major contributor to decreased average life expectancy, which is shortened by approximately 15 years.[136] Tumors typically increase in number with the rising age. About half of all cases of NFM are caused by a sporadic mutation in parental germ cells or during fetal development.[131–133] Schwannomas are the main tumor type of NFM2 and classically appear bilaterally on the vestibular nerves.[133,137] NFM1 is also known as *von Recklinghausen disease.* Compared with type II, type I is more common (one per 3000 births)[132] and usually identified in younger children. It is associated with mutations in the *NF1* gene, which produces a protein called neurofibromin, the complete function of which is not yet understood. However, it is suspected to be a tumor suppressor. Diagnostic criteria for NFM1 include the presence of two of the following features: six or more café-au-lait spots, two or more fibromas, freckling in the axillary or inguinal region, optic pathway glioma, two or more Lisch nodules, specific osseous lesions, and a first-degree relative with NFM1.[132] Infants usually appear normal at birth, but initial café-au-lait spots appear by the age of 3 years in 95% of affected individuals (Fig. 11.4).[138] Cognitive impairment is the most common

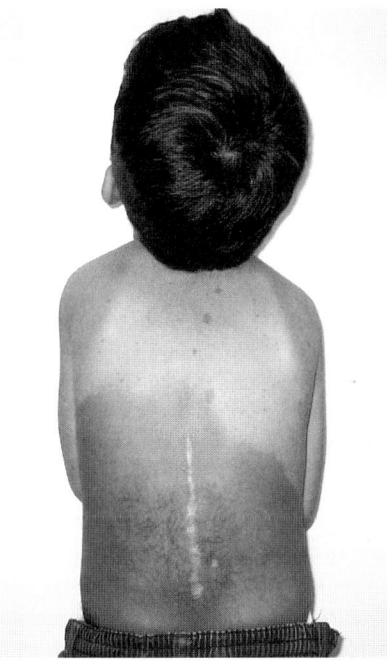

Fig. 11.4 A 4-year-old boy with neurofibromatosis and the characteristic café-au-lait spots on his trunk.

neurological complication of NFM1[138] and is postulated to be caused by altered expression of neurofibromin in the brain and/or by brain lesions, which appear hyperintense on MRI.[138] These focal areas of high signal intensity on T2-weighted MRI, known as *unidentified bright objects* (UBOs), are seen in 60% of children and young adults with NFM1. These lesions—commonly found in the basal ganglia, internal capsule, thalamus, cerebellum, and brain stem[135,139]—tend to disappear in adulthood and often do not cause other overt neurological symptoms.[135] Fewer than 10% of these individuals are mentally retarded, but about 30% to 60% of affected children have mild and nonprogressive learning disabilities.[135,140] Poorer social skills and differences in personality, behavior, and quality-of-life perception have been reported in children with NFM1 compared with children without the disorder.[132]

In older children and adolescents, pain, itching, and stinging can occur from cutaneous neurofibromas. In approximately half of all patients, neurological motor deficits occur from plexiform neurofibromas when the growth puts pressure on peripheral nerves, spinal nerve roots, and the spinal cord.[138] One percent to 5% of children aged 0 to 6 years develop symptoms associated with optic pathway glioma.[132,135] Neurofibromatous vasculopathy interferes with arterial and venous circulation in the brain.[132,138,141] Hydrocephalus occurs in some individuals.[132,135] Hypertension is common and may develop at any age,[132] and cardiovascular disease is a major cause of premature death.[136,138,142] Headaches are a commonly reported symptom in children, adolescents, and adults with neurofibromatosis.[132,134,143,144]

Scoliosis may develop in 10% of patients and is rapidly progressive from ages 6 to 10 years, or it may manifest in a milder form without vertebral anomalies during adolescence.[132] Other skeletal deformities include pseudarthrosis of the tibia and fibula, tibial bowing, craniofacial and vertebral dysplasia, rib fusion, and dislocation of the radius and ulna.[132] Differences in leg length[132] have also been noted and may contribute to scoliosis. NFM2 occurs less frequently than NFMI (one in 25,000 to 40,000 births)[7] and is caused by a mutation in the gene encoding the protein neurofibromin 2, also called *Merlin*. Merlin is produced in the nervous system, particularly in Schwann cells that surround and insulate the nerve cells of the brain and spinal cord. Although type II shares characteristics with type I, it is commonly characterized by tumors of the eighth cranial nerve (usually bilateral), meningiomas of the brain, and schwannomas of the dorsal roots of the spinal cord. Contrary to first descriptions of NFM1 and NFM2, café-au-lait spots are seldom a singular feature of NFM2[133]; rather, signs and symptoms of tinnitus, hearing loss, and balance dysfunction usually appear during adolescence or in early 20s.[131,133] Problems with visual acuity caused by strabismus and refractive errors are common in young children.[145] NFM2 may be underrecognized in children up to 10 years of age because early hearing loss and tinnitus are present in only 20% of cases; otherwise only singular features of the condition are observed. Infants may have cataracts, and children may demonstrate unilateral facial paralysis, eye squinting, mononeuropathy (foot or hand drop), meningioma, spinal tumor, or cutaneous tumor. It is recommended that children of parents with NFM2 should be considered to be at 50% risk for NFM2 and screened from birth.[124]

Autosomal Recessive Disorders

An unaffected carrier of a disease-causing trait is *heterozygous* for the abnormal gene (possessing one normal and one mutated copy of the gene). If both parents are unaffected carriers of the gene, each of their offspring has a 25% risk of exhibiting the disorder.[21] Consanguinity involving close relatives increases the chance of passing on autosomal recessive traits.[21] Certain types of limb defects, familial microcephaly, and a variety of syndromes are passed on through autosomal recessive

genes. Four examples of autosomal recessive disorders affecting children in therapy settings are presented in this section: cystic fibrosis (CF), Hurler syndrome, phenylketonuria (PKU), and spinal muscle atrophy (SMA).

Cystic fibrosis. CF is one of the most common autosomal recessive disorders and is more often seen in Caucasians, affecting one in 2000 to 4000. The CF gene has been mapped to chromosome 7 and its protein product, CF transmembrane regulator (CFTR).[21] CFTR is involved in the regulation of chloride channels of the bowel and lung, which are dysfunctional in patients with CF. Although CF has markedly variable expression, the overall median survival time has improved from about 6 years of age in the 1940s to an average of 36 years of age in 2006.[146] In addition to the phenotypical features of CF, diagnosis of CF is made when two or more disease-causing mutations exist on the CTFR gene.[146] Newborn screening tests for CF are required in all states in the United States.[147]

Fibrotic lesions of the pancreas cause pancreatic insufficiency in the majority of patients, which leads to chronic malnutrition. Ten percent to 20% of newborn infants with CF also have intestinal tract involvement with a meconium ileus. The sweat glands are commonly affected; high levels of chloride found in the sweat are the basis for the sweat chloride test used in diagnosis. The most serious impairment in CF is obstruction of the lungs by thick mucus, which leads to chronic pulmonary obstruction, infections that destroys lung tissue, and eventual death from pulmonary disease in 90% of these individuals.[21]

Improved survival rates in recent decades are the result of improved antibiotic management, aggressive chest physical therapy, and pancreatic replacement therapy. Postural drainage, percussion, vibration, and breathing exercises are key components of the management program provided by the therapist and caregivers.[148] Modern and less labor-intensive devices such as those that provide positive expiratory pressure (PEP device) may not be as effective at clearing secretions as conventional chest physiotherapy,[148] but patient and caregiver compliance with a regular program may be improved.[149] Attention to diet is important, and every attempt should be made to maintain a routine exercise program with a goal of helping the children be more active to improve their respiratory status and prevent secondary impairments of adolescence and adulthood, such as stress incontinence in young women caused by excessive coughing,[150,151] chronic back pain, and osteopenia and osteoporosis.[152] New gene therapy research in the United Kingdom to treat CF appears promising; however, application of its results has not been approved to date.[153]

Massery[150] describes the relationship between respiration, postural control, and secondary impairments in the musculoskeletal and neuromuscular systems that develop in individuals with CF. She addresses the threefold problems faced by such patients: (1) lung dysfunction leading to increased respiratory demand, (2) increased workload of respiration as a deforming force on the immature musculoskeletal frame, and (3) resultant impaired motor strategies for postural control during physical activity. Patients were once widely cautioned to avoid overexertion and fatigue with exercise, but as they are living longer, more evidence supports the benefits of regular, even vigorous exercise for children and adults with CF. Guidelines for exercise frequency and intensity have been published by the Association of Chartered Physiotherapists in Cystic Fibrosis.[154]

Hurler syndrome (mucopolysaccharidosis I, severe type). Hurler syndrome is an inborn error of metabolism that results in the abnormal storage of mucopolysaccharides in many different tissues of the body.[104] The incidence is estimated to be 1 in 100,000 live births for the severe forms[7] and 1 in 500,000 for milder forms.[155] *IDUA* is the only gene currently known to be associated with this multisystemic disorder.[155]

Infants born with Hurler syndrome are usually normal in appearance at birth, may have inguinal or umbilical hernias,[155] and may have higher birth weights than their siblings. Symptoms of this progressively debilitating disease usually appear during the latter half of the first year of life,[155] with the full disease picture apparent by 2 to 3 years of age.[155] Diagnosis is made by identification of deficiency in lysosomal enzymes.[155,156] Premature death, usually from cardiorespiratory failure, occurs within the first 10 years of life.[155]

Characteristic physical features are caused by the storage of glycosaminoglycans (GAGs)[155] and include a large skull with frontal bossing, heavy eyebrows, edematous eyelids, corneal clouding, a small upturned nose with a flat nasal bridge, thick lips, low-set ears, hirsutism, and gargoyle-like facial features. Growth retardation results in characteristic dwarfism.[155] Some individuals with the physical characteristics of Hurler syndrome have normal intelligence, but most have progressive and profound intellectual disability.[155]

Spastic paraparesis or paraplegia and ataxia have been observed in individuals with Hurler syndrome.[21] Commonly reported orthopedic deformities include flexion contractures of the extremities, thoracolumbar kyphosis, genu valgum, pes cavus, hip dislocation, and claw hands as a result of joint deformities.[54] Defective ossification centers of the vertebral bodies result in spinal deformity, complications of nerve entrapment, atlanto-occipital instability, and restricted cervical range of motion.[155] Conductive and sensorineural hearing loss is common.[155] Delayed motor milestones have been noted as early as 10 months of age,[156] with severe disabilities occurring with increasing age. Adaptive equipment is often needed, and most children with Hurler syndrome become wheelchair users in their later years.[156]

Phenylketonuria. PKU is the result of one of the more common inborn errors of metabolism. Mutations of the *PAH* gene located on chromosome 12 cause a deficiency in the production of phenylalanine hydroxylase.[157] Without this enzyme there is no conversion of phenylalanine to tyrosine, resulting in an abnormally excessive accumulation of phenylalanine in the blood and other body fluids.[157,158] If untreated, this metabolic error results in mental and growth retardation, seizures, and pigment deficiency of hair and skin.[159] PKU is most prevalent among individuals of northern European ancestry, with a frequency of one in 10,000 to 15,000 births in the United States.[157] It is estimated that one of every 50 individuals is heterozygous for PKU.[21]

Children born with PKU are usually normal in appearance, with microcephaly and delayed development becoming apparent toward the end of the first year. Parents usually become concerned with the child's slow development during the preschool years.[159] If PKU is untreated, the affected child may go on to develop hypertonicity (75%), hyperactive reflexes (66%), hyperkinesis (50%), or tremors (30%)[160] in addition to intellectual disability. IQ levels generally fall between 10 and 50, although rare cases of untreated individuals with normal intelligence have been reported.[159]

A simple blood plasma analysis, which is mandatory for newborn infants in all 50 US states,[147] can detect the presence of elevated phenylalanine levels in nearly 100% of cases.[158] This test is ideally performed when the infant is at least 72 hours old. If elevated phenylalanine levels are found, the test is repeated and further diagnostic procedures are performed. Placing the infant on a low phenylalanine diet (low protein) can prevent the intellectual disability and other neurological sequelae characteristic of this disorder.[159] Follow-up management by an interdisciplinary team consisting of a nutritionist, psychologist, and appropriate medical personnel is advised in addition to special diet. Individuals with poor compliance with the recommended diet have a greater risk of osteopenia in adulthood.[158]

Spinal muscle atrophy. SMA (5q SMA) is characterized by progressive muscle weakness due to degeneration and loss of the anterior horn cells in the spinal cord and brain stem nuclei.[161,162] Diagnosis of SMA is based on molecular genetic testing for deletion of the *SMN1* gene (named for "survival of motor neuron 1"), located at 5q13. Another gene, *SMA2,* can modify the course of SMA. Individuals with multiple copies of *SMA2* can have less severe symptoms or symptoms that appear later in life as the number of copies of the *SMN2* gene increases.[163] The overall disease incidence of SMA is 5 in 10,000 live births.[163]

The clinical classifications of SMA are still evolving.[161,162,164] At present, four subtypes (I to IV) are well accepted, and a fifth, type 0, is being explored. The subtypes are based on age at symptom onset and expectations for maximum physical function, the latter being more closely related to life expectancy.[164]

SMA type 0 is characterized by extreme muscle weakness apparent before 6 months of age that likely had a prenatal onset.[153,154] Some infants have a prenatal history of decreased fetal movements during the third trimester.[153]

SMA type I, otherwise known as *Werdnig-Hoffmann disease* or *acute infantile SMA*, has an onset before 6 months of age.[161,164] Incidence is estimated to be one in 20,000 live births. It is characterized clinically by severe hypotonicity, generalized symmetrical muscle weakness, absent deep tendon reflexes, and markedly delayed motor development. Intellect, sensation, and sphincter function, however, are normal.[161] Children usually cannot sit without support and have poor head control.[164] They have a weak cry and cough as well as problems with swallowing, feeding, and the handling of oral secretions.[162] The diaphragm is spared, but combined with weakness in intercostal muscles, infants exhibit paradoxical breathing, abdominal protrusion, as well as a bell-shaped trunk with chest wall collapse.[162] Overall, this pattern of chest wall weakness and poor respiratory function contributes to the greatly increased susceptibility to pulmonary infection, which usually results in death before the age of 2 years.[162,163]

SMA type II, otherwise known as *intermediate* or *chronic infantile SMA*, has an onset at age 6 to 18 months and is associated with delayed motor milestones.[164] Seventy percent of children diagnosed with SMA type II are alive at 25 years of age.[161]

Children with SMA type II can usually sit independently if placed but cannot stand unsupported.[162] Bulbar weakness with swallowing difficulties, poor weight gain, and diaphragmatic breathing are common.[163] Finger trembling is almost always present.[161,162] Joint contractures are present in most individuals. Severe kyphoscoliosis that requires bracing and/or surgery often develops, but patients are at risk of postanesthesia complications.[162] Respiratory failure is the major cause of morbidity and mortality. Nocturnal oxygen desaturation and hypoventilation occur before daytime hypercarbia and are early indications of the need for ventilator support.[162]

SMA type III is characterized by onset of symptoms in childhood after 18 months.[161] It is also known as *juvenile SMA* or *Kugelberg-Welander syndrome*. These individuals have a normal life-span and usually attain independent ambulation and maintain it until the third or fourth decade of life.[161] Lower extremities are often more severely affected than the arms. Strength is often not sufficient for stair climbing, and balance problems are common.[161] Muscle aches and joint overuse symptoms are frequently reported.[162]

SMA type IV typically has an onset beyond 10 years of age and is associated with a normal life expectancy and no respiratory complications.[162,164] Individuals maintain ambulation during the adult years.[162]

Variants of SMA occur in individuals with similar phenotypes and clinical diagnostic features on EMG testing that are not associated with the deletion of *SMN1*.[164] Genetic testing for *SMN* gene deletion achieves up to 95% sensitivity and nearly 100% specificity.[162] For cases that remain unclear, a clinical diagnosis may be accomplished through

EMG and muscle biopsy, which reveal neurogenic atrophy. Key physical signs are common: symmetrical weakness in the more proximal musculature versus distal and lower extremity weakness that is greater than in the arms.[162] Traditional strength measurements are not practical for children with SMA. The Gross Motor Function Measure[165] has excellent reliability on studies of gross motor evaluation in this population.[162,166] Consensus guidelines on pulmonary care, including assessment, monitoring, and treatment; feeding and swallowing and gastrointestinal dysfunction and nutrition; and orthopedic management have been published by the Standard of Care Committee for Spinal Muscle Atrophy.[162] In 2004, at the University of Massachusetts Medical School, it was discovered that the drug nusinersen (Spinraza) could treat the symptoms of SMA by correcting *SMN2* exon 7 splicing. Twelve years later, in December 2016, the drug was approved for patient use.[167] Before 2016 there were no drugs to effectively treat the symptoms of SMA.[168,169] Studies of long-term treatment efficacy of the drug will be important, with a remaining concern regarding its affordability.

Sex-Linked Disorders

The third mechanism for transmission of specific gene defects is through sex-linked inheritance. In most sex-linked disorders, the abnormal gene is carried on the X chromosome. Female individuals carrying one abnormal gene usually do not display the trait because of the presence of a normal copy on the other X chromosome. Each son born to a carrier mother, however, has a 50:50 chance of inheriting the abnormal gene and thus exhibiting the disorder. Each daughter of a carrier mother has a 50:50 chance of becoming a carrier of the trait.[21] Four syndromes that result in disability are discussed in this section: hemophilia, fragile X syndrome (FXS), Lesch-Nyhan syndrome (LNS), and Rett syndrome (RS).

Hemophilia. Hemophilia is a bleeding disorder caused by a deficient clotting process. Affected individuals will have hemorrhage in joints and muscles, easy bruising, and prolonged bleeding from wounds. The term *hemophilia* refers to hemophilia A (coagulation factor VIII deficiency) and hemophilia B or Christmas disease (coagulation factor IX deficiency). There are numerous other clotting diseases, and some that were once referred to as hemophilia are now genomically distinguished. For example, von Willebrand disease has a distinctly different genetic basis from hemophilia; it follows an autosomal recessive or autosomal dominant pattern and involves mutation of the von Willebrand factor (VWF) gene, located on chromosome 12. VWF plays a role in stabilizing blood coagulation factor VIII.[170] Hemophilia A and B occur as X-linked recessive traits owing to mutations of genes *F8* and *F9,* respectively, both of which are located on the X chromosome.[171]

Hemophilia A is reported to affect 1 in 4000 to 5000 males worldwide.[171] Hemophilia B is less common, affecting 1 in 20,000 males worldwide.[171] Hemophilia can affect females, though in milder form. The severity and frequency of bleeding in hemophilia A are inversely related to the amount of residual factor VIII (less than 1%, severe; 2% to 5%, moderate; and 6% to 35%, mild).[171] The proportions of cases that are severe, moderate, and mild are about 50%, 10%, and 40%, respectively.[172] The joints (ankles, knees, hips, and elbows) are frequently affected, causing swelling, pain, decreased function, and degenerative arthritis. Similarly, muscle hemorrhage can cause necrosis, contractures, and neuropathy by entrapment. Hematuria and intracranial hemorrhage, although uncommon, can occur even after mild trauma. Bleeding from tongue or lip lacerations is often persistent.[21]

Hemophilia is usually diagnosed during childhood, with the most severe cases diagnosed in the first year of life: bleeding from minor mouth injuries and large "goose eggs" from minor head bumps are the most frequent presenting signs in untreated children.[171] Children are especially vulnerable to bleeding episodes owing to the nature of their physical activity combined with periods of rapid growth.[171]

Treatment includes guarding against trauma and replacement with factor VIII derived from human plasma or recombinant techniques.[21] In the late 1970s to mid-1980s it was estimated that half of the affected individuals in the United States contracted hepatitis B or C or human immunodeficiency virus (HIV) infection when treated with donor-derived factor VIII. The initiation of donor blood screening and use of heat treatment of donor-derived factor VIII have almost completely eliminated the threat of infection.[21] Although replacement therapy is effective in most cases, 30% of treated individuals with hemophilia A and 3% of those with hemophilia B have neutralizing antibodies that decrease its effectiveness.[171] Before treatment with clotting factor concentrates was available, the average life expectancy was 11 years[171]; currently, excluding death from HIV, life expectancy for those with severe hemophilia who receive adequate treatment is 63 years.[171] Factor replacement therapy is credited for increasing the ease and safety of vigorous exercise and sports participation for such individuals.[173] The benefits of regular exercise are the same as those for unaffected individuals and outweigh the risks in treated persons.[174] A 2002 pilot study by Tiktinsky and colleagues[174] found decreased episodes of bleeding in a population of young adults with a long-term history of resistance training that began in adolescence.

Fragile X syndrome. FXS is the most common sex-linked inherited cause of intellectual disability, affecting 1 in 4000 males and one in 8000 females.[175] Males manifest a more severe form than females. A fragile site on the long arm of an X chromosome is present, with breaks or gaps shown on chromosome analysis. A region of the X chromosome, named *FMR1,* normally codes for proteins that may play a role in the development of synapses in the brain. Mutations of this region are errors of trinucleotide repeats, in which the number of CGG triplets at this region is expanded, thereby making the gene segment unable to produce the necessary protein.[175]

Developmental milestones are slightly delayed in affected males.[175] Eighty percent of males are reported to have intellectual disability, with IQs of 30 to 50 being common but ranging up to the mildly retarded to borderline range.[175] *Penetrance* (the proportion of individuals with a mutation that actually exhibit clinical symptoms) in the female is reported to be only 30%.[21] Other impairments include epilepsy, emotional lability, attention-deficit/hyperactivity disorder (ADHD), and clinical autistic disorder in 30% of males.[175,176] Life-span is normal for individuals with this condition.[175]

Lesch-Nyhan syndrome. Also known as *hereditary choreoathetosis,*[177] LNS leads to profound neurological deterioration. First described in 1964 by Lesch and Nyhan,[178] it is associated with a mutation in the *HPRT1* gene on the X chromosome. This gene codes for an enzyme called hypoxanthine guanine phosphoribosyltransferase, which allows cells to recycle purines, some of the building blocks of DNA and ribonucleic acid (RNA).[179] Without this gene's normal function, there is an overproduction of uric acid (hyperuricemia),[179] which accumulates in the body. High uric acid levels are thought to cause neurological damage.[177,179]

The prevalence of LNS is 1 in 380,000 individuals.[179] Females born to carrier mothers have a 25% chance of inheriting the mutation. There are rare reports of females demonstrating this syndrome as a result of X chromosome inactivation. Most female carriers are considered to be asymptomatic, but some may have symptoms of hyperuricemia in adulthood.[179]

LNS is detectable through amniocentesis, and genetic counseling is advisable for parents who have already given birth to an affected son.[180]

The prenatal and perinatal course is typical for affected individuals. Hypotonia and delayed motor skills are noticeable by the age of 3 to 6 months.[179] Dystonia, choreoathetosis, and opisthotonus indicative of extrapyramidal involvement emerge during the first few years of life.[179] Many children are initially diagnosed with athetoid cerebral palsy when pyramidal signs such as spasticity, hyperreflexia, and abnormal plantar reflexes emerge.[179] Most children never walk. A hallmark of the disease is severe and frequent self-injurious behaviors such as lip and finger biting, which emerge in almost all affected children by their third year.[179] Because of the extreme self-mutilation that characterizes this disorder, it has been questioned whether these children have normal pain perception.[181] Although they have the abnormal catecholamine metabolism seen in other patients with congenital pain insensitivity,[182] behaviors documented in children with LNS suggest that they do sense pain, demonstrated by their apparent relief when they are restrained from hurting themselves. Children may actually request the restraining device[183] even when the device may be one that would not physically prevent biting, such as a glove or bandaid.[179] A reported survey of parents of children with LNS indicated that parents often find behavioral programming techniques helpful in modifying aggression toward self or others.[183] However, there is no consensus on the best kind of behavioral treatments, as any reward, either positive or negative, may increase the frequency of self-injury.[184] Some parents have reported that they elected tooth extraction as a means to prevent biting. Other impairments in children with LNS include severe dysarthria and dysphagia. Bilateral dislocation of the hips may occur as a result of the spasticity.[179] Growth retardation is also apparent, along with moderate to severe intellectual disability. Individuals may have gouty arthritis and kidney and bladder stones.

Blood and urine levels of uric acid have been decreased successfully through the administration of allopurinol, with a resultant decrease in kidney damage. With current management techniques, most individuals survive into the second or third decade of life.[179]

Rett syndrome. RS is inherited in an X-linked pattern and affects females almost exclusively, as it is most often lethal in boys before 2 years of age. Males may inherit RS with an extra X chromosome in many or all of the body's cells.[185-188] The estimated incidence is one in 15,000 to 20,000 females[189] It has been reported that 99% of all cases of RS are the result of sporadic mutations.[188,190] Most cases of RS, called *classic RS,* are caused by mutations in the *MECP2* gene, which is responsible for directing proteins critical for normal synaptic development; however, it is unclear how these mutations lead to all the signs and symptoms of the syndrome.[188,191] Several variants of RS exist; they have overlapping features with classic RS but may have a much milder or more severe course.[188]

Classic RS is characterized by apparently normal development during the first 6 months of life, followed by a short period of developmental plateau and then rapid deterioration of language and motor skills typically occurring at 6 to 18 months of age.[188,192] Most girls survive into adulthood.[188] The hallmark of the syndrome is that during the period of regression, previously acquired purposeful hand skills are also lost and replaced by stereotypical hand movements. These nonspecific hand movements have been described as hand wringing, clapping, waving, or mouthing. Virtually all language ability is lost, although some children may produce echolalic sounds and learn simple manual signing. Evidence of minimal receptive language skills may be observed. Autistic behaviors, inconsolable crying and screaming, and bruxism are common features of individuals with RS.[188] Almost all individuals with RS function in the range of severe to profound intellectual disabilities.

Head circumference is normal at birth, and its increase may decelerate in early childhood, but microcephaly is not a consistent feature of RS.[188] Retarded growth and muscle wasting are observed in most girls, likely associated with poor food intake and gastrointestinal problems.[188]

Almost one-fourth of girls with RS never develop independent ambulation skills; otherwise the onset of walking is usually delayed until about 19 months of age.[193] Initially hypotonia may be evident, but with advancing age, spasticity of the extremities develops.[194] Increased muscle tone is usually observed first in the lower extremities, with continued greater involvement than in the upper extremities. Peripheral vasomotor disturbances, especially in the lower limbs, are often noted.[188]

Scoliosis, which is often severe enough to require surgical correction, occurs in most girls by adolescence, characterized by a long C-shaped thoracolumbar curve, kyphoscoliosis, and an early onset of posterior pelvic tilt and abducted shoulder girdles.[193,195-199] Heel cord tightening and hip instability have also been identified as areas of potential concern.[195] Abnormal EEG and seizures occur in 70% of individuals with RS in the first 5 years of life. Cranial CT results are normal or show mild generalized atrophy. Breathing dysfunction, including wake apnea and intermittent hyperventilation,[196] is also associated with RS. Interventions reported in the literature have focused on splinting,[200] behavioral modification techniques to teach self-feeding skills,[201] aquatic therapy,[202] occupational therapy,[203] music therapy,[204] physical therapy,[188,197,198,204] and the first two combined in a dual-intervention approach.[205]

Mitochondrial Deoxyribonucleic Acid Disorders

In addition to the nuclear genome, humans have another set of genetic information within their mitochondria. Nuclear genes exist in pairs of one maternal and one paternal allele. In contrast, there are hundreds or thousands of copies of mtDNA in every cell. mtDNA is small, circular, and double-stranded. It has been well studied and was mapped long before the human nuclear genome. mtDNA contains 37 genes responsible for normal function of the mitochondria in all body cells.[206] Humans inherit mtDNA maternally. It is highly susceptible to mutation, and the molecule has limited ability to repair itself. Tissues that have a high demand for oxidative energy metabolism, such as brain and muscle, appear to be most vulnerable to mtDNA mutations.[17] Normal and mutated versions of mtDNA can coexist within a patient's body, but when a certain critical number of mutations exist, the body's tissues will show clinical signs of dysfunction. These disorders affect the metabolic functions of the mitochondria, such as the generation of adenosine triphosphate, the body's energy currency. Many patients with point mutations of mtDNA exhibit symptoms in early childhood; these mutations may be the most frequent cause of metabolic abnormality in children.[17] The minimum minimal birth prevalence of childhood mitochondrial respiratory chain disorders is reported to be 6.2 per 100,000. [18,207-209] Medical intervention for mitochondrial encephalomyopathies cannot treat the underlying disease, but rehabilitative therapies have been reported to be of value.[210,211] An example of a childhood disorder that can result from an mtDNA mutation is Leigh syndrome.

Leigh Syndrome

Leigh syndrome or subacute necrotizing encephalomyopathy may also be transmitted by X-linked recessive and autosomal recessive inheritance. Approximately 20% of all cases of Leigh syndrome are caused by mitochondrial mutations.[212] The discussion in this section focuses on characteristics of mtDNA-associated Leigh syndrome.

Leigh syndrome has an onset in infancy, typically at 3 to 12 months of age. Initial features may be nonspecific, such as a failure to thrive and persistent vomiting.[212,213] It is a progressive disorder caused by lesions that can occur in the brain stem, thalamus, basal ganglia, cerebellum, and spinal cord. Common clinical features include seizures, epilepsy, muscle weakness, peripheral neuropathy, speech and feeding difficulties, gastrointestinal and digestive problems, and heart problems. Most affected children have hypotonia, movement disorders such as chorea, and ataxia. Life expectancy is 2 to 3 years; death most often results from respiratory or cardiac failure.[212]

Multifactorial Disorders

Multifactorial disorders are believed to be a result of the combined effects of mutations in multiple genes as well as environmental factors.[21] Environmental factors may be those that have an impact on a developing fetus, such as prenatal diet, or those that have an impact on humans as we age, such as cigarette smoking. Disorders in this category can result in congenital malformations such as spina bifida and clubfoot. An in-depth discussion of spina bifida can be found in Chapter 13. Management information on clubfoot can be found in pediatric textbooks that include orthopedic information.[214-217]

Many diseases such as cancer can result when the environment interacts with genetic variations that exist in all humans.[21] Scientists are exploring genetic contributions to premature births,[218,219] the leading cause of infant mortality and morbidity.[220,221] It is most likely a result of multiple genetic and environmental determinants that tend to run in families.[218,219] Premature infants are at higher risk of neurological, musculoskeletal, and respiratory problems than are term infants. Management of infants with low birth weight is discussed in Chapter 9 of this text.

BODY STRUCTURE AND FUNCTION PROBLEMS COMMON TO MANY PEDIATRIC GENETIC DISORDERS

Specific examples of genetic disorders in children were presented in the foregoing section. Although there are many disorders that physical and occupational therapists may see often, others are rare and may only be suspected based on clustered problems of body structure, function, and activity limitations. Decisions about which interventions to implement and the expected outcomes will be largely influenced by the diagnosis of the specific disorder, once attained. Many genetic conditions share in common a short list of primary problems that will negatively affect the child's physical movement and daily activities and participation, both immediately and in the long term. Table 11.2 summarizes the problems common to many genetic disorders that are most relevant for physical or occupational therapists.

The term *pediatric movement disorders* (PMDs) in the scientific literature is no longer a generic term; instead, these conditions are now defined and classified largely as a result of the work of the NIH Taskforce on Childhood Movement Disorders.[222] PMDs are classified based on movement phenomenology such as hyperkinetic movement (e.g., dystonic or tics).

PMDs have one or more of the characteristics of abnormal posturing, unintended excessive movement, movement at unintended or inappropriate time, dysfunction in the target, and velocity of an intended movement.[223,224] The knowledge of a genetic causation of PMDs is growing since the definitions of movement disorders have been clarified and their phenotypes are better understood. Specific genes are implicated in movement disorders based on how the movement appears; for example, a mutation in the PPRT2 gene (chromosome 16) is responsible for many instances of paroxysmal kinesigenic dyskinesia (PKD).[225]

Hypertonicity

Abnormalities of tone may result from dysgenesis or injury to developing motor pathways. Hypertonia is common to many motor disorders and is defined as "abnormally increased resistance to externally imposed movement about a joint."[226] Examples of externally imposed movement are passive movement by the therapist or changes in ankle and knee position resulting from ground reaction forces during ambulation. Children with hypertonus generally display stiff or jerky movements that are limited in variety, speed, and coordination. Controlled, voluntary movements tend to be limited to the middle ranges of a joint. Total patterns of flexion or extension may dominate, with limited ability for selective joint movements. The motor development of children with hypertonicity may be further complicated by the retention of primitive reflexes, which can result in stereotyped movements associated with sensory input.[226]

Sanger and colleagues[226] proposed a classification system to objectively define and distinguish different types of hypertonicity. Three general types of hypertonicity—spasticity, dystonia, and rigidity—may occur alone or in combination. Spasticity is a velocity-dependent increased resistance to muscle stretch that may occur above a given threshold of speed and/or joint angle and may depend on the direction of joint movement. Dystonia is also an involuntary alteration in the pattern of muscle activation during voluntary movement or maintenance of posture. The observable disorder is demonstrated by intermittent muscle contractions causing twisting or repetitive movement, postures, or both.[226] Dystonia may be triggered by attempts at voluntary movement or to prevent the movement of a joint (e.g., to prevent knee buckling in stance). The pattern and magnitude of the abnormal muscle activity may change with the child's arousal, emotional state, and tactile contact.[226] Rigidity is a form of hypertonus in which the speed of movement and joint angle do not affect the quality of the movement. Stiffness caused by diminished tissue length and extensibility of muscles and connective tissue is not included in the recent definitions of hypertonus but may exist alongside hypertonicity.[226,227]

Children may learn to use stereotypical patterns of movement and hypertonus to achieve functional goals by activating the muscle synergies of a reflex without sensory feedback.[228] If a goal of therapy is to facilitate functional movement that is not dominated by persistent reflexes, it is critical to practice new motor patterns to accomplish the functional activity for which that reflex is being used. The focus of therapy activities must be on active movement of the child and not on passive inhibition techniques of abnormal reflexes for the sake of "normalization" of tone and movement.[228-231]

Hypotonicity

In contrast to hypertonia, low tone or hypotonia is not clearly defined. The "floppy" infant or child is commonly characterized as having hypermobility of joints that lack resistance to passive movement, with diminished antigravity movement and postural stability. Hypotonia may occur because of central or peripheral nervous system dysfunction, as is the case in newborns with PWS and toddlers with SMA type II, respectively. Many genetic disorders are revealed in newborns based on the common features of severe, global hypotonia and low Apgar scores.[232] Retrospective studies of newborns report key features of absence of antigravity movements and decreased reflexes. The presence of fetal hypokinesia and/or polyhydramnios is reported to be predictive of neonatal hypotonia in many cases.[233] In full-term neonates with hypotonia, studies report that 30% to 60% of cases are associated with a genetic disorder. A clinical neurological examination such as described by Dubowitz and the use of dysmorphic data bases can identify the majority of cases.[233,234] First-line genetic testing is indicated in neonates with hypotonia plus facial dysmorphism or signs of peripheral hypotonia (e.g., as seen in SMA).[233]

Martin and colleagues[235] surveyed physical and occupational pediatric therapists and reported that the majority of therapists do not use formal examination methods to quantify hypotonia directly; instead, they use measurements for various expressions of hypotonia, most often muscle strength and developmental milestones. This study also confirmed that most therapists agree that children with hypotonicity have diminished postural control and thus tend to lean on supports to maintain a position. Examples of this behavior are locking out weight-bearing joints and assuming positions that provide a broad base of support to maximize their stability (Fig. 11.5). Although retention of primitive reflexes is less likely in children with hypotonia compared with those with hypertonia, delays in the development of postural reactions are a major concern. Limited strength and lack of endurance are often concerns with children who have hypotonicity. Hypotonicity and joint laxity are often associated with motor delay; however, therapists should not assume that hypotonia and joint laxity are absolutely predicative of persistent motor delay.[236] For example, many premature infants, with or without a genetic disorder, have global hypotonia at birth that resolves and does not cause long-term functional impairment.[236,237] Hypotonicity is a persistent problem in many children with developmental delay. Therapists may address hypotonia and problems of postural control with a variety of treatment modalities and techniques, including aquatic therapy,[238] hippotherapy,[239] and neurodevelopmental therapy.[240]

Hyperextensible Joints

Hyperextensible joints are commonly observed in children with hypotonicity and are noted in many children with a variety of genetic disorders, representing different underlying organ structure problems. Activities should be modified to avoid undue stress to these joints and the surrounding ligaments, tendons, and fascia. For example, positions that allow the knee or elbow joints to lock into extension should be modified so that weight bearing occurs through more neutral alignment. Varying the placement of toys and support surfaces, providing physical assistance, and using adaptive equipment can help modify weight-bearing forces to achieve more neutral alignment.[241] For example, if hyperextensibility of ligaments leads to excessive pronation in stance (Fig. 11.6), the use of ankle-foot orthoses may provide enough support to the structures to allow functional activities in standing (see the discussion of orthotics in Chapter 32). For a child who stands with knee hyperextension, a vertical stander may allow that child to stand and play at a water table with her or his classmates for extended periods with the knees in a more neutral position. Rather than restricting a child's repertoire of upright positions, it is preferable to modify an activity or provide external support to enable a child to participate fully (Fig. 11.7).[242]

Contractures and Musculoskeletal Deformities

Skeletal anomalies and deformities are associated with many genetic disorders. The therapist should be aware of factors that can contribute to the development of deformities to prevent or minimize such problems. The physical or occupational therapist may work with orthopedists, prosthetists, and orthotists to detect and prevent the progression of a variety of conditions.

Conditions that cause hypertonicity or spasticity are well known to place children at risk for joint contracture.[243] Children with hemophilia are at great risk of joint contractures associated with hemarthroses and intramuscular hemorrhages.[244] Spinal deformities, such as lumbar lordosis and thoracic kyphosis and scoliosis, are also common concerns in children with hypertonia or hypotonia. Although joint contractures are less likely to occur in a child with hypotonicity, habitual positioning may lead to soft tissue restrictions. For example, children with hypotonia often adopt a constant position of wide abduction, external rotation, and flexion at the hips ("frog" or "reverse W" position)[245]; in these children, soft tissue contractures can develop at the hips and knees. Children whose hips are maintained in a position of adduction, flexion, and internal rotation are at a risk for hip subluxation or dislocation.[245]

Deformation of the anterior chest wall and shoulder girdles may result from primary problems in the cardiopulmonary system in children with CF. When coupled with hypotonicity and poor postural control, the anterior chest wall muscles tighten as a result of the long-term rounded, internally rotated shoulders and protracted scapulas, in which case therapeutic interventions should target improving chest wall and scapulothoracic mobility as well as strengthening postural muscles (Fig. 11.8).[246–248] In general contractures and deformities are a concern for most children who display a limited variety of postures and movements. While choosing treatment techniques, therapists should consider the nature of the disorder that places the child at risk for contractures; disorder-specific techniques can be found in textbooks on pediatric occupational and physical therapy.[214,249]

Respiratory Problems

A genetic risk for respiratory distress in infancy has been suggested by reports of family clusters.[250] Furthermore, comparison of short- and long-term respiratory function in infants with respiratory distress syndrome suggests that if all other factors of nutrition, previous mechanical ventilation, and gestational development are comparable, genetic risk may account for cases of chronic and potentially irreversible respiratory failure.[250]

Respiratory problems are often observed in children with limited mobility. If the mobility impairments are the result of hypotonicity or hypertonicity, impaired respiration may be a result of chest and skeletal deformities. Many infants with genetic disorders are born prematurely and are more susceptible to respiratory problems than infants born at full term.[218,219,245] Prolonged mechanical ventilation and other medical procedures may increase the time neonates spend in the supine position, thus increasing the risk of gravity-induced deformity of the rib cage and inefficiency of the respiratory musculature.[246,251,252]

Some children may find it difficult to tolerate one position for an extended time owing to respiratory difficulties. For these children, frequent changes of position and use of adapted positioning devices may be necessary. Premature infants in the neonatal intensive care unit may benefit from regular prone positioning to facilitate restorative sleep,[252–254] improved arterial oxygen saturation,[255] and improved respiratory synchrony.[256] Children with respiratory problems may require mobilization techniques, deep breathing, chest expansion exercises, and postural drainage. In the case of children with CF, a comprehensive program of respiratory care is the primary therapeutic goal.[257]

Developmental Delay

Genetic disorders that affect neuromuscular, somatosensory, and cognitive function are frequently associated with developmental delays in children. The genetic basis for multisystem syndromes such as Down syndrome or LNS can be identified by cytogenetic and molecular techniques. Congenital malformations, hearing impairment, and mental or growth retardation are examples of common components of developmental delay that often have a genetic basis.

Developmental delay is typified by the failure to meet expected age-related milestones in one or more of five areas: physical, social and emotional, intellectual, speech and language, and adaptive life skills. Developmental milestones that are typically assessed in the first 5 years of life are listed in Box 11.2.

Physical and occupational therapists can observe the interaction between each of the five areas of development in an infant or child. For

TABLE 11.2 Characteristic Features of Selected Genetic Conditions

Genetic Condition	Typical Age at Diagnosis	Craniofacial Dysmorphism	Musculoskeletal Involvement	Neuromuscular System Involvement and Tone	Cardiopulmonary Involvement
Trisomy 21	Prenatal or infancy	Yes	Joint laxity and instability	Hypotonia	Yes
Trisomy 18	Prenatal, neonatal	Yes	Yes	Hypotonia	Yes
Turner syndrome	Infancy, adolescence; girls	Yes	Short stature, hip dislocation, scoliosis		Yes
Klinefelter syndrome	Adolescence; adulthood; males	Yes	Yes	Varies with age	
Cri-du-chat syndrome	Infancy	Yes	Yes	Hypotonia	Yes
Prader-Willi syndrome	Infancy	Yes	Scoliosis	Hypotonia	Secondary to obesity
Angelman syndrome	Infancy	Microcephaly		Hypotonia and seizures, ataxia	
Acute lymphoblastic leukemia	Childhood		Bone pain and muscle cramps		
Osteogenesis imperfecta	Varies with type and severity		Multiple fractures and muscle weakness		Yes
Tuberous sclerosis complex	Infancy, early childhood		Yes, cyst formation	Hypertonia; seizures	Yes, cyst formation
Neurofibromatosis type 1	Infancy, childhood		Yes		
Cystic fibrosis	Infancy		Chest wall deformity, muscle and bone pain		Yes
Hurler syndrome	Infancy	Yes	Yes	Yes	Yes
Spinal muscle atrophy type II	Infancy		Yes	Hypotonia	Yes
Hemophilia type A	Childhood or earlier if severe		Joint pain and hemarthroses		
Fragile X syndrome	Childhood	Yes	Joint laxity		Yes
Lesch-Nyhan syndrome	Infancy		Gouty arthritis	Varies	
Rett syndrome	Late infancy to early childhood		Scoliosis	Hypotonia, ataxia, seizures	

example, a child with severe hypotonia who has limited movement experiences will not develop a well-adapted sensory system. Children with problems processing sensory information often withdraw from social interaction, through which they would otherwise find opportunities to develop speech, language, and social skills. Dynamic systems theory[258] explains the relationship among all of these developing components in a child; language does not develop independently of gross motor skills, and the ability to feed or dress oneself is as related to social, emotional, and intellectual development as it is to fine motor skills.

Suspicion of developmental delay often leads to physician referral. An accurate medical diagnosis is important as it facilitates knowledgeable surveillance for potentially associated health problems. A delayed diagnosis can preclude timely implementation of beneficial medical, therapeutic, and educational services. Children who are identified to be at risk for developmental delay may be referred to EI programs.

Other Systemic Involvement	Other Disease Processes	Sensory Dysfunction	Motor Delay	Cognitive Delay	Hallmark Feature(s)
	Alzheimer disease, sleep apnea, obesity	Vision, hearing	Yes	Yes	Facial features, simian crease
Yes		Yes	Yes	Yes	Life-span <1 year
Distal lymphedema; reproductive system		Hearing			Webbed neck appearance and short stature
Endocrine and reproductive system			Yes	Yes	Intellectual disability; course of gonadal development
		Vision			"Cat cry"
Reproductive system	Morbid obesity	Vision	Yes	Yes	Hypotonia, obesity
			Yes	Yes	Happy demeanor, sleep disorders
	Osteopenia, osteoporosis				Lethargy, fever, respiratory infections
	Dentinogenesis	Hearing (type I)			Multiple fractures
Skin lesions, adenomas; renal disease		Vision	Yes	Yes	Sebaceous adenomas, seizures
Café-au-lait spots and cutaneous neurofibromas; vasculopathy		Vision			Café-au-lait spots, neurofibromas
Gastrointestinal system; urinary stress incontinence in females	Osteoporosis, osteopenia				Lung and digestive dysfunction
Yes		Vision, hearing	Yes	Yes	Progressive craniofacial abnormalities and developmental deterioration
Yes			Yes		Progressive loss of peripheral motor function
Skin bruising					Bleeding, bruising, joint pain, and loss of motion
		Yes		Yes	Intellectual disability, autism
Urogenital system		Yes	Yes	Yes	Self-injurious behavior, gouty arthritis
		Yes	Yes	Yes	Regressive developmental delay; stereotypical, purposeless hand movements

Examples of assessment techniques and interventions for children with developmental delay can be found in textbooks on pediatric physical therapy.[259,260]

Behavioral Phenotypes in Genetic Syndromes

Study of the cognitive and behavioral aspects of individuals with certain genetic syndromes has given rise to the term *behavioral phenotype*. Certain clusters of behavior that characterize a given syndrome can aid in the early recognition and diagnosis of a syndrome and guide in intervention. Aspects of behavioral phenotypes include social interaction, sleeping patterns, mood, attention, motivation, adaptive and maladaptive strategies, intellect, and memory.[261–265]

Down syndrome, PWS, AS, FXS, and LNS are examples of genetic disorders discussed in this chapter with delineated behavioral phenotypes.[262,263] Compulsive overeating in children with PWS, sleep disturbances in children with AS, and self-injury in children with LNS are

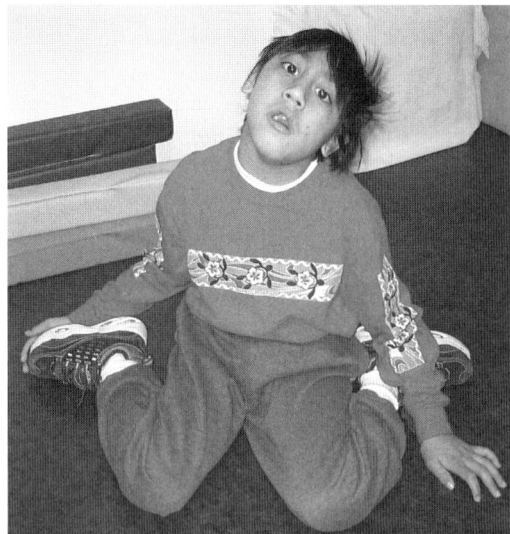

Fig. 11.5 An 8-Year-Old Boy With Hypotonia Associated With a Chromosomal Translocation Error. Note the broad base of support in this "W" sitting position.

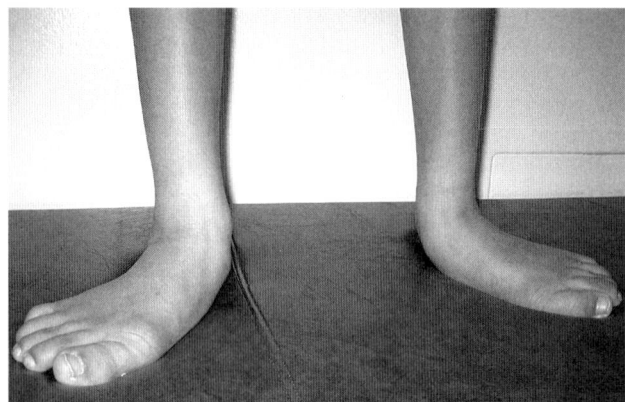

Fig. 11.6 Excessive bilateral pronation and flat feet associated with hyperextensibility in an 8-year-old boy with global hypotonia.

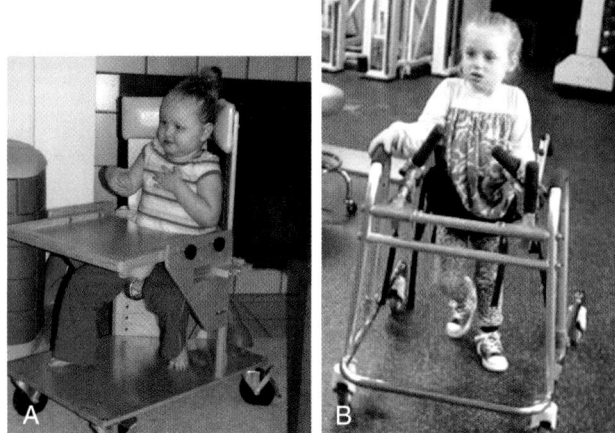

Fig. 11.7 Equipment Adapted to Promote Participation in Upright Activities for Children With Trunk Weakness and Poor Postural Control. **(A)** The corner chair gives this child with Rett syndrome the proper back support; toys can be placed within her reach on the tray. **(B)** This particular gait trainer allows appropriate patterns of weight shifting to occur while providing her with stability in the pelvis and lower trunk.

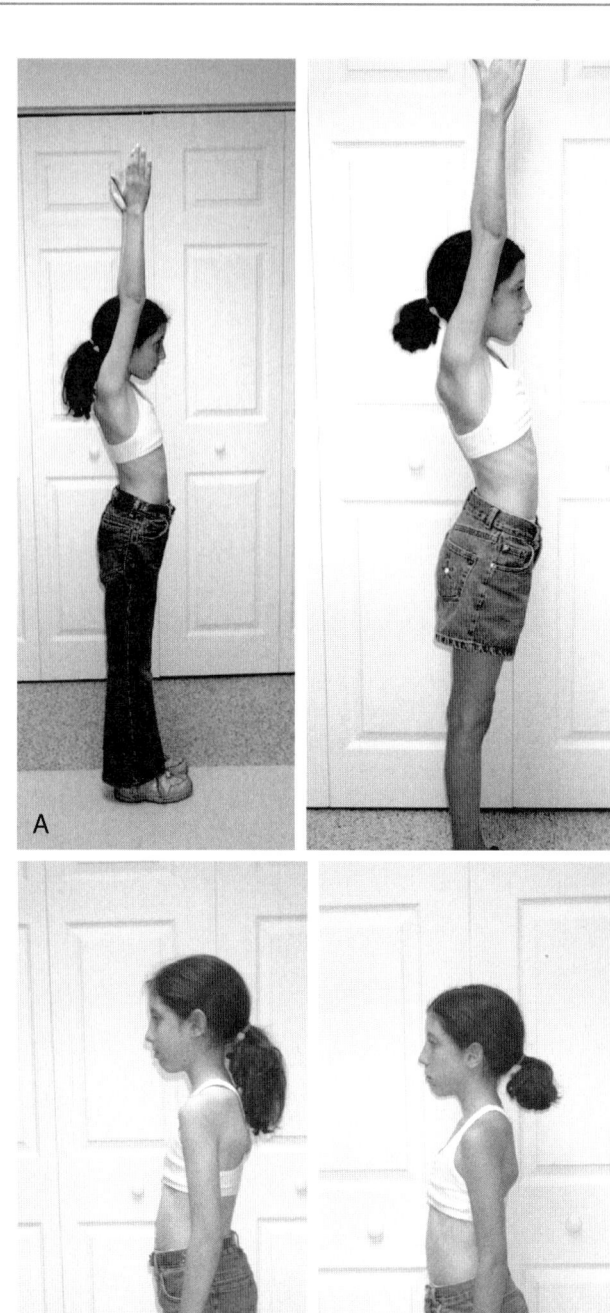

Fig. 11.8 (A) Note improved post-intervention scapular position and improved glenohumeral range of motion. **(B)** Note improved post-intervention reduction of forward-head posture and reduction of rounded shoulders.

BOX 11.2 Failure to Meet Developmental Milestones

By 1 Month

Sucks poorly and feeds slowly

Lower jaw trembles constantly even when infant is not crying or excited

Does not respond to loud sounds or bright light

Does not focus on and follow a nearby object moving side to side

Rarely moves

Extremities seem loose and floppy or very stiff

By End of Third Month

No Moro reflex

Does not notice own hands by 2 months

Does not grasp and hold objects

Eyes cross most of the time or eyes do not track well together

Does not coo or babble

By End of Fourth Month

Head flops back when infant is pulled up to sitting by his or her hands

Does not turn head to locate sounds

Does not bring object to mouth

Does not smile spontaneously

Inconsolable at night

By End of Fifth Month

Persistent tonic neck reflexes

Cannot maintain head up when placed on stomach or in supported sitting position

Does not reach for objects

Does not roll in both directions

By End of Seventh Month

Reaches with one hand only

Cannot sit with help by 6 months

Does not follow objects at a distance

Does not bear some weight on legs

Does not laugh; does not try to attract attention through actions

Refuses to cuddle; shows no affection for caregiver

By End of Twelfth Month

Does not creep on all fours

Cannot stand when supported

Does not search for toy hidden while he or she watches

Says no single words (e.g., "mama" or "dada")

Does not use gestures such as waving hand or shaking head; does not point to objects or pictures

By End of Second Year

Cannot walk by 18 months

Failure to develop heel-toe walking pattern after several months of walking

Does not speak at least 15 words by 18 months

Does not use two-word sentences by 2 years

Does not know the function of common objects (brush, telephone, spoon) by 15 months

Does not imitate actions or words; does not follow simple instructions

By End of Third Year

Frequent falling and difficulty with stairs

Persistent drooling or unclear speech

Inability to build a tower of more than four blocks

Difficulty manipulating small objects

Cannot copy a circle

Cannot communicate in short phrases

No pretend play

Little interest in other children

Extreme difficulty separating from caregiver

By End of Fourth Year

Cannot throw a ball overhand

Cannot jump in place with both feet

Cannot ride a tricycle

Cannot grasp a crayon between thumb and fingers; cannot scribble

Resists dressing, sleeping, using the toilet

Does not use sentences of more than three words; does not use "me" and "you" appropriately

Ignores other children or people outside the family

Does not pretend in play; no interest in interactive games

Persistent poor self-control when angry or upset

By End of Fifth Year

Does not engage in a variety of physical activities

Has trouble eating, sleeping, using the toilet

Cannot differentiate between fantasy and reality

Seems unusually passive or aloof with others

Cannot correctly give her or his first and last names

Does not use plurals or past tense when speaking

Does not talk about daily experiences

Does not understand two-part commands

Cannot brush teeth efficiently

Cannot take off clothing

Cannot wash and dry hands

Cannot build a tower of six to eight blocks

Does not express a wide range of emotions

Seems uncomfortable holding a crayon

---

behavioral problems that can have a significant negative impact on quality of life for children and their families. Although children with Down syndrome have fewer maladaptive behaviors than most children with intellectual disabilities,[261,263,265] they have been shown to abandon challenging tasks sooner than other children at similar developmental levels in exchange for peer social interaction.[264] Furthermore, this strength of sociability in children with Down syndrome contributes to the child's learning through modeling and peer collaboration. A knowledgeable, observant therapist can use peer groups to motivate and model for a child with Down syndrome, but he or she should also recognize that the child may be distracted by other children and default to a social strategy, thus avoiding the task at hand.[264]

MEDICAL MANAGEMENT AND GENETIC COUNSELING

The physical or occupational therapist should have general knowledge of both medical management of children with genetic disorders and genetic counseling for family members. This information allows the therapist to answer the family's general questions and refer family members to the appropriate persons for more specific information.

Medical Management

Early detection of genetic disorders has improved the health and survival of individuals with certain genetic disorders such as PKU, hemophilia, and CF. Medical treatment for the other disorders is not curative but rather palliative or directed at specific associated anomalies.

Surgical Intervention

The congenital heart defects present in many individuals with Down syndrome can in most instances be corrected by cardiac surgery.[26] Orthopedic surgery in the form of insertion of intramedullary rods in the tibia or femur may minimize the recurrence of repeated fractures associated with OI.[123,265] Surgical correction of dystrophic scoliosis may be warranted in individuals with NFM,[119] RS,[193,196,198,199,204] or Werdnig-Hoffmann disease[162] if the deformity is severe and bracing is not successful. Radiographic screening for atlantoaxial instability in children with Down syndrome can be initiated beginning at 2 years of age.[22] If atlantoaxial instability is excessive or results in a neurological deficit, a posterior fusion of the cervical vertebrae is recommended.[36] Surgical removal of obstructive or malignant tumors is advisable in certain cases of NFM and removal of cerebral nodular growths for the control of seizures in individuals with tuberous sclerosis.[128] Surgical interventions such as gastric bypass, small intestinal bypass, and jaw wiring have been attempted for weight control in children with PWS but have had limited success.[90,97]

Pharmaceutics

Second-generation bisphosphonates can reduce fracture frequency, improve bone quality, and improve outcomes after orthopedic surgery in children and lessen the severity of osteoporosis in adults.[123] Antibiotics and pneumoeustachian tubes to lessen the frequency and severity of otitis media can reduce the incidence of hearing loss in individuals with Down syndrome[26] and Turner syndrome.[66] The use of appetite-regulating drugs for individuals with PWS has had equivocal results. Reproductive hormone therapy can promote pubertal development in girls with Turner syndrome[66,69] and boys with Klinefelter syndrome.[76,266] Growth hormone has been shown to improve stature in girls with Turner syndrome.[66] The use of anticonvulsants is an important part of seizure management for individuals with RS[193,197] and tuberous sclerosis.[129] Allopurinol has been used for individuals with LNS to prevent urological complications, although it has no effect on the progressive neurological symptoms.[179] The use of large, potentially toxic amounts of vitamins and minerals (the orthomolecular hypothesis) has been proposed for children with many different types of developmental disabilities. This approach has been rejected for children with Down syndrome on the basis of the results of several investigations. In addition, supplementation of individual metabolites such as 5-hydroxytryptophan or pyridoxine for children with Down syndrome is ineffective.[267]

Pharmacogenetics is a new field of scientific research that helps provide a biochemical explanation for why some patients respond well to a medication and others with the same condition being treated do not. "Personalized medicine" is an approach whereby doctors may make decisions regarding which medications, dosages, and combinations with other drugs to prescribe based on the analysis of selected genes in their patients.[21]

The Age of Precision Medicine

Advancements in cell therapy are rapid; therefore the information describing them in this section are likely to be quickly outdated.

The purpose of gene therapy is to correct defective genes responsible for disease by replacing missing or mutated genes, changing gene regulation, or enhancing the "visibility" of disease genes to improve the body's immune response. Gene therapy trials have been approved for use in humans only on somatic cells. A vector carries the gene product to the person's cells; vectors may be either an altered virus, stem cells, or liposomes.[268]

The oversight of gene therapy falls under the US Department of Health and Human Services, which oversees agencies that, in turn, are responsible for establishing research protocols (National Institutes of Health [NIH]), evaluating investigational gene products (US Food and Drug Administration [FDA]), monitoring ethics (Recombinant DNA Advisory Committee), and educating human subjects (Office for Human Research Protections).[269] The clinical development of a gene product that could be widely dispensed must include four phases: phase 1 consists of regulatory approval of the protocol and then human pharmacology focusing on safety and tolerability and pharmacokinetics; phase 2 examines the effectiveness in terms of dose and regimen and target populations; phase 3 determines a basis for licensure and marketing of the product; and phase 4 establishes therapeutic use in a wider population.[269] A list of approved cellular and gene therapy products can be found on the US FDA's website. The interested reader can obtain an up-to-date listing of current gene therapy protocols from the NIH's Genetic Modification Clinical Research Information System (GeMCRIS) on the World Wide Web at www.gemcris.od.nih.gov/Contents/GC_HOME.asp.

In light of the limited medical treatment strategies available for children with genetic disorders, the physical or occupational therapist must be concerned with maximizing the child's developmental or functional potential within the limitations imposed by the lack of possible cures and the prospect of the shortened life-span that characterizes many of these disorders. When deterioration of skills is expected, therapy must be directed at maintaining current functioning levels, minimizing decline, and minimizing caregiver support as much as possible.

Genetic Counseling

Developmental, physical, or occupational therapists must have an understanding of the modes of inheritance of the various genetic disorders and information about the services that can be offered through genetic counseling. Although the physician has primary responsibility for informing the parents about the availability of genetic counseling, the close professional and personal relationships that therapists often develop with families may prompt family members to seek this type of information from the therapist.

Although a physical or occupational therapist cannot fill the role of a qualified genetic counselor, it is important that therapists be aware of the availability and location of genetic counseling services so that they may be assured that parents of a child with a genetic disorder have this information. Most major university-affiliated medical centers provide genetic counseling.

Process of Genetic Counseling

Six steps or procedures in genetic counseling were introduced in the 1970s by Novitski; they included descriptions of various genetic tests and a clinical interview.[270] The desired outcome of genetic counseling is to make an accurate medical diagnosis of the child's disorder. In the case of a suspected chromosomal abnormality, this usually involves determining the karyotype of the child and possibly the karyotypes of the parents. Other diagnostic procedures may include a medical examination, FISH, DNA studies, biochemical studies, muscle biopsy, and other laboratory tests.

A pedigree or family tree is constructed of all known relatives and ancestors of both parents.[270] Pedigree information includes the age at death and cause of death of ancestors, a history of stillbirths and spontaneous abortions, and a history of appearance of any other genetic defects or unknown causes of intellectual disability. The country of origin of ancestors is also important because certain genetic defects, such as PKU, are far more prevalent in families of a particular ethnic origin. Once the defect has been identified and a pedigree constructed, Novitski[270] advises that further information be obtained from one of the comprehensive resource texts on genetic disorders. Informing family members about the characteristics of the disorder and its natural history may diminish fears of the unknown.

The third procedure in genetic counseling is to estimate the risk of recurrence of the disorder.[271] In specific gene defects, the probability of recurrence is fairly straightforward, with a risk of 25% for autosomal recessive disorders and a 50% risk for each male child in sex-linked disorders. These percentages, however, do not hold true in cases of spontaneous mutations. In cases of chromosomal abnormalities such as Down syndrome, karyotyping is mandated to determine whether the child has the translocation type of Down syndrome. In that case the risk of recurrence is much greater than with a history of standard trisomy 21 Down syndrome.

Informing parents of the probability of recurrence is the next procedure. Novitski[270] points out the common misunderstanding that if a risk is one in four for a child to be affected, as in an autosomal recessive disorder, many parents assume that if they have just given birth to a child with the disorder, the next three children should be normal. It is important to explain that each subsequent child faces a one in four risk of inheriting the disorder regardless of how many siblings with the disorder have already been born. Estimating the risk of multifactorial disorders is a complex process. Although these conditions tend to cluster in families, there is no clear-cut pedigree pattern. The risk of recurrence of a multifactorial disorder is typically low, but if a couple has had two children with the same condition, the recurrence risk is presumed to be higher, with either a high genetic susceptibility or a chronic environmental insult suspected.

The fifth step in genetic counseling is for the parents to decide on the course of action they will take for future pregnancies once the counselor has presented all available facts to them.[271] Some parents may choose not to have any more children; others may elect to undergo prenatal diagnostic procedures for subsequent pregnancies. These decisions rest entirely with the parents and may be influenced by their individual religious or ethical preferences.

Follow-up counseling and review of the most recent advances in medical genetics are the final steps in the genetic counseling procedure.[270] Genetic counseling can play an important role in opening channels of communication among parents as well as other family members and their friends; connecting parents and siblings to support groups; and helping families to address their grief, sadness, or anger.[272] The effect of a child's disability on the family may modify the parents' earlier decision regarding whether to have more children. Recent medical advances may allow a more certain prenatal diagnosis of specific genetic disorders.[273,274]

Early Detection of Genetic Conditions

Diagnosis of many genetic disorders is made clinically, as in observation of a congenital malformation; however, many serious conditions are not immediately apparent after birth. Detection of genetic conditions is performed through various screening procedures, followed by specific diagnostic testing to confirm a suspected disorder. With technological advancements in genetics, these procedures have been expanded for the unborn and the newborn. Couples planning to have children can be tested for specific genetic disorders before conception or embryonic implantation.[275] Health care professionals and parents should be informed about both the positive and the negative aspects of using this new knowledge and technology. The American College of Medical Genetics has published lists of the more common reasons for genetics referral as guidelines for health care providers working with infants, children, or couples planning to have children.[276]

Newborn Screening

Routine newborn screening is required in the United States and is performed on whole populations for common disorders. The purpose of screening is the early identification of infants who are affected by a certain condition for which early treatment is warranted and available. Of the 4 million newborn infants screened each year, approximately 3000 have detectable disorders.[277] Currently all 50 states require screening for three disorders: PKU, congenital hypothyroidism, and galactosemia.[147] Some populations known to be at higher risk of certain disorders may be screened automatically, or individuals may elect state-specific screening.[277] Most states screen for eight or fewer disorders.[278] Tandem mass spectrometry (MS/MS) is a laboratory technique that allows for the identification of several metabolic disorders using a single analysis of a small blood sample drawn from the neonate. Many states use MS/MS for newborn screening for various disorders and have expanded their list of those that are mandated and those that are part of limited pilot programs.[279] Some genetic screening is performed primarily for research purposes when the disorder is not preventable, for example, type I diabetes. Screening for type I diabetes is available in some states, and early reports are that 90% of parents consent to the test.[280]

Benefits of newborn screening are earlier definitive diagnosis and medical intervention for the affected child. Concerns about expanded newborn screening include hasty medical decisions before conclusive evidence is available and parental stress because of a lag time between screening and definitive results. A study by Waisbren and colleagues[281] conducted on parents of children screened for biochemical genetic disorders recognized that parents generally reported less stress the earlier a diagnosis could be made. However, in the same study, in cases in which the test yielded a false-positive result, parents reported a higher stress index and their children were twice as likely to experience hospitalization (usually the emergency department) than in mothers of children with normal screening results.[281] In the case of a positive screening result, infants will typically undergo more definitive genetic testing.

Genetic Testing in Infants and Children

Many genetic disorders can be diagnosed by clinical criteria specific to that disorder. If a diagnosis cannot be made on the basis of the patient's clinical presentation, then genetic testing may be warranted. The number of human genes being studied for disorders, as of time of this edition, is 16,454. In more than 516 labs, there are 55,913 tests for 11,414 known conditions.

Specific information can be found at https://www.ncbi.nlm.nih.gov/gtr. In the United States, the standards and methods of all laboratories performing clinical genetic tests are governed at the federal level.[275]

Prenatal Testing

Tests to diagnose a genetic disorder in a developing fetus can be placed into two broad categories: invasive and noninvasive procedures. Currently, in contrast to the most common invasive procedures, noninvasive methods typically cannot permit a definitive diagnosis, but they can be performed with less risk to the fetus. Invasive procedures are recommended in cases of high risk for a serious disorder, when definitive diagnosis could lead to treatment, and to allow parents to make decisions about the pregnancy.[282] The ethical implications for prenatal testing are many. Parents are often given information that requires a sophisticated understanding of biology and medicine to fully clarify the implications and results of a diagnostic procedure. For example, amniocentesis can detect many chromosomal abnormalities, but the functional outcome of some disorders can have great variety.[283]

Invasive procedures. The most common prenatal diagnostic procedure is amniocentesis, which is used to detect early genetic disorders in the fetus at 11 to 20 weeks of gestation.[282] This method involves inserting a long, slender needle through the mother's abdominal wall and into the placenta to extract a small amount of amniotic fluid.[284] Laboratory tests of amniotic fluid reveal all types of chromosome abnormalities and a number of specific gene defects, including LNS, and some disorders of multifactorial inheritance, such as neural tube defects. This procedure carries a risk of miscarriage of about 0.5% to 1.7%,[285] and the risk increases the earlier that it is performed.[282]

Chorionic villus sampling involves extracting and examining a portion of the placental tissue. It has nearly a 99% detection rate for chromosomal abnormalities[282] and can be definitive earlier than amniocentesis; however, the risk of severe limb defects (amniotic band syndrome) increases the earlier that it is performed. The miscarriage rate with this procedure is estimated to be 0.5%.[282]

Noninvasive procedures. Ultrasonographic examination of a fetus has been used to identify congenital malformations since 1956. It is currently offered to most women in the United States. It is currently believed that there is no inherent risk from this procedure. First-semester sonography is performed mainly to confirm the gestational age, identify multiple pregnancy, and measure nuchal thickness (NT). NT is a measure of the subcutaneous space between the skin and the cervical spine in the fetus; increased NT is often associated with trisomies. Second-trimester ultrasonography can detect problems in the quantity of amniotic fluid, large fetal structural defects, and certain smaller defects associated with a genetic disorder. A definitive diagnosis is not made on the basis of the presence of small defects alone; rather, the findings are considered along with the other risk factors present.[286] Again, there are ethical questions about the risk to the parents (emotional stress and uncertainty) versus the benefits of early detection.

Tests of maternal serum screening done at about 15 to 20 weeks of gestation can detect chromosomal abnormalities, but their accuracy depends on many factors including gestational age, maternal weight, ethnicity, multiple pregnancy, maternal type I diabetes, and maternal smoking.[282] Finally, it is possible to perform cytogenic analysis of fetal blood cells, which can be isolated from a sample of the mother's blood; however, this requires expensive equipment and expertise.[282]

Assisted Reproductive Technology and Preimplantation Genetic Diagnosis

Couples who want to conceive often seek genetic counseling if one or more parents is aware of a familial genetic condition, if they are having difficulty conceiving, and commonly in cases of advanced maternal or paternal age. More than 1 million babies have been born worldwide as a result of in vitro fertilization (IVF).[287] IVF has enabled couples with fertility problems to conceive and more recently has been used to diagnose a genetic disease or condition in an embryo when it has differentiated into just eight cells.[288] Chromosomal abnormalities are the most commonly detected aberrations, and approximately 100 single-gene disorders have been diagnosed.[288] The ultimate purpose of preimplantation genetic diagnosis is to implant only mutation-free embryos into the mother's uterus; however, infants conceived with assisted reproductive technology (ART) are two to four times more likely to have certain types of birth defects than children conceived naturally.[287] The reasons for the increased risk of birth defects is unknown, but it may be that ART results more often in multiple births, which are at higher risk regardless of the use of ART.[287] Intracytoplasmic sperm injection (ICSI) is another form of ART used often in cases of paternal infertility. Male infertility caused by azoospermia or oligozoospermia is associated with several genetic factors, such as paternal sex chromosome aneuploidy in the case of Klinefelter syndrome.[79,289] Preimplantation genetic testing is

optional in the United States but recommended in cases of family history and in men with nonobstructive azoospermia.[289]

Ethical, Social, and Legal Issues in Genetics

Advancements in genetics have led to important ethical questions about testing and screening for genetic disorders during the course of a couple's family planning and after the birth of their child. Ethical debates about genetic testing are inevitable. The persistent ethical issue in newborn screening surrounds mandatory or voluntary approaches taken by the states.[8] All states require newborn screening, usually without parental consent for the tests. Thirty-three states have newborn screening statutes or regulations that allow exemptions from screening for religious reasons, and 13 additional states have newborn screening statutes or regulations that allow exemptions for any reason. The majority of states have statutes that contain confidentiality provisions, but these provisions are often subject to exceptions.[278]

In pediatric medicine, parents are traditionally presumed to be best suited to decide whether to pursue genetic testing. Organizations such as the American Academy of Pediatrics (AAP) have argued that parental autonomy should not be absolute in cases of life-threatening situations coupled with clear medical treatment benefit, but the AAP supports efforts to make informed parental consent a standard in the United States. Furthermore, the AAP does not support the broad use of carrier screening in children or adolescents or the position that newborn screening should be used to identify carrier status in parents of newborns identified as having disorders through newborn testing.[8] The American Society of Human Genetics has recommended that family members not be informed of misattributed paternity revealed through testing for the purpose of screening for disorders and that informed consent should include cautions regarding the unexpected finding of a different disease.[290]

Pediatricians and other health care professionals should be prepared to equip families with the appropriate information to use in the decision making process regarding genetic testing. From a medical standpoint, Ross and Moon[291] propose a decision algorithm that weighs the risks and benefits. A decision to pursue genetic testing would be advised if the child were symptomatic, had a suspected genetic condition, or was from a high-risk family; if early diagnosis would decrease morbidity or mortality; and if the testing method were considered ethical and would lead to a beneficial treatment. Last, practitioners and researchers should be prepared to educate families on the protections and limitations of the Genetic Information Nondiscrimination Act of 2008 (GINA). This federal law, which sets a nationwide level of protection for US citizens, does not preempt state law, which usually provides broader safeguards. GINA prohibits health insurers from using the results of *predictive* genetic testing done for an individual to determine policy rates for that individual or for persons in a similar population; this includes information discovered in the course of medical testing and research. However, it does not protect a person's right to insurance for a genetic illness that is diagnosed. GINA prohibits insurers from requesting or requiring that person to undergo a genetic test. It prohibits employers from requesting, requiring, or using a person's genetic information in making employment decisions, including information about the employee's family's genetic information. GINA does not apply to decisions about life, disability, or long-term care insurance, nor does it apply to members of the military.[292]

INTEGRATING GENETICS INFORMATION FOR PRACTICAL USE IN PEDIATRIC CLINICAL SETTINGS

Therapists in all settings frequently find it challenging to keep up with practice issues and the growing body of knowledge and evidence in rehabilitative medicine. In clinical settings where most of a therapist's day is spent in actual hands-on treatment, the wealth of information that is available may seem burdensome and practically inaccessible. Patients and their families will present the therapist with many questions about medical interventions, diagnostic procedures, and research. Although therapists know that a working knowledge of all of these areas is important, often time and access to resources are limited.

Pediatric therapists know the importance of collaboration with other professionals, including a type of collective knowledge about the child and his or her diagnosis, impairments, functional limitations, and quality-of-life issues identified by the family. A 1998 survey of individuals from six different health professions, including physical therapists, revealed that most professionals are not confident in their education and working knowledge in the field of genetics.[293] Additional studies have indicated that there are not enough genetic counselors[281,291] to meet the growing needs of patients and families and that patients often express the most stress and dissatisfaction because their primary care physician does not appear to be informed about their child's disorder.[281,294] See Case Study 11.1, Part 1.

Basic Knowledge and Skills Competence for Physical and Occupational Therapists

The National Coalition for Health Professional Education in Genetics (NCHPEG) is an organization of individuals from approximately 120 health professions. They have proposed basic competencies for all health care professionals.[15] With a working knowledge about genetics,

---

CASE STUDY 11.1, PART 1 Therapists' Role in the Early Recognition and Clinical Diagnosis of Genetic Disorders

This case study series portrays how basic knowledge and skills competence in genetics are essential for therapists in the delivery of services for pediatric patients with genetic disorders. Two female patients with presenting signs of developmental delay received physical therapy services before and after receiving a definitive diagnosis.

Screening for Genetic Disorders at Initial Visit

Developmental delay is a common classification for infants and young children entering into physical therapy services before a definitive diagnosis of a particular genetic disorder has been made. Family history and course of pregnancy are key areas for the physical therapists to consider during ongoing assessment. The sensitive nature of this information requires that appropriate trust and rapport have been established between practitioner and family.

For the female patients discussed in this case, no remarkable information was revealed to indicate that a genetic disorder was suspected: Each of the girls was the first-born child and lived with her biological parents, in whom there was no previous family history of a genetic disorder. This was the first pregnancy for the mothers of both girls. The mothers each became pregnant in their late 20s without the assistance of reproductive technology, and they received the recommended course of prenatal care without specialized prenatal testing. The course of the mothers' pregnancies and deliveries was unremarkable, as was the neonatal period for the children.

Both girls were Caucasian, with blond hair, blue eyes, and no notable dysmorphism. Figs. 11.9A and B show the two girls. The first child was 16 months old and the second 14 months before given a medical diagnosis.

Medical Records Review

	Dylen: Contrasting Features	Danika: Contrasting Features	Features of Both Girls
0–6 Months of Age			
Parental concerns	Vomiting and abnormal eye movements		Low muscle tone and slow motor development.
Tests and measures	Normal brain MRI scan and EEG at 3 months	No tests	
Development			Normal head control. Purposeful reach, grasp, and object release. Good eye contact and "happy" disposition. Some babbling and one-syllable sounds.
6–8 Months of Age			
Parental concerns	Tongue thrusting and episodic nystagmus; parents suspect seizures	Sleep disturbances; visual disturbance suspected	Both girls are slow to achieve independent sitting and crawling.
Tests and measures			
Development	Pivots in prone position at 8 months. Sits without support at 8 months.	Not yet sitting	Delayed trunk control. Both girls roll over by 7 months.

EEG, Electroencephalogram; *MRI*, magnetic resonance imaging.

Pediatric therapists should recognize that marked developmental delay and global hypotonia are two features common to many genetic disorders. However, in the case of both girls, the urgency of a genetics referral was lessened by the following factors: no dysmorphic features, healthy neonatal development, absence of family history of genetic disorders, and no other major presenting risk factors (e.g., no prior loss of pregnancies, young maternal age, and normal course of pregnancy).

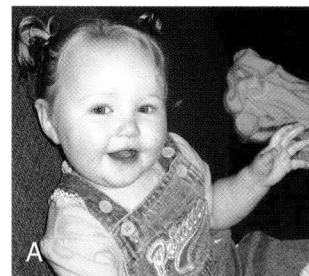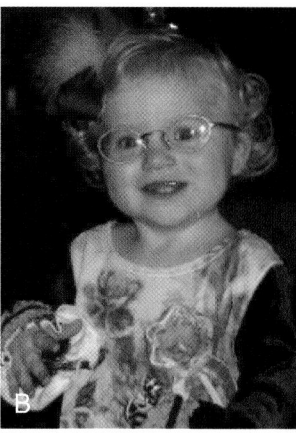

Fig. 11.9 (A) Dylen at 16 months of age, approximately the age she was diagnosed with Rett syndrome. **(B)** Danika at 14 months of age, approximately the age at which she was diagnosed with Angelman syndrome.

therapists can develop competence in eliciting and accessing genetic information from subjective interviews with proper patient consent, can learn how to protect patient privacy while making appropriate recommendations to genetics professionals, and can understand the social and psychological implications of genetic services.[293,295]

Professional education for physical[11] and occupational therapists[296] faces challenges to prepare practitioners who meet the minimum competencies set forth by NCHPEG.[15] Most physical therapists responding to the survey by Long and colleagues[293] reported that they received most of their information through nonscientific media and that they had limited or no education in genetics. Some of the barriers to the implementation of genetics content in professional programs include lack of faculty qualified to teach the content and time limitations within a didactic program.[11] Continuing education courses for practicing clinicians are in short supply. Physical therapists have identified needs for continuing education in genetics to include topics such as the role of genetics in common disorders such as cancer and heart disease, an overview of human genetics, what treatments were available, and how to direct patients to information resources. Although occupational therapists were not part of Long's study, it is felt that colleagues would stress similar needs.[293]

Service Delivery for Children With Genetic Disorders and Their Families

For therapists to be supportive of families they are working with, they must acknowledge the importance of family priorities, respect the family's cultural values and beliefs,[297–299] include families as integral team members, and promote and deliver services that build on family and community resources.

This section includes strategies for supporting families of children with genetic disorders, assessment strategies, the construction of therapeutic goals and objectives, and guiding principles for pediatric interventions.

Family-Centered Service

Family-centered service is both a philosophy and an approach to service delivery that is considered to be a best practice in EI and pediatric rehabilitation.[300–302] Children with genetic disorders have complex, long-term needs that can be addressed by a family-centered service delivery model. At the core of this model is the manner in which therapists interact with the children and their families—the therapist's mindfulness, attentiveness, and respectfulness—elements that are as important as the actual interventions delivered.[303,304] Therapists educated in the family-centered approach are also able to understand the impact of

disability on a family as well as the value of support systems such as family and community.[272]

Bailey and colleagues[272] highlight the particular needs of families who have children diagnosed with genetic disorders; such families must have productive partnerships with health care providers. Therapists should not be reluctant to learn about a rare condition from parents, as many are not "passive recipients of information" but rather "coproducers" of what and how information available may be used in their child's care.[272,305] Parents can be trusted to be a reliable source in the recognition of their child's condition and needs,[306] but in some instances the therapist's role may be to steer families to accurate information or assist with interpreting information that they have discovered. For example, the term *untreatable condition* may be misinterpreted by parents to mean that there are no reasonable interventions that might benefit their child (see Case Study 11.1, Part 4).

The *Relational Goal-Oriented Model* (RGM) of service delivery links the "what" with a more in-depth consideration of the "how" (how service providers and organizations can optimize both the process and outcomes of service delivery).[307] The role of the family in the child's life and the importance of the insights of parents into their child's abilities and needs[308] are crucial. Three important aspects of caregiving—information exchange, respectful and supportive care, and partnership or enabling—are foundational to family-centered care.[309] Family-centered service recognizes that each family is unique, that the family is the constant in the child's life, and that the family members have expert knowledge of the child's abilities and needs. The family works together with service providers to make informed decisions about the services and supports that the child and family receive. The strengths and needs of all family members are considered in family-centered service.[310] In the interactional exchange between the child/family and therapists, understandings occur, commitments and decisions are made, the child and family receive affirmation and support, and information is translated into meaningful, usable knowledge through the process of communication.[311,312] Developing mutual trust and open communication between the child, the family, and the physical and occupational therapists as well as other practitioners is at the core of clinical practice.

Therapists working with children must recognize and acknowledge the multitude of tasks that all families work to accomplish. In addition to tasks specifically related to caring for a child with a disability, families must perform functions to address the economic, daily care, recreational, social, and educational and vocational needs of both individual members and the family as a whole.

As Turnbull and Turnbull[313] have cautioned, each time professionals intervene with families and children, they can potentially enhance or hinder the family's ability to meet important family functions. For example, intervention that promotes a child's social skills can be an important support to positive family functioning. On the other hand, intervention that focuses on the child's deficits can have a negative impact on how the family perceives that child and the place of the child in the family. The RGM emphasizes the importance for therapists to join with parents to provide responsive and flexible therapy services in accordance with changing family needs and circumstances.[314]

The *Life Needs Model*[302,307] acknowledges the need for therapists to work collaboratively with service providers in other disciplines to improve community participation and quality of life for children and youth with disabilities, based on the expressed needs of the child and his or her family members. Helping the family to identify a support group is often useful for adjustment and continuing encouragement in coping with issues. Support groups can be found at www.geneticalliance.org, a comprehensive website provided by the Alliance of Genetic Support Groups. Family empowerment mediates relationships between family-centered care and improvements in children's behaviors[315] and directly affects families' satisfaction with services for their children and their well-being.[316]

Assessment Strategies

Knowledge of a child's diagnosis can aid in the selection of appropriate assessment tools and can alert the therapist to any potential medical problems or contraindications associated with the specific syndrome that might affect the assessment procedures (tests and measures). Therapists must be careful, however, not to develop preconceived opinions about a child's capabilities on the basis of how other children with similar diagnoses have performed. It is critical to remember that there is wide behavioral and performance variability among children within each genetic disorder. For example, wide variability in the achievement of developmental milestones has been reported among children with Down syndrome.[317]

The assessment process includes many components that in certain areas are specific to the practice of either physical or occupational therapy. For the physical therapist, use of the *Guide to Physical Therapist Practice*[318] is recommended as a framework to identify appropriate tests and measures for impairments or disabilities. For the occupational therapist a useful reference is the assessment section of the textbook *Occupational Therapy for Children*.[249]

Typically a therapist's assessment begins with movement observation and analysis followed by testing of the neuromuscular status of the child, such as primitive reflexes, automatic reactions, and muscle tone. For children with orthopedic involvement, assessment of muscle strength, joint range of motion, joint play, and soft tissue mobility is also important. An assessment of the child's developmental level and functional ability should be completed. Such assessments can be used to discriminate between typical and delayed development, to identify the constraints interfering with the achievement of functional skills, and to guide the development of treatment goals and strategies. Most developmental assessment tools fall into one of the following categories: (1) discriminative, (2) predictive, and (3) evaluative measures.[319] Each of these three types of developmental assessment tools yields a different type of information. It is important to understand these differences and the intended purpose of each type of assessment to ensure that evaluation tools are used appropriately. A list of tests and measures commonly used by pediatric physical therapists is given in Table 11.3.

Discriminative Assessment

A discriminative assessment is used to compare the ability of an individual with the ability of members of a peer group or with a criterion selected by the test author.[319] Such instruments provide information necessary to document children's eligibility for special services but rarely provide information useful for planning or evaluating therapy programs.[320] Norm-referenced tests such as the Alberta Infant Motor Scale,[321] the Bayley Scales of Infant Development (motor and mental scales),[322] and the Peabody Developmental Motor Scales[323] are examples of tests used with infants and young children to verify developmental delay or to assign age levels. The Test of Infant Motor Performance is used to identify the risk of developmental delay in infants from 32 weeks postconception to 16 weeks after term.[324] An example of a norm-referenced assessment tool for older children is the Bruininks-Oseretsky Test of Motor Proficiency.[325]

It may be possible to detect improved motor performance by administering a developmental test used to identify children who have motor delays. Such tests, however, usually cannot detect small increments of improvement because there are relatively few test items at each age level and developmental gaps between items are often large.

In assessing whether intervention has been effective, the use of most discriminative tools does not examine a child's performance of functional activities in natural environments.[320]

Predictive Assessments

Predictive measures are used to classify individuals according to a set of established categories and to verify whether an individual has been classified correctly.[319] Measures designed to predict future performance are often used to detect early signs of motor impairment in infants who are at risk for neuromotor dysfunction.[320] Knowledge of developmental milestones and the ability to identify typical and atypical movement at various ages is paramount to the therapist's competency in administering a structured assessment such as those used to predict future disability in children. Prechtl and others[326] have described how assessment of "general movements" in infants can be used to identify children with cerebral palsy.[327] The Movement Assessment of Infants[328] was designed to assess muscle tone, reflex development, automatic reactions, and volitional movement and has value in predicting future neurodevelopmental problems in high-risk infants when administered during the first year of life.[329,330] The Test of Infant Motor Performance[324] and the Alberta Infant Motor Scale[321] are other instruments commonly used to predict poor motor outcomes.

Evaluative Assessments

An evaluative measure is used to document change within an individual over time or change occurring as the result of intervention.[319] Helping Babies Learn[331] is a curriculum-referenced test that provides information about a child's developmental progress relative to a prespecified curriculum sequence.

To determine whether a child's ability to perform meaningful skills in everyday environments has improved, a functional assessment should be used. Functional assessments focus on the accomplishment of specific daily activities rather than on the achievement of developmental milestones. Emphasis is placed on the end result in terms of the achievement of a functional task, although the form or quality of the movement should never be ignored by the therapist. Assistance in the form of people or devices is incorporated into the assessment of progress, with the measurement of progress focusing on the achievement of independence.[332] Qualitative aspects of movement that have important functional implications—such as accuracy, speed, endurance, and adaptability—are also considered.

Functional assessments can be used to screen, diagnose, or describe functional deficits and to determine the resources needed to allow the child to function optimally in specific environments (e.g., school, home). Another use of functional assessments is to evaluate the nature of the problem and the specific task requirements limiting function to develop educational plans and teaching strategies.[332] A final use of functional assessments is to examine and monitor for changes in functional status. Such assessments can be used for program evaluation and for determining the cost-effectiveness of services or programs. (See Chapter 7 for additional information regarding evaluation tools.)

The Functional Independence Measure (FIM) is an example of a functional assessment. The FIM assesses the effectiveness of therapy on functional dependence in the areas of self-care, sphincter control, mobility, locomotion, communication, and social cognition.[333] Seven levels of functional dependence ranging from needing total assistance to complete independence are used to determine an individual's status. An adaptation of the FIM places greater emphasis on functional gains as opposed to the level of care. The WeeFIM[334] has been developed for use with children through the age of 6 years.

The Pediatric Evaluation of Disability Inventory (PEDI) is a functional assessment that focuses on the domains of self-care, mobility,

TABLE 11.3 Pediatric Tests and Measures and What They Measure

Developmental Screening Tools

Name of Tool	Age Range		References
Ages and Stages Questionnaires	1 month to 5 years	Parent-completed tool	Rydz D, Shevell M, Majnemer A, et al. Developmental screening. *J Child Neurol.* 2005;20(1):4–21. Squires J, Bricker D, Twombly E. *Ages and Stages Questionnaires: Social-Emotional (ASQ-SE).* Baltimore, MD: PH Brookes Publishing Co; 2002. www.pbrookes.com
Parent Evaluation of Developmental Status	Birth to 8 years	Parent-completed tool	Glascoe FP. *Collaborating With Parents: Using Parents' Evaluation of Developmental Status (PEDS) to Detect and Address Developmental and Behavioral Problems.* Nolensville, TN: PEDStest.com, LLC; 2013. *www.pedstest.com.*
Child Developmental Inventory (CDI)	Used with high-risk infants' follow-up	Parents' observations	Doig KB, Macias MM, Saylor CF, et al. The Child Development Inventory: a developmental outcome measure for follow-up of the high-risk infant. *J Pediatr.* 1999;135(3):358–362.
Infant Development Inventory (part of the CDI)	Birth to 18 months	Parents' observations	Doig KB, Macias MM, Saylor CF, et al. The Child Development Inventory: a developmental outcome measure for follow-up of the high-risk infant. *J Pediatr.* 1999;135(3):358–362.
Bayley Infant Neurodevelopmental Screener	3–24 months	Pediatrician or health care provider	Weiss LG, Oakland T, Aylward GP. *Bayley-III Clinical Use and Interpretation.* Boston, MA: Academic; 2010.
Denver Developmental Screening Test	Birth to 6 years	Pediatrician or health care provider	Bryant GM, Davies KJ, Newcombe RO. The Denver Developmental Screening Test. Achievement of test items in the first year of life by Denver and Cardiff infants. *Dev Med Child Neurol.* 1974;16(4):475–484.

Screening for developmental delay in primary care is inconsistent and often insufficient to direct the family physician. The American Academy of Pediatrics recommends surveillance at all well-child visits combined with screening for developmental delay at 9, 18, 24, or 30 months of age using a **standardized developmental screening tool.** Two of the most extensively evaluated parent-completed tools are the Parent Evaluation of Developmental status (PEDS) and Ages and States Questionnaires (ASQ). The literature supports screening for developmental delay with parent-completed tools rather than directly administered tools. (Mackrides and Ryherd, 2011)[334a]
The following are suggested developmental screening tools.

Developmental Tests for Measuring Activity (According to the International Classification of Functioning, Disability, and Health (ICF) Model)

Tests/Tools	Description	References
Gross Motor		
Alberta Infant Motor Scales (AIMS)	Identifies motor delays and measures changes in motor performance over time; birth to 18 months.	Piper MC, Darah J. *Motor Assessment of Developing Infant.* Philadelphia: WB Saunders; 1993.
Bruininks-Oseretsky Test of Motor Proficiency (BOTP-2)	Identifies motor abilities and can be used for program planning, to monitor change over longer periods of time for child with mild disabilities; 4.5–14.5 years of age.	Bruininks RH. *Bruininks-Oseretsky Test of Motor Proficiency: Examiners' Manual.* Circle Pines, MN: American Guidance Service; 1978.
Gross Motor Function Measure (GMFM)	Measures change in gross motor function over time; especially children with cerebral palsy; 5 months to 16 years.	Russell D, Rosenbaum PL, Cadman DT, et al. The gross motor function measure: a mean to evaluate the effects of physical therapy. *Dev. Med Child Neurol.* 1989;1:341–352.
Motor Function Measure	Developed to assess children with neuromuscular diseases. Measures three dimensions: standing and transfers, axial and proximal motor function, and distal motor function.	Bérard C, Payan C, Hodgkinson I, et al. A motor function measure for neuromuscular diseases. Construction and validation study. *Neuromuscul Disord.* 2005;15:463–470.
Peabody Developmental Motor Scales, 2nd ed.	Identifies gross and fine motor delays; used to monitor program; birth to 5 years.	Folio MR, Fewell RR. *Peabody Developmental Motor Scales: Examiner's Manual.* 2nd ed. Austin, TX: Pro-Ed; 2000.
Test of Infant Motor Performance (TIMP)	Provides early identification of motor delays; assesses postural control for early skill acquisitions; 32 weeks to 4 months.	Campbell SK, Hedeker D. Validity of the Test of Infant Motor Performance for discriminating among infants with varying risk for poor motor outcome. *J Pediatr.* 2001;139:546–551.

TABLE 11.3 Pediatric Tests and Measures and What They Measure—cont'd

Tests/Tools	Description	References
Multi-Domain Tests		
Activities Scale for Kids	Permits 5- to 15-year-old children and youth to accurately self-report their physical functioning; sensitive to small amount of change.	Young NML, Williams JI, Yosida KK, et al. Measurement properties of the activities scale for kids. *J Clin Epidemiol.* 2000;53:125–137.
Battelle Developmental Inventory, 2nd ed.	Identifies developmental level and monitor changes over time; birth to 8 years.	Newborg J, Stock JR, Wnek L, et al. *Batelle Developmental Inventory.* Allen, TX: DLM; 1998.
Bayley Scales of Infant Development III	A standard series of measurements originally developed by psychologist Nancy Bayley used primarily to assess the development of infants and toddlers aged 1 to 42 months.	Johnson S, Moore T, Marlow N. Using the Bayley-III to assess neurodevelopmental delay: which cut-off should be used? *Pediatr Res.* 2014;75(5):670–674.
Brigance Inventory of Early Development, rev. ed.	Identifies students' present level of performance and monitors progress. Diagnoses delays, disabilities, giftedness, and other exceptional features.	https://www2.curriculumassociates.com/products/detail.aspx?title=brigied2.ca; Curriculum Associates, LLC-Brigance IED II (2010).
Canadian Occupational Performance Measure (COPM)	Outcome measure in the areas of self-care, productivity, and leisure. Any age.	Law M, Paptiste S, McColl MA, et al. The Canadian occupational performance measure for occupational therapy. *Can J Occup Ther.* 1990;57:82–97.
Functional Independence Measure for Children (WeeFIM)	Measures changes in mobility and activities of daily living; used for program evaluation and rehabilitation outcome assessment; 6 months to 7 years.	Granger CV, McCabe MA. *Uniform Data System for Medical Rehabilitation: WEEFIM II System Clinical Guide.* Buffalo, NY; Uniform Data System for Medical Rehabilitation; 2004.
Harris Infant Neuromotor Test (HINT)	Screening tool to detect early signs of cognitive and neuromotor delays; birth to 12 months.	Harris S, Dabniels L. Reliability and validity of the Harris Infant Neuromotor Test. *J Pediatrics.* 2000;139:249–253.
Hawaii Early Learning Profile (HELP-Strands)	Comprehensive, ongoing, family-centered curriculum based assessment of progress for infants and toddlers (birth to 3 years and their families). Curriculum-based assessment tools that identify needs, monitor growth and development, and establish a plan to address assessment results.	VORT Corporation. Hawaii Early Learning Profile (HELP), first published in 1995. Note: No MCID available. No research articles available using HELP as primary outcome measure.
Movement Assessment Battery for Children (Movement ABC-2)	Identifies and describes impairments in motor performance of children and adolescents, 3 to 16 years of age.	Brown I, Lalor A. The Movement Assessment Battery for Children—second edition (MABC-2): a review and critique. *Phys Occup Ther Pediatr.* 2009;29(1):86–103.
Pediatric Evaluation of Disability Inventory (PEDI)	Measures self-care and mobility performance in the home and community; 6 months to 7.5 years.	Haley S, Coster WJ, Ludlow LH, et al. *Pediatric Evaluation of Disability Inventory (PEDI) Version 1: Development, Standardization, and Administration Manual.* Boston, MA: Infant Research Group, Dept. Of Rehabilitation Medicine at New England Medical Center; 1992.
PEDI-CAT (Computerized version)	Outcome measure of the PEDI, using computer adaptive test in children with cerebral palsy.	Shore BJ, Allar BG, Miller PE, et al. Measuring the reliability and construct validity of the PEDI-Computer Adaptive Test (PEDI-CAT) in children with cerebral palsy. *Arch Phys Med Rehabil.* 2018;100:45–51.
POSNA (Pediatric Musculoskeletal Functional Health Questionnaire)	Useful for a wide variety of ages and diagnoses; ideally suited for orthopedic surgeons to assess the functional health and efficacy of treatment of their patients at baseline and follow-up.	Daltroy LH, Lian MH, Fossel AH, et al. The POSNA pediatric musculoskeletal functional health questionnaire: report on reliability, validity, and sensitivity to change. Pediatric Outcomes Instrument Development Group. Pediatric Orthopedic Society of North America. *J Pediatr Orthop.* 1998;18(5):561–571. Miller DJ, Cahill PF, Janickl JA, et al. What's new in pediatric orthopedic quality, safety, and value? A systematic review with result of the 2018 POSNA quality, safety, and value initiative (QSVI) challenge. *J Pediatr Orthop.* 2018;38:646–651.
School Function Assessment (SFA)	Measures function in the school environment, kindergarten to sixth grade.	Coster QW, Deeney T, et al. *School Function Assessment.* San Antonio, TX: Therapy Skill Builders; 1998.
Toddler and Infant Motor Evaluation (TIME)	Identifies children with mild to severe motor problems; measures sensory development; monitors progress over time; 4 month to 3.5 years.	Miller IJ, Roid GH. *Toddler and Infant Motor Evaluation: A Standardized Assessment.* Tucson, AZ: Therapy Skill Builders; 1997.

Continued

TABLE 11.3   Pediatric Tests and Measures and What They Measure—cont'd

Functional Balance Tests

Test and Measures	What It Measures	Reference
Early clinical Assessment of Balance (ECAB)	Consist of items from the PBS and the Movement Assessment for infants; ECAB measures of head, trunk, sitting, and standing postural control for children up to 7 years and 11 months of age.	McCoy S, Bartlett D, Yocum A, et al. Development and validity of the early clinical assessment of balance for young children with cerebral palsy. *Dev Neurorehabil.* 2014;17(6):375–383.
5-Repetitions Sit-to-Stand	Measures time to complete five consecutive cycles of sit-to-stand.	Wang TH, Liao HF, Peng YC. Reliability and validity of the five-repetition sit-to-stand test for children with cerebral palsy. *Clin Rehabil.* 2011;26(7):664–671
Functional Reach Test (FRT)	Measures distance one or both hands can reach forward while maintaining standing balance.	Norris RA, Wilder E, Norton J. The functional reach tests in 3 to 5 year-old children without disabilities. *Pediatr Phys Ther.* 2008;20:47–52.
Pediatric Balance Scale (PBS)	Provides 14 different activities to test balance from simple (sitting to standing) to relatively more complex (retrieving object from the floor).	Franjoine MR, Darr N, Held SL et al. The performance of children developing typically on the pediatric balance scale. *Pediatr Phys Ther.* 2010;22: 350–359.
Pediatric Reach Test (PRT)	Measures distance one hand can reach forward and laterally while maintaining sitting or standing balance.	Bartlett D, Birmingham T. Validity and reliability of a pediatric reach test. *Pediatr Phys Ther.* 2003;15(2):84–92.
Segmental Assessment of Trunk Control (SATCO)	Measures the ability to maintain trunk control while sitting in a steady, active, and reactive state of sitting; the test determines the highest level of trunk support at which child loses postural control.	Butler P, Saavedra S, Sofranac M, et al. Refinement, reliability, and validity of segmental assessment of trunk control. *Pediatr Phys Ther.* 2010;22(3): 246–257.
Timed Floor to Stand (TFTS)	Measures the time it takes to get up from the floor, walk 3 m, turn around, and walk back to sit down in the same spot on the floor.	Weingarten G, Lieberstein M, Itzkowitz A, et al. Timed floor to stand-natural: reference data for school age children. *Pediatr Phys Ther.* 2016;28(1):71–76.
Timed Up and Down Stairs (TUDS)	Measures the time it takes to ascend one flight of stairs, turn around in the landing, and descend the same flight of stairs.	Zaino CA, Marchese VG, Westcott SL. Timed Up and Down Stairs Test: preliminary reliability and validity of a new measure of functional mobility. *Pediatr Phys Ther.* 2004;16(2):90–98.
Timed Up and Go (TUG)	Measures time it takes for an individual to get up from a seat, walk 3 m, turn around, and walk back to sit down on the same seat.	Steffen TM, Hacker TA, Mollinger L. Age- and gender-related test performance in community dwelling elderly people: Six-Minute Walk Test, Berg Balance Scale, and Timed Up and Go Test and gait speeds. *Pediatr Phys Ther.* 2002;82(2):128–137.

These Standardized Balance Tests are simple and quick yet are good indicators of falls risk.
The first three test static and dynamic balance as well as leg strength. These also take less than 5 minutes to complete.

Fall Screening Tests

Timed Up and GO Test	Measures time it takes for an individual to get up from a seat, walk 3 m, turn around, and walk back to sit down on the same seat.	Steffen TM, Hacker TA, Mollinger L. Age and gender-related test performance in community dwelling elderly people: Six-Minute Walk Test, Berg Balance Scale, and Timed Up & Go TEST and gait speeds. *Pediatr Phys Ther.* 2002;82(2):128–137.
Single Leg Stand	Measures static standing ability (balance with feet fixed).	Bohannon R, Larking P, Cook A, et al. Decrease in timed balance test score with aging. *Phys Ther.* 1984;64:1067–1070.
Single Chair Rise	Measures ability of person to rise from a chair.	Guralnik JM, Simonsick EM, Ferucci L, et al. A short physical performance battery assessing lower extremity function: association with self-reported disability and prediction of mortality and nursing home submission. *J Gerontol.* 1994;49:M85–M94.

Other Balance Measures for Assessments and/or Outcomes

Timed Chair Rise ×5	Measures ability of person to rise from a chair repeated (five times).	Whitney SL, Wrisley DM, Marchetti GF, et al. Clinical measurement of sit-to-stand performance in people with balance disorders: validity of data for the Five-Times Sit-to-Stand Test. *Phys Ther.* 2005;85:1034–1045.
Chair rise in 30 s	Measures how many times a person can rise to stand from chair for 30 s.	Rikli R, Jones J. Development and validation of a functional fitness test for community-residing older adults. *J Aging Phys Act.* 1999;7:129–161

TABLE 11.3 Pediatric Tests and Measures and What They Measure—cont'd

Test and Measures	What It Measures	Reference
Tandem stand	Assesses static balance with narrow base of support. Person stands with one toes of foot touching the heel of another foot.	Gurlnik JM, Ferruci L, Simonsick EM, et al. Lower-extremity function in persons over the age of 70 years as a predictor of subsequent disability. *N Engl J Med.* 1995;332(9):556–561.
360 degrees turn protocol	A measure of dynamic balance. Person turns in a complete circle, 360 degrees.	Berg KO, Wood-Dauphinee SL, Williams JI, et al. Measuring balance in the elderly: validation of an instrument. *Can J Public Health.* 1992;83(suppl 2):S7–S11.
Four Square Step Test	Tests more advance dynamic balance.	Dite W, Temple VA. A clinical test of stepping and change of direction to identify multiple falling older adults. *Arch Phys Med Rehabil.* 2002;83:1566–1571.
Alternate Step Test	Modified version of Berg Balance stool stepping test.	Tiedemann A, Shimada H, Sherrington C, et al. The comparative ability of eight functional mobility tests for predicting falls in community-dwelling older people. *Age Ageing.* 2008;37:430–435.
Tandem Walk Test	Walk heel to toe along a 10-foot line as quickly as possible without loosing balance.	Bickley LS, Szilagyi PG, Bates B. *Bates' Guide to Physical Examination and History Taking.* 11th ed. Philadelphia, PA: Lippincott Williams & Wilkins; 2013:717.

Walking/Ambulation Tests

Tests (Listed Alphabetically)	What It Measures	References
Dynamic Gait Index	Evaluates the ability to walk while performing different tasks and/or responding to different gait demands.	Marchetti GF, Whitney SL. Construction and validation of the 4-item dynamic gait index. *Phys Ther.* 2006;86(12):1651–1660.
Energy Expenditure Index (EEI)	Measures the energy cost or efficiency of walking with a comfortable speed or a fast speed for 2 to 3 minutes.	Rose J, Gamble JG, Lee J, et al. The energy expenditure index: a method to quantitate and compare walking energy expenditure for children and adolescents. *J Pediatr Orthop.* 1991;11(5):571–578.
Functional Mobility Scale (FMS)	Qualifies use of assistive devices for three distances using a six-point ordinal scale; the three distances represent mobility at home (5 m), school (50 m), and in the community (500 m).	Graham HK, Harvey A, Rodda J, et al. The Functional Mobility Scale (FMS). *J Pediatr Orthop.* 2004;24(5):514–520.
50-Foot Walk Test	Provides two measures; the amount of time it takes to walk 30 feet and the maximum amount of time to walk 50 feet that is acceptable to the classroom teacher.	Unver B, Kalkan S, Yuksel E, et al. Reliability of the 50-Foot Walk Test and 30-s chair stand test in total knee arthroplasty. *Acta Ortop Bras.* 2015;23(4):184–187.
Perceived Exertion Scales	Pictorial scales that seek a person's self-perception of the effort he or she is putting in to complete a tasks, can be used in conjunction with the other tests listed in this walking document.	Borg GA. Perceived exertion: a note on "history" and methods. *Med Sci Sports.* 1973;5(2):90–93
6-Minute Walk Tests	An endurance test that measures the distance walked in 6 minutes.	McDonald C, Henrickson E, Han J, et al. The 6-minute Walk Test: a new outcome measure in Duchenne Muscular Dystrophy. *Muscle Nerve.* 2010; 41(4):500–510.
30-Second Walk Tests	A simple test that measures the distance walked in 30 seconds.	Van Brussel M, Helders P. The 30-second Walk test norms for children. *Ped Physical Therapy.* 2009;21(3):244
Timed Floor to Stand (TFTS)	Measures the time it takes to get up from the floor, walk 3 m, turn around, and walk back to sit down in the same spot on the floor.	Weingarten G, Kaplan S. Reliability and validity of the timed floor to stand test-natural in school-aged children. *Pediatr Phys Ther.* 2015;27(2): 113–118.
Timed Up and Down Stairs (TUDS)	Measures the time it takes to ascend one flight of stairs, turn around in the landing, and descent the same flight of stairs.	Zaino CA, Marchese VG, Wescott SL. Timed Up and Down Stairs Test: preliminary reliability and validity of a new measure of functional mobility. *Pediatr Phys Ther.* 2004;16(2):n90–98.
Timed Up and Go (TUG)	Measures time it takes for an individual to get up from the seat, walk 3 m, turn around, and walk back to sit down on the same seat.	Steffen TM, Hacker TA, Mollinger L. Age- and gender-related test performance in community dwelling elderly people: Six-Minute Walk Test, Berg Balance Scale, and Timed Up & Go Test, and gait speeds. *Phys Ther.* 2002;82(2):128–137.

and social cognition.[335] The PEDI incorporates three measurement scales: (1) the capability to perform selected functional skills, (2) the level of caregiver assistance that is required, and (3) identification of environmental modifications or equipment needed to perform a particular activity. The PEDI has been standardized and normed and is intended for use with children whose abilities are in the range of a typical 6-month-old to 7-year-old child.

The final example of a functional assessment is the School Function Assessment (SFA).[336] The SFA is designed to measure a student's performance in accomplishing functional tasks in the school environment. It is composed of three sections that focus on (1) the student's participation in major school activities, (2) the task supports needed by the student for participation, and (3) the student's activity performance. The SFA is standardized and was conceptually developed to be reflective of the functional requirements of a student in elementary school. See Case Study 11.1, Part 2.

Family-Driven Goals and Objectives
Therapy Goal Orientation

Goal orientation is a second fundamental feature of effective service. The earlier section on relation-based practice described how relationships between child, family, and therapists are fundamental in providing effective intervention. Goal orientation encompasses both joint goal setting by (1) parents, caregivers, and families and (2) therapists and other service providers[337] and the pursuit of meaningful child-, parent-, and family-selected goals.[338] Goals of parents and families are to create a supportive environment for their child, provide opportunities for growth and belonging, and help their child to live as adaptive and independent a life as possible.[307] Family-centered care incorporates trusting relationships in which the therapist demonstrates respect for the family's values, beliefs, and goals rather than imposing a plan of care on the child and family that aims to correct "deficiencies."

After a child's strengths and needs have been evaluated and the family's objectives identified, therapy goals and objectives can be developed. In the past, establishment of these goals has primarily been the responsibility of professionals and often did not incorporate the needs and desires of the family. More recently, however, professionals have recognized the value of having families guide the process of establishing intervention goals and objectives.[339,340] This shift toward collaborative goal setting and family-centered care has occurred largely as a result of the belief that families should determine their vision of the future for their children and that professionals should act as consultants and resources to help families achieve that vision. The stress that caregivers experience with the everyday care of a child can reduce compliance with a home therapeutic program,[341] which further supports the notion that parents should be jointly involved with therapists to determine goals and the means by which to attain identified outcomes.[342] When parents and families contribute to the planning process, they are more likely to believe in goals that are set and to play a role in ensuring that relevant strategies are implemented.[307] They gain a sense of control over their child's services, supports, and resources, and this contributes to their personal and family's well-being.[343] For children living in the United States, these goals are developed within the context of individualized service plans.

Individualized Service Plans

In the United States, the Individuals with Disabilities Education Act (IDEA) requires public schools to develop an Individualized Education Plan (IEP) for every student with disability. An IEP is designed to meet the unique educational needs of a student with disabilities as defined by federal regulation 34 CFR 300.320.[344] Under IDEA 2004, a free appropriate public education (FAPE) is provided that is individualized to a specific student with a disability and that emphasizes special education and related services to prepare the student for further education, employment, and independent living (20 U.S.C. 1400 et seq, 20 U.S.C. 1400 © [5][A][i]).

Beginning with the enactment of US Public Law 94-142 in 1975[345] and several important legislative revisions in 1990 (IDEA),[345–347] 1991

CASE STUDY 11.1, PART 2 Assessment Strategies

	Dylen: Contrasting Features	Danika: Contrasting Features	Features of Both Girls
9–13 Months of Age			
Tests and measures			Both girls have abnormal EEG findings.
			Alberta Infant Motor Scale score: below fifth percentile.
			PEDI: Composite independence in functional skills less than 12% with total caregiver assistance.
Development	Regression in motor skills: sitting, rolling, and fine motor	Sits alone at 11 months	Dylen demonstrates skill regression; Danika slowly attains motor skills.
	Babbling vocalization		
	Emergence of truncal and extremity ataxia		
Other objective findings	Cold feet with reddened appearance; normal BP and HR	Emergence of hand-flapping behaviors	Both girls have small head circumferences.

BP, Blood pressure; *EEG,* electroencephalogram; *HR,* heart rate; *PEDI,* Pediatric Evaluation of Disability Inventory.

Another role of the therapist is to use assessment instruments that will help establish a baseline of motor and self-help skills and to monitor for progress or regression; the Alberta Infant Motor Scale and the PEDI, respectively, were initially used for these purposes. Last, the results of these tests and outcomes of intervention are interpreted and conveyed to the family and the child's pediatricians. In the case of both girls, delays in motor, language, and self-help skills persisted, and ultimately both girls and their families were referred for genetic evaluation. Both girls received 1 to 2 hours of physical therapy weekly in their natural environment. The Peabody Developmental Motor Scales were added to monitor progress, guide goal development, and justify the need for continued EI services.

TABLE 11.4   Comparison of Required Components of the Individualized Education Plan and Individualized Family Service Plan

Content	IFSP IDEA Part C (34CFR303.344)	IEP IDEA Part B (34CFR300.320 THROUGH 300.324)
Information about child's status	A statement of child's present levels of physical, cognitive, communication, social or emotional, and adaptive development (physical development includes vision, hearing, and health status)	A statement on child's present levels of academic and functional performance
Family information	Statement of family's resources, priorities, and concerns related to enhancing the child's development	Information regarding parent's concerns can be documented in the present information about the child's status
Outcomes	Statement of measurable outcomes expected to be achieved for child and family and the criteria, procedures, and time lines used to determine the degree of progress toward outcomes and whether modification or revisions of outcomes or services were necessary	Statement of measurable annual goals, including academic and functional goals Include a description of how child's progress toward annual goals will be measured and process to report child's progress to parents
Services	Statement of specific Early Intervention (EI) services necessary to meet child's needs; include frequency, intensity, method of service delivery, location of services and natural environments	Statement of specific special education and related services to be provided, modifications, and supplementary aids to be provided to child
Schedule of services	Projected dates for initiation of services, anticipated duration	Projected date for beginning and ending date of service; any modification needed; frequency, location, and duration of services
Service coordinator	Identification of the service coordinator	No comparable requirement
Transition plan	Procedures and steps for transition from EI to preschool services under Part B Establish transition plan: 90 days to 9 months before third birthday	Procedures needed for postsecondary goals related to training, education, employment, and, where appropriate, independent living skills To be in effect when child turns 16 years of age
Transfer of rights	N/A	Must include statement that child has been informed about reaching the age of majority
Other		Explanation of any time the child will not participate along with nondisabled children

IDEA, Individuals with Disabilities Education Act; *IEP*, Individualized Education Plan; *IFSP*, Individualized Family Service Plan.

(PL 102-119), 1997 (PL 105-17), and 2004 (PL 108-446, Individuals with Disabilities Education Improvement Act of 2004),[348] physical and occupational therapists working in public school settings are required to establish long-term annual goals and short-term therapy objectives within the framework of each child's educational needs. The document that defines a child's educational needs, including therapy services, from preschool through 12th grade is the IEP. Similar requirements are in effect for infants and preschool-aged children, documented in the individualized family service plan (IFSP). An IFSP must be written after a multidisciplinary assessment of the strengths and needs of the child has been completed. This assessment must include a family-directed assessment of the supports and services necessary to enhance the family's capacity to meet the needs of their child with a disability.[347,348] A comparative listing of the components of an IEP and IFSP is given in Table 11.4.

Functional Objectives

The development of behaviorally written, measurable therapy objectives is crucial for monitoring the effects of intervention in a child with a genetic disorder. Many of the clinical symptoms listed in the descriptions of genetic disorders given earlier in the chapter may be monitored through systematic, periodic data-keeping procedures. One example is the monitoring of functional hand skills in girls with RS (see Case Study 11.1, Part 2). Periodic vital capacity measures for a child with OI or a child with Werdnig-Hoffmann disease can reflect progress toward a goal of maintaining respiratory function.

In the past, therapy objectives typically focused on a child's deficits. For example, delays in achieving motor milestones are often used to identify gaps in development, and therapy objectives are written and programs established to address these deficits. When the child meets an objective, new deficits are identified and new objectives developed. A different model for goal development that is consistent with a family-centered intervention philosophy is the "top down" approach, described by Campbell[349] and later by McEwen[350] and Effgren.[216] In this model, the child and family identify a desired functional outcome that is the driving factor for the therapeutic intervention plan. An example of this approach is seen in goal attainment scales. Goal attainment scaling (GAS) is an individualized, criterion-referenced measure of small, clinically important changes in a child's functional performance over time.[351,352] Similar to behavioral objectives, GAS requires (1) the identification of observable goals, (2) reproducibility of conditions under which performance is measured, (3) measurable criteria for success, and (4) a time frame for goal achievement. In contrast to behavioral objectives, however, GAS identifies five possible outcomes with accompanying score values. By using five possible levels of attainment, it can be determined whether a child has made progress despite not having achieved the expected outcome or whether progress has exceeded the expected outcome. Case Study 11.1, Part 3, is an example of use of a goal attainment scale to assess a parent and child functional objective of sitting up on the floor to play with toys.

Both girls had poor postural control with muscular weakness and hypotonia that limited the activity of sitting. The parents of both girls expressed a desire that their daughters would be able to sit up and play with toys on the family room floor. The table illustrates the use of GAS for the goal of seated play with toys. In the course of care, Danika made good progress toward the goal depicted in this scale; however, Dylen did not, and in fact demonstrated regression. Dylen's poorer outcome was indicative of the diagnosis of Rett syndrome (RS), which was revealed later. The family's goals for Dylen were revised, and the GAS was still a suitable framework.

Score	Attainment Level in Time Frame (INSERT) _____	Criterion-Referenced Goals Within Each Range (Time Frame: 3 Months)
−2	Much less than expected outcome with therapy	(Child name) ring-sits on the floor supported on 1 or 2 hands plus 25% physical assistance for balance support and guided reach and grasp of toys placed near her lap.
−1	Less than expected outcome with therapy	(Child name) ring-sits on the floor with standby assistance and uses both hands to play with toys placed near her lap.
0	Expected outcome with therapy	(Child name) ring-sits on the floor with supervision, reaches, and retrieves toys placed in front of her at arm's length away.
+1	Greater than expected outcome with therapy	(Child name) sits on floor independently and plays with toys placed at arm's length in front and to sides of her.
+2	Much greater than expected outcome with therapy	(Child name) sits on floor independently and retrieves toys placed slightly out of reach in front, to sides, and 45 degrees behind her and returns to upright for play.

Rather than focusing on a child's deficits, such outcome-focused objectives provide a more positive and supportive context for therapy and at the same time address the family's needs and priorities. This approach to developing therapy goals and objectives in ways that support positive family functioning is also an important aspect of delivering therapy services to children and their families.

General Intervention Principles

Several general treatment principles guide the delivery of therapy services to children with genetic disorders and are detailed in this section. Special considerations for treatment of a child with a specific genetic condition may be found in the preceding section. The reader is also referred to Chapter 8 for information on interventions in neurological rehabilitation.

Focus on Activities and Participation

The goal of any therapeutic program for children should be to improve the quality and quantity of their participation in society. Achievement of basic motor skills such as sitting, standing, and walking is an outcome that can be measured with commonly used clinical tools, but whether or not children actually apply new skills on a regular basis (participation) is more difficult to capture objectively.[353] Therapists must possess knowledge, skills, and tools if they are to assess and treat children in all domains defined by the World Health Organization (see Case Study 11.1, Part 1). With the purpose of improving participation in the end, pediatric therapists employ a variety of intervention strategies to increase opportunities that can help children to achieve independence and enjoyment of activities at home and school and in the community

Many of the classic therapeutic approaches for children with neurological disorders incorporate techniques targeting impairments of body structure and function, such as abnormal muscle tone or joint alignment, to improve movement quality.[240] Motor learning science and task-oriented models of neurological rehabilitation are based on the rationale that control of movement arises from appropriate practice of skills within the context of functional activities and enriched environments.[353–356] Intervention therefore is aimed at teaching motor problem solving (adaptability to varied contexts),[357] developing effective compensations that are maximally efficient, and providing practice of new motor skills in functional situations. Rather than teaching individuals to perform movement patterns in a controlled therapy setting, this approach focuses on the learning that must take place for an individual to function independently of a therapist's guidance.[353,355] Environmental adaptations can take many forms and include assistive technology that aids in the attainment of functional outcomes such as independence in self-help skills, communication, and mobility.[358] For example, children with Down syndrome commonly have hypotonia, joint laxity, and delayed walking. Orthotics such as supramalleolar orthoses may be used to improve underlying joint and postural instability,[359] and treadmill training has been shown to diminish delays in walking.[360]

Modern neurophysiological approaches use hands-on physical guidance with the child during movement practice of functional skills and activities. The inhibition of certain movements and facilitation of others are based on the rationale that less used movements will be eliminated in the pruning process of the developing brain and frequently used movement patterns will be reinforced[240,353,361]; therefore approaches of this nature may be beneficial for infants and very young children with movement disorders.

Learning and performance of an activity seldom require just one component of function (e.g., mobility, language, cognition); therefore it should be understood and expected that improvements in one domain may indirectly, but significantly, have a positive impact on another. For example, Damiano[361] stresses the benefits of a lifetime of regular movement activity, with or without adaptations, on the overall development of children. Regardless of treatment techniques, it is a widely accepted principle that children learn new skills best when they are taught and practiced within the context in which they will be used.[362]

Delivery of Services in Natural Environments

The term *natural environment* refers to places and settings in which infants and children typically spend their day.[347] The movement toward integrating therapy into classroom settings is one example of providing services in a natural environment.[363–365] In an integrated model of service delivery, therapists work in the classroom with teachers, rather than removing students to an isolated therapy room to provide services. Therapists work closely with the teacher to establish common goals for the student and to devise programs that will allow therapeutic activities to be interwoven into a variety of activities throughout the day in a natural manner.

Another example of providing therapy in a natural environment is providing home-based services for infants and young children. Home-based programs are "normal" options for young children because the natural environment for most infants and toddlers is the home—either their own home or that of a day care provider.[363–365] For children who are medically fragile, it is the preferred option for therapy.[366,367] For other families, transportation to a center-based program may be difficult because of the expense or length of travel required.

Incorporating Therapy Activities Into Daily Routines

Therapists must work collaboratively with families to develop sessions that incorporate therapeutic activities into the family's daily routine (e.g., during play, dressing, bathing, meals). Rather than practicing narrowly defined tasks in a controlled clinic environment, therapy activities should be interwoven into a variety of activities throughout the day in a natural manner. Practicing skills in the context of daily routines allows the child to learn to adapt to the real-life contingencies that arise during a functional task.[355] In addition, activities become more meaningful to both the child and the family (Fig. 11.10).

Use of Assistive Technology Devices

The Assistive Technology Act of 2004 defines an assistive technology device as any item, piece of equipment, or product system—whether acquired commercially, modified, or customized—that is used to increase, maintain, or improve functional capabilities of individuals with disabilities (29 U.S.C. Sec 2202[2]).[368]

As noted previously, an important aspect of providing developmental therapy services is the use of assistive technology devices to

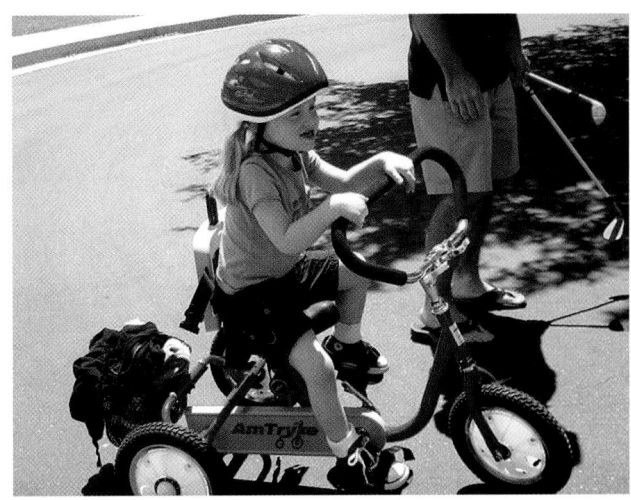

Fig. 11.10 This child with Angelman syndrome enjoys riding her adaptive tricycle to the park with her family.

maximize a child's functional abilities, level of independence, and inclusion in school and community activities with peers. Examples of assistive technology include mobility devices, augmentative communication devices, and adapted computer keyboards. Assistive technology also includes adaptive devices such as splints, bath chairs, prone standers, and other positioning equipment that can be used to provide optimal body alignment and minimize the risk for contractures or deformities while encouraging a greater variety of movement patterns. Such devices can be constructed from readily available materials or obtained commercially. The developmental physical or occupational therapist works with the family and other team members to select, construct, or order assistive devices and to assist caregivers in the use of the devices.

Case Study 11.1, Part 4, demonstrates how these general treatment principles are applied to a particular child receiving therapy services. The case example also shows how the family's priorities and needs are considered and supported in the planning and delivery of services.

CASE STUDY 11.1, PART 4   Focus on Activities and Participation in Meaningful Environments and Routines

Both families were referred by their respective physicians for genetic counseling and evaluation on the suspicion of Angelman syndrome (AS) based on the cluster of developmental delay, features of blue eyes and blonde hair, head circumference, and abnormal EEG findings. Danika received an earlier referral to a geneticist at 14 months of age; subsequent test results confirmed the diagnosis of AS by the time she was 16 months old. The course of medical diagnosis for Dylen was confounded by her presenting signs of frequent, intense vomiting coinciding with suspicion of seizure activity. Dylen did not receive genetic testing until she was 30 months of age. In the cases of both girls, their documented response to therapy and course of motor development were weighed by their respective physicians in their course of care and referral for genetics evaluation. AS was ruled out first for Dylen, and subsequent testing confirmed a diagnosis of RS.

During the period immediately after their child's diagnosis, the parents in each family shared many questions and new knowledge with the treating therapist. Both families accessed local and national family support groups and were encouraged to learn of activities that their children would likely enjoy. The partnership between the therapists and the families was strengthened by clarifying that "untreatable condition" means that neither condition could be remedied by medical intervention and by focusing on the families' values and priorities.

Both girls had limited postural endurance in sitting and standing that was anticipated to persist for several months. Adaptive equipment for these activities was employed for both girls to allow them to participate in functional upright activities (see Fig. 11.7). Danika enjoyed aquatic activities and tricycling, whereas she merely tolerated hippotherapy. Dylen was found to enjoy movement activities more when music was played during treatment.

Continued

	Dylen: Contrasting Features	Danika: Contrasting Features	Features of Both Girls
14–36 Months of Age			
Diagnosis; body organ or structure and function	Rett syndrome; gastroesophageal reflux	Angelman syndrome; sleep disorder	Global developmental delay, seizures, hypotonia
Activities, limitations, and development	Motor skills plateaued at 9 months' chronological age, followed by period of skills regression to 6 months' developmental level	Ambulatory with assistive devices Persistent absence of expressive language but learns to respond to her name Expresses pleasure with giggles and subtle, jerky motions Uses raking motion to pick up small foods	Attends special education preschool
Physical therapy interventions	Movement-oriented activities with music	Aquatic therapy	Postural strengthening, sensorimotor activities
Assistive and adaptive equipment	Adaptive seating provides best opportunities to interact with others in learning environment	Walks indoors and outdoors with a gait trainer (see Fig. 11.7B) and shorter distances with a conventional posterior four-wheeled walker	Gait trainer Adaptive tricycle Bilateral ankle-foot orthoses
Participation of child and family			Support group events: walk, ride, stroll

SUMMARY

This chapter has addressed several chromosomal abnormalities and specific gene defects that are most likely to be seen in children in a typical developmental therapy setting. The inclusion of family members in all aspects of therapy has been stressed, along with the need to consider family goals, priorities, and resources in the development and implementation of therapy services. The importance of developing functional goals and delivering services in natural environments has also been emphasized. Finally, many diseases or conditions have a genetic component that must be considered in the course of medical management. Physical and occupational therapists should expand their working knowledge of genetics to appropriately refer patients for genetic services. Readers are encouraged to consult the companion references for knowledge resources.

REFERENCES

To enhance this text and add value for the reader, all references are included on the companion Evolve site that accompanies this textbook. This online service will, when available, provide a link for the reader to a Medline abstract for the article cited. There are 383 cited references and other general references for this chapter, with the majority of those articles being evidence-based citations.

Vocabulary

Chromosomal microarray-a first-tier, high-resolution, diagnostic test using probes or markers to analyze small portions of DNA from known location on each of 46 chromosomes. The markers will help detect very small imbalances of chromosomal material such as duplications and deletions of specific DNA segments and help determine the cause of a health condition.

Clustered Regularly Interspace Short Palindromic Repeats (CRISPR)-technological genomic editing tool acting as a molecular scalpel; applied to a strand of DNA at a specific site for the purpose of altering the protein product of the targeted section of nucleotides.

De novo mutation-a genetic alteration present for the first time in one family member as a result of a variant/mutation in a germ cell of either parent. Also called a *de novo variant*, *new mutation*, and *new variant*.

Diploid-cells having a inherited, paired chromosomes. All human somatic cell are diploid. Gametes are haploid cells.

DNA sequencing- The process of determining the order of nucelotides in DNA to identify genetic variants that cause disease.

Epigenetics-study of how genes are expressed phenotypically without a change in the original genetic code, due to influence on gene regulation and expression via the action of the "epigenome."

Epigenome-derived from Greek work "epi" (above) the genome: the epigenome is not part of DNA itself, but rather is a chemical compound attached to the DNA that regulates the function of the gene: the what, when, and where. The epigenome can be passed on from cell to cell during cellular division, generationally.

Gametes-a mature haploid male (sperm) or female (egg/ova) germ cell.

Gene-Environment Interaction-a different effect of an environmental exposure on disease risk in persons with different genotypes. Gene-environment interaction explains in part the genetic disorders collectively called *multifactorial disorders*.

Gene replacement therapy (GRT)-experimental technique to use vectored genes to treat or prevent disease by replacing a mutated gene with a healthy copy, inactivating a mutated gene, or introducing a new gene into the body.

Genome (Human) complete set of nucleic acid sequences in a human's DNA, organized into 23 chromosome pairs, within the human cell nuclei (nuclear genome) and in smaller DNA molecules (mitochondrial genome) found within mitochondria cells.

Genetics-the study of the structure, function, and heritability of a single gene.

Genomics-the study of the interrelationship between all genes of an individual's genome and resultant impact on growth and development.

Genome-wide Association Studies (GWAS)-research method to identify genes involved in human disease. Method searches the genome for small variations called single nucleotide polymorphisms (SNPs) that occur more frequently in people with a particular disease than without.

Germline DNA-genetic information, genes, that exists in gametes/germ cell (sperm, ova). Germline DNA is the inherited source of DNA that exists in all other cells in the body. Mutation of a germ cell can be passed via human sexual reproduction to offspring.

Germline mutation-a genetic change occurring in the gamete of an individual and not the somatic cells of the same individual; therefore, germline mutations that may result in a genetic condition can be passed to offspring without it being present in either parent (circumstance for a de novo mutation).

Haploid cell-cell containing half the chromosomes required in human sexual reproduction to produce a new human zygote/offspring. Sperm and ova are haploid cells.

Hyperkinetic movements: excess movement including tics, stereotypies, dystonia, chorea, tremor, and myoclonus.

Inborn errors of metabolism (IEM)-inherited disorders in which the body cannot properly turn food into energy; a pediatric movement disorder may be the predominant symptom of an hat IEM.

Monogenic disease aka single gene disorder- Disease thought to be caused by a mutation in a single gene or one or both inherited chromosomes. Examples are cystic fibrosis (CF) and Duchenne muscular dystrophy (DMD). Even though caused by a single gene, the phenotype can vary (e.g. severity of the disease) due to differences in the patient's environment and genetic variations elsewhere in the individual's genome.

Multfactorial genetic disorders-disorders that do not follow a predictable pattern of inheritance or expression due to a combination of genetic factors and external factors such as diet, lifestyle, exposure to chemicals, and other toxins. Example conditions are certain forms of cancer, Alzheimer disease, and eczema.

Next-generation (gene) sequencing (NGS)-aka *massively parallel or deep sequencing*. This term is a catch-all phrase to describe the most modern methods to sequence nucleotides in DNA. Currently, advances in NGS allow an entire human genome to be sequenced in only a single day as opposed to the traditional and more expensive, time-consuming, Sanger sequencing method. There are three types of NGS: 1) whole-genome sequencing (WGS), 2) whole-exome sequencing (WES) and 3) targeted sequencing.

Nucelotide-building block of DNA and RNA. A nucleotide consists of a base plus molecule of sugar and one phosphoric acid. DNA contain four different nitrogenous bases: Thymine, Cytosine, Adenine, Guanine.

"Pediatric movement disorders" (PMD) (field of medical study)-a classification of movement disorders that appear in pediatric age. PMD includes movements that cannot be fully initiated, modulated, or interrupted voluntarily. Involuntary movements caused by epileptic, cerebellar, pyramidal, and neuromuscular disorders are excluded. PMDs are divided into *primary disorders (movement is only symptom) and secondary (other predominate symptoms, e.g. developmental delay)*. Two classifications of PMD: hyperkinetic and hypokinetic. PMD are defined as one or more of the following: dysfunction in target and velocity of intended movement, abnormal posturing, presence of unintended excessive movement, normal movements occurring at unintended or inappropriate times.[224]

Phenomenology of movement-the interpretation of the appearance of an individual's movement. For example, classifying a child's movement as *hyperkinetic* based on the appearance of dystonia or tremor.

Phenotypic pleiotropy-the phenomenon of a single gene affecting multiple traits in a single individual.

Precision medicine/Personalized medicine- a model of customized treatments based on the individual patient's unique genetic make up, environment, and lifestyle.

Mechanotransduction-mechanism by which mechanical perturbation (e.g exercise) influences genetic expression and cellular behavior

Single nucleotide polymorphism (SNP)-a genetic variation in a nucleotide, occurring in a specific position in the genome that is identified to commonly occur people. *Polymorphism* refers to the fact that at the specific nucleotide position on a gene, there are "poly" or "many" variations, of A, C, T, or G at the site.

Somatic cell-diploid human cells other than gametes. Changes/mutations in somatic cells are not passed via human sexual reproduction to offspring.

Somatic cell genome editing-modification to genes in the cells of a living person, such as in medical practice of *gene therapy.*

Targeted next- generation gene sequencing-gene sequencing that focuses on specific regions of the genome based on relatively few specific genes that are commonly linked by pathological mechanisms or known clinical phenotype. An example of targeted gene sequencing is a dystonia gene panel.

TaskForce on Childhood Movement Disorders –created by NIH in 2001, this taskforce of professionals worked to define consistent terminology across disciplines to describe and classify terms spasticity, dystonia, rigidity, and other pediatric movement disorders. The taskforce was comprised of professionals from developmental pediatrics, neuology, neurosurgery, orthopedic surgery, physical therapy, occupational therapy, physical medicine and rehabilitation, neurophysiology, muscle physiology, and biomechanics.[222,223]

Tic-movement that is repeated, individually recognizable, intermittent. Often brief, suppressible, and may be associated with premonitory urge.

United Nations Educational, Scientific, and Cultural Organization (UNESCO)-agency of the United Nations (UN). UNESCO has 195 member states and in 2003 adopted the International Declaration on Human Genetic Data in response to concern over the use of human genetic data contrary to individual human rights and freedom. www.unesco/org/new/en/social-and-human-sciences/themes/bioethics/human-genetic-data

Variants of unknown significance (VOUS)-an genetic variant identified in genetic testing with unknown clinical significance.

Whole-exome sequencing-sequencing that evaluates only the protein-coding portions of a gene.

Whole-genome sequencing-sequencing that evaluates the entire genomic content of an individual.

Zygote-a human zygote is the fertilized egg cell resulting from union of female and male gametes (egg and sperm).

12

Learning Disabilities and Developmental Coordination Disorder

Lenin C. Grajo, Julia Guzman, Stacey E. Szklut, and Darbi Breath Philibert

OBJECTIVES

After reading this chapter the student or therapist will be able to:

1. Define the characteristics that typically identify a child with learning disabilities.
2. Articulate accepted definitions and terminology used in the field of learning disabilities.
3. Describe the proposed causes of learning disabilities.
4. Describe the clinical presentation of subgroups within the learning-disabled population.
5. Identify members of the specialist team and service provision types for children with learning disabilities.
6. Describe the characteristics of the child with developmental coordination disorder.
7. Identify areas of evaluation to assess motor deficits effectively in the child with a learning disability.
8. Articulate theoretical development and intervention techniques applicable to children with learning disabilities and motor deficits.
9. Describe the lifelong ramifications for the individual with learning disabilities.

KEY TERMS

developmental coordination disorder
learning disabilities
life-span disability
model of disablement
motor learning

neurodevelopmental treatment
nonverbal learning disabilities
praxis
sensorimotor
verbal learning impairments

AN OVERVIEW OF LEARNING DISABILITIES

Clinical Presentation

Learning disabilities are not a singular disorder but a group of varied and often multidimensional disorders.[1] Difficulties in learning may manifest themselves in various combinations of impairments in language, memory, visual-spatial organization, motor function, and the control of attention and impulses.[2,3] The characteristics of a child with a learning disability are often diverse and complex. Each child presents a different composite of system problems/impairments and functional deficits, preventing participation in activities and societal limitations. Table 12.1 summarizes some of the clinical and behavioral manifestations in children with learning disabilities.

The most commonly recognized performance difficulties in learning are associated with academic success. Fletcher and colleagues[11] argued that learning disabilities should be characterized as "unexpected" because the child is not learning up to expectations despite adequate instruction. Typically, the areas of deficits are observed in verbal learning, including difficulties with reading, the acquisition of spoken and written language, and arithmetic. Impairments in nonverbal learning are equally important and more recently recognized. The three primary areas affected by nonverbal learning disorders include visual-spatial organization, social-emotional development, and sensorimotor performance.[12] Accompanying behavioral manifestations may include problems with self-regulatory behaviors, such as lack of attention, hyperactivity, and poor impulse control. Difficulties in social perception and social interactions may also be observed.[12,13] These learning and behavioral difficulties may be isolated (e.g., academic, motor, or behavioral), combined (e.g., academic and motor), or global (academic, motor, and behavioral).[14] In addition to verbal and nonverbal disabilities, specific motor impairments also can be present and affect academic achievement or daily life tasks.[15,16]

Definition

The heterogeneity of persons with learning disabilities has made consensus on a single definition difficult. Many disciplines describe learning disabilities according to their own frames of reference. Medical professionals tend to relate the deficit to its cause, particularly to cerebral dysfunction. Terms historically used include *brain injured,*[17] *minimal brain dysfunction,*[2] and *psychoneurological disorder,*[18] all implying a neurological cause for the deviation in development. However, educational professionals prefer to describe the child's difficulties in behavioral or functional terms. Educators view children with learning disabilities as "children who fail to learn despite an apparently normal

TABLE 12.1	**Common Clinical and Behavioral Manifestations of Learning Disability in Children**
Clinical and Behavioral Manifestation	**Description**
Deficiencies in rapid automatized naming and reading difficulties[4]	Language-based phonological deficits do not account for many of the reading difficulties in children with a learning disability (LD). Many children have slower speeds of processing information as seen in assessments of rapid automatized naming of common objects (e.g., letters, colors, numbers, pictures of objects).
Cognitive processing difficulties[5]	Children with LD demonstrate deficiencies in the following cognitive areas related to learning and language acquisition: • Syntactic awareness—the ability to understand the basic grammatical structure of language used. • Working memory—the ability to retain information in short-term memory while processing new information. • Morphological awareness—Morphemes are the smallest units of meaning within words; they help to make word pronunciation predictable and preserve the semantic relationship between words.[6] Morphological awareness is the conscious awareness of the morphemic structure of words and the ability to reflect on and manipulate this structure. • Orthographic processing—the awareness of the structure of the words in a language
Memory difficulties[7]	Many children with learning disabilities may demonstrate difficulties in complex divided attention and inability to monitor activities making multitasking challenging; children with LD may demonstrate limited processing and storage demands often manifesting as carelessness, forgetfulness, or lack of attention to details.
Mathematical difficulties[8]	Many children with LD may have slower acquisition of counting knowledge and arithmetical skills.
Language-learning difficulties[9]	Many children with LD may demonstrate late acquisition of first word; may require more and multiple exposures to expand vocabulary; reliance of shorter and simple words to communicate; poor articulation and atypical speech patterns; and restricted range of communicative intent.
Social cognition deficits[10]	Children with LD may demonstrate challenges with social adjustment, slower processing of social cues and information, challenges with social and emotional interpretation, problem-solving skills, role-taking abilities.

capacity for learning."[19] Current terminology within the academic environment includes *reading disorder, mathematics disorder, disorder of written expression,* and *intellectual disabilities.*[20,21] The lack of consensus for one accepted definition continues to affect consistency in diagnosis, research, and intervention for persons with learning disabilities.

After multiple revisions, the National Joint Committee on Learning Disabilities (NJCLD), which represents several professional organizations, proposed the following definition:

Learning disability is a general term [for a condition] that:
• Is intrinsic to the individual . . . [the term] refers to a heterogeneous group. (Each individual with learning disabilities presents with a unique profile of strengths and weakness.)
• Results in significant difficulties in the acquisition and use of listening, speaking, reading, writing, reasoning, or mathematical abilities. (These difficulties are evident when appropriate levels of effort by the student do not result in expected performance, even when provided with effective instruction.)
• Is presumed to be due to central nervous system dysfunction and may occur across the life-span. (They persist throughout life and may change in their presentation and severity at various stages of life.)
• May occur concomitantly with other impairments or other diagnoses. (For example, difficulties in self-regulation and social interaction may exist separately or result from the learning disability. Individuals with attention-deficit disorders, emotional disturbances, or intellectual disabilities may experience learning difficulties, but these diagnoses do not cause or constitute them.)
• Is not due to extrinsic factors. (Such as insufficient or inappropriate instruction, or cultural differences.)[22]

This definition identifies a proposed cause but does not provide a clear exclusion statement regarding what learning disabilities may not result from. A positive component of this definition is the lifelong nature of the condition. In addition, by including the behavioral manifestations of regulatory and social difficulties, a more complete picture of functional problems for the individual with learning disabilities is presented. This could assist in the creation of more comprehensive and life-spanning programs of service and ultimately help in the recognition and remediation of functional and societal limitations.

The definition used in educational settings was initially passed in Public Law 94-142 and later incorporated into the Individuals with Disabilities Education Act (IDEA) (Section 602.26).

Children with learning disabilities are defined by IDEA as follows:
• Individuals with a disorder in one or more of the basic psychological processes involved in understanding or using spoken or written language. (This emphasizes the receptive and expressive difficulties a student may demonstrate.)
• Those who are experiencing difficulties in the ability to listen, think, speak, read, write, spell, or do mathematical calculations. (These highlight the academic difficulties the student may experience.)
• Those who may have conditions such as perceptual disabilities, brain injury, minimal brain dysfunction, dyslexia, and developmental aphasia.
• Those who have a learning problem that does not result from other disabilities such as motor deficits, emotional disturbances, or environmental, cultural, or economic differences.

This description does not specifically address cause but does highlight psychological processes versus neurological impairments. The primary disability focus is on language, which may exclude difficulties in learning that involve nonverbal reasoning. This definition does not mention regulatory, reasoning, and social perception difficulties that may contribute to understanding the student's complete profile. On a foundational level, this definition formed the basis for creating academic programs and delineating appropriate services for children with learning disabilities.

IDEA mandates that all children will have free and appropriate education and authorizes aid for special education and educationally relevant services for children with disabilities. IDEA influences how children with learning disabilities are identified and classified. The 1997 amendments of IDEA, by promoting the early identification and provision of services, redirected the focus of special education services by adding provisions that would enable children with disabilities to make greater progress and achieve higher levels of functional performance.[23]

The IDEA 2004 amendments eliminate a previous requirement that students must exhibit a severe discrepancy between intellectual ability and achievement for eligibility. This "severe discrepancy" policy often mandated that children would have to experience failure for several years to demonstrate the requisite degree of discrepancy.[24] The current goal is to identify ways of serving students more quickly and efficiently once they begin to show signs of difficulty.[24] Congress also indicated specifically that (1) intelligent quotient (IQ) tests could not be required for the identification of students for special education in the learning disabilities category and (2) states had to allow districts to implement identification models that used Response to Instruction (RTI).[25] The RTI models suggest that the learning difficulty may be intrinsic to the child, inherent in the instruction, or a combination of both. The models propose systematically altering the quality of instruction and repeatedly measuring the child's response to that instruction. Inferences can then be made about the child's deficits contributing to learning difficulties.[26]

IDEA 2004 also limits the schools from finding a student eligible for special education services if the learning problems are determined to be caused by a lack of appropriate instruction. The law currently encourages schools to use scientific, research-based interventions to maximize a student's opportunity for success in the general education setting (least restrictive environment [LRE]) before being placed in special education. IDEA encourages educators to stress the importance of identifying individual differences and patterns of ability within each child and adjust the educational methods accordingly. Academic achievement relies heavily on the effectiveness of the teacher and the instructional techniques. Studies indicate that learning disabilities do not fall evenly across racial and ethnic groups, with a higher incidence of special education services needed for black, non-Hispanic children.[27] The No Child Left Behind (NCLB) Act challenges states and school districts to become more accountable for improving educational standards by intensifying their efforts to close the achievement gap between underachieving students and their peers.

In 2015 the Every Student Succeed Act (ESSA) replaced the NCLB. By law, ESSA requires state plans to include a description of how the state will implement the following[28,29]:

- Academic standards
- Annual testing
- Goals for academic achievement
- Ways that schools will be held responsible for student achievement
- Plans for supporting and improving struggling schools, including professional development for educators and support for English learners

Despite the ESSA mandate, a systematic analysis by the NCLD[29] has found that groups of students, including students with disabilities, low-income students, and students learning English, are frequently neglected.

Classifications

The two most widely used classification systems are those of the American Psychiatric Association (APA) (*Diagnostic and Statistical Manual of Mental Disorders* [DSM])[30] and the World Health Organization (WHO) (International Classification of Diseases [ICD]).[31] Educational professionals prefer the DSM classification for its academic relevance. A variety of specific academically related disorders are outlined in the DSM. The latest edition, DSM-V,[32] defines specific learning disorders (SLDs; often referred to as learning disorder or learning disability; see note on terminology) as a neurodevelopmental disorder that begins during school age, although may not be recognized until adulthood. Learning disabilities refers to ongoing problems in one of three areas, reading, writing, and math, which are foundational to one's ability to learn.

The classification system commonly used by therapists is the ICD. The ICD codes are state-mandated diagnostic codes used for billing and information purposes. In the recently revised ICD-11,[33] learning disability is categorized under a "Mental, Behavioral, and Neurodevelopmental disorder." Specifically, learning disability is labeled as a developmental learning disorder and is "characterized by significant and persistent difficulties in learning academic skills, which may include reading, writing, or arithmetic." In addition, ICD-11 describes developmental learning disorders as "not due to a disorder of intellectual development, sensory impairment (vision or hearing), neurological or motor disorder, lack of availability of education, lack of proficiency in the language of academic instruction, or psychosocial adversity."[34]

Incidence and Prevalence

In the United States the National Center for Learning Disabilities[35] reported that 1 in 5 children has learning and attention issues and 1 in 16 children will have Individualized Educational Plans (IEPs) for specific learning disabilities. From this subset, it has been reported that in fourth grade, 27% without disabilities, 69% with disabilities, and 85% with specific learning disabilities fall below basic levels of literacy.[35] In 2015 to 2016, the number of students aged 3 to 21 receiving special education services was 6.7 million, or 13% of all public school students. Among students receiving special education services, 34% had specific learning disabilities.[36]

Perspectives on the Causes of Learning Disabilities

Learning disability is a diverse diagnosis with varied manifestations; therefore searching for a single cause would be inadequate. Historically, researchers have studied causative factors including (1) brain damage or dysfunction caused by birth injury, perinatal anoxia, head injury, fetal malnutrition, encephalitis, and lead poisoning; (2) allergies; (3) biochemical abnormalities or metabolic disorders; (4) genetics; (5) maturational lag; and (6) environmental factors, such as neglect and abuse, a disorganized home, and inadequate stimulation.[37-39]

Current sources agree that possible causes of learning disabilities can include problems with pregnancy and birth (e.g., drug and alcohol use, low birth weight, anoxia, and premature or prolonged labor) and incidents occurring after birth (e.g., head injuries, nutritional deprivation, and exposure to toxic substances such as lead).[40-42] Genetic and hereditary links also have been observed, with learning difficulties often seen across generations within families.[42] The emotional and social environment have also been considered as a contributing factor to learning disabilities.[21]

Children with learning disabilities frequently display a composite of neuropsychological symptoms that interfere with the ability to store, process, or produce information. These symptoms typically include disorders of speech, spatial orientation, perception, motor coordination, and activity level. Researchers have attempted to identify areas of the brain that may be responsible for these functional limitations. Tools being used include empirical measures of physiological function such as electroencephalography, event-related potentials (ERPs), brain electrical activity mapping (BEAM), regional cerebral blood flow (rCBF), positron emission tomography (PET), and functional magnetic resonance imaging (fMRI). These measures expand the understanding of brain functioning but are best used in conjunction with data on functional and behavioral manifestations.

Research findings on brain structure have documented that certain functions are specialized within each hemisphere, and this specialization is optimal for efficient learning.[43,44] The left hemisphere processes information in a sequential, linear fashion and is more proficient at analyzing details. Academically, this hemisphere is responsible for recognizing words and comprehending material read, performing mathematical calculations, and processing and producing language.

The right hemisphere processes input in a more holistic manner, grasping the overall organization or the "gestalt" of a pattern.[45,46] This type of organization is advantageous for spatial processing and visual perception. Functionally, the right hemisphere synthesizes nonverbal stimuli, such as environmental sounds and voice intonation, recognizes and interprets facial expressions, and contributes to mathematical reasoning and judgment. Over time these differences in left and right brain processing have become accepted and are commonly labels of cognitive style (i.e., left-brained versus right-brained learner).

A strict left-right dichotomy is oversimplified because it does not take into account many aspects of functional brain organization.[45,47] Both hemispheres must work together for a variety of specific academic outcomes such as reading and mathematical concepts. In addition to the communication that occurs between the hemispheres via the corpus callosum, essential communication within the hemispheres is also present. Intrahemispheric communication is critical for developing higher level cognitive functions such as memory, language, visual-spatial perception, and praxis.[48] Research suggests that children with learning disabilities show different patterns of cerebral organization than normal children.[45,47] However, brain plasticity is the basis for designing and implementing a variety of intervention techniques aimed at improving processing.

Subgroups

In early attempts to classify learning disabilities, Denckla and Rudel[49] determined that approximately 30% of the 190 children they assessed by neurological examination could be classified into three recognizable subgroups. The other 70% exhibited an unclassifiable mixture of signs. Of the 30%, the first subgroup was classified as children having a *specific language disability*. These children, who were failing reading and spelling, showed a pattern of inadequacy in repetition, sequencing, memory, language, motor, and other tasks, all of which require rote functioning. The second group had a specific *visual-spatial disability*. These children had average performance in reading and spelling with delayed arithmetic, writing, and copying skills. The children in this subgroup all had social and/or emotional difficulties. The third group manifested a *dyscontrol* syndrome. These children had decreased motor and impulse control, were behaviorally immature, and were average in language and perceptual functioning.

Grouping children with learning disabilities based on patterns of academic strengths and weakness is as important as grouping them based on neuropsychological or cognitive measures. With an academic classification the heterogeneity of learning disabilities can be more clearly recognized and learning modalities can be adjusted to the individual child. For example, a child with a specific reading difficulty could be experiencing deficits in word recognition,

fluency, or comprehension. Through identification of the specific areas of weakness in reading, intervention can be individualized to improve academic performance.[11]

Based on historical and current trends the following general subgroups will be explored: verbal learning impairments, nonverbal learning disabilities (NVLDs), motor coordination deficits, and social and emotional challenges.

Verbal Learning Impairments

Verbal learning impairments typically include dyslexia, dyscalculia, and dysgraphia. Harris[20] classifies these deficits in functional terms, with dyslexia including disorders of reading and spelling, dyscalculia denoting a mathematics disorder, and dysgraphia describing a disorder of written expression. These learning disorders may occur individually or concurrently. Each of these verbal learning impairments will significantly influence academic performance.

Dyslexia (developmental reading disorder). Dyslexia is a learning impairment in which the ability to read with accuracy and comprehension is substantially less than expected for age, intelligence, and education and that impairs academic achievement or daily living.[30] The International Dyslexia Association adopted the following definition in 2002: "Dyslexia is a specific learning disability that is neurological in origin. It is characterized by difficulties with accurate and/or fluent word recognition and by poor spelling and decoding abilities. These difficulties typically result from a deficit in the phonological component of language that is often unexpected in relation to other cognitive abilities and the provision of effective classroom instruction. Secondary consequences may include problems in reading comprehension and reduced reading experience that can impede the growth of vocabulary and background knowledge."[50] Table 12.2 summarizes a multidimensional perspective to common characteristics of dyslexia.

Dyslexia is the most common learning disorder, affecting as many as 80% of individuals identified as learning disabled.[51] Prevalence rates range from 10% to 15% of the school-aged population,[50] with the highest noted estimate of 17.4%.[52] Historically, dyslexia was considered more common in boys than in girls, but data indicate an equal distribution between the sexes.[53] Boys are more likely to act out as a result of having a reading difficulty and are therefore more likely to be identified early. On the other hand, girls are more likely to try to "hide" their difficulty, becoming quiet and reserved.[25]

Causes of dyslexia can be both genetic and neurobiological.[21,25,50] Genetic causation has been linked to chromosomes 1, 2, 3, 6, 11, 13, 15, and 18.[54] There is a strong inheritability of the genetic links for dyslexia. Statistics suggest that 30% to 50% of children with dyslexia have a parent with the disorder.[55] Neuroanatomical abnormalities, atypical brain symmetry, and disruptions in neural processing have been observed in children with reading disorders.[21,25,53,56] Anatomically, the measurements that best discriminate between children with and without dyslexia are the right anterior lobe of the cerebellum and the area involving the inferior frontal gyrus of both hemispheres.[25] Dynamic investigations using functional brain imagining techniques (PET, fMRI, and the newer ultrafast echo planar imaging [EPI]) are providing significant information on brain functioning during cognitive tasks such as reading and picture naming.[21,53]

Reading skills consist of a combination of visually perceiving whole words and phonetically decoding letters, morphemes, and words.[57] Individuals with reading disorders exhibit brain activation patterns that provide evidence of an imperfectly functioning system for segmenting words into phonological (language) parts and linking the visual representations of letters to the sounds they represent.[52] These disruptions of the posterior reading system result in increased reliance on ancillary systems during reading tasks, including the frontal lobe

TABLE 12.2 Signs of Possible Reading Difficulties

Sensory and Behavioral Signs

1. Has short attention span for semistructured and highly structured reading tasks.
2. Easily distracted by extraneous stimuli in the environment and zones out during reading performance.
3. Avoids and indicates dislike for structured reading and writing tasks.
4. Complains of fatigue; shows visible signs of increased arousal and stress during structured reading tasks.
5. Gives up easily, whines and cries when encountering challenging words and texts during reading.
6. Squirms/fidgets on seat during reading tasks.

Performance Skills

1. Does not track words in text with eyes.
2. Skips words and lines during reading.
3. Does not attempt to sound out letters and words.
4. Confuses /b/, /d/, /p/, /q/ during reading.
5. Reverses letters and numbers consistently during writing.
6. Performance of near and far point copying is usually slow and laborious. Copies only one or two letters at a time.
7. Complains that letters look the same or moving when reading.

Reading Participation

1. Does not initiate reading at home and school.
2. May like being read to but will hesitate reading to someone.
3. Prefers easier books or books with more pictures and less words.
4. Prefers silent reading on his or her own over reading with and to others.
5. Gives up easily on reading sheets and homework.
6. Dislike for school and will have multiple reasons to get excused from class (e.g., frequent need to go to the restroom; feeling sick all the time; aggressive behaviors and hostility; defiance).
7. Glances over pictures and does not seem to process words and sentences during silent reading.
8. Slow, effortful, dysprosodic reading.
9. Gets left behind or lost during group reading.

and right hemisphere posterior circuitry. This suggests that the child with dyslexia may be compensating for poor phonological skills with other perceptual processes, helping to explain why individuals with dyslexia can develop reading skills, although they often remain slow and nonautomatic.[53]

Dyscalculia (mathematics disorder). Dyscalculia is a learning impairment in which mathematical ability is substantially less than expected for age, intelligence, and education and that impairs academic achievement or daily living.[30] Difficulties occur with comprehending a variety of math concepts, including number quantities, money, time, and measurement. This disorder also involves difficulties with computations and problem solving of specific math functions, which affects the ability to understand, remember, or manipulate numbers or number facts.[25] This heterogeneous disorder may involve both intrinsic and extrinsic factors.[58] Intrinsic factors are hypothesized to include deficits in visual-spatial skill, quantitative reasoning, sequencing, memory, or intelligence. Extrinsic factors can be a combination of poor instruction in the mastery of prerequisite skills as well as attitude, interest, and confidence in the subject.

Characteristics of dyscalculia include the following[59]:

- Confusing numbers and math symbols ($+, -, \times, \div$)
- Inconsistent ability in addition, subtraction, multiplication, and division

- Problems sequencing numbers, or transposing them when repeated
- Difficulty with abstract concepts of time and direction
- Poor mental math ability
- Difficulty with money, budgeting, balancing checkbooks, and financial thinking (e.g., checking change or estimating the cost of items in a shopping basket)
- Problem reading analog clocks
- Trouble keeping score during games and playing games with flexible rules of scoring such as poker

Prevalence of dyscalculia is 5% to 6% in the school-aged population, with a nearly equal male-to-female ratio.[21,60] Geary[61] concludes that individuals with arithmetic disabilities currently appear to constitute at least two subgroups: those with only mathematical disorders and those with concomitant reading disorders and/or attention-deficit disorder.

Although there is evidence that this disorder is familial and heritable, much less research on its cause is provided than on the causes of most other learning disorders. Dyscalculia shares genetic influences with reading and language measures. The association between dyslexia and dyscalculia seems to be largely genetically mediated.[21,60] Other risk factors for development of dyscalculia include prematurity and low birth weight. In addition, environmental deprivation, poor teaching, classroom diversity, and untested curricula have been linked to cause.[60]

The neurological cause of dyscalculia was initially hypothesized to be right hemisphere dysfunction because of the strong relation of visual-spatial skills to numerical computation.[62] Additional research supports the involvement of both hemispheres because mathematics computation involves a complex relation of spatial problem solving, sequential analysis, language processing, and memory.[60] Specifically involved are portions of the parietal and frontal lobes.[21] In an effort to compensate, individuals with dyscalculia can recruit alternate brain areas, but this substitution often results in inefficient cognitive functioning.[60]

Dysgraphia (disorder of written expression). Dysgraphia is a learning impairment in which writing ability is substantially less than expected for age, intelligence, and education that impairs academic achievement or daily living.[30] The DSM, fourth edition (DSM-IV) diagnosis of "disorder of written expression" depends on recognition of "writing skills substantially below those expected given the person's chronological age, measured intelligence, and age appropriate education" that "significantly interferes with academic achievement or activities of daily living (ADLs) that require composition of written texts."[30] Children with dysgraphia have specific difficulties in the ability to write, regardless of the ability to read. This may include problems using words appropriately, putting thoughts into words, or mastering the mechanics of writing. Classifications of dysgraphia can include penmanship-related aspects of writing (e.g., motor control and execution), linguistic aspects of writing (e.g., spelling and composing), or a combination.[63] This heterogeneous disorder is frequently found in combination with other academic, learning, and attention disorders.[20,25]

Characteristics of dysgraphia include the following[64]:

- Poor legibility: irregular letter size and shapes, poor spacing
- Mixing uppercase and lowercase letters; unfinished letters
- Spelling difficulties
- Fatigues quickly or complains of pain when writing
- Decreased or increased speed of copying or writing
- Needs to say words out loud while writing
- Struggles with organizing thoughts on paper
- Difficulty writing grammatically correct sentences and organized paragraphs

- Large gap between knowledge base and ability to express ideas in writing
- Awkward pencil grip

Limited data are available on the prevalence of dysgraphia. Although 10% to 30% of school-aged children struggle with handwriting, we cannot assume they have been diagnosed with dysgraphia.[65] Difficulties in written expression are frequently underidentified and can be masked by reading disorders or considered to be attributable to poor motivation. Studies have suggested that dysgraphia may be as common as reading disorders and may occur in 3% to 4% of the population.[20,63]

Dysgraphia has been suggested to be a neurological processing disorder that seldom occurs in isolation and can result from a number of other dysfunctions, including attention deficit, auditory or visual processing weakness, and sequencing problems.[21,66] The complex nature of written expression makes finding the cause difficult. Writing involves integration of spatial and linguistic functions, planning, memory, and motor output. This suggests involvement of both the left and right hemispheres for skill in decoding, spelling, formulating, and sequencing ideas, and producing work in correct spatial orientation, all coupled with rules of punctuation and capitalization.

Nonverbal Learning Disability

NVLDs (or NLDs) are considered by some to be a neuropsychological disability. Although this condition has been identified for more than 30 years, it has not yet been included as a diagnostic category in the DSM.[67] The pioneer in the field, Dr. Byron P. Rourke, first identified in 1985 this separate and distinct learning disability. In 1995 he defined nonverbal disability as "a dysfunction of the brain's right hemisphere—that part of the brain which processes nonverbal, performance-based information, including visual-spatial, intuitive, organizational and evaluative processing functions."[68] Nonverbal learning disorders affect both academic performance and social interactions in children. Three primary areas affected by NVLDs include visual-spatial organization, sensory-motor integration, and social-emotional development. The social and emotional difficulties for individuals with nonverbal learning disorders are paramount, leading some researchers to label this a *social-emotional learning disability*.[20,69] NVLDs are generally identified by a distinct pattern of strengths and deficits, with excellent verbal and rote memory skills and poorly developed sensory-motor and graphomotor ability, executive functioning, and social interactions.[20,70,71]

Characteristics of NVLDs include the following[21,67,72]:
- Higher verbal IQ compared with performance (nonverbal) on the Wechsler Intelligence Scale for Children (WISC)
- Develops speech, language, and reading skills early
- Strong vocabulary and spelling
- Ability to memorize and repeat a massive amount of information provided it is in spoken form
- Learns better and faster through hearing information rather than seeing it
- Difficulties with constructional and spatial planning tasks
- Fine and gross motor difficulties affecting printing and cursive writing, physical coordination, and balance
- May exhibit limited facial expression, flat affect, unchanging voice intonation, and robotic speech
- Poor interpretation of emotional responses made by others
- Trouble reading and understanding facial expressions, gestures, and voice intonations
- Nuances of spoken language, such as hidden meanings, figures of speech, jokes, and metaphors, are interpreted on a concrete level

- Struggles with conversation skills, dealing with new situations, and changing performance in response to interactional cues
- Difficulties in problem solving and understanding cause-effect relationships
- Poor awareness of social space
- Can be intrusive and disruptive

NVLDs make up 5% to 10% of all individuals with learning disabilities.[73] NVLD is frequently overlooked in the educational arena because children with this disorder are highly verbal and develop an extensive vocabulary at a young age. Well-developed memory for rote verbal information positively influences early academic learning of reading and spelling. Yet these students will have difficulty performing in situations where adaptability and speed are necessary, and their written output will be slow and laborious.[70] Nonverbal learning disorders are therefore challenging to identify at younger ages but become progressively more apparent and debilitating by adolescence and adulthood. The challenges in early identification, the absence from the DSM-V, and the different views held by psychological and educational disciplines often result in lack of awareness of, accurate diagnosis of, and appropriate service provision for these students.

Little is known about possible genetic or environmental causes of NVLD. There are no family, twin, adoption, segregation, or linkage studies available.[21] Pennington[21] proposes that both Turner syndrome and fragile X syndrome in females appear to be possible genetic causes of NVLD. Similarities include deficits in executive functions, increased difficulties in math versus reading and spelling, functional structural language but impaired pragmatic language, and social anxiety and shyness.[21] Differential diagnosis is essential because NVLD can occur in conjunction with dyscalculia, attention deficit, adjustment disorder, anxiety and depression, emotional disturbances, and obsessive-compulsive tendencies.

Motor Coordination Deficits

Children with learning disabilities may or may not manifest motor coordination problems. Conversely, some children have motor and coordination problems but do not experience learning difficulties. Children with motor deficits typically have difficulty acquiring age-appropriate motor skills and move in an awkward and clumsy manner. Difficulties in daily functional tasks and performance areas (e.g., school and leisure skills) are common. Motor deficits can result from a wide variety of neurological, physiological, developmental, and environmental factors. These impairments can manifest in diverse ways depending on the severity of the disorder and the areas of motor and social performance affected. This will be discussed at length in the next section.

Social and Emotional Challenges

Behavioral patterns or disorders associated with learning disabilities include frustration, anxiety, depression, attention deficits, conduct problems, and global behavior problems. Ames[74] stressed that no single behavior pattern is prevalent in children with learning disabilities. Children with learning disabilities not only struggle in the classroom but experience difficulties in the social arena as well.[75] Issues in learning and related behaviors affect one another in a complex manner, leaving us to wonder which is the cause and which is the symptom.

Frustration, deflated self-esteem, and other social and emotional difficulties tend to emerge when instruction does not match learning styles.[76] This frustration mounts as the child notices classmates surpassing them, and this often results in exasperation with trying to keep up. The pressure then becomes for the child to "try harder," when ironically most do not understand just how hard the child is trying. The dissatisfaction in not meeting the teacher's expectations is often overshadowed by the inability to succeed in personal goals and a lack of self-worth. This can result in the development of internal perfectionism to deal with the lack of competence, with the belief of the child that he or she should not make mistakes.[77]

Anxiety is another response that may occur with persistent difficulties in understanding and successfully completing schoolwork. This occurs when the child feels out of control and lacks the ability to plan and execute strategies for success.[76] The mismatch between ability, expectations, and outcomes can cause frustration, disappointment, and stress, triggering a range of emotions and behaviors that interfere with everyday functioning in multiple environments.[76]

Other emotional difficulties are noted in attention. When a lesson is taught in a manner that is too complex, the child may become inattentive. Attention problems can influence behavior, often relating to difficulties with impulse control, restlessness, and irritability, affecting learning and peer interactions. These issues frequently coincide with frustration, anger, and resentment, which may manifest as a conduct problem (e.g., verbal and nonverbal aggression, destructiveness, and significant difficulties interacting with peers). Children with learning disabilities often become discouraged and fearful, are less motivated, and develop negative and defensive attitudes. These patterns of behavior can worsen with age, contributing to juvenile delinquency.[3] Low self-esteem and depression are common during school years and tend to escalate around age 10 years.[78]

Poor academic progress, additional prompting needed from teachers, and negative attention for disruptive behaviors can cause children with learning disabilities to perceive themselves as being "different."[79] Lack of success in school experiences can influence the development of positive self-perception and can have powerfully negative effects on self-esteem.[76] A self-defeating cycle may be established: the child experiences learning problems, school and home environments become increasingly tense, and disruptive behaviors become more pronounced. These responses, in turn, further affect the child's ability to learn. Lack of success generates more failure until the child anticipates defeat in almost every situation.

Assessment and Intervention

Specialists

Evaluation and intervention for children with learning disabilities should involve an interdisciplinary team, owing to the varied nature of presenting problems. Most children with learning disabilities are seen by a group of professionals, the makeup of which depends on the purpose, location, philosophical orientation, or availability of resources of a particular program. Box 12.1 lists the different professionals and specialists who might participate in assessment or remediation of children with learning disabilities. The types of professionals are grouped into the four categories of education, medicine and nursing, psychology, and special services; they have been listed only once, although some professions could be categorized in multiple ways.

Therapists should be familiar with the roles of the various medical specialists and of primary care physicians. Psychologists have two distinct and often separate roles in the care of children with learning disorders. The first role is in identification of learning strengths and weaknesses. Psychological testing is often essential in the recognition of specific learning problems and may be done by clinical psychologists, school psychologists, or clinical neuropsychologists who specialize in diagnosis of learning disorders. The second role of psychologists is to provide mental health services and support systems to address academic, social-emotional, and behavioral issues. Counseling and behavior management can also be provided by a psychiatrist, behavioral specialist, or social worker. School adjustment or guidance

---

BOX 12.1 Types of Specialists Working With Children With Learning Disabilities

Education
Classroom teacher
Special educator
Guidance counselor
Learning disability specialist
Educational diagnostician
Reading specialist
Physical educator
Adaptive physical educator

Medicine and Nursing
Family physician
Pediatrician
Pediatric neurologist
Psychiatrist
School nurse
Biochemist
Geneticist
Endocrinologist
Nutritionist
Ophthalmologist or optometrist
Otologist or ear, nose, and throat specialist

Psychology
Clinical psychologist
Neuropsychologist
School psychologist
Child psychologist

Special Services
Occupational therapist
Physical therapist
Speech and language pathologist
Audiologist
Vision specialist
Social worker
Recreational therapist
Music therapist
Vocational education specialist

---

counselors offer support and advice on specific academic difficulties, social conflicts, and affective issues.

Physical educators, adaptive physical educators, physical therapists (PTs), occupational therapists (OTs), and speech therapists also may be involved in the assessment of motor deficits and related areas. Overlap in the areas assessed may occur. The unique training of each professional influences both the selection of tests and the qualitative aspects of assessment based on observations of a child's performance. Although the evaluations may appear similar, differences among professions are apparent in orientation and rationale when interpreting dysfunction.

Planning an assessment protocol can prevent unnecessary duplication of testing and provide comprehensive information related to the referral concerns. The referral concerns and the functional difficulties the child is experiencing drive the assessment. Communication of information between professionals and the parents will generate a comprehensive picture of the child's areas of strength and weakness, necessary for effective intervention planning. Case Study 12.1 illustrates the concept of a comprehensive pediatric assessment.

CASE STUDY 12.1 Joan

History: Joan is a 5-year-old, female, kindergarten student who is undergoing a complete psychological, neurological, educational, social, occupational, physical, speech, and language therapy school reevaluation. Joan received outpatient services including OT 1× week for 60 min and PT 1× week for 60 min for remediation of severe motor coordination and planning problems, as well as concerns with her graphomotor (ability to write) and visual perceptual skills for a year, but she no longer receives outpatient services. Joan was noted to have strabismus of both eyes. As per school records, Joan failed a hearing screening on her left ear.

Family Concerns: Joan is the third child of an intact family. She has two older brothers who excelled in sports. Joan's mother is concerned about her daughter's gross motor development and stated that Joan was "slower to walk, run, and jump than her other children." She followed her pediatrician's advice for outpatient therapy until her insurance benefits ran out. Joan's mother expressed that because she is the youngest child and her only daughter, she did not enroll Joan in extracurricular sports because of fear that she would get hurt and because, unlike her other children, "Joan is clumsy and awkward—not a graceful child." Joan's mom reported that her daughter has difficulty completing everyday day tasks such as dressing, writing, using playground equipment, and participating in sports activities with her peers and has agreed to a complete battery of assessments. As per parent report, Joan does not like to rough-house with her brothers and only likes indoor, sedentary play activities.

Clinical Observations at School: Joan demonstrated left-hand dominance. Her upper extremity range of motion and muscle tone were in the low end of normal limits. Her sitting posture was functional; however, because of the height of the table, Joan slumped in the chair, could not reach the floor, and frequently shifted positions. Joan stabilized using her right hand when necessary. She was able to cross midline, use both hands simultaneously, and transfer objects from one hand to another. Joan was able to cut a circle but held the scissors with an immature thumb down (inverse) grasp. Joan initiated a coloring activity with a tight grasp of the crayon in her left hand. She demonstrated heavy pressure on a writing utensil and broke the tip of a mechanical pencil. Joan presented with fair motor planning skills; she had difficulty sustaining certain postures such as standing on her tiptoes with her arms overhead or standing on one foot for more than 2 s. She also had some difficulty imitating positions even after demonstration.

Written Work: Joan is able to spell her first and last name; however, she writes her first name in mirror writing (i.e., the writing runs in the opposite direction to normal with individual letters reversed). She can print uppercase and lowercase letters of the alphabet but does not have uniform top-to-bottom letter formation. She has difficulty writing on the writing line with letters floating above and below the writing line when copying the alphabet and words.

Standardized Examination
The Beery-Buktenica Development Test of Visual Motor Integration, Sixth Edition (VMI)
The VMI measures a student's ability to reproduce shapes of increasing complexity following a developmental sequence. It is designed to assess the extent a student can integrate his or her visual and motor abilities (visual-motor integration). Summary of Joan's scores and impressions:

	Raw Score	Standard Score	Percentile	Inter-pretation
Motor integration	15	89	23	Below average
Visual perception	14	88	21	Below average

Joan has decreased visual spatial awareness, which interferes with the spacing between her words, following lines, and the organization of her written work on

paper. She formed letters with incorrect directionality, skipped lines, and frequently lost her place when copying. Joan's visual perceptual limitations interfere with legibility of her writing. Joan has fine motor and visual perceptual deficits that impact the quality of her written work. She was referred to a developmental optometrist to assess her visual motor and visual perceptual skills.

Bruininks-Oseretsky Test of Motor Proficiency, Second Edition (BOT-2)
Bruininks-Oseretsky Test of Motor Proficiency, Second Edition (BOT-2) is used to measure motor performance in fine and gross motor functioning. The test assesses eight areas including fine motor precision, fine motor integration, manual dexterity, bilateral coordination, balance, running speed and agility, upper-limb coordination, and strength. For the purpose of this assessment, Joan was evaluated using the short form of the assessment in the areas of fine motor precision, fine motor integration, bilateral coordination, balance, and upper-limb coordination.

Listed as follows are raw score and point score totals of Joan's evaluation:

Subtest 1: Fine Motor Precision	11
Subtest 2: Fine Motor Integration	6
Subtest 3: Manual Dexterity	5
Subtest 4: Bilateral Coordination	12
Subtest 5: Balance	6
Subtest 6: Running Speed and Agility	6
Subtest 7: Upper Limb Coordination	10
Subtest 8: Strength	6
Total Point Score	62
Standard Score	**40 Below Average**
Percentile	**16th Below Average**
Standard Deviation	**−2.0**

Fine Manual Control: This motor-area composite measures control and coordination of the distal musculature of the hands and fingers, especially for grasping, drawing, and cutting.

The Fine Motor Precision subtest consists of activities that require precise control of finger and hand movement. The objective of the subtest is to measure ability to draw, fold, or cut within a specified boundary. The Fine Motor Integration subtest requires the examinee to reproduce drawings of various geometric shapes that range in complexity from a circle to overlapping pencils. Sample's score is consistent with individuals who, when copying from pictures, can accurately draw a variety of geometric shapes such as a triangle and a wavy line, as well as more complex designs such as a five-point star and overlapping pencils.

Manual Coordination: This motor-area composite measures control and coordination of the arms and hands, especially for object manipulation. The Manual Dexterity subtest uses goal-directed activities that involve reaching, grasping, and bimanual coordination with small objects. Emphasis is placed on accuracy; however, the items are timed to differentiate levels of dexterity more precisely. The Upper-Limb Coordination subtest consists of activities designed to measure visual tracking with coordinated arm and hand movement.

Body Coordination: This motor-area composite measures control and coordination of the large musculature that aids in posture and balance. The Bilateral Coordination subtest measures the motor skills involved in playing sports and many recreational games. The tasks require body control, and sequential and simultaneous coordination of the upper and lower limbs. The Balance subtest evaluates motor-control skills that are integral for maintaining posture when standing, walking, or reaching.

Strength and Agility. This motor-area composite measures control and coordination of the large musculature involved in locomotion, especially in recreational and competitive sports.

Personal Strengths and Weaknesses. A personal strength or weakness is indicated when an examinee's motor-area composite standard score is either substantially higher or substantially lower than his or her other motor-area composite standard scores. For Joan, Fine Manual Control represents a relative strength and Body Coordination represents a personal weakness. Based on the information obtained through the chosen subtests, it can be concluded that Joan has overall below average fine and gross motor development for her age range.

The Sensory Processing Measure

The Sensory Processing Measure is an assessment tool used to gauge presence of sensory processing issues, praxis, and social participation in elementary school-aged children. This assessment tool provides a unique and all-encompassing perspective of a child's sensory functioning in the environments of the home, school, and community were used to evaluate fine motor skills. The assessment covers behaviors from the main sensory systems including visual, auditory, tactile, proprioceptive, and vestibular functioning. It is essential to look at these different environments because symptoms or behaviors may manifest in differently in different environments.

Subtest	Raw Score	T-Score	Interpretive Range
Social participation	30	71	Definite difference
Vision	18	64	Some problems
Hearing	14	64	Some problems
Touch	24	68	Some problems
Body awareness	30	75	Definite dysfunction
Balance/motion	17	60	Some problems
Planning and ideas	30	77	Definite dysfunction
Total	162	78	Definite dysfunction

SPM Description and T-Score (Teacher) Average = 40T–59T, Some Problems = 60T–69T, Definite Difference = 70T–80T NOTE: Additional observations are included (Parent and Occupational Therapist). As noted above, Joan has a definite sensory dysfunction in the areas of social participation, body awareness (difficulty grading the proper amount of force), and planning and ideas (frequently bobbles or drops items she is carrying and shows poor organization of materials in on or around her desk). These areas of dysfunction may be affecting her social participation and school performance.

School-Based Service Delivery Models

The model of service delivery for each individual child should be developed to facilitate the student's ability to be successful in the learning environment. A continuum of services exists to enable interventionists to be responsive to all children's needs. The continuum includes consultation, integrated or supervised therapy, and direct service.[80] Unfortunately, a lack of available resources can influence what type and frequency of services are provided. In creating a plan that truly addresses the issues hindering a child's learning within the academic setting, the team must work together to fabricate relevant and inclusive goals.

IDEA currently requires that all children in special education be educated in the LRE. The law requires that students with disabilities be educated to the extent appropriate with their peers, within the inclusion classroom. Removing the child from the classroom for special education and intervention is discouraged unless it is absolutely necessary for the student to learn effectively. Although the model of inclusion can be effective for many children, it requires members of the team to work closely together with the regular education teacher. This collaborative effort ensures an understanding of the child's special learning needs and incorporation of therapeutic procedures into the regular classroom to facilitate the best learning environment.

Bricker[81] contends that adhering strictly to this model can be detrimental to certain students, and each case must be looked at individually. The LRE should be determined after assessing the specific needs of the child. If services in a regular classroom, coupled with supplemental aids and services, do not meet the needs of the child, an alternate environment should be considered. The first adaptation might be to have the child participate for the majority of the day in the regular classroom and leave for special instruction for part of the day. In some educational settings, children with learning disabilities are given full-time instruction in a special classroom with a small group of other children with learning disabilities. A special education teacher or a learning disability specialist is in charge of the classroom. The most specialized environment would be a private school only for children with learning disabilities.

LEARNING DISABILITIES AND MOTOR DEFICITS OR DEVELOPMENTAL COORDINATION DISORDER

Developmental coordination disorder (DCD) is a term that was first introduced in the DSM in 1987 to define a condition that has affected children for more than a century.[82] It is defined as a failure of acquisition of skills in both gross and fine movements, not based on impaired general learning or lack of opportunity to gain motor skills as peers.[83] The APA and the WHO both have inclusive and exclusive criteria in their definition. For APA, the inclusive criteria include "impairment in the development of motor coordination, which can be manifested in delays in milestones such as standing and walking; inferior performance in sports activities; and untidy handwriting."[84] Exclusive criteria include a motor deficit not due to another diagnosed condition. In addition, if a significant learning difficulty is present, the motor difficulties should supersede the cognitive limitations. The WHO definition overlaps with the APA definition by noting that a child would need to score two standard deviations below the mean on a standardized test of motor impairment and be accompanied by limitations of academic performance and/or ADLs.[85] In addition, there should be no concurrent neurological disorders, and those with an IQ below 70 should be excluded from diagnosis. Studies in DCD have shown that children perceive themselves as less competent than their peers, not only in the domain of physical competence but also in self-esteem and social acceptance.[82]

Approximately half of children with learning disabilities have motor coordination problems.[86] Motor deficits are often the most overt sign of difficulty for the child with learning disabilities. Lowered academic achievement within any or all areas of learning (reading, spelling, writing) is also seen in children with DCD.[15,30] A study by Jongmans and colleagues[86] indicates that children with concomitant perceptual-motor and learning problems are more severely affected in motor difficulties than those with only DCD or who are only learning disabled. At times, extreme discrepancy in competence over a range of motor skills exists, with strengths in some motor areas and significant weaknesses in others. Presentation of difficulties may change over time depending on developmental maturation, environmental demands, and interventions received.

An International Consensus Meeting on Children and Clumsiness was held in 1994 with expert educators, kinesiologists, OTs, PTs, psychologists, and parents. These experts discussed a common name to identify "clumsy" children with movement, coordination, and motor planning difficulties. The term *DCD*, as first described in DSM-III,[30] was identified to distinguish these children from those with severe motor impairments (such as those with cerebral palsy or paraplegia) and children with normal motor movements. A child with DCD often exhibits difficulty with motoric academic tasks such as handwriting and gym class, self-care skills such as dressing and using utensils, and leisure activities including playground games and social interactions.[87]

Definition

The DSM-5[32] classifies DCD as a discrete motor disorder under the broader heading of neurodevelopmental disorders. The specific DSM-5 criteria for DCD are as follows:

- Acquisition and execution of coordinated motor skills are below what would be expected at a given chronological age and opportunity for skill learning and use; difficulties are manifested as clumsiness (e.g., dropping or bumping into objects) and as slowness and inaccuracy of performance of motor skills (e.g., catching an object, using scissors, handwriting, riding a bike, or participating in sports).
- The motor skills deficit significantly or persistently interferes with ADLs appropriate to the chronological age (e.g., self-care) and impacts academic or school productivity, prevocational and vocational activities, leisure, and play.
- The motor skills deficits cannot be better explained by intellectual disability or visual impairment and are not attributable to a neurological condition affecting movement (e.g., cerebral palsy, muscular dystrophy, or a degenerative disorder).

Clinical Presentation

DCD is a childhood disorder characterized by poor coordination and clumsiness. Typically, there is no easily identifiable neurological disorder accompanying this lack of motor skills required for everyday life.[88] Characteristics can be seen in developmental areas such as gross motor, fine motor, visual motor, self-care, and social-emotional areas. Children tend to develop at a slower rate and require more effort and practice to accomplish age-level tasks. The salient features are coordination difficulties that include decreased anticipation, speed, reaction time (RT), and quality and grading of movement.[89,90] These children often have difficulties analyzing the task demands of an activity,

interpreting cues from the environment, using knowledge of past performance, and transferring and generalizing skills.[91]

Coordination difficulties are most apparent when complex motor activities are attempted. Physical education class often presents major problems. For example, a 9-year-old boy described his motor problems as follows: "When the gym teacher tells us to do something, I understand exactly what he means. I even know how to do it, I think. But my body never seems to do the job."[92]

Development of gross and fine motor skills, coupled with the child's ability to master body movements, enhances feelings of self-esteem and confidence. Through persistence in mastering the varied challenges of motor exploration the child builds self-reliance. The frustrations and accomplishments enhance confidence and the ability to take risks. By engaging in group activities children develop essential social skills, including how to compromise, work as a team, and deal with conflicts and different personality styles.

Poor motor coordination often results in significant social and emotional consequences. When a child is poorly coordinated, she or he is often teased and shunned from group play. This may lead to anxiety and avoidance of participation in games, as children frequently judge themselves to be both physically and socially less competent.[93] Anxiety may be more prevalent in adolescence, most notably in boys.[94] Because they are often unsuccessful in group participation, difficulties with navigating the changing demands of cooperative play and negotiating with others and reluctance to advocate for themselves often result. Boys with learning and motor coordination problems have been found to demonstrate significantly less effective coping strategies in all domains of functioning compared with a normative sample.[95] Feelings of incompetence, depression, or frustration are common and can be lifelong problems.[96,97] The impact of motor coordination difficulties on social behavior is exemplified by this statement from a child with learning disabilities and motor deficits:

Gross motor characteristics of DCD include the following:
- Diminished core strength and postural control
- Delayed balance reactions
- Often falling, tripping, and bumping into things; acquiring more than the usual number of bruises
- Motor movements that are performed at a slower rate despite practice and repetition[90]
- Motor milestones that may be achieved in the later range of normal development
- Poor anticipation (do not use knowledge of past performance to prepare)
- Notably different quality of running and ball skills from typical peers
- Difficulty learning bilateral tasks such as riding a bicycle, catching a ball, and jumping rope
- Possible hesitance with and avoidance of new or complex motor tasks (e.g., playground equipment, gym class)
- Possibly poor safety awareness
- Inability to smoothly turn and position body when going up ladder to a slide or to get into a chair
- Possible sedentary activity level; may prefer to engage in solitary play
- Tendency to not play games by the rules
- Often, avoidance of team sports such as T-ball and soccer
  Fine motor characteristics of DCD include the following:
- Diminished wrist and hand strength
- Maladaptive or immature grasp patterns
- Possible use of excess or not enough pressure
- Poor refinement of small motor movements with hands (qualitatively, the child looks like he or she is wearing a pair of gloves when trying to manipulate small objects)

- Often dropping or breaking items
- Delayed dressing skills (buttons, zippers, fasteners, shoelaces)
- Trouble with eating utensils (scooping, piercing)
- Difficulty with tool use (e.g., scissors, pencils, stapler, hole punches)
- Writing that is laborious and often illegible
- Impaired drawing ability characterized by poor motor control, with wobbly lines, inaccurate junctures, and difficulty coloring within the lines
- Decreased ability with pasting, gluing, manipulating stickers and other art materials
- Difficulty with constructive, manipulative play (e.g., block building, Tinkertoys, Legos)
- Often the presence of associated articulation deficits, possibly because of the fine motor nature demanded for articulation
  Visual motor characteristics of DCD include the following:
- Difficulty with visually guided motor actions (i.e., eye-hand and eye-foot coordination)
- Hesitancy or decreased safety on stairs
- Trouble with timing needed for kicking, hitting, and catching ball
- Difficulty with hopscotch and four squares
- Poor judgment of spatial relationships (knowing where the body is in space)
- Delayed development of prepositional and directional concepts
- Difficulty with spatial planning tasks such as puzzles, building models, and constructional toys
- Handwriting that is often labored, with spacing and sizing problems evident; letters may be irregular, illegible, and poorly organized on the page
  Self-care characteristics of DCD include the following:
- Slowness to develop independence in ADLs
- Overreliance on parents to help with self-care skills
- Clothes that are often on backward or crooked
- Struggles with cutting fingernails, putting on makeup, tying necktie, using a hair dryer
- Difficulty blowing nose with tissue, putting on Band-Aid
- Trouble putting toothpaste on toothbrush
- Messy eater, spills often, does not recognize food on face
- Difficulty pouring from a container, opening lunch box, unwrapping sandwich, opening containers, peeling fruit
- Trouble packing a bag, backpack, or suitcase
- Difficulty sequencing daily routines
  Social and emotional characteristics of DCD include the following:
- Often emotionally immature
- May exhibit behavioral difficulties such as acting out or becoming class clown
- May be more introverted and anxious
- Can appear fiercely competitive, hating to lose, complaining that rules are unfair
- Can be self-deprecating, calls self "stupid"
- Often easily frustrated
- May experience depression and feelings of incompetence
- Has difficulty making and maintaining friendships, plays alone
- Has feelings of low self-worth, poor self-esteem[98]
- Perceived by others as lazy, overprotected, or immature[99]
- Adolescents may have fewer social pastimes and hobbies than peers

Prevalence

The prevalence fluctuates between 4% and 5% in mainstream primary schools[83,85] to 6% of the population,[100] and more recently, up to 10% worldwide.[101] Prevalence is directly related to the way the assessment is used and the establishment of cut-off points. Gender differences have been examined on numerous occasions, and the consensus is that the condition is more prevalent in boys than girls, with a ratio of 2.[85]

Perspectives on the Causes of Developmental Coordination Disorder

There is no single explanation for the cause of DCD. Neurological dysfunction, physiological factors, genetic predisposition, and prenatal and perinatal birth factors have been proposed to explain the basis of DCD.[99,102] It is recognized that DCD is heritable and is genetically distinct from attention-deficit/hyperactivity disorder (ADHD), although the comorbidity rate is up to 50%.[21] Comorbidity is high with other diagnoses, including autism spectrum disorders,[88] as well as a variety of developmental learning problems such as math disability, reading disability, specific language disabilities, spelling and writing disabilities, and so on. Correlation has also been noted between preterm infancy and low birth weight with characteristics of DCD. The heterogeneity of DCD makes finding a unitary cause difficult. Children with DCD present wide variability in both locus of specific problems and functional disabilities. Further complicating an understanding of the cause is that the intervention for the child with DCD is driven by competing treatments.[103]

Few studies have been conducted to look at brain images in children with DCD, with no particular patterns of abnormality observed.[99] Hadders-Algra[104] has suggested that DCD is a result of damage at the cellular level in the neurotransmitter and receptor systems, rather than a specific region of the brain. Resulting coordination difficulties can be from a combination of one or more impairments in proprioception, motor programming, timing, or sequencing of muscle activity.

Possible physiological origins of motor coordination deficits have highlighted multisensory processing. Ayres,[105] in her theory of sensory integration, suggested that the integration among sensory systems is imperative for refined motor performance in children. She proposed that normal development depends on intrasensory integration, particularly from the somatosensory and vestibular systems. Lane[106] outlines the role of vision, combined with vestibular and proprioceptive inputs, as a foundation to motor performance. In combination, these systems sustain postural tone and equilibrium, provide awareness and coordination of head movements, and stabilize the eyes during movement in space.

More recently, Piek and Dyck[107] found support for the correlations between DCD and deficits in kinesthetic perception, visual-spatial processing, and multisensory integration.[107] In general, it is thought that reduced rates of processing information and deficits in handling spatial information may underlie the deficits in motor control.[88] Obviously more work is needed on the cause of DCD.

Subtypes of Developmental Coordination Disorder

Various approaches have been used to investigate subtypes of DCD, including classification by underlying causes, clinical and descriptive approaches, and statistical clustering.[108] Initial attempts at classifying subtypes within DCD support the heterogeneity of this group of children.[109] Work by Dewey and Kaplan[110] suggests that children with DCD may be classified into subgroups based on distinctions in motor planning and motor execution deficits. They identified three subgroups: children who exhibited deficits in motor execution alone, those whose primary deficits were in motor planning, and children who exhibited a generalized impairment in both areas.

Macnab and colleagues[111] identified five different profiles of children with DCD. They used measures of kinesthetic acuity, gross motor skill, static balance, visual perception, and visual motor integration. Two distinct groups emerged, with children exhibiting generalized visual deficits and generalized dysfunction in all areas. Generalized gross motor deficits did not emerge as a distinct subgroup, because the third group demonstrated a discrepancy between static balance and complex gross motor tasks, and the fourth group had poor performance on running but performed well on kinesthetic acuity. Other groups included children with deficits in visual motor and fine motor problems. These results suggest that a subtype based on motor execution or planning problems alone may be too general.

Diagnosis

A two-step approach to assessment using the Movement Assessment Battery for Children (M-ABC)[112] is the preferred standardized measure for motor impairment. The M-ABC checklist is used as a guide to examine the effects on daily living.[85] The M-ABC is the most widely used instrument and contains a standardized normative referenced test, plus a criterion-referenced test. The diagnosis of DCD is made for those scoring at or below the fifth percentile checklist.[85] The M-ABC consists of three subtests: manual dexterity, ball skills, and static and dynamic balance. Each subtest is given a score and totaled for an overall impairment score. A higher numerical score is indicative of a higher level of impairment.[82]

DCD may co-occur with other disorders such as ADHD, dyslexia, and autism spectrum disorders. There is also evidence suggesting that one-third of children with speech and language impairment are likely to have DCD as well.[83] Because of the heterogeneous nature of the disorder, it is often underrecognized by health care professionals. In a survey of the physicians from Canada, the United States, and the United Kingdom, only 41% of pediatricians and 23% of general practitioners had knowledge of the condition. Furthermore, only 23% of the pediatricians and 9% of the general practitioners surveyed had ever diagnosed DCD.[113] A systematic review involving school-aged children showed significantly greater odds of developing DCD among children who had very low birth weights (<1500 g) or were very preterm (<32 weeks) than among age-matched controls born at term with normal birth weights.[113]

Neurophysiology

There is no clear etiology for DCD; however, it is a recognized as a central processing disorder.[101,114–116] Some early studies have considered the neural mechanisms potentially implicated in DCD. However, the underlying neural processes remain unclear and the heterogeneous nature of the disorder further confounds attempts to find an underlying cause. The cerebellum is believed to be more implicated than peripheral mechanisms in the pathophysiological mechanisms of DCD.[115] The behavioral manifestations of lack of postural control and lack of coordination suggest involvement of cerebellum, basal ganglia, and frontal and parietal lobes.[101] The cerebellum might also be involved in the pathophysiology of DCD, because a disruption of the cerebellocerebral network has been given as an explanation for DCD.[115] In skilled action, cerebellar and parietal areas process information and their outputs are integrated into one smooth movement. The posterior parietal cortex appears to also be involved with a faulty "feedforward mechanism" where the person cannot create an efference copy of a motor plan and thus has an "efference copy deficit."[115] The use of visual information sources in the guidance of goal-directed behavior was studied by de Oliveira and Wann[117] through visual pursuits. The DCD subjects showed an impaired internal model with inadequate forward or predictive model of movement and difficulties in skilled movement when near and far visual information were present; therefore it is possible that integration of cerebellar and parietal areas was inadequate.[117]

Assessment of Motor Impairments

A variety of professionals may be involved in a comprehensive assessment of motor deficits. Pediatric OTs and PTs are often the core team assessing functional motor concerns. Areas assessed by pediatric OTs and PTs often overlap, so communication is essential to ensure that testing is not replicated. Ideally, performance will be evaluated in multiple environments and include components of skill, functional performance areas, and social and societal participation. Specific recommendations should include activities to enhance performance in the environments in which the child functions.

Clinical judgment of the therapist is important in designing an assessment protocol and synthesizing information to create a complete profile of the child. A variety of standardized and nonstandardized evaluation tools should accompany structured clinical observations and caretaker interviews. Observations of the child can yield more readily usable information than a standardized score,[118] enabling the therapist to view the child in natural routines, self-directed activities, and unstructured play. The interview process is essential to gather information about the child's interactions and participation. This process paints a verbal picture of the child to help us to understand levels of functioning and participation in a variety of environments. Other crucial information obtained is how the child's difficulties are affecting the ability to parent or teach the student.[118]

Before choosing an evaluation tool the therapist should be aware of the intended purpose of this measure. Tools used to assess children with DCD are used for distinct purposes: identify impairments, describe severity of impairments, or explore activity or participation limitations.[91] The choice of evaluations may also be determined by the setting, frame of reference of the therapist, and functional concerns of the child. A therapist should be familiar with all aspects of test administration and scoring for evaluation tools and should comply with the training requirements described in the test manual. Test construction, reliability, and validity for assessing DCD should be considered. Appendix 12.A provides an overview of standardized tests available for the assessment of motor dysfunction in children with learning disabilities. Uses and limitations of the individual tests and test batteries are listed.

Identification of subtle motor difficulties is critical and challenging. These subtle motor difficulties initially can be undetected, leading to unrealistic expectations of age-level motor performance. The child's difficulty with skilled, purposeful manipulative tasks or with finely tuned balance activities may not be readily apparent in the classroom or may be perceived as lack of effort. Children with DCD may be able to perform certain motor tasks with a level of strength, flexibility, and coordination that is qualitatively average but must use increased effort and cognitive control for sustained success.

Levels of performance in gross and fine motor testing may fall in the borderline range. Careful observations are of paramount importance because the child's deficits are often qualitative rather than quantitative. A child might have age-appropriate balance on testing but lack ability in weight shifting and making quick directional changes, which affects the ability to participate in extracurricular activities such as soccer or baseball. When assessing children with subtle motor deficits, it is important to realize that many evaluation tools have been developed for children with moderate to severe neurological impairments.

Children with DCD do not exhibit obvious evidence of neuropathological disease (i.e., "hard" neurological signs such as a cerebral lesion). Subtle abnormalities of the central nervous system are frequently noted by the presence of "soft" neurological signs. Deficits associated with soft neurological signs include abnormal movements and reflexes, sensory deficits, and coordination difficulties. Evaluation of soft neurological signs is typically part of an examination by a

BOX 12.2   Common Soft Neurological Signs Used in Assessment of Children With Learning Disabilities and Motor Deficits

Minor Neurological Indicators

Left-right discrimination
Finger agnosia
Visual tracking
Extinction of simultaneous stimuli
Choreiform movement
Tremor
Exaggerated associated movements
Reflex asymmetries

Coordination

Finger-to-nose touching
Sequential thumb-finger touching
Diadochokinesia
Heel to shin
Slow controlled motions
Postural-motor measures
Muscle tone
Schilder's arm extension posture
Standing with eyes closed (Romberg test)
Walking a line
Tandem walking (forward and backward)
Hopping, jumping, skipping
Ball throw and catch
Imitation of tongue movements
Pencil and paper tasks
Fine motor tasks (stringing beads, building block towers)

Sensory Indicators

Graphesthesia
Stereognosis
Localization of touch input

pediatric neurologist, although therapists can assess these areas in conjunction with standardized testing. Box 12.2 lists soft neurological signs frequently used to assess this population.

Researchers suggest that a high percentage of children with learning disabilities exhibit certain soft neurological signs. An early study reported that 75% of 2300 children with positive total "neurological soft sign" ratings had the symptom of poor coordination.[119] More recently, 169 children aged 8 to 13 years were assessed for a relation between soft neurological signs and cognitive functioning, motor skills, and behavior. Those children with a high index for soft neurological signs were found to have significantly worse scores in each domain.[120] The relationship between neurological soft signs and DCD is difficult to validate without more current systematic research; however, they are indicators that intervention may be needed.[121]

In general, a composite of soft neurological signs is more predictive of dysfunction than single signs. Children without notable motor difficulties can frequently exhibit one or more soft signs, therefore identification of a single sign must be interpreted cautiously. Neurological signs involving complex processes were found to be the most predictive. The clinician needs to be familiar with typical developmental patterns, as certain soft neurological signs such as motor overflow, right-left confusion, visual tracking difficulties, and articulatory substitution are expected at younger ages and mature in quality over time.

Compiling a complete picture of motor deficits in children with learning disabilities involves assessing the following complex skills: (1) postural control and gross motor performance, (2) fine motor and visual motor performance, (3) sensory integration and sensory processing, (4) praxis and motor planning, and (5) physical fitness. Each of these interrelated functions is described in this chapter as an area of clinical assessment.

Postural Control and Gross Motor Performance

Muscle tone and strength. Low muscle tone and poor joint stability have been identified as characteristic of some children with learning disabilities. On observation, the child with low tone may look "floppy" and may have an open-mouth posture, lordotic back, sagging belly, and knees positioned closely together; muscles may be poorly defined and feel "mushy" or soft on palpation, and joints may be hyperextensible. A common method for assessing muscle tone and proximal joint stability involves placing the child in a quadruped position and observing the ability to maintain the position without locking of the elbows, winging of the scapula, or sagging (lordosis) of the trunk. The therapist can determine joint stability by asking the child to "freeze like a statue." The therapist then provides intermittent pushes to the trunk, assessing the child's ability to remain in a static position.

Children with low tone may develop patterns of compensation called *fixing patterns*. These patterns often include elevated and internally rotated shoulders, internally rotated hips, and pronated feet. The child compensates for low tone by using the stable joint positions and holding himself or herself stiffly for increased stability. These patterns may resemble those of children with slightly increased tone. Careful observation and palpation of muscles will help to differentiate fixing patterns from increased muscle tone. Judgments of muscle tone are primarily made through clinical observations and felt in a hands-on assessment.

Manual muscle testing can provide detailed information about impairment in strength of individual muscles but is not regularly used in assessing children with learning disabilities, unless concerns of a possible degenerative disease exist. More appropriately, the child's functional ability should assess strength to move against gravity during activities. Within developmental assessments, the therapist is observing range of motion against gravity in skills such as reaching, climbing, throwing, and kicking. The therapist also can have the child hold positions against gravity to assess strength and endurance (e.g., prone extension and supine flexion).

Early postural reflexes. Early reflexes are essential for the development of normal patterns of motor development. These reflexes facilitate movement patterns that become integrated into purposeful motions. If they are not fully integrated, qualitative differences in muscle tone, postural asymmetries, transitional movement patterns, bilateral coordination, and smooth timing and sequencing of motor tasks may be observed. Residual reactions (e.g., asymmetrical tonic neck reflex [ATNR] and symmetrical tonic neck reflex [STNR]) that might be noted in children with DCD are subtle and most often are seen in stressful, nonautomatic tasks. McPhillips and Sheehy looked at incidence of primitive reflex patterns and motor coordination difficulties in children with reading disorders.[122] The group with the lowest reading scores had a significantly higher rate of ATNR and motor impairments when compared with good readers. Assessment for persistence of primitive reflex patterns in children with learning disabilities should emphasize impact on functional aspects of performance.

The effect of lack of integration can be observed during tasks such as writing at a table or gross motor activities such as using ball skills and jumping rope. Persistence of these primitive reflexes may be seen in the child's inability to sit straight forward at the table. The ATNR influence might be observed by a sideways position at the table with the arm on the face side used in extension. During ball games the child may have diminished ability to throw with directional control because head movements will influence extension of the face-side arm. If the STNR is not fully integrated the child is often unable to flex the legs while sitting at a desk looking down at his or her work (neck flexion). Although residual reflex involvement may affect performance of these tasks, many other components are involved that require consideration.

Righting, equilibrium, and balance. Righting and equilibrium are dynamic reactions essential for the development of upright posture and smooth transitional movements. Righting reactions help to maintain the head in an upright alignment during movement in all directions. Equilibrium reactions occur in response to a change in body position or surface support to maintain body alignment. In simpler terms, equilibrium reactions get us into a position, and righting reactions keep us in that position. Together these reactions provide continuous automatic adjustments that maintain the center of gravity over the base of support and keep the head in an upright position.

Righting and equilibrium reactions are best assessed on an unsteady surface such as a tilt board or large therapy ball. These reactions occur in all developmental positions, and complete assessment will consider a range of positions during functional performance in gross and fine motor activities. To test equilibrium, the child's center of gravity is quickly tipped off balance. The equilibrium response is one of phasic extension and abduction of the downhill limbs for protection and of flexion of the uphill body side for realignment. In daily actions, most of the righting reactions are subtle and occur continuously to slight changes in body position. Subtle shifts of the support surface can be made to assess the child's ability to maintain the head and trunk in a continuous upright position. Righting and equilibrium reactions are the basis for functional balance and postural control.

To balance effectively, we use visual information (about the body and external environment), proprioceptive information (about limb and body position), and vestibular information (about head position and movement) to initiate an appropriate corrective response.[123] Balance reactions occur as a response to changes in the center of gravity that stimulate the vestibular receptors (utricles and semicircular canals). This stimulation causes muscles to activate, allowing balance to be maintained in static and dynamic activities (e.g., sitting in a chair, walking, standing on a bus). When the vestibular system works in conjunction with vision and information from the muscles (proprioception), balance is easier and more refined. Considering the impact of these sensory systems working together is important during assessment. The therapist should test the child's balance with the child's eyes open and closed and observe differences in ease and quality of performance. Standing with eyes closed relies more on vestibular and proprioceptive input, and difficulty may indicate that the child depends heavily on the visual system for balance. To further assess this sensory interaction, balance should also be observed on steady and unsteady surfaces (e.g., dense foam or a tilt board) with and without visual orientation. Traditional tests of balance include (1) the Romberg position—standing with feet together and eyes closed, (2) Mann position—standing with feet in tandem with eyes closed, and (3) standing on one leg with eyes open and eyes closed.

Postural control. Postural control is dependent on muscle tone, strength, and endurance of the trunk musculature, as well as automatic postural reactions required to maintain a dynamic upright position. A child has adequate postural control when he or she can maintain upright positions, shift weight in all directions, rotate, and move smoothly between positions. These areas are often deficient in children with DCD, affecting both gross and fine motor performance.

The child may fatigue quickly and fall often during gross motor play. Other body parts may be used for additional support because of weak postural musculature—for example, placing the head on the ground when crawling up an incline or sticking out the tongue when climbing or pumping a swing. In sitting, a child with diminished postural control will fatigue quickly, either leaning on his or her hands for additional support or moving frequently in and out of the chair. These compensations affect the child's ability to perform fine motor tasks or maintain attention for cognitive learning because so much effort is exerted on sitting up. Observing the effects of fatigue is important because both sitting and standing postures may deteriorate over the course of a day. The problem stems from motor programming problems versus muscle power.

Gross motor skills. *Gross motor coordination* refers to motor behaviors related to posture and locomotion, from early developmental milestones to finely tuned balance. Children with learning disabilities and DCD may attain high degrees of motor skill in specific activities. Motor accomplishments frequently remain highly specific to motor sequences or tasks and do not necessarily generalize to other activities, regardless of their similarities. When variation in the motor response is required, the response often becomes inaccurate and disorganized.

Although children with DCD can sit, stand, and walk with apparent ease, they may be awkward or slow in rolling, transitioning to standing, running, hopping, and climbing. Skilled tasks such as skipping may be accomplished with increased effort, decreased sequencing and endurance, and associated movements.

Evaluation of gross motor skills should include both novel motor activities and age-appropriate skills. For example, the child can be asked to imitate a hopping sequence or maneuver around a variety of obstacles. Skills that have been accomplished can be varied slightly (e.g., hopping over a small box). Age-appropriate social participation tasks, such as tag and dodge ball, can be observed for qualitative difficulties in timing and spatial body awareness. Developmentally earlier skills also should be observed to assess the quality of performance. *Bruininks-Oseretsky Test of Motor Proficiency, Second Edition* (BOT-2)[124] and the *Peabody Developmental Motor Scales*[125] are examples of tools for standardized assessment of gross motor skills (see Appendix 12.A).

Coordination Deficits

Three subtypes of DCD have been identified: ideomotor, visual-spatial and constructional, and mixed dyspraxia.[101] The principal areas of impairment of the three subtypes were digital perception, imitations of gestures, digital praxis, Lego blocks, visual spatial structuration, visual motor integration, and coordination between upper and lower limbs. The accuracy of goal-directed movements, motor organization, and control of motor actions has been studied.[101,117] Individuals with and without DCD do not differ in their ability to engage in motor imagery, and evidence suggests both groups used motor imagery (as opposed to visual imagery) because performance was better in simple rotations.[117]

O'Brien and colleagues[116] examined the mechanisms underlying motor coordination in children with DCD. The processing of visual, auditory, and vibrotactile information was explored in children 6 to 7 years and 9 to 10 years with and without DCD. Because motor deficits of children with DCD include poor balance and postural control, difficulty with eye-hand coordination, longer movement times, and problems with sequencing, the authors studied patterns of choice RT to analyze the speed in which children process input and initiate a response. Thirty-six children were matched in the study (20 control and 16 with DCD), and their RT was analyzed to see the differences between spatially compatible and spatially incompatible RTs using the anatomical and spatiotemporal mapping hypotheses. Spatial compatibility refers to conditions in which the location of the stimulus corresponds with the location of the response (i.e., same side), and spatially incompatible conditions are those in which the stimulus and expected response are in opposite sides.[116] According to the anatomical mapping theory, ipsilateral responses should be faster than contralateral responses because they do not require transfer of information to the opposite hemisphere. The spatiotemporal mapping refers to the spatial relationship between the stimulus and the response; thus the RT would be shorter when the stimulus is in spatial proximity to the response.[116] In the experiment, the children were asked to depress a switch with the index finger of each hand to respond as soon as they saw, felt, or heard a visual, auditory, or vibrotactile stimulus presented in blocked schedules of 15 trials under each condition. The authors found no differences between the group of 8- to 10-year-old children (with and without DCD) under the compatible or incompatible conditions. However, the 6- to 7-year-old children with DCD had significantly longer RTs than their counterparts without DCD under incompatible conditions. Overall, RTs for children with DCD were slower than were those of their peers without DCD under all sensory conditions (visual, auditory, and vibrotactile). In this study, the spatiotemporal mapping theory gained support as the primary mechanism children use when responding to simple visual, auditory, and vibrotactile input.[116]

Visuospatial Deficits

Children with DCD tend to rely more on visual than on proprioceptive information in organizing responses and often fail to anticipate or use perceptual information in preparing responses.[116] Because DCD is a prominent motor function and visuospatial disorder, several studies have adopted the hypothesis that the basal ganglia, the parietal lobe, and the cerebellum may be implicated in its pathogenesis.[101,115,117] Children with DCD have been found to respond slower in visuospatial cueing tasks than children in control groups. Wang and colleagues.[126] found that children with DCD, as compared with typically developing children, exhibited slower RTs when responding to spatially cued targets, suggesting that a dysfunctional corpus callosum may be the cause of DCD.

The mechanisms underlying the deficit in visuospatial working memory (VSWM), a higher-order skill related to the ability to allocate attentional resources despite distraction or interference, have been investigated. Electrophysiology was used to compare brain activity while performing a VSWM task in children with DCD and typically developing children, resulting in children with DCD exhibiting weaknesses in VSWM.[101] These results suggest that the component associated with resource allocation for attention and memory tasks showed smaller amplitude in the children with DCD, thus possibly explaining the longer processing time for information.[101]

Fine Motor and Visual Motor Performance

Fine motor skills. Fine motor coordination involves motor behavior such as discrete finger movements, manipulation, and eye-hand coordination. A child with DCD often demonstrates multiple fine motor concerns. Areas of difficulty typically include grasp and manipulation of small objects and dexterous hand skills, such as buttoning or putting coins into a vending machine. Assessment should include both standardized assessments and structured observations of functional performance.

A complete fine motor assessment should include observations of proximal trunk control to distal finger movements. Trunk control and shoulder stability affect the accuracy and control of reaching patterns and create a stable base from which both hands can be used to perform bilateral skills. The assessment of distal control considers wrist stability, development of hand arches, and separation of the two sides of the

hand, all providing a foundation for the control of distal movement. Qualitative observations of distal fingertip control include finger motions to move objects into and out of the palm of the hand and rotate an object within the hand.

Although standardized assessments such as BOT-2[124] and the *Peabody Developmental Motor Scales*[125] have fine motor sections, they do not measure manipulative components described previously. Combining qualitative observations during a variety of fine motor tasks with knowledge of typical development is important. Soft neurological signs, including diadochokinesia (rapid alternation of forearm supination and pronation), sequential thumb-to-finger touching, and stereognosis (identifying objects and shapes without visual input) can provide further qualitative information.

Eye-hand coordination, visual motor integration. Eye-hand coordination is the ability to use the eyes and hands together to guide reaching, grasping, and release of objects. This can include larger motions such as catching and throwing a ball to more refined tasks such as putting pennies in a bank or buttoning a shirt. Coordination of the eyes and the feet (eye-foot coordination) is important for skills such as ascending and descending stairs and kicking a ball. Children with DCD often exhibit difficulties in one or more of these areas. Qualitatively, they demonstrate poor coordination in the timing and sequencing of their actions. Evaluations such as BOT-2[124] and the Movement ABC[112] have subtests that assess eye-hand coordination in a standardized way. Supplemental clinical observations include the assessment of ball skills, fine motor tasks such as stringing beads and building block towers, and written accuracy tasks of drawing or coloring within a boundary.

Visual motor tasks involve the ability to reproduce shapes, figures, or other visual stimuli in written form. This skill is multidimensional, involving perceiving a visual image, remembering it, and integrating it to a written response. Visual motor integration is the foundational skill needed for handwriting. In addition, handwriting involves combination of fine motor control, motor planning, and sensory feedback to be accurate and legible. Children who have difficulties with handwriting commonly produce sloppy work with incorrect letter formations or reversals, inconsistent size and height of letters, variable slant, and irregular spacing between words and letters.

Assessment of visual motor skills can be completed through standardized measures such as the *Developmental Test of Visual Motor Integration* (BEERY VMI, Sixth Revision) or the *Motor-Free Visual Perception Test, fourth edition.*

The production of handwritten work can be assessed by using the Evaluation Tool of Children's Handwriting (ETCH),[127] the *Minnesota Handwriting Assessment* (MHA), and Handwriting Without Tears: The Print Tool.[128] Handwriting and drawing samples provide valuable information regarding functional abilities in written production.

Sensory Processing

It has been proposed that the term *sensory processing* be used for the assessment and diagnosis of sensory challenges impairing daily routines.[129] The process begins with *registration* or recognition of incoming sensory input *("What is it?")*. The incoming information is quickly scanned for relevance in a process called *sensory modulation* *("Is it important?")*. Sensory modulation determines the appropriate action for a situation and regulates arousal. Our system needs to respond strongly and quickly if our hand moves near a hot stove but should not respond as strongly if we are unexpectedly bumped. *Discrimination* of sensory input involves discerning subtle differences in sensation to learn about the qualities of objects and refine body movements within space. When we are receiving clear information from our sensory receptors, we can understand and label what is happening (e.g., sour-sweet, hot-cold, soft-firm, heavy-light, up-down, fast-slow). Efficient sensory registration, modulation, and discrimination result in organized social and motor behavior.

Children with DCD often experience sensory processing difficulties. Diminished registration of sensation can result in poor body and environmental awareness, low arousal levels, and delayed postural reactions and motor coordination. These children may be sedentary or seek out strong sensation. *Sensory modulation* difficulties manifest primarily in emotional and behavioral responses. Behaviors often include oversensitivity, with aversive or exaggerated responses to sensation. These children struggle to remain regulated during typical daily events and may avoid uncomfortable sensations, demonstrate behavioral disorganization, seek strong, potentially unsafe input, become aggressive, or have tantrums. They often have difficulty performing in situations involving integration of multiple inputs (e.g., cafeteria, gym class, playground, team sports). Sensitivity to movement input can also cause the child to avoid playground equipment or become nauseated during car rides. Delayed *sensory discrimination* typically results in poor body awareness that may underlie qualitative motor difficulties observed in children with DCD. They often exhibit poor motor coordination and planning, deficient safety awareness, and poor grading of force, as well as timing and sequencing difficulties. These children may avoid complex motor challenges, team sports, and playground activities. Discrimination difficulties can also affect the acquisition of prepositional concepts (up, down, left, right, in front of, behind, next to). The child who has difficulty discriminating information from the body typically exhibits deficits in skilled actions involving balance, timing movements in space, bilateral and eye-hand coordination, fine motor control, and handwriting.

Clinical observation of a child's responses to a variety of sensory inputs and the ability to organize multiple inputs provides essential information regarding the integration of sensory input. Sensory modulation dysfunction is not easily identified with standardized, skill-based measures because of its physiological basis. Caregiver questionnaires, such as the Sensory Processing Measure[130,131] and the Sensory Profile,[132,133] can provide valuable information on modulation and regulation. Other tests, such as BOT-2[124] and the Movement ABC-2,[112] can provide qualitative observations in addition to quantitative measures of motor skill.

Gross and fine motor tasks that involve postural and ocular responses, bilateral motor coordination, planning, and sequencing reflect efficient sensory processing. Soft neurological signs, coupled with observations of play (e.g., playground, gym class, recess), can provide qualitative information on sensory discrimination and planning. The *Clinical Observations of Motor and Postural Skills* (COMPS) assessment tool[134] is a set of six standardized clinical observations and soft signs that can be useful in identifying motor deficit with a postural component.

Praxis and Motor Planning

Praxis involves the ability to plan and carry out a new or unusual action when adequate cognitive and motor skills are present. The components of praxis include *ideation* or generating an idea of how one might act in the environment, *planning* or organizing a program of action, and *execution* of the action sequence. Motor planning involves the same components relative to a novel motor task.

Children with praxis difficulties, or dyspraxia, may exhibit a paucity of ideas. The child may enter a room filled with toys or equipment and have limited capacity to experiment and play. Other children with dyspraxia may move from one activity to the next without generating effective plans for participating in or completing tasks. Lack of

variation and adaptation in play can be another indication of planning problems. Observations of typically developing children show continuous modifications in play, with spontaneous adaptations to motor sequences, making explorations varied and increasingly successful. Children with dyspraxia often have difficulties in situations characterized by changing demands, such as unstructured group play. Transitions also may be difficult because they involve the creation or adaptation of a plan. Frustration and difficulties with peer interactions frequently are part of the composite.

Observations of motor planning deficits may include trouble figuring out new motor activities, disorganized approaches, resistance, or inability to vary performance when a task is not successful, and awkward motor execution. Poor planning abilities can lead to the child being adult dependent, hesitant, or resistant to trying new activities. At times, children with dyspraxia also may exhibit poor anticipation of their actions. They can quickly engage in play with the equipment but demonstrate little regard for safety (e.g., kicking a large ball across the room where other children are playing). Movements are often performed with an excessive expenditure of energy and with inaccurate judgment of the required force, tempo, and amplitude.[135] Such children typically require more practice and repetition to master more complex, sequential movements. Frequently, children with planning problems recognize the differences between their performance and that of other children the same age, which significantly affects their self-esteem.

Manifestations of poor motor planning ability are apparent in many daily tasks. Dressing is often difficult. Children are not able to plan where or how to move their limbs to put on clothes. Problems are often demonstrated in constructive manipulatory play, such as building with toys, cutting, and pasting. Similarly, learning how to use utensils, such as a knife, fork, pencil, or scissors, is difficult. The child with dyspraxia often also has problems with handwriting.

Clinical observations can add valuable information regarding the child's ability to see the potential for action, organize and sequence motor actions for success, and anticipate the outcome of an action.

Physical Fitness

Physical fitness involves a person's ability to perform physical activities that require aerobic fitness, endurance, strength, or flexibility. Factors influencing fitness include motor competency, frequency of exercise, physical health, and genetically inherited ability. Physical fitness can encompass health-related and skill-related fitness.[136] Cardiorespiratory endurance, muscular strength and endurance, flexibility, and body composition are components of health-related fitness and important to monitor. Agility, speed, and power are the skill-related fitness components and are needed for the acquisition of motor skills and sports and recreational activities.[137]

Children with DCD often have performance difficulties in games and athletic activities. They are often less active than typical peers and withdraw from physical activity. As a result, the level of physical fitness, strength, muscular endurance, flexibility, and cardiorespiratory endurance may be poorly developed. Hands and Larkin[136] found that body mass index (BMI) in children with motor difficulties was higher than in a control group of typical peers.[136] The percentage of overweight and obese 10- to 12-year-olds was found to be significantly higher in a DCD group than in typically developing peers.[138] This increased weight may further increase their movement difficulties.

In a study of 52 children aged 5 to 8 years with DCD, Hands and Larkin[136] revealed significantly lower scores on tests for cardiorespiratory endurance, flexibility, abdominal strength, speed, and power than the age- and gender-matched controls. Another study of 261 children aged 4 to 12 years found similar disparities for children with DCD, with poor performance in fitness tests, with the exception of flexibility.[138] These disparities in fitness were found to increase with age between the two groups.[138]

One task of the PT is to differentiate between poor physical fitness resulting from low motor activity as opposed to problems of low muscle tone, joint limitations, decreased strength, and reduced endurance. The low motor activity is a neurological sign and leads to a developmental lag or deviation in motor function. Collaboration among the physical educator, the adaptive physical educator, and the PT is critical. The President's Challenge is a physical fitness test administered twice a year in schools across the country. Children complete five events that assess their level of physical fitness in strength, speed, endurance, and flexibility. The test was founded in 1956 by Dwight Eisenhower to encourage American children to be healthy and active, after a study indicating that American youths are less physically fit than European children.[139] Standardized assessments of gross motor functioning, such as BOT-2,[124] that assess strength, speed, and endurance can provide information related to a child's fitness level.

INTERVENTION FOR THE CHILD WITH LEARNING DISABILITIES AND MOTOR DEFICITS OR DEVELOPMENTAL COORDINATION DISORDER

Creating an Intervention Plan

Using the information gathered throughout the assessment process, the therapist synthesizes areas of strength and weakness to develop an intervention plan. If impairments, activity limitations, and participation restrictions exist that affect the child's successful performance, intervention may be warranted. For example, children with DCD might demonstrate impairments in coordination or balance that underlie activity limitations in catching or throwing a ball, which create participation restrictions in playing baseball with peers.[140] Determining the child's functional difficulties and identifying the severity of the impairment will be important to justify service and guide the service delivery model and type of intervention. For children with DCD who have greater impairment and activity limitations, individualized treatment may be more beneficial, whereas those with less involvement may thrive with group intervention.[141]

Interpreting test data, integrating findings, identifying functional limitations, and creating goals is a complex process. Initial impressions of the child's areas of difficulty may result in the recommendation for further examination before outlining refined goals relevant to functional performance. Collecting additional assessment information may involve observations in other environments or during functional daily tasks, and/or formal testing. The end product is the creation of statements that delineate the type and quality of behavior desired as a result of remediation. In other words, the therapist must set treatment goals to be achieved through intervention.

Setting goals for the child with learning disabilities with motor deficits must be done by considering a variety of factors:
1. Referral information and age of the child
2. Medical, developmental, and sensory processing history
3. Parents' and teachers' perception of the child's strengths and concerns about functional impairments
4. Educational information
   a. Major difficulties experienced in school
   b. How motor problems are interfering with the child's daily participation
   c. Current services being received
5. Child's peer relationships, play and leisure activities, and self-esteem

6. Therapists' observations and assessment of the child through informal and formal evaluation, both standardized and nonstandardized
7. Functional expectations and abilities at home and school

Goals for the child should be stated in terms of long-term and short-term objectives. Goal setting ideally involves establishing specific, measurable, attainable, realistic, and time-targeted objectives. Short-term objectives are generally composed of three parts: (1) the *behavioral statement* is what will be accomplished by the child; (2) the *condition statement* provides details regarding how the skill or behavior will be accomplished; and (3) the *performance statement* denotes how the skill or behavior will be measured for success. The most important consideration is ensuring that the goals and objectives chosen are relevant to the child's functional daily performance and are meaningful to the team, including the family, working with the child. Case Study 12.2 provides an example of functional objectives.

Models of Intervention

Improvements in motor deficits can be achieved through a variety of models of intervention, both indirect and direct. Indirect intervention involves working with key people in the child's life to help them facilitate the child's delineated goals. An indirect model can occur through consultation, specialized instruction, and coaching. Direct intervention involves the therapist working directly with the child on specific goal areas or skills.

Mild deficits, subtly affecting participation in activities, may be addressed through a consultative (indirect) approach. This model of service provision incorporates the use of another team member's expertise to be responsible for the outcome of the child.[80,142] The therapist may suggest environmental or task adaptations to facilitate more successful participation. Consultation with parents would be appropriate for the goal of riding a bicycle without training wheels. Parents may not understand the complexity of the task and may be focused only on the end product, which can cause frustration for all involved. To facilitate confidence and success, the therapist might recommend environmental modifications such as beginning on an open stretch of grass or dirt, with no other people around to decrease the child's anxiety. Breaking the task down into incremental steps for the parent and child (i.e., practicing getting on and off bike, balancing on still bike, gliding, braking, steering, pedaling) can allow success at each step.

Within a school setting, environmental adaptations might include changing the height or position of the desk or decreasing extraneous visual and auditory distracters. Task accommodations could include using a special grip to facilitate more refined pencil grasp or allowing more time for written work. In these instances, the teacher would be responsible for carrying out the program and determining its effectiveness. Communication between the therapist and teacher encourages problem solving and changing action plans over time. Kemmis and Dunn[143] demonstrated positive outcomes on a variety of functional classroom goals when an OT and teacher met weekly throughout the school year in what they called a "collaborative consultation approach." Using this model, they achieved 63% (134 of 213) of their outlined goals. This collaborative effort supports the shared responsibility for identifying the problem or weakness of the child, creating practical solutions, implementing the intervention as the solution, and altering the plan as necessary for increased effectiveness.[80]

Another model of indirect therapy involves teaching members of the team to implement treatment strategies. Specialized instruction or coaching allows the therapist to support a child within the natural environment by working with care providers who are with the child every day. The aim is to educate key people in the child's life to coach the child within the context of teachable moments.[144] These moments,

CASE STUDY 12.2 Jaiden

History: Jaiden is an 8-year-old child who emigrated from Russia 2 years ago and receives English as second language and small group academic instruction. He currently attends the third grade in a regular education classroom. Jaiden has a diagnosis of attention-deficit/hyperactivity disorder (ADHD) and secondary diagnoses of specific developmental reading disorder, low muscle tone, mixed receptive/expressive language disorder, fine motor impairment, and lack of coordination. Jaiden expressed that his least favorite class is gym. He also refuses to participate in after-school sports, as per his classroom teacher.

Examination: During classroom observation, Jaiden was engaged in completing previously assigned coursework. He interacted with a peer sitting next to him and would frequently be inattentive to the work to be completed. He required significant prompting and constantly adjusted his posture or stood when asked to complete seated work. Jaiden is reported to be very active, miss oral directions, and appears not to hear when called by name. He also has difficulty functioning if there is noise nearby. In addition, Jaiden is reported to come too close to peers when talking and tends to touch people and objects around him. His behavioral observations indicate that he is inefficient in his approach to tasks, takes long to complete tasks, and makes tasks more complicated than needed. He also seems more curious than other students as per his classroom teacher.

The administration of the Children's Assessment of Participation and Enjoyment (CAPE) was attempted to assess Jaiden's interest in various activities, more specifically to guide instruction and intervention. Although he was presented with cards visually representing the various activities (alone and with others, indoors-outdoors), he was not able to complete the standardized assessment because he often changed topics and had difficulty returning to task. His habit of inadvertently changing his focus of attention and conversation is observed to sometimes interfere with every day activities and may contribute to his difficulties with learning, behavior, discipline, and sustaining positive social participation.

Body Awareness/Proprioceptive Processing: Jaiden displayed difficulty with symmetrical and asymmetrical upper extremity positioning even when given verbal cues and a demonstration. Jaiden also displayed poor task approach and motor sequencing.

Fine Motor Skills: Jaiden is right-hand dominant and used an atypical grasp with this index finger wrapped on the pencil and his thumb in hyperextension. Jaiden requires adaptations and a pencil grip for writing assignments. His upper extremity range of motion was within normal limits, and his muscle tone was low throughout his body. Jaiden's sitting posture was functional. Jaiden stabilized adequately using his left hand when necessary. As observed through activities, he was able to cross midline, use both hands simultaneously, and transfer objects from one hand to another. Typical development of grasp was observed, with intact and voluntary release, intact in-hand manipulation, and accurate reaching for objects. Proprioception, or the sense of body in space, was adequate for grasp and release. Tactile input, the sensation of touch, was observed within normal limits.

Visual Perceptual Skills: Jaiden's skills of visual tracking, visual regard, spatial relations, and figure ground are intact. Jaiden is able to distinguish right from left on body and understand basic directional terms. Jaiden had difficulty copying complex forms/shapes such as a star or overlapping forms. He also wrote his letters of his name out of sequence, J A I D N E.

Written Work: Jaiden was able to identify starting and stopping points on paper. He was able to print in designated spaces and work from left to right. Jaiden's writing is legible, but he has difficulty adhering to the writing line, his letters rest above the line, or he does not form descending letters below the line. Jaiden has difficulty with letter formation especially letters that involve diagonal strokes such as "x" or "y." He also reversed letter "q" and wrote his name out of sequence. Jaiden had difficulty reading the sentence he was asked to copy. As per school records, his reading level is below the first grade level.

When determining appropriate behavioral objectives for Jaiden, looking at the areas of functional relevance such as pleasure and safety in gross motor play, peer interactions, and independence in age-appropriate activities of daily living is critical. These areas of concern for Jaiden were consistent with those of his parents. His parents wanted him to feel more competent and less frustrated in play, at home, and at school.

One of the long-term goals was *improve Jaiden's planning and coordination abilities to increase his confidence and success in gross motor activities*

Jaiden was interested in learning to ride a bicycle, and his parents were hopeful that he could become more confident at the neighborhood playground. These objectives would measure the development of improved proficiency in discrimination of his body in space, postural control balance reactions, and motor planning. The following objectives were written:

1. Jaiden will independently climb the ladder and come down the slide without exhibiting fear, bumping into other children, or falling.
2. Jaiden will develop the ability to ride his bicycle without training wheels in straight lines and will learn to turn corners.

To address improvement in independence for self-care:

1. Jaiden will put on his coat independently in correct orientation and successfully zip it 4 out of 5 times.
2. Jaiden will successfully tie his shoes without assistance in a timely manner.

To address greater success in peer interactions:

1. Jaiden will participate in a structured game, following the rules, for 10 min.
2. Jaiden will play outside with the children in the neighborhood without conflict for at least 1 hour.

The OT believed that through remediation of sensory discrimination and motor deficits Jaiden could develop improved motor competence and planning abilities. This would lead to greater success in peer interactions and improved feelings of self-confidence.

If the OT or PT is working as a member of a team within the school, behavioral objectives will have implications for the child's performance in the school environment. Within the school system, statements of goals and specific objectives are included in the Individualized Educational Plan (IEP). Other areas related to gross and fine motor skills and peer interactions also were influential to Jaiden's success at school. Specific objectives written pertaining to school would have functional outcome measures chosen from tasks within the school environment such as gym class, playground interactions, and classroom expectations.

---

when a child is interested and working on acquiring a new skill, occur throughout the day and in many different environments.[145] This allows for therapeutic consistency and repeated practice, thereby increasing the chances for skill acquisition within the context of daily routines.

With this model, the therapist observes children and adults doing familiar routines and collaborates with the adults to enhance those routines in varied environments.[146] When implementing an intervention strategy, the therapist might teach another adult to guide specific, developmentally appropriate skill sets with the child or problem solve to create strategies for greater success. Over time, parents and other caregivers are empowered to look at a toy, an activity, or an experience and find ways to adapt it to increase successful involvement and skill development. Successful coaching can enhance parent-child relationships indirectly by helping parents to feel more comfortable and competent in their abilities to meet their child's needs.[147]

Direct intervention involves designing individualized treatment plans and carrying them out with the child individually or in a small group. This approach can focus on developing the foundations that underlie motor performance such as sensory processing, postural control, and motor planning. Specific skills, such as shoe tying or bike riding, can be practiced with the therapist as well, breaking these tasks down into component skills. Through combining approaches, adapting methods over the course of therapy, and responding to the changing needs of the child over time, progress is achieved more effectively.[103] Best practice dictates that direct therapy should always be provided in conjunction with one of the other service models to ensure generalization of skills to natural settings.[80] Without the use of other models, therapists cannot be confident that changes observed in the isolated setting are affecting the child's overall performance.

Intervention Approaches

According to the *International Classification of Functioning, Disability and Health* (ICF),[148] interventions should be directed toward several distinct goals:

- To remediate impairment
- To reduce activity limitations
- To improve participation

Two intervention approaches—bottom up and top down—have been developed. When using a bottom-up approach, therapy focuses on the missing or faulty underlying performance skills and client factors that prevent movement skills such as sensory-motor or perceptual motor techniques relying on the visual system. In contrast, a top-down approach focuses on specific performance by providing practice or problem-solving conditions in a variety of contexts. Cognitive motor refers to conditions where the child must identify a specific motor problem or problem solving where the child must evaluate the feasibility of the task.[114] The top-down approach or functional skill training based on the dynamical systems theory has gained acceptance as more successful when taking into account contextual and environmental factors and use a motor learning approach at the level of the task. Task specific in a meaningful environment. Interventions should directly target the person's ability to transfer and generalize new skills. Some key elements of the top-down approach include practice of the skills, practice in variable environments and contexts, and consistent provision of feedback.[149]

Interventions focused on treating at the ICF level of remediating impairments generally target the improvement of processing abilities (e.g., visual, proprioceptive, and vestibular) or performance components (e.g., balance and strength). The tenet is that by strengthening these foundational skills the child will develop greater success in appropriate activities and participation. This type of intervention is referred to as a "bottom-up" approach and is based on neuromaturational or hierarchical theories.

Intervention focuses on increasing the child's ability to take part in the typical activities of childhood.[91] These treatment methods assume that skill acquisition emerges from interaction among the child, the task, and the environment.[103] Intervention is contextually based, occurring in everyday situations and focusing on the activities and tasks inherent to that situation. Problem solving, preparatory activities, and skill training may be used together to increase successful participation. This type of approach may minimize the challenges of learning new skills for a child who cannot easily generalize learning to new situations.

The intervention methods presented in this chapter for remediation of motor deficits in the child with learning disabilities include motor learning approaches (e.g., cognitive orientation to daily occupational performance [CO-OP])[150]; sensorimotor treatment techniques; motor skill training approaches (e.g., ecological intervention[151]); and

physical fitness. None are mutually exclusive, and each requires a level of training and practice for competence, as well as experience in normal development. Most therapists synthesize information from different intervention techniques and use an eclectic approach, pulling relevant pieces from a variety of intervention modalities to best meet the needs of each child.

Therapeutic interventions to improve general coordination usually result in small gains. The main reason is because therapy lacks scientific foundation as the etiology of DCD is unknown.[85,114] The relevance of research into the underlying causes of DCD is important for designing therapeutic treatment and to advance current knowledge about movement coordination. Most ADLs involve the coordinated use of visual information that is gathered before and during the execution of actions.

Children with DCD experience motor difficulties in a broad range of ADLs, such as mobility, personal hygiene, feeding, and dressing; handwriting and crafting; ball skills; and riding a bike.[152] The five most common interventions cited in the literature are those designed to facilitate self-care tasks, task-specific approaches, interventions aimed at facilitating play, the CO-OP, and motor learning theories.[153] The ICF, the universal framework for health-related conditions, defines ADL as functional motor activities that are performed during daily life, "self-care and self-maintenance," "productivity and schoolwork," and "leisure and play."[152] A systematic review divided intervention into four categories: task-oriented intervention; traditional occupational therapy or physical therapy; process-oriented therapies; and chemical supplements.[83] The task-oriented interventions were aimed at learning specific motor skills that are particularly difficult for the child, and the process-oriented therapies focused on more global functions (e.g., sensory integration or visual-motor perception).[154] The largest effect sizes were shown for task-oriented interventions and for occupational or physical therapy with only a weak effect for process-oriented approaches. Therefore a referral to an OT or a PT to focus treatment on performing everyday tasks is recommended.[85] Although there is no conclusive evidence of which intervention is better, a metanalysis[155] found that top-down approaches seem more efficacious than bottom-up and that home programs are superior to one-one interventions. Lastly, interventions that allow for more practice, occurring 3 to 5 times per week, yield better outcomes than intervention occurring less often. From motor learning research, there are three principles arise: practice distribution, feedback, and goal setting. Practice is the most important principle, and massed practice is best during initial stage of learning. Children should receive extensive repetition and practice of the same skill until achieving a rudimentary level of mastery and followed by a varied practice schedule knowing that mastery of skill may take longer in children with DCD. Positive feedback should be specific to allow the child to correct errors and encourage practice. Feedback should be immediate at first attempts of the skill and gradually faded to encourage the child's independence. Finally, goals must be small, progressive, and achievable to provide the child a sense of competency.[114]

The CO-OP measure is a client-centered approach that focuses on (1) skill acquisition, (2) cognitive strategy development and discovery of domain-specific strategies for problem solving, and (3) generalization and transfer where the child can use the skills and strategies for other daily tasks.[155] The CO-OP is a four-step self-talk strategy where the child must verbalize his or her own goals. A therapist helps the child to talk himself or herself through a solution to a motor problem and the child is active and cognitively involved in both problem solving and the learning of the skill.[114]

Motor Learning Theories

Motor learning refers to the process of acquiring, expanding, and improving skilled motor actions. The basic treatment premise of motor learning theories is that improvement in movement skills is elicited through appropriate practice and timely feedback. Motor learning has taken place when a permanent change in the child's ability to respond to a movement problem or achieve a movement goal has occurred, regardless of the environment.[156] Therefore therapists measure learning through tests that measure retention and transfer of skills.[157]

The closed-loop theory of Adams[158] is recognized as the first comprehensive explanation for motor learning. Adams believed that the central nervous system, based on sensory feedback, controls the execution of movement. He proposed that once a movement has occurred, errors are detected and compared with existing "memory traces." With practice, these memory traces become stronger and the accuracy of the movement increases, thus emphasizing learning through feedback.

In 1975 Schmidt contributed the idea of "open-loop" motor learning, which emphasized the ability to produce rapid action sequences in the absence of sensory feedback (e.g., hitting a baseball). He proposed that new movements were created from previously stored motor programs (schemas) of similar movements, as opposed to feedback from individual motor actions.[159] Schemas comprise general rules for a specific group of actions that can be applied to a variety of situations.[160] When a motor action occurs, the initial movement conditions, parameters used, outcomes, and sensory consequences of the action are stored in memory. With each goal-directed movement, specific parameters are used (e.g., force needed to pour juice into a glass) and consequences occur (e.g., spillage or not). Repeated actions using different parameters and creating different outcomes create data sets that help to refine the motor program, reducing errors and improving anticipation or feedforward information.[160] Schmidt's[159] schema theory contributed to current theories of motor learning principles regarding practice schedules and feedback about outcome of movements, known as *knowledge of results* (KR).

Based on the knowledge of motor skill development in children with DCD, four key variables are important to consider in targeted intervention. They include stage of the learner, type of task, scheduling of practice, and type of feedback.

Three stages of the learner have been proposed[161,162]: the *cognitive stage, associative stage,* and *autonomous stage.* As a child learns and develops new motor actions, he or she progresses through the various stages at different rates, depending on the complexity of the skill. The *cognitive stage* is the initial phase of learning in which there is large variability as the child gets the general idea of the movement.[140] Awkward body postures are observed, errors are often made, and awareness of what needs to be improved or changed does not exist. (Consider when a young child attempts to throw a ball; the throw is a gross movement, the projection of the ball varies, and the movement appears uncoordinated.) As practice continues, the degree of accuracy increases, which is characteristic of the *associative stage.* Fewer errors are made, and error information is used to correct the movement patterns. (As the child continues to throw the ball, the ball may get closer to the target, with improved coordination observed.) During the *autonomous stage,* the skill is performed fluently and automatically, without as much effort or thought. Improvements in accuracy continue and errors are detected, with corrections made automatically. (The child can now throw a ball at a target and hit the target with coordinated, accurate movements, such as pitching; however, if a child were introduced to throwing a curve ball, the stages would start over.)

The type of task is a mechanism to classify motor skills in a dimensional fashion. Task components contribute to intervention decisions. The types of tasks are *gross motor* or *fine motor; simple* or *complex; discrete, serial,* or *continuous;* and *environment changing* or *stationary.* Gross and fine motor tasks are classified according to the type of muscle groups required.[163] *Gross motor skills* use large muscles and

tend to be fundamental skills (e.g., walking and running). *Fine motor skills* tend to require greater control of small muscles and usually have to be taught (e.g., handwriting, cutting). Task complexity refers to the level of difficulty and amount of feedback required. *Simple* tasks, such as reaching, require a decision followed by a response. A *complex* task, such as cutting out a picture, requires continual monitoring and feedback until completion. Tasks can require simple single actions or the coordination of sequential motions for completion. A single *discrete* movement has a clear beginning and ending, such as activating a button. *Serial* movements require a series of distinct movements combined to achieve the outcome, such as writing a sentence. *Continuous* movements, such as running, contain movements that are repetitive. Tasks that are discrete or serial can be practiced in parts, but continuous tasks usually need to be practiced as a continuous segment.

Environmental variations can greatly increase the complexity of the task, requiring higher levels of feedforward information and feedback. In an unstable or *changing* environment, the child has to learn the movement and monitor the environment to adapt to changes—for example, running on an uneven surface. The more predictable and stable the task and environments are, the easier it is to learn and replicate motor skills. Tooth brushing is an example of a task that generally occurs in a *stationary* environment. Home and classrooms can be stable, in that many elements within these settings are fixed and do not change. The size and shape of chairs, location of toys on the floor, and movements of other children are considered "variable features" within these stable environments. These variable features require a greater amount of motor control because the child must adjust movements and actions to the changing demands. Therapists generally practice in stable environments and therefore must ensure that the children are able to function under varied circumstances encountered in daily life situations.

Practice is believed to increase learning of a skill or movement. Variations in practice can occur in the order tasks are performed, in the environment where the tasks are practiced, and by changing aspects of the task. Practice schedules can be developed based on the practice techniques (*blocked* or *random*) or how task learning is approached (*component* or *whole task*). *Blocked* practice means the task is repeatedly rehearsed, sometimes focusing on one aspect of a technique or a specific motor sequence (e.g., hitting a golf ball off a tee with the same club). Repetitive, blocked practice often leads to improved immediate performance, particularly in situations that are stable. *Random* practice involves performing a number of different tasks in varied order or using several different aspects of technique (e.g., hitting golf balls from a tee, sand trap, and rough with the appropriate club). Random practice encourages learners to compare and contrast strategies used in performing the task, which positively influences performance in changeable environments.

If a task is discrete or contains multiple parts, breaking it down into *components* for blocked practice may be beneficial. For success in changeable situations in which the task component is integrated into skilled action, *whole-task* practice is essential—for example, practicing shooting basketballs, then practicing while moving or running toward the basket. When generalization is the goal, practice sessions can progress from stable (shooting from specific positions on the court) to a changeable environment (such as shooting basketballs with a person trying to block the shot). Opportunity and variety in practice appear to improve motor learning, particularly when skills are practiced in a random manner. Practice should therefore be varied and occur in multiple environments (e.g., home and school) to maximize motor learning.

Different types of feedback also affect the process of learning. *Intrinsic* feedback is received from any of the child's internal sensory systems and is usually not perceived consciously unless external direction draws attention to it (e.g., when a child performs a task with his or her tongue sticking out). *Extrinsic* feedback is received from an outside source observing the results of an action and can be provided in the form of knowledge of performance (KP) or KR. KP focuses on movements used to achieve the goal, whereas KR focuses on the outcome.

Therapists tend to provide excessive feedback, especially when task performance is below what is expected. Low frequency and fading feedback, progressively decreasing the rate at which feedback is provided, appear to be most effective in facilitating learning.[135] One proposed reason is that with less feedback the individual can more readily engage in the processes that enable learning versus focusing on external cues. During intervention, feedback should not be provided for every movement or task execution. It is more beneficial to offer children the opportunity to self-evaluate and correct their own performance. The therapist can provide feedback as necessary to encourage successful task completion and reduce frustration. Verbal feedback can be general or specific. Children with DCD often lack the skills required to analyze task demands, interpret environmental cues, use KP to alter movements, or adapt to situational demands.[164] They therefore do not interpret and use sensory or performance feedback as well as children who are developing typically.[157] Motor observations of the child with DCD often reveal clumsiness, difficulty judging force, timing, and amplitude of motions, and deficits in anticipating the results of a motor action. Reactions, movements, and response times are typically slower,[165] thus the type of task and the method of teaching should be considered when recommending participation in sports and leisure activities.[140] Children with DCD can become successful in repetitive sports, such as swimming, skating, skiing, and bicycling. However, ball-related sports, such as hockey, baseball, tennis, football, and basketball, tend to be more difficult and frustrating owing to the high level of unpredictability and frequent changes in the direction, force, speed, and distance of the movement.[140]

When using the motor learning model of practice, the therapist should incorporate a variety of teaching techniques, including verbal instructions, positioning, and handling, as well as observational learning (demonstrations).[157] The task and environment should be structured with extrinsic and intrinsic feedback provided, using a practice schedule that is optimal for the type of task.[166] Children with DCD benefit from experiential and guided learning when practice is performed so that each repetition of the action becomes a new problem-solving experience. To test whether motor learning has occurred, the therapist must create opportunities for demonstration of retention (repeating what was learned in a previous session), transfer (perform a different but closely related task), and generalization (perform a learned task in a new environment).

One method of intervention based on the principles of motor learning is the CO-OP, a frame of reference developed as a treatment approach specifically for children with DCD.[150] In this cognitive-based approach, the therapist focuses on the movement goal and facilitates the child's identification of the important aspects of the task, examines the child's performance during the task, identifies where the child is having the most difficulty, and problem solves alternative solutions.[166] Rather than using verbal instructions, this approach uses guided questions to help the child discover the problems, generate solutions, and evaluate his or her attempts in a supportive environment. Furthermore, the therapist solicits verbal strategies from the child that can help to guide the motor behavior, such as typical verbal cues that the therapist tends to provide during intervention.

To benefit from the CO-OP approach, the child must have sufficient cognitive and language ability to rate the level of his or her

performance and satisfaction of self-identified goals using the *Canadian Occupational Performance Measure* (COPM).[167] The basic objectives of this approach include skill acquisition, cognitive strategy development, and generalization or transfer of skills into daily performance. CO-OP is delivered over 12 one-on-one sessions, each lasting approximately 1 hour. The therapy process is divided into five phases: preparation, assessment, introduction, acquisition, and consolidation. Children are taught to talk themselves through performance issues using an approach of Goal-Plan-Do-Check. Domain-specific strategies are used to enhance performance, with the purpose of helping the child to see how he or she can set goals, plan actions, talk through doing, and check outcomes. Using this frame of reference, therapists help the child to acquire occupational performance skills using a metacognitive problem-solving process.[150]

Research on the CO-OP model of motor learning. Current beliefs regarding the nature of motor learning for children with DCD suggest that assessment of participation, versus impairments, should be used to determine change over time.[157] By increasing the child's ability to participate in childhood activities, secondary deficits such as loss of strength and endurance might be prevented. Relatively new intervention strategies that use contemporary motor learning principles emphasize the role of cognitive processes (top down) in development of specific skills. The CO-OP model uses this approach to help children achieve their functional goals.[150]

Research on the effectiveness of this approach to improve motor skills and functional performance is limited but shows promise. Polatajko and Cantin[168] reviewed three articles describing four studies and concluded that there was convergent evidence for the effectiveness of the CO-OP approach for children with DCD.

An exploratory study completed in 1994 by Wilcox as part of his graduate work was discussed by Polatajko and colleagues.[169] This initial single case study included 10 children aged 7 to 12 years who were referred to occupational therapy for motor problems. Using a global problem-solving approach to intervention, this study sought to identify whether children with DCD could use these strategies to acquire skills of their choice, and, once learned, whether the skills were maintained and performance in other areas enhanced. Children selected skills that were challenging and meaningful for them, such as shuffling playing cards, applying nail polish, making a bed, and writing legibly. Each of the 10 children made gains in the chosen activity, with 29 of the 30 targeted skills showing improvement.

A pilot study compared the CO-OP model to a traditional treatment approach with a group of 20 children aged 7 to 12 years. Findings indicated that the CO-OP model of intervention produced larger gains on client-selected goals. Improvements in self-ratings of performance and satisfaction were greater than in the comparative group. Although informal, the follow-up data suggested that children maintained their acquired skills and applied strategies to other motor goals.

Limitations in making conclusions regarding the effectiveness of this treatment are mandated by the small number of research studies, primarily carried out by the same research group. Mandich and colleagues[103] suggest that larger studies with control groups are needed. Suggestions for future research include identification of the salient features of this treatment approach, as well as determining the generalization and skill transfer to other settings.

Sensorimotor Intervention

Sensorimotor activities provide the foundation for the development of play in children.[170] The first level of play (i.e., sensorimotor) is pleasurable, intrinsically motivated activity that involves the exploration of sensation and movement.[170] As children react with adaptive motor responses to the array of sensations from their bodies and the environment, central nervous system organization occurs. The assumption that the organization of sensory and motor experiences is essential to effective motor performance is the premise of sensorimotor intervention.[171] Treatment encourages the child to actively engage in a variety of sensory-rich, motor-based activities, to enhance functional motor performance.[169] Evolution of sensorimotor intervention has not revolved around a single, unified theory but has incorporated a variety of theoretical foundations.[172]

The goals of sensorimotor intervention are outcome based, with emphasis on the development of age-appropriate perceptual-motor and gross motor skills. The therapist chooses activities that meet the child's developmental levels, promote sensory and motor foundations, and encourage practice of appropriate motor skills. For the child having difficulty keeping up with the skilled activities in gym class such as rope jumping, components of these activities will be encouraged, with emphasis on sequencing and timing. The therapist may use a heavier jump rope or wrist and ankle weights to provide more sensory information for improved task performance.

In sensorimotor intervention, tasks are chosen for their innate sensory and motor components. The child is directed to activities that encourage the use of the body in space to complete a structured motor sequence. Activities incorporate sensory components such as movement (vestibular), touch (tactile), and heavy work for the muscles and joints (proprioception). Play interactions are considered important to encourage sensorimotor integration within the context of meaningful interactions with persons and objects.[170] Children may propel themselves prone on a scooter board through an "obstacle maze" while looking for matching shapes, for example. This activity provides tactile, proprioceptive, and vestibular sensory input and encourages the development of postural strength and endurance while addressing perceptual skill development.

Research on sensorimotor intervention. Sensorimotor intervention is a widely accepted modality, used by 92% of school-based therapists as a foundation for improving handwriting.[173] The activities used and goals addressed in treatment are extremely varied, because all functional motor skills involve some level of sensory and motor organization. Activities can range from horseback riding to using a vibrating pen when learning how to write letters. Owing to the enormous variation in intervention strategies and outcome measures, operationalizing treatment to make comparisons between research studies can be difficult. In a recent systematic review, Polatajko and Cantin[168] found five studies that met their criteria for using sensorimotor intervention. In those five studies, both the techniques used (e.g., therapeutic riding, movement therapy, educational kinesiology) and the populations addressed (autism, sensory modulation disorder, DCD) varied greatly. This review suggested that evidence for the effectiveness of sensorimotor intervention was "inconclusive," with the heterogeneity of diagnoses and functional problems limiting the ability to interpret efficacy.[168]

Overall, relatively few studies have investigated the efficacy of sensorimotor integration. In an early comparison study, DeGangi and colleagues[174] found that children provided with structured sensorimotor therapy made greater gains in sensory integrative foundations, gross motor skills, and performance areas such as self-care than children who engaged in child-centered activity. More recently, Chia and Chua[175] used sensorimotor intervention in a random controlled study of 14 children with learning disabilities and DCD. Intervention consisted of providing sensory stimuli and facilitating a normal motor response while remediating impairments in posture and muscle weakness. Positive results in neuromotor functioning were noted. In a second study, Inder and Sullivan[176] used educational kinesiology techniques in four single-subject design experiments. Positive gains were

documented in some aspects of sensory organization and in an overall decrease in the number of falls children had.

Four studies have explored the effects of sensorimotor remediation on handwriting. Those programs that used sensorimotor interventions over only a short period of time did not yield positive results. Sudsawad and colleagues[177] compared the effects of kinesthetic-based intervention with handwriting practice with 45 first graders over a 4-week period. They found neither group to make significant improvements in handwriting and suggest that there is no support that kinesthetic training improves handwriting legibility for this age. In 2006, Denton and colleagues[178] compared sensorimotor intervention with therapeutic practice in 38 school-aged children with handwriting difficulties over 5 weeks. These authors noted moderate improvements in handwriting with therapeutic practice and a decline in ability in the sensorimotor group. They suggest that, although sensorimotor foundations did improve with sensorimotor intervention, there is no indication that these foundations affect the development of handwriting. Their findings suggest that structured therapeutic practice using motor learning principles has a much stronger impact on the development of handwriting.

Two studies that investigated the combined effects of sensorimotor intervention and higher-level teaching strategies did demonstrate a positive impact on handwriting.[179,180] Peterson and Nelson[179] found that low socioeconomic first graders who received 20 sessions of occupational therapy combining sensorimotor, biomechanical, and teaching-learning strategies made significant gains over those receiving academic instruction alone. Weintraub and colleagues[180] compared a control group with two treatment conditions (task-oriented approach versus combination of sensorimotor and task orientation). Immediately after treatment and at a 4-month follow-up, significant gains in handwriting were observed in both treatment groups compared with the control group. The authors support the use of "higher-level" teaching strategies to improve the skill of handwriting.

Motor Skill Training

Motor skill training involves learning skills and subskills functionally relevant to the child's daily performance. Tasks are taught in a sequential manner by developmental ages or by steps from simple to complex. Skill training can occur for a wide variety of gross, fine, and visual motor tasks, as well as ADLs. An assortment of theoretical models and techniques may be used based on the child's impairment and activity and participation deficits.

Motor skill training can involve both indirect and direct facilitation of specific motor tasks. Activities that include balance, locomotion, body awareness, and eye-hand coordination can improve functional skills such as being able to sit at a desk within the classroom and complete written work, as well as success in recess games such as basketball. Specific skills such as dribbling and foul shooting can also be specifically taught and practiced. The goal is to provide a great variety of motor activities at the child's developmental motor level to promote motor generalizations for more successful participation.

An example of this approach is Sugden and Henderson's[151] "ecological intervention," which is a method of skill training for children with DCD. In this model the therapist, called a *movement coach,* provides instruction to many individuals who interact with the child on how to develop specific targeted skills. All caregivers are actively involved in goal development and achievement. By having a variety of individuals work together across daily life environments, children more quickly become skilled.[151] This approach also develops the caregivers' ability to understand the demands of specific tasks and to help facilitate the child's performance in all settings.

Physical Fitness Training

As previously reviewed, children with DCD are at great risk of low levels of physical fitness. The benefits of fitness and physical activity in minimizing disease and maximizing overall wellness are well documented. Deleterious effects resulting from DCD or factors associated with it include but are not limited to fatigue, hypoactivity, poor muscle strength and endurance, decreased flexibility, poor speed and agility, and diminished power.

Specific muscular training may be needed to undo the effects of reduced activity.[181] Poor muscle strength, especially in the abdominal area, can lead to musculoskeletal issues such as back pain because posture and pelvic alignment require adequate muscle strength. Children with DCD often require specific instruction to perform muscle strengthening activities (e.g., sit-ups, push-ups) with appropriate form. Decreased flexibility and muscle tightness in the lower extremities can contribute to difficulties in running, jumping, and hopping. Flexibility can be encouraged with a regimen of stretches specific to the areas of tightness. Gentle and regular stretching can be incorporated into warmups during sessions or physical activities.

Fitness can improve and be maintained when children participate in regular, preferably daily, physical activity. These activities often require more structure and direction for children with movement difficulties. As therapists, our overall goal should be to educate children about the value and enjoyment of regular activity.[181] Hands and Larkin[181] suggest the following plan to ensure children with DCD learn or rediscover the joy of movement:

- Educate children to understand and monitor their bodies' responses to exercising (e.g., heart rate increases when they run).
- Assist them in finding developmentally appropriate activities they will enjoy with some success.
- Encourage them to maintain a healthy, active lifestyle by encouraging participation in lifelong activities such as swimming, cycling, golf, sailing, yoga, or weight training.

In sports and leisure activities, the emphasis should be on participation and fitness rather than competition. Encourage activities that do not require constant adaptation, because children with DCD tend to be more successful in sports that have a repetitive nature to the movements (e.g., swimming, running, skating, skiing).[142,183] Sports that have a high degree of spatial challenge or unpredictability, such as baseball, hockey, football, and basketball, are less likely to be successful for children with DCD.[182] Activities that are taught through sequential verbal guidance, such as karate, may be easier to learn.[140]

PTs and OTs can have a positive impact on participation in fitness activities for children with DCD. A summary of key suggestions,[91] including the following, can assist with encouraging involvement in community sports and leisure activities:

- Provide frequent encouragement and reward effort.
- Encourage participation, rather than competition; emphasize fun, fitness, and skill building.
- Use a variety of teaching methods to demonstrate new skills (one-on-one instruction, verbal cues, demonstration).
- Provide hand-over-hand instruction during the early acquisition phase.
- Break down skills into smaller, meaningful parts.
- Keep the environment as predictable as possible.
- Modify or adapt equipment for safety (e.g., use foam balls instead of hard balls).
- Focus on the enjoyment, not the product.
- Encourage multiple roles in some activities (e.g., referee, scorekeeper, time keeper).
- Recognize the child's strengths and reinforce social interaction.

Encouraging and facilitating participation in a healthy lifestyle can aid in ending the vicious cycle of withdrawal, diminished opportunities for physical development, and decreased fitness and strength over time, a pattern very commonly seen in children with DCD.[91]

LEARNING DISABILITIES AND DEVELOPMENTAL COORDINATION DISORDER ACROSS THE LIFE-SPAN

Learning disabilities persist into adulthood and present lifelong challenges. Continuing issues with attention, cognition, emotional adjustment, and interpersonal skills can affect education, employment, family life, and daily routines. Adolescents and adults with learning disabilities frequently struggle with the concentration and organization needed to effectively manage daily routines and finances, vocational education or training, job procurement and retention, and finances.[183,184]

A recent longitudinal study[185] demonstrated that IQ scores remain stable from childhood to adulthood, as do deficit areas. Therefore poor readers remain poor readers, poor spellers remain poor spellers, and delayed math skills persist. In addition, adults who had affective illness or mood disorders as children have a significant risk of recurrent episodes (e.g., depression, bipolar disorder). An early 20-year longitudinal study of individuals with learning disabilities cited a rate of 42% for adult psychological disturbance (e.g., depression, alcohol abuse, anxiety disorders), compared with 10% in the general population.[186]

More recently, Seo and colleagues[187] found more optimistic results in their comparison of outcomes for individuals age 21 and 24 with and without documented learning disabilities. No significant differences were found in postsecondary school achievement or employment rates and earned income, although the 21 year olds with learning disabilities did receive significantly more public aid, such as food stamps, social security, and unemployment. The learning-disabled group did not have increased incidence of committing crimes or feeling victimized as young adults. Emotional health[185] and strong social relationships[188] are crucial for success; therefore children should be supported to develop healthy social connections and personal talents.

Several attributes have been identified as predictors of success for adults with learning disabilities.[188,191] A combination of internal and external factors supports the individual in the belief that he or she can take control, evaluate needs, and develop appropriate coping strategies, while knowing when to seek additional help.[189] The ability to be proactive, set goals, and persevere is a key internal element to attaining success. Understanding one's learning disability, with recognition of strengths and limitations, affords more thoughtful choices in life roles. Self-esteem and confidence are promoted with external emotional support and positive feedback from family, friends, teachers, work colleagues, and employers.

The persistent motor coordination difficulties attributed to DCD further affect perceptions of competence[97,190] and successful accomplishment of daily life skills.[191] Raskind and colleagues[186] found that physical status, including motor impairment, was an important variable in determining success in adulthood. Slowness and variability in movement continue to be a pervasive feature, causing difficulties in tasks that require sequencing and dual-task performance, such as driving a car.[191] Adults with DCD report higher levels of difficulty with motor-related tasks such as self-care and handwriting.[192] Compared with adults with dyslexia, a greater number of adults with DCD continue to live at home with their parents, have fewer spare-time activities, and are more socially isolated.[192,193]

Learning disabilities with motor impairments appear to have a persistent effect on a sense of competence and self-concept.[15,193] Many individuals develop negative perceptions of themselves as they experience frustration and ineffectiveness. They set lower aspirations, further reinforcing the cycle of failure. A combination of ADHD and DCD was found to be the most important predictor of poor psychosocial functioning in early adulthood.[194] Higher incidence of drug and alcohol abuse, affective disorders, crime conviction, and unemployment have been documented. Without adequate support, adults with DCD have difficulties reaching their potential. They may benefit from counseling about their condition, vocational assessment, and guidance to assist with finding a suitable work environment, time management and organizational strategies, workplace and academic accommodations, and behavioral management.

SUMMARY

Learning disabilities are heterogeneous and multidimensional in their presentation. Research continues to work on identifying the causes and the associated functional deficits of learning disabilities, as well as developing effective intervention techniques. The variability of the group suggests a spectrum of neurological processing difficulties. As physiological measures of brain function improve, our theoretical understanding increases.

Assessment and teaching methods continue to be refined to identify underlying deficits and effective remediation strategies. The current trend is to recognize issues inherent in the child (i.e., a true learning disability) versus issues from inadequate or ineffective instruction. Early identification of difficulties and systematic alteration of instruction methods are advocated to serve students more quickly and efficiently. The challenge for the clinician is to recognize the multitude of components that interact to impede functional abilities and social participation for the child with learning disabilities.

Children with learning disabilities frequently manifest motor coordination problems. These motor deficits may be subtle and difficult to identify in a neurological evaluation or standardized testing. With better awareness and assessment measures, more children are being identified and diagnosed with DCD. Many theoretical models have been developed in an attempt to explain the qualitative motor deficits observed in children with learning disabilities and to provide constructs to develop intervention programs. Continued formal research and careful documentation of clinical outcomes are needed to synthesize therapeutic approaches that best meet the individual needs of the child.

Identification, advocacy, teaching, and remediation are important aspects of the OT's and PT's roles. The goal is to formulate an intervention program that best addresses the underlying deficits in foundation skills and the functional weaknesses in daily life tasks. The experienced interventionist will combine knowledge from many areas of theoretical development and remediation to facilitate the best performance in each child.

It is clear that learning disabilities and DCD both persist across the life-span and can have a multitude of detrimental effects. All areas of daily life performance can be affected, including social and emotional functioning, self-care, education, vocation, and interpersonal relationships. Both intrinsic factors (perseverance, insight, sense of control) and extrinsic factors (emotional support, mentoring, positive feedback) play a role in the ultimate success of the individual with learning and motor challenges. Our role as a pediatric therapist is to provide the necessary extrinsic support and effective intervention to alleviate the deleterious effects of living with a disability.

REFERENCES

To enhance this text and add value for the reader, all references are included on the companion Evolve site that accompanies this textbook. This online service will, when available, provide a link for the reader to a Medline abstract for the article cited. There are 203 cited references and other general references for this chapter, with the majority of those articles being evidence-based citations.

A Summary of Standardized Motor Tests

BRUININKS-ORESTSKY TEST OF MOTOR PROFICIENCY, SECOND EDITION (2005)[124]

Authors

Robert H. Bruininks, PhD, and Brett D. Bruininks, PhD

Source

American Guidance Service, Inc., Circle Pines, MN 55014

Ages

4 to 21 years

Administration

Individual. Complete form: 45 minutes to 1 hour. Short form: 15 to 20 minutes.

Equipment

Test kit needed

Description

The *Bruininks-Oseretsky Test of Motor Proficiency, Second Edition* (BOT-2) is the most recent revision of the Oseretsky Test of Motor Proficiency, first published in Russia in 1923. The Bruininks-Oseretsky Test is designed to provide information on a wide range of motor skills and is sensitive enough to identify mild to moderate motor control problems. In this revision the authors worked to improve the test item presentation, quality of the test kit, and functional relevance of test content. They also expanded the norms through age 21 and improved the test items for 4- to 5-year-olds. The BOT-2 yields standard scores, scaled scores, and percentile ranks, separately for males and females, and combined. Age equivalency scores are also available. The test assesses motor functioning in eight areas:

1. Fine Motor Precision: Functionally relevant drawing, paper folding, and cutting item that focuses on assessment of precise finger control. These items are untimed, and they focus on qualitative refinement.
2. Fine Motor Integration: Copying geometric shapes of increasing complexity as accurately as possible. These items are untimed, as they focus on precision.
3. Manual Dexterity: Goal-directed activities that involve reaching, grasping, and bimanual coordination with small objects (pennies, pegboard, card sorting, and stringing beads). Emphasis is placed on speed and accuracy (dexterity), and all items are timed.
4. Bilateral Coordination: Items that measure skill in sequential and simultaneous coordination of the upper and lower extremities. Includes both familiar tasks (e.g., jumping jacks and finger pivots

["itsy-bitsy spider"]), as well as novel tasks (e.g., tapping feet and fingers with opposite sides of the body).
5. Balance: Static and dynamic balance items measure motor control for maintaining posture when standing, walking, and making transitional movements in space (e.g., reaching for a plate on a shelf). Assesses three areas that affect balance: trunk stability, static and dynamic postural control, and use of visual cues.
6. Running Speed and Agility: Four activities to assess speed and agility (shuttle run, hopping on one and both feet, stepping over balance beam).
7. Upper-Limb Coordination: Items that involve visual tracking and coordinated hand and arm movements (eye-hand coordination). Tasks include catching, throwing, and dribbling, with one or both hands together.
8. Strength: Assesses trunk and upper and lower extremity strength necessary for effective gross motor performance in daily activities.

CONSTRUCTION AND RELIABILITY

The Bruininks-Oseretsky Test has been carefully standardized on 1520 subjects from 38 states, stratified across sex, ethnicity, socioeconomic, and disability status. Sample sizes were larger in the younger age ranges because children develop more rapidly than adolescents. Three measures of reliability were determined for subtests, composites, short form, and complete form: internal consistency, test-retest, and interrater. In general, all were high, with best reliability shown when the complete form was used.

Comment

The BOT-2 appears to be one of the better standardized tests of motor performance. The 1978 version has been one of the most widely used tests to assess motor proficiency and has been used in research to identify motor deficits in individuals with DCD.[195,196] It offers various levels of testing and screening with a comprehensive "complete form" that provides the most reliable measure of overall motor proficiency. The short form can be used for screening, to determine if further evaluation is necessary. In addition, only those single subtests or composites that are relevant to the child's areas of difficulty can be administered. When qualifying a student for special education, it is suggested that this thorough assessment be used. In this revision the authors focused on including a variety of tasks that are engaging and goal directed, assessing both quantitative and qualitative aspects of motor performance. When testing children with motor dysfunction, careful attention must be paid to qualitative performance on individual items. A child may demonstrate the ability to complete a test item, but qualitatively it is accomplished with increased effort, decreased refinement, and speed.

MOVEMENT ASSESSMENT BATTERY FOR CHILDREN, SECOND EDITION (2007)[112]

Authors

Sheila E. Henderson, David A. Sugden, and Anna L. Barnett

Source

Harcourt Assessment, Proctor House, 1 Proctor Street, London, WC1V6EU

Ages

3 to 16 years

Administration

Individual; 20 to 30 minutes

Equipment

Test kit required

Description

The *Movement Assessment Battery for Children, Second Edition* (Movement ABC-2) is a recent revision of the M-ABC, which was originally developed from the Test of Motor Impairment (TOMI)–Henderson Revision. The Movement ABC-2 is a norm-based assessment of gross and fine motor performance whose main intent is to identify and describe children with movement difficulties. The test was also designed for intervention planning, program evaluation, and research. There are three components of the Movement ABC-2: the standardized evaluation, a checklist of competency in specific daily motor behaviors, and a companion manual for program planning (Ecological Approach to Intervention).[151] The evaluation tool yields standard and percentile scores, with two determined cut-off points delineating definite movement difficulties and children at risk. The age ranges have been expanded, and the test is divided into three age brackets: children aged 3 to 6 years, 7 to 10 years, and 11 to 16 years. The test items vary in each age range, with increased complexity and skill required in the older age bands. There are eight tasks assessing three areas of coordination: manual dexterity, ball skills, and static and dynamic balance.

1. Manual Dexterity: Speed and dexterity with the preferred hand. Includes two manipulative tasks such as coins in a bank, stringing beads, pegs in a pegboard, threading lace, and turning pegs and nuts and bolts, as well as a written maze.
2. Ball Skills: Eye-hand coordination is assessed with two beanbag and ball tasks emphasizing aiming at a target and catching.
3. Static and Dynamic Balance: One task of static balance with eyes open, and two tasks of dynamic balance that emphasize spatial precision and control of momentum.

Construction and Reliability

The standardization sample included 1172 children in the United Kingdom. A stratified sampling was done to ensure that representative proportions of age, gender, race, and ethnicity, and parent educational level were included. Before the main study, testing was done around the world and revealed no culture-specific problems. The researchers consider this revision to be similar enough to the M-ABC that the studies used with that test remain relevant. Test-retest reliability for consistency of individual item scores fell within a range deemed acceptable, from 0.64 to 0.86. The mean of 0.77 was achieved for the test as a whole. Interrater reliability was excellent, exceeding 0.95.

Comment

This revision is the culmination of a lengthy program of research and development begun in 1966 by two groups of researchers. The Movement ABC-2 offers some additional advantages: (1) the checklist helps teachers to identify children with movement problems, and (2) information is provided for a cognitive-motor approach to intervention across environments. The test items are easy to administer and score. Although the manual provides a clear picture of what the task looks like, there are no standardized verbal instructions given in this revision. Scoring is based on a traffic light system, with the red zone (at or below 5th percentile) indicating significant movement difficulty, amber zone (6th to 15th percentile) delineating children at risk, and the green zone (above 15th percentile) indicating the absence of movement difficulties. Percentile scores are useful for parents and teachers because they are easily understood, but therapists should recognize that they do not form an equal interval scale, tending to cluster near the median of the normal curve. Therefore, for subtest raw scores near the median, a change of 1 point to the raw score could result in an increase of 8 percentile points, whereas at either end of the normal curve this might only translate to 2 percentile points.

PEABODY DEVELOPMENTAL MOTOR SCALES, SECOND EDITION (2000)[125]

Authors

M. Rhonda Folio and Rebecca R. Fewell

Source

Pro-Ed, 8700 Shoal Creek Boulevard, Austin, TX 78757

Ages

Birth to 5 years

Administration

40 to 60 minutes (test items may be scored by direct observation or by parent or teacher report)

Description

An early childhood motor development program that provides, in one package, both in-depth assessment and training or remediation of gross and fine motor skills. The assessment is composed of six subtests that measure interrelated motor abilities that develop early in life. The *Peabody Developmental Motor Scales, Second Edition* (PDMS-2) can be used by OTs, PTs, diagnosticians, early intervention specialists, adapted physical education teachers, psychologists, and others who are interested in examining the motor abilities of young children. The PDMS was designed for use with children who show delay or disability in fine and gross motor skills. Test items are similar to those on other developmental scales, but only motor items are included. Items are scored on a 3-point scale: 0 for unsuccessful, 1 for partial, and 2 for successful performance. Age-equivalent scores, motor quotients, percentile rankings, and standard scores are provided. Scoring software for the PDMS-2 is available to convert the PDMS-2 scores into standard scores, percentile ranks, and age equivalents and generate composite quotients. The software also can be used to compare PDMS-2 subtest performances and composite performances to identify intraindividual differences and provide a printed report of the student information, including treatment goals and objectives.

Subtests

1. Reflexes: This eight-item subtest measures a child's ability to automatically react to environmental events. Because reflexes typically

become integrated by the time a child is 12 months old, this subtest is given only to children from birth through 11 months.

2. Stationary: This 30-item subtest measures a child's ability to sustain control of his or her body within its center of gravity and retain equilibrium.

3. Locomotion: This 89-item subtest measures a child's ability to move from one place to another. The actions measured include crawling, walking, running, hopping, and jumping forward.

4. Object Manipulation: This 24-item subtest measures a child's ability to manipulate balls. Examples of the actions measured include catching, throwing, and kicking. Because these skills are not apparent until a child has reached the age of 11 months, this subtest is given only to children aged 12 months and older.

5. Grasping: This 26-item subtest measures a child's ability to use his or her hands. It begins with the ability to hold an object with one hand and progresses up to actions involving the controlled use of the fingers of both hands.

6. Visual-Motor Integration: This 72-item subtest measures a child's ability to use his or her visual perceptual skills to perform complex eye-hand coordination tasks such as reaching and grasping for an object, building with blocks, and copying designs.

Composites

1. Gross Motor Quotient: This composite is a combination of results on the subtests that measure the use of the large muscle systems:
   - Reflexes (birth to 11 months only)
   - Stationary (all ages)
   - Locomotion (all ages)
   - Object manipulation (12 months and older)
2. Fine Motor Quotient: This composite is a combination of results on the subtests that measure the use of the small muscle systems:
   - Grasping (all ages)
   - Visual-motor integration (all ages)
3. Total Motor Quotient: This composite is formed by a combination of results on the gross and fine motor subtests. Because of this, it is the best estimate of overall motor abilities.

Construction and Reliability

Reliability coefficients were computed for subgroups of the normative sample (e.g., individuals with motor disabilities, African Americans, Hispanic Americans, girls, and boys), as well as for the entire normative sample. The normative sample consisted of 2003 persons residing in 46 states and was collected in the winter of 1997 and spring of 1998. Normative samples relative to geography, sex, race, and other critical variables are therefore representative of the current US population.

A test-retest reliability of 0.84 for the Gross Motor Scale and of 0.73 for the Fine Motor Scale (0.89 Total Motor) was reported based on a sample of 30 children from Austin, Texas, in the age range of 2 to 11 months. A second group of 30 children from Nacogdoches, Texas, aged 12 to 17 months, was tested with a test-retest reliability of 0.93 for the Gross Motor Scale and 0.94 for the Fine Motor Scale (0.96 Total Motor). These values are of sufficient magnitude for a tester's confidence in the test scores' stability over a period of time. The correlation coefficients between the PDMS and the PDMS-2 for criterion-prediction validity in the Gross and Fine Motor Quotients exceed 0.80, which supports the equivalency of the tests.

The PDMS-2 scores were correlated with those of the *Mullen Scales of Early Learning: AGS Edition* (MSEL:A) when both tests were administered on the same day to 29 children, aged 2 months to 66 months, in Evansville, Indiana. The relations of the PDMS-2 and MSEL:A demonstrated that Gross and Fine Motor Quotients exceed 0.80, high enough

to support the equivalency of the tests. When the concurrent validity of the age equivalent and standard scores of the Bayley Scales of Infant Development II (BSID-II) Motor Scale and PDMS-2 were calculated, the standard scores show poor agreement and had low concurrent validity, particularly the BSID-II Motor Scale and the PDMS-2 Locomotion Subscale.[197] The differences in the scores of these two tests warrant concern when using one test to make clinical decisions for service eligibility.

Comment

The PDMS-2 is primarily useful for children with mild to moderate motor deficits, such as a child with learning disabilities or a child with developmental delay. The test does not discriminate among children with moderate to severe motor disability because they fall far below the standard scores given. The skill categories are unevenly distributed and have too few items at some age levels to be meaningful. Despite the drawbacks, the PDMS-2 is probably the most valuable motor scale test currently available for preschool children.

CLINICAL OBSERVATIONS OF MOTOR AND POSTURAL SKILLS, SECOND EDITION (2000)[134]

Authors

Brenda N. Wilson, MS, OT(C), Nancy Pollock, MSc, OT(C), Brenda Kaplan, PhD, and Mary Law, PhD, OT(C)

Source

Therapro Inc., 225 Arlington Street, Framingham, MA 01702

Ages

5 to 11 years

Administration

Individual; 15 to 20 minutes

Equipment

Test kit required for ATNR measurement tools. Stopwatch and mat needed for certain items.

Description

The *Clinical Observations of Motor and Postural Skills* (COMPS) is a standardized screening tool using six clinical observations suggested by Ayres[105,198] of "soft neurological signs" to identify motor problems with a postural component. Historically, the clinical observations used by therapists have not had standardized administration or objective scoring and they have not taken into account the child's age and changes in abilities as the child matures. The authors felt it was important to objectify these observations and relate performance to age, as neuromotor maturation is very rapid in this age group. The test is designed to measure cerebellar function, postural control (stability), and motor coordination (mobility). Motor planning and sequencing are not intended to be measured directly, and repetition of directions, therapist prompting, and item practice are meant to separate motor performance from the cognitive aspects of planning. The test has six test items:

1. Slow Movements: Assesses the ability to move arms in a slow and symmetrical manner. Scoring is based on quality of performance, speed, and symmetry.
2. Rapid Forearm Rotation: A test of diadochokinesis; score is based on the number of forearm rotations accurately completed in 10 seconds.

3. Finger-Nose Touching: Measures proprioceptive mechanisms of motor control by switching midtask from eyes open to eyes closed. Scoring is based on accuracy, fluidity of motion, and force of touch.
4. Prone Extension Posture: The child holds a position of extension against gravity. Scoring is based on the duration of ability to hold position, quality of extension, and effort.
5. Asymmetrical Tonic Neck Reflex: The degree of inhibition of this reflex is looked at by measuring elbow flexion with manual head turn in a quadruped position. This test is also useful for identifying poor postural stability through observations including needing a wide base of support to sustain the position and locking elbows for stability.
6. Supine Flexion Posture: The child holds a position of flexion against gravity. Scoring is based on the duration of ability to hold position, quality of extension, and effort.

Construction and Reliability

Standardization of the test was done in two cities (Calgary and Hamilton) on a sample of 123 children, 67 who demonstrated DCD and 56 with no known motor problem. Test-retest reliability, interrater reliability, internal consistency, and construct validity were completed with a sample of 132 children with and without DCD. Test-retest reliability over 2 weeks was 0.98, and interrater reliability for pediatric OTs was 0.87. The internal consistency was high, indicating that the test discriminates well between children with and without motor problems, although the sample size was small.

Comment

The COMPS is a useful standardized tool for identifying subtle motor problems in children and was designed for and tested on children with DCD. The COMPS was not designed for children with known neurological or neuromotor problems such as intellectual delay, cerebral palsy, or epilepsy. It can be used as a screening tool for motor dysfunction, to assist in determining intervention approaches that would be beneficial for the child, and possibly to measure change over time. Children with motor performance problems can score within normal limits on the COMPS, and children who demonstrate low scores may not be exhibiting functional difficulties. The association between these clinical observations and functional performance is not always clear; therefore it is essential to gather information regarding the child's current functioning from observation and interview.

SCHOOL FUNCTION ASSESSMENT (1998)[199]

Authors

Wendy Coster, PhD, OTR/L, Theresa Deeney, EdD, Jane Haltiwanger, PhD, and Stephen Haley, PhD, PT

Source

Pro-Ed, 8700 Shoal Creek Boulevard, Austin, TX 78757-6897
Website: https://www.proedinc.com

Ages

5 to 12 years

Administration

Individual; untimed. Individual scales may be completed in 5 to 10 minutes.

Equipment

Record form; rating scale guides

Description

The *School Function Assessment* (SFA) is a judgment-based, criterion-referenced assessment to evaluate and monitor a student's performance on functional tasks that support school participation. This measure was designed to facilitate collaborative program planning for students with a variety of physical and cognitive disabilities. The SFA measures a student's ability to perform activities within the school setting that support participation in the academic and social aspects of an elementary program (grades K-6). Functional skills such as moving around the school, using classroom materials, interacting with peers, and caring for personal needs are included. The instrument is best completed by school professionals who are familiar with the student's typical performance. Task items are written in measurable, behavioral terms that can be used directly in the student's IEP. Criterion cut-off scores are provided for use in determining eligibility for special services. The SFA contains three parts:

1. Participation: Rates the student's involvement in six major school activity settings: regular or special education classroom, playground or recess, transportation, bathroom and toileting activities, transitions to and from class, and mealtime or snack time.
2. Task Supports: Identifies and rates the assistance and adaptations currently provided to the student for both physical and cognitive and behavioral tasks. Two types of task supports are examined separately: assistance (adult help) and adaptations (modifications to the environment or program, such as specialized equipment or adapted materials).
3. Activity Performance: Examines the student's performance of specific school-related functional activities. Physical tasks include travel, maintaining and changing positions, recreational movement, manipulation with movement, using materials, setup and cleanup, eating and drinking, hygiene, clothing management, going up and down stairs, written work, and computer and equipment use. Cognitive/behavioral tasks include functional communication, memory and understanding, following social conventions, compliance with adult directives and school rules, task behavior and completion, positive interaction, behavior regulation, personal care awareness, and safety.

Construction and Reliability

A sample of 678 students in two groups participated in the standardization of SFA. One group included children with special needs (363 students). These students had a variety of disabilities, including motor impairment, communication impairment, emotional or behavioral difficulties, and cognitive limitations. The second group included 315 students in regular education programs. Internal consistency was excellent at 0.92 to 0.98, indicating that items in a scale relate to one another and measure the same construct. Test-retest reliability was 0.82 to 0.98.

Comment

This assessment is unique in its focus on activity and participation levels, versus identifying impairments. It helps school personnel to recognize and ameliorate functional limitations that are affecting successful school participation. The comprehensiveness of assessment and functional IEP-ready goals makes it a useful tool to qualify and develop programs for children in need of special education services. Complete instructions are contained in the assessment booklet. Therefore the respondent does not need to refer to a manual to complete items, easing data collection. The manual is then used to compute transformed scores and interpret results.

BEERY-BUKTENICA DEVELOPMENTAL TEST OF VISUAL-MOTOR INTEGRATION, SIX REVISION (2010)[200]

Authors

Keith E. Beery, PhD, Norman A. Buktenica, and Natasha A. Beery

Source

Pearson Clinical Assessments, 19500 Bulverde Rd #201, San Antonio, TX 78259

Ages

2 to 99 years

Administration

Individual or group; 5 to 15 minutes

Equipment

Protocol booklets (test forms), No. 2 pencil

Description

The *Beery-Buktenica Developmental Test of Visual-Motor Integration* (BEERY VMI) was developed for early screening and intervention of visual-motor deficits. It tests the ability to integrate visual and motor abilities by presenting 30 geometric forms of increasing difficulty to copy. A booklet is provided; below the design is a blank space in which the child replicates the form. A shorter format including the first 21 items is best suited for children aged 2 to 7 years. Items are judged pass or fail on criteria given in the manual, and scores are reported in standard scores and percentiles. Age equivalents are also available. If the child has significant difficulty completing the test or scores below the average range, this may be indicative of a visual-motor integration delay. To further assess where the difficulties lie, two additional tests are available to assess visual perception and motor coordination separately.

1. Visual Perception: Visual perception is assessed by limiting the motor response to pointing. The child matches geometric forms to a stimulus. Administration takes approximately 3 minutes.
2. Motor Coordination: Motor accuracy is assessed on a task of drawing within a double-lined path. Administration takes approximately 5 minutes.

Construction and Reliability

The BEERY VMI is based on a significant amount of research on visual-motor integration, coordination, and development. The test has been normed five times between 1964 and 2003, with a total of more than 11,000 children. For this revision the Visual Perception and Motor tests were standardized on the same sample of 2512 children. This test has an extensive range of age-specific norms, with 600 children for the age range of 2 to 6 years. Test-retest reliability is high for the three test components, ranging from 0.90 to 0.92. Various studies of interrater reliability, internal consistency, and concurrent and construct validity are reported in the manual. Comparisons to other tests assessing visual-motor integration supported the validity the BEERY VMI.

Comment

The VMI provides a quick and easy method to assess the development of a child's ability to copy geometric forms. The uses are varied, including identification of significant difficulties with visual-motor integration and determination of an effective intervention program, as well as use as a research tool. For complete assessment of the child with learning disabilities and DCD, it is best used in conjunction with other tests of gross motor, fine motor, visual perception, and eye-hand coordination. This culture-free, nonverbal assessment is suitable for children with diverse educational, environmental, and language backgrounds. New to this addition are teaching materials to promote visual-motor integration for children from birth through elementary school. These include *My Book of Letters and Numbers; My Book of Shapes;* a laminated wall chart of basic gross motor, fine motor, and visual developmental milestones; and a checklist for parents of over 200 developmental "stepping stones" to help parents observe skill development and track progress.

MOTOR-FREE VISUAL PERCEPTION TEST, FOURTH EDITION

Authors

Ronald P. Colarusso, EdD, and Donald D. Hammill, EdD

Source

Western Psychological Services. 625 Alaska Avenue, Torrance, CA 90503
Website: https://www.wpspublish.com

Ages

4 to 80+ years

Administration

Individual; 20 to 25 minutes

Equipment

Protocol booklets (test forms), manual

Description

The *Motor-Free Visual Perception Test, Fourth Edition* (MVPT-4) is an assessment tool that seeks to evaluate visual-perceptual skills and identify potential deficits in children and adults aged four and older. This assessment provides an overall picture of an individual's visual perception skills and does not offer detailed information in regard to specific areas that may be lacking. The five areas of visual perception included in the test items are spatial relationships, visual discrimination, figure-ground, visual closure, and visual memory.[201] During administration, the evaluator reads the instructions for the test plate, and the child either points to the response that they choose or recites the corresponding letter.

Construction and Reliability

Data was collected from 2012 to 2014 on a nationally stratified sample of more than 2700 individuals. This assessment is internally consistent with the average Cronbach's alpha value of 0.80. A value of 0.80 indicates that the assessment is internally consistent. Significant positive relationships between test and retest standard scores also verify the reliability of the MVPT-4.[201] It has been concluded that the MVPT-4 measures all aspects of visual-perceptual skills in which it intends to measure, therefore confirming validity.[201]

Visual Perceptual Abilities Assessed

- Visual discrimination—discriminates dominant features of objects, including position, shape, and form.
- Spatial relationships—perceive the positions of objects in relation to oneself and other objects, including perception of pictures, figures, and patterns that are disoriented in relation to each other, such as figure reversals and rotations.

- Visual memory—recognize a previously presented stimulus item after a brief interval.
- Figure-ground—distinguish an object from background or surrounding objects.
- Visual closure—perceive a whole figure when only fragments are presented.

Comment

Before administering the MVPT-4, the chronological age of the client and reason for the selection of this specific assessment should be recorded. The client should feel like he or she is in a safe and comfortable environment. All directions and expectations should be explained in simple terms, and there should be an opportunity for the client to ask questions. The assessment may begin when the examiner feels that the client understands the procedure and expectations. If another person needs to be in the room to make the client feel comfortable, this is appropriate as long as they sit out of sight and do not engage in conversation. During this test, the examiner can observe the client's behaviors including their ability to focus, attend to the task, and stay seated. Notes about the client's behavior can be documented on the score sheets comments section. If lack of attention and other behaviors are preventing the client from successfully completing the assessment, the assessment should be discontinued and resumed at a later time.[201]

EVALUATION TOOL OF CHILDREN'S HANDWRITING (1995)[127]

Author

Susan J. Amundson

Source

O.T. Kids, PO Box 1118, Homer, AK 99603

Ages

First through sixth grades (6 to 11 years)

Administration

Individual

Equipment

Protocol booklet, task sheets and wall charts, stopwatch, No. 2 pencil

Description

The Evaluation Tool of Children's Handwriting (ETCH) is designed to evaluate manuscript and cursive writing for components of legibility and speed. Specific components of the child's handwriting, including letter formation, spacing, size, and alignment, are included for assessment. The following tasks are presented in order:

1. Lowercase alphabet letters (from memory)
2. Uppercase alphabet letters (from memory)
3. Numeral writing (from memory)
4. Near point copying (visual model)
5. Far point copying (visual model)
6. Dictation (verbal)
7. Sentence composition (independent)

A quick reference card is included with standardized directions and timing criteria. Written and illustrated scoring criteria have been designed to assist the evaluator in determining the legibility of letters and numbers. The primary focus of scoring is whether the written material is readable.

Construction and Reliability

Based on the efforts of numerous occupational therapy practitioners, students, and professors, the ETCH itself has evolved through scientific investigation. Pilots of the ETCH were designed by using adaptations of written tasks from existing tools. Three editions of the ETCH have been sampled by practitioners working in school systems, with feedback given on the examiner's manual, ease of administration and scoring, item selection, scoring procedures, and face validity of the instrument. When the ETCH was published, it lacked normative and psychometric information. Since that time, test reliability, validity, and normative data of the ETCH are being compiled through various research studies. Eight studies of handwriting speed are included for reference in the manual. The most recent examination of test-retest reliability studies[202] identified adequate stability of total word (0.95), letter (0.88), and number (0.84) scores. Individual letter, word, and number subtests were not as stable and should be used cautiously in interpretation of problems. Interrater reliability ranged from 0.63 to 0.94 for individual manuscript items and 0.64 to 0.97 for cursive. Overall, the total word reliability is more stable than task scores, ranging from 0.90 to 0.98.

Comment

The ETCH assesses functional writing skills that are relevant to academic performance. The varied tasks allow the examiner to identify areas of strength and weakness in written performance, including legibility components, speed, and composition models (visual, verbal, and memory). Information received from the ETCH is qualitative at this point because of the lack of normative samples. The author suggests that the ETCH be used in conjunction with observations of the child's writing activity in natural environments, such as classroom and home, as a determination of difficulties in functional written performance.

MINNESOTA HANDWRITING ASSESSMENT (MHA)

Author

Judith Reisman, PhD, OTR, FAOTA

Source

Pearson Clinical Assessments, 19500 Bulverde Rd #201, San Antonio, TX 78259

Ages

6 to 8 years

Administration

Individual or group; Initial Timed Portion: 2.5 minutes to establish rate score. Additional time given if test not completed in 2.5 minutes.

Total: 7 to 10 minutes (scoring time dependent on administrator's familiarity with scoring procedures)

Equipment

Test sheets, pencil, manual, stop-watch, ruler, red pen

Description

The Minnesota Handwriting Assessment (MHA) is a near-point copy test. Students are asked to copy words onto a marked lined paper. This assessment helps to identify students with handwriting difficulties through an objective analysis and normative rating system. It can also provide baseline data to document treatment effectiveness by specifically focusing on the students' rate of completing the writing task legibility (speed), alignment, size, and spacing.

Construction and Reliability

Normative data was provided for a large sample ($n = 2186$) of typically developing children in grades one and two (aged 6 to 8 years; 78 to 103 months).[203] The sample of students was from 11 US states. An effort was made to obtain an ethnically diverse sample by soliciting a mix of students from both urban and rural school districts across several states. However, the sample does not reflect the ethnic composition of students in the general population. Special education students, mainstreamed into the regular classroom, were included (4% of the total sample). Diagnostic information for special education students was not provided. Sample by gender was on average 49% female and 51% male. Interrater and intrarater reliability for total MHA scores are reported to be excellent (Pearson correlation .77 to .88). Test-retest reliability was assessed in a sample of 99 grade two students with testing readministered after 5 to 7 days and found to range from poor to adequate (legibility, 64%-alignment, 86%) for total rate scores. Adequate intraclass correlation coefficients of test-retest reliability were also reported.[203]

Comment

Time efficient to use in classroom—children do not have to miss significant class time to take it.

It is a fairly objective assessment with a detailed manual with samples for guidance. The MHA is based on normative data and can measure treatment effectiveness with pretesting and posttesting. The limitations are the long and detailed scoring and some components subject to interpretation.

THE PRINT TOOL[128]

Authors

Jan Olsen, OTR, and Emily Knapton, OTR/L

Source

Handwriting Without Tears, 8001 Mac Arthur Boulevard, Cabin John, MD 20818
Email: janolson@hwtears.com; website: https://www.hwtears.com

Ages

6 years old and older

Administration

Individual; administration for handwriting sample takes 15 minutes, scoring approximately 30 minutes

Equipment

Student booklet and pencil, or a writing sample can be collected from school; evaluation score sheet; transparent measuring tool for accurate scoring; comprehensive scoring overview; handwriting remediation plan forms to develop goals; and strategies for remediation

Description

The Print Tool is a formal printing assessment to use in evidence-based remediation programs. The Print Tool is used to evaluate handwriting skills, plan intervention, and measure progress in students experiencing handwriting difficulty. A student's ability to print dictated letters and numbers is assessed. Evaluation scores for each specific skill area assessed help identify the student's strengths and needs. The Print Tool provides general remediation suggestions and specific strategies to be carried out with the author's remedial Handwriting Without Tears curriculum. This tool can be used in all school and therapy settings and with all curricula. Eight handwriting components for capitals, lowercase letters, and numbers are considered:

1. Memory: remembering and writing dictated letters and numbers
2. Orientation: Facing letters and numbers in the correct direction
3. Placement: Putting letters and numbers on the baseline
4. Size: How big or small a child chooses to write
5. Start: Where each letter or number begins
6. Sequence: Order and stroke direction of the letter or number parts
7. Control: Neatness and proportion of letters and numbers
8. Spacing: Amount of space between letters in words and between words in sentences

Construction and Reliability

The Print Tool has been recently released. Standardization has not been completed; however, suggested age-related expectations are provided in the manual. Data collection is in process for standardization in the future.

Continuing education is recommended to understand the complete process of observing, scoring, and compiling a remediation plan with The Print Tool. A Level 1 Certification is offered by the Handwriting Without Tears organization. Both the assessment and the award-winning Handwriting Without Tears curriculum were developed based on the authors' many years of successful practice in evaluating and remediating handwriting problems. The Handwriting Without Tears program is a structured remedial program geared toward different age and skill levels. It is multisensory, developmentally based, and easy to implement. Support is provided via the Handwriting Without Tears website.

13

Spina Bifida: A Neural Tube Defect*

Yasser Salem and Ellen M. Godwin

OBJECTIVES

After reading this chapter the student or therapist will be able to:
1. Identify the various types of spina bifida.
2. Recognize the incidence and etiology of spina bifida.
3. Identify the clinical manifestations of myelomeningocele, including neurological, orthopedic, and urological sequelae.
4. Understand medical management in the newborn period and beyond.
5. Determine physical and occupational therapy evaluations, including manual muscle testing, range of motion, sensory testing, reflex testing, muscle tone assessment, developmental and functional and mobility assessments, and perceptual and cognitive evaluations.
6. Determine the major physical and occupational therapy goals and appropriate therapeutic management for each of the following stages: (a) before surgical closure of sac, (b) after surgery during hospitalization, (c) early infancy, (d) preambulatory, (e) toddler through preschool age, (f) primary school age through adolescence, and (g) transition to adulthood.
7. Identify psychological adjustment to spina bifida.

KEY TERMS

Chiari malformation
crouch-control ankle-foot orthosis
diastematomyelia
hydrocephalus
lipomeningocele

myelodysplasia
myelomeningocele
neural tube defects
reciprocating gait orthosis
sacral agenesis

spina bifida
spina bifida cystica
spina bifida occulta
standing A-frame
tethered spinal cord

INTRODUCTION

Spina bifida, a congenital spinal cord injury, is a complex disability that results from a failure of the caudal neural tube to fuse early in embryonic development. This congenital condition predisposes many areas of the central nervous system (CNS) to not develop or function adequately. In addition, all areas of development (physical, cognitive, and psychosocial) that depend heavily on central functioning will likely be impaired. The clinician must therefore be aware of the significant impact this neurological defect has on motor function as well as on a variety of related human capacities.

A developmental framework, the *Guide to Physical Therapist Practice,*[1] and the International Classification of Functioning, Disability and Health (ICF) have been used to aid in understanding the sequential problems of the child with spina bifida. The developmental model, however, must always stay in line with the functional model for adult trauma because the problems of the congenitally involved child rapidly evolve into limitations in the functional activities and participation in the life of the injured adult. By concentrating on the present while keeping an eye on the future, appropriate management goals can be achieved.

OVERVIEW AND PATHOGENESIS

Spina bifida occurs in utero and is present at the time of birth. Understanding how this malformation develops requires an appreciation of normal nervous system maturation.

Overview of Neural Tube Formation

The nervous system develops from the external layer of the zygotic disc called the ectoderm in a process called neurulation. During embryonic development, a longitudinal thickening of the ectoderm, which is called the neural plate, will differentiate into the brain and spinal cord to form the CNS. The neural plate is a trough-shaped differentiation of the ectodermal layer of the embryonic disc. The neural plate is a vertically oriented, topographically flat sheet of cells; its wide end lies rostrally and becomes the brain, whereas the slim end lies caudally and becomes the spinal cord. A midline groove (central or ventricular zone) divides the neural plate into right and left halves (marginal zones). The central zone contains cells, neuroblasts, and glioblasts and the marginal zone contains the processes of cells of the ventricular zone. The edges of the neural plate (neural folds) fold gradually, creating and deepening the neural groove. By the 20th day of gestation, the neural plate is an oblong structure that is wide at its rostral area (future brain) and slim caudally (future spinal cord). On day 21 of gestation, the edges continue to grow dorsally toward each other until they meet, fusing to create a hollow cylinder called the neural tube. Along the site of fusion, cell surface coats consisting of glycoproteins are deposited

---

*Videos for this chapter are available at studentconsult.com.

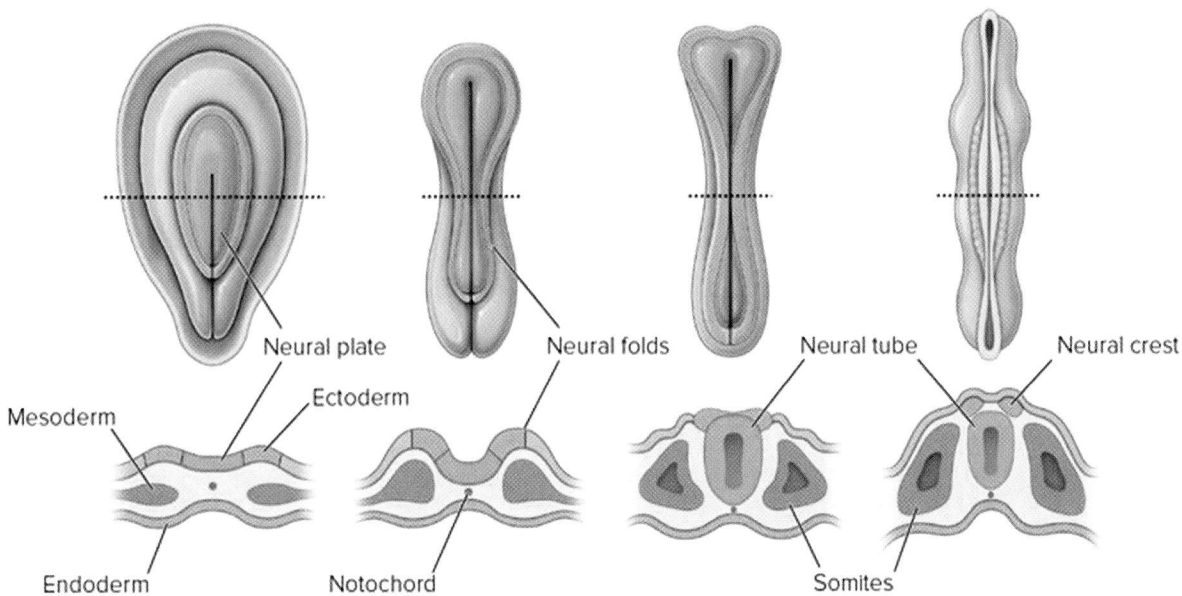

Fig. 13.1 Neural Tube Formation. (From Lundy-Ekman L. *Neuroscience: Fundamentals for Rehabilitation.* 4th ed. Elsevier.)

as a glue to hold the folds in place until more permanent cell-to-cell contacts can be established.

The neural tube closes first in the future cervical region. The closure proceeds rostrally and caudally, like zippering, leaving an opening at the rostral (cranial) end called the anterior neuropore and an opening at the caudal end called the posterior neuropore. The anterior and posterior neuropores close on days 24 and 27 of gestation, respectively (Fig. 13.1).

By day 26, the neural tube differentiates into two concentric circles. The mantle layer (inner wall) contains cell bodies and will become gray matter. The marginal layer (outer wall) contains processes of cells, whose bodies are located in the mantle layer. The marginal layer develops into white matter, consisting of axons and glial cells.

At the junction between the neural plate and remaining ectoderm lies a narrow strip of cells that develop from the ectoderm, called the neural crest, that will generate a variety of adult structures, including most neurons of the peripheral nervous system (PNS). When the neural crest has developed, the neural tube and the neural crest move inside the embryo. The neural crest detaches from the lateral edge of the neural plate and assumes a location anterolateral to the neural tube. The overlying ectoderm is destined to become the epidermal layer of skin and closes over the tube and neural crest.

As the nervous system continues to develop, the rostral end of the neural tube differentiates into a series of vesicles that constitute the major brain regions and the caudal end of the neural tube forms the spinal cord. The neural crest differentiates to form most of the PNS neurons, with the rest arising from nearby ectoderm.

Neural Tube Defects

It is generally accepted that neural tube defects (NTDs) are caused by the failure of the neural tube to close, although it has also been suggested that a closed tube may reopen in some cases.[2,3] A variety of defects results from the failure of the neural tube to properly close. Failure of closure of the neural tube may occur at several sites and the clinical types of NTDs differ depending on the site at which closure fails.[3]

The types of NTDs include anencephaly, spina bifida, encephalocele, craniorachischisis, and iniencephaly. The latter two types are rare, but they tend to occur with disproportionate frequency in areas that

have a high rate of NTDs, such as northern China.[4] The most dysraphic disorders occur at the location of the anterior or posterior neuropores, resulting in anencephaly, encephalocele, or spina bifida.

Craniorachischisis is the most severe type of NTD in which the neural tube does not fuse. In this condition, either the none of neural tube closes, which leaves the entire spinal cord open, or the tube is partially closed, which leaves the spinal cord partially open. Craniorachischisis comprises 10% of NTDs, in which the entire neural tube remains open from midbrain to low spine.[3]

Iniencephaly is an uncommon but severe form of NTDs with severe defect of the cervical spine. Iniencephaly involves bifid neural arches, with retroflexion of the skull and an extremely short neck. Most cases involve occipital encephalocele. It seems to be more common in females.[3]

Failure of fusion of the cranial end of the neural tube results in a condition known as *anencephaly*. In this defect, there is minimal development of the brain, including an absence of development of the forebrain.[5] In most cases, the brain stem may be fairly intact, but the cerebellum may be absent. A failure of the anterior neuropore to close results in a failure of development of the surrounding meninges and skull to form over the incomplete brain, leaving the brain and brain stem exposed (Fig. 13.2). Considerable facial abnormalities are commonly seen in these children. This NTD is not compatible with life. Most fetuses with this condition die before or shortly after birth, and almost none survive for more than few days.

Failure of the neural tube to close completely at the cranial level results in crania bifidum, a defect in the cranium. An encephalocele is a herniation of intracranial contents through a defect in the cranium. The cystic structure may contain only meninges (meningocele), meninges and brain structures (meningoencephalocele), or meninges, brain structures, and a part of the ventricular system (meningohydroencephalocele) (Fig. 13.3). Encephaloceles may occur anywhere along the center of the skull from the nose to the back of the neck. Encephaloceles are most common in the occipital region, but they may also occur between the forehead and the nose or at the top of the head. Encephalocele can be asymptomatic but can also be fatal, depending on the extent of brain damage.[3]

Defects in the closure of the posterior neuropore cause a range of malformations known collectively as spina bifida (Fig. 13.4). The

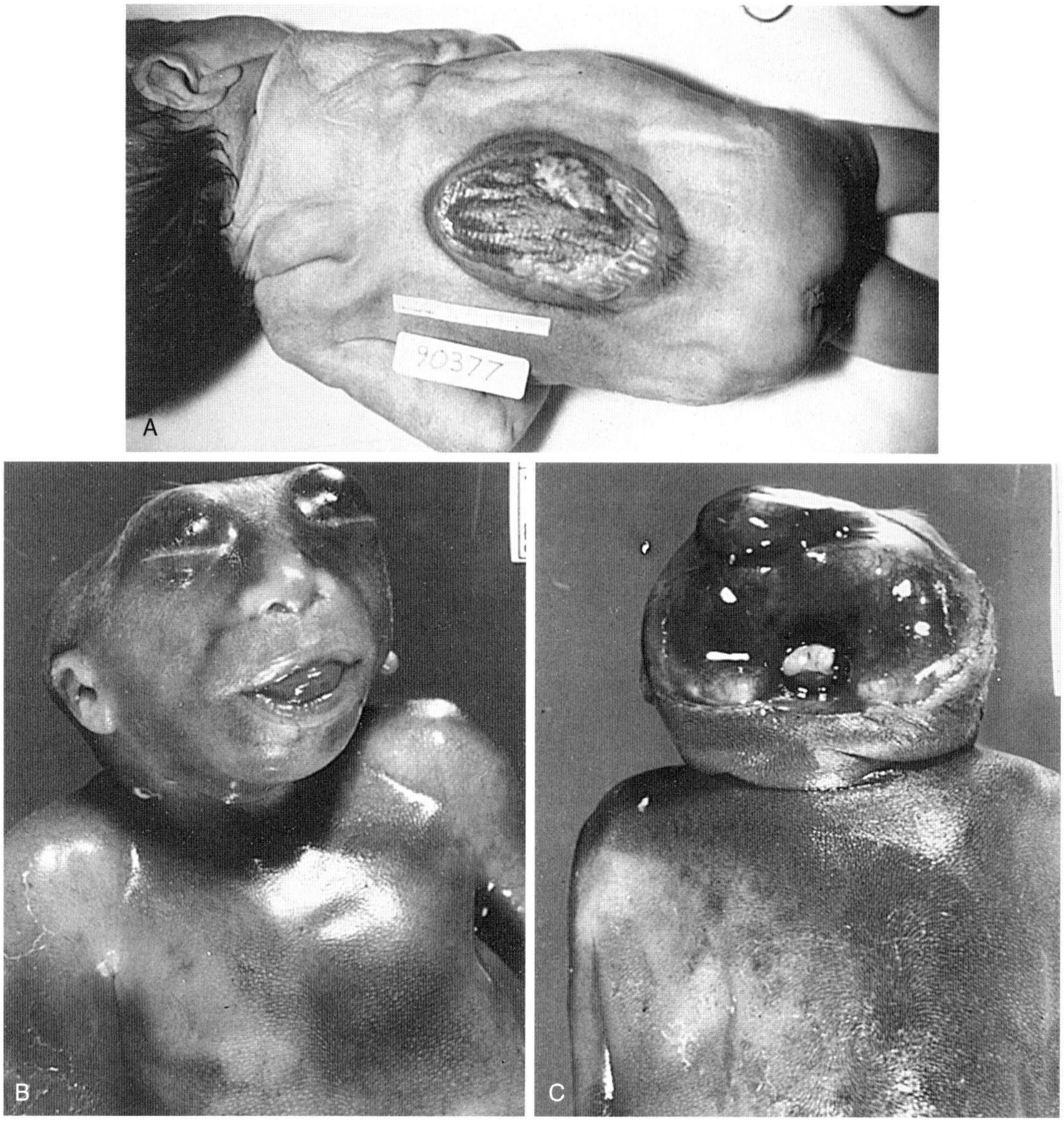

Fig. 13.2 **(A)** Spina bifida in a newborn. **(B** and **C)** Anencephaly showing absence of the cranial vault. (From *Pathophysiology: The Biologic Basis for Disease in Adults and Children,* 6th ed. McCance – Elsevier.)

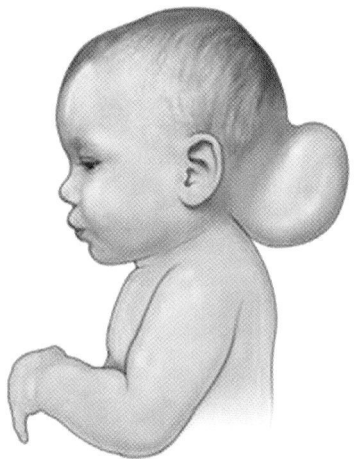

Fig.13.3 **Encephalocele.** (From *Neurologic Rehabilitation: Neuroscience and Neuroplasticity in Physical Therapy Practice,* Nichols Larsen – McGraw Hill.)

defect always involves a failure of the vertebral arches at the affected levels to form completely and fuse to cover the spinal cord. In most cases, the malformation is covered with skin, but the site may be marked by unusual pigmentation, hair growth, telangiectases (large superficial capillaries), or a prominent dimple. The defect can be open myeloschisis and is considered the most severe form of spina bifida. Spina bifida is the most common of the NTDs.

TYPES OF SPINA BIFIDA

Spina bifida results from a failure in neural tube closure and closure of the overlying posterior vertebral arches (dysraphism). The extent of the defect may result in one of two types of spina bifida: occulta or cystica. The terms *spina bifida, myelodysplasia,* and *myelomeningocele* are frequently used interchangeably.

Spina bifida occulta is characterized by a failure of one or more of the vertebral arches to meet and fuse in the third month of gestation. The spinal cord and meninges are unharmed and remain within the vertebral canal (Fig. 13.5A). The bony defect is covered with skin that

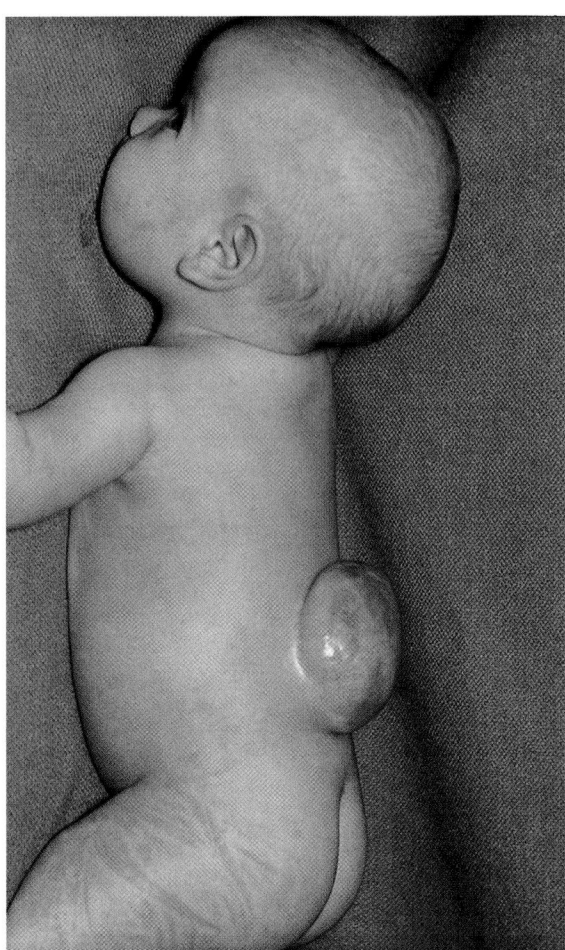

Fig. 13.4 Meningomyelocele in an Infant. (From *Neuroscience Fundamentals for Rehabilitation.* 4th ed. Lundy-Ekman.)

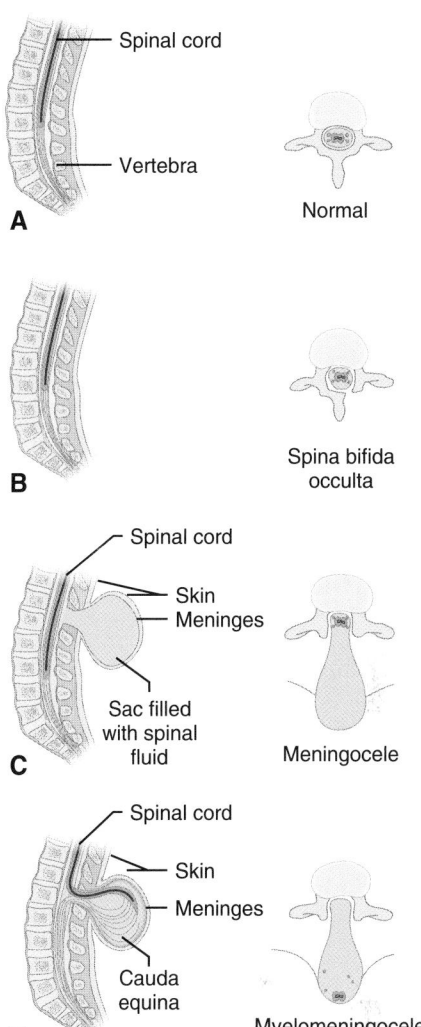

Fig. 13.5 Types of Spina Bifida. (A) Normal anatomical structures. **(B)** Spina bifida occulta. **(C)** Meningocele. **(D)** Myelomeningocele. (From *Pathology Implications for the Physical Therapist.* 4th ed. Goodman. Elsevier.)

may be marked by a dimple, pigmentation, or patch of hair.[6] The most common site for this defect is the lumbosacral area, and it is usually associated with no disturbance of neurological or musculoskeletal functioning. Most individuals with spina bifida occulta are unaware that they have this defect.

Spina bifida cystica results when the neural tube and overlying vertebral arches fail to close appropriately. Cystic protrusion of the meninges or the spinal cord and meninges occurs through the defective vertebral arches and produces a cystic sac.

The milder form of spina bifida cystica, called *meningocele,* involves protrusion of the meninges and cerebrospinal fluid (CSF) only into the cystic sac (see Fig. 13.5B). The spinal cord remains within the vertebral canal, but it may exhibit structural abnormalities.[7] Clinical signs vary (according to the extent of spinal cord anomalies) or may not be apparent. This is a relatively uncommon form of spina bifida cystica.

A rare but more severe form of spina bifida cystica, called *myelocele* or *myelocystocele, or terminal myelocystocele,* is present when the central canal of the spinal cord is dilated (syringocele) and surrounded by an expanded dural sheath, producing a large, skin-covered cyst. The neural tube appears to close normally but is distended from the cystic swelling. The CSF may ceaselessly expand the neural canal. Most born with myelocystocele have no neurological deficit; however, prompt medical attention is mandatory for repair of the cyst.[8,9]

The more common and severe form of the spinal bifida is known as *myelomeningocele,* in which both spinal cord and meninges are

contained in the cystic sac (see Fig. 13.5C). Within the sac, the spinal cord and associated neural tissue show extensive abnormalities. In incomplete closure of the neural tube (dysraphism), abnormal growth of the cord and a convoluted pathway of neural elements interrupt the normal transmission of neural impulses. The result is a variable sensory and motor impairment at the level of the lesion and below.[6] In an open myelomeningocele, nerve roots and spinal cord may be exposed, with dura and skin evident at the margin of the lesion. Exposure of the open neural tube to the amniotic fluid environment leads to neuroepithelial degeneration, with massive loss of neural tissue by the end of pregnancy.[10]

Although spina bifida cystica can occur at any level of the spinal cord, myelomeningoceles are most common in the thoracic and lumbosacral regions. Myelomeningocele occurs in 94% of the cases of spina bifida cystica, and two-thirds of open lesions involve the thoracolumbar junction.[6]

Other forms of spinal dysraphism include diastematomyelia, lipomeningocele, and sacral agenesis. Diastematomyelia is present in 30% to 40% of patients with myelomeningocele and is secondary to partial or complete clefting of the spinal cord.[11] Lipomeningocele, another form of spina bifida cystica, is usually caused by a vertebral defect associated with a superficial fatty mass (lipoma or fatty tumor) that merges with the lower level of the spinal cord. No associated hydrocephalus is present, and neurological deficit is generally minimal; however, problems with urinary control and motor control of the lower extremities may be noted.[12] Neurological tissue compromise may be caused by a tethered spinal cord; therefore early lipoma resection is indicated for cosmesis and to minimize neurological sequelae.

Lumbosacral or sacral agenesis may occur and is caused by an absence of the caudal part of the spine and sacrum. Children with this form of dysraphism may have narrow, flattened buttocks, weak gluteal muscles, and a shortened intergluteal cleft. The normal lumbar lordosis is absent, although the lower lumbar spine may be prominent. Calf muscles may be atrophic or absent. The pelvic ring is completed with either direct opposition of the iliac bones or with interposition of the lumbar spine replacing the absent sacrum. These children may have scoliosis, motor and sensory loss, and visceral abnormalities, including anal atresia, fused kidneys, and congenital heart malformations. Management is started early and is symptomatic for each system.[13]

INCIDENCE, ETIOLOGY, PREVENTION, AND ECONOMIC IMPACT

Incidence

Statistics about the incidence of spina bifida vary considerably in different parts of the world. Spina bifida and anencephaly, the most common forms of NTDs, affect about 300,000 newborns each year worldwide.[14] In the United States, the most recent annual prevalence estimates that 1460 babies are born with spina bifida, and[15] the incidence is currently 2.48 per 10,000, down from approximately 7.23 per 10,000 births from 1974 through 1979 (before the folic acid mandate[16–18]). Current worldwide folic acid fortification programs have resulted in a decreased incidence of spina bifida,[19,20] with annual decreases of 6600 folic acid–preventable spina bifida and anencephaly births reported since 2006.[21] There was a 31% decline in spina bifida prevalence rates in the immediate postfortification period (October 1998 through December 1999[17,19]). Additionally, there was a continued decline in spina bifida prevalence rates from 1999 to 2004 of 10%.[22] Studies have also demonstrated that decline has varied by ethnicity and race from prefortification to optional fortification to mandatory fortification in the United States.[17,22] Initially after fortification, the largest decline in prevalence was noted in Hispanic and non-Hispanic white races or ethnicities. Despite this initial decline, postfortification prevalence rates remain the highest in infants born to Hispanic mothers and less in infants born to non-Hispanic white and non-Hispanic black mothers.[22] In addition to periconceptual folate supplementation, it is thought that incidence has decreased subsequent to food fortification in several countries, decreased exposure to environmental teratogens, and increased and more accurate prenatal screening for fetal anomalies.[14]

The incidence of spina bifida has declined since the advent of amniocentesis and the use of ultrasonography for prenatal screening. The diagnosis of spina bifida is one of the common indications for birth termination.

Spina bifida is thought to be more common in females than in males,[23] although some studies suggest no real sex difference.[7] A study of the association of race and sex with different neurological levels of myelomeningocele found the proportions of whites and females to be significantly higher in patients with thoracic-level spina bifida.[8] A significant relation has also been noted between social class and spina bifida: the lower the social class, the higher the incidence.[24,25]

Etiology

A multifactorial genetic inheritance has been proposed as the cause of spina bifida, coupled with environmental factors of which nutrition, including folic acid intake, is key. Genetic factors seem to influence the occurrence of spina bifida. Cytoplasmic factors, polygenic or oligogenic inheritance, chromosomal aberrations, and environmental influences (e.g., teratogens) have all been considered possible causes.[10,21] Many studies identified an increased risk of NTD-affected pregnancy to be associated with epidemiological findings such as maternal and paternal ages and occupations, maternal reproductive history, including maternal country of birth and country of conception, nutrition, including folic acid and vitamin B12 deficiency, hyperthermia during early pregnancy, hyperglycemia or diabetes or obesity, and maternal use of medications during early pregnancy.[26]

Genetic considerations, such as an Rh blood type, a specific gene type (HLA-B27), an X-linked gene, and variations in the many folate pathway genes have been implicated, but not conclusively.[27,28] Malformations are attributed to abnormal interactions of several regulating and modifying genes in early fetal development.[29] Disturbance of any of the sequential events of embryonic neurulation produces NTDs, with the phenotype (i.e., spina bifida, anencephaly) varying depending on the region of the neural tube that remains exposed.[10] Environmental factors combined with genetic predisposition appear to trigger the development of spina bifida, although definitive evidence is not available to support this claim.[30]

A family history of spina bifida is one of the strongest risk factors.[23] The chances of having a second affected child are between 1% and 2%, whereas in the general population, the percentage drops to one-fifth of 1%.[31,32] Although these factors are related to the incidence of spina bifida, the cause of this defect remains in question.

It is generally accepted that inadequate maternal intake of natural folate, or its synthetic form, folic acid, before and during early pregnancy, is associated with an increased risk of spina bifida.[23,26] Several studies have shown that the failure to consume folic acid supplements or folic acid-containing multivitamins increases the risk of having an affected child by two- to eightfold.[33] The risk of having a child affected by an NTD is indirectly related to both maternal folate and folic acid intake as well as to maternal folate status. Folate is important in nucleic acid synthesis and in the biosynthesis of methionine through the conversion of homocysteine to methionine. Disruptions in folate metabolism can result in increased homocysteine concentrations, which are teratogenic to the neural tube. The precise mechanism underlying the association between NTDs and folate has not been established.

Vitamin B12, which is metabolically related to folate, might also be associated with NTDs. Studies have shown that deficient or inadequate maternal vitamin B_{12} status is associated with a significantly increased risk for NTDs.[34–36]

Environmental conditions such as hyperthermia in the first weeks of pregnancy or dietary factors such as maternal consumption of canned meats, blighted potatoes, or tea have been implicated but not substantiated.[37,38]

Maternal diabetes is another factor related to the incidence of spina bifida.[39] Women with pregestational diabetes are at increased risk of having a child with spina bifida and other types of birth defects.[23] In these women, the risk of nervous system malformation including spina bifida is two- to tenfold higher than the risk in the general population. The mechanism underlying this teratogenic effect has not been established, but it is clearly related to the degree of maternal metabolic control.[40]

Other factors associated with NTDs include maternal exposure to anticonvulsant drugs during early pregnancy. Many anticonvulsant drugs such as valproic acid are known teratogens. An increased risk of spina bifida is associated with exposure to valproic acid or carbamazepine alone, or in combination with each other or other anticonvulsants.[41,42] This risk is increased for women who are taking more than one anticonvulsant.

Women who use these drugs for indications other than epilepsy (e.g., bipolar disease, migraine, chronic pain) are also at higher risk of having a child with spina bifida if they become pregnant while taking these drugs.[23,41,42] The mechanism by which valproic acid and carbamazepine increase the risk of spina bifida has not been established.

Prevention

Historically, nutritional deficiencies, such as of folic acid and vitamin A, have been implicated as a cause of primary NTDs.[43–46] Fifty to 70% of NTDs can be prevented if a woman of childbearing age consumes sufficient folic acid daily before conception and throughout the first trimester of pregnancy. As a result of research findings in support of folic acid implementation, the US Public Health Service has mandated folic acid fortification since 1998 as a public health strategy. Prenatal vitamins, especially folic acid, are recommended to discourage the condition's development. Current fortification programs are preventing about 22,000 cases, or 9% of the estimated folic acid–preventable spina bifida and anencephaly cases.[21] At this time, folic acid supplementation and fortification provide the only means of primary prevention for spina bifida and other NTDs.[23]

Economic Impact

Health care use and costs for children with spina bifida are significantly greater than those of unaffected children.[47] The lifetime cost to society per affected person with spina bifida is estimated to be over $600,000.[48–50] One-third of this amount comprises direct medical costs with the remainder being indirect costs, including special educational and caregiver needs and the loss of employment potential.[48] In addition to medical management costs per child, there are additional costs that affect both the family and society across the life-span and are variable and often related to differential market forces and social welfare policies.[50]

A study published in 2012 that examined the associated costs during the first year of life among children with spina bifida indicated that the estimated hospital cost per infant is $39,059[47] and the total medical expenditures during the first year is more than $50,000.[51] The majority of expenditures during infancy were from inpatient admissions secondary to surgeries concentrated during this time period for those with spina bifida.[51] After infancy, average medical care expenditures during 2003 ranged from $15,000 to $16,000 per year among different age groups of persons with spina bifida. Incremental expenditures associated with medical care were not stable, but decreased with increasing age, from $14,000 per year for children to $10,000 per year for adults aged 45 to 64 years.[51] These data were published in 2007 and reflect costs collected during 2002–2003. With a dynamic economy, it is likely that these values underestimate the cost to society today. Infants born with spina bifida who developed hydrocephalus had Medicaid health care expenditures 2.6 times higher than infants born with spina bifida who did not develop hydrocephalus.[52]

A study examining hospitalizations during the first year of life among children with spina bifida reported that the average number of hospitalizations per infant is 2.4, while the average total days of hospitalization is 25.2, and approximately 18% of the infants were hospitalized more than three times during the first year of life.[47]

CLINICAL MANIFESTATIONS

Weakness and Paralysis

Determining the extent of neurological impairment is not as straightforward as assumed and requires thorough and careful examination and evaluation of the infant. At birth, two main types of motor dysfunction in the lower extremities have been identified. The first type involves a complete loss of function below the level of the lesion, resulting in a flaccid paralysis, loss of sensation, and absent reflexes. The extent of involvement can be determined by comparing the level of the lesion with a chart delineating the segmental innervation of the lower limb muscles and the examination findings. Orthopedic deformities may result from the unopposed action of muscles above the level of the lesion. This unopposed pull may lead to hip flexion, knee extension, and ankle dorsiflexion contractures, depending on the level of the lesion.

When the spinal cord remains intact below the level of the lesion, the effect is an area of flaccid paralysis immediately below the lesion and possible hyperactive spinal reflexes distal to that area. This condition is quite similar to the neurological state of the severed cord seen in traumatic injury. This second type of neurological involvement again results in orthopedic deformities, depending on the level of the lesion, the spasticity present, and the muscle groups involved.

Muscle Tone Abnormalities

Abnormality in muscle tone is a common feature observed in children with spina bifida. In these children, muscle tone can range from flaccidity to normal tone to spasticity. A mixture of spasticity and hypotonia may be observed in some children with spina bifida. Normal muscle tone has been reported in a small number of children with spina bifida. The majority of children with spina bifida will have lower motor neuron lesions. Children with lower level spina bifida present with signs and symptoms of lower motor neuron lesions including areflexia, hyporeflexia, flaccidity, or hypotonia. Children with higher level spina bifida present with signs and symptoms of upper motor neuron (UMN) lesions including spasticity. Children with Chiari II malformation, hydrocephalus, tethered cord syndrome (TCS), or cervical hydromyelia may present with spasticity, which has also been reported to occur in the upper extremities of many children with shunting. The relationship between muscle tone and function is not clearly understood and is controversial. Problems related to spasticity may include the potential for contractures, difficulty maintaining or changing positions, and the presence of exaggerated primitive reflexes. Difficulties associated with flaccidity may include inability to generate muscle force, inability to bear weight on the flaccid limb, deformities, poor limb posture, and other secondary disorders such as decreased bone strength. Determining the type of muscle tone abnormality and severity may help in decision making regarding treatment, such as braces, and teaching compensatory strategies for functional skills.

Sensory Impairment

Children with spina bifida have impaired sensation below the level of the lesion. The sensory loss often does not match exactly the lesion and radiological levels and needs to be carefully assessed. Sensory loss includes pain, temperature, kinesthetic, proprioceptive, and somatosensory information. Sensory deficits manifest in several ways. The child may be hyposensitive or not sensitive to sensory input, startling or withdrawing from light touch or painful stimuli. Because of sensory deficits, children will often have to rely heavily on vision and other sensory systems to substitute for this loss.

Sensory loss (level) correlates with outcomes in terms of mobility, continence, major complications, and overall disability as well as with deaths caused by renal failure. Sensory deficits may produce serious functional consequences. Impairment in sensation may result in significant motor deficits such as impaired balance and coordination. Sensory deficits can compromise safety and make the child vulnerable to injury if their response to painful or damaging stimuli is impaired. It is important that the child and parents be aware of these deficits and of possible ways to compensate or substitute for them, such as relying on vision. Sensory deficits should be considered when creating awareness about safety and prevention of associated disorders such as skin breakdown and pressure ulcers.

Hydrocephalus

Hydrocephalus is common in children with spina bifida, developing in 80% to 90% of children with myelomeningocele.[32,53] Hydrocephalus is a pathological enlargement of the brain ventricles as a result of increased amounts of CSF. CSF is produced by the choroid plexus in each brain ventricle. CSF passes through the ventricular system, exiting the fourth ventricle and entering the subarachnoid space, which is continuous around the brain and spinal cord. After passing through the subarachnoid space, the CSF reaches the arachnoid villi in the superior sagittal sinus and flows into the venous system. Absorption of CSF is via the arachnoid villi that are associated with venous sinuses as well as lymphatics that are associated with cranial and spinal nerves.

Hydrocephalus in patients with spina bifida results from a blockage of the normal flow of CSF between the ventricles and spinal canal. Excessive pressure in the ventricles exerted by CSF compresses the nervous tissue, which causes brain damage and may result in disproportionally large head size in newborns or infants. The pressure may interfere with the function of the adjacent structures and can cause a range of impairments in brain function.

In newborns and infants, the most obvious effect of the buildup of CSF is an abnormal increase in head size, which may be present at birth because of the great compliance of the cranial sutures in the fetus, or may develop postnatally.[54] Other signs of hydrocephalus include bulging fontanels or a tense soft spot (fontanel) on top of the head. Frontal lobe functions are also involved in causing disorders in emotion, planning, spatial awareness, and intellectual function. Hydrocephalus may result in a downward gaze of the eyes (sunsetting of the eyes) from compression of the oculomotor nerve. Symptoms may also include vomiting, sleepiness, irritability, seizures, abnormal muscle tone, weakness, sensory deficits, and poor feeding and growth.

In older children and adults, signs and symptoms may include abnormal enlargement of the head, headache, seizures, nausea and vomiting, blurred or double vision, sleepiness, lack of sleep, lethargy, poor appetite, weakness, sensory deficits, abnormalities in muscle tone, poor balance and coordination, and urinary incontinence.

Internally, a concomitant dilation of the lateral ventricles and thinning of the cerebral white matter are usually present. Without reduction of the buildup of CSF, increased brain damage and death may result. Surgical treatment for hydrocephalus can restore and maintain normal CSF levels in the brain. It is very important for all individuals (doctors, nurses, therapists, teachers, etc.) working with children with spina bifida to watch for any signs and symptoms of hydrocephalus, particularly in children with shunts due to shunt malfunction. These signs and symptoms include a high-pitched cry, sudden changes in appetite/sucking or feeding, unexplained and recurrent vomiting, unwillingness to move the head or lay down, breathing difficulties, seizures, unexplained weakness, changes in muscle tone, difficulty walking, decreased balance, or unexplained poor school performance.

Chiari Malformation

Chiari II, also known as Arnold-Chiari II malformation, is a common presentation in children with myelomeningocele, with a 99% chance of having an associated Chiari II (Fig. 13.6).[11] This malformation is a congenital anomaly of the hindbrain that arises in the fifth week of gestation as a consequence of abnormal neurulation.[55] This complex anomaly involves downward displacement of the cerebellum and herniation of the medulla, and at times the pons, fourth ventricle, and inferior aspect of the cerebellum, through the foramen magnum into the upper cervical canal. The herniation usually occurs between C1

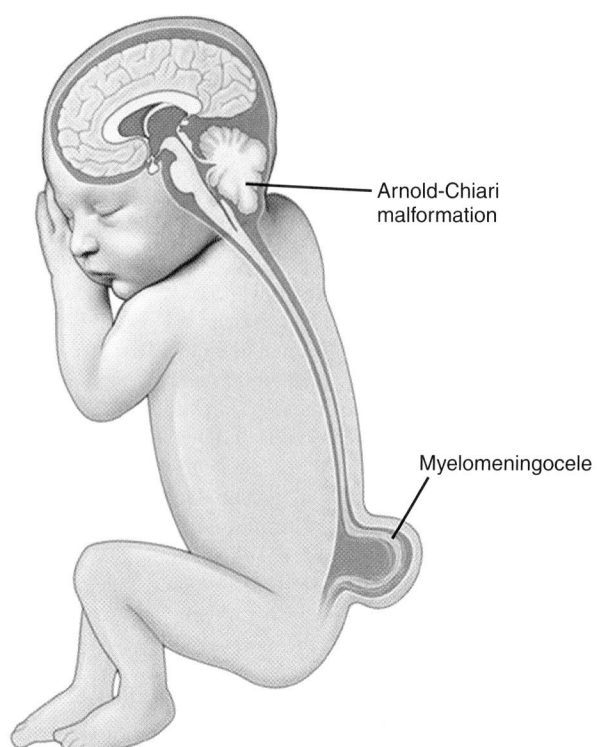

Fig. 13.6 Myelomeningocele and Arnold-Chiari II Malformation. (From *Neurologic Rehabilitation: Neuroscience and Neuroplasticity in Physical Therapy Practice*, Nichols-Larsen – McGraw Hill.)

and C4, but may extend down to T1.[11,56,57] In those with Chiari II malformations and spina bifida, there is a significant reduction in cerebellar volume while, within the cerebellum, the anterior lobe is enlarged and the posterior lobe is reduced.[58] Cardinal features of the Chiari II malformation include myelomeningocele in the thoracolumbar spine, venting of the intracranial CSF through the central canal, dysgenesis of the corpus callosum, hypoplasia of the posterior fossa, herniation of the hindbrain into the cervical spinal canal, and compressive damage to cranial nerves.[55] The abnormal configuration of the brain in Chiari II malformation often results in hydrocephalus, a blockage of the normal flow of the CSF in the ventricular system. Hydromyelia and syringomyelia are seen in patients with Chiari II malformation (Fig. 13.7).

Not all Chiari II malformations are symptomatic. The severity can vary dramatically, and signs and symptoms can vary from no symptoms to severe, potentially debilitating, or life-threatening symptoms. Chiari II malformations may present with a spectrum of signs and symptoms related to brain stem compression and lower cranial nerve dysfunction. As a result of a symptomatic Chiari II malformation, problems with respiratory and bulbar function may be evident in a child with spina bifida.[6] Paralysis of the vocal cords occurs in a small percentage of patients and is associated with respiratory stridor. Apneic episodes also may be evident, although their direct cause remains in question. Children with spina bifida may also exhibit difficulty in swallowing and have an abnormal gag reflex.[6] Problems with aspiration, weakness and cry, and upper-extremity weakness may also be present in children with a symptomatic Chiari II malformation.[59,60] Thus depending on the orthopedic deformities present and the neurological involvement, severe respiratory involvement is possible in the affected child. These symptoms may be caused by significant compression of the hindbrain structures or dysplasia of posterior fossa contents, which can also occur in patients with Chiari II malformation.[11,61] This complex hindbrain malformation is a common cause of death in children with myelomeningocele, despite surgical intervention and aggressive medical management.[62]

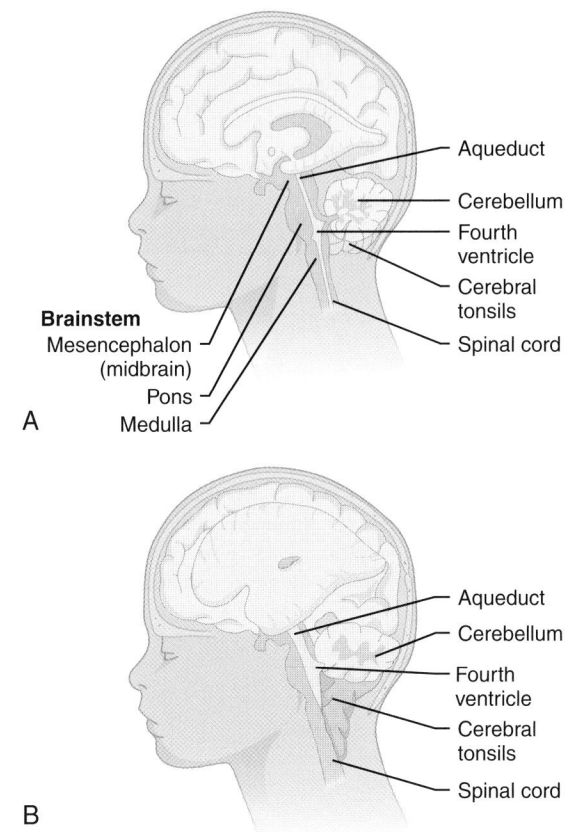

A
Brainstem
Mesencephalon (midbrain)
Pons
Medulla

Aqueduct
Cerebellum
Fourth ventricle
Cerebral tonsils
Spinal cord

B

Aqueduct
Cerebellum
Fourth ventricle
Cerebral tonsils
Spinal cord

Fig. 13.7 **(A)** Normal Brain with Patent cerebrospinal fluid (CSF). **(B)** Arnold-Chiari malformation type II with enlarged ventricles. (From *Pathology: Implications for the Physical Therapist.* 4th ed. Goodman, Elsevier.)

Occipital headaches felt near the base of the skull radiating to the neck and shoulders are a common symptom in older children, which can be brought on or worsened by coughing, straining, or sneezing. Signs and symptoms may include abnormalities affecting the eyes, including blurred vision, double vision, abnormal sensitivity to light, nystagmus, and pain behind the eyes. Vertigo, dizziness, ringing in the ears (tinnitus), and bilateral hearing impairments can also develop. Additional symptoms associated with a Chiari malformation may include muscle weakness, balance deficits, poor coordination and paresthesia, and tingling or burning sensations in the fingers, toes, or lips.

Some children never require treatment for a Chiari malformation. Severe brain stem Chiari II malformation may be reversed after repair and lower rates of hydrocephalus are noted after fetal closure.

Association Pathways

Diffusion tensor tractography studies of association pathways in children with spina bifida have revealed characteristics of abnormal development, impairment in myelination, and abnormalities in intrinsic axonal characteristics and extraaxonal or extracellular space. An imaging study in children with spina bifida indicated that there is a pattern of thinning associated with hydrocephalus with an overall reduction in white matter and increased neocortical thickness in the frontal regions, suggesting long-term disruption of brain development in children with spina bifida that extends far beyond the NTD in the first weeks of gestation.[63] Other studies indicated changes or abnormalities in the tectum.[64–66] These changes in diffusion metrics observed in children with spina bifida are suggestive of abnormal white matter development and persistent degeneration with increased age.[67]

Hydromyelia

Hydromyelia is sometimes used interchangeably with syringomyelia, the name for a condition that also involves the development of syrinx, or a fluid-filled cavity within the spinal cord. Hydromyelia is commonly seen in patients with myelomeningocele, and studies have reported that 17% to 80% of patients with myelomeningocele have hydromyelia.[11,68,69] Hydromyelia is usually defined as an abnormal widening (dilatation) of the central canal of the spinal cord, with an accumulation of CSF within the central spinal canal. Hydromyelia signifies dilation of the center canal of the spinal cord, whereas hydrocephalus signifies dilation of the ventricles of the brain. This can progress with increased pressure to the surrounding tissues. The area of hydromyelia may be focal, multiple, or diffuse, extending throughout the spinal cord. Hydromyelia does not seem to be present at birth or in early infancy, rather, it appears later on.[70] Adults with SB remain at risk for developing a syrinx anywhere along the spinal cord.[71] The hydromyelia may be a consequence of untreated or inadequately treated hydrocephalus with resultant transmission of CSF through the obex into the central canal, with distention as a result of increased hydrostatic pressure from above.[11,72] The increased collection of fluid causes the fluid cavity to expand. It may displace or cause pressure necrosis of the nerve fibers inside the spinal cord leading to muscle weakness and scoliosis, resulting from loss of input to the paraspinals.

In a majority of patients, syringomyelia or hydromyelia are asymptomatic,[71,72] but in other cases, symptoms may be fatal.[71] Syringobulbia is of particular concern and may contribute to sleep disordered breathing and sudden death.[71] A wide variety of symptoms can occur, depending upon the size and location of the fluid cavity. Common symptoms of hydromyelia include rapidly progressive scoliosis, upper-extremity weakness, spasticity, ascending motor loss in the lower extremities, dissociated segmental sensory disturbances, bladder dysfunction, and pain.[11,72,73]

Magnetic resonance imaging (MRI) with contrast (gadolinium) is a key tool for the diagnosis of hydromyelia. Not all children develop symptoms from hydromyelia that require treatment.[74] Aggressive treatment of hydromyelia at the onset of clinical signs of increasing scoliosis is mandatory and may lead to improvement in or stabilization of the spinal curve in 80% of cases. In cases where hydrocephalus or Chiari malformation are causing the hydromyelia, the surgeon will treat the underlying cause and the syrinx will usually shrink or disappear. Surgical interventions may include revision of a CSF shunt, posterior cervical decompression, or a central canal to pleural cavity shunt with a flushing device.[11,61] Surgical treatment of hydromyelia has a very good outcome.

Tethered Cord

Tethered spinal cord is defined as a pathological fixation of the spinal cord in an abnormal caudal location (Figs. 13.8 and 13.9). This fixation

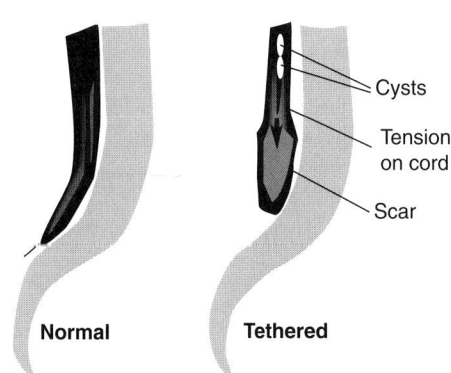

Cysts
Tension on cord
Scar

Normal   **Tethered**

Fig. 13.8 Tethered Cord in Myelodysplasia. (From Staheli LT. *Practice of Pediatric Orthopedics.* Philadelphia: Lippincott Williams & Wilkins; 2001.)

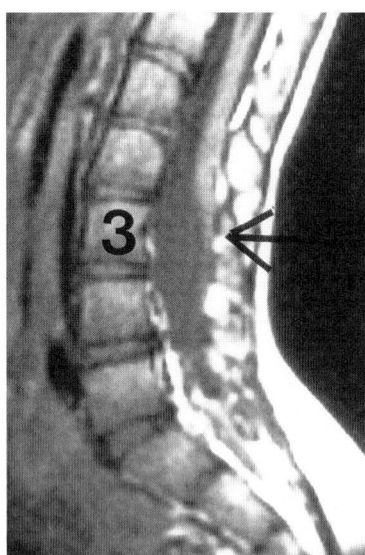

Fig. 13.9 Magnetic resonance image showing a tethered spinal cord at L3. (From Lundy-Ekman L. *Neuroscience: Fundamentals for Rehabilitation.* 4th ed. Elsevier.)

produces mechanical stretch, distortion, and ischemia with daily activities, growth, and development.[75] Ischemic injury from traction of the conus directly correlates with degree of oxidative metabolism and degree of neurological compromise. In addition to ischemic injury, traction of the conus by the filum may also mechanically alter the neuronal membranes, resulting in altered electrical activity.[76–80] The abnormal attachments cause an abnormal stretching of the spinal **cord** that limits its movement within the spinal column and may cause strain on the spinal cord during normal movements. This abnormal attachment is associated with progressive stretching and increased tension of the spinal cord as a child ages, potentially resulting in a variety of symptoms. The progression of neurological signs and symptoms is highly variable due to variation in growth rate of the spinal cord and the spinal column. In some individuals, symptoms can develop at birth, infancy, or early childhood (EC). Some patients may not develop symptoms until adulthood. The most commonly reported triggers in adult patients with repaired SB myelomeningocele are falls, back trauma, heavy lifting, and vaginal childbirth.[71] The presence of TCS should be suspected in any patient with abnormal neurulation (including patients with myelomeningocele, lipomeningocele, dermal sinus, diastematomyelia, myelocystocele, tight filum terminale, and lumbosacral agenesis).

The specific symptoms, severity, and progression vary from one individual to another. Presenting symptoms may include decreased strength (often asymmetrical), development of lower-extremity spasticity, back pain at the site of sac closure, early development or an increasing degree of scoliosis (especially in the low lumbar or sacral level[81–83]), or a change in urological function.[62,84,85] Ten to 30% of children will develop TCS after repair of a myelomeningocele. Essentially all children with a repaired myelomeningocele will have a tethered spinal cord, as demonstrated on MRI. Diagnosis of TCS is made based on clinical criteria. The six common clinical presentations of TCS are increased weakness (55%), worsening gait (54%), scoliosis (51%), pain (32%), orthopedic deformity (11%), and urological dysfunction (6%).[86] This clinical spectrum may be primarily associated with these dysraphic lesions or may be caused by spinal surgical procedures.[75] The cord may be tethered by scar tissue or by an inclusion epidermoid or lipoma at the repair site.[11] In individuals with no or minimal symptoms, surgery may not be indicated, and the symptoms should be monitored for progression. Surgery soon after symptoms emerge

appears to improve chances for recovery and can prevent further functional decline. Surgery is recommended to prevent or reverse progressive neurological symptoms. The primary goal of surgery is to detach the spinal cord where it is adherent to the thecal sac, relieving the stretch on the terminal portion of the cord. Surgery to untether the spinal cord (tethered cord release [TCR]) is performed to prevent further loss of muscle function, decrease the spasticity, help control the scoliosis,[82,87] or relieve back pain.[88,89]

The responses to treatment for TCS vary from one person to another. The effectiveness of a TCR may be demonstrated by an increase in muscle function, relief of back pain, and stabilization or reversal of scoliosis.[82,87,89] It has been reported that scoliosis response to untethering and progression of scoliosis after untethering vary with the location of tethering,[82,89] as well as Risser grade[90] and Cobb angle.[91] Those with Risser grades 3 to 5 and Cobb angle less than 40 degrees are less likely to experience curve progression after untethering. Those with Risser grades 0 to 2 and Cobb angle greater than 40 degrees are at a higher risk of recurrence.[76,91] Spasticity, however, is not always alleviated in all patients.[92] Selective posterior rhizotomy has been advocated for patients whose persistent or progressive spastic status after tethered cord repair continues to interfere with their mobility and functional independence.[62,68]

Orthopedic Deformities

There are both congenital and acquired orthopedic deformities seen in patients with spina bifida. The orthopedic problems that occur with myelomeningocele may be the result of (1) the imbalance between muscle groups; (2) the effects of posture, positioning, and gravity; and (3) associated congenital malformations. Decreased sensation and neurological complications also may lead to orthopedic abnormalities.[93]

Besides the malformation of vertebrae at the site of the lesion, various spinal deformities may be present including hemivertebrae; deformities of other vertebral bodies and their corresponding ribs may also be present.[93,94] Lumbar kyphosis may be present as a result of the original deformity (congenital). In addition, as a result of the bifid vertebral bodies, the misaligned pull of the extensor muscles surrounding the deformity, as well as the unopposed flexor muscles, contributes further to the lumbar kyphosis. As the child grows, the weight of the trunk in the upright position may also be a contributing factor.[94] Scoliosis may be present at birth because of vertebral abnormalities or may become evident as the child grows older. The incidence of scoliosis is lower in low lumbar or sacral level deformities.[94,95] Scoliosis may also be neurogenic, secondary to weakness or asymmetrical spasticity of paraspinal muscles, TCS, or hydromyelia.[95] Lordosis or lordoscoliosis is often found in the adolescent and is usually associated with hip flexion deformities and a large spinal defect.[7,94] Many of these trunk and postural deformities exist at birth but are exacerbated by the effects of gravity as the child grows. They can compromise vital functions (cardiac and respiratory) and should therefore be closely monitored by the therapist and family.

The type and extent of deformity in the lower extremities depend on the muscles that are active or inactive. In total flaccid paralysis, in utero deformities may be present at birth, resulting from passive positioning within the womb. Talipes equinovarus (clubfoot) and vertical talus (which produces a "rocker-bottom" deformity) are two of the most common foot abnormalities. Knee flexion and extension contractures also may be present at birth. Other common deformities are hip flexion, adduction, and internal rotation, usually leading to a subluxed or dislocated hip. Although many of these problems may be present at birth, preventing positional deformity (such as the frog-leg position), which may result from improper positioning of flaccid extremities, is of the utmost importance. Orthopedic care varies throughout the course of the child's life. One of the main goals of orthopedic care of a patient with spina bifida is to correct deformities that may prevent the patient from using orthoses to ambulate in childhood. Additionally, monitoring of spinal balance and the status of the hips is required. Changes in clinical orthopedic management have evolved to establish evidence-based interventions.[96]

Osteoporosis

Osteoporosis and osteopenia are often present in patients with spina bifida mostly related to the limited opportunities for weight bearing and upright mobility. The higher the level of neurological involvement, the greater the risk. Early mobilization and weight bearing can aid in decreasing osteoporosis.[94,97] Because the paralyzed limbs of the child with spina bifida have increased amounts of unmineralized osteoid tissue, they are prone to fractures, particularly after periods of immobilization, especially spica casting.[98–100]

Bowel and Bladder Dysfunction

Myelomeningocele is likely the most common congenital diagnosis for the development of a neurogenic bladder in children.[101] Because of the usual involvement of the sacral plexus, nearly all patients with myelomeningocele have some degree of neurogenic bladder, and children with spina bifida commonly deal with some form of bowel and bladder dysfunction.

Spinal control of bladder, bowel, and sexual functions originates in the sacral spinal cord levels S2 to S4. When the bladder is empty, efferent sympathetic signals from spinal levels T11 to L1 inhibit contraction of the bladder wall and maintain contraction of the internal sphincter. When the bladder fills, the fullness of the bladder stretches the bladder wall and afferent fibers send signals to the reflex center in the sacral spinal cord about the fullness status. This information is then conveyed to the brain. When the condition is appropriate, the higher brain centers initiate emptying the bladder by sending signals to the urination center in the sacral spinal cord, which send signals to the parasympathetic neurons to stimulate contraction of the bladder wall and relaxation of the internal sphincter. Simultaneously, the pontine center sends signals to the spinal cord to facilitate neurons that inhibit the external sphincter and inhibit pelvic floor muscles. Bowel control is similar to bladder control. Stimulation of stretch receptors in the wall of the rectum stimulates emptying of the bowels by sending signals to the bowel center in the sacral spinal cord, which sends signals to alert the higher brain centers about the fullness status. If appropriate, the higher brain centers send signals to the bowel control centers in the sacral spinal cord to relax the sphincter and empty the bowels.

The level of spinal level lesion determines the type of bladder and bowel dysfunction. Lesions above the sacral spinal cord (the control center of the bladder and bowel) result in UMN bladder or bowel. The lesion interrupts descending efferent signals to the bladder and bowel centers but does not interrupt the sacral level reflexive control of the bladder and bowel. Disruption of the higher center control results in lack of inhibition of the bladder and bowel reflexive action, leading to hyperactive bladder and bowel. In this lesion, the bladder and bowel will not receive the signals from the higher center to empty. Reflexive emptying may occur automatically whenever the bladder and bowel are stretched by a certain volume. In this case, the bladder and bowel often expel or "squirt" small volumes at inconvenient times. The UMNL results in hypertonic, hyperreflexive bladder and bowel with reduced capacity. Failure to store or to empty the bladder with reduced capacity make those individuals prone to kidney damage.

Injuries at the sacral level are considered to be lower motor neuron lesions. This type of lesion results in damage to the reflexive bladder and bowel emptying and flaccid paralysis with the bladder and bowel being hypertonic. In this lesion, the reflexes are absent, so there is no spontaneous emptying of the bladder or bowel. The bladder and bowel are flaccid. Urine or stool will fill the bladder or bowel without emptying. When the bladder or bowel overfill with urine or stool and cannot stretch any further, urine or stool leak or dribble out. This emptying is often incomplete. Individuals will often experience dampness from urine or smearing of stool. The continual filling without emptying leads to an overfilling of the bladder and bowel, which can cause infection.

The effects of bladder and bowel dysfunctions pose a serious medical condition with serious medical complications that require long-term management. Besides various forms of incontinence, incomplete emptying of the bladder remains a constant concern because infection of the urinary tract and possible kidney damage may result.[102] Regulation of bowel evacuation must be established so that neither constipation nor diarrhea occurs. Negative social aspects of incontinence can be minimized by instituting intervention that emphasizes patient and family education and a regular, consistently timed, reflex-triggered bowel evacuation.[103]

Bladder and bowel dysfunctions can have serious health complications, including death. They have negative influences on self-esteem, social activities, and quality of life, imposing significant limitations on a person's activity and participation in daily activities.[104] Urinary and fecal incontinence forms a major barrier to attending school, obtaining employment, and sustaining relationships.[105]

Cognitive Impairment and Learning Issues

Children with spina bifida have a rather different cognitive profile than typically developing children.[106,107] Impairments in the cognitive profile is related to both Arnold-Chiari II malformation and hydrocephaly. The Arnold-Chiari II malformation and hydrocephaly affect the development of brain structures of the hindbrain, midbrain, ventricular system, and subcortical gray matter. These deficits lead to impairments in the cognitive domains of executive functioning, visual-spatial working memory, intelligence, language, and learning.

Although children with spina bifida without hydrocephalus may have normal intellectual potential, children with hydrocephalus, particularly those who have shunt infections, are likely to have below-average intelligence.[108–110] These children often demonstrate learning disabilities and poor academic achievement.[111] Even those with a normal IQ show moderate to severe visual-motor perceptual deficits.[112] The inability to coordinate eye and hand movements affects learning and may interfere with activities of daily living (ADLs), such as buttoning a shirt or opening a lunchbox.[113] Difficulties with spatial relations, body image, and development of hand dominance may also be evident.[6,113] Children with myelomeningocele demonstrate poorer hand function than age-matched peers. This decreased hand function appears to be caused by cerebellar and cervical cord abnormalities rather than hydrocephalus or a cortical pathological condition.[114]

Prenatal studies have shown that the CNS as a whole is abnormally developed in fetuses with myelomeningocele.[115–118] The impairment of intellectual and perceptual abilities has been linked to damage to the white matter caused by ventricular enlargement.[6] This damage to association tracts, particularly in the frontal, occipital, and parietal areas, could account for the often severe perceptual-cognitive deficits noted in children with spina bifida.[67,119] Lesser involvement of the temporal areas may account for the preservation of speech, whereas the semantics of speech, which depends on association areas, is impaired. The "cocktail party speech" of children with spina bifida can be deceptive because they generally use well-constructed sentences and precocious vocabulary. A closer look, however, reveals a repetitive, inappropriate, and often meaningless use of language not associated with higher intellectual functioning. Research on learning difficulties in children with spina bifida and hydrocephalus suggests that many of these children experience difficulties. Tasks and skills affected include memory, reasoning, math, handwriting, organization, problem solving, attention, sensory integration, auditory processing, visual perception, and sequencing.[116–118]

Integumentary Impairment
Latex Allergy

Children with spina bifida have a higher risk of allergic reaction to latex. Latex allergy and sensitivity have been noted with increasing frequency in children with myelomeningocele, with frequent reports of intraoperative anaphylaxis.[120–125] These children have also been reported to have a higher than expected prevalence of atopic disease.[126] A 1991 Food and Drug Administration Medical Bulletin estimated that 18% to 40% of patients with spina bifida demonstrate latex sensitivity,[120,127] with others reporting an incidence of 20% to 67%.[121,128,129] Within latex is 2% to 3% of a residual-free protein material that is thought to be the antigenic agent.[124] Frequent exposure to this material results in the development of the immunoglobulin E antibody. Children with spina bifida are more likely to develop the immunoglobulin E sensitivity because of repeated parental or mucosal exposure to the latex antigen.[130] Exposure to latex occurs when products containing rubber come in contact with a person's skin or mucous membranes such as the eyes, mouth, genitals, bladder, or rectum. Skin contact produces less severe reactions such as raised, pinkish, itchy bumps (welts), which develop suddenly and last a few days, but leave no visible trace. In addition, the powder from balloons or gloves can absorb particles and become airborne, causing reactions when breathed by a latex sensitive person. The most potent and life-threatening reaction is entry into the vascular system, which can lead to changes in blood pressure and circulation (anaphylactic shock). Latex-containing products include rubber gloves, therapy balls, some baby bottle nipples and pacifiers, spandex, dental dams, elastic or rubber bands, balloons, adhesive bandages, wheelchair tires, exercise bands, some urinary catheters, some enema tubing, art supplies, beach toys, and chewing gum. Because of the risk of an anaphylactic reaction, exposure to any latex-containing products should be avoided. Latex-free gloves, toys, therapy balls, treatment mats, and exercise bands are now widely available and should be considered for standard use in all clinics treating children with spina bifida. Spina bifida, even in the absence of multiple surgical interventions, may be an independent risk factor for latex sensitivity. Foods reported to be highly associated with latex allergy include avocado, banana, chestnut, and kiwi.[131] Latex-free precautions from birth are more effective in preventing latex sensitization than are similar precautions instituted later in life.[131–133] Latex sensitization decreased from 26.7% to 4.5% in children treated in a latex-free environment from birth.[132]

Pressure Ulcers

Children with spina bifida are at high risk of developing skin injury. Various types of skin breakdown have occurred in 85% to 95% of all children with spina bifida by the time they reach young adulthood.[134] The most common causes of skin injury include lack of sensation and presence of paralysis that results in prolonged sitting in one position. Common areas at risk for pressure sores and decreased skin integrity include the heels, feet, buttocks, lower back, kyphotic or scoliotic prominences, and perineum. Deformities, particularly spinal deformity, may alter sitting balance and puts them at risk for uneven pressure loading on insensate skin with resultant skin ulcers.[135]

A pressure ulcer develops when excessive and prolonged pressure is applied to the skin and soft tissues, usually over a bony prominence, and injures the skin and deep tissues. The pressure can result in reduced capillary flow, preventing oxygen from reaching tissues under the area of pressure. This may cause ischemia, cell death within the

deeper tissues, and eventually, tissue necrosis. Excessive pressure may manifest itself early as reactive hyperemia or sore, a blister, and later, as an open sore or overt necrosis. Chronic, untreated sores may lead to osteomyelitis and eventual sepsis.[126] The amount of pressure and length of time the pressure is in place will increase the severity of the lesion and ulcer. Persistent posture, such as sitting in one position, is a risk factor for skin breakdown and ulcers over the ischial tuberosity. Spinal deformity also alters their sitting balance and puts them at risk for uneven pressure loading on insensate skin and resultant skin ulcers.[135] Pressure sores often result in loss of time from school and work and can lead to financial hardship from medical treatment and hospitalizations. These negative consequences can largely be prevented with attention to education and instruction of the child and family. The goal of such education is to foster an understanding of the causes of skin breakdown and the necessary meticulous attention to skin care that must be carried out on a regular basis. Other common injuries include burns and trauma to insensate feet, emphasizing the importance of health education and guidance in prevention of secondary disability.[55]

Growth Nutrition and Obesity

Children with spina bifida face multiple challenges throughout their life-span. Arnold-Chiari II malformation, hydrocephalus neurogenic bowel, neurogenic bladder, and lack of activities are common associated disorders that have implications for growth and nutrition.

Nutritional intake and weight gain and loss have been found to be problematic in children with myelomeningocele. Early on, infants with spina bifida may have feeding issues as a result of an impaired gag reflex, swallowing difficulties, and a high incidence of aspiration.[6,60] Altered oral-motor function has been attributed to the Chiari II malformation.[136] These impairments may lead to nutritional issues and delayed growth and weight gain. Speech, physical, and occupational therapists (OTs) working as a team are often needed to address these issues.

Conversely, obesity can be a significant issue for children with spina bifida, particularly when the child gets older and moves into teenage years and adulthood. This problem is complex and multifactorial.[137] Mobility limitations and decreased energy expenditure result in lower physical activity levels. In addition, decreased lower limb mass diminishes the ability to burn calories, which leads to weight gain and makes it challenging for a child to achieve and maintain a healthy weight. Decreased caloric intake as well as a lifelong engagement in rewarding and physically challenging physical activities are necessary to enhance weight control and prevent obesity.

The presence of obesity may put the child at risk for additional associated problems such as high blood pressure, high blood sugars (diabetes), and high cholesterol.

Obesity may limit the child's ability to walk, transfer, and move, resulting in reduced mobility and decreased physical activity. This can limit the child's independence in self-care.

Being obese and overweight increases pressure on the skin. This may increase the risk of pressure ulcers for children in wheelchairs. Increased weight increases the amount of pressure on skin in the seating position and thus places the child at more risk for development of pressure ulcers.

Obesity may limit the child's ability to breathe and expand his chest, thereby increasing the risk for development of deformities, particularly scoliosis, as well as increasing the breathing difficulty associated with scoliosis.

Dysphagia and Swallowing

Chiari malformation and hydrocephaly may result in direct pressure upon cranial nuclei or cranial nerves by the herniated cerebellar tonsils and/or cause traction on the cranial nerves as they pass around the herniated tissue to ascend to the neural foramina. This may affect coordination of the muscles involved in sucking, swallowing, and breathing patterns in infants and can result in neurogenic dysphagia. Additionally, hypotonicity and poor sitting posture, along with the Arnold-Chiari II malformation and hydrocephaly, may put infants with spina bifida at a higher risk for feeding issues.

Anthropometrics

Children with myelomeningocele are short in stature. Growth in these children may be influenced by growth-retarding factors as a result of a neurological deficit such as tethered cord.[138] Endocrine disorders and growth hormone deficiency have also been found to contribute to short stature in this population.[139] As a result of complex CNS anomalies (midline defects, hydrocephalus, and Arnold-Chiari malformation), these children are at risk for hypothalamopituitary dysfunction leading to growth hormone deficiency.[140,141] Treatment with recombinant human growth hormone has proven successful in fostering growth acceleration in these children.[140,142,143]

Obtaining an accurate length/height measurement in children with spina bifida may be challenging secondary to contractures, scoliosis, and body structure differences. In addition to the 2000 Centers for Disease Control and Prevention (CDC) growth charts, spina bifida growth charts may be used in conjunction with the CDC growth charts to evaluate growth in a child with spina bifida.[144] The disease-specific charts include growth data according to lesion level and ambulatory status.

Linear growth usually slows down around 2 years of age, but weight gain may continue trending or increase at a faster rate due to decreased activities. Children with spina bifida have earlier growth spurts and higher rates of precocious puberty; however, their final adult height is shorter in relation to their peers.[145]

The lack of activity and ambulation results in a low level of total energy expenditure and needs, which can make it a challenge for a child to achieve and maintain a healthy weight. Children with spina bifida have been shown to maintain their weight with an energy intake meeting 80% of the Recommended Dietary Allowance (RDA).[146]

Psychosocial and Emotional issues

Psychological and social issues in children with spina bifida seem to be affected by deficits in cognitive function and clinical manifestations such as neurological deficits, mobility deficits, and urological disorders. The consequences of the cognitive deficits seem to affect the social life of these individuals.[147,148] Considering all the clinical manifestations resulting from this congenital neurological defect, social and emotional difficulties will arise for these children and their families. These will be considered appropriate when discussing the stages of recovery and rehabilitation from birth through adolescence.

MEDICAL MANAGEMENT

A patient with spina bifida requires a lifelong commitment by the patient, his or her family, and the health care personnel involved in the treatment. The medical goal is to maintain stable neurological functioning throughout the patient's lifetime.[121] The wide range of extensive impairments and long-term disabilities in patients with spina bifida present a considerable challenge to the management of these patients. Patients with spina bifida require extensive and long-term medical needs due to medical conditions and neurological presentation, as well as the long-term aberrations of normal neurological, urological, and musculoskeletal function associated with the condition. Patients with spina bifida require interdisciplinary treatment. The medical treatment will vary based on the age, type, and severity of the

clinical presentations. Medical and surgical management may start prenatally, including fetal surgery, and will be important throughout the individual's life. Fetal or neonatal surgeries are followed by monitoring. Because of the neurological, orthopedic, and urological complications associated with spina bifida, some patients may require surgeries at a later age.

Prenatal Testing and Diagnosis

The majority of cases with spina bifida can be diagnosed during pregnancy. Ultrasonography can be used for early detection of spina bifida during pregnancy.[149] A common blood test, maternal serum alpha-fetoprotein (AFP), is offered during the second trimester (16th to 20th week of pregnancy) to screen for NTDs, including spina bifida and anencephaly. Positive findings of AFP in the amniotic fluid or a positive sonography can be followed by detailed sonography or amniocentesis to diagnose spina bifida. The presence of significant levels of AFP in the amniotic fluid has led to the detection of large numbers of affected fetuses,[150] and maternal serum AFP levels have been effective in detecting approximately 80% of NTDs.[151] Prenatal screening can be most effective when a combination of serum levels, amniocentesis or amniography, and ultrasonography is used.[152–154] Although this screening is not yet performed routinely, it is suggested for those at risk for the defect. Additionally, the fetal karyotype test can be used to identify or rule out chromosomal anomalies.

When a diagnosis of spina bifida confirmed, ultrasonography is used to detect any brain cranial abnormalities including the presence of Chiari II malformation. Ultrasonography can be used to assess spontaneous leg movements, spine and lower extremity deformities, and other physical defects.[155] Prenatal MRI, with ultrafast T2-weighted sequences, can also be used to characterize the Chiari II and other brain malformations.[156]

Prenatal Care

NTDs, including spina bifida, are among the common indication for birth termination. Most fetuses with spina bifida that are not electively terminated receive no treatment until after birth.

If it is determined that the unborn baby has a confirmed diagnosis of spina bifida, both fetus and mother should be referred to a high-risk pregnancy specialist for further evaluation and follow up. A series of ultrasounds will be performed throughout pregnancy to monitor the fetus' progress and detect any other brain anomalies or lower limb deformities. A chromosomal analysis may be recommended to identify chromosomal abnormalities. Other tests, including a fetal MRI, may be recommended to detect cranial abnormalities and other associated disorders such as Chiari II malformation.

Knowledge of the defect allows for preparation for cesarean birth and immediate postnatal care. This includes mobilization of the interdisciplinary team that will continue to care for the child. For parents who decide to carry an involved fetus to term, adjustment to their child's disability can begin before birth, which includes mobilizing their own support system. Education from an integrated team regarding what will follow after delivery and neurosurgical closure is imperative to aid families in decision making and to allow families to assess and understand the child's disability and future care options.

Advances in the field of prenatal medicine that affect spina bifida management and outcome include in utero treatment of hydrocephalus and in utero surgical repair to close the myelomeningocele. This challenging surgical procedure is practiced in only a few specialty centers and so far has been shown to offer palliation of the defect, at best.[157] Treatment such as this, in conjunction with prenatal diagnosis, has been shown to have a positive impact on the incidence and severity of complications associated with spina bifida.[158–165] Limitations of current postnatal treatment strategies and considerations of prenatal treatment options continue to be explored. Ethics, timing of repair, and surgical procedures are all being investigated. In addition, continued assessment of outcomes from those who have undergone presurgical management requires continued exploration. The Management of Myelomeningocele Study (MOMS) was initiated in 2003 as a large randomized clinical trial designed to compare the two approaches to the treatment of infants with spina bifida (prenatal or fetal surgery versus postnatal surgery) to determine if one approach was better than the other. The primary end point of this trial was the need for a shunt at 1 year, and secondary end points included neurological function, cognitive outcome, and maternal morbidity after prenatal repair. Results demonstrated that prenatal surgery significantly reduced the need for shunting and improved mental and motor function at 30 months. Reduced incidence of hindbrain herniation at 12 months and successful ambulation by 30 months were also reported. While prenatal surgery was associated with improved function and reduced need for shunting, maternal and fetal risks, including preterm delivery and uterine dehiscence at delivery, were reported.[166]

Neurosurgical Management

The key early priorities in the management of spina bifida are to repair the spinal cord and spinal nerves, to protect the exposed nerves and structures from additional trauma, and to prevent infection from developing in the exposed nerves and tissue through the spinal defect (Fig. 13.10). Timing of the surgical closure and repair is important and may occur prenatally or soon after birth to minimize the risk of neural damage and infection. The aim of either surgery is to replace the nervous tissue into the vertebral canal, cover the spinal defect, and achieve a watertight sac closure.[167] This early management has decreased the possibility of infection and further injury to the exposed neural cord.[43,167,168]

Fetal surgery may be performed in utero, particularly for the child myelomeningocele, usually during weeks 19 to 25 of pregnancy. Postnatal surgery is usually recommended 24 to 48 hours after birth. Fetal surgery is performed within the uterus and involves opening the mother's abdomen and uterus and repairing the spinal cord of the fetus. The benefits of fetal surgery include less exposure of the vulnerable spinal nerve tissue to the intrauterine environment, thus reducing the damage to the spinal cord. Additionally, fetal surgery may decrease the risk of fetal hindbrain abnormalities, thus decreasing the severity

TABLE 13.1	Signs and Symptoms of Shunt Malfunction
Infants	Bulging fontanel
	Swelling along the shunt tract
	Prominent veins on scalp
	Downward eye deviation ("sunsetting")
	Vomiting or change in appetite
	Irritability or drowsiness
	Seizures
	High-pitched cry
Toddler	Headache
	Vomiting or change in appetite
	Lethargy or irritability
	Swelling along the shunt tract
	Seizures
	Onset of or increased strabismus
Older child	All the above, plus:
	Deterioration in school performance
	Neck pain or pain over myelomeningocele site
	Personality change
	Decrease in sensory or motor functions
	Incontinence that begins or worsens
	Onset of or increased spasticity

of certain complications such as Chiari II and hydrocephalus, and in some cases may decrease the possibility of needing treatment for hydrocephalus and shunt implantation. The major risks to the fetus are those that might occur if the surgery stimulates premature delivery, such as brain hemorrhage, organ immaturity, or death. Delivery may need to occur at a high-risk pregnancy center. Cesarean section is the preferred method of deliver to avoid trauma to the spinal sac and minimize the amount of damage to the infant's exposed spinal nerves that may occur during vaginal delivery. A child born with meningocele or myelomeningocele usually requires care in the neonatal intensive care unit (NICU).

Progressive hydrocephalus may be evident at birth in a small percentage of children born with myelomeningocele. A greater majority, however, have hydrocephalus 5 to 10 days after the back lesion has been closed.[167,169–171] With the advent of computed tomography (CT), early diagnosis of hydrocephalus can be made in the newborn without the need for clinical examination.

Although clinical signs are not always definitive, hydrocephalus may be suspected if (1) the fontanels become full, bulging, or tense; (2) the head circumference increases rapidly; (3) a separation of the coronal and sagittal sutures is palpable; (4) the infant's eyes appear to look downward only, with the cornea prominent over the iris ("sunsetting sign"); and (5) the infant becomes irritable or lethargic and has a high-pitched cry, persistent vomiting, difficult feeding, or seizures (Table 13.1).[32,54,172]

If the results of CT confirm hydrocephalus, a ventricular shunt is indicated to control excessive CSF buildup and further brain damage. This procedure involves diverting the excess CSF from the ventricles to another site for absorption. In general, two types of procedures—the ventriculoatrial (VA) and ventriculoperitoneal (VP) shunt—are currently used, the latter being the most common (Fig. 13.11). The shunt apparatus is constructed from Silastic tubing and consists of three parts: a proximal catheter, a distal catheter, and a one-way valve. As CSF is pumped from the ventricles toward its final destination,

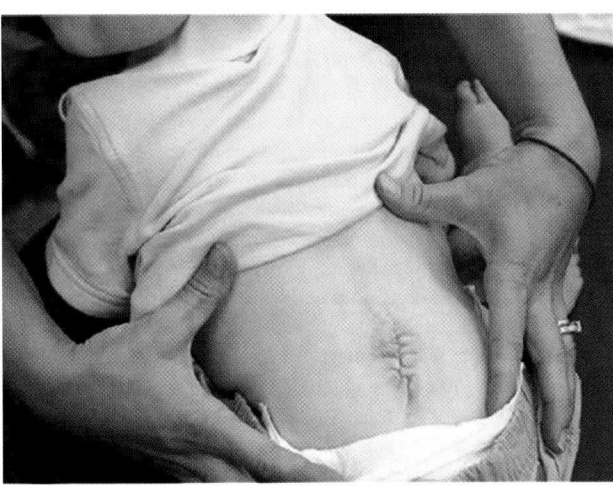

Fig. 13.10 Postsurgical Repair Scarring. (From *Neurologic Rehabilitation: Neuroscience and Neuroplasticity in Physical Therapy Practice,* Nichols Larsen – McGraw Hill.)

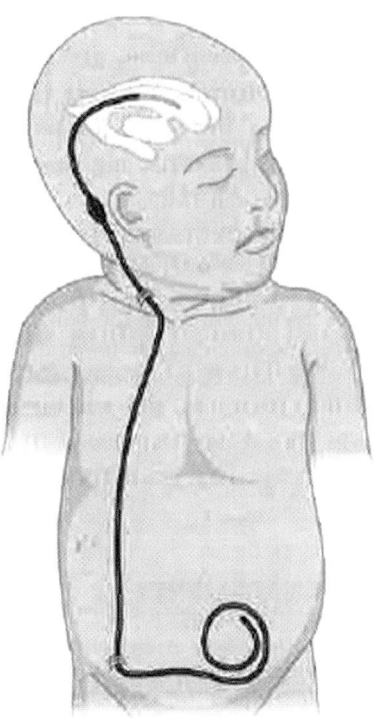

Fig. 13.11 Ventriculoatrial shunt. (From Goodman C, Fuller K. *Pathology Implications for the Physical Therapist.* 4th ed. Elsevier–Saunders; 2014.)

backflow is prevented by the valve system. In this manner, intracranial pressure is controlled, CSF is regulated, and hydrocephalus is prevented from causing damage to brain structures. An alternate means of controlling hydrocephalus may be the use of endoscopic third ventriculostomy (EVT). EVT is a procedure that, in selected patients with obstructive hydrocephalus, allows egress of CSF from the ventricles to the subarachnoid space. This can decompress the ventricles and allow normal intracranial pressures and brain growth. This procedure is typically reserved as a last resort.[173]

Management strategies in the care of shunted hydrocephalus vary.[174] Shunt complications occur frequently and require an average of two revisions before age 10 years.[53] The most common causes of complications are shunt obstruction and infection.[6,175] Revising the blocked end of the shunt can clear obstructions. Infections may be handled by external ventricular drainage and courses of antibiotic therapy followed by insertion of a new shunting system.[6] The problem of separation of shunt components has been largely overcome by the use of a one-piece shunting system. The single-piece shunt decreases the complications of shunting procedures. Shunt revision is usually required as the child grows by installing a larger one.

Surgical treatment for hydromyelia usually has good outcomes; it may include treating the underlying cause such as revision of a CSF shunt, posterior cervical decompression, or a central canal to pleural cavity shunt with a flushing device.[11,61]

Asymptomatic tethered spinal cord will require monitoring for any changes in the clinical signs and symptoms. Conservative treatments such as medications, alternative therapies, rest, and physical therapy may provide temporary relief from pain. The only successful intervention is untethering surgery. Surgery for tethered spinal cord is generally performed if there are clinical signs or symptoms of deterioration such progressive or severe pain, loss of muscle function, deterioration in gait, or changes in bladder or bowel function. The surgery for untethering the cord involves releasing the spinal cord and clearing it from the scarred tissues attached to it. Early surgery on a tethered spinal cord may allow the child to return to his or her baseline level of functioning and prevent further neurological deterioration.

Prophylactic antibiotic therapy 6 to 12 hours before surgery and 1 to 2 days postoperatively is effective in controlling infection for both sac repair and shunt insertion.[69] This brief course of antibiotics has not led to resistant organisms. Prophylactic antibiotic therapy has been prescribed since the introduction of clean intermittent catheterization (CIC) to minimize treatment and prevention of urinary tract infections in children with spina bifida. Long-term use of antimicrobial prophylaxis is associated with increased bacterial resistance. Recent studies indicated that routine antibiotic prophylaxis may not be necessary and discontinuation of antibiotic prophylaxis for urinary tract infections is associated with reduced bacterial resistance to antibiotics in children with spina bifida.[176,177] The main cause of death in children with myelomeningocele remains increased intracranial pressure and infections of the CNS. With the use of antibiotics, shunting, and early sac closure, the survival rate has increased from 20% to 85%.[54,110,121]

Urological Management

Initial newborn workup should include a urological assessment. The urology team aims to preserve renal function and promote efficient bladder management. An early start to therapy helps preserve renal function for children with spina bifida.[178] Initially, a renal and bladder ultrasound is performed to assess those structures.[115] Urodynamic testing can be performed to determine any blockage in the lower urinary tract. Functioning of the bladder outlet and sphincters, as well as ureteric reflux, can also be evaluated. These tests, plus clinical observations of voiding patterns, help the urologist classify the infant's bladder function. If the bladder has neither sensory nor motor supply, a constant flow of urine is present. In this case, infection is rare because the bladder does not store urine and the sphincters are always open.[179]

If no sensation but some involuntary muscle control of the sphincter exists, the bladder will fill, but emptying will not occur properly. Overflow or stress incontinence results in dribbling urine until the pressure is relieved. Because of constant residual urine, infection is a potential problem and kidney damage may result.[179] When some voluntary muscle control but no sensation is present, the bladder will fill and empty automatically. The child can eventually be taught to empty the bladder at regular intervals to avoid unnecessary accidents.

Regardless of the type of bladder functioning, urodynamics should be performed on a yearly basis in order to check for infection and bladder and kidney function. This is important as urine retention in the bladder can cause urine to backflow into the kidneys, thereby damaging them. Urodynamic tests can include urine tests, blood tests, and ultrasound of the bladder and kidneys. Cystogram and cystoscopy can be applied as needed. On the basis of clinical findings and urodynamic test results, the urologist will suggest the appropriate intervention.

The goals of an effective bladder program are to reduce common problems such as hydronephrosis, overfull bladder, urinary tract infection, bladder and kidney calculi, reflux, and bladder accidents.

A bladder retraining program may include establishing a routine, diet, and healthy life style. Establishing routines involve schedules for eating, drinking, and for emptying the bladder. It is best to limit or avoid caffeine, fizzy drinks, and alcohol, as these can irritate the bladder. Manual stimulation using Crede technique (pushing on bladder with your fingertips) can help voiding.

In principle, all newborn patients are put on CIC, oxybutynin, and chemoprophylaxis immediately after closure of the back.[180] CIC involves inserting a fine tube into the urethra to drain urine out of the bladder. This CIC program may start immediately after closure of the back. Of course, it is still a matter of discussion whether it is necessary to perform CIC from birth onward in all children.[180] This program of CIC is typically done every 3 to 4 hours to prevent infection and maintain the urological system.[181–184] Parents are taught this method and can then begin to take on this aspect of their child's care. At the age of 4 or 5 years, children with spina bifida can be taught CIC and can become independent in bladder care at a young age. Achieving this form of independence adds to the normal psychological development of these children. Early CIC helps eliminate overflow incontinence and maintaining safe pressures in the lower urinary tract has also reduced the need for bowel augmentation of the bladder from 90% to less than 5%.[180] Although CIC is not possible for all children with spina bifida, it remains the method of choice for bladder management.

Indwelling catheterization is a form of long-term catheterization that can be used if CIC is not successful. This involves inserting a fine tube through the urethra up into the bladder. This can be attached to either a valve or a drainage bag. The catheter will need to be replaced every few weeks. A suprapubic catheter is an alternative form of long-term catheterization and involves a small surgical procedure to place a tube directly into bladder through the abdomen. This can be attached to either a valve or a drainage bag.

Intravesical injection of botulinum toxin (Botox) into the detrusor muscle is performed as an outpatient procedure using a cystoscope under anesthesia. This injection can be repeated safely. This approach is a good temporary measure to enhance bladder capacity and decrease intravesical pressures.

Neuromodulation modifies the innervation of the bladder. Neuromodulation includes nonoperative measures such as transurethral electrical bladder stimulation by providing consistent stimulation of the efferent fibers of the sacral nerve roots or by providing rhythmic contractions of the pelvic floor; minimally invasive procedures such as implantation of a sacral neuromodulation, which is a reversible implanted (pacemaker) device; as well as operative measures that reconfigure sacral nerve root anatomy.[181,185] Xiao Procedure is a new procedure in which the proximal stump of the ventral root of L5 is anastomosed to the distal stump of the S3 ventral root. Early research studies about this procedure were promising, but recent studies showed that this procedure is ineffective.

The most common type of urinary diversion is the creation of a urostomy or Ileal Conduit. This involves creating a stoma using a piece of the small bowel (usually the small intestine) which will be repositioned to serve as a passage, or conduit, for urine from the ureters to a stoma. This stoma will come through the abdomen into an external pouch.[186–188] A Mitrofanoff is a continent stoma created by using a small piece of the appendix or small bowel to form a conduit between the bladder and skin surface. An opening is created low on the abdomen or through the belly button, and a catheter is inserted into the opening when needed to empty the bladder.[186–187] Traditional bladder reconstruction includes bladder augmentation by enlargement of the bladder with a piece of intestine to increase bladder capacity and lower intravesical pressures.

Most individuals with spina bifida will have common bowel problems including lack of control, constipation, impaction, diarrhea, and bowel accidents. Bowel management and training programs should be started early. Medications, digital stimulation, laxatives, stool softeners, suppositories, enemas and irrigation, and attention to fiber content in the diet are all of value in establishing a bowel management program. Similar to a bladder retraining program, a bowel retraining program may include establishing a routine, diet, and healthy lifestyle. Establishing routines involves maintaining schedules for eating, drinking, and for emptying the bowel. A balanced diet with plenty of fiber and enough fluid consumption helps regulate the bowel and keep stools at the right consistency to avoid constipation.

If a bowel management program is not effective, surgical treatments may be needed. The Antegrade Colonic (Continence) Enema (ACE) can be used for patients with fecal incontinence, severe constipation, or lack of anal control. This procedure is an important adjunct in the case of adults and children with problems of fecal elimination in whom standard medical therapies have failed.[189,190] This procedure involves creating a stoma, usually from the appendix or the small intestine. Similar to the bladder stoma, a connection is formed between the bowel and the skin. A small artificial opening is created in the umbilicus or lower abdominal wall. A catheter can be inserted into the stoma, and a washout solution is injected to carry out a controlled bowel movement. Colostomy involves diverting one end of the large bowel through an opening in the abdominal wall; a pouch is placed over the opening to collect stools. Colostomy is usually the last resort if other methods have not been successful.

ORTHOPEDIC MANAGEMENT

Children with spina bifida present with multiple orthopedic disorders. Some of these conditions are seen at birth or occur early in life, and some occur secondary to existing disorders. Careful evaluation and management of these patients should occur as part of a team approach given the variety and complexity of the medical conditions and comorbidities associated with spina bifida. The primary goals for orthopedic management should be to minimize deformity and maximize function and mobility, while limiting complications.[99]

Orthopedic management of the newborn with a myelomeningocele will generally concentrate on the feet and hips. Soft tissue release of the feet may take place during surgery for sac closure. Casting the feet (Fig. 13.12) and performing early aggressive taping are also effective in the management of clubfoot deformities.[191,192] Short-leg posterior splints (ankle-foot orthoses [AFOs]) may be used to maintain range of motion (ROM) and prevent foot deformities.

The orthopedist will also evaluate the stability of the hips. In children with lower-level lesions, attempts to prevent dislocation are made by using a hip abductor brace (Fig. 13.13A) or a total-body splint (see Fig. 13.13B) for a few months after birth. With higher-level lesions, dislocated hips are no longer treated because they do not appear to have an effect on later rehabilitation efforts.[172,193–195]

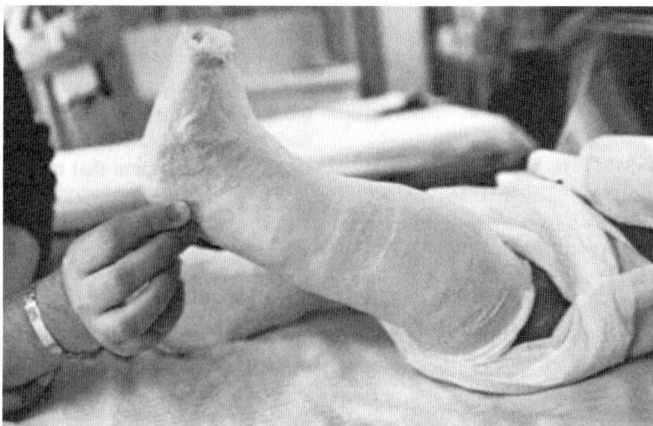

Fig. 13.12 Plaster cast of the foot and ankle to reduce clubfoot deformities.

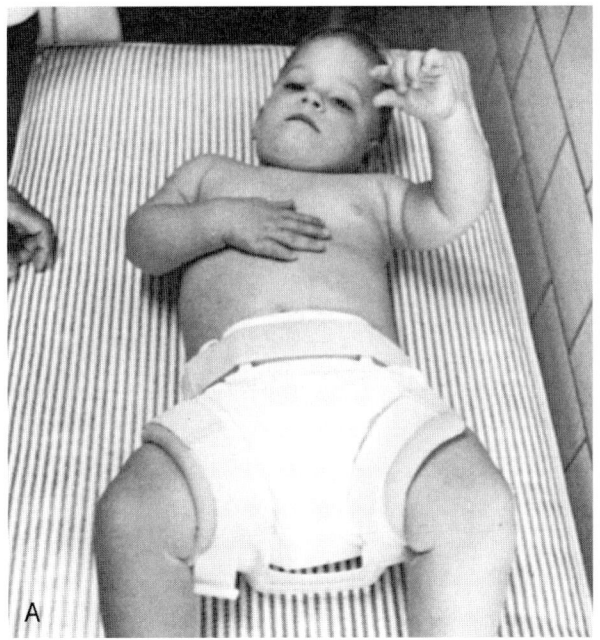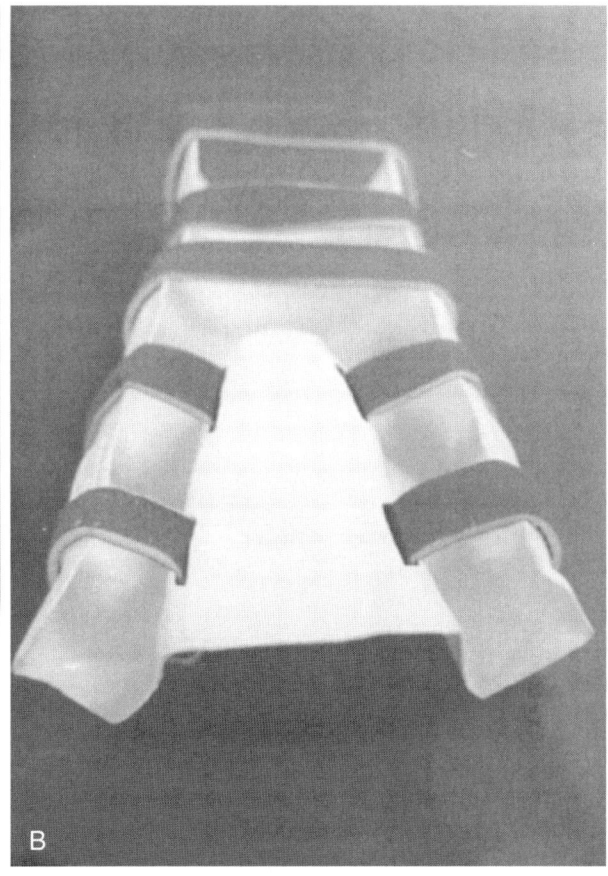

Fig. 13.13 (A) Hip abductor brace. **(B)** Total-body splint.

Orthopedic management needs to be ongoing throughout the child's lifetime, with continued assessment of orthopedic deformities and the need for surgical intervention. Important management issues relevant to function that the physical therapist (PT) should be aware of may include hip dislocation, knee valgus stress, scoliosis, foot deformities, fractures, osteoporosis, and postoperative management (Fig. 13.14).

Hip Dislocation

Hip dislocation is commonly seen in children with spina bifida. Dislocation is probably related to paralysis, muscle imbalance, lack of sensation, and joint development, as well as contractures in muscles and soft tissues around the hip joint.[93,196] If not treated properly, contractures can lead to pelvic obliquity and compensatory spinal abnormality.[93] Hip dislocation in children with spinal bifida can be paralytic or teratological. Paralytic hip dislocation is a common and complicated problem that may occur at any level of neurological deficit.[197]

In the past, surgeries were aimed at the maintenance of hip reduction as indicated by radiographic realignment.[99] Transfer of the iliopsoas tendon along with open reduction and capsular plication was the most common surgery in children with spina bifida in order to achieve and maintain reduction of paralytic hip dislocations.[99]

Concerns developed regarding whether the radiological success of hip reduction led to restricted ROM and pathological fractures, thereby compromising the functional result. Subsequent studies of functional results found that the presence of a concentric reduction did not lead to improved hip ROM or the ability to ambulate. Additionally, several studies reported a high rate of complications leading to decrease in ambulatory function, limited ROM, re-dislocation, and

pathological fractures in children treated surgically for the reduction of hip dislocation. Although hip reduction surgery may reduce the dislocated hip, the result must be weighed in terms of the potential for complications and functional decline.[99]

Current treatment goals for those with hip dislocation focus on functional outcomes versus maintaining radiographical realignment. Thus current treatment focuses on maintaining level pelvis and free motion of the hips. Reports stressed that the preservation of muscle strength, specifically of the iliopsoas and quadriceps, is more relevant to determining potential for adult ambulation than the status of the hip joint.[99]

The most important factor in determining ability to walk is the level of neural involvement and not the status of the hip.[99,194,198–200] A level pelvis and good hip ROM are more important than hip relocation. In general, surgical hip procedures include surgical hip reduction, soft tissue procedures, or osseous procedures. Surgical hip reduction is used to stabilize the hip and prevent further subluxations. Soft tissue procedures seek to balance muscle forces and prevent contractures. These may include transfer of iliopsoas to greater trochanter, transfer of external oblique muscle combined with adductor tenotomy or transfer of adductors to the ischium, or tenotomy of iliopsoas and adductor muscles to relieve the muscle balance of the hip. Osseous procedures are aiming to correct deficiency of the acetabulum as well as to correctly center the femoral head in the acetabulum. These procedures may include Shelf procedure, Pemberton osteotomy, or Chiari osteotomy. Femoral osteotomy may be performed to correct rotational and angular deformity.

In those with a thoracic lesion with both hips unstable or who are unable to walk, surgeries to reduce hips are not indicated. Treatment

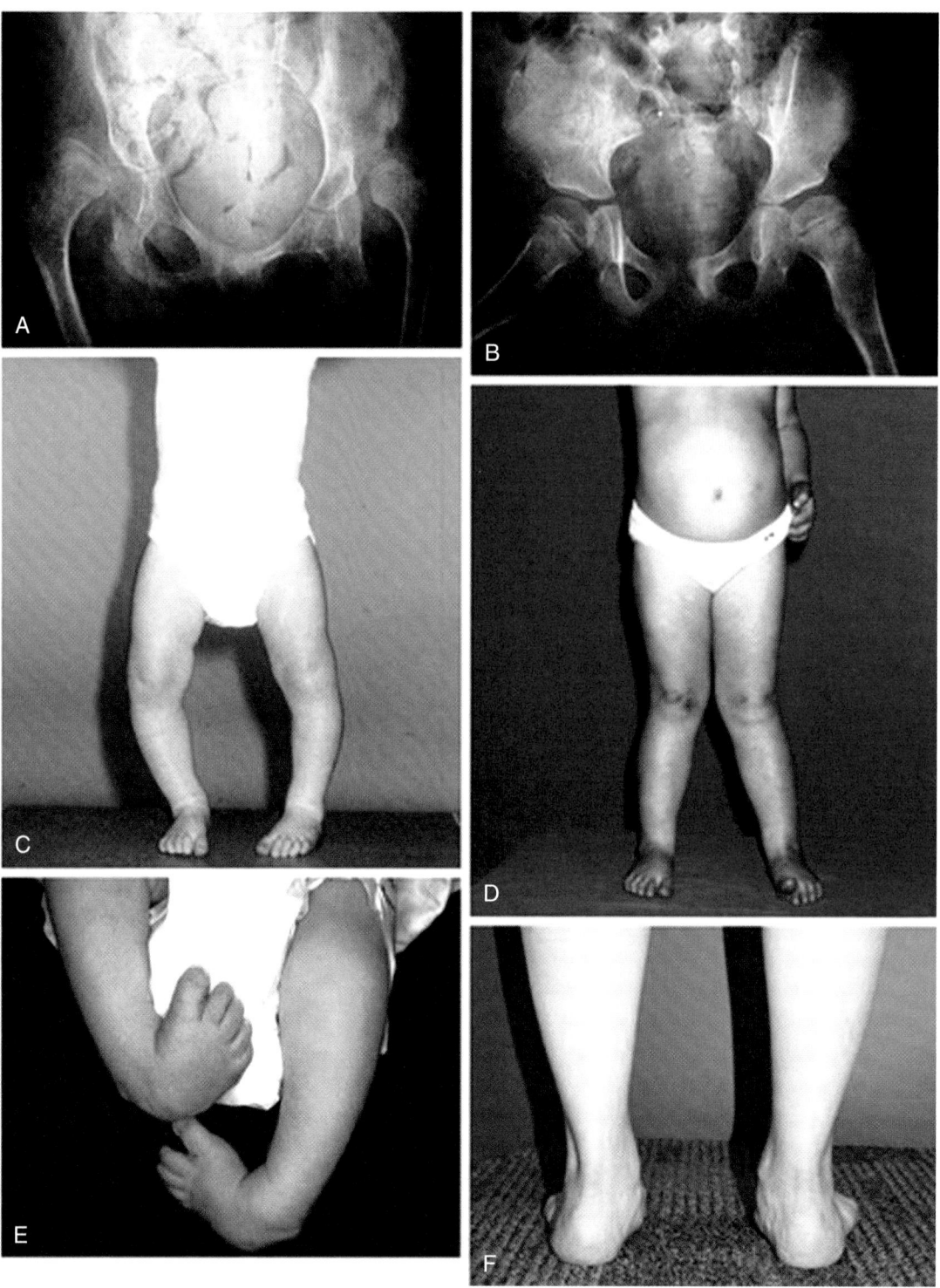

Fig. 13.14 Lower Limb Deformities. (A) Hip dislocation, **(B)** hip dysplasia and subluxation, **(C)** Genu varus, **(D)** Genu valgus, **(E)** Equinovarus, **(F)** Calcaneal valgus. (From *Campbell's Physical Therapy for Children Expert Consult.* 5th ed. Figure 14.)

should be directed at preventing or releasing the contractures. Similarly, in those with lumbar lesions and asymmetry caused by contracture, treatment will be directed at releasing the contracture and no attempts will be made to reduce the hip. This can be accomplished by exercises, positioning, or anterior hip release for hip flexion contractures. Muscle transfers alone usually are not effective in producing stability of the hip in these children. Hip dislocations in those with

lower lumbar (L4 or below) or sacral level lesions should be considered as lever-arm dysfunction, and surgical hip relocation is indicated.[96,197–199] Reduction of the hip in these children is aimed at the prevention of progressive subluxation, which will ultimately interfere with walking. Osteotomy can be indicated to avoid future leg length discrepancy or pelvic obliquity. Immobilization after hip dislocation may lead to a frozen, immobile joint from an open reduction procedure, re-dislocation from a lack of significant dynamic forces available for joint stability around the hip joint, and an increased fracture risk. Recently, a questionnaire called the Spina Bifida Hips Questionnaire (SBHQ), which was developed to evaluate the ADLs important to children with spina bifida and dislocated hips along with their families, has demonstrated construct validity as well as reliability.[201]

Knee Valgus Stress

Many children with spina bifida who walk have excessive trunk and pelvic movement, knee flexion contractures, and rotational malalignment that may lead to excessive knee valgus stress. Valgus knee deformity is frequently seen in low-lumbar and sacral-level patients leading to instability, pain, and arthritis in adulthood. The most common deformities leading to this problem are rotational malalignment of the femur and femoral anteversion in association with excessive anterior tibial torsion. The knee valgus deformity is influenced by increased lateral truck sway, weak hip abductor muscles, and internal hip rotation in combination with increased knee flexion and valgus foot deformity.[202]

These deformities should be addressed via surgical correction, as excessive knee valgus stress can lead to knee pain and arthritis in adulthood.[96,99,202,203] Surgical correction of excessive rotational deformities has been shown to lead to a significant improvement in knee stress and pain and may prevent the onset of late degenerative changes.[204] If knee valgus is associated with knee flexion contracture or hindfoot valgus, the surgical correction of these deformities is required at the same setting. In addition to physical therapy and exercises, the use of assistive aids, bracing, or a combination of both should be encouraged to increase stance-phase stability, decrease stress in the knee joint, and maintain long-term joint viability.[203,205]

Rotational Deformities

Rotational deformities of the lower extremities are frequently seen in both ambulatory and nonambulatory patients with spina bifida. Femoral torsion may be present at birth in newborns and does not seem to decrease with growth due to abnormal gait and activity level; it may be secondary to foot deformities. Tibial torsion may be congenital secondary to clubfoot or other foot deformities; it may also be secondary to muscle imbalance or associated foot deformity.

For the nonambulatory children, torsional problems are largely cosmetic. For the ambulatory child, torsional deformities in the lower extremity can be addressed using Torsional Splints attached to an AFO, often referred to as a twister cable. In the long term, significant rotational deformities may be addressed surgically with de-rotational osteotomy.

Scoliosis

The prevalence of scoliosis in spina bifida is estimated to be as high as 50%.[206] Increasing scoliosis can lead to the loss of trunk stability when curves are greater than 40 degrees and when associated pelvic obliquity becomes 25 degrees or more. Scoliosis can progress to affect sitting[207] and standing balance. It may affect the ability to sit, stand, and walk and interferes with positioning in the wheelchair. Surgical intervention, often recommended to prevent further progression, may improve or further impair sitting balance, ambulation, and performance of ADLs.[208] Various authors have reported that although surgery can improve curves by up to 50%, surgical morbidity must be considered, with complications possibly being as high as 40% to 50%. Functional benefits are largely unsubstantiated owing to poorly constructed studies.[209] Wai[210,211] suggests that spinal deformity may not affect overall physical function or self-perception. After surgical correction, it may take up to 18 months to appreciate functional improvement, and walking may be

difficult for those who were just exercise ambulators before correction. Although surgical repair of scoliosis does improve quality of life in patients with cerebral palsy and muscular dystrophy, this has not been demonstrated in those with spina bifida.[212] Interventions such as chair modifications to shift the trunk to improve balance in the coronal plane and reduce pelvic obliquity and truncal asymmetry should be considered as a first option, before surgical correction.[208,212]

Back Pain

Back pain needs to be efficaciously evaluated in those with spina bifida who report experiencing it. Knowing when the patient experiences pain, what increases pain, what positions exacerbate pain, and what region of the body is affected can help lead to appropriate referral, testing, and management. Knowing if your patient has a shunt, spinal rods, and/or a Chiari malformation will also be important to your assessment and management. Pain in the neck, shoulders, and upper back with associated weakness and/or abnormal sensory findings should be evaluated by the treating neurosurgeon to rule out shunt malfunction. Spinal rods that have broken or that are breaking through the skin may also be a source of pain in this area. Pain not caused by rods, a shunt, Chiari issues, or a syrinx may have a mechanical cause and could be a result of poor posture, tension, or weight gain. A patient who reports low back pain may have a symptomatic tethered cord if the patient is also reporting changes in gait, increased tripping or falling, bladder changes, and/or pain shooting down the legs. Manual muscle testing (MMT) and urodynamic testing are appropriate at this point and should be compared with baseline testing findings. Mechanical low back pain may be a result of abnormal gait mechanics, asymmetrical strength, and use of older orthotics that no longer fit. Assessment of seating and support systems, including cushions, and gait mechanics with the use of orthotics and ambulatory aids are mandatory to increase stability and redistribute balance over stressed joints, maximizing reduction of the patient's pain and discomfort. Strengthening, particularly of the gluteal muscles, for those who are ambulatory may also be indicated. In addition, programs aimed at weight reduction may be necessary to alleviate stress and pain to preserve long-term viability of tissues. In addition, for women, the chest may cause tension on the upper back, and breast reduction has been advocated for some to relieve this tension.[213–215]

Foot Deformity

Almost all children with spina bifida will experience problems with foot deformity. Foot deformities are caused when muscle weakness leads to abnormal positioning in utero or may occur from ongoing muscle imbalance, postural effects of gravity, and growth. Foot deformities include calcaneus, equinus, varus, valgus, clubfoot, vertical talus, or a combination of deformities. A plantigrade foot in neutral position is essential for optimal walking, and a well-positioned foot may protect against skin breakdown. Foot deformity can cause difficulty with shoe wear and bracing.

The goal of treatment of the foot in spina bifida should be a flexible and supple foot. An insensate flail foot often becomes rigid over time, and foot management can become complicated by pressure sores. Up to 95% of patients will use an orthosis, and a supple flail foot will be easier to manage over time. Surgeries that are extraarticular with avoidance of arthrodesis, as well as simple tenotomies versus tendon releases and lengthenings, may best manage outcomes for bracing and ambulation.[96] Clubfoot or equinovarus deformities may be managed with early and intensive taping in the newborn period, known as the *French method*,[216,217] as well as by stretching and casting and surgical intervention. The Ponseti method, advocated by some, has also been reported to have positive outcomes; however, the significant investment in time and commitment by the family for frequent cast changes may affect the ability to carry out other ADLs without disruption.[197] Recurrent clubfeet are difficult to treat, but a talectomy with calcaneo-cuboid fusion may be used for recurrent clubfeet.[218] In those with li-pomas, foot deformity that may be acquired over time is best managed in a similar manner as in equinovarus deformities. Maintaining a supple and plantigrade foot with adequate muscle balance and using soft tissue correction through tendon lengthening, tendon transfer, and plantar fascial release are recommended until 8 years of age. After that time, deformities may become more rigid and may necessitate more bony procedures.[219]

Valgus deformity can also occur at the ankle joint and can be easily treated with guided growth principles in a growing child, which allows for gradual correction of the deformity by tethering the medial side of the growth plate.[220,221] Severe hindfoot valgus can be treated by medial displacement osteotomy of the calcaneus in children with spina bifida. This allows preservation of motion with osteotomies opposed to arthrodesis of joints.

Calcaneus deformity is not very common but may occur in patients with unopposed anterior tibialis activity, leading to excessive pressure on the heel area with subsequent risk of skin breakdown. Tendon transfer or release do not seem to be successful. Long standing calca-neal deformity may be addressed with triple arthrodesis (fusing the three joints about the hindfoot).

Osteoporosis, Osteopenia, and Fracture

Osteoporosis (thinning of the bone) and osteopenia (low bone min-eral density [BMD]) in the legs and spine have been described in children and teens with spina bifida. These conditions increase the risk of fracture, increase the time for healing after fracture, and may lead to back pain. A study by Valtonen and colleagues in 2006 documented the occurrence of osteoporosis in adults with spina bifida. This condition is often not recognized.[222] Medical factors may contribute to increase the risk of osteoporosis, osteopenia, and fracture, such as physical in-activity, lack of physical loading and weight bearing due to lack of ambulation or inability to ambulate, decreased vitamin D, diminished exposure to sunlight, urinary diversion, renal insufficiency, hypercalci-uria, medication for epilepsy, and oral cortisone treatment for more than 3 months.[97,223,224] It can be assumed that patients with meningo-myelocele are at potential risk for development of osteoporosis at a younger age because of flaccidity, impaired walking ability, and subse-quent low physical loading of the lower limbs. Older age and higher levels have been associated with increased numbers of fractures in spina bifida.[222] The optimal strategies for prevention and treatment of osteoporosis in this population have not been established. Further research is required to see if the methods used to prevent and treat osteoporosis in individuals without spina bifida also work for teens and adults who have spina bifida. Considering the effects of prolonged immobilization on independence in daily activities and quality of life, there should be no disagreement that all efforts are necessary to pre-vent these fractures. Furthermore, osteoporotic fracture may lead to a vicious cycle of immobilization, decreased bone density, and repeated fractures.[222] Annual incidence of fracture is 0.029% in adolescents and 0.018% in adults.[225]

Management of bone fragility in children with disabilities has been limited to conservative measures such as standing program, loading and weight-bearing activities, and calcium and vitamin D intake. Those measures may not be enough to treat osteoporosis. The effects of standing programs on bone density are unclear,[226,227] although stand-ing with the use of a standing frame or vibration therapy appear to in-crease BMD in other children with disabilities.[228,229] Studies have shown promising results of regular functional electric stimulation–assisted

training, but this is often nearly impossible to carry out in daily life.[230] Additionally, the period of immobilization after a surgical intervention should be reduced, if possible, and weight bearing should be allowed as soon as possible. Management should include attention to nutri-tional factors, in particular, adequate intake of calcium and vitamin D.[231] However, constipation secondary to neuropathic bowel is a fre-quent problem in patients with spina bifida, and supplementation with calcium may exacerbate it.[229] Antiresorptive drugs may be used for adults with low BMD. Parathyroid hormone therapy would be an al-ternative if the patient fails to gain adequate BMD. This therapy is not used in children and adolescents due to the risk of osteosarcoma. Bisphosphonates may be used to increase bone strength in children with osteoporosis, but its use should be weighted along with the seri-ous side effects.[229]

The prevention of fractures should be among the major goals in the rehabilitation of people with meningomyelocele. The assessment of BMD is worthwhile in nonambulatory children and patients with risk factors for osteoporosis, because low BMD is a known risk factor for fractures.[223]

Postoperative Management

Care should be taken to avoid postoperative complications such as skin breakdown and postimmobilization fractures in the postoperative pe-riod. To decrease the risk of nonunion and allow for early mobilization and weight bearing, one should consider rigid internal fixation versus Kirschner wire fixation. After surgery, immobilization in a custom-molded body splint rather than a hip spica cast is preferred. Postop-erative physical therapy should begin as soon as wounds are stable and healing is occurring. Therapy should focus on ROM (active and pas-sive) and early weight bearing. Crawling should be strictly forbidden for a minimum of 3 to 4 weeks postimmobilization to reduce the risk of fracture.[99]

EVALUATION

Since assessment is important for guiding clinical management and for evaluating therapeutic outcomes, thorough assessment of patients with spina bifida is essential. Assessment allows for detailed identifications of impairments, functional limitations, and disability. Assessment identi-fies the patient's strength, challenges, and needs. Assessment is a guide to treatment and lays the foundations for planning of future manage-ment. In attempting to evaluate the child with spina bifida, a number of evaluations can be chosen, each designed to test specific yet perhaps unrelated components of function. The following section discusses those test procedures as well as the specific standardized tests that would best define the complexity of the problem.

Assessing Muscle Strength

Loss of muscle strength is one of the main impairments in children with spina bifida. Therefore assessment of muscle strength and timely detection of muscle weakness is critical and should be assessed regularly in the growing child to monitor any changes in strength. Ac-curate and reliable strength measures are essential in early and ongoing management of a child with spina bifida.[232]

Assessing the muscle strength of children, in general, and young children with spina bifida, in particular, can be a challenge. Several alternatives to MMT have been advocated to evaluate motor function in children. MMT is used worldwide with children with spina bifida. Alternate methods to MMT for strength assessment of children with spina bifida include hand-held dynamometry (HHD), isokinetic strength testing, somatosensory evoked potentials, and electromyogra-phy. Muscle contour and symmetry can be used as a subjective method to assess muscle strength in some children. Observation of significant muscle atrophy and limb contour can be indicative of significant muscle strength.

In the newborn, infant, very young child, or a child who is not able to understand or follow directions, the traditional form of MMT is not appropriate or possible. Therefore alternate methods to assess muscle strength in this population are necessary. Observation of infant spontaneous movements, such as leg kicking and responses to stimuli, can be used to assess strength in the newborn or infant. Observation of the infant or young child performing typical movement activities or functional tasks can be used to assess strength. This may include observing the child moving their hand to reach for a toy, kicking their leg against gravity, or using the hip flexors during creeping.

In the newborn, testing may be done in the first 24 to 48 hours before the back is surgically closed. In this case, care must be taken not to injure the exposed neural tissue during testing. Prone and side lying to either side are the most convenient and safe positions for evaluation during this time. Subsequent testing is done soon after the back has been closed and as indicated throughout childhood.

In evaluating the newborn, the importance of alertness is essential. A sleeping or drowsy infant will not respond appropriately during the evaluation. The infant must be in the alert or crying state to elicit the appropriate movement responses. Testing hungry or crying infants provides an advantage because they are likely to demonstrate more spontaneous movements in these behavioral states. The cumulative effect of a variety of sensory stimuli may be more effective in bringing the infant to alertness than using one stimulus in isolation. For example, the infant may be picked up and rocked vertically to allow maximum stimulation to the vestibular system and to help bring the child to an alert state. In addition, the therapist may talk to the child to help him or her fixate visually on the therapist's face. Tactile stimuli above the level of the lesion further add to the child's level of arousal, thus contributing to more conclusive test results. In this way, the CNS receives an accumulation of information from a variety of sensory systems rather than relying on transmission from one system that may be weak or inefficient.

As the child is aroused, spontaneous movements can be observed and muscle groups palpated. Additional methods to stimulate movement may be necessary. For example, tickling the infant generally produces a variety of spontaneous movements in the upper and lower extremities. Passive positioning of children in adverse positions may stimulate them to move. For example, if the legs are held in marked hip and knee flexion, the infant may attempt to use extensor musculature to move out of that position. If the legs are held in adduction, the child may abduct to get free. Holding a limb in an antigravity position may elicit an automatic "holding" response from a muscle group when spontaneous movements cannot be obtained in any other way.

In grading muscle strength, differentiation between spontaneous, voluntary movement, and reflexive movement is important. After the severing of a spinal cord, distal segments of the cord may respond to stimuli in a reflexive manner. This results from the preservation of the spinal reflex arc and is known as *distal sparing*. If distal sparing of the spinal cord is present, the muscles may respond to stimulation or muscular stretch with reflexive, stereotypical movement patterns. The quality of this reflexive movement will be different from that of spontaneous movement and must be distinguished when testing for the level of voluntary muscle functioning.

Muscle strength is generally graded for groups of muscles and can be graded by using either a numerical scale (1 to 5), an alphabetical designation (Fig. 13.15), or simply by noting presence or absence of muscular contraction by a plus or a minus on the muscle test form. The last method may be sufficient initially, but as the child matures, a more definitive muscle grade should be determined.

By use of an MMT form that lists the spinal segmental level for each muscle group, an approximate level of lesion can be determined from the test results (see Fig. 13.15). Because the spinal cord is often damaged asymmetrically, MMT does not always accurately reflect the level of the lesion. If reflex activity is also noted on the form, the presence of distal sparing of the spinal cord can be determined. Muscle testing of the newborn gives the clinician an appreciation of muscle function and possible potential for later ambulation, as well as an awareness of possible deforming forces. For example, if hip extensors or abductors are not functioning, then the action of hip flexors and adductors must be countered to prevent future deformities.

Muscle testing of the toddler or young child may require some of the techniques previously described. In addition, developmental positions can be used to assess muscle strength in an uncooperative youngster. For example, strength of hip extensors and abductors can be assessed as a child attempts to creep up steps or onto a low mat table. With addition of resistance to movements, fairly accurate muscle grades can be determined. To elicit hip flexor action in sitting, it is useful to place an interesting toy or object on the child's ankle or between the toes, as the child will often lift the leg spontaneously to reach for it. Ingenuity and creativity are prerequisites for muscle testing in the young child. Reliability of MMT in children with spina bifida younger than 5 years is difficult, but has been demonstrated in a clinic setting where all therapists were trained in specific MMT techniques to ascertain consistency in testing.[233] By the age of 4 or 5 years, muscle grades can generally be determined by traditional testing techniques, although the reliability of the test results will increase with the age of the child.[234] In most clinics, MMT is used to assess strength and changes in strength over time. Reliability of MMT may be called into question when trying to assess meaningful, detectable changes in power against gravity. If that is the case, a HHD can be used to test muscles with a grade of 3 or greater. Excellent intertester reliability of HHD for children with spina bifida has been reported.[232]

Muscle testing is indicated before and after any surgical procedure and at periodic intervals of 6 months to 1 year to detect any change in muscle function. Timely detection of any loss in strength is critical, as the child may encounter increased weakness resulting from tethering of the spinal cord or shunt malfunction as they grow. The level of innervation should not decrease throughout the life of the child with spina bifida. In the growing child or adolescent, an increasing weakness resulting from shunt malfunction, tethering of the spinal cord, or hydromyelia frequently can be substantiated by a muscle test of the lower extremities. The MMT is also valuable in determining the motor level so that potential future functional level can be determined (Fig. 13.16).

Muscle Tone Assessment

Over recent years, a controversy has developed with regard to the clinical significance of assessing muscle tone. Determining the severity and type of muscle tone abnormality is important to determine the type of bracing as well as serve as a baseline to determine whether neurological deterioration from Chiari II or hydrocephaly is occurring.

Children with spina bifida may present with a mixture of hypotonia and hypertonia. Tone examination should consider the presence of reflexive movements. In older children, examination should consider the difference between spasticity and stiffness resulting from contractures.

The most common method for assessment of muscle tone is passive movement of the limb. The Ashworth scale, Modified Ashworth scale, and Tardieu scale are commonly used scales to rate the severity of spasticity. Pendulum test can be also used to assess the type and severity of muscle tone abnormality. The severity, type, and distribution of muscle tone abnormalities should be noted.

THE CHILDREN'S MEMORIAL HOSPITAL
PHYSICAL / OCCUPATIONAL THERAPY

MUSCLE EXAM - MM

PATIENT NAME _____ M.R. # _____

ATTENDING M.D. _____ PT. D.O.B. _____

DIAGNOSIS _____

_____

DATE: _____

P.T. NAME: _____

	*	LEFT	RIGHT	*	COMMENTS: (Include ROM limitations, spasticity, reflexive movements, etc.)
ILIOPSOAS (L₁ - 2)					
SARTORIUS (L₁. 3)					
HIP ADDUCTORS (L₂ - 4)					
TENSOR FASCIA LATA					
GLUTEUS MEDIUS (L₄ - S₁)					
GLUTEUS MAXIMUS (L₅ - S₁)					
QUADRICEPS (L₂ - 4)					
MEDIAL HAMSTRINGS (L₄ - S₂)					
LATERAL HAMSTRINGS (L₄ - S₁)					
ANTERIOR TIBIALIS (L₄ - L₅)					
POSTERIOR TIBIALIS (L₄ - L₅)					
PERONEUS LONGUS (L₅ - S₁)					
PERONEUS BREVIS (L₅ - S₁)					
GASTROC - SOLEUS (S₁ - S₂)					
EXT. HALLUCIS LONGUS (L₅ - S₁)					
FLEX. HALLUCIS LONGUS (S₁ - S₂)					
EXT. DIGITORUM LONGUS (L₄ - S₁)					
EXT. DIG. B. (L₄ - S₁)					
FLEX. DIGITORUM LONGUS (L₄ - S₁)					
FLEX. DIG. B. (L₄ - S₁)					
LUMBRICALES					

*INDICATE INCREASE (↑) OR DECREASE (↓) IN STRENGTH IN COMPARISON TO PREVIOUS TEST DATED _____

PLEASE NOTE ANY SIGNIFICANT INFORMATION ON OTHER MUSCLE GROUPS UNLISTED ABOVE (i.e., EHB; Flex. HB; Internal or External Rotators)

X	PRESENT	UNABLE TO BE GRADED
N	NORMAL	COMPLETE RANGE OF MOTION AGAINST GRAVITY WITH FULL RESISTANCE
G	GOOD	COMPLETE RANGE OF MOTION AGAINST GRAVITY WITH MODERATE RESISTANCE
G-	GOOD MINUS	COMPLETE RANGE OF MOTION AGAINST GRAVITY WITH SOME RESISTANCE
F+	FAIR PLUS	COMPLETE RANGE OF MOTION AGAINST GRAVITY WITH SLIGHT RESISTANCE
F	FAIR	COMPLETE RANGE OF MOTION AGAINST GRAVITY
F-	FAIR MINUS	INCOMPLETE (GREATER THAN 1/2 WAY) RANGE OF MOTION AGAINST GRAVITY
P+	POOR PLUS	LESS THAN 1/2 WAY AGAINST GRAVITY OR FULL ROM GRAVITY ELIMINATED PLUS SL RESISTANCE
P	POOR	COMPLETE RANGE OF MOTION WITH GRAVITY ELIMINATED
P-	POOR MINUS	INCOMPLETE RANGE OF MOTION WITH GRAVITY ELIMINATED
T	TRACE	CONTRACTION IS FELT BUT THERE IS NO VISIBLE JOINT MOVEMENT
O	ZERO	NO CONTRACTION FELT IN THE MUSCLE

FORM 354042790

Fig. 13.15 Muscle Examination Form Using Alphabetical Designation. (Courtesy Josefina Briceno, PT, Children's Memorial Hospital, Chicago.)

Sensory Testing

The primary aim of sensory testing is to determine the lowest level of normal sensation. Full sensory tests are not possible until the child has acquired sufficient cognitive and language abilities to respond appropriately to testing. Sensory testing of the infant and young child is simplified to determine the level of sensation as accurately as possible with a minimal amount of testing. As sensory level does not necessarily correlate with the level of the lesion and radiological level, there may be a skip in sensory loss at some sensory level. Because of this skip of sensory loss, it is necessary to test all dermatomes and multiple areas within a given dermatome to ascertain an accurate dermatomal level.

In general, sensory testing is best carried out with the child in a quiet state. In newborns and infants, many aspects of sensory function

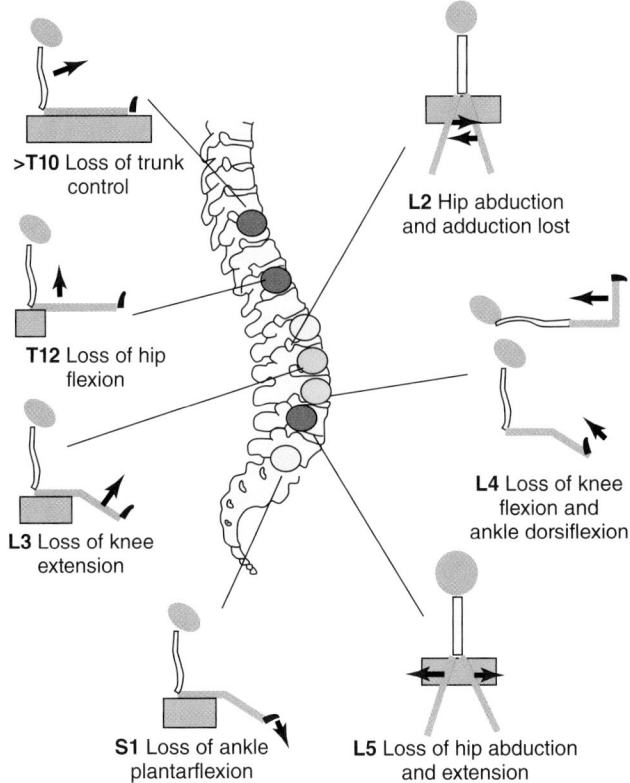

Fig. 13.16 Weakness Related to Level of Spinal Defect. (From Staheli LT. *Practice of Pediatric Orthopedics.* Philadelphia: Lippincott Williams & Wilkins; 2001.)

>T10 Loss of trunk control

L2 Hip abduction and adduction lost

T12 Loss of hip flexion

L3 Loss of knee extension

L4 Loss of knee flexion and ankle dorsiflexion

S1 Loss of ankle plantarflexion

L5 Loss of hip abduction and extension

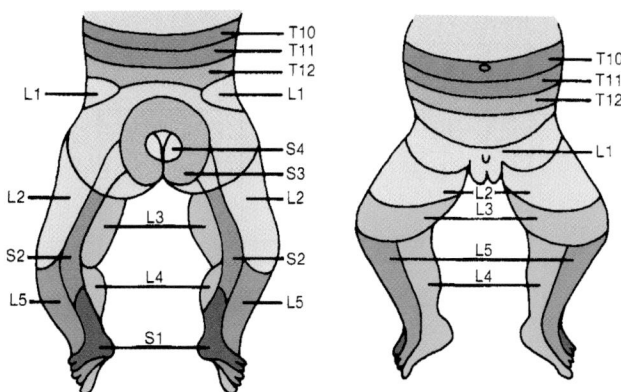

Fig. 13.17 Lower-limb Dermatomes. (From Brocklehurst G. Spina bifida for the clinician. *Clin Dev Med.* 1976;57:53.)

are observed simultaneously with motor function and during play. Sensory testing in newborns and infants is usually limited to basic testing while assessing for motor output as a potential response to a stimulus. Light touch or tickling usually precipitates a withdrawal of the foot. Response to touch can be determined by looking for a withdraw of the trunk or limb in response to a light tickle or pinch. Proprioception can be grossly assessed by moving the limb into an awkward position and watching the child's response to it. Vibration sense can be observed using a tuning fork, and the infant or newborn will usually withdraw a limb in response. Noxious stimuli such as nail bed pressure, pinching of the skin, or pinprick should also elicit a facial grimace, cry, or withdrawal.

In the newborn, beginning at the lowest level of sacral innervation, the skin is stroked with a pin or other sharp object until a reaction to pain is noted. Although none of these methods is fail-safe, they may be helpful in adapting a muscle test to a newborn or young infant. Repeated evaluation may be necessary to get an accurate picture of muscle function.

Because of dermatome innervation, the pin is usually drawn from the anal area across the buttocks, down the posterior thigh and leg, then to the anterior surface of the leg and thigh, and finally across the abdominal muscles. Reactions to be noted are a facial grimace or cry, which indicates that the painful sensation has reached a cortical level Care must be taken to see that each sensory dermatome has been evaluated. Results can be recorded by shading in the dermatomes where sensation is present (Fig. 13.17).

A newborn sensory evaluation is usually done before surgical closure of the spinal meningocele. Although sensory and motor levels can be determined as previously described, the infant's general condition should be considered in interpreting test findings. Any medication

taken by the mother during labor and delivery may influence the neonate's performance and should therefore be noted. In addition, the physiological disorganization normally seen in all infants during the first few days after birth may also affect testing.[235] At best, this presurgical evaluation establishes a tentative baseline, but significant changes in the infant's neurological status in the first few weeks of life should not be surprising to the clinician.

In the young child from 2 to 6 years of age, light touch sensation and position sense can be tested in addition to pain sensation. Again, to elicit an appropriate response and reliable test results, the ingenuity of the therapist will be required. Using games such as "Tell me when the puppet touches you" may be more effective for the young child than traditional testing methods. Sensory dermatome mapping using the chart in Fig. 13.17, or a similar form such as the WeeSTeP once the child with spina bifida gets older, can aid in establishing sensory level as well as insensate areas that may be at high risk of injury.[236]

From age 6 years through adolescence, formal and full sensory testing can be carried out and additional sensory tests of temperature and two-point discrimination may be added. Traditional methods are usually sufficient to ensure reliable testing, but a more behavioral approach may be indicated, depending on the individual's cognitive functioning.

After testing, a survey of the sensory dermatome chart should indicate whether sensation is normal, absent, or impaired. MMT, including myotome testing and sensory testing (dermatomes), can assist in determining the spinal level of function (Fig. 13.18).

Range of Motion Assessment

Assessment of joint ROM is a standard examination for children with spina bifida, since development of contractures is a common presentation in these children. ROM is an important component of functional tasks and a key determinant for function in children with spina bifida. Development of contracture may preclude the development of motor milestones. It is necessary to identify the available ROM, as it is necessary for developing the plan of care, such as establishing an exercise program to promote ROM and flexibility, and preventing or delaying development of contractures. ROM can help determine functional abilities and predict future functional abilities. It may also help determine the type and timing of assistive devices and surgical interventions that address contractures.

Several methods can be used to examine ROM, including goniometry, visual observation, still photographs, or computerized motion analysis systems. In clinical practice, the use of goniometry and structured visual observation are the most common methods to assess ROM. Accurate examination is typically assessed using universal

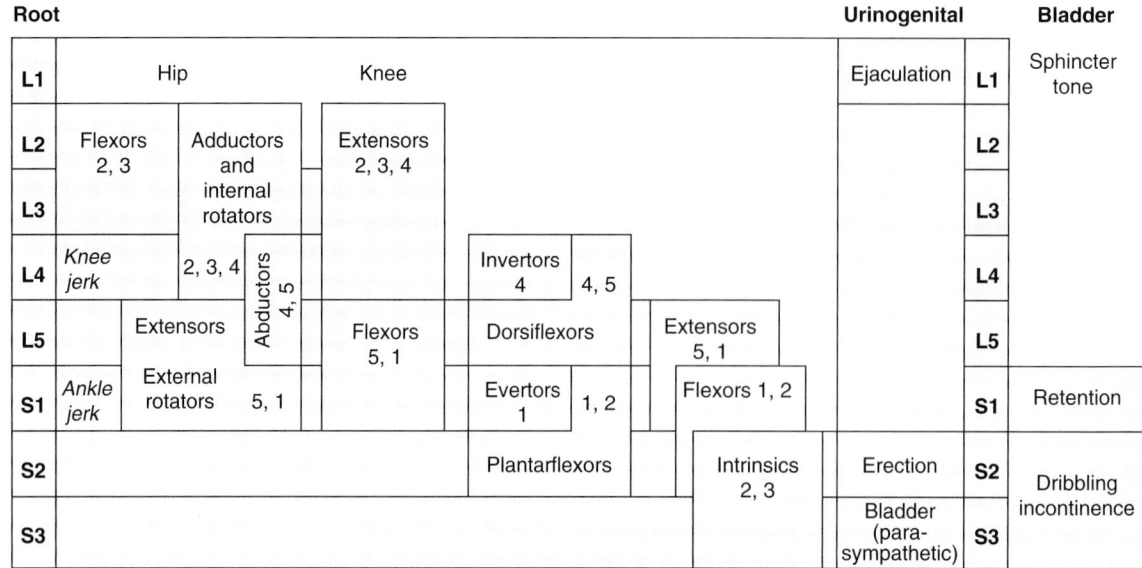

Root								Urinogenital		Bladder
L1	Hip			Knee				Ejaculation	L1	Sphincter tone
L2	Flexors 2, 3	Adductors and internal rotators		Extensors 2, 3, 4					L2	
L3									L3	
L4	*Knee jerk*	2, 3, 4	Abductors 4, 5		Invertors 4	4, 5			L4	
L5		Extensors		Flexors 5, 1	Dorsiflexors		Extensors 5, 1		L5	
S1	*Ankle jerk*	External rotators	5, 1		Evertors 1	1, 2	Flexors 1, 2		S1	Retention
S2					Plantarflexors		Intrinsics 2, 3	Erection	S2	Dribbling incontinence
S3								Bladder (para- sympathetic)	S3	

Fig. 13.18 Segmental Nerve Supply of the Lower Extremities. (From Stokes M. *Physical Management in Neurological Rehabilitation.* London: Elsevier; 2004.)

goniometer. Visual observation can be also used as screening for ROM or when a very quick assessment is needed. Moreover, ROM can be assessed using structured observation of functional motor skills and some handling/positioning. For example, squatting position is a good indication of passive ROM of hip and knee flexion. ROM examination should be performed with hands placed close to the joint being moved to prevent unnecessary stress to soft tissues and joint structure.

A complete ROM evaluation of the lower extremities is indicated for the newborn with spina bifida. Examination in newborns should take into consideration the normal physiological flexion that is greatest at the hips and knees. In the normal newborn, these apparent "contractures" of up to 35 degrees are eliminated as the child gains more control of extensor musculature and kicks more frequently into extension.

Hip adduction should not be tested beyond the neutral position because of the risk of hips dislocation, which are often unstable or dislocated. ROM should be done slowly and without excessive force to avoid fractures, so often experienced in paralytic lower extremities. ROM should be checked with the same frequency as MMT. Active ROM of the upper extremities can be assessed by observation and handling the infant. A formal ROM evaluation for the upper extremities is not usually indicated. A baseline ROM and tone assessment of the upper extremities should be completed.

In the child with spina bifida, contractures may be evident at multiple joints at birth because of unopposed musculature (Fig. 13.19). Common limitations in ROM in neonates with spina bifida include tightness of hip flexors, hip adductors, ankle dorsiflexors, and evertors (Tappit-Emas, 1999). These contractures are primarily due to lack of unopposed forces from weak or paralyzed antagonist muscles. For example, tightness and contractures of the hip flexors is common in children with L2 to L4 motor level. This can be due to unopposed forces from weak or paralyzed hip extensors. Hip flexion and knee flexion contractures are common in older children with spina bifida. In addition to the muscle imbalances, contractures and tightness can be due to poor positioning. Passive and active ROM continue to be monitored with documentation of changes that are noted over time.

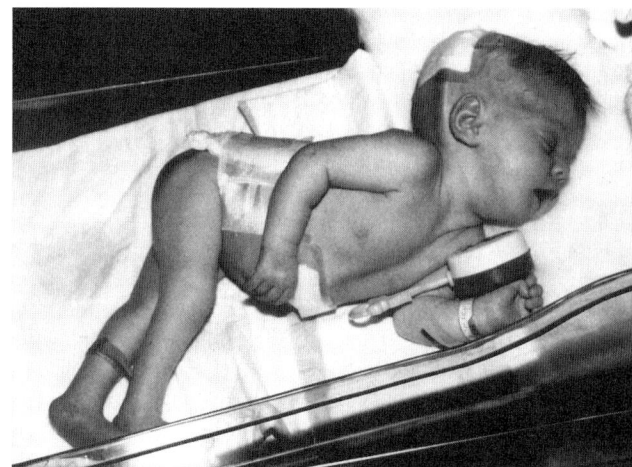

Fig. 13.19 Infant With Myelomeningocele With Contractures. (From Molnar GE, Alexander MA. *Pediatric Rehabilitation.* Philadelphia: Hanley & Belfus; 1999.)

Reflex Testing

There are different type of reflexes that can be tested including deep tendon, neonatal, and developmental reflexes. The evaluation of deep tendon reflexes may be used to assess the function of the afferent (sensory) neurons and the efferent (motor) neurons, and to differentiate between children with UMN lesion and children with lower motor neuron lesion. A reflex hammer is used to measure deep tendon reflexes. Routinely evaluated reflexes include the patellar tendon reflex (L2 to L4), Achilles tendon reflex (S1 to S2), and anal reflex (pudendal nerve, S3 to S4). Deep tendon reflexes are evaluated bilaterally.

Neonatal and developmental reflexes testing is used to check for the presence of normal reflex activity and to check for the integration of primitive reflexes and the development of more mature reactions. In the newborn, for example, strong rooting and sucking reflexes are expected. In the child with spina bifida, because of possible involvement of the CNS as previously described, these reflexes may be depressed or absent. Because these reflexes play an integral part in obtaining nutrients for the infant, their value is obvious. On the other hand, primitive reflexes that persist past their expected span may also indicate abnormality. For example, if the asymmetrical tonic neck reflex persists past 4 months, it will limit the infant's ability to bring the hands to midline for visual and tactile exploration.

As the primitive reflexes initially needed for survival and to experience movement become integrated, they are replaced by more mature and functional reactions. Righting and equilibrium reactions help the child attain the erect position and counteract changes in the center of gravity. Because these reactions depend on an intact CNS, as well as a certain level of postural control, they may be delayed, incomplete, or absent in the child with spina bifida. For example, a child with a low thoracic spinal cord lesion may show an incomplete equilibrium reaction in sitting. This may be caused by the lack of a stable postural base or by lack of initiation of the reaction centrally. Both the neurological and muscular components of these reactions must be considered. Reflex testing for the child with spina bifida may not be as intensive as that for a child with cerebral palsy. It may, however, provide a check on the progress of normal development, and as such, reflect the integrity of the CNS. In general, persistent presence of primitive reflexes beyond the age of 2 years and absent development of postural reflexes (righting and equilibrium reactions) may be negative indications for ambulation.

Development and Functional Assessment

Besides being aware of a child's sensory and motor levels, assessing the functional level is also important. Two important questions need to be asked: "Does the child demonstrate normal components of posture and movement synergies?" and "What is the child's level of function and mobility?" Several developmental and functional evaluations can be used with the child with spina bifida. The following are some suggestions for evaluation approaches and specifically designed tests to assist in assessment of this area.

Initially, a developmental sequence may be used to assess how a child is functioning. In each position used, both posture and movement are evaluated. The goals in using this type of assessment are to determine what a child can and cannot do, the quality of the action, and what is limiting the child. The progression begins in the supine position, rolling to prone, prone on elbows, prone on hands, up to sitting, on hands and knees, kneeling, half-kneeling, standing, and walking. Both the ability to attain and the ability to maintain the positions should be assessed.

The way in which a task is accomplished is as important to evaluate as the accomplishment itself. For example, in rolling, is head righting sufficient to keep the head off the supporting surface? From the hands-knees position, can reciprocal crawling be initiated without the lower extremities being held in wide abduction? Can the child pull to stand easily by using trunk rotation? Assessing the quality of the child's abilities will assist the clinician in determining where therapeutic measures should begin and what the goals of such intervention will be. Standardized assessments may provide the families with guidelines and a record of motor skills over time.

There are no standardized functional or motor assessments specific to those with spina bifida. Some assessments look at development relative to standardized norms and may guide the family and therapist in determining treatment goals and challenges. This information may be invaluable in determining bracing needs and other equipment needs as well as timing of various interventions. If a standardized assessment is desirable for the infant with spina bifida, the Alberta Infant Motor Scale (AIMS) might be appropriate. The AIMS[237] is designed to

measure motor development from birth to 18 months of age. It is a 58-item observational test of infants in supine, prone, sitting, and standing positions. Each item includes detailed descriptions of the weight-bearing surface, the infant's posture, and antigravity movements expected of the infant in that position. The AIMS requires minimal handling of the infant and can be completed in 20 to 30 minutes. The test was normed on a cross-sectional sample of 2200 infants in Alberta, Canada. Interrater and test-retest reliability are high (0.95 to 0.99), as is concurrent validity with the Peabody Developmental Motor Scales (PDMS) (0.99) and the Bayley Scales of Infant Development (0.97).[238] For the child with spina bifida, the AIMS could be used to assess current motor development and track progress in motor development over time. The AIMS is also useful in determining the percent of delay in motor development in an infant, which is often needed to determine eligibility for early intervention services under IDEA (Individuals with Disability Education Act).

The Milani-Comparetti Motor Development Screening Test for Infants and Young Children may also be useful in assessing the functional level of the child with spina bifida. This screening examination is designed to evaluate motor development from birth to 2 years of age (Fig. 13.20). It requires no special equipment and can be administered in 4 to 8 minutes. The test evaluates both spontaneous behavior and evoked responses. Spontaneous behavior includes postural control of the head and body in various positions as well as a sequence of active movement patterns. Primitive reflexes, righting, and equilibrium reactions constitute the evoked responses. The Milani-Comparetti test was normed on a sample of 312 children from Omaha, Nebraska. Interrater reliability percent of agreement was 89% to 95%. Test-retest reliability percent agreement was 82% to 100%. Predictive validity of the test has not been well established.[239] The Milani-Comparetti test should assist the clinician in evaluating each child's underlying postural mechanisms and his or her ability to attain the erect position. The test manual provides information on special examination procedures and scoring. It should be noted that the Milani-Comparetti is a screening tool and a more detailed assessment of motor performance should also be performed.

The Ages and Stages Questionnaire (ASQ) is a screening assessment that assesses developmental and social-emotional delays during crucial early ages of life. This test is available in English and Spanish and can be completed in 10 to 15 minutes.[240] It was developed and validated on 15,138 children in all 50 states and several US territories. The test-retest reliability (0.92), interrater reliability (0.93), validity (0.82 to 0.88), sensitivity (0.86), and specificity (0.85) have been well documented.[240] This test provides parents and providers with a checklist to easily assess change over time.

The PDMS-2 is another standardized assessment that may prove helpful in evaluating a child with spina bifida.[241] The PDMS-2 consists of six gross and fine motor subtests for children from birth through 6 years of age. The test takes 45 to 60 minutes to complete or 20 to 30 minutes per subtest. The two scales allow a comparison of the child's motor performance with a normative sample of children at various age levels. A stratified sample of 2003 children from 46 states in the United States was used to develop PDMS-2 test norms. Test-retest and interrater reliability are high. Content, construct, and concurrent validity have been well established. Although the child with spina bifida and activity limitations would not be expected to succeed on many of the gross motor items at the later age levels, the scale still serves as a reminder of expected gross motor performance at each age. Children with higher levels of neurological impairment will have more difficulty completing the test items. The fine motor scale offers a chance to assess fine motor performance of children with congenital spinal cord injury. This area has been frequently overlooked in children with myelomeningocele. Fine motor

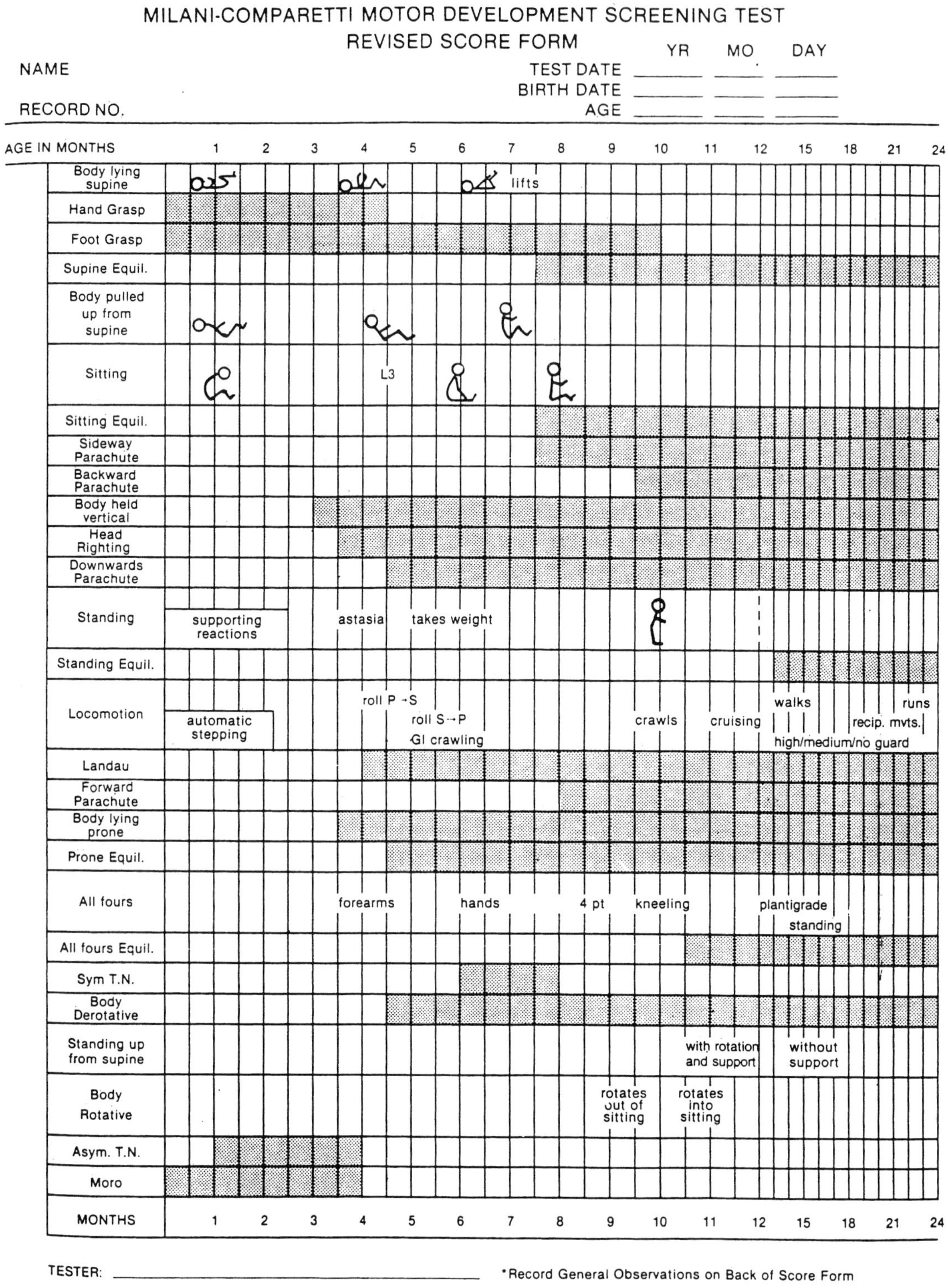

MILANI-COMPARETTI MOTOR DEVELOPMENT SCREENING TEST
REVISED SCORE FORM

NAME

RECORD NO.

TEST DATE ___ ___ ___
BIRTH DATE ___ ___ ___
AGE ___ ___ ___

YR MO DAY

AGE IN MONTHS	1	2	3	4	5	6	7	8	9	10	11	12	15	18	21	24
Body lying supine								lifts								
Hand Grasp																
Foot Grasp																
Supine Equil.																
Body pulled up from supine																
Sitting				L3												
Sitting Equil.																
Sideway Parachute																
Backward Parachute																
Body held vertical																
Head Righting																
Downwards Parachute																
Standing	supporting reactions			astasia	takes weight											
Standing Equil.																
Locomotion	automatic stepping			roll P→S / roll S→P / GI crawling						crawls	cruising	walks / high/medium/no guard		recip. mvts.	runs	
Landau																
Forward Parachute																
Body lying prone																
Prone Equil.																
All fours				forearms		hands		4 pt	kneeling			plantigrade standing				
All fours Equil.																
Sym T.N.																
Body Derotative																
Standing up from supine										with rotation and support		without support				
Body Rotative									rotates out of sitting	rotates into sitting						
Asym. T.N.																
Moro																
MONTHS	1	2	3	4	5	6	7	8	9	10	11	12	15	18	21	24

TESTER: _____ *Record General Observations on Back of Score Form

Fig. 13.20 Milani-Comparetti Motor Development Screening Test Revised Score Form.

development, however, may be affected because of congenital abnormalities in brain development associated with myelomeningocele or related to tethering of the spinal cord that can result in fine motor paresis. In addition, the PDMS-2 offers guidelines for administering the test to children with various activity limitations.[241]

The Bruininks-Oseretsky Test of Motor Proficiency, second edition (BOT-2), can be used to evaluate the higher functioning ambulatory child with lower lumbar or sacral level spina bifida.[242] Fine manual

control, manual coordination, body coordination, and strength and agility subtests can be used to assist in evaluating areas of fine motor control, balance, and coordination difficulties. This test has been standardized on a sample of 1520 subjects from age 4 through 21 years.[242]

The Movement Assessment Battery for Children, second edition (Movement ABC-2), can be used to identify children who are significantly behind their peers in motor development, assist in planning an intervention program in either a school or a clinical setting, and measure change as a result of intervention or can serve as a measurement instrument in research involving motor development. This tool may be useful to assess children with lower lumbar and sacral level myelomeningocele, as well as children with lipomeningocele. The Movement ABC identifies and evaluates the movement problems that can determine a child's participation and social adjustment at home or school. The Movement ABC Checklist provides classroom assessment of movement difficulties, screening for "at risk" children (aged 5 to 12 years), and systematic monitoring of treatment programs. It provides a comprehensive assessment for those identified as "at risk" (3 to 16 years, 11 months), yielding both normative and qualitative measures of movement competence, manual dexterity, ball skills, and static and dynamic balance.[243]

The Pediatric Evaluation of Disability Inventory (PEDI) is a comprehensive assessment of function in children aged 6 months to 7 years.[244] The PEDI measures both capability and performance of functional activities in three areas: self-care, mobility, and social function. Capability is a measure of the functional skills for which the child has demonstrated mastery. Functional performance is measured by the level of caregiver assistance needed to accomplish a task. A modifications scale provides a measure of environmental modifications and equipment needed in daily functioning. The PEDI has been standardized on a normative sample of 412 children from New England. Some data from clinical samples ($N = 102$) are also available. Interrater reliability of the PEDI is high as demonstrated by high intraclass correlation coefficients (ICCs = 0.96 to 0.99). Concurrent validity of the PEDI with the WeeFIM (child's version of the Functional Independence Measure) was also high ($r = 0.80$ to 0.97).[244] The PEDI can be administered in approximately 45 minutes by clinicians or educators familiar with the child or by structured interview of the parent. The PEDI should provide a descriptive measure of the functional level of the child with myelomeningocele as well as a method for tracking change over time. The PEDI has had a rich tradition in helping to document functional development. Computer Adapted Test (PEDI-CAT) is a revised version of the PEDI. In addition to the original three domains, a responsibility domain has been added. The PEDI-CAT has been validated from the patient's birth through twenty years old.

Another assessment of motor performance that may be commonly used with the school-aged child with spina bifida is the School Function Assessment (SFA). The SFA is standardized and was conceptually developed to reflect the functional abilities and needs of a student in elementary school. The three areas assessed include the student's participation in school activities, task supports required by the student for participation, and the student's activity performance.[245,246] It was designed to facilitate collaborative program planning for students with a variety of disabling conditions. The instrument is a judgment-based (questionnaire) assessment that is completed by one or more school professionals who know the student well and have observed his or her typical performance on the school-related tasks and activities being assessed. Items have been written in measurable, behavioral terms that can be used directly in the student's Individualized Educational Plan (IEP).[245]

Finally, the Functional Mobility Scale (FMS) was originally developed a tool to describe the functional mobility of children with cerebral palsy,[247] and has recently been applied to children with spina bifida.[248] The scale assesses a child's mobility at three distances: 5, 50, and 500 m. These distance are to represent, home, school, and community ambulation. The child is scored on a 6-point scale based on the ability to ambulate on level or unlevel surfaces and the type of assistive device needed at each distance. A score is given for each distance and has been found to distinguish groups of children with various levels of disability. The FMS was standardized on a group of 310 children in Australia and was found to have high levels of interrater and intrarater

reliability (ICC's of 9.0 to 9.5). Its construct, content, and concurrent validity was established with comparisons to the Pediatric Outcomes Data Collection Instrument (PODCI), Child Health Questionnaire, and mobility up timers ($r = 0.81$ to 0.89)

Gait Analysis

Instrumented three-dimensional computerized gait analysis (IGA) was initially used to evaluate children with cerebral palsy beginning in the 1980s. Since that time, the use of IGA has increasingly been used to evaluate children with spina bifida. The body of knowledge of the use of IGA in the management of children with spina bifida has steadily increased.

The use of gait analysis has helped physicians and other health care providers gain a better understanding of the impact of orthopedic impairments on function and has caused a shift in the focus of orthopedic management from focusing on radiological changes to functional outcomes.[99] IGA affords a better understanding of the complex gait patterns of children with spina bifida to determine factors leading to changes in gait, including changes in alignment, muscle length, muscle torque, and symmetry. Intervention strategies for orthopedic surgery, orthotics, and rehabilitation can be planned and assessed with more accuracy. This is especially important in the assessment of individuals with rotational deformities. Gait analyses have also been useful in establishing a database of trends in kinetics and kinematics for various levels of spina bifida and the development of classification schemes.[249] Children with lumbar and sacral level lesions are most suitable for assessment with IGA due to their greater ambulation capabilities. Access to gait analysis laboratories and issues with insurance coverage have been a limitation in the use of IGA in the management of children with spina bifida and other disabilities, but is improving.

Perceptual and Cognitive Evaluations

When evaluating a child with spina bifida, some assessment of perceptual and cognitive status is important to include. The appropriate assessment depends largely on the age of the child. The assessment may be performed by the physical, occupational, or speech therapist, depending on the setting.

For the newborn from 3 to 30 days old, the Brazelton Neonatal Behavioral Assessment scale may be adapted to assess the infant's organization in terms of physiological response to stress, state control, motoric control, and social interaction.[235] Ideally, the infant should be medically stable and free from CNS-depressant drugs before evaluation. Generally, this evaluation will occur after the back lesion has been closed and a shunt has been positioned to relieve the hydrocephalic condition.

Although test results may not have prognostic value because of the plasticity of the nervous system at this young age, they supply the clinician with information concerning the current status of the child. This information can be conveyed to the infant's caregivers—both medical personnel and parents—so that strengths can be appreciated and weaknesses anticipated and handled appropriately. Helping parents identify that their infant has their own unique characteristics and assisting them in dealing with these characteristics does a great deal to strengthen already precarious parent-infant bonding.

PHYSICAL THERAPY MANAGEMENT

Given the range of impairments seen in patients with spina bifida, there is a clear need for coordinated interdisciplinary approach. Intervention for the patients with spina bifida involves multiple systems, including neuromuscular, musculoskeletal, integumentary, and psychosocial systems. The goal of management of these children is to achieve maximal independence in mobility and to maximize their function, quality of life, and community participation. Intervention should be unique for each patient and may vary based on the severity of the lesion, level of the lesion, presence of associated disorders, and patient's age. Intervention for patients with spina bifida needs to be individualized to fit the patient and family' needs. Intervention activities may focus on enhancing participation across immediate and expanded environments such as home, daycare, preschool, school, and community.

Before Closure of Myelomeningocele

Physical therapy management of the infant before Closure of Myelomeningocele is limited by his or her medical condition (Table 13.2). Therapists are called to the NICU or stepdown unit on a regular basis in large tertiary care centers to carry out preoperative MMT and help ascertain functional motor level. Physicians (neurosurgeons and orthopedic surgeons) on the spina bifida care team rely on this assessment to guide their discussion with the families regarding care and prognosis. When carrying out the preoperative MMT, great care must be taken to avoid contaminating an open sac, which is usually covered with a Telfa nonadherent dressing or a wet sterile dressing that must be kept moist with a saline solution. PTs as part of the NICU team may also provide suggestions for the positioning and handling of the infant during the course of their NICU/nursery stay.

After Surgery, During Hospitalization, and Transitioning to Home

A major goal during this stage is to prevent contractures and maintain ROM while giving stimulation to provide as normal an environment as possible.

TABLE 13.2	**Summary of Treatment Planning and Rehabilitation Related to Significant Stages of Development**	
Stage of Recovery	**Major Physical Therapy Goals**	**Physical Therapy Management**
Newborn to Toddler (Preambulatory Phase)		
Stage 1: Before surgical closure of myelomeningocele—newborn	Determine functional motor level	Preoperative manual muscle testing
Stage 2: After surgery, during hospitalization—newborn to infant	Confirm functional motor level Prevent contracture and deformity Encourage normal sensorimotor development	Postoperative manual muscle testing ROM exercises taught to hospital personnel and family Positioning in prone and side lying Provide toys of various colors, textures, and shapes Graded auditory and visual stimuli: music boxes, squeaky toys, brightly colored objects Therapeutic handling to encourage good head and trunk control
Stage 3: Condition stabilized— infant to toddler	Confirm functional motor level Encourage normal development sequence	Manual muscle testing once or twice per year Work in sitting on head righting and equilibrium reactions Eye-hand coordination activities Early weight bearing on lower extremities Encourage prone progression Weight shifting in standing frame Comprehensive home program
Toddler Through Adolescent (Ambulatory Phase)		
Stage 4: Toddler through preschool	Confirm functional motor level Begin ambulation Continue development in cognitive and psychosocial areas Collaborate on goals with other team members	Manual muscle testing once or twice per year Choose appropriate orthotic device Gait training Development and strengthening of righting and equilibrium reactions Consider referral to EI program Public preschool program Continue home program Open communication with other team members
Stage 5: Primary school through adolescence	Confirm functional motor level Reevaluate ambulation potential Maintain present level of functioning Prevent skin breakdown as child becomes more sedentary Promote independence in self-care skills Remediate any perceptual-motor problems Provide appropriate adaptive devices Promote self-esteem and social-sexual adjustment	Postoperative manual muscle testing Replace orthotic device as necessary Wheelchair prescriptions as necessary Teach locomotion activities Maintain strength in trunk and extremities Teach skin care Work with team members to teach dressing, feeding, hygiene, and bowel and bladder care Provide program and activities for sensorimotor integration Check for fit and proper use of adaptive devices Collaborate with other team members in counseling efforts

EI, Early intervention; *ROM,* range of motion.

Therapeutic intervention after surgical back closure during this stage is often limited by the infant's neurological and orthopedic status. Physical therapy in postoperative and intensive care units addresses infant positioning needs and provides parent and family education.

Handling and positioning procedures must avoid adding pressure on the operated site. The prone position helps prevent fluid around the spinal cord from leaking out through the incision and allows for optimal positioning of the leg without any pressure or tension on the operated site. Lying prone is also recommended for the child with hip dysplasia. Some neurosurgeons may permit partial side lying to allow for position changes and to facilitate feeding. Feeding can start when the child is stable and alert after surgery. Holding the child upright against the body may be introduced gradually to help with feeding, and cuddling the child in this position can provide comfort. Once the incision is healed, the child can be positioned normally. Positioning the head below the heart level should be avoided for children with hydrocephalus to avoid increased intracranial pressure.

ROM exercises, positioning, and handling should be taught to the nursing staff and to the family before discharge. ROM exercises should be performed slowly and carefully. Excessive hip flexion or adduction should be avoided to prevent hip subluxation or dislocation.

A normal sensory experience should be presented to the child in spite of the hospital setting. Because of their medical conditions, hospitalized infants often experience early separation from their parents. Teaching the family to handle the child as described may enhance parent-infant bonding. Adequate bonding is essential for normal psychosocial development to occur.

In treating the newborn after surgery, great care must be taken to avoid contaminating the surgical dressing, which usually consists of Xeroform Petrolatum Gauze (3% bismuth tribromophenate in a special petrolatum blend on fine mesh gauze) covered with Telfa. The Xeroform dressing is nonadherent but clings and conforms to all body contours. This postoperative dressing remains on for 2 weeks.

Newborn Through Early Infancy

After discharge, the child should be monitored closely by the spina bifida team, which may include a neurosurgeon, an orthopedist, a urologist, a nurse clinician, a PT, an OT, an orthotist, and a social worker. Before discharge, a definitive home program as well as referral to the local Early Intervention (EI) program should be given to the family because the child will most likely require ongoing therapy, including both PT and OT. Other professionals who may be involved in the child's EI program may include speech and language pathologists (SLPs), developmental therapists (DTs), social workers, and psychologists.

Range of Motion Exercises

ROM is a key determinant for function throughout rehabilitation. Adequate ROM is necessary for functional excursions of the muscle and joints, and for maintaining normal posture and alignment. Sufficient ROM is also necessary to prevent the development of contractures, deformities, and secondary disorders.

ROM exercises should be performed daily, with hands placed close to the joint being moved and holding briefly at the end of the range, thereby preventing unnecessary stress to soft tissues and joint structure. Exercises should be performed carefully for the child with hip instability or with very low muscle tone to avoid subluxation or dislocation. Positions beyond neutral or excessive hip flexion should be avoided, particularly for the child with hip instability. Range should be increased slowly and without excessive force to avoid fractures that are so often experienced in paralytic lower extremities.

Therapists should take into consideration that normal physiological flexion is greatest at the hips and knees, and that these apparent "contractures" do not require intervention. In children with spasticity, therapists should use special care when performing ROM exercises and stretching on the muscles that are spastic or tend to develop contractures, particularly hip flexors and adductors, knee flexors, and ankle plantar flexors. If clubfeet or other foot deformities are present, soft tissue stretching may be indicated. Stretching should begin distally on the soft tissue of the forefoot and proceed proximally toward the calcaneus. This is done to take advantage of the pliability of soft tissue structures and to minimize future fixed deformity. In addition, taping may be used to maintain optimal ROM and alignment between periods of stretching.

In the home, ROM exercises can be carried out while the child is being held over the adult's shoulder or prone in the adult's lap. These positions allow closeness between the caregiver and infant, thus encouraging maximal relaxation and interaction between them. ROM exercises can be incorporated into the child's routine alongside feeding and diaper changes. This approach makes it easy for the parents to remember to do them.

Handling and Positioning

Positioning should focus on normal alignment and facilitating normal development and social skills. Positioning and handling should encourage symmetry and avoid the effects of tonic reflexes such as asymmetrical tonic neck reflex. Handling should use a variety of movement and postures to facilitate functional activities and sensorimotor development. Positioning and handling should also be taught to the family.

When the child is not being handled, resting positions can be used to maintain ROM and enhance development. The prone position is the most advantageous because it prevents hip flexion contractures and encourages the development of extensor musculature as the child lifts his or her head. Side lying, which allows the hands to come to midline and generally encourages symmetrical posture, can be used for alternate positioning. As much as possible, the supine position should be avoided because the child is most dominated by primitive reflexes and the effects of gravity in this position. For example, for the child with spina bifida with CNS involvement, the effects of the tonic labyrinthine reflex combined with paralytic lower extremities may make movement from the supine position extremely difficult. Before initiating activities in the supine position, the therapist should obtain medical clearance.

Positioning of the lower extremities should consider the existing limitations in ROM, muscle tone, or deformities such as clubfoot or the common contractures and deformities seen in children with spina bifida. Forced leg swaddling should be avoided to minimize the risk of hip subluxation. The presence of hydrocephalus and the increased risk of developing pressure sores are other factors to consider when positioning and handling a child with spina bifida.

Sensorimotor Training

Developing normal sensorimotor experiences is one of the treatment goals for young infants. Sensorimotor activities facilitate the emergence of motor and developmental skills, mobility, play, and social skills. Sensorimotor activities encourage behaviors such as reaching, handling toys, rolling, and other developmental skills. Sensorimotor training involves activities that promote normal alignment, joint stability, trunk rotation, dissociation between body segments, spatial and perceptual awareness, weight bearing, and weight shifting and transition from one position to another.

A normal sensory experience should be presented to the child early in infancy, including while in the hospital setting. Toys of various colors, textures, and shapes should be made available. Musical mobiles hung low enough for the child to reach provide a variety of sensory experiences. Stimuli such as squeaky toys or the human face and voice can be used to encourage visual and auditory tracking. Controlled stimulation relevant to the infant's neurological state, rather than overstimulation, should be the rule. Depending on the age of the child, appropriate learning situations must be presented to provide the child with as normal an environment as possible for perceptual and cognitive growth.

Facilitation of Normal Development

During the stage of early child development, the primary emphasis should be on attaining good head and trunk control, eliciting appropriate righting reactions, facilitating the ability to sit, and promoting early mobility. The normal developmental sequence may guide the progression of motor activities, ultimately preparing the child to assume the upright posture.

One of the first skills to develop is head control, including ability to hold the head upright and move and maintain head positions. Head control may be difficult if the head size is large due to hydrocephalus. Rolling may be difficult or delayed in some children with spinal bifida due to large head size and weakness and paralysis in the trunk and lower extremity muscles. Creeping and crawling are also delayed due to weakness and paralysis of the trunk and lower extremities, which results in the lack of ability to stabilize and bear weight on the lower extremities.

Therapists may focus on the facilitation of developmental skills. For example, the child can be seated on the therapist's lap, facing the therapist, and alternately lowered slowly backward and side-to-side. This action helps stimulate head righting and to strengthen the neck and abdominal muscles. Weight shifting in various positions and through therapeutic handling is important to enhance the development of early head and trunk control. Developmental handling may be limited by surgical interventions that limit mobility.

Active movements such as reaching to toys in different directions from different developmental positions help stimulate head and trunk control and facilitate trunk elongation. Reaching activities from sitting (supported or unsupported) to toys in different directions may assist in head control, trunk elongation and rotation, and development of sitting control.

Infant to Toddler (Preambulatory)

In this stage of rehabilitation, the major emphasis is on preparing the child mentally and physically for upright standing and mobility. In addition, routine MMT should be performed every 6 to 12 months to reassess functional motor level and to ascertain that no change in status has occurred. Goals of preventing contractures and maintaining ROM will remain throughout the child's life. Standing and ambulation become more difficult and often impossible in the presence of contracture and deformities. If possible, prone positioning during play and sleeping assists greatly in stretching tight musculature, particularly hip flexors. Resting splints for the lower extremities or a total-body splint can be used as necessary to position and maintain ROM and alignment.

Developmental strategies should be aimed at facilitating movement and motor control. Assuming that the child has previously gained good head and trunk control, the next step is developing sitting equilibrium reactions. Independent sitting is typically delayed and may not occur until the age of 1 to 2 years old. This may be due to weakness and paralysis in the trunk and lower extremities, large head size, and lack of trunk mobility following surgery. Back surgery and a tendency to develop scoliosis may limit the child's ability to shift the pelvis in

response to equilibrium stimulation. This may contribute to delayed sitting and impact upright sitting posture. Reaching activities that involve weight bearing and weight shifts from a variety of sitting postures can be used to facilitate sitting. Activities that develop equilibrium reactions from sitting can be used to promote sitting. As the child learns to sit independently, the child will learn to reach in different directions, and this will facilitate accommodation to equilibrium shift. As sitting balance improves, fine motor and eye-hand coordination activities should be introduced. Upper-extremity functioning is often overlooked in the child with spina bifida, whose problems appear to be concentrated in the lower extremities. However, most children with spina bifida show decreased fine motor coordination, and this problem should be addressed when developmentally appropriate. The normal infant begins to reach and grasp by 6 months of age; therefore the child with spina bifida must be given ample opportunities to practice and perfect these same skills at an early age. Because many children with spina bifida may be receiving PT as their primary service through EI in these early months, referral to and consultation with an OT at this age are highly recommended.

Following a normal developmental sequence, the child with spina bifida will usually begin some form of prone progression as trunk and upper-extremity stability improve. This is a significant phase of development because it allows for the development of a sensorimotor base as the child expands environmental horizons. During this phase of high mobility, insensate skin must be checked for injury frequently and often must be protected by heavier clothing. This may help prevent any major skin breakdown, which could significantly delay the rehabilitation process. A scooter board may provide the child with spina bifida opportunities to explore the environment. "Soft tummy" versions of the scooter boards are available for the child with sensitive skin. For some children with high-level lesions in whom prone mobility is not safe or practical for long distances, a Star Car (Tash), Ready Racer (Tumble Forms), PlasmaCar, or similar mobility equipment may be used. These provide the child with a means of exploring the environment safely and independently.

Emphasis on head and trunk control and strengthening exercises in a variety of sitting postures is important in this early preambulatory phase. Development of adequate strength and motor control for trunk righting, equilibrium reactions, and protective reactions will ultimately lead to improved sitting balance. Hands-free sitting with good balance is the optimal goal in this stage to allow for independence and freedom in play skills. In addition, hands-free sitting is a necessary precursor to ambulation with lower-extremity bracing and often is the determinant in deciding if a child will use a standing frame or will become a functional ambulator.

Early weight bearing is also of utmost importance, both physiologically and psychologically. The upright position has beneficial effects on circulation and renal and bladder functioning as well as on the promotion of bone growth and density. Psychologically, weight bearing in an upright posture allows a normal view of the world and contributes to more normal perceptual, cognitive, and emotional growth. One way to achieve this weight bearing is in the kneeling position. This is developmentally appropriate because children 8 to 10 months old frequently use kneeling as a transition from all fours to standing.

Because young infants are frequently held in the standing position and bounced on their parents' laps, this form of weight bearing on the lower extremities is appropriate from birth onward. Failure to promote weight bearing in this manner may deprive the child with spina bifida of the normal experience of standing at a very early age. When standing these children, care must be taken to see that the lower extremities are in good alignment and that undue pressure is not exerted on them.

This way they experience normal weight bearing while minimizing the risk of fractures.

Also, in this phase of preambulation, transitions from one position to another should be assessed and facilitated. Teaching the child strategies for transitions will enhance his or her optimal functional independence. Compensations may be taught to substitute for weakened musculature. In addition, adaptive equipment and mobility devices may be recommended to enhance acquisition of age-appropriate milestones. Providing appropriate facilitation of mobility at a level similar to that of a child's peers is important for psychosocial growth and development.

Once the child is able to crawl, the child will attempt to pull to standing. This skill requires integration of many factors, including strength in the trunk and upper and lower extremities, and some level of standing balance and ability to bear weight on the lower extremities. The ability to pull to a standing position is typically delayed and may not occur until the child is 3 years of age. When the child attempts to pull to a standing position or would be expected to do so normally (at 10 to 12 months of age), the use of a standing device is indicated. Generally, a standing frame is the first orthosis chosen. This is a relatively inexpensive tubular frame to which adjustable parts are attached. Because it is not custom made, it can be fitted fairly quickly, although adjustments may be necessary to accommodate spinal deformities. This standing device offers support of the trunk, hips, and knees and leaves the hands free for other activities. Time spent in the standing frame should be increased gradually. This allows the child to adjust to the upright position in terms of muscle strength, endurance, blood pressure, and pressure on skin surfaces. Parents may assist in providing activities that focus on standing ability and tolerance. Parents can help facilitate the child's tolerance to standing using different activities, such as coloring while standing. Proper alignment should be taken into consideration while standing to avoid developing deformities.

In typical development, while standing, children will attempt to shift weight in preparation for cruising and walking. Cruising along an object such as a chair or sofa is the next step in development. Initial cruising is controlled by arm strength but also requires balance, strength, and the ability to shift and bear weight on the lower extremities. The control of cruising will shift gradually from the upper to lower extremities in preparation for independent ambulation. After children have built up a tolerance for standing, they may be taught to move in the device by shifting their weight from side to side. Initial shifting of weight onto one side of the body is necessary to allow the other side to move forward. This preliminary weight shift is also a prerequisite for developing equilibrium reactions in the standing position and will thus prepare the child for later ambulation. As the child shifts weight, the trunk musculature on the weight-bearing side should elongate and on the nonweight-bearing side should shorten as muscle strength allows. This normal reaction to weight shifting also includes righting of the head and should be closely monitored by the therapist for completeness. Activities may focus on standing tolerance and ability to shift weight. Parents can help facilitate cruising using different play skills such as reaching to toys in different standing postures.

A therapy program must be designed to meet the individual's needs in each area. Age alone does not determine the appropriateness of therapeutic goals. Goals that are not suited for the child's cognitive and emotional needs, in addition to physical needs, will not facilitate best outcomes. For example, an 18-month-old may have the physical capabilities to ambulate independently with crutches and braces. The child may not, however, have the cognitive skills necessary to learn a four-point gait or be ready emotionally to separate from his or her mother for intensive therapy sessions. A more realistic goal may be to let the child walk holding onto furniture (cruising) while a wheeled walker for more independent ambulation is slowly introduced. Another alternative to using a conventional walker is to encourage the child to play with push toys such as grocery carts and baby buggies.

During this preambulatory stage, therapy goals may be accomplished through a comprehensive home program, with frequent checks to note progress or problems and to change the program accordingly. For the more involved child, increased frequency of direct intervention may be indicated to achieve optimal developmental progress. A telehealth program can assist in adherence to home program.

The program must be reevaluated often and have goals changed if conditions such as shunt malfunctions or fractures occur. The warning signs for shunt dysfunctions are generally those previously described for suspected hydrocephalus. In addition, swelling along the shunt site may indicate a malfunction. Swelling and local heat or redness of a limb are the usual signs of a fracture. The limb may also look misaligned, and the child may develop a fever. As previously mentioned, these fractures generally heal quickly with proper medical intervention and minimally interrupt rehabilitation efforts.

Toddler Through Preschool (Ambulatory Phase)

This period in development marks the end of infancy and the beginning of childhood. For the typically developing child who has developed a strong sensorimotor foundation, physical development is marked by increased coordination and refinement of movement patterns. In addition, a great variety of motor skills will be achieved as the typically developing child learns to throw, catch, run, hop, and jump. This is also a period of great cognitive growth, as children's use of mental imagery and physical knowledge of their environments expand. Concepts of size, number, color, form, and space are all developing. Emotionally, most children are becoming more independent and begin to break away from the sheltered environment of the home. They are now more interested in interacting with others and become social beings to a greater extent.

All these changes in physical, cognitive, and emotional development will be evident in the child with spina bifida, although the degree depends on the extent of the functional limitations and their effect on the child's ability to participate in life. The characteristics of normal development must be understood so that cognitive, emotional, and motor behaviors can be nurtured and enhanced in the child with spina bifida.

Goals for this stage, as for any other stage, must address physical, cognitive, and emotional development. The most obvious goal at this stage is to help the child who is already standing to progress to an ambulatory status. Even the child with a low thoracic lesion can usually manage some form of ambulation.

Thus far, the child has learned to shift weight in the standing frame. By rotating the trunk toward the weighted side, the non-weight-bearing side can be shifted forward (Fig. 13.21). By reversing the weight shift, the opposite side can be moved forward and a type of "pivoting forward" progression can be accomplished. To maintain balance while shifting, the child may initially use a two-wheeled walker. The therapist may help initiate weight shift and trunk rotation by alternately pulling the arms forward.[250] Once the child has gained this form of mobility, the type of permanent bracing chosen will depend on the level of the lesion and a variety of other factors.

The overall goal for ambulatory training is to promote efficient, independent mobility with the least amount of bracing while maintaining optimal joint integrity. Ambulatory potential as well as choice of bracing depends on many factors, including neurosegmental level of the lesion, motor power at the neurosegmental level, stability in neurological condition, extent and degree of orthopedic deformity, balance, age, height, weight, sex, motivation, spasticity and tone abnormalities, type,

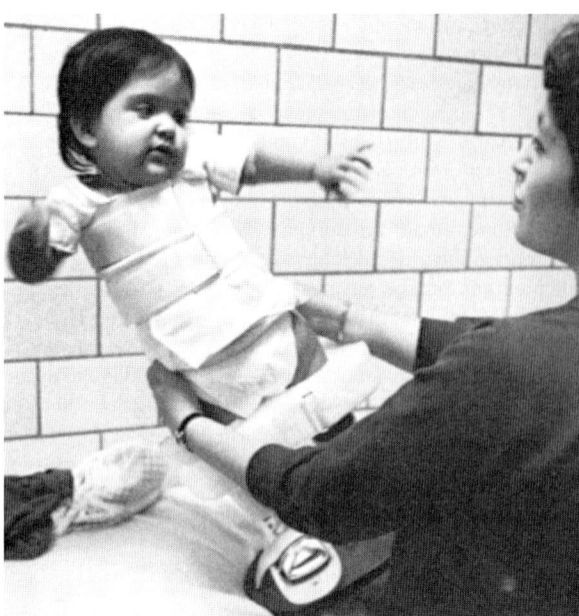

Fig. 13.21 Weight Shift and Forward Rotation in Standing Frame.

design and effectiveness of the orthosis, effectiveness of PT intervention, environmental factors, upper-extremity strength and control, and cognitive level.[208,251] The best prognosis for ambulation is most often seen in the child who is not shunted and has good cognition, good quadriceps power, no deformity, a stable neurological condition, and hands-free sitting balance. Factors that may limit the potential for ambulation include hydrocephalus, high-level lesions, kyphosis or kyphoscoliosis, and unstable neurology.

Developmental progression preceding ambulation in spina bifida shows a high degree of variability.[252] A study on motor development and ambulation in children with spina bifida reported that those with greater muscle power of the lower limb muscles ambulated earlier and more frequently.[252] This study also reported that walking starts in some children during the first year of life and is seen increasingly more frequently until 6 years of age.[252] Those engaged in physical therapy programs aimed at achieving the specific goal of walking are also likely to make earlier strides toward ambulation, although this has not been formally studied. Those who have been enrolled in early body weight supported treadmilll training (BWSTT) programs as infants have demonstrated early stepping responsiveness, and it has been suggested that BWSTT training intervention could promote muscle strengthening and take advantage of neural plasticity to promote development of the neuromuscular patterns necessary to support the onset of gait. There is also potential to improve bone density, cardiovascular function, and the integrity of lower spinal sensorimotor function. Infants with spina bifida demonstrate developmental delay as early as 3 months of age, and BWSTT intervention during the first postnatal year has the potential to reduce this delay and promote earlier onset of gait in the population with spina bifida.[253] Efficacy of enhanced sensory inputs during treadmill stepping in children with spina bifida has also been examined. Increasing friction by using Dycem matting and enhancing visual flow by using a checkerboard pattern on the treadmill belt both appear to be more effective than the standard black treadmill belt in eliciting stepping.[254] A study on stepping responses in infants with spina bifida reported a decrease in number of steps per minute compared with typically developing peers (14.4 vs. 40.8 steps per minute) and a decrease in frequency of alternating steps.[255] In contrast to these interlimb coordination differences, the study reported that

within-limb step parameters in infants with spina bifida were quite similar to those in children who were typically developing.[255]

For thoracic and high-level lumbar lesions, a parapodium is often chosen. The parapodium was developed by the Ontario Crippled Children's Centre in 1970 and is similar to the standing frame except that hinges at the hips and knees allow for sitting and standing.[250] It also can be adjusted for growth and can accommodate orthopedic deformities. As with the standing frame, proper alignment of the parapodium is critical. The therapist, in conjunction with the orthotist, should check for correct standing alignment. The prevention of additional orthopedic deformities, development of good muscular control, and normal body image depend on a well-fitting orthosis.

After a pivoting gait has been learned with the parapodium, a swing-to or swing-through gait can be attempted. By 4 to 5 years of age, a swing-through gait, with the child using Lofstrand crutches, can usually be accomplished. Variations of the parapodium allow for easier locking and unlocking of hip and knee joints. A swivel or pivot walker also may be attached to the footplate. Another type of orthosis for the child with a thoracic or high lumbar lesion is the Orthotic Research and Locomotion Assessment Unit (ORLAU) swivel walker. It consists of modular design similar to that of the standing frame, with a chest strap and knee blocks attached to swiveling footplates.[256] Rather than the whole base moving forward, as when weight is shifted in the parapodium, in the swivel walker each footplate is spring-loaded and is able to swivel forward independently, thereby allowing for independent balance on one foot. The ORLAU swivel walker is manufactured in the United Kingdom, and assembly kits may be ordered; however, availability is limited.[257] Another parapodium in use is the Rochester parapodium. Separate hip and knee joints allow a variety of free movement for sitting and bending down. The lower portion remains rigid and supportive when hips are flexed. Therefore a child can bend and pick up objects from the floor, and the unlockable hip and knee joints will relock automatically on extension.

There is a perception that although children with myelomeningocele use orthoses effectively, very few continue ambulation into adulthood. Two studies of patients with thoracic-level myelomeningocele[258] demonstrated that the ORLAU can be used effectively into the adult years. Both studies noted a 58% to 59.4% compliance rate. Patients in the studies who started using the ORLAU after 11 years of age continued use for 3 to 24 years. Children who do not ambulate had a fivefold increase in pressure sores and twice the number of fractures compared with those who did ambulate.[258] Vigorous walking programs should be considered to assist long-term health.[258]

Both the parapodium and swivel walker have had some problems with instability, ease of application, and cosmesis. New designs attempt to correct these problems.[259] Nevertheless, existing limitations in the parapodium and swivel walker, particularly energy cost of walking, slow rate of locomotion, and cosmesis, have limited their use, primarily to the younger child. These devices, however, remain an effective means of preventing musculoskeletal deformities caused by long-term sitting, wheelchair positioning, and general immobility. They also enhance social-emotional development gained from the upright position.[256,260]

Another option for the child with a higher-level lesion and good sitting balance is the reciprocating gait orthosis (RGO). This brace consists of bilateral long-leg braces with a pelvic band and thoracic extension, if necessary. The hip joints are connected by a cable system that can work in two ways: If the child has active hip flexors, he or she can activate the cable system by shifting weight and flexing the non-weight-bearing extremity. This brings the weight-bearing extremity into relative extension in preparation for the next step. Without hip flexors, the child extends his or her trunk over one extremity, thus positioning it in relative extension. By virtue of the cable system, the non-weight-bearing extremity moves into flexion, thus initiating a step. Several types of the RGO are in use, including the dual-cable LSU[261] and the horizontal-cable type. Most recently, the Isocentric Reciprocating Gait Orthosis (I-RGO) (Center for Orthotics Design, Campbell, CA) has been used for children with high-level spina bifida. It has a more cosmetic and efficient design compared with the dual-cable LSU or horizontal cable–type RGO. This cableless brace has two to three times less friction and is therefore more energy efficient. The brace stabilizes the hip, knee, and ankle joints and balances the person, enabling him or her to stand hands free without the use of crutches or a walker (Fig. 13.22). Leg advancement for walking occurs through use of hip flexor or lower abdominal muscle contraction or through use of active or passive trunk extension. In a study of 15 patients with lesions from T10 to L3, use of the RGO produced favorable results. It was used effectively by 13 of the 15 patients. Initial use of the RGO was initiated at 5 years, and 8 of the 15 discontinued use at 10 years of age. During the period of use, four became community ambulators, nine were household ambulators, and two remained nonfunctional (standing only). Average daily use ranged from 6 hours for those ambulating in the community to 30 minutes for those who were nonfunctional ambulators. Six of the 15 had no quadriceps power yet were able to functionally use the RGO for ambulation. Strong motivation and realistic goals are important to successful use.[262]

A more common means of maintaining the upright position has been through the use of long- or short-leg braces. Polypropylene braces and carbon-reinforced braces are considerably lighter than metal bracing and therefore reduce the energy cost of walking for the child with spina bifida. They allow close contact and can be slipped into the shoe rather than worn externally, thus affording the patient a better-fitting, more cosmetic orthosis.

The type of orthosis chosen (long-leg, with or without pelvic band, or short-leg) depends on the level of the spina bifida and the muscle power within that level (Table 13.3). Because lesions are frequently incomplete, muscle strength must be accurately assessed before bracing is prescribed. Independent sitting balance with hands free also is a prerequisite for use of long- or short-leg braces. Even children with L3 to L4 lesions who demonstrate incomplete knee extension may be able to use a short-leg brace with an anterior shell rather than requiring long-leg bracing.[263] This crouch-control AFO (CCAFO) will prevent a crouching gait pattern by improving knee extension during gait (Fig. 13.23).[264] Another alternative to a standard solid ankle AFO may be the carbon fiber spring AFO. This brace provides dynamic assist, supports the patient through the entire stance phase, and increases energy return during the third rocker phase of push-off, simulating the natural push-off action.[265] For children demonstrating excessive knee valgus caused by hip adduction, use of a Ferrari KAFO (FKAFO) may be considered.[266] The PT must work in conjunction with the orthopedist and orthotist to have each child fitted with the minimal amount of bracing that allows for joint stability and a good gait pattern.

Children with lower-level lesions (L5 to S1) who use below-knee bracing often develop the ability to or choose to ambulate without assistive devices. However, recent studies have shown that crutch use may decrease excessive pelvic motion, which results in reducing abnormal joint forces.[202,205] The use of crutches may prevent abnormal joint forces, maintain joint integrity, and decrease the risk of additional orthopedic complications.

The literature has suggested that the long-term use of crutch-assisted ambulation may result in long-term pathology. In patients with higher lumbar lesions (L3 to L4) who use Lofstrand crutches, the dynamics and kinematics of upper-extremity function were explored during swing-through and four-point reciprocal modes of gait. Although there were better joint kinematics in the shoulder and other upper-extremity joints during swing-through gait, kinetics were more problematic with increased force and torque in shoulder and wrist joints in those using a swing-through gait. Whereas the swing-through gait allows a potentially faster mode of ambulation, long-term use of this pattern may lead to increased upper-extremity pathology. Careful monitoring of all joints, including upper-extremity joints, during gait reassessment should be considered in order to deter and manage these potential issues that may compromise overall joint integrity and function.[267]

The excessive femoral torsion present in all newborns at birth does not decrease with growth and development in the child with spina bifida because of abnormal gait and activity.[99] Children ambulating with AFOs often show excessive rotation at the knee because of the lack of functioning lateral hamstrings. Rather than going to a higher level of bracing, a twister cable can be added, which often decreases the rotary component during gait.[99] Twister cables can be heavy-duty torsion or more flexible elastic webbing, depending on function. Typically, the young child who is just beginning to pull to stand and remains reliant on floor mobility as the primary means of mobility should have elastic twisters prescribed to allow for ease of creeping and transitions. The older and more active child will require heavy-duty torsion cables. Rotational stresses may eventually lead to the onset of late degenerative changes around the knee. A tibial derotation osteotomy may be indicated to prevent these changes from occurring.[99,204,268]

For children with low lumbar or sacral lesions who have at least fair strength in their dorsiflexors and plantar flexors, a University of California Biomechanics Laboratory (UCBL) or polypropylene shoe insert to control foot position is often the only bracing needed. These

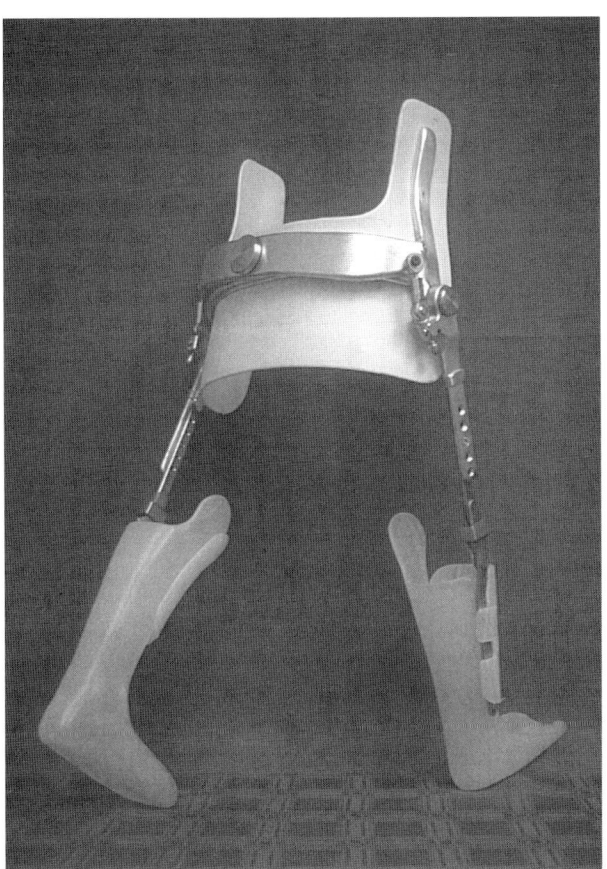

Fig. 13.22 Reciprocating Gait Orthosis.

TABLE 13.3   Common Gait Patterns and Levels of Assistance Required in Myelomeningocele

Level of Lesion	Muscle Performance	Recommended Level of Assistance and Bracing	Ambulatory Progression
T8–L1 and above	Flaccid LEs with fair to poor trunk	Parapodium: ORLAU, Toronto, Rochester Assistive devices often unnecessary with ORLAU but may improve function with Toronto or Rochester braces	
L1–L2	Flaccid LEs with hip flexors present	Parapodium with progression to RGO RGO, ambulating with hips locked	Begin ambulating with a walker, progress to forearm crutches Four-point or swing-through gait
L3–L4	Fair quadriceps with weak or absent hamstrings	HKAFOs may be used with severe lordosis because of weak or absent gluteal musculature and decreased trunk control or to control rotation and abduction and adduction. If quadriceps are less than fair strength, KAFOs may be needed As the patient progresses he or she may be cut down from KAFOs to AFOs; AFOs may be used with or without twister cables	Begin ambulating with a walker, progress to forearm crutches Four-point gait Begin ambulating with a walker and progress to forearm crutches. In some rare cases the patient may progress to no assistive device at all depending on the gait pattern With increased use of trunk reversal, the patient should be returned to forearm crutches to allow for a pattern that is more cosmetic and energy efficient Four-point gait pattern
L5	Good hip flexors and quadriceps; fair anterior tibialis; weak gluteus medius and maximus, toe extensors and gastrocsoleus	AFOs with or without twisters depending on gluteal strength AFO is used to prevent a crouch gait pattern from weak gastrocsoleus	Forearm crutches or no assistive devices Four-point gait
S1	Good hip flexors, quadriceps, gluteus medius, and toe extensors; weak gluteus maximus and gastrocsoleus	AFO	Generally, no assistive device is used unless decreased balance reactions or excessive lateral trunk flexion is present
S2–S3	Good hip flexors, quadriceps, gluteus medius and maximus, and gastrocsoleus	Often no bracing needed	Often no assistive devices needed

AFO, Ankle-foot orthosis; *HKAFO,* hip-knee-ankle-foot orthosis; *KAFO,* knee-ankle-foot orthosis; *LE,* lower extremity; *RGO,* reciprocating gait orthosis.

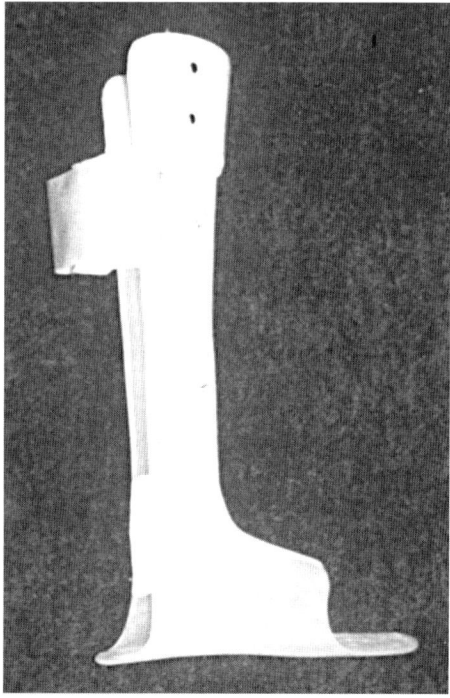

Fig. 13.23 Crouch Control Ankle-foot Orthosis.

inserts fit snugly inside the shoe and help control calcaneal and forefoot instabilities. A supramalleolar orthosis (SMO) will also fit easily inside the shoe but will provide additional medial and lateral support and stability that an insert would not provide. Even though a child may be able to ambulate without an assistive device or bracing, consideration must be given to the stresses that occur at the joints that, over time, may lead to orthopedic deformity. The greatest risk of joint instability often occurs at the knee. Barefoot walking versus use of an AFO has shown increased instability, joint stress, and pain at the hip and knee as well as increased energy expenditure.[269–271] Even though children may be able to ambulate without the use of crutches, comparison of gait kinetics and kinematics of walking with crutches has shown a significant decrease of valgus forces at the knee and better overall alignment of the lower extremities.[205] Treatment aimed at strengthening the gluteus medius and maximus to aid in increasing pelvic stability and reducing kinematic compensations can also be important in the management of patients with lesions at this level to enhance their efficiency during ambulation.[272,273]

Gait training, begun as the child first starts to stand, can now continue in a more formalized manner. By using the appropriate orthosis and assistive devices (walker, crutches, or cane), each child must be helped to achieve the most efficient and effective gait pattern possible (see Table 13.3). As a part of gait training, the child should be taken out of the bracing and "challenged" so that righting and equilibrium reactions can be developed to their maximum. For example, having a child maintain balance while sitting on a ball or another movable surface (tilt board, trampoline) requires the participation of all available musculature, especially abdominal and trunk extensor muscles (Fig. 13.24). Strengthening available musculature is a primary objective in this phase of treatment. Slow gains in muscle strength are often the result of continued emphasis on strengthening during physical therapy. In addition to trunk muscles, the gluteus medius, gluteus maximus, and quadriceps are often targeted. Prone activities such as picking up toys while over a Swiss ball or moving around while prone on a scooter board require use of these muscles while providing an enjoyable exercise for the child. Therapists may use therapeutic equipment, such as the Lokomat, and LiteGait or robotic devices to assist in walking and gait training. Participation in hippotherapy and aquatic therapy programs at this age can also be beneficial. These treatment approaches can be used to improve muscle strength in general and the gait pattern when bracing is reapplied. Regardless of the strengthening activities chosen, the pediatric therapist has the special task of using creativity to involve the child in therapeutic play activities. The ideas for creative activities are limitless but essential for combining therapy with age-appropriate cognitive abilities.

Studies examining the effects of strength and endurance training in those with spina bifida[274–276] have demonstrated enhanced functional outcomes. These studies included individuals in wheelchairs as well as ambulators. Interventions aimed at strengthening those with spina bifida, including electrical stimulation,[277,278] behavioral treatment,[279,280] and motor skills training,[279] have been reported. The evidence supporting strengthening, using exercise, electrical stimulation, and motor

skills training, was recently examined in a systemic review.[281] This review synthesized six studies supporting interventions in strengthening.[275,277–282] The level of evidence for the studies was determined using the American Academy of Cerebral Palsy and Developmental Medicine Levels of evidence.[283] The total number of subjects in all of the six studies was 26 subjects. All six studies reported improvements in strength; however, only three noted statistically significant results. Although the evidence suggests the possibility of being able to increase muscle strength using these modalities, in this population one must interpret the results with caution owing to lack of rigor, small subject populations, and variability across studies.

Upper extremity strengthening exercises may be necessary for those with spina bifida. Upper extremity strength training can help maintain the ability to perform functional skills including transfer, pushing wheelchair, and use of assistive devices for walking such as walking and crutches. Upper extremity strength training can also help increase cardiovascular endurance and prevent injuries associated with overuse.

Spina bifida is a congenital-onset condition that requires intervention by the PT from infancy through adolescence. Most of the impairments and functional deficits described throughout this chapter last throughout a lifetime. Health providers familiar with the complexity of the secondary impairments should follow up with individuals with spina bifida on a regular basis. Physical therapy plays an important role in screening for potential problems and providing recommendations for maintenance of mobility and health-related fitness as well as promoting activity and participation for children with spina bifida. OTs within the school systems often provide interventions within the area of integration of perceptual function. However, additional research needs to be done to guide "best practice," as there is little support for those interventions that expert clinicians deem beneficial in the habilitation of these patients.

Obesity affects the ability for interaction and participation at multiple levels across the life-span of those with spina bifida. Obesity may affect independence in transfers and ambulation, self-care and mobility, as well as in personal social interactions at all ages. Some children may lose the ability to ambulate if they have excessive weight gain without a comparable gain in muscle strength. Often, the child with spina bifida may be the last to be asked to participate and/or the child's inability may affect his or her ability or willingness to participate in physical games and activities with peers. Obesity puts more pressure on skin, thereby increasing the already high risk of skin breakdown. It may make it difficult for the child to reach private areas of the body, thus interfering with hygiene. Equipment and orthotic needs can also be complicated by increases in weight gain and obesity as the child ages.

Studies using dual-emission x-ray absorptiometry (DEXA) have shown that those with spina bifida have significantly decreased lean body mass as compared with controls.[284] Children with spina bifida likely have lower metabolic rates secondary to decreased muscle mass and decreased ability to burn calories. Those with higher-level lesions often have greater issues with obesity owing to decreased lower-extremity muscle activity, decreased physical activity, and decreased overall muscle mass. Adult wheelchair users have been shown to require 1500 fewer calories per day, and overall nutritional intake should be lower for those with spina bifida than their typically developing peers.[285 287] A weight management program is recommended for both the ambulatory and wheelchair users. Interventions to address physical inactivity and obesity may include increased physical activity, regular exercise, behavioral modifications, nutrition education programs, and attention to weight control. Exercise programs targeting upper-extremity resistance combined with aerobic activities such as swimming and arm-cycling

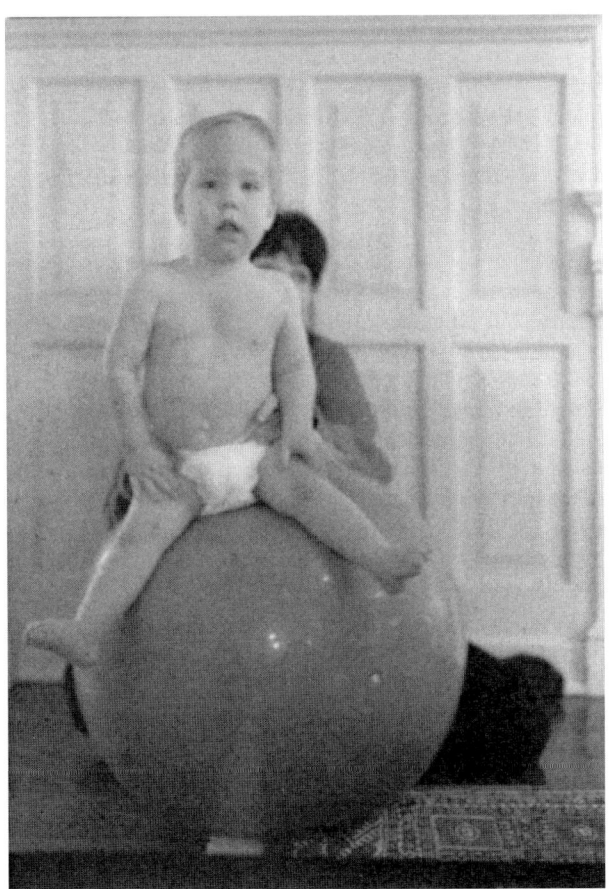
Fig. 13.24 Balance and Strengthening Exercises Done on a Movable Surface.

using arm-ergometry can be helpful in addressing obesity in those with spina bifida. Adolescents with spina bifida who used an upper-extremity cycling program that was integrated with video gaming three times per week for 16 weeks improved oxygen uptake and maximum work capability.[284,288,289]

Sensory limitations may impede progress during early ambulation training. Because of limited kinesthesia and proprioception, available sensory systems must be augmented, and the child must be taught to substitute with nonimpaired sensory systems. Impaired kinesthesia in children with spina bifida impedes their ability to anticipate changes in terrain and poses a safety problem. Vision may be the most relevant system that allows them to scan and preplan for changes in their walking environment. The parents and child should learn that the child is at risk of injuring a limb as the child cannot feel painful stimuli that might injure that limb. The parents and child should be educated to frequently check the position of the limb and observe the skin for any sign of irritation. They will also need to learn to check water temperature and use extra caution around extremely hot or cold objects. Tight or restrictive clothing and shoes should be avoided. Sensory deficits impact function and should be considered when teaching a child functional skills. Adding weight to the limb (ankles) or walker may supplement proprioceptive awareness and facilitate gait training.

Gait training and muscle strengthening are not the only consideration of the therapist. How cognitive and psychosocial development can be enhanced during this stage of the child's development is also important. One appropriate solution is to place the child in a center-based EI program. Although these programs may vary in the services they provide, most usually include age-appropriate play activities and some type of parental counseling. In addition, many offer therapeutic intervention from physical, occupational, and speech therapists. This intervention may occur in groups or individually and typically occurs in the child's natural environment.

In addition to the socialization that center-based EI programs provide for the child with spina bifida, they also teach the child age-appropriate ADLs, such as dressing and undressing. At this age, ADL skills are more appropriately taught in a group setting than individually. For many children the EI program, along with individualized therapy, is sufficient to enhance development in the physical, cognitive, and psychosocial realms.

Presently, when children reach the age of 3, public school education becomes available to them. The preschool or EC program continues to offer the same fundamental benefits as the EI program. It is the role of the EI therapist to communicate the specific needs of each child entering the public school system. In this way, continuity in the child's rehabilitation program is preserved.

The spina bifida team, usually headed by a pediatrician or clinical nurse specialist, continues to follow the child closely during this stage. The neurosurgeon checks shunt functioning and performs revisions as necessary. The orthopedist supervises bracing efforts to prevent and correct deformities in the spine and lower extremities. Well-child care and general medical treatment are the responsibility of the pediatrician on the team. The urologist continues to monitor renal functioning while keeping the child dry and free of infection. At this stage, the clinical nurse specialist will usually teach bowel and bladder training to the child and family. This clinician generally initiates this training according to age-appropriate developmental guidelines.

Bladder training usually consists of transferring the job of CIC from the parents to the child. Children as young as 3 years, but certainly by the age of 5 years, can learn CIC in a short period.[290] Children may first practice on dolls with male and female genitalia. Next, using mirrors to understand their own genital anatomy, they are able to accomplish the technique on themselves. CIC in conjunction with

pharmacotherapy is useful in achieving continence in children with spina bifida.[181] Another method of bladder training recently being used is intravesical transurethral bladder stimulation. This technique has allowed children with neurogenic bladder to rehabilitate their bladder function so that they can detect bladder fullness and generate effective detrusor contractions, leading to improved continence.[115,291]

Bowel training can be achieved through proper diet, regular evacuation times, and appropriate use of stool softeners and suppositories.[115] Constipation (and resulting bypass diarrhea) can be prevented by proper habit training and use of fiber supplements. Stool softeners (not laxatives and enemas) and suppositories should be used to keep the stools soft and help stimulate evacuation. Finally, toilet training, which amounts to scheduled toileting in time with the stool stimulants, usually achieves bowel continence. Surgical procedures, such as the Malone ACE procedure,[102] may be necessary when other interventions have failed. The Malone ACE procedure, performed in conjunction with a Mitrofanoff procedure to gain urinary continence, can help these patients attain a better quality of life. Consistency at each step along the way is the key to successful bowel training. A therapist may be called on to assist the parents and child in achieving independence in this ADL.

Other members of the team, such as the psychologist, social worker, and dietician, continue to function in their appropriate roles, interacting with the child and family as necessary. PTs and OTs, as members of the team, must collaborate with the efforts of other team members in the creation of their treatment plans.

Mobility and bladder and bowel dysfunction in toddlers and school-aged children represent ongoing stressors for parents of children with spina bifida. It has been noted by many that spina bifida represents a considerable challenge to all family members, particularly mothers. Family climate, parents' partner relationships, and social support networks play a considerable role in balancing stress and psychological adjustment for parents. Awareness of available systems of support for the patient and family as well as resources to which parents and their children can be referred for psychological and social support as needed are important for all health care practitioners.[292,293]

Primary School Through Adolescence

The primary school years and adolescence is a period when there is less rapid growth than earlier childhood and ends with a period of rapid physiological growth. Children in the 6- to 10-year age group are interested in a wider variety of physical activities as they challenge their bodies to perform. The adolescent, however, is going through a period of great sexual differentiation as primary and secondary sexual characteristics develop more fully.

Cognitively, children are able to solve problems in a more sophisticated manner, although they revert to illogical thinking with complex problems. As they reach adolescence, they become capable of hypothetical reasoning and their thought processes approach those of adults.

Emotionally, the 6- to 10-year-old is in a period of relative calm. Children are interested in schoolwork and are eager to produce. This is a period during which they are developing relationships outside of the family and beginning to assume an identity and autonomy. Problem-solving and decision making skills are at the crux of this time period. However, it is also challenging to promote independence and minimize self-reliant behaviors. Social passivity may ensue as "learned helplessness" behaviors emerge. Therefore professionals, including both PTs and OTs, should begin targeting independent function early and before adolescence.[294] Relevant family education regarding this issue should be inherent in all care plans, and independent behaviors should be promoted from very early on. Engagement in family decision making and opportunities for active problem solving have been linked to increased positive self-esteem and ego development.[295] During this time period, children with spina bifida are at risk for developmental delays in social functioning.[294]

School-aged children and adolescents are building the skills of the future, preparing them for adult work. This is a prime time to introduce and teach new skills while fostering increased autonomy and independence. Autonomy is difficult for the youngster with spina bifida. Motor skills impeding progress toward autonomy vary for each child and are dependent on the level of spina bifida as well as on any cognitive impairment. However, it has been observed that the motor skills hardest to attain are those that involve motor planning and that the process skills hardest to attain are those related to adaptation of performance and initiation of new steps. Thus guidance to learn not only how to do things but how to get things done is important.[296]

Interventions targeting independence have been embedded into various settings, including after school, adapted sports, and summer camps. O'Mahar and colleagues[297] report on one such camp program focused on campers 7 to 14 years of age the program emphasized individualized collaborative (i.e., parent and camper) goal setting, group sessions with psychoeducation and cognitive tools, and goal monitoring by the camp counselor. Campers reported significant gains in individual goals, management of spina bifida responsibilities, and independence.[297]

Children with spina bifida and disabilities, in general, do not participate in physical, recreational, and social activities to the same degree as typically developing children. Decreased participation in physical, recreational, and social activities is greater when children with spina bifida 6 to 12 years of age have medical issues such as a shunt for hydrocephalus and bowel and bladder issues. Participation for children with spinal bifida has been found to decline with age. School-aged children participate less than preschoolers, and adolescents participate less than school-aged children. Preschool is a time of intense learning in all domains—physical, intellectual, and social. As children get older, their physical participation declines. Thus the school-age years may be a time to encourage participation in physical and recreational activities. Participation in physical activities often foster social interaction, which is also needed at this age.[298]

Usually at this age, if it has not occurred previously, the evaluation of future ambulation potential occurs. The child whose larger size and limited abilities make ambulation more difficult each day frequently warrants this evaluation. Strength does not increase in the same proportion as body weight.[299] Ambulation, although possible for the young child, may be impossible for that same person as a young adult.

As the energy cost of walking becomes too high, the use of a wheelchair for locomotion often becomes appropriate. To a teenager whose emotional needs include a strong peer identity, transitioning to a wheelchair may foster increased independence owing to improved ability to participate and engage with peers. Appropriate alternatives may be to delay the decision to use a wheelchair full time or limit ambulation to short distances or to those places most important to the child. Again, goals must be tailored to the child's needs and encompass his or her whole being.

Although no guidelines include every patient, children with thoracic-level lesions are rarely ambulators by the late teens.[195,300,301] Those with upper lumbar lesions may be household ambulators with long-leg bracing but will require wheelchairs for quick and efficient mobility as adults. With low lumbar lesions, most adults can become community ambulators. Patients with sacral-level lesions are usually able to ambulate freely within the community. Many require minimal bracing and ambulate without assistive devices.[99,195] It must be remembered that ambulatory status is not determined by level of the lesion alone. The muscle power available; degree of orthopedic deformity; age, height, and weight of the patient; and, of course, motivation are also determining factors.[85,99,193,302]

For children and adolescents who continue to ambulate with orthoses, in accordance with the child's growth spurts, frequent adjustment or reordering of bracing will be necessary. Continual reevaluation of orthotic needs may reveal that the level of bracing may decrease as the child grows and becomes stronger; the opposite development is also a possibility. Ambulatory children must be taught to assess their skin for pressure areas or abrasions from orthoses and shoes. Those with sacral level lesions must be cautious with their choice of shoes/footwear.

Because a large number of older children with spina bifida will become full-time wheelchair users, potential problems connected with a sedentary existence must be properly managed. Skin care, always a concern for the child with spina bifida, becomes a priority for the constant sitter. Well-constructed foam, gel, or air-cell seat cushions are essential for distributing pressure evenly. Children should be taught frequent weight shifting within the chair to relieve pressure area as well as to use mirrors for self-inspection of the skin twice daily. Clothing should not be constricting but should be heavy enough to protect sensitive skin from wheelchair parts. Children must also be taught to avoid extremes of temperature and environmental hazards, such as radiators, sharp objects, and abrasive surfaces. The therapist must reinforce the importance of skin care to prevent setbacks in the rehabilitation process that may result when skin breakdown develops.

Children with higher-level lesions may need spinal support to prevent deformities. A polyethylene body jacket or thoracolumbosacral orthosis (TLSO) can be used to provide this support and, hopefully, prevent the progression of any paralytic deformities. Whatever type of device or wheelchair padding is used, the therapist must check to see that weight is distributed equally through both buttocks and that the spine is supported as needed. Part of the therapeutic intervention is to provide strengthening exercises or activities to be done out of the supporting orthosis. This is necessary to maintain existing trunk strength and to preserve the child's present level of function.

Generally, in late childhood or early adolescence, orthopedic deformities that have been gradually developing may require surgical intervention. Progressive scoliosis or kyphosis may require internal fixation when conservative methods fail.[303] Lengthening or release of tight or contracted muscles at the hip and knee is often required.[195] The iliopsoas, adductors, and hamstrings are frequently the offending muscles. These surgeries, followed by strengthening exercises and gait training, often add to the ambulatory life of the child with spina bifida. For example, in a child who displays an extreme lordotic posture, hip flexion contractures may be present and surgical lengthening of the tight muscles may be required to allow improved biomechanical alignment for standing and balance. A postoperative therapeutic program might include periods of prone lying to prevent future contractures and strengthen hip and pelvic musculature, core, and abdominals for stability and support to develop and maintain improved standing alignment. Gait training will be necessary to incorporate improved posture and alignment into the gait pattern.

Of primary importance during this stage is preparing the child for independence in ADLs, which may be broken down into self-care, locomotion-related, and social interaction activities. In conjunction with the nurse, PT, and OT, self-care skills of dressing, eating, and food preparation; general hygiene; and bowel and bladder care can be addressed. Because the adolescent is so concerned with achieving independence, he or she is more likely to comply with a regimen of strengthening exercises if shown how they relate to functional independence. A creative therapist may, for example, incorporate trunk

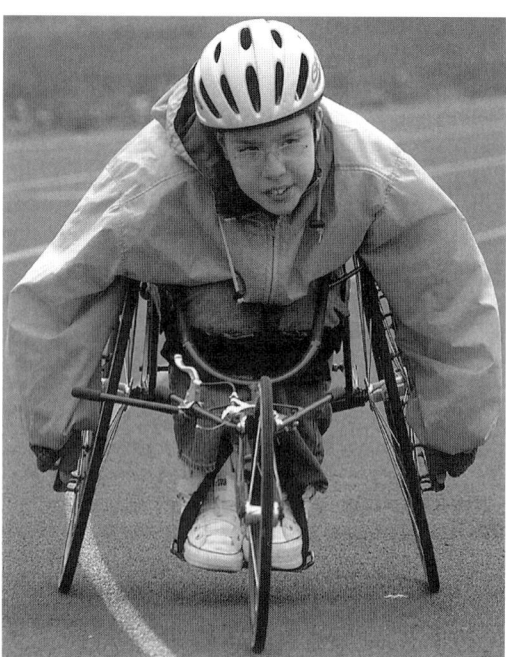

Fig. 13.25 Participation in Wheelchair Racing. (Courtesy Su Metzel.)

stability and upper-extremity strengthening work in activities such as making popcorn or getting ready for a dance. In addition, fostering social and recreational independence through adaptive sports and fitness programs and leisure activities should not be overlooked. Participation in adaptive sports can aid immensely in improving strength, endurance, and self-esteem. Community adaptive recreational programs may include T-ball, martial arts, swimming, tennis, basketball, skiing, bowling, and many other common sports and leisure activities (Figs. 13.25 through 13.27).

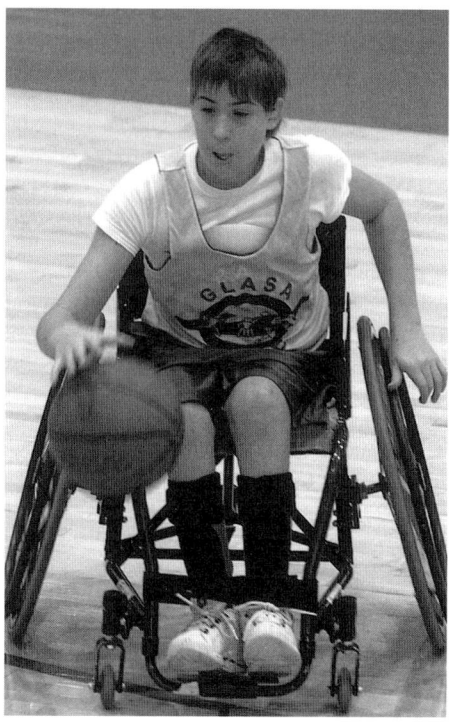

Fig. 13.26 Participation in Wheelchair Basketball. (Courtesy Su Metzel.)

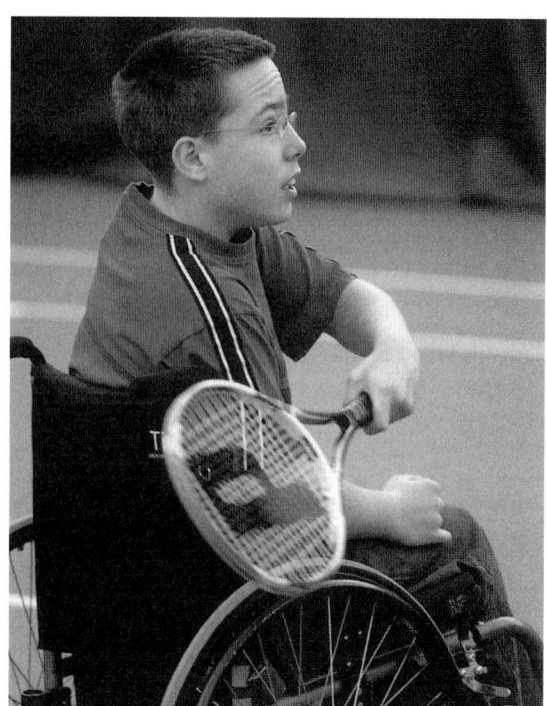

Fig. 13.27 Participation in Adaptive Tennis. (Courtesy Su Metzel.)

Locomotion activities should include all gait-related skills, such as falling down, getting up, and ambulation on various terrains and stairs. Transfers of all types should also be included in locomotion activities. Again, a creative therapeutic program helps make achievement of skills more palatable. For example, school-aged children may enjoy a competitive relay race situation in which each child falls, gets up, walks across the room, and sits down in a chair safely. This type of activity combines gait-training activities with group socialization and may meet a variety of goals (motor and psychosocial) at the same time.

The achievement of independence in ADLs for the child and adult with spina bifida does not depend solely on the level of paralysis. Also, important are psychosocial and environmental factors. Mean ages for the achievement of various ADL activities have been developed and may assist the therapist in establishing realistic therapeutic goals in this area.[304]

Often during this stage of rehabilitation, the therapist is asked to assist in assessing cognitive function. The perceptual and cognitive evaluations previously discussed may be administered and the results interpreted for parents and school personnel.

Also, as previously discussed, children with spina bifida have a general perceptual deficit that can manifest itself in a variety of ways. First, the child may have difficulty recognizing objects and the relations that they have to one another. He or she may therefore perceive the world in a distorted manner and have reactions that are unstable and unpredictable. These perceptual difficulties will most likely affect academic learning, and the child may associate failure with the learning process. At times, difficulties in attaining independence in ADLs may also be linked to perceptual problems. The perceptual difficulties of the child with spina bifida may result in emotional difficulties for the older child and adolescent, as they are not achieving independence to the same extent as their typically developing peers.[113]

Remedial programs that use a multisensory approach to developing perceptual skills, such as the Frostig Program for the Development of Visual Perception, have been effective in improving the visual perception of children with spina bifida.[113] Programs of this type are most effective when remediation begins early—preferably at or before the time the child enters school. Developmental optometry examination and remediation programs focusing on vision training may also be of benefit.

Children with spina bifida may also have difficulties with tasks requiring sensorimotor integration. Children requiring sensory integration therapy should be referred to a therapist certified in this area, most often OTs. Many appropriate activities for sensorimotor integration may be adapted from Ayres[305] or Montgomery and Richter, and are now being carried out in sensory gyms by certified therapists both physical and occupational.[306]

Regardless of the school setting chosen for the child, the therapist should be able to serve the classroom teacher as a consultant. Advice on adaptive seating and therapeutic goals appropriate for the classroom help ensure that the rehabilitation process will continue in the classroom as well as promote optimal conditions for learning.

When a child is moving from the preschool to the elementary school setting, the support of the therapeutic team is essential and invaluable. The teacher's expectations, as created by the therapist, regarding the child's special needs and abilities, often spell the difference between success and failure of complete academic and psychosocial integration within the school setting. Even though the child may no longer require direct therapeutic intervention, periodic consultation, including site classroom visits, is recommended to prevent minor problems from developing into major ones. For example, bowel and bladder accidents can be avoided by scheduling regular times for toileting. The teacher may be able to make minor adjustments in the teaching schedule to accommodate this scheduling. The PT should consult with and educate the teacher and classroom staff on how a child's braces and adaptive equipment operate to enable the teacher and staff to assist the child as needed.

The psychological perspective of the child colors therapeutic goals in this stage. As the child nears adolescence, these psychosocial aspects become of paramount importance. Although the therapist should not take on the role of the psychologist, collaborative efforts in the area of counseling will be necessary. Questions will arise many times during physical and occupational therapy sessions, requiring factual answers that the therapist can and should provide.

TRANSITIONS TO ADOLESCENCE

The consequences of the physical, medical, and cognitive effects of spina bifida extend into young adulthood and have an impact on quality of life.[307] Adolescence is a stormy emotional period. Adolescents remain in turmoil as they seek their identities through sexual, social, and vocational activities. As their value systems develop, they feel less ambivalence between remaining children and striving for independence.

Adolescents with spinal bifida are often unable to perform everyday tasks in an efficient and independent manner due to both lower motor abilities as well as lower processing abilities. Difficulties with motor planning and how to adapt body position impede the ability to accomplish a task efficiently. Processing skills hardest to achieve include adapting performance to the situation and the initiation of new steps. Therefore for the child with myelomeningocele, adolescence may not be the optimal time to introduce new skills leading toward self-care and independence. This needs to be introduced at a much younger age and consistently as the child develops. Adolescents with spina bifida need the opportunity not only to learn skills but how do get things done. It is important to inform parents and caregivers of children with spina bifida from an early age to provide the opportunity to practice skills as well as autonomy in the performance of everyday activities.[296]

TRANSITION TO ADULTHOOD

The transition to adult health care has lagged behind the medical advancements that have increased the number of survivals into adulthood.[308] As the individuals transition into adulthood, a unique set of challenges arise. Eighty-five percent of infants born with spina bifida will reach their adult years. Adults with spina bifida continue to present with unique long-term medical challenges. The health of adults with spina bifida can vary widely based on age, level of lesion, number and severity of comorbidities, functional skills achieved in childhood, degree of self-care skills, amount of family and community support, and access to medical care.[71]

Adults with spina bifida are at risk for the same secondary complications as children, but also have potential health concerns from the longitudinal effects of paralysis, weakness, sensory loss, hydrocephalus, immobility, neurogenic bowel and bladder, bone and joint deformity, and contractures and abnormal peripheral circulation.[71] In addition, there are potential complications from the lingering effects of childhood procedures such as ventricular shunting, urinary and continence procedures, and orthopedic surgeries.[71] A prospective study reported the 25-year outcomes and medical needs of an original cohort of patients with spina bifida in a multidisciplinary clinic. Eighty-six percent of those patients had CSF diversion, with 95% who had undergone at least one shunt revision. For those who underwent a TCR, 97% experienced an improvement or stabilization in their preoperative symptoms. Forty-nine percent had scoliosis, with 43% requiring a spinal fusion. More than 80% of the young adults had social bladder incontinence. Twenty-three percent had at least one seizure. Approximately $\frac{1}{3}$ were allergic to latex, and six patients had experienced a life-threatening allergic reaction. Eighty-five percent of the individuals attended or had graduated from high school and/or college. The results of this study indicate that late deterioration is common in individuals with spina bifida. One of the greatest challenges today is establishing a network of care for these adults with spina bifida.[121]

For the adolescent with spina bifida, the transition to adulthood includes a new set of expectations. Independent mobility expands to driving or arranging public transportation and getting to the correct destination in unfamiliar surroundings for leisure and recreation, continued education, or job opportunities. Self-care includes performing ADLs but expands to household management and financial responsibilities. Social relationships expand to include long-term partnerships with friends and business contacts; encounters with equipment vendors, insurance professionals, and medical providers; and may include hiring, firing, and directing personal health care assistants.

For some adults with spina bifida, living independently in society is a difficult goal to reach. Approximately 50% to 70% of adults with spina bifida live with family or in an assisted-living arrangement. The individual with spina bifida continues to require assistance with management of and resources related to medical, rehabilitative, and social-emotional needs throughout adulthood.[215,309–311] Secondary impairments span a wide range of domains, but management of secondary health conditions is a priority in reducing mortality, deterioration of general health, and further impairments throughout the adult years. Renal, respiratory, and cardiac complications have been identified as frequent causes of death.[215] Living with the long-term consequences of spina bifida places increased demands on the musculoskeletal system, and the effects of aging can appear earlier than usual. Osteoporosis, increased risk of fractures, risk of osteoarthritis, muscular pain from overuse of the upper extremities with use of crutches and longer-distance wheelchair propulsion over all terrains, increased transitions for self-care management and routines, and abnormal stresses placed on the knee from weak hip abductors and calf muscles can lead to degenerative changes and joint pain. Obesity and weight gain resulting from a more sedentary lifestyle and hypertension, heart disease, and diabetes are common problems with aging.[312] Thinner and less elastic skin that is susceptible to breakdown, insufficient pressure relief and poor tissue perfusion, incontinence and perspiration, wound infections after surgical procedures, burns and bumps that occur to insensate limbs, and long-term immobilization during hospitalizations have been major sources of decreased skin integrity.[215,312,313]

Muscular strength, flexibility, balance, and endurance decrease during the aging process. Changes in the CNS affect memory, reaction time, and attention span. An increased risk of depression and anxiety has been documented in several studies that measure quality of life in the adult with spina bifida.[215,309,314] Secondary conditions in adults with spina bifida have been linked to admission rates to hospitals that are nine times higher than in the nondisabled population. Adults with spina bifida also have medical expenditures that are three to six times greater than those of adults without spina bifida.[215]

Additional unmet needs reported by adults with spina bifida are related to functional mobility, household management, and active recreation. Being independent with regard to mobility has been the most important determinant in quality-of-life surveys.[22,314] A review of the literature over the past few years has indicated high unemployment rates for people with disabilities. For those with spina bifida, 47% of adults were in competitive employment, 15% were in sheltered or supported employment, and 38% were unemployed or had never been employed.[315] Limited mobility accounts for only part of the high unemployment rate. Accessibility into public buildings is another factor that limits employment opportunities. Tight doorways, steep ramped entrances and exits, inefficient workstations, and unreliable public transportation all play a role in a lower employment rate. Universal design (broad-spectrum solutions that produce products and environments that are usable and effective for everyone), construction of newer buildings with attention to adjustable work tables for computers and equipment access for people with different body proportions, as well as wider doorways, lower counters, doors that open electrically, and bathroom modifications (for both manual and power wheelchair users) with Americans with Disabilities Act (ADA) specifications for building modifications will improve universal access for all people with and without disabilities. Modifications of bathrooms that accommodate wheelchair and crutch users, including different height grab bars and roll-in shower arrangements, sloping landscape for entrances and exits, and room modifications with lower counters and closet access, to name a few considerations, may enhance travel and leisure time and recreational opportunities. A study that reviewed life-span issues of people with childhood-onset disabilities reported that more than 50% requested more information on their specific medical condition and the consequences of this condition on adulthood recreation.[314]

Most adults with spina bifida use some form of assistive technology (AT) that plays a significant role in increasing independence at home and in the community.[309] A study on the use of AT among individuals with spina bifida indicated that 35% use bracing, 23% use walking devices, and 57% to 65% use lightweight wheelchairs (both manual and power assisted[309]). Mobility equipment needs change as people age. Therapists have expertise in adaption and modification and can recommend solutions for decreased mobility. Physical changes in the workplace and home to decrease excessive stress on joints while maintaining flexibility and musculoskeletal alignment for efficiency without pain may also be required. Evaluating the individual needs of the patient and locating and selecting the types of technology that may enhance the adult's personal care management and improve efficiency in household tasks may make the difference in helping the patient have a more satisfying quality of life. Cell phones, computer access, and watch

timers for pressure relief and personal care routines can all assist memory and organizational skills.[309]

AFO is the most frequent used orthosis for children with spina bifida. AFOs often help improve alignment and walking and prevent contractures and deformities dependent on the level of lesion. Some AFOs are made with carbon springs that store energy. Other leg and feet braces can be used to stabilize weak muscles and prevent malalignments. Crutches can be used to minimize the amount of weight bearing on the legs and hips. Crutch tips that can be changed to accommodate different surfaces (e.g., with spikes attached for snow and ice), forearm crutches with hand grips and forearm cuffs that distribute weight and reduce joint stress to shoulders and wrists, powered add-on devices for manual wheelchairs to reduce stress on painful shoulders, adjustable furniture, wrist rests, footrests, and arm supports to ensure correct posture and reduce cervical and lumbar strain are examples of current and experimental AT that may promote greater independence. Specific devices are supported by the individual needs assessment of the patient by the therapist and education in the device's maintenance for appropriate use and durability. It is beyond the scope of this chapter to discuss specific equipment items in detail.

The transition to adult health care has lagged behind the medical advancements that have increased the rate of survival into adulthood.[308] As individuals transition into adulthood, a unique set of challenges arise. Transitioning to health care providers can be challenging due to reduced family support, concerns with executive skills, and lack of access to knowledgeable adult care providers. Although some pediatric spina bifida clinics provide services to the adult population, many other clinics have age limits. Additionally, changes in insurance policies as the patient reaches certain age may require that the patient move to different providers or hospitals. One of the challenges to health care is finding access to health care providers who provide services for adults with special needs, in both the primary care setting and medical subspecialties.[38,308]

Resistance to health care transitioning is multifaceted and may come from the patient, family, or both. Transitioning to adult health care may involve leaving multidisciplinary care clinics to care from multiple specialists with less multidisciplinary or coordinated care. Lack of coordinated medical care is a significant issue as the adolescent transitions into adulthood. This may result in a lack of follow-up and missing treatment visits. Transition may be delayed due to lack of initiatives or motivation or anxiety about the change in providers. Decreased intellectual functions in some individuals with spina bifida may affect provider, parent, and patient readiness to transfer responsibility of important health care activities and decisions.[316] Resistance may also come from parents who may feel that a transition to adult care would begin to exclude them from the dynamics of care and decision making processes.

Lack of clinical guidance on how to transition from long-term pediatric providers to adult care may cause patients to miss routine primary care or subspecialty appointments.[316] A study on adult with spina bifida from 19 to 64 years of age reported that that 75% of the participants could not name their primary care physician and had not seen a medical professional in over a year.[215] In adulthood, lack of regular care or experiences care in adult care individuals with spina bifida may result in increased preventable secondary complications and higher rate of emergency department admission.

Transitioning from adolescence to adulthood involves acquiring adult life skills and experiences to manage health care tasks and decisions, as well as developing and learning a new role as a recipient of care in an adult setting.[316] It is possible that transitioning to adult care may provide patients with feelings of autonomy and independence in their abilities to manage care.

The transition to adulthood should be gradual and should include a coordinated approach involving the patient, family, and significant individuals involved in the patient's care.[316] The recommended age for starting the discussion on transition is 14 years but may occur earlier.[308] Discussions about the timing of the transfer of care should take place early among the patient, family, and pediatric provider and not during an acute medical crisis. A good support system including family support and motivation can facilitate the transition to adult health care.

Although some pediatric spina bifida clinics provide services to the adult population, many other clinics have age limits. Additionally, changes in the insurance policy as the patient reaches a certain age may require the patient to move to different providers or hospitals. Transitioning health care providers can be challenging due to reduced family support, concerns with executive skills, and lack of access to knowledgeable adult care providers.

Transitioning to adult health care may involve leaving multidisciplinary care clinics to care from multiple specialists with less multidisciplinary or coordinated care. One of the many challenges to adults with spina bifida is finding access to health care providers who provide services for adults with special needs, in both the primary care setting and medical subspecialties.[38,308] Lack of coordinated medical care and clinical guidance on how to transition from long-term pediatric providers to adult care may cause patients to miss routine primary care or subspecialty appointments.[316] A study on adult with spina bifida from 19 to 64 years of age reported that that 75% of the participants could not name their primary care physician and had not seen a medical professional in over a year.[215] In adulthood, lack of regular care may result in increased preventable secondary complications and higher rate of emergency department admission.

Five key elements have been identified as necessary elements for the successful transition from pediatric to adult medical care.[215] These include (1) early preparation and education of the individual and family, (2) flexible timing of the transition, (3) introduction to the transition clinic, (4) interested adult center providers, and (5) a coordinated transfer of care approach among the individual, family, pediatric primary care providers, and adult specialists. The barriers include child health care providers refusing to "let go," reluctance to leave a family-centered care program, and adult care providers having limited knowledge about or interest in caring for these individuals. Finding a primary care physician or physiatrist who can assist with identifying a team of health care specialists for referrals as needed is a major concern for this adult population. The Spina Bifida Association of America publishes a health guide for adults living with spina bifida, based on feedback from adults across the United States. The *Health Guide* was sponsored by a grant from the National Center for Birth Defects and Developmental Disabilities and the Centers for Disease Control and Prevention.

Spina bifida is a congenital-onset condition that requires intervention by the therapists from infancy through adolescence. Most of the impairments and functional deficits described throughout this chapter last throughout the patient's lifetime. Health providers familiar with the complexity of the secondary impairments should follow individuals with spina bifida on a regular basis. Both PTs and OTs play an important role in screening for potential problems and providing recommendations for the maintenance of mobility and health-related fitness. Optimal management of the adult with spina bifida involves more than the sum of the subspecialties. This requires interdisciplinary, coordinated care among all of the providers and health professionals. Optimal management involves assessing individual's strengths, weaknesses, and needs to anticipate future challenges and opportunities.

Sexuality and Reproductive Issues

There are limited studies of gynecological and sexual issues in patients with spina bifida. Generally managing the bladder and bowel is very important for sexual function and good hygiene.

Women with spina bifida and hydrocephalus may have early onset puberty and menarche.[71] Hydrocephalus may impact neuroendocrine function and the abnormal fetal development of the neurological system in spina bifida. Generally, the sexual capacity of the female with spina bifida is near normal. A woman with spina bifida has potential for a normal orgasmic response, is fertile, and can bear children.[317] High-dose folic acid supplementation is recommended prior to conception and during early gestation. The pregnancy, however, may be considered high risk, depending on existing orthopedic abnormalities. There have been some reports of congenital anomalies, but pregnancy outcomes are generally good.[318] Cesarean sections are common due to the neuromuscular and musculoskeletal changes of the perineum and contractures and deformities of the hips and lower extremities. The challenges of neuromuscular impairments, immobility, contractures, and deformities may impact menstrual hygiene. Several factors may impact sexual activity, especially positioning and sensation such as bladder and bowel function and hygiene, urinary or colon conduit and stoma, skin integrity, neuromuscular impairments, immobility, contractures, and deformities.

Affected males are frequently sterile and have small testicles and penises. The majority may have issues with erectile dysfunction. Their potential for erection and ejaculation depends on the level of the lesion. In general, the higher the neurological lesion level, the less likely the individual is to have typical function. Erection may be preserved in males with higher lesion level compared to individuals with lower motor neuron lesion. In many cases psychological problems may be a primary cause of sexual failure. Sexuality is not merely a process involving the genitalia; it also depends on a positive body image and a feeling of self-esteem that is nurtured from birth.[319]

Although great advances in medical management of children with myelomeningocele have been made, a contrasting lack of improvement related to sexual function and reproductive issues exists. Five factors have contributed to delayed social and sexual growth in these adolescents: (1) severity of the mental impairment, (2) poor manual dexterity, (3) lack of education, (4) overprotective parents, and (5) limitations in health care personnel's ability to address sexuality with individuals with physical disabilities and their families.[320] Either the parents or the child/patient may bring up questions about sexuality. Parents of children with spina bifida realize the need to teach their children about sexuality, but they often feel inadequate about doing so and are reluctant to bring up questions to health care professionals.[321] The therapist must be open, informed, and able to provide resources to both parents and children.

Adolescents and adults with spina bifida show great concern with regard to self-esteem and sexual function.[322] Some of these concerns appear directly related to efficient bowel and bladder management.[323] Strategies to cope with bowel and bladder difficulties, as previously outlined, combined with appropriate emotional support from family and medical personnel help alleviate this concern.

PSYCHOSOCIAL ADJUSTMENT TO SPINA BIFIDA

Because of the congenital nature of spina bifida, psychological adjustment is somewhat different from adjustment to a traumatic spinal cord injury or other disabilities that occur later in life. The psychological adjustment to this congenital disability must be considered from the perspective of the parents, the family, and, of course, the child.[324]

Although there is considerable variability in the degree to which children with spina bifida, their parents, and their siblings experience stress and adjustment difficulties, children with spina bifida are at risk for higher rates of stress and adjustment problems.[325] Parents of children with spina bifida may appear resilient, although they experience more stress than the parents of typically developing children.[325]

A longitudinal study concerning the psychological aspects of spina bifida showed that the parents go through a series of steps in the adjustment process. From birth to approximately 6 months of age, parents experience shock and bewilderment. Information given during this time may be disregarded, rejected, or misinterpreted. Health care professionals must therefore be prepared to repeat the same information to parents on several occasions during the first few years of the rehabilitation process. The period of the first 6 to 18 months of the child's life may be the most stressful for parents. Frequent hospitalizations during this time place increased pressure on the whole family. Parents are now able to fully comprehend the implications of their child's functional limitations and inability to participate in life. They begin to worry about the future and the impact of the disability on the rest of the family structure. The period from the age of 2 years through the preschool years is relatively peaceful. The parents are more concerned with toilet training, social acceptability, and general information on child rearing. They seem less aware of their child's cognitive limitations as he or she continues to develop into a relatively happy, well-adjusted child.

By the age of 6 years, children are becoming more aware of their limitations and parents are concerned about problems that may arise as their children enter elementary school. The child's psychological adjustment depends partly on the severity of his or her motor problems but primarily on the attitude of the parents and family and on the environmental conditions to which the child is exposed.[326,327]

Because of their disabilities, children with spina bifida are often denied small tasks or chores that promote a sense of responsibility. To promote emotional growth and psychological well-being, caregivers must be persuaded to let go. Children with spina bifida must develop responsibility and independence by being given the chance to interact and even compete with their peers. During adolescence, concerns regarding independent living situations and vocational placement must be addressed. With a foundation of strong support systems fostering emotional maturity, the future can be bright for the child with a congenital spinal cord injury.

Adults with spina bifida, like their younger counterparts, have difficulties in psychological adjustment and in fully engaging in the community. Depression and increased anxiety are common symptoms in those individuals. These symptoms may contribute to spending more time at home and less time outside and in social and community participation. The lesion level, functional abilities and skills, shunting, urinary and continence procedures, orthopedic surgeries, associated disorders and complications, and family support are among the key factors that contribute to psychological adjustment difficulties. In addition, there are other factors that may impose challenges to psychological adjustment in adults with spina bifida; The transition from pediatric health care to adult health care may be challenging. Individuals with spina bifida are less likely to attend college. They have less vocational opportunities and a lower employment rate compared with typically developing individuals. They form romantic relations at a lower rate and report a lower quality of life that tends to decline from adolescence to young adulthood. The participation in leisure and recreational activities tends to be low in adults with spina bifida. Appropriate emotional family support and psychological support, activities that provide social supports such as group exercises, and physical activities may assist in alleviating the psychological symptoms of depression and anxiety and may increase community engagement and participation.

REFERENCES

To enhance this text and add value for the reader, all references are included on the companion Evolve site that accompanies this textbook. This online service will, when available, provide a link for the reader to a Medline abstract for the article cited. There are 327 cited references and other general references for this chapter, with the majority of those articles being evidence-based citations.

14

Traumatic Spinal Cord Injury*

*Myrtice B. Atrice, Paula M. Ackerman, Kristen Webber, Elizabeth Pharo,
Elizabeth Sasso-Lance, and Rebecca Hammad*

OBJECTIVES

After reading this chapter the reader will be able to:

1. Describe the demographics, etiology, and mechanism of injury of spinal cord injury.
2. Discuss the acute medical management of people with spinal cord injury.
3. Describe the secondary conditions of spinal cord injury, the appropriate interventions, and the impact of complications on the rehabilitation process.
4. Identify the basic components of the examination process.
5. Identify patient problems based on the examination, establish appropriate goals, and plan individualized treatment programs for patients with a spinal cord injury.
6. Describe adaptive equipment available to increase function.
7. Discuss progression of each individual and the process of discharge planning throughout the rehabilitation process.
8. Describe functional expectations for individuals with complete spinal cord injuries.
9. Identify equipment needs for a given spinal cord injury lesion.
10. Describe various principles of neuroplasticity to promote recovery after spinal cord injury.

KEY TERMS

American Spinal Injury Association (ASIA) autonomic dysfunction
autonomic dysreflexia
body weight supported treadmill training (BWSTT)
bulbocavernosus reflex
complete lesion
deep vein thrombosis (DVT)
discomplete
dual diagnosis
Functional Independence Measure (FIM)
incomplete lesion
intermittent catheterization
locomotor training
lower motor neuron

mobile arm support (MAS)
neuroprosthetics
orthostatic hypotension
paraplegia
pressure injury
pulmonary embolism (PE)
robotic exoskeleton
spinal cord injury (SCI)
spinal shock
tenodesis
tetraplegia
upper motor neuron
venous thromboembolism (VTE)

Spinal cord injury (SCI) is a catastrophic condition that, depending on its severity, may cause dramatic changes in a person's life. SCI usually happens to active and independent people who at one moment are in control of their lives and in the next moment are paralyzed. Loss of sensation and loss of bodily functions can lead to dependence on others for even the most basic needs. To reduce negative impact, individuals with SCI need a well-coordinated, specialized rehabilitation program to assist them in maximizing the development of skills necessary to live a satisfying and productive postinjury life.[1-2]

A successful rehabilitation program requires a team of health care professionals who work in collaboration to address alterations in body function, increase the individual's independence in all daily activities, ensure long-term health and wellness, and return the individual to the highest level of community participation specific to that individual's life situation. Ideally, the team should include a physician, a case manager, an occupational therapist, a physical therapist, a recreational therapist, a prosthetist or orthotist, a nurse, a speech-language pathologist, a dietician, an assistive technologist, a respiratory care practitioner, a psychologist, a social worker, a vocational counselor, a rehabilitation engineer, and a chaplain.[3-5] The most important element determining success in any rehabilitation program is

---

*Videos for this chapter are available at studentconsult.com.

the patient's and caregiver's active participation throughout the rehabilitation process.

This chapter provides a general overview for the management of individuals with SCI throughout inpatient and postacute phases of the rehabilitation continuum. The information is intended to aid health care professionals in the treatment of individuals with SCI by providing guidelines to maximize each individual's return to their preinjury lifestyle.

SPINAL CORD LESIONS

SCI occurs when the spinal cord is damaged as a result of trauma, disease processes, vascular compromise, or congenital neural tube defect. The clinical manifestations of the injury vary depending on the extent and location of the damage to the spinal cord.

Tetraplegia

Tetraplegia (preferred to *quadriplegia*) refers to impairment or loss of motor and/or sensory function as a result of damage to the cervical segments of the spinal cord. Function in the upper extremities (UEs), lower extremities, and trunk is affected. It does not include brachial plexus lesions or injury to peripheral nerves outside the neural canal.[6]

Paraplegia

Paraplegia refers to impairment or loss of motor or sensory function as a result of damage to the thoracic, lumbar, or sacral segments of the spinal cord. Depending on the level of the damage, function may be impaired in the trunk and/or lower extremities. Also, the term paraplegia can be used to refer to cauda equina and conus medullaris injuries but not to lumbosacral plexus lesions or injury to peripheral nerves, which are considered outside of the central nervous system.[6]

Complete, Discomplete, and Incomplete Lesions

In a complete lesion, sensory and motor function in the lowest sacral segments (S4-S5) is absent postinjury.[7] The American Spinal Injury Association (ASIA) classification for this type of injury is the ASIA Impairment Scale (AIS) A. The ASIA Impairment Scale is determined by completion of the International Standards for Neurological Classification of Spinal Cord Injury (ISNCSCI) assessment.[6]

Discomplete injury is a relatively new term in SCI research and practice. It is defined as a lesion that is "clinically complete but which is accompanied by neurophysiological evidence of residual brain influence on spinal cord function below the level of the lesion."[8] Studies of people whose spinal cord injuries were considered complete under ASIA standards have shown that in a large percentage (84%), there was residual brain influence on the spinal cord below the level of the lesion.[8] The current gold standard for testing, the ISNCSCI, does not examine this aspect of SCI.

With incomplete lesions, there is detectable residual sensory or motor function below the neurological level and specifically in the lowest sacral segment. According to ASIA standards, any sensation in the anal mucocutaneous junction or deep anal pressure[6] indicates that the lesion is incomplete. If only sensation is preserved, the injury is classified as AIS B. If motor function in key muscles is maintained to some degree, patients may achieve level AIS C, D, or E classification. This testing will be reviewed further in this chapter.[6,9]

DEMOGRAPHICS

The number of people living in the United States today with SCI is between 247,000 and 358,000.[10] The incidence of SCI in the United States is approximately 17,700 new cases per year, 78% of which are

TABLE 14.1 Spinal Cord Injury Demographics

Mean age at injury	43 years
Gender	
Male	78%
Female	22%
Race/Ethnicity	
Non-Hispanic White	60.6%
Non-Hispanic Black	21.9%
Hispanic Origin	12.8%
Asian	2.7%
Other	1.3%
Native American	0.7%
Causes of Injury	
Motor vehicle accident	38.3%
Falls	31.6%
Violent acts	13.8%
Sports injuries	8.2%
Medical or Surgical	4.6%
Other	3.5%
Common Injury Sites[10]	
Incomplete tetraplegia	47.2%
Incomplete paraplegia	20.4%
Complete paraplegia	20.8%
Complete tetraplegia	11.5%
Normal	0.08%

Data from National Spinal Cord Injury Statistical Center. *Spinal Cord Injury: Facts and Figures at a Glance.* February 2018, Birmingham, AL, 2018, University of Alabama, National Spinal Cord Injury Statistical Center. Available at https://www.nscisc.uab.edu/Public/Facts%20 and%20Figures%20-%202018.pdf

males.[10] The average age at the time of SCI has increased steadily from 29 years to 43 years since the mid-1970s.[10] Vehicle crashes and falls are the top two causes of SCI and account for close to 70% of new cases each year. Table 14.1 lists additional demographics.

In 2015, the average length of inpatient stay was 45 days (11 days in an acute care facility and 34 days in rehabilitation). This was a slight decline from 2005, where the average length of inpatient stay was 50 days (12 days in an acute care facility and 38 days in rehabilitation), and a substantial decline from the 1970s when the average length of inpatient stay was 122 days (24 days in an acute care facility and 98 days in rehabilitation). The average yearly health care and living expenses vary according to severity of injury. In the first year, individuals with high tetraplegia spend an average of $1,102,403 (up from $829,843 in 2005), whereas individuals with paraplegia spend an average of $537,271 (up from $303,220 in 2005).[10] Approximately 30% of individuals living with SCI are rehospitalized, with the average rehospitalization lasting 22 days. Genitourinary disease is the leading cause of hospitalization, followed by skin, respiratory diseases, digestive, circulatory, and musculoskeletal issues as other leading causes. Additionally, the life expectancy for patients with SCI continues to increase but is still below the national average of persons without SCI. Mortality rates are significantly higher during the first year after injury, especially for severely injured persons. According to the National SCI Database, the leading causes of death after an SCI are pneumonia, pulmonary emboli, and septicemia.

SEQUELAE OF TRAUMATIC SPINAL CORD INJURY

As stated previously, most spinal cord injuries occur as a result of trauma, be it motor vehicle accidents, falls, violence, or sports-related injury. The degree and type of forces that are exerted on the spine at the time of the trauma determine the location and severity of damage to the spinal cord.[11] Injuries to the vertebral column can be classified biomechanically as flexion or flexion-rotation injuries, hyperextension injuries, and compression injuries.[12] Penetrating injuries to the cord are usually the result of gunshot or knife wounds.[12]

Spinal cord damage can also be caused by nontraumatic mechanisms. Circulatory compromise to the spinal cord resulting in ischemia causes neurological damage at and below the involved cord level. This can be caused by a thrombus, swelling, compression, or vascular malformations and dysfunction. Degenerative bone diseases can cause compression of the spinal cord by creating a stenosis of the spinal canal and intervertebral foramina. Stenosis can also result from the prolapse of the intervertebral disc into the neural canal. The encroachment of tumors or abscesses within the spinal cord, the spinal canal, or the surrounding tissues also can lead to SCI. Congenital malformation of the spinal structures, as in spina bifida, can compromise the spinal cord and its protective layers of connective tissue. Some of the more common diseases and conditions that result in compromise of the spinal cord include Guillain-Barré syndrome, transverse myelitis, amyotrophic lateral sclerosis, and multiple sclerosis.[9]

After the spinal cord has sustained trauma, cellular events occur in response to the injury and are classified in three phases of progression: acute, secondary, and chronic responses. The acute process begins on occurrence of an injury and continues for 3 to 5 days.[13] Abrupt necrosis or cell death can result from both mechanical and ischemic events. The impact of an SCI often causes direct mechanical damage to neural and other soft tissues as well as severe hemorrhaging in the surrounding gray and white matter, resulting in immediate cell death.[14–15] In the next few minutes after the insult, injured nerve cells respond with trauma-induced action potentials, which lead to increased levels of intracellular sodium. The result of this influx is an increase in osmotic pressure, or movement of water into the area. Edema generally develops in as many as three levels above and below the original insult and leads to further tissue deconstruction.[13,15,16] Increased levels of extracellular potassium and intracellular concentrations of calcium also result in an electrolyte imbalance that contributes to a toxic environment.[17–19] Abnormal concentrations of calcium within the damaged cells disrupt their functioning and cause breakdown of protein and phospholipids, leading to demyelination and destruction of the cell membrane.[18] The cascade of these events consequently contribute to a dysfunctional nervous system.

During this acute phase, evidence of spinal shock and neurogenic shock may be present. Spinal shock may begin 30 to 60 minutes after spinal trauma and is characterized by flaccid paralysis and absence of all spinal cord reflex activity below the level of the spinal cord lesion.[20] The length of time this condition lasts can range from about 24 hours after injury to several weeks.[21–22] Spinal shock represents a generalized failure of circuitry in the spinal neural network and is thought to be directly related to a conduction block resulting from leakage of potassium into the extracellular matrix.[23] Accurately determining the completeness of the lesion may be difficult until spinal shock is resolved. The signs of spinal shock resolution are controversial; however, the return of reflexes may be a good indication.[21] Neurogenic shock, on the other hand, refers to a life-threatening condition. It consists of hypotension, bradycardia, and peripheral vasodilatation caused by severe central nervous system damage resulting in loss of sympathetic stimulation to the blood vessels and unopposed vagal activity. This is common in patients with a SCI at the level of T6 or higher. An important goal of treatment in the first week after sustaining an SCI is to maintain a mean arterial pressure (MAP) of 85 to 90 mm Hg.[2,24–26]

The secondary phase of the injury occurs within the course of minutes to weeks after the acute process and is characterized by the continuation of ischemic cellular death, electrolytic shifts, and edema. Extracellular concentrations of glutamate and other excitatory amino acids reach concentrations that are six to eight times greater than normal within the first 15 minutes after an injury.[19] In addition, lipid peroxidation and free radical production also occur.[27] Apoptosis (a secondary programmable cell death) occurs and involves reactive gliosis. There is also an important immune response that adds to the secondary damage that may be a result of a damaged blood-brain barrier, microglial activation, and increased local concentrations of cytokines and chemokines.[28] The lesion enlarges from the initial core of cell death, expanding from the perilesional region to a larger region of cell loss.

In the chronic phase, which occurs over a period of days to years, apoptosis continues both rostrally and caudally. Receptors and ion channels are altered, and with penetrating injuries, scarring and tethering of the cord occurs. Conduction deficits persist due to demyelination, and permanent hyperexcitability develops with consequential chronic pain syndromes and spasticity in many individuals with SCI.[29] Changes in neural circuits result from alterations in excitatory and inhibitory inputs, and axons may exhibit some limited regenerative and sprouting responses.[19]

CLINICAL SYNDROMES

Some incomplete lesions have a distinct clinical picture with specific signs and symptoms. An understanding of the various syndromes can be helpful to the patient's team in planning the rehabilitation program. However, using a syndrome for classification is not recommended due to the fact that many clinical cases present as a variation of a syndrome versus presenting as a true syndrome. Additionally, there are no clear objective guidelines by which to define an incomplete injury from a syndrome.[30] Fig. 14.1 depicts the anatomy of the spinal cord,[9] which can be referred to as the various syndromes are described.

Central Cord Syndrome

Central cord syndrome is the most common of the SCI syndromes and accounts for about 9% of traumatic SCIs in adults.[31–32] In adults 45 to 50 years of age, hyperextension injuries in the presence of cervical spondylosis or spinal stenosis is the most common cause during a low impact accident or injury. Younger patients are more likely to have a flexion-compression injury during a high impact accident or injury, causing fracture or disc herniation.[9] However, it is suggested that injury occurs in the white matter of the lateral corticospinal tracts with diffuse axonal injury, and there is sparing of the central gray matter. Additionally, Wallerian degeneration may occur in axons nearby the injury site causing neurological impairment.[31]

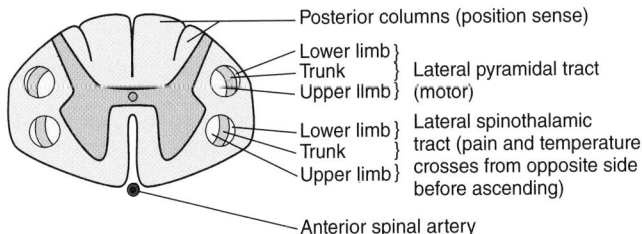

Fig. 14.1 Cross-Sectional Anatomy of the Spinal Cord.

Although the prognosis for functional recovery is good for individuals with central cord syndrome, the pattern of recovery is such that intrinsic hand function is the last thing to return. Most people with central cord syndrome will recover some level of ambulatory function, and over half will experience spontaneous voiding and bladder emptying. Slightly under half may gain some form of hand function.[9,31]

Brown–Séquard Syndrome

Occasionally, as a result of penetrating injuries (gunshot or stab wounds), only the lateral half of the spinal cord is damaged. Brown–Séquard syndrome occurs in 1% to 4% of traumatic SCIs and is characterized by ipsilateral loss of motor function and position sense and contralateral loss of pain and temperature sensation several levels below the lesion.[9,31] The prognosis for recovery is good. Nearly all patients attain some level of ambulatory function, 80% regain hand function, 100% have bladder control, and 80% have bowel control.[9] While rare in its pure form, this syndrome more commonly presents with features of central cord syndrome, sometimes called Brown–Sequard–plus syndrome.[6]

Anterior Cord Syndrome

Anterior cord syndrome, also known as anterior spinal artery syndrome, occurs in 2.7% of traumatic SCIs, and is often caused by flexion injuries in which bone or cartilage spicules compromise the anterior spinal artery, thereby impairing the blood supply to the anterior two-thirds of the spinal cord. Motor function and pain and temperature sensation are lost bilaterally below the injured segment, whereas light touch and proprioception are preserved. The prognosis is extremely poor for return of bowel and bladder function, hand function, and ambulation.[6,9]

Posterior Cord Syndrome

Posterior cord syndrome is rare, with an incidence of less than 1%. This results from compression by disc or tumor, infarction of the posterior spinal artery, or vitamin B12 deficiency.[32] Clinically, proprioception, stereognosis, two-point discrimination, and vibration sense are lost below the level of the lesion; and motor function and pain and temperature sensation are preserved.[9,32] Additionally, patients presenting with posterior cord syndrome may have bowel and bladder continence, allowing for increased functional return home.[33]

Cauda Equina Syndrome

Damage to the cauda equina involves the lumbosacral nerve roots, often sparing the cord itself. This syndrome is commonly caused by a burst fracture of a lumbar vertebrae or a centrally herniated disc and results in a lower motor neuron lesion that is usually incomplete. This lesion results in flaccid paralysis with no spinal reflex activity present. Sensation may be partially or completely lost, and sacral reflexes will be absent, affecting the lower urinary tract, distal bowel, and sexual function.[9,34] Bladder outcomes worsen the longer the cauda equina is compressed.[35] Due to the potential of lumbosacral nerve roots to regenerate, there is a more favorable prognosis for recovery.[32]

Conus Medullaris Syndrome

Typically caused by trauma and tumors, this syndrome is similar to cauda equina syndrome; however, the injury is more rostral and may involve the cord and be related to an L1-L2 bony injury. Clinically the presentation may appear mixed with characteristics of both upper and lower motor neuron lesions due to possible involvement of both the conus and the nerve roots. Sacral reflexes may be preserved depending on the level of the lesion and therefore may be overactive or acontractile.[6,9,34]

DUAL DIAGNOSIS: CO-OCCURRING BRAIN AND SPINAL CORD INJURY

Incidence reports of co-occurring brain and SCI range from 15% to 70%.[36–37] The significant variation in reporting of this co-occurrence is due to the diagnostic factors utilized by physicians immediately following injury. When imaging is the primary resource used to determine co-occurrence of brain injury with SCI, rates range from 16% to 24%. When posttraumatic amnesia is added as a diagnostic factor, rates increase to 42% to 50%.[38–40] According to the International Classification of Diseases, codes to classify brain injury are based on loss of consciousness and posttraumatic amnesia. Despite the frequency of co-occurring brain and SCI, this dual diagnosis tends to be undiagnosed or undocumented and therefore is often not adequately addressed during SCI rehabilitation.[38–41]

Co-occurring traumatic brain injuries are missed when the SCI or any other injury is prioritized for lifesaving needs.[38] Frequently, the initial paramedic and emergency department reports do not include information regarding the loss of consciousness and duration of posttraumatic amnesia. This lack of reporting leads to an underdiagnosis of brain injury. Unless significant cognitive deficits or a medical status change indicate the need for further diagnostic testing, the patient progresses through the continuum of care without a formal diagnosis of brain injury.

The rehabilitation team often notes signs, symptoms, and behaviors of brain injury in their documentation and team meetings. The rehabilitation process involves working with a team over an extended period of time, novel task training, and a holistic approach, which increases the likelihood that the patient will endorse behaviors, signs, and symptoms of brain injury. If the patient with a co-occurring brain and SCI is not managed and identified properly, they are commonly misperceived as being noncompliant, unable to learn, and/or having poor coping abilities, poor motivation, or a bad attitude.[41–42]

Patients with co-occurring brain and SCI require a longer inpatient rehabilitation length of stay to reach expected outcomes based on their SCI level. This allows for the opportunity to learn adaptive and compensatory techniques, which are typically acquired by their non brain–injured peers. If length of stay is not adjusted, evidence indicates that this population will experience a significant reduction in short- and long-term functional outcomes.[41–44] This population will endorse difficulties in functional motor tasks such as transfers, bed mobility, dressing, etc., due to poor motor planning, spatial awareness, and decreased executive functioning.[41,43–44] The therapy team should utilize the Rancho Los Amigos Brain Injury Severity Scale (Rancho Level) to guide the introduction of errorless learning versus errored learning.

Successful progression of the patient with a co-occurring brain and SCI requires the rehabilitation team to understand how the patient's cognitive status (Rancho Level) influences their stage of motor learning. Refer to the Box 14.1 for more information on the Rancho Los Amigos Brain Injury Severity Scale. Correctly identifying the stage of motor learning and crafting therapy to meet the patient's stage maximizes long-term functional gains (Box 14.2). Errorless learning is the ideal method for patients who meet criteria suggesting Rancho VII or less, because they are in the cognitive stage and just emerging to the associative phases of learning. Error-based learning (also known as trial and error learning) should occur later in the rehabilitation process, with individuals who are categorized as Rancho VIII or greater. It is important to note that continuing with errorless learning with patients who have the capacity to progress through the associative and autonomous stages of motor learning will result in reduced functional gains.[43–46]

BOX 14.1 Rancho Los Amigos Brain Injury Severity Scale

I	No Response	Completely unresponsive to stimuli
II	Generalized Response	Inconsistent and nonpurposeful response to stimuli
III	Localized Response	Specifically, but inconsistently to stimuli
IV	Confused-Agitated	Behavior is bizarre and nonpurposeful relative to immediate environment
V	Confused-Inappropriate	Responds to simple commands fairly consistently
VI	Confused-Appropriate	Goal directed behavior but is dependent on external input or direction
VII	Automatic-Appropriate	Appears oriented and appropriate within hospital and home setting, goes through routine automatically
VIII	Purposeful-Appropriate	Recalls and integrates past and recent events, responsive to environment

Fulk GD. Traumatic brain injury. In: O'Sullivan SB, Schmitz TJ, eds. *Physical Rehabilitation.* 5th ed. Philadelphia, PA: F. A. Davis Company; 2007:895–935).

BOX 14.2 Stages of Motor Learning

Stage	Patient Presentation	Ideal Environment for Patients in Stage
Cognitive Stage	Understanding the task is compromised and task performance has lots of variability	Quiet environment, extra time, and external cues
Associative Stage	Performance is refined but some errors or variability persist, internal cues from the learner are present	Environment can be distracting
Autonomous Stage	Performance of tasks achieved with few errors	Learning can be assessed formally with standardized measures

From Pohl PS. *Motor Learning. Topics in Physical Therapy: Neurology. An APTA Professional Development Home Study Course.* APTA; January 2002.

Proper management of patient with co-occurring brain and SCI requires a holistic approach, increased length of stay, and carefully crafted approach to learning. Establishing a patient-centered approach to care, adapting the environment, and the activity based on the patient's presentation are essential. In addition to these basic alterations, individuals working with an adult population with co-occurring brain and SCI need to be mindful to avoid language that may be perceived as patronizing, such a pet names, slowed speech, overly simplistic sentence structure, etc., to maintain the dignity of the patient and their family. With a comprehensive approach, patients with co-occurring brain and spinal cord injuries can make significant progress toward independence postinjury.

MEDICAL MANAGEMENT

Medical treatment for the acute SCI includes anatomical realignment and stabilization interventions, pharmacological management to

BOX 14.3 Principal Elements for Initial Medical Management of the Patient With Acute Traumatic Spinal Cord Injury[1,47–48,50–52]

- Resuscitate (maintain the airway)
- Immobilize at the scene—Emergency Medical Services (EMS)
- Rapid transport to the nearest spinal cord injury care facility
- Maintain airway and maintain mean arterial pressure (MAP)
- Steroids not recommended—consider steroids ONLY within the first 8 h post injury
- Radiographical assessment (computed tomography is initial study of choice)
- Immediate realignment of the spine; closed vs. open reduction
- Immobilize-external or internal orthosis
- Maintain MAP perfusion
- Magnetic resonance imaging for mass lesion, extent of cord injury
- Operative decompression early. Delay only for medical stabilization

lessen/prevent further neurological trauma and enhance neural recovery,[47–49] as well as to support all organ systems affected by this potentially catastrophic event (Box 14.3).

Immobilization/Transportation

The injured person should be triaged and immobilized at the accident scene by trained emergency medical personnel and transported to a level one trauma center. Immobilization is recommended for all trauma patients with a cervical spine or SCI or with a mechanism of injury having the potential to cause further damage. Immobilization for persons with penetrating injuries is not recommended due to increased mortality from delays in resuscitation. Additionally, immobilization is not recommended for trauma patients who are awake, alert, not intoxicated, without neck pain, without any abnormal sensory or motor changes, and are without any additional significant associated injuries. Once stabilized, transportation to a specialized SCI treatment center is recommended.[1,51–52]

Surgical Stabilization

In the emergency department, definitive radiological assessment and neurological assessment are the key factors to determine the medical course. Specific diagnostic studies are used to determine the severity, type, and degree of spine instability. Indications for surgical intervention include, but are not limited to, signs of progressive neurological involvement, type and extent of bony lesions, and degree of spinal cord damage.[53]

Cervical Spine

In the presence of instability and neurological compromise, surgical stabilization is usually indicated after a thorough radiological and neurological assessment. High-quality computerized tomography (CT) imaging is the recommended radiological assessment. The ISNCSCI examination is the preferred neurological assessment tool.[6] If high-quality CT is not available, routine 3-view cervical spine series (anteroposterior, lateral, and odontoid views) is recommended. Common surgical procedures include posterior and anterior approaches or a combination of both.[54] Fig. 14.2 shows radiographs of a person who had an anterior cervical fusion at C3-C4. Unstable compression injuries are usually managed by a posterior procedure except when there is a deficient anterior column. Anterior approaches are indicated for patients with evidence of residual anterior spinal cord or nerve root compression and persistent neurological deficits.

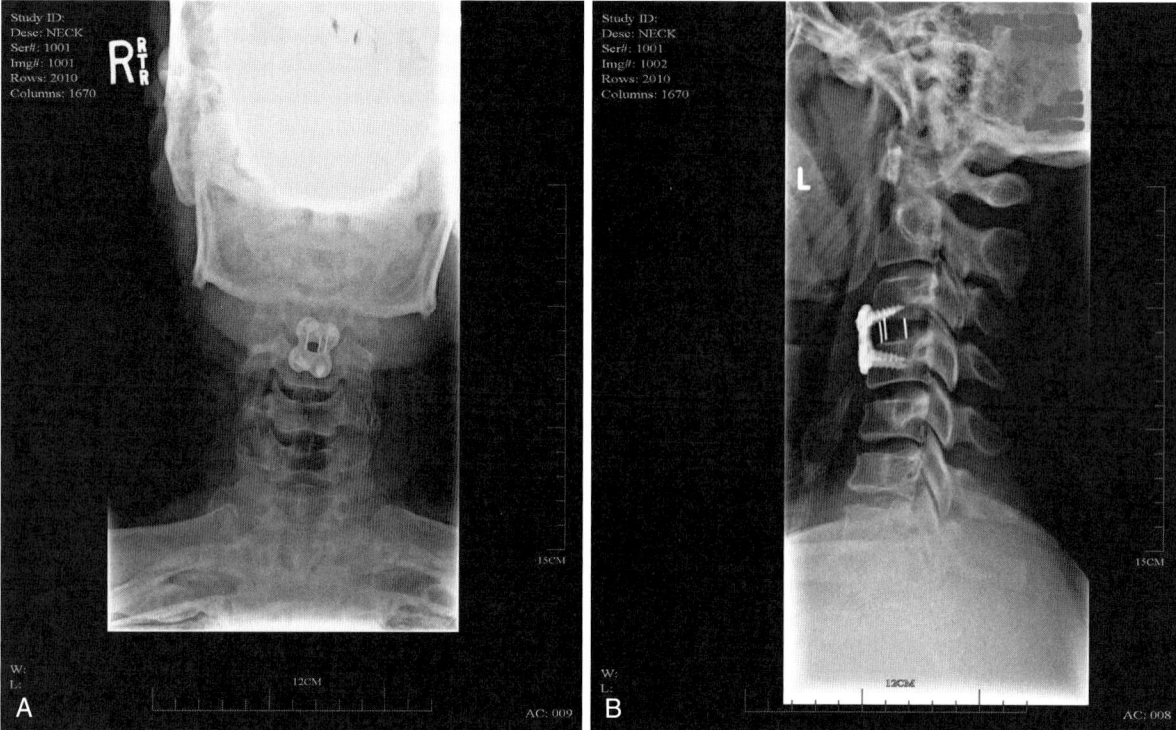

Fig. 14.2 (A) Radiograph of a person who had an anterior cervical fusion at C3-C4. **(B)** Lateral radiological view of anterior fusion C3-C4.

After cervical surgical stabilization, the use of a cervical orthosis is recommended. Examples of these orthotic devices are Philadelphia collar (Fig. 14.3), Miami collar, sternal-occipital-mandibular immobilizer (SOMI) brace (not pictured), and Aspen collar (Fig. 14.4). These orthotic devices are used until there is radiographical evidence of solid bony fusion, which usually takes 6 to 8 weeks, and/or at the physician's discretion.[55] When surgery is not indicated but external stabilization is needed to provide immobilization, halo vest immobilization may be used for closed reduction of the cervical spine.[1,56] The halo orthotic device restricts more movement in the upper cervical spine compared with the lower cervical spine. The halo device consists of three parts: the ring, the uprights, and the jacket (Fig. 14.5). The ring fits around the skull, just above the ears. It is held in place by four pins that are inserted into the skull. The uprights are attached to the ring and jacket by bolts.[1] The jacket is usually made of polypropylene and lined with sheepskin. This equipment is left in place for up to 12 weeks until bony healing is satisfactory.[55] The advantage of using the halo device is the ability to mobilize the patient as soon as the device has been applied without compromising spinal alignment. This allows the rehabilitation program to commence more rapidly. It also allows for delayed decision making regarding the need for surgery.

The disadvantage of the halo device is that pressure and friction from the vest or jacket may lead to altered skin integrity.[55] Special attention must be given to ensure the skin remains intact. During more active phases of the rehabilitation process, the halo device may slow functional progress because of added weight and interference with the middle-to-end range of upper-extremity movement. In a small percentage of patients, there are complications of dysphagia and temporomandibular joint dysfunctions associated with wearing the halo device.[55]

It should be noted that cervical traction using Gardner Well Tongs (not pictured) has been used much less in the last 25 to 30 years due to

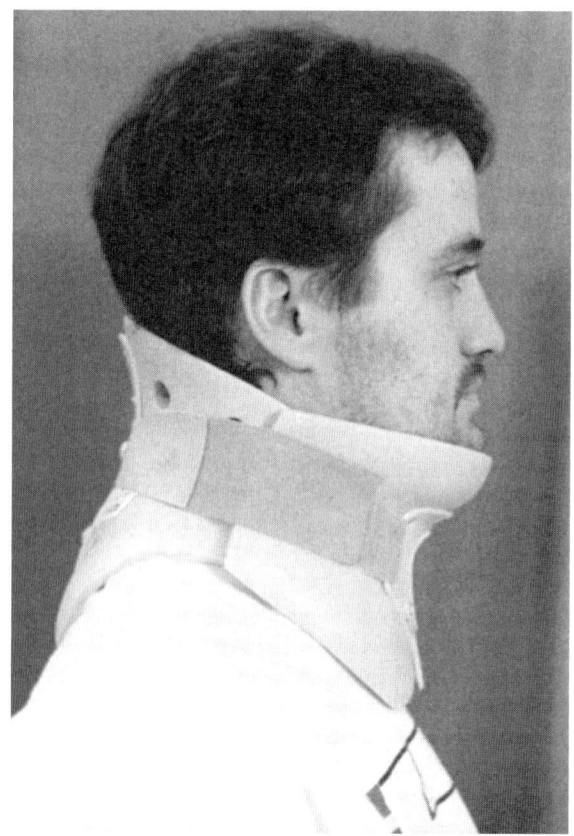

Fig. 14.3 Philadelphia Collar. It is fabricated of polyethylene foam with rigid anterior and posterior plastic strips; it is easily applied via Velcro closures, and it limits flexion, extension, and rotary movements of the cervical spine.

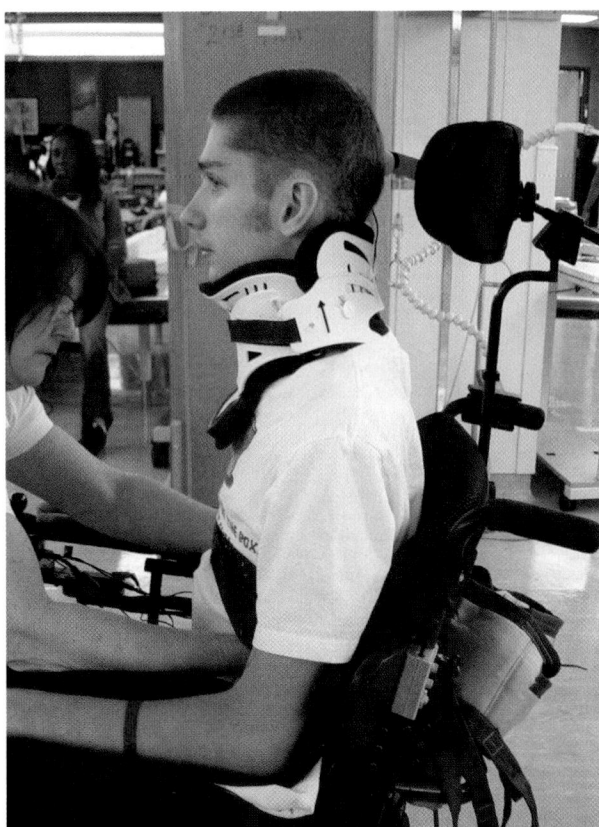

Fig. 14.4 The Aspen collar (formerly known as the Newport collar) encircles the neck, is somewhat open, and provides cervical motion restriction. It is rigid yet flexible at its edges to conform to each patient's anatomy. Pads and shells are removable and washable.

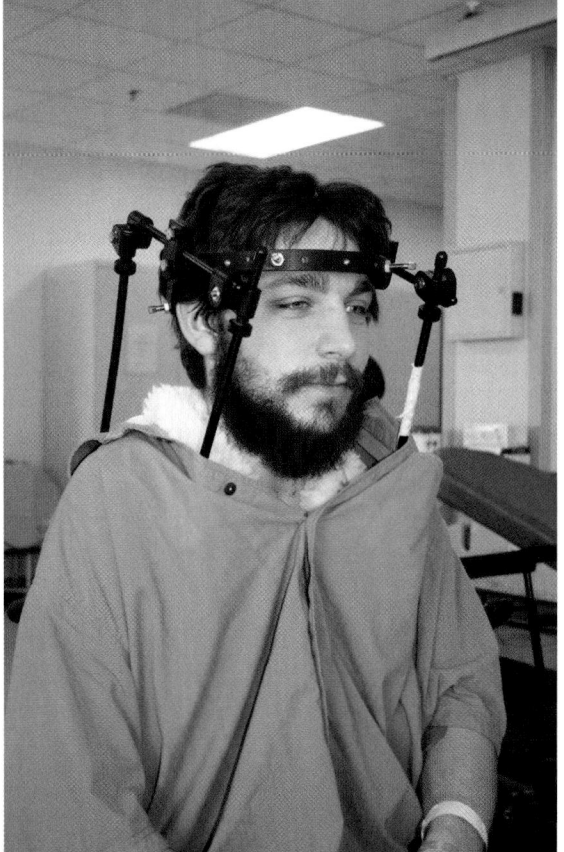

Fig. 14.5 Halo Orthosis. Basic components are the halo ring, distraction rods, and jacket (jacket not pictured).

improved surgical techniques but may be indicated when surgery is delayed due to life-threatening trauma in other areas of the body. The reader should be aware that the management of the pediatric SCI patient is more specialized and will not be addressed in this chapter.

Thoracolumbar Spine

Thoracic level SCIs account for approximately 35% of all SCI.[57] Internal fixation of the thoracolumbar region is necessary when stability and distraction cannot be maintained by other means. The timing of surgery has been a topic of debate. However, the consensus is that surgery should occur as soon as the patient is hemodynamically and respiratorily stable within the first 24 to 48 hours after the injury.[58-59] The surgical approach may be either anterior, posterior, or a combination of both based on the patient's radiological and neurological assessments. A commonly used thoracic stabilization procedure is transpedicular screws (Fig. 14.6). Surgeons may use the Thoracolumbar Injury Classification and Severity Score (TLICS) as well as the American Orthopedic Spine Group recommendations in the decision making process for surgical intervention.[48,60]

The goals of the operative procedures at any spinal level are to reverse the deforming forces by decompression, restore proper spinal alignment, and stabilize the spine.[54,61] All these procedures have advantages and disadvantages. The surgeon, patient, and family must be involved in the decision making process to select the most appropriate method of treatment. Assuring spinal stability sets the stage for a successful therapeutic rehabilitation process.[62]

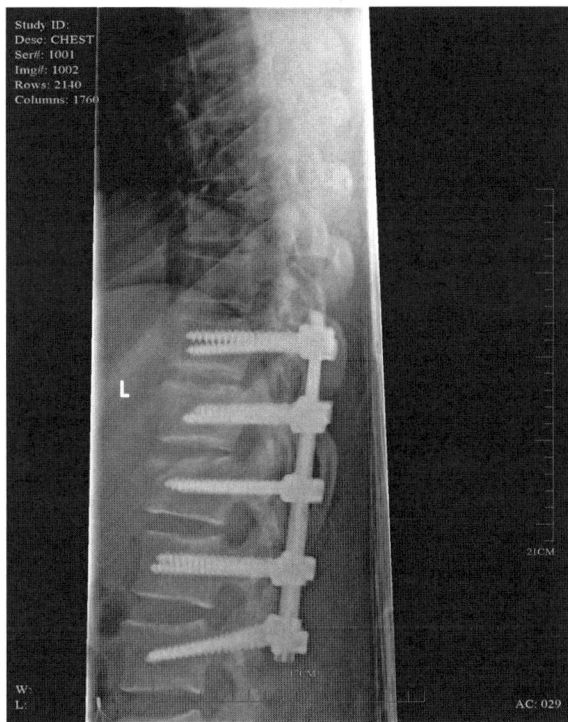

Fig. 14.6 Radiograph of Transpedicular Screws. (Courtesy Dr. H. Herndon Murray, Assistant Medical Director, Shepherd Spinal Center, Atlanta, Georgia.)

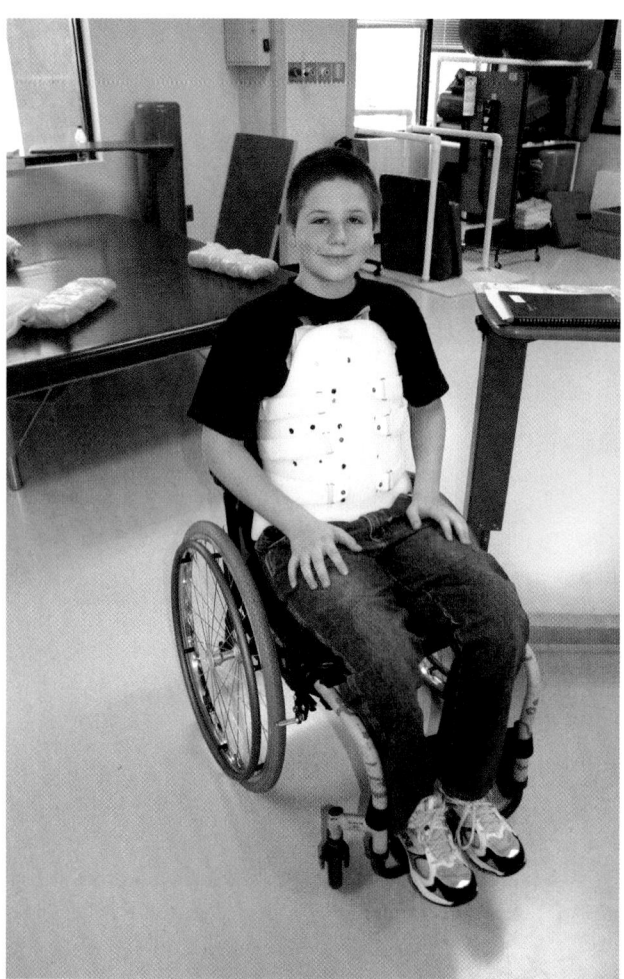

Fig. 14.7 Custom Thoracolumbosacral Orthosis. This molded plastic body orthosis has a soft lining. It controls flexion, extension, and rotary movements until healing of the bone has occurred.

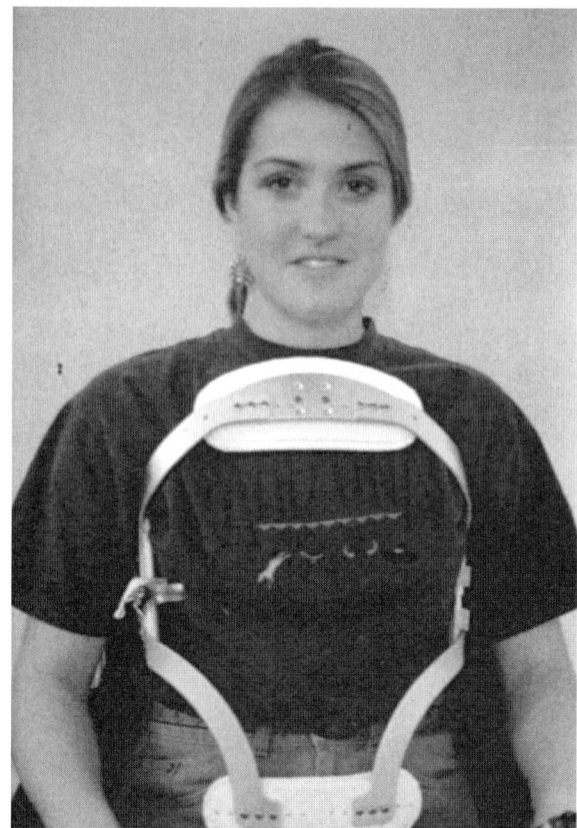

Fig. 14.8 Jewett Hyperextension Brace. A single three-point force system is provided by sternal pad, suprapubic pad, and thoracolumbar pad. Forward flexion is restricted in the thoracolumbar area.

Postoperatively, an external trunk support may be necessary to limit excessive vertebral motion and to maintain proper thoracic and lumbar alignment. This may be achieved by a custom thoracolumbosacral orthosis (Fig. 14.7),[63] Jewett brace (Fig. 14.8), or other appropriate orthotic device at the discretion of the surgeon. Spine precautions may be warranted following surgical intervention to allow for a complete fusion to take place and to minimize the possibility of surgical failure. The use of and specificity of postoperative precautions vary and are surgeon specific.

Clinical Trials and Ongoing Research

Much scientific work has been done in an effort to manage the cascade of cellular events following the primary SCI injury. The results of previous large phase II and III landmark investigations[47,50,52] aimed at neuroprotection[47,50,52] have been discredited through several meta analyses over the past decade. However, there is some consensus that the use of corticosteroids within the first 8 hours of injury is supported by level III scientific evidence and should be considered in appropriate instances. Knowledge[50] gained from past research has laid the foundation for ongoing investigations. Present research includes but are not limited to studies aimed at neuroprotection, neuroregeneration, spinal

cord stimulation, cell-based therapies, and the use of biomaterials (Table 14.2).[51,64]

THERAPEUTIC REHABILITATION CONTINUUM OF CARE

Therapeutic rehabilitation can be effectively delivered beginning in an acute-care setting at the time of injury and continuing on through a lifetime of care. Rehabilitation teams may use one of three models: multidisciplinary, interdisciplinary, and transdisciplinary.[66] The standards set forth by the Commission on Accreditation of Rehabilitation Facilities (CARF) suggest that the interdisciplinary model of team structure is optimal in the rehabilitation setting.

The continuum of care may be divided into several phases that include medical management (previously described), acute care (including the intensive care unit), inpatient rehabilitation, and post-acute services (including day program rehabilitation, outpatient rehabilitation, and home health). The continuum also includes returning the patient into wellness programs and community reentry outreach programs. The progression of a patient through the rehabilitation process will vary greatly from one person to the next. The patient may also move back and forth throughout the continuum of care.

Inpatient (Acute Care and Rehabilitation)

Inpatient rehabilitation begins during the critical and acute-care stages after an SCI. The primary emphasis of early rehabilitation is to lessen

TABLE 14.2 Summary of Current Topics in Spinal Cord Injury Research Related to Regeneration, Restoration, Recovery, and Neuroprotection (USA)[65]

Category	Intervention	Goal	Description	Example/Location
Regeneration	Biological: autologous human Schwann cells[65a]	Safety; repair myelin to improve axon function and improve neural plasticity	Schwann cells harvested from the sural nerve of the participant will be autologously transplanted into the epicenter of the participant's spinal cord injury	Miami project: Safety of Autologous Human Schwann Cells (ahSC)
	Biological: human embryonic stem cells[65b]	Safety; neurological recovery	Use stem cells to promote partial repair of spinal cord tissue	Asterias Biotherapeutics: Biological AST-OPC1
	Device: neural-spinal scaffold[65c]	Safety; facilitate repair of the spinal cord	An investigational bioresorbable polymer scaffold that is designed for implantation at the site of injury within a spinal cord contusion to provide structural support to the spared spinal tissue and a matrix to facilitate endogenous repair	InVivo Therapeutics: Inspire Study for Neuro-Spinal Scaffold
Restoration	Device: brain-machine interface[65d–f]	Safety of individual and efficacy of electrodes, improve function and restore movement	Brain-machine interface (BMI) technology is based on the finding that with intact brain function, neural signals are generated even though they are not sent to the arms, hands, and legs. By implanting electrodes in the brain, individuals can be trained to send neural signals, which are interpreted by a computer and translated to movement	University of Pittsburgh, University of Miami
	Device: implantable neuroprosthetic[65g]	Restore grasp and trunk function	Network of implantable systems to help increase functional independence	Cleveland, Ohio
	Drug and device[65h]	Develop new approaches to restore upper limb function	Paired pulse induced spike-timing dependent plasticity (STDP) enhances synaptic strength between residual corticospinal tract (CST) axons and spinal motoneurons (SMNs) resulting in temporary improvements in upper-limb function in humans with incomplete cervical SCI. Motor training will be combined with paired-pulse STDP stimulation to further enhance plasticity and behavioral recovery	Veterans Administration Office of Research Drug: Seromycin, Dextromethorphan; Device STDP
Recovery	Noninvasive brain stimulation:[65i–l] (electrical)	Restoration of upper-extremity (UE) function	Transcranial direct current stimulation (tDCS) or transcranial pulsed current stimulation (tPCS) provides regional brain polarization for neuromodulation; low voltage to increase brain excitability in order to make brain and nervous system respond to training or with activity	Shepherd Center, Burke Medical Research Institute: transcranial pulsed and direct current stimulation (tPCS and tDCS)
	Transcutaneous spinal cord stimulation (TSCS)[65m]	Improve muscle activity and function	Transcutaneous electrical stimulation applied over the cervical or thoracic spinal cord to target upper or lower extremities	Kennedy Krieger, University of Washington (UE), Shepherd Center (LE)
	Epidural spinal cord stimulation[65n,o]	Facilitate volitional movement, stepping	Establish the disinhibitory effect of spinal cord stimulation	University of Minnesota, University of Louisville
	Acute intermittent hypoxia (AIH)[65p]	Improve lower-extremity (LE) function and walking	Subjects breath lower levels of oxygen to trigger a cascade of events in the SC, which improve sensitivity and circuitry necessary for breathing and walking	Spaulding Rehabilitation Hospital; AIH

Continued

TABLE 14.2   **Summary of Current Topics in Spinal Cord Injury Research Related to Regeneration, Restoration, Recovery, and Neuroprotection (USA)—cont'd**

Category	Intervention	Goal	Description	Example/Location
Neuroprotection	Drug[65q,r]	Preserve neuro tissue and improve recovery	Administered early after injury to help prevention of cell death associated secondary injury that progresses after initial trauma	University of Miami, Ohio State University
	Diet: Ketogenic[65s]	Determine if ketogenic diet vs. standard diet significantly improves motor, sensory, and gut function	Determine if ketogenic diet (high fat, low carb) can be a neuroprotection against secondary injury cascade	University of Birmingham

U.S. National Library of Medicine. Published: January 1, 1993. Updated July 5, 2018. Available at: www.clinicaltrials.gov. Accessed September 4, 2018.

the adverse effects of neurotrauma and immobilization. This focus may last from a few days to several weeks, depending on the severity and level of injury and other associated injuries. Although therapeutic intensity may be limited, patients may begin participating in early therapy, which should include—but should not be limited to—out-of-bed activities, gaining upright tolerance, range-of-motion (ROM) exercises, early strength training, skin management, and education. Goals during this phase should focus on the prevention of secondary conditions and preparation of the patient for full rehabilitation participation. Discharge planning and caregiver training is initiated by the treatment team in this phase in order to ensure a smooth transition back into the community. Comprehensive discharge planning typically looks at discharge location, supervision or care needs, community resources, circle of support, advocacy, and insurance benefits for postacute referrals.

As the acute phase progresses, out-of-bed activities are tolerated for longer periods of time and the patient begins to work toward specific long-term goals. In accordance with Medicare guidelines for inpatient rehabilitation, the patient is able to participate in therapeutic programs a minimum of 3 hours a day.[67–68] The intensity of therapy may continue to be limited according to unresolved medical issues. As medical issues resolve and endurance improves, the patient will progress to a higher and more active level of participation. During inpatient rehabilitation, the patient gains varying levels of independence in activities of daily living (ADLs) and functional mobility. Community outings are used to refine advanced skills, identify further needs, and foster community reintegration and participation. Other aspects of rehabilitation during this phase are continuation of caregiver training, home exercise programs, assistive technology (AT) referrals, home and school or work evaluation, driving and dependent passenger evaluations, delivery and fitting of discharge equipment, and referrals for continued services.

Postacute Rehabilitation

Postacute rehabilitation and discharge from an inpatient rehabilitation program mark only the beginning of the lifelong process of adjustment to changes in physical abilities, community reintegration, and participation in life activities. Due to the shortened lengths of hospitalization and the reduction of inpatient and outpatient insurance benefits, services provided after discharge are becoming increasingly important. A direct consequence of shorter hospitalization results in patients who have more acuity, greater care needs, and fewer skills attained in the inpatient rehabilitation program before entry into

the postacute arena. Services provided after inpatient discharge may include home health services, day program, single-service outpatient therapy visits, wellness programs, and routine follow-up visits and services.

Home health referrals are often selected when home services are needed or when the medical acuity requires ongoing nursing assessment. The benefits of receiving care in the home allow for ADL and mobility training in that specific environment, whereas day program or outpatient therapy typically has more equipment and tools for skill progression. Common day program or outpatient therapy treatment programs have included advanced transfer training, advanced wheelchair skills, locomotor training, progression of ADL, home exercise programs, and finalization of durable medical equipment (DME).

There are a variety of outpatient rehabilitation options for individuals, and depending on the facility, the programs may be described as day program, outpatient therapy, or single-service outpatient therapy visits. One common thread for virtually all outpatient settings is that the patients are medically stable and do not require skilled nursing services during the night. The "day program" concept has emerged to meet the demand for more comprehensive rehabilitation services. The primary purpose of these services is to provide a coordinated effort for the patient to return to full reintegration into the community, with the focus on performance of functional skills, and on the transference of these skills into the community. Other outpatient rehabilitation options are "single-service," which indicates the patient has goals specific to a single discipline, such as physical therapy, occupational therapy, or speech therapy. Goals within each discipline are met, and there is a lesser degree of coordination of services. Wellness programs have emerged as an option for promotion of lifelong health. Typically, these programs are offered as a self-payment option and may not be tied directly to functional goals related to ADLs or mobility performance.

Regardless of what services the patient is referred for after the inpatient discharge, patients may progress from one option to another or may be appropriate to move in and out of services in a less linear fashion. Each stage of rehabilitation requires an examination of the patient's body function and structure, activity, participation levels, and personal and environmental factors. This is known as the International Classification of Functioning, Disability and Health (ICF), which is a framework from the World Health Organization.[69]

EXAMINATION AND EVALUATION OF BODY FUNCTION AND STRUCTURE

Regardless of where the patient begins the rehabilitation process, an examination is completed on admission. The examination and evaluation will assist in establishing the diagnosis and the prognosis of each patient as well as determining the appropriate therapeutic interventions. The patient and caregivers participate by reporting activity performance and functional ability.[55,70] Any pertinent additions to the history stated by the patient should be described. The patient's statement of goals, problems, and concerns should be included. The main areas of the examination are outlined here.

History

The history should include general demographics, social history, occupation and employment status, pertinent growth and development, living environment, health history and history of current condition, functional status and activity level, completed tests and measures, medications, family history, reported patient and family health status, and social habits.[71] Reviewing the medical chart is a vital step and should be conducted prior to hands on examination. If the history suggests a loss of consciousness or brain injury, the clinician should consider the possibility of compromised cognition and should include appropriate tests and measures during the examination.

Systems Review

The physiological and anatomical status should be reviewed for the cardiopulmonary, integumentary, musculoskeletal, and neuromuscular systems. In addition, communication, affect, cognition, language, and learning style should be reviewed.[71]

Tests and Measures

Depending on the data generated during the history and systems review, the clinician performs tests and measures to help identify impairments, activity limitations, and participation restrictions as well as to establish the diagnosis and prognosis of each patient. Tests and measures that are often used for persons with SCI are included in Box 14.4. For more detail related to specific tools, refer to the *Guide to Physical Therapist Practice (http://www.apta.org/Guide/)*,[72] *ANPT Outcome Measures Recommendations (EDGE)*, *Rehab Measures Database*, or *Spinal Cord Injury Rehab Evidence (SCIRE)*.[73–74]

Neurological Examination

American Spinal Cord Injury Association Examination

It is recommended that the ISNCSI be used for the specific neurological examination after an SCI.[6] See Fig. 14.9 for the ASIA motor and sensory examination form. Assessment of muscle performance allows for specific diagnosis of the level and completeness of injury. The examination of muscle performance includes each specific muscle and identifies substitutions from other muscles.

Along with the strength of each muscle, the presence, absence, and location of muscle tone should be described. The Modified Ashworth Scale is a common tool used to describe hypertonicity.[61,75] The patient's sensation is described by dermatome. The recommended tests include (1) sharp-dull discrimination or temperature sensitivity to test the lateral spinothalamic tract, (2) light touch to test the anterior spinothalamic tract, and (3) proprioception or vibration to test the posterior columns of the spinal cord. Sensation is indicated as intact, impaired, or absent per dermatome. A dermatomal map is helpful and recommended for ease of documentation.

BOX 14.4 Tests and Measures

Body System and Structure
Aerobic capacity and endurance
Anthropometric characteristics
Circulation (arterial, venous, lymphatic)
Cognitive functioning
Integumentary integrity
Joint integrity and mobility
Motor function
Muscle performance, including abnormal muscle tone
Neurological examination, including cranial and peripheral nerve integrity
Orthotic, protective, and supportive devices
Pain
Skeletal integrity and posture
Range of motion
Reflex integrity
Sensory integrity
Ventilation and respiration
Diagnosis of impairment and disabilities

Activity or Participation
Assistive and adaptive devices assessment
Community, social, and civic life (including educational level and work/school status)
Environmental barriers
Gait, locomotion, and balance
Self-care, domestic life, and home management

FUNCTIONAL EXAMINATION FOR ACTIVITY

It is recommended that a complete functional assessment is performed on initial examination and thereafter, in order to document progress. A myriad of standardized tools exists to assess functional skills that address home, community, and institutional mobility and ADL functional skills. The Functional Independence Measure (FIM) is one of the more commonly used tools that is currently applied for many impairment diagnostic groups, including SCI.[76] Another tool that is recognized as a primary outcome measure to assess functional recovery for the patient with SCI is the Spinal Cord Injury Independence Measure III (SCIM III).[77] This tool was specifically designed for the functional assessment of individuals with SCI. The SCIM III has been shown to be valid, reliable, and easily administered.[78–80] Other tools, such as the Quadriplegia Index of Function (QIF)[81] and the Craig Handicap Assessment and Reporting Technique (CHART),[82] are options. Additional assessments for patients with SCI are described in Table 14.3.

GOAL SETTING FOR ACTIVITY AND PARTICIPATION SKILLS

Goal setting is a dynamic process that directly follows the examination. Each activity limitation identified should be addressed with specific short- and long-term goals. The clinician must interpret new information continuously, which leads to continuing reevaluation and revision of goals.[71] Goals should always be individualized and directed by the patient and should be established in collaboration with the treatment team, the patient, and the caregiver, along with realistic consideration of anticipated needs on return to the home environment. Factors to consider in the goal-setting process include age, body type, associated

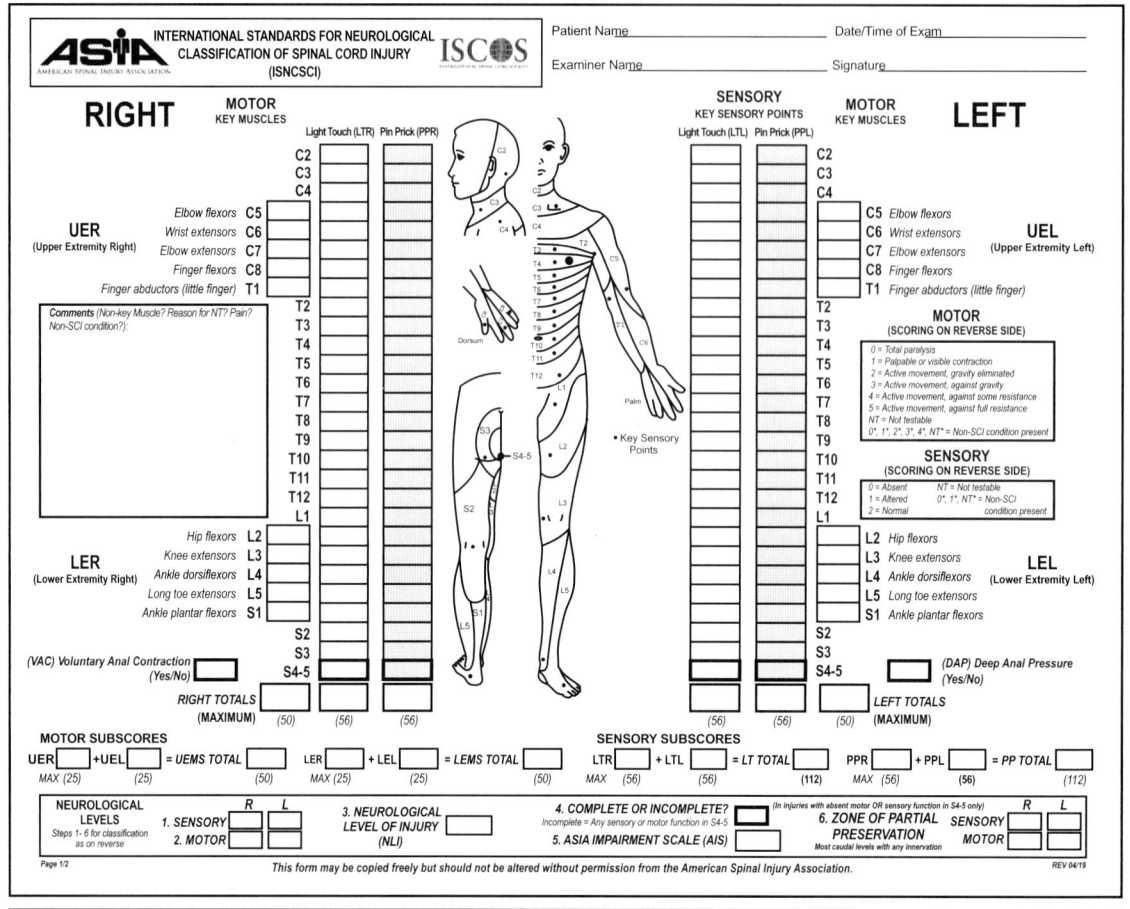

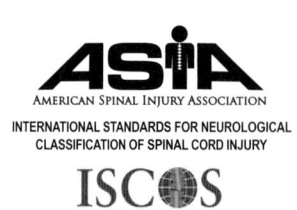

Fig. 14.9 American Spinal Injury Association Motor and Sensory Evaluation Form.

TABLE 14.3   Assessment of Function Summary

Overall Functional Assessments	Description
Spinal Cord Injury (SCI) Functional Assessments	
Spinal Cord Injury Independence Measure (SCIM)[83]	Designed for the functional assessment of individuals with spinal cord injury in the categories of self-care, respiratory, sphincter management, and mobility skills
Quadriplegia Index of Function (QIF)[84–85]	Assesses function for individuals with tetraplegia in the categories of transfers, grooming, bathing, feeding, dressing, wheelchair mobility, bed activities, bowel, bladder, and knowledge of personal care
Capabilities of upper extremity (CUE) instrument[86]	Assesses the action of grasp, release, and reaching in individuals with tetraplegia by measuring reaching and lifting, pulling and pushing, wrist action, hand and finger actions, and bilateral action
Walking Function Assessments	
Spinal cord injury functional ambulation inventory (SCI-FAI)[87]	Observational gait assessment that assesses gait, assistive device use, and walking mobility
Walking Index for Spinal Cord Injury (WISCI)[88]	An ordinal scale describing walking function that takes into consideration level of independence, assistive device use, and lower-extremity orthotic use
Six-minute walk test[89]	An endurance walking test that measures the distance walked over a 6-min period of time
Ten-meter walk test[90]	Measures walking speed by measuring how fast an individual walks a distance of 10 m
Timed Up-and-Go Test[90]	Assesses standing, walking, turning, and sitting
Wheelchair Function Assessments	
Wheelchair circuit[91]	Assesses the performance of various wheelchair propulsion skills by measuring ability, performance time, and physical strain for eight standardized skills
Wheelchair assessment tool[92]	Measures the ability and time to perform 6 mobility and wheelchair skills for individuals with paraplegia
Wheelchair skills test[93]	Assesses the ability to perform 50 separate skills in the areas of wheelchair handling, transfers, maneuvering the wheelchair, and negotiating obstacles
Obstacle course assessment of wheelchair user performance[94]	Assesses the wheelchair user's performance in 10 difficult environmental situations
Wheelchair users functional assessment (WUFA)[95]	A 13-item assessment of wheelchair skills in individuals who primarily use a manual wheelchair for their mobility
Wheelchair physical functional performance (WC-PFP)[96]	Assesses the ability to complete various tasks from the wheelchair by measuring upper body strength, upper body flexibility, balance, coordination, and endurance
Functional evaluation in a wheelchair[97]	Assesses functional performance from a manual and/or power wheelchair via a self-administered questionnaire

injuries, premorbid medical conditions, additional orthopedic injury, cognitive ability, psychosocial issues, spasticity, endurance, strength, ROM, funding sources, family and social roles, work and school status, and level of participation or motivation.

Long-term goals for the rehabilitation of patients with SCI reflect functional outcomes and are based on the strength of the remaining innervated or partially innervated musculature. Short-term goals identify components that interfere with functional ability and are designed to "address these limiting factors while building component skills"[55] of the desired long-term goals.

Functionally based goals are established in the following areas: bathing, bed mobility, bladder and bowel control, communication, environmental control and access, feeding, dressing, gait, grooming, home management, ROM and positioning, skin care management, transfers, transportation and driving, wheelchair management, and wheelchair mobility. Refer to Table 14.4 for anticipated goals for each level of injury. Information presented in this table should be

recognized as general guidelines because variability exists. These guidelines are most usefully applied to patients with complete SCI. Goal setting for individuals with incomplete SCI is often more challenging, given the greater variability of patient presentations and the uncertainty of neurological recovery. As with any patient, continual reevaluations provide additional insight into functional limitations, progression, and potential, thereby directing the goal-setting process. In addition to specific functional goals and expectations, other factors impacting goals should be considered, such as caregiver training, home, work, or school modifications, and community reentry.

Rehabilitation teams may elect to hold a goal-setting or interim conference for each patient, during which team members, including the patient, have the opportunity to discuss the long-term goals that have been established. It may be useful to request that the patient sign a statement acknowledging his or her understanding of, and agreement to, all long-term goals.

TABLE 14.4   Functional Expectations for Complete Spinal Cord Injury Lesions

Functional Component	Outcome Potential	Anticipated Equipment to Achieve Outcomes
C1-4		
Sitting tolerance	80–90 degrees for 10–12 h per day	Power wheelchair with power tilt, recline Wheelchair cushion
Communication Mouth stick writing	Minimal assistance	Mouth sticks and docking station
ECU	Setup	ECU
Page turning	Minimal assistance to setup	Book holder
Computer operation	Minimal assistance to setup	Computer
Call-system use	Setup	Call system or speaker phone
Cuff-leak speech (ventilator dependent)	Up to 6 h	
Feeding	Dependent, but verbalizes care	
Grooming	Dependent, but verbalizes care	
Bathing	Dependent, but verbalizes care	Reclining shower chair
Dressing	Dependent, but verbalizes care	
Bowel management	Dependent, but verbalizes care	
Bladder management	Dependent, but verbalizes care	
Bed mobility Rolling side to side Rolling Supine, prone Supine to and from sitting Scooting Leg management	Dependent, but verbalizes care	Four-way adjustable hospital bed to assist caregiver with task
Transfers Bed Tub, toilet Car Floor	Dependent, but verbalizes care	Overhead lift system Hydraulic lift Slings
Power wheelchair mobility Smooth surfaces Ramps Rough terrain Curbs	Modified independent Modified independent Modified independent Dependent, but verbalizes	Power wheelchair with power recline or tilt system Lap tray Armrests, shoulder supports, and lateral trunk supports
Manual wheelchair mobility Smooth surfaces Ramps Rough terrain Curbs Stairs	Dependent, but verbalizes	Manual reclining or tilt wheelchair with same options as power wheelchair
Skin Weight shift Padding, positioning Skin checks	Modified independent with power wheelchair Dependent, but verbalizes Dependent, but verbalizes	Recline or tilt wheelchair Wheelchair cushion Pillow splints, resting splints Mirror
Community: ADL-dependent passenger evaluation	Dependent, but verbalizes	Modified van
ROM exercises to scapula, upper extremity, lower extremity, and trunk	Dependent, but verbalizes	
Exercise program	Independent for respiratory and neck exercises	Portable or bedside ventilator (C1-3 only)

TABLE 14.4   Functional Expectations for Complete Spinal Cord Injury Lesions—cont'd

Functional Component	Outcome Potential	Anticipated Equipment to Achieve Outcomes
C5		
Sitting tolerance	90 degrees for 10–12 h per day	Power recline or tilt wheelchair Wheelchair cushion
Communication		
Telephone use	Modified independent	Telephone adaptations
ECU	Setup	ECU
Page turning	Setup	Book holder, wrist support with cuff
Computer operation	Supervision	Computer
Writing, typing	Setup	Long Wanchik brace
Feeding	Minimal assist to setup	Mobile arm support Adaptive ADL equipment
Grooming		
Wash face	Minimal assistance to setup	Mobile arm support
Comb or brush hair	Minimal assistance	Wrist support with adapted cuff
Oral care	Minimal assistance to setup	Adaptive ADL equipment
Bathing	Dependent, but verbalizes care	Upright or tilt shower chair
Dressing	Dependent, but verbalizes care	
Bowel management	Dependent, but verbalizes care	
Bladder management	Dependent, but verbalizes care	Automatic leg bag emptier
Bed mobility		
Rolling side to side	Dependent to maximal assistance	Four-way adjustable hospital bed to assist caregiver with care
Rolling		
Supine, prone		
Supine to and from sitting		
Scooting		
Leg management		
Transfers		
Bed	Dependent to maximal assistance for level transfers, verbalizes unlevel transfers	Overhead or hydraulic lift and slings
Tub, toilet		Possible transfer board
Car		
Floor		
Power wheelchair mobility	Recommended mode of locomotion	Power wheelchair with power recline or tilt system
Smooth surfaces	Modified independent	
Ramps	Modified independent	Recommend lap tray
Rough terrain	Modified independent	Armrests, shoulder supports, and lateral trunk supports
Curbs	Dependent, but verbalizes	
Manual wheelchair mobility		
Smooth surfaces	Dependent to minimal assistance for short distances on smooth surface	Upright or reclining wheelchair with special back and trunk supports
Ramps	Dependent, but verbalizes care	Consider manual wheelchair with power assist pushrims
Rough terrain	Dependent, but verbalizes care	
Curbs	Dependent, but verbalizes care	
Stairs	Dependent, but verbalizes care	
Skin		
Weight shift	Modified independent with power wheelchair Maximal assistance to dependent with manual wheelchair	Recline or tilt wheelchair and wheelchair cushion
Padding, positioning	Dependent, but verbalizes	Pillow splints or resting splints
Skin checks	Dependent, but verbalizes	Mirror
Home management		
Prepare snack	Maximal to moderate assistance	Wrist support with cuffs Adaptive ADL equipment

Continued

TABLE 14.4 **Functional Expectations for Complete Spinal Cord Injury Lesions—cont'd**

Functional Component	Outcome Potential	Anticipated Equipment to Achieve Outcomes
Community ADL		
Drive van	Independent	Highly adapted vehicle
Dependent passenger evaluation	Dependent	Modified van
ROM exercises to scapula, upper extremity, lower extremity, and trunk	Dependent, but verbalizes	
Exercise program		Airsplints or light cuff weights
Upper extremity and neck	Minimal assistance	E-stim unit
C6		
Sitting tolerance	90 degrees for 10–12 h per day	
Communication		
Telephone use	Modified independent	Adaptive ADL equipment
Page turning		Tenodesis splint
Writing, typing, keyboard		Short opponens splint
Feeding	Modified independent	Adaptive ADL equipment
Grooming	Minimum assistance to modified independent	Adaptive ADL equipment Tenodesis splint
Bathing		
Upper body	Minimal to modified independent assistance	Upright shower chair
Lower body	Moderate assistance	Various bathing equipment
Dressing		
Upper body	Modified independent	Adaptive ADL equipment
Lower body (bed)	Maximum to minimal assistance	
Bowel management	Maximum to modified independent	Dil stick Adaptive ADL equipment
Bladder management	Male: moderate assistance to modified independent	Tenodesis
	Female: moderate assistance to dependent	Adaptive ADL equipment
Bed mobility		
Rolling side to side	Independent to minimal assistance	Four-way adjustable hospital bed or regular bed with
Rolling		loops or straps; or no equipment
Supine, prone		
Supine to and from sitting		
Scooting		
Leg management	Minimum assistance to dependent	
Transfers		
Bed	Minimal assistance	Transfer board
Tub, toilet	Moderate assistance	
Car	Maximal to moderate assistance	
Floor	Dependent, but verbalizes procedure	
Power wheelchair mobility	Recommended mode of locomotion	Power upright wheelchair for weak C6
Smooth surfaces	Modified independent	
Ramps	Modified independent	
Rough terrain	Modified independent	
Curbs	Dependent, but verbalizes	
Manual wheelchair mobility		Ultralight upright wheelchair (recommended as primary only if scapulae grades are 3 or better)
Smooth surfaces	Modified independent	May need adaptations to facilitate more efficient propulsion (i.e., push pegs and plastic-coated handrims)
Ramps	Modified independent	
Rough terrain	Moderate to minimal assistance	
Curbs	Dependent, but verbalizes procedure	Consider manual wheelchair with power assist pushrims
Stairs	Dependent, but verbalizes procedure	

TABLE 14.4   Functional Expectations for Complete Spinal Cord Injury Lesions—cont'd

Functional Component	Outcome Potential	Anticipated Equipment to Achieve Outcomes
Skin		
Weight shift	Modified independent	Upright wheelchair with push handles
Pad, positioning	Moderate to minimal assistance	Mirror
Skin checks	Moderate to minimal assistance	
Home management		
Light home management	Minimal assistance	Various adaptive ADL equipment
Heavy home management	Dependent to moderate assistance	
Community ADL		
Driving vehicle	Modified independent	Modified vehicle
ROM exercises to scapula, upper extremity, lower extremity, and trunk	Minimal assistance	Leg lifter to assist with lower-extremity ROM
Exercise program	Minimal assistance	Cuff weights Air splints E-stim unit
C7-8		
Sitting tolerance	90 degrees for 10–12 h per day	
Communication		
Telephone use	Modified independent	Adaptive ADL equipment
Page turning		
Writing, typing, keyboard		
Feeding	Modified independent	Adaptive ADL equipment
Grooming	Modified independent	Adaptive ADL equipment
Bathing		
Upper body	Modified independent	Upright shower chair
Lower body	Modified independent	Various bathing equipment
Dressing (upper and lower body)	Modified independent for upper-body dressing	Adaptive ADL equipment
In bed	Minimal assistance to modified independent	
In wheelchair	for lower-body dressing	
Bowel management	Modified independent	Dil stick
Bladder management		
Bed	Male: modified independent	Various bladder management or adaptive ADL equipment
Wheelchair	Female: moderate assistance to modified independent	
	Male: modified independent	
Bed mobility		
Rolling side to side	Modified independent	Leg lifter
Rolling		
Supine, prone		
Supine to and from sitting		
Scooting		
Leg management		
Transfers		
Bed	Modified independent	Transfer board
Tub, toilet	Modified independent	May not need transfer board for even surfaces
Car	Minimal assistance for loading wheelchair	
Floor	Maximal assistance	
Power wheelchair mobility		
Smooth surfaces	Modified independent	Power upright wheelchair
Ramps	Modified independent	
Rough terrain	Modified independent	
Curbs	Dependent, but verbalizes	

Continued

TABLE 14.4   Functional Expectations for Complete Spinal Cord Injury Lesions—cont'd

Functional Component	Outcome Potential	Anticipated Equipment to Achieve Outcomes
Manual wheelchair mobility		
Smooth surfaces	Modified independent	Upright wheelchair
Ramps	Modified independent	
Rough terrain	Modified independent	
Curbs	Minimal to moderate assistance	
Stairs	Maximal assistance	
Skin		
Weight shift	Modified independent	Upright wheelchair with push handles
Pad, positioning	Minimal assistance to modified independent	
Skin checks	Minimal assistance to modified independent	Mirror
Home management		
Light home management	Modified independent	Various ADL equipment
Heavy home management	Moderate assistance	
Community ADL		
Driving vehicle	Modified independent	Modified vehicle
ROM exercises to scapula, upper extremity, lower extremity, and trunk	Modified independent	Leg lifter to assist with lower-extremity ROM
Exercise program	Modified independent	Cuff weights or e-stim unit
Paraplegia		
Sitting tolerance	90 degrees for 10–12 h per day	
Communication	Independent	
Feeding	Independent	
Grooming	Independent	
Bathing		
Upper body	Independent	Upright tub chair
Lower body	Modified independent	Long-handled sponge and hand-held shower hose
Dressing (upper and lower body)	Adaptive ADL equipment	
In bed	Modified independent	
In wheelchair	Modified independent	
Bowel management	Modified independent	Dil stick if positive bulbocavernous reflex
		Suppositories if negative bulbocavernous reflex
Bladder management	Modified independent	
Bed mobility		
Rolling side to side	Modified independent	
Rolling		
Supine, prone		
Supine to and from sitting		
Scooting		
Leg management		
Transfers		
Bed	Modified independent	May need a transfer board
Tub, toilet		
Car		
Floor		
Upright wheelchair		
Manual wheelchair mobility		Upright wheelchair
Smooth surfaces	Modified independent	
Ramps		
Rough terrain		
Curbs	Moderate assistance to modified independent	
Stairs (three or four)		

TABLE 14.4 Functional Expectations for Complete Spinal Cord Injury Lesions—cont'd

Functional Component	Outcome Potential	Anticipated Equipment to Achieve Outcomes
Ambulation Smooth surfaces Ramps Rough terrain Curbs Stairs	Depends on level of injury Modified independent for T12 injuries and below Will vary with higher thoracic injuries	Appropriate orthotics and assistive device(s)
Skin Weight shift Pad, positioning Skin checks	Modified independent	Mirror
Home management Light home management Heavy home management	Modified independent Modified independent	Various adaptive ADL equipment
Community ADL Driving vehicle	Modified independent	Hand controls for vehicle
ROM exercises to left extremity and trunk	Modified independent	Leg lifter to assist with lower-extremity ROM
Exercise program	Modified independent	Cuff weights and e-stim if any weakened lower-extremity muscles

ADL, Activity of daily living; *ECU*, environmental control unit; *ROM*, range of motion.

EARLY REHABILITATION AND COMPLICATION PREVENTION

Early rehabilitation of the patient with SCI begins with prevention. Of individuals living with SCI, 70% will have at least one complication or secondary condition (nonneurological) during their inpatient rehab stay; those with high cervical injuries (C1-4) are 2.2-times more likely to have at least one.[98] Preventing secondary conditions speeds entry into the rehabilitation phase and improves the possibility that the patient will become a productive member of society.

Table 14.5 describes an overview of the primary complications that can arise after an SCI. In this table, known causes and common management activities are reviewed. Tests and measures commonly used to determine the complication and the recommended medical and/or therapeutic interventions are listed in the table. Although various reports of incidences are published, the largest database is the Model Spinal Cord Injury Care Systems report.[99] Because of their high incidence and potential effect on long-term outcomes, the following conditions[98] require further discussion: skin compromise, loss of ROM or joint contractures, respiratory compromise after SCI, and urinary tract infections (UTIs).

Preventing and Managing Pressure Injury and Skin Compromise

After SCI and during the period of spinal shock, patients are at greater risk for the development of pressure injury.[115] The use of backboards at the emergency scene and during radiographic procedures contributes to potential skin compromise; therefore immediate concern for tissue death, especially at the sacrum, should be taken into account. Recently, padded spine boards have become available and are recommended to reduce the risk of skin complications. In addition to this immediate risk factor of immobility associated with severe injury, completeness of injury and age can increase the risk of pressure

injury[116,117]; some studies show a relationship between pneumonia and the incidence of skin compromise.[116]

Preventive skin care begins with careful inspection and a risk assessment.[101,115] Soft tissue areas over a bony prominence are at greatest risk for acquiring a pressure sore.[101,115] Key areas to evaluate include the sacrum, ischia, greater trochanters, heels, malleoli, knees, occiput, scapulae, elbows, and prominent spinous processes. A turning schedule should be initiated immediately. Even if the patient has unstable fractures or is in traction, he or she can be turned and positioned with flat pillows using the logroll technique. Even small changes off the sacrum and coccyx are helpful. The patient's position in bed should be initially established for turns to occur at least every 2 hours.[101] This interval can be gradually increased to 6 hours with careful monitoring for evidence of skin compromise. A reddened round area over the bone that does not disappear after 15 to 30 minutes is the hallmark start of a pressure sore, and action to avoid or minimize pressure in the area must be taken immediately to avoid progression. Turning positions include prone, supine, right and left side-lying, semi prone, and semi supine positions.[118] Secondary injuries such as fractures and the presence of vital equipment, such as ventilator tubing, chest tubes, and arterial lines, should be considered when choosing turning positions. The prone position is the safest position for maintaining skin integrity but may not always be feasible. Additionally, skin integrity and body type should be considered. Someone with fragile skin may require more frequent turns or weight shifts; an obese individual with excess skin folds may be at risk for moisture buildup, whereas someone with little soft tissue may have increased pressure on bony areas. A history of smoking or diabetes are other examples that impact skin health.[101,115]

Pillows or rectangular foam pads may be used to bridge off the bony prominences and relieve potential pressure. This is especially helpful above the heels. Padding directly over a prominent area with a firm pillow or pad may only increase pressure and should be avoided. Great care should be taken for regular checks if this bridging technique is used in the trunk or buttocks region while the patient is in bed,

TABLE 14.5   Complications After Spinal Cord Injury

Complication	Cause	Diagnostic Tests and Measures	Medical Treatment or Intervention	Therapeutic Intervention
Cardiopulmonary				
Pneumonia Atelectasis	Bacterial or viral infection, prolonged immobilization, prolonged artificial ventilation, and general anesthesia	Radiographical studies and diagnostic bronchoscopy	Antibiotics, bronchodilator therapy, therapeutic bronchoscopy, suctioning	Chest physical therapy: percussion, vibration, postural drainage, mobilization, and inspiratory breathing exercises
Ventilatory failure	Weakness or paralysis of the inspiratory muscles and unchecked bronchospasm	Pulmonary function tests (PFTs), arterial blood gases (ABGs), end-tidal CO_2 monitoring, and pulse oximetry	Artificial ventilation and supportive therapy, management of underlying cause (e.g., pneumonia), and oxygen therapy	Airway and secretion management treatment as above, early mobilization once stabilized, and biofeedback to assist with ventilator weaning as appropriate
Venous thromboembolism, including deep vein thrombosis (DVT)[a]	Venous stasis, activation of blood coagulation, pressure on immobilized lower extremity, and endothelial damage[61,100]	Doppler studies, leg measurements, extremity visual observation and palpation, and low-grade fever of unknown origin	Subcutaneous heparin[61,100] Prophylactic anticoagulation can decrease incidence to 1.3%[61,100] Vena cava filter for failed anticoagulant prophylaxis	Early mobilization and range of motion (ROM) for prevention, centripetal massage for prevention, compression garments, education about smoking cessation, weight loss, and exercise; avoid constricting garments and monitor overly tight leg bag straps and pressure garments (PVA 2016)
Pulmonary embolus	Dislodging of DVT	Ventilation-perfusion lung scan, signs and symptoms, including chest pain, breathlessness, apprehension, fever, and cough	Vena cava filter Anticoagulation therapy	None
Orthostatic hypotension	Vasodilation and decreased venous return and loss of muscle pump action in dependent lower extremities and trunk[61]	Monitor blood pressure with activity and changes in position and observation for signs and symptoms	Medications to increase blood pressure and fluids in the presence of hypovolemia	Gradient compression garments: Ace wraps, abdominal binders, and appropriate wheelchair selection to prevent rapid changes in position early in rehabilitation
Apneic bradycardia	True origin unknown; believed to be caused by sympathetic disruption resulting in vagal dominance in response to a noxious stimulus or hypoxia[61,100]	Electrocardiogram Heart rate Respiratory rate	Hyperventilation	Remove noxious stimulus
Integumentary System				
Pressure injury	Prolonged external skin pressure exceeding the average arterial or capillary pressure[101]	Wound measurements, staging classification, and nutritional assessment[101]	Nutritional support as needed, surgical or enzymatic debridement, surgical closure, muscle flap, skin flap or graft, and antibiotics as appropriate	Irrigation and hydrotherapy, dressing management, and electrotherapy[101]
Shearing	Stretching and tearing of the blood vessels that pass between the layers of the skin[101]	See pressure injury	See pressure injury	Add protective padding during functional activities, skill perfection, and correct handling techniques
Moisture	Excessive sweating below the level of injury, urinary and bowel incontinence, and poor hygiene	See pressure injury	See pressure injury, treat possible urinary tract infection, and medications for bladder incontinence	Protective barrier ointments and powders establish effective bowel and bladder programs, educate for improved hygiene, and refine activity of daily living (ADL) skills

TABLE 14.5   Complications After Spinal Cord Injury—cont'd

Complication	Cause	Diagnostic Tests and Measures	Medical Treatment or Intervention	Therapeutic Intervention
Neuromuscular and Musculoskeletal				
Spasticity	Upper motor neuron lesion[61] Deep tendon reflex spasticity scale evaluation	Ashworth or Modified Ashworth Scale Baclofen pump insertion[102]	Antispastic pharmacological agents: baclofen, diazepam (Valium), dantrolene Surgical intervention: myelotomy, rhizotomy, peripheral neurotomy[61] Botox injection	Prolonged stretching; inhibitive positioning or casting Cryotherapy, weight-bearing exercise, and aquatic therapy
Flaccidity	Lower motor neuron lesion. Most often in injuries at L1 level and below	Deep tendon reflexes (would be absent)	None	None for treating flaccidity; however, secondary treatments that need to be considered include positioning to improve postural support, education for skin protection, and bracing and splinting to maintain joint integrity
Autonomic dysreflexia	Triggering of an uncontrolled hyperactive response from the sympathetic nervous system by a noxious stimulus; noxious stimuli may include bowel or bladder distention, urinary tract infection, ingrown toenail, tight clothing, and pressure sore	Sudden rise in systolic blood pressure of 20-40 mm Hg above baseline observation of signs and symptoms: Sweating above level of injury Goosebumps Severe headache Flushing of skin from vasodilation above level of injury[61,103]	Catheterization of the bladder, irrigation of indwelling catheter, pharmacological management if systolic blood pressure is greater than 150 mm Hg Remove ingrown toenail if present	Immediately position the patient in upright position, identify and remove noxious stimuli, check clothing and catheter tubing for constriction, and perform bowel program if fecal impaction is suspected
Contractures	Muscle imbalance around joint; prolonged immobilization, unchecked spasticity, pain	Goniometric measurements	Tendon release; Botox injection for isolated spasticity	ROM functional use of extremity, casting or splinting, achieving and maintaining optimal postural alignment
Heterotopic ossification (HO)	Unknown	Alkaline phosphatase levels (increase after 6 weeks)[104,105]; observation[106] for sudden loss of ROM, local edema, heat, erythema, and nonseptic fever	Etidronate disodium (Didronel): use prophylactically or during inflammatory stage Surgical resection	Maintain available ROM; avoid vigorous stretching during inflammatory stage; and achieve and maintain optimal wheelchair positioning
Osteoporosis and joint changes degenerative	Bone demineralization	Bone scan	None; calcium supplement for prevention	Weight-bearing techniques: amount and type unknown, specific to spinal cord injury
Spinal deformities	Muscle imbalance or weakness around spinal column; poor postural support; and asymmetrical functional activities	Posture evaluation and seating evaluation	If severe: surgical fixation and thoracic orthosis	Restore postural alignment, avoid repetitive asymmetrical activities, and control spasticity
Genitourinary and Gastrointestinal				
Urinary tract infections	Presence of excessive bacteria in urine	Urinalysis, urine culture and sensitivity, temperature	Antibiotics	Monitor fluid intake and educate for proper technique during bladder care
Gastroduodenal ulcers, gastrointestinal bleeding	Acute: disruption of central nervous system, abdominal trauma or stress response to neuroendocrine system[107] Chronic: impairment of autonomic nervous system[103]	Hematocrit and hemoglobin; observation of gastrointestinal fluids	Surgical intervention; restore normal gastrointestinal function	Establish effective bowel program, establish high-fiber diet, and provide education and stress management

Continued

TABLE 14.5   Complications After Spinal Cord Injury—cont'd

Complication	Cause	Diagnostic Tests and Measures	Medical Treatment or Intervention	Therapeutic Intervention
Neurogenic bowel[108]	Refer to bowel management section	Positive bulbocavernosus reflex: indicates reflexic bowel	Oral laxative, suppositories, and enemas	Establish comprehensive bowel program
Other				
Thermoregulation problems	Interruption between communication with autonomic nervous system and hypothalamus Lack of vasoconstriction and inability to shiver or perspire[61]	Body temperature	Cooling or warming blanket if extreme	Education about risk and proper protection from elements; behavior modification, and education for proper hydration and appropriate clothing
Pain	Radicular pain originating from the injury,[109] kinematic or mechanical pain, direct trauma, and referred pain[61,111]	Pain scales, functional assessment,[110] and taxonomy	Immobilization and rest, pain medications, injections for pain, or antiinflammatory measures	Restore ideal alignment and posture, thermal modalities and electromodalities, manual therapy as well as improve movement patterns
Edema	Dependent position of extremity with loss of muscle pump; venous insufficiency; IV infiltrate; lymphatic system overload; trauma i.e., fracture; and systemic edema i.e., organ failure	Rule out VTE; circumferential measurements; volumeter; pitting scale	Medications to increase fluid return; review of medications contributing to edema	Elevation of extremity above heart; gradient compression garments; and complete decongestive therapy (CDT) with certified lymphedema therapist
Cardiometabolic Syndrome (exists when 3 of the following risk factors present): central obesity, hypertriglyceridemia, low-plasma high-density lipoprotein cholesterol (HDL-C), hypertension, and fasting hyperglycemia[112]	Decrease in physical activity, hypercaloric diet, and changes in metabolism[112]	Screen for metabolic syndrome: • Waist circumference • Lipid profile • Plasma glucose • Blood pressure[113]	Prescription medications exist to treat hyperglycemia, hypertension, dyslipidemia, and obesity	Lifestyle interventions including diet, exercise, behavioral modifications, smoking cessation, and nutritional counseling[112–114]

[a]Consortium for Spinal Cord Medicine Clinical Practice Guidelines. *Prevention of Venous Thromboembolism in Individuals with Spinal Cord Injury.* Washington, D.C., 2016, Paralyzed Veterans of America.
[b]Consortium for Spinal Cord Medicine Clinical Practice Guidelines. *Neurogenic Bowel Management in Adults with Spinal Cord Injury.* Washington, D.C., March 1998, Paralyzed Veterans of America.

owing to eventual shifting of the foam. In the presence of an open wound cutouts and donut-type cushions should be avoided, as the edges of the cushion would increase pressure on the already compromised area.[101]

Keeping the head of the bed as low as tolerated minimizes the risk for shearing and excessive sacral pressure. For individuals not able to turn themselves, or who are not appropriate for rigorous turning schedules (e.g., patients with unstable fractures), an active support surface such as an alternating pressure mattress is recommended. Low air loss, alternating pressure, or even air-fluidized mattresses are available for those who require the head of the bed to be elevated more than 30 degrees for prolonged periods and have other extenuating conditions such as multiple wounds, recent skin flap surgery, respiratory distress, diabetes, and/or low prealbumin.[101]

While the patient is sitting, a customized seating system with appropriate pressure redistribution (relief) cushion is ideal to provide optimal postural support while preventing increased areas of pressure.[101] Wheelchair footrest height should be assessed, as increased footrest height can lead to increased pressure under the ischial tuberosities[119]; a pressure relief (weight shift) schedule should be established and strictly enforced. Bathroom equipment also should be appropriately padded, and the patient should be able to perform weight shifts. To encourage compliance with weight shifts, options such as using timers, personal technology devices, and patient education on the need for weight shift schedules are utilized.[119]

Although pressure is one of the most prevalent causes of skin compromise, other forces may lead to problems, including friction, shearing, excessive moisture or dryness, infection, and bruising or bumping during activities. This is especially true of patients with SCI because of altered thermoregulation, changes in mobility, decreased or absent sensation, and incontinence of bowel and bladder. In addition, as patients begin to learn functional skills, they may have poor motor control and impaired balance, and must be carefully monitored to avoid injury. Other SCI-related considerations for risk are incontinence, as it may cause moisture buildup on the skin; nutrition, as adequate fluid and nutrition is needed to maintain skin health; and vascular integrity, as blood flow also impacts skin health. When making recommendations for equipment that a spinal cord injured individual needs, skin integrity, appropriate pressure relief, and reduction of heat and moisture should always be considered.[101,115]

Should skin compromise occur, the first intervention is to identify and remove the source of the compromise. Modifications to the seating system or changing to a more pressure-reducing mattress system or cushion may be necessary. Examination and treatment will then need to focus on healing the wound and preventing other secondary conditions that may occur as a result of potential immobility and delayed physical rehabilitation. The reader is encouraged to refer to The National Pressure Ulcer Advisory Panel for educational and clinical resources.[115]

Treatment interventions may include hydrotherapy, specialty wound dressings, electro-modalities, and thermal modalities to increase circulation.[55,101] Mechanical, autolytic, enzymatic, or surgical debridement may be necessary to obtain and maintain a viable wound bed. If the wound does not heal, surgical interventions with myocutaneous or muscle flaps may be necessary for closure. Coordinated return-to-sit programs or protocols after such medical interventions are necessary to prevent opening of the surgical site. Such surgical procedures are costly and significantly delay functional rehabilitation.

After closure and healing of the wound, education becomes a priority to maintain skin integrity. The patient must adhere to a more rigorous skin check program as rehabilitation continues, giving special attention to the affected area. Education for a nutritious diet and teaching patients to advocate for themselves is critical. Problem-solving equipment and lifestyle issues that may affect their skin condition will reduce the recurrence rate. Alcohol, tobacco, and drug use (both recreational and prescription) should be managed for long-term success. Prevention of skin compromise is critical and cannot be stressed enough to health care providers, patients, and caregivers.[101]

Prevention and Management of Joint Contractures

The development of a contracture may result in postural misalignment or impede potential function. Daily ROM exercises, proper positioning, and adequate spasticity management may help prevent contractures. Contracture prevention includes the use of splints (Fig. 14.64) for proper joint alignment, techniques such as weight bearing, ADLs, and functional exercises. Patients exhibiting spasticity may require more frequent ROM intervention.[118]

Adaptive Shortening or Adaptive Lengthening of Muscles

Although isolated joint ROM should be normal for all patients, allowing adaptive shortening or adaptive lengthening of particular muscles is recommended to enhance the achievement of certain functional

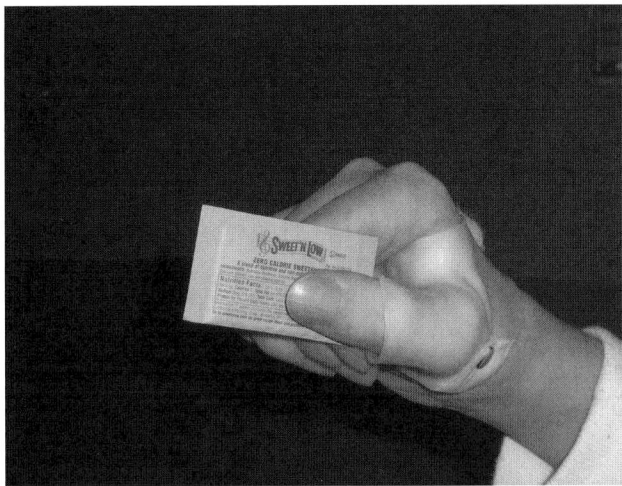

Fig. 14.10 Tenodesis Grasp Utilizing a Short Opponens Splint.

skills.[118] Likewise, unwanted shortening or lengthening of muscles should be prevented. The following section reviews a few examples of these concepts as they relate to SCI.

Tenodesis is described as the passive shortening of the two-joint finger flexors as the wrist is extended. This action creates a grasp, which assists performance of ADLs (Fig. 14.10).[102,118] A patient with mid to low tetraplegia may rely on adaptive shortening of these long finger flexors to replace active grip.[118] If the finger flexors are stretched across all joints during ROM exercises, the achievement of some functional goals may be limited as their tenodesis may be ineffective if they become overstretched. ROM to the finger flexors should be applied only while the wrist is in a neutral position. There is controversy over shortening of the flexor tendons. Some clinicians argue that the patient can develop a fixed flexion contracture of the proximal interphalangeal joints (IP), interfering with future surgical attempts to restore finger function. It is recommended to promote tenodesis functioning via adaptive shortening while maintaining joint suppleness.

In the presence of weakened or paralyzed elbow extensors, patients are at risk of flexion-supination contracture due to the unopposed strength of the elbow flexors. The shortening of the elbow flexors in a supinated position will limit participation in ADL function and transfer skills (Fig. 14.11). Contracted elbow flexors (which contribute to supination) in a patient with an SCI level of C6 can cost this patient his or her independence. Likewise, the rotator cuff and the other scapular muscles should be assessed for their length-tension relationships and their ability to generate force. Normal length of these muscles should be maintained. For example, achieving external rotation of the shoulder (active and passive) is critical for patients with low-level tetraplegia. Shortening of the subscapularis, an internal rotator, and other structures can quickly result in a decrease in motion, limiting bed mobility, transfers, feeding, and grooming skills.

Appropriate length of lower extremity (LE) and trunk muscles are also important for function. Hamstrings should be lengthened to allow 110 to 120 degrees of a straight leg raise. If adequate hamstring length does not exist, it is important to make modifications to prevent overstretching of the low back muscles during functional activities. The combination of lengthened hamstrings and adaptive shortening of the back-extensor muscles provides stability for balance in the short- and long-sitting positions. Balance in short sitting aids in the efficiency of transfers and bowel and bladder management while balance in long sitting assists with lower-extremity dressing and other ADLs. It is also

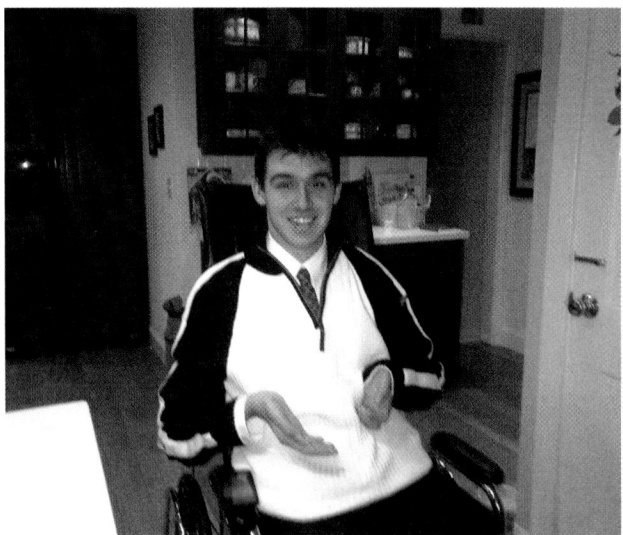

Fig. 14.11. Supination Contraction of a Patient With C5 Level of Injury.

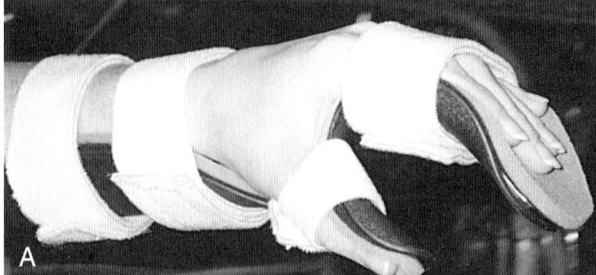

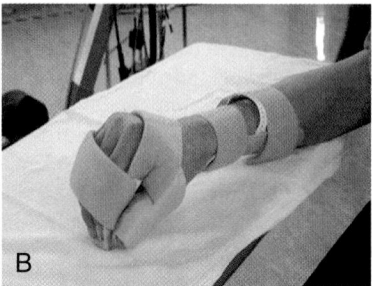

Fig. 14.12 **(A)** Resting hand splint. **(B)** Volar intrinsic plus splint maintains alignment of the wrist and fingers to promote metacarpophalangeal flexion for tenodesis grasp.

important to maintain functional ROM in hips, knees, and ankles as limited ROM in any of these joints can impact the ability to achieve standing and ambulation goals.

Splinting to Prevent Joint Deformity

Deformity prevention is the first goal of splinting.[120] Patients with cervical spinal cord injuries may have lost normal neural input to musculature in their wrists and hands. Other patients may have partial motor control, which may lead to muscle imbalances and loss of ROM. In the absence or weakness of elbow extensors, a bivalve cast or an elbow extension splint at night may be beneficial to prevent joint contractures. At the wrists, a volar wrist support is commonly used initially and may be progressed to a longer-term option of a definitive wrist orthosis or custom wrist orthosis fabricated by an orthotist. Other splints often used for deformity prevention of the hands include resting hand splints with proper positioning to maintain the support of the wrist and web space (Fig. 14.12A).[121] Another hand-based option is the intrinsic plus splint (see Fig. 14.12B), which places the metacarpophalangeal (MP) joints between 70 and 90 degrees of flexion and decreases intrinsic hand muscle tightness. The intrinsic plus splint position promotes joint motility for tenodesis and is the preferred position.

Another goal of splinting in the SCI population is to increase function. Patients with tetraplegia at the C5 level rely on an orthosis to be independent with communication, feeding, and hygiene. They must have joint stability and support at the wrist and the hand to perform these skills. The splint is often adapted with a utensil slot or cuff so the patient can effectively perform the skills mentioned previously.

Patients who are not strong enough to use their wrists for tenodesis may require splinting to support their wrists until they can perform wrist extension against gravity. Long opponens splints can be used to position the thumb for function and support the weak wrist (Fig. 14.13). Once the wrist muscles strengthen, the long opponens splint can be cut down to a hand-based short opponens to maintain proper web space and thumb positioning while maximizing tenodesis.

As mentioned previously, patients with injuries at the C6 level can use their wrists for a tenodesis grasp.[102,122,123] Critical components of the splint assessment for these patients are the positioning of the thumb, web space, and index finger observed during the grasp. It is recommended that the patient's hand be positioned with the thumb in

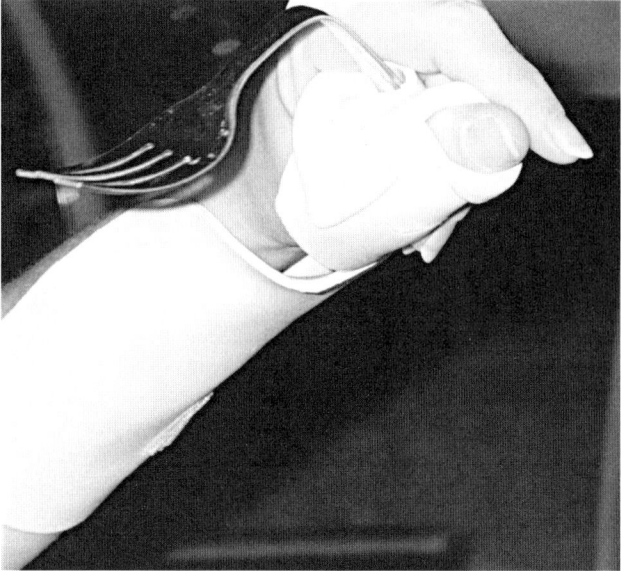

Fig. 14.13 Long Opponens Splint.

a lateral pinch position because this is the most commonly used prehension pattern to pick up objects. Patients who are not splinted may not have the proper positioning to pick up objects because their tenodesis is "too tight" or "too loose."

Patients with C8 to T1 injuries or patients who have incomplete injuries may have "clawing" or hyperextension of the metacarpophalangeal joints. This is caused by finger extensor musculature that is stronger than finger flexor musculature.[102] To prevent this, a splint can be made to block the metacarpophalangeal joints and promote weak intrinsic muscle function. Depending on the extent of the imbalance, these splints can be used during function or worn only at night. Alternatively, the splinting position of composite finger extension (MPs and IPs simultaneously) with wrist extension may be considered for a prolonged stretch.

Cost, time, material, and clinician experience are important considerations when deciding between custom and prefabricated splints. A well-fitting, prefabricated splint can be as effective as a custom-fabricated splint in certain situations. Custom splints require additional resources and clinician expertise. One way to minimize time spent in the fabrication of splints is to use a good pattern and premade straps. Finally, educating the patient on the splint-wearing schedule, skin checks, and splint care is important for preventing skin breakdown.

Treatment for Joint Deformity

If a joint contracture occurs despite preventive measures, more aggressive treatments are necessary. This may include more aggressive use of splinting, plaster or fiberglass casting techniques, or injections of neurolytics, such as botulinum toxin type A (Botox).[124–126] When splinting is not effective, casting may be indicated. The patient with minimal ROM limitations may require only one cast. The patient with significant limitations may require multiple casts, called serial casting. This process involves the application of several casts that are removed and reapplied over a period of weeks to increase extensibility in the soft tissues surrounding the casted joint.[127] With each cast, the involved joint is placed at submaximal ROM.[128] Once the cast is removed, the joint should have an increase of approximately 7 degrees of ROM.[128] This process continues until the deformity is minimized or resolved. The final cast is fabricated into a bivalve splint by cutting the cast into a top half and bottom half and adding strapping. The bivalve splint acts as a positioning device to promote ROM gains made during serial casting. It can be easily applied and removed (Fig. 14.14). Casting contraindications include the following: skin compromise over the area to

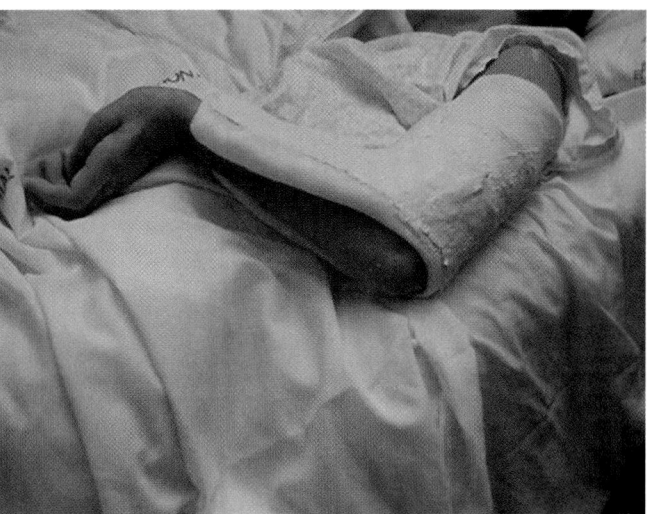

Fig. 14.15. Dropout Cast.

be casted, heterotopic ossification, edema, decreased circulation, severe fluctuating hypertonicity, and inconsistent monitoring systems.

The elbow, wrist and hand, and finger joints are the most common joints casted for patients with SCI. Long-arm casts are used when elbow and wrist contractures must be managed simultaneously. In the case of a pronation or supination contracture, a long-arm cast would also be the cast of choice as the elbow and wrist joint must be included to impact forearm rotation. Dropout casts are used with severe elbow flexor or extensor contractures, but the patient should be in a position in which gravity can assist (Fig. 14.15). Forearm based wrist-hand and individual finger casts are indicated for contractures that prevent distal upper-extremity function. Most commonly, a patient will have a wrist flexion-extension contracture or have finger flexor-extensor tone and will require a cast to use the tenodesis or individual fingers for fine motor skills. Casting is an expensive and labor-intensive treatment modality, but if indicated and used appropriately it can assist a patient in regaining lost joint ROM needed for increased independence and function.

Botox may be used in conjunction with casting. In a study conducted by Corry and colleagues[125] tone reduction was evident when botulinum toxin type A was used; however, ROM and functional improvement varied among subjects. Pierson and co-workers[126] found that, with careful selection, subjects who received Botox had significant improvements in active and passive ROM. Research indicates that patients who have flexor spasticity without fixed contracture will benefit the most.

Surgical intervention may be recommended by an orthopedic physician in severe cases of joint contracture.[129] Some of the more commonly used surgical options include joint manipulation under anesthesia, arthroscopic surgical releases, open surgical releases, and rotational osteotomy.

Prevention and Management of Respiratory Complications

Individuals with a SCI are susceptible to respiratory complications. While level of injury, age, and trauma are leading variables, those with high cervical injuries will be 3.3-times more likely to develop a respiratory condition.[98] This population is more likely to have pneumonia, atelectasis, or some other respiratory condition. Pneumonia frequently leads to death in this population (National Spinal Cord

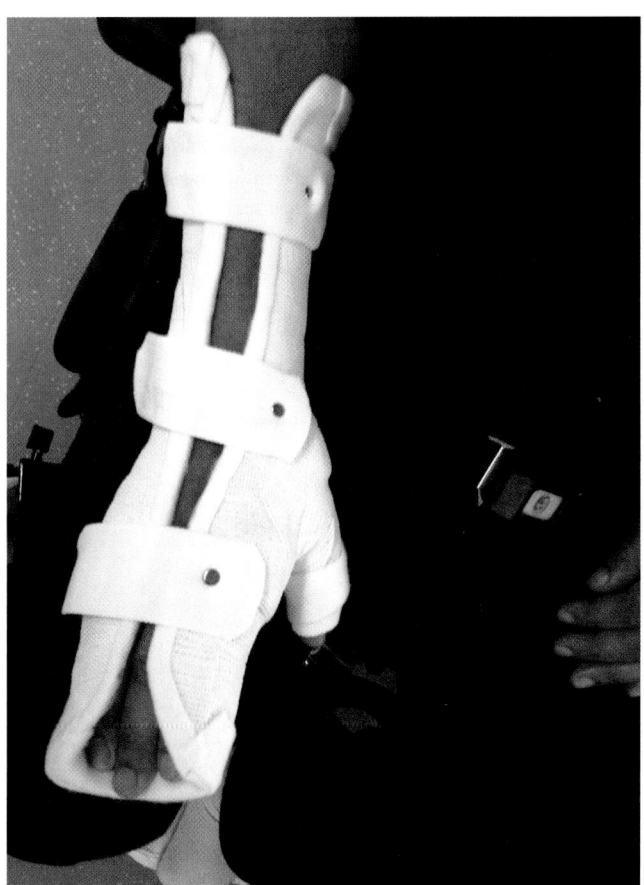

Fig. 14.14. Bivalve Splint.

Injury Statistical Center). Atelectasis can occur in the presence of diaphragmatic paralysis, and the most common location is in the left lower lobe.[130] Early management must focus heavily on preventing pulmonary complications and maximizing pulmonary function so the patient may perform physical activities. The clinician should first determine which ventilatory muscles are impaired. The primary ventilatory muscles of inspiration are the diaphragm and the intercostals. The diaphragm is innervated by the phrenic nerve at C3 through C5. The intercostals are innervated by the intercostal nerves positioned between the ribs. If the diaphragm is weak or paralyzed, its descent will be lessened, reducing the patient's ability to ventilate. Overall dysfunction of these muscles will lead to respiratory insufficiency, increased airway resistance, and impaired secretion clearance. Additionally, if dysphagia is present in someone who has an SCI, it can lead to increased risk of infection.[98]

Accessory muscles of ventilation are primarily located in the cervical region. The accessory muscles are used to augment ventilation when the demand for oxygen increases, as during exercise. Accessory muscles may also be recruited to generate an improved cough effort.[130] The most commonly cited accessory muscles are the sternocleidomastoids, the scalenes, the levator scapulae, and the trapezius muscles. The erector spinae group may also assist by extending the spine, thus improving the potential depth of inspiration.

The abdominals are the primary muscles used for forced expiration in such maneuvers as coughing or sneezing. The latissimus dorsi, the teres major, and the clavicular portion of the pectoralis major are also active during forced expiration and cough in the patient with tetraplegia.[131] Alterations in the function of these muscles will have an impact on the patient's ability to clear secretions and produce loud vocalization. Gravity plays a crucial role in the function of all ventilatory muscles. Neural input to the diaphragm increases in the upright position in persons with intact nervous systems. As one moves into an upright position, the resting position of the diaphragm drops as the abdominal contents fall. The diaphragm is effectively shortened, which makes generating a strong contraction more difficult. However, with intact abdominal musculature, a counter pressure is produced and adequate intraabdominal pressure is maintained, allowing the diaphragm to perform work. If weakness or paralysis of the abdominal wall is present, the patient may need a binder or corset to maintain the normal pressure relationship.[118,130,132] Unless the SCI has affected only the lowest sacral and lumbar areas, some degree of ventilatory impairment is present and should be addressed in therapeutic sessions.

Many treatment techniques are available to address the myriad causes of ventilatory impairment. Decreased chest wall mobility and the inability to clear secretions should always be addressed. Maintaining chest wall mobility is needed to prevent contractures and lung restrictions. With high cervical injuries, the risk of bulbar involvement increases—this impacts secretion clearance. Interventions may include inspiratory muscle training, chest wall mobility exercises, and chest physical therapy.[118,133–135]

Inspiratory Muscle Training

Inspiratory muscle training may be used to train the diaphragm and the accessory muscles that are weakened by partial paralysis, disuse from prolonged artificial ventilation, or prolonged bed rest. In the presence of significant impairments, it is generally recommended that training be initiated in the supine or side-lying position and progressed to the sitting position when tolerated. When training a moderately weak diaphragm, gentle pressure during inspiration may be used to facilitate the muscle (Fig. 14.16). Accessory muscle training may be facilitated with the patient in the supine position while a slight stretch is placed on these muscles.[132–135] The stretch is accomplished by shoulder abduction and external rotation, elbow extension, forearm supination, and neutral alignment of the head and neck.[133–135] A more challenging position incorporates upper thoracic extension. The clinician's hands are placed directly over the muscle to be facilitated. The patient is instructed to breathe into the upper chest (Fig. 14.17). As the treatment progresses, the diaphragm may be inhibited for short training periods by applying pressure over the abdomen in an upward direction. Care must be taken to avoid excessive pressure to prevent occlusion of vital arteries.

As the inspiratory muscles strengthen, resistive inspiratory devices may be used. Inspiratory devices are relatively inexpensive and most function similarly. Most devices have a one-way valve that closes when the patient inspires, forcing him or her to breathe either through a small aperture or against a spring-loaded resistance. Although evidence fully supporting this intervention remains inconclusive,[136] some researchers have shown improvements in total lung capacity[137] and improved endurance measures.[138] The diaphragm may also be trained by using weights on the abdominal wall with the patient in the supine position. However, muscle trainers appear to promote more of an endurance effect than the use of abdominal weights.

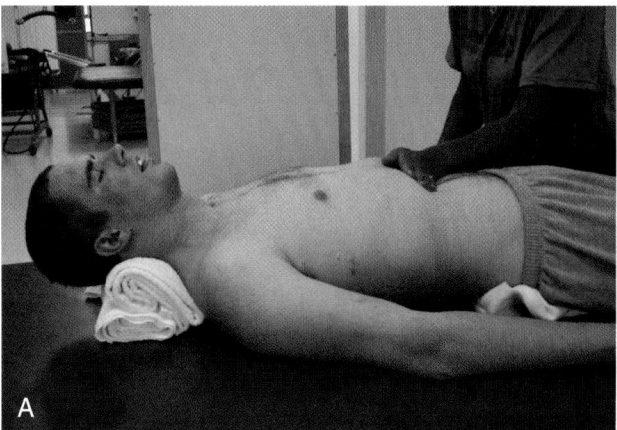
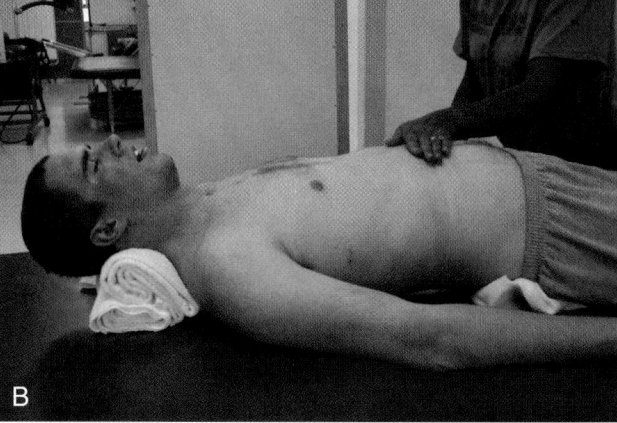

Fig. 14.16 Diaphragm Facilitation. (A) Hand placement and patient positioning to facilitate the diaphragm and inhibit accessory muscle activity. **(B)** Firm contact is maintained throughout inspiration. The lower extremities are placed over a pillow in flexion to prevent stretching of the abdominal wall.

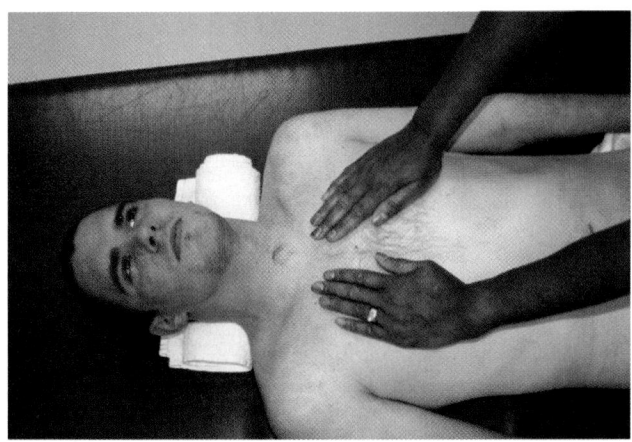

Fig. 14.17 Accessory Muscle Facilitation. Hand placement and patient positioning.

Diaphragm and Phrenic Nerve Pacing

When the primary inspiratory muscles are no longer volitionally active as a result of SCI, the diaphragm can be stimulated directly or by phrenic nerve pacing. These interventions are most commonly indicated when the lesion is at or above the C3 level.[139–142] Assessing the viability of the phrenic nerve will indicate whether stimulation will produce an optimal contraction of the diaphragm and whether it will be painful to the patient.[130,142] Transdiaphragmatic pacing, in which electrodes are placed laparoscopically on the diaphragm, is also an option.[143] Transdiaphragmatic pacing is less invasive than direct phrenic nerve pacing, may be implanted and initiated on an outpatient basis, and may result in improved outcomes. Both of these procedures require a reconditioning program that involves extensive caregiver and patient training. Complications could include myopathic changes of the diaphragm, phrenic nerve compression, or infection.[140] Many patients require some residual use of mechanical ventilation even after maximal tolerance has been achieved so as not to over fatigue the phrenic nerve. Other researchers are also considering pacing intercostal muscles[144] or using a combination of diaphragmatic and intercostal pacing. There is limited evidence comparing the outcomes associated with these devices in isolation or in combination therapies.

Glossopharyngeal Breathing

Glossopharyngeal breathing is another way of increasing vital capacity in the presence of weak inspiratory muscles. Moving the jaw forward and upward in a circular opening and closing manner traps air in the buccal cavity. A series of swallowing-like maneuvers forces air into the lungs, increasing the vital capacity. This technique has been reported to increase vital capacity by as much as 1 L.[134,145] Additionally it may improve voice volume.[130] Although this technique is rarely used to sustain ventilation for long periods of time,[145] it may be used in emergency situations and to enhance cough function. The patient with high tetraplegia should attempt to master this skill.

Secretion Clearance

Ventilatory impairment, the leading cause of rehospitalization in people with tetraplegia, occurs when the patient cannot produce an effective cough to clear secretions.[146] Factors such as artificial ventilation and general anesthesia hamper secretion mobilization. With artificial ventilation, patients may require an artificial airway.[130] The presence of this airway in the trachea is an irritant, and the patient subsequently produces more secretions. A description of various types

and parameters of ventilation is beyond the scope of this chapter. Clinicians working with patients requiring artificial ventilation are referred to other publications.

Secretions are most commonly removed by tracheal suctioning, unassisted coughing, assisted coughing, or mechanical insufflation–exsufflation. Insufflation–exsufflation utilizes rapidly alternating pressures to deliver a breath followed by an exhalation that sucks the air out, and is believed to be the most effective method of clearing secretions.[130,147] A recent case study investigated the use of abdominal electrical stimulation to assist with insufflation–exsufflation and found it may be more effective than insufflation–exsufflation alone in clearing secretions. To date, conclusive research determining which single technique or combination of techniques achieves the best outcome is not available. Insufflation–exsufflation may result in fewer complications and is reported to be more comfortable to the patient. Postural drainage, percussion or clapping, and shaking or vibration are used to assist with moving secretions toward larger airways for expectoration.[11,118]

Assisted coughing is typically used with people who are unable to generate sufficient effort to clear secretions independently. It also helps with basic postural drainage.[130] The assistant places both hands firmly on the abdominal wall. After a maximal inspiratory effort, the patient coughs and the assistant simply supports the weakened wall. A gentle upward and inward force may be used to increase the intraabdominal pressure, yielding a more forceful cough (Fig. 14.18).[127] Excessive pressure over the xiphoid process should be avoided to prevent severe injury.

Patients may learn independent coughing techniques. In preparation for a cough, the patient positions an arm around the push handle of the wheelchair, opening the chest wall to enhance inspiratory effort. The other arm is raised over the head and chest during inspiration. This procedure is followed by a breath hold, strong trunk flexion, and then a cough (Fig. 14.19). Another technique for independent coughing is accomplished by placing the forearms over the abdomen and delivering a manual thrust during cough. This technique is more difficult and may not provide an inspiratory advantage.

Urinary Tract Infection

UTIs are one of the most prevalent complications associated with spinal cord injuries, with an overall incidence of 62% within the first year of injury.[148] Since individuals with SCI often need some form of catheterization—indwelling or intermittent—it is often catheter insertion that introduces bacteria into the bladder, and it is the indwelling catheters that are associated with higher risk compared to intermittent ones.[149,150] A type of external catheter—a condom catheter frequently used with males—can be associated with increased incidence of a UTI if not changed at least every other day.[150] Once in the urinary system bacteria multiply in a short period of time.[149]

Important factors leading to UTI in the SCI population is method of voiding, vesicoureteral reflux, high pressure voiding, large postvoid residuals, presence of stones, outlet obstruction, and the ability to fully empty the bladder. Indwelling catheters lead to a decrease in the mucosal lining, thereby interfering with the function of the mucus, which leads to increased bacteria adhering to the bladder wall. If the bladder is not fully emptied and becomes distended, ischemia can occur in the bladder wall, which impairs its natural defense mechanisms against bacteria.[149] Additionally, high bladder volumes (over 500 mL) can lead to distention and therefore monitoring fluid intake and frequency of emptying is crucial.[151] For these reasons it is important to choose the least invasive method of draining the bladder that is most feasible for the level of injury and functional status of the patient.[149,150]

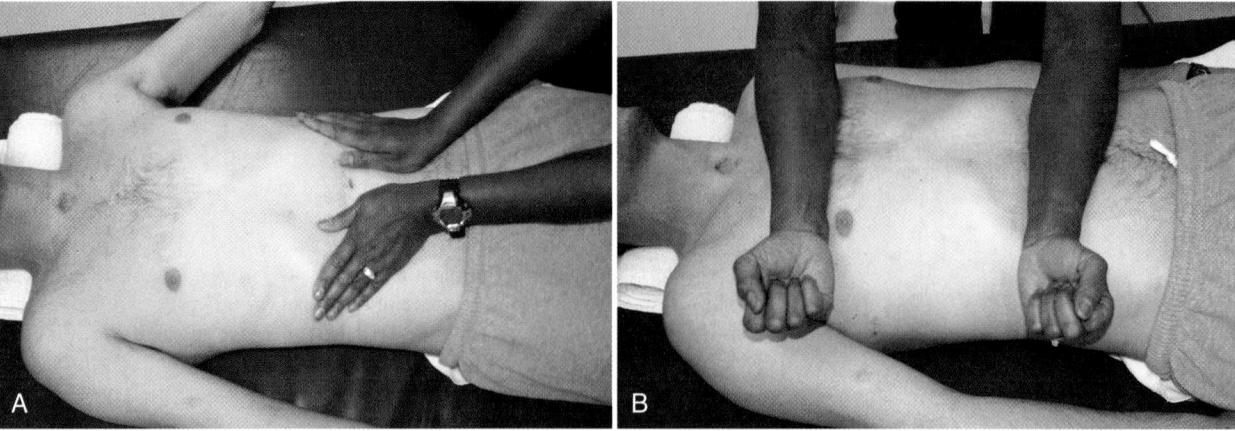

Fig. 14.18 Assisted Coughing. **(A)** Hand placement for the Heimlich-like technique. **(B)** Anterior chest wall assisted coughing. The inferior forearm supination promotes an upward and inward force during the cough.

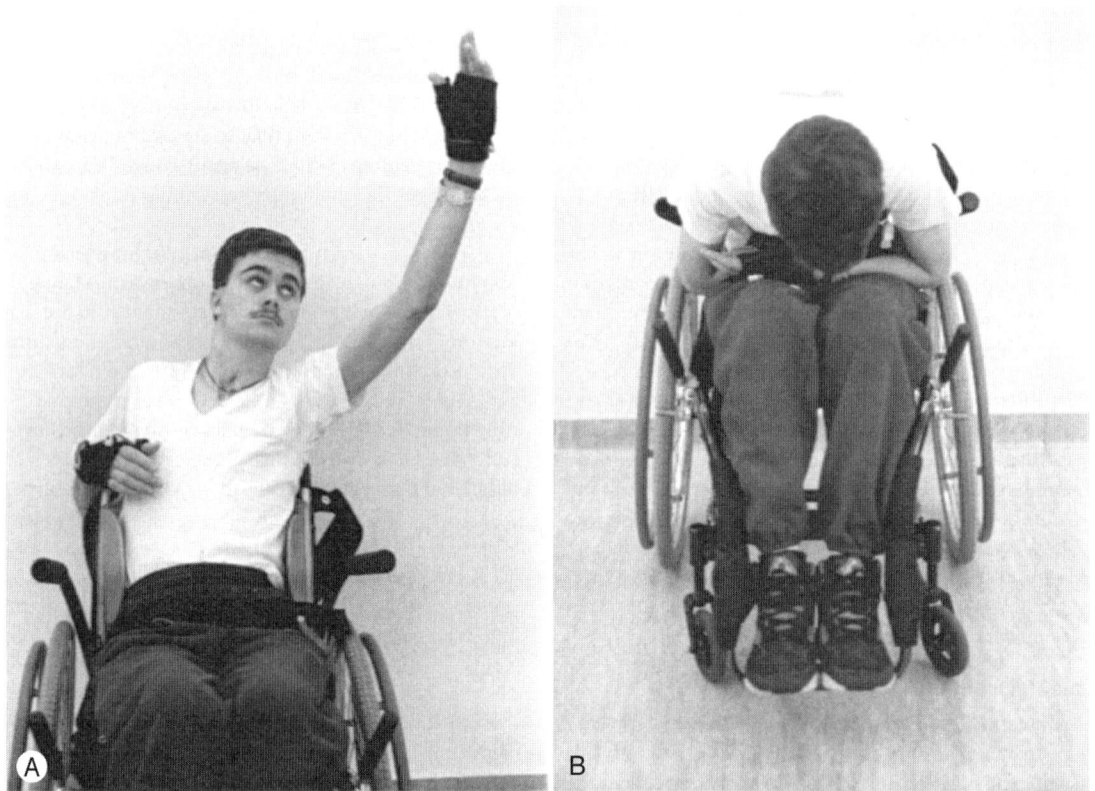

Fig. 14.19 Self-Produced Assisted Coughing. **(A)** Full inspiratory position. **(B)** Expiratory or cough position.

Early Mobilization

Getting the patient upright as soon as possible promotes self-mobility and should be planned carefully. An appropriate seating system for pressure relief and support should be chosen. Most patients require a reclining wheelchair with elevating footrests or tilt-in-space wheelchairs when they are first acclimating to the upright position.[118] The patient is transferred initially to a reclining or tilting back position and progressed to an upright position as signs and symptoms of medical stability allow. The patient should be monitored for evidence of orthostatic hypotension. Dizziness or lightheadedness is most common. Ringing in the ears and visual changes also may occur. Changes in mental function may indicate more serious hypotension, and the

patient should be reclined immediately. Assessing blood pressure before and during activities provides an objective measurement of the patient's status.

Because of paralysis, the abdominal wall may not support the internal organs and viscera. In these cases, an abdominal binder or corset should be applied to all patients with lesions above T12 to assist in venous return[55,133]; as discussed, this will enhance ventilatory function. If the patient has a history of vascular insufficiency or prolonged bed rest, wrapping the lower extremities with elastic bandages while applying the greatest pressure distally may be beneficial.

Abdominal binders and corsets are fitted so that the top of the corset lies just over the lower two ribs. The bottom portion is placed

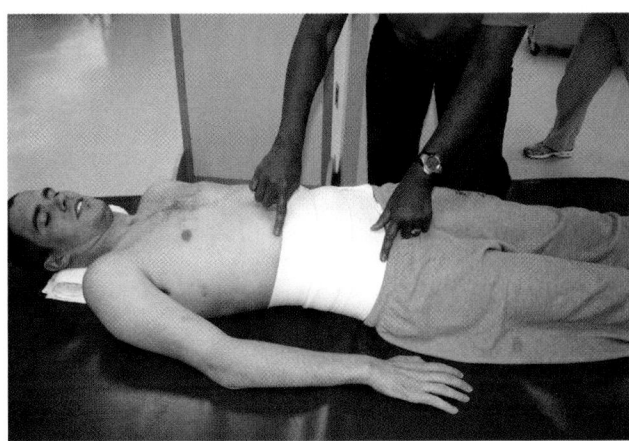

Fig. 14.20 Abdominal Binder. Correct placement is over the anterior-superior iliac spine and at the level of lower rib cage. Custom corsets may be used if an elastic binder does not provide adequate support to enhance vital capacity.

over the anterior iliac spine and iliac crest (Fig. 14.20). The corset or binder should be adjusted slightly more tightly at the bottom to assist in elevating the abdominal contents.[118] Properly fitting the abdominal binder is essential. If it is placed too high or allowed to ride up, ventilation may be impaired by restriction of chest wall excursion. If placed too low, it will not provide the necessary abdominal support.[55,134]

The patient can be transferred initially with a manual or mechanical lift. Lift systems may be advantageous because they allow total control of the patient and give the assistant more time to ensure that monitoring devices, lines, or tubes attached to the patient remain intact. Lift systems may be freestanding hydraulic lifts or electronic devices, or may be mounted on the ceiling.

Once the patient is out of bed, a weight shift or pressure relief schedule is immediately established. Initially, weight shifts are performed at 30-minute intervals and modified according to skin tolerance. A timer may be issued to ensure reminders for weight shifts. This is particularly important if the patient has cognitive deficits. The skin is inspected thoroughly before and immediately after out-of-bed activities. Total sitting time is progressed according to tolerance.

REHABILITATION: ACHIEVING FUNCTIONAL OUTCOMES

Once secondary conditions are managed and the patient is able to tolerate out-of-bed activities, more aggressive functional training begins. The following information will address special considerations for functional progression related to SCI.

Optimal neck, shoulder, and upper-extremity strength and ROM are important factors to consider in order to maximize functional outcomes. Neck musculature is typically painful and restricted in cervical injuries, especially after surgical procedures. Most patients will have a cervical orthosis in place postoperatively to prevent rotation and flexion and extension. Cervical spine mobility may be so limited that correcting a forward head posture is the first goal. Soft tissue massage, manual therapy, and other modalities may be beneficial. When cleared by the physician, the patient can begin more aggressive neck exercises.

The key muscle groups to consider include the musculature of the shoulder, scapula, and thoracohumeral muscles, which allow for humeral flexion, adduction and abduction, shoulder internal and external rotation, and scapular movements. Patients with high cervical injuries have the potential for the development of tight upper trapezius muscles, shoulder subluxations, capsule tightness, nerve root injury, or radicular pain.[152] Upper trapezius inhibitory taping or scapular taping to relax the tight muscles and facilitate the weak scapular musculature is often beneficial. If the injury level is above C7, the scapular musculature may not be fully innervated, and thus positioning in the proper alignment and strengthening the innervated musculature are essential. Some individuals require positional aides, such as slings or custom orthosis, to avoid humeral displacement or subluxation. The clinician will use findings from manual muscle testing and the goniometric examination to determine the appropriate stretching, strengthening, and positional interventions. Patients may need to begin with gravity-eliminated exercises using air splints, bilateral slings, skateboards, and functional electrical stimulation (FES).[152,153]

Activities of Daily Living and Instrumental Activities of Daily Living

ADLs include skills such as communication, feeding, grooming, bathing, dressing, bladder and bowel management, sexual health, home management, and community reentry. Instrumental activities of daily living (IADLs) encompass multistep activities to care for self and others,[154] such as parenting, household management, and financial management. Depending on the level and severity of the SCI, patients will achieve varying levels of independence. Most of the ADL areas discussed in this section will address skill levels with a complete injury. Activities should be graded differently for an incomplete injury after completion of ISNCSCI examination and manual muscle testing. For purposes of this discussion we will use terms used in the FIM.

Patients with complete high-level tetraplegia (C1 to C4) will be dependent in most ADLs and IADLs; therefore the focus of ADL training is to verbalize how to safely perform all skills. Patients with low-level tetraplegia (C5 to C8) may achieve some level of independence, but this will vary according to the amount of intact musculature and the patient's body shape and weight, age, and motivation level. The ability of these patients to achieve maximum independence in all areas of ADLs may be accomplished with appropriate orthoses or adaptive equipment.[155] See Table 14.4 for functional expectations and Table 14.6 for orthotic indications.

Patients with complete injuries at the C5 or C6 level have unique challenges regarding return to ADL participation. These patients must have biceps function and adequate elbow ROM before any ADL goals can be achieved. To achieve these goals, patients need to work toward supporting their body weight with simultaneous extension of the shoulder, elbow, and wrist (otherwise known as propping; Fig. 14.21A to C). Elbow positioning devices such as pillow splints, casts, or resting splints enhance alignment. Other orthotics to consider for maximizing function include definitive wrist supports and mobile arm supports (MASs)[156] or short opponens splints if the patient has wrist extension. Appropriate wheelchair positioning with lap trays, armrests, wedges, or lateral trunk support is important to maximize function for persons with C5 or C6 injuries.[155]

Patients with a complete C7 or C8 level of injury generally achieve ADL goals with less adaptive equipment and task-specific training. With the presence of triceps, ADL skills are easier to achieve. Most patients, given the right body type, will be able to achieve these goals with only minimal assistance from a caregiver.[155]

Patients with complete paraplegia usually achieve total independence with communication, feeding, and grooming. These patients may need adaptive equipment to perform some of these IADL and

TABLE 14.6 Upper-Extremity Orthotics

Splint	Level of Spinal Cord Injury	Rationale
Dynamic Orthotics		
Mobile arm support (ball-bearing feeder)	Weak C5 Incomplete injuries Also indicated with shoulder weakness (internal-external rotator muscle grades 2– to 3/5; bicep-supinator muscle grades 2-/5)	Function Assists in reaching in horizontal and vertical planes Increases functional ROM and strength Independence with feeding and hygiene after setup Provides support to allow correct movement patterns
Overhead rod and sling	Weak C5 Incomplete injuries Also indicated with shoulder weakness (internal-external rotator muscle grades 3 to 3+/5; bicep/supinator muscle grades 3/5)	Function Increases functional ROM and strength Independence with wheelchair driving after setup Independence with feeding and hygiene after setup Provides support to allow correct movement patterns
Static Splints, Casts, and Orthotics		
Resting hand splint[121]	C1-C7	Position Prevent joint deformity Preserves web space Preserves balance with intrinsic and extrinsic musculature
Intrinsic plus splint[121]	C1-C7	Position Same as resting hand splint but places finger MP joint in more flexion Long term, allows better tenodesis alignment of first digit and thumb
Elbow extension splints, bivalve cast	C5-C6	Position Prevents elbow contracture from muscle imbalance and/or hypertonicity
Rolyan Tone and Positioning (TAP) splint (prefabricated)	C5-C6	Position Provides constant low stretch Use with muscle imbalance and/or mild hypertonicity
Dorsal wrist support splints	C5	Function (e.g., slot for utensils) and position Prevents severe wrist drop and ulnar deviation If positioning is needed long term, may consider permanent splint fabricated by orthotist
Long opponens splint	C5	Position and function Can be dorsal or volar Prevents wrist drop and ulnar deviation Preserves web space and supports thumb, reducing subluxation Slot may be fabricated for function
Wrist cock-up splint	C5 Incomplete injuries	Position and function Supports wrist in slight extension Allows finger movement for incomplete injuries
Short opponens splint	C6-C7	Position and function Supports thumb to prevent subluxation Improves tenodesis and prehension
Tenodesis brace or splint[102,122,123]	C6-C7	Function Enhances natural tenodesis in either tip-pinch or lateral pinch May consider permanent splint fabricated by orthotist
MP block splint[102]	C8-T1	Position Prevents "claw hand" or hyperextension of the MP joints Protects weak intrinsic musculature

MP, Metacarpophalangeal; *ROM*, range of motion.

ADL skills; however, they should be able to be performed without assistance from another person. Endurance is a major concern for the patient's independence while performing ADLs. Some skills require a considerable amount of time and effort. If endurance becomes a factor, patients should choose to perform some activities while receiving assistance for other skills that are too challenging or time-consuming.[155]

Feeding

Patients with complete C1 to C4 tetraplegia are dependent in feeding; therefore verbalization of this skill is essential. Patients with complete C5 SCI with weak shoulders and biceps musculature require a dynamic orthosis to support the UE during feeding. The most common orthoses used are the MAS[156,157] (Fig. 14.22) and the deltoid aid. Patients

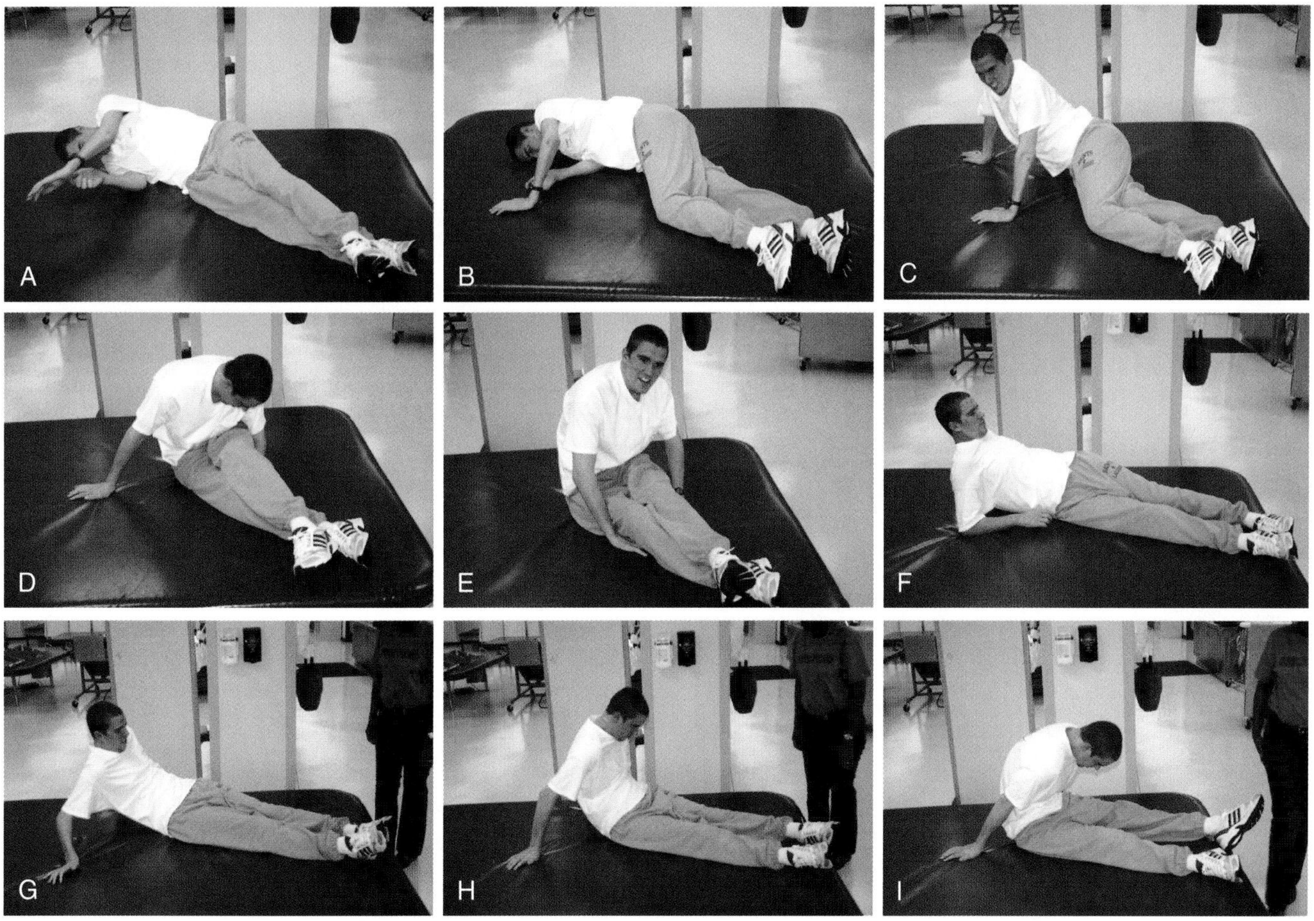

Fig. 14.21 Bed Mobility and Coming to Sit. (A) The patient rolls from supine to side-lying position. **(B)** He progresses to supporting his weight through the downside elbow and shoulder. **(C)** He pushes up onto extended arms. **(D)** While shifting his weight onto the left arm, he unweights the right arm and hooks his right hand behind his right knee, gaining enough leverage to push and pull himself toward upright in a long sitting position. **(E)** He continues to shift his weight to the right until he gains a balanced sitting position with his weight forward over his extended legs. Supine to sitting: **(F)** and **(G)** Starting from a supine position on a bed or a mat, the arms are extended and the hands positioned under the buttock or in the curve of the back (lumbar spine); the head is lifted, and leverage is used to pull up until the upper body weight is supported on bilateral elbows. **(H)** The weight is shifted from right to left or vice versa, and the elbows are extended to support the upper body weight. **(I)** While the elbows are kept extended, the hands are carefully walked forward until balanced long sitting has been achieved.

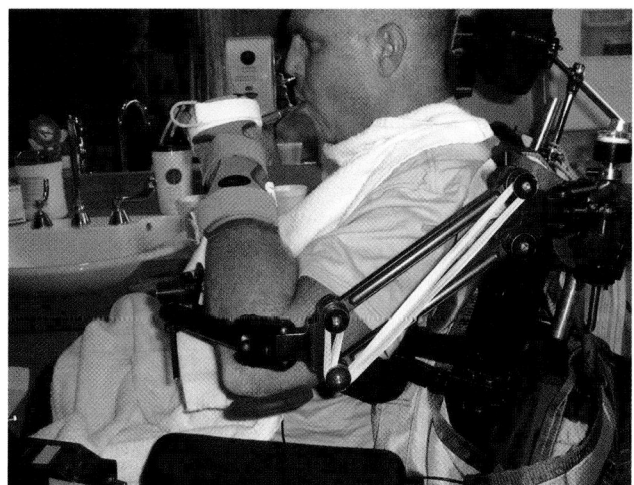

Fig. 14.22 Mobile Arm Support Used During Feeding.

with low-level tetraplegia may not have weakness in the shoulder impacting feeding, but they may have weak wrist function. This weakness can be addressed with dorsal wrist supports with a built-in functional cuff, whereas the patient with no finger function can use a tenodesis grasp for managing objects or to hold a feeding utensil. A universal cuff can be worn on the hand to hold feeding utensils (Fig. 14.23A). The patient with weak finger function can use built-up handles on the utensils. There are also commercially available utensils such as those in Fig. 14.23B. Cutting with decreased hand function is addressed with adapted equipment such as rocker knives.

Grooming

The basic components of grooming are washing the face, combing or brushing the hair, performing oral care, shaving, and applying makeup. More advanced grooming activities may include nail care, donning and doffing of contact lenses, or other hygiene tasks specific to the individual. Individuals with complete C1 to C4 tetraplegia are dependent; therefore verbalization of this skill is essential. Patients with

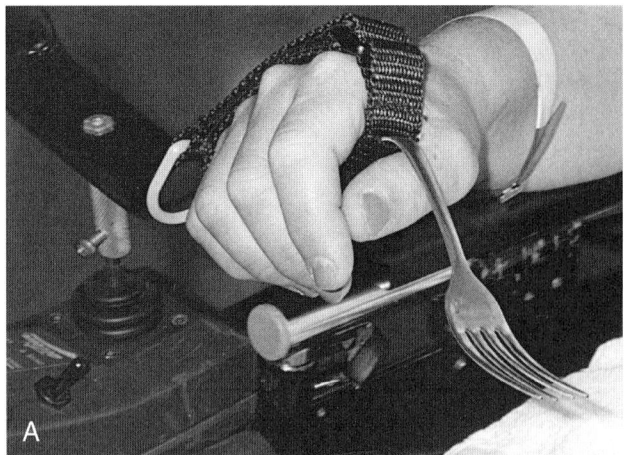

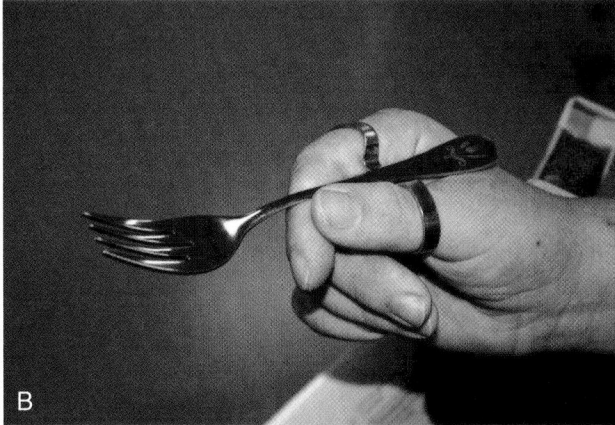

Fig. 14.23 **(A)** Universal cuff used for feeding. **(B)** Dining with Dignity is one commercially available type of flatware for individuals with impaired grip.

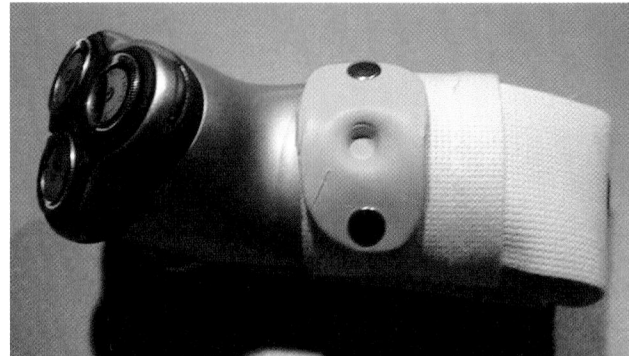

Fig. 14.24 Simple Razor Adaptation That Helps Turn Razor On and Off With a Grosser Motor Movement.

complete C5 injuries perform these skills with some assistance but may require orthotic devices, such as a mobile arm support (MAS) and a splint for wrist support. Patients with complete low-level tetraplegia may need cuffs or built-up grips on razors, brushes, and toothpaste to be independent (Fig. 14.24). All patients require a bathroom that is carefully designed and set up to allow for wheelchair access and chair-level functioning. Patients with tetraplegia often rely on the support of the elbows as an assist, so sink height and durability should be considered. The proper positioning and adaptive equipment will be the difference between independence and dependence in these skills (Figs. 14.25 and 14.26).

Bathing

Bathing includes washing and rinsing the UEs, LEs, and the trunk. Patients with complete C1 to C4 tetraplegia are dependent in bathing; therefore verbalization of this skill is essential. Patients with complete C5 injury can range from requiring maximal assistance to being dependent in bathing. Arm support and positioning for C1-5 tetraplegia is essential to ensure that shoulder integrity is maintained.[155] Prolonged poor positioning in shower chairs or bathing equipment can result in humeral displacement, capsule tightness, nerve root injury, or radicular pain.[152] Patients with complete low-level tetraplegia bathe with moderate assistance to total independence with use of adaptive devices. Patients with paraplegia are typically independent in bathing but may need adaptive devices. After examination of the patient's upper-extremity strength, balance, spasticity, body type, skin integrity, endurance, and home accessibility; the therapy team can determine the appropriate bathing equipment and setup for the patient (Fig. 14.27).

Patients with limited upper-extremity and trunk strength may need straps to assist with trunk support and adaptive cuffs to control the hand-held shower head. Basic bathing safety should be taught to all patients. Bathing safety includes checking the water temperature with a known area of intact sensation; skin checks before and after bathing; weight shifts throughout the routine; and skin protection during the transfers. These precautions are necessary to prevent burns and skin breakdown during the bathing process.[155]

Dressing

Dressing includes dressing and undressing the UEs and LEs with clothing that fits the patient's premorbid lifestyle. Patients with complete C1 to C5 tetraplegia are dependent; therefore verbalization of this skill is essential. This verbalization should focus on how to direct the caregiver in shoulder protection techniques. Independence in this skill for patients with low tetraplegic and paraplegic injuries may depend on where the skill is performed (e.g., mat, bed, or wheelchair). Patients with low-level tetraplegia can perform upper body dressing and undressing independently with equipment such as a button hook, hook and loop fasteners (Velcro), or adapted loops. Initially, lower-body dressing is performed in bed (Fig. 14.28) versus the wheelchair because of endurance, strength, and body type issues. Patients with paraplegia are expected to dress with total independence in the bed, but they may need equipment such as a leg lifter or a long-handled shoe horn for dressing in the wheelchair (Fig. 14.29). Mastering dressing in the wheelchair is ideal for independence in the community.[155]

Bladder Management

Bladder management includes selecting and performing the bladder program, clothing management, body positioning, setup and equipment cleanup, urine disposal, and body cleanup. Patients often enter the rehabilitation program with an indwelling catheter as their bladder management program. The indwelling catheter should be removed as soon as possible to reduce the risk for chronic UTIs.[149] Following removal of the indwelling catheter, the rehabilitation team implements dependent intermittent catheterizations until the patient gradually takes over their bladder routine. Some patients require more extensive review of their bladder function prior to establishing successful bladder management. In these cases, physicians utilize water or video urodynamic studies to determine the patient's bladder status and to determine optimal bladder training programs.

The neurologically intact individual manages bladder function through the use of sensory messages sent via S2-S4 nerve roots, which triggers a reflex starting a cascade allowing for bladder control. Following an SCI, this communication between the bladder, spinal cord, and

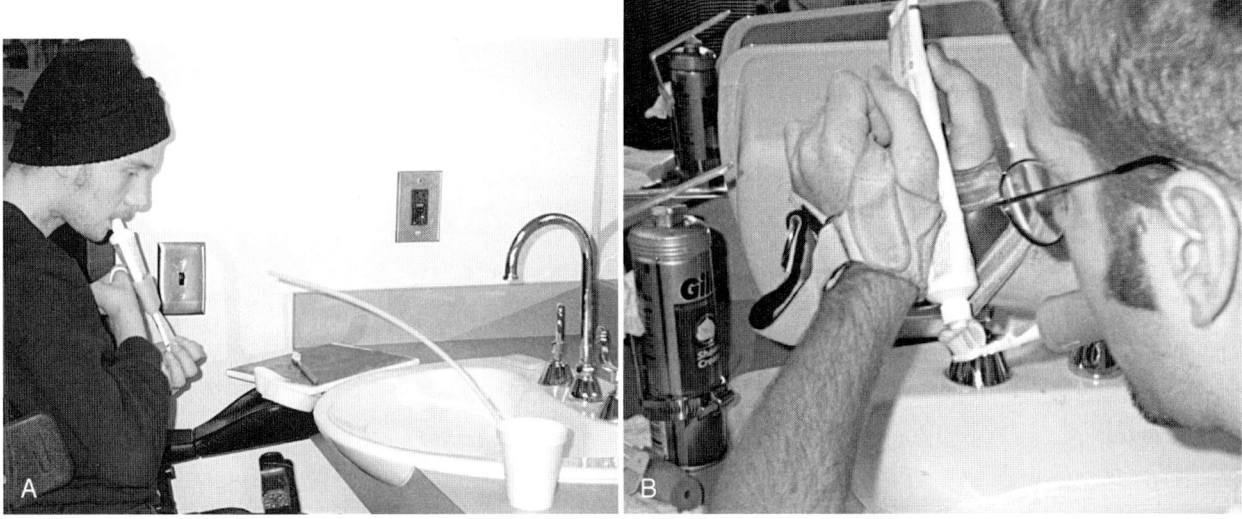

Fig. 14.25 **(A)** A patient with a C5 spinal cord injury is able to brush his teeth with use of a cuff, adapted long straw, and proper wheelchair positioning at the sink. **(B)** Patient with C6 spinal cord injury uses bilateral tenodesis to support toothpaste while holding a toothbrush in his mouth.

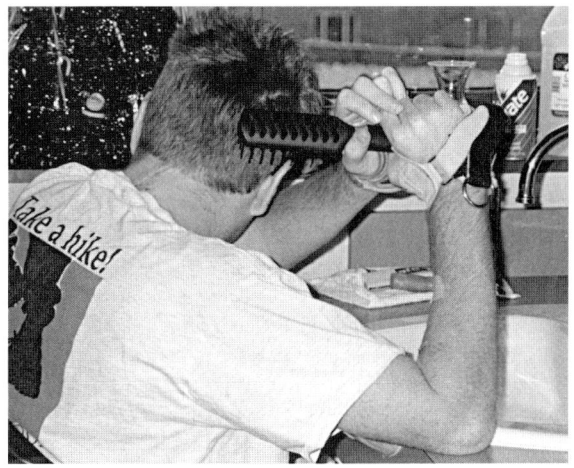

Fig. 14.26 Sink height can be important in assisting this patient with C6 spinal cord injury to brush his hair.

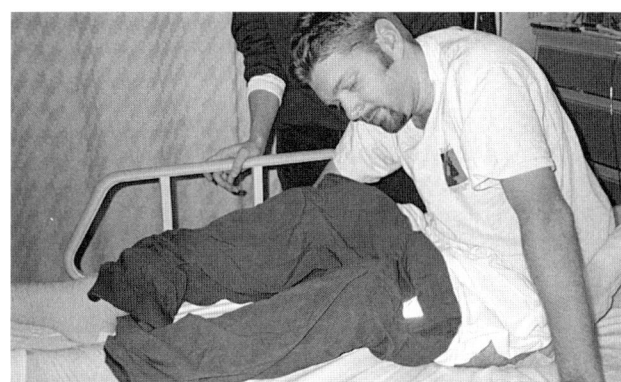

Fig. 14.28 Patient with low-level tetraplegia maintains balance while performing lower-extremity dressing in bed.

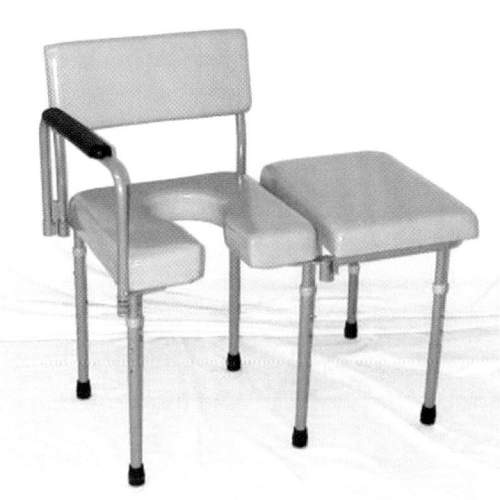

Fig. 14.27 Adjustable height shower and commode chair with 2-inch padded watercrest seat with optional armrest, backrest, and transfer arm.

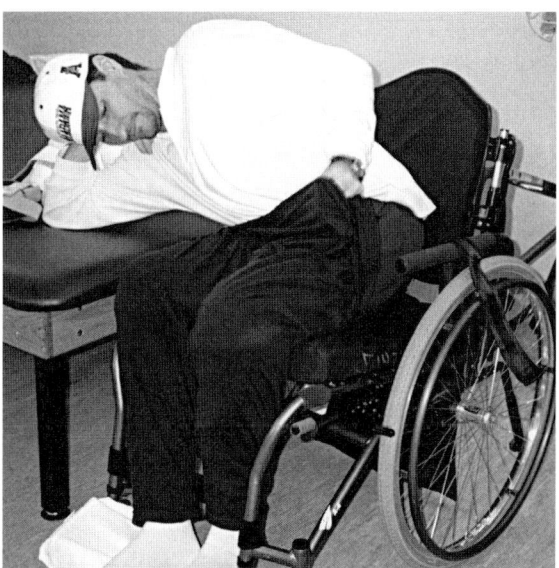

Fig. 14.29 Early practice when dressing in the wheelchair may involve leaning on a surface to assist with this skill.

brain is disrupted, resulting in one of two different possible bladder presentations based on the level of SCI.

On the basis of injury level, patients have either a reflexive bladder (upper motor neuron lesions) or an areflexive bladder (lower motor neuron lesions).[118] The reflexive bladder reflexively empties when the bladder is full. The therapeutic goals for managing the reflexive bladder include low-pressure voiding and low residual urine volumes. The nonreflexive bladder will not empty reflexively and needs to be manually emptied at regular intervals. The goals for managing the areflexive bladder include establishing a regular emptying schedule and continence between emptying. Management of an areflexive bladder includes performance of intermittent catheterizations.[158]

Typically, patients with complete C1 to C5 tetraplegia are dependent in their bladder programs. An automatic leg-bag emptier can assist with the elimination component of the bladder skill. The patient will be dependent in the other components of bladder management; therefore verbalization of this skill is essential. Male patients with injuries at C6 level and below have the potential to complete the majority of bladder management. Several factors influence the patient's potential for independence including catheter selection, hand function, body habitus, urethral integrity, and adaptive equipment. Patients with limited hand function often utilize adaptive devices, such as orthoses, to assist with catheter insertion, adaptive scissors to open bladder packages, flip-top openers, and leg bag loops (Fig. 14.30).[155,159]

Among patients with a paraplegic level of injury, intermittent catheterization is the most commonly used modality. A 2016 study found that patients who were determining how to transition from indwelling catheters to intermittent catheterizations primarily relied on their clinical team to determine the type of catheter and devices for performance.[160] Female patients with paraplegia will most likely need to begin their training in bed with a mirror to obtain the most ideal position. If finger sensation is intact, touch technique can be taught to eliminate reliance on a mirror. The majority of male patients with paraplegia require minimal use of adaptive equipment during bladder management at bed or wheelchair level. Some people with SCI may decide to have a suprapubic catheter placed or a bladder augmentation procedure as a lifestyle choice. Each method of bladder management has advantages and disadvantages requiring patients to balance factors such as the potential for secondary complications from renal and urinary health, convenience, comfort, expense, and quality of life.[161]

Bowel Management

The goal of bowel management is to have the patient able to predictably induce regular elimination. As described under bladder management, the level of injury will assist in telling if the patient will have either a reflexive bowel or a nonreflexive bowel.[118] The bulbocavernosus reflex (BCR) is elicited by pinching the dorsal glans penis or by pressing the clitoris and palpating for bulbocavernosus and external anal sphincter contraction.[162] If the patient has a positive BCR, this is indicative of a reflexive bowel. With a reflexive bowel, tone of the internal and external anal sphincter is present although the patient will not feel the need to have a bowel movement. Voluntary anal contraction and relaxation are not possible, but the nerve connection between the colon and the spinal cord are still intact, allowing the patient to reflexively eliminate stool. This can be done with chemical or mechanical stimulation.[162]

Flaccid bowel programs are much more difficult to regulate because there is no internal or external anal sphincter tone. Timing and diet are critical for the success of this program. A suppository may be required to assist with the process, and in this situation the rectum should be emptied before suppository insertion.[163] If the established bowel program is not followed consistently, involuntary bowel movements or impaction may occur.

Bowel management training must begin as soon as the patient is medically stable. The components of bowel management include clothing management, body positioning, setup and cleanup of equipment, performance of the bowel program, disposal of feces, and cleanup of self. To establish the most effective bowel training program, the interdisciplinary team must work together. The team will need to discuss patient medications that may affect the bowels, the time of day when the patient plans to perform the program, the physical appropriateness related to scapular strength and endurance, and all equipment that will be used.

Patients with injury above the C6 level will be dependent in performing the bowel program; however, they should be independent in the verbalization of the technique. Patients with limited hand function (C6 to C7) may require a digital bowel stimulator and a suppository inserter with an adapted cuff or splint (Fig. 14.31). In addition, a roll-in shower chair or upright shower or commode chair with a padded cut out in the seat will allow the patient to reach the buttock area to perform the stimulation. For this level of injury, it may be advantageous to perform the bowel program in conjunction with the shower to conserve energy with transfers. For individuals with paraplegia, full independence is expected for completion of all bowel management skills. These programs are typically performed on appropriate

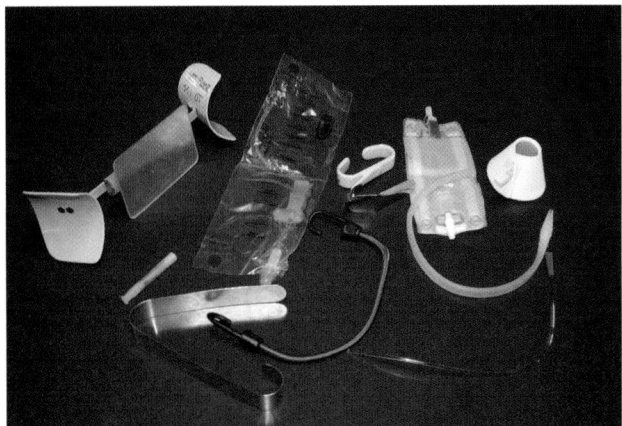

Fig. 14.30 Bladder management supplies may include knee spreader with mirror, sterile catheter kit, catheter inserter, leg bag with tubing and adapter, catheter, "HouseHold" for positioning, bungee cord to hold pants, pants holder, small prelubricated female catheter.

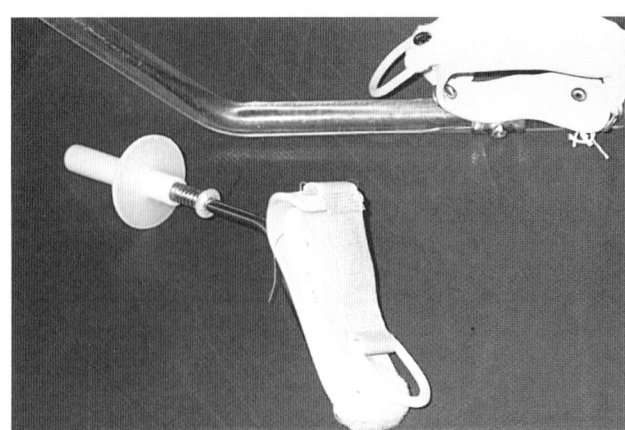

Fig. 14.31 Dil Stick and Suppository Inserter With Adaptive Cuffs.

BOX 14.5 Guidelines for Bowel Program

1. Perform the bowel program at the same time each day.
2. Follow a diet high in fiber (25–35 g recommended).
3. Drink at least 8 glasses of water per day.
4. Drink a hot liquid 30 min before initiating the bowel program.
5. Perform the bowel program in an upright position.
6. Consider premorbid bowel schedule.

bathroom equipment or the bed. Weight shifts and body positioning are essential during the patient's bowel routine to prevent skin breakdown from occurring.[155]

To increase the effectiveness of the bowel program the patient should follow the guidelines identified in Box 14.5.

Sexual Health

Sexuality is how people experience and express themselves as sexual beings and is a normal part of being human,[164] so it is not surprising that people with SCI place a high priority on resuming sexual functions after their injury.[165] After SCI, men may experience impairments in penile erection, ejaculation, orgasm, and fertility. Women with SCI may experience impairments in the ability to become aroused or achieve orgasm and/or may have decreased vaginal lubrication.[164] Addressing sexual functions is a high priority for both men and women after SCI.[165] Table 14.7 lists the relationship of the level of spinal injury to sexual function. Treatment of sexual dysfunction should be a coordinated effort among the patient, appropriate health care professionals, and the identified significant other. Sexual counseling, educational programs, and medical management provide opportunities to address the areas of sexual dysfunction, alternative behaviors, precautions, and other related areas.[166]

Depending on the level and completeness of the SCI, most men can attain an erection either through psychogenic (via T11 to L2 pathways) or reflexogenic pathways (S2 to S4)[167]; however, these erections are often not reliable or adequate for sexual intercourse. The first-line treatment for erectile dysfunction after SCI is the use of phosphodiesterase type V inhibitors such as sildenafil (Viagra), tadalafil (Cialis), and vardenafil (Levitra). Other treatments include intracavernosal

TABLE 14.7 Relation of Level of Spinal Injury to Sexual Function

Injury Level	Sexual Function
Cauda equina/conus	Males Usually no reflex erections Rare psychogenic erection Ejaculation occasionally occurs Females Vaginal secretions often absent Patients generally fertile
Thoracic/cervical	Males Reflex erections predominate (usually short duration) Psychogenic erections generally absent Ejaculation occasional Females Vaginal secretions present as part of genital reflex Fertility preserved Sensation of labor pain absent

(penile injectable) medications, mechanical methods (e.g., vacuum devices and penile rings), and, as a last resort, surgical penile implants.[164]

Male orgasm and ejaculation are likely to occur together; however, after SCI an orgasm may not always lead to ejaculation, or there may be retrograde ejaculation into the bladder.[168] A study by Sipski and colleagues showed that 78.9% of men with incomplete upper motor neuron SCI achieved orgasm as compared with 28% of men with complete upper motor neuron injuries ($P < .001$), whereas 0% of men with lower motor neuron injuries affecting their sacral cord achieved orgasm.[168]

"Will I ever be able to become a father?" is a common question of men after SCI. Pregnancy rates in partners of men with SCI are lower than in the general population, but there is a good chance (greater than 50%) that men with SCI can become biological fathers with advances in reproductive assisted technology. Roughly 2 weeks after an SCI, semen quality declines[169] to levels approaching those observed in males with chronic SCI.[170] There is evidence that bladder management with clean intermittent catheterization may improve semen quality over other methods of bladder management.[171] The two most common methods of sperm retrieval are vibrostimulation (less invasive) and electroejaculation. These methods are successful for persons with lesions above T10. If these methods are not successful, there is an option of surgical aspiration. Depending on the semen quality, a progression from intravaginal insemination, intrauterine insemination, in vitro fertilization (IVF), to IVF plus intracytoplasmic sperm injection is recommended.[164]

Women with SCI require access to integrated care starting with sexual wellness visits, child planning classes, and preconception through postpartum care.[172] Research is currently lacking regarding reproductive aging in women with SCI; what is clear from the literature thus far is the need for women with SCI to receive education regarding the importance of accessing care following injury.[173] Timing of sexual health education following injury should begin during the rehabilitation process and continue throughout the patient's life. Health care providers need to be mindful to ensure all females receive information on sexual health regardless of age, marital status, and level of disablement following spinal injury or dysfunction.[174]

Women need to be educated on how to screen the health care provider for wheelchair access into the clinic, treatment room, and transfer status onto the exam table.[174–176] A 2013 study found that the subspecialty of gynecology had the highest rate of inaccessible practices.[177] It is up to the rehabilitation team to ensure female patients receive the knowledge necessary to access quality care. For example, pelvic exams following injury should not be performed in the patient's wheelchair since pelvic positioning significantly impacts the quality of a pelvic exam.[178] The therapy team should work with female patients to determine transfer techniques and options, altered positioning for exams, and topics to cover with their health care providers throughout their life-span.

Immediately following injury, amenorrhea may up last up to 4 to 5 months. This delay allows health care providers to review menses management techniques without the challenge of discharge. Some women choose to limit menses via pharmacological interventions; others manage with tampons, menstrual cups, pads, or period panties. Careful consideration should be placed on the likelihood of eliciting autonomic dysreflexia, caregiver burden, and skin integrity when determining interventions. Following injury, the women's hand function, lifestyle, comfort, and personal preferences need to be considered to maximize quality of life.

Despite delay in return to menstruation, it is believed that fertility in women is unaffected by SCI.[179] Women need to be educated regarding contraceptive options following injury. Women are able to conceive; however, there are increased risks to pregnancy, which may include bladder problems, spasticity, pressure sores, autonomic dysreflexia, and problems with mobility.[172,180] As noted previously, women need close collaboration with their health care providers prior to and throughout pregnancy to ensure safety.

In addition to addressing wellness visits following injury, women need specific education regarding intimacy and relationships. Women with SCI may have impairment in arousal and orgasm. The vagus nerves are thought to facilitate the presence of vaginal–cervical perception of orgasm. Preservation of T11 to L2 sensory dermatomes is associated with psychogenically mediated genital vasocongestion and lubrication.[181] There is some evidence that supports the use of sildenafil in women to partially reverse subjective sexual arousal difficulties.[164] For women who have a lower motor neuron lesion, vaginal secretions are often absent, and an artificial lubricant is recommended. Safe transfers, positioning, and devices should be reviewed to ensure sexual function, responsiveness, and expression needs are met. It is important that health care providers maintain professional boundaries when addressing sexual issues and consider the age of injury onset, previous sexual experiences, and baseline sexual knowledge. Sexual education and counseling should occur in accordance with patient-centered care.[182]

Home Management

Home management may be divided into two components: light home management and heavy home management. Light home management includes managing money, preparing a snack in the kitchen, doing laundry, and making the bed. Heavy home management includes shopping for groceries, preparing a complex meal in the kitchen, dusting, and vacuuming. The clinician should discuss the role the patient would like to assume at home. The patient may want to resume previous home management roles or may want to discuss changing roles with a family member or caregiver to have energy for other skills.

Patients with C1 to C5 tetraplegia will be dependent in home management. Patients with limited or no hand function will need adaptive kitchen devices, adapted utensils, and adapted cleaning equipment. Preplanning activities may be essential for independent function with patients at all levels of injury. Patients with hand function may require extended handles on equipment and must incorporate energy conservation techniques.

Parenting

Research has shown the importance of parenting behavior and attitude on children's ability to adjust to various circumstances. However, this adjustment is not affected by the disability status of a parent.[183,184] Patients with C1 to C5 tetraplegia may be dependent in the physical aspects of parenting. Patients with low-level tetraplegia are able to participate in the more physical aspects of parenting with some level of adaptations, such as a wheelchair-accessible table with sides to change an infant.[185] Parenting skills for a patient with paraplegia depend on the environment and the specific activity being performed as well as the mobility of the individual. Therapists can provide advice and ideas to assist with the selection of parenting and baby equipment as well as being a resource in discussing and adapting equipment options such as slide-down cribs, adjustable-height high chairs, carrying slings or supports, and baby strollers that can be more easily pushed with one hand.[185,186]

Assistive Technology

AT can be helpful in letting people resume more independent lives in areas of self-care, work, and recreation. AT is defined by the 1998 Technology-Related Assistance for Individuals with Disabilities Act

(Public Law 105-394). It defines AT devices as "any item, piece of equipment, or product system, whether acquired commercially, modified, or customized, that is used to increase, maintain, or improve functional capabilities of individuals with disabilities." Hedrick and colleagues[187] found that in both civilians and veterans the most frequently used AT devices were (1) manual mobility and independent living devices (e.g., manual wheelchairs, manual exercise equipment, manual motor vehicle control devices, such as a steering knob, walkers, and reachers); (2) powered mobility and independent living devices (e.g., power lifts, power doors, motorized wheelchairs, power-assisted motor vehicle operation devices); (3) prosthetics and orthotics (static and dynamic, e.g., splints, mentioned earlier); (4) alternative computer access devices, which may be as simple as a typing splint to as complex as brain control; and (5) speech-generating devices, formerly known as *augmentative and alternative communication devices.*

Many specialty facilities that treat large numbers of SCI patients will have specialized therapists called Assistive Technology Practitioners (ATPs), Seating and Mobility Specialists (SMS), Certified Driver Rehabilitation Specialist (CDRS), and/or AT departments to specifically assess, select, and train in the use of device(s)—specifically seating, driving, and electronic access.[188] ATPs have a broad scope of practice regarding technology implementation for consumers with disabilities. ATPs, SMS, and CDRS demonstrate extensive experience in each specialty field, pass certification exams, and may come from many backgrounds including rehabilitation, education, and engineering.

Not every team has access to someone with a specialized certification; thus consideration should be given by the primary therapist in the evaluation phase to include what are the patient's primary needs at this time and moving forward for safety, quality of life, and independence. For example, when considering the wheelchair, a therapist must first consider the physical needs of the patient and then look at the environmental context. Considering where the patient will use the chair and how it will get there, looking at the "big picture" rather than only the mobility device is essential for success. How will the wheelchair be transported? Can the wheelchair be locked down so the patient may drive in a van or be a dependent passenger? Can the patient load the manual chair into his or her car (Fig. 14.32)? All of these details need to be considered as the patient makes a final decision on chair type and specialization.

There are specially trained practitioners called *driving rehabilitation specialists* who specialize in recommending equipment and transportation of the patient as a passenger in addition to providing driver education and driver training. They help to evaluate and to assist with making correct vehicle modifications and adaptive equipment choices for the patient as a driver. There are over 700 specialists who identify as driving rehabilitation specialists represented in the United States and Canada. Certified Driver Rehabilitation Specialist Certification (CDRS) is a credential offered by the Association of Driver Rehabilitation Specialist (ADED) representing advanced experience and expertise in diverse areas within the field. Those that hold a CDRS credential have passed a formal certification exam, have proven their capacity for providing the full spectrum of driver rehabilitation services, are held to the ADED Best Practice Guideline and Code of Ethics, and recertify every 3 years. Currently there are 370 active CDRS in the United States and Canada. A professional can be found on the Association for Driver Rehabilitation Specialists.[189,190]

When considering a sedan, these specialists will evaluate the patient to see how he or she operates primary and secondary vehicle controls, opens and closes the door, transfers into the vehicle, and stores, secures, and retrieves the wheelchair. If the patient is unable to perform any of those tasks, then a van may be an option. Modifications

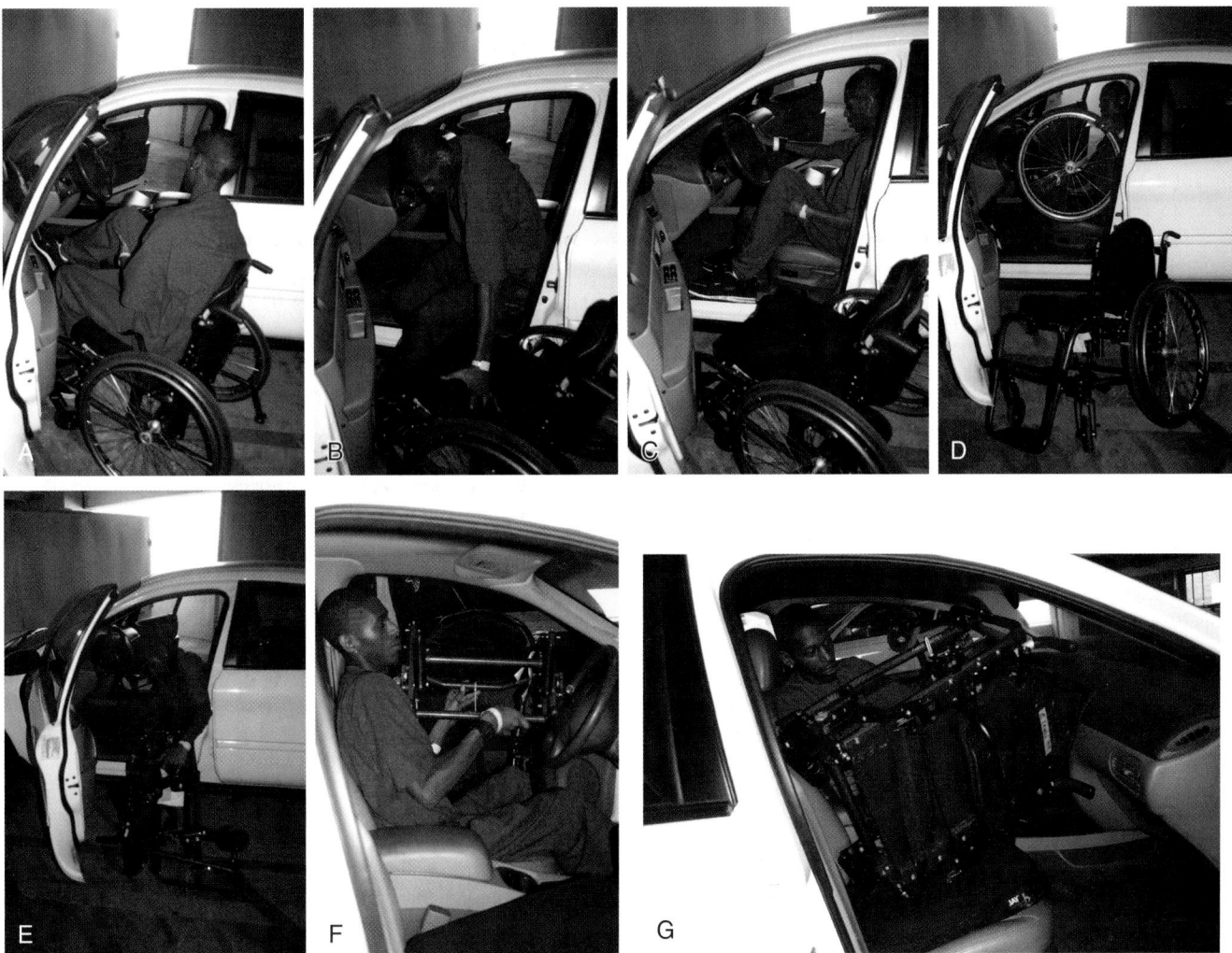

Fig. 14.32 Car Transfer. Most patients with a paraplegic level of injury are modified independent (FIM level 6) in the performance of a car transfer. The patient approaches the car on the driver's side and opens the door. **(A)** After stabilizing the wheelchair, he may place his foot or feet into the car or leave them on the footrest or the ground. **(B)** He performs a depression-style transfer onto the seat of the car; **(C)** positions his lower extremities appropriately inside the car; and **(D)** prepares to get the wheelchair into the car by removing the wheels (quick release) and cushion and placing these on the floor in the front passenger area or in the back seat. **(E** to **G)** The rigid model of the wheelchair is folded and transferred across the patient onto the passenger seat. Transferring out of the car is the reverse process, beginning with getting the wheelchair out of the car and reassembling it.

can allow a person to transfer to the van's driver seat or to drive from the wheelchair. The driving control technology that is available to compensate for reduced strength or ROM includes steering systems, hand controls, and reduced effort and zero effort steering and braking. The rehabilitation specialist will provide a comprehensive evaluation to determine the patient's ability to drive. That evaluation will consider visual, perceptual, and functional abilities as well as reaction time and behind-the-wheel assessment. In both sedan and van selection, it is always best to recommend that the patient consult the driving rehabilitation specialist before purchasing and modifying the vehicle.

Technology is ever changing; therefore the patient may need assistance to access many electronic devices, such as computers, digital readers, televisions, lights, call systems, cell phones, music systems, and smart home systems. Many patients require extensive assistance to understand and integrate their task-specific products into their smart

home devices. Smart home devices fall under the blanketed domain of home automation or domotics.[191] From 2011 to 2016 the market experienced rapid growth in the domain of home automation with the first devices with full voice activation hitting the market. Both phone and home speaker systems allow for one touch or voice activation for device use following set up. Despite significant improvements in access with these advances, patients with diaphragmatic compromise, dysarthric speech, poor dentition, and/or consonant deletion due to a regional accent struggle with voice activation and commands. As smart home systems progress for the general population, the cost of device and versatility of the products improve for individuals with disabilities. Although working toward home automation can be the goal for those with disabilities, the professionals assisting with device set up and maintenance need to consider the unique challenge of integrating devices across platforms. Patients need to be educated regarding how to troubleshoot their home automation systems, who to contact if issues occur, and vulnerabilities that may result from one device updating when others do not.

The most popular and inexpensive way to access a computer is speech recognition software. For patients who are unable to utilize voice activation with a computer, dexterity is required to operate many standard devices. There are off-the-shelf adaptations using universal designs to enable persons with limited dexterity to use technology, including touch screen or keyboard on screen allowing for pointer and mouth-stick use. A person with a higher tetraplegic level of injury can use alternative methods to access a computer, such as pneumatic controls (sip-and-puff devices), eye gaze system, or bite-switch options.[192] Shortcut keystrokes are a way for most users to limit the burden of keyboard use while also eliminating the need for a mouse.

Often considered a "last-choice communication system" it is important to note that Brain-Computer Interfaces (BCIs) have advanced significantly in since 2014. BCIs translate brain signals into computer commands in real-time via electroencephalographic signals, magneto-encephalography, electrocorticography, intracortical microelectrode recording of action potentials, or through imaging such as functional magnetic resonance imaging, or functional near-infrared spectroscopy.[193] The *Journal of Brain-Computer Interface* published its first issue in 2014, and the journal continues to report on a broad range of BCIs that replace, restore, enhance, supplement, or improve brain output.[193] At this time, the majority of BCI studies have focused on proof-of-principle; whereas actual BCI use has been limited to a handful of case studies. Investigators note that the most promising area of BCI use is not in-home computer access or home automation, but instead it is part of neurorehabilitation.

It is easy for therapists to become swept up in the latest technology when determining how to improve their patients' access and quality of life. When introducing AT and adaptive equipment to the patient, therapists should focus on utilizing the most basic form of technology with the shortest learning period. Often, patients are introduced to and utilize technology for a limited time before moving into different equipment or attempting to complete a task in a new way. For example, patients with C3 to C4 injuries, depending on neck strength and ROM, can use equipment such as mouth sticks for pushing cell phone buttons from the wheelchair in addition to the head rest buttons or a sip-and-puff switch (Fig. 14.33). Patients with C5 injuries begin to use their biceps, deltoids, and internal and

external rotator strength to interact with their environment. Positioning of the buttons, devices, or mounts for devices is important for these patients, who may or may not be using an MAS. Adaptive splinting for support at the wrist can allow these patients to use their upper arms in writing, typing, turning pages, and using computers (see Fig. 14.13). Patients with wrist function but no finger function can use utensil holders with a pointer to "dial" a phone number, for example, or can use their natural tenodesis to grasp and manipulate objects. For injuries at the T1 level and below, interaction with the environment in all areas should be independent.

Additive Manufacturing

Commonly referred to as 3D printing, additive manufacturing (AM) is the creation of an object by building it layer by layer. AM printers have become more accessible in hospitals and clinics as AM printer price decreases, size varies, and production quality improves.[194] AM allows for complete freedom in design through the use of computer aided design (CAD) software that works by scanning the patient to allow for device creation based on their unique characteristics.[194] The CAD software divides the computer generated object into layers. The AM machine then prints out each layer of the device in the material selected by the creator. AM is currently used in rehabilitation for individuals following SCI for orthoses, prostheses, and AT fabrication.

Preliminary studies of AM fabrication devices in rehabilitation highlight the use of this technology for complete customization, rapid manufacturing time, and an inexpensive durable material. A 2014 feasibility study revealed that an AM created prosthetic hand cost $50 to fabricate, compared to the traditionally obtained device, which cost over $4,000.[195]

It is important to note that AM does not have a developed reimbursement model at this time, due to perceived issues in quality control between products, risk management, and liability. All of these topics require investigation before insurance authorization standards are established. Despite the lack of funding, AM is beginning to be widely used in the rehabilitation model as a cost effective and personalized solution to orthoses, prostheses, and AT fabrication.

Mobility

Bed Mobility and Coming to Sit

The components of bed mobility include rolling side to side, rolling supine to prone, coming to sit, and scooting in all directions while either long or short sitting. Initial training for bed mobility is usually conducted on the mat, as it is easier to learn on the firmer surface. When skills on the mat are mastered, the patient can be progressed to a less firm surface, such as the bed. Bed mobility is a challenging skill for patients with tetraplegia to learn because of their limited upper-extremity strength (see Fig. 14.21A to C).[55,118,196] To accommodate the loss of upper-extremity musculature, compensatory strategies and assistive devices, such as bed loops, may be used (see Fig. 14.21F to I). Patients with paraplegia often master bed mobility skills quickly and much more easily than patients with tetraplegia because of their intact upper-extremity musculature.[55,118]

Pressure Relief in the Upright Position

The patient with high tetraplegia achieves independent pressure relief in the wheelchair through appropriately prescribed specialty controls. For example, a pneumatic control switch may be used to activate the tilt mode of a power wheelchair (Fig. 14.34). When the patient is unable to operate a specialty switch, an attendant control may be used. When powered options are not feasible because of cognitive deficits, financial limitations, or other reasons, a manual recliner (Fig. 14.35A)

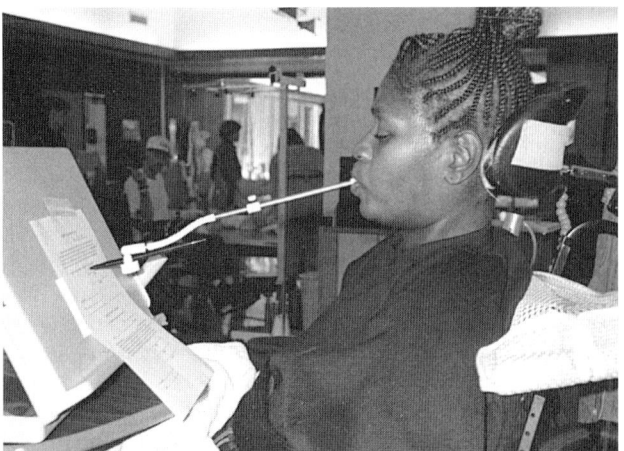

Fig. 14.33 Mouth stick writing can be accomplished with the patient upright in the wheelchair and with the support of a bedside table and bookstand.

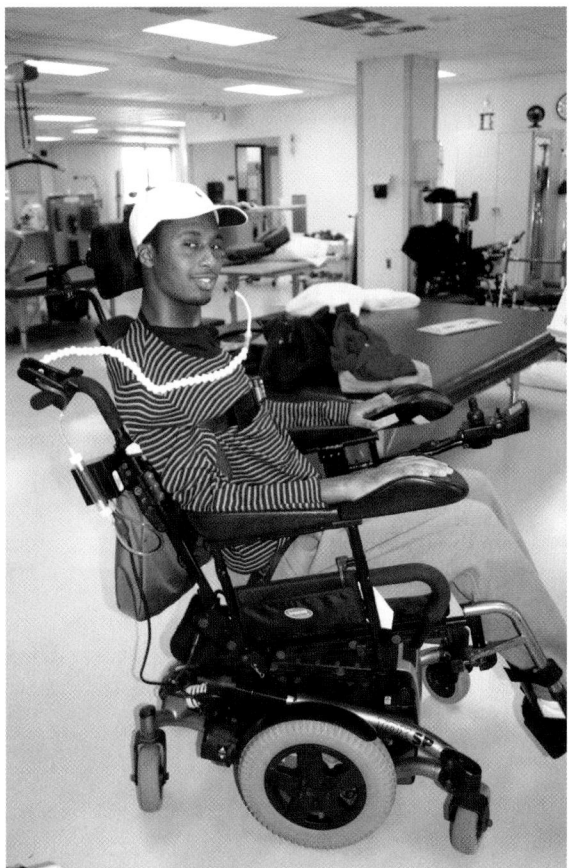

Fig. 14.34 The pneumatic control (sip-and-puff straw) is usually ordered on a power reclining or tilt-in-space wheelchair for patients with injury levels above C6. The straw is removable, and several are supplied with the wheelchair. The straw is attached to a flexible arm, and it is adjustable to different heights and angles to fit the needs of the patient.

or tilt wheelchair (see Fig. 14.35B) is recommended. When patients are dependent in performing pressure relief, they can be taught to instruct others in this skill. Patients with mid- and low-level tetraplegia are taught to perform a side or forward lean technique for pressure relief if the strength of the shoulder musculature is appropriate (Fig. 14.36). Traditionally, patients with paraplegia are often taught to perform pressure relief by performing and maintaining a pushup (depression) (Fig. 14.37). However, evidence suggests that the use of alternative methods should also be encouraged for these individuals because they may considerably reduce upper limb (UL) mechanical loads while being just as effective.[197,198] It is important for individuals with SCI to reduce UL loads whenever possible in order to preserve UL function and prevent overuse injury. The forward lean and side to side methods of performing a weight shift have been proven to be effective alternatives to a depression pressure relief in order to preserve skin and soft-tissue integrity among individuals with SCI.[197,198]

The appropriate time to maintain the change in position is usually 60 seconds at intervals of 30 to 60 minutes. The treatment plan should include instructing the patient in ways to ensure that the schedule for pressure relief is maintained in all settings. The use of watches, clocks, timers, and attendant care may be necessary.

Wheelchair Transfers

The physical act of moving oneself from one surface to another is described as a *transfer*. Wheelchair transfers may be accomplished in many different ways. The type of transfer used by a patient is determined by the injury level, residual limb function, assistance needed, patient preference, and safety of the transfer. When performing transfers, both the patient and the person assisting must give attention to the use of appropriate body mechanics.

Dependent transfers may be accomplished with an electric (power) patient lift, manual hydraulic patient lift, manual pivot, transfer board, or manual dependent lift, which may require two or three people. A transfer using an overhead power patient lift is the least physically challenging for the caregiver; however, these lifts are costly and are not

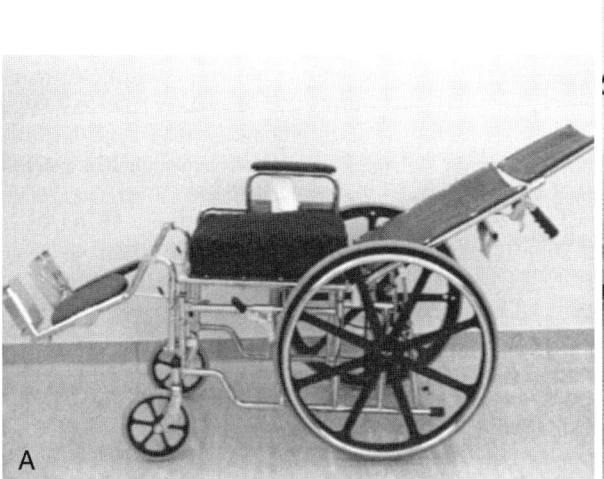
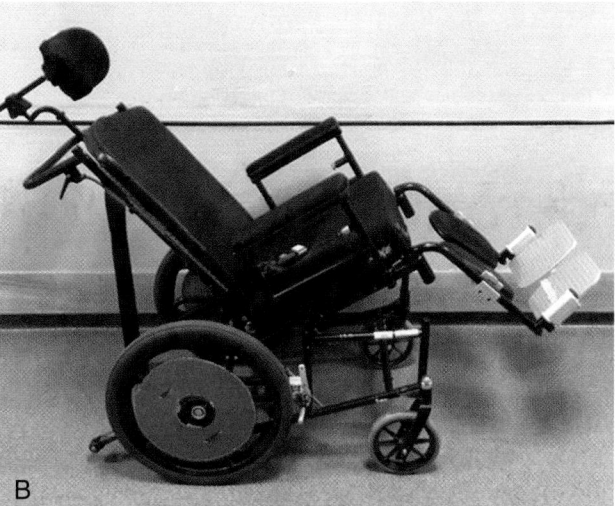

Fig. 14.35 (A) The manual reclining wheelchair is a piece of durable medical equipment that is prescribed on a temporary or a permanent basis. The back of the wheelchair fully reclines, and the legrests elevate to allow for effective pressure relief while the patient is out of bed. Other features of the wheelchair are desk armrests, which may be adjustable in height; a removable headrest; and removable legrests. The wheelchair folds and may be transported in a vehicle. **(B)** The manual tilt in space wheelchair is an alternative to the manual reclining wheelchair and may be preferred especially in cases where increased muscle tone in hip extensors is present. The 90/90 hip position is better maintained in this wheelchair, which can decrease the need for repositioning.

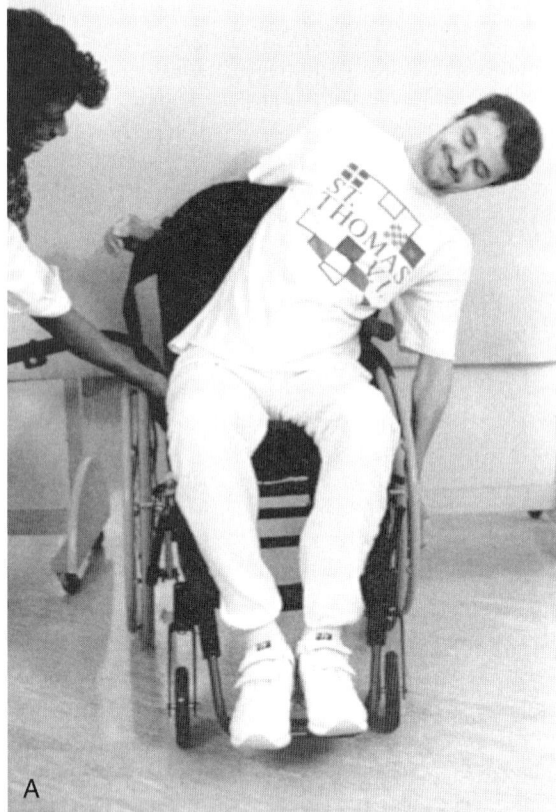

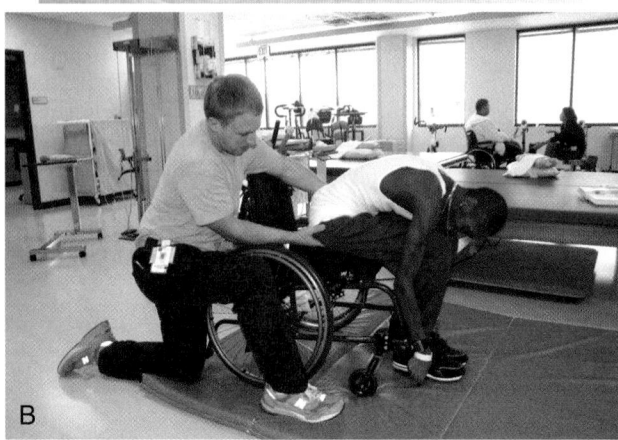

Fig. 14.36 (A) Pressure Relief: Side Lean. The tetraplegic patient with a C6- to C7-level injury may use a side lean to achieve pressure relief over the ischial tuberosities. The patient hooks one upper extremity around the push handle or back post of the wheelchair on one side and leans away from the hooked upper extremity until the ischium on the hooked side is clear of the wheelchair cushion. The position is maintained for 1 minute and repeated on the other side. **(B) Pressure Relief: Forward Lean.** The forward lean method of pressure relief is used for many different injury levels. The subject must have adequate range of motion at the hips and in the lumbosacral spine to allow the ischia to clear the wheelchair cushion at the end range position.

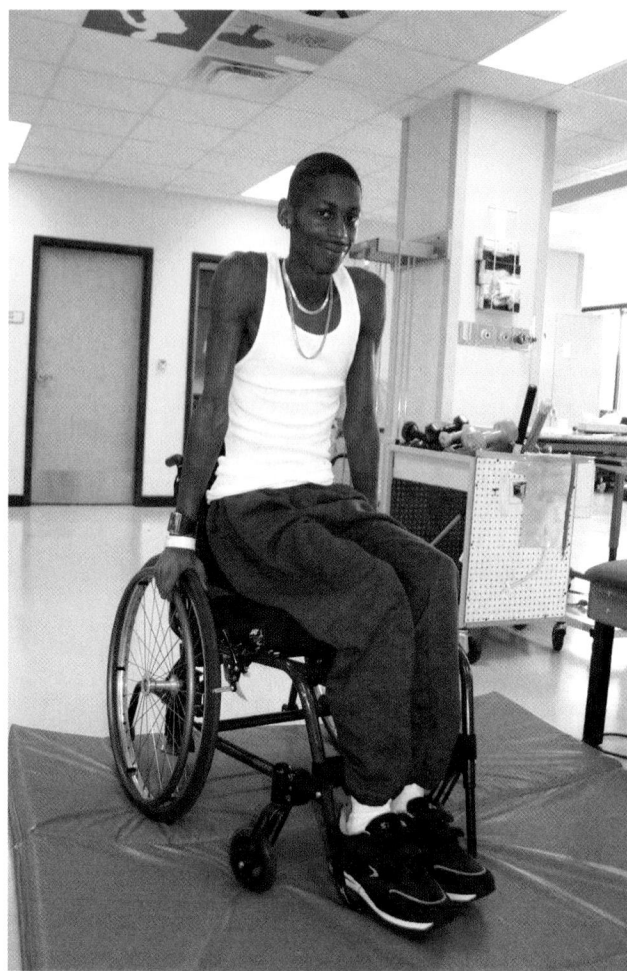

Fig. 14.37 Pressure Relief: Depression. This method of pressure relief is consistent with a full pushup in the wheelchair. Most patients with a paraplegic level of injury and some patients with a low tetraplegic injury level are able to perform this method of pressure relief.

easily transportable. The use of a manual hydraulic patient lift may be desirable if funding is not available for a power lift or the transfer needs to be done in an outdoor environment (i.e., car transfer). However, the hydraulic patient lift may not be the method of choice due to bulkiness, difficult storage, and transport. Pivot transfers or manual lifts may be used based on patient/caregiver preference or when

patients are smaller in stature and other, more costly, lift systems are not available to the individuals.

Transfers can be performed with the use of a transfer board, depression style, or via the stand or squat-pivot method. The mechanics of teaching an assisted transfer to a patient with C7 tetraplegia is depicted in Fig. 14.38. To use compensation for movements such as transfer, momentum forces create movement by teaching patients to swing their head in the opposite direction from where they want the hips to go. Also, head and eye gaze relationships are important for balance and rolling whereby arm swing creates momentum and the body will follow the eyes and head when learning this skill. The patient is taught to position the wheelchair, position the transfer board, use correct body mechanics to get the best leverage to effect movement in the desired direction, remove the board, and position his or her body appropriately.[55,199]

Wheelchair transfers are performed on many different surfaces. The training procedure begins with the easiest transfer and progresses to the more difficult transfer. Instructions for wheelchair transfers usually begin on level surfaces and progress to uneven surfaces as individual strength and skill allow.[55] Given these two principles, the following list is an example of how one might proceed with transfer training:
1. Mat transfer (see Fig. 14.38)
2. Bed transfer

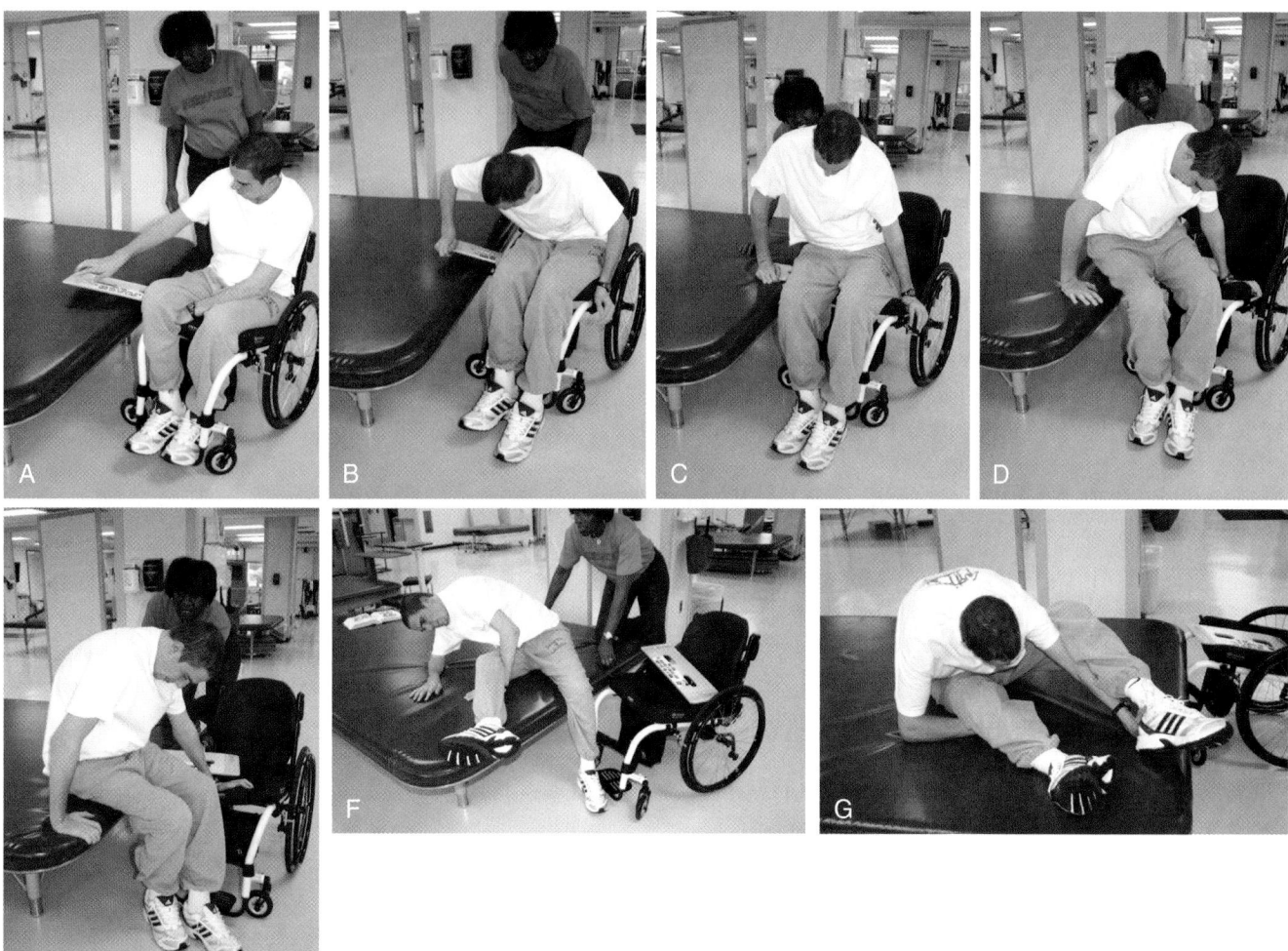

Fig. 14.38 Wheelchair to Mat Transfer Using a Transfer Board. **(A)** The patient positions the wheelchair at a 20- to 30-degree angle to the surface to which he is transferring and positions the board with or without assistance. **(B)** The patient moves forward in the wheelchair to clear the tire in preparation for lateral movement on the transfer board. **(C)** To achieve the appropriate mechanical leverage, the patient is instructed to twist the upper body and look over the trailing shoulder **(D)**. He pushes and lifts to affect movement across the board. **(E)** When the patient has achieved a safe position on the transferring surface, the transfer board is removed. **(F and G)** The patient is helped to get his feet onto the surface.

3. Toilet transfer
4. Bath transfer
5. Car transfer (see Fig. 14.32)
6. Floor transfer (Figs. 14.39 to 14.41)
7. Other surfaces (e.g., armchair, sofa, theater seat, and pool)

Wheelchair Mobility Skills

Instructions in the safe and appropriate use of the wheelchair may begin before getting the patient out of bed by orienting the patient to the wheelchair and its component parts.

Ideally, a power reclining or tilt wheelchair is supplied for patients with C1 to C5 tetraplegia to promote maximal independence. The most common drive-system options available for these patients include, but are not limited to, chin drive, pneumatic systems (see Fig. 14.34), and head control (Fig. 14.42). A patient with mid- to low-level tetraplegia may be instructed in the use of both power and manual upright wheelchairs. The patient with paraplegia is instructed in the use of a manual upright wheelchair unless there are extenuating

circumstances. For example, a power wheelchair is appropriate for a patient who is 50 years old and has severe rheumatoid arthritis.

There are wheelchair options that combine the benefits of a manual wheelchair with a power-assist component (Fig. 14.43).[200–202] This option may be best suited for patients who have some upper-extremity weakness, joint degeneration, upper-extremity pain from propelling a manual wheelchair, or reduced exercise capacity or endurance. This type of wheelchair could potentially delay secondary injuries of manual wheelchair users. Both power and manual wheelchair mobility training begins on level surfaces. When a patient is instructed on how to propel a manual wheelchair, it is suggested that a semicircular pattern be used to reduce the trauma to the UEs. Wheelchair gloves are beneficial in reducing friction over the palms of the hands during propulsion (Fig. 14.44). Research evidence is available that demonstrates the safety and superior efficacy of a formal approach to wheelchair skills training of wheelchair users and their caregivers. The Wheelchair Skills Program is one example of such a program and is available free on the Internet.[203] This program includes useful evaluation

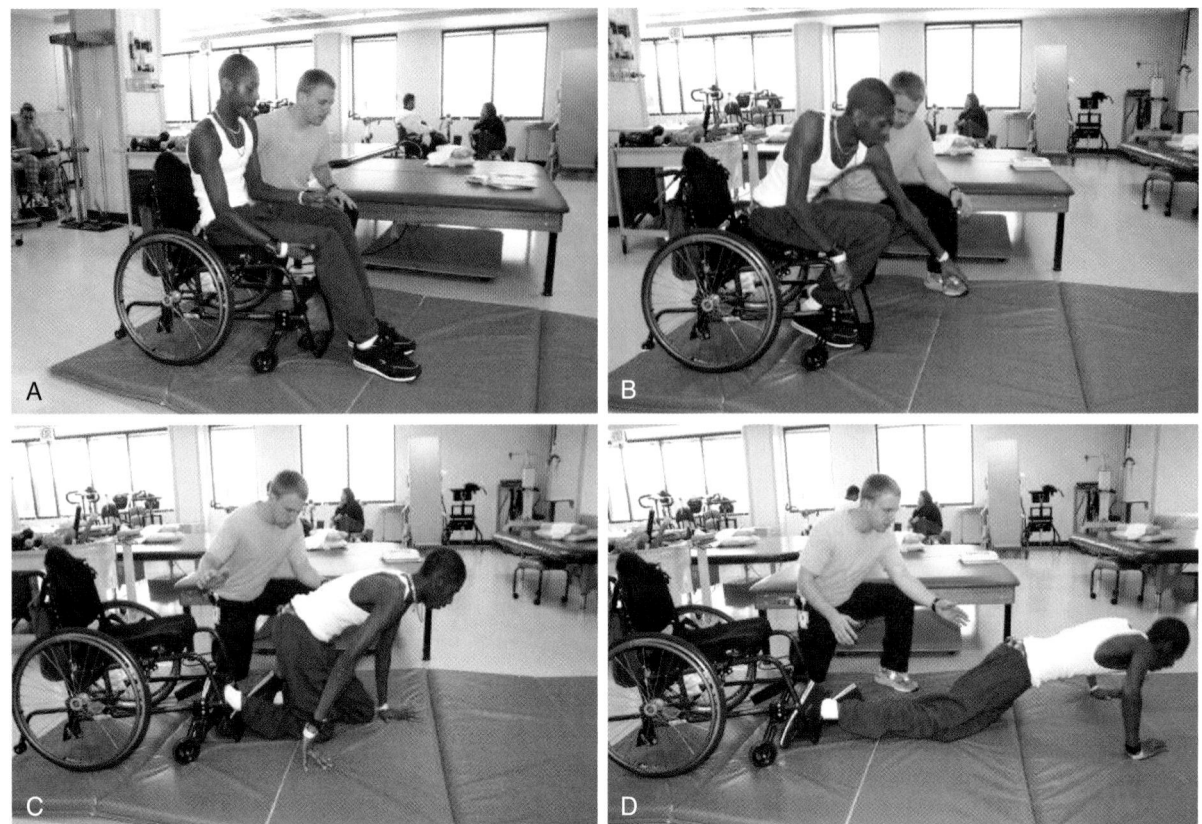

Fig. 14.39 Floor Transfer. The independent performance of a floor transfer is a goal for most patients who have a paraplegic level of injury. The patient may use different techniques to get onto the floor. Forward floor transfer: **(A)** The patient positions his feet off the footrest and moves forward onto the front edge of his cushion. **(B)** He reaches for the floor, first with one hand then with both, and **(C)** lowers his knees to the floor. **(D)** He advances his hands forward until his body is clear of the wheelchair.

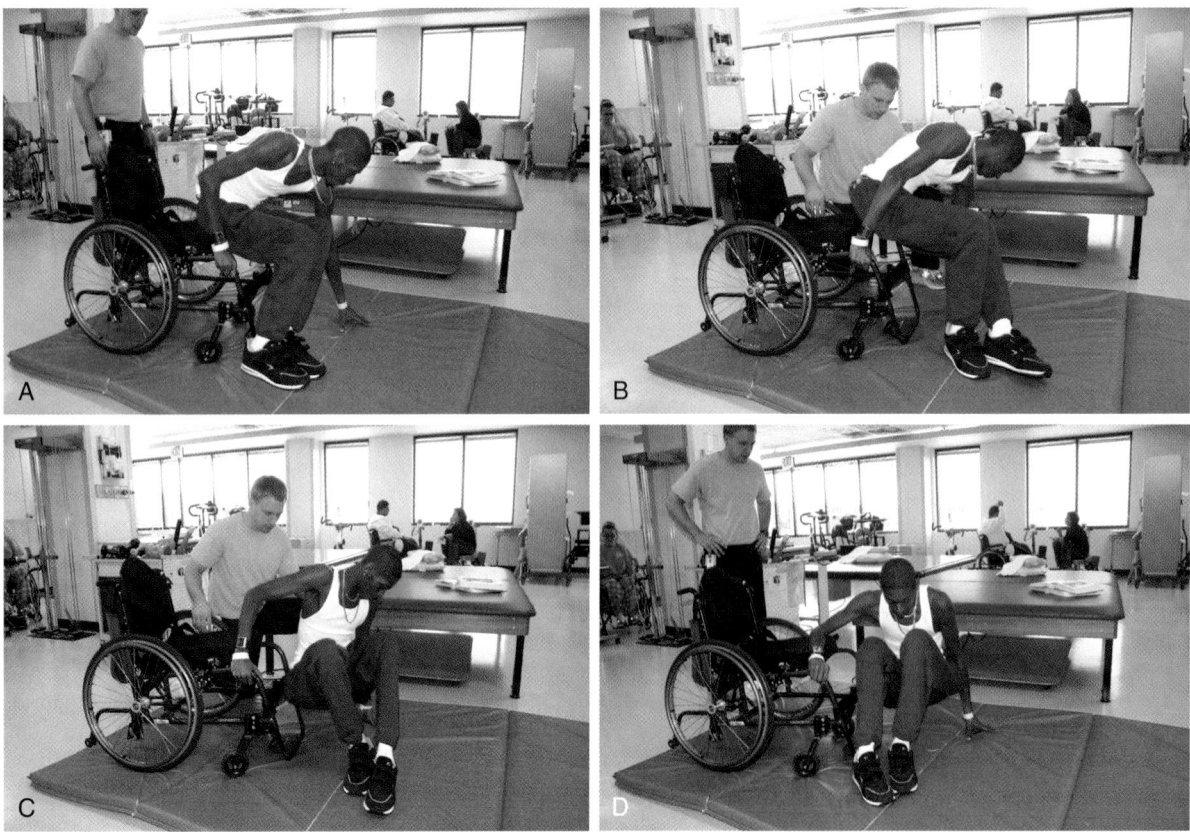

Fig. 14.40 Floor Transfer Sideways. After moving to the front of the wheelchair seat, **(A)** the patient leans to the left and reaches for the floor and **(B)** shifts his weight toward the left arm. **(C** and **D)** He balances his weight between both arms and in a very controlled manner lowers his body to the floor.

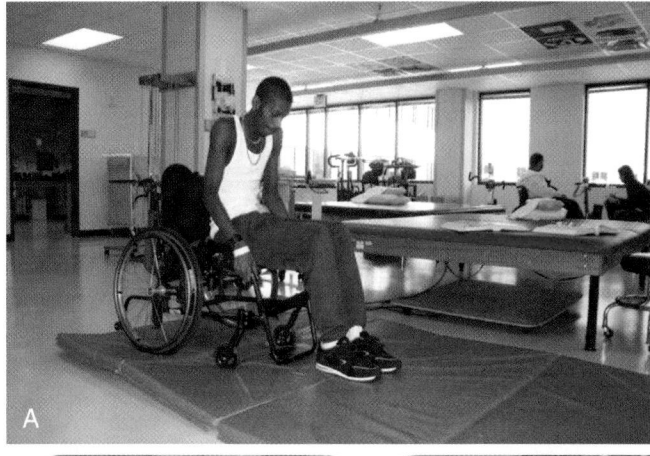

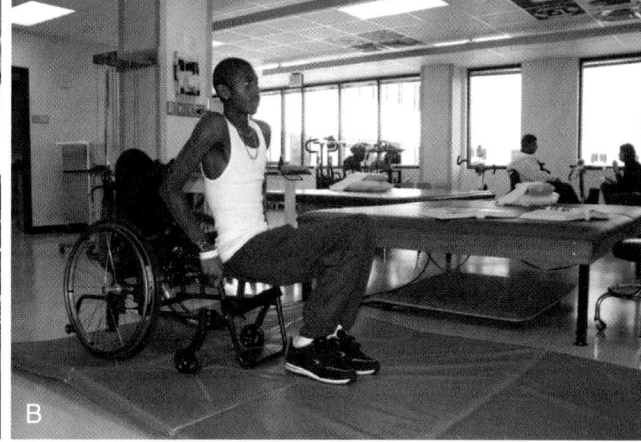

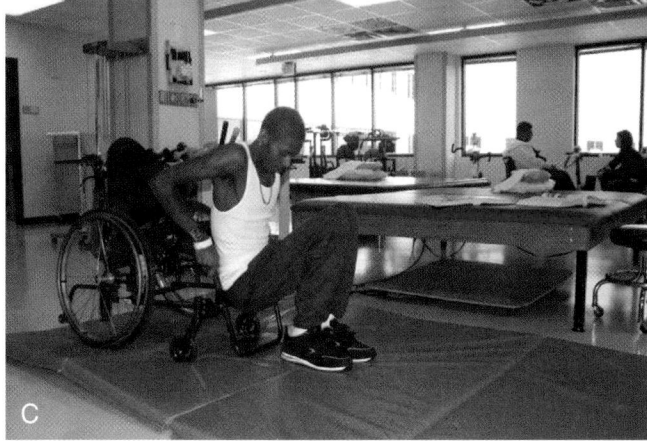

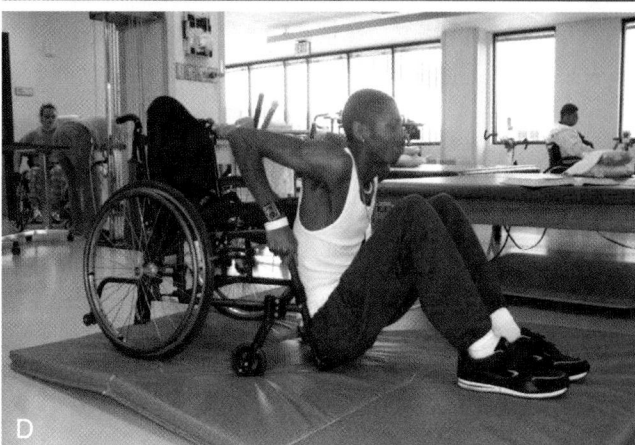

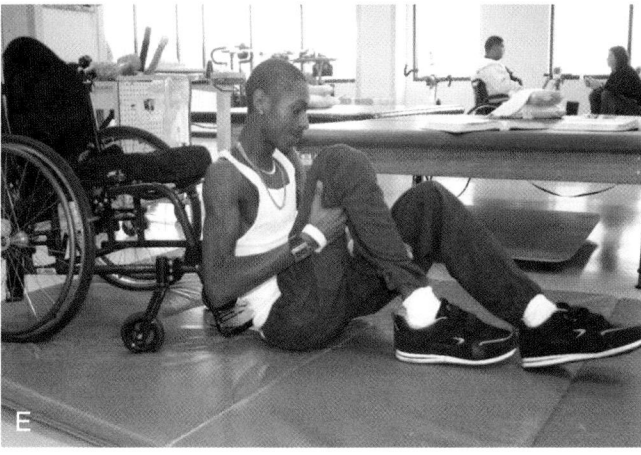

Fig. 14.41 Forward Lowering Floor Transfer. (A) This transfer method begins from a balanced position on the front edge of the wheelchair seat with feet on the floor. (B) Hips are lifted off the seat forward enough to (C) lower the buttocks to the footrest. Note that this requires significant strength and control through the upper body as well as (D) excellent range of motion in shoulder extension and a reasonably loose anterior shoulder capsule. (E) Legs are moved forward for balance. Also, a small pillow or cushion (not shown here) can be used to pad the footrest to protect the patient's skin.

and training tools to help practitioners translate this research evidence into clinical practice.[204,205]

Wheelchair mobility training may progress toward more difficult skills as follows:
1. Mobility on level surfaces in open areas
2. Setup for transfers
3. Mobility in tight spaces
4. Mobility in crowded areas
5. On and off elevators
6. Up and down ramps
7. Through doors
8. Wheelies (Fig. 14.45)
9. Negotiation of rough terrain
10. Up and down curbs and steps (Figs. 14.46 and 14.47)

Equipment

In SCI rehabilitation, the use of equipment is necessary to achieve the expected outcomes. Clinicians work closely with the physician and other team members, including the rehabilitation technology supplier, to determine the most appropriate equipment to meet individual needs. It is important to have access to trial equipment so the patient has the opportunity to practice with equipment similar to what will be prescribed. Ideally the rehabilitation technology supplier should be accessible to the rehabilitation team to allow for necessary adjustments

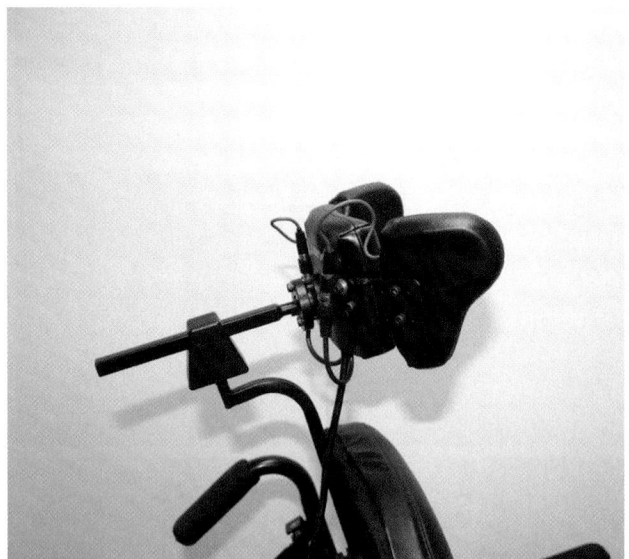

Fig. 14.42 Head array is a headrest and head control for driving wherein the position of the head activates the drive control of the wheelchair. It is appropriate for persons with high cervical injuries. The head array switches can be adjusted to the individual's specific needs relative to their active range of motion and control of their head. The switches are embedded in the headrest panels and not only control driving but can also control the activation of other devices for environmental control. The side panels of the headrest can be straight or curbed depending on the needs of the patient. Additionally, the head array can be sized for either adult or pediatric patient.

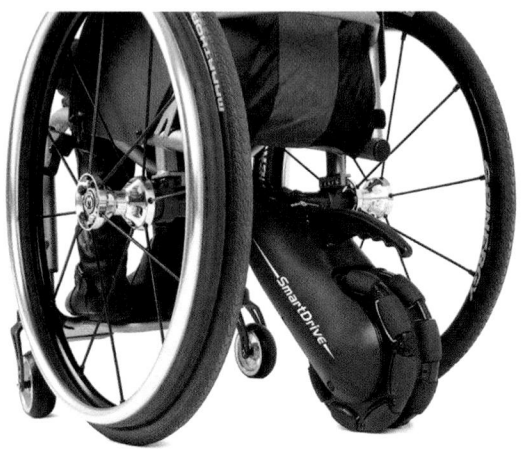

Fig. 14.43 Smartdrive. Courtesy of Permobil.

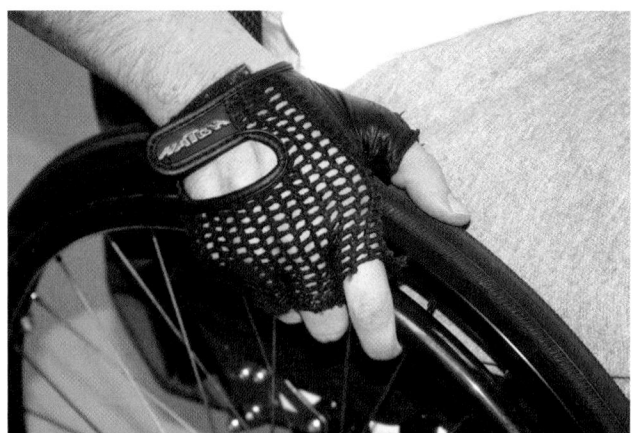

Fig. 14.44 Para Push Gloves. Wheelchair gloves, mesh back, open fingers, and leather-padded palm. Usually appropriate for patients with paraplegia-level injuries. Available from multiple suppliers.

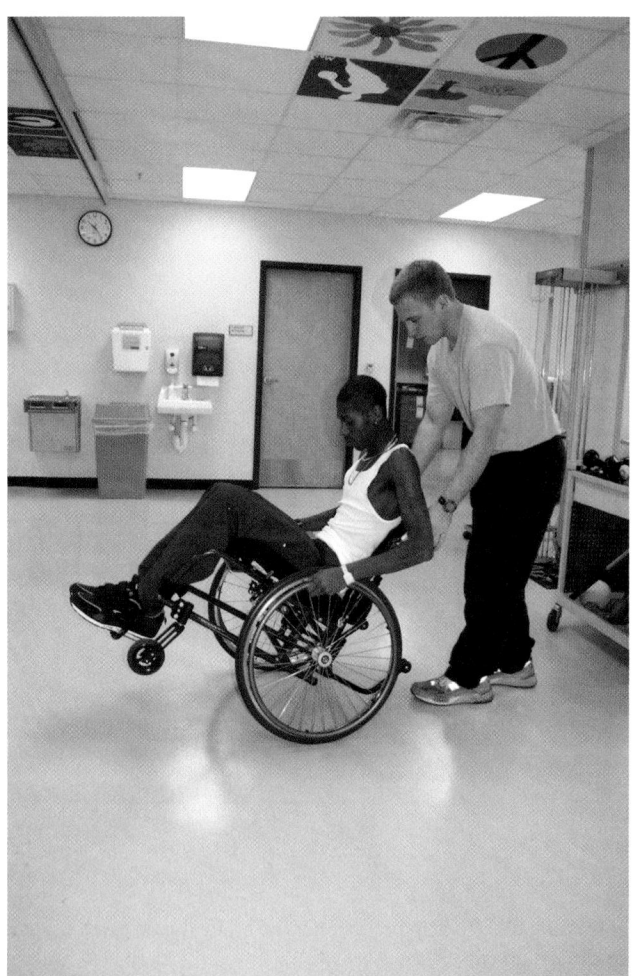

Fig. 14.45 A wheelie is a functional mobility skill that enhances functional independence. The performance of a wheelie is a precursor to negotiating steep ramps, curbs, steps, and rough terrain.

to the equipment. In addition, rehabilitation technology suppliers should be knowledgeable and responsible for educating rehabilitation professionals regarding new products. When possible, all equipment should be ordered from a single supplier to reduce confusion when the need for repairs arise. To ensure that the most appropriate piece of equipment is prescribed, the following must be considered: durability, function, transportability, comfort, cost, safety, cosmesis, and acceptance by the user.[206] Generally, the higher the injury level, the more costly the equipment based on the technology involved. Table 14.8 lists equipment according to injury level.

Equipment should be ordered as soon as possible so the patient can be fitted before discharge. Shorter lengths of stay make early equipment ordering difficult. For example, a patient may not have 3/5 wrist extension to be fitted with a tenodesis brace but with strengthening over time would be an excellent candidate. Clinicians need to negotiate

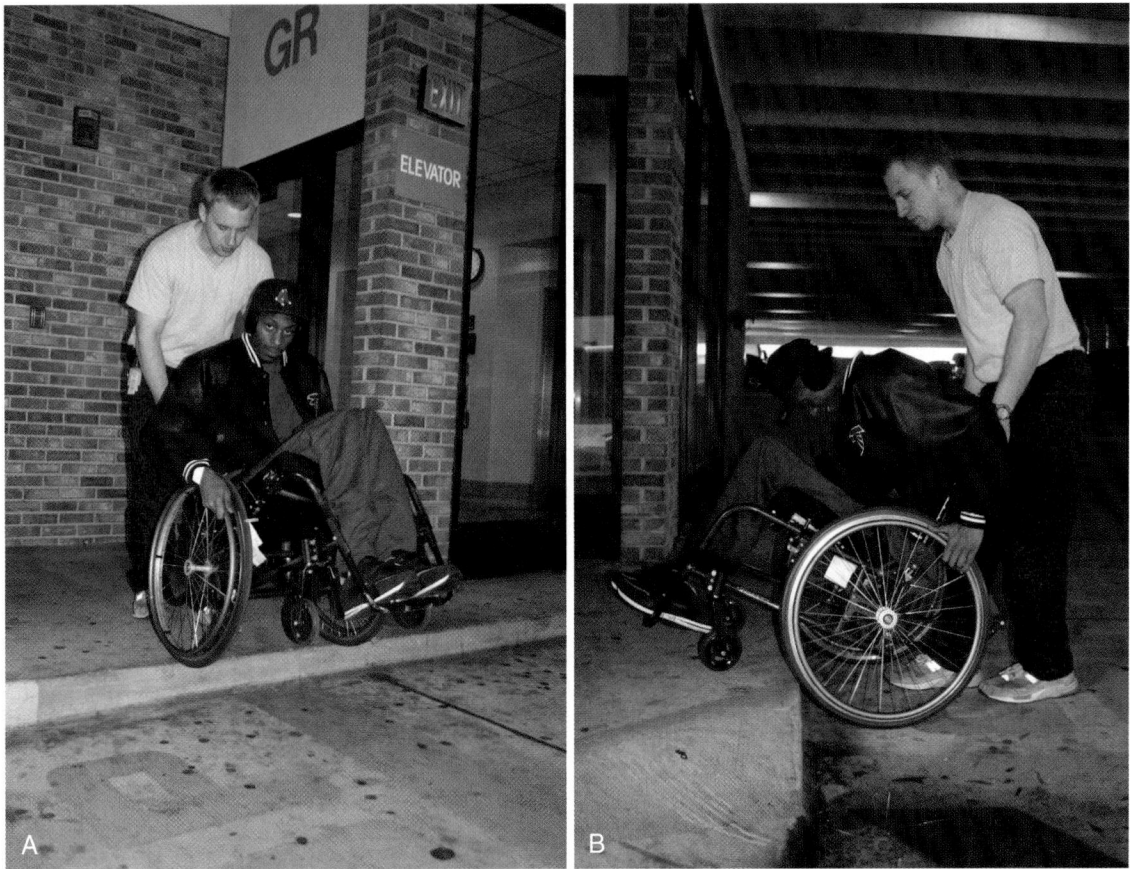

Fig. 14.46 (A) Descending a curb is an advanced wheelchair mobility skill. This man with AIS A, T12 paraplegia assumes the balanced wheelie position and approaches the curb in a forward position. The wheelie position is maintained as he rolls off the curb. **(B)** Climbing a curb with assistance is also an advanced skill. This is the same man as in A. He "pops" into a wheelie and advances his wheelchair to move his casters up onto the curb. He then reaches back to his wheel, leans forward, and pushes as the helper assists by lifting the back of the chair. A more advanced skill would be to perform this activity by approaching the curb with speeds fast enough to gain momentum, "pop" a wheelie, and advance up and over the curb in one continuous movement (not shown). The curb height, strength, level of injury, and body composition of the patient are determining factors for speed requirements.

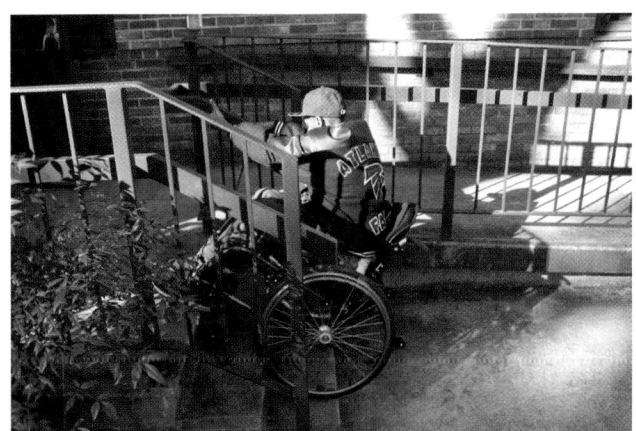

Fig. 14.47 Descending Steps Using One Handrail. This patient with AIS A, level T12 approaches the steps backward, using the handrail on his right with both hands, and lowers himself down three steps. This is one of several methods that may be used to negotiate steps.

with the funding source so that equipment may be ordered in the outpatient setting. Equipment required for the SCI population is costly and requires extensive review by third-party payers before funding is approved or denied. Many health care policies do not cover the funding of needed equipment. As a result of these factors, many patients are discharged without the equipment they need. Lack of appropriate equipment may result in (1) a feeling of loss of control, (2) contractures and postural deformities, (3) skin breakdown, (4) a loss of skills learned in rehabilitation, (5) poor self-image, and (6) increased dependence on others.[55,207]

Seating Principles

Many individuals spend 8 to 12 hours or more per day in their wheelchairs after an SCI. Consequently, proper seating of these patients may be the most important intervention clinicians provide. The seating process should be addressed on admission, continually throughout the rehabilitation program, and regularly after discharge to help prevent and minimize complications. The wheelchair is an integral part of the patient's self-image and in many ways will help define personal

TABLE 14.8 Equipment Needs Correlated to Injury Level

Injury Level	Equipment	Cost (in $)	Injury Level	Equipment	Cost (in $)
C1–C3	Ventilator (bedside)	8,000–12,000		Mobile arm support	500–1,000
	Ventilator (portable for wheelchair)	8,000–12,000		Upper-extremity orthotics	700–1,200
	Power tilt or recline wheelchair	17,000–26,000	C6	Power upright wheelchair	7500–20,000
	Manual recline wheelchair for transport	2,000–3,000		Manual wheelchair	2,000–6,000
	Wheelchair cushion	450–600		Power assist wheels (Fig. 14.63)	6,000
	Reclining commode or shower chair	2,500–4,000		Wheelchair cushion	450–600
	eADL control devices (TV, lights, fans)	400–1,000 (less if you have voice)		Bedside table	225
				ECU	6,000–1,0000
	eADL (thermostat, door locks, and openers)	200–7,000		eADL as listed above	
	ECU	6,000–10,000		Electric hospital bed	2,000–4,000
	Call system	100–500		Specialized mattress	800–10,000
	Bedside table	225		Commode or shower chair	500–1,500
	Fully electric hospital bed	2,000–4,000		ADL equipment	900–1,500
	Specialized mattress	3,500–4,0000		Tenodesis splint	1,700
	Access to a computer–accessories	1,000–2,000		Transfer board	100–200
	Computer and accessories	1,500–3,000		Hand control for car	500–2,500
	Communication devices	5,000–20,000		Bowel-bladder equipment	125–250
	Overhead power lift	6,000–15,000	C7–C8	Power upright wheelchair	7,500–15,000
	Hydraulic lift for transfers	1,200–2,000		Manual wheelchair	2,000–6,500
C4–C5	Power tilt or recline wheelchair	17,000–26,000		Wheelchair cushion	450–600
	Manual wheelchair for transport, i.e., K-4	1,500–2,000		Bedside table	225
	Lap tray	500–1,000		ECU	250–1,000
	Wheelchair cushion	450–600		Electric hospital bed	2,000–3,000
	Bedside table	225		Specialized mattress	600–10,000
	ECU	6,000–10,000		Commode or shower chair	1,500
	eADL control devices (TV, lights, and fans)	75–1,000		Hand controls for car	300–1,500
	eADL (thermostat, door locks, and openers)	200–7,000		ADL equipment	300–1,000
	Call system	100–500		Transfer board	100–200
	Fully electric hospital bed	2,000–4,000		Bowel and bladder equipment	125–250
	Specialized mattress	3,500–40,000	Paraplegia	Manual upright wheelchair	3,500–4,000
	Commode or shower chair	1,500–3,000		Wheelchair cushion	450–600
	Communication devices	5,000–20,000		Raised or padded commode seat (cutout)	200–400
	Access to computer (accessories only)	1,000–2,000		Tub bench	220
	Access to computer (computer and accessories)	1,500–3,000		Hand controls for car	500–1,000
				ADL equipment	100–300
	Call system	100–500		Bowel and bladder equipment	50–250
	ADL equipment	400–1,400		Lower-extremity orthotics (if ambulation is a goal)	4,000–6,000
	Hydraulic lift for transfers	1,400–2,000			
	Overhead power lift	4,000–15,000			
	Overhead power lift (not in ceiling)	4000–5000			

ADL, Activity of daily living; *eADL*, electronic activities of daily living; *ECU*, environmental control unit.
Based on 2017–2018 Atlanta, Georgia, retail prices.

lifestyle.[208] Goals for seating the patient with an SCI are identified in Box 14.6.

Every seating session begins with a thorough examination, as described earlier. Trial simulations are essential to determine how the patient will function and maintain posture over time in the seating system. Simulations help to avoid costly mistakes. The patient must be involved in the decision making process to ensure that the seating system will work.

Individuals with SCI are at high risk of pressure injury due to lack of mobility and impaired sensation. Great care should be taken to reduce pressure over bony prominences and to distribute pressure over as large an area as possible or to offload the pressure from the bony prominences.[209] Pressure-distributing or off-loading cushions should be evaluated clinically and with pressure-sensing devices to determine the optimal wheelchair cushion for each individual.

BOX 14.6 Goals for Seating the Patient With Spinal Cord Injury

1. Maximize functional independence
2. Improve pressure distribution and relief of pressure
3. Optimize comfort
4. Enhance the quality of life
5. Optimize good postural alignment and sitting balance
6. Compensate for fixed deformities
7. Allow for transportation of the mobility system

The following are basic seating concepts of proper postural alignment:
- Neutral pelvic alignment
- Symmetrical alignment of the trunk and neck
- Neutral head positioning over the pelvis
- Maintenance of a horizontal gaze
- Maintenance of ankle in neutral alignment with full support of the foot
- Maintenance of the thighs in neutral abduction and adduction with full contact with the cushion
  - Neutral shoulder positioning to avoid shoulder elevation, protraction, or retraction and to provide adequate upper-extremity support.[208] Elbow angle that approximates 100–120 degrees when the hand is resting at the top of the wheel or pushrim[202]

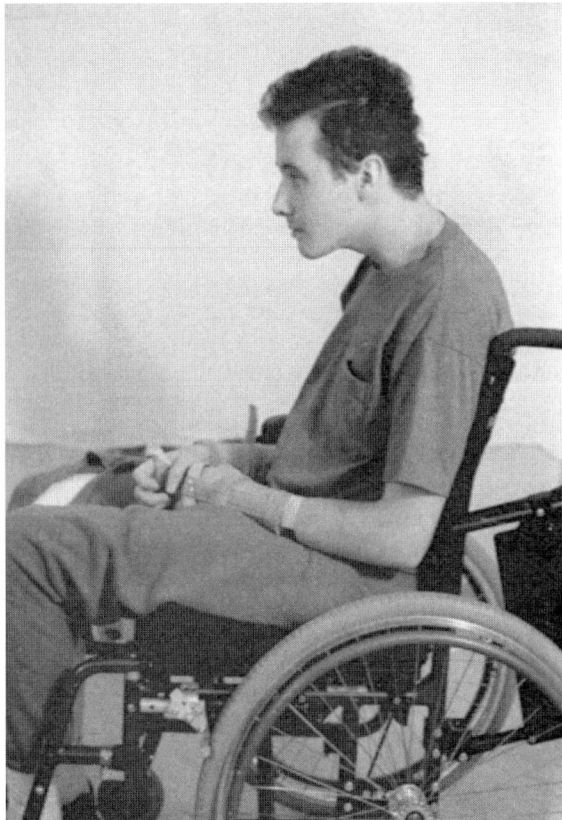

Fig. 14.48 Example of Typical Kyphotic C-Curve Posture in the Patient With Tetraplegia.

Many patients with muscle paralysis of the trunk find that the effects of gravity in a sitting position pull the head and upper torso forward and over the pelvis, resulting in a long kyphosis or a C-curved posture (Fig. 14.48).[210] Two resulting problems are increased weight bearing on the sacrum and development of a thoracic kyphosis, leading to neck hyperextension in an effort to maintain a horizontal gaze.[208,210] This position is also assumed by patients to improve their balance. This occurs when the seat-to-back angle is closed and the patient feels as if he or she is falling forward. Unfortunately, this poor sitting posture is quickly learned and difficult to correct. This posture can often be prevented by tilting the wheelchair slightly backward while maintaining a fixed seat-to-back angle (Fig. 14.49). In this position, the effects of gravity augment sitting balance and facilitate good spinal alignment. Education regarding proper positioning, the use of a sacral block, a firm wheelchair seat and back, and properly applied pelvic positioning devices also aid in preventing the kyphotic posture.

Asymmetrical muscle strength, asymmetrical spasticity, and preferential use of one UE over another often result in poor trunk alignment. The use of lateral trunk supports, lateral pelvic supports, and properly applied seat belts may aid in maintaining a symmetrical trunk posture.[208]

Strong muscle spasms, combined with the effects of gravity, may cause the person with severely impaired mobility to slide down in the wheelchair, resulting in increased pressure on the sacrum and shearing of the skin. For these patients, a manual wheelchair with adjustable seat and back angles can be used to improve stability. Power wheelchairs with power tilt systems allow users to reposition themselves and use the power tilt for improved stability.

Optimal pressure distribution is achieved by maximizing the surface area, allowing immersion into the seat cushion, and promoting a symmetrical posture. The width of the seat should be equal to or slightly more than that of the widest body part, with recent weight changes, body type, and other factors taken into consideration. The seat depth should come within 1 to 2 inches of the popliteal fossae, except when it interferes with LE management of the wheelchair; that is, foot propulsion. The height of the back should reflect the patient's motor function and seated stability. If the back is too high, it can create postural instability and restrict functional activities such as wheelchair

propulsion and wheelies. Patients with tetraplegia who use the push handles of the wheelchair to hook while performing functional activities may require custom modification of the wheelchair back (Fig. 14.50).

The size, weight, and portability of the wheelchair seating system affect the individual's lifestyle. The patient's home or work environment must be evaluated closely for accessibility so the wheelchair seating system can be used effectively in those environments. The buildings must be structurally sound and spacious to accommodate heavy-power wheelchair systems. The means of transportation of the wheelchair (car vs. van) may determine whether a rigid or folding wheelchair frame is indicated. Transit options and tie-down systems must be considered for safe transportation. The manual wheelchair must be adjusted to make it as efficient as possible to propel to reduce stress on upper-extremity joints. Many manual wheelchairs are lightweight (less than 35 pounds) and have multiple adjustments and choices of tires and casters, which make manual wheelchair propulsion more efficient. Reducing rolling resistance, positioning the rear axle for maximum propulsion stroke efficiency, and teaching efficient propulsion techniques reduce shoulder musculature fatigue and upper-extremity injury. Rear wheel size and rear seat to floor height should be selected so that when the wheelchair user is seated, he or she is able to touch the rear axle with the middle finger. This position increases the range of contact during propulsion. In addition, shifting the distribution of the user's weight back over the rear axle (usually accomplished by moving the rear wheel axle forward) reduces the percentage of weight on the front casters, making propulsion more efficient.[204,211] This adjustment reduces the rear stability of the wheelchair, so the use of anti-tip bars and/or training in wheelie maneuvers is essential.

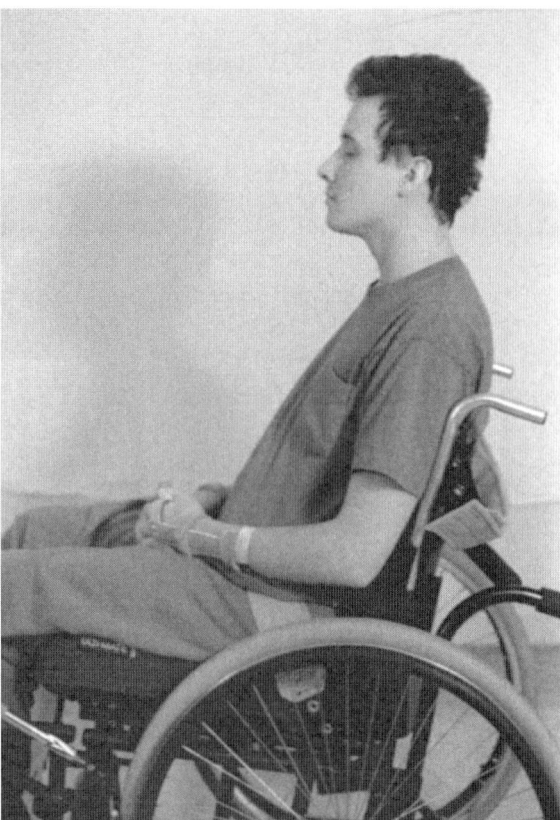

Fig. 14.49 Example of Corrected C-Curve Posture.

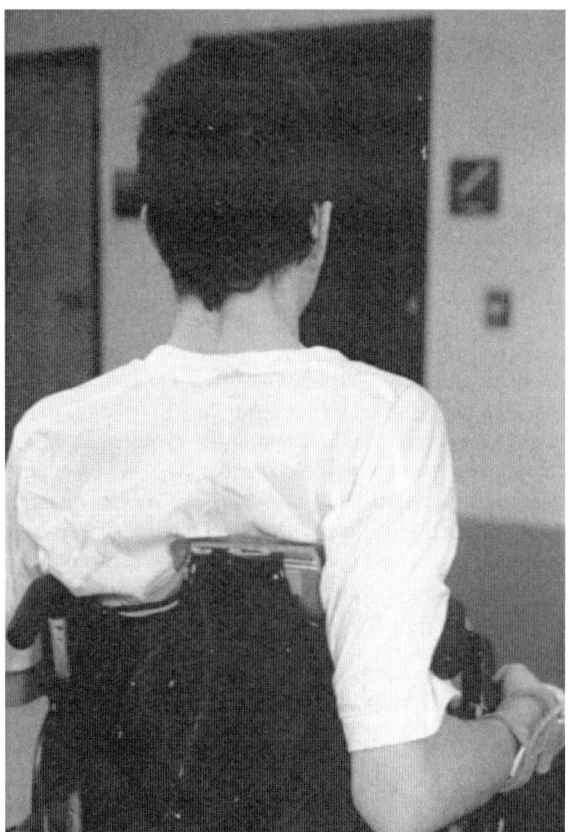

Fig. 14.50 Example of custom modification of a wheelchair back to allow a patient with tetraplegia to hook the push handle with one upper extremity.

Finally, along with wheelchair fit, the esthetics of the wheelchair can affect the individual's self-image and therefore the reentry into the community. This should be considered when assisting the patient to make wheelchair seating decisions.

Return to Walking

"Will I ever walk again?" is a question often asked during SCI rehabilitation. The team must be empathetic toward and acknowledge the patient's goals for ambulation, and the topic should be discussed openly. The professionals involved in the care of the patient must be careful not to take hope away from the patient as hope is important to maintain positive outcomes and coping skills during the rehab phase. It is also important for clinicians to consider the potential for continued recovery of function when addressing ambulation with people with SCI, especially with those newly injured. Varying amounts of recovery are possible after an SCI due to the potential for neuroplastic and activity-dependent changes to occur.[212] These concepts will be discussed later in the chapter.

When ambulation is an appropriate goal, the treatment program may be short and relatively uncomplicated for some and extremely laborious for others. Treatment techniques may include therapeutic exercise, biofeedback, neuromuscular stimulation, locomotor training, balance training, standing, and various other pre-gait and gait activities. The walking disposition of patients with incomplete SCI is challenging due to the complexity of problems and the varying degree of impairments. These patients may have pain, ROM limitations, ventilator pump dysfunction, weakness, spasticity, as well as sensory and balance dysfunction. In addition, their premorbid physical condition and body type must also be considered. Musculoskeletal asymmetries, such as muscle shortening on the stronger side and lengthening on the weaker side, may be present and may lead to pelvic obliquity and scoliosis.

Locomotor and Gait Training

The term locomotor training has been widely used over the years to refer to interventions directed at walking function and gait. Although the terms are often used interchangeably, it is important to differentiate between locomotor training and traditional gait training.[213]

Locomotor training is based on the principles derived from basic science using spinalized cats and body weight support treadmill training (BWSTT) systems in the 1980s.[214-218] It is then progressed to human subjects with increasing popularity in the 1990s and 2000s (Fig. 14.51A).[219-224,] Much of the theory behind this rehabilitation approach is based on activating intrinsic connections of spinal cord circuitry to elicit the appropriate patterns of muscle activation for walking called central pattern generators (CPGs).[225] Research involving the cat model has provided the most conclusive and descriptive evidence for the presence and activity of CPGs,[226] including the ability to produce locomotor output in spinalized animals.[227]

Locomotor training requires repetition and adherence to specific training principles and sensory cues with the goal of generating locomotor output by activating the neural circuits. The principles include (1) maximizing LE weight bearing, (2) optimizing sensory cues appropriate for task, (3) optimizing posture and kinematics for each motor task, and (4) maximizing recovery and minimizing compensation.[228]

In contrast, gait training specifically addresses learning to walk again, and often uses orthotics and or assistive devices to help compensate for strength impairments due to paresis or paralysis.[213]

Although locomotor training started with BWSTT, there have been several other equipment options that have recently been developed to help assist with the delivery of locomotor training. Some of the other

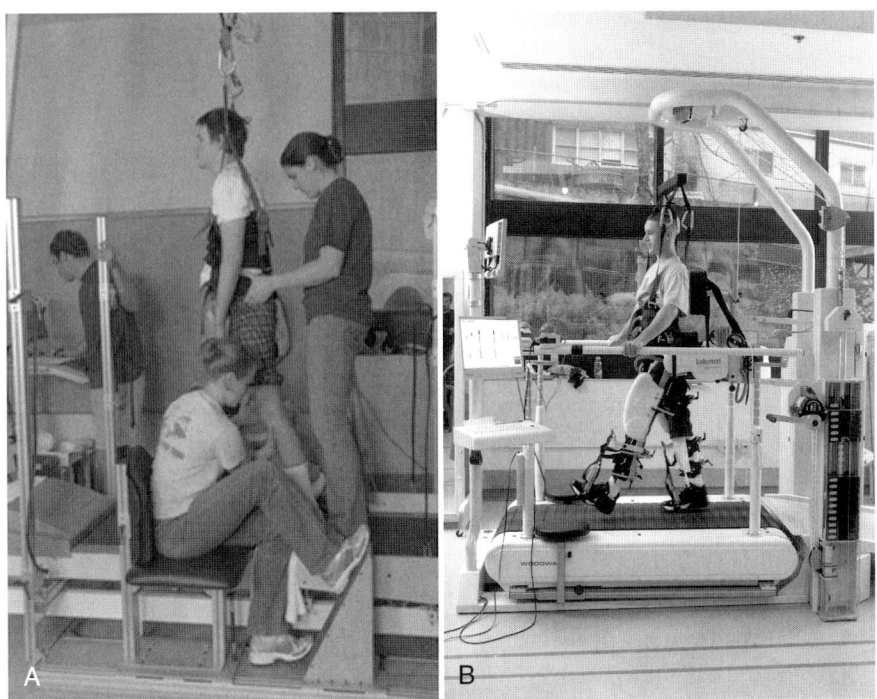

Fig. 14.51 (A) Manual treadmill. Treadmill training with body-weight–supported and manual assistance is being completed on the TheraStride Innoventor, which combines a treadmill and support harness system with software that measures variables of gait training, including speed, weight supported, and amount of time walked. Two or three therapists are needed to provide assistance at the trunk and lower limbs to facilitate an appropriate gait pattern. **(B)** Robotic treadmill. The Lokomat by Hocoma is a robotic-assisted treadmill that provides adjustable body-weight support and gives clinicians the ability to adjust gait-specific parameters when completing training with patients who have mobility deficits.

interventions may include body weight support overground systems, robotic body weight support treadmill systems, and exoskeletons. Many of these devices offer a less burdensome alternative to facilitate walking in people with SCI while reducing therapist strain.[222,229] Over the last several years, much research has been done looking at the effectiveness of these various types of locomotor training for people with SCI. However, many questions remain regarding the efficacy of specific intervention choices and timing for this population. In a randomized controlled trial, Dobkin and colleagues reported that after 12 weeks of equal administration of locomotor training using treadmill training with manual assistance and conventional overground gait training, no differences in walking abilities were reported in patients with incomplete SCIs with either intervention.[223] Field-Fote and Roach[230] conducted a randomized controlled trial (RCT) evaluating walking speed. Sixty-four participants with chronic incomplete SCI and minimal walking function were randomly assigned into one of four different stepping groups using bodyweight support including treadmill training with manual assistance, treadmill training with electrical stimulation, overground training with stimulation, and treadmill training with robotic assistance. After 12 weeks of training, the effect size for speed and distance was greatest with overground training, but differences among the four groups were not statistically significant.[222] Finally, a Cochrane Review published in 2012 that reviewed five RCTs and looked at the effects of locomotor training on improvement in walking function for people with traumatic SCI concluded that there is insufficient evidence that any one locomotor training strategy improves walking function more than another for people with SCI.[231]

Although these studies demonstrate that no conclusive results have been found determining that one method of locomotor training is

superior to another, it is important not to dismiss the potential benefits that each type of locomotor training may offer in certain situations. Determining the best method must be based on several different factors including the patient's available resources, spasticity level, general health conditions, body anthropometry, strength, ability to initiate movement, tolerance to upright posture, skin condition, and ROM. These considerations may make one type of locomotor training or training device more beneficial and or more feasible than another. Many clinicians and centers choose to use a multifaceted treatment approach offering a variety of types of locomotor training when available and appropriate. If various types of locomotor equipment are not available, the clinician can still utilize the principles and theories of locomotor training to capitalize on activity-dependent neuroplasticity and attain favorable results.[230]

It is also important to acknowledge that most of the large studies evaluating the benefits of locomotor training have studied individuals with chronic injuries that have some degree of walking function. In many instances, locomotor training equipment, including robotic, manual treadmill, and overground bodyweight support systems, enable newly injured individuals with minimal ability to stand, weight bear, or walk very early on after injury. Clinicians must acknowledge the current evidence, but then use clinical judgment and an understanding of the resources available to determine the best treatment approach for recovery of walking. This should be done on an individualized basis making sure to address patient's specific goals and postdischarge environment.

Regardless of what type of training is used, or what tools or technology may or may not be available to help administer it, recovery of walking function can and should be considered with patients with

SCI. Prior to initiating locomotor training, an individual should be able to tolerate being vertical with a stable blood pressure. Also, skin should be intact for any locomotor device that contacts the skin (i.e., a harness or a robotic device). If skin is not intact, an alternate locomotor training device should be used.

Orthotics: Traditional and Powered

Ideally, each patient's neurological recovery potential is maximized before or while brace prescription takes place. It is imperative that advanced rehabilitation strategies that facilitate neural plasticity and recovery of function (i.e., walking and or task specificity training) are utilized throughout the rehabilitation process. However, if it is determined that an orthotic (compensatory approach) is necessary to maximize safety and function with discharge to home and the community, a team approach to orthotic prescription is desirable to meet the needs of patients with SCI. Even if orthotic devices enable these patients to become independent with standing or walking, the energy costs, joint deterioration, and muscle stresses over the life expectancy of each individual need to be considered. Orthotic prescription should be approached systematically. The patient's goals, funding, premorbid and current health status, social support, and the environment to which they are returning should be considered. A basic clinical algorithm for the selection of orthoses for persons with neurological impairment has been proposed by researchers at Rancho Los Amigos Medical Center. This algorithm is referred to as the Rancho ROAD-MAP (Recommendations for Orthotic Assessment, Decision Making, and Prescription).[232] Successful brace prescription uses the minimum amount of bracing to achieve the maximum amount of function. It also anticipates changes in each patient's clinical picture. For example, braces may be manufactured with joints built into the plastic, or joints that begin as fixed, and are later cut to allow articulation. Some models of knee-ankle-foot orthoses (KAFOs) can be altered to become ankle-foot orthoses (AFOs).[55]

Factors that affect orthotic selection are cost, injury level, residual motor function, experience bias of the clinician, patient's medical status, skin and cardiovascular integrity, and patient's acceptance. Generally, the hip-knee-ankle-foot orthosis (HKAFO) is used when selected motions of the hip need control or the benefits of the reciprocating gait orthosis are desired, as is the case with the pediatric population or with adults with SCI higher than T10. In the absence of gluteal muscles, use of a KAFO is typically indicated when the quadriceps muscle strength is less than 3/5. AFOs are indicated in the presence of knee and or ankle instability and weakness and to control the joints.[233]

With traditional orthoses, the energy cost for ambulation is highest for persons with complete paraplegia who use a swing-through gait pattern with spreader bar, and lowest for persons who use bilateral AFOs or a combination of an AFO and a KAFO. Even individuals requiring only bilateral AFOs have a gait efficiency of less than 50% of normal, underscoring the importance of the hip extensor and abductor muscles required for functional ambulation. These gluteal muscles are often severely or completely paralyzed in this population.[234,235]

The energy cost of ambulation for a person with paraplegia is progressively reduced when more residual motor function is present in the lower extremities. Conversely, the individual with incomplete tetraplegia has higher energy costs for ambulation despite spared lower-extremity function because of upper- and lower-extremity weakness (Boxes 14.7 and 14.8 and Figs. 14.52 to 14.56).[234–238a]

Materials and components of bracing continue to evolve. Carbon fiber is becoming more common in bracing due to being lightweight and flexible but also supportive. However, the trade-off is that carbon fiber is not easily modified/customized.[55]

BOX 14.7 Categories of Ambulation and Average Walking Speed (Perry 1995)

1. Standing only
2. Exercise—ambulates short distances
3. Household—ambulates inside home or work, uses wheelchair much of the time (<0.4 m/s)
4. Limited community-independent on all surfaces; does not use wheelchair (0.4–0.8 m/s)
5. Full community ambulation (>0.8 m/s)

BOX 14.8 Lower-Extremity Orthoses[233]

Hip-Knee-Ankle-Foot Orthoses
Reciprocating gait orthosis (RGO) (see Fig. 16.50)
Bilateral knee-ankle-foot orthoses (KAFOs) with pelvic band

Knee-Ankle-Foot Orthoses
Scott-Craig KAFOs (see Fig. 14.53)
Conventional KAFOs (metal uprights)
Polypropylene KAFOs (see Fig. 14.54)
Hybrid KAFOs (see Fig. 14.54)

Ankle-Foot Orthoses
Conventional ankle-foot orthoses (AFOs) (metal)
Custom polypropylene AFOs
Carbon-fiber AFO (see Fig. 14.56)
Solid ankle AFO (see Fig. 14.55A)
Custom polypropylene AFOs, articulated ankle (see Fig. 14.55B)

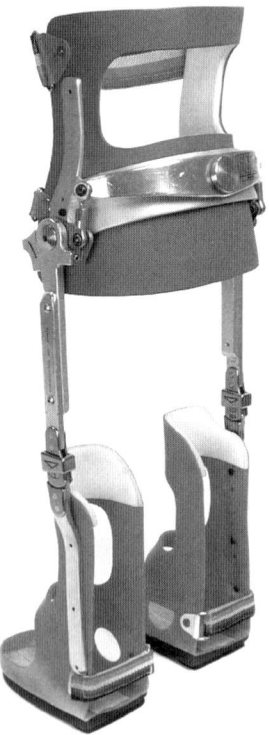

Fig. 14.52 The reciprocating gait orthosis (RGO), although generally used with children, is also used with adults. Its main components are a molded pelvic band, thoracic extensions, bilateral hip and knee joints, and lower limb segments that may be of polypropylene construction with a solid ankle. The RGO uses a dual cable system to couple flexion of one hip with extension of the other.

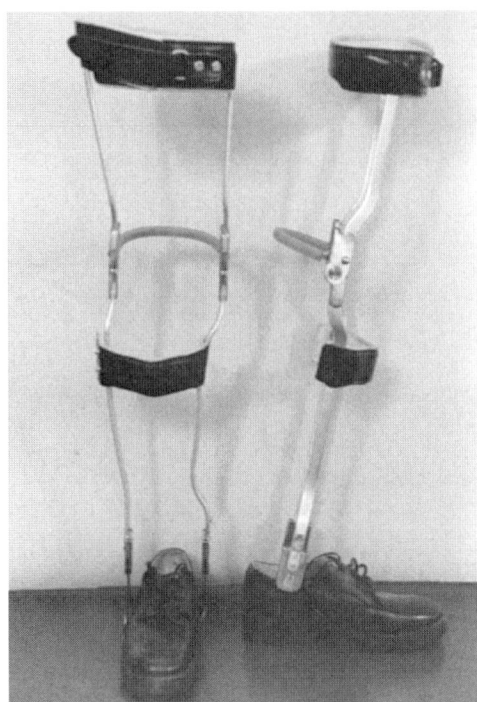

Fig. 14.53 Scott-Craig knee-ankle-foot orthosis is a special design for spinal cord injury. The orthosis consists of double uprights, offset knee joints with pawl locks and bail control, one posterior thigh band, a hinged anterior tibial band, an ankle joint with anterior and posterior adjustable pin stops, a cushion heel, and specially designed longitudinal and transverse foot plates made of steel.

As technology continues to advance, so do the components manufactured for orthotics. One example is the development of stance control knee joints for KAFOs. Traditionally, KAFOs kept the knee locked into full extension throughout swing and stance phase of the gait cycle, thus restricting normal hip/knee flexion during swing phase. However, stance control knee joints allow the knee to unlock during the swing phase and lock during the stance phase, thus functioning in a more normal reciprocal pattern. Research indicates that there are clear indications of the benefits to stance control orthosis systems including greater knee flexion and greater ground clearance in swing, relief of joints on the sound limb, reduction in compensatory movements and energy consumption, as well as improved patient satisfaction.[239]

The philosophy regarding the use of orthoses for ambulation for individuals with complete paraplegia varies greatly among clinicians. In the past, some clinicians have encouraged ambulation for these individuals, whereas others strongly discourage it, given that only a small percentage of persons with complete paraplegia continue to use bilateral KAFOs after training has been completed.[236,238] However, with the evolution and development of LE robotic exoskeletons or powered orthoses (discussed later in section), individuals with little or no LE movement may now safely ambulate in a more energy efficient capacity.[240,241] When the philosophy of the clinician is to use a traditional nonpowered orthosis for patients who do not have functional motor control below their level of injury, criteria should be established so that both the patient and the clinical staff are consistent in their expectations and approach to ambulation.

If the decision is made to order braces after a trial period training with BKAFOs and stability aids (a walker or forearm crutches), specific goals should be discussed and established. Goals range from standing and exercise ambulation to community ambulation. Most persons

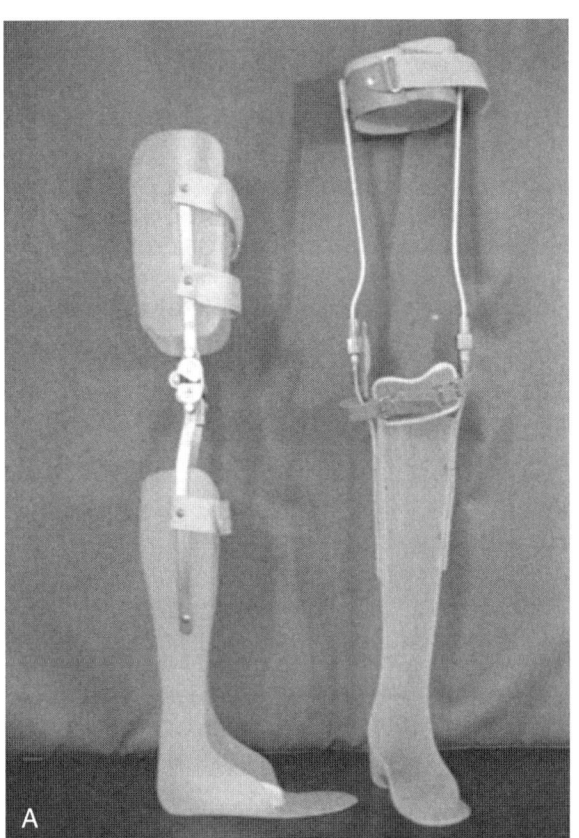

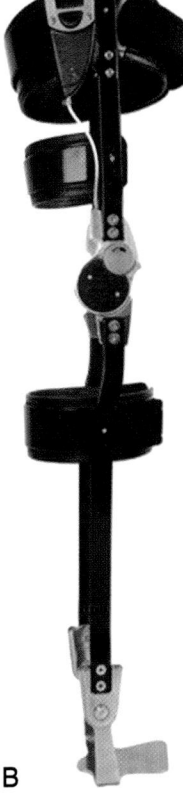

Fig. 14.54 (A) Polypropylene knee-ankle-foot orthosis (KAFO) and combination plastic and metal KAFO. **(B)** Stance-control KAFO knee joint. This joint combines the stability of a locked knee during the stance phase of walking but allows flexion of the limb for the swing phase of gait. A locked knee makes it much harder to clear the leg over the ground. Some long-leg brace users are perfect candidates for the stance-control KAFOs. These devices, through a few different types of joint mechanisms, create a locked knee when the leg is supporting the weight of the body but unlock when the leg is lifted to allow for easy advancement of the leg as it is allowed to bend. For the right patients, this allows them as much mobility to get around as it does stability.

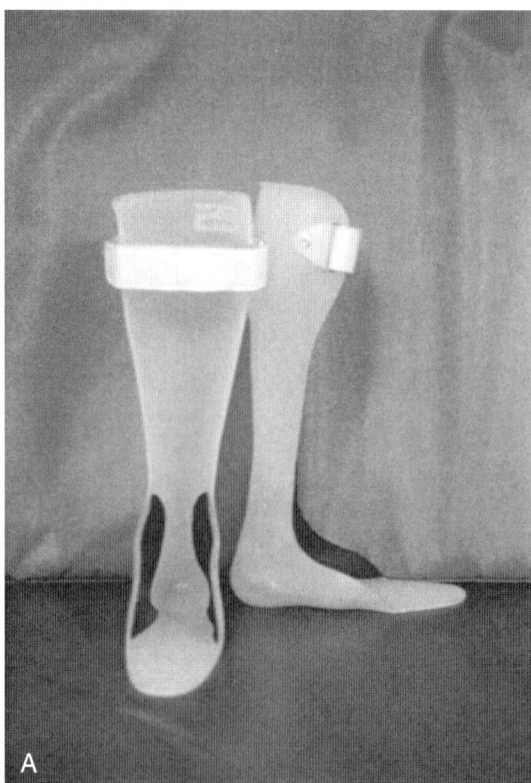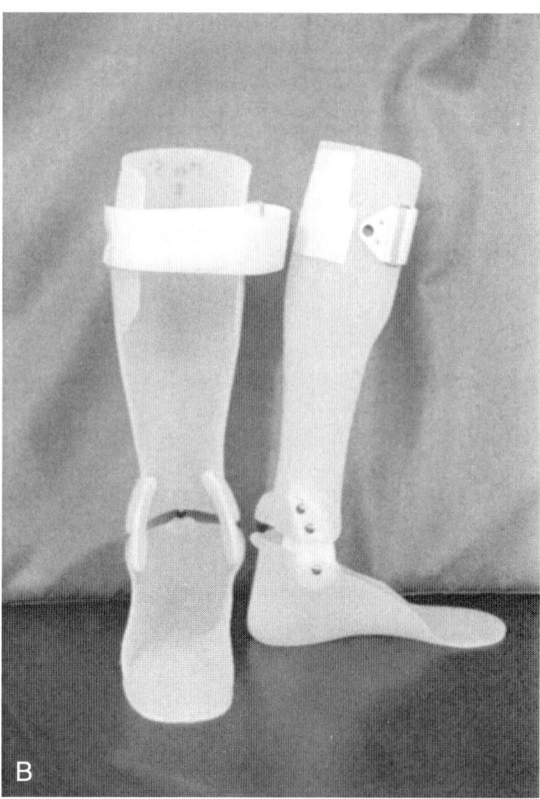

Fig. 14.55 **(A)** Custom-made solid ankle-foot orthoses (AFOs) in 5 degrees of dorsiflexion with full footplates. **(B)** Custom-articulated AFOs with adjustable Oklahoma ankle joints.

with complete injuries L2 or higher achieve only exercise ambulation because of the energy expenditure required for functional community ambulation.

Current research indicates that the energy cost of ambulation for individuals with complete lesions at T12 or higher is above standard anaerobic thresholds and cannot be maintained over time. This study also concluded that ambulation for these individuals using a swing-through gait pattern is equivalent to "heavy work."[234–238] Consequently, it is understandable why BKAFOs often end up unused after a short time as they may be too tiring to use regularly. A functional alternative to BKAFO walking for persons with complete paraplegia are robotic exoskeletons. Evans and colleagues demonstrated that persons with paraplegia can alter the amount of exertion to walk with a robotic exoskeleton for either mobility or exercise.[242]

Robotic exoskeletons are becoming more widespread as an option for personal use (to take home) and for use in rehabilitation settings as an option for gait retraining. There are currently four different exoskeletons that are US Food and Drug Administration (FDA) approved for clinical use (exercise) in the United States (Ekso, Indego, ReWalk, and Rex), three of which may be used for gait or locomotor training. See Table 14.9 for details. Each inclusion criteria, diagnosis for use, and device operation are very different.

Exoskeletons for Rehabilitation

Initially exoskeleton use was only for people with paraplegia. However, recent expansion of FDA approval now allows for people with low cervical (C7) injuries and stroke to use exoskeletons in clinical settings. An Institutional Review Board (IRB) approved research settings, people with levels of injury as high as C5 have successfully stood and walked with exoskeletons using an appropriate stability aid and physical assistance.[243] Exoskeletons can be used on a variety of indoor and outdoor surfaces, and some even have capabilities for stair climbing.[244] Exoskeletons may be used as a mobility device, for exercise, or as a gait retraining intervention to help promote recovery and facilitate neuroplasticity.[242,245–247]

Exoskeletons for Personal Use

There are currently two FDA-approved exoskeletons (Indego and ReWalk) approved for personal use in one's home and community in the United States. For safety reasons, current FDA guidelines require a trained support person (companion) to be present with the user at all times while in the device. People with SCI may choose to use exoskeletons for personal use for exercise and/or mobility. From a health and wellness standpoint, there are several benefits supported in the literature to standing and walking to include, but not limited to, pain reduction, improvements in bowel and bladder function, improved spasticity, and potential benefits in bone health.[248] Exoskeletons are not covered by Centers for Medicaid and Medicare Services (CMS) or most private insurance companies. A few workers compensation companies have covered the cost of the device and training. The Veterans Administration is covering the cost of the device and training for those who qualify to use (meet manufacturer qualifications) either the Indego or the ReWalk system. Prior to coverage of exoskeleton home use for the private sector, much more evidence supporting medically necessary versus medically beneficial will have to be substantiated.

It is important that users and clinicians realize that exoskeletons are not intended to replace wheelchairs, but rather to provide users with an alternate means of mobility. One main reason for this is that the wheelchair is more efficient due to speed. The average walking speed for someone using an exoskeleton is 0.26 m/s.[249–251] This can vary significantly based on the exoskeleton used; the user's physical presentation, level, and completeness of injury; and the user's proficiency

TABLE 14.9 Exoskeleton Chart

Company	Parker Hannifin	ReWalk Robotics Inc.	Ekso Bionics Inc.
FDA approval (US)	Rehab and Personal	Rehab and Personal	Rehab
Device weight	26 lbs (12 kg)/30 lbs (13.5 kg)	51 lbs (23 kg)/66 lbs (30 kg)	55 lbs (25 kg)
Indication for use	SCI Rehab C7 (AIS A-D) and below, SCI Personal T3 (AIS A-D) and below, Stroke Rehab	SCI Rehab T4 (AIS A-D) and below, SCI Personal T7 (AIS A-D) and below	SCI Rehab C7 (AIS D) and below SCI, T4 (AIS A-D) and below SCI; Stroke Rehab
Variable power assist	0%–100% support at each right and left lower extremity as well as to separate out hip or knee joint	Walking current able to be modified dependent on the weight and spasm of the patient	0%–100% support for either the right or left lower extremity. Does not isolate hip or knee
Walking surfaces	Level and unlevelled surfaces; 8 degrees incline	Level and unlevelled surfaces; 8 degrees incline	2 degrees incline
Fall detection/mitigation	Yes	No	No
Functional gait speed	Exercise and Community	Exercise and Community	Exercise
Potential to wear in wheelchair (w/c)	Often (modularity: 5 components)	No; size prevents wear in standard W/Cs	No; size prevents wear in standard W/Cs

Parker Hannifin offers two Indego devices, one for personal use and another for rehabilitation technology. The device above is for the purposes of rehabilitation. Courtesy of Parker Hannifin Corporation, Courtesy of ReWalk Robotics, and Courtesy of Ekso Bionics.

using the exoskeleton. To be considered a limited community ambulator for someone with SCI, walking speeds need to be approximately 0.40 m/s to 0.8 m/s, and greater than 0.8 m/s to ambulate without an assistive device or to be considered a full community ambulator.[252,253] Walking speeds necessary to cross a street is range from 0.44 m/s to 1.32 m/s.[254,255] Until recently, exoskeleton-enabled gait speeds were not fast enough to support community ambulation. However, the development of a new controller for one of the exoskeleton devices enables users to accomplish faster speeds. With only a few training sessions, all subjects achieved walking speeds above limited community thresholds, and some of the subjects achieved within 1 standard deviation of full community ambulation.[256] With additional training sessions, it is reasonable to assume that the appropriate patients could achieve walking speeds approaching 1.2 m/s or greater.

RECOVERY AND RESTORATION

For many years SCI rehabilitation focused on compensatory strategies; however, clinicians and researchers have made the case for recovery more popular for nearly 20 years. When considering restoration and recovery versus compensation it is important to understand the science that supports the clinical interventions seen today. This section will focus on applying the science of neuroplasticity to clinical interventions.

PRINCIPLES OF NEUROPLASTICITY

For recovery to occur, the nervous system needs to adapt. Evidence shows that the nervous system is plastic,[257,258] and that neurons can rearrange their anatomical and functional connectivity in response to environmental input, thereby achieving new or modified outputs. Possible mechanisms are the balance between inhibitory and excitatory synaptic connections are improved, silent connections are aroused, new dendrites sprout, the number or size of synapses increases, or new neurons are "born" (neurogenesis). Regardless of which occurs, clinicians need to capitalize on it— and how they train these new connections is the art of the clinician applying the science. There are 10 *Principles of Neuroplasticity* (see Box 14.9) that can guide the clinician on treatment planning.[257]

Clinicians and researchers use various terms to describe high-volume and high-intensity approaches for treating deficits induced by neurological paralysis[257,259]: *use-dependent plasticity*, experience-dependent plasticity, *activity-dependent plasticity, activity-based restorative therapies (ABRT), activity-based therapies, and activity-based rehabilitation*. Regardless of the term used, the goal is to use rehabilitation therapies to facilitate recovery. This can be done by applying the principles of neuroplasticity in order to achieve activation of the spinal circuitry located above and below the level of injury.[260] Those who

BOX 14.9 Principles of Experience-Dependent Plasticity[257]

Principle	Description
Use it or lose it.	Failure to drive specific brain functions can lead to functional degradation.
Use it and improve it.	Training that drives a specific brain function can lead to an enhancement of that function.
Specificity.	The nature of the training experience.
Repetition Matters.	Induction of plasticity requires sufficient repetition.
Intensity Matters.	Induction of plasticity requires sufficient training intensity.
Time Matters.	Different forms of plasticity occur at different times during training.
Salience Matters.	The training experience must be sufficiently salient to induce plasticity.
Age Matters.	Training-induced plasticity occurs more readily in younger brains.
Transference.	Plasticity in response to one training experience can enhance the acquisition of similar behaviors.
Interference.	Plasticity in response to one experience can interfere with the acquisition of other behaviors.

Kleim JA, Jones TA. Principles of experience-dependent neural plasticity: implications for rehabilitation after brain damage. *J Speech Lang Hear Res.* 2008;51:S225-S239.

subscribe to this type of intervention may follow the five key components to ABRT: weight-bearing activities, FES, task-specific practice, massed practice, and locomotor training.[259] There is some overlap between these key components and the 10 *Principles of Neuroplasticity*; however, not all components can be extrapolated to *all* activities. For instance, when needing to accomplish UE tasks, locomotor training

may not be the intervention of choice. However, repeated reaching activities may utilize these principles and be key to helping a patient reach a functional goal.[261] Clinicians should keep activities specific and purposeful to the end goal.

The use of technology can facilitate training by applying these principles and/or key concepts. For example, a device may allow longer training time (repetition) or maintain an intensity level that would otherwise be a physical burden on a clinician. There are many types of rehab technologies to choose from with the goal of promoting the positive effects gained in training (Table 14.10).[55,262] When implementing these devices, the therapist must have knowledge of the impairment being treated, how to safely use the device while capitalizing on its benefits, and how to coach the patient to be an active participant in the training.[263] Maintaining active participation provides afferent stimulation, which is key for harnessing neuroplasticity.[261] It is important for the clinician to be mindful that the use of technology alone will not cause neuroplastic changes to occur. The technology must be thoughtfully and skillfully applied throughout the treatment session. Additionally, one should consider the desired output and what other modes of afferent input are needed. For example, with locomotor training the stance limb requires adequate loading to elicit hip flexion on the contralateral limb for stepping needs.[259,263,264]

While positive outcomes are always the goal, one must recognize the potential for maladaptive changes.[257,258,263,305] For instance, increased recruitment of excitatory spinal interneurons may enhance spasticity, which in turn may potentially have a negative effect on function.[258] Undirected synaptic plasticity could lead to an imbalance of inhibitory and excitatory activity.[263] Again, careful and thoughtful application of neuroplastic principles and interventions can help avoid these maladaptive changes and lead to positive outcomes.

TABLE 14.10 Summary of Rehabilitation Technologies for Spinal Cord Injury

Types of Devices (Examples)	General Info	Indications	Options	Potential Benefits
Multichannel[265–269] FES,[270,271] Cycles[260,272] Sadowsky, Johnston • Restorative Therapies (RT 300 series) (Fig. 14.57) • MyoLyn MyoCycle • Hasomed RehaMove[273,274]	Muscle groups assigned to specific channels; e-stim delivered with timed and sequenced revolutions with or without motor support; and frequency, pulse duration, and amplitude adjustable	Strengthening, endurance training, muscle conditioning, and reciprocal patterning	Upper and lower extremity cycling; options to include trunk musculature; active or passive cycling; some devices are designed for supine bed use; and able to use channels for other activities	Maintenance or increase in muscle bulk, increase in blood flow, reduction in muscle spasms, maintenance of ROM, and maintenance of bone density
Other multichannel FES devices[274,275]: • RT 200 seated elliptical, RT 600 stepper, RT Xcite • Hasomed RehaMove Cycle	Device has more than 2 channels; able to assign channels to multiple muscle groups at once	Strengthening of multiple muscle groups at once, repeated mass practice, and task specificity to increase endurance with an activity	FES to extremities and trunk; some are portable; may have preprogrammed settings for specific activities; and different devices offer different	Task specific muscle retraining in conjunction with functional activity or ADL and enables increased muscle fibers to be used during activity
Neuroprosthetics/Neuromuscular Reeducation devices[276–279] • Bioness H200 (Fig. 14.61) and L300 (Fig. 14.58) • Walk-aide (Fig. 14.59) • MyoPro[280–282]	Wearable device in the form of prosthetic that delivers e-stim or power to provide assistance and used primarily for gait training, functional activities, and/or ADLs	Muscle retraining, foot drop, repeated mass practice, and task specificity to increase endurance with an activity	Reaching and/or grasping, gait; exercise modes; wireless; and clinic or personal use	Task specificity; repetition; muscle strengthening; and structural support or joint protection
Body Weight Support Tracking Systems[283,284] • Aretech Zero-G • Bioness Vector	Overhead harness system; reduces percentage of weight bearing through patient's LEs while supporting trunk	Gradual introduction to weight bearing, standing, or ambulating; basic or dynamic balance training	Computer interface; static or dynamic systems; able to use over ground or over treadmill; prevent falls; and track progress	Initiate weight bearing, balance, and upright earlier; reduced effort to patient, therapist/team; increased safety; and low fear of falling

TABLE 14.10 Summary of Rehabilitation Technologies for Spinal Cord Injury—cont'd

Types of Devices (Examples)	General Info	Indications	Options	Potential Benefits
Body Weight Support Treadmill Systems[285] (Robotic, Manual[286–289]) • Hocoma Lokomat[285–287] • Aretech Zero-G Lite • Motorika Optimal G • P&S Walkbot • Healthsouth Auto-ambulator	Patient is suspended by harness over treadmill; robotic system includes exoskeleton that attaches to patient's LEs and can assist or guide stepping pattern; manual system utilizes team of trained staff to guide pelvis in weight shifts and LEs in stepping pattern	Impaired gait, proprioception or motor control; decreased standing endurance; weight bearing restrictions; weakness; spasticity; and weight bearing	Robotic—computer interface; adjustability of gait pattern; stability vs. motion at pelvis; manual feature; interactive programs or virtual reality; track progress/ outcomes; decreased number of staff needed. Manual—computer interface assists therapist with setting amount of body weight support and tracking speed and endurance parameters	Assist in providing locomotor training: repeated mass practice; task specificity; increase endurance and/or speed with stepping; decrease level of assistance with stepping; improved trunk/postural training in upright position; increased circulation of LEs; improved bowel/bladder function; and improved respiratory function
Gaming & Computer Interface Devices • Virtual Reality Headsets • Wii • PlayStation • Xbox • Hocoma Armeo[290,291]	Gaming device used in the home; has various activities from sports to first person action	Balance, activity specific intervention, gross and fine motor options	Can add games/activities; and various controller options dependent on device (ex: motion sensor, head control, and multiplayer w/single controller)	Able to track changes; patient can visibly see progress; inexpensive and easy to use in the home
Whole Body Vibration (Fig. 14.62)[292–295] • Wave • Powerplate • Vibeplate	Vibration is delivered through a plate the patient can utilize at various positions (standing, sitting w/feet on plate, prone w/UEs on plate, etc.); evokes reflex contractions; can mimic resistance or aerobic training; can also be fatiguing to muscles; can reduce H-reflex depending on frequency	Stimulate motor unit recruitment; increase strength output; modulation of spasticity	Ideal devices allow adjustable amplitude and frequency to suit therapeutic goal; various sizes available for portability and to meet patient needs	Priming of neural circuits to enhance training (i.e., in prep for repeated tasks); decrease spasticity, which negatively impacts function or the ability to participate in tasks designed to capitalize on neuroplasticity
Robotics • AMES[296–297] • Alter G Bionic Leg[298] • Erigo[299–300] • LE Exoskeleton[248] (Ekso, Indego, ReWalk)	*Motorized* device attaching to a limb with the purpose of guiding and/or assisting movement	Passive or assisted limb movement; repetition of movement; afferent input for a desired output; decrease pain or spasticity; strength training; and functional training	May have e-stim or vibration associated with device; sensor driven movement; vary degree of assist. Various types: somatosensory augmentation, intention-based robotic limb, passive or active-assist devices, exoskeletal walking devices designed to be used with assistive device for overground walking[296–297]	Increased independence with ADLs or mobility; exercise; repetition; and general and/or early mobility
Manipulandum • ReJoyce[301–302]	Hand strengthening and training disguised as games—functional ROM, functional tasks, and placement tasks	For hand strength and fine motor training, endurance, and task specificity training	Difficulty modulated based on performance; computer contains outcome measure and progress tracking; can be used in conjunction with other interventions (i.e., e-stim), can be used in the home; and therapist can supervise and track remotely	Continued training in the home; functional and neuroplastic improvements in ARAT and GRT (—Action Research Arm Test and Grasp Release Test)[302–304]

ADL, Activities of daily living; *FES*, functional electrical stimulation; *LE*, Lower extremity; *ROM*, range of motion.

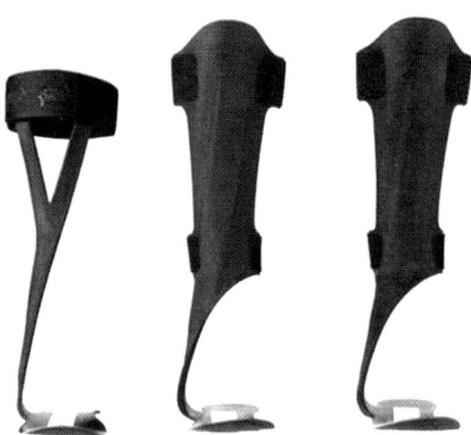

Fig. 14.56 Allard Braces. The Allard family of ankle-foot orthoses (AFOs) include a prefabricated shell that can be customized by the trained orthotist to the specific needs of the patients. These dynamic orthoses are constructed of carbon composites, which accounts for their strength as well as their light weight. There are three different AFOs in the series: Ypsilon, ToeOFF, and BlueRocker. The AFOs are intended to be used with a custom foot orthotic.[238a]

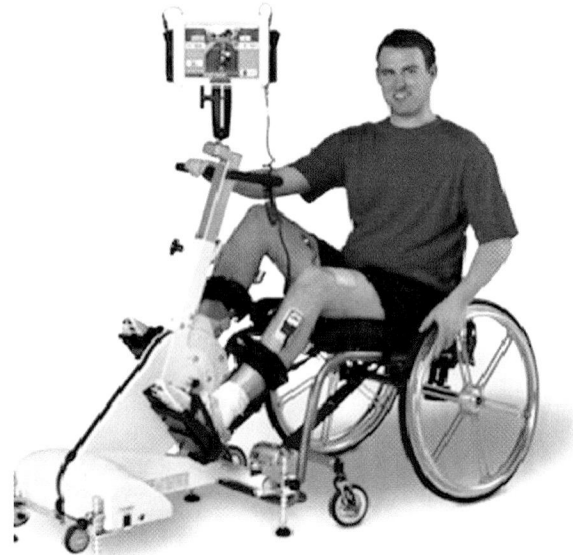

Fig. 14.57 RT300-SL leg functional electrical stimulation (FES) system is a portable FES cycle that can be easily accessed from the patient's wheelchair. Adhesive electrodes can be applied to a variety of lower-extremity muscles including the quadriceps, hamstrings, gluteals, tibialis anterior, and gastrocnemius. These muscles are stimulated at the appropriate time to facilitate a cycling motion using a lower-extremity ergometer. FES bike software has the capability to store patient-specific parameters between sessions and patients. Courtesy of Restorative Therapies.

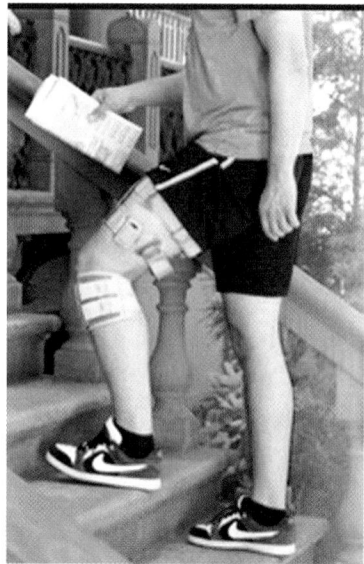

Fig. 14.58 Bioness L300 system is a neuroprosthetic device that contains an orthotic cuff and electrodes. It fits just below the knee to supply FES to the lower leg, targeting the peroneal nerve to cause dorsiflexion. An additional thigh cuff (L300 Plus) can be added to help assist with knee flexion and extension and provide additional support. Courtesy of Bioness, Inc.

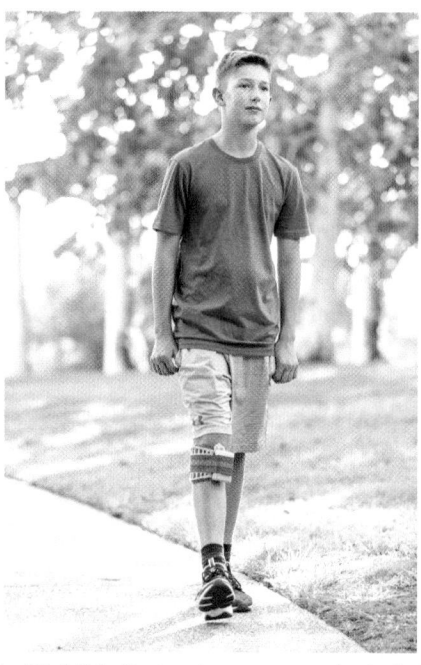

Fig. 14.59 The WalkAide System is a neuroprosthetic device that contains an orthotic cuff and electrodes. It fits just below the knee to supply functional electrical stimulation (FES) to the lower leg, stimulating the appropriate muscles and causing dorsiflexion. It is activated by a tilt sensor mechanism and relies on the angle of the tibia for appropriate timing of the FES to assist with foot drop. Courtesy of Hanger, Inc.

UPPER-EXTREMITY RESTORATION

Improving hand and upper-extremity function plays a critical role in achieving independence with ADLs. Surgical restoration of hand grasp, lateral pinch, or elbow extension in a patient with tetraplegia can be an option through tendon transfers.[306,307] Typically, before individuals are considered for surgery, their neurological function has reached a plateau, they are psychologically stable, and they have functional goals.[307] Individuals seeking restorative surgery to the UE, to provide another function lost from paralysis, undergo a

preoperative evaluation using the International Classification for Surgery of the Hand in Tetraplegia (ICSHT).[308] This classification provides information about the number of voluntary muscles available for surgical transfer and whether the person has cutaneous sensation in the thumb. A physical assessment is included to evaluate UE active range of motion, passive range of motion, and strength. The presence of UE contractures and/or poorly managed spasticity may limit an individual's candidacy.[309] Before any surgical interventions, therapy may be recommended to ensure that the individual is a candidate for tendon transfer procedures.[307] Postoperative rehabilitation varies on the basis of specific procedures and may consist of 2 months or more, with strength improvements continuing for up to 1 year postoperatively.[310] Tendon transfer procedures may be an option to improve UE function.

Regardless of the procedure, the therapist can tap into neuroplasticity principles and interventions mentioned above to assist with what might be considered a transition to potential recovery. Retraining the nervous system along with the musculoskeletal system helps patients reach their goals for independence.

HEALTH PROMOTION AND WELLNESS

Health promotion and wellness are something that should be introduced and presented throughout the continuum of care and do not necessarily require someone to be enrolled in a specific health and wellness program. Education on wellness should include:

- Prevention of chronic diseases and secondary conditions
- Physical activity
- Nutrition
- Injury prevention
- Psychological support

Individuals with spinal cord injuries are living longer due to improvements in medical management, but this has also led to increased incidence of chronic diseases, such as cardiovascular disease (CVD) and comorbid endocrine disorders in persons with SCI.[112,311,312] CVDs are a major cause of morbidity and mortality among aging people with SCI (C),[113] with the prevalence of heart disease being 17.1% for people with SCI compared to 4.9% for individuals without SCI.[313] Heart disease is the fourth leading cause of death among people with SCI aged 40 to 70 years.[314]

The terms cardiometabolic syndrome (CMS) or metabolic syndrome are terms widely reported to describe a clustering of risk factors that are often reported after SCI and worsen the risk of cardiovascular disease (CVD) prognosis. Cardiometabolic syndrome is said to exist if three of the five following risk factors are present: central obesity, dyslipidemia (specifically low high-density lipoprotein cholesterol), elevated triglycerides, hypertension, and insulin resistance.[112] Although there is no single definitive cause for the development of CMS after SCI, there is a high likelihood that physical deconditioning along with a hypercaloric diet are major contributors.[112]

Physical deconditioning and a sedentary lifestyle after SCI has ranked individuals with SCI at the lowest end of the human fitness spectrum,[315] and recent reports find that 50% of people with SCI have no leisure-time physical activity, and 15% of those that do report physical activity do not meet the minimal threshold for meaningful health benefits.[114,316] There are many reasons why someone with an SCI may find it difficult to engage in physical activity including muscle paralysis, physical, financial, and transportation barriers.[114,317] However, there are a variety of exercise interventions (to be discussed later in this section) that are available to people with SCI and can promote clinically relevant improvements in health, fitness, and overall function.[114] It is also important to note that as a health professional, encouraging and educating patients on the importance of exercise and prescribing appropriate exercise programs that minimize barriers is critical to the patient engaging in exercise. Research has demonstrated that a health professional's recommendation to exercise is the single most important determinant for the adoption of an active lifestyle.[318]

Although critical, exercise is only one piece of the healthy lifestyle puzzle. There are physical, nutritional, and behavioral modifications that need to be made for someone to lead a healthy lifestyle. Research has shown that physical activity alone does not offset the caloric excess of someone who is not eating a health-conscious diet,[319,320] and caloric restriction may be the most important of all three components in preventing diabetes or prediabetes.[319,320] People with SCI require a reduction in calories to prevent weight gain due to decreases in muscle mass with an associated increase in fat mass as well as lower levels of physical activity.[113,321] As a result, obesity is extremely prevalent among people with chronic SCI with prevalence rates for overweight and obesity ranging from 55.0% to 95.7% of the population.[322] This is why appropriate nutrition and caloric levels to maintain stable body mass as well as behavioral support to assist with following a healthy diet are so important in helping someone consistently engage in a healthy lifestyle.[112]

Recent evidence resulting from a National Institute of Health multisite RCT demonstrated significant weight reduction (58%) and decreased incidence of type 2 diabetes from a 1 year structured lifestyle intervention as part of a diabetes prevention program consisting of moderate-intensity physical activity, an energy restricted Mediterranean-style diet, and behavioral approaches.[319] This lifestyle intervention program was also applied to people with SCI, further demonstrating the importance of all three components of a healthy lifestyle.[112,319]

Physical Activity and Exercise Interventions

Physical activity after SCI has been shown to improve muscle strength, endurance, mobility, the ability to fall asleep, self-image, and blood lipid profiles, as well as decrease the risk of premature death. In addition, exercise has been shown to decrease anxiety, loneliness, depression, stress, heart disease, blood pressure, respiratory illness, diabetes, obesity, and other medical complications.[323] Current evidence has established two guidelines for physical activity for adults with SCI: (1) for cardiorespiratory fitness and muscle strength and (2) for cardiometabolic health benefits. See Box 14.10 on physical activity guidelines. It is important to note that both guidelines recommend a lower frequency and duration than the 150 min/wk advised for the general population.[324]

Exercise programs for individuals with SCI must take into consideration the musculoskeletal, respiratory, cardiovascular, and autonomic nervous system changes that occur after SCI. Components of an exercise program should include flexibility, muscular strength, and cardiovascular endurance; and an appropriate exercise prescription should address exercise mode, intensity, duration, and frequency. It is important to find a type of exercise that is enjoyable for each individual so that it can be easily integrated into his or her lifestyle, as a variety of exercise interventions exist that may lead to improvements in health, fitness, and overall function.[114]

Exercise programs, both in the clinic and home, may or may not incorporate specialized equipment. The types of equipment available for exercise testing or training in persons with SCI are well documented in the literature. Arm crank ergometers, wheelchair ergometers, circuit resistance training (CRT), wheelchair treadmills,

---

BOX 14.10 Physical Activity Guidelines for Adults With Spinal Cord Injury[324]

Fitness guideline for cardiorespiratory fitness and muscle strength benefits

- 20 min of moderate to vigorous intensity aerobic exercise 2×/wk
- 3 sets of strength exercises 2×/wk for each major functioning muscle group, at a moderate to vigorous intensity

Cardiometabolic health guideline—for cardiometabolic health benefits

- 30 min 3×/wk of moderate to vigorous intensity aerobic exercise

Martin Ginis KA, van der Scheer JW, Latimer-Cheung AE, et al. Evidence-based scientific exercise guidelines for adults with spinal cord injury: an update and a new guideline. *Spinal Cord.* 2018; 56(4):308-321. doi:10.1038/s41393-017-0017-3.

lower-extremity cycling with FES, overhead bodyweight support systems, as well as field test protocols are among the more widely used equipment in the clinic.[325]

When volitional extremity movement exists, exercise utilizing those available muscles should be used to improve cardiovascular and metabolic health in individuals with SCI. Specifically, there is evidence that arm-crank ergometry, wheelchair propulsion, hand cycling, and CRT can improve cardiovascular fitness, metabolic health, and physical capacity measures in individuals with SCI.[114] Exercise equipment varies in expense, and each clinic must choose the method that best fits its treatment setting and budget. Home exercise programs may be established with equipment such as weights and cuff weights, elastic bands and tubing, and hand cycles. However, regardless of what equipment is being used, careful consideration and individualized attention to available muscle strength and proper kinematics is required prior to prescribing exercise. One type of exercise does not fit all people with SCI, and therefore modifications often need to be made in order to accommodate various types of injuries, presentations, and postural deformities in order to maximize benefit and minimize injury, especially an overuse injury.

Overuse syndromes are common among long-term wheelchair users. When any type of exercise program is established, factors that are specific to SCI should be considered.[326] Long-term wheelchair use can lead to an increased incidence of carpal tunnel syndrome, elbow or shoulder tendonitis, early onset of osteoarthritis, and rotator cuff injuries. The motion and resistance of the upper-extremity muscles during wheelchair propulsion can lead to an overdevelopment of anterior shoulder muscles, scapular protraction, and posterior shoulder weakness. This musculature imbalance may lead to elevation and internal rotation of the humeral head that may cause pain as a result of impingement. Injuries can be prevented or slowed if individuals perform a proper warm-up with stretching and flexibility exercises, wear protective equipment (e.g., helmet and padded gloves), alternate modes of exercise, get proper rest between exercise sessions, and establish exercise programs to help prevent or correct muscle imbalances.

CRT is one type of exercise program that is specifically designed to help strengthen weak muscles that are critical to function in people with SCI (upper trunk and shoulder complex) while stretching the muscles that tend to be tight (chest and back).[327] In addition to the strengthening and stretching components, it also incorporates cardiovascular endurance exercise. The cardio components can be accomplished using low-resistance, high-speed arm cranking, or simply spinning arms in the air with no equipment.[327,328] As a result, CRT is one simple method of exercise for people with SCI that can address several fitness goals at once. It can be used performed in a rehab setting, in a more traditional gym, or even in a home setting.[329] Research has shown that a CRT program, using alternating strengthening exercises and low-resistance, high-speed arm exercise can be beneficial in improving muscle strength, endurance, and anaerobic power of middle-aged men with paraplegia while also significantly reducing their shoulder pain.[326] CRT has also been shown to increase peak oxygen consumption and cardiorespiratory endurance in patients with chronic paraplegia.[327,330] (See Box 14.11 for description of the program.)

Whether it is through an established health and wellness program or an individualized health and wellness plan, a person living with an SCI has the potential to increase quality of life, improve ADLs, decrease secondary conditions, decrease depression, and decrease the number of related hospitalizations. It is a goal that integration to wellness programs for individuals with SCI will become a standard in all facilities, and individual health professionals will address health and wellness as part of routine care.

BOX 14.11 Circuit Resistance Training Program[114,328,330]

Exercises	Instructions
Arm ergometer/arm spinning Military press Horizontal rows Chest fly Preacher curls Latissimus pull-down Seated dips	• Sets of resistance exercises will be performed in pairs • 10 repetitions of each exercise (6 s movement each rep) • 2 min of endurance exercise (arm ergometer or spinning); cadence of 50 rpm (no resistance) interposed between pairs • 2 more sets resistance exercises performed. • Resistance and endurance exercises are alternated until subjects have rotated through each resistance station 3 times for a total of 3 sets • ≤15 s rest between stations

Perform CRT 3× week on nonconsecutive days. Each session lasts about 40–45 min. Start with warm-up and end with cool down of approximately 4 min of arm ergometer or arm spinning.

EDUCATION

Education of the patient and caregivers is an integral part of the rehabilitation process. Formal education includes group and individual instruction and family and caregiver training. Patients and caregivers are taught the following: preventive skin care, bowel and bladder programs, safe ways to perform all ADL tasks, nutritional guidelines, thermoregulation precautions, pulmonary management, cardiopulmonary resuscitation, management of autonomic dysreflexia, equipment management and maintenance, transfer techniques, wheelchair mobility, ambulation, proper body positioning, ROM exercises, ADL basics, and leisure skills. Home programs are taught to maintain or increase strength, endurance, ROM, and function. Energy conservation techniques and proper body mechanics are incorporated into all aspects of training.

Patients are formally tested on their knowledge, and remedial instruction should be provided in deficient areas. Caregivers should be formally evaluated on their abilities to safely provide care to the patient. Supervised therapeutic outings and passes allow the patient, caregivers, and the team to identify problem areas and provide additional education in those areas.

PSYCHOSOCIAL ISSUES

The immediate reaction to the onset of SCI is physical shock accompanied by anxiety, pain, and fear of dying. The response to such an injury varies greatly and depends on the extent of the injury, the premorbid activity level, the style of coping with stress, and family and financial resources. There may be great sensory deprivation from immobilization, neurological impairment, and the monotony of the hospital routine. Several psychological theories have been proposed to describe responses and coping mechanisms. The process of coping with these changes is referred to as *adjustment* (see Chapter 5).

Rehabilitation personnel are becoming more aware of the need to teach not only functional skills but also psychosocial and coping skills to the patient and significant others. Education in the following areas facilitates the adjustment process: creative recreation, financial planning, negotiating community barriers, social skills, managing an attendant, creative problem solving, accessing community resources, fertility and child care options, assertiveness, sexual expression, vocational planning and training, and the use of community transportation. These skills may be introduced in the inpatient rehabilitation setting but will be developed further in the home and community environments. True adjustment and adaptation begin after discharge from rehabilitation.[331,332]

DISCHARGE PLANNING

Discharge planning begins from the time the patient is being considered for admission and continues through the rehabilitation program. It is a continuous process that includes the patient, family, treatment team, and community resources, with the goal being successful community reintegration and a perceived good quality of life. The rehabilitation team must identify the specific needs of the patient and must structure the program to enhance the chance of success. Lengths of stay are getting shorter in response to pressure from third-party payers to contain costs. This requires the discharge planning process to be expedited so that procurement of needed equipment, completion of architectural modifications, and referrals to postacute services and community resources occur in a timely manner.

ARCHITECTURAL MODIFICATIONS

Architectural barriers in the home, transportation system, workplace, or school may prevent access to opportunities. The architectural changes required by the person with SCI for independence in the home and community depend on the degree of impairment, financial resources, and patient and family acceptance of modifications or equipment. The clinician should discuss equipment options with the patient and family on the basis of the degree of modification they plan to make to their home. Thinking creatively about low-tech adaptations should be considered part of the therapist's role. Problem solving with and by the patient is vital to the process of identifying alternatives as ideas for the future (Fig. 14.60).

Many available resources describe the dimensions of the basic wheelchair and specifications for making homes and facilities accessible to wheelchair users. See Appendix 14.A at the end of this chapter for resources on architectural modification. When architectural modification recommendations exceed the scope of the clinician, referral to an AT Practitioner may be necessary. If families are considering building a home to meet their needs, universal design principles should be integrated into the plans to ensure access and aging in place for the patient and their family.

APPENDIX 14.A Selected References: Architectural Modification

The IDeA Center. *Center for Inclusive Design and Environmental Access.* Buffalo, NY. Available at: http://idea.ap.buffalo.edu/. Accessed November 1, 2019.[333]

National Research Center on Home Modification. Los Angeles, CA. Available at: https://homemods.org/resources/. Accessed October 4, 2018.[334]

Davies TD, Lopez CP. *Accessible Home Design Book: Architectural Solutions for the Wheelchair User.* Vol. 2. Paralyzed Veterans of America; 2006.[335]

Center for Inclusive Design and Environmental Access. Steinfeld E. *Inclusive Housing: A Pattern Book, Design for Diversity and Equality.* W.W. Norton & Company, Inc.[336]

The Center for Universal Design. *Removing Barriers to Health Care.* Chapel Hill, NC: 2017. Available at: https://fpg.unc.edu/node/6264.[337]

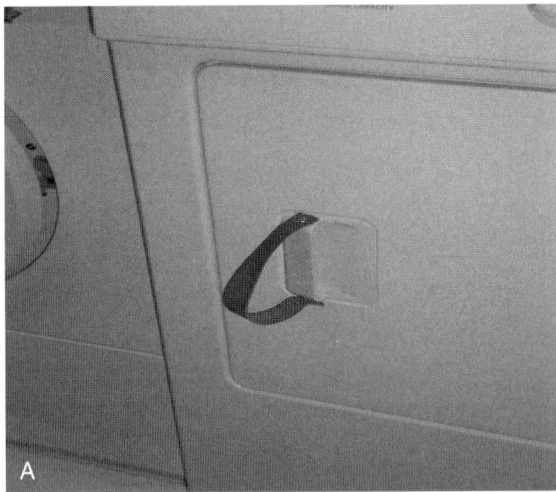
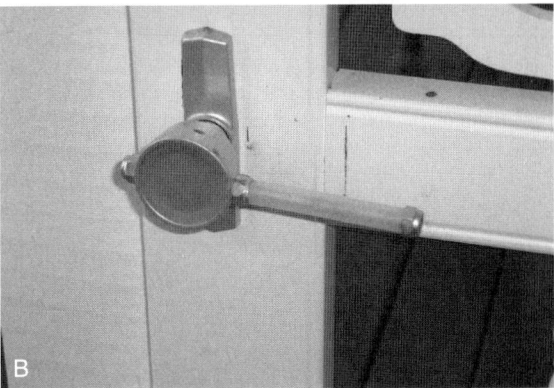

Fig. 14.60 Low-Tech Home Adaptations. **(A)** A strap is added to make a clothes dryer door accessible. **(B)** A hole is drilled and a handle added to a screen door knob.

COMMUNITY REINTEGRATION

Successful community reintegration after SCI includes returning to preinjury social roles and, more specifically, returning to work, school, and/or leisure interests. Public school systems have a legal obligation to provide an appropriate school setting for a child with a disability. Rehabilitation teams may assist with school reentry by adding school visitations and education for faculty or peers. School accessibility can be assessed, and the patient and therapists can have an opportunity to share appropriate information about the new impairments before reentry into the school system. Also, rehabilitation programs that are CARF accredited must offer academic programs. School reentry programs may enhance communication between academic rehabilitation faculty and school, bridging the gap for return. Students returning to college may need assistance developing problem-solving skills related to campus accessibility, Americans with Disabilities Act (ADA) rights, campus transportation options, and self-advocacy for sports adaptations. Figs. 14.60 to 14.64 represent the range of solutions utilized by clinicians to address patient needs. Solutions to address patient needs can range from functional electrical stimulation, power assisted mobility, vibration therapy to address tone and muscle recruitment, and positioning devices.

Rehabilitation programs must also emphasize returning to work throughout the process. For patients who have sustained a traumatic SCI and are included in SCI model systems data, 57.7% report being employed at the time of the accident. Only 12.4% are employed at the 1-year anniversary, but by the 20-year anniversary, 33.1% are

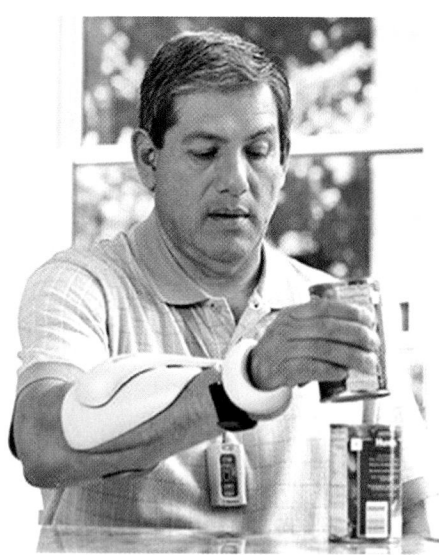

Fig. 14.61 The Bioness H200 system is a neuroprosthetic device that contains an orthosis for the upper extremity and electrodes. It fits to the wrist and forearm and targets opening and closing of the hand and fingers. The device can be used in an exercise mode or to perform functional tasks. Courtesy of Bioness, Inc.

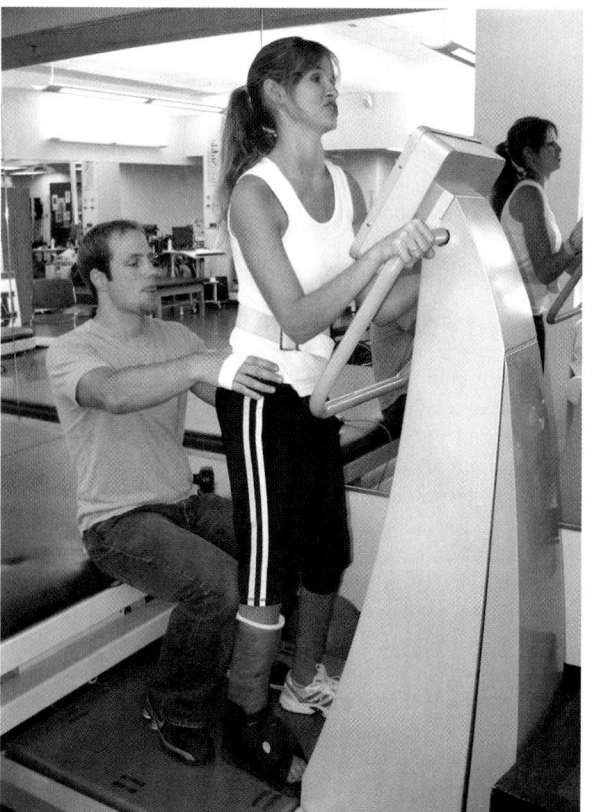

Fig. 14.62 Vibration therapy is a modality with a wide range of purposes including tone or spasticity management and muscle recruitment.

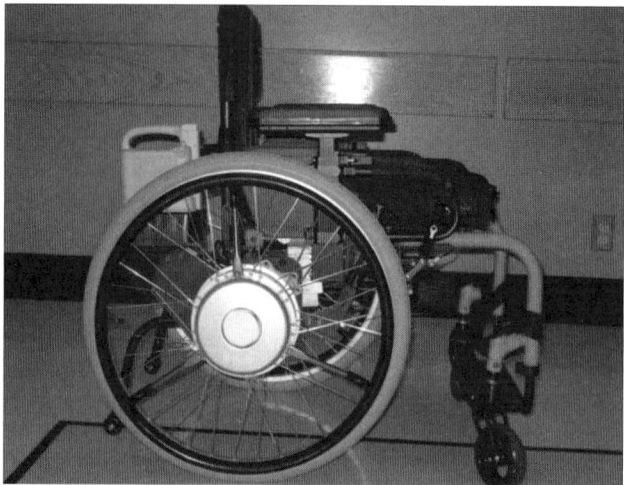

Fig. 14.63 Power assist wheels added to a manual wheelchair meet the needs of users who may need supplemental support in the community while also requiring the ease of transportation that a manual chair provides. Power assist wheels help users with energy conservation and shoulder maintenance long term.

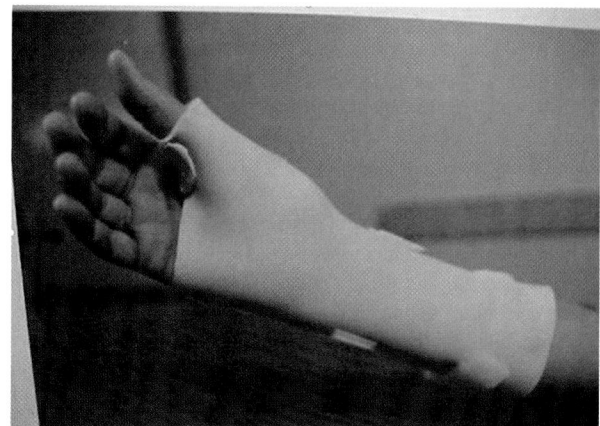

Fig. 14.64 A volar based forearm thumb spica splint can help maintain soft-tissue length and thumb integrity while providing the user with the ability to complete fine motor tasks with digits II-IV.

employed. Many individuals can return to their previous jobs after SCI.[338] The ADA of 1990 (PL 101-336) prohibits businesses with 15 or more employees from discrimination against "qualified individuals with disabilities" with respect to the terms, conditions, or privileges of employment.[339] Job site and job responsibilities may need to change to accommodate the new impairments, allowing the patient to fully participate. For those who are unable to perform previous jobs or who were unemployed before injury, many programs exist for training in vocational skills. The Department of Rehabilitation Services (DRS) evaluates patients for skills and functional abilities and provides funding for those qualifying for job training, job site modification, and the purchase of essential equipment that may include transportation. Services offered by the DRS vary from state to state. Each state agency has a list of resources available in the community, such as rehabilitation technology, independent living centers, and job training and placement programs. Individuals should refer to their state DRS for assistance with employment.

Engaging in sports and other leisure skills can open doors for patients returning to the community. Participating in sports and leisure, whether learning a new skill or adapting something previously enjoyed, may boost physical capacity and enhance self-worth. Adapted sporting activities found in the United States include power soccer, quad rugby, wheelchair basketball, tennis, swimming, and snow skiing, to name a few. The Paralympics provide competitive venues for elite athletes, and many road races across the United States have opened the doors for wheelchair athletes to compete alongside able-bodied runners. A handful of colleges and universities have developed adapted sports teams and are beginning to offer student scholarships.

CONCLUSION

Comprehensive treatment of the individual with SCI can be very challenging. Health care reform issues force the rehabilitation team to explore new cost-efficient options to continue to provide high-quality rehabilitation. New medical and rehabilitation interventions provide the clinician with a plethora of interventions to improve functional recovery and to promote neurological recovery after SCI (see Table 14.9). Scientists continue to research ways to prevent and/or cure paralysis and loss of function after SCI; however, until those goals have been achieved the best defense against SCI is to prevent the injury from occurring. Programs that target the top mechanisms for traumatic SCI, such as ThinkFirst, are aimed at helping individuals of all ages learn to reduce their risk of SCI by educating them to make safe choices. Creation of innovative apps called AutoCoach that teach parents how to teach their teens to drive, Distracted Driving programs and laws, and continued efforts to educate the community through mass media campaign on key concepts such as "Buckle up, Drive safe and sober, Arrive alive, Wear a helmet, Check the water before you dive," are important elements in the effort to reduce the number of new spinal cord injuries.[340,341]

CASE STUDY 14.1 C5-C6 Fracture

The patient, a 23-year-old man, was injured when he dove into the shallow end of a swimming pool while at a party. He had hit his head on the bottom of the pool but never lost consciousness. His friends noticed he did not come to the surface, and they dove in and brought him to the surface so he could breathe. When the emergency medical services personnel arrived at the scene, the patient was complaining of neck pain and was unable to move his trunk and legs. A cervical collar was applied, and he was placed on a spine board for transportation to the closest emergency medical center.

On arrival, the physician ordered radiographs of the spine, skull, and chest, which revealed a C5-C6 fracture and subluxation. Physical examination revealed the following: patient awake and alert, absent deep tendon reflexes below the C5 level (indicative of spinal shock), absent sensation below the nipple line, and no volitional movement in the upper or lower extremities except for shoulder shrugs, elbow flexion, and trace wrist extension.

Within 2 hours of the initial injury, 30 mg/kg of methylprednisolone, was administered intravenously. Additional emergency department treatment consisted of starting an intravenous catheter, inserting a Foley catheter, administering oxygen by means of a nasal cannula, and continuing immobilization in the cervical collar. CT scans of the cervical spine confirmed the initial diagnosis of fractures. The patient was admitted to the intensive care unit. Approximately 36 h after his accident, the patient underwent a wiring and fusion internal fixation from C5-C7 using an anterior approach. The patient was placed on deep vein thrombosis prophylaxis. Arrangements were made for transfer to a model SCI center on day 5.

On admission to the SCI center, the patient was taken to the rehabilitation unit and evaluated by the attending physician. Referrals were made to the rehabilitation team, including dietary services, occupational therapy, physical therapy, psychological services, respiratory therapy, social services, speech therapy, therapeutic recreation, and vocational counseling. The nursing staff initiated strict turning times with appropriate padding and positioning to prevent pressure ulcers and pulmonary complications.

The therapy evaluations, including the ISNSCI exam, were completed within 24 hours of admission and revealed the following neurological findings: the biceps were 5/5 and wrist extensors were 3/5. All other key muscles of the UE were absent. The motor neurological level was C6 bilaterally, and the AIS was an A. There was no sensory sparing below the C6 level of injury.

The patient's physical therapy (PT) sessions focused heavily on bed and mat mobility activities, balance activities in long sitting and short sitting and in supported and unsupported positions, w/c skills, and transfer activities. He also focused on strengthening his shoulder, neck, and biceps muscles. The patient was prescribed a manual wheelchair with power assist wheels in the seating clinic and was modified independent with propulsion on smooth surfaces and over rough terrain. He was dependent with bed transfers. During all PT sessions, care was taken to preserve functional tenodesis.

Because he had a complete SCI, most skill acquisition strategies focused on teaching compensatory movements, using momentum and a "head-hip" relationship to learn new movement. The foundation is that movement strategies are often opposite from able bodied movement where the head commonly leads the movement and the body *generally* follows in the same direction. To use compensation for movements such as transfer, momentum forces create movement by teaching patients to swing their head in the opposite direction to where they want the hips to go. Also, head and eye gaze relationships are important for balance and rolling, whereby arm swing creates momentum and the body will follow the eyes and head when learning this skill.

The patient required minimal assistance in meal preparation and was able to eat with modified independence using utensils with built-up handles. He was able to dress his upper body with the use of a button hook and zipper pull. He was modified independent in all grooming skills and could bath his UE and trunk. He required maximum assistance to bathe his lower extremities, but he used a long-handled sponge to help to access hard-to-reach areas. The patient was modified independent in written communication skills with adapted writing equipment (built up pens/pencils or short splint). His occupational therapy (OT) sessions use similar strategies, teaching compensation techniques for movement and using adaptive equipment.

Questions

Would you describe the movement strategies the patient uses to perform mobility skills as using compensation or using recovery focused movement patters?
Compensation—the patient has a complete C6 SCI. He is many years status post (s/p) injury, and his neurological recovery has reached a plateau. He currently is using compensatory movement patterns using substitutions, momentum, and residual strength to complete mobility tasks.

When performing mobility skills, such as scooting and transfers, why is it important to preserve tenodesis?
Tenodesis preserves compensatory grasp, which is important for other ADL skills, such as dressing, grooming, and eating, and allows functional grasp for other mobility skills.

Question

What compensatory strategy(s) is the patient using to accommodate for UE paralysis during (a) rolling; (b) coming to sit;and (c) long sitting?
(a) *External rotation of the shoulder and supination of the forearm to accommodate for loss of triceps function; also, patient used neck flexion to reduce the amount of weight on the bed surface during rolling*
(b) *Flexion of the trunk; external rotation of the shoulder and scapular depression; use of the head to allow momentum simultaneously with the arm movements*
(c) *For prop sitting, the patient used external rotation of the shoulder to allow the elbow to be in a locked position, wrist in extension with fingers flexed to preserve tenodesis*

Question

Describe forward chaining techniques and how they may be used as a training technique during dressing.
Forward chaining training includes taking a task, breaking that task into steps, and training the patient one step at a time beginning with step 1, then 2,

Continued

CASE STUDY 14.1   C5-C6 Fracture—cont'd

then 3.... Once the patient has mastered each individual step, then the final goal is to have the patient complete all steps together in a single instance for task success.

With dressing, first have the patient learn to handle the pants, especially if they do not have all muscles of the UE innervated. Second, work on managing pants over one foot and then the other foot utilizing different techniques to un-weight the ankles for success of the task. Third, pull the pants to upper thighs and then get the pants over the hips by shifting weight back and forth to accomplish this task. Finally work with fasteners. Successful completion of the task is indicated when all steps of lower body dressing can be accomplished at one time.

Question

Based on the technology chart you reviewed, what devices would you consider incorporating into this patient's plan of care and why?

A UE neuroprosthetic such as the Bioness H200—to provide electrical stimulation to the muscles of the hand to maintain intrinsic muscle mass and to work on opening/closing of the hand. This would hopefully assist in the long-term use of the hand for functional activities and to improve use of tenodesis grip.

FES cycling for UE and LE—to provide reciprocal extremity motion, afferent input below the level of injury, provide muscle pumping (especially to the legs) to assist with circulation. Including the trunk muscles will help with sustaining muscle tone for postural maintenance.

REFERENCES

To enhance this text and add value for the reader, all references are included on the companion Evolve site that accompanies this textbook. This online service will, when available, provide a link for the reader to a Medline abstract for the article cited. There are 341 cited references and other general references for this chapter, with the majority of those articles being evidence-based citations.

Neuromuscular Diseases

Diane D. Allen

OBJECTIVES

After reading this chapter the student or therapist will be able to:

1. Describe the basic pathology, clinical course, and medical treatment of amyotrophic lateral sclerosis and Guillain-Barré syndrome.
2. Describe the current rehabilitative goals and interventions for each condition.
3. Describe the "safe" parameters for exercise related to disuse atrophy and overwork damage.
4. Apply intervention concepts discussed in this chapter to other neuromuscular diseases.

KEY TERMS

amyotrophic lateral sclerosis (ALS)

disuse atrophy

dysarthria

dysphagia

Guillain-Barré syndrome (GBS)

noninvasive (positive-pressure) ventilation (NIV)

overwork damage

percutaneous endoscopic gastrostomy (PEG)

polyradiculoneuropathy

Neuromuscular diseases encompass disorders of *upper* or *lower motor neurons* (UMNs, LMNs) or the muscles they innervate. This chapter traces the connections among the central nervous system (CNS), peripheral nervous system (PNS), and musculoskeletal system through the disordered functioning associated with two neuromuscular diseases: amyotrophic lateral sclerosis (ALS), which damages UMNs and LMNs including cranial nerves; and Guillain-Barré syndrome (GBS), which compromises LMNs and sensory neurons of the PNS, including the autonomic nervous system (ANS).

To review the normal connections, UMNs originate in the motor cortex of the brain as cells also known as *Betz* or *pyramidal cells*. Axons from these UMNs collect together and descend as the *corticobulbar* and *corticospinal* tracts to synapse with LMNs located in the *bulbar* area of the brain stem (pons and medulla: signaling motor functions through cranial nerves [V and] VII-XII) and *ventral horn* of the spinal cord (anterior portion of the spinal gray matter: signaling motor functions of the neck, trunk, and limbs; Fig. 15.1). Axons from the LMNs collect together and exit the CNS as nerve roots from the brain stem or spinal cord. In the spinal canal, the motor or *ventral* nerve roots join with incoming sensory fibers forming the *dorsal* roots; when bundled together, the motor and sensory fibers become *spinal nerves* exiting the spinal canal. Spinal nerves collect together to form *peripheral nerves*, bundles of fibers traveling to muscles or sensory receptors. The axons of the LMNs in these peripheral nerves then synapse with muscle fibers. LMNs are also known as α *motor neurons* because they have relatively large diameter axons. One axon of a lower (α) motor neuron plus all the muscle fibers it innervates equals a *motor unit* (Fig. 15.2). The motor unit responds to excitation by propagating

a signal along the axon and contracting all of the muscle fibers associated with it. Muscle contraction stimulates sensory receptors in the muscles, tendons, joints, and skin, depending on the type and force of contraction. These receptors send signals through sensory fibers of the peripheral nerves (running in the same nerve bundle as the axons of the LMNs) to communicate the result of muscle contraction and movement to the CNS, both locally within the spinal cord and to higher neural levels for processing. Depending on the site of the pathology, neuromuscular diseases can be classified as neurogenic or myopathic. ALS and GBS are neurogenic disorders: they affect the neurons, not the muscles directly.

With motor neurons involved in both disorders, movement abilities can show several types of deficits. Using the conceptual model of the six dimensions of movement,[2] *strength* and *endurance* are primary losses, with *flexibility* and *speed* deficits secondarily resulting from these. The movement dimensions of *adaptability* and *accuracy* may be affected to a greater or lesser extent. See Fig. 15.3 for a movement ability plot or MAP showing the relationship of possible deficits in the six dimensions of movement with ALS or GBS.[3] Changes in movement ability can make themselves apparent in limbs, trunk, neck, face, eyes, or oral cavity.

Weakness is a primary symptom in both disorders (with loss of *strength*), with decreases in the individual's ability to generate force in the affected muscles. Loss of muscle strength can result in not only limb and trunk dysfunction but also speech, swallowing, and respiratory difficulties. Fatigue is another primary deficit (with loss of *endurance*); neurogenic disorders tend to result in *central fatigue* (deficit in ability to recruit and activate motor units) in contrast with myopathic

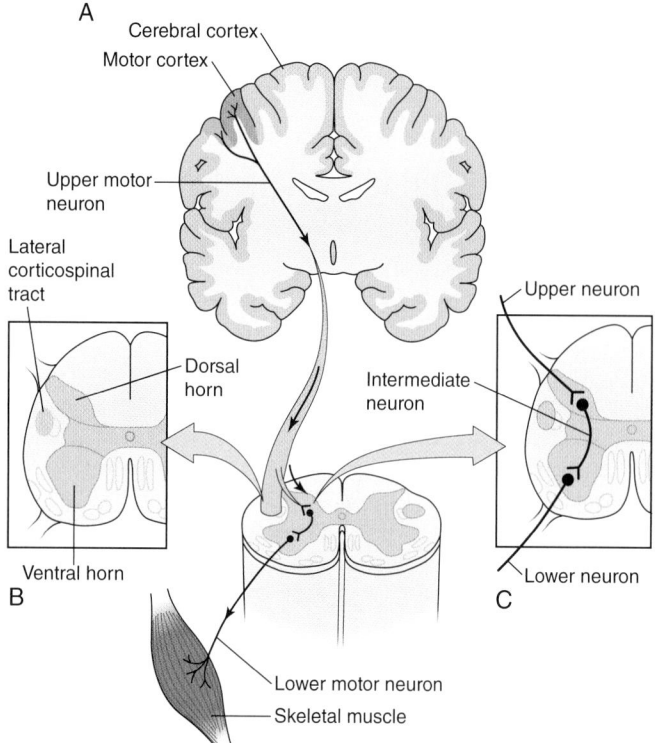

Fig. 15.1 Upper and Lower Motor Neurons. (A) The origin of the upper motor neurons in the motor cortex, showing an uncrossed portion of their pathway to the lateral corticospinal tract and spinal cord to synapse with lower motor neurons. Lower motor neurons originate in the nuclei of the motor cranial nerves (not depicted) and ventral horn of the spinal cord, and carry the neural signal to skeletal muscles. **(B)** Cross-section of the spinal cord showing the location of the lateral corticospinal tract on one side of the body. **(C)** Pathway of an upper motor neuron showing the connection with lower motor neurons in the ventral horn. (Modified from Blatzheim K. Interdisciplinary palliative care, including massage, in treatment of amyotrophic lateral sclerosis. *J Bodyw Mov Ther.* 2009;13:328–335.)[1]

disorders that tend to induce *peripheral fatigue* (deficit in ability of muscle fibers to contract forcefully).[4]

Secondary movement problems include loss of flexibility and speed of movement. *Flexibility* may be affected if muscles develop *spasticity* (with UMN involvement in ALS) and show resistance to quick stretch. Other flexibility issues or loss of range of motion (ROM) arise secondarily if resistance to movement, painful muscle spasms, or immobility because of weakness and fatigue result in stiff muscles and joints. *Speed* is affected as force production diminishes and stiffness impedes movement; individuals will have more difficulty putting on a burst of speed. Muscles may also adapt to weakness and disuse by changing the ratio of slow- and fast-twitch muscle fibers (with fewer fast-twitch fibers), further affecting the ability to move fast at will.

Adaptability, the ability to sense obstacles or changes in the environment and change the course of a movement in response,[2] may be affected with primary sensory loss in GBS. Adaptability may be secondarily affected when the strength dimension is so dysfunctional (ALS or GBS) that the muscles cannot change the course of a movement (to keep a body upright), even if sensory information (about a perturbation) reveals a need for it. *Accuracy,* the ability to move in a coordinated fashion with the right timing and direction for the task, may also show secondary deficits related to weakness (ALS and GBS). Accuracy shows primary deficits as ataxia in some forms of GBS (Miller-Fisher syndrome) that are more likely to have dysfunction of the neurons carrying proprioceptive information from the muscle spindles.

The International Classification of Functioning, Disability and Health (ICF) model[5] provides a framework for understanding the effects of devastating diseases such as ALS and GBS (Fig. 15.4). Movement disorders with neuromuscular diseases *(health condition)* affect not only the *body structures* of motor nerves and muscles and *body functions* commensurate with the movement dimensions of strength, endurance, and flexibility, but also the *activities* and *participatory* roles that an individual has in life. Activities such as walking may undergo limitations when the lower extremity muscles are weak; participation in work or leisure activities may undergo restrictions when walking

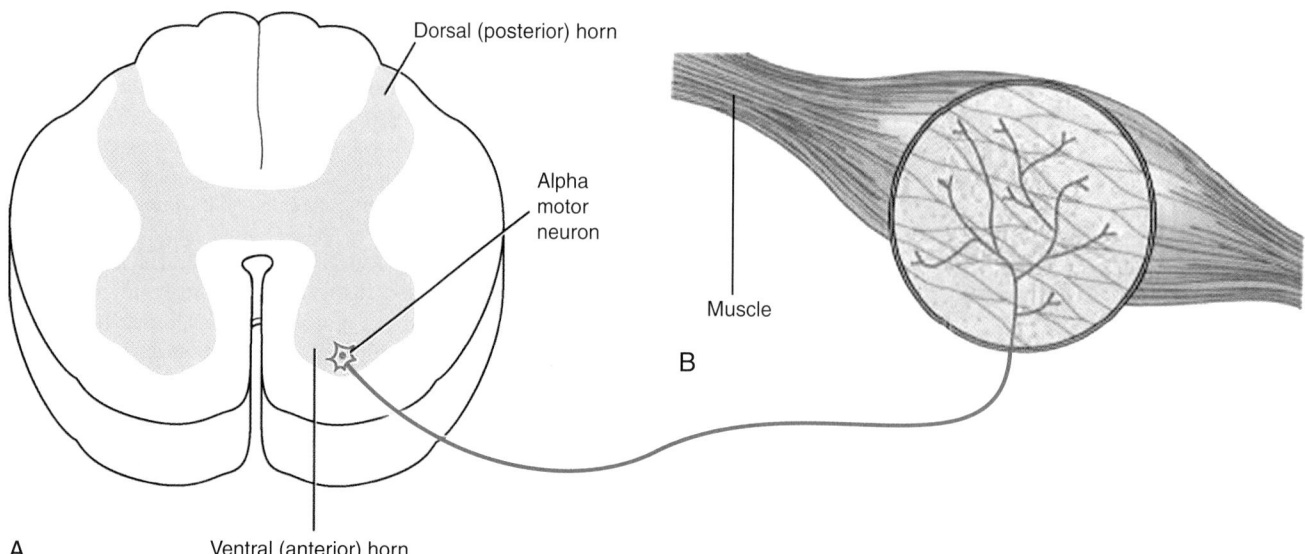

Fig. 15.2 One Motor Unit: α motor neuron **(A)** and muscle fibers innervated by it **(B)**. (Modified from Allen DD, Widener GL. Tone abnormalities. In: Cameron MH, ed. *Physical Agents in Rehabilitation.* 5th ed. St. Louis, MO: Elsevier; 2018.)

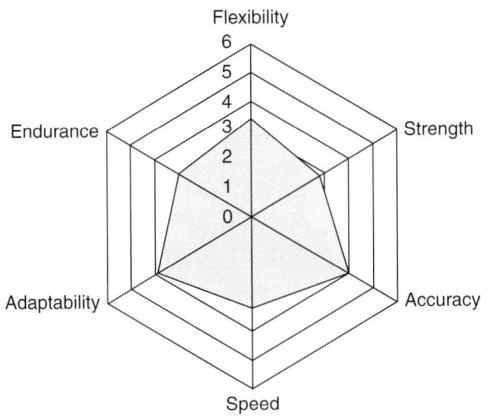

Fig. 15.3 Movement Ability Plot (MAP)[3] depicting movement dimensions[2] likely to be most affected by amyotrophic lateral sclerosis (ALS) or Guillain-Barré syndrome (GBS) when a patient is moderately impaired: strength and endurance are primary, but other movement dimensions will also be affected. Scale from logits is transformed to 0 (cannot do even with assistance—may be the case with severe impairment in ALS or GBS) to 6 (moves competitively, as in a professional athlete).

deteriorates. *Environmental* and *personal* factors will influence how the individual responds to the impairments of body structure and function within the activities and participatory roles that individual engages in. As the medical and rehabilitative management of these disorders proceeds, patients' individual needs will require assessment to ensure that, together with the patient (and family), the rehabilitative team can help optimize quality of life at whatever stage of the disease process the patient presents.

AMYOTROPHIC LATERAL SCLEROSIS

Etiology, Incidence, and Medical Diagnosis

ALS, the most common form of *motor neuron disease* in adults and frequently called *Lou Gehrig disease* in the United States, is a relentless, degenerative, terminal disease affecting both UMNs and LMNs. The name comes from two concurrent events. "Amyotrophy" indicates the muscle atrophy and weakness resulting from massive loss of lower (α) motor neurons originating in the spinal cord and motor cranial nerve nuclei in the lower brain stem. "Lateral sclerosis" indicates the demyelination and gliosis (i.e., "scarring" with hypertrophy and a dense

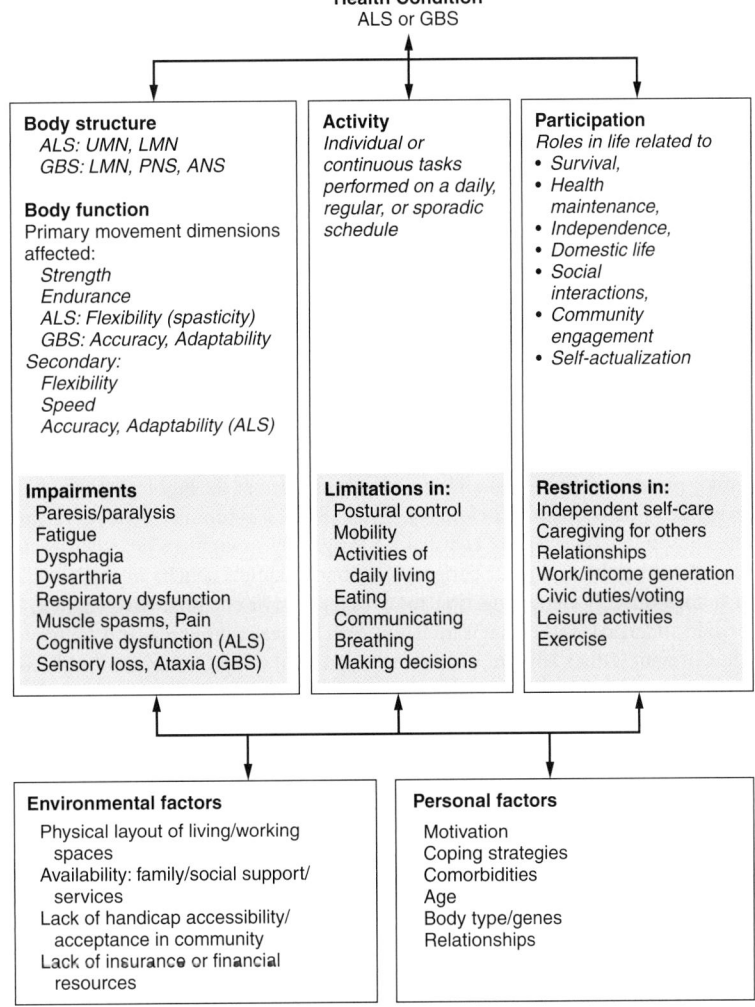

Fig. 15.4 Framework for relating the effects of ALS or GBS to function based on the International Classification of Functioning, Disability and Health[5] and the Six Dimensions of Movement.[2] *ALS,* Amyotrophic lateral sclerosis; *GBS,* Guillain Barré Syndrome; *PNS/ANS,* peripheral/autonomic nervous system; *UMN/LMN,* upper/lower motor neurons. (Adapted from *International Classification of Functioning, Disability and Health: ICF.* Geneva, Switzerland: World Health Organization; 2001.)

fibrous network of neuroglia) of the corticospinal tracts (that run laterally in the spinal cord) and corticobulbar tracts resulting from degeneration of the *Betz cells* (also known as *pyramidal cells*) in the motor cortex, the cell bodies of the UMNs. With both UMNs and LMNs affected, people typically experience rapid degeneration, become dependent for all care, and (without mechanical ventilation) die of respiratory failure within 3 to 5 years after symptom onset. A notable exception to this rule was Dr. Stephen Hawking, who lived with ALS for over 50 years before his death in 2018, working and contributing to society even while dependent on mechanical ventilation and assistance for all motor functions.

The cause of ALS is unknown. Numerous theories have proposed genetic, infectious,[6] environmental, and autoimmune etiologies. Some authors suggest that ALS and other neurodegenerative disorders are related to TDP-43 proteinopathy, which links ALS to frontotemporal lobar degeneration (FTD), a disease that affects cognitive function but typically spares memory.[7] Ninety percent of cases of ALS are sporadic without a known genetic component; however, approximately 5% to 10% seem to have a complex genetic basis coded on *ALS1* through *ALS8* and other mutations that are associated with frontal lobe dementias. Twenty percent of genetic causes of ALS are considered to be related to mendelian mutations in the superoxide dismutase–1 (SOD1) gene *(ALS1)*. Other factors considered in the genesis of ALS are vascular endothelial growth factors, toxicity (e.g., from heavy metals such as lead, selenium, and mercury) leading to motor neuron death, oxidative stress, and mitochondrial dysfunction related to microglial inflammation[8,9] and environmental factors.[10] Controversy regarding the role of physical activity as a risk factor[11] or a factor associated with earlier onset of ALS versus neuroprotection against ALS[12] has evidence on both sides.[13] Factors such as trauma and multiple traumatic brain injuries, associated with greater risk for ALS,[12] confound the evidence regarding the association of ALS with vigorous sport activity. Some evidence indicates that ALS is the consequence of multiple interactions among these factors, and that none of them alone is the direct cause.[14,15]

Because ALS has no specific biomarkers identified, the differential diagnosis requires extensive work up, ruling out other possibilities and allowing time to monitor progression. Cervical or lumbar myelopathy, syringomyelia, multiple sclerosis, primary lateral sclerosis, diseases associated with LMN pathology, heavy metal toxicity, paraneoplastic syndromes, myopathies, and Lyme disease must be excluded before the diagnosis of ALS is made.[16] Creatine phosphokinase levels are elevated in approximately 70% of patients and tend to be higher in patients with limb onset ALS rather than bulbar onset.[17] Genetic testing to identify the mutations in the copper/zinc (Cu/Zn) SOD1 gene is available when a family history of ALS is present. Other laboratory tests, such as identification of biochemical markers in the blood and cerebrospinal fluid (CSF), are used to exclude other neurological diseases. Testing CSF may have an additional benefit. A meta-analysis of 10 articles examining elevated levels of neurofilaments (reflective of ongoing destruction of axons) in the CSF revealed a pooled sensitivity and specificity at 81% and 85%, respectively, for association with motor neuron disease (9 out of 10 articles specified ALS), indicating potential diagnostic accuracy in people already showing symptoms.[18] Electromyography (EMG) and nerve conduction studies can be helpful to confirm the presence of widespread LMN disease (with neurogenic and fibrillation potentials and/or sharp waves) without peripheral neuropathy or polyradiculopathy. Neuroimaging studies can rule out conditions such as cervical myelopathy and myelitis[19] that may have clinical signs similar to those of ALS.[20] To date, while multiple laboratory tests, genetic testing, and imaging studies are performed, they are used more to rule out other possibilities than to rule in ALS.

Clinical diagnosis of ALS requires a pattern of observed and reported symptoms of both UMN and LMN disease and persistent declines in physical functions that cannot be attributed to other disorders. Because of the overlap of symptoms with other neuromuscular disorders, misdiagnosis is not uncommon.[21] The World Federation of Neurology (WFN) has developed suggested diagnostic criteria (the El Escorial criteria, refined by the Awaji[22] criteria to identify specific EMG interpretations), indicating suspected, possible, laboratory-supported-probable, probable, and definite ALS for patients with ALS entering clinical research trials.[23] The categories have sometimes been simplified, labeling just three: possible, probable, and definite ALS. (The WFN ALS website [www.wfnals.org] provides up-to-date criteria used for clinical studies.) Essentially, a patient with "definite" ALS must show concomitant UMN and LMN signs in multiple spinal regions (regions designated as cervical, thoracic, lumbosacral) or in two spinal regions plus bulbar signs and show evidence of progression over a 12 month period.[19,23] The category of "possible" ALS can be interpreted as a diagnosis of ALS if progressing LMN signs are present in two or more body regions, even without UMN signs, yet apparent as long as other diseases have been ruled out; the literature suggests that UMN *pathology* is present before clinical signs become apparent.[19]

ALS has an incidence of approximately 2 to 3 cases per 100,000 Caucasians, with somewhat lower incidence in Asians and African Americans.[14] Mean age at onset is 57 years, with two-thirds of patients aged 50 to 70 years old at time of onset.[24] Men are affected approximately 1.3 to 1.5 times more frequently than are women, although gender differences decrease with late onset of disease (aged 70+).

Clinical Presentation

For an overall view of the clinical presentation of a person with ALS as categorized by the ICF model, review Fig. 15.4. The predominant body function impairments of ALS are weakness and fatigue (affecting movement dimensions of strength and endurance[2]), with muscle atrophy and fasciculation indicating body structure effects on LMNs and spasticity indicating body structure effects on UMNs (see Fig. 15.1). Activity limitations and participation restrictions progress as the impairments of weakness and fatigue become more severe, but an individual's clinical presentation will depend on environmental and personal factors as well, such as economic resources and coping mechanisms (see Fig. 15.4).

Some less prominent or prevalent body function impairments were originally thought to be exclusionary criteria for ALS: ocular motor abnormalities, deficits in sphincter control (especially bladder), sensory loss, or cognitive involvement. With longer survival facilitated by mechanical ventilation and better tools to examine pathology, these signs and symptoms are no longer considered spared, but merely resistant or delayed.[25] For example, in a review of literature on ocular motor pathology in ALS, Sharma and colleagues[25] speculate that the ontogenetically older and more complex pathways of the ocular motor system protect it somewhat from ALS pathology. The nuclei for cranial nerves III, IV, and VI do not receive direct monosynaptic connections from the motor region of the cortex like other motor neuron pools in the brain stem or spinal cord. Also, the predominant neurotransmitters are different (fewer glycinergic and muscarinic cholinergic receptors in the ocular motor nuclei) and the oculomotor neurons contain a higher ratio of calcium-binding proteins (important for maintaining lowering levels of intracellular calcium, thought to be a source of excitotoxicity in ALS) than in motor neuron pools typically affected in ALS.[25] In addition to ocular motility, signs of neurogenic bladder have been reported in about 40% of patients,[26] and progressive functional deficit in sensation have been recorded in ALS, perhaps related to ongoing immobility.[27]

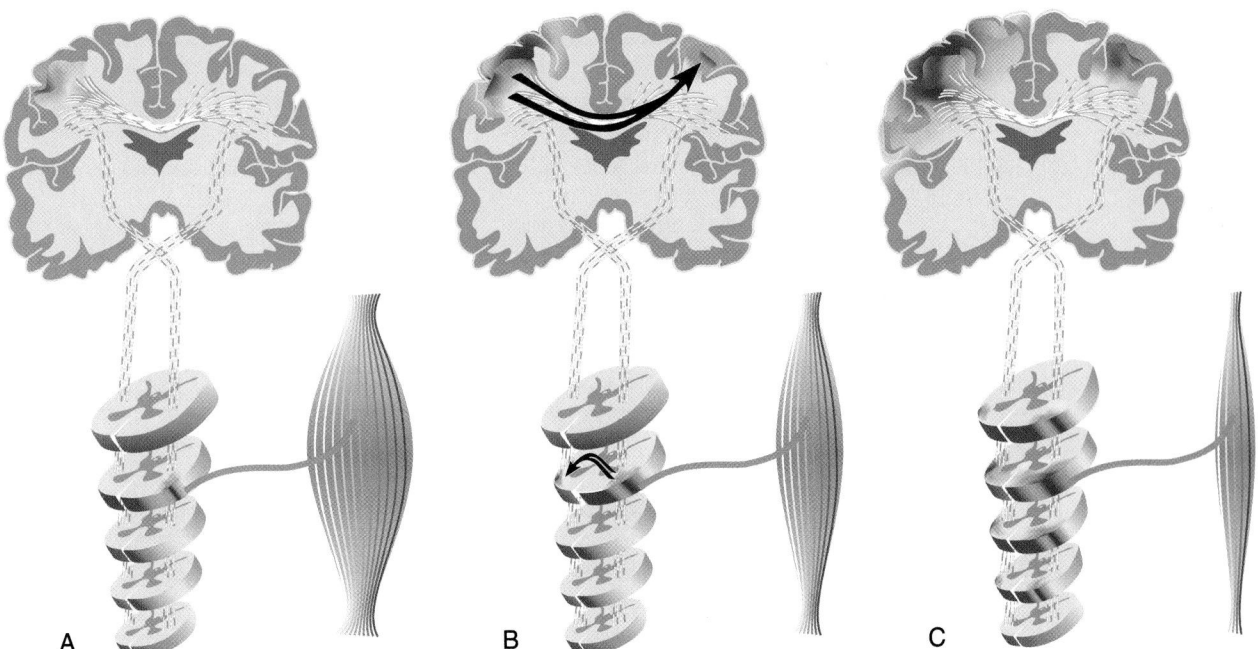

Fig. 15.5 Possible Pattern of Degeneration in Amyotrophic Lateral Sclerosis. **(A)** Onset in cortex or spinal cord; **(B)** interhemispheric and interneuronal connections in the cortex and spinal cord spread the disease from the site of onset to contralateral motor neurons; **(C)** degeneration continues in areas adjacent to sites of onset, affecting additional muscles in the same limbs and in additional regions. (Figure from Walhout R, Verstraete E, van den Heuvel MP, et al. Patterns of symptom development in patients with motor neuron disease. *Amyotroph Lateral Scler Frontotemporal Degener.* 2018;19:21–28.)

Similarly, cognitive deficits have been noted in ALS. A small subgroup of patients with both familial and sporadic forms of ALS has been identified as having concomitant evidence of FTD, with pathology in cortical areas outside of the cortical motor regions. These patients show lower scores on executive cognitive functions, word finding, and phrase length.[28] As people can exhibit a combination of ALS and FTD, the evidence suggests that a common cause may be possible.[29] Because of these findings, therapists should be aware of the possibility of cognitive deficits in their patients with ALS, manifested as a decrement in planning, organization, and language problems.[30] Such patients may have more difficulty following through on medication and therapeutic recommendations, and their families may need more support. Unassociated with overall cognitive impairment, some deficits in action knowledge as opposed to object knowledge have been noted in patients with ALS, correlating with atrophy in the motor and premotor cortex.[31]

Although impaired strength and endurance predominate in ALS, the appearance of weakness (paresis to paralysis) and fatigue are heterogeneous. Some people have limb (spinal) onset; others have cranial nerve (bulbar) onset.[32] Many start with a single limb involved (flail arm or flail leg) at first, with different neural roots and nerves affected within that limb. Some may present with progressive muscular atrophy (LMN predominant); others present with primary lateral sclerosis (UMN predominant). During initial diagnostic visits, patients frequently report to their physicians a profound sense of fatigue or the loss of exercise tolerance. Because the onset of ALS is insidious, most patients are not aware of the strength changes, or they have adjusted to the changes until they have difficulty with a functional activity such as tying shoes, climbing stairs, or stumbling with a fall. Physical examination usually demonstrates more widespread and extensive weakness and atrophy than reported by the patient. By the time most patients report weakness, they have lost approximately 80% of their motor neurons in the areas of weakness. Relative preservation of function despite so much tissue damage demonstrates both the reserve and the plasticity of the nervous system (or the mindset of the individual patient who delays reporting changes) in the drive to adapt to meet functional goals. As the disease progresses, weakness spreads to include musculature throughout the body.

ALS progression varies with several distinct patterns according to the primary area of onset.[33] Lower-extremity onset is slightly more common than upper-extremity onset, which is more common than bulbar onset. With leg onset, the next area of symptoms tends to be the contralateral leg, then the ipsilateral and contralateral arm before bulbar symptoms appear, especially if a distinct indication of both UMN and LMN disease is present (Fig. 15.5). A significant diagnostic feature of the pattern of disease is the asymmetry of the weakness and the sparing of some muscle fibers, even in highly atrophied muscles. For example, a patient may have weakness of the right intrinsics and shoulder musculature or weakness of the left anterior tibial muscles. Bulbar symptoms are presaged by tongue fasciculations and weakness, facial and palatal weakness, and swallowing difficulties, which result in dysphagia and dysarthria. Table 15.1 lists bulbar and respiratory impairments and activity limitations in ALS. Pseudobulbar signs (sometimes referred to as pseudobulbar palsy or affect) are sometimes present in ALS, manifested by exaggerated laughing or crying beyond what seems to be appropriate to the situation.[34] Despite the pattern of onset, the eventual course of the illness is similar (with variations in timing) in most patients, with an unremitting spread of weakness to other muscle groups leading to total paralysis of limb, trunk, and diaphragm musculature and muscles innervated by the cranial nerves. Death is usually related to respiratory failure, occurring within 3 years of symptom onset in approximately 50% of patients.[35] With mechanical ventilation, up to 10% of people with ALS live longer than 10 years.[36]

TABLE 15.1 Common Physical Findings with Bulbar Palsy

Body Structure—Innervation	Observation	Body Function Impairment	Activity Limitation
Tongue—Cranial Nerve (CN) XII	Fasciculations at rest; atrophy; difficulty articulating during speech	Strength: paresis to paralysis affecting range of motion and force in the anterior-posterior (protrusion-retraction), superior-inferior (touch palate), and lateral directions Speed: impaired ability to perform rapid motion Endurance: fatigues quickly	Dysarthria (spastic/flaccid/mixed): imprecise consonants *t, d, l, k, sh, soft g*; slowed lateral motion, "ta-ta-ta" or "la-la-la" Inability to manipulate food bolus or avoid pocketing of food in cheeks Inability to lick lips or popsicle Unable to sustain effort to continue a conversation or complete a regular meal
Lips—CN VII	Lips slack Smile uneven, partial or absent Leakage of food or saliva	Strength: impaired to absent lip closure, pursing, suction action Endurance: if lip closure successful with effort, fatigues quickly	Dysarthria (imprecise consonants *p* and *b; f, v*) Inability to whistle or kiss Inability to use a straw or fully clear a spoon or fork Drooling
Palate—CN V, X, IX	Uvula movement impaired during phonation (say "ahhhh"); changes in resonance of speech	Strength: unsustained or slow palatal elevation Endurance: fatigues with effort	Dysarthria (hypernasal speech; imprecise *k* and hard *g*) Impaired nasopharyngeal reflex on swallowing Choking; aspiration
Muscles of mastication, Masseter, temporalis—CN V	Atrophy; mouth hangs open	Strength: weak or no-longer-palpable contraction Endurance: chewing fatigue	Elimination of foods that require chewing Mouth breathing with drying of secretions
Pterygoids—CN V	Jaw does not move side to side or protrude	Strength: weak or absent	Cannot stick chin out
Tongue, lips, jaws combined	Slowed speaking rate Speech intelligibility drops	Strength: impaired Endurance: highly fatigable	Speaking rate over 160 words per minute (wpm) = Normal, presymptomatic* 120–160 wpm = Early changes in speech intelligibility <120 wpm = Rapid decline in speech intelligibility
Trapezius—CN XI Sternocleido-mastoid—CN XI	Cannot shrug shoulders Cannot lift head from supine	Strength: progressive weakness Endurance: highly fatigable	Inability to comb hair Inability to perform facial grooming May need neck collar to help support head when upright
Vocal cords, CN X	Breathy voice (if flaccid); strained or tense voice (if spasticity present), other changes in phonation during speech	Strength: progressive loss of vocal cord closure (weak—> flaccid) Flexibility: tight (if spasticity present) vocal cords Endurance: highly fatigable (if weak)	Impaired oral communication Impaired singing Impaired inspiration (if spasticity present)
Extraocular muscles—CN III, IV, VI	Fixed gaze or nonconvergent eye movement	Strength: progressive weakness to paralysis	Generally occurs after other bulbar and head/neck muscle loss so no compensatory head movement available: limitation of gaze Diplopia if strength loss is asymmetrical
Respiratory Group Diaphragm—C3-C5	Shortness of breath Low voice volume	Strength: progressive weakness Endurance: highly fatigable	Diminished vital capacity Poor breath control; impaired ability to sniff or blow Difficulty sustaining a vowel
Intercostal and abdominal muscles—T1-T11 Accessory muscles of respiration—CN VII, XI, XII, C5-C8	Weak cough	Strength: progressive weakness Endurance: highly fatigable	With vital capacity moderately impaired, change in speech phrasing; at severely impaired, one syllable per breath, short of breath when swallowing

*Bandini A, Green JR, Wang J, Campbell TF, Zinman L, Yunusova Y. Kinematic features of jaw and lips distinguish symptomatic from presymptomatic stages of bulbar decline in amyotrophic lateral sclerosis. J Speech Lang Hear Res. 2018;61:1118-1129.

Once ALS has been diagnosed, knowing the natural history of the progression of ALS should help in the institution of medical and supportive treatment planning and interventions. Disease-specific standardized scales have been developed that help chart the course of ALS. Hillel and colleagues[37] developed the ALS Severity Scale (ALSSS) for rapid functional assessment of disease stage. Their ordinal scale allows clinicians and therapists to score patients in four categories, with 10 points possible for each: speech, swallowing, and lower-extremity and upper-extremity function (Box 15.1). A multistage scale of severity

BOX 15.1   Amyotrophic Lateral Sclerosis Severity Scale

Lower Extremities, Upper Extremities, Speech, Swallowing

Lower Extremities (Walking)

Normal

| 10 | Normal ambulation | Patient denies any weakness or fatigue; examination reveals no abnormality |
| 9 | Fatigue suspected | Patient experiences sense of weakness or fatigue in lower extremities during exertion |

Early Ambulation Difficulties

| 8 | Difficulty with uneven terrain | Difficulty and fatigue when walking long distances, climbing stairs, and walking over uneven ground (even thick carpet) |
| 7 | Observed changes in gait | Noticeable change in gait; pulls on railings when climbing stairs; may use leg brace |

Walks With Assistance

| 6 | Walks with mechanical device | Needs or uses cane, walker, or assistant to walk; probably uses wheelchair away from home |
| 5 | Walks with mechanical device and assistant | Does not attempt to walk without attendant; ambulation limited to less than 50 ft; avoids stairs |

Functional Movement Only

| 4 | Able to support | At best, can shuffle a few steps with the help of an attendant for transfers |
| 3 | Purposeful leg movements | Unable to take steps but can position legs to assist attendant in transfers; moves legs purposefully to maintain mobility in bed |

No Purposeful Leg Movement

| 2 | Minimal movement | Minimal movement of one or both legs; cannot reposition legs independently |
| 1 | Paralysis | Flaccid paralysis; cannot move lower extremities (except, perhaps, to close inspection) |

Upper Extremities (Dressing and Hygiene)

Normal Function

| 10 | Normal function | Patient denies any weakness or unusual fatigue of upper extremities; examination demonstrates no abnormality |
| 9 | Suspected fatigue | Patient experiences sense of fatigue in upper extremities during exertion; cannot sustain work for as long as normal; atrophy not evident on examination |

Independent and Complete Self-Care

| 8 | Slow self-care | Dressing and hygiene performed more slowly than usual |
| 7 | Effortful self-care performance | Requires significantly more time (usually double or more) and effort to accomplish self-care; weakness is apparent on examination |

Intermittent Assistance

| 6 | Mostly independent | Handles most aspects of dressing and hygiene alone; adapts by resting, modifying (e.g., use of electric razor), or avoiding some tasks; requires assistance for fine motor tasks (e.g., buttons and ties) |
| 5 | Partial independence | Handles some aspects of dressing and hygiene alone; however, routinely requires assistance for many tasks such as applying makeup, combing, and shaving |

Needs Attendant for Self-Care

| 4 | Attendant assists patient | Attendant must be present for dressing and hygiene; patient performs the majority of each task with the assistance of the attendant |
| 3 | Patient assists attendant | The attendant directs the patient for almost all tasks; the patient moves in a purposeful manner to assist the attendant; does not initiate self-care |

Total Dependence

| 2 | Minimal movement | Minimal movement of one or both arms; cannot reposition arms |
| 1 | Paralysis | Flaccid paralysis; unable to move upper extremities (except, perhaps, to close inspection) |

Speech

Normal Speech Processes

| 10 | Normal speech | Patient denies any difficulty speaking; examination demonstrates no abnormality |
| 9 | Nominal speech abnormalities | Only the patient or spouse notices speech has changed; maintains normal rate and volume |

Detectable Speech Disturbance

| 8 | Perceived speech changes | Speech changes are noted by others, especially during fatigue or stress; rate of speech remains essentially normal |
| 7 | Obvious speech abnormalities | Speech is consistently impaired; rate, articulation, and resonance are affected; remains easily understood |

Intelligible With Repeating

| 6 | Repeats message on occasion | Rate is much slower, repeats specific words in adverse listening situation; does not limit complexity or length of messages |
| 5 | Frequent repeating required | Speech is slow and labored; extensive repetition or a "translator" is commonly used; patient probably limits the complexity or length of messages |

Speech Combined with Nonvocal Communication

| 4 | Speech plus nonverbal communication | Speech is used in response to questions; intelligibility problems need to be resolved by writing or a spokesperson |
| 3 | Limits speech to one-word responses | Vocalizes one-word responses beyond yes and no; otherwise writes or uses a spokesperson; initiates communication nonvocally |

Continued

BOX 15.1   Amyotrophic Lateral Sclerosis Severity Scale—cont'd

Loss of Useful Speech

2	Vocalizes for emotional expression	Uses vocal inflection to express emotion, affirmation, and negation
1	Nonvocal	Vocalization is effortful, limited in duration, and rarely attempted; may vocalize for crying or pain
X	Tracheostomy	

Swallowing

Normal Eating Habits

10	Normal swallowing	Patient denies any difficulty chewing or swallowing; examination demonstrates no abnormality
9	Nominal abnormality	Only patient notices slight indicators such as food lodging in the recesses of the mouth or sticking in the throat

Early Eating Problems

8	Minor swallowing problems	Reports some swallowing difficulties; maintains essentially a regular diet; isolated choking episodes
7	Prolonged times, smaller bite size	Mealtime has significantly increased and smaller bite sizes are necessary; must concentrate on swallowing thin liquids

Dietary Consistency Changes

6	Soft diet	Diet is limited primarily to soft foods; requires some special meal preparation
5	Liquefied diet	Oral intake adequate; nutrition limited primarily to liquefied diet; adequate thin liquid intake usually a problem; may force self to eat

Needs Tube Feeding

4	Supplemental tube feedings	Oral intake alone no longer adequate; patient uses or needs a tube to supplement intake; patient continues to take significant (>50%) nutrition orally
3	Tube feeding with occasional oral nutrition	Primary nutrition and hydration accomplished by tube; receives less than 50% of nutrition orally

No Oral Feeding

2	Secretions managed with aspirator and/or medications	Cannot safely manage any oral intake; secretions managed with aspirator and/or medications; swallows reflexively
1	Aspiration of secretions	Secretions cannot be managed noninvasively; rarely swallows

Adapted with permission from Hillel AD, Miller RM, Yorkston K, et al. Amyotrophic lateral sclerosis severity scale. *Neuroepidemiology*. 1989;8: 142–150.

has also been proposed based on milestones common among 1471 patients with ALS in one treatment center.[38] Patients in stage 1 (mild disease) have symptom onset, with noticeable or functional involvement in one region (bulbar, upper limb, lower limb, or diaphragmatic); at stage 1, individuals are functionally independent in ambulation, activities of daily living (ADLs), and speech. Stage 2a is when most people get diagnosed; stage 2B is when a second region shows clinical involvement. Stage 3 is when a third region is involved; the patient has (moderate) deficits in function in three regions or a moderate to severe deficit in one region and mild functional loss in two other regions. Stage 4A indicates need for gastrostomy because of eating difficulties; 4B indicates need for respiratory support (usually noninvasive ventilation).[38] The ALS Functional Rating Scale (ALS FRS) and the ALSFRS-Revised consist of 13 items with response options of 0 (unable) to 4 (normal performance) that assess how well people are functioning across various systems; this scale is frequently used clinically and in clinical trials to document status and changes (Box 15.2).[39] Mitchell and Borasio provide more information on the natural history of ALS.[34]

Along with the primary impairments of weakness and fatigue affecting body structure and function in ALS, patients also have progressive limitations in activity and participation.[40] Activity limitations result in gradual loss of independence in community and then household tasks. Mechanical and electronic adaptive devices can help extend independence in some ADLs past the initial strength losses. Participation limitations result in progressive isolation from the community and family unless extraordinary efforts are made to implement an evolving communication system, usually using electronic interfaces.

Medical Prognosis

In almost all cases ALS progresses relentlessly and leads to death from respiratory failure. The rate of progression seems to be consistent within each patient but varies considerably among patients. Patients with an initial onset of bulbar weakness (dysarthria and dysphagia) and respiratory weakness (dyspnea) tend to have a more rapid progression to death than patients whose weakness begins in the distal extremities.[34] Reports vary in terms of long-term prognosis, depending on medical care and choices regarding mechanical ventilation, but death usually follows within 2 to 4 years after diagnosis. Diagnosis is often delayed 1 to 2 years after the onset of symptoms when the clinical presentation of symptom progression is recognized by a physician. A small number of patients live for 15 to 20 years.[21]

Years of survival after diagnosis may change as drug therapies are developed.[41] In addition, increasing numbers of patients are electing to prolong life with home-based mechanical ventilation as opposed to palliative or comfort care only.

Medical Management

ALS has no known cure and few effective disease-slowing treatments. Mitchell and Borasio[34] summarize the results of trials of many putative ALS-modifying pharmaceuticals. Riluzole has the longest history as an approved treatment of ALS. Riluzole, a glutamate inhibitor, provides very modest improvement over a placebo in both bulbar and limb function, but not in actual strength of muscles.[42] According to meta-analyses of randomized controlled trials (RCTs), riluzole extends lifespan an average of 2 to 3 months.[42] The side effects were minimal in some studies, but fatigue and weakness have been noted in 26% and 18% of patients taking riluzole compared with a placebo.[43] In 2017, the

BOX 15.2 Amyotrophic Lateral Sclerosis Functional Rating Scale Revised

Date:........................ Name Patient:.. Date of Birth:................................

Patient's number .... Right-/left-handed

Item 1: SPEECH
4 ☐ Normal speech process
3 ☐ Detectable speech disturbance
2 ☐ Intelligible with repeating
1 ☐ Speech combined with nonvocal communication
0 ☐ Loss of useful speech

Item 2: SALIVATION
4 ☐ Normal
3 ☐ Slight but definite excess of saliva in mouth; may have nighttime drooling
2 ☐ Moderately excessive saliva; may have minimal drooling (during the day)
1 ☐ Marked excess of saliva with some drooling
0 ☐ Marked drooling; requires constant tissue or handkerchief

Item 3: SWALLOWING
4 ☐ Normal eating habits
3 ☐ Early eating problems—occasional choking
2 ☐ Dietary consistency changes
1 ☐ Needs supplement tube feeding
0 ☐ NPO (exclusively parenteral or enteral feeding)

Item 4: HANDWRITING
4 ☐ Normal
3 ☐ Slow or sloppy: all words are legible
2 ☐ Not all words are legible
1 ☐ Able to grip pen, but unable to write
0 ☐ Unable to grip pen

Item 5a: CUTTING FOOD AND HANDLING UTENSILS
    Patients *without* gastrostomy → Use 5b if >50% is through g-tube
4 ☐ Normal
3 ☐ Somewhat slow and clumsy, but no help needed
2 ☐ Can cut most foods (>50%), although slow and clumsy; some help needed
1 ☐ Food must be cut by someone, but can still feed slowly
0 ☐ Needs to be fed

Item 5b: CUTTING FOOD AND HANDLING UTENSILS
    Patients with gastrostomy →5b option is used if the patient has a gastrostomy and only if it is the primary method (more than 50%) of eating.
4 ☐ Normal
3 ☐ Clumsy, but able to perform all manipulation independently
2 ☐ Some help needed with closures and fasteners
1 ☐ Provides minimal assistance to caregiver
0 ☐ Unable to perform any aspect of task

Item 6: DRESSING AND HYGIENE
4 ☐ Normal function
3 ☐ Independent and complete self-care with effort or decreased efficiency
2 ☐ Intermittent assistance or substitute methods
1 ☐ Needs attendant for self-care
0 ☐ Total dependence

Item 7: TURNING IN BED AND ADJUSTING BED CLOTHES
4 ☐ Normal function
3 ☐ Somewhat slow and clumsy, but no help needed
2 ☐ Can turn alone, or adjust sheets, but with great difficulty
1 ☐ Can initiate, but not turn or adjust sheets alone
0 ☐ Helpless

Item 8: WALKING
4 ☐ Normal
3 ☐ Early ambulation difficulties
2 ☐ Walks with assistance
1 ☐ Nonambulatory functional movement
0 ☐ No purposeful leg movement

Item 9: CLIMBING STAIRS
4 ☐ Normal
3 ☐ Slow
2 ☐ Mild unsteadiness or fatigue
1 ☐ Needs assistance
0 ☐ Cannot do

Item 10: DYSPNEA
4 ☐ None
3 ☐ Occurs when walking
2 ☐ Occurs with one or more of the following: eating, bathing, dressing (ADL)
1 ☐ Occurs at rest: difficulty breathing when either sitting or lying
0 ☐ Significant difficulty: considering using mechanical respiratory support

Item 11: ORTHOPNEA
4 ☐ None
3 ☐ Some difficulty sleeping at night due to shortness of breath, does not routinely use more than two pillows
2 ☐ Needs extra pillows in order to sleep (more than two)
1 ☐ Can only sleep sitting up
0 ☐ Unable to sleep without mechanical assistance

Item 12: RESPIRATORY INSUFFICIENCY
4 ☐ None
3 ☐ Intermittent use of BiPAP
2 ☐ Continuous use of BiPAP during the night
1 ☐ Continuous use of BiPAP during day & night
0 ☐ Invasive mechanical ventilation by intubation or tracheostomy

Interviewer's name..

ALS Functional Rating Scale Revised (ALS-FRS-R). Version: May 2015

Amyotrophic Lateral Sclerosis Functional Rating Scale—Revised; Form adapted from Cedarbaum JM, Stambler N, Malta E, et al. The ALSFRS-R: a revised ALS functional rating scale that incorporates assessments of respiratory function. BDNF ALS Study Group (Phase III). *J Neurol Sci.* 1999;169:13–21. Form available online: https://www.encals.eu/wp-content/uploads/2016/09/ALS-Functional-Rating-Scale-Revised-fill-in-form.pdf.

Federal Drug Administration (FDA) approved the use of edaravone, a free radical scavenger, in the early disease stages of ALS; further research is needed to determine whether this drug is associated with improvement in quality of life.[44]

Animal studies reveal some promise. In a mouse model of ALS, cell-therapy researchers targeted both the motor neurons and astrocytes and the microglia that surround them, noting an additive effect on life-span and motor function.[45] This study confirms that the pathology in the genetic strains of ALS stems from both the mutant gene expression in motor neurons and in the hostile cellular environment provided by the microglia. Unfortunately, the study of animal models may relate to the genetic forms of ALS (about 10% of cases) but does not translate well to the sporadic forms. A 2016 Cochrane review of cellular treatments in humans with ALS found no completed RCTs, although several trials were under way.[36] Jaiswal in 2017[15] highlighted the promise of stem cell research for humans: induced pluripotent stem cells can be prepared in vitro to differentiate as motor neurons with ALS, to create "disease in a dish." Microglia and astrocytes can also be created. With substantial amounts of human cells to work on, promising replacement cellular therapies can be tried, repeated, and modified before in vivo trials begin.

The popular press has reported on nutritional cures for ALS, including regular use of vitamin E. However, Orrell and colleagues[46] found insufficient evidence to support clinical use of vitamin E supplements in ALS as an additive to riluzole treatment or as adjunctive therapy, although no apparent contraindication was found to taking the supplement. Vitamin D supplementation was associated with a reduction in functional decline in preliminary studies.[47] Other nutritional and nonpharmaceutical supplements have had some success in animal models of ALS, but this has not yet been confirmed in humans.[48]

Cannabis has been studied for its effect on spasticity in patients with multiple sclerosis and spinal cord injury, but evidence in ALS is limited. In a study of 131 people with ALS, 13 used cannabis, with reports of reduction in spasticity, pain, and depression.[49] A systematic review cites moderate-quality evidence indicating that tetrahydrocannabinol (THC) is probably ineffective in reducing muscle cramps in ALS.[50] As with many other approaches, more high-quality research is needed.

Because of the apparent hopelessness of the diagnosis, many physicians, especially those not associated with major medical centers having neuromuscular disease units, do not refer patients with ALS for rehabilitative or support services. However, few primary care physicians or neurologists have extensive experience in the care of patients and families coping with ALS because of the low incidence of the disease. Referral of patients with ALS to a multidisciplinary clinic typically extends the patient's life-span, especially patients with bulbar onset of ALS.[35,42,51]

Although the overall disease course has not been halted, several specific impairments have been addressed through medical and pharmaceutical interventions. The following subsections discuss medical management of muscle spasms and pain, dysphagia, dysarthria, and respiratory dysfunction.

Muscle Spasms and Pain

Some patients experience muscle cramps and spasms related to UMN pathology, and up to 73% of patients complain of pain, typically in the later stages.[34] Muscle soreness and nonspecific aching are common, perhaps resulting from immobility or small traumas to paralyzed muscles during caregiving procedures or injudicious overexertion. A Cochrane systematic review in 2013 found no randomized or quasi-RCTs of drug therapy for pain in ALS, although the authors noted several case series reporting the use of acetaminophen, nonsteroidal antiinflammatory drugs (NSAIDs), or opioids.[52] In a more recent study, 46% of 80 patients with motor neuron disease (71 with ALS) reported chronic pain (daily for over 3 months), with muscular origins being the most frequent source.[53] Neuropathic pain was absent. In this study, analgesics or antiinflammatories usually resulted in good relief of pain.[53] Because many patients have compromised respiratory function, the physician must take great care when prescribing pain medication that depresses respiratory drive, especially opiates, which are often used when antispasmodics or antiinflammatory pain medications no longer work.[35] Patients should be instructed to keep a daily reporting log of the effectiveness of prescribed medication so that the dosage can be adjusted if necessary.

Stretching and massage may prove helpful for nocturnal muscle cramps.[35] Some patients may respond to medications such as quinine or baclofen to relieve symptoms, but evidence of effectiveness is currently low quality in ALS.[50]

In addition to muscle spasms, spasticity may affect function in many patients. In a review of studies on the treatment of spasticity in ALS, Ashworth and colleagues[54] found only one randomized study addressing spasticity: a moderate-endurance exercise regimen decreased spasticity at 3 months after initiation of the program. Kesiktas and colleagues[55] report that in a controlled study of spasticity in patients after *spinal cord injury*, adding hydrotherapy to a program of medication and exercise decreased severity of spasticity-related spasms and decreased the amount of medication required. A similar response could be hypothesized in patients with ALS. Medications such as baclofen (sometimes administered via implanted intrathecal baclofen pump), tizanidine, dantrolene sodium, and diazepam are useful for some patients with spasticity. Because each has a different action and side effects, the medications may have to be adjusted to find the right dosage and combination for the individual. In some patients with severe cramping, botulinum toxin injections might be helpful, but they must be carefully administered to prevent further weakness and loss of function. Note that spasticity, as a sign of UMN loss, may appear in some patients, but then may diminish or disappear as LMN disease in ALS eventually stymies the ability of the nervous system to increase tone in the muscles.

Dysphagia

Dysphagia, defined as difficulty swallowing liquids, foods, or saliva, contributes to deficits in nutrient intake in the patient with advancing ALS,[56] and must be dealt with aggressively. Dysfunction with chewing, manipulation of food, and swallowing is associated with weakness of the lips, tongue, palate, and mastication muscles.[57] One study of 86 consecutive patients with ALS determined that 79% had dysphagia; they tended to be underweight, with dysfunction of both oral and pharyngeal phases of swallowing and more difficulty with thin liquids.[58] This means that most patients with dysphagia also have severe problems with management of their saliva (sialorrhea). If a patient has difficulty transporting saliva back to the oropharynx for swallowing, choking and drooling are common. Drooling, in particular, is disconcerting to the affected person, who must constantly wipe the mouth or have someone do it for him or her. Embarrassment associated with lack of control of saliva or management of food intake can result in social isolation.[57] As the progressive loss of swallowing develops, patients are at extreme risk for aspiration. Combined with dysfunction of the respiratory muscles, aspiration can be deadly.

Direct rehabilitation to address the action of eating and swallowing is rarely described in the literature, and little has been reported regarding objective measures of its benefit.[59] General techniques include attention to head position and posture when eating, changing bolus size and swallowing frequency, using sensory augmentation, and changing the consistency or texture of foods and drinks. Tongue strengthening has been piloted, with direct changes in tongue strength and endurance, but little effect on swallowing safety.[59]

When swallowing becomes a burden, secretions are often thickened because of dehydration. Viscosity of saliva can best be treated by hydration and, in some cases, pharmaceuticals. Medications such as decongestants, tricyclic antidepressants, and anticholinergic agents can help control the amount of saliva, provided the patient is well-hydrated.[60] A randomized pilot study compared radiotherapy and botulinum A toxin injections into salivary glands to control drooling and found little difference between them; neither works well when the patient has severe dysphagia.[61]

Although dietary treatment is not known to be effective in changing the course of ALS, rapid weight loss in ALS (>10% original body mass index) has been linked to more rapid loss of function; thus a nutritious diet must be maintained to meet caloric, fluid, vitamin, and mineral needs. Seventy-three percent of patients with ALS in mid stages have difficulty bringing food to the mouth, making them dependent on others for their dietary needs. Because of the time it takes to be fed, many patients decrease their intake. In a study of 370 patients with ALS at clinical stages 2, 3, and 4, Lee and colleagues[56] found that energy intake was less than total daily energy expenditure at all stages, but especially at stage 3. The authors conclude that nutrition support should be started at least before stage 3.[56] Nutrition support should include a dietary consultation to determine the choice and progression of solid and liquid foods and supplements.[62] Appel and colleagues[62] describe nutritional plans to maintain nutrient intake and hydration in patients with motor neuron diseases.

Patients who are no longer able to consume nutrients orally because of motor control problems and recurrent aspiration may need a percutaneous endoscopic gastrostomy (PEG) for feeding, depending on the patient's wishes for long-term care.[63] Some evidence exists that the PEG should be performed early in the disease process to prevent severe weight loss and aspiration.[64] Plus, a PEG must be placed (if at all) before the forced vital capacity (FVC) drops below 50%, because the PEG placement procedure generally includes intubation; if the FVC is too low, clinicians may not be successful at weaning the patient off the ventilator once the PEG is placed. Mixing nutritional issues with respiratory life support complicates the decision making process for the patient and family. Although a PEG may not appreciably lengthen survival time,[65] quality of life may improve if patients have less fear of choking or aspiration and further weight loss is inhibited. Receiving nourishment from a PEG does not prevent the person from taking food orally if desired.

Dysarthria

Dysarthria, defined as impairment in speech production, is the result of abnormal function of the muscles and nerves involved in talking. It is manifested by dyscoordination of the tongue and lips, larynx, soft palate, and respiratory system. Speech impairments are the initial symptom in most patients with bulbar involvement; however, a survey of 38 ALS clinics in the northeast region of the United States indicated that formal speech testing is performed at only 18% of sites.[66] Evaluation of speaking rate and sentence intelligibility have been particularly advocated; speaking rates less than 120 words per minute are associated with a more rapid decline in intelligibility.[66] Speech intelligibility is compromised by hypernasality, imprecise consonants and vowels, abnormalities of speed and cadence of speech, and reduced vocal volume.[67] Speech is further compromised by inadequate breath control for normal phrasing. A possible option to help patients with severe hypernasality is a palatal lift prosthesis to augment velopharyngeal function.[68,69] Because little can be done medically to delay the loss of speech control, early referral to a speech therapist is essential. Numerous augmentative and alternative communication systems are now available, the simplest being voice amplifiers, dry erase boards, communication boards, and text to speech apps on devices such as tablets or phones. More complex (and costly) systems include computer-based head or eye tracking text-to-speech systems that can be modified as patient status changes. The type of communication system should be chosen upon consultation among the patient-caregiver and rehabilitation team.[70]

Up to 95% of people with ALS eventually lose their speech function, with devastating effects on quality of life.[67] In the advanced stages of ALS, if a patient has a tracheostomy for respiration and has lost all motion in bulbar muscles as well as limb and trunk musculature, communication may rely on eye movements. This is called "locked-in state" because cognition and emotion are assumed to be relatively intact. Some brain-computer interface technologies have assisted with communication in this state. If eye movement is also lost, the condition is called "completely locked-in state." Functional near-infrared spectroscopy (recording changes in oxygenation of the brain) as the entry point for brain-computer interface has been tried in people with ALS to at least give capability for automatic yes/no responses to questions.[71] Future research may continue to expand on the technology currently under investigation.

Respiratory Management

Respiratory failure is the primary cause of death in patients with ALS. Progressive respiratory failure is related to primary diaphragmatic, intercostal, abdominal, and accessory respiratory muscle weakness (see Table 15.1).[72] Respiratory failure should be anticipated and discussed early following the diagnosis of ALS (as patients and families are ready), so that patients and their caregivers can express their wishes and develop an advanced directive for care in the terminal phase of the disease.[73]

Physiological tests used to indicate respiratory dysfunction include vital capacity (VC), sniff nasal pressure, *maximal inspiratory pressure* (MIP), and nocturnal oximetry.[21] VC (commonly reported as percentage predicted) has been measured in various ways; measuring *slow vital capacity* (SVC, recording volume upon slow exhalation after maximal inspiration as opposed to *forced vital capacity* [FVC] that requires fast and effortful exhalation) has been advocated in ALS because it requires less effort and thus can continue to be assessed through more of the disease process.[74] However, FVC remains the usual indicator of the need for ventilation: when the measure drops below 75% (of normal expected) FVC, the individual should be monitored for respiratory failure; 50% (of normal expected) FVC indicates need for ventilatory assistance.[75] Some researchers have explored instituting assisted respiration intermittently at earlier stages (77% FVC).[76] Clinical signs of increased respiratory dysfunction are dyspnea with exertion or lying supine, hypoventilation, weak or ineffective cough, increased use of auxiliary respiratory muscles, tachycardia (also a sign of pulmonary infection with fever and tachypnea), changes in sleep pattern, daytime sleepiness and concentration problems, mood changes, and morning headaches.[77]

In early stages of patient care, physical therapists (PTs) may help manage respiratory dysfunction by providing postural drainage with cough facilitation (suctioning if necessary), especially during acute respiratory illnesses. The patient and care providers should also be taught breathing exercises, chest stretching, and incentive spirometry techniques, as well as postural drainage techniques if the caregivers are prepared to provide such support. Although breathing exercises consisting of resisted inspiratory muscle training can facilitate functional respiration, even practicing unresisted breathing for 10 minutes three times a day has been shown to result in improved function.[78] Breathing techniques such as diaphragm training have shown little benefit, perhaps because patients have difficulty changing their pattern of breathing even with the training. Overall, inspiratory muscle training in ALS, although showing some effect on survival time in one out of the four studies reviewed, requires further research with standardized protocols and timing.[79] An assessment of the home environment is imperative to identify sleeping positions and energy conservation techniques that can make breathing easier and be incorporated into the patient's daily life.

As respiratory symptoms increase, some advocate the intermittent use of oxygen at 2 L/min or less; the down side of supplemental oxygen

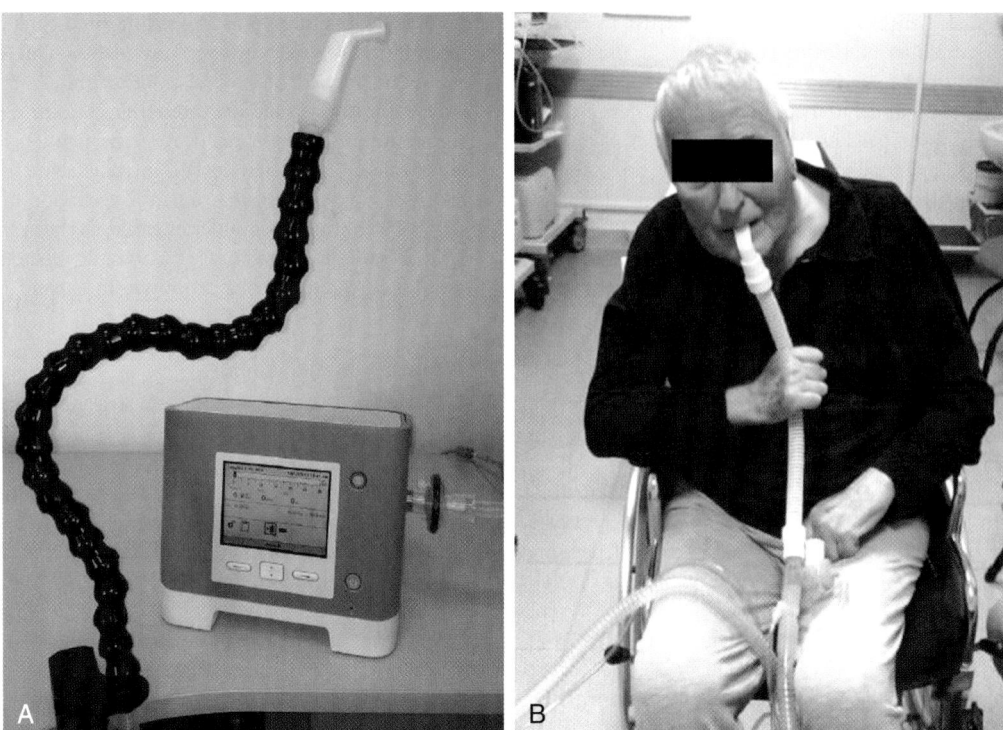

Fig. 15.6 Example of Mouthpiece Ventilation Interface for Noninvasive Ventilation. **(A)** Mouthpiece, flexible tubing, mechanical ventilation unit; **(B)** patient with amyotrophic lateral sclerosis using mouthpiece interface for noninvasive ventilation (NIV) during the day. This patient requires NIV 24 hours a day. He uses a nasal interface at night. (From Garuti G, Nicolini A, Grecchi B, et al. Open circuit mouth-piece ventilation: concise clinical review. *Rev Port Pneumol.* 2014;20:211–218.)

is possible suppression of the respiratory drive with potentially poorer outcomes. When hypoventilation with a decline in oxygen saturation becomes common during sleep, resulting in morning confusion and irritability, patients have the option to initiate use of noninvasive, intermittent positive-pressure ventilation (abbreviated NIV or NIPPV). NIV provides greater inspiratory than expiratory pressure to decrease the effort of breathing, and can be administered by mask, contoured nasal delivery systems, or a mouthpiece[80] interface (Fig. 15.6). Some evidence indicates that early use of NIV can increase survival time by several months and increase quality of life.[81] Moderate-quality evidence indicates that the length of survival with NIV depends on bulbar function: if bulbar function is less than moderately impaired, median additional days was 205; if bulbar function is poor, NIV neither prolongs survival nor improves quality of life, although sleep function may improve.[76] When a patient can no longer benefit from NIV, a decision must be made about initiating invasive ventilation by tracheostomy[82] or to switch to palliative care.[83] (See also Miller and colleagues[84] for a discussion of practice parameters in the decision making process related to ventilatory support.) Although in the initial stages of ALS most patients indicate they would not want prolonged ventilator dependence at home, patients may change their minds as they adapt to the disease restrictions or they and family members may retain hope for the future despite functional losses.[85] A small study of patients who started tracheostomy intermittent positive-pressure ventilation (TIPPV or TIV) demonstrated increased long-term survival (2 to 64 months).[73] In another series of 70 patients on long-term TIPPV, 50% of the patients were living after 5 years; however, 11.4% of these patients had entered a "locked-in" state.[86] Decisions about long-term ventilator use should be made by the patient and involved family

members or partners, with input from the interdisciplinary team caring for the patient. Discussions of preferred long-term care options should be revisited as the patient's condition changes.

If a patient decides that home ventilation is a reasonable option, those involved in the decision might benefit from visiting another patient who is using in-home mechanical ventilation (HMV). Because the decision for home mechanical ventilation (HMV: NIV or TIPPV) also affects the life of the patient's spouse, children, and extended family, who may be responsible for some aspects of home care or whose lives may be affected by the presence of in-home nurses or attendants, the decision for HMV should not be taken lightly. Extensive preparation, ongoing support, and respite options for caregivers are necessary if HMV is to be successful. Success of HMV also depends on such variables as third-party payment for home care equipment and nurse or attendant staffing, working status of the partner or spouse, age and physical fitness of the spouse and children, pre-ALS family psychosocial interactions, and financial factors. HMV should be viewed as long term, often extending for more than 1 year. Initiation of HMV results in a reasonable perceived quality of life for the patient, yet caregivers report that their quality of life may be lower than the patient's because of the burden of care that must be provided.[87]

With chronic respiratory insufficiency, the patient and family must be involved in the long-term care decisions related to instituting mechanical assistance (invasive ventilation) under either emergency situations or in response to gradual deterioration. This discussion should occur before respiratory failure develops in patients. Acute respiratory failure can happen quickly and is generally frightening; few patients or family members are prepared to forego intubation and artificial ventilation during the emergency unless they have settled the issue early.

Patients and caregivers should understand that not making a decision about mechanical ventilation, noninvasive or invasive, is a decision to support mechanical ventilation.[88]

Physicians and health care workers who work with the patient and family must be aware of their own feelings and beliefs about prolonging life and the value of quality of life. For example, a healthy physician or therapist who values control and an active lifestyle may envision a life on a ventilator as intolerable and pass that value on to the patient, who may or may not have the same needs. The patient's decision, or change in decision, must be respected by the medical team involved in care. In medical centers that use a team approach, patients and families may find support by meeting with counselors or peers with ALS who are making or have made decisions about long-term ventilator care.

Therapeutic Management of Movement Dysfunction Associated With Amyotrophic Lateral Sclerosis

Perhaps because of the multitude of issues to consider when managing the impairments and limitations associated with ALS, evidence suggests that patients treated by a specialized ALS multidisciplinary team (typically including physician, PT, occupational therapist, speech language pathologist, respiratory therapist, nurse coordinator, and social worker)[89] fare better than do those treated by single-source providers,[90] or general neurology clinics.[43] One study reported a 2-year post-diagnosis mortality rate of 24% with multidisciplinary care compared to about 50% after 18 months in historical controls.[91] However, a systematic review of the evidence for multidisciplinary care advantages in this population concluded that the evidence is of low quality, so far,[92] with no controlled trials identified as of 2017.[50] Whether administered through an ALS-specific multidisciplinary team or not, therapeutic management will necessitate examination of the patient's current status, evaluation of the deficits in relation to patient preferences and needs, and establishment of a plan based on mutually determined and realistic goals. In addition to the team members listed previously, the plan may eventually involve nutritionists, orthotists, pulmonologists, gastroenterologists, assistive technology experts, home modification/designer experts, psychologists, and palliative-care providers.[89]

The rate of the patient's disease progression, the areas and extent of involvement, and the stage of illness must be considered. A patient at the initial stages (independent) will have different needs than a patient at later stages (dependent) whether or not the patient has chosen to have assisted ventilation. NIV or tracheostomy ventilation may extend life-span, but typically individuals have a markedly reduced mobility level. The goal at all stages is to focus on what the patient needs to optimize health and increase quality of life. With guidance and environmental adaptations, patients with slowly progressing weakness may be able to continue many of their ADLs for an extended number of months or years. In the final stages of the disease, when the patient is bedridden, programs to increase long-term strength or endurance evolve into programs to improve patient-caregiver communication and handling for daily tasks. At this stage, interventions such as stretching may not effectively control contracture development. However, patients who are dependent on all mobility may still benefit from positioning and ROM exercises to decrease muscle and joint pain related to immobility. The prescription of assistive devices and training of caregivers will be needed through much of the final stage. The efficacy of therapeutic interventions will be related to the timing of interventions, the motivation and persistence of the patient in carrying out the program, and support from family members or caregivers. Objective documentation using standardized outcome measures will help justify the usefulness of therapeutic interventions at each stage of this disease. For examples of rehabilitation team roles at three different stages of ALS, see the review with case studies by Majmudar and colleagues.[89]

Assessment

Rehabilitation professionals specifically address body function impairments, activity limitations, and participation restrictions related to ALS (see Fig. 15.4), along with environmental and personal factors, using standardized measures where possible.[93]

The extent of the therapeutic assessment by any one rehabilitation professional will depend on whether the clinician is working as a member of a rehabilitative team or as an independent or clinic-based therapist receiving a referral to evaluate and treat. PTs and OTs working as team members may have a more circumscribed role related to gross motor function and ADLs, with other consultants focusing on bulbar, respiratory, and environmental adjustments. The therapist working in a facility without a neuromuscular disease clinic or in a community or rural environment, however, should be aware of the need to carry out a broad-based assessment. In addition to standard neuromuscular, musculoskeletal, and functional-level examinations within the specific discipline of PT or OT, the therapist should also evaluate the patient's stated or observed functional problems relative to bulbar and respiratory impairments, environmental barriers to independence, and caregiver education.

If possible, before the patient's initial visit, the therapist would benefit from contacting the patient and requesting that he or she keep an activity log for several days. If an early contact is not possible, the therapist can assign that task during the initial session. The log should include 15-minute time increments in which the patient or caregiver can record what she or he was doing during a specific period. The log should also indicate whether the patient was experiencing fatigue or pain during the activity and how the patient perceived her or his respiratory status. An example of a completed activity log is shown in Fig. 15.7. The patient's sense of fatigue with repetitive muscle activity or functional tasks should be specifically tracked.

Primary deficits. Weakness and fatigue will be the primary deficits (see Fig. 15.3), with spasticity or other problems following depending on the location of strength loss. Muscle weakness and the experience of fatigue will require separate measures.[94] In the literature, strength has been assessed with manual muscle testing (MMT) or maximal voluntary isometric contract (MVIC) against a strain gauge or dynamometer. Multiple muscles may be tested by uniformly trained therapists and averaged together using MMT numbers along with minus and plus scores (e.g., 4−, 4, 4+) to convert scores to a 0 to10 scale; the result is both reproducible and sensitive to change in ALS. Equally reproducible is the Tufts Quantitative Neuromuscular Evaluation (TQNE) that measures muscle strength of 10 muscle groups bilaterally using standardized positions and a strain gauge or dynamometer, along with pulmonary function and timed motor tasks. The TQNE provides reliable measurement but requires large equipment space and frequent position changes, which can be very resource intensive and fatiguing for patients.[95] For testing of single muscles or a few muscles to determine change with intervention, a quantitative measure is recommended, such as hand-held dynamometry testing or grip or pincher strength testing, with standardized protocols to maximize reliability.

Fatigue may occur at any stage, whatever the patient's strength or physical capabilities.[96] Fatigability is typically greater in people with ALS than without ALS, and can be assessed with a Rate of Perceived Exertion (RPE) scale following activity, the change in maximal strength produced (dynamometer recording or MVIC) after strenuous activity, or the deficit in number of meters walked in minute 6 versus minute 1 of a 6-Minute-Walk-Test (6MWT). Perception of fatigue can be assessed using self-report measures such as a visual analogue scale for fatigue (VAS-F) or questionnaires covering different dimensions of fatigue such as the Fatigue Severity Scale (FSS).[97]

Name: _____ C. J. _____   DATE: _5 - 10 - 00_
                                      DAY: _Saturday_

DAILY ACTIVITY LOG

Instructions: 1) In column I write in what you are doing during the 24 hour period. You may draw a line or an arrow to indicate when the activity occurs for more than one 15 minute time period.

2) In column II indicate whether you are lying down, sitting, standing, or moving actively (walking, etc.) during the activity.

3) In column III on a 10 point scale, indicate how fatigued you feel while performing the activity (No fatigue = 0, extreme fatigue = 10.)

4) In column IV indicate where you feel pain if any and score the intensity on a 10 point scale (No pain = 0, extreme pain = 10.)

Try to fill out your log three or four times a day so you don't forget what you have been doing. An example is shown below.

	I	II	III	IV	
	What are you doing?	What position are you in	Fatigue level	Pain	
	Type of activity	(lying, sitting, standing, moving)	0 – 10	Location	Intensity 0 – 10
5:30 AM	Sleep	lying	0		
45					
6:00					
15					
30	Bathroom	Standing	2	neck	3
45	Shave, etc				
7:00					
15	Breakfast	sitting	3	neck	3
30					
45					
8:00	Reading	sitting	3	neck	3
15				shoulder	
30					
45	Walk	standing, walking	4	neck	2
9:00					
15	nap				
30		lying	2	neck	4
45				hips	1
10:00	Reading/TV	sitting	4	neck	3
15				hips	
30					
45	Walk	standing, walking	5	hips	3
11:00					

Fig. 15.7 Example of a Log for Monitoring Activity Level of Patients With Amyotrophic Lateral Sclerosis.

Initial examination. A typical initial examination of a patient's movement and function includes the following components. Different rehabilitation personnel will target this list depending on the standards of their discipline, such as the comprehensive list of examination components in the Guide to Physical Therapist Practice.[98] Considerations specific to an examination in ALS are shown in Box 15.3. The extent of the examination in any one session depends on the patient's condition and the patient's or caregiver's ability to participate.

- **Patient History.** The chart review or history should extract the patient's medical and activity records, especially time since diagnosis, time course, and rate of disease progression to date, current

medications, concurrent medical issues, current activities and participation, and any symptoms related to them. The history should focus on current and recent activities and participation signifying patient's lifestyle, ADL tasks, hobbies or interests, and work focus; primary complaints, including weakness, fatigue, muscle spasms, pain, respiratory status, safety, or speech and swallowing issues; psychosocial support issues (family, caregivers, and agencies); the patient's and family members' understanding of ALS and the likely progression and prognosis; and the patient's current concerns and goals. This last item is critically important: the focus of attention should be on the patient's and family's current concerns and goals, rather than on the therapist's knowledge of issues expected in the future.

- **Systems Review.** Screening for multisystem involvement should include checking vital signs at rest, skin integrity, bony abnormalities, sensory integrity, communication ability, and the ability to follow multistep commands. Cognitive screening may include measures such as the Mini-Mental Status Exam (MMSE) because of the possibility of ALS-FTD. When gross screening shows systems with deficits, more extensive examination may be indicated, or the patient may be referred to appropriate health care professionals.

- **Tests and Measures.** Body functions to be tested include movement ability (with attention to the six dimensions of movement[2] appropriate to the region of the body with deficits), pain, cognitive function (if needed), and specific impairments such as dysarthria, dysphagia, and respiratory function. Measures should also be used to document relevant activity limitations, participation restrictions, and environmental and personal factors affecting function at the current stage of the disease process. Any Clinical Practice Guidelines regarding core sets of outcome measures should be followed as appropriate.[99] Tests and measures generally include:
  - Baseline testing of muscle strength (MMT or hand-held dynamometer testing, grip strength, 5 times sit-to-stand test—also used to assess transfers),[99] endurance (6MWT, time tolerating activity, self-report questionnaires for fatigue), flexibility (ROM, muscle tone), speed (timed tasks), and accuracy and adaptability as needed. Therapists may observe and document any areas of atrophy or fasciculations.
  - Assessment of functional activity level (using a standardized test or assessment tool whenever possible) to include, as appropriate: transfers, gait, upper-extremity function, postural control, eating, toileting, and assistive devices. Suggested tools include the ALSFRS-R,[39] the ALSSS,[37] timed walk test (25-foot walk test or 10-m walk test), Timed Up and Go test,[100] 6MWT,[101] and 9-Hole Peg Test. Of the generic walking measures, the 6MWT has been validated in ALS.[101] Although weakness may affect balance during gait, patients with ALS have not shown deficits in postural control during quiet stance despite significant paresis or tone changes, possibly because sensation is relatively preserved.[102] However, generic postural control tools may be useful, such as the Berg Balance Test (when the patient can stand dynamically) or the Function in Sitting Test (when standing is no longer possible but unsupported sitting is available). The Barthel Index or Functional Independence Measure (FIM) could be used for testing of independence in ADLs.
  - Documentation of pain (onset, type, site, and intensity; use body chart and subjective pain scale); identify what makes pain worse or better. Sensory testing may also be required.
  - Assessment of bulbar and respiratory function (review Table 15.1). Perform cranial nerve screening tests; observe facial, lip, tongue, and jaw movements; look for atrophy or fasciculations in the tongue; and palpate muscles of mastication.

BOX 15.3 Considerations Specific to the Examination of Patients With Amyotrophic Lateral Sclerosis

Chart Review, Patient History
Time since onset, time since diagnosis
Initial symptoms
Disease progression rate
Comorbidities
Current medications and medical management
Lifestyle, activities, participation, preferences
Support system, caregivers available
Living environment
Current concerns and goals

Systems Review
Skin integrity (for redness or decubitus ulcers in patients who are immobile): visually inspect pressure points (bony prominences that might develop pressure sores) in supine, side-lying and sitting positions
Communication (augmentation required?)
Cognition (in case of overlapping frontotemporal degeneration)
Vital signs
Sensation

Tests and Measures
Visual inspection to identify symmetry of muscle bulk, fasciculations, function
Movement ability of body region(s) with deficits
  Flexibility: Range of motion, muscle tone (spasticity)
  Strength: Identify patterns/progression of weakness/paralysis
  Accuracy: Observe/record ataxia/dysmetria in upper and lower extremities; perform rapid alternating movements as appropriate
  Speed: Timed tasks in motions where primary movers have against-gravity capability.
  Adaptability: Ability to change movement as obstacles or the environment changes
  Endurance: Questionnaires for experienced fatigue, circumstances; test fatigability
Cranial nerves (bulbar vs. ocular-motor; motor and sensory)
Balance, static and dynamic, sitting and standing (if testable)
Functional status (activities of daily living, participation in life, eating, bowel and bladder function, ambulation) in the patient's natural environment or simulated circumstances
Pain: Intensity, type, and location (use body chart); what aggravates/eases?
Dysarthria, dysphagia, and respiration (screen for changes, refer to specialists)
Environmental adaptations and equipment relevant to current and projected status
Quality of life, including subdimensions such as sleep, well-being
Psychosocial systems: Identify patient and family concerns, self-efficacy. Refer for social worker evaluation of financial resources, day-to-day living problems (e.g., transportation and child care), support systems, and coping strategies

Document breathing patterns at rest and with exertion; listen to breath control during speech. For an in-depth evaluation of bulbar function, the patient should be referred to an ear, nose, and throat clinic, speech-language pathologist, or communications disorders clinic, unless full evaluation is available in a comprehensive ALS clinic.

- Assessment of quality of life or subdimensions such as sleep, well-being, and life satisfaction using generic measures that have been validated in other neuromuscular populations. The Nottingham Health Profile and SF-36 have been recommended in this population.[96]
- Assessment of the patients' environment with a focus on energy conservation and safety at current and future functional capabilities. Assessment of adaptive equipment needs and modifications. Documentation of personal factors (motivation and coping skills) affecting function and availability of psychosocial support is especially necessary as the disease progresses.

In evaluating the results of the examination, the therapist should synthesize data to define the following, all of which are necessary for developing goals with the patient:

- Rate of the patient's disease progression to date
- Distribution of weakness, atrophy, and spasticity; respiratory factors leading to hypoxemia; ease of fatigability; and bulbar involvement
- Stage of the disease
- Any preexisting impairments and/or activity limitations

Goals of Therapeutic Intervention

Intervention goals and the recommended exercise and activity program designed by PTs or OTs must be based on the patient's personal goals. Goals are often a difficult area for therapists to discuss with the patient because the disease is progressive despite intervention. Patients, therapists, and physicians may tend to assume that because nothing can be done to "cure" the disease, not making additional demands on a patient who is already coping with daily loss is somehow kinder. Some believe that exercise programs may create false hopes that exercise will delay progression. Others believe (mistakenly) that exercise will hasten progression.[103] The literature on rehabilitation in neuromuscular disorders, however, suggests that patients with ALS can benefit from carefully designed exercise and activity programs. Active participation in determining goals for therapy can provide the patient and the family with some sense of control over a difficult situation.[16] A standardized tool such as the Movement Ability Measure[104,105] (MAM or MAM-CAT,[106] validated in musculoskeletal and neuromuscular populations and recommended as a scale of patient-reported mobility[107]) can assist the patient and therapist to identify together the movement dimensions the patient prioritizes, so that therapy and home exercises can emphasize what the patient values most[106] (Fig. 15.8). Other tools that help engage the patient in treatment planning include Goal Attainment Scaling[108] (used in diverse populations, including neurological), Canadian Occupational Performance Measure,[109] and the Patient-Specific Functional[110] Scale (used more in musculoskeletal populations).

The broad general goals for both patient and therapist are related to maintaining maximal independence in daily living and a positive quality of life for as long as possible. More specific therapeutic goals are (1) maintenance of mobility and independent functioning (sometimes with training in new strategies and motions to perform locomotion and other functional tasks given current status), including safe mobility for patient and caregiver; (2) maintenance of maximal muscle strength and endurance within limits imposed by ALS; (3) prevention and minimization of secondary consequences of the disease, such as contractures, adhesive capsulitis, thrombophlebitis, deep vein

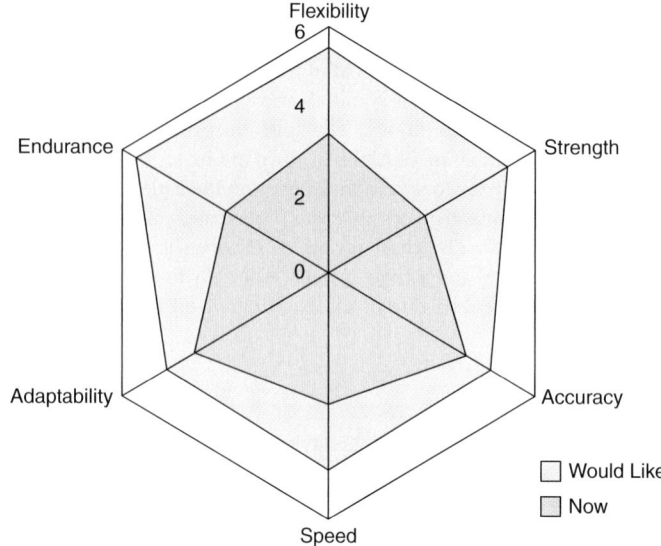

	Now	Would Like	Gap
Flexibility	3.4	5.5	−2.1
Strength	2.8	5.2	−2.4
Accuracy	4.0	4.7	−0.7
Speed	3.2	4.8	−1.6
Adaptability	3.9	4.7	−0.8
Endurance	3.0	5.6	−2.6
Total	20.3	30.5	−10.2

Fig. 15.8 Movement ability plot from the self-report Movement Ability Measure (MAM)-CAT[106] tool depicting the gaps between the movement ability an individual has *now* and the ability the individual *would like* to have. Dimensions with the largest gap (endurance at −2.6, with strength and flexibility closely following) should be the focus of the episode of care. Scale from logits is transformed to 0 (cannot do even with assistance) to 6 (moves competitively).

thrombosis (DVT), decubitus ulcers, and respiratory infections[16]; (4) management of energy conservation techniques and respiratory comfort; (5) determination of adaptive equipment needs to include mobility, self-help and feeding devices, augmentative communication units, and hygiene equipment that supports both patient and caregiver[16]; and (6) minimizing or preventing pain.[111]

Therapeutic Considerations

To prevent more rapid functional loss than expected from the natural history of the disease, both the patient and therapist must delicately balance the level of activity between the extremes of inadequate and excessive exercise. Exercise has been recommended for the general public for its many benefits.[112] Inadequate exercise may result in loss of strength and endurance from disuse, as well as secondary problems such as loss of ROM, muscle cramping, and pain. Excessive exercise may result in excessive fatigue and consequent inability to perform ADLs during recovery periods. Overuse injury with excessive volume and/or intensity of exercise may also lead to unnecessary pain, fatigue, and loss of strength. The next two sections review the evidence for the optimal amount of activity or exercise.

Disuse atrophy. Because ALS is typically diagnosed in older adults, patients may not have maintained their aerobic fitness or muscle strength before the onset of this disorder. Newly diagnosed patients also commonly report that they had markedly decreased their activity level in the months before diagnosis because of a sense of fatigue or increasing clumsiness from progressive weakness. If the patient led a sedentary lifestyle before diagnosis, the additional decrease in activity level after the onset of ALS can lead quickly to marked cardiovascular deconditioning and disuse weakness. The disuse weakness lowers muscle force production and reduces muscle endurance.

Exercise intolerance or overwork damage. Observers during the poliomyelitis epidemic of the 1940s and 1950s reported that muscle activity or overwork exercise led to a loss of muscle strength.[113] During that epidemic, physicians and therapists noted that patients with poor- and fair-grade muscles who exercised repeatedly or with heavy resistance after reinnervation often lost the ability to contract the muscle at all.[114] However, controlled testing of this observation suggests that overwork damage occurs in mostly denervated muscles, not in all muscles. In a seminal study in rats, Reitsma[115] noted that *vigorous exercise* damaged muscles if less than one-third of motor units were functional. If more than one-third of the motor units remained, exercise led to hypertrophy, a beneficial result. One mechanism of potential overwork damage is inhibition of the collateral sprouting of intact axons to re-innervate "orphaned" muscle fibers when other axons degenerate (Fig. 15.9). Yuen and Olney[116] provided evidence that collateral sprouting of intact axons can partially reinnervate orphaned muscle fibers in ALS. This reinnervation process creates macromotor units (more motor fibers innervated per motor neuron) and is sensitive to overload: in a rat model of partially denervated muscles, highly intensive activity reduced the ability of adjacent axons to sprout when fewer than 20% of intact motor units remained.[117] Reduction in sprouting does not occur when denervation is more moderate.[117] In a mouse model, vigorous exercise had no adverse effect on the course of ALS.[118] Lui and Byl[119] systematically reviewed the literature reporting exercise effects in animal models of ALS and calculated an effect size of 1.39 (where numbers over 0.8 are considered large) in favor of exercise. The few negative effects they noted were associated with either very high–intensity exercise or a slow rate of exercise (slower than usual activity for animals when unrestricted in activity). These results reflect the responses of animal models of disease rather than humans, so would need to be interpreted with caution.[119]

Normal functional reserve in healthy adult ventilation means that only 70% of maximal voluntary ventilation is used during exercise testing.[77] Adequate reserves likely allow patients with ALS to maintain a normal ventilatory response, but may mask early losses of respiratory function. Close monitoring is warranted even with moderate exercise. Some of the specific mechanisms of exercise intolerance in neuromuscular diseases include inspiratory muscle weakness, expiratory insufficiency from diminished elasticity, disrupted sleep (frequently from respiratory impairment), vocal cords that go into spasm with forceful exhalation, inadequate muscle activation, and central fatigue.[77]

Researchers have expressed concern about the possible relation between high-resistance exercise and muscle fiber degeneration in humans with motor neuron disease.[120] Because of early concerns about stressing substantially denervated muscles, Sinaki and Mulder[121] published recommendations in 1978 that patients with ALS not engage in any vigorous exercise and focus instead on exercise associated with walking and daily activities. On the other hand, McCrate and Kaspar[122] reviewed the possible mechanisms by which exercise protects nerves from more rapid degeneration. Thus the controversy continues. Evidence regarding the positive benefits of exercise in ALS has been accumulating, with fewer adverse effects than some expected.

Evidence of the benefits of exercise. Few controlled trials have been published regarding exercise in ALS, and most enroll small sample sizes because the disease is relatively rare.[123] However, an examination of the protocols and inclusion criteria of their subjects may still provide useful information for the clinician.

Resistive exercises are necessary for improving strength. Aksu and colleagues[124] compared a supervised versus home exercise protocol in 26 ambulatory ALS patients. They noted that supervised breathing exercises, stretching, manually applied resistance exercise with PNF,

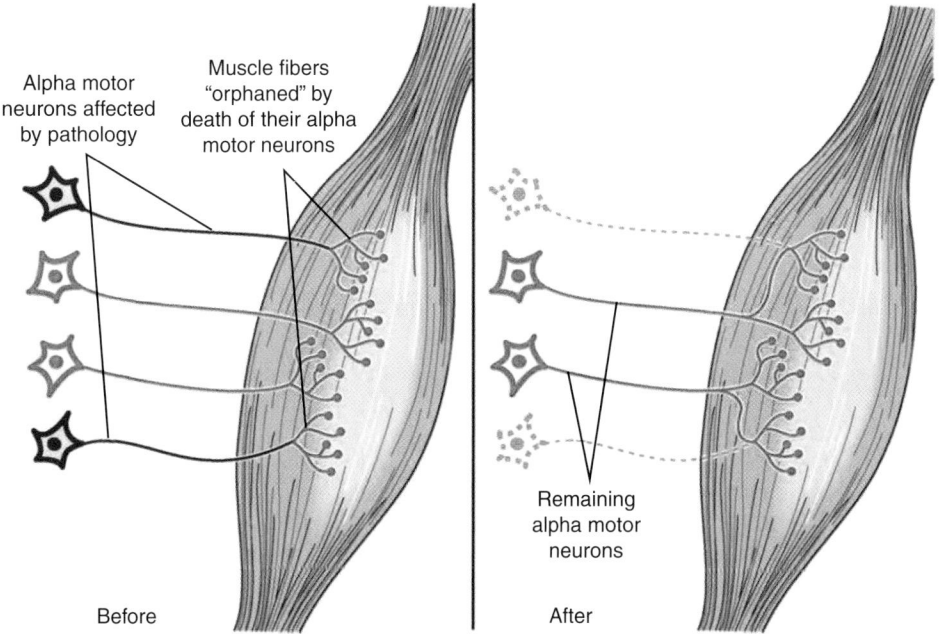

Alpha motor neurons affected by pathology

Muscle fibers "orphaned" by death of their alpha motor neurons

Remaining alpha motor neurons

Before

After

Fig. 15.9 After degeneration of some α motor neurons, adjacent α motor neurons may undergo collateral sprouting to re-innervate orphaned muscle fibers, creating macromotor units. (Adapted from Allen DD, Widener GL. Tone abnormalities. In: Cameron MH, ed. *Physical Agents in Rehabilitation: An Evidence-Based Approach to Practice.* 5th ed. St. Louis, MO: Elsevier; 2018.)

and functional mobility training 3 days a week for 8 weeks resulted in small gains in function in the first 4 weeks and a slower decline over the subsequent 10 months compared with home-based breathing, stretching, and active ROM exercises. The groups were not randomly allocated but were not significantly different in the measured variables at baseline.[124] In an RCT, Drory and colleagues[125] assigned 25 patients with ALS to a group continuing their normal daily activities or a group participating in a daily program of moderate exercise individualized for each patient. The primary exercise focus was to have muscles of the trunk and limbs work against "modest" loads while undergoing significant shortening (not lengthening or eccentric contractions). The exercises were completed twice daily for 15 minutes at home with phone contact by the treating therapist every 14 days. Data were evaluated for 3 and 6 months after initial assessment. All patients showed continued disease progression; however, in all cases, at the 6-month assessment patients who exercised showed positive effects in maintenance of muscle strength, less fatigue, less spasticity, less pain, and higher functional ratings.[125] In another RCT, Dal Bello-Haas and colleagues[126] prescribed moderate load and moderate-intensity resistance exercises individually to patients in the early stages of ALS. The exercise group had significantly less decline in function, small improvements in strength, and no reported adverse effects, compared with patients who performed stretching exercises alone.[126] A Cochrane review designated the quality of these two RCTs as "fair" to "adequate," and class II level evidence.[127]

In a more recent RCT, Lunetta and colleagues[128] found that supervised exercise, especially those who had resistive plus aerobic exercise at 60% power daily for 2 weeks each month over 6 months, resulted in better ALSFRS-R scores than the 30 people with ALS who had twice weekly home care. Merico and colleagues[129] conducted a pilot RCT of endurance and resistance training in 38 ambulatory individuals with ALS. Fifteen received standard neuromotor rehabilitation that specifically

excluded eccentric and concentric muscle contractions. Twenty-three participants received individualized, progressive programs of submaximal, time-based isometric contraction of muscles testing 3, 4–, or 4 on the MMT scale, and moderate aerobic exercise using ergometer or treadmill according to the subject's level of disability. Both groups received intervention 1 h/day, 5 days/week, for 5 weeks. The specific exercise group had improved strength, oxygen consumption, and function compared to the other group.[129] Jensen and colleagues[130] conducted a study in which five ambulatory subjects with ALS were their own controls, with 12-week lead in period followed by 12 weeks of resistance training two to three times per week. The resistance was increased progressively for 10 major muscle groups (six per session), from 3 sets of 12 repetitions at a load of 15-repetition maximum (RM) to conclude at 2 sets of 5 repetitions at 6 RM. For these five subjects, strength decline did not slow during training; at biopsy, some type II muscle fibers hypertrophied, but others atrophied.[130] The subjects mostly had shorter disease duration prior to study involvement (4 at less than 12 months) and higher ALSFRS-R function scores (average 40 points) than in other studies, which may have affected response to this treatment. Table 15.2 summarizes the studies of exercise published since 2000 in ALS. As a side note, preliminary evidence suggests that creatine supplementation may increase isometric power in patients with ALS over the short term.[131]

Few researchers have considered rehabilitation to increase endurance in neuromuscular disorders.[112,134] Endurance training for longer than 10 to 15 minutes in patients with ALS may be restricted by central fatigue, the decreased ability to recruit all motor units or develop high discharge rates,[135] and not merely alterations in oxygen supply or muscle metabolism. In healthy individuals, exercise has the potential to improve motor unit activation, blood supply, muscle metabolism, and chemical imbalances and thus has promise in ALS. In addition to studies of strengthening or combined exercises, studies focusing on aerobic exercise have reported positive results. Braga and colleagues[133]

TABLE 15.2 Summary of Exercise Studies Since the Year 2000 in Amyotrophic Lateral Sclerosis

Author	Study Population (Sample Size): Research Design	Duration of Training	Training Modality	Training Protocol	Response(s)
Drory et al., 2001[125]	ALS disease duration 20 months (25): RCT assigned to treatment or control groups	24 weeks	Moderate load, trunk and limbs, concentric contractions	Twice daily, 15 min per session	Treatment group: Maintenance of strength, less fatigue, less spasticity, less pain, higher function
Aksu et al., 2002[124]	ALS (26): Convenience assignment to treatment and control groups	8 weeks	Breathing exercises, PNF, stretching vs. stretching, ROM, and breathing exercises	3 days/week supervised vs. home	Treatment group: Increased ROM, strength; function sustained better
Dal Bello-Haas et al., 2007[126]	Early stage ALS (27): RCT, allocated to resistance exercises plus stretch or just stretch groups	24 weeks	PT-prescribed resistance exercises performed at home to patient tolerance	3 days/week resisted exercise plus stretch vs. just stretch group	Treatment group: Slowed decline and small strength gains
Sanjak et al., 2010[132]	ALS (9; 6 completed study): Pilot study	8 weeks	Repetitive rhythmic exercise performed for 30 min total, 5 min ex followed by 5 min rest	3 times per week, 60-min session with 6 intervals of 5 min	Improved Rating of Perceived Exertion, ALSFRS-R; gait variables improved
Lunetta et al., 2016[128]	ALS disease duration <24 months, ALSFRS-R average 38 (60): RCT, monitored ex vs. usual care group	6 months with a 1 year follow up	Ex group divided into 3 groups: (a) resisted ex 3 sets of 3 repetitions at 60% power plus cycloergometer; (b) resisted ex; (c) passive ex; usual care received passive ex and stretching	Ex: daily 20-min sessions for 2 weeks each month; usual care: 20 min 2 days per week at home	Treatment group: ALSFRS-R (especially motor portion) was better, especially ex group (a) at end of treatment and at 1 year; survival and respiratory support did not differ

TABLE 15.2 Summary of Exercise Studies Since the Year 2000 in Amyotrophic Lateral Sclerosis—cont'd

Author	Study Population (Sample Size): Research Design	Duration of Training	Training Modality	Training Protocol	Response(s)
Jensen et al., 2017[130]	ALS, ambulatory without assistance, ALSFRS-R average 40, disease duration <12 months (4/5): case series	12 weeks lead in; 12 weeks training	Progressive resistance for 10 major muscle groups: 3 sets of 12 repetitions at 15 RM to 2 sets 5 repetitions 6 RM	Training: 2–3 times per week, 6 muscle groups each session	Training period: No attenuation of strength loss; mixed increase in hypertrophied and atrophied type II fibers
Braga et al., 2018[133]	ALS disease duration <12 months, ALSFRS-R = 39 (48): controlled trial, allocation to groups based on geographical residence	6 months	Both groups had standard care exercises daily, with ROM, limb relaxation, trunk balance, gait training. Group 1: Also had treadmill exercise with training intensity (moderate) defined by cardiopulmonary exercise testing (CPET)	Daily standard exercises to perceived fatigue. Group 1 added twice weekly CPET regulated moderate intensity ex	Group 1 had better respiratory measures at peak effort: Oxygen uptake peak, metabolic equivalent, carbon dioxide output, and minute ventilation
Merico et al., 2018[129]	ALS disease duration 30 months, ALSFRS-R = 35 (38): RCT, 23 completed ex group; 15 completed standard rehabilitation	5 weeks	Ex group: 3 repetitions isometric contraction held for 80% of time of max contraction plus aerobic ex at 65% max heart rate adjusted for age; standard group: stretching, active mobilization, muscle reinforcement	5 days/week, 1 h each day	Treatment group: Improved in strength, oxygen consumption, FIM test; standard group improved in FIM test but not as much

ALS, Amyotrophic lateral sclerosis; *ALSFRS-R*, ALS Functional Rating Scale-Revised; *ex*, exercise; *FIM*, Functional Independence Measure; *max*, maximum; *PNF*, proprioceptive neuromuscular facilitation; *PT*, physical therapist; *RCT*, randomized controlled trial; *RM*, repetitions maximum; *ROM*, range of motion.

provided standard care exercises to two groups of patients with ALS with disease duration averaging less than 9 months, adding moderate intensity (level determined by cardiopulmonary exercise testing) treadmill walking two times per week to group 1. Group 1 showed better ALSFRS-R scores than Group 2 at 6 months, and slope of functional decay was not as steep. Sanjak and colleagues[132] conducted a treadmill study of nine patients with ALS who already required assistive devices to walk, six of whom completed the study. The frequency was three times a week for 8 weeks, with 30 minutes of walking split up into 5-minute intervals of exercise and rest. Improvements in ALSFRS-R score, FSS, and gait measures were noted in the first 4 weeks and retained at 8 weeks. A systematic review of studies focusing on reducing fatigue (perception of tiredness or decreased ability to contract muscles at maximum force) describe three studies in ALS indicating possible improvements with modafinil (a drug that reduces sleepiness),[136] respiratory exercise versus sham intervention, and repetitive transcranial magnetic stimulation (rTMS).[137] Signs of fatigue after any exercise must be monitored carefully. If a patient shows evidence of significant, persistent weakness after institution of an exercise program or persistent morning fatigue after exercise on the previous day, the therapist must carefully redesign the patient's exercise program and activity level and increase the frequency of monitoring the patient's program.

In addition to strength and endurance benefits from exercise, ongoing moderate exercise programs may also help decrease persistent pain and muscle stiffness that often accompany weakened, overtaxed muscle groups.[138] Factors such as spasticity, age at onset of ALS, prior levels of fitness and activity, and psychological factors, including past responses to extremely challenging situations and satisfaction with social support, must also be considered when prescribing rehabilitation for this population. See Box 15.4 for factors to consider when prescribing exercise in the early stages of ALS.

BOX 15.4 Considerations for Exercise Prescription

Based on evidence and current practice, exercise prescription in the early stages of ALS (and recovery stages of GBS) should address the following[111]:

1. Include both a formal exercise program and enjoyable physical activities to improve compliance.
2. Include activities with opportunities for social development and personal accomplishment.
3. Strengthening programs should use moderate resistance rather than high resistance, and focus on muscles that have at least antigravity strength (3/5 on MMT).
4. Endurance programs should be monitored for signs of fatigue, more so when continuous activity lasts longer than about 15 min. Activity programs should include rest periods.
5. Patients should ensure that they have adequate oxygenation and carbohydrate loads[112] as well as adequate fluids before exercising.
6. Muscle strength must be monitored to assess for possible overwork weakness; in unsupervised programs, patients must watch for signs and symptoms that indicate overwork, including postexercise fatigue that interferes with daily activities, feeling weaker or pain beyond 30 min after exercise, having excessive soreness 24–48 h after exercise, and experiencing severe muscle cramping, heaviness in the extremities, or prolonged shortness of breath.[139] Therapists should check with an independently exercising patient regularly to assess whether any deterioration in strength may be from progression of the disease or overwork weakness.
7. The program must be adjusted as the disease progresses.

ALS, Amyotrophic lateral sclerosis, *GBS*, Guillain-Barre syndrome; *MMT*, manual muscle testing.

Therapeutic Interventions

Sinaki[140] has described three phases and six substages of ALS with recommended exercise levels (Box 15.5). These phases and stages provide an orderly structure for describing therapeutic interventions, although patients may not fit precisely within the stages. Bulbar signs may have progressed to a different stage than motor ability in the limbs, for example, and respiratory dysfunction can occur on its own

time schedule. However, recommending a progression of interventions from independence to partial independence to dependence may be particularly helpful to therapists who do not have the opportunity to work with large numbers of patients with ALS.

Most patients need specific guidance about what types of activities and exercises they should do.[86] Although many physicians may suggest to patients that they increase their activity level, their suggestions are

---

BOX 15.5 Exercise and Rehabilitation Programs for Patients With Amyotrophic Lateral Sclerosis According to Stage of Disease

Independent (Phase I)

Stage 1

Patient Characteristics

Mild weakness

Clumsiness

Ambulatory

Independent in activities of daily living (ADLs)

Treatment

Continue normal activities or increase activities if sedentary to prevent disuse atrophy

Begin program of range-of-motion (ROM) exercises (stretching, yoga, tai chi)

Add strengthening program of gentle resistance exercises to all musculature with caution not to cause overwork fatigue

Provide psychological support as needed

Stage 2

Patient Characteristics

Moderate, selective weakness

Slightly decreased independence in ADLs, such as:
- difficulty climbing stairs
- difficulty raising arms
- difficulty buttoning clothing

Ambulatory

Treatment

Continue stretching to avoid contractures

Continue cautious strengthening of muscles with manual muscle testing (MMT) grades above F+ (3+); monitor for overwork fatigue

Consider orthotic support (e.g., ankle-foot, wrist, thumb splints)

Use adaptive equipment to facilitate ADLs

Stage 3

Patient Characteristics

Severe selective weakness in ankles, wrists, and hands

Moderately decreased independence in ADLs

Easy fatigability with long-distance ambulation

Ambulatory

Slightly increased respiratory effort

Treatment

Continue stage 2 program as tolerated; use caution not to fatigue to point of decreasing patient's ADL independence

Keep patient physically independent as long as possible through pleasurable activities such as walking

Encourage deep breathing exercises, chest stretching, postural drainage if needed

Prescribe wheelchair, standard or motorized, with modifications to allow eventual reclining back with head rest, elevating legs

Partially Independent (Phase II)

Stage 4

Patient Characteristics

Hanging-arm syndrome with shoulder pain and sometimes edema in the hand

Wheelchair dependent

Severe lower-extremity weakness (with or without spasticity)

Able to perform ADLs but fatigues easily

Treatment

Heat, massage as indicated to control spasm

Preventive antiedema measures

Active assisted passive ROM exercises to the weakly supported joints; caution to support, rotate shoulder during abduction and joint accessory motions

Encourage isometric contractions of all musculature to tolerance

Try arm slings, overhead slings, or wheelchair arm supports

Motorized chair if patient wants to be independently mobile; adapt controls as needed

Stage 5

Patient Characteristics

Severe lower-extremity weakness

Moderate to severe upper-extremity weakness

Wheelchair dependent

Increasingly dependent in ADLs

Possible skin breakdown as a result of poor mobility

Treatment

Encourage family to learn proper transfer, positioning principles, and turning techniques

Encourage modifications at home to aid patient's mobility and independence

Electric hospital bed with antipressure mattress

If patient elects home mechanical ventilation (HMV), adapt chair to hold ventilator unit

Dependent (Phase III)

Stage 6

Patient Characteristics

Bedridden

Completely dependent in ADLs

Treatment

For dysphagia: soft diet, long spoons, tube feeding, and percutaneous gastrostomy

To decrease flow of accumulated saliva: medication, suction, and surgery

For dysarthria: palatal lifts, electronic speech amplification, and eye-pointing electronics

For breathing difficulty: clear airway, tracheostomy, and ventilator if patient elects HMV

Medications to decrease impact of dyspnea

Modified from Sinaki M. Exercise and rehabilitation measures in amyotrophic lateral sclerosis. In: Yase Y, Tsubaki T, eds. *Amyotrophic Lateral Sclerosis: Recent Advances in Research and Treatment*. Amsterdam: Elsevier Science; 1988.

seldom specific. Examples of exercise advice that patients have recalled are "Try to move around as much as possible," "Walk some more," and "Be active, but don't overdo it." Because changing their typical exercise pattern is difficult for most patients, even when they know doing so is important, referral for a physical therapy consultation can be helpful for movement-related issues.[141]

Independent: Phase I, Stages 1 to 3. A program to increase activity must be specifically designed, with input from the patient about willingness to participate and knowledge of the patient's environmental situations and social support systems. In the early stages of the disease, patients should be encouraged to continue as many of their usual and valued prediagnosis activities as tolerated. For example, a golfer should continue to golf for as long as possible. Walking the course should be encouraged if it is not too fatiguing. When walking or balance becomes difficult on uneven terrain, the golfer can use a golf cart, decrease the number of holes played, move to a par three course, or hit balls at a driving range. If upper-extremity weakness is a major problem that interferes with swinging the club for distance shots, the player can continue playing the greens or on putting courses. Some people who play golf may need adaptations to club handles with nonskid material such as Dycem (Dycem Non-Slip products, http://www.dycem.com) or Scoot-Gard (Vantage Industries Product) to prevent the club from rotating on impact. Similar progressions could be imagined for patients with other activity interests.

Patients with newly diagnosed ALS who had a sedentary lifestyle before diagnosis should be encouraged to increase their activity level as fatigue status and rate of disease progression allow. This may include activities that require muscular effort within or around the home, such as sharing household and gardening tasks or beginning a walking program around the neighborhood. After diagnosis, some patients begin searching for in-home exercise devices such as bicycles and rowing machines. As with healthy persons who plan to start an exercise program after the purchase of exercise equipment, patients with ALS often do not use the new equipment consistently if they did not do so before a diagnosis. The search for a "perfect" exercise machine may reflect the patient's desperation to do something tangible. Without taking away the patient's motivation to exercise, therapists can encourage participation in physical activity and/or exercise programs that do not require expensive equipment, such as walking or working out using video-guided exercise routines. A media-savvy therapist can make a video for each patient that includes stretching and gentle exercise programs that elicit muscle contractions from all functional muscle groups (by using inexpensive elastic bands or small weights) with follow-up breathing, "warm down," and relaxation exercises. Patients could follow a program of isometric contractions of the major muscle groups held for 6 seconds each and isotonic elastic band exercises at submaximal levels to maintain and improve muscle strength, with progression established by the therapist. Patients who are limited by fatigue should exercise for short periods several times a day rather than attempting to exercise all muscle groups in one session.

For most patients in the early stages of ALS, pleasurable, natural activities such as swimming, bowling (using a lighter ball if shoulder strength is a problem), walking, bicycling (three-wheeler may be needed or in-home stationary bicycle, either of which must be evaluated for easy mounting and dismounting), or tai chi can be recommended. Some patients prefer to exercise alone, whereas others will gain confidence and companionship by joining a group activity. Listening to the patient's desires related to group activities is important. The dropout rate is high among those who have been pressured to participate. Some spouses or family members are supportive of the patient's activity needs and will join the patient in his or her regimen.

If possible, the spouse and family members should be engaged in the treatment planning process.

The therapist must observe patients completing their entire recommended activity program. The patient's response to the program must be monitored because fatigue from exercise sessions can interfere with the ability to carry out other normal daily activities. If patients become too exhausted at the end of a session, they may learn to fear exercise and may become depressed about the decreased activity status. This depression may lead to decreased activity and further deconditioning

Partially independent: Phase II, Stages 4 and 5. When the patient is partially independent, the goal of physical and occupational therapy intervention should be to help the patient adapt to limitations imposed by weakness, fatigue, or spasticity, an increasingly compromised cardiorespiratory status, and possible musculoskeletal pain secondary to weakness or muscle imbalance. This transition stage is often disturbing for patients because the decrease in function and independence becomes clear; therapists should accentuate what the person can do and how accommodations can be made to help maintain independence. After a full physical assessment of the patient's motor status similar to the initial evaluation, the patient, family members, and therapists (including a PT, OT, and speech-language pathologist if a team approach is possible) should discuss treatment options and adaptive devices that can help the patient remain as independent as possible. Majmudar and colleagues[89] and Connors and colleagues[142] provide lists of commonly used adaptive equipment that might provide helpful ideas.

During the transition from independence to partial independence, many patients show significant weakness of both upper- and lower-extremity musculature, but they each have their own pattern and rate of progression of weakness and onset of spasticity, bulbar, and respiratory symptoms. A typical patient at this time may have marked weakness of the intrinsic muscles, shoulder muscle weakness (in some cases "hanging arm" syndrome) with shoulder pain, and generalized lower-extremity weakness (in some cases more severe distally). Patients may be able to walk within the home environment, but many patients have precarious balance; they may fall easily because of muscle weakness. Getting up from a fall will be more difficult when the weakness affects antigravity muscles such as the gluteus maximus, quadriceps, and plantarflexors. At this stage, most patients report fatigue with minimal work and have to rest frequently when carrying out ADLs. ROM can deteriorate quickly in this phase of the disease, requiring daily stretching for the calf, quadriceps, hip adductors, trunk lateral flexors, shoulder (to prevent adhesive capsulitis), and long finger flexors.[40] Moderate resistive exercise as described by Drory and colleagues[125] (see Table 15.2) can have a modest effect in reducing spasticity.

Patients at this point, even if ambulatory, may consider using a wheelchair outside the home to conserve energy.[111] Factors to consider in choosing a wheelchair include extent of insurance coverage or financial assistance programs for purchase of wheelchair (some policies or programs may provide only one type of wheelchair or only one wheelchair, either motorized or manual); transportability of the wheelchair from home to community and work (few motorized wheelchair brands fold for stowing in a car trunk, and few families can afford to purchase a van with a ramp or lift that will allow the patient to drive or be driven while in a motor chair); reclining potential of chair back, tilt of the seat, and headrest (preferably electric) to allow the patient to shift weight and rest while in the chair during later stages of the disease; seat elevator; elevating leg rests to avoid prolonged sitting with the legs in a dependent position; for power w/c, adaptable electronic controls that can be modified for changes in hand function; removable arm rests for ease of transfer; headrest or extension; potential mounting area for portable ventilator equipment if needed; and ease with which caregiver can help patient with chair mobility transfers.[111] Chairs should have lumbar support and appropriate cushioning to prevent pressure ulcers.[139]

At this stage, patients with more advanced bulbar symptoms begin to experience dysarthria and may need guidance in dealing with communication issues. In a study of communication strategies in ALS, Murphy[143] indicated four major reasons for communication: to identify needs or request help, share information, respond politely in social situations, and maintain social closeness. The primary focus of communication for the study participants was to maintain social closeness. Although few patients had any instruction in ways to deal with communication problems, most patients and caregivers created ways to make themselves understood, such as giving cues about the topic and context, creating a "shorthand" language, and checking with the dysarthric speaker to ensure that the listener understands the patient correctly. A number of patients in the study who had significant dysarthria commented that attempting to communicate socially was extremely tiring. Therapists who are guiding patients with energy conservation techniques should be aware of the exhaustion that can be associated with communication. See Box 15.6 for a number of strategies recommended by the American Speech-Language-Hearing Association[144] that can be used by the person with ALS to deal with the effects of dysarthria. Also in this stage, some patients and families may need support to identify adapted feeding systems (special utensils, adapted plates, adjustable tables) and hygiene equipment if transfers in the family bathroom are problematic.[142]

BOX 15.6 Recommended Strategies for the Individual With Dysarthria

- Reduce background noise in the room
- Face the person while talking
- Use short, simple phrases rather than long, complicated ones
- Take the time to say what needs to be said; do not allow people to rush conversation
- Make extra use of body language, such as gestures and facial expressions, and use writing to supplement speech, if possible
- Do not worry about saying things correctly; if the basic message being conveyed is understood, then that is enough

American Speech-Language-Hearing Association. Dysarthria. Available at: www.asha.org/public/speech/disorders/dysarthria.htm. Accessed November 23, 2018.

Mr. Turner in Case Study 15.1 was cared for in a neuromuscular disease clinic, so he benefited from input from multiple specialists working as a team to help him maintain his independence. Unfortunately, many patients do not have the benefit of such a coordinated treatment environment. Therefore when necessary, the therapist must be in a position to provide input on adaptive and safety devices and bulbar issues if other specialist input is not available. Therapists working in smaller communities and rural areas most likely need to be chameleon-like to play many therapeutic roles when working with the patient with ALS.

CASE STUDY 15.1   Mr. Turner

Transitioning to Partial Independence

Mr. Turner is a 45-year-old man who first noticed symptoms about 15 months ago. As progression continued and medical testing ruled out other possibilities, he was diagnosed 7 months ago with ALS. He was started on a schedule of visiting a regional ALS clinic every 3–4 months. This is his second visit.

Mr. Turner lives at home with his wife, who works full-time, and two teenage children. Mr. Turner is a computer programmer for an engineering firm. Since his diagnosis, Mr. Turner has been able to continue his full-time work schedule, although he states that he is no longer able to touch type and can type with the index fingers only. He has noticed that his shoulders and neck hurt (4 out of 10 on a numeric pain rating scale) after an hour at the computer. In the last 2 weeks he has found it fatiguing to walk to the office dining area for lunch (approximately 100 m), and he fears that he will be knocked down when walking in crowds. He dropped his lunch tray last week, which was embarrassing, so he decided to eat in his office, even though he misses the socialization and opportunity to discuss work issues with his colleagues.

Mr. Turner has been able to continue most of his nonwork activities, although he is no longer able to operate his sailboat independently and is having trouble maintaining his balance when playing golf. He now uses a cart and plays only nine holes. He states that his wife and children are supportive and that they have made some changes in the home environment to accommodate his increasing weakness. He also revealed, however, that his children seem frustrated with him because he is so much slower than he was before the illness.

On assessment, Mr. Turner showed marked wasting of hand intrinsic muscles. He was unable to abduct or flex either shoulder past 90 degrees. His right shoulder showed considerable atrophy, especially of the deltoid and supraspinatus muscles. All other upper-extremity movements were weakened but in the G− (4−/5 MMT) range. His neck posture was forward: neck extension was F+ (3+) and neck flexion was G− (4−/5). Scapular winging was noted bilaterally. No spasticity or loss of passive ROM was evident in the upper extremities. Lower-extremity musculature showed generalized weakness at the F (3/5) to F+ (3+/5) range, with left musculature weaker than right, marked wasting of the anterior and posterior compartment muscles of the lower legs, and a cavus foot position bilaterally. Spasticity of the hip adductors and hamstrings was noted (Modified Ashworth Scale grade 2), but no passive ROM loss was detected in the lower extremities. Most obvious during gait was inadequate dorsiflexion for heel strike and no propulsion during heel-off. He showed a bilateral corrected gluteus medius pattern on weight bearing. He showed uncontrolled genu recurvatum in mid- to terminal stance during gait, using gluteus maximus thrust to lock the knee for stability. He had great difficulty ascending and descending the four steps to enter his home. There were no stairs to negotiate at work.

Until this appointment, Mr. Turner had not been willing to discuss the use of adaptive equipment or a wheelchair. During prior clinic visits his decisions were supported and he was told that when he was ready, therapists would work with him and his family to help with equipment decisions.

Mr. Turner also showed some early bulbar signs. He noted that he sometimes had to catch drool when working intensely, and that his pillow was moist in the morning. Tougher and bulkier food sometimes got stuck in his throat; he pocketed some food in the cheek area that he had to make a conscious effort to move out with his tongue. Swallowing was still adequate for eating all foods; however, he had had a few coughing episodes when drinking coffee and wine. He showed no increased use of accessory musculature when breathing and had no reports of respiratory distress. His cough was adequate to clear secretions. His FVC was 90% and ALSFRS-R score was 36 (out of 48). Body weight has remained steady over the last 7 months despite decreasing activity.

CASE STUDY 15.1 Mr. Turner—cont'd

Goals

With input from the therapist, Mr. Turner and his wife identified the following general goals:

1. Increase mobility while conserving energy.
2. Control fatigue and pain of upper extremities and neck during computer work.
3. Maintain maximal muscle strength and ROM (patient reported that he felt stiff).
4. Identify safety issues within the home and work environment and adjust household and work environment to prepare for the time when Mr. Turner could not ascend and descend stairs safely.

Treatment Plan

A treatment plan was developed to achieve the following:

1. Increase mobility. Because of his increased walking difficulties, Mr. Turner decided to use a four-wheeled walker with a seat attachment at home. He had hand grip weakness, but elected against using forearm troughs because of their bulk. He used bicycle type (hand) brakes on the walker. For his work-site, he selected a motorized wheelchair so that he could maintain his independence at work. Although he found that he could push an ultralight manual chair, his upper-extremity strength was clearly decreasing. Mr. Turner decided that he preferred a lightweight foldable power wheelchair to an electric scooter because of the financial cost of switching devices when the scooter no longer provided adequate postural support. As Mr. Turner was still ambulatory in the community and at home, insurance would not pay for the power wheelchair at this time; the therapist was able to connect him with the regional ALS group, and he was able to borrow one from the ALS loan closet to keep at work.

   Because Mr. Turner's family had no vehicles to transport the electric wheelchair easily, the ALS Society also loaned the family a manual wheelchair for home use. Although not ideal, it was functional. Mr. Turner's teenagers made some inexpensive adjustments to adapt the chair for a headrest, and repainted the chair to his specifications.

   Because Mr. Turner wanted to keep as active as possible and use his walker within the home, he was fitted with light-weight bilateral ankle-foot orthoses (AFOs) to assist with ankle dorsiflexion during swing phase of gait. Straps were simple overlap style because Mr. Turner had poor thumb and grasp control.

2. Decrease fatigue and pain of neck and upper extremities. Mr. Turner was taught some simple ROM exercises of the neck and arms to perform every half hour while working at the computer. In a simulated work environment, the therapist noted that Mr. Turner had a forward head position when working at a computer similar to his workstation. The height of the computer was adjusted to decrease his neck strain, and the desk height was adjusted to allow his wheelchair to fit under the desk so that his arms could rest fully on the surface. He felt immediate relief with the adaptations. He was also fitted for a soft neck collar to wear when he felt he needed more neck support. (As his condition worsened, he learned to rest his head on the headrest of his chair and recline slightly for a few minutes every 15 min.)

3. Maintain maximal muscle strength and ROM. Mr. Turner was taught as many self-ranging maneuvers as possible, which he was encouraged to do in small segments frequently throughout the day. For example, his series of motions included neck rotations, side bends, and flexion and extension within strength limits; upper-extremity motions including shoulder flexion and abduction to maintain or improve the 90 degrees he had at assessment; hip flexion, abduction, and rotation; full knee extension; and all ankle motions. When using the walker, Mr. Turner was encouraged to extend each hip fully and to stretch his heel cords. Mrs. Turner and their children were taught to administer full ROM exercises, including trunk rotations, with special attention to ranging of the shoulders to prevent impingement. Simple massage techniques were also taught to all family members who felt comfortable with the task.

Mr. Turner had been active before the onset of ALS, and he liked to exercise. He rented a portable pedaling unit to attach to a chair at home. He pedaled two to four times a day, with no additional resistance, to the point at which he felt fatigue (usually 3 to 5 min at this stage). He carefully monitored his soreness and fatigue level after exercise and increased and decreased his pedaling depending on how he felt immediately and 2 days after exercise. Mr. Turner felt invigorated by this exercise, which he usually did while watching television. He was also taught a series of simple elastic band exercises for his upper extremities, with tensile strength adjusted according to his ability to contract his muscles without severe fatigue. Mr. Turner was also shown a series of isometric exercises for all major muscle groups to do at least once during the work day. Because he had some foot and ankle edema, he was encouraged to wear lightweight pressure stockings while sitting. Mr. Turner also had access to a swimming pool, and he was encouraged to carry out walking and upper-extremity exercises in the pool as long as another adult was with him in the water at all times.

4. Assess environment of home and work. Occupational therapy input was requested to help with work efficiency and placement of tools for ADLs to avoid wasting energy. Mr. Turner's OT made several visits to his worksite and home to identify adaptations of the environment for safety and independence. His wheelchair was eventually adapted with universal joint arm troughs to decrease his effort during self-feeding and basic upper-body hygiene. Ramps were recommended for home entry, and safety rails were placed in the bathroom. Mr. Turner was able to transfer to a shower chair, and the shower head was replaced with a hand-held unit.

   A speech pathology consultation was also requested. Using information from the PT's MMT, the speech pathologist carried out a thorough bulbar evaluation and provided information about swallowing techniques. The speech therapist focused on ways to decrease drooling and instructed Mr. Turner and his wife how to prepare foods with textures that were easily swallowed and manipulated.

Transitioning to Dependence

Within 7 months (to 14 months post diagnosis), Mr. Turner was no longer able to continue working despite workplace adaptations. The electric wheelchair was brought home for regular use when sitting or "strolling" around the neighborhood; the manual wheelchair was only used for brief excursions to a store or community event when a family member could push it. He could still walk short distances in the house with his walker and get dressed on his own, but he got breathless with dressing. His speech was beginning to be affected with slowing and effort to attain normal volume. He lost 10 pounds, so he was referred to the dietician for information about how to maintain nutritious calorie intake. The speech pathology consultant recommended ways to conserve energy when speaking, and to make eating more enjoyable and efficient—for example, advising him on ways to cope with food pocketing (tongue mobility was beginning to be impaired) by using techniques such as hand pressure on the cheek to push food back to the center of the mouth. At home, he became more dependent for household tasks, using a knife and fork, and managing saliva. OT recommended aids such as reachers, utensil adaptors to facilitate grip, rubber pen grippers, key adaptors to permit turning, and thumb abduction splints to assist in pincer grasp. At this point, his ALSFRS-R was 30 (63% of normal) and FVC was 70%.

As his ALS continued to progress over the next 7 months (to 21 months post diagnosis), Mr. Turner was able to use ADL tools for a while but gradually gave them up as he lost more hand strength. He also lost functional ambulation. He had to rely on others for more of his daily self-care although he could still assist if given time. Transfers required moderate assistance using a stand and pivot technique. Despite nutritional support, Mr. Turner lost another 15 pounds because of frustration with the length of time it took to eat. His ALS FRS-R had dropped to 23, and FVC was at 60%.

Continued

Mr. Turner had great difficulty adjusting to physical dependence. Initially Mr. Turner angrily resisted his wife's attempts to help him with eating and dressing tasks. This began to alienate her and the children until a family meeting was held with their medical social worker and PTs and OTs. All family members had the opportunity to express their frustrations. A major irritation to the children was what they perceived to be their constant waiting for their father to complete a task. Mrs. Turner was most irritated when Mr. Turner yelled at her when she attempted to help, even though he frequently expressed anger about his clumsiness. Mr. Turner sadly admitted that he was having increasing difficulty with his ADLs and was sometimes too tired after dressing to participate in family activities. At the end of the meeting, the family had worked out a compromise plan. Mr. Turner would continue to do as much as possible for himself. He would specifically ask for help from Mrs. Turner when he wanted it so she did not get caught in his anger about needing help. He preferred that the children not have to take any role in his personal care and hygiene at this point but realized that he might need their help later. Visiting nurse support was requested twice a week to help with bathing, and the OT was requested to make another home visit to develop strategies to help with toileting needs. Mr. Turner felt comfortable with his wife and children carrying out ROM exercises. A PT home episode of care (4 visits spread out over 3 weeks) was arranged to review the ROM exercise and positioning program, as well as respiratory exercises, postural drainage techniques, and family review of body mechanics.

By 28 months post diagnosis, Mr. Turner required assistance for feeding, all self-care, and turning in bed. With an augmented communication system, Mr. Turner was able to continue control over his expressive, cognitive, and emotional life. He could read and text (slowly) on a computer/tablet once set up so his minimal hand power could be facilitated to tap for page turning and cursor movement. Mr. Turner was dependent for all physical needs but could help direct his care, instructing caregivers in the best ways to position him for comfort. Nursing assistants were provided through his insurance 14 h a day from 6:30 a.m. to 8:30 p.m. He had a condom catheter and was assisted onto a bed pan for bowel movements. His weight stabilized because the nursing assistants could feed him at short intervals throughout the day. He could be assisted (using a Hoyer lift) into his powered wheelchair for a couple of hours at a time, two to three times a day, but spent more of his day in bed because of fatigue. He had a hospital bed with a special mattress for comfort; the head and knees could be elevated and he could be propped on pillows to change his position. Family members provided

care from 8:30 p.m. until midnight. Mr. Turner was able to activate a bell after midnight to call for help if needed. In addition, his wife and children followed a schedule to turn him every 3 h throughout the night. Nighttime responsibilities were taking a heavy toll on his wife, who worked full time, and the children, who were in high school and community college. His ALSFRS-R was 17, and FVC had dropped to 50%. Although he had mechanical cough assistance when needed, Mr. Turner had resisted starting respiratory assistance with NIV. However, in the following months he began NIV for longer periods of time and finally progressed to tracheostomy intubation.

When Mr. Turner became ventilator dependent at 35 months post diagnosis, he required attendance 24 h daily. Fortunately the family was able to pay for an attendant to remain at Mr. Turner's bedside throughout the night, although the family members all felt that they had no privacy. The family was committed to having Mr. Turner remain at home until his death, but all agreed that they needed occasional respite. Thus several week-long hospitalizations were made to give the family a break in the constant care needs.

Although Mr. Turner had elected HMV with a tracheostomy, he also had signed a durable power of attorney for health care, indicating that he did not want treatment for infections and that palliative care for comfort should direct his treatment. He had a strong lust for life, but he had come to accept his impending death. He did not have strong religious views, but he had talked with all his caregivers and therapists about his concerns related to death. He freely expressed his fear of "nonbeing." Because his caregivers and therapists were willing to talk about his and their own feelings, Mr. Turner came to believe that he would live on in the minds, hearts, and behaviors of those he had known. This idea seemed to give him great comfort. He particularly liked to talk to others about special times they had had together and how their interactions had affected each other. To help Mr. Turner process his death, his family, friends, and medical team put together an album of pictures and statements about their time together. Mr. Turner frequently liked to have his wife read through the book with him. His family continued to carry out his ROM exercises and massage because Mr. Turner had indicated that the treatments provided him physical comfort and the spiritual closeness he needed with his family. His primary treatment during the last few days consisted of morphine to decrease his respiratory discomfort. At about 36 months post diagnosis with ALS (about 3.6 years post symptom onset), Mr. Turner died at home in his sleep from a respiratory illness.

Dependent: Phase III, Stage 6. PTs and OTs are usually less involved in care when the patient becomes dependent; nursing personnel become more active. During this phase, therapists make home visits to support caregivers and respond to questions about pain control, bed mobility, positioning to prevent pressure ulcers, ROM, and equipment adaptations.[40,111,139] Therapists should be sure to teach all caregivers some basic body mechanics to use during lifting and patient care activities. If possible, caregivers should be taught how to safely move the person with ALS from the bed to a reclining wheelchair or other reclining chair, perhaps with a Hoyer lift or other assistive devices, during specific times of the day so that the person can continue to be part of the family activities. However, the ease of caregivers in transferring and caring for the person in the wheelchair must also be considered. Although some patients want to be in the midst of family activities even when dependent on HMV, other patients feel uncomfortable with their dependency and appearance and are reasonably content to stay in their room with television and visits from family members. This highly personal decision by patients must be respected. The therapist should review ROM procedures with family and professional caregivers and provide splinting or positioning devices if spasticity or paralysis leads

to caregiving difficulties (e.g., excessive adductor tone and contractures interfering with hygiene and bowel care) or tissue damage and pain. If nursing care providers do not give advice on pressure relief beds or mattresses of air or foam,[139] therapists should be prepared to do so. Unfortunately, many insurance providers and Medicare may not fund special mattresses, and they can be costly. Therapists may also need to review postural drainage techniques with caregivers.

Of greatest importance in the dependent stage, and sometimes in earlier stages, is the patient's ability to communicate. In the earliest manifestation of dysarthria, therapists train patients to slow the speech rate and cadence, exaggerate lip and tongue movements, and manage phrasing through breath control. Although spouses and caregivers can often interpret their partner's or patient's severely dysarthric speech (see earlier discussion of partial independence), most patients who use NIV or invasive ventilation for a prolonged period need to find nonverbal methods to communicate. If severe bulbar impairments precede extremity paralysis, paper and pencil, alphabet and word boards, and adapted computer keyboards can be used with minimal upper-extremity or finger strength for pointing. The American Speech-Language-Hearing Association provides suggestions for developing communication boards with the specific language most appropriate for the patient's situation.[144] For example, the board may be designed with commonly needed sentences, words used in the person's daily life, and the alphabet. As the person's ability to finger point decreases, the language board can be redesigned. A laser pointer strapped to the head may assist a patient in continuing to use a communication board using head/neck movements. When no extremity movement is possible, subtle neck movements or pressures, eye gaze, eye blink, upper facial movements, and electroencephalographic activity can be harnessed to operate communication devices. Learning to use more intensive brain-computer interfaces, however, takes months of intense training and may not provide a reasonable system for communication for most patients with ALS.[71,145]

Some patients with hypernasality benefit from using an orthodontic palatal appliance. Patients with a tracheostomy may benefit from use of a Passy-Muir (Irvine, CA) speaking valve tracheostomy tube. These devices require recommendation by communication specialists. As speech quality deteriorates and sound projection wanes, the spouse or caregiver can use an electronic speech amplifier to magnify the patient's speech. Speech pathologists and therapists have information on commercially available amplifying devices that are often used by persons with hearing problems but can be used by hearing people to amplify the speech of a person with severe weakness of phonation.

When selecting a communication device, therapists must work closely with the patient and family members to ensure that the system is compatible with patient skills and communication needs and preferences. Expensive systems commonly lie unused because of simple factors such as lack of proximity to the patient, interference of the unit with personal care, increased caregiver workload to manage the unit, and slowness of communication processing. The best systems are tailored to the precise needs of the patient; however, many patients do not have the financial or insurance support to purchase the device, and many patients in the end stages of ALS do not have the time to wait for systems designed for their specific needs. In such cases, commercially manufactured systems may be most appropriate.

Some patients and caregivers learn to communicate effectively with simple eye gaze, eye blinking, and clicking techniques with Morse code or self-developed codes. At minimum, patients with no ability to communicate or move must have some system to communicate emergency needs with their caregivers; for example, looking to the right means "help" and looking to the left means "pain." Therapists should help patients develop alternative modes of communication before intelligible speech becomes impossible.

In addition to communication systems, environmental control systems can be programmed to turn on and off television, lights, and other electronic units with the same type of switching units used for communication (e.g., eye blink, infrared beam, and head movement pressure). Unfortunately, these devices are often expensive and may not be available to all patients. Financial support is often not extended for high-tech equipment by third-party payers because of the patient's limited life expectancy. The ability to communicate and call for help, however, is of paramount importance with completely dependent patients.

By the dependent stage, most patients have significant problems eating and maintaining nutrition, although these problems may manifest in earlier stages. Patients often report choking or coughing after swallowing liquids or problems moving food around in the mouth or to the back of the throat for swallowing. These problems are best handled medically and can be assessed with videofluoroscopy or videoendoscopy. The aggressiveness of treatment intervention depends on the patient's preference and whether she or he still wants to attempt any oral feeding (e.g., syringe feeding and oral gastric tubes) or wishes to have a PEG or another alternative to oral feedings implemented. Therapists, however, can help patients and caregivers develop strategies that improve eating and nutrition, such as adjusting eating position, changing head and neck alignments, adding thickeners to liquids, and adjusting portion sizes and texture of foods.[16]

Psychosocial Issues in Amyotrophic Lateral Sclerosis
From the Clinicians' Perspective

Giving the bad news of a terminal diagnosis is difficult for even the most experienced clinician. In dealing with the diagnosis of ALS, most physicians now believe that the diagnosis, prognosis, and possible patterns of progression should be shared with the patient and family or partners and caregiving friends. Only by knowing the truth can patients and families deal openly with one another and make plans for the future. McCluskey and colleagues[146] suggest that those giving the medical or therapeutic diagnosis should attend to best practice parameters when giving bad news, such as creating the appropriate setting, identifying patient and caregiver needs, asking what patients and caregivers want to know, providing knowledge, exploring feelings of the patients and caregivers, and formulating a strategy for dealing with the situation. Patients and family members seldom remember what they are told when first given a terminal diagnosis. They do, however, remember how the information was given. Therefore information should be given honestly but with a sense of hope.

All information need not be given at the time of diagnosis. Rather, the patient and family can be exposed to more in-depth information over a number of sessions when they have the opportunity to ask questions that occur during the assimilation process. Therapists, especially those working in isolation from a comprehensive clinic, should also follow these guidelines by providing information, helping the patient and family to identify goals, and establishing a plan for intervention. Patients should know that the goals will have to be adjusted and plans reset as the disease process continues. If patients and families know that they can contact the therapist for support and advice, many of the negative aspects of the illness can be confronted in a positive manner. Preferably, an appointment for a follow-up visit will be set so patients and family members feel that contact with the care provider is expected.

Information about transitions related to nutrition, communication, and respiratory functions should be delivered to patients and families in time to make thoughtful decisions rather than just before or during a time of crisis, such as after a choking episode or during respiratory arrest. Care should also be taken to respect the cultural and spiritual views of the patient and family.[83] Preferably, patients and family members will prepare an advance medical directive that should be reviewed with the physician at least every 6 months.

Therapists treating patients who do not have access to a multidisciplinary ALS clinic should remember that they are often the person who works most closely with the patient, and they should plan on spending enough time with the patient and family to respond to concerns and help with problem solving. Patients and families will progress through the adjustment process with different responses and at different rates; they may move through a continuum of coping strategies, ranging from cognitive approaches, characterized by asking many questions and reviewing the most current research, to the extreme of marked denial and disinterest in participating in any medical or therapeutic recommendations.

Therapists should be aware of their own biases and knowledge base as they communicate with patients and families about consequential decisions like PEG and NIV use; physicians and allied health professionals can differ in their attitudes regarding these interventions.[147] Therapists may need to consult with specialists on an ALS team

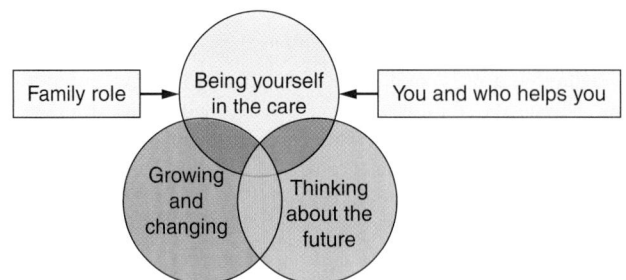

Categories	Focused codes
Being yourself in the care	Defending autonomy, continuing life as before, doing what you need, changing habits
Growing and changing	Nurturing the mind, growing with the disease, inquiring about the disease, accepting the illness
Thinking about the future	Spending time for yourself, life beyond tracheostomy, being aware of death, controlling the disease, the meaning of time
You and who helps you	Deciding, controlling the care, depending physically, finding the right person, being a burden
Family role	Being grateful, distinguishing roles, discovering parents, adjustment in couple dynamics

Fig. 15.10 Themes generated regarding self-care from patients with motor neuron disease. (From Bassola B, Sansone VA, Lusignani M. Being yourself and thinking about the future in people with motor neuron disease: a grounded theory of self-care processes. *J Neurosci Nurs.* 2018;50:138–143.)

regarding guidelines for decision making and potential benefits to patients of these interventions, but may also need to share with the physicians what they have heard regarding the patient's perspective during their more extensive interaction with the individual patient/caregiver or family in the home.

Patients' Attitudes and Fears

To investigate ways that patients take care of themselves psychologically, Bassola and colleagues[148] used a grounded theory approach to examine interview responses from 21 patients with motor neuron disease (9 had ALS). Common themes included control of decision making related to present and future adherence to medical recommendations, and acknowledgement of the need to change as the disease progresses (Fig. 15.10).[148] Patients wanted to process and respond in their own way, in their own time. Patients cite the importance of both family and caregivers; a healthy relationship with each is critical,[148] especially when family relationships and caregiving roles overlap.

Purtilo and Haddad[149] identified four major fears of the patient who has a terminal condition: fear of isolation, fear of pain, fear of dependence, and fear of death itself. Such fears add stress for the patient and family. Patients with progressive diseases often see their social contacts decrease. Mr. Turner in Case Study 15.1 was concerned when he was no longer able to join his colleagues in the company cafeteria. After he received his motorized wheelchair, he was able to continue his social contacts until his bulbar symptoms progressed to a point that he chose not to eat in public. When Mr. Turner lost the ability to speak and had to use his computerized speech system, he noticed that fewer colleagues stopped by his office to talk because of the slowness of the communication process. Although he understood the problem, Mr. Turner mourned the loss of friendship and his loss of standing as a competent computer expert. Because of his need for social contact, Mr. Turner continued to work until he could no longer tolerate the sitting position. His fear of isolation increased when he became homebound. Although colleagues came for visits regularly at first, as Mr. Turner progressed to a near locked-in state, only a few close friends came by for brief visits. Mr. Turner's greatest fear was being separated

from his family and abandoned to hospital care with inconsistent staffing patterns. Fortunately, in his community, Mrs. Turner was able to set up visitations from several church members, clerics, and hospice volunteers.

Fear of uncontrolled *pain* is common among people with terminal diseases. Patients need assurance that their pain will be controlled. Fortunately, today pain medications can be administered in many forms, dosages, and frequencies that can be tailored to the patient's specific needs. In a study of the final month of life with ALS, caregivers reported that a major emphasis of care was to eliminate as much pain and discomfort as possible, even if it shortened the patient's life.[150] Keeping a pain log of intensity, type, location, and time of pain may provide the physician with information necessary to best prescribe dosages. Many patients with ALS do experience significant pain from musculoskeletal sources, persistent spasms or spasticity, and pressure sores. Most of these problems can be handled with appropriate pain medications, muscle relaxants, careful positioning, frequent ROM exercises, and tissue massage. Massage may help decrease cortisol levels, decreasing anxiety and increasing mental relaxation along with any local musculoskeletal effects.[1] Undertreated and uncontrolled pain is associated with a patient's seeking information on assisted suicide.[151] Some patients who expressed interest in assisted suicide options did not follow up because of religious beliefs and concerns about possible loss of life insurance coverage for surviving family members.[152]

A major concern of patients with ALS is the *dependence* necessary, with increasing reliance on the help of others as the patient loses functional ability. Because the process is gradual, most patients have the opportunity to make adjustments. Increasing reliance on others and resulting privacy issues tend to be uncomfortable for patients who have always valued self-control and independence. Some patients are also concerned about their increasing dependence on others because of increased burden of care on spouses or other caregivers.[153] Concern for others sometimes prompts patients to choose hospital, nursing home, or in-patient hospice care over home care during the terminal stage of the disease. Not all patients with terminal illness react the same way during the dying process. Throughout the process, patients and family members may cycle back and forth through a range of different emotional and coping reactions: depression, anger, hostility, bargaining, and acceptance and adaptation (order is not implied).[149]

How the patient coped with life's difficulties before the illness and her or his prior relationship patterns often direct how the patient will deal with the terminal illness. One man and his family who decided early in life to "try for happiness" relate the continued vibrancy of life despite his ALS and near total dependence for all physical needs (watch the video: https://www.youtube.com/watch?time_continue=2&v=2OVUFqgvm_Q; read the story: https://paloaltoonline.atavist.com/a-vibrant-life).[154] This individual has written a book using an eye-gaze device, in which an infrared reader scans the movement of his pupils. The patient can track a digital keyboard on his computer monitor and click with an on-screen mouse (read the story: https://paloaltoonline.atavist.com/powered-by-passion).[155] Other patients and the significant others in their lives may choose a different coping response, or cycle through multiple responses as each functional loss forces additional changes.

Depression. Health care providers and family members often have great difficulty coping with a patient who is depressed; they may make repeated efforts to "talk the person out of" their sadness or hopelessness. Medical professions must be able to distinguish between depression that can be destructive and the mourning or grieving process that is a necessary and vital response to dealing with loss. In both states the person may feel a level of withdrawal, sadness, apathy, loss of interest in activities, and cognitive distortions. In a clinically depressed state, however, the patient experiences an accompanying loss of self-esteem.

A person in mourning rarely experiences the loss of self-esteem essential to a diagnosis of clinical depression. A person who grieves for what is lost but who has retained agency (ability to make decisions for themselves) may make plans for the impending death. Such behaviors are positive coping strategies. On the other hand, depressive symptoms expressed as hopelessness, uncontrolled suffering, and perceived burden on caregivers may lead to feelings of worthlessness; such feelings are more closely related to a choice for treatment discontinuance of feeding or ventilatory support.[152]

Diagnosis of depression is complicated by pseudobulbar affect (emotional lability with exaggerated laughing and crying), which is manifested by approximately 50% of patients with ALS. This emotional lability is not under complete control of the patient and is often misunderstood by family members and caregivers. Although current treatment is antidepressant medications, underlying clinical depression may or may not be present that would respond to higher doses of antidepressant medication and counseling.[43]

Pressuring a patient who appears depressed to see a mental health clinician can lead to loss of trust if the patient is not comfortable talking about feelings or confiding in a counselor. OTs and PTs and other persons involved in the direct care of a patient who is dying may find that their patients feel safer talking with nonprofessional counselors or psychotherapists about the burden of their care on family members or their own impending death. Rehabilitation personnel should therefore be aware of local options for in-home support services, palliative care, and end-of-life options and services and be prepared to listen to the patient's concerns if the patient expresses the need for emotional support.

The existence of depression and potential associated cognitive impairment has been discussed as a factor reducing a patient's decision making capability in the right-to-die debate.[156] In ALS, however, a patient's wish to die may not be directly related to depression and may not be related to cognitive or behavioral impairments. In a study of 247 patients with ALS, average disease duration of 1 year, 62 expressed

a wish to die (25%), and only 37% of those 62 patients (i.e., 23 patients out of 247) had clinical depression.[156] Such evidence must be considered, along with individual circumstances, in any discussion regarding life-saving interventions or physician-assisted death participation (where legal).

Family Members as Caregivers in Amyotrophic Lateral Sclerosis

Often in the concern for the patient's needs, health care professionals pay little attention to the effect a person's degenerative illness has on other members of the family. ALS significantly affects the person's extended family because the patient gradually becomes increasingly dependent on family members, partners, or caregiving friends for physical care, social arrangements, cognitive stimulation, and emotional support. For some families, the spouse may have to take on additional work, return to work, or, in the case of some older homemakers, join the workforce for the first time to deal with the financial stresses that occur when chronic illness invades the family unit. Family members must also absorb the former family duties of the dependent person. For example, a spouse or child may have to handle all the cooking, cleaning, or other household chores or work to help support the family. Once the patient becomes dependent, the caregiver may need to reduce or discontinue employment to take care of the patient. All family members may need to become involved in the physical care of the increasingly dependent person with ALS. Caregivers frequently influence the decision making process throughout management of ALS, but especially when considering the use of tracheostomy and invasive ventilation (TIV).[85] A study comparing ALS caregivers in Japan and America noted that caregivers in both countries were more likely to say yes to TIV than the patients they cared for.[85]

Children of patients with ALS also have to deal with major changes in their lifestyle. Although they may love their parent who is sick, at some level most can become frustrated with factors such as the need to provide physical care to parents. This is a difficult problem especially for children who have not had a positive relationship with that parent. Children living in the home of a parent who is dying of ALS also express frustration about the lack of privacy in their home when nursing personnel and attendants are present, interruptions in family and personal life plans, embarrassment because of the parent's appearance and dependency, lack of attention from the caregiving and working parent, and fear of financial crises (e.g., possible loss of home and no financial support for college).

The entire family is affected by the sick person's increasing dependency, behavioral or cognitive changes, and impending death. In a small study of 11 family caregivers, many caregivers felt frustrated and resentful because their lives were consumed with the caregiving responsibilities. Most caregivers had adjusted to some degree after 2 to 4 years. Caregivers who adjusted most successfully learned to take time for themselves without guilt and to tap their social support systems for help.[157] Fortunately, most families manage to cope with the process—the major contributing factor being the coping ability of families before the illness.

To be really effective, the therapist working with the patient with ALS must be prepared to help families and caregivers find appropriate ways of coping with the emotional, social, and physical stress of caregiving. For example, therapists should present, without pressing, adaptive equipment options to patients when they first start to show impairment in functional ability. If shown how the equipment will help them maintain independence, most patients are receptive to its use. Even when presented in a positive way, however, a wheelchair or adaptive devices may be resisted long after the adaptations would facilitate mobility and ADLs. Therapists must be attentive to patients' feelings and fears at this time because use of a wheelchair (or other specific equipment) heralds to many patients the "beginning of the end."

Other factors that affect the family of a patient with ALS include medical insurance and differing levels of long-term care coverage. Some families are fortunate to have excellent coverage that provides extensive home nursing support, whereas other families are unable to cope with the financial stresses and must accept public assistance during the final stages of the disease. As opposed to Germany and Japan, which provide long-term nursing care insurance, in the United States financial stress on patients with ALS can reach more than $150,000 per year for ventilation support at home.[88] Financial burden significantly impacts patient and caregiver decisions. (Resources are available for end-of-life issues e.g., www.nlm.nih.gov/medlineplus/endoflifeissues.html#cat1.)

GUILLAIN-BARRÉ SYNDROME

Pathology, Incidence, and Medical Diagnosis

GBS, also known as acute inflammatory demyelinating polyradiculoneuropathy (AIDP), is the most common form of the broad spectrum of acute or subacute conditions causing generalized paralysis. GBS is an immune-mediated disease that affects nerve roots and peripheral nerves, leading to motor neuropathy and flaccid paralysis with possible sensory and ANS effects.[158] Unlike ALS, GBS makes itself apparent very quickly, progressing to complete paralysis (in some cases) within days to weeks instead of years. Fortunately, GBS usually has a good prognosis, with most patients returning to their prior functional status by 1 to 2 years after onset. Note, however, that "prior functional status" does not mean that no impairments remain; prognosis will be discussed in a later subsection.

Purely motor forms and mixed motor and sensory forms of GBS have been identified.[159] The motor subtype, *acute motor axonal neuropathy* (AMAN), has a good prognosis, although recovery of ambulation may take longer than in AIDP[160]; this subtype is more common in Asia and South America. Less common subtypes include *acute motor and sensory axonal neuropathy* (AMSAN), which has a less positive prognosis (and may be a severe variant of AMAN)[161]; *Miller-Fisher syndrome*, with primarily cranial nerve (especially oculomotor) symptoms, ataxia, and areflexia[162]; and *chronic inflammatory demyelinating polyradiculoneuropathy* (CIDP), which causes progressive or relapsing and remitting numbness and weakness.[163] AIDP may be relabeled as *acute onset CIDP* in about 5% of individuals[164] who experience a new *relapse* (episode of deterioration) after 8 weeks from onset of weakness, or if three or more relapses occur within that first 8 weeks. Most references to GBS can be assumed to describe the AIDP and AMAN varieties; Miller-Fisher syndrome, AMSAN, and CIDP are typically called out specifically if research findings include or address them.

The incidence of GBS is approximately 1 to 4 cases per 100,000 persons. Lower incidence is noted in younger ages (0.62 cases per 100,000 person-years for 0- to 9-year-olds, increasing by a highly variable 20% with every 10-year increase in age)[165] and in Western countries compared with Asia. AIDP is one subtype of the disease, accounting for 90% of the cases in North America and Europe.[166] Epidemiological studies show that males are affected by GBS up to twice as often as are females[167]; a meta-analysis of incidence studies in North America and Europe showed an incidence in males that was 1.6 that of females.[165]

Approximately 27% of patients with GBS have no identified preceding illness; however, more than two-thirds had symptoms of an infectious disease approximately 2 weeks before the onset of GBS symptoms. In the motor form (AMAN) and in Miller-Fisher syndrome, serum antibodies have been found against specific *gangliosides*,

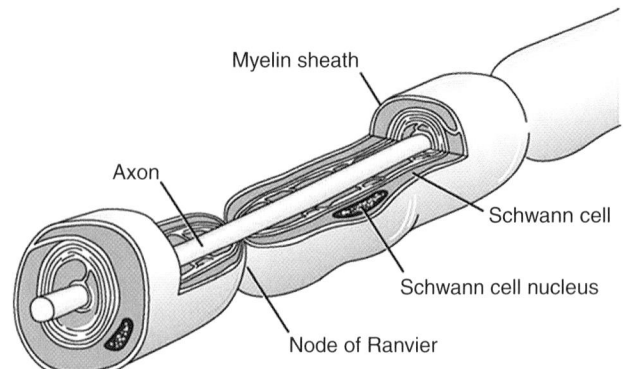

Fig. 15.11 Myelin Formed by Schwann Cells on the Axon of an α Motor Neuron. (Reproduced from Allen DD, Widener GL. Tone abnormalities. In: Cameron MH, ed. *Physical Agents in Rehabilitation: An Evidence-Based Approach to Practice.* 5th ed. St. Louis, MO: Elsevier; 2018.)

lipids that reside on neuronal membranes and assist with cell function.[162] Research has identified a specific lipid in *Campylobacter jejuni* that mimics normal human gangliosides in AMAN; following this infection, the antibodies developed to attack the bacterial lipid also bind to normal gangliosides. The new compounds activate axon-destroying *complement*,[168] the cascade of immune system events that triggers macrophage proliferation and inflammation. Associations with additional infectious agents have been recorded, with differing propensities to activate myelin- or axon-destroying complement (e.g., *Mycoplasma pneumoniae*, influenza A, cytomegalovirus, Epstein-Barr, and *flavivirus*).[169] The flaviviruses include both Dengue and Zika; a meta-analysis of the incidence of GBS in confirmed cases of Zika virus reveals an incidence of 1.23%, much more prevalent than in the noninfected population, although still somewhat rare.[169]

GBS pathology may be easier to grasp after a brief review of normal anatomy. In healthy peripheral nerves, a myelin sheath formed by Schwann cells wraps around the axon of α motor neurons to insulate the axon (Fig. 15.11). This insulation speeds electrochemical conduction of the neural signal using a process known as "saltatory conduction" because transmission jumps past insulated sections, from node to node *(nodes of Ranvier)*, the spaces between myelin sheathing (Fig. 15.12). In GBS, an infection or triggering event activates the immune system's *complement* cascade. The cascade of events in the complement (a specific series of molecules and actions that *complement* other immune system responses to identified threats) breaks up

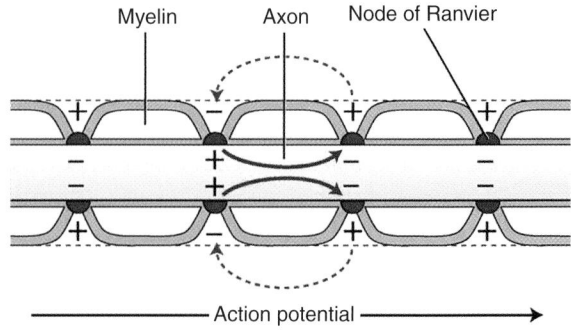

Fig. 15.12 Saltatory Conduction Along a Myelin-Wrapped Axon. (Reproduced from Allen DD, Widener GL. Tone abnormalities. In: Cameron MH, ed. *Physical Agents in Rehabilitation: An Evidence-Based Approach to Practice.* 5th ed. St. Louis, MO: Elsevier; 2018.)

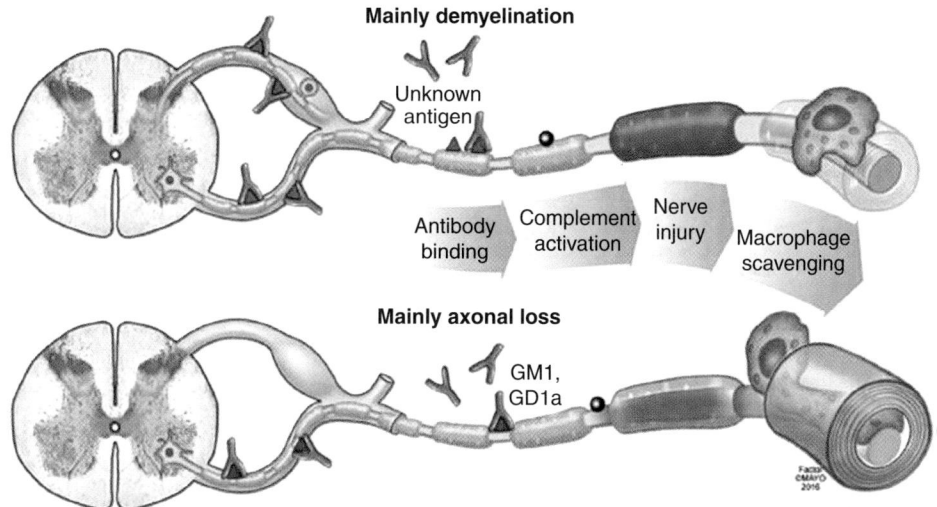

Fig. 15.13 Guillain-Barré Pathogenesis. In the demyelinating subtype, no specific antigen has been identified, but complement activation destroys myelin and macrophages proliferate to clean up myelin debris. In the axonal subtype, gangliosides GM1 and GD1a on the neuronal membrane have been identified as the normally occurring molecules that various bacterial and viral antigens mimic. Antibodies bind to these molecules at the nodes of Ranvier (between myelin sheathing) and activate the complement sequence from there. Macrophages clean up debris from membrane and axon destruction, leaving the myelin relatively intact. (Reproduced[168] from Wijdicks EFM, Klein CJ. Guillain-Barré syndrome. *Mayo Clin Proc.* 2017;92:467–479.)

myelin (in AIDP) or damages axons in spinal roots and peripheral nerves (in AMAN) by attacking the neuronal membrane (resulting in disruption of voltage-gated sodium channels)[161] at the nodes of Ranvier or axon terminals close to the muscle fibers. The cascade promotes inflammation and attracts macrophages to come in and clean up the fragments (Fig. 15.13).

In AIDP, damage to the myelin sheath disturbs saltatory propagation of the action potential, resulting in slowed conduction velocity or complete *conduction block* (difference in amplitude of signal when comparing proximal versus distal stimulation along a peripheral nerve). Partial conduction block is most often seen in the early stages of GBS, and the conduction block increases through the *progressive stage* of the disease (usually about 4 weeks). The most common conduction block findings are in the peroneal nerve, followed by the tibial nerve. Proximal conduction block is evident more often than distal conduction block. In axonal neuropathy (AMAN), conduction block can be more severe, and the number of functional motor units is decreased (Fig. 15.14).[170]

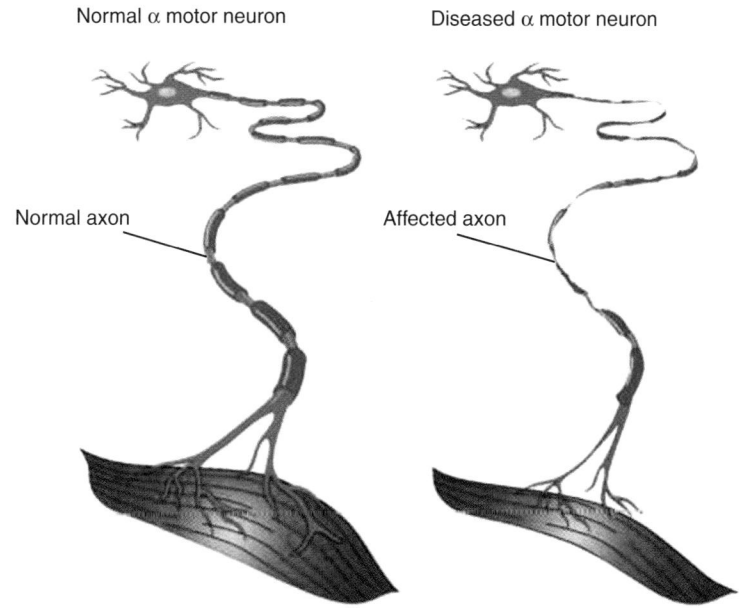

Fig. 15.14 Normal Neuron and Degenerated α Motor Neuron in Pathological Conditions. (Adapted from http://www.brainstorm-cell.com/assets/ALS-Neurons.jpg.)

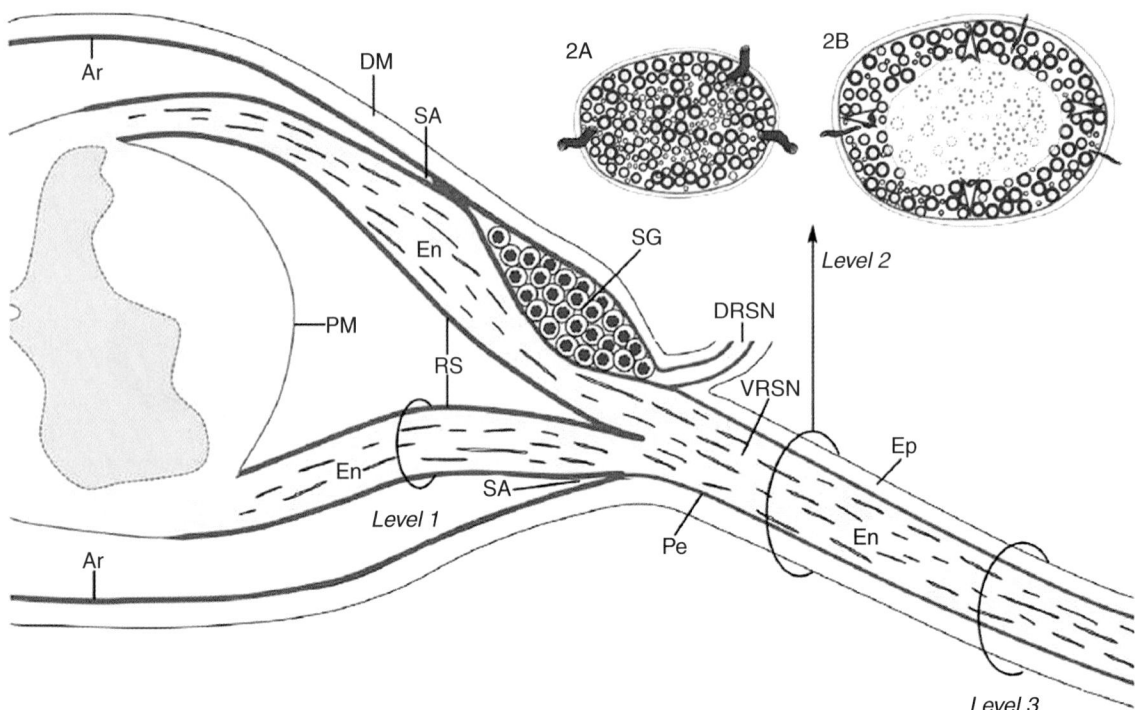

Fig. 15.15 Membranes and anatomy of spinal nerves (including the ventral ramus *[VRSN]* and dorsal ramus *[DRSN]*) and nerve roots (including the spinal ganglion *[SG]*, also known as the dorsal root ganglion). The nerve membranes, in order, are endoneurium *(En)*, perineurium *(Pe)*, and epineurium *(Ep)*. The En persists along spinal nerves and nerve roots to their junction with the spinal cord. The Ep is continuous with the dura mater *(DM)* beginning at the subarachnoid angle *(SA)*. The Pe continues past the SA, mostly between the DM and arachnoid *(Ar)* membranes, but part of it becomes an inner layer of the root sheath *(RS)*. The external layer of the RS is formed by the arachnoid membrane turning back on itself at the SA. Where the roots join with the spinal cord, the RS becomes part of the pia mater *(PM)*. Inflammation, edema, and demyelination or axonal injury in early Guillain-Barré can occur at levels 1, 2, or 3: nerve root, spinal nerve (including ventral and dorsal rami), or peripheral nerve, respectively. In axonal subtypes, Figs. (2A) and (2B) show the spinal nerve (level 2) with transperineurial blood vessels in the normal cross-section (2A), and with edema that pushes axons away from each other, constricting vessels against the compliance limits of a relatively inelastic Pe (*arrows*, 2B), resulting in ischemia and further injury. Edema can also constrict the passage of the spinal nerve as it emerges through the intervertebral foramen (proximal to the DRSN). (Figure modified from Berciano J. Spinal nerve involvement in early Guillain-Barré syndrome; the Haymaker and Kernohan's Legacy. *J Neurol Sci.* 2017;382:1–9.)

Some researchers have noted in early GBS (the *acute stage*, within 10 days of onset) that inflammatory edema in the *endoneurium* and *epi-perineurium* (membrane layers that cover the nerve) may cause compression and constriction of transperineural blood vessels, resulting in ischemia of the axons (Fig. 15.15). When axons are compressed or deprived of blood flow, they show *Wallerian-like degeneration* (the portion of the axon distal to the lesion degenerates—away from the cell body) and the surrounding myelin of degenerating axons can collapse. When complement activation only affects myelin (in AIDP), the axons are left intact and can remyelinate, typically in a matter of weeks.[171] However, when axons degenerate, recovery depends on axonal regeneration from intact elements of the neurons, which takes months and may be incomplete.[135] In acute axonal motor neuropathy, the immune system and complement affect the axon directly, leaving the myelin intact.[172] Some evidence indicates that axonal loss is related to longer-lasting or permanent muscle weakness.[173]

The diagnosis of GBS requires both clinical and supportive medical tests. Progressive weakness involving multiple nerve root and nerve distributions *(polyradiculoneuropathy)*, usually symmetrical, developing over a couple of days or weeks, accompanied by hypo- or areflexia, generally triggers medical tests such as examination of CSF and electrodiagnostic tests of neural conduction.[166] Characteristic CSF will show *albumino-cytological dissociation*: increased protein (from the fragments of axons and myelin) with no elevation of white blood cells. Motor and sensory neural conduction tests are generally performed at

BOX 15.7 Common Diagnostic Features of Guillain-Barré Syndrome

A. Motor weakness
  1. Progressive symptoms and signs of motor weakness that develop rapidly (1–2 weeks)
    a. Relative symmetry of motor involvement
    b. Typical progression of weakness from legs to arms; may start in proximal leg muscles, limiting stair climbing or rising from sitting position; may self-limit to upper and/or lower extremities or may extend to full tetraplegia with respiratory and cranial nerve involvement. Facial and oropharyngeal muscle involvement noted in about 50% of cases
  2. Muscle stretch reflexes depressed or absent in at least distal tendon responses
  3. In Miller-Fisher syndrome, diplopia and ataxia may be present
B. Mild sensory symptoms or signs, particularly paresthesias and hypoesthesias in stocking/glove patterns; these may precede motor signs by 1–2 days
C. Autonomic dysfunction such as tachycardia and arrhythmias, vasomotor symptoms: extreme blood pressure fluctuations and response to drug therapy may be the presenting signs. Acute autonomic dysfunction typically resolves during the plateau phase
D. Absence of fever at onset of symptoms; recent history of flulike illness common
E. Laboratory test results characteristically show elevation of cerebrospinal fluid protein with normal white blood cell counts (cerebrospinal fluid cells at 10 or fewer mononuclear leukocytes per cubic millimeter of cerebrospinal fluid)
F. Electrodiagnostic testing, nerve conduction velocities of motor nerves usually slower and may reveal a conduction block, but may take 2 weeks to develop. Electromyography in paralyzed muscles may show fibrillation
G. Serum testing may reveal antibodies to specific gangliosides, specific viral or bacterial infection; may rule out drug or toxins in the blood
H. Recovery usually begins 2–4 weeks after plateau of disease process

From references 161, 162, and 168.

multiple motor and sensory sites, frequently including the median, ulnar, tibial, peroneal, and sural nerves; abnormalities indicating potential GBS include slowed velocity, lower amplitude of signal, longer latency distally or in the F response, and decrease in compound motor action potential.[160] No test is completely definitive: CSF abnormalities may take up to 2 weeks to develop,[174] and electrodiagnostic tests may continue to be normal for several weeks after onset; up to 20% of patients never have abnormalities apparent on nerve conduction testing.[166] CSF may rule out other diagnoses if cytology suggests carcinomatous origins or active infection. Serum samples may be tested for recent infection with *Campylobacter jejuni*, cytomegalovirus, or other viruses, especially if patients report having had a course of febrile diarrhea, sore throat with headaches, or upper respiratory infection in the 4 weeks preceding symptoms. The diagnostic criteria for GBS were developed and modified by the US National Institute of Neurological Disorders and Stroke and are provided in Box 15.7.[161]

Clinical Presentation

For an overall view of the clinical presentation of a person with GBS as categorized by the ICF model, review Fig. 15.4. The predominant body function impairments of GBS are weakness and fatigue (affecting movement dimensions of strength and endurance[2]), with muscle atrophy and fasciculation indicating body structure effects on LMNs with their motor units (review Figs. 15.1 and 15.2).[175] Because the affected body structures include nerve roots, spinal nerves, and peripheral nerves (review Fig. 15.15), sensory neurons and neurons transmitting information to and from the ANS can also show deficits. Sensory

dysesthesias and autonomic malfunction (*dysautonomia*) can range in severity from annoying pins and needles to life-threatening cardiac arrest. Activity limitations and participation restrictions occur at onset, worsening through the acute stage (about 10 days) and any further progression to the *nadir* (peak) of motor impairment (2 to 8 weeks after onset), depending on the severity of weakness and fatigue, stabilizing during the plateau (2 to 4 weeks), and improving from the beginning of recovery (2 to 3 months post onset to several years). As with ALS, an individual's clinical presentation will depend partly on environmental and personal factors, such as economic resources and coping mechanisms.

Onset

The initial symptoms of GBS may be acute onset of severe midline back pain or sensory paresthesias with tingling progressing from the distal limbs more proximally. Individuals may also complain of a "tight band" feeling.[168] Weakness develops, either as the initial symptom or within 1 or 2 days of sensory signs, frequently in proximal muscles first. Individuals may notice trouble climbing stairs or rising from a chair. Motor signs drive the course of the disease in both children and adults: rapidly evolving, relatively symmetrical ascending (legs to arms) weakness or flaccid paralysis. Motor impairment at the nadir may vary from mild weakness (may be worse in distal lower-extremity musculature)[166] to total paralysis of the peripheral, axial, facial, and extraocular musculature. Tendon reflexes are usually diminished or absent. Because development of motor signs can be rapid and ANS symptoms can develop without warning, cardiac arrest or respiratory failure can occur fairly suddenly. Most patients are hospitalized with monitoring of cardiorespiratory function through the nadir in case cardiac pacemaker, intubation, or less invasive mechanical ventilation becomes necessary.

Respiration

One-third of patients may require assisted ventilation because of paralysis or weakness of the diaphragm, intercostals, and accessory inspiratory musculature, or weakness of abdominal musculature (affecting forceful cough) and diminished recoil of the thorax with stiffness developing over a period of time.[168] Impaired respiratory muscle strength may lead to an inability to manage aspiration and to decreased VC, tidal volume, and oxygen saturation. Secondary complications such as infections or organ system failure lead to death in 3% to 6% of patients with GBS, with higher rates of 10% or 20% when individuals have severe comorbidities.[168]

Guillain-Barré Syndrome Disability Scale

The GBS disability scale (also referred to as the Hughes scale)[160] is commonly used to track the clinical course of GBS although authors differ slightly in the descriptors they use for different grades[166] (Box 15.8). A grade of 2 on the GBS disability scale (walks without device) is frequently the target of acute care therapies. Therapy is considered more effective than the alternative if individuals take less time from the onset of symptoms to reach the level of walking without assistance (grade 2), or if a higher proportion of patients walk without assistance by 4 weeks. The GBS disability scale focuses on activity limitations resulting from weakness, especially related to respiration and walking. While used frequently to record status of a patient, the psychometrics of this scale have not been reported, and it has low sensitivity to small changes in impairments or activities.[176]

Weakness

The primary deficit driving the course of GBS is *loss of muscle strength*. Strength is typically tested at individual muscles with a manual muscle

BOX 15.8   Guillain-Barré Syndrome Disability Scale[160,166]

0 = Normal (healthy)

1 = Minimal signs and symptoms, able to run (minor symptoms or signs of neuropathy but capable of manual work)

2 = Ambulates independently (at least 5 m across an open space but incapable of manual work/running)

3 = Able to walk 5 m with aid (stick, appliance, or support)

4 = Bed bound (or wheelchair)

5 = Requires assisted respiration (for any part of the day or night)

6 = Death

test (MMT: 0 to 5, with 5 being normal and 0 meaning unable to contract). However, the clinical course of strength loss and recovery does not show random deficits in individual muscles but is fairly symmetrical and related to distal versus proximal musculature. In many studies, strength testing has been standardized for recording the clinical course in GBS based on MMT scores across multiple muscle groups. MMT scores across specific distal and proximal muscle groups of the bilateral upper and lower extremities are summed to form the Medical Research Council (MRC) strength assessment.[166] MRC for GBS designates six pairs of muscles[177] (although some authors report assessment across four pairs of proximal and distal muscles)[166]: shoulder abductors, elbow flexors, wrist extensors, hip flexors, knee extensors, and ankle dorsiflexors.[178] Each of 12 (or 8) muscles is scored from 0 to 5 using the MMT definitions, with 60 (or 40) indicating the top score for normal strength across the tested muscle groups. Using 40 as the top score (for the sum across eight muscles), authors have categorized motor deficit as mild (MRC 31 to 40), moderate (MRC 11 to 30), and severe (MRC 0 to 10).[166] Mild motor deficit may be translated as most muscles testing as 4 to 5/5 on MMT; moderate indicates that most muscles test as a 2 to 3/5, and severe indicates that muscles test as 0 to 1/5. Others divide the MRC (60) into "decade" groups[177] of scores: 51 to 60, 41 to 50, 31 to 40, 21 to 30, and less than 21. A modification of the MRC proposes a new scoring system of 0 to 3 for each muscle to improve reliability among physicians (who performed the MRC in the data used) who were shown to be inconsistent in their use of the 0 to 5 MMT scale.[178] In the new scoring system, the scores would indicate normal strength (3), slight weakness (2), severe weakness (1), and paralysis (0). The modified scoring has not yet become the standard practice.

Note that the MRC scores include the upper and lower extremities, but do not assess axial muscles or cranial nerve weakness. Axial muscles typically have deficits that align with limb muscle weakness; muscles innervated by cranial nerves may be more or less affected than limb musculature in patients with GBS.

Approximately 50% of patients develop some *cranial nerve involvement*, primarily facial muscle weakness, although patients may also develop paresis or paralysis in oropharyngeal (bulbar involvement in AIDP or AMAN) and oculomotor (most frequently in Miller-Fisher syndrome) muscles.[168] Bulbar signs are occasionally the presenting motor symptoms. When bulbar signs are present, dysarthria and dysphagia are likely, which is similar to that seen in ALS but without spasticity in the tongue or larynx (see Table 15.1).

Fatigue

Fatigue is common in GBS and can be both a primary and secondary effect. Primary fatigue may result from increased central effort required to activate partially denervated muscles and diminished ability to recruit sufficient motor units to maintain peripheral contractions.[96] Fatigue is inevitable when muscles weakened through the disease process must work at a higher percent of their maximal strength for ordinary daily tasks. However, in a consensus statement combining literature review and expert opinion, authors agree that at least part of the cause of fatigue in GBS is the forced inactivity[179] consequent to muscle weakness. Thus secondary fatigue may occur with deconditioning. Most measures of fatigue do not distinguish between these sources, but management differs so distinction is useful. Fatigue experienced in the early stages of the disease is assumed to be primary fatigue: it is related to the severity of weakness, and intervention usually requires reduced activity to minimize overuse of partially denervated muscles. Fatigue experienced after reinnervation of muscles is assumed to be secondary fatigue: it is not related to severity of the initial illness, and intervention can utilize the overload principle or progressively challenging activities.

Severe fatigue (undifferentiated as to primary or secondary fatigue) is present in 38% to 86% of patients with GBS, depending on the cutoff point used to define severity and the age of the sample, with a positive correlation between severe fatigue and greater age.[180] Fatigue tends to be long-lasting: up to 42% claim they still have severe fatigue after 20 years[181] post onset of GBS. In a study comparing people "well-recovered" from GBS and healthy controls, maximal voluntary contraction was only slightly less than healthy controls, but a sustained contraction showed less peripheral fatigue and more central activation failure (indicating inability to maintain recruitment at MVC level even though the muscles had not yet fatigued) in the first minute in GBS.[182] The people with GBS also rated their experience of fatigue as significantly higher before the exercise, and tended to increase after the exercise, while the fatigue of healthy controls did not. The authors interpreted these findings as indicative of a possible change in muscle fiber type, and the loss of some motor units compared to pre-GBS status. A limited number of recovered motor axons in GBS would mean that the dropout of only a few motor units during sustained contraction would signal a relatively large central activation failure.[182]

Other Signs and Symptoms

ANS involvement, sensory deficits, and pain are also frequently seen to a greater or lesser extent in the clinical course of GBS.[183]

ANS symptoms are noted in about 50% of patients; both motor and sensory autonomic neurons may be affected. *Dysautonomia* may manifest as orthostatic hypotension, blood pressure instability, cardiac arrhythmias, and sometimes bowel and bladder dysfunction. It is relatively common in patients with GBS requiring ventilatory support and can compromise management of respiratory function or result in cardiac arrest (an emergency situation). Blood pressure fluctuation may result from demyelination of the vagus cranial nerve.[168] One study of 34 patients with GBS still showed some abnormal drop in blood pressure upon standing several years after GBS onset, although none of them complained of orthostatic problems.[184] Other typical ANS symptoms may result in peripheral pooling of blood (with consequent orthostatic hypotension), poor venous return, *ileus* (absence of contractile activity in the intestines), and urinary retention. In patients with paraplegia or tetraplegia at the nadir of GBS, approximately one-fourth had problems with urinary retention caused by detrusor areflexia or overactivity, overactive urethral sphincter, and disturbed bladder sensation.[167] However, bladder symptoms are generally slower to develop than other motor symptoms and tend to resolve more quickly. In fact, severe bowel or bladder dysfunction at initiation of symptom onset reduces the possibility that the diagnosis is GBS.[166]

One author states that other dysautonomic symptoms such as residual impotence[176] "settle with time."

Sensory symptoms such as distal hyperesthesias, paresthesias (tingling, burning), numbness, and decreased vibratory or position sense are common. The sensory disturbances often have a stocking-and-glove pattern rather than a dermatomal distribution of loss. Although the sensory problems are seldom disabling,[168] they can be disconcerting and upsetting to patients, especially when interpreted as pain during the acute stage. Uncomfortable *dysesthesias* are thought to result from the imbalance of sensory input from intact smaller, unmyelinated sensory fibers versus input from impaired larger, myelinated fibers. In some cases, response to pinprick, light touch, and vibration and proprioception may remain fairly normal or only mildly impaired (especially in GBS designated as the motor neuronal type, or AMAN) despite other sensory symptoms.

Pain associated with GBS can have heterogeneous origins, both *nociceptive* and *neuropathic*, and a careful evaluation is needed to treat it effectively. For example, nociceptive pain may stem from inflammation at the nerve roots and peripheral nerves or entrapment when the spinal nerve develops edema at the exit through the intervertebral foramen (review Fig. 15.15).[185] Neuropathic pain can arise from either central or peripheral sensitization in GBS, having been identified in the animal model of experimental autoimmune neuritis (EAN), which shows symptoms of polyradiculoneuropathy similar to GBS in humans.[174]

Pain was identified as a significant presenting symptom in the historical articles describing GBS[168]; in a more current study, pain reached its peak in the 2 weeks preceding the onset of weakness in about one-third of cases.[174] When pain presents as the first symptom of GBS, it is typically symmetrical, and at the midline of the back or in the gluteals, quadriceps, and hamstrings; lower leg and upper-extremity muscle pains are less common initially. This pain has been described as acute and worsening with activity or strenuous exercise; it is thought to reflect inflammation and entrapment of nerve roots. Because acute low back pain may have similarities to this initial pain, therapists who work with patients presenting with acute severe back pain must be alert to differentiating signs and symptoms: GBS initial pain develops quickly (over a few days) but is not associated with known injury or stress (which are frequently identifiable in low back pain); patients may also have paresthesias (pins and needles) in stocking and glove patterns rather than following nerve roots; patients with GBS may have vibratory perception loss, or multiple decreased tendon reflexes. Further, GBS will rapidly evolve with an onset of weakness either prior to pain or within days of its onset.

Pain experienced beyond the initial presentation is also common. A majority of patients with GBS (54% to 89%) report having significant pain during the acute stage of the disease, and 38% still report pain after 1 year post onset of weakness.[174]

Multiple pain types can occur simultaneously or sequentially in GBS.[185] Pain may manifest as paraesthesia or causalgia, with acute *hyperesthesias* or sensitivity to touch or air movement[186]; unless controlled pharmacologically, hyperesthesias can interfere with nursing care and limit therapy interventions. Muscle aching or cramping pain can last for days in weakened muscles (<3/5 MMT score) that have been overworked beyond capacity. Joint pains can occur as a result of lack of movement or overstretching when muscles are flaccid on one side of an unsupported joint. Some pain reported during convalescent stages has been described as "stiffness."

Secondary complications and residual deficits. Secondary problems can develop from severe weakness, pain, and the corresponding lack of activity. The possibility of DVT and pulmonary embolus must be monitored, especially in people who are not moving around as much as they did before disease onset; prophylactic treatment is sometimes used.[187] Pressure ulcers and pulmonary infections are also common secondary complications in GBS although most can be prevented with careful medical management.[164] Other complications can occur related to the severity of symptoms, side effects of mechanical ventilation or immunotherapy, autonomic dysfunction, or postinfection disorders.[188]

In 8% to 16% of those with GBS, individuals may show a reversal of direction of recovery, with relapse after a plateau or after movement starts to recover[183] in the first 8 weeks. This relapse may be called *treatment-related fluctuation*; some authors advise a second course of immunotherapy treatment, but the research regarding its effectiveness in such cases is lacking.[189]

Residual deficits in about 20% of people 1 year and more after onset of GBS can range from minimal impairments to impairments that limit activity and participation and prohibit return to prior levels of function. Many former GBS patients may prefer to avoid further medical scrutiny after a year plus of intense focus on their impairments. However, some residual deficits years post GBS onset may be successfully addressed with an intensive episode of rehabilitation.[190]

Medical Prognosis

Most patients have a *fulminating* course of GBS, in which the *disease develops suddenly and severely*. Many progress to maximal paralysis within 1 to 2 days of onset, 50% of patients reach the *nadir* (the point of greatest severity) within 1 week, 70% by 2 weeks, and 80% by 3 weeks. In some cases the process of increasing weakness continues for 1 to 2 months. If function continues to deteriorate, or if deterioration begins again after 8 weeks, the condition may be rediagnosed as acute onset of the chronic form of GBS, or CIDP. The acute and progressive stages of the acute forms of GBS are generally followed by a *plateau*, during which no further deterioration is evident, but no motor recovery has yet begun.

The *onset of recovery* varies, with most patients showing gradual recovery of muscle strength starting 2 to 4 weeks after the condition has plateaued. Once begun, recovery is typically protracted, with the most gains in the first year, but additional gains possible several years after the onset of symptoms.

The *extent of recovery* also varies, with about 33% claiming they are completely cured within a mean of 230 days (about 8 months) after onset of GBS.[191] Approximately 80% become ambulatory within 6 months of onset of symptoms. However, 50% to 67% of patients may show neurological deficits remaining at 1 year (e.g., loss of power,[191] diminished or absent tendon reflexes), but only about 15% have residual loss of function.[176] The most common long-term deficits are weakness of the anterior tibial musculature and, less often, weakness of the foot and hand intrinsic, quadriceps, and gluteal musculature. Motor and sensory disturbances may still affect work, home functioning, and leisure activities 1 to 5 years after onset. Fatigue or poor endurance is also noted as a long-term consequence of GBS, possibly attributable to deconditioning and muscular fatigue during the recuperative process.[180] Vajsar and colleagues[192] report that fatigue and poor exercise tolerance were common persisting symptoms in children who otherwise appeared to have fully recovered from acute GBS. Different studies show significant proportions of patients with continuing symptoms at 1, 2, 10, and 20 years: 43% were still affected psychologically[191] (mood changes, anxiety, and depression), and 14% were dependent in ADLs at 1 year, 17% were unable to work at 2 years,[193] 52% had some limitation in walking at 10 years,[194] and 10 out of 24 individuals noted severe fatigue 20 years[181] after GBS onset. Three percent to 5% of patients die of secondary cardiac, respiratory, or other systemic organ failure.[167]

Note that the chronicity of remaining impairments following acute GBS does not change the diagnosis to the chronic form of GBS or CIDP; CIDP depends on a relapsing course, where renewed deterioration results in worsening of symptoms after recovery begins.

Although not the focus of most studies on the long-term impact of GBS, *sensory deficits* (impaired response to pinprick, light touch, and vibration and proprioception in combination with other sensory losses) are an ongoing problem for some patients 1, 3, and 6 years after recovery from acute GBS. In a study of 90 patients who completed a survey at homecoming and 12 months after initiation of the disease process, 36% still had disturbed sensation in the arms and 60% had disturbed sensation in the legs[191] at 1 year. Similar percentages were noted in a different study of 122 individuals at 3 and 6 years after GBS onset.[195] The muscle aches and cramps experienced by some of these patients appeared to be related to sensory rather than persistent motor dysfunctions as usually thought. Sensory and persistent nociceptive abnormalities may be related to the smaller size of the neuronal fibers carrying information from the periphery to the spinal cord: one study in GBS showed that small myelinated fibers (A-δ fibers) are more likely than larger myelinated fibers to have myelin and axon impaired simultaneously,[196] potentially leading to prolonged recovery times.

Factors associated with a poor prognosis include severity of muscle weakness (especially tetraplegia), the need for respiratory support, cranial nerve involvement associated with loss of eye movement and swallowing, rapid rate of progression from onset, length of time to nadir, older age at onset, history of gastrointestinal illness, and recent cytomegalovirus infections.[167] In a study of 76 patients with GBS who had been in the intensive care unit (ICU), mechanical ventilation was associated with more morbidities and fatalities, although one of those who had been ventilated for over a year was eventually able to ambulate independently.[197] In a derivation cohort of 397 patients with GBS in Europe, the factors associated with slower recovery (inability to walk unaided 10 m at 1, 3, and 6 months after hospital admission) were increased age, lower combined strength score, and previous course of diarrhea.[198] In separate research, the Erasmus GBS Outcome Score[199] was developed that predicts whether a person will be able to walk independently at 6 months; the prognostic variables include age, preceding diarrhea, and the GBS disability score at 2 weeks. Individuals who have the Miller-Fisher type of GBS have a better prognosis, with complete recovery from eye muscle weakness, areflexia, and ataxia in 60% to 100% of patients after 6 months[183] with no more than supportive care.[200] A varying percentage (25% to 50%) of individuals with Miller-Fisher syndrome progress to developing limb weakness or bulbar symptoms that overlap with the more typical GBS presentation; in these cases, individuals may benefit from the addition of immunotherapy as part of their medical management although specific research in this subgroup is sparse.[183]

Medical Management

Medical treatment depends on the rate of progression and degree of paralysis and other symptoms. In mild cases of GBS showing limited weakness and sensory dysfunction, spontaneous recovery may occur with only monitoring over time. In moderate to severe cases, medical management is critical: early institution of immunotherapy can limit the progression of neural damage, and excellent supportive care can prevent secondary problems.[164] If an individual has rapid onset of pulmonary and cardiac manifestations of dysautonomia[187] or acute respiratory compromise, medical management can save a life.

Life Support

When an individual presents with rapid progression of severe weakness, hospitalization is the likely choice to provide supportive care and

Measure	Categories	Score
Days between onset of weakness and hospital admission	>7 days	0
	4–7 days	1
	≤3 days	2
Facial and/or bulbar weakness at hospital admission	Absence	0
	Presence	1
MRC sum score at hospital admission	60–51	0
	50–41	1
	40–31	2
	30–21	3
	≤20	4
EGRIS		0–7

Fig. 15.16 Erasmus Guillain-Barré Respiratory Insufficiency Score Model. Elements of the Erasmus Guillain-Barre Respiratory Insufficiency Score (EGRIS) predicting the need for mechanical ventilation in the first week of hospitalization. An EGRIS of 2 is associated with a probability of .08 of requiring mechanical ventilation in the first week; an EGRIS of 7 is associated with a .91 probability. *MRC*, Medical Research Council, the summed manual muscle test scores of a designated six pairs of limb muscles, each muscle scored 0 to 5, with 5 being normal. (Reproduced from Walgaard C, Lingsma HF, Ruts L, et al. Prediction of respiratory insufficiency in Guillain-Barré syndrome. *Ann Neurol.* 2010;67:781–787.)

monitoring. The individual may be monitored every 1 to 3 hours[164] for onset of respiratory insufficiency and continuously for cardiac arrhythmias and extreme BP fluctuations (exceeding 85 mm Hg). Monitoring for dysautonomia generally continues until the patient has discontinued ventilatory support, had tracheostomy removed, or begun to recover without needing either intervention.[179] Walgaard and colleagues[177] developed a model (Erasmus Guillain-Barré Respiratory Insufficiency Score [EGRIS]) to predict those who are more likely to require ventilatory assistance based on measures typically gathered upon hospital admission. EGRIS was developed on a cohort of 397 patients in Europe: 20 (5%) were intubated prior to hospitalization, 83 (22%) during the first week, and 16 (4%) during the second week of hospitalization. EGRIS included MRC (summed score from MMT of six pairs of bilateral muscles), rate of initial disease progression (by the number of days between weakness onset and hospitalization), and facial/bulbar weakness (Fig. 15.16).[177]

Patients who progress to respiratory deficiency must be treated in an intensive care environment where adequate respiratory function can be maintained, secondary infections can be prevented or limited, and metabolic functions can be carefully monitored. The patient is typically intubated for mechanical ventilation if functional VC falls below 20 mL/kg (or <60% of predicted value[161,201]) or PO$_2$ value falls below 75 mm Hg[202]; if VC, inspiratory, or expiratory pressures fall by more than 30% from baseline; if the patient has bulbar dysfunction (especially with aspiration); or if the patient is increasingly dyspneic even if VC is above the cutoff level.[202] Intubation is considered invasive ventilation and may be performed with an endotracheal tube or via tracheostomy.[82] One consensus document noted that tracheostomy can be delayed for 2 weeks to see if pulmonary function tests improve with just the endotracheal tube. If function does not improve in that time, transition to tracheostomy intubation may be performed to increase patient comfort and airway safety, and make weaning easier.[179,203] Twenty-five percent of patients who experience respiratory failure will develop pneumonia. Even if daytime respiration seems adequate, night-time respiratory insufficiency (sleep-disordered breathing) should be suspected if patients have persistent sleepiness or fatigue.[180]

Psychological Support

Patients with GBS who are in the ICU on ventilation, with varying levels of paralysis and sensory dysfunction, will require management to address psychological and communicative concerns. Patients may feel trapped and out of control if severe paralysis and respiratory equipment hinder them from expressing their needs. These patients can usually hear well, and most can see what is happening around them. They benefit from being oriented to time, having the health care personnel explain all procedures, and having some means of obtaining help. In one study, patients without vocal communication or means of activating a call light were trained to hold their breath for 12 seconds to trigger the apnea alarm of the ventilator, set at 12 seconds, to indicate when they needed additional pain medication.[186] Therapists can work with the ICU staff to provide the patient with other forms of communication, such as eye blink, clicking, and communication boards designed for their needs. Having some form of communication and knowing that they will not be left alone will help prevent traumatic stress reactions.[187]

Immunotherapy

As monitoring and supportive care get underway, one of two specific immunotherapy-based treatments will usually begin. Both have good evidence-based support to decrease the duration of ventilator dependence and time to the beginning of recovery if initiated within 2 weeks of symptom onset. In *plasma exchange* (also known as *plasmapheresis*), the blood plasma is purified (to decrease the concentration of pathological autoantibodies)[200] by extracting the blood and processing it outside of the body, and then reinjecting it.[188] In essence, blood is extracted through a vein, the blood plasma is separated from cells using membrane filtration or centrifugation and removed; the cellular component is reinfused along with a replacement solution consisting of fresh frozen plasma, albumin or saline, or doubly-filtrated auto-plasma to maintain the individual's blood volume during the process. One plasma volume is exchanged on five separate occasions, usually every 2 days.[188] In *intravenous immunoglobulin* (IVIg), human plasma from over 1000 donors is purified, marketed, and injected into a vein of the patient. The injected immunoglobulin seems to neutralize pathogenic antibodies, inhibit complement activation, and modify macrophage activity.[200]

Moderate evidence supports plasma exchange as decreasing recovery time and improving outcome at 1 year compared to supportive care alone.[204] Plasma exchange is most beneficial if begun within the first week of diagnosis and can be beneficial up to 30 days after diagnosis.[204] Plasma exchange is also cost-effective as used in patients with mild, moderate, or severe courses of GBS.[166,205] IVIg is somewhat safer and easier to administer than plasma exchange: IVIg requires only one peripheral vein for injection (plasma exchange requires two, one of which must accept a high flow volume, and possibly insertion of a central venous line), no special equipment for plasma separation or purification, and no specifically trained personnel to complete the procedure. IVIg speeds recovery by the same amount of time as plasma exchange in adults and is more effective than supportive care in children.[206] High-quality evidence supports IVIg use in adults with GBS; the quality of evidence is slightly less high to support its use in children with GBS.[189] Evidence comparing IVIg with plasma exchange is mixed. In one randomized comparison, plasma exchange resulted in better muscle strength, disability levels, and biochemical indicators

at 2 weeks after intervention.[207] In a trial in which treatment was applied according to economic level of the patient, the group receiving IVIg (the more costly alternative in many health care settings perhaps because of the need for processing plasma from 1000s of human donors) outperformed the group receiving plasma exchange in length of ICU stay, time to beginning of recovery, and weaning off of mechanical ventilation.[208] In a retrospective study comparing outcomes of 1166 patients with GBS, disability outcomes were equivalent at 2, 6, and 12 months, although those with IVIg (with a relatively higher economic status) had a shorter hospital stay on average.[166] Adding IVIg to plasma exchange does not improve time to recovery any more than either treatment alone.[206] Thus the standard therapy for any patient with GBS having a 2 or higher disability score (walking is impaired) is to treat with *either* plasma exchange *or* IVIg, but not both. The American Academy of Neurology has published practice parameters guiding the dosage of these immunological interventions.[209]

Pharmacotherapy for Pain

Gabapentin and carbamazepine, both anticonvulsant drugs, have each been used successfully to decrease neuropathic pain in people with GBS in the ICU, with advantages for those taking gabapentin in decreasing pain and minimizing demand for fentanyl (used as a supplementary analgesic).[186] Although corticosteroids have been used to decrease the inflammatory process in GBS since the 1960s, an RCT showed no significant reduction in pain with methylprednisolone,[174] and a review of studies showed that corticosteroid treatment alone does not hasten recovery from GBS.[210] If pain is more related to muscle and joint aching, acetaminophen or other simple analgesics and NSAIDs may suffice[179] for short-term relief.

Other Supportive Management

Additional supportive treatment generally includes enteral nutrition for those with dysphagia, bladder catheterization for severely affected patients along with pharmacological agents for ileus, antibiotics for pulmonary infections, and heparin or other medications as prophylaxis against DVT. Although no studies have been published in GBS, heparin and support stockings have evidence supporting their effectiveness at reducing risk of DVT in other populations of nonambulatory acutely ill or postoperative patients[179] and are recommended by consensus. Pressure ulcers can usually be prevented with air mattresses, regularly scheduled turning and repositioning of the patient, and use of padding over pressure points[186] such as elbows, knees, and heels.

So far, no pharmaceutical agents have been helpful in alleviating fatigue in this population. In a study of the use of amantadine to relieve severe fatigue in 74 patients with GBS randomly allocated to treatment or placebo groups, the groups showed no difference in any of the primary or secondary measures recorded.[211]

Medical management for CIDP, the chronic form of GBS, has its foundation in the management choices for the acute onset of GBS, with IVIg as a first line medication. Because of the long-term nature of the relapsing and chronic impairments, corticosteroids have also been used successfully in many patients.[212] Articles that focus specifically on CIDP provide information about other differences in medical management for this relapsing form of the disease[213,214] but were not reviewed for this chapter. A case report of a patient with CIDP from the perspective of the PT has also been published.[215]

Therapeutic Management of Movement Dysfunction Associated With Guillain-Barré Syndrome

Therapeutic management of the movement deficits associated with GBS includes supportive management during the acute and progressive phases, prevention of long-term medical comorbidities during the plateau, and staged rehabilitation throughout recovery.[201] Unfortunately, direct evidence and controlled trials to support rehabilitation is sparse in GBS,[179] and clinicians must make assumptions based on similarities with other populations (e.g., poliomyelitis and peripheral neuropathies) at various stages. With the assumption that the patient will have significant return of function within months, rehabilitation professionals must help maintain the integrity of functioning systems, address pain and other complaints, teach compensatory strategies, and appropriately promote increasing activity as patients regain mobility. The immediate needs of the patient will change as the patient moves through the acute stage, the plateau at the nadir, the beginning of recovery, and later recovery stages of GBS before and after muscles attain antigravity (3/5 MMT) strength. Transitioning between the therapeutic goals required at each stage necessitates careful examination of the current status, progression of the disease, and needs of the patient.

In direct contrast to ALS, the stages of GBS frequently start with hospitalization and progress through to clinical and outpatient care. Hospitals and ICUs are where a multidisciplinary team is typically most available. If a patient moves to an inpatient rehabilitation unit, multidisciplinary care hopefully continues, with team planning and common goal setting with the patient as the prime decision maker. In this setting, functional improvement can occur, as recorded using Functional Independence Measure (FIM) scores, and this improvement is retained 6 months later.[216,217] Unfortunately, as patients transition to home care and independence, they may have less access to some of the disciplines they need to address lingering impairments. Research assessing the effects of a multidisciplinary team in GBS is lacking,[218] with only one controlled trial identified.[190] Low-quality studies show that inpatient rehabilitation is effective in improving function and decreasing disability, but the data are only available from the beginning recovery stages, not in the protracted time frames in which many people with GBS experience impairments. When multidisciplinary resources are not available, each clinician must be prepared to screen for important components of patients' needs and intervene and refer appropriately. Clinicians must also advocate for patients who have not received an order for physical therapy, for example, either as an inpatient or after discharge, because of the disability that remains for some who are independent in basic functions.[219]

Examination

Rehabilitation professionals will specifically address body function impairments, activity limitations, and participation restrictions related to GBS (see Fig. 15.4), along with environmental and personal factors, using standardized measures where possible. A typical examination of a patient's movement and function includes the following components. As in ALS, different rehabilitation specialists will target assessment depending on the standards of their discipline, modifying from comprehensive lists such as that found in the Guide to Physical Therapist Practice.[98] Considerations specific to GBS are shown in Box 15.9. The extent of the examination in any one session depends on the patient's condition and ability to participate.

- **Patient History.** Chart review and history taking should extract the course of the disease across what time period, along with any recent illness (especially gastrointestinal or respiratory tract infection in the 4 weeks preceding symptom onset), recent vaccinations, preexisting neuromotor or other medical conditions, current concerns, and the patient's immediate goals.
- **Systems Review.** Screening tests can help determine whether cranial nerves or sensory and autonomic systems are involved along

---

BOX 15.9   Considerations Specific to the Examination of Patients With Guillain-Barré Syndrome

Chart Review, Patient History

Patterns and sequence of symptom onset

Recent illness, vaccination, or injury

Prior episodes of sensorimotor problems

Comorbidities

Current medical management

Patient complaints and preferences

Systems Review

Vital signs critical: Blood pressure resting and immediately after activity (prone, sitting, standing, if possible); heart rate resting and immediately after activity, dysrhythmias

Body temperature stability; respiration stability

Skin integrity (for redness or decubitus ulcers in patients who are immobile): visually inspect pressure points (bony prominences that might develop pressure sores) in supine, side-lying, and sitting positions

Communication (augmentation required?)

Comorbidities

Tests and Measures

Visual inspection to identify symmetry of muscle bulk, fasciculations, and function

Stretch reflexes

Movement ability of body region(s) with deficits

    Flexibility: Range of Motion (use a form for serial recording)

    Strength: Manual muscle testing, carefully identifying pattern of weakness (testing should be muscle specific as possible rather than assessing muscle groups only; recommend use of a standardized form for serial recording of muscle testing)

Accuracy: Observe/record ataxia/dysmetria in upper and lower extremities, trunk, neck, bulbar areas; perform rapid alternating movements as appropriate

Speed: Timed tasks in motions where primary movers have against-gravity capability

Adaptability: Ability to change movement as obstacles or the environment changes

Endurance: Questionnaires for experienced fatigue, circumstances; test fatigability

Cranial nerve testing/screening, especially oculomotor

Balance, static and dynamic, sitting and standing (if testable)

Functional status (activities of daily living, participation in life, eating, bowel and bladder function, and ambulation) in the patient's natural environment or simulated circumstances

Sensation: Pattern and type of sensory loss or changes (e.g., paresthesias, anesthesia, and hypoesthesias)

Pain: Intensity, type, and location (use body chart); what aggravates/eases?

Psychosocial systems: Identify patient and family concerns in acute circumstances and projections about long-term issues. Refer for social worker evaluation of financial resources, day-to-day living problems (e.g., transportation and child care), support systems, and coping strategies

Quality of life, including sleep, well-being

Environmental adaptations and equipment relevant to current and projected status

Electrodiagnostic testing: Nerve conduction velocity; electromyography. (These studies to be performed by a clinician skilled in the procedures. This may be a physical therapist, physician, or technician depending on facility.)

with motor systems in the trunk and limbs. Checking vital signs (heart rate, blood pressure, respiratory rate, and ease of breathing) at rest and immediately after activity, assessing skin integrity especially in immobile patients, screening cranial nerve performance, and noting communication ability are all important components. Additional testing of sensation (and documentation on a body chart, for example) or autonomic systems may be required if the screening tests indicate a potential problem. Cognition may be screened. Referral to appropriate health care professionals may be indicated.

- **Tests and Measures.** Body functions to be tested include the six dimensions of movement,[2] pain, sensation, and specific impairments such as dysarthria, dysphagia, and respiratory function. Both primary and secondary effects should be recorded, along with relevant activity limitations, participation restrictions, and environmental and personal factors affecting function. Any Clinical Practice Guidelines regarding core sets of outcome measures should be followed as appropriate.[99]
  - Strength (a primary target of GBS) and flexibility (a secondary effect of loss of movement) require serial documentation to track the patient's course of progression or improvement. MMT, dynamometry, grip strength, or isokinetic testing may be useful in various stages to test strength; goniometry is typically used for ROM testing and flexibility. Patterns of weakness associated with contractures (such as significantly decreased voluntary movement or asymmetries of strength on the two sides of a joint) may be noted, and the appropriate level of passive or active stretching can be planned. Full MMT and joint ROM assessment may require several sessions in the initial stages. Following the initial assessment or after the recovery stage begins, a few specific muscles and joints may be selected to test for changes weekly (e.g., the muscles designated for the MRC summed score; grip strength; sternocleidomastoids, deltoids, triceps, flexor carpi ulnaris, lumbricals, iliopsoas, gluteus medius, anterior tibialis, and flexor hallucis longus; and shoulders, fingers, and ankles).
  - Endurance can be recorded using amount of activity tolerated (with specific symptoms noted before rest is required), time on a task (e.g., "tolerated 6 minutes of sitting before requiring rest in a reclining position," or "able to sustain a muscular force for 15 seconds before strength deficit"), perceived exertion (RPE scale), or work performed in a designated time period (meters walked in 6 minutes). Physical measures of endurance may be called fatigability measures. Self-report measures of fatigue include questionnaires such as the FSS, Fatigue Impact Scale (FIS), Modified Fatigue Impact Scale (MFIS),[176] or the VAS-F.[180] Note that several factors may interfere with complete assessment of strength, flexibility, and endurance in the acute and progressive stages. Patients who report considerable pain during handling or active movement may not tolerate standard procedures, or may be unwilling or unable to cooperate with testing. Fatigue and respiratory difficulties may also preclude complete strength assessment in a single session. Fatigue in the initial stages may result from increased effort to activate weakened muscles and inability to maintain force generation for function.[96] As recovery begins, fatigue can also be related to deconditioning.
    - Pain may be tracked by level and type on a visual analogue scale (VAS-pain), numeric rating scale (NRS-pain), and body chart, or the Dallas Pain Questionnaire.[176] Tracking pain can help distinguish between weakness and loss of ROM related to pathological condition, immobility, or pain. Pain should also be tracked to observe response to intervention.

- Sensation should be assessed using proprioception tests (e.g., through passive movement at index finger and big toe)[184] as well as light touch (e.g., Semmes-Weinstein monofilaments) and vibratory (e.g., biothesiometry; 128 Hz tuning fork at base of finger and thumb)[184] measures.
- Other dimensions of movement may be assessed. *Accuracy* should be assessed if signs of ataxia are observed, such as when the individual has the Miller-Fisher type of GBS. Rapid alternating movements of the hands or feet are common tasks that are timed for 10 repetitions, or counted for number of repetitions in a 10 second period. Ataxia can also be assessed using a standardized tool such as the Scale for the Assessment and Rating of Ataxia (SARA), which contains eight performance-based items rated on an ordinal scale, with higher numbers indicating more severe ataxia.[220] The SARA has positive psychometric features when used in other neurological populations such as multiple sclerosis.[221] *Adaptability* may be observed as the ability to resume a task when a trajectory is perturbed; if the individual is ambulatory, the Functional Gait Assessment[99] standardizes assessment of adaptability. *Speed* of movement can be recorded by timing the completion of functional tasks.
- Functional tests (at the activity level of the ICF model) may include standardized scales of independence in ADLs or balance, tests of manual dexterity, and temporal measures of gait, although few standardized measures are specifically validated in GBS. Chehebar and colleagues[201] compared three standardized functional scales: the GBS disability scale, Barthel Index, and the FIM. The GBS disability scale is specific to this population and is widely used in research, but with scores only ranging from 0 to 6, it does not have the granularity to reflect small changes. The Barthel Index and FIM are able to document change in other neurological populations; while the Barthel Index is more economic and practical, neither is detailed enough to direct clinical decision making for individual patients.[201] The FIM has reflected improved independence in patients with GBS following inpatient rehabilitation[216]: in 1079 older adult patients with GBS, the average improvement in mobility was 144%; in self-care it was 84.1%; and in cognition it was 51.7%. The FIM has shown sensitivity in detecting disability in people with GBS and improvement correlates with decreased requirement for mechanical ventilation.[176] Other functional tests recommended in GBS include the Canadian Occupational Performance Measure and the Modified Rankin Scale.[176] Balance tests may include the Function in Sitting Test (standardized for low-level patients post-stroke), the Berg Balance Scale[176] (for those able to stand upright), Tinetti Assessment Tools, or the more advanced Functional Gait Assessment[99] that uniquely documents adaptability while walking. Tests of manual dexterity could include the Box and Block Test of Manual Dexterity[176] and the 9-Hole-Peg Test. Measures of gait could include the 10 m or 25-foot walk test (25FWT), Timed-Up-and-Go (TUG), 6MWT, digital gait analysis,[222] or measures of stride length and cadence.
- *Dysarthria*, *dysphagia*, and *respiration* should be tested in the acute and progressive stages and thereafter if the individual had these impairments acutely. Review Table 15.1 for items to consider; unlike ALS, patients with GBS rarely show spasticity and may have sensory loss in the face in addition to motor losses. A simple estimate of VC can be done at bedside. If, after taking a large breath, the patient can count out loud only to 10, the total VC is approximately 1 L and intubation may be considered.[223] Some clinicians recommend cervical auscultation to listen to swallowing sounds during the acute phase of GBS, and listening

to breath sounds for indications of aspiration. With evidence of swallowing difficulties and possible aspiration, the patient should be referred for comprehensive testing with videofluoroscopy. Other referrals for bulbar evaluation may be considered to an ear, nose, and throat specialist, speech-language pathologist, or communication disorders clinic unless full evaluation is available in the facility or at a comprehensive neurology clinic.

- Quality-of-life measures (at the participation level of the ICF model) have not been generated that are specific to people with GBS. Health-related quality-of-life measures used in related populations (neuromuscular diseases) include the Nottingham Health Profile and the SF-36, which have the advantage of including a fatigue component labeled as "energy" and "vitality," respectively.[96] Recommended measures may also include the Sickness Impact Profile,[224] Rotterdam 9-item scale (regarding disadvantages during specific tasks), and the Handicap Assessment Scale.[176] A new measure has been developed for inflammatory neuropathies, the IN-QoL,[225] that was shown to be responsive to change in GBS. It may be useful in future trials. Assessment of environmental factors might include the Environmental Status Scale, which assesses restriction in participation.[176]

Forsberg and colleagues[226] provide a comprehensive list of tests they administered in a prospective study of 42 patients followed for 2 years after the onset of GBS. At 2 weeks post onset, 40 of 42 patients had submaximal scores on total muscle strength, grip strength, balance, and gait speed testing. At 2 months, total muscle strength was still most affected, whereas 25% of the patients had regained maximal grip strength, balance, and gait speed (designated as 1.4 to 1.5 m/s). By 2 years, more than half of the subjects still lacked the maximum total muscle score, and 40% claimed fatigue. Sensory deficits were claimed by up to 36% of patients at 2 years.[226] Thus tests of strength, balance, gait speed, fatigue, and perception of sensory deficits remain relevant 2 years post diagnosis of GBS.

Changes in the patient's condition should be monitored with serial MMT, ROM assessments, sensory testing, and functional status examinations. Before the patient is discharged from the hospital or rehabilitation unit, therapists should complete an assessment of the patient's home environment so that appropriate safety and adaptive equipment can be in place in time for the patient's return home.

Intervention Goals

General goals for the care of the patient with GBS, to be specified with reference to the patient's status and preferences, include the following:

- Facilitate resolution of respiratory problems, communication difficulties, and dysphagia.
- Minimize pain and desensitize dysesthesias.
- Prevent contractures, decubitus ulcers, and injury to weakened or denervated muscles.
- Optimize strength and endurance through judiciously progressive resistance and aerobic exercise while monitoring overuse and fatigue.
- Prescribe and update as necessary appropriate adaptive equipment, wheelchairs, and orthoses to optimize function.
- Resume psychosocial roles at optimal level and improve quality of life.

Therapeutic Interventions

In a Cochrane review focused on people with peripheral neuropathies, no randomized or quasi-RCTs of exercise or rehabilitation were identified for patients with GBS as of September 2009.[171] Since then, one RCT has been conducted.[190] In addition several intervention studies have been reported that do not have randomization and may only compare to healthy controls (Table 15.3). Many of the therapeutic recommendations therefore come from consensus of experts based on clinical experience with GBS and disorders that result in similar impairments and activity limitations.

TABLE 15.3 Summary of Exercise Studies Since the Year 2000 in Guillain-Barré Syndrome

Author	Study Population (Sample Size): Research Design	Duration of Training	Training Modality	Training Protocol	Response(s)
El Mhandi et al., 2007[227]	GBS first week of recovery stage (6): Pragmatic cohort study; healthy controls (6)	3–4 weeks inpatient, 4–10 weeks outpatient and home exercise program	Individualized inpatient and outpatient rehabilitation: muscular reinforcement and active mobilizations	Outpatient consisted of 2–3 physical therapy sessions per week	Outcomes assessed at 6, 12, and 18 months after recovery began: increase in MVIC and isokinetic strength noted at all time periods in knee, elbow, shoulder, and ankle muscles
Graham et al., 2007[228]	GBS >1 year after nadir (10), CIDP stable for 6 months, (4); healthy controls (8): case-control intervention study	12 weeks	10 min warm up at below 60% of peak heart rate, 20 min of aerobic ex at 65%–85% of peak heart rate, isometric strengthening exercises sustained 10-s maximal isometric contractions, functional activity practice, major muscle group stretches	3 times a week for 36 sessions, unsupervised, community-based strengthening, aerobic, functional exercise program	Improvements at end of program were retained at 6-month follow-up: Overall Disability Sum Score improvement, physical function score of SF-36, Fatigue Severity Score, Anxiety, Depression; both patients and healthy controls showed moderate increases at end of program in isometric muscle strength of trained muscles, able to exercise at peak load for longer duration

TABLE 15.3 Summary of Exercise Studies Since the Year 2000 in Guillain-Barré Syndrome—cont'd

Author	Study Population (Sample Size): Research Design	Duration of Training	Training Modality	Training Protocol	Response(s)
Garssen et al., 2004[182]; Bussman et al., 2007[229]	GBS with fatigue, stable for 3 months (16); CIDP with fatigue, stable (4); healthy controls (10): case control intervention study	12 weeks	Bicycle exercise training for patients but not controls	3 times per week, supervised; 5 min of warm up (65% of maximum heart rate) and 30 min of cycling (70%–90% max heart rate); 5–10 min of cool down	20% fatigue severity reduction, improvement in fatigue impact, anxiety, depression, physical component of SF-36, isokinetic muscle strength elbow and knee
Khan et al., 2011[190]	GBS, chronic phase (79): RCT, individuals assigned to high intensity or lower intensity treatment groups	Up to 12 weeks	Experimental group: multidisciplinary training, three 1-h sessions consisting of half-hour blocks of PT, OT, psych, speech, social; control: home based program of maintenance ex and education for self management plus 30 min activity (walking, stretching)	Experimental group: 2–3 times per week for 12 weeks; control: 2 times a week	Assessment at 12 months: Treatment group had significantly higher scores on FIM (mobility, self-care, continence) and relationships than controls

CIDP, Chronic inflammatory demyelinating polyradiculoneuropathy; *ex*, exercise; *FIM*, Functional Independence Measure; *GBS*, Guillain-Barré syndrome; *max*, maximum; *MVIC*, maximal voluntary isometric contract; *OT*, Occupational Therapist; *PT*, physical therapist; *RCT*, randomized controlled trial; *ROM*, range of motion.

Respiratory dysfunction, communication difficulties, dysphagia. Depending on the facility, PTs may be involved in the respiratory care of patients with GBS. PTs may conduct chest percussion, breathing exercises, resistive inspiratory training, or strict protocols to prevent overfatigue of respiratory muscles while weaning patients from mechanical ventilation.[176] A therapist working in a clinic or small community hospital may be the first person to note a patient's changing respiratory status during an evaluation and treatment session for muscle weakness or acute back pain. That therapist must be prepared to alert medical staff about the need to test oxygen saturation levels and VC. Likewise, if the patient has mild symptoms at admission, the patient may not seem to require intensive care. If the patient is not continuously monitored for autonomic function, the therapist should be on the lookout for rapid onset or life-endangering symptoms requiring emergent intervention.[230]

Goals of treatment for respiratory impairment are related to increasing ventilation or oxygenation, decreasing oxygen consumption, controlling secretions, and improving exercise tolerance. See Irwin and Tecklin[223] for coverage of treatment programs and techniques appropriate for the GBS patient with acute or residual respiratory dysfunction.

When patients have endotracheal intubation, communication can be difficult and frustrating, especially if general paralysis also hinders writing or pointing to a communication board. The rehabilitation team can help develop and execute alternative means of communication. If phonation is effortful, supported posture in an upright and aligned position may help coordinate breathing and speech. Readers are also referred to Box 15.6 for recommended strategies to manage dysarthria and effortful speaking.

In the more severe cases of GBS, cranial nerve involvement can lead to dysphagia and vocal cord paralysis. Therapeutic goals are the prevention of choking and aspiration and the stimulation of effective swallowing, eating, and oral speech.

In many facilities, speech pathologists, or OTs are responsible for establishing a dysphagia treatment program. However, all health care personnel may need to participate in preventing aspiration, by helping patients maintain an upright position for 30 to 60 minutes after feeding through a tube or promoting effective swallowing and eating with upright positioning and head tilted slightly forward. The act of chewing and swallowing is complex and requires coordinated reflexive and conscious action. Intervention is focused on positioning, head control, and oral-motor coordination (e.g., sucking an ice cube, stimulating the gag response, facilitating swallowing with quick pressure on the neck and thyroid notch timed with intent to swallow). A conscious swallowing technique is introduced with thick liquids and progressed to thinner liquids after the patient's oral-motor coordination response is enough to control movement of fluids. Once the patient has good lip closure, fluids should be introduced one sip at a time from a straw cut to a short length to minimize effort. Semisoft, moist foods are gradually introduced (pasta, mashed potatoes, squash, gelatin). Any crumbly or stringy foods (coffee cakes, cookies, snack chips, celery, and cheeses) should be avoided, and the patient should not attempt to talk or be interrupted during eating until choking episodes no longer occur and swallowing is comfortable and consistent. Feeding training should occur during frequent, short sessions to prevent fatigue. Therapists should be prepared to use the Heimlich maneuver if choking occurs or have a suction machine available at bedside. Readers are referred to the section on medical management of ALS for additional suggestions on dysphagia management.

Pain. Pain may be a major factor limiting the patient's passive or active motion, and the treatment team should determine the best approach to alleviate pain. Medical management alone may not reduce pain to 0, and many studies examine the effects of pharmacological agents only in the acute and active rehabilitation stage. No studies have examined interventions for pain in the later recovery stage (3 months and following). A combination of positioning and passive to active movement may be helpful, but no controlled trials have provided evidence to support nonpharmacological treatments for pain in GBS.

Sensory treatments may be of benefit to reduce the experience of pain. Transcutaneous electrical nerve stimulation (TENS) might be an adjuvant treatment option to help with desensitization in patients whose pain is not controlled with passive movement or pain medications.[176] Another option is capsaicin,[231] the active ingredient in chili peppers, which when applied topically interacts with the sensory neurons to relieve pain from peripheral neuropathies. Therapists, wearing gloves, may apply a topical anesthetic until the area is numb. The capsaicin is then applied topically. The capsaicin remains on the skin until the patient starts to feel the heat, at which point it is promptly removed using soap and water. Because the nerves are overstimulated by the burning sensation, the sensory gateway is unable to report pain for an extended period.[231] A high-concentration capsaicin patch has been studied with good results in people with peripheral neuropathies with other etiologies, but not in GBS.[232]

Some patients who experience extreme sensitivity to light touch, such as from movement of sheets, air flow, and intermittent touch contact, benefit from a "cradle" that holds sheets away from the body. Some find relief if the limbs are wrapped snugly with elastic bandages, which provide continuous low pressure while warding off light and intermittent stimuli. Alternatively, the patient's pain response can be desensitized through methodical stimulation with frequent, consistent stimuli to the affected area for short durations to allow acclimatization.[176]

A randomized pilot study of yoga using meditation, relaxation, and breathing techniques 5 days a week for 3 weeks resulted in improved self-reported sleep in patients with GBS, but no difference in pain, anxiety, depression, or functional scales compared with a group that had the same inpatient rehabilitation without the yoga.[233] In fact, both groups had significant reduction in average pain on a numeric pain rating scale. Thus it may be that usual multidisciplinary rehabilitation itself is partly responsible. The authors reported that both groups received pharmacotherapy, physiotherapy (ROM, stretching, strengthening with weights, breathing exercises, and gait training), and occupational therapy (ADL training, hand function training, trunk stability training, and education about transfer techniques).[233]

Contractures, decubitus ulcers, and injury to weakened or denervated muscles

Positioning. A consensus statement arising from a review of the literature plus expert opinion for a group of scientists and clinicians specializing in GBS recommended that rehabilitation should focus on proper limb positioning, posture, orthotics, and nutrition.[179] Positioning and passive ROM to prevent contractures and decubitus ulcers is particularly important in the acute stage.[234]

Positioning to prevent pressure sores starts within the first few days of hospitalization, especially for the patient who has complete or nearly complete paralysis along with loss of sensation. A positioning program for the dependent patient is the first line of defense against decubitus ulcers and pulmonary infection, with turning at least every 2 hours for both pressure relief and lung drainage. The rehabilitation team may assist nursing personnel in determining positions that do not excessively stress vulnerable (flaccid) joints and create pictures to place by the bed to assist persons on each shift to follow the prescribed schedule and positions. In addition, the patient may have a special mattress or mattress unit that constantly changes the pressure within the mattress to shift the patient's position or is designed to spread pressure over wide surfaces. Patients who are slender or who have lost

significant muscle mass from GBS-induced atrophy will have prominent bony surfaces; the therapist may need to fashion foam "doughnuts" or pads or use sheepskin-type protection for pressure relief. Nerves are especially vulnerable to pressure in this state; the ulnar, peroneal, and cutaneous femoral nerves should all be protected with padding and positioning to avoid compression.[176] Patients who have muscle pain may prefer to have their hips and knees flexed. If so, the patient must be taken out of the flexed position for part of each hour to avoid muscle shortening.

As part of a complete positioning program, therapists should consider how best to maintain the physiological position of the hands and feet. Research has shown that mild continuous stretch maintained for at least 20 minutes is more beneficial than stronger, brief stretching exercises. Thus the use of splints for prolonged positioning is superior to the use of short bursts of intermittent, manually applied passive stretching to attain functional range. Although some facilities still use a footboard to control passive ankle plantarflexion, most therapists now use moldable plastic splints that can be worn when the patient is in any position. Because ankle-foot splints often prevent visual inspection of the heel position, care must be taken to ensure that the heel is firmly down in the orthosis and that the strapping pattern is adequate to secure the foot. The strap system must be simple enough to be positioned properly by all staff and family members caring for the patient. The ankle-foot splint should extend slightly beyond the end of the toes to prevent toe flexion and skin breakdown from the toes rubbing on sheets. Care should be taken not to compress the peroneal nerve with the splint as it crosses the fibula, a particularly vulnerable area after the loss of muscle mass in the lower legs from the GBS. Wrist and hand splints may be prefabricated, resting-style splints, or molded to meet the patient's specific needs. Because spasticity is not typically a problem in the patient with GBS, a simple cone or rolled cloth may be adequate to maintain good wrist, thumb, and finger alignment for short-term immobility.

Range of motion. With paralysis in GBS comes the risk of muscle shortening and joint contractures.[179] ROM is the best defense against such impairments. To be effective, the ROM program must start within the first couple of days of hospitalization and include both accessory and physiological motions to increase circulation; provide lubrication of the joints; and maintain extensibility of capsular, muscle, and tendon tissue. Special attention should be paid to 2-joint muscles (hamstrings and gastrocnemius), which are at greater risk for shortening.[176] Passive ROM exercises to the ends of normal range for all extremity joints, fingers and toes, neck, and trunk should be performed twice daily—more frequently if the patient has no active movement. Patients can be instructed to perform the ROM exercises themselves if they can move actively without pain or fatigue; during the acute stage of declining strength, they should be observed during ROM activities to ensure adequacy of the range and any changes in quality of movement. If the patient cannot complete movement through full range independently, a therapist or well-instructed and monitored caregiver can assist the patient in moving to the end of range. This may not be easy if the patient has pain with touch or motion. Knowing whether to "push through the pain" or stay within the limits of pain is often a great dilemma for the therapist. The therapist needs to find a balance between working for full joint range and reacting to the patient's reports of pain. If the ends of ranges become stiff, stretch should be slow and sustained at the endpoint for 10 to 30 seconds. Orthotic devices might assist in maintaining prolonged stretch at the end ranges of some joints.

Some patients will prefer to position their limbs so muscle and tendons are in the shortened range in an attempt to decrease muscle pain. This may lead to capsular contractures. The therapist should note changes in "end feel" over time when testing ROM of each joint to determine if capsular and ligamentous structures are also becoming more restricted as the muscle and tendon tissue shortens. Patients who have intact sensation of pain and temperature may respond positively to the use of heat (up to approximately 45°C or 113°F) before stretching to decrease muscle pain and facilitate tissue elongation before stretching. For safety reasons, heat should not be used on a patient with a sensory deficit that inhibits ability to distinguish differences in temperature.

Injury prevention. Denervated and weakened muscles can be injured easily; the therapist is responsible for ensuring that ROM activities are done with appropriate support of the limb to prevent sudden overstretching and possible damage of joint structures. Instruction to caregivers regarding passive ROM activities must include details such as externally rotating the shoulder during abduction to prevent impingement and ensuring that the subtalar joint is in the neutral position during dorsiflexion to avoid overstretching of the midfoot. In inpatient settings where the patient is treated by a changing staff of therapists or nurses or by family members, a positioning schedule with diagrams, a splinting plan, and ROM recommendations should be presented in poster format at the patient's bedside to facilitate consistent treatment.

ROM can usually be maintained with standard positioning and ROM programs. Nevertheless, some patients, especially those who have severe extremity and axial pain early during the disease process and those who have been quadriplegic and ventilator dependent for prolonged periods, may develop significant joint contractures despite preventive interventions. As with patients with spinal cord or severe head injuries, heterotopic ossification can occur with immobility-related hypercalcemia.[179] Early mobilization was associated with therapeutic decreases in serum calcium levels in one study.[179] Aggressive ROM (but not hard or abrupt movements that may injure the muscle) may impede the effects of heterotopic bone overgrowth that can have a severe impact on ROM. Once heterotopic ossification has been identified, treatment includes modification of ROM exercise to use only the pain-free arc for active and passive motion.[176]

Massage may play a positive role in maintaining muscle tissue mobility and tissue nutrition while limiting the amount of intramuscular fibrosis development. The use of massage in patients with GBS has not been reported; however, it may be a useful adjunct to ROM exercises in patients who do not have marked hypersensitivity to touch, significant muscle pain, or a history of DVT. Patients with or without a history of DVT who are immobile for long periods or who have concomitant cardiac illnesses may have marked pooling of fluids with swelling of the distal limbs and orthostatic hypotension.[179] After medical clearance, edema-specific massage and limb-elevation techniques may be useful if tolerated by the patient. Early active ROM exercises creating "muscle pumping" contractions in muscles with at least fair strength (3/5 MMT) can help prevent uncomfortable edema.

Optimizing Strength and Endurance While Monitoring for Overuse and Fatigue

Although most patients with GBS recover from the paralysis, the course and rate of recovery may vary significantly among patients. With such a variable natural course, it is difficult to tell whether any particular exercise program has a positive effect unless compared against a control group. However, few controlled studies have been conducted to examine exercise in GBS. No controlled evidence exists to indicate that active exercise can change the rate of progression of the disease or regrowth of myelin or axons, although it may improve function through increased strength and aerobic capacity once muscles are reinnervated (see Table 15.3). Despite the lack of evidence, consensus recommendations[197] and "usual care" as described for the control

groups for GBS medical intervention trials support rehabilitation. In addition, several case reports have described improvements with various rehabilitation programs.[235–237] Individualized programs have been advocated consisting of gentle strengthening, isometric, isotonic, isokinetic, manual resistive, and progressive resistive exercises.[179] The major goal of exercise and physical activity throughout the course of GBS must be to maintain the patient's musculoskeletal system in an optimal ready state, prevent overwork, enhance circulation and cardiorespiratory endurance within the limits of active movement, and pace the recovery process to obtain maximal function as reinnervation occurs. Once reinnervation occurs (generally after a muscle exceeds 3/5 on a MMT), progressive resistance exercises at moderate intensities (50% to 70% of 1 repetition maximum [1RM]), use of the overload principle, and progressive challenge can be built in to the rehabilitation program as tolerated.

As was discussed in the section on therapeutic considerations for patients with ALS, a muscle that has significant denervation is more likely to respond to exercise with overwork fatigue. Strenuous exercise and fatigue during this early period have been associated with recurring episodes of a temporary loss of function. Thus the current opinion for patients with GBS is that excessive exercise during denervation and early reinnervation (when only a few functioning motor units are present) can lead to further damage rather than to the expected exercise-induced hypertrophy of muscle.

Exercise from onset through the plateau. When motor function is still deteriorating, and cardiovascular variables fluctuate with dysautonomia, resisted and aerobic exercise cannot be well monitored for their effects. Negative response (overwork damage) may be confused with progression of the disease. Thus, exercise in the acute and progressive stages may be limited to ROM (of all joints, including back and neck) performed actively by the patient (with mild deficits) or with assistance by the therapist (for patients with moderate or severe deficits). As the disease reaches its nadir, activity remains limited. Once weakness stops progressing, passive maintenance of ROM remains important for all muscles and joints not moving actively.

Once the plateau is reached (no further deterioration noted for several days and medical issues stabilized), tentative progression can be tried. The therapist might start by asking for a voluntary contraction of a muscle or muscle group during breathing (e.g., diaphragm), positioning, or ROM, and increasing experience of upright positioning. During the plateau, patients can move with appropriate assistance as long as it is without pain or excessive fatigue.[176] Slings or adaptive devices may help support the weight of a limb to continue active movement in a gravity-eliminated plane for those muscles that have lost antigravity strength (<3/5 MMT).

Beginning of recovery. As strength begins to return after the plateau, therapists must prescribe limited repetitions of low-resistance activities, with strict avoidance of antigravity strain on the muscles until strength reaches the 3/5 (Fair) range of MMT. In the beginning of recovery, short periods of exercise should be frequent. As reinnervation occurs and denervated motor units become responsive, the early process of muscle reeducation may follow progressions used in recovery stages after poliomyelitis or in the technique called "rhythmic initiation" described in proprioceptive neuromuscular facilitation (PNF). Using this technique to encourage active contraction of the muscle the therapist should demonstrate the expected movement to the patient. The therapist then passively moves the patient's limb while the patient observes. After gaining a clear picture of what movement is expected, the patient is encouraged to contract muscles, first "helping" with the movement, then taking over as able. Once the patient can move smoothly through the entire motion independently, the therapist may apply gradually stronger resistance; the therapist can determine when resistance is too strong if the patient's movement becomes less smooth through the whole motion or stops on the way. If the sensory and pain status of the patient permits, facilitation techniques such as skin stroking, brushing, vibration, icing, tapping, and verbal and visual cueing may be used in conjunction with the muscle reeducation process. The patient is taught to reassess his or her movements and make corrective responses.

Functional activities should be appropriate for the muscle grade of the active muscle or muscle group. For example, if the patient's deltoid muscle has a poor (2/5) grade on MMT (full ROM with gravity eliminated), the patient should be cautioned not to attempt to elevate her or his arm against gravity (e.g., to shave or comb one's hair). Patients may exercise when the limb weight is supported (using overhead slings, powder boards, pool exercises) to allow the patient to move actively through a full range in the gravity-eliminated position until he or she can take slight resistance in that plane of movement. Children, teenagers, or adults with impaired judgment often need a strict schedule of rest and activity. Work simplification and energy conservation strategies may be useful to improve function in the beginning recovery stages of GBS.[176]

Active repetitions can be added very slowly, with frequent rest periods and monitoring to avoid fatigue. Activity should be halted at the first point of fatigue or muscle ache; abnormal sensations (tingling, paresthesias) that persist for prolonged periods after exercise may also indicate that the exercise or activity level was excessive. Any progression of resistance or repetitions of strengthening exercises at the below 3/5 level should be instituted in one session, and the results monitored for 30 minutes (for fatigue that prevents daily activities) and for 3 to 5 days for overwork weakness, muscle spasms, or soreness; if adverse response is minimal, exercises may remain at that level until additional assessment reveals that exercises may be progressed further.[176] If additional weakness or soreness ensues, the additional activity should be regressed to a prior level for several days, with reinitiation at a lower level of resistance or number of repetitions, followed by a more gradual increase.

Patients and staff need to be reminded that prolonged sitting in bed or in a wheelchair, even when supported, may tax the axial musculature, including the neck. A program of gradual sitting should be instituted, with the final goal being independent, unsupported sitting with functional equilibrium reactions. In busy hospitals, a schedule of sitting, resting, and specific activity should be posted in clear view at the patient's bedside.

In the initial stages of *upright activity* after any period of bed rest, therapists must progress upright tolerance very carefully because 19% to 50% of people with GBS show orthostatic hypotension along with dysautonomia. A program to improve tolerance to upright position can be started in the ICU if the patient is on a type of standing bed. If a standing bed is not available, a sitting program can be initiated as soon as it is tolerated. A progressive standing program can be instituted when the patient's respiratory system and ANS are no longer unstable and the patient can be moved to a tilt table or standing frame. Caution should be taken to stabilize the patient's limbs fully to maintain alignment and to limit activity in muscles that have strength below the fair range (3/5 MMT). When beginning training, some patients benefit from using an abdominal binder or foot-to-thigh compression stockings (if tolerated without provoking dysesthesia) to counter the pooling of fluids. Because of the relation between poor hydration and hypotension, therapists must ensure the patient is well hydrated before beginning upright or standing tolerance programs.[176]

In patients with Miller-Fisher syndrome, *ataxia* may be a significant feature hindering movement as recovery begins. No specific rehabilitation literature has yet been published in this variant of GBS, but progressions for ataxia in multiple sclerosis or cerebellar disease[238] may

be useful. Therapeutic management may address dysmetria of the limbs, trunk, or neck or stabilize the trunk during gait training. Providing augmented sensation through vibratory stimulation, the wearing of substantial limb weights or small torso weights may be effective in helping to stabilize the core for more controlled movement of distal musculature.[238] Diplopia resulting from oculomotor deficits may be addressed with variable use of an eye patch, at first to minimize annoyance and balance disturbance, but also to practice eye movement in each eye separately before practicing convergent movements.

Activity progression during active recovery. As strength increases, additional resistance may be applied to muscles showing good recovery (4/5 MMT) while avoiding strain on muscles that have not yet reached the same level, frequently the most distal musculature. Functional tasks may be practiced specifically. For example, a patient may score full independence on a Barthel Index and have minimal disability remaining at 10 months post onset, but have pain on heel contact during gait that limits his activity. In a case report describing such a patient, part-practice of components of gait with closed chain and eccentric lower extremity exercise progressing to lunging, jumping, running, and practice of throwing from a wobble board were useful in improving gait performance and participation according to digital and subjective measures.[222] Even when strength has returned throughout, rehabilitation and exercise may need to continue to address fatigue that may persistently affect each of the ICF levels: body function and structure, activity, and participation.[180] For an outline of treatment progression for a patient with severe GBS during the acute stage from week 1 through week 12, see Table 15.4.

As the patient gains strength, clinicians should direct isolated movements into functional activities to add salience and provide more normal distractions to encourage automaticity of function. For those patients who experience significant losses in proprioception after GBS, sensory reintegration activities and high repetitions of task practice may help redevelop motor engrams that are based on the altered sensory perception. Aerobic training may be instituted to improve physical fitness, functional outcome, and quality of life, and decrease fatigue.[176]

As reinnervation progresses and strength and exercise tolerance increases, the therapist may choose to use facilitative exercise techniques. In a case report following 2 months of inpatient rehabilitation for a man with GBS, home physical therapy 3 days per week successfully promoted proximal muscle stability for function using neurodevelopmental sequencing; practiced activities progressed from supine and prone to function in quadruped and kneeling.[237] PNF[239] with manual resistance of prescribed patterns could also be useful to promote recruitment of maximal desired contraction in specific muscle groups. Although PNF techniques are excellent for eliciting maximal contraction, care must be taken not to overwork the weaker components of PNF movement patterns. A positive aspect of PNF techniques is that they can be tied in with functional patterns such as rolling, which is necessary for bed mobility; transitions to quadruped, kneeling, sitting, and standing; and gait.

As muscles regain antigravity strength, independent function becomes possible, although movement may still be slow and function may require assistive devices. Patients will likely progress from inpatient to home to outpatient services, with necessarily less frequent therapy sessions. More of their exercise and physical activity will need to be performed unsupervised, under their own initiative or in community programs or gyms. A successful "home" program is one in which the patient knows the purpose of each exercise and understands the reason for the level of intensity; the patient must value the activity's end goal and be able to perform each exercise effectively in their own environmental context. Standardized tools that engage the patient in

TABLE 15.4 Outline of First 12 Weeks for Patients With Moderate to Severe Guillain-Barré Syndrome: Medical Status and Treatment

Timing	Medical Status	Treatment[a]
Week 1	Intubation with endotracheal tube Ventilator dependent Complete cranial nerve paralysis Tetraplegia	Postural drainage every 3 h around the clock Passive ROM exercises to all joints; communication and nutrition programs instituted; other support as needed Splinting (molded plastic) of hands and feet to maintain functional position Positioning, splinting, and ROM program schedule posted at bedside
Weeks 2–5	At 2 weeks, transition to tracheostomy if pulmonary function no better than when intubated	Postural drainage decreased to two times each shift (every 8 h) Passive ROM exercises, physiological and accessory motions, gentle stretching of intercostal musculature, trunk rotations Continue splinting and positioning program; continue communication and nutrition programs, modifying as needed Family education: family members taught gentle physiological ROM techniques, with attention to correct shoulder patterns and simple massage techniques
Weeks 6–7	Ventilator set on intermittent ventilation Weaning to use ventilator only at night by end of week 7 No active muscle contractions except eye opening and lip movements Dysphagia	Postural drainage two times each shift (every 8 h) Continue ROM program, splinting, and positioning Begin to build tolerance of upright sitting with good trunk alignment Begin facilitation of active facial and tongue muscle activity in patterns necessary for swallowing, eating, and speaking; speech pathology, occupational therapy for oral training Family members active in care as they choose, helping with ROM, splinting, and positioning schedule
Weeks 8–12	Palpable muscle activity in neck, trunk, proximal musculature of upper and lower extremities	Postural drainage one time each shift Chest stretching, breathing exercises Dysphagia program in collaboration with speech consultant Muscle reeducation program with electromyographic biofeedback (if MMT 3/5 or better); gravity-eliminated exercises using suspension slings attached to bed Tilt-table standing program to increase tolerance to upright (wearing positioning splints if necessary) Collaborate with occupational therapist for treatment in wheelchair with suspension slings to facilitate active arm motion in gravity-limited position Exercise, rest, positioning schedule posted Family, patient educated about stimulating activity level to prevent fatigue, overuse of reinnervating muscles

[a]Treatment depends on rate of recovery.
MMT, Manual muscle testing; *ROM*, range of motion.

goal setting may be useful: the MAM[104,105] (or MAM-CAT,[106] validated in musculoskeletal and neuromuscular populations and recommended as a scale of patient-reported mobility),[107] Goal Attainment Scaling[108] (used in diverse populations, including neurological), Canadian Occupational Performance Measure[109] (known in the OT literature), or the Patient-Specific Functional[110] Scale (used more in musculoskeletal populations). A tool such as the MAM-CAT may assist the patient and therapist to identify together the movement dimensions the patient prioritizes so that therapy and home exercises can emphasize what the patient values most (see Fig. 15.8).[106]

In the months (and years) that follow inpatient rehabilitation, the course of therapy may be intermittent as long as any GBS-related deficits continue, with episodes of care interspersed with periods of independent activity progression. Episodes of care might include examining current status, updating exercise prescription, reviewing use of orthotic and assistive devices, suggesting strategies for optimizing function, supervising any new exercises or activities to ensure competence, and encouraging the patient or client in maintaining health and fitness. The main goal of each episode of care will depend on the patient's own preferences for activity and participation, with consideration of age-appropriate norms, any comorbidities, and the pre-GBS level of function.

Documenting relapses. Throughout the recovery period, therapists should carefully document any serial negative changes or plateaus in motor, sensory, or respiratory impairments or functional status that may herald a relapse. Documentation is critical so that new personnel in each new setting do not miss a change that has been ongoing prior to transfer or discharge. Although 65% to 75% or more of patients with GBS show a return to clinically normal motor function, 2% to 5% of patients have a recurrence of symptoms similar in onset and pattern to the original illness. Recurrence of symptoms should trigger immediate reassessment of physical status, potential medical referral, and monitoring for worsening cardiorespiratory signs.

Addressing residual deficits in later stages of recovery. The possibility of lingering endurance deficits should be considered as patients and therapists address long-term plans. Patients may appear to have reached full recovery of strength but still report fatigue that limits return to work or activities that require sustained maximal effort.[240]

Determining the source of fatigue in a late stage of GBS may be complicated by differences in measures of experienced fatigue (subjectively reported) versus physiological fatigue (central or peripheral reduction in voluntary muscle force production) and the weak relationship between these in many neuromuscular disorders.[241] In addition, cardiovascular fitness may continue to be compromised after recovery from GBS weakness. Fitness compromise may be caused by altered muscle function, but may also be related to cardiovascular deconditioning from an imposed sedentary lifestyle.[192] Several researchers have discussed the effect of endurance exercise training in the later recovery stage of GBS. Fehlings and colleagues[242] tested muscle strength and endurance in a group of children at least 2 years after acute onset of GBS. Although the children appeared essentially recovered, endurance of the arm muscles was lower than that of the lower extremities. They hypothesized that the typical walking, running, and cycling activities that the children participated in were sufficient to improve strength and endurance of lower-extremity muscles, but that upper extremities were not challenged to the same degree. The authors recommended that children be encouraged to participate in activities such as swimming to improve upper-extremity endurance. Controlled tetherball and volleyball activities are also appropriate to engage upper-extremity endurance.[242] Tuckey and Greenwood[236] reported positive results of aerobic treatment with partial body-weight support (PBWS) treadmill exercise for a patient with severe GBS. Garssen and colleagues[243] reported a 20% reduction in fatigue levels, along with improved physical condition and strength, after a 12-week intensive bicycling exercise program for patients several years after the onset of GBS. On the other hand, Bussman and colleagues[229] showed that the change in physical fitness (as assessed using measures of oxygen uptake and peak power output) with a 12-week exercise program was only weakly associated with changes in activity (recorded with an activity monitor) or perceived physical functioning (coefficients $<.30$). Associations with perceived mental function, however, were much stronger (coefficients of change scores were .54 to .57). Thus exercise programs may have a significant effect on psychological variables along with physical measures; clinicians and patients should be sure to document these outcomes of a course of exercise. Tools used in the Bussman and colleagues[229] study included self-report questionnaires such as the cognitive portion of the FIS and the Hospital Anxiety and Depression Scale.

Improvements in strength and endurance after GBS may continue for months to years. A prospective study following six patients for 18 months after onset of GBS recorded continuing improvement of muscle strength on average throughout the assessment period, and yet the average strength of major muscle groups had not yet reached that of healthy controls.[227] Although the traditional thought has been that little clinical improvement occurs after 2 to 3 years, Bernsen and colleagues[244] found that 21% of the patients in a study of 150 patients after recovery from acute GBS reported improvement after 2.5 to 6.5 years, although the authors thought the perception of improvement was related to improved sensory function. Of interest for future research and clinical decision making are the long-term consequences of GBS and how the normal aging process will affect patients who have some mild residual effects—for example, whether some patients will develop increasing weakness over time similar to persons with postpolio syndrome.

Adaptive Equipment and Orthoses

Judicious use of orthotic devices and adaptive equipment should be considered an integral part of the rehabilitation process. The purpose of the orthotic and adaptive devices is twofold: (1) to protect weakened structures from overstretch and overuse and (2) to facilitate ADLs within the limits of the patient's current ability. The purpose of adaptive equipment and orthotics is similar in ALS; thus articles that have discussed these devices could be helpful in GBS as well.[89,142] Orthotic devices and adaptive equipment should be introduced and

discontinued on the basis of serial evaluations of strength, ROM, and functional needs. For example, a hospitalized patient who has poor (2/5) middle deltoid strength may practice upper-extremity activities such as eating while using suspension slings. A thumb position splint may be used temporarily to aid thumb control in grasping tasks.

Most patients will need a wheelchair for several months until strength and endurance improve. As strength returns, patients recovering from severe paralysis may need to change from use of a wheelchair with a high, reclining back with a headrest to use of a lightweight, easily maneuverable chair. A quandary for the therapist is to predict how long a wheelchair will be necessary and whether it should be rented or purchased as the patient progresses through different stages of recovery. While moving from wheelchair mobility to independent ambulation, patients will usually progress from parallel bars to a walker with a seat to allow frequent resting, and then to crutches or a cane. Because wheelchairs, walkers, crutches, and canes, especially custom appliances, are expensive and not always covered by insurance, the therapist should carefully consider the cost and benefit to the patient during the recovery process.

Although most patients with GBS are able to walk within 8 months of onset, many show a prolonged residual weakness of calf and, most commonly, anterior compartment musculature, requiring the use of an AFO. The decision whether to use a prefabricated orthosis or custom appliance is not always simple. Several temporary orthotic measures can be considered. For example, if the patient shows good gastrocnemius-soleus strength with mild weakness of the dorsiflexors, a simple elastic strap attached to the shoelaces and a calf band may be sufficient to prevent overuse of the anterior compartment muscles. An old-fashioned, relatively inexpensive spring wire brace, which can be attached to the patient's shoes to facilitate dorsiflexion, is a good choice for patients who report skin hypersensitivity when wearing a plastic orthosis.

Most therapy units today have access to varied sizes of plastic, fixed-ankle AFOs that can be used until a decision is made to have the patient fitted with custom AFOs. A system of prefabricated AFOs with adjustable ankle motion joints has been developed that allows the therapist to limit plantarflexion and dorsiflexion to the specific needs of the patient. For patients with reasonable control of plantarflexion and dorsiflexion but with lateral instability because of peroneal weakness, a simple ankle stirrup device such as the AirCast Air-Stirrup Ankle Brace (AirCast, Summit, NJ) can be used temporarily to provide lateral ankle stability. Although few patients with GBS need knee-ankle-foot orthoses (KAFOs) on a long-term basis, inexpensive air splints or adjustable long-leg metal splints to control knee position are sometimes helpful when working on weight bearing in the standing position and during initial gait training.

Psychosocial Roles and Quality of Life

Patients with GBS have a significantly reduced health-related quality of life compared with control subjects at approximately 1 year after onset, associated with decreased functional scores and changes in work status.[217] Although physical training may improve functional scores and work capabilities, Bussmann and colleagues[229] found little correlation between physical fitness and actual mobility. They hypothesized that training can result in physical changes but also influence psychological components, such as positive mood and self-confidence, more closely linked to quality of life.

Psychosocial Issues

Although most patients with GBS have a good recovery over a period of 2 or more years, the acute stage of the disease can be frightening, especially to patients who progress to complete paralysis and respiratory failure. Nancy, in Case Study 15.2, reported that she was terrified during the time she was totally paralyzed (including eyelid movement) and on a respirator. She said that nurses, doctors, and hospital staff seemed to assume she could not hear because she was unable to respond in any manner. In her words:

They acted like I was already dead, and I thought I would be from the way they were talking. The thing I hated the most was when the night nurses from the registry would come in and ask how to

make the ventilator work! I felt panicked. Can you imagine having your life depend on a machine and knowing that the person who was supposed to make it work had no idea what to do if a tube came unconnected? They were always worried about my blood pressure. Who wouldn't have high blood pressure in that situation! The thing I liked about my therapists was that they told me what they were going to do even when I couldn't respond. They didn't just start doing things or pulling on me like other people did.

CASE STUDY 15.2 NANCY

Onset, Acute Stage

Nancy, a 16-year-old girl with a history of repeated hospitalizations for asthma, was admitted to the hospital with tingling in the hands and feet and mild respiratory distress. Because staff thought her asthma attacks had a significant emotional component, her repeated complaints of paresthesias, muscle pain, and weakness were largely ignored or attributed to anxiety attacks. The day after admission, Nancy began staggering while walking and became extremely agitated and hysterical, screaming that she was dying and could not breathe. A medical assessment showed evidence of wheezing with a normal chest radiograph and decreased VC. She was uncooperative during strength testing, although strength was estimated to be within normal limits except for approximately Fair (3/5) strength of the dorsiflexors and everters and Good (4/5) strength of the plantar flexors. She became extremely upset when her feet were touched.

Because of her psychological history, she was referred for psychiatric assessment and was placed on an anxiolytic medication. Two hours later she had a full respiratory arrest and was intubated and maintained on mechanical ventilation. Over the next 3 days she developed flaccid tetraplegia, and within 5 days she had complete cranial nerve involvement. During the acute stage, she was catheterized because of urinary retention and was treated for a bowel obstruction.

Nancy's physical therapy treatment began in the ICU. Formal strength testing was inappropriate. She received passive ROM twice daily from physical therapy; passive ROM was full but felt stiff at ends of ranges in the wrist, fingers, and ankles. The goals were to assist in respiratory care, prevent joint contractures, and prevent stasis ulcers during the period of immobility. Although her postural drainage treatment was performed using respiratory therapy techniques in conjunction with aerosol medication by intermittent positive-pressure ventilation (IPPV), PTs began a course of chest stretching techniques in coordination with a fastidious ROM program performed twice a day by a therapist and on the evening and night shifts by a nurse. A pressure relief mattress was ordered for her bed. The nursing staff changed her position every 2 h despite the pressure relief mattress that altered pressure under her as she lay supine or partially turned to the left or right. To prevent contracture development, an OT fabricated bilateral wrist and finger splints; a PT molded ankle splints to maintain 90 degrees of dorsiflexion with neutral eversion-inversion. A positioning and ROM schedule in poster form with pictures of positions and ROM patterns was posted at Nancy's bedside.

Because Nancy reported severe hypersensitivity to light touch or to any passive movement of her limbs, a cradle was placed on the bed to prevent sheets from touching her and to prevent air flow changes from irritating her skin. She was fitted for above-knee light pressure stockings, which seemed to decrease her sensitivity to light touch.

Progression, Plateau, and Beginning of Recovery

Deterioration of motor ability slowed and then plateaued with full tetraplegia, dependence, and cranial nerve involvement at approximately 10 days after

onset. Within another week, Nancy started a gradual return of respiration, but weaning from the ventilator was complicated by infections. She was successfully weaned at 29 days, after several episodes of pneumonia. After extubation, she still had swallowing and speech problems.

Because weaning from the ventilator was difficult, the PT played more of a role in education and breathing instruction than was typical (the respiratory therapists collaborated so that the PT could do the instructing during twice daily ROM activities). The PT instructed Nancy, the staff, and her family in appropriate breathing exercises to be performed every 1 or 2 h. Because her parents wanted to be involved with her care, they were taught ROM techniques with special attention to correct shoulder ROM techniques. The PTs continued to follow Nancy twice a day to ensure that accessory motions were completed with physiological motions. Moist hot packs were used effectively before ROM exercises for 1 week to minimize severe muscle pain.

As part of her positioning program, Nancy was placed in a supported semisitting position while intubated. As muscle control returned, a muscle reeducation program was initiated that focused initially on the head and trunk and then on the upper and lower extremities. Exercise periods were limited to 15 min twice a day. She would have benefited from more frequent short sessions; however, this was not possible. Her parents were shown how to guide her active exercise program cautiously so that she was able to exercise more frequently at low repetitions. When each muscle group reached an MMT grade of Fair (3) or greater, Nancy was allowed to use the muscles in functional activities with specified limitations in activity duration. When she was able to tolerate upright sitting and had some bed mobility, Nancy was transferred to a Nelson bed in which she could begin a gradual standing weight-bearing program.

A speech therapist worked with Nancy in the ICU to help her relearn safe swallowing patterns and to reintroduce her to different-textured foods. A dietician had been working with Nancy throughout her hospitalization to ensure adequate nutrition while intubated, and she worked closely with the speech therapist to progress Nancy's diet as she became able to handle liquids and solids.

After being weaned from the ventilator and transferred to the general floor, Nancy was brought to the physical therapy department for treatment, which was frequently done in conjunction with occupational therapy. As strength increased, she began a program of resisted exercise. Trunk and upper- and lower-extremity PNF patterns were used as the primary exercise technique; however, great caution was used to avoid overworking weak muscle groups evoked during use of the PNF pattern. A full mat program with rolling and coming to sitting was also instituted. OTs focused on graduated use of Nancy's upper extremities, first using overhead slings attached to a wheelchair and later using a lap board to support her weakened shoulder musculature while practicing hand activities.

Nancy remained in inpatient rehabilitation for a further week after extubation. Upon discharge at 36 days after onset, swallowing and speech problems

Continued

CASE STUDY 15.2   NANCY—cont'd

were resolved. Sensation was normal for perception of temperature changes and deep pressure. Proprioception was diminished at the ankle, knee, and fingers. Paresthesias and hypoesthesias, aggravated by light touch, were present in a glovelike pattern in both hands and a stocking pattern in both feet, although much improved compared to the acute stage. At discharge, both the PT and OT made a home visit with the hospital social worker and parents to determine what home adaptations and support services would be necessary. Nancy was provided with an ultralight rental wheelchair through her insurance for use until a final determination was made for long-term need. Nancy was also fitted with prefabricated adjustable AFOs, which were purchased through the physical therapy department. At 3–6 months post onset, a determination would be made about expected recovery of her persistently weakened dorsiflexors. If Nancy appeared to need AFOs for a prolonged period, a set of custom molded AFOs would be ordered.

Home Work

After less than 2 months of hospitalization, Nancy was discharged home to return for daily outpatient rehabilitation.

Follow-up of Nancy's outpatient therapy showed that she continued to make gradual recovery over the next 1.5 years. She returned to school 3 months after rehabilitation discharge (about 5 months post onset) using a wheelchair. She graduated to a walker, then to forearm crutches, and finally to independent ambulation. She refused to be seen using a walker at school, so she continued to use the wheelchair at school until she was independent on crutches.

Nancy continued to wear bilateral AFOs but was weaned from full-time use approximately 14 months after discharge (16 months post onset). During the weaning process, Nancy wore her AFOs at school while walking and for any walking distance over four city blocks or if she heard her feet begin to slap from fatigued dorsiflexors. By 16 months, Nancy showed no evidence of overuse weakness after her regular activities, although she had difficulty with endurance activities in her physical education classes. When hiking, she carried her AFOs to use when she expected a long downhill trek to prevent overwork from eccentric muscle activity. By age 19 years—3 years post onset—Nancy had returned fully to her normal activity level.

Psychosocial issues, continued. Skirrow and colleagues[245] remind clinicians that the "intensive care patient is plunged into a world of machines that flash and beep; of tubes and wires that seem to spring from almost every orifice; and of mind-numbing sedative and analgesic medications." Evidence is increasing that patients treated in acute trauma rooms or ICUs can have posttraumatic stress disorder (PTSD). Particularly vulnerable are patients who have had previous traumatic experiences. PTSD places patients at marked risk for increased startle responses, extreme vigilance or anticipation of painful events, sleep disorders, terrifying dreams, and dissociative flashbacks after leaving the ICU; sometimes these symptoms may be left untreated for years after the experience.[246] Patients discharged from prolonged ICU experiences, especially those who had respiratory failure, have an increased incidence of anxiety, depression, and panic disorders years after discharge.

In a nursing study of patient experiences in the ICU, researchers found that patients often felt anxious, apprehensive, and fearful. The patients expected ICU nurses to be experienced and technically adept; patients who felt most secure despite traumatic ICU experiences felt that the nurses were vigilant to their needs and offered personalized care,[187] a point clearly made by Nancy's comments about her perceptions while intubated. Although one might expect ICU staff to be tuned in to patient needs, the highly technical nature of modern ICUs may attract personnel less focused on individual patient care, or it may prevent caring staff from attending to the little kindnesses that are so comforting to critically ill patients. Baxter[246] suggests that caregivers in the ICU orient patients to what is being done, to approach the patients within their field of vision, and to minimize unexpected noises and sudden touching.

Although most patients recover well from GBS, 3 to 6 years after onset of GBS 38% of patients in a Dutch study had to make a job change to accommodate their physical status, 44% had to alter their leisure activities, and nearly 50% described ongoing psychosocial changes.[244] Similar findings were reported in a study of Japanese patients recovering from GBS.[247,248] Regularly scheduled rehabilitation checkups and multiweek episodes of care to update the exercise program may reduce the lingering impairments, but such extensive clinical follow-up is rarely reported.

The effect of GBS on caregivers and family members is not as discussed in the literature on GBS as it is in ALS. However, sudden catastrophic illness of one member of a family inevitably affects all members.

A spouse, partner, or parent may have feelings of shock, denial, and helplessness if a patient's nadir involves dependent tetraplegia and mechanical ventilation. In Case 15.2, this manifested in the parents' desire to help with ROM activities at bedside. The financial toll can also be profound even with health insurance, with lost work or study time and the cost of nonmedical caregivers (such as babysitters for other children). For the small percentage of patients with GBS who have a fatal course or persistent severe deficits, counseling and other support may be of help to family members.

Summary of Therapeutic Management in Guillain-Barré Syndrome

In summary, the rehabilitation program for a person with GBS must be graded carefully according to the stage of illness and needs of the patient. In the acute care environment when respiratory deficits are present, the initial emphasis is directed toward support of maximal respiratory status through postural drainage, chest stretching, and breathing exercises. Because of prolonged bed rest and immobility related to weakness, passive, accessory, and physiological ROM must be maintained with around-the-clock efforts. Splinting or positioning devices are recommended to maintain functional positions during prolonged periods of immobility. A gradual program to increase upright tolerance is begun when respiratory and autonomic functions have stabilized. Therapists must keep in mind the potential to damage denervated muscles with aggressive strengthening programs when developing a rehabilitation plan and a home-based conditioning program. Perhaps as a result of cautious exercise programs, cardiovascular conditioning appears to lag significantly behind strengthening, so endurance training should specifically follow the return of strength. Adaptive equipment and orthoses should be used as needed to protect weakened muscles, facilitate normal movement, and prevent fatigue during the reinnervation process. Once MMT reaches 3 to 4/5, however, strengthening can begin to ramp up with progressive resistance. Strengthening and endurance exercise parameters do not need to remain at such a cautious level. At this point, most patients with GBS have been discharged. Although a rehabilitation program has been found to make a measurable difference in patients' recovery,[190] many patients do not receive follow-up care.[249] Therefore therapists should be assertive in ensuring that their patients with GBS have ongoing contact with rehabilitation specialists who can guide the recovery process and minimize remaining impairments.

CHAPTER SUMMARY

In this chapter, discussion of two different diseases reveals the varied effects of neuromuscular pathology on a person's day-to-day function. ALS is an adult-onset degenerative disease of the UMN and LMN; GBS is an inflammatory autoimmune process affecting LMN, PNS, and ANS of children and adults. In these conditions, the therapist must design a therapy program that will provide the patient with the impetus to become or remain as active as possible without causing possible muscle damage from excessive exercise demands or overwork.

Therapists must be aware of their own feelings and reactions to patients with severe neuromuscular diseases. Working with patients with GBS is usually a positive experience because most patients attain full or nearly full recovery despite severe disability during the acute illness and a long recovery period. Working with patients with degenerative terminal diseases such as ALS, however, draws deeply on the therapist's emotional and spiritual strength. A typical response of health care professionals is to view these patients' conditions as hopeless and to assume that the patients must also perceive their existence as hopeless, depressing, and without value. Research does suggest an increased incidence of depression and demoralization in patients with degenerative, terminal diseases compared with populations with no diagnosed diseases. Other research, however, has indicated that many patients perceive their own life satisfaction much more positively than professionals would believe. Therapists must tap into patients' positive energy to design treatment programs that respect patients' goals and life plans within the context of their environment.

Limited evidence exists to document the effectiveness of rehabilitation for patients with neuromuscular diseases. Determining the most appropriate exercise and therapeutic intervention programs therefore requires diligent examination of the dysfunctions and needs of the individual patient and assessment of the effects of interventions appropriately adapted from use in other populations. Because few medical-clinical facilities see a large enough sample of patients with these diagnoses, therapists must align with their professional organizations to institute nationwide, multisite research studies to provide clear evidence of effectiveness of therapy in these populations.

ACKNOWLEDGMENTS

The author acknowledges the contribution of Ann Hallum, PT, PhD, author of previous editions of this chapter. Thank you, also, to Andrew J. Lui, PT, DPT, who graciously reviewed and made clinical suggestions on the ALS portion of this chapter.

REFERENCES

To enhance this text and add value for the reader, all references are included on the companion Evolve site that accompanies this textbook. This online service will, when available, provide a link for the reader to a Medline abstract for the article cited. There are 249 cited references and other general references for this chapter, with many of these references systematic reviews gathering the best available evidence of effective clinical practice.

Beyond the Central Nervous System: Neurovascular Entrapment Syndromes*

Bradley W. Stockert and William J. Garcia

OVERVIEW

The purpose of this chapter is twofold. The first purpose is to develop the concept that the entire nervous system forms a continuous tissue tract. This concept is central to the idea that movements of the trunk and/or limbs can have a profound biomechanical and physiological impact on the peripheral nervous system (PNS) and central nervous system (CNS). Mobility of the nervous system and some of the responses of the system to movement in normal and sensitized states are discussed.

The second purpose is to develop in the reader an understanding of the neurovascular entrapment syndrome. This is an underrecognized impairment present in some patients with a wide variety of diagnoses; for example, nonspecific arm pain, repetitive strain injury, carpal tunnel syndrome (CTS), and thoracic outlet syndrome (TOS). Standard medical care frequently fails with these patients. A theoretical model for the development and perpetuation of neurovascular entrapment syndrome is presented. Background information regarding the syndrome is provided, and the appropriate screening tools for assessment of the impairment are discussed. Treatment suggestions and a case study are presented at the end of the chapter.

PERIPHERAL NEUROANATOMY

The PNS is generally regarded as the portion of the nervous system that lies outside the CNS (i.e., the brain and spinal cord).[1,2] The major components of the PNS include motor, sensory, and autonomic neurons found in spinal, peripheral, and cranial nerves. Although this partitioning is valid from an anatomical perspective, it often leads to a lack of appreciation as to the truly continuous nature and integrative function of the nervous system as a whole. The concept that the entire nervous system is a continuous tissue tract reinforces the idea that limb and trunk movements can have physiological and mechanical effects on the PNS and the CNS, which are local and global.

The nervous system is composed of two functional tissue types. One type of tissue is concerned with impulse conduction. This functional category includes nerve cells and Schwann cells. The second type provides support and protection of the conduction tissues—that is, the connective tissues.

Three levels in the organization of a peripheral nerve have been described (Fig. 16.1).[2,3] At the innermost level the nerve fiber is the conducting component of a neuron (nerve cell). A connective tissue layer called the *endoneurium* surrounds each nerve fiber. The endoneurium surrounds the basement membrane of the neuron and plays an important role in maintaining fluid pressure within the endoneurial space. There are no lymphatic channels within the endoneurial space, and the pressure within this space increases with compression of the neuron.[4]

The second level of organization consists of a collection of many nerve fibers (a fascicle) surrounded by a layer of connective tissue called the *perineurium*.[2,3] The perineurium acts as a selective barrier to diffusion and as such exerts significant control over the local movement of fluid and ions. This connective tissue layer acts like a pressurized container; that is, extrusion of the contents occurs if the membrane is cut. The compartment enclosed by the perineurium does not contain lymphatic channels.[4] This may be a problem during inflammatory states when edema is present deep to the perineurium. The perineurium is the last connective tissue layer to rupture in tensile testing of peripheral nerves.[5] The outermost connective tissue layer of a peripheral nerve is called the *epineurium*. The epineurium surrounds, protects, and enhances gliding between the faniculi. Lymphatic channels are found within the epineurial compartment.

All three connective tissue layers are interconnected—they are not separate and distinct, but are continuous tissue layers.[2,3] Each of the connective tissue layers contains free nerve endings from the nervi nervorum. As a result, all three connective tissue layers are a potential source of pain. In addition, all three layers are continuous with the homologous connective tissue layers of the CNS—that is, the dura mater and the epineurium.

The vascular supply for peripheral nerves is designed to provide uninterrupted blood flow regardless of the position of the trunk and limbs. Extrinsic vessels provide blood flow to segmental vessels that, in turn, supply an extensive intrinsic (intraneural) vasculature within the PNS. These segmental vessels branch off of the extrinsic vessels and enter peripheral nerves in areas of low nerve mobility relative to the surrounding tissue. The intrinsic vasculature supplies all three connective tissue layers within the PNS. Arterioles and venules are found in the epineurial and perineurial spaces, but only capillaries are found in the endoneurial compartment.

Peripheral nerves are regularly subjected to compression and elongation (stretching), which have been shown to raise intraneural pressure. Compression and elongation decrease the diameter of the intrinsic blood vessels, increase the intraneural pressure, and result in a reduction in blood flow within the nerve. Compressive forces of 20 to 30 mm Hg have been shown to adversely affect intraneural blood flow,[6] while compressive forces of 50 to 70 mm Hg have been shown to result in complete arrest of blood flow,[7] which results in damage to myelin and axons.[6] A strain (elongation) of 6% to 8% has been shown to decrease intraneural blood flow by 50% to 70% in the sciatic nerve of rats.[4,8,9] A strain of 15% in the sciatic nerve of a rabbit has been shown to result in complete arrest of blood flow,[7] and the same strain produces an 80% reduction in blood flow in the rat sciatic nerve.[9] Strains of 11% or greater are produced by some of the positions used in neurodynamic tests of the upper limb.[6] Significant increases in intraneural pressure and concomitant decreases in intraneural blood flow have been shown to adversely affect neuronal conduction.[7,10,11]

---

*Videos for this chapter are available at studentconsult.com.

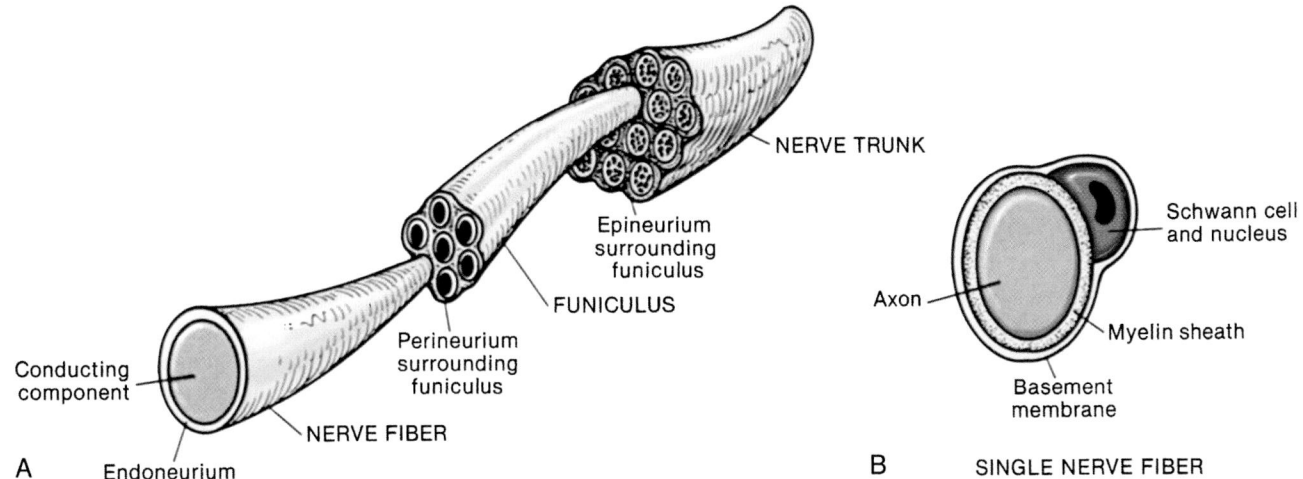

Fig. 16.1 Three Levels of Organization of a Peripheral Nerve or Nerve Trunk. **(A)** Nerve trunk and components. **(B)** Microscopic structure of nerve fiber.

Intraneural blood flow in the median nerve at the wrist can be assessed with Doppler sonography and used in the diagnosis of CTS.[12]

The cytoplasm in cells moves and has thixotropic properties; that is, the viscosity of cytoplasm is lower when it is continuously moving.[4] In neurons, the movement of the cytoplasm from the cell body through the axons (anterograde movement) occurs at two speeds. Fast axoplasmic flow occurs at a rate of about 100 to 400 mm/day and is used to carry ion channels and neurotransmitters (i.e., materials required for normal impulse conduction) to the nerve terminals. Slow axoplasmic flow occurs at a rate of about 6 mm/day and is used to transport cytoskeleton proteins, neurofilaments, and other materials used to maintain the physical health of the cell. A third flow occurs in the opposite direction (retrograde) at a rate of about 200 mm/day. Retrograde transport carries unused substances and exogenous materials taken up at the terminus (e.g., neurotrophic factors). The material carried back to the cell body by retrograde transport has been shown to influence activity in the cell nucleus.[4]

Compression raises intraneural pressure, which has a negative impact on the flow of cytoplasm.[4] Anterograde and retrograde flow of axoplasm is impaired with 30 mm Hg compression on the nerve, hypoxia, or a strain of 11% or greater.[13–15] Prolonged or intense exposure to compression can result in conduction abnormalities, endoneurial edema, fibrin deposition, demyelination, and axonal sprouting. Each of these events increases the likelihood of developing adhesions and abnormal impulse-generating sites (AIGSs).[4] (The negative impact of AIGSs is discussed in the section on adaptive responses to pain.)

MOBILITY OF THE PERIPHERAL NERVOUS SYSTEM

Several types of tissues (e.g., bone, fascia, and muscle) surround peripheral nerves as they "travel" to target tissues. Peripheral nerves can be thought of as passing through a series of tissue tunnels composed of various biological materials. The composition of the tissue tunnel changes with the passage of the nerve from the vertebral column (an osseous tunnel) to the target tissue (e.g., from an osseous tunnel to a soft tissue and/or fibro-osseous tunnel). A "mechanical interface" exists at the junction between the nerve and the material adjacent to the nerve that forms the tissue tunnel. Movement of the trunk and/or limbs can cause three types of movement to occur in the peripheral nerves: *unfolding, sliding, and elongation.*[16]

When there is little or no tension in a peripheral nerve, the axon typically contains undulations (folds). As tension is applied the axon

will *unfold* so that the undulations disappear. *Sliding* can be defined as movement between the nerve and the surrounding tissues at the mechanical interface (extraneural movement). Sliding by itself does not cause significant elongation or tension to develop within the nerve, so intraneural pressure remains relatively unchanged. Ultrasound studies have shown that the median, ulnar, sciatic, and tibial nerves undergo extraneural movement (sliding) with movement of the upper and lower limbs, respectively.[17–20]

Elongation of the nerve occurs when tension is applied to a nerve, and there is little or no unfolding and sliding at the mechanical interface. Elongation causes movement to occur between the neural elements and connective tissue layers (intraneural movement). Elongation decreases the diameter of the nerve, resulting in an increase in the intraneural tension and pressure.[16] An increase in intraneural pressure has been shown to decrease the flow of blood and axoplasm, resulting in altered neural function (see previous section). Elongation within the median and ulnar nerves has been shown to occur with movements of the upper limb.[6]

Both extraneural and intraneural movements may occur simultaneously within a nerve, but they may not be uniformly distributed. When a body moves, some parts of the PNS will undergo primarily extraneural movement (sliding) with little or no development of tension, while other areas will undergo intraneural movement (elongation), which results in an increase in intraneural tension and pressure. As a consequence, some areas within a nerve slide, developing little or no tension, whereas other areas of the same nerve elongate significantly, increasing the amount of intraneural tension.[6] In areas repeatedly exposed to high amounts of tension (e.g., the median nerve at the wrist) the nerves are found to contain a higher-than-average amount of connective tissue.[16]

If one considers the entire nervous system as a continuous tissue tract, then the idea that movement and/or tension developed in one region of the nervous system can be distributed and dissipated throughout the entire nervous system becomes apparent.[21,22] The inability of a component within the nervous system to dissipate and/or distribute movement and tension can lead to abnormal force development and lesions elsewhere in the continuous tissue tract.[23]

PERIPHERAL NERVE ENTRAPMENT

Seddon's classification of nerve injury is based upon mechanical trauma.[24] Schaumberg[2] modified this paradigm into an anatomically based scheme containing three classes of injury (Table 16.1). Injuries

TABLE 16.1 **Classification of Acute Traumatic Peripheral Nerve Injury**			
Anatomical Classification	**Class I**	**Class II**	**Class III**
Previous nomenclature	Neuropraxia	Axonotmesis	Neurotmesis
Lesion	Reversible conduction block resulting from ischemia or demyelination	Axonal interruption but basal lamina remains intact	Nerve fiber and basal lamina interruption (complete nerve severance)

Modified from Schaumberg HH, Spencer PS, Thomas PK. *Disorders of Peripheral Nerves.* Philadelphia: FA Davis; 1983.

in class II and III are caused by macrotrauma, which results in some disruption to the integrity of the nerve fiber. The following discussion of entrapment is focused on microtrauma in which there is no breach in the anatomical integrity of the nerve fiber (class I). Mechanical microtrauma resulting in nerve entrapment can occur with excessive or abnormal friction, compression, and/or tension (elongation).[2]

Tissue tunnels, peripheral nerves, and the mechanical interfaces between them are all vulnerable to mechanical microtrauma—that is, abnormal friction, compression, and/or tension.[2,16] Some peripheral nerves are exposed to bony hard interfaces (e.g., the lower cords of the brachial plexus at the first rib), which are potential sources of abnormal friction. Inflammation and swelling within a tissue tunnel can produce compression of a nerve, for example, the median nerve within the carpal tunnel. The point at which a nerve branches limits the amount of gliding (extraneural movement) available at that location, and increases the amount of local intraneural tension developed with movement (e.g., the tibial nerve in the popliteal fossa).[2,16]

Microtrauma can produce an intraneural lesion that causes a decrease in intraneural flow of blood and axoplasm, demyelination, and/or conduction defects.[2,16] If the lesion occurs in the connective tissues of the nerve, there may be pain, inflammation, proliferation of fibroblasts, and scar formation (fibrosis). Ultrasound studies have shown that the median nerve in patients with CTS is enlarged by approximately 30%.[25] An intraneural scar decreases the compliance of the nerve and increases the amount of intraneural pressure and tension generated with elongation.[22] Intraneural lesions can impair or completely block the ability of the nerve to conduct action potentials.[2,16,26] Partial or complete conduction blocks can result in abnormal sensation, loss of motor function, autonomic dysfunction, and atrophy of target tissue (e.g., muscle and/or skin). However, several forms of physical activity/exercise, including swimming and treadmill training, have been shown to improve recovery from peripheral nerve injury in animal models (crushed sciatic nerve) using a variety of outcome measures.[27–31] There is no consensus about the best time to start any form of exercise following peripheral nerve injury although one study suggested earlier intervention was beneficial.[28]

Microtrauma can produce an extraneural lesion.[2,16,22,26] The damage in an extraneural lesion occurs in the tissue surrounding the nerve—that is, at the mechanical interface. Swelling within the tissue tunnel can produce compression of the nerve. Fibrosis can produce adhesions at the mechanical interface leading to a decrease in sliding of the nerve. A decrease in the ability of a nerve to slide within a tissue tunnel will result in an abnormal increase in intraneural tension and pressure as movement is imposed on the nerve. The increase in local intraneural tension can produce abnormal changes in the conduction of action potentials, and the tension will be distributed in an aberrant pattern throughout the continuous tract of the nervous system. The resultant abnormal distribution of tension predisposes the nervous system to the development of lesions at other sites.[16]

Friction, compression, and tension can produce microtrauma, which results in intraneural and extraneural pathology.[2,16] For example, fibrosis can produce a combined pathological state that results in

a substantial reduction in the ability of a nerve to slide within the tissue tunnel and a substantial increase in intraneural tension during nerve elongation as the compliance of the nerve is decreased. Movement of the median nerve at the carpal tunnel has been shown to occur with movements of the upper limb.[17–20] Longitudinal and transverse movements of the median nerve at the carpal tunnel have been shown to be reduced in the presence of microtrauma (i.e., CTS,[25,32] nonspecific arm pain,[33,34] and whiplash injury).[34]

Intraneural and extraneural lesions result in an abnormal distribution of sliding and tension throughout the nervous system with movement of the trunk and/or limbs. The abnormal distribution of tension within a nerve increases the probability of a second lesion or abnormality developing within the nerve. This situation led Upton and McComas[35] in 1973 to first use the term "double crush injury." (This term should be considered a misnomer because a "crush" does not necessarily occur.) For example, entrapment of the median nerve at the carpal tunnel can cause the development of abnormal tension in cervical spinal nerves, resulting in a lesion at that site. Upton and McComas[35] have shown that a lesion at the carpal tunnel increases the risk of having a second neural lesion in the cervical region.

PATHOGENESIS OF NEUROVASCULAR ENTRAPMENT

Neurovascular entrapment can occur at any point along the continuous tract of the nervous system. The carpal tunnel, a common site of entrapment, has been studied and provides a framework of information regarding the pathogenesis of neurovascular entrapments. Sunderland[36] has reasoned that a change in the normal pressure gradients within the carpal tunnel can lead to compression of the median nerve. In order to maintain homeostasis in the carpal tunnel and the median nerve, blood must flow into the tunnel, then into the nerve and back out of the tunnel. For blood flow to occur in the median nerve the blood pressure must be highest within the epineurial arterioles, and becomes progressively lower in the capillaries and epineurial venules and lowest within the extraneural space of the carpal tunnel. Any increase in the pressure of a single compartment has the potential to disrupt the normal pressure gradients and impair the flow of blood within the compartments of the carpal tunnel and the median nerve. Impaired intraneural blood flow can lead to localized hypoxia, edema, inflammation, and fibrosis.[36]

An increase in pressure within the carpal tunnel can occur for a variety of reasons—for example, synovial hyperplasia, thickening of tendons, venous congestion, inflammation, and/or edema. Venous blood flow within a nerve will be impaired, and venous stasis will develop if pressure within the extraneural space of the carpal tunnel becomes greater than the pressure within the epineurial venules. Because blood pressure within venules is relatively low, partial occlusion of blood flow can begin to occur in the carpal tunnel with pressures as low as 20 to 30 mm Hg.[16,37] Intraneural blood flow in the median nerve at the wrist can be detected with Doppler sonography.[12]

The pressure within the extraneural space of the carpal tunnel is normally about 3 mm Hg (range of 2 to 10 mm Hg) with the wrist in a neutral position.[4,38] The pressure can rise to over 20 mm Hg with the wrist in full flexion, and pressure can rise to over 30 mm Hg when the wrist is placed in 90 degrees of extension[39] or with the functional task of using a computer mouse to drag or point at an object.[40] Studies have shown that the pressure within the carpal tunnel in someone with CTS can be 30 mm Hg or more with the wrist in neutral, and can increase to about 100 mm Hg when the wrist is in 90 degrees of flexion[4,13,14] or extension.[13,38] Compressive forces of 20 to 30 mm Hg have been shown to adversely impact intraneural blood flow,[6] whereas compressive forces of 50 to 70 mm Hg have been shown to result in complete arrest of blood flow[7] and cause demonstrable damage to myelin and axons.[6] Motor and sensory abnormalities begin to manifest at about 40 mm Hg, and complete blockade of the median nerve has been shown to occur at 50 mm Hg.[41] The pressure found in the carpal tunnel of people with CTS is clearly adequate to disrupt the normal flow of blood, axoplasm, and action potentials within the median nerve, causing severe impairment to normal nerve functions.

Sunderland[36] proposed that venous congestion or stasis within the carpal tunnel will lead to localized hypoxia, edema, and fibrosis. Hypoxia causes capillary endothelial cells to deteriorate and local C fibers to secrete substance P and calcitonin gene–related peptide,[4] which in turn causes mast cells to release histamine and serotonin.[42,43] Together these chemical mediators augment the inflammatory state and cause the endothelial cells of capillaries to further deteriorate by becoming flatter, larger, and leakier, enhancing exudation and edema.

Deterioration of the capillary endothelium results in exudation and the formation of a protein-rich edema in the interstitial space. Protein-rich edema stimulates proliferation of fibroblasts, resulting in fibrosis. This intensifies the abnormal pressure gradients, resulting in more tissue hypoxia; that is, a positive feedback or self-perpetuating cycle of pathology is initiated. Intraneural fibrosis decreases compliance of the nerve, and extraneural fibrosis results in the formation of adhesions at the mechanical interface between the nerve and the tissue tunnel. Fibrosis causes a nerve to become stiffer and less mobile, resulting in an abnormal increase in tension when movement is imposed on the nerve.

This set of circumstances (described above) may be referred to as a *neurovascular entrapment syndrome,* and it has the potential to cause the development of problems elsewhere in the system—that is, a double crush injury (see previous section). Upton and McComas[35] studied 115 subjects with CTS or ulnar impingement at the elbow. They found that 81 of the 115 subjects also had evidence of a neural lesion at the neck. Because all nerves essentially travel within tissue tunnels, the potential exists for this scenario to occur elsewhere in the continuous tissue tract of the nervous system (e.g., the thoracic outlet).[5,16,44]

ADAPTIVE RESPONSES TO PAIN

A thorough discussion of the pain associated with neurovascular entrapment is beyond the scope and intent of this chapter. The topic of pain management is discussed in Chapter 30 of this book. However, we would like to describe the development of hyperexcitable states and AIGSs in neurons as well as their role in the development of pain associated with neurovascular entrapment.

"Normal" or physiological pain occurs when peripheral nociceptors are subjected to a stimulus that is at or above the threshold for firing. "Abnormal" or pathological pain can occur when there is a change in the sensitivity (threshold) of the somatosensory system.[45]

Devor[46] wrote that "the crucial pathophysiological process triggered by nerve injury is an increase in neuronal excitability."

Neurons that become inflamed, hypoxic, and/or demyelinated can enter a hyperexcitable state.[2,46–54] A neuron in a hyperexcitable state can begin to discharge spontaneously and/or develop a sustained rhythmic discharge after stimulation. In addition, hyperexcitable neurons can develop mechanosensitivity,[48] chemosensitivity,[4] and/or thermal sensitivity,[52] all of which can result in the production of allodynia, a form of pathological pain.[34,46,50,52,54,55] These changes in the behavior of a nerve can occur in the absence of detectable degeneration.[47–49] The changes in impulse generation and neuronal sensitivity are characteristics of an AIGS.[4] A hyperexcitable state and an AIGS can develop with the mechanical microtrauma and inflammation often associated with peripheral nerve pathology that result from compression, tension, and friction.[2,46,55,56] A variety of chemical mediators have been implicated in the development of a hyperexcitable state in a neuron; for example, neurotrophins,[57,58] histamine,[59] and other inflammatory mediators.[60] These chemical mediators are thought to act through changes in gene expression,[52,57,58] changes in voltage-gated sodium channel expression,[52] and a reduction in anterograde axoplasmic transport.[51,59]

The dorsal root ganglion appears to play a significant role in the pain associated with peripheral nerve pathology.[45,48] Mechanical microtrauma and inflammation of peripheral nerves can cause the dorsal root ganglion to become hyperexcitable (sensitized).[48] The change in sensitivity allows what were weak, subthreshold stimuli to evoke pain and suprathreshold stimuli to evoke exaggerated pain (hyperalgesia). In addition, the dorsal root ganglion can develop mechanosensitivity, chemosensitivity, and thermal sensitivity, resulting in allodynia.[52] This change in sensitivity reflects a change in the physiology of the nerve and may be a component in the development of enhanced central sensitivity to pain and the development of a chronic pain state.[45]

As noted previously, the PNS and CNS represent a continuous tissue tract. The pain and symptoms associated with musculoskeletal injury and/or peripheral nerve pathology can include changes that are the result of an alteration in the autonomic nervous system, which is considered part of the continuous tissue tract of the nervous system.[2,61] For example, catecholamines do not normally elicit pain. However, if a nerve is injured or if there is local inflammation, the catecholamines can induce pain (chemosensitivity) and maintain or enhance pain in inflamed tissues.[4]

Some patients who are treated for musculoskeletal injuries have signs that may be related to autonomic dysreflexia.[44] Wyke[62] demonstrated that stimulation of nociceptors in spinal joints resulted in reflex changes in the cardiovascular, respiratory, and endocrine systems. Dysregulated breathing has been documented in patients with chronic pain.[63] Patients with nonspecific arm pain have a reduced sympathetic vasoconstrictor response in the hand of the affected limb.[64] Thermal asymmetry has been documented in the hands of patients with neurogenic TOS.[65] Feinstein and colleagues[66] showed that injecting saline solution into the thoracic paraspinal muscles caused pallor, diaphoresis, bradycardia, and a drop in the blood pressure. These cardiovascular and respiratory changes are often associated with an alteration in the output from the autonomic nervous system.[44,61,67]

In patients with cumulative trauma disorder (CTD), signs of abnormal autonomic nervous system output can include (1) vasomotor reflexes leading to cool, pale skin,[64] (2) changes in the pattern of sweating (hypohidrosis and/or hyperhidrosis), (3) trophic changes in the skin, (4) hyperactive flexor withdrawal reflexes, and/or (5) paradoxical breathing patterns.[44] Edgelow has described paradoxical breathing as the predominant use of the scalene muscles for ventilation during quiet breathing versus normal ventilation, which is predominantly a function of the diaphragm.[44] Edgelow found that paradoxical breathing is present in most patients with CTD of the upper extremity.[44] A better appreciation of the contribution of the autonomic nervous system to the pathology and symptoms present in some patients with neurovascular entrapment may enhance the effectiveness of their treatment.

CLINICAL EXAMINATION AND TREATMENT OF NEUROVASCULAR ENTRAPMENT

For an effective evaluation of a patient with a neurovascular entrapment problem, the whole person must be addressed and involved in the evaluation and treatment processes. This approach requires the therapist to consider a biopsychosocial approach versus a biomedical approach. In this case, the therapist becomes the evaluator, teacher, and guide for the patient. Traditionally, a biomedical approach has been taken with disorders such as neurovascular entrapment. In a biomedical model, the patient's disability and impairments are seen as a direct correlation to the tissue pathology.[68] The biopsychosocial model addresses the whole patient and provides a means for the therapist to consider the biomedical factors (underlying tissue) and psychosocial factors influencing a patient's symptoms.[68] Utilization of this approach has become more accepted in physical therapy practice, along with the understanding that pain is often influenced by a patient's emotional well-being, thoughts about their condition, cultural beliefs, and environmental influences.[68] Given the impact that neurovascular entrapment symptoms can have on a patient, it is imperative that a clinician understand the interplay between the biomechanical impairments and any underlying psychosocial issues. Neurovascular entrapment can occur in both the upper extremity and lower extremity; however, the most common examples seen by therapists are TOS and CTS. The clinical examination discussed will highlight the specifics regarding neurovascular entrapment of the upper extremity.

Patients with neurovascular entrapment often present with severe and irritable symptoms; therefore a detailed subjective examination is necessary to understand the behavior of the symptoms and the impact the symptoms are having on the patient's life. Initial goals of the subjective exam include determining if the patient is appropriate for physical therapy, developing a hypothesis list regarding potential sources of the patient's symptoms, and determining the extent and vigor of the objective examination. The subjective exam should begin with the patient completing a detailed body chart that outlines the specific area of symptoms and the patient's description of the symptoms. A body chart provides the clinician a thorough picture of symptom location and the potential relationship between areas of symptoms. The patient's description of the symptoms may provide the clinician with potential hypotheses regarding pain mechanisms and potential neurovascular involvement. The patient with primarily *neurological symptoms* may have pain that is described as sharp or burning with numbness or paresthesia, and spasms or weakness in the extremity.[69,70] *Vascular symptoms* may be due to either arterial or venous compression. *Arterial symptoms* may include pain in the distal portion of the extremity (vs. pain proximally at the shoulders or neck), swelling, complaints of stiffness or heaviness of the extremity, coldness of the distal extremity, pallor, and paresthesia (likely due to ischemia).[69-71] Symptoms that originate from venous compression are likely to be described as feelings of stiffness or heaviness of the extremity, asymmetrical extremity edema, paresthesia, and limb discomfort/pain.[69-71]

Understanding pain mechanisms and the overlap between these mechanisms can be helpful for both the clinician and patient. It is

beyond the scope of this chapter to discuss in detail each of these mechanisms and the body of evidence supporting them. However, a brief explanation is appropriate when treating patients with painful conditions. Pain mechanisms have been classified based on the dominant neurophysiological mechanism.[72-74] Classification of pain mechanisms is a useful way for clinicians to identify the likely neurophysiological source of symptoms. The three main pain classifications are *nociceptive, peripheral neuropathic,* and *central sensitization.* Smart and colleagues[72-74] have identified common signs and symptoms to assist clinicians in classifying pain mechanisms in patients with low back pain with and without leg symptoms. *Nociceptive pain* is classified by distinct symptoms and signs: pain localized to the area of injury/dysfunction, clear and proportionate mechanical/anatomical aggravating and easing factors. Symptoms are usually intermittent with movement or mechanical provocation; no dysesthesias are present, and there is no night pain, and no description of burning or shooting symptoms. If the patient assumes antalgic postures to relieve pain, the odds of pain being nociceptive are reduced.[74] The strongest predictor of nociceptive pain is pain localized to the area of injury/dysfunction with an odds ratio (OR) of 69.[74] *Peripheral neuropathic pain* consists of three signs and symptoms: pain referred in a dermatome or cutaneous nerve distribution, a history of nerve injury (pathology or mechanical compromise), and pain or symptoms are provoked with mechanical tests such as neurodynamic testing (e.g., straight leg raise).[73] Symptoms that are in a dermatomal or cutaneous distribution have an OR of 24, suggesting that if symptoms are in a dermatomal or cutaneous nerve distribution the patient is 24 times more likely to have neuropathic pain.[73] *Central sensitization* is pain that is typically present outside of tissue pathology and is associated with an increase in sensitivity of the CNS. Four signs and symptoms have been associated with central sensitization: pain that is disproportionate and nonmechanical, and is unpredictable in terms of aggravating and easing factors; pain that is disproportionate to the extent of injury or pathology; the presence of maladaptive psychosocial factors; and diffuse nonanatomical areas of pain or tenderness to palpation.[72] The OR for disproportionate pain with nonmechanical/unpredictable aggravating factors is 30.69. It is important for clinicians to understand that patients are likely to present with varying amounts of each of these pain mechanisms regardless of acuity of the injury. For example, a patient may present with a 2-week onset of symptoms that appears to be CTS and have symptoms that are 70% peripheral neuropathic, 20% nociceptive, and 10% central sensitization. Understanding and classifying pain allows the clinician the ability to better plan the objective examination and treatment plan. Establishing symptom behavior by obtaining aggravating and easing factors and the 24-hour behavior of the symptoms provides further insight into the patient's presentation and the clinician's potential hypotheses. A discussion of which activities, postures, and positions/movements produce the patient's symptoms—including the amount of time to onset and location/intensity of symptoms, followed by positions, movements, or activities to settle the symptoms—can aide in determining whether the neural or vascular system is a potential source of the problem and determining the level of tissue irritability. When an extended period of time is required for symptoms to ease after very little activity provokes the symptoms, then irritability may be deemed high. Motor changes of relevance to the potential problem of neurovascular entrapment include complaints of dropping things, weakness, or an inability to perform motor tasks that were done previously without difficulty. Key components that should be discussed with the patient include history of trauma, repetitive activities, sustained static or tension postures (e.g., computer keyboard work), or physical activities performed with a high level of cognitive demand, as seen in a pianist. In addition, the progression of the symptoms or complaints should be determined. The history should include a discussion of general health and screening questions for relevant medical conditions such as asthma, diabetes, and hypothyroidism. Chapter 6 of this text provides more detail regarding medical screening and a differential diagnosis to ensure patients are appropriate for evaluation and intervention.

Health-related quality of life or patient-reported outcome measures are useful in patient management to assess multiple domains such as physical ability, psychological, emotional, and social well-being. Condition specific measures can be utilized for neurovascular entrapments, such as The Michigan Hand Outcomes Questionnaire for patients with CTS.[75] For conditions such as TOS, condition-specific measures do not currently exist; therefore clinicians may choose more generic measures such as the Neck Disability Index or the Disabilities of the Arm, Shoulder, and Hand (DASH).[76] The Fear Avoidance Beliefs Questionnaire was developed to measure fear and avoidance of activity in patients with low back pain; however, it has now gained acceptance for usage in conditions outside of low back pain, to screen for depression risk factors. The depression screening questions consist of a cluster of three questions that have established likelihood ratios (LR), +LR of 9.1 and −LR 0.05.[77] Use of these tools in daily practice provide the

clinician with a broader view of the patient's self-rated function and insight into potential psychosocial barriers to treatment. Health-related quality of life measures provide reliable, valid, and responsive tools to measure the outcome of interventions.[78]

Objective Examination

The objective examination in patients with neurovascular entrapment can be complex, and the clinician needs to utilize tests and measures that help rule out potential competing diagnoses. The differential diagnosis for a suspected neurovascular entrapment of the upper extremity includes cervical spine referral/radiculopathy, brachial plexus injury, rotator cuff pathology, glenohumeral joint dysfunction, lateral epicondylalgia, medial epicondylalgia, complex regional pain syndrome (CRPS I or II), systemic disorders, and upper extremity deep vein thrombosis.[70]

Given the extensive differential diagnosis list, both the subjective and objective exams will be comprehensive. The clinician must gauge the patient's level of irritability during the subjective exam to determine the vigor of the objective exam, thereby avoiding excessive or unintentional provocation of the patient's symptoms. Table 16.2 provides the suggested modifications to a standard biomechanical

TABLE 16.2 Suggested Modifications to a Standard Biomechanical Evaluation

Nerve Mechanosensitivity Testing
Upper Limb Neural Dynamic Test (active and passive)[4]

Right position:	_____	causes/increases symptoms
Left position:	_____	causes/increases symptoms

Nerve Palpation[4]

Median	Right/left	causes/increases symptoms
Radial	Right/left	causes/increases symptoms
Ulnar	Right/left	causes/increases symptoms

Neurological Examination

Myotomes	Right	Left
Deep tendon reflexes[76]	Biceps Brachioradialis Triceps	(0=absent, 1=diminished, 2=average, 3=exaggerated, 4=clonus/very brisk)

Sensation-Dermatome/Peripheral Nerve Field

Light touch	Right	Left
Sharp/dull	Right	Left

Upper Motor Neuron Testing

Hoffman's:	Present/Absent
Clonus:	Present/Absent
Babinski:	Present/Absent

Special Tests
Tinel Sign[79,80]

Supraclavicular region:		Right	Left
Elbow:		Right	Left
Wrist:	Median	Right	Left
	Ulnar	Right	Left

Continued

TABLE 16.2   Suggested Modifications to a Standard Biomechanical Evaluation—cont'd

Adson Test[79,81]   *(Change in Pulse Pressure/Provocation of Symptoms)*
Right:

Left:

Wright Test[79]   *(Change in Pulse Pressure/Provocation of Symptoms)*
Right:

Left:

ROOS Test[79]   *(Provocation of Symptoms)*
Right: (time)

Left: (time)

Hyperabduction Test[79]   *(Change in Pulse Pressure/Provocation of Symptoms)*
Right:

Left:

Phalen Test[80]   *(Provocation of Symptoms)*
Right:

Left:

Median Nerve Compression Test[80,81]   *(Provocation of Symptoms)*
Right: (time)

Left: (time)

Breathing Pattern (Ability to Relax the Scalene Muscles With Quiet Breathing)
Normal or dysfunctional pattern

Palpation Findings
(Tenderness: Normal = 0; Mild = 1+; Moderate = 2+; Severe = 3+)

Scalene muscles:	Right:	Left:
Subclavius:	Right:	Left:
Pectoralis minor:	Right:	Left:

Vascular Integrity
Temperature of hands (ambient room temperature)

Right: (index)	(digiti minimi)
Left: (index)	(digiti minimi)

examination of the upper quarter necessary to rule in/out potential neurovascular entrapment. The clinician must adjust the examination based on the patient's unique presentation and the irritability of the condition. Generally, it is recommended that the examination proceed from active movement produced by the patient to passive assessment. When possible, testing maneuvers should be performed by the patient so that he or she can learn to self-assess his or her status before and after treatment procedures. This self-assessment gives the patient control, thus decreasing the fear of movement or reinjury. The concept of the patient gaining control of the problem(s) is fundamental and must be integrated into the initial patient contact for development of an effective self-management approach. Without an effective self-management strategy, the patient is at risk for recurrent problems and the development of a chronic condition. The objective examination

scheme presented here is considering neurovascular entrapment of the upper extremity. Emphasis will be placed on CTS and TOS; however, the sequence of the examination can remain the same for the lower extremity by replacing the regions examined and the special tests utilized.

Observation is initially completed in sitting; the patient's head on neck posture should be assessed while looking for deviations of the head in the frontal and sagittal planes. The clinician should take note of rounded shoulders and an increase in thoracic kyphosis as these changes in posture may increase tension on the brachial plexus.[69] The scapular position should be assessed at rest and dynamically with active motion of the upper extremities.[70] Observation includes evaluating the integrity of the vascular system in the extremities. The hands, or feet, should be inspected for discoloration, and the skin temperature

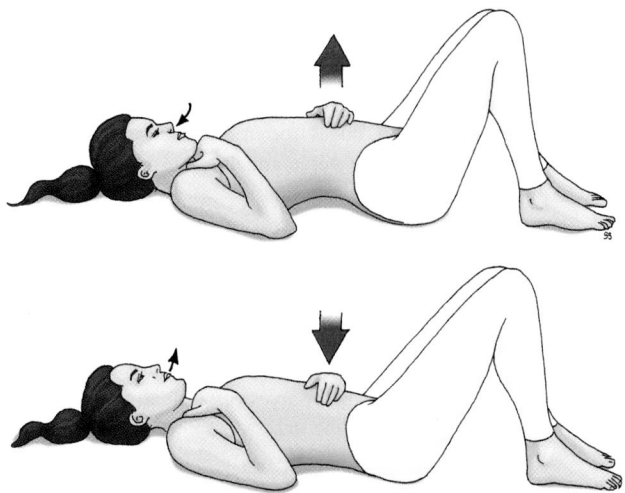

Fig. 16.2 Diaphragmatic Breathing. As the patient inhales, the stomach should rise and the lordosis in the low back should increase. During exhalation the stomach should fall and the back should flatten against the floor.

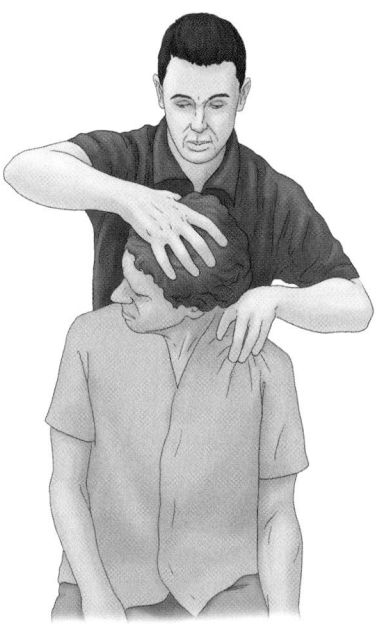

Fig. 16.3 Demonstration of clinician performing the cervical rotation and lateral flexion (CRLF) test on a patient.

should be determined in each of the peripheral nerve territories present in the affected limb. *Hand temperature* is assessed with an infrared hand-held thermometer. Thermal measurements are made of the second digit (innervated by the upper roots of the brachial plexus) and fifth digit (innervated by the lower roots). Temperature is assessed during rest, diaphragmatic breathing, walking on a treadmill, and repeated movements of the upper extremities. A normal response is an increase in temperature in response to these activities. A cooling response is considered abnormal. Cool, cyanotic skin can be an indication of arterial insufficiency or sympathetic dysreflexia in the area, whereas swelling can be an indication of inflammation and venous or lymphatic insufficiency. The hands should be inspected for the presence of atrophy, which can be present as a result of neurovascular entrapment. Observation of the patient's breathing pattern at rest and in the supine position should be performed.

The normal *breathing pattern* at rest is primarily diaphragmatic (Fig. 16.2). However, patients with neurovascular entrapment often demonstrate a breathing pattern at rest that relies predominantly on the scalene muscles. The scalene breathing pattern mechanically narrows the thoracic outlet area, thus potentially perpetuating a neurovascular entrapment syndrome in the area. The scalene breathing pattern may be a sign of protective posturing. The *breathing pattern* is further assessed by palpating the scalene muscles in the area between the inferior border of the sternocleidomastoid and is superior to the clavicle. This procedure is best done while the patient performs relaxed inhalation. The scalene muscles are normally quiet during relaxed inhalation. Contraction of the scalene muscles and elevation of the sternum are considered to be abnormal during quiet inhalation. Patients are instructed to breathe with the "belly" only (diaphragmatic breathing). If they are unable to do this, breathing is considered to be paradoxical.

Active/passive range of motion testing includes a screening of the upper quarter and should include the cervical spine, shoulder, elbow, wrist, and hands. The depth of assessment is based on the need to rule in or out the competing disorders. During the active and passive range of motion assessment, the examiner measures the quality and quantity of the motion as well as the joint end feel during passive motion testing. Range of motion is objectively documented using a goniometer or inclinometer at the initial assessment and is compared at follow-up

visits.[70] In patients with suspected TOS, first rib mobility can be assessed via a combined movement test of cervical rotation and lateral flexion (CRLF).[82] Fig. 16.3 demonstrates the CRLF with the patient in sitting, the uninvolved side is assessed first to establish a baseline followed by the involved side. The test is considered positive if a bony block is experienced, limiting the lateral flexion portion of the test.[82]

Resisted testing using standard manual muscle testing procedures can be utilized to identify muscle imbalances/weakness in the shoulder, scapula, elbow, wrist, and hand.[83] Strength can be assessed using a 0 to 5 classification or a hand-held dynamometer. Motor function of the cervical spine, specifically the longus capitis and longus colli, is completed as described by Jull and colleagues[84] This method of assessment and treatment targets the deep neck flexor muscles and reduces recruitment of the sternocleidomastoid and scalene muscles, which can become overactive in patients with neurovascular entrapment conditions such as TOS or CTS. The reliability of hand-held dynamometer use in the upper extremity is limited with only testing of the elbow demonstrating acceptable intrarater reliability.[85]

Hand strength (grip strength) assessment is done as a standard part of the objective exam for patients suspected of having neurovascular entrapment. Many patients with suspected neurovascular entrapment of the upper extremity complain of changes to grip strength, and in cases of an advanced condition demonstrate atrophy of the hand intrinsic muscles. Grip strength is commonly assessed with a grip dynamometer, and the average of three trials per hand is recorded.[76]

Neurological examination is a thorough process that includes sensory testing, motor, and deep tendon reflexes (DTRs) assessment in the upper extremities. Standard assessment of sensation includes light touch and pin-prick testing. Sensation loss in conjunction with motor deficits and normal or abnormal DTRs may be indicative of neurological TOS. Sensation loss in the median nerve distribution may be indicative of CTS. Reduction of DTRs (hyporeflexia) may be due to cervical spine involvement, which suggests further examination if present. Hyperreflexia may indicate upper motor neuron involvement and should be followed up with clinical tests such as Babinski, Clonus, and Hoffman's.

Neurodynamic testing beyond the standard neurological examination is used to assess the sensitivity of neural tissue.[86] Neurodynamics of the upper extremity are assessed with the use of upper limb neural dynamic (ULND) tests as described by Butler.[4] Passive neck flexion is examined to assess dural sensitivity, whereas the straight leg raise test is used to assess the sensitivity of the sciatic nerve and sacral plexus. Reliability of ULND testing has been reported to be 0.54 for the median nerve, 0.44 for the radial nerve, and 0.36 for the ulnar nerve.[87] In addition to these passive neural dynamic tests performed by the examining therapist, the patient is instructed to complete the neurodynamic maneuvers actively.

Self-neurodynamic tests are encouraged prior to the passive techniques in all patients; however, it is highly encouraged in patients who have high severity. Care must be taken to educate the patient to stop at the first sensation of tension and not to linger with the arm in any self-test position that provokes symptoms. The self-neurodynamic tests are performed by guiding the patient through a series of positions using the upper extremity (Fig. 16.4). This is an active test that the patient, the medical provider, and the physical therapist can use as an indicator of upper quarter neural sensitivity. The test provides immediate feedback regarding the patient's response to an exercise or other form of intervention. The test results can be used as an indicator of a change in patient status. The test is an important tool that helps the patient recognize and manage symptom flares. The self-neurodynamic test is one of the self-assessment tools that encourage the patient to take control of his or her treatment. The provided example (see Fig. 16.4) demonstrates a self-neurodynamic test of the median nerve. A modification to this test in an irritable patient can include instructing the patient to turn his or her head to the involved side and/or having the patient look at the palm of the hand prior to initiating the test. Once the upper extremity is in the tension position, the patient is instructed to look straight ahead, adding additional tension to the test maneuver. Testing of the radial and ulnar nerves can be carried out in a similar fashion with the components of the active test mimicking the standard passive test. (Please refer to the references at the end of this chapter for more information on neural dynamic tests.)

Palpation is used to determine whether tenderness or tightness is present in the soft tissues. Palpation of the subclavius, pectoralis minor, and scalene muscles is significant because of the relationship these muscles have with the subclavian vein, brachial plexus

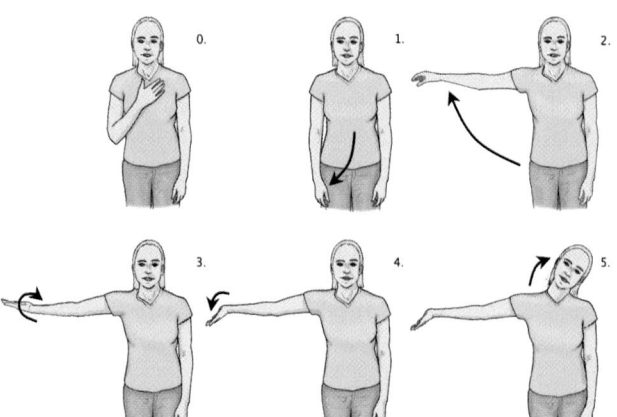

Fig. 16.4 Demonstration of Arm Self-Neurodynamic Test Positions. The arm self-neurodynamic test is an active upper extremity neural dynamic test.

components, and subclavian artery, respectively. The results of palpation should be correlated to the neurological and vascular changes found elsewhere in the extremity. Nerve palpation is a means to examine mechanosensitivity of the nerve in addition to ULND testing.[4] The reliability of nerve palpation ranges from moderate to substantial, 0.59 (0.46, 0.72).[87] Palpation of the nerve and the self-neurodynamic are often the preferred methods of examination of mechanosensitivity in the irritable patient.

Accessory mobility testing of the cervical and thoracic spine is commonly necessary for patients with TOS and/or CTS. Impairments identified in corresponding levels to the upper extremity (C5 to C7) may have an impact on neurovascular disorders when taking a "double crush" syndrome into consideration. The joints of the shoulder, elbow, wrist/hand are assessed passively for accessory mobility as indicated.[76] For further information regarding accessory mobility testing of the cervical and thoracic spine, refer to Magee.[16,76]

Special tests in the upper extremity can be utilized to contribute to the process of ruling in/out neurovascular entrapments. The number of special tests available for CTS and TOS are extensive with varying diagnostic utility given the range in sensitivity (Sn), specificity (Sp), and LRs. It is beyond the scope of this chapter to discuss all the tests available; however, the tests with the best diagnostic utility will be discussed. Given the potential confusion between a diagnosis of CTS and TOS, tests that differentiate between the two conditions are recommended.[70] Typically, tests for TOS assess a change in or the obliteration of the pulse. The reliability of a change in pulse is poor; therefore it is recommended that symptom provocation be assessed as well as a change in the patient's pulse. There are several clinical tests for TOS; however, Gillard and colleagues identified a cluster of tests that can be used to rule in/out TOS. Adson maneuver, Wright's, ROOS, hyperabduction test, and Tinels are the five clinical tests that make up the cluster identified by Gillard. Tinels is conducted at the supra and infraclavicular region with symptom provocation assessed. During Wright test and the hyperabduction test, it is recommended that the clinician monitor both the pulse and symptoms. Five positive tests yield a +LR of 5.3 while five negative tests yield a −LR of 0.19.[79] A combination of clinical tests for TOS is valuable for ruling in/out the condition.

Clinical tests for CTS are primarily provocative tests directed at the carpal tunnel. Phalen test is the most widely accepted test used in the clinic. The patient sustains a position of wrist flexion while holding both forearms vertical for 60 seconds. Phalen's has a reported Sn of 0.59 to 0.64 and Sp of 0.75 to 0.93.[80,81] The negative predictive value (NPV) for Phalen's is 0.65, and the positive predictive value (PPV) is 0.91.[80] Tinels is utilized on the median nerve as it enters the carpal tunnel. Tinels has a reported Sn of 0.41, Sp of 0.90, an NPV of 0.56, and a PPV of 0.83.[80] The compression test or pressure pain provocation test is performed using sustained pressure at the carpal tunnel × 1 minute. The test has an Sn range of 0.14 to 0.42 and an Sp range of 0.96 to 0.99.[80,81] The NPV for the pressure provocation test is 0.58 and PPV is 0.97.[80] Given the current range in the diagnostic tests for TOS and CTS, it is important that the clinician consider all exam findings from the subjective and objective exam along with the results of the special tests when attempting to rule in/out a neurovascular disorder.

Symptom Patterns Characteristic of Neurovascular Entrapment

1. Symptoms often present as severe and irritable with a combination of pain mechanisms including nociceptive, peripheral neuropathic, and central sensitization.
2. Function is markedly reduced in the target task (injury-producing activity) and activities of daily living.

3. The patient reports feeling that his or her emotions are in a state of "being out of control."

The examination scheme is designed to evaluate for the presence of a neurovascular entrapment syndrome; however, the examination should be planned out to match the patient's current presentation and tissue irritability. The common signs in addition to the more traditional musculoskeletal signs are reassessed after intervention and serve as guides in determining the effectiveness of treatment.

Common Signs of Neurovascular Entrapment

1. Abnormal hand temperature within the following parameters:
   a. Cold hands defined as in the 70°F range at rest and during activity at the target task
   b. Asymmetry between the temperatures of the second digit and the fifth digit, with the fifth digit being colder[88]
2. Abnormal breathing pattern: accessory, chest, or paradoxical rather than diaphragmatic.
3. Abnormal mobility and sensitivity of the nervous system: specifically, the dura, the brachial plexus, the sciatic nerve, or sacral plexus.
4. Sensory dysfunction of the involved hand.
5. A combination of positive diagnostic tests to help rule in the condition.

This combination of symptoms and signs can identify a neurovascular component of the patient presentation. Improvements in these signs and symptoms serve as markers that identify treatment effectiveness—namely, a decrease in pain, an improvement in function, and a feeling of being more in control.

Neurovascular Entrapment Interventions

Treatment must follow the same principles that guide the examination; that is, the patient is taught self-assessment techniques and strategies to encourage active self-control of their treatment and activities of daily living. The patient may use any of the following self-assessment techniques, as appropriate, to guide the course of treatment: pain scale, hand temperature, active neurodynamic test, or grip strength test. Any treatment or activity that increases symptoms, and any protective posturing or tension is modified or discontinued.

Maximizing a positive treatment response requires a unique partnership between the physical therapist and the patient that facilitates a therapeutic alliance and the patient's feeling of being in control. The feeling of being in control is thought to have a positive impact on the response to treatment. The patient–therapist relationship is enhanced by providing simple, clear explanations of the condition.[89] Treatment should reflect the individual needs of the patient and their preferences.[89] By doing this, the therapist is likely to improve the patient's compliance with their program and active participation in the rehabilitation process. The patients are provided with self-assessment tools and treatment options. They are taught methods for self-assessment of the immediate impact of each intervention. They are taught to assess their responses to the core program on the basis of signs and symptoms as indicated above (pain scale, hand temperature, active neurodynamic test, or grip strength test).

Our intention is not to present every component of a total treatment program, but rather to highlight those core components that address common impairments identified in patients with neurovascular disorders. Treatment is initiated by addressing breathing patterns if an abnormal breathing pattern is observed, such as a scalene breathing pattern. The patient is guided through a series of breathing exercises designed to improve the circulation to the extremities, calm the nervous system, and retrain the diaphragm and scalene muscles, if appropriate. The breathing exercises are progressed through the use of foam rollers (Fig. 16.5), which are used to increase the mobility of the spine

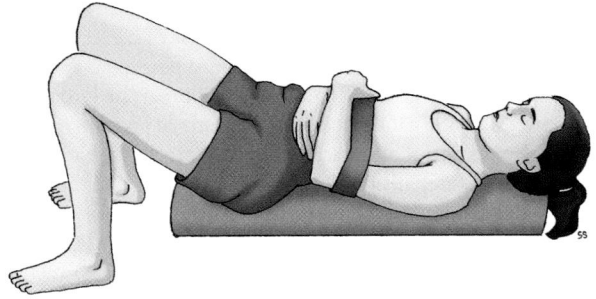

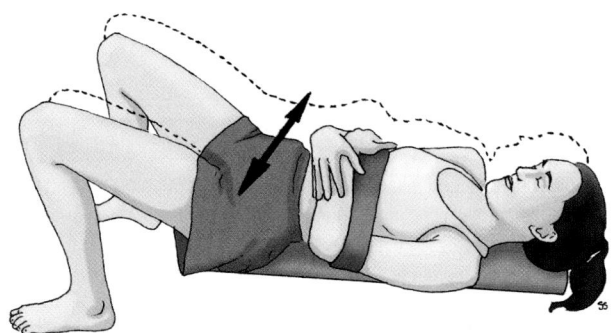

Fig. 16.5 Foam Roller Exercise for Mobilization of the Spine. The roller is placed underneath the spine with the patient in the supine position. The patient gently rolls from side to side to increase mobility of the spine.

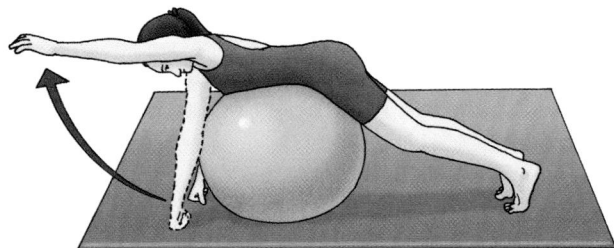

Fig. 16.6 Patient in a Quadruped Position on a Therapy Ball With the Chin Tucked and the Neck Straight. The patient can lift an upper or lower extremity to provide a challenge to the muscles that stabilize the spine.

and rib cage. The breathing exercises are combined with functional movements of the trunk and extremities in a manner that mobilizes the nervous system. In Fig. 16.5, a strap was utilized to support the involved extremity. Once the patient is able to manage the symptoms, their treatment can progress to stabilization exercises with a gym ball (Fig. 16.6).

Core Components of Treatment

Intervention is prioritized based on the patient's tissue irritability. Beyond addressing abnormal breathing patterning, it is recommended to initiate treatment at the most proximal impairments. Specific muscle reeducation for the longus capitis and longus colli of the cervical spine is accomplished utilizing Jull's protocol.[84] The patient is taught to minimize mechanical stress to the cervical and thoracic spine through instruction in body mechanics. Manual therapy techniques to address impairments at the cervical and thoracic spine are also utilized, and the patient is taught self-mobilization techniques, as appropriate, for use at home. Manual therapy interventions and patient generated exercises commonly target the first rib and scalene musculature as these structures can impact neurovascular tissue in patients with TOS and even CTS. If scapula dyskinesis is identified during the active motion portion of the examination and use of correction techniques alter the patient's symptoms, then scapula position is addressed in the rehabilitation process.[90] Scapula control is progressed from basic setting exercises for the patient to obtain the optimal position followed by progression to control of the scapula with humeral active motion.[90]

Hand temperature, neurodynamic impairments, and breathing dysfunctions are addressed by training the patient to perform relaxed diaphragmatic breathing with spinal motion (see Fig. 16.2). The expected outcomes are to normalize hand temperature and to increase range of motion of the involved extremity while decreasing sensitivity of the nervous system. Adverse neurodynamics are also addressed by treating soft tissue impairments identified along the course of the nerve with utilization of slider techniques. Slider techniques produce the largest amount of nerve excursion with minimal strain compared to tensioner techniques.[91] Coppieters and Alshami,[92] in a cadaver study of nerve gliding, noted increased strain on the median nerve in positions of wrist extension combined with elbow extension. Addressing the interfacing soft tissue along with slider techniques can contribute to a reduction in neuromechanosensitivity of the involved extremity. Low cardiovascular endurance is addressed by having the patient begin a progressive aerobic conditioning program of walking. The goal of treatment should not only focus on improving the clinical signs and symptoms found on examination, but also the patient's overall functional status. Continual reassessment of key clinical indicators throughout treatment, and reassessment of the patient-reported outcome measures, inform the patient and clinician how to progress each element of the entire rehabilitation program.

CASE STUDY

The following case example describes brief components of this patient's initial physical therapy examination and treatment. This presentation is not meant to describe a complete case but rather to illuminate key concepts in the clinical reasoning behind the physical therapy examination, the assessment, and the plan of care in a patient with signs and symptoms of neurovascular entrapment.

Patient Description

The patient was a 50-year-old male who was left-hand dominant. He presented with a 12-week history of tingling and pain in his left hand. The symptoms were located in the palmar aspect of the hand and included the thumb, index, and long fingers. The body chart demonstrates the location and description of the patient's symptoms (Fig. 16.7). He denied any specific injury to the left hand and stated the symptoms had progressed over the past 12 weeks. The symptoms were described as constant and variable and were worse at night. The patient was unable to work as a carpenter and martial arts instructor due to these left-hand symptoms.

The patient reported the following *aggravating factors*: (1) Playing drums would increase left-hand symptoms within 5 minutes. (2) Unable to play the guitar due to left-hand symptoms within 2 to 3 minutes. (3) Diminished left-hand coordination/dexterity. The patient noted consistently dropping items from his left hand. *Easing factors* for the patient's symptoms included shaking his left hand or avoiding the use of the left hand. *24-hour behavior*: Sleep was interrupted due to left-hand tingling. The patient indicated that left-hand symptoms were more intense at night and required frequent position changes. He reported waking every 2 hours and his ability to return to sleep varied. He complained of feeling fatigued due to lack of regular sleep. Symptoms in the morning and during the day were largely dependent on the use of his left hand.

Past history included neck pain that was diagnosed as a C6 disc herniation 12 years ago. He indicated multiple upper extremity injuries from martial arts training and three bicycle accidents. The current symptoms in his left hand had not been experienced in the past.

Clinical Reasoning

Diagnostic hypothesis is based on the subjective examination findings:
1. Potential C6/7 referral due to past history of neck pain and location of symptoms
2. Potential carpal tunnel syndrome (CTS) due to location and description of symptoms
3. Potential median nerve entrapment proximally with altered neural dynamics
4. Nonmusculoskeletal condition:
   a. Night symptoms require further screening

Physical Examination

In sitting, the patient demonstrated an increase in thoracic kyphosis without evidence of head on neck deviations. The patient's breathing pattern appeared normal at rest while sitting. Based on the patient's body chart and symptom description, the nervous system was considered a potential source of symptoms. (See Table 16.2 for suggested modifications to a biomechanically based musculoskeletal examination to use when the nervous system is considered a significant source of dysfunction.)

The patient was instructed to complete active motions to the limit of his range and indicate the onset of symptoms during movement testing. The physical examination was planned to help rule in/out competing hypotheses such as the cervical spine and CTS. The general health screen and basic vital sign assessment assisted in reducing the suspicion of a nonmusculoskeletal source of symptoms. The patient was asked to complete a functional test mimicking guitar playing. Modification of cervical position did not produce symptoms; however, manual cervical traction provided relief of the patient's left-hand symptoms.

Active cervical range of motion revealed motion loss with left rotation and lateral flexion with a firm end feel compared to right rotation and lateral flexion. Limitations in left rotation and lateral flexion produced local neck pain; however, these movements did not aggravate his left-hand symptoms. Grip strength was tested using a grip dynamometer and revealed a significant side-to-side difference, with the right at 105 pounds and the left at 75 pounds.

Neurovascular examination revealed reproduction of the patient's left-hand symptoms with direct palpation of the median nerve proximally at the humerus. Neurodynamic testing emphasizing the median nerve, both active and passive, reproduced the patient's left-hand symptoms. Special tests utilized to rule in/out CTS, including Phalen, Tinel, and the compression test at the carpal tunnel, all reproduced the patient's symptoms.

Based on the patient's past history, cervical motion loss with left rotation and lateral flexion, and relief of symptoms with manual traction, an accessory mobility test of the cervical spine was conducted. This test revealed hypomobility of the C6 and C7 motion segments as well as T1 to T3 motion segments. The left-hand symptoms were not reproduced during accessory mobility testing.

Clinical Reasoning

Diagnostic hypothesis is based on physical examination findings:
1. Carpal tunnel syndrome
2. Double crush syndrome
3. Altered neural dynamics based on the presence of:
   a. Provocation of distal symptoms with direct palpation of the median nerve
   b. Active and passive neurodynamic test of the median nerve produces left hand symptoms

Intervention

The patient was taught a neural dynamic self-assessment technique that primarily sensitized the median nerve. He was instructed to use this test to evaluate his response to activity. If he had a negative response to an exercise or activities of daily living—as evidenced by an increase in symptoms or a decrease in the range of his arm self-test—he was instructed to modify or discontinue the activity and perform a self-treatment that restored his tension-free range.

Given the physical examination findings and hypothesis regarding a double crush pathology, manual therapy was deemed appropriate. The patient was treated with left downglide mobilizations into tissue/joint resistance directed at C6 and C7, followed by manual cervical traction. Immediate reassessment of median nerve palpation and upper limb neurodynamic testing revealed reduction in symptoms and improvement in mobility. Active cervical left rotation was unchanged. Instruction in self-traction with a towel was provided as part of his home exercise program, including instruction to use his self-test before and after traction (Fig. 16.8).

A slider exercise was implemented and directed primarily at the median nerve. An active slider exercise was chosen for excursion of the median nerve with minimal tensile stress. The slider exercise was followed by instruction in exercise on the foam roller. The intention of the foam roller exercise was to help mobilize his thoracic spine to improve his cervical posture on his own. After the slider and foam roller exercise, he maintained improvement in the tension-free range of his left arm self-test. The patient was instructed to complete these exercises 3 to 4 times per day and consistently monitor for changes in his signs and symptoms. Education included positioning for sleep at night, the use of a towel roll to support the cervical spine, and the use of a body pillow for arm support. Given the relief experienced with traction, the patient was encouraged to utilize towel traction prior to bed in an attempt to reduce symptoms and to improve sleep.

The plan for future visits should include continued use of manual therapy intervention targeting hypomobility of the cervical and upper thoracic spine as needed. Exercise progression should be based on the patient's symptoms and neural irritability. Progression of his exercise program should include scapula stabilization prone on a therapy ball (see Fig. 16.6), postural strengthening, and functional grip. Simulated work tasks, ergonomic improvements, and progression to recreational activities should be addressed, including emphasis on continued self-assessment of the response of the nervous system to the progression of activity.

Discussion

This case illustrates the importance of evaluating the role of the nervous system in patients with signs and symptoms associated with repetitive use of the upper extremity. In this case example the patient's problem was chronic without a specific injury. On further investigation he reported cervical symptoms in the past that needed to be explored given the potential relationship to his current complaint. The cervical symptoms could have delayed his recovery if not appropriately assessed on initial examination. As discussed earlier in this chapter, Upton and McComas[35] first reported the double crush phenomenon, and this case demonstrates the relationship between lesions at the carpal tunnel and the cervical spine. It is likely that the patient's past cervical involvement at the C6 level contributed to the restricted neural mobility along the median nerve; however, one is only able to theorize about the order of these lesions. Pain mechanisms for this patient were classified as primarily peripheral neuropathic with a nociceptive component. There was no evidence of central sensitivity based on the signs and symptoms presented by Smart and colleagues.[72] The most significant finding is that treatment directed at the cervical spine impacted the distal symptoms and reduced the neural sensitivity. There can be a wide spectrum of presentations of neurovascular entrapments ranging from subtle signs and symptoms of nervous system involvement to dramatic, life-altering, complex problems in patients who have undergone multiple medical and surgical interventions without obtaining symptom relief. The key to success in treating patients with neurovascular entrapments is recognizing the signs and symptoms of subtle nervous system involvement early. Neural sensitization[4] and possible processing changes in the central nervous system[72,73] necessitate evaluation of the nervous system as a potential source of symptoms in patients with symptoms

of repetitive use. If the issues of nervous system irritability and sensitization are not addressed during evaluation and throughout treatment, then the risk for increasing the patient's symptoms and continuing the cycle of nervous system hypersensitivity is high.

The indicators that this patient may have had a nervous system dysfunction were his description of symptoms, aggravating factors that included repetitive use, and the pattern of his symptoms. The indicators of nervous system dysfunction on physical examination were the restricted upper limb neural dynamic test (active and passive) and symptomatic response to palpation of the median nerve. Another objective indicator not assessed initially that may have further guided the treatment could have been measuring the temperature of the patient's hands.[88]

A key concept to keep in mind is the role of education in treating patients with a problem such as neurovascular entrapment. Patient–clinician communication is extremely important when dealing with all patients, but the clinician's communication skills are especially challenged when dealing with a patient who has a neurovascular entrapment. Describing the dysfunction of a neurovascular entrapment to the patient in succinct, nonmedical terminology can be quite difficult, but it is a critical step in the patient encounter to help him or her develop an understanding of what is wrong so he or she can engage in self-treatment. Teaching patients self-assessment tools restores their control, allowing them to guide their own treatment and to be more responsible for their own well-being.

Questions

1. How vigorous should the objective exam be in a patient with suspected neurovascular entrapment?

   Answer: The objective or physical exam vigor is based on the patient's tissue irritability. This is established during the subjective exam and is monitored over the course of the physical exam. In this patient case, the patient's symptoms were worse at night and resulted in the patient waking every 2 h. This piece of information alone could lead the clinician to suspect a higher level of irritability; however, when one considers that during the day the patient is able to complete functional tasks without significant worsening in the intensity of his symptoms, then irritability is considered low. Classifying the patient's irritability as minimal allowed the examination to proceed with active and passive movements to the limits of available motion while monitoring symptom onset/response. If the patient had presented with irritability that was classified as moderate to high, then the examination would have been altered, instructing the patient to move just to the onset of symptoms. The number of examination items was not limited in this patient case given the low irritability and the desire to rule in/out CTS. If the irritability was classified as moderate to high, then the number of examination items would have been reduced with emphasis placed instead on symptom control.

2. How would you instruct a patient to do an active self-test of the arm?

   Answer: I say to the patient "I am going to ask you to place your arm in a sequence of positions. I want you to stop when you feel tightness anywhere in your arm or if you feel an increase or change in your symptoms. We will redo the self-test after we have done some exercises. That way you can decide which exercise helps you the most." After the patient has completed one form of treatment followed by a reassessment self-test, then I help the patient interpret the symptom response. "If your self-test result was worse (less arm range or increased pain), it means that your nervous system was moved too far and is more sensitive. This means that the exercise we tried is too vigorous for you at this time. If your self-test result was better (greater range, less pain), then this exercise was helpful and was calming to your nervous system. The self-test is something you can always use to help you evaluate whether an exercise or activity is going to be appropriate or too vigorous for your arms."

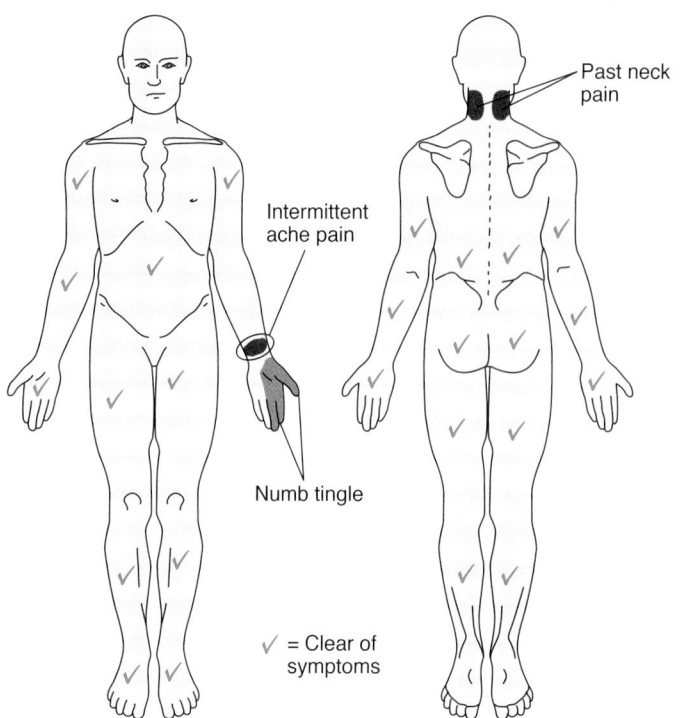

Fig. 16.7 Body Chart With Symptomatic Areas Marked by the Patient in the Case Study.

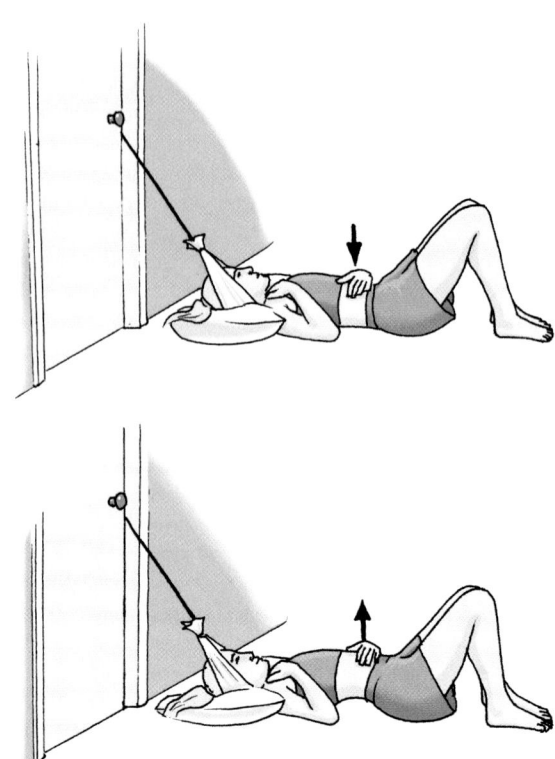

Fig. 16.8 Towel Traction Unit. Through arching of the low back, the amount of traction is increased slightly. Through flattening of the low back, the amount of traction is decreased slightly.

ACKNOWLEDGMENTS

The authors wish to acknowledge and extend their deep appreciation to Peter Edgelow and Laura Kenny for their work on previous versions of this chapter. They both contributed significantly to the development of many of the ideas presented. We are honored and thankful for the opportunity to have known and worked with them.

REFERENCES

To enhance this text and add value for the reader, all references are included on the companion Evolve site that accompanies this textbook. This online service will, when available, provide a link for the reader to a Medline abstract for the article cited. There are 92 cited references and other general references for this chapter, with the majority of those articles being evidence-based citations.

17

Multiple Sclerosis

Gail L. Widener and Kristin Horn

OBJECTIVES

After reading this chapter the student or therapist will be able to:

1. Describe the pathological processes, prevalence, and clinical presentation of people with multiple sclerosis.
2. Compare and contrast the subtypes of multiple sclerosis and the common disease progression in each.
3. Discuss the medical management of the disease and the disease symptoms, including diagnosis and treatment.
4. Describe the concept of variability and how it applies to people with multiple sclerosis, pathology, medical management, and rehabilitation.
5. Describe how the International Classification of Functioning, Disability and Health provides a common language for describing the impact of disease on people with multiple sclerosis and how it provides a framework for rehabilitation management.
6. Describe the outcome measures that can be used to examine people with multiple sclerosis that cover body system problems (impairments), functional skill and activity limitations, participation restrictions, and quality of life.
7. Develop a rehabilitation plan of care using evidence-based interventions to maximize patient function and quality of life.

KEY TERMS

autoimmune disease
axonal damage
clinically isolated syndrome
demyelination
disease-modifying therapy
exacerbation
immune system

inflammation
lesion
neurodegeneration
neuroprotection
plaques
primary progressive
progressive relapsing

radiologically isolated syndrome
relapse
relapsing remitting
remission
secondary progressive

OVERVIEW OF MULTIPLE SCLEROSIS

Multiple sclerosis (MS) is a progressive disease of the central nervous system that can impact the brain, spinal cord, and optic nerve. Because there is no known cure for the disease, rehabilitation is fundamental to management of the various symptoms and dysfunctions that occur. One key aspect of this disease for rehabilitation clinicians to understand is variability. This applies to how the disease initially manifests, how it progresses, and the medical and rehabilitation interventions used to slow disease progression and enhance function. The clinical presentation and disease progression of each person with MS will be unique. This requires clinicians to assess each patient/client individually and collaborate with them to determine the optimal plan of care.

Incidence and Prevalence

MS is one of the most common causes of nontraumatic disability in young people and adults[1] and is the most common inflammatory condition of the central nervous system (CNS). It is reported that approximately 400,000 people in the United States and over 2.5 million people worldwide have the disease.[2] People are most commonly diagnosed between 20 to 50 years of age, with the average age around 31.[1]

However, MS can be diagnosed in people of almost any age. Approximately 3% to 5% of all people with MS are diagnosed before their 18th birthday, with an estimated 10,000 children and adolescents with MS in the United States.[3–5] Another 15,000 people aged 18 years or less have symptoms consistent with MS.[2]

MS is found in people who reside above the northern or below the southern latitude of 40 degrees with greater frequency than in those who live closer to the equator (Fig. 17.1). Given the increased sun exposure of people living closer to the equator, lack of vitamin D is being investigated as a potential factor contributing to disease development[6]; there is a reduced relapse rate noted with higher blood levels.[7] Other environmental risk factors include smoking, obesity,[8] and exposure to infectious agents: Epstein-Barr virus and infectious mononucleosis are currently considered the most likely candidates.[9,10] Additionally, genetics may play a role in the development of MS. An identical twin with MS means that the other twin will have a 25% chance of diagnosis, suggesting something beyond genetics. Having a first-degree relative with MS will increase the risk of disease from 1 in 750 to 1 in 40.[2] Currently, the most likely genetic factor linked to MS is a form of the HLA-DRB1 gene.[11]

Women are affected 1.5 to 2.5 times more frequently than men.[12] Men are, however, more likely to have a more aggressive disease progression and a worse prognosis.[13,14] It has been generally accepted that

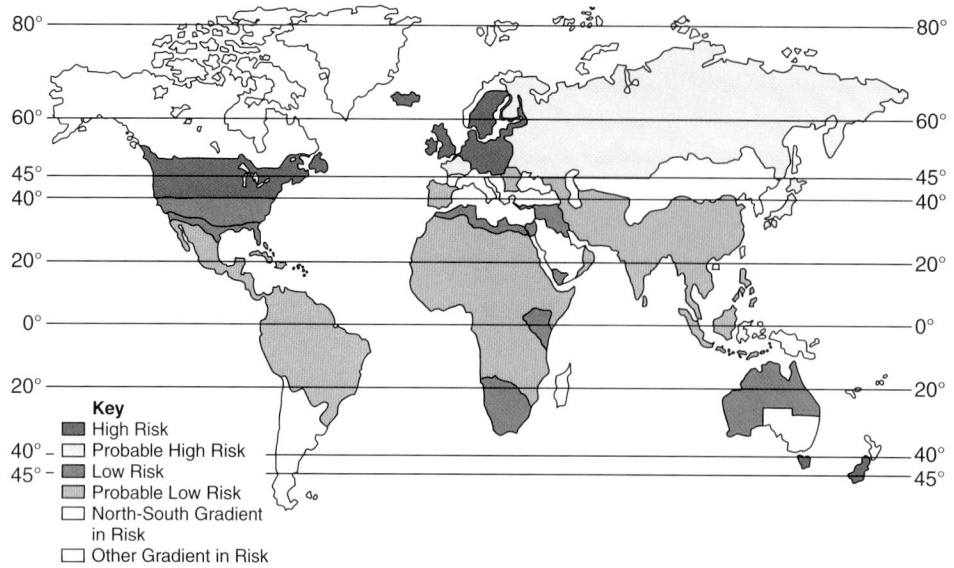

Fig. 17.1 World Distribution of Multiple Sclerosis. (From Multiple Sclerosis Resource Center, www.msrc.co.uk.)

Caucasians with Northern European ancestry have the greatest incidence of MS, whereas people of Asian, African, or Hispanic ethnicity are at lower risk. However, these findings may represent a significant bias as few studies have looked at the incidence and prevalence of MS in many parts of the world, including Africa, Asia, and the Middle East,[15] which may put the longitudinal hypothesis into question. A recent investigation in the US found that African Americans have a greater incidence than whites, with black females having the highest incidence.[16] African Americans develop MS at an earlier age,[17] have more frequent relapses and become disabled earlier than Caucasians,[18] and have a greater risk of developing progressive disease.[19] These factors suggest that tissue destruction occurs earlier and progresses more rapidly in this population.[18] Additionally, African Americans with MS have poorer responses to disease modifying medications.[20] In contrast,

Inuits, Yakutes, Hutterites, Hungarian Romani, Norwegian Lapps, Australian Aborigines, and New Zealand Maoris do not appear to develop MS.[21] Overall, being diagnosed with MS may be related to age, sex, genetics, geography, or ethnic background.

Subtypes of Multiple Sclerosis

Several MS disease phenotypes or subtypes have been identified (Fig. 17.2). Importantly, the course of the disease is highly variable regardless of the subtype of MS.

The initial neurological episode or attack is typically identified as the *clinical isolated syndrome* (CIS). Symptoms must last for at least 24 hours and can be monofocal or multifocal. If lesions are present on magnetic resonance imaging (MRI), there is a high risk of developing MS. In one group of people with CIS followed for 20 years, 63% were

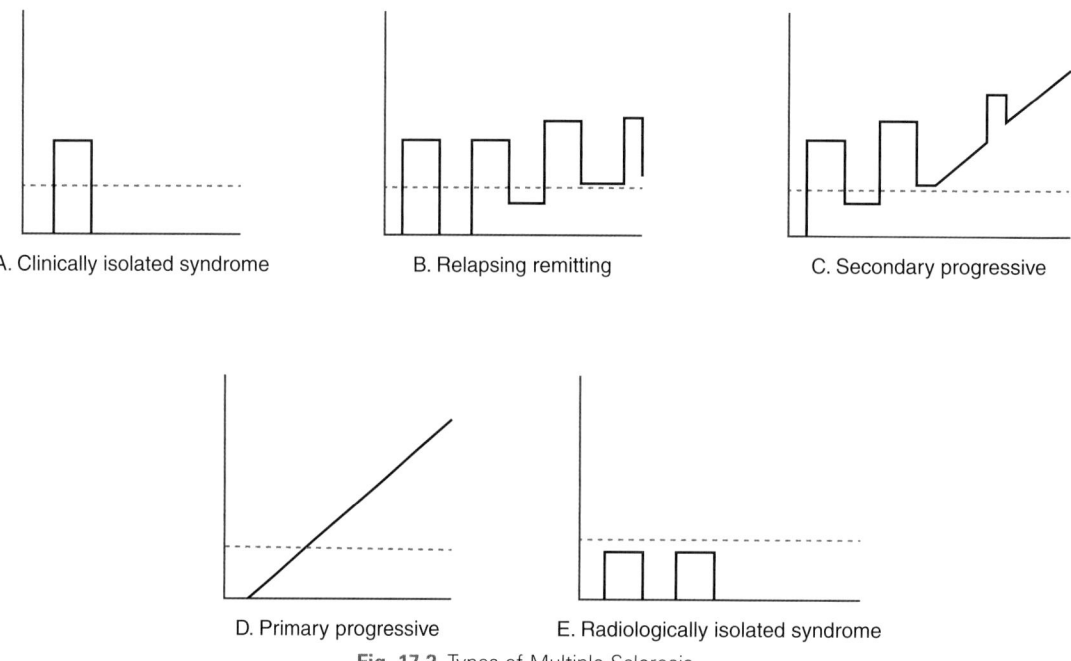

A. Clinically isolated syndrome   B. Relapsing remitting   C. Secondary progressive

D. Primary progressive   E. Radiologically isolated syndrome

Fig. 17.2 Types of Multiple Sclerosis.

eventually diagnosed with definite MS.[10] The newly revised McDonald criteria for diagnosing MS22 encourages the identification of lesions on MRI that indicate prior disease activity, thus allowing earlier diagnosis (see Fig. 17.2A).

Relapsing remitting MS (RRMS) (see Fig. 17.2B) represents about 85% of people with MS, characterized by exacerbations (attacks, relapses) that can last days to months and are typically followed by periods of less active disease or remissions. During remissions, function can return to prerelapse levels, but most frequently recovery is not complete. Attacks normally occur with a frequency of one or two per year. Approximately 90% of people with RRMS transition to *secondary progressive* MS (SPMS) 10 to 15 years after diagnosis (Fig. 17.2C).[11,23]

With *SPMS*, relapses may occur early but gradually lessen over time and convert to a steady progression of increasing disability and disease severity. It is thought that the clinical disability associated with SPMS results from the neurodegeneration that occurs as a result of tissue injury that accumulates from early in the disease process. In addition to less inflammation, there is a greater amount of brain atrophy in people with SPMS compared with RRMS. Fig. 17.3 shows the natural history of RMS and SPMS, comparing the change in brain volume with increasing clinical disability and disease burden.[24]

Primary progressive MS (PPMS) is less common, affecting only 10% to 15% of people with MS. From disease onset, progression results in a gradual worsening of symptoms without relapses. People tend to be older when diagnosed (late 30s or early 40s), have fewer abnormalities on brain MRI, and respond less favorably to standard MS drug therapies. Progressive myelopathy is commonly associated with PPMS (see Fig. 17.2D).

The term *radiologically isolated syndrome* (RIS) is used to describe a group of individuals whose imaging studies (MRI) strongly suggest the presence of MS; however, they have no clinical manifestations of the disease (see Fig. 17.2E). These individuals are typically identified after MRI has been prescribed for an unrelated concern, such as headaches. Small studies indicate that about a third of these people develop MS within 5 years; there is an increased risk of developing MS in individuals with asymptomatic lesions in the spinal cord.[25]

There is a push to categorize people with MS as either relapsing (RMS) or progressive (PMS), with primary or secondary as two types of progressive disease.[23]

Pathology

Multiple sclerosis is an incurable autoimmune disease resulting from dysregulation of the immune system, both T-cells and B-cells. Initiation of immune system dysregulation may occur in response to genetic and environmental factors discussed above.[8] The disease is characterized by inflammation, demyelination, axonal injury, and death that are present in lesions throughout the CNS.[15,26] Initially, MS was thought to be a disease of the white matter (WM) or myelinated parts of the neurons; however, the gray matter (GM), primarily neuron cell bodies, is significantly involved from early in the disease. Areas of demyelination and axonal damage interfere with normal conduction of neural signals, leading to a disruption of function.

Early in the course of the disease, lesions are composed of proinflammatory immune system components that produce demyelination, axonal injury, and loss of oligodendrocytes, referred to as *active* disease. Astrogliosis activated by the damaged neurons produces gliotic scarring called *plaques*. Plaques are visualized as sclerosis in postmortem brain tissue, hence the name multiple sclerosis. Active disease is followed by periods of remission in which acute inflammation is reduced (*inactive disease*). Axonal remyelination occurs but is highly variable and in RMS is related to recovery of function during periods of remission. Treatment in the initial stages of the RMS disease is aimed at reducing inflammation and immune system dysfunction with disease-modifying therapies (DMTs).

Later in the course of the disease inflammation becomes more diffuse while demyelination and axonal loss continue, suggesting a greater neurodegenerative process.[27] In most individuals, disease progression becomes more constant with a lack of exacerbation. Owing to the lack of inflammation, DMTs are less effective in progressive forms of the disease.

Brief Description of the Common Clinical Manifestations

MS can affect the optic nerve and any tissue within the brain or spinal cord, so almost any neurological symptom can result. Individual assessments are required to identify the problems present. The following list, however, constitutes the most common problems encountered by people with MS.

Due to the heterogeneous nature of the disease, symptoms are widespread according to the part or parts of the CNS that are affected. Common symptoms include fatigue, weakness, spasticity, sensory impairments (vision, somatosensation, vestibular, and hearing), pain, bladder or bowel dysfunction, tremor, incoordination or ataxia, sexual dysfunction, disorders of emotion, dysarthria, and dysphagia. Dysfunctions related to the disease include mobility and balance impairments and cognitive deficits. The most commonly reported problems in RMS are paresthesia, fatigue, and weakness, while PMS includes balance dysfunction and fatigue.[28] The symptoms most related to a reduced health-related quality of life for people with relapsing disease are balance dysfunction, spasticity, and depression while spasticity, paralysis, weakness, and pain have the greatest impacts in PMS.[28]

MEDICAL MANAGEMENT

Diagnosis

Historically, people with MS would wait for a diagnosis for a year or more—sometimes even longer. Although there are no definitive tests that diagnose MS, the addition of MRI has accelerated diagnosis. In 2001 the International Panel on the Diagnosis of Multiple Sclerosis

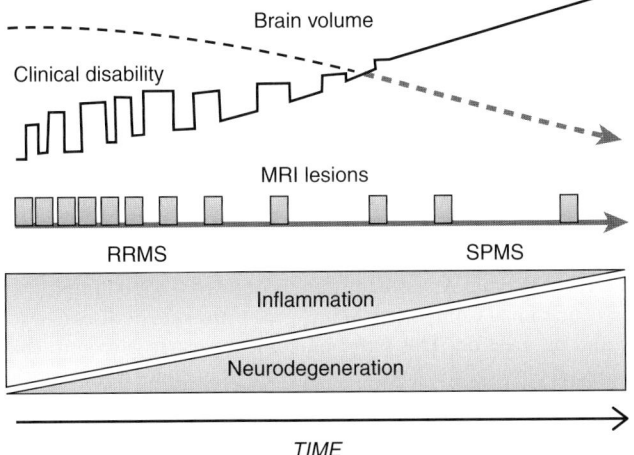

Fig. 17.3 Natural history of relapsing remitting multiple sclerosis *(RRMS)*—conversion to secondary progressive multiple sclerosis *(SPMS)*. Figure shows the typical clinical course of RRMS with conversion to SPMS. Magnetic resonance imaging *(MRI)* activity *(gray line and boxes)* indicates the inflammatory lesions; they occur more frequently early in the disease and occur with greater frequency than in clinical disability *(solid black line)*. Brain volume indicated by the stippled line shows brain atrophy increasing as the inflammatory component of the disease slows and is replaced by neurodegeneration.

updated criteria to include MRI, visual evoked potentials, and cerebrospinal fluid (CSF) analysis published as the McDonald criteria.[22] Revisions to these criteria occurred in 2005 and 2010, with the latest iteration in 2017.

Key requirements for MS diagnosis in the 2017 McDonald criteria include dissemination of lesions in the CNS in space and time. Demonstration of dissemination in space on clinical exam or MRI plus the presence of oligoclonal bands found in CSF enable the diagnosis of MS. Additionally, lesions on MRI with clinical sequelae can be used to demonstrate the presence of disease in space or time in patients with supratentorial, infratentorial, or spinal cord lesions. Cortical lesions can be used to indicate dissemination in space.

Due, in part, to the increased use of paraclinical assessments (MRI, CSF, and evoked potentials) the diagnosis of MS is occurring earlier, and treatment is begun more quickly with the hope that this will result in a slower accumulation of clinical disability or even reduction in the total disability experienced by individuals with MS. Even with the improved technological measures used to facilitate diagnosis, an accurate clinical history is critical. Historically, diagnosis of MS often required many years with the onset of more than one clinical episode of MS. Often patients recall episodes of transient symptoms that did not last long enough to require attention by a primary care provider.

MRI studies have shortened the time taken to diagnose MS. Although T2-weighted MRI images show MS lesions as hyperintense and identify new or active inflammatory lesions, MRI has been shown (Fig. 17.4) to overestimate clinical relapses. Conventional MRI with T1 weighting identifies older lesions (with less inflammation) as hypointense (black holes) and can identify brain atrophy. T1 imaging demonstrates a stronger correlation with clinical status and disease severity than the lesion load found with T2 weighting. Gadolinium-enhanced T1-weighted MRI images also show active inflammatory MS lesions as hyperintense (white). Lesions identified on MRI that are characteristic of MS include periventricular, cortical or juxtacortical, and infratentorial lesions, as well as and lesions that span 1 to 2 segments in the spinal cord.[22] Therefore the presence of both old and new lesions on MRI fulfills the criterion of dissemination in time.

Two additional paraclinical tests can be used to aid in the diagnosis of MS and differentiate it from other diseases and conditions. The first is analysis of CSF. This requires a lumbar puncture in which CSF is gathered and analyzed to identify *oligoclonal bands* indicating the presence of immune system proteins (immunoglobulins) or active inflammation. The majority of people with MS have oligoclonal bands; however, because people with other diseases or conditions also have oligoclonal bands, the test is not specific for MS. The lack of oligoclonal bands at diagnosis has been related to a slower progression of the disease and increased time to reach markers of disability such as walking with an assistive device.

Evoked potentials record the nervous system's response to stimulation of a specific sensory pathway (visual, auditory, vestibular, or general somatosensory). Evoked potentials use an externally evoked sensory stimulus to activate the specific sensory system while the timing of the response to the stimulus is monitored. Demyelination and axonal degeneration cause a slowing of signal transmission along stimulated neurons and therefore will increase the time it takes to respond to the presented stimulus. Damage to the optic system is a common first symptom in MS, and therefore visual evoked potentials are often helpful in diagnosis.

Quantifying Disease Severity

Evidence supporting many interventions for individuals with MS has been researched according to how severely an individual is impacted by the disease. Severity of disease and progression can be monitored by ongoing clinical assessments, MRI imaging, and the use of several outcome measures. The Kurtzke Disease Severity Scale,[29] an outcome measure, was initially developed to allow primary care providers a way to measure clinical disability and monitor disease progression. It has been replaced by the Expanded Disability Status Scale[30] (EDSS) (Table 17.1). The EDSS is an 11-point ordinal scale completed by a physician or physician extender, with 0 indicating no disability and 10 indicating death caused by MS. The scale addresses 8 functional systems (pyramidal, cerebellar, brain stem, sensory, bladder/bowel, visual, cerebral [mental], and ambulatory status).[31] Mild disease severity is related to EDSS scores of 0 to 3, moderate disease 4 to 6.5, and severe disease indicated by scores greater than 6.5. Scores greater than 4 are primarily determined by ambulatory status. Using a unilateral assistive device such as a cane or crutch equals an EDSS score of 6.0, while a 6.5 indicates the need for bilateral assistance. Levels beyond 6.5 indicate a progressive nonambulatory status. The National MS Society (NMSS) Task Force on Clinical Outcomes Assessment also recommends the Multiple Sclerosis Functional Composite (MSFC)[32] as a measure of disease severity and progression. This set of outcome measures is used to chart change in physical and cognitive function. It includes three tests that measure upper-extremity function (Nine-Hole Peg Test [NHPT]), lower-extremity function and mobility (25-Foot Timed Walk [25FTW]), and cognitive function (Paced Auditory Serial Addition Test [PASAT]). In the past, the EDSS and MSFC outcome measures have been used extensively in research evaluating the impact of various pharmaceuticals or rehabilitation interventions on people with MS. Disease severity can also be measured by therapist observation of ambulation (Disease Steps)[33] or via patient self-report (Patient Determined Disease Steps)[34] with both of these measures having high correlations with the EDSS.

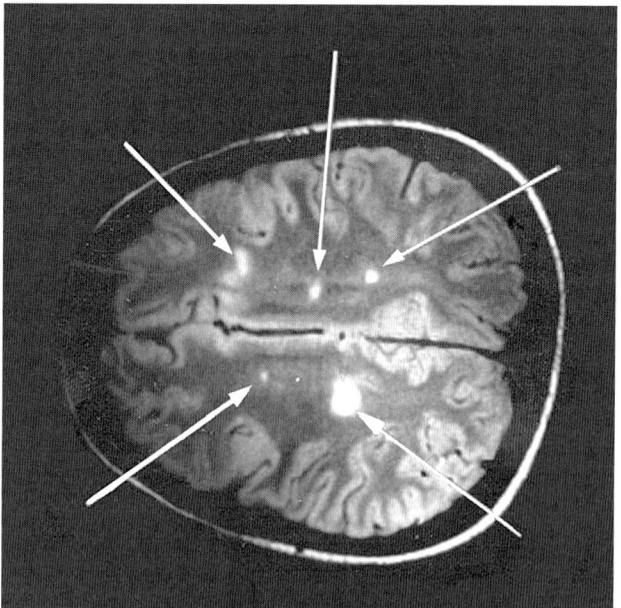

Fig. 17.4 T2-weighted magnetic resonance imaging scan of plaques associated with multiple sclerosis. Plaques are indicated by *arrows*. (From Frey H, Lahtinen A, Heinonen T, et al. Clinical application of MRI image processing in neurology. *Int J Bioelectromagnet.* 1999;1[1].)

TABLE 17.1 Expanded Disability Status Scale

Score	Description
0	Neurologically normal
1.0	No disability, minimal signs in one FS
1.5	No disability, minimal signs in more than one FS
2.0	Minimal disability in one FS
2.5	Mild disability in one FS or minimal disability in two FS
3.0	Moderate disability in one FS, or mild disability in 3 or 4 FS. No walking impairments
3.5	Moderate disability in one FS and more than minimal disability in several others. No walking impairment
4.0	Significant disability and self-sufficient and able to be up and about 12 h a day. Able to walk without aid or rest 500 m
4.5	Significant disability and up and around much of the day, able to work a full day, may have some limitation of full activity or require minimal assistance. Able to walk without aid or rest 300 m
5.0	Disability severe enough to limit full day activity and ability to work a full day without special requirements. Able to walk without aid or rest 200 m
5.5	Disability severe enough to limit full day activity. Able to walk without aid or rest 100 m
6.0	Requires assistance to walk—one cane or crutch, etc. Able to walk 100 m with or without rest
6.5	Requires two walking aids—canes, crutches, walker, etc. Able to walk about 20 m without rest
7.0	Unable to walk more than 5 m with or without aid. Essentially restricted to wheelchair (WC) for mobility. Can independently propel self in WC, perform transfers. Able to be up and about for about 12 h a day
7.5	Unable to take more than a few steps. Restricted to WC and may need aid in transferring. Can wheel self and cannot carry on in a standard WC for a full day, may require a motorized WC
8.0	Essentially restricted to bed, chair, or dependent in WC. May be out of bed for much of the day. Retains many self-care abilities. Generally, has effective use of arms
8.5	Essentially restricted to bed much of the day. Has some arm function and retains some self-care abilities
9.0	Confined to bed. Can still communicate and eat
9.5	Confined to bed and totally dependent. Unable to communicate effectively or eat/swallow
10.0	Death due to MS

FS, Functional systems (FS include pyramidal, cerebellar, brain stem, sensory, bladder/bowel, visual, cerebral, and ambulatory status); *MS,* multiple sclerosis; *WC,* wheelchair.

Modified from https://www.mstrust.org.uk/a-z/expanded-disability-status-scale-edss. Accessed September 2018.

Medical Management of Disease

Disease-Modifying Therapeutics

Disease-modifying therapeutics (DMTs) are aimed at reducing immune system dysfunction, thereby reducing damage to neural tissue and long-term disability for people with RMS. There are several different medications that act on various components of the immune system with the intention of modifying the course of the disease (Table 17.2). These drugs can be injected, taken orally, or infused. In general, most of the drugs are approved for use with RMS and have been shown to reduce the number of attacks experienced. These drugs are often used off-label for other forms of MS. Measurement of therapeutic effectiveness includes relapse rate, progression of disability (EDSS), and quantitative evidence of lesions on MRI. All DMTs have side effects (see Table 17.2), and some of them are very serious. Medications with more serious side effects are generally used if drugs with fewer side effects have failed or produced breakthrough relapses. It is common that people will try several DMTs before finding the one they best tolerate.

Ocrelizumab is a new drug that targets B-cells and is the first to be approved by the FDA for use with PMS. Several of the DMTs are typically used with RMS and PMS when there is evidence of inflammation in the form of relapses or active disease on MRI, but they appear to be less effective if inflammation is no longer present.

Management of Acute Relapses (Antiinflammatory Medications)

High-dose corticosteroids (such as prednisone or methylprednisolone) are used to reduce the inflammatory response during exacerbations for people with RMS. These drugs are generally given over 3 to 5 days via IV (Solu-Medrol) or orally (Deltasone). An additional medication is injection of HP Acthar Gel, a purified form of adrenocorticotropic hormone. Lastly, plasmapheresis can be used for severe relapses that do not respond to the other forms of treatment. Although no medications have demonstrated effectiveness in people with PMS, anecdotal evidence suggests that intermittent pulses of intravenous methylprednisolone can help slow progression of clinical disability in some patients.[24]

TABLE 17.2 Disease Modifying Therapeutics for Multiple Sclerosis

Disease Modifying Agent	Indication	Common Side Effects	Disease Modifying Agent	Indication	Common Side Effects
Injectable Medications (All Can Have Infusion Site Reactions)			**Infused Medications (All Can Result in Infusion Reactions)**		
IFN β-1a (Avonex, Rebif) IFN β-1b (Betaseron, Extavia)	RMS	Flulike symptoms Injection-site reactions Depression Elevated liver enzymes	Alemtuzumab (Lemtrada)	RMS	Infections (urinary, respiratory, viral, and fungal) Itching Pain and paresthesia Dizziness Diarrhea Vomiting
Glatiramer acetate (Copaxone, Glatopa)	RMS	Systemic reactions/immediate postinjection Elevated liver enzymes			
Peginterferon β-1a (Plegridy)	RMS	Hepatotoxicity Depression or suicidal thoughts	Mitoxantrone (Novantrone)	RMS SPMS	Cardiotoxicity Treatment related leukemia Infections Alopecia Amenorrhea Nausea
Daclizumab (Zinbryta)	RMS	Withdrawn from worldwide market 2018			
Oral Medications					
Dimethyl fumarate (Tecfidera)	RMS	Flushing Diarrhea Nausea Pain Elevated liver enzymes	Natalizumab (Tysabri)	RMS	Hepatotoxicity Muscle weakness Headache Fatigue Pain Infections Depression
Fingolimod (Gilenya)	RMS	Flulike symptoms Increased liver enzymes Headache Diarrhea Pain Cough	Ocrelizumab (Ocrevus)	RMS PMS	Itching and hives Rash Fatigue Dizziness Shortness of breath and coughing Tachycardia Headache Pain
Teriflunomide (Aubagio)	RMS	Liver damage Diarrhea Nausea Influenza Alopecia Peripheral neuropathy			

PMS, Progressive multiple sclerosis; *RMS,* remitting multiple sclerosis; *SPMS,* secondary progressive multiple sclerosis.

Prognosis

More aggressive forms of MS are related to greater number of relapses in the first 2 years postdiagnosis, short intervals between first and second relapses, incomplete recovery from first attack and poor recovery from relapses, male sex, African American descent, older age at disease onset, initial symptoms involving the cerebellum or motor systems, or multifocal involvement at onset.[35,36] Paraclinical factors related to more destructive disease include greater disease burden on MRI, evidence of brain atrophy, and low serum levels of vitamin D.[25] Previous research had reported that people with MS have a suicide rate that is twice that of the general population, with recently diagnosed younger males at greatest risk (Feinstein 2017).[36a] A systematic review[37] found that suicide in MS was only slightly higher than an age-matched cohort. In general, people with MS live about 6 to 7 years less than healthy cohorts.[38,39]

MULTIDISCIPLINARY MANAGEMENT OF CLINICAL MANIFESTATIONS

Overview

Physical rehabilitation has changed over the past 20 years for people with MS. Increasing evidence[40–42] indicates that patients respond well to exercise that was previously thought to be too fatiguing or led to increased relapses in this population. Such evidence provides guidance for those who can apply exercise appropriately. Appropriate application, however, varies from patient to patient. The myriad locations and combinations of CNS lesions in MS, along with the differences in individual lifestyles and genetic makeup, result in variable clinical presentations. No one approach represents the gold standard for rehabilitation management. Thus clinicians must assess the preferences and needs of each individual before negotiating with the patient/client the best interventions to prescribe.

Rehabilitation for people with MS occurs in every setting: inpatient hospital, outpatient clinics, skilled nursing facilities, home care, and community-based support or exercise groups. With the current health care climate of decreasing access to and reducing coverage for rehabilitation, therapists and the interprofessional team must be able to make evidence-based decisions for intervention effectiveness to insurers as well as patients. Effective interventions across settings and disciplines achieve the goals of optimal physical and cognitive functioning, safety, and quality of life for the individual with MS.

Throughout the episode of care, the patient/client's preferences and goals should guide rehabilitation—from assessment through intervention. An important framework for patient/client assessment is the

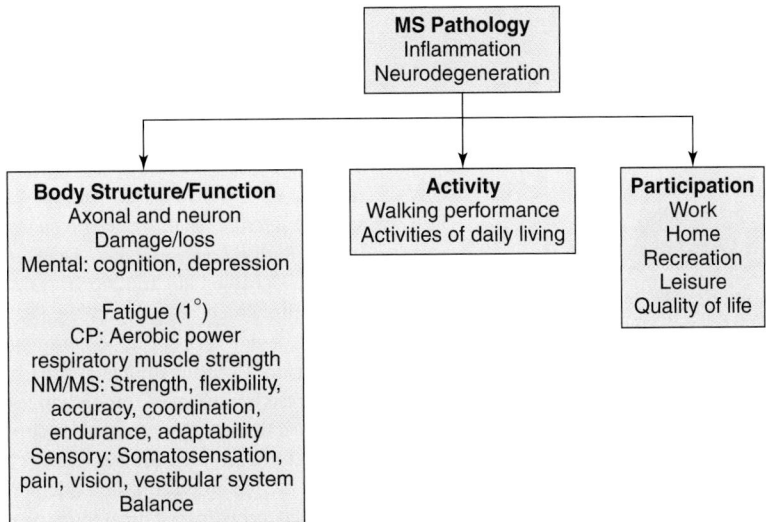

Fig. 17.5 Common Problems That Occur in People With Multiple Sclerosis. *CP,* Cardiopulmonary; *MS,* musculoskeletal; *NM,* neuromuscular.

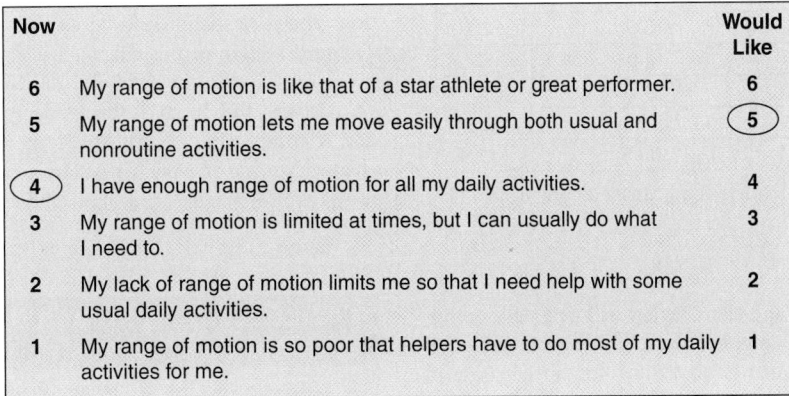

Fig. 17.6 Sample Questions From the Movement Ability Measure.

International Classification of Functioning and Health: ICFH model (2001). See Chapter 1 for a complete description of this model. Fig. 17.5 describes the common problems that occur in people with MS.

Understanding the patient or patient's perspective is critical to achieving best results from rehabilitation. Several tools exist for documenting patients' preferences and have been used with MS; the Goal Attainment Scale (GAS),[43] the Canadian Occupation Performance Measure (COPM),[44] and the Patient-Specific Functional Scale (PSFS).[45] A more broad-based assessment of movement ability is the Movement Ability Measure (MAM) developed and validated by Allen (2007a and 2007b).[45a,45b] This measure includes the six dimensions of movement—flexibility, strength, endurance, speed, accuracy, and adaptability—based on the Movement Continuum theory.[46] This self-report instrument records a patient's current and preferred movement ability in the performance of daily activities during home, work, and leisure. See Fig. 17.6 for a sample of the questions for flexibility. Examining patient-identified gaps between current and preferred abilities should guide therapists' assessment and interventions. In people with MS, these gaps correlate strongly with measures of physical performance, with the dimension of speed showing the greatest overall gap.[47] Fig. 17.7 illustrates the Movement Ability levels and gaps from an individual with MS.

To be most effective, rehabilitation must *challenge* each individual with sufficient *intensity* and *repetition*, be *specific* to the goals of the patient/therapist, and be *salient* to the patient. Application of these five concepts are critical to produce a relatively permanent change in the capacity to perform physical activities and skilled movement via physiological adaptation. To determine the correct dosage of intervention, assessment must be finely tuned to the individual's abilities and needs. Whenever possible, the goal should include restoration of impaired function rather than simply compensation for lost abilities as was common in the past. This section reviews and describes a multidisciplinary approach to addressing the common dysfunctions that occur with MS. It includes assessment tools for examining the patient's and patient's status, frameworks for applying rehabilitative techniques and interventions, and special considerations for rehabilitation in this population.

Assessment

The initial interview should include a quick screen or questioning about the body systems and areas that are commonly impaired in people with MS and the problems commonly encountered: motor strength, coordination, spasticity, sensory disruption (vestibular, visual, and somatosensory), bladder control, depression, and cognition. If impairments are present, there is a strong likelihood of negative impact on the patient's ability to perform activities of daily living (ADLs) or participate in meaningful life roles related to work, home, and leisure.

Special Dysfunctions Associated With Multiple Sclerosis

All patients with MS must be asked if they have fallen in the last 6 months because of the high fall rate in this population.[48–50] Results

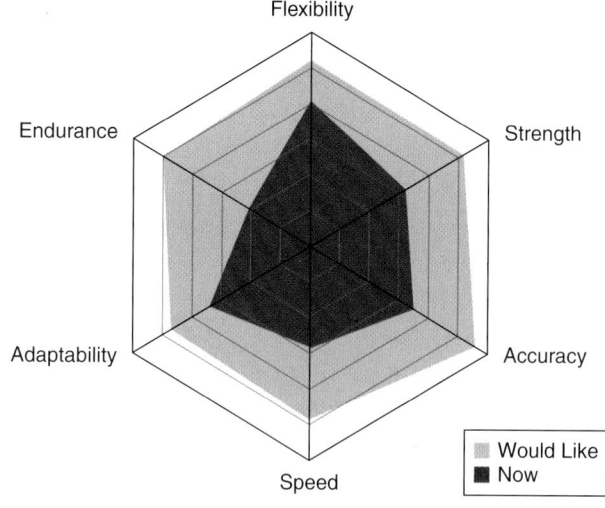

Dimension	Now	Would Like	Gap
Flexibility	4.1	5.2	−1.1
Strength	3.2	5.2	−2
Accuracy	3.5	5.6	−2.1
Speed	2.8	4.8	−2
Adaptability	3.4	4.7	−1.3
Endurance	2.1	5	−2.9
Total	**19.1**	**30.5**	**−11.4**

Fig. 17.7 Example of Patient Determined Gaps on the Movement Ability Measure.

should trigger a referral to the patient's primary care provider for follow-up. See Table 17.3 for signs and symptoms that may indicate a referral to another health care professional.

The physical examination should start with testing the patient's ability to perform functional activities that the patient or his or her caregivers have identified as problematic. Activities may include performance of transfers, gait, ADLs, or cognitive tasks as well as the specific activities that the person states are impaired in his or her work, home, and recreational life. Examining the movement analysis of patient-identified key functional tasks will likely give the therapist insights into which body, structure, and function impairments are influencing the patient's ability to complete the task in an optimal manner.

To gain a greater understanding of a patient's prognosis and current presentation and track changes throughout the rehabilitation program, therapists may consider choosing a couple of outcome measures. Outcome measure selection is unique for each individual and should be dependent on the patient's chief complaints and therapist-identified problematic areas. It is recommended that both subjective and objective outcome measures are included to gain a greater understanding of patient perspective and presentation. Comprehensive lists of standardized tests and measures for impairment, activity limitations, and participation restrictions and QOL are provided in Chapter 7. The next section of this chapter will focus on the tests and outcome measures found to be valid and reliable in the examination of individuals with MS. In 2011, the Academy of Neurologic Physical Therapy, a component of the American Physical Therapy Association, charged a group of experts in MS to recommend outcome measures for use in clinical practice, education, and research. The recommendations

of the patient/client interview and chart review will help develop hypotheses about which potential impairments might be contributing to the patient's or patient's presentation and difficulty participating in meaningful life roles. These hypotheses can help guide the therapist's examination plan. The examination needs to be designed to observe the problematic tasks identified by the individual and test the therapist's hypotheses about the causes of these activity limitations or participation restrictions.

During the assessment, examiners must determine if the problems identified by the patient (or those found by the assessor) fit within their scope of practice or whether the patient requires a referral to an appropriate health care professional. The Patient Health Questionnaire-2[51] is a two-question depression screening tool found accurate for adolescents, adults, and older adults in the general population.[52] See Fig. 17.8. A score of 3/6 indicates that major depression is likely, particularly in groups at higher risk for depression (such as people with MS), and

TABLE 17.3 **Common Referrals for People With Multiple Sclerosis**	
Signs/Symptoms	**Appropriate Health Professional Referral**
Changes in vision	Neuroophthalmologist/optometrist
Bladder dysfunction (nocturia, urgency, frequency, retention)	Neurologist, urologist, neurourologist, and pelvic physical therapist
Increase/change in spasticity/muscle tone	Neurologist
New onset of potential exacerbation	Neurologist
Depression/anxiety/other mental health manifestations	Psychologist
Balance deficits, falls, weakness	Physical therapist

Patient Health Questionnaire-2: Screening Instrument for Depression				
Over the past two weeks, how often have you been bothered by any of the following problems?	Not at all	Several days	More than one-half the days	Nearly every day
Little interest or pleasure in doing things	0	1	2	3
Feeling down, depressed, or hopeless	0	1	2	3

Fig. 17.8 Patient Health Questionnaire-2. (Adapted from Patient Health Questionnaire [PHQ] Screeners. http://www.phqscreeners.com. Accessed October, 2018.)

Recommendations for Patients With Multiple Sclerosis

Highly Recommended Measures	Recommended Measures	
12-item MS walking scale	Activities-specific balance	Hauser ambulation index
6-minute walk test	Confidence scale	Maximal inspiratory & expiratory pressure
9-hole peg test	Box & blocks test	
Berg balance scale	Disease steps	VO$_2$ max and VO$_2$ peak[†]
Dizziness handicap inventory[†]	Dizziness handicap inventory*	Modified fatigue impact scale
MS functional composite[†]	Dynamic gait index	MS functional composite*
MS impact scale (MSIS-29)	Fatigue scale for motor & cognitive functions	MS international quality of life questionnaire
MS quality of life (MS QoL-54)		MS quality of life inventory[†]
Timed 25 foot walk	Four square step test	Rivermead mobility index
Timed up & go (TUG) with cognitive & manual	Functional assessment of MS	Short form health survey of medical outcome study (SF-36)[†]
	Functional independence measure*	
	Functional reach	Trunk impairment scale*
	Goal attainment scale	Visual analog scale (fatigue)
	Guy's neurological disability scale	

*Inpatient rehab only.
[†]Outpatient rehab only

Fig. 17.9. APTA MSEDGE Recommended Outcome Measures.

of this group were published in 2014 and are included in Fig. 17.9.[53] Through a modified Delphi process, this group chose outcome measures based on an extensive review of the literature concerning psychometric properties and clinical utility of outcome measures in people with MS. The critical review and recommendations for each outcome measure were entered into the Evaluation Database to Guide Effectiveness (EDGE) form and are available at: https://www.google.com/search?q=APTA+MS+EDGE&ie=utf-8&oe=utf-8&patient=firefox-b-1. Measures were chosen for use in people across the span of EDSS levels; across the ICF constructs of (1) body structure and function, (2) activity, and (3) participation; in settings in which patients with MS are managed—inpatient, outpatient, and at home; and use of the outcome measures in clinical practice, education, and research. Ratings of the outcome measures ranged from 1 to 4 with 4 representing the highest recommendation and 1 indicating not recommended due to low clinical utility, poor psychometric properties, and or the measure was not tested in MS.

Assessing Impairments and Activity

In general, standardized methods of examining muscle strength and endurance, somatosensation, vision, coordination, cardiovascular status and endurance, posture, muscle tone, reflexes, fatigue pain, and cognition are useful in examining individuals with MS. As with many neurological conditions, abnormal posturing or pain may necessitate using nonstandardized test positions or methods that must be noted in the patient documentation. If a patient is unable to attain the normal test position while performing a muscle strength test, the assessed strength is documented along with the position in which the muscle or muscle group was tested. Functional movement analysis is used to assess patients' and patient's ability, strategies, and the quality of movements used to perform ADLs such as transfers, bed mobility, and gait. Outcome measures standardize the assessment of activity or task performance and are an excellent way to document change in ability over time.

Spasticity. Therapists can use several tools to assess spasticity in people with MS. Clinicians typically measure spasticity using the Modified Ashworth Scale.[54] The numerical rating scale (NRS)—spasticity[55] is good scale for assessing change over a single session or intervention. These two scales have been shown to have a moderate correlation in people with MS (Anwar, 2009).[55] Clinicians should be aware that because spasticity is typically measured while the patient is at rest in the MAS protocol, the scores may not reflect the degree to which spasticity may be interfering with movement. Careful observation of the patient's movements may also inform the clinician about how spasticity is affecting the patient's physical function. Several spasticity self-report measures are recommended by the MS EDGE Taskforce and might be more valuable to assess change in the perception of the impact of spasticity on function over time, such as across an episode of care (see Fig. 17.9).

Ataxia and incoordination. Few standardized tests have been developed to specifically measure ataxia. The Scale for the Assessment and Rating of Ataxia (SARA)[56,57] and the International Cooperative Ataxia Rating Scale (ICARS)[58] are examples of standardized tests that clinicians may use to assess an individual's ataxia. Both the SARA and ICARS have good psychometric properties and have been tested in people with MS.[59] The ICARS includes four subsection assessments of posture and gait, limb ataxia, dysarthria, and the oculomotor system. The maximum score is 100 with higher scores indicating greater disability. While the ICARS has shown high correlation with EDSS, the clinical utility of the SARA may be greater due to its brevity.[59] The SARA does not include an ocular motor examination; therefore clinicians should be sure to include these tests in other portions of their evaluation. Due to cerebellar damage or loss of somatosensation and proprioception, people with MS can also experience uncoordinated movement.

Tests of nonequilibrium coordination are designed to measure the presence of dysmetria or dysdiadochokinesia, both of which occur in patients with MS. However, these tests (including finger to nose and heel to shin) are somewhat subjective and are therefore difficult to use to demonstrate improvement pre- and post-intervention. However, using a stopwatch during these tests can increase the objectivity of the measurements. Counting the number of repetitions of a given activity performed in a set amount of time (e.g., how many alternating fore-arm supinations and pronations can be performed in 30 seconds), or recording the time it takes to complete a set number of repetitions of a given activity (e.g., how long it takes to complete five alternating supination-pronation movements), can quantify otherwise subjective impressions. Refer to Chapter 7 for additional assessment tools.

Vestibular dysfunction. The vestibular system can be affected by MS both centrally (lesions in the vestibular nucleus, cerebellum, or sensory pathways)[60] or peripherally with conditions such as benign paroxysmal positional vertigo.[61] The techniques used to assess vestibu-lar disorders are similar to those discussed in Chapter 21. Computer-ized platform posturography (CPP) assessment is reliable and valid for people with MS and can identify vestibular dysfunction.[62] It is important to keep in mind that people with MS will often have additional problems that might require modification of the vestibular intervention—for example, heat intolerance, additional visual or somatosensory deficits, spasticity, and motor weakness.

Fatigue. Identifying if and when fatigue occurs in individuals with MS is important to assessment and the structuring of intervention. Questions should address the type of fatigue, whether mental or physical; when during the day it occurs; whether it is related to physical or mental exertion; and what the person with MS does, if anything, to relieve it. In addition, fatigue-related self-report scales can help the rehabilitation professional gain an understanding of the perceived impact that fatigue may be having on a patient with MS. Two of the commonly used self-report scales recommended by the MS EDGE Taskforce are the Modified Fatigue Impact Scale (Fisk 1994)[63] and the Fatigue Scale for Motor and Cognitive Function.[64] These measures may also aid the therapist in determining if the intervention had any impact on the patient's perceived level of fatigue.

Cognition. Cognitive deficits common to people with MS include deficits in learning and memory, information processing speed, and executive functions such as planning, organization, and initiation.[65] In MS, delays in processing speed are connected to learning impairments.[66] The Paced Auditory Serial Addition Test (PASAT)[67] is recommended by an expert panel of the National MS Society as a test for disease-related cognitive impairments in people with MS. Components of the PASAT specifically assess working memory and processing speed.

Balance. Balance is foundational to upright movement and is produced by a complex interaction among sensory inputs, central processing, and motor responses. It can be discussed under both body structure and function or activity. In either case balance dysfunction has been identified in people with MS with minimal as well as more advanced disability.[68,69] Cameron and Lord[70] report the three most common problems with balance to be delayed response to postural perturbations, increased body sway while standing quietly, and an inability to move outside the base of support.

Some balance tests focus on stationary or static tasks that allow observation of body sway in standing, including single-leg stance test, Romberg test with eyes open or eyes closed, tandem stance, and CPP; others add movement and challenge dynamic balance. Other tests challenge anticipatory balance (reactions to perturbations related to self-generated movement) or reactive balance. The MS EDGE Task-force recommends Berg Balance Scale and Functional Reach Test to assess balance. See Fig. 17.9. Frzovic and co-workers[71] found that single-leg stance, tandem stance, response to external perturbations, and the Functional Reach Test were able to distinguish people with MS from healthy controls.

Developed by Horak and colleagues,[72] the Balance Evaluation Sys-tems Test (BESTest) is an instrument examining complex balance dis-orders that includes the six domains that underlie orientation and postural stability: biomechanical constraints, stability limits and

verticality, transitions and anticipatory postural reactions, reactive postural responses, sensory orientation, and stability in gait. The BESTest has been shown valid and reliable for people with MS.[73] The authors suggest that total test scores should be used because several of the subsections of the test showed ceilings effects. There is an abbrevi-ated version of the BESTest, the mini-BESTest,[74] that covers four of the six systems, focusing on dynamic balance. These promising tests may offer the clinician a better way of identifying which components of orientation and postural control are dysfunctional and which may allow more targeted interventions. A systematic review of the use of the miniBESTest demonstrated it to be reliable, valid, and responsive in community-dwelling elders, people with Parkinson disease, and people post-stroke.[75]

CPP provides an objective assessment of sensory contributions to balance dysfunction in people with MS,[76] which is reliable in people with MS.[77,78] The Sensory Organization Test (SOT) is useful in identifying the relative sensory contributions (visual, vestibular, and proprioceptive) to stationary balance and response to perturba-tion. Understanding the sensory conditions under which the patient loses balance and falls assists the therapist in providing exercises that will challenge those conditions in a safe and controlled manner. For example, the patient who relies heavily on visual input to main-tain balance (conditions with eyes closed in the SOT) would be prescribed exercises and activities that challenge the vestibular and proprioceptive systems, such as standing on foam while the eyes are closed. An additional measure that may be more assessable for clinical use is the Nintendo Wii Balance Board (WBB).[79] Keune and co-workers found excellent internal consistency and reliability when testing individuals with MS for 4 minutes on the WBB, 4 months apart. They found that WBB had consistent results with both the Timed Up and Go test and the Berg Balance Scale (BBS) and showed increased body sway in people with EDSS scores greater than 3.

Two self-report measures of balance ability and confidence are Activity-specific Balance Confidence scale (ABC) and the Dizziness Handicap Inventory (DHI). Both have been used extensively in MS. Cattaneo and colleagues[80] found that both the ABC and DHI tools discriminated between fallers and nonfallers and were therefore good predictors of fall status in people with MS. Refer to Chapter 20 for additional information on balance.

Gait. Gait can be measured in myriad ways depending on the goal of the assessment. Speed, distance, and quality may all be important to the patient and therapist. Observational gait analysis is the gold standard for clinical measurement of gait quality. Although motion-analysis laboratories are able to provide detailed kinetic and kinematic assessment of joint angles and gait cycle, it is costly and typically not available in most clinical settings. Instrumented mats can provide cli-nicians with temporal and spatial gait parameters such as step length, step width, cadence, and single-leg support and double-leg support times. Although this is less costly than motion analysis, it may still be out of reach for many clinics. Gait speed and velocity can also be mea-sured by having the patient walk a given distance while being timed. These walks can occur at a self-selected pace or as fast as the person can walk safely. See Fig. 17.9 for recommended gait assessment measures. Gijbels and co-workers[81] report that the 6-Minute Walk Test (6MWT) was better at predicting habitual walking in people with mild to moderate MS than the 25-Foot Timed Walk (25FTW). However, the 25FTW may be more sensitive to change when compared with the EDSS.[82] The 6MWT distance was reduced in peo-ple with MS compared with healthy controls and was inversely related to disability.[83]

The Multiple Sclerosis Walking Scale–12 (MSWS-12)[84,85] is a 12-item patient-rated questionnaire that measures the perception of the impact of MS on walking ability and is recommended by the MS EDGE Taskforce.

Upper-extremity tests of function. Movement impairments of the upper extremities can result in decreased ability to perform ADLs and other functional activities. Standardized tests such as the Box and Block Test (BBT)[86] or the Nine-Hole Peg Test (NHPT)[87] provide objective data about unilateral manual dexterity or the ability to manipulate objects. Both tests are inexpensive but do require some equipment and a stopwatch. The NHPT is part of the MSFC and therefore has been used extensively in evaluating people with MS.

Assessing Quality of Life and Participation.

For people with MS, participation restrictions are associated most strongly with cognitive deficits and to a lesser amount with walking, balance, and upper extremity dysfunctions.[88] The following are participation and quality of life (QOL) measures commonly used in people with MS. See Fig. 17.9 for a list of the measures recommended by the MS EDGE Taskforce. An individual's perceived ability to participate may also be included in some QOL outcome measures that are included in the following sections.

QOL measures are patient-report tools that evaluate the value a person places on his or her abilities and limitations and how these affect the individual's social, emotional, and physical well-being. Many of these tools include questions that address an individual's perception of how well he or she is able to fulfill life roles and how the disease affects this participation. In a meta-analysis of exercise training on QOL in people with MS, Motl and Gosney[89] found that disease-specific measures of QOL detected larger changes than generic QOL measures. The two highly recommended outcome measures are the Multiple Sclerosis Quality of Life–54 (MSQOL-54)[90] and the MS Impact Scale–29. While both have strong psychometrics, the MS Impact Scale is easier to score and is a shorter questionnaire for patients/clients to take.

The MSQLI was developed by the Consortium of Multiple Sclerosis Centers Health Research Subcommittee in 1997. It is composed of 10 components covering issues important in MS. It includes the Health Status Questionnaire, Modified Fatigue Impact Scale, MOS Pain Effects Scale, Sexual Satisfaction Survey, Bladder Control Scale, Bowel Control Scale, Impact of Visual Impairment Scale, Perceived Deficits Questionnaire, Mental Health Inventory, and MOS Modified Social Support Survey. It takes about 45 minutes to administer the complete set of questionnaires and does not provide a sum score for all tests.

There is good test-retest reliability for the MSQLI even in people with MS and cognitive dysfunction.[91] A shortened version of the tool exists, but the psychometric properties have not been thoroughly tested. The MS EDGE task force document recommends that the MSQLI be used only in the outpatient MS population.

Interventions

Benefits of Exercise in Multiple Sclerosis

Exercise is an important intervention given that people with MS are less physically active than their healthy peers.[92] Exercise is one of the interventions that have shown consistent benefits for people with MS, similar to healthy adults and people with other neurological dysfunctions. The literature examining the impact of exercise on impairments, activity, and participation/quality of life for people with MS has exploded in the past 10 years. A recent review reiterated that exercise is safe and well tolerated in this population.[93]

The benefits of exercise have been determined by both systematic review and meta-analysis. Meta-analysis has confirmed the benefits of exercise on the impairments of aerobic capacity,[94] lower extremity muscle strength,[95] fatigue,[96] and depression[97]; reduced activity limitations such as walking performance[98] and balance[99]; and confirms that it positively impacts quality of life.[100,101] Systematic reviews have also revealed that exercise reduced fatigue,[102] improved cognition,[103] and improved health-related quality of life.[95]

In addition to the benefits outlined above, Motl and Pilutti[104] reviewed the growing evidence that exercise may play an additional role as a disease-modifying treatment. They reported that potential slowing of disease progression and reducing relapse rate,[105,106] a reduced progression of walking disability,[107,108] and decreased lesion volume on MRI.[98,109–111] However, according to a recent systematic review, the impact of aerobic or resistance training on markers of inflammation have shown equivocal results.[112] The authors hypothesize that the reason for a lack of results may be due to two main factors: the low level of fitness in people with MS compared with a healthy cohort and training periods of less than 8 weeks duration in most of the studies.

While evidence supporting the benefits of increased physical activity and exercise is clear, in order for people with MS to achieve the best result, exercise prescription must be tailored to the individual's needs. Appropriate assessments must be completed to link deficits in underlying capacity and movement with the necessary exercise intervention. Table 17.4 presents a summary of the exercise guidelines for aerobic, resistance, and flexibility training for people with MS based on

TABLE 17.4   Aerobic, Resistance, and Flexibility Training Guidelines for People With Multiple Sclerosis

	Aerobic	Resistance	Flexibility
Mode	Cycling, walking, swimming, elliptical, etc.	Free weights, weight machines, body weight, resistance bands, and pulleys	Static stretching
Intensity	Moderate intensity 64%–75% HR_{max}; (12–15/20 RPE) Start lower if sedentary	60%–80% 1 RM (use ≥3 RM to estimate 1 RM) Start lower if sedentary or older	Static stretch to point of mild discomfort or tightness Do not cause pain
Duration	10–60 min of accumulated moderate activity Use interval or intermittent training for people with heat sensitivity	10–15 repetitions/set 1–2 sets per session At least 2–5 min rest between sets	30–60 s stretches 2–4 repetitions
Frequency	2–5 times/week	2–3 times/week	5–7 times/week 1–2 times/day

HR_{max}, Heart rate maximum; *RM*, repetition maximum; *RPE*, rate of perceived exertion.
Recommendations based on White 2004, Dalgas 2012, Latimer-Cheung 2013, and ACSM's Guidelines for Exercise Testing and Prescription 2018.

guidelines from White and Dressendorfer,[113] Dalgas and colleagues[105] Latimer-Cheung and colleagues[95] and the American College of Sports Medicine.[114] When beginning an exercise program, the initial prescription should be based on the goals of the individual, the initial level of fitness, familiarity with the type of exercise, and the individual's preferences for type of exercise. As with every exercise intervention, the intensity, duration, and frequency should be gradually increased with the individual's tolerance. For people with MS that have heat intolerance, intermittent exercise and shorter exercise bouts, interspersed with periods of rest that allow heat to dissipate, will allow a greater volume of exercise to be performed.[115,116] Cooling before exercise has improved physical performance in people with MS.[117]

To make physiological or neuroplastic changes, exercise interventions need to be tailored to individuals with MS. This means that the exercise program needs to be meaningful to the individual, practiced at a high intensity with sufficient repetition, as challenging or difficult as the individual can tolerate, and specific to the changes that need to be made for the person to achieve his or her goals.

Multidisciplinary Management of Multiple Sclerosis Symptoms

Fatigue. Fatigue is one of the most frequent and disabling symptoms associated with MS and is best managed with a multidisciplinary team composed of physicians, physical therapists, occupational therapists, and nurses. As described earlier, the causes of fatigue can be divided into two basic categories: primary and secondary. Primary fatigue related to demyelination and neurodegeneration may have fewer options for treatment. Secondary fatigue caused by deconditioning, comorbidities such as thyroid disease, depression, poor nutrition, heat intolerance, sleep disturbance, and medications may be more easily managed.

Pharmaceutical combined with rehabilitation interventions have been recommended for management of fatigue.[118,119] While amantadine (Symmetrel) and modafinil (Provigil) have been frequently prescribed to help manage fatigue, newer research has cast doubt on the effectiveness of modafinil. A meta-analysis comparing the effects of amantadine, modafinil, and rehabilitation interventions found that rehabilitation produced stronger, longer-lasting reduction in patient-reported fatigue and fatigue severity than pharmacological agents.[120]

Several rehabilitation strategies for fatigue management have been reported and show promise[118]; however, few research studies have demonstrated effectiveness in randomized controlled trials or in comparisons among approaches. Interventions for fatigue management include cooling devices and garments, energy conservation education training, exercise, and a multifaceted class aimed at teaching people with MS how to manage their fatigue. One study found that the cooling suits used in the home improved fatigue and participant's independence in ADLs.[121] Another study found that 60 minutes of neck or head cooling resulted in improved 6MWT times.[122] The use of cooling is recommended in the Multiple Sclerosis Council's Clinical Practice Guidelines on fatigue (MSC Clinical Practice Guidelines) and by expert opinion.

People with both RMS and PMS of mild to moderate disability can benefit from exercise to reduce self-reported fatigue. Exercise shows promise as an intervention that can improve fatigue for people with MS, but to date, no one type of exercise—resistance, aerobic, mixed, or other (e.g., yoga or balance training)—has been proven most effective.[95,96,102] Most reviewed studies have a small number of participants, do not pre-define people with fatigue, and generally only include people with mild to moderate levels of disability and frequently no control or comparison groups. Specific guidelines about the correct dosage of exercise needed to reduce fatigue are still lacking.[123]

Energy conservation is defined by the fatigue and MS guidelines of the Multiple Sclerosis Council for Clinical Practice Guidelines[124] as energy effectiveness, and includes an analysis of individuals' home, work, and leisure activities and the environments in which they occur to develop activity modifications designed to reduce fatigue. This can include a variety of strategies such as reducing energy expenditure through activity and modification, workspace organization, and improving efficiency of movements; balancing work and rest periods; delegating tasks; evaluating standards and prioritizing activities; and using assistive technologies that conserve energy usage.[125] In a systematic review, energy conservation was effective at making immediate improvements in the physical, social function, and mental health subscales of the Fatigue Impact Scale.[126]

Assistive devices may reduce energy expenditure while performing ADLs. Using wheeled mobility (such as wheelchairs or scooters) for longer-distance outings (to the shopping mall, an extended event, on vacation) can conserve energy and extend the time a person can participate in activities of importance to him or her. However, therapists should be aware that using assistive devices such as walkers or crutches actually increases energy expenditure for elderly people,[127] and therefore the need for improved support must be balanced with the increased energy demands that an assistive device might add.

Spasticity. Spasticity, present in up to 80% of people with MS, is more common in the lower extremities. It commonly impacts walking, stair climbing, sexual activity, and sleep.[128] While often interfering with physical function, spasticity can also add support to weakened limbs, allowing more effective mobility. Therefore spasticity management must include a thorough assessment of the impact of the spasticity on an individual's function. The goal of medical management of spasticity is to maintain full range of motion (ROM) of muscle and soft tissue structures to allow maximal physical function and proper hygiene. Haselkorn and colleagues[129] developed the clinical practice guidelines for managing spasticity in people with MS for the Multiple Sclerosis Council. To date, this is the most comprehensive set of guidelines developed. They indicate that successful management includes both pharmaceuticals and rehabilitation strategies.

Medical management of spasticity includes the use of first-line oral pharmacotherapy agents including baclofen (Lioresal), tizanidine (Zanaflex), or gabapentin (Neurontin).[130] Adjuvant therapies are recommended if the previous drugs are unsuccessful and include diazepam (Valium) or dantrolene (Dantrium).[130] Nabiximols or cannabis extracts (such as Sativex) can be used in addition to the drugs previously mentioned.[130] Many of these drugs, since they are given as oral agents, can have negative side effects that interfere with movement and increase fatigue, both of which can impact daily life and rehabilitation.

Management of focal or more severe spasticity may include local anesthetics such as lidocaine, bupivacaine, etidocaine, all of which are short-acting with side effects of CNS and cardiovascular toxicity and hypersensitivity. Neurolysis treatment with phenol or alcohol is longer acting; however, these agents can have the side effects of pain, swelling, fibrosis, and dysesthesias. Focal spasticity affecting functional muscle groups can also be effectively treated with neuromuscular blocking agents, including alcohol, phenol, or botulinum toxin. Blocks last 1 to 3 months with relatively few side effects.[131] Clinical practice guidelines[129] recommend that neuromuscular blocks be performed by appropriate specialists in conjunction with a rehabilitation program.

Refractory spasticity is defined as unsuccessful treatment with oral medications and/or rehabilitation. In this situation two other options exist: surgery or placement of an intrathecal baclofen pump (ITB).[130] Intrathecal pumps, inserted into the spinal cord, allow adjustable drug delivery. Baclofen, the drug of choice for the intrathecal pump, can be given in higher doses; use of the pump avoids the side effects often encountered when the drug is taken orally. Other surgical procedures include tendon lengthening or tendon transfer and are performed to maintain adequate hygiene or prevent or correct contractures and therefore preserve function.

Several rehabilitation strategies to manage spasticity are available, including ROM, stretching tight or spastic muscles, strengthening opposing muscles, electrical stimulation, and education. Although none of these interventions is supported by strong research evidence, many are used routinely in clinical practice. Other approaches (cold therapy, light pressure, or stroking) are recommended for use in conjunction with stretching or ROM programs. Regardless of the technique employed, educating individuals and caregivers about the importance of adhering to a spasticity management program is essential. The Multiple Sclerosis Council for Clinical Practice Guidelines[129] recommends, based on expert opinion, stretching a muscle with spasticity for at least 60 seconds or using braces or splints to provide a prolonged stretch. A group-delivered self-management program based on the MSC guidelines found that people with MS who completed the *Spasticity: Take Control* program compared to a usual care group had significant improvements in the self-reported impact of spasticity, even though scores on the MAS remained unchanged.[132]

Nilsagård and co-workers[133] found subjective reports of improved spasticity after a single session of cooling, although no statistically significant differences in spasticity measures were found. Stationary bicycling may improve blood flow to lower extremity spastic muscles by increasing alternate contraction and relaxation of muscles, which may increase the delivery of oxygen and removal of lactate from continuously contracting muscles and reduce pain. However, while a 4-week unloaded cycling program reduced the impact of spasticity on participants self-reported function, physiological measurement of spasticity did not change.[134]

Pain. The occurrence of pain in people with MS is often underestimated. Pain can be acute, as in optic neuritis, trigeminal neuralgia, or Lhermitte syndrome, or chronic, as in dysesthesias in the limbs or joints or mechanical pain related to abnormal positions or repeated movements that cause abnormal wear and tear on the musculoskeletal system. Therefore both nociceptive and neuropathic pain can be present. It is important to discern the type of pain in order for the most appropriate treatment to be rendered. The classes of drugs used to treat pain are anticonvulsants, antidepressants, cannabinoids, dextromethorphan/quinidine, and opioids/opioid antagonists.[135]

Nociceptive pain can often be treated with analgesics (acetaminophen, nonsteroidal antiinflammatory drugs [NSAIDs], or opioids) and is generally more amenable to physical therapy. Neuropathic pain generally requires pharmacological intervention, although an interdisciplinary team approach may be valuable. First-line medications for neuropathic pain that occurs in the spinal cord are calcium channel blockers (gabapentinoids) or *N*-methyl-D-aspartate (NMDA) antagonists (ketamine). Treatment of trigeminal neuralgia is opioid drugs such as antidepressants (nortriptyline, duloxetine) or anticonvulsants (gabapentin, pregabalin).[135] Refer to Chapter 30 on pain management for additional information.

Occupational and physical therapists can address poor body mechanics and weakness and poor movement patterns with retraining, and soft collars may help reduce Lhermitte syndrome. However, little evidence supports these interventions.[136] In a systematic review of nonpharmacological management of pain in people with MS, Jawahar[137] found that low frequency (4 Hz) transcutaneous electrical nerve stimulation was found to be most beneficial for reducing neuropathic pain. Other interventions included in the review were education, yoga and exercise, and robotic assisted gait training. While the evidence was lacking in most cases, the educational interventions of cognitive restructuring and self-hypnosis showed the greatest reduction in pain scores.[137]

Cognitive-behavioral therapy has been successful in managing chronic pain in many populations using both in-person and online delivery systems[138]; however, little evidence exists for using it in people with MS. A recent pilot study suggests that a self-management program of telephone-supported home-based cognitive behavioral therapy (CBT) may be effective for people with MS.[139]

Balance and postural control. Balance is foundational to the ability to stay upright and perform dynamic movements. Balance dysfunction is a frequent problem in people with MS and results in a person limiting his or her participation in home, work, and leisure activities—even for people using wheelchairs or scooters. Poor balance along with cane use and poor performance on tests of balance and ambulation are associated with an increased risk of falls.[140–142] Other fall risk factors that have been identified include fear of falling, male sex, poor concentration or forgetfulness, and urinary incontinence.[140,143] Rehabilitation is the primary intervention used to improve balance in people with MS. However, factors contributing to falls such as urinary urgency/incontinence can also be addressed through specific pelvic floor rehabilitation and pharmacological interventions and will be discussed later in this section.

Rehabilitation programs must be based on a thorough understanding of the impairments and personal and environmental factors that may be contributing to the balance dysfunction. In a recent systematic review Gunn and colleagues found that exercise interventions produced changes in balance ability with moderate effect sizes, but did not change falls outcomes.[48] Several exercise strategies were used to improve balance including specific balance and gait training, aerobic and resistance exercise, and combined programs.[48,144]

An additional technique that shows promise for improving balance and reducing falls in people with MS uses small amounts of weight applied strategically at the torso in response to identified balance loss. In torso weighting using the balance-based torso-weighting method (BBTW), a trained clinician assesses the directional loss of balance and asymmetry when the standing patient is perturbed with nudges and maximal rotational force at the shoulders and pelvis. Small amounts of weight (generally less than 1% to 1.5% of body weight) are then placed on a vestlike garment to counter the balance loss. The lightly weighted vest can then be worn during the performance of activities in therapy or daily for home, work, or leisure activities.[145] While wearing the orthotic, people with MS showed improved body sway compared to a no-orthotic condition and compared with healthy age-matched controls.[146] Another study showed that the weighted condition produced fewer falls and improved balance during the Sensory Organization test, a type of computerized dynamic platform posturography.[147]

Although no systematic reviews have been performed, results from recent randomized controlled trials suggest that customized vestibular rehabilitation programs, such as the Balance and Eye-Movement Exercises in Persons with Multiple Sclerosis (BEEMS),[148] result in improvements in balance, fatigue, and quality of life.[148,149] These programs incorporate comprehensive approaches to ensure that balance and eye movements are continually challenged by systematically narrowing the base of support, moving from static to more dynamic movements, and integrating eye movement challenges.

Regardless of the type of exercise, the critical component of successful programs is maintaining a high level of challenge to the individual, thereby forcing physiological adaptations.

Mobility. People with MS rate gait as one of the most important bodily functions.[150] Gait is often adversely affected in people with MS.

Approximately 40% to 75% of people with MS report gait difficulties, with many claiming it is the most challenging aspect of the disease.[151,152] Gait disturbances have been reported in people with MS even before mild disability occurs and deficits that increase with faster walking speeds.[153] Lesions in the brain and spinal cord produce a wide variety of potential impairments that can adversely affect gait.[92] Physical rehabilitation is the primary intervention used to manage mobility dysfunctions. However, one medication is FDA-approved for use to improve walking ability in people with MS: dalfampridine (Ampyra). In clinical studies dalfampridine demonstrated the ability to improve walking speed in people with MS.[154] However, changes in the quality of gait or movement were not measured. A recent study showed that after 2 years of using dalfampridine, participants have improvements in the 25TWT, 6MWT, and the MSWs-12, indicating that this drug could be an effective option to improve walking ability in MS.[155]

A review article by Kelleher and colleagues[156] revealed that imbalance, fatigue, spasticity, incoordination, muscle weakness, and sensory system impairments were all reported to negatively affect ambulation ability. Therefore addressing each of these impairments has the potential to improve gait. A variety of rehabilitative methods can improve ambulation. Snook and Motl[107] performed a meta-analysis of exercise studies aimed at improving walking mobility in people with MS and found that larger effects were associated with supervised exercise training, programs of less than 3 months duration, and mixed samples of people with RRMS and progressive MS. A meta-analysis of the impact of aerobic and resistance exercise training on walking ability found that exercise made significant improvements to walking speed and endurance, but had little impact on Timed Up and Go (TUG) scores.[98]

Several systematic reviews have shown an association with improved aerobic capacity and muscle strength while reporting a smaller yet meaningful impact on mobility.[40,95] Guidelines for exercise in people with MS have been developed (see Table 17.4). Based on these studies, exercise should be an important component of interventions designed to promote improved mobility in people with MS. Additionally, high-intensity resistance training programs are being explored in people with MS, and while there are some mixed results, high-intensity training shows promise in improving walking as well as other aspects of individual's function.[157,158]

Task-specific gait training has been evaluated in people with MS. Treadmill training has been investigated in several small, pilot, or case studies with promising results of improved QOL, energy expenditure, and gait parameters.[159,160] A systematic review found little evidence to support either treadmill training or robot-assisted training due to the small, heterogenous samples.[161] A more recent analysis of robot-assisted gait training shows some promise in people with MS, with a modest impact on walking endurance compared to conventional walking training.[162]

Torso weighting, using the BBTW method, has also shown improvements in walking ability in people with MS. In a randomized controlled trial in people with MS who reported gait abnormalities, wearing the weighted orthotic increased their gait speed compared with no weight controls and improved TUG scores compared with a standard weighted control.[163] In a separate study, researchers found that the gait parameters of velocity, cadence, time in single limb support improved in people with MS when wearing the BBTW orthotic compared to the no-weight condition, and became closer to values found in age-matched healthy controls.[164]

When people with MS do not respond to therapeutic interventions to restore function, mobility assistive devices such as canes, crutches, walkers, wheelchairs, and scooters are used to enhance mobility through compensation. Mobility-assisted technology (MAT) can improve function in people with moderate to severe impairments of ambulation and may reduce activity limitations and participation restrictions by reducing fatigue and enhancing energy conservation to allow greater involvement in work, family, social, vocational, and leisure activities. Other MAT technologies include functional electrical stimulation (FES), neuroprostheses, and orthotics. FES is applied to specific muscles or muscle groups to activate weak muscles. Some of these stimulators can be built into a neuroprosthesis that can be set up for use during exercising or walking.[165] In a single group, pre-post study, increased gait velocity and improvement on the MSWS-12 and the MSIS-29 were reported after wearing a neuroprosthesis for two weeks that facilitated dorsiflexion during the swing phase of gait.[166]

Orthotics such as the ankle-foot orthosis (AFO) or hip flexion assist orthosis (HFAO)[167] can compensate for muscle weakness in the lower extremity, improve foot and knee positioning, and reduce energy expenditure. Therapists often work cooperatively with orthotists to ensure proper fit. Use of wheeled mobility devices such as a manual wheelchair, power wheelchair, or scooter requires a formal evaluation by an occupational or physical therapist with justification that it is required for mobility at home at least on a part-time basis. Therapists must take a long-term view of the projected needs of the patient when prescribing wheeled mobility, as most insurance companies will replace this equipment only every 5 years.

Tremor. Tremor in MS has been self-reported in 25% to 58% of patients.[168] People with tremor reported as mild or greater were more likely to retire early, be unemployed, and have higher levels of disability compared with MS patients without tremor. Pharmacological management was common in over 50% of individuals with mild to severe tremor. Individuals with more severe tremor are more likely to report benefits from using pharmacological interventions. The most commonly used drugs for symptomatic management of tremor are benzodiazepines and anticonvulsants.[168] Cannabinoids, B-blockers, antispasmodics, mood stabilizers, ethanol, and Alzheimer's dementia treatment have also been reported.[168] Please refer to Table 17.2. GABA agonists were reported as the most successful in reducing tremor. Surgical interventions, including stereotaxic thalamotomy and deep brain stimulation, have been studied, but the evidence to support the effects on functional status and disability is lacking. The effectiveness of other options including physical therapy, tremor-reducing orthoses, and extremity cooling have yet to be proven beneficial in clinical trials.[169]

Bowel and bladder management. Urinary incontinence and retention are common and often embarrassing problems for people with MS. A systematic review of interventions for the treatment of lower urinary tract symptoms in patient with MS notes that 80% to 100% of people will have symptoms at some time, and 70% categorize the impact of bladder or urinary problems on their lives as "high" or "moderate."[170] Physical therapy can help decrease incontinence leakage episodes and improve quality of life through pelvic floor muscle training and biofeedback by physical therapists with specialized training in pelvic floor rehabilitation.[171,172] Patients may also be advised to avoid bladder irritants including caffeine and alcohol, and to maintain proper hydration. Persistent problems may require pharmacological intervention or catheterization, although unwanted side effects and increased risk of infection make these choices less desirable for many. A few medications have been shown to be helpful: anticholinergic agents are used to manage detrusor overactivity or dyssynergia, and underactivity is treated with cholinomimetic agents.[173]

Bowel dysfunction has been estimated to occur in 39% to 73% of people with MS, with constipation and fecal incontinence as the primary dysfunctions.[174] Assessment of bowel dysfunction using the Wexner Constipation and Incontinence scale[175] and using a 2-week bowel diary will facilitate an understanding of the problem and its significance to the individual.[176] People with constipation are encouraged to combine adequate fluid intake with dietary fiber or to take medications that increase bulk formation, soften stool, or stimulate stool expulsion; prucalopride is also prescribed.[176] When bowel problems persist, people are encouraged to follow a regular bowel management program that entails establishing routines for mealtimes, fluid intake, and uninterrupted periods after meals for bowel elimination.[173,176,177] Additional interventions can include biofeedback, transanal irrigation, sacral neuromodulation, and surgery (colostomy or ileostomy).[176]

Cognitive impairments. Strategies for managing cognitive impairments include compensation techniques such as memory notebooks, diaries, calendars, and computer-assisted programs for memory, attention, or other executive functions. Neuropsychologists, speech-language pathologists, and occupational therapists can all direct cognitive rehabilitation programs. Strategies for coping with cognitive impairments are often shared with the other members of the health care team for reinforcement with patients. A recent cross-sectional investigation found a weak correlation in people with MS with poorer cognition and a lower aerobic capacity.[178]

Direct interventions addressing specific cognitive tasks have been reported, but the results are mixed, with the best support for verbal learning and memory.[179,180] Cognitive behavioral therapy, exercise, and education programs are promising psychosocial interventions to improve coping and lessen cognitive symptoms.[181] The evidence is promising with small effects of fitness, physical activity, or exercise on cognition.[103] In a systematic review Maitra[182] found that cognitive behavioral therapy programs performed by occupational therapists were positively correlated with improvement in Functional Independence Measure (FIM) scores.

Depression is very common in people with MS, yet it is infrequently identified or treated.[183] Therapy can include supportive psychotherapy and medication given individually or in combination. To date two pharmacological therapies have shown the most promise in reducing cognitive deficits (L-amphetamine sulfate and donepezil), and neither has serious adverse effects.[184] There is growing evidence to support psychological interventions for people with mild to severe MS-related cognitive deficits, aimed at alleviating depressive symptoms and helping people cope with and adjust to their impairments.[179,180,185] Refer to Chapter 27 for additional information regarding interventions with individuals with cognitive impairments.

Dysarthria and dysphagia. Dysarthria is reported in up to 40% of people with MS. It is the disruption of muscular control in the central and peripheral speech mechanisms, which leads to abnormalities of speed, range, timing, strength, sound, and accuracy of speech movements.[186] Speech language pathologists (SLPs) address dysarthria by determining interventions that take into consideration the stage of the disease and speech quality. Typical programs may include exaggerating articulation, increasing voice volume, and increasing strength of oral musculature. The SLP will collaborate with other therapists to encourage follow-through with these programs to improve verbal communication during therapy sessions. Exercise programs designed to increase expiratory muscle strength have not been successful in improving voice quality or production but have shown increased respiratory muscle strength.[187]

Dysphagia or difficulty with chewing and swallowing is noted in 15% to 20% of people with MS[188] and becomes more prevalent in people with MS as the disease progresses.[189] SLP and occupational therapists facilitate proper swallowing with exercises that will improve posture to prevent aspiration and strengthen muscles of mastication. Other interventions may include diet modifications and education for the patient and his or her family or caregivers. Dieticians may be consulted to facilitate proper food choices.

Special considerations. Several special considerations for this population have been incorporated into the sections above, including patient preference, fall risk, fatigue, spasticity, and heat intolerance. Consideration of these factors must be incorporated into planning interventions and during the execution of a therapy session. Patient/client preferences must be integrated into the plan of care. For example, if a patient prefers fishing to soccer, for example, therapy might target overhead casting for an upper extremity limitation rather than throwing a soccer ball, and maintaining balance on an unstable surface (in a rocking boat) rather than while kicking a ball. Adapting exercises and physical activities to the patient's or patient's identified values and limitations should increase motivation to incorporate activities into an ongoing lifestyle. If a patient has a high fall risk, close guarding, a harness system, or partial body-weight supported activities overground or on a treadmill should help mitigate the risk while still practicing responses to increasing balance challenges. Pre-activity cooling might help reduce spasticity or heat intolerance, along with prolonged stretch for muscles with spasticity. If the patient/client is easily fatigued, the clinician might incorporate intermittent exercise/activity, introducing brief mandatory rests as soon as the first degradation of movement quality is noted.

Each of these special considerations along with other patient/client characteristics can affect response to treatment. Effectiveness of rehabilitation has been mixed for many types of interventions, frequently because the sample of people with MS is heterogeneous.[157] Average response to an intervention will seem nil or small if one group responds with an increase on an outcome and another group cancels out that effect because it responds not at all or with a decrease. The objective of comparing characteristics of different groups is to determine which characteristics are associated with positive response to that intervention.

One important consideration for therapists is movement variability. Traditionally, skilled movement is less variable than unskilled movements. However, *optimal movement variability*[190] theoretical perspective suggests that both too little variability and too much variability can indicate potential problems. Therefore successful interventions require therapists to facilitate the development of an optimal movement variability, somewhere between too much and too little. Using nonlinear tools to describe the structure of variability over time during a quiet standing task in people with MS, Hunt and colleagues[191] noted a strong, significant correlation between the direction of change with an intervention and the baseline level of movement variability. For participants at the higher end, with more random patterns of center-of-pressure movement, their nonlinear values decreased with intervention. For participants at the lower end, with more repetitive center-of-pressure patterns of movement, their nonlinear values increased with intervention. If the optimal movement variability was somewhere in the middle, then both groups converged on the more optimal value with intervention.[191]

When attempting to achieve optimal movement variability, therapists must consider the patient's abilities and the types of activities that are likely to challenge them to increase or reduce movement. If patients are constraining movement so tightly that they cannot respond to environmental changes or challenges, the objective is to increase variability in their movements. Intervention for people in this group might include unpredictable environmental challenges that will encourage error detection and self-correction of their movements.[190] If patients' movements are random such that they have difficulty accomplishing target tasks consistently, the objective is more regularity in their movement patterns. Interventions for this group might include facilitating co-contraction proximally for enhanced stability, extrinsic feedback about performance, repetition of tasks within the constraints of environmental factors (such as the use of a walker or other device), substituting different sensory modalities (vision) for an individual that has deficits (somatosensation), and reducing task complexity by limiting the number of joints moving simultaneously.[192]

SUMMARY

This chapter has focused on the pathology, clinical presentation, multidisciplinary management, and rehabilitation of people with MS. Understanding the type of MS, clinical disability, and severity of the disease will help therapists determine the best assessment and intervention strategies to manage the rehabilitation program. Using the ICF framework will facilitate the assessment of the impairments, activity limitations, and participation restrictions affecting each patient or client. In addition, assessing the environmental and personal factors present will help tailor the program to the patient's needs. Using outcome

measures that are valid and reliable for people with MS will assist the therapist's understanding of the entire range of impairments, activity limitations, participation restrictions, and QOL issues patients are facing in their everyday life. Therapists need to link the findings from examination and collaborate with the patient to set appropriate goals for therapy. Lastly, to achieve the best outcomes therapists should design interventions that are salient to the patient, have sufficient repetition and intensity, be specific to the goals, and be challenging enough to focus the individual's attention.

CASE STUDY 17.1 Initial Interview

Mrs. P. is a 54-year-old woman with a 28-year history of MS. She was first diagnosed with relapsing disease after her first daughter was born and remembers having a lot of trouble walking, Mrs. P. is concerned about her trunk weakness, back pain, and difficulty with walking; she often stumbles. She reports having fallen twice in the past year when she lost her balance and was unable to catch herself. One fall was at home, and one in the backyard. Therefore she has been using a single-point cane, especially on days when she feels off balance. Mrs. P. is limited to 10 minutes of walking and standing secondary to fatigue and difficulty balancing. She is overweight (BMI 29) and reports some bladder incontinence and heat sensitivity. Mrs. P. is a homemaker with 4 children; the youngest is 6. Leisure activities include playing the piano, singing, doing the Wii balance exercise for 10 min several times a week, and walking 10 min on a treadmill at 2.5 mph after using a cooling vest twice a week. After her treadmill walking, she feels fatigue for 3 to 4 h. Recently she has noted having more difficulty with singing and at times feels out of breath. Mrs. P's goals are improved posture, better breath control, no back pain, the ability to walk without stumbling or using a cane, and the ability to keep up with her children and her busy life.

Assessment

Mrs. P.'s Disease Steps classification is 3 (she uses a cane intermittently and is able to walk for 100 feet without it), and her EDSS score is 6.0. Vital signs are within normal limits (WNL) at rest and for exercise. This patient is cognitively intact and reliable in her response to questions. Her active and passive ROM is WNL throughout her extremities, trunk, and neck. She has selective motor control with normal tone. Manual muscle tests of bilateral upper extremity (UE) were normal, with the lower extremity (LE) 4/5 except for right hip flexion 3+/5, hip extension-abduction and plantarflexion 3/5. Abdominals 2/5, back extensors 3/5 (able to lift trunk against gravity through full range with difficulty and unable to take resistance). Sensation to light touch (LT), pain, and proprioception are intact throughout except for bilateral (B) feet, noted to have diminished sensation to LT. In sitting her posture is extremely slumped (from 30 to 45 degrees when fatigued) with notable thoracic kyphosis. She requires standby assist from supine to prone secondary to trunk weakness and instability. She requires use of B UEs in weight bearing to move from sitting to standing. During observational gait analysis, she demonstrates an asymmetrical step length with the left longer than the right and a right heel strike that is notably loud or audible. Her TUG score is 8 s using B UEs to stand up. The 25FTW is 5.6 s. The 6MWT was 324 m with one short rest. BBS was 45/56, putting her at risk of falls. Standing perturbation tests reveal loss of stability with an anterior nudge (posterior loss of balance [LOB]), posterior nudge (anterior LOB), and lateral and upper and lower trunk (LOB to opposite side). Rotational resistance tests to the right upper and lower trunk result in a stepping response, and the patient is unable to maintain stability, resulting in a stepping response. Results of rotational resistance tests to left upper and lower trunk are normal. The ABC scale score was 60% and the MSWS-12 score was 38/60 (63%).

Plan of Care and Goals

Mrs. P. had weakness in B LEs, balance problems, and an unsteady gait with at least two falls in the past 6 months. The ABC and MSWS-12 score were also low.

All of these results indicate that her gait and balance dysfunctions were interfering with her functional mobility and QOL. The physical therapy plan of care included balance and gait training, improved posture and time standing, and increased muscle strength, endurance, and cardiovascular fitness. Goals included a decreased fall risk with an improved BBS score of 54/56, increased MSWS-12 of 85%, and improved B LE and trunk strength (4/5 in all muscle groups), improved endurance to walk 450–500 m in 6 min without rest, decreased back pain to 0 to 1/10 on most days in 12 to 24 weeks. Additionally, the patient was referred to a PT with a specialty in women's health to manage her urinary incontinence.

Intervention

BalanceWear orthotic applied with placement of 1.5 pounds of weight to the torso to address the perturbation and rotational asymmetries (posterior right upper and lower trunk and anterior near navel) improved her reactive balance control. After applying the BW orthotic with the rigid component back pain resolved immediately; she felt better breath control and trunk support. The BBS score increased to 51/56, a significant improvement. TUG score remained the same, but she no longer needed her UE to stand up. Her posture also improved to 50% less kyphosis. During gait while weighted, a softer (inaudible) right heel strike was noted, and her step length was even and her 25FTW decreased to 4.8 s. Mrs. P. expressed that she felt much steadier and more balanced with the BalanceWear orthotic and was thrilled to have no back pain.

Mrs. P. was seen in a managed care setting and was able to make significant progress with her physical therapy program. She was seen in physical therapy (1×/week × 1 month, 2×/week × 2 months, 1×/month × 3 months) to improve her posture, strength, balance, and fitness. Breath-control exercises using her diaphragm were implemented to improve singing, monitoring progress with an inspiratory spirometer. Because this patient understood the principles of exercise, she was advised to perform the specific exercise until she experienced a decrease in the quality of movement or the muscles fatigued. A general stretching program was initiated, including specific stretches to improve her posture in sitting and standing. For strengthening exercise she started with one set of 8 to 15 reps; resistance was increased by 2% to 5% when 15 reps were efficient for major muscle groups including hip flexion-extension-abduction, heel raises for plantarflexion, rowing (shoulder retraction) with yellow Thera-Band in standing, curl-ups in hook-lying, and quadruped weight shifts, which were performed 2× to 3×/week. To address her deconditioning, an interval treadmill-training program was implemented on alternating days. Recommendation was to maintain the intensity of 2.5 mph at 64% to 75% of HRmax and do intervals of four blocks of 3 minutes with 1- to 2-min rest breaks in between and to continue to use the cooling vest before exercise. She was instructed to increase the blocks she was performing up to 7 as she tolerates. She continued with the Wii balance program, increasing to 30 min on the days she was not doing the treadmill. On those days she also performed specific balance exercises in the corner, beginning with her eyes open (single-leg stance; tandem stance). Mrs. P. was advised to use the BalanceWear orthotic for 2 h during functional activities and walking and to perform her exercises with it every other day. If she became less steady, she was advised to wear the orthotic an additional 1–2 h per day.

RESOURCES

Many websites are available to assist therapists and their patients with MS to understand the disease and find resources to help them manage the disease.

American Occupational Therapy Association
  800-377-8555
  www.aota.org

American Physical Therapy Association (APTA)
  800-999-2782
  www.apta.org

APTA Neurology Section, MS EDGE Outcome Measures taskforce
  www.neuropt.org/professional-resources/neurology-section-
    outcome-measures-recommendations/multiple-sclerosis

Multiple Sclerosis Association of America
  msaa@msaa.com
  www.mymsaa.com.

National Multiple Sclerosis Society
  nat@nmss.org
  https://www.nationalmssociety.org

Multiple Sclerosis Foundation
  support@msfocus.org
  https://www.msfocus.org

Rehabilitation Measures Database
  www.rehabmeasures.org

REFERENCES

To enhance this text and add value for the reader, all references are included on the companion Evolve site that accompanies this textbook. This online service will, when available, provide a link for the reader to a Medline abstract for the article cited. There are 192 cited references and other general references for this chapter, with the majority of those articles being evidence-based citations.

18

Disorders of the Basal Nuclei

Erin Vestal, Angela Rusher, Kristin Ikeda, and Marsha Melnick

OBJECTIVES

After reading this chapter the student or therapist will be able to:
1. Describe the circuitry of the basal nuclei.
2. Relate the anatomy and physiology of the basal nuclei to its roles in sensorimotor and cognitive processes.
3. Use the information on anatomy, physiology, and pharmacology to explain the signs and symptoms seen in classic disease states— for example, Parkinson disease, Huntington disease, and dystonia.
4. Develop an evaluation plan for patients with diseases of the basal nuclei.
5. Develop an intervention plan for patients, with the rationale for treatment methods.
6. Determine treatment effectiveness, especially in the case of degenerative disease.

KEY TERMS

basal nuclei
dystonia

Huntington disease
Parkinson disease

This chapter considers the degenerative, metabolic, hereditary, and genetic disorders that typically have their onset in adulthood, including Parkinson disease, Parkinsonian syndromes, Huntington chorea, Wilson disease, dystonias, heavy metal poisoning, and drug intoxication. Owing to the wide variety of diseases with their wide variety of causes, the concentration is on understanding the clinical problems and commonalities that exist within this grouping. The predominant area of the brain affected by these disorders is the basal nuclei: this group of central nervous system (CNS) structures is therefore discussed in some detail.

THE BASAL NUCLEI

The most commonly seen disorders affecting the basal nuclei include Parkinson disease, Huntington chorea, and dystonias, including drug-induced dyskinesias. All of these medical diagnoses involve impairments in muscle tone, movement coordination and motor control, and postural stability and the presence of extraneous movement. Taken together, these disorders now affect approximately 1 million people in the United States and more than 10 million people worldwide.[1–3]

To understand how this area of the brain can account for such a wide variety of symptoms, the anatomy, physiology, and neurochemistry of the basal nuclei structures must be considered.

Anatomy

The dorsal or sensorimotor basal nuclei are composed of three nuclei located at the base of the cerebral cortex—hence their name. These nuclei are the caudate nucleus, the putamen, and the globus pallidus. Two brain stem nuclei, the substantia nigra and the subthalamic nucleus, are included as part of the basal nuclei because they have a close

functional relation to the forebrain nuclei. In addition, connections between the basal nuclei and the pedunculopontine nucleus (PPN) are important in regulating underlying tone. Other parts of the basal nuclei, the ventral basal nuclei, are intimately related to the limbic system. The anatomical location of the various parts of the basal nuclei is shown in Fig. 18.1.

The caudate nucleus and the putamen are similar structures embryologically, anatomically, and functionally and, together, are often referred to as the neostriatum—a term derived from the word *striate*— and used to denote pathways from and to the caudate and putamen. An older term, *corpus striatum*, refers to the caudate, putamen, and globus pallidus. The various connections and interconnections of this system are discussed on the basis of these definitions.

Afferent Pathways

Functionally, the basal nuclei can be divided into an afferent portion and an efferent portion (Fig. 18.2). The afferent structures are the caudate and putamen. They receive input from the entire cerebral cortex, the intralaminar thalamic nuclei, and the centromedian-parafascicular complex of the thalamus as well as from the substantia nigra and the dorsal raphe nucleus, both located within the brain stem. The projections from the cortex are systematically arranged so that the frontal cortex projects to the head of the caudate and putamen and the visual cortex projects to the tail. In addition, the prefrontal cortex projects mainly to the caudate, whereas the sensorimotor cortex projects mainly to the putamen.[4–7] Projections from the cortical regions that represent the proximal musculature, and those from the premotor regions, may be bilateral.[5,6,8–11] These close and profuse connections between the cortex and the basal nuclei suggest a close interfunctional relationship. The projections from the thalamus to the caudate-putamen are also somatotopically arranged. The heaviest projections

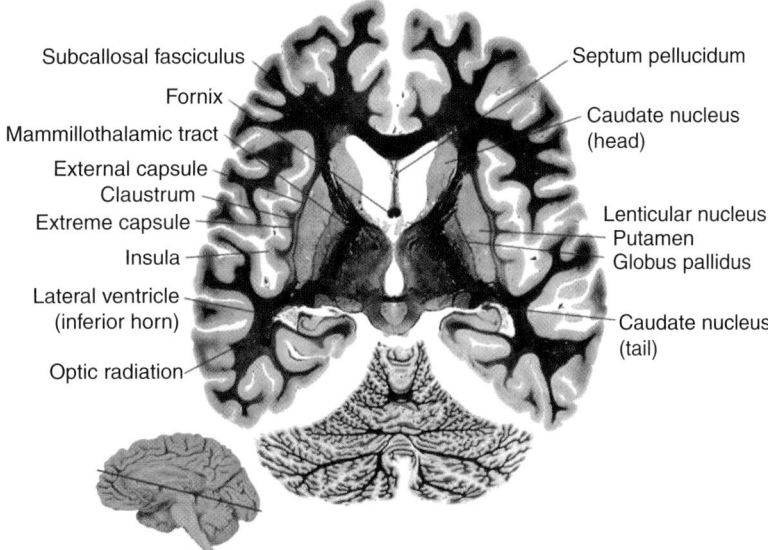

Fig. 18.1 A Coronal Section of the Anatomical Location of Various Parts of the Basal Nuclei. (Reprinted from Nolte J. *The Human Brain: An Introduction to Its Anatomy.* St. Louis: CV Mosby; 1981.)

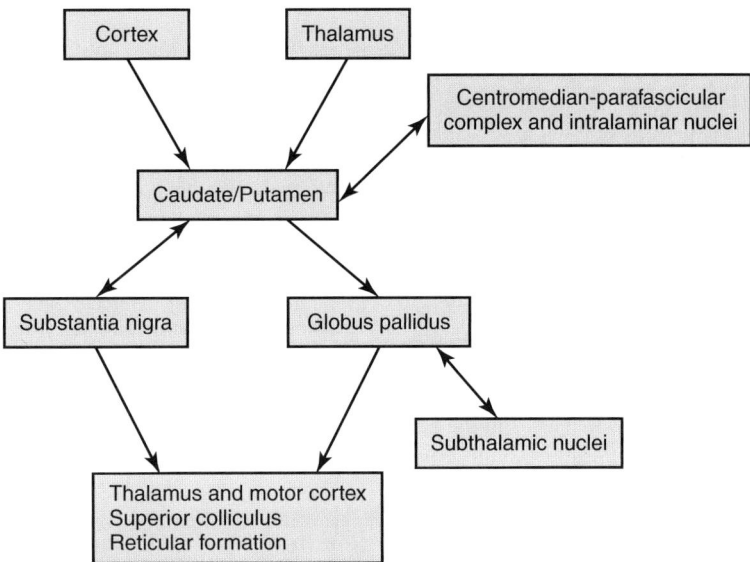

Fig. 18.2 Afferent and efferent portions of the basal nuclei.

are from the centromedian nucleus, and these nuclei also receive massive input from the motor cortex.[6,7–11]

The somatotopic arrangement of the cortico-striatal–thalamic-cortical pathways is maintained throughout the loop. This finding has led to an important functional hypothesis that the basal nuclei form parallel pathways subserving specific sensorimotor and associative functions.[4] The putamen is linked to the sensorimotor functions and the caudate to the associative, including cognitive functions.[8,11]

As knowledge of the circuitry of the basal nuclei has advanced, so has the knowledge regarding the microscopic structure. The caudate-putamen looks somewhat homogeneous because of the

predominance of one cell type. Careful analysis using precise staining methods has demonstrated the appearance of patches within these nuclei. It is hypothesized that this organization is important for the ability of the basal nuclei to modulate ongoing sensory input and choose the appropriate motor response.[11] The intrinsic structure of the caudate-putamen also suggests that at least nigral input occurs in a way that could immediately modulate the input coming from the cortex.[12,13]

Efferent Pathways

The input that has been processed in the caudate-putamen is sent to the globus pallidus (pallidum) and substantia nigra (nigra), which constitute the efferent portion of the basal nuclei. The globus pallidus and substantia nigra are each divided into two regions. The globus pallidus has an external and an internal region; the substantia nigra consists of the dorsal pars compacta and the ventral pars reticulata. Embryologically and microscopically, the internal segment of the globus pallidus and the pars reticulata of the substantia nigra are similar. These two regions are the primary efferent structures for the basal nuclei. The projections from the caudate and putamen to the pallidum and nigra maintain a somatotopic arrangement.[9,14,15] From these structures the information is transmitted to the thalamus and then to the cortex, still maintaining somatotopy. The superior colliculus, the PPN, and other, less-defined brain stem structures (perhaps the reticular formation) also receive pallidal and nigral output. All output of the basal nuclei has then been processed through the globus pallidus and/or the substantia nigra before proceeding to other areas of the brain (see Fig. 18.2).

Pathways to the Motor System

Information processed in the basal nuclei can influence the motor system in several ways, but no direct pathway to the alpha or gamma motor neurons of the spinal cord exists. The first route is the projection to the ventroanterior and ventrolateral nuclei of the thalamus, which then project predominantly to the premotor cortex. Another pathway is through the superior colliculus and then to the tectospinal tract. Pathways exist from the globus pallidus and substantia nigra that terminate in areas of the reticular formation (e.g., the PPN) and therefore may influence the motor system through the reticulospinal pathways. Research also supports the connection of the basal nuclei and the cerebellum and thus these two regions of the brain have the opportunity to further integrate movement responses.[16] This includes support for the cerebellar-basal nuclei connection contributing to the Parkinsonian tremor and dystonia.[17–19]

The basic circuitry of the basal nuclei comprises two loops.[6] The loops for the sensorimotor system are shown in Fig. 18.3. The direct loop is the loop that begins in the motor regions of the cortex and projects to the putamen and then directly to the globus pallidus, the internal segment, and on to the thalamus. The indirect pathway adds the subthalamic nucleus between the globus pallidus, external segment, and internal segment before sending the signal on to the thalamus. The subthalamic nucleus also receives direct input from the premotor and motor cortex as well as from the pallidum.[20,21] The darkened neurons represent inhibitory connections, and the open neurons represent excitatory connections. In general, the direct pathway, by disinhibition, activates the thalamocortical pathway; the indirect pathway inhibits the thalamocortical system. The role of these loops in normal and diseased states is clarified in the discussion of the physiology and pharmacology of the basal nuclei.

In summary, input from the motor cortex, all other areas of the cortex, parts of the thalamus, and the substantia nigra enter the basal nuclei through the caudate and putamen. Here they are processed and sent on to the globus pallidus and substantia nigra. The appropriate "gain" of the system is adjusted, for example, how large a movement is necessary or how much postural stability is needed. The information is sent to the muscles by way of the thalamus and motor cortex, the superior colliculus, and/or the reticular formation.

Physiology

The caudate and putamen are composed of neurons that fire slowly; the globus pallidus neurons fire tonically at high rates. The

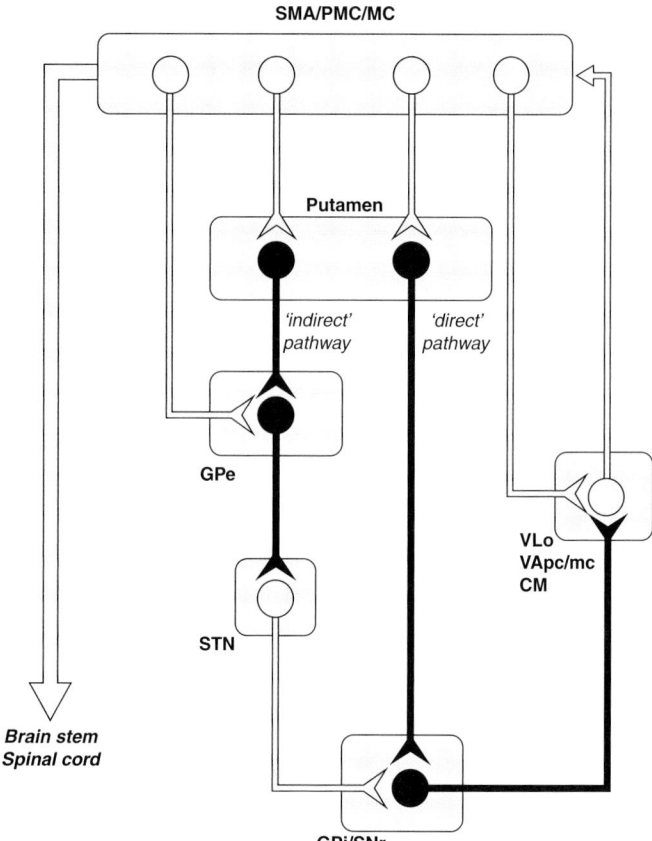

Fig. 18.3 Diagram of the sensory motor portion of the basal nuclei depicting the direct and indirect pathways. Black circles represent inhibitory neurons; open circles represent excitatory neurons. *CM*, Centromediannucleus of the thalamus; *GPe*, globus pallidus external segment; *GPi*, globus pallidus internal segment; *MC*, motor cortex; *PMC*, premotor cortex; *SMA*, supplementary motor cortex; *SNr*, pars reticularis of the substantia nigra; *STN*, subthalamic nucleus; *VApc/mc*, ventral anterior pars parvocellularis and pars magnocellularis of the thalamus; *VLo*, ventral lateralis pars oralis nucleus of the thalamus. (Reprinted from Alexander GE, Crutcher MD. Functional architecture of basal nuclei circuits: neural substrates of parallel processing. *Trends Neurosci.* 1990;13:266–271.)

low firing rates of the caudate-putamen are partially a result of the nature of thalamic inputs. Input from the cortex seems to have priority over input from the thalamus and substantia nigra. These data indicate that the cortex is instrumental in regulating the responsiveness of caudate and putamen neurons.[22] In turn, basal nuclei stimulation may prepare the cortex for subsequent inputs; this might be especially important when a response must be withheld until an appropriate stimulus occurs, such as keeping the foot on the brake until the light turns green.[22,23–25] Mink hypothesized that basal nuclei inputs to the cortex activate only the most necessary pathways and inhibit all unnecessary pathways (Fig. 18.4).[26]

The pattern of neuronal firing in the direct and indirect pathways also suggests that the basal nuclei modify input to the cortex. The neurons of the efferent portion of the basal nuclei respond with either phasic increases or phasic decreases in activity, which, in turn, will affect the activity in the thalamus and hence the cortex. A decrease in

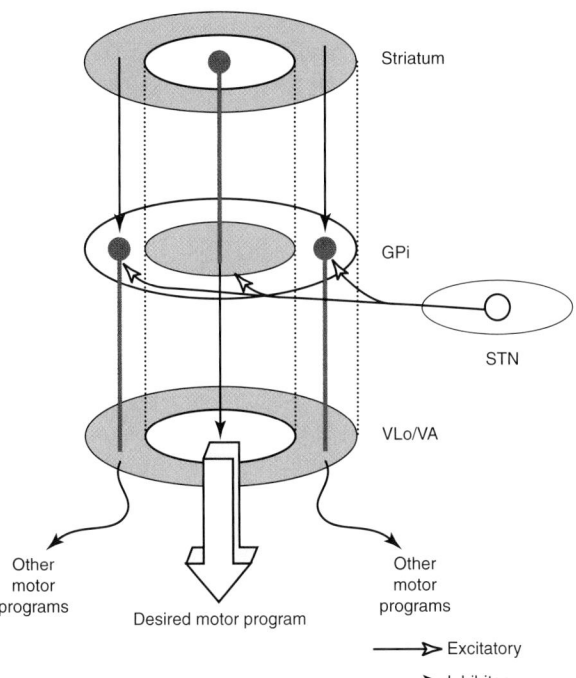

Fig. 18.4 The net effect of basal nuclei circuitry to produce an area of excitation (the desired program) surrounded by an area of inhibition (all other unnecessary programs). *GPi*, Globus pallidus internal segment; *STN*, subthalamic nucleus; *VLo/VA*, ventral lateralis oralis/ventral anterior. (Adapted from Mink JW. The basal nuclei: focused selection and inhibition of competing motor programs. *Prog Neurobiol.* 1996;50:381–425.)

activity of the internal segment of the globus pallidus removes inhibition to the thalamus and thus enables cortical activation. Whether the two pathways are activated concurrently or whether different activities activate the two pathways separately is not yet known; either way, the basal nuclei would have a role in cortical activation and modulation. One of the current views in relationship to disease processes is that an underactive direct pathway and/or an overactive indirect pathway would lead to decreased activation of the cortex and hence bradykinesia and akinesia, whereas an overactive direct pathway and/or underactive indirect pathway would lead to the presence of extraneous movements (see Fig. 18.3).[5,27]

How do these pathways relate to everyday function? Rigidity could be explained by too much muscle activity (through the pathways from the basal nuclei to the PPN and on to the spinal cord). Akinesia and bradykinesia typical of individuals with Parkinson disease are caused by insufficient excitation or too many conflicting patterns of movement. Increased extraneous movements are characteristic of basal nuclei diseases and can be attributed to the dysfunctions within these pathways. If the amount of muscle activity and the sequence and timing of activation are inappropriate, the individual will have difficulty in selecting the environmentally appropriate behavior.[26–29] Aldridge and colleagues found that the basal nuclei were modulated dependent on the purpose of the impending movement.[28]

Relationship of the Basal Nuclei to Movement and Posture

Lesion experiments; single and multiple unit recordings in awake, behaving animals; careful observations of the sequelae of human

disease processes; and the results of functional magnetic stimulation studies in humans have provided some answers regarding the precise role of the basal nuclei in movement and posture.

Automatic Movement

The earliest view of the basal nuclei came from Willis in 1664. He hypothesized that the corpus striatum received "the notion of spontaneous localized movements in ascending tracts … Conversely, from here tendencies are dispatched to enact notions without reflection [automatic movements] over descending pathways."[30] Willis possessed great insights in the discussion of the signs and symptoms of basal nuclei disease. Magendie in 1841 demonstrated that removal of the striatum bilaterally produced compulsive movements, whereas removal of only one striatum produced no visible effect.[31] Studies by Nothnagel[32] demonstrated that lesions of the nigra tended to produce immobility. With the advent of the use of electrical stimulation in the late-19th century, further information on the function of the basal nuclei was gathered. Stimulation of the caudate nucleus did not (and does not) produce movement of muscles or limbs, as occurs with stimulation of the motor cortex; however, at higher levels of current, total-body patterns and postures were usually evoked. The earliest stimulation of the caudate nucleus produced an increase of flexion of the head, trunk, and limbs and tonic contraction of the facial muscles.[28] These early studies are mentioned because of the insights they provide for the symptoms of the disorders of today.

Motor Problems in Animals

Contemporary experiments using lesion paradigms show a wide variety of motor problems in a variety of animals. Hypokinesia, a decrease or poverty of movements, a decreased amount of exploration of novel environments, and a tendency to assume a fixed posture are the most common problems after a lesion in the basal nuclei. These motoric dysfunctions are seen regardless of the method by which the lesion is made: pharmacological, surgical, or by stimulation. In essence, movements are altered in scale (related to the gain), take longer for completion, and take place under altered conditions of antagonistic muscle interactions (e.g., contraction).[33–41]

Movement Initiation and Preparation

The hypothesis that the basal nuclei are involved in movement initiation and preparation has been an area of some research disagreement. A "readiness potential," recorded from the scalp of human beings before movement and thought to reflect basal nuclei activity, is more apparent in complex than in simple movements, for example, before dorsiflexion with gait but not before dorsiflexion when sitting.[42–45]

Neuronal recordings from awake, behaving animals found that units in the basal nuclei alter their activity before changes in the electromyographic activity of the prime movers of the task.[46–52] Studies recorded from multiple units in animals moving freely in their home environment suggest that neurons in the caudate-putamen and in the substantia nigra are activated in sequential, purposeful movements.[28] More recent functional magnetic resonance imaging (fMRI) studies emphasize the role of the mesial premotor cortex and its role as part of the cortico-basal nuclei-thalamo-cortical network for motor planning and movement initiation. This includes the role of the substantia nigra during motor planning caused by the dopaminergic gating of motor sequences.[53]

Postural Adjustments

The basal nuclei have been implicated in the process of posture and postural adjustments. People with diseases of the basal nuclei assume flexed or other fixed postures as the disease progresses (Fig. 18.5). In addition, these individuals have decreased postural stability and are therefore at risk for falls. Animal experiments indicate that a deficit exists in determining response based on one's own body position, or "egocentric localization."[54–56] This deficit decreases the ability of a person with basal nuclei disease to modify a postural response to the precise environmental demands.

Martin,[57] in his extensive studies of individuals with Parkinson disease, was the first to describe severe disturbances in posture, especially when vision was occluded. Melnick and colleagues[58] showed that a decrease in static postural adjustments in persons with Parkinson disease could be seen early in the disease process.[59] Bloem and colleagues[60–62] and Visser and colleagues[63] meticulously studied the reflexes involved in postural adjustments and described deficits in the longer loop reflexes but not in the short latency reflex associated with the stretch reflex.

Others have investigated the interactions of the sensory systems involved in balance in those with Parkinson disease.[63–67] Bloem and colleagues[61] and Visser and colleagues[63] concluded that postural instability was caused by a decrease in proprioception. In a recent review of proprioception and postural stability and motor control,

Nicola and colleagues also describe the kinesthetic and proprioceptive deficits in people with Parkinson disease. Nicola and colleagues concluded that there was a "failure" in the body map similar to the failure in egocentric localization described previously.[55,59] A decrease in the ability to use proprioceptive and kinesthetic information to properly scale the input and response also contributes to a loss of balance reactions.

Perceptual and Cognitive Functions

The basal nuclei are not solely motor systems. The previous paragraphs demonstrate the role of the basal nuclei in sensory integration, but they are also involved in cognitive functions and responses associated with reward.[37,38,48,50,68] Researchers have found that learned movements are more affected by basal nuclei lesions than reflexes, neurons in the basal nuclei are responsive to some sensory input, especially proprioceptive input, and neurons in other parts of the basal nuclei are responsive to reward and anticipation of the reward.[29,69,70] Klockgether and Dichgans,[71] as well as Jobst and colleagues,[72] found that patients with Parkinson disease likewise had impairments in kinesthesia and that as a person moved a limb further from the body's center, kinesthetic sense decreased. Schneider and colleagues[73] found that animals that developed parkinsonian symptoms from a neurotoxin had deficits in operantly conditioned behavior. They suggested that the decrease in performance resulted from a "defect in the linkage" between a stimulus and the motor output centers. These sensory difficulties may be important factors in evaluation and treatment of basal nuclei diseases, especially those associated with dystonia.

The basal nuclei appear to be involved in the process of withholding a response until it is appropriate.[74] A deficit in alternation of response may be the result of a tendency toward perseveration of a previously reinforced cue.[75] Additional deficits exist in remembering or relearning tasks requiring a temporal sequence.[76] Graybiel[29] integrated the behavioral findings with information from her anatomical and chemical studies to suggest that the basal nuclei are important in providing behavioral flexibility. She hypothesizes that the basal nuclei are involved in procedural learning that leads to the development of habits. These habits become routine and are easily performed without conscious effort; we are free to react to new events in our environment and to think. Graybiel and colleagues have performed electrophysiological experiments that explain this learning process, and these studies demonstrate great plasticity in basal nuclei networks.[77,78] This enables the individual to select the proper movements in the proper environmental context. These cognitive dimensions are important to remember when developing a plan of care for a patient with basal nuclei dysfunction.

The ability to perform cognitive activities involves integrating sensory information and, on the basis of this information, making an appropriate response. Humans with basal nuclei disease may show problems in perceptual abilities, including deficits in tasks that involve perception of interpersonal and intrapersonal space.[79] The basal nuclei seem to have a sensory integrative function as evidenced by experiments that show a multisensory and heterotopic convergence of somatic, visual, auditory, and vestibular stimuli.[29,69] Segundo and Machne,[70,80] as well as Nicola and colleagues,[55] hypothesized that the function of the basal nuclei was not subjective recognition of the stimuli but rather in the regulation of posture and movements of the body in space and in the production of complex motor acts.

For movements to be properly controlled and properly sequenced, the two sides of the body need to be well integrated. There is

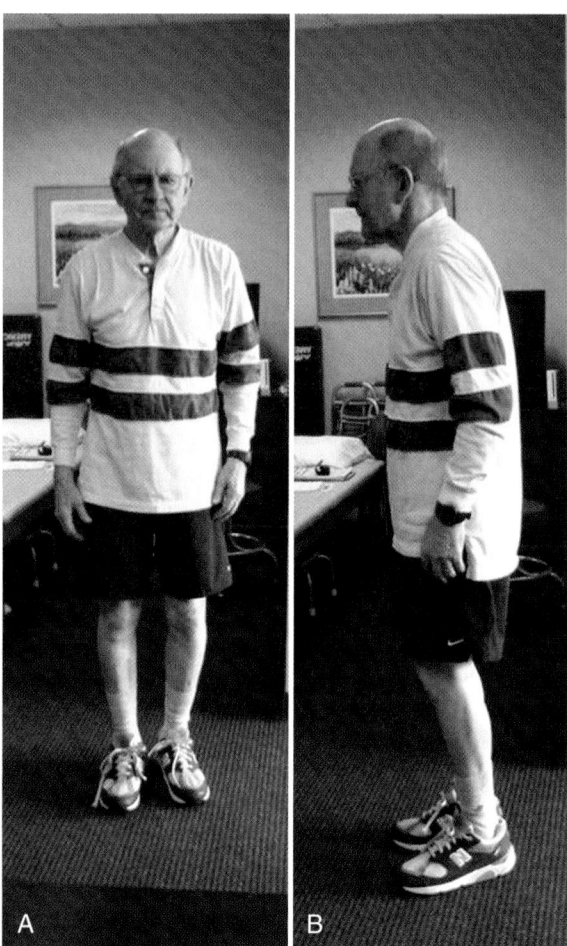

Fig. 18.5 Typical posture of a patient with Parkinson disease from the front **(A)** and from the side **(B)**. Note the flexed spine, mild flexion at the hips and knees, and excessive dorsiflexion with weight predominantly on the heels. Patient was at Hoehn and Yahr stage 2.5.

anatomical evidence that suggests some means of bilateral control for the basal nuclei. A lesion of one caudate nucleus or nigrostriatal pathway produces a change in the unit activity of the remaining caudate.[76,81] Studies of the dopaminergic pathway also indicate interactions between the two sides of the body.[81] For this reason one may find deficits in function even on the "uninvolved" side of an individual with disease or lesion of the basal nuclei. It is also possible that diseases of the basal nuclei may go unnoticed until damage is found bilaterally.

This summary of experimental results on the function of the basal nuclei illustrates several points. At least in some general way the basal nuclei are involved in the processes of movement related to preparing the organism for future motion and future reward. This may include preparing the cortex for approximate time activation, setting the postural reflexes or the gamma motor neuron system, organizing sensory input to produce a motor response in an appropriate environmental context, and inhibiting all unnecessary motor activity. Owing to the multilevel involvement of the basal nuclei in movement, it is crucial that clinicians carefully observe all aspects of movement (simple and complex) with and without interference of sensory cues or performance of dual tasks as well as postural tone during examination, treatment, and the responses to treatment.

Neurotransmitters

Before a detailed analysis of the diseases of the basal nuclei can be considered, a brief description of the neurotransmitters of this region is necessary. The most prevalent diseases discussed in this chapter indicate a deficit in specific neurotransmitters. The pharmacological treatment of Parkinson disease and, in the future, perhaps other "Parkinson's plus" or "basal nuclei plus" diseases, is based on these neurochemical deficits. The basal nuclei possess high concentrations of many of the suspected neurotransmitters: dopamine (DA), acetylcholine (ACh), γ-aminobutyric acid (GABA), substance P, and the enkephalins and endorphins. This discussion, however, includes only the first three neurotransmitters. A diagram of the basal nuclei pathways, which includes the neurotransmitters, is shown in Fig. 18.6.

DA is the major neurotransmitter of the nigrostriatal pathway and is produced in the pars compacta of the substantia nigra. The axon terminals of these dopaminergic neurons are located in the caudate

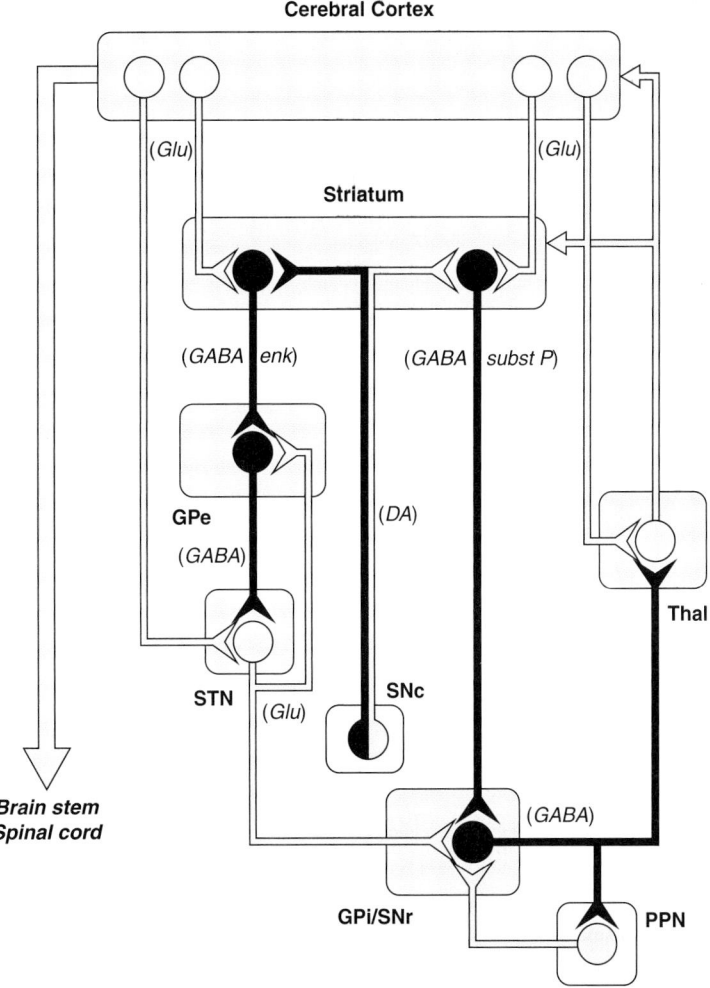

Fig. 18.6 The Neurotransmitters of the Direct and Indirect Pathways of the Basal Nuclei. Black circles represent inhibitory neurons; *open circles* represent excitatory neurons. *DA,* Dopamine; *enk,* enkephalin; *glu,* glutamate; *GABA,* γ-aminobutyric acid; *GPe,* globus pallidus external segment; *GPi,* globus pallidus internal segment; *PPN,* pedunculopontine nucleus; *SNr,* pars reticularis of the substantia nigra; *STN,* subthalamic nucleus; *subst P,* substance P; *Thal,* thalamus. (Reprinted from Alexander GE, Crutcher MD. Functional architecture of basal nuclei circuits: neural substrates of parallel processing. *Trends Neurosci.* 1990;13:266–271.)

nucleus and putamen. DA appears to be excitatory to the neurons in the direct pathway (GABA and substance P neurons) and inhibitory to the neurons in the indirect pathway (GABA and enkephalin neurons).[1] This dual effect means that a loss of DA will lead to a loss of excitation in the direct pathway and an excess of excitation of the indirect pathway, leading to a powerful decrease in activation of the thalamocortical pathway.

Several DA receptors exist; however, their chemical interactions permit the continued use of D1 and D2 receptor classes.[6] The role of DA may modulate the effects of other neurotransmitters such as glutamate. Many new drugs (called the *dopamine agonists*) influence only one of these receptors. Recent experiments have been trying to determine which behaviors are mediated by which DA receptor in the hope that this research may lead to more effective drug treatment with fewer side effects.

Because various drugs and chemicals can act as agonists (similar to) and antagonists (blocking the action of) of DA, they are used in treating disease involving the basal nuclei. Agonists include amantadine, apomorphine, and a class of drugs called the *ergot alkaloids* (e.g., bromocriptine). Amphetamine, which prevents the reuptake of DA, can enhance the effect of any DA present in the system. Antagonists include haloperidol, clozapine, and antipsychotic drugs of the phenothiazine class. With time these drugs may deplete the basal nuclei of DA and therefore cause Parkinson disease or tardive dyskinesia. Similar effects on the DA system are observed in a single dose of methamphetamine.[82]

ACh is believed to be the neurotransmitter of the small interneurons of the caudate and putamen. It is presumed to inhibit the action of DA in this region and classically must be "in balance" with DA (and GABA). Dopaminergic axon terminals are found on cholinergic neurons. Substances that increase dopaminergic activity decrease release of ACh and vice versa.[83] The antagonists of ACh, such as belladonna alkaloids and atropine-like drugs, were one of the first class of drugs used in the treatment of Parkinson disease. ACh antagonists are still used as adjuncts to treatment for patients with Parkinson disease. As some of the drugs to treat dementia are ACh agonists, care must be used when these are prescribed for the person with basal nuclei dysfunction, especially Parkinson disease.

GABA is an inhibitory neurotransmitter that is found throughout the brain. In the basal nuclei, it is synthesized in the caudate nucleus and putamen and transmitted to the globus pallidus and substantia nigra.[84] GABA in the basal nuclei may permit movement to occur by allowing a distribution of neuronal firing. It may also provide a means of feedback inhibition in the efferent parts of the basal nuclei so that the program of activity is not repeated unless needed.[84] Individuals with Huntington disease have a deficiency of this chemical. Although agonists of GABA exist (e.g., muscimol and imidazole acetic acid), a successful drug for the treatment of Huntington disease has not yet been found. This may be a result of either the ubiquitous nature of GABA or the very complex circuitry and interrelationships that exist among GABA, ACh, and DA.

In addition to the transmitters discussed, co-transmitters may be found in the basal nuclei. Two such co-transmitters are cholecystokinin and neurotensin. The interactions of these co-transmitters may alter the sensitivity of DA receptors. Fuxe[85] suggests that the interactions of co-transmitters may alter the "set point" of transmission in synapses. They may therefore be important in supersensitivity, which is one of the side effects of DA therapy.

Lastly, the neurotransmitter from the cortex to the caudate nucleus and putamen is glutamate. Studies are ongoing to investigate glutamate antagonists as a treatment for Parkinson disease. Glutamate

receptors use calcium, and in the future, drugs affecting calcium channels may also have a therapeutic effect.

SPECIFIC CLINICAL PROBLEMS ARISING FROM BASAL NUCLEI DYSFUNCTION

Parkinson Disease

Parkinson disease is a diverse disorder with a long list of motor and nonmotor symptoms. It is a slowly progressing degenerative disease defined by a decrease in the DA stores of the substantia nigra and associated with striatal Lewy bodies (intracellular inclusions) and α-synuclein deposition. It is DA that gives the substantia nigra its coloration (and hence its name); therefore the lighter the nigra, the greater the DA loss. The term Parkinsonism is often used and is an umbrella term that refers to a group of disorders that produce abnormalities of the basal nuclei. Primary Parkinsonism is known as idiopathic Parkinsonism and what people are referring to when using the term Parkinson's. Secondary Parkinsonism has a determined etiology including tumors, viruses, and drugs. While no two people will experience the exact combination of symptoms, there are some commonalities. It was first described by Parkinson in 1807 as a disease characterized by rigidity, bradykinesia (slow movement), micrography, masked face, postural abnormalities, and a resting tremor.

Parkinson disease is among the most prevalent of all CNS degenerative diseases. Presently, there are an estimated 1 million people in the United States with this disease, with approximately 60,000 new cases each year; the incidence is 4.5 to 20.5, and the prevalence is 31 to 347 per 100,000 (refer to the list of websites at the end of this chapter). Incidence increases with advancing age, and it is estimated that one in three adults over the age of 85 will have this disease.[1] Four percent are diagnosed before the age of 50 years. The personal and societal burden of Parkinson disease is estimated at 25 billion a year in the United States alone and includes the cost of treatment, the burden of caregiving, and the cost of lost earnings in patients below the age of 65 years.[86]

The cause of Parkinson disease remains unknown, and the consensus is that it is multifactorial.[87,88] Some evidence indicates involvement of environmental factors and that interaction of environment and aging lead to a critical decrease in DA. Several investigators have found a link between growing up in a rural area and Parkinson disease, with connections to pesticide and insecticide exposure, as well as elements in well water.[89–95] Accumulation of free radicals, cell death to excitatory neurons from toxins, and dysfunction of nigral mitochondria have all been implicated in the pathological process. The genetics of Parkinson disease was in debate for many years, but it is now known that at least 10% to 15% percent of all cases of Parkinson disease are familial. Recent studies have discovered the presence of altered autosomal dominant (α-synuclein, LRRK2), autosomal recessive (PARK7, PINK1, PRKN), and altered risk factor modifier genes that may put you at risk of developing the disease. Research is still underway regarding genetic links, but it is believed that a complex interaction between genetic and nongenetic-factors is the cause of PD; thus a family history may be an important risk factor.[94,96–100] Beyond genetics, there is new research investigating the link between early symptoms of Parkinson disease and the nerve cells lining the digestive tract. Large toxic amounts of the alpha-synuclein protein—hallmark of Parkinson disease–have been found in the gut of people who developed Parkinson disease. There is also evidence that people who have a vagotomy (one or more branches of the vagus nerve are cut) have a lower risk of developing PD, supporting the brain-gut connection.[101] So the debate continues, with most neurologists agreeing that the multifactorial approach will yield the best opportunity to develop a cure.

Symptoms

Bradykinesia, akinesia, and complex motor planning. Bradykinesia (a decrease in motion) and akinesia (a lack of motion) are characterized by an inability to initiate and perform purposeful movements. They are also associated with a tendency to assume and maintain fixed postures. All aspects of movement are affected, including initiation, alteration in direction, and the ability to stop a movement once it has begun. Spontaneous or associated movements, such as swinging of the arms in gait or smiling at a funny story, are also affected. Bradykinesia is hypothesized to be the result of a decrease in activation of the supplementary motor cortex, premotor cortex, and motor cortex.[102] The resting level of activity in these areas of the cortex may be decreased so that a greater amount of excitatory input from other areas of the brain would be necessary before movement patterns could be activated. In the individual with Parkinson disease, an increase in cortically initiated movement even for such "subcortical" activities, such as walking, supports this hypothesis. Automatic activities are cortically controlled, and each individual aspect seems to be separately programmed. Associated movements in the trunk and other extremities are not automatic, which means that great energy must be expended whenever movement is begun.[103]

Bradykinesia and akinesia affect performance of all types of movements; however, complex movements are more involved than simple movements, such as dorsiflexing the foot at toe-off in walking as opposed to dorsiflexing the foot in a seated position.[70,104–107] In addition, patients with parkinsonism have increased difficulty performing simultaneous or sequential tasks, over and above that seen with simple tasks. Parkinsonian patients must complete one movement before they can begin to perform the next, whereas control subjects are able to integrate two movements more smoothly in sequence. This deficit has been shown in a variety of tasks, from performing an elbow movement and grip to tracing a moving line on a video screen. The patient with Parkinson disease behaves as if one motor program must be completely played out before the next one begins, and there is no advance planning for the next movement while the current movement is in progress.[105–109] Morris and colleagues demonstrated a similar phenomenon in walking. Patients with parkinsonism were unable to perform walking while carrying a tray with a glass of water and had even more difficulty when walking and reciting a numerical sequence.[110,111]

Sequential movements become more impaired as more movements are strung together; for example, a square is disproportionately slower to draw than a triangle and a pentagon more difficult than a square.[4,107] These results indicate that patients with Parkinson disease have difficulty with transitions between movements. Transitional difficulties are more impaired in tasks requiring a series of different movements than tasks requiring a series of repetitive movements. For example, an individual will have less difficulty continually riding a stationary bike than movement requiring transitions such as coming from a chair to standing, walking, and turning a corner. Therefore treatment must include complex movements with directional changes to ensure that the patient is safe outside the treatment setting.

Bradykinesia is not caused by rigidity or an inability to relax. This was demonstrated in an electromyographic analysis of voluntary movements of persons with Parkinson disease.[112] Although the pattern of electromyographic agonist-antagonists burst is correct, these bursts are not large enough, resulting in the inability to generate muscle force rapidly enough. Even in slow, smooth movements, these individuals demonstrated alternating bursts in the flexor and extensor muscle groups. This type of pattern, expected in rapid movements that require the immediate activation of the antagonist to halt the motion, interferes with slow, smooth, continuous motion. Other researchers have

found an alteration in the recruitment order of single motor units.[113,114] These alterations included a delay in recruitment, pauses in the motor unit once it was recruited, and an inability to increase firing rates. These people would therefore have a delay in activation of muscles, an inability to properly sustain muscle contraction for movement, and a decreased ability to dissipate force rapidly.[26,113,115] Such changes may account for perceived decreases in strength that are seen in persons with Parkinson disease. They are also important to remember in both treatment planning and the efficacy of treatment efficiency.

Rigidity. The rigidity (increased resistance to passive movement) of Parkinson disease may be characterized as either "lead pipe" or "cogwheel." The cogwheel type of rigidity is a combination of lead-pipe rigidity with tremor. In rigidity, there is an increased resistance to movement throughout the entire range in both directions without the classic clasp-knife reflex so characteristic of spasticity. Procaine injections can decrease the rigidity without affecting the decrease of spontaneous movements, confirming that rigidity is not the same phenomenon as bradykinesia.[116,117]

Rigidity is not caused by an increase in gamma motor neuron activity, a decrease in recurrent inhibition, or a generalized excitability in the motor system.[118] Long- and middle-latency reflexes are enhanced in Parkinsonism, and the increase in long-latency reflexes approximates the observable increase in muscle tone. Short-latency reflexes (i.e., deep tendon reflexes), on the other hand, may be normal in persons with Parkinson disease.

Tatton and others[119] found differences in certain cortical long-loop reflexes in normal and drug-induced Parkinsonian monkeys, which led them to speculate that the "reflex gain" of the CNS may lose its ability to adjust to changing environmental situations. For example, in normal people, the background level of motor neuron excitability is different for the task of writing from the task of lifting a heavy object; in individuals with Parkinson disease, motor neuron excitability would be set at the same level. Similarly, in the normal individual, there would be a difference in excitability if the environmental demands were for excitation or inhibition of a muscle; for the individual with Parkinson disease, there would be similar motor neuron excitability regardless of task demands. Furthermore, this lack of modulation may mean that the person with Parkinsonism perceives himself or herself to be moving farther than he or she is actually moving. It is also consistent with a decrease in system flexibility and an inability to adjust to equilibrium perturbations.[60,62,65]

An important aspect of rigidity is that it might increase energy expenditure.[120] This would increase the patient's perception of effort on movement and may be related to feelings of fatigue, especially postexercise fatigue.[121]

Tremor. In those diagnosed with Parkinson disease, about 70% will experience a tremor at some point in the disease. The tremor observed in Parkinson disease is present at rest, usually disappears or decreases with movement, and has a regular rhythm of about 4 to 7 beats per second; however, it may worsen with intense emotions, fatigue, or anxiety. Tremor often occurs unilaterally and then progresses bilaterally in the hands, described as "pill rolling", but can also appear as a postural tremor, or in other parts of the body including the lower lip, jaw, or leg. The electromyographic tracing of a person with such a tremor shows rhythmical, alternating bursting of antagonistic muscles. Tremor can be produced as an isolated finding in experimental animals that have been treated with drugs, especially DA antagonists. DA depletion, however, is not the sole cause of tremor. It appears that efferent pathways, especially from the basal nuclei to the thalamus, must be intact because lesions of these fibers decrease or abolish the tremor.[122] Tremors can be severely disabling, affecting all aspects of activities of daily living (ADLs) requiring fine motor control such as eating, drinking, dressing, shaving, and writing. Upper extremity tremors are what lead many people to seek initial treatment and diagnosis.

Postural Instability. Postural instability is a serious problem in Parkinsonism that leads to increased episodes of falling, with the sequelae of falls contributing to morbidity. More than two-thirds of all patients with Parkinsonism fall, and more than 10% fall more than once a week.[123] People with Parkinson disease have a ninefold risk of recurrent falls compared with age-matched control subjects.[61,124-128] Patients have an increased likelihood of falling as the duration of the disease increases. Drug treatment is not usually effective in reducing the incidence of falls. Deep brain stimulation (DBS) and exercise, on the other hand, have been shown to be effective in increasing functional skills and/or motor performance that, in turn, may decrease the number of falls.[129-132] Large randomized clinical trials have been performed to determine the efficacy of exercise and will be discussed later in the chapter.[133]

Although the pathology of postural instability is unknown, several hypotheses exist. One explanation for postural instability is ineffective sensory processing. Several investigators have found deficits in proprioceptive and kinesthetic processing.[57,72,115,134] For example, Martin[57] found that labyrinthine equilibrium reactions were delayed in patients with Parkinson disease. Studies of the vestibular system itself, however, have shown that this system functions normally. Pastor and colleagues[135] studied central vestibular processing in patients with Parkinson disease and found that the vestibular system responds normally and that patients can integrate vestibular input with the input from other sensory systems. This group hypothesized that the parkinsonian patients had an inability to adequately compensate for baseline instability. This theory is in partial agreement with studies by Beckley, Boehm, and others[60,62,65] demonstrating that patients with Parkinson disease were unable to adjust the size of long- and middle-latency reflex responses to the degree of perturbation. These patients are therefore unable to activate muscle force proportional to displacement. Melnick and colleagues[58] found that subjects with Parkinson disease were unable to maintain balance on a sway-referenced force plate. Glatt[136] found that patients with Parkinson disease did not demonstrate anticipatory postural reactions and, in fact, behaved exactly as a rigid body with joints. In a variety of studies, Horak and colleagues[137,138] reported similar findings and found defects in strategy selection as well; patients with Parkinson disease chose neither a pure hip strategy nor a pure ankle strategy but mixed the two in an inappropriate and maladaptive response. Investigators have found that antiparkinsonian medications could improve background postural tone but did not improve automatic postural responses to external displacements.[60,62,65,137] Other studies have demonstrated deficits in proprioceptive perception—what has been termed an "impaired proprioceptive body map." Patients with Parkinson disease did not alter anticipatory postural adjustments in response to step width changes, unlike control subjects.[139] Increased step width requires increased lateral reactive forces to unload the stance leg. The lack of ability to prepare for these extra forces may indicate that narrow stance width, start hesitation, and freezing of gait are compensatory mechanisms to proprioceptive loss.[134] Likewise, when patients could not see their limbs, they had difficulty moving the foot to a predetermined location in response to perturbation. Control subjects had no difficulty.[140,141] Taken together, it appears that postural instability results from inflexibility in response repertoire; an inability to inhibit unwanted programs; the interaction of akinesia, bradykinesia, and rigidity; and some disturbance in central sensory processing.

Gait. The typical Parkinsonian gait is characterized by decreased velocity and stride length.[142-143] As a consequence, foot clearance is decreased, which places the individual at a greater fall risk.[144] In many patients, especially as the disease progresses, speed and shortening of stride progressively worsen as if the individual is trying to catch up with his or her center of gravity; this is termed *festination*. Forward festination is called *propulsion;* backward festination is known as *retropulsion.* One hypothesis is that festinating gait is caused by the decreased equilibrium responses. If walking is a series of controlled falls and if normal responses to falling are delayed or not strong enough, then the individual will either fall completely or continue to take short, running-like steps. The abnormal motor unit firing seen with bradykinesia may also be the cause of ever-shortening steps. If the motor unit cannot build up a high enough frequency or if it pauses in the middle of the movement, then the full range of the movement would decrease; in walking this would lead to shorter steps. Festination may also be the result of other changes in the kinematics of gait.

The changes in gait kinematics include changes in excursion of the hip and ankle joints (Fig. 18.7). Instead of a heel-toe, the patient may have a flat-footed or, with disease progression, a toe-heel sequence. The flat-footed gait with poor weight shifting decreases the ability to step over obstacles or to walk on carpeted surfaces. The use of three-dimensional gait analysis has shown that there is a decrease in plantarflexion at terminal stance. Changes are also seen in hip flexion, which may alter ankle excursion; however, qualitative aspects of the timing of joint excursion appear intact. Fig. 18.7 illustrates the joint angles in a 55-year-old patient with Parkinson disease compared with adults without basal nuclei dysfunction.[145]

Impaired gait and postural instability are the two impairments that contribute to the greatest activity limitations to persons with Parkinsonism. The inability to ambulate safely and the high fall risk of these patients are the major elements contributing to mortality and preventing independence in home and work as the disease progresses.

Perception, attention, and cognitive deficits. Especially in recent years, researchers have tried to address the cognitive and perceptual impairments of people with Parkinson disease.[134,146-149] The learning and perceptual deficits are hypothesized to be caused by a decrease in cortical excitation from the caudate nucleus,[108] whereas the movement deficits are hypothesized to be caused by a decrease in putaminal excitation of the cortex. Cognitive involvement can also include memory loss, confused thinking, and dementia. Parkinson disease medications may worsen these cognitive impairments.

The deficits are of frontal lobe function and include an inability to shift attention, an inability to quickly access "working memory," and difficulty with visuospatial perception and discrimination. Research attention has focused on the specific deficits of parkinsonian patients compared with patients with Alzheimer's disease, patients with frontal lobe damage, and those with temporal lobe damage.[146,149,150] The perceptual deficits of all groups appear to increase with progression of the disease process. In general, patients have difficulty in shifting attention to a previously irrelevant stimulus, learning under conditions requiring selective attention, or selecting the correct motor response on the basis of sensory stimuli.[151-153] There is also evidence that DA is involved in selection of responses that will be rewarding.[55] These impairments will affect treatment strategies.

Learning deficits also have been found in patients with Parkinsonism; procedural learning has been particularly implicated, as would be indicated based on the physiology of the system. Procedural learning is learning that occurs with practice or, as defined by Saint-Cyr and colleagues,[154] "the ability gradually to acquire a motor skill or even a cognitive routine through repeated exposure to a specific activity constrained by invariant rules." In their tests, patients with Parkinson disease did very poorly on those related to procedural learning, but their declarative learning was within normal limits. Pascual-Leone and colleagues[108] studied procedural learning in more detail. They found

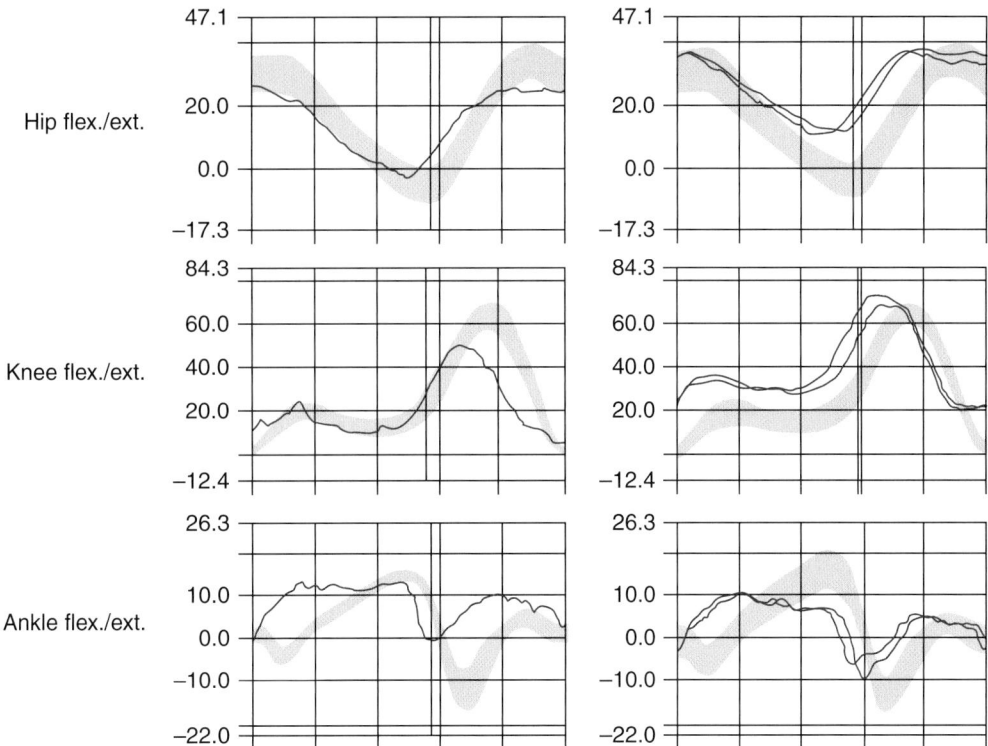

Fig. 18.7 Angles of Excursion During Gait in a Patient With Parkinson Disease. *Shaded areas* are mean ± standard deviations for adults *without* Parkinson disease; *black lines* represent a patient *with* Parkinson disease. Movement shown for right- and left-lower extremities. Note decreases, especially in left lower extremity for extension and bilateral decreased plantarflexion.

that patients with Parkinson disease could acquire procedural learning but needed more practice than control subjects did. They also found that the ability to translate procedural knowledge to declarative knowledge was more efficient if it occurred with visual input alone rather than the combination of visual input with motor task. This may be a rationale for more therapy, not less.

Nonmotor symptoms. Nonmotor symptoms are consistently seen in patients with Parkinson disease and may be attributable to dopaminergic pathways outside the basal nuclei. Braak and colleagues[155,156] hypothesized that Parkinson disease actually begins with DA deterioration in the medulla and progresses rostrally. Often, the first signs are loss of sense of smell, constipation, vivid dreams (rapid-eye movement [REM] behavior disorder), and orthostatic hypotension.[157] Orthostatic hypotension may cause some dizziness and requires coordination of medications for other medical problems. L-Dopa and DA agonists may lower blood pressure. These symptoms alone do not indicate Parkinson disease, but combined they may indicate risk. Physical therapy may be most effective when started early, so researchers are trying to learn more about these early symptoms.

Other nonmotor symptoms that decrease quality of life include incontinence in men and women, sexual dysfunction, excess saliva, weight changes, and skin problems. Urinary incontinence may increase the risk of hospitalization and mortality.[158] Nonmotor symptoms that can interfere with and complicate physical and occupational treatment include fatigue, fear, apathy, anxiety, and depression. Referrals to medical professionals for these symptoms are imperative.

Sleep disorders are widespread in Parkinson disease and include more than just REM sleep disorder.[156] The patient may experience daytime drowsiness and decreased sleep at night, as well as the presence of restless leg syndrome.[159] Daytime drowsiness may be a side

effect of medication; however, it can also be exacerbated after therapeutic exercise, so a cool-down period is necessary before the patient sits down and relaxes.

Another side effect of medication is the presence of hallucinations. Many patients report seeing very ugly creatures or monsters, and when such hallucinations occur in the therapeutic session, they can be most uncomfortable for the therapist and the patient. These hallucinations also make it difficult for the patient to use adjunct treatments such as computer games and virtual reality activities. These and other nonmotor symptoms often predominate as the disease progresses,[156] contributing to severe disability, impaired quality of life, and shortened life expectancy.

Stages of Parkinson Disease

Staging of Parkinson disease uses the Hoehn and Yahr scale (Table 18.1).[160] Originally developed as a 5-point scale, in recent years 0, 1.5, and 2.5 measurements have been added. The 1.5 and 2.5 ratings have not been validated, but because their use is so common, the latest recommendation is to continue using them while the validity is studied.[161]

In stage 1 of the disease, initial motor symptoms, often a resting tremor or unilateral micrography (bradykinesia of the upper extremity), is present. Stage 2 progresses with rigidity and bradykinesia bilaterally, and postural alterations and axial symptoms begin to occur. This commonly starts with an increase in neck, trunk, and hip flexion that, accompanied by a decrease in righting and balance responses, leads to a decreased ability to maintain the center of gravity over the base of support.

While these postural changes are occurring moving into stage 3, so does an increase in rigidity, which is most apparent in the trunk and

TABLE 18.1 Hoehn and Yahr Staging Scale for Parkinson Disease

Stage	Progression of Symptoms
0	No signs of disease.
1	Unilateral symptoms only.
1.5	Unilateral and axial involvement.
2	Bilateral symptoms. No impairment of balance.
2.5	Mild bilateral disease with recovery on pull test.
3	Balance impairment. Mild to moderate disease. Physically independent.
4	Severe disability, but still able to walk or stand unassisted.
5	Needing a wheelchair or bedridden unless assisted.

The Hoehn and Yahr scale is commonly used to describe how the symptoms of Parkinson disease progress. The original scale included stages 1 through 5.[162] Stage 0 has since been added, and stages 1.5 and 2.5 have been proposed to best indicate the relative level of disability in this population.[163]

proximal and axial musculature. Trunk rotation becomes severely decreased; there is no arm swing during gait and no spontaneous facial expression; and movement becomes more and more difficult to initiate. Movement is usually produced with great concentration and is perhaps cortically generated, thereby bypassing the damaged basal nuclei pathways. This great concentration then makes movement tiring, which heightens the debilitating effects of the disease, requiring assistive devices to ambulate in stage 4.

Eventually the individual becomes wheelchair bound and dependent. In the late and severe stages of the disease, especially without therapeutic attention for movement dysfunctions, the patient may become bedridden and may demonstrate a fixed trunk-flexion contracture regardless of the position in which the person is placed. This posture has been called the "phantom pillow" syndrome because, even when lying supine, the person's head is flexed as if on a pillow.

Throughout this progressive deterioration of movement, there is also a decrease in higher-level sensory processing. In addition, the patient can perform only one task at a time. Reports of dementia range from 30% to 93% in patients with Parkinson disease.[164] The presence of dementia in this population may indicate involvement of the ACh or noradrenergic mesolimbic system. In this case, treatment with anticholinergic drugs may increase a tendency toward dementia, especially in older patients. Sometimes, cognitive deficits are inferred because of slowed responses, spatial problems, sensory processing problems, and a masked face.

The most serious complication of Parkinson disease is bronchopneumonia. Decreased activity in general and decreased chest expansion may be contributing factors. Aspiration pneumonia can also contribute to mortality because patients may experience dysphagia and dysarthria. The mortality rate is greater than in the general population, and death is usually from pneumonia.

Pharmacological Considerations and Medical Management

The knowledge that the symptoms of Parkinson disease are caused by a decrease in DA led to the pharmacological management of this disease. Because DA itself does not cross the blood-brain barrier, levodihydroxyphenylalanine (L-dopa), a precursor of DA that does, has been used to treat Parkinson disease since the late 1960s.[162,165–166] An inhibitor of aromatic amino acid decarboxylation (carbidopa) is usually

given with L-dopa to prevent the conversion to DA before entering the brain. The decarboxylase inhibitor allows a reduction in dosage of L-dopa itself, which helps decrease the cardiac and gastrointestinal side effects of DA.

Amantadine is another drug that has been effective in the treatment of patients with Parkinson disease. Although the mechanism of action of this antiviral medication is unknown, it is thought to include a facilitation of release of catecholamines (of which DA is one) from stores in the neuron that are readily releasable. It is often administered in combination with L-dopa.

Treatment of Parkinson disease with L-dopa in these various combinations is extremely helpful in reducing bradykinesia and rigidity. It is less effective in reducing tremor and the postural instability. Because Parkinson disease involves the nigral neurons, the receptors and the neurons in the striatum (which are postsynaptic to dopaminergic neurons) remain intact and, initially, are somewhat responsive to DA.[163,167] With time, however, the receptors appear to lose their sensitivity, and the prolonged effectiveness (10 years or more) of L-dopa therapy is questionable.[168–170] A further complication of L-dopa therapy is the development of involuntary movements (dyskinesias) and the "on-off" phenomenon—a short-duration response resulting in sudden improvement of symptoms followed by a rapid decline in symptomatic relief and perhaps the appearance of dyskinesias and/or dystonias.[171,172] With time the "on" effect becomes of shorter and shorter duration.[168,171,173,174] Controlled-release or slow-release L-dopa may decrease these side effects. The effectiveness of L-dopa does not appear to be closely correlated with the stage of the disease.

The use of L-dopa alone or in combination with carbidopa has not provided a cure or even prevented the degeneration of Parkinson disease.[173,174] As more has become known about the DA receptor, specific agonists have been developed. Ropinirole, pramipexole, pergolide, and bromocriptine are examples of DA receptor D2 agonists that are used alone or with L-dopa. The agonists are thought to decrease the wearing-off effects as well as decrease the dyskinesias that occur with long-term L-dopa use, but L-dopa remains the most effective medication. It is quite likely that newer D2 and/or D2-D1 (DA receptor D1) agonists will be developed. Pharmacological interventions also include drugs that prevent the breakdown of DA (e.g., catechol-O-methyltransferase [COMT] inhibitors) and/or its reuptake. Entacapone is an example of a COMT inhibitor.[175]

Another approach to pharmacological treatment of individuals with Parkinson disease was developed from research on a designer drug that contained the neurotoxin 1-methyl-4-phenyl-1,2,3,6-tetrahydropyridine (MPTP). It was found that the conversion of MPTP to the active neurotoxin MPP+ could be prevented by monoamine oxidase inhibitors such as deprenyl and pargyline.[71,173] Deprenyl, rasagiline, and selegiline are now used before the initiation of, or in conjunction with, L-dopa and carbidopa.

Another treatment alternative is surgery performed in precise areas of the basal nuclei, known as *stereotaxic surgery*. Stereotaxic surgery is an old technique that has made a comeback based on the new knowledge of basal nuclei connectivity and improvements in the procedural instrumentation. Initially, one of the structures of the basal nuclei was lesioned with freezing or high-frequency stimulation. Today, the globus pallidus internal segment or the subthalamic nucleus is stimulated with implanted electrodes. This technique is known as *DBS*. DBS has now been approved by the US Food and Drug Administration (FDA). An advantage of DBS over permanent lesions is that DBS is reversible and is safer for bilateral surgeries. Stimulation of the globus pallidus internal segment or subthalamic nucleus has been shown to decrease all symptoms; subthalamic nucleus stimulation is also effective in reducing dyskinesias and may lessen the amount of medication taken.[176–178] Effects of stimulation are greater for symptoms manifested in the "off" state. DBS has been demonstrated to improve rigidity, bradykinesia, and akinesia, as well as gait[59,178–182] and balance.[58,183] It has also been demonstrated to improve movement velocity and speed of muscle recruitment for activity.[181,183] The proposed mechanism of action is interference with the abnormal neuronal firing.[184,185] In a randomized, controlled clinical trial, DBS was more effective in reducing symptoms and increasing quality of life than medication.[186,187] This group also found that although some side effects were worse (e.g., brain hemorrhage), the total number of adverse reactions was greater in the medication group. Whether stimulation of the subthalamic nucleus is neuroprotective, that is, prevents further degeneration, is presently under investigation. Thalamic stimulation is used for decreasing tremor. Therapists may find that intense treatment immediately after these surgeries may be able to take advantage of neural plasticity.

Fetal transplantation of the substantia nigra to the caudate nucleus remains under investigation. A double-blind, placebo-controlled trial was completed with mixed results.[184,188–190] Studies continue, including those of dose, cell type, and placement of cells. Recently, however, there was a report of Lewy-body inclusions in grafted cells 14 years after the transplant.[191] The authors concluded that Parkinson disease was an ongoing process and that what caused the disease initially also affected the grafted cells.

Examination of the Patient With Parkinson Disease

Examination of an individual with Parkinson disease should assess impairments and functional activities and draw correlations of impact on participation in the individual's life. Additionally, information regarding quality of life and the patient's perception of their function and disease is extremely valuable. The use of objective outcome measures for the different International Classification of Functioning Disability and Health (ICF) domains is strongly recommended, with population specific cut-offs that correlate with function and predictors of future events (i.e., falls). It is essential to perform outcome measure testing at initial exam, with re-assessment at regular intervals to assess changes, modify interventions as appropriate, and allow for open, updated communication with patients, family, and physicians.

When assessing the overall clinical presentation of a person with Parkinson disease, the Hoehn and Yahr scale (see Table 18.1) is the most commonly and widely used to describe the severity of the disease. It is based on clinical features and functional disability, assigning a numerical value of dysfunction as it relates to unilateral or bilateral involvement, and whether postural stability is compromised.[160,161] Progression through the Hoehn and Yahr scale has prognostic implications—stage 3 has been correlated with increasing physical and cognitive impairment scores despite medication adjustments and therefore a marked deterioration in quality of life;[161] however, it should be understood that this tool is not linear and does not include nonmotor functions. Because the scale provides an overall assessment of impairment and disability combined, clinicians should use it to create a general clinical picture of their patient and, as such, help guide their interventions and decision making.

The Movement Disorder Society Sponsored-Unified Parkinson's Disease Rating Scale (MDS-UPDRS) is the most widely used clinical rating scale for Parkinson disease. The scale assesses both nonmotor and motor symptoms associated with the disease, including nonmotor experiences, motor experiences of daily living, motor examination, and motor complications.[188,189,191,192] The tool gathers information from the clinician's exam, as well as from patient/caregiver response. It is sensitive in terms of detecting change in function and disability as the disease progresses (especially in the earlier stages of the disease), while having a high correlative value with the Hoehn and Yahr scale.[161,193] Another clinical scale is the Core Assessment Program for

Surgical Interventional Therapies in Parkinson's Disease (CAPSIT-PD), which includes timed tests for motor evaluation and neuropsychological testing.[194–196] This scale was designed to provide minimal requirements and standardize assessments for those undergoing surgical intervention, and is used during the evaluation and consideration of a patient being considered for DBS surgery. Knowledge of these scales will help the therapist communicate with other health care professionals.

When completing an examination of a patient with Parkinson disease, subjective and quality of life questionnaires, in combination with functional activities assessment, will provide the most valuable information to guide treatment planning and goal setting. The Parkinson's Disease Questionnaire (PDQ)-39 is a self-reported questionnaire that assesses how the disease impacts function and well-being. It is the most frequently used measure to assess health status in people with Parkinson disease and is recommended for all stages of the disease.[197] The abbreviated PDQ-8 takes one item from each of the eight dimensions of the PDQ-39. Both the PDQ-39 and PDQ-8 are valid and reliable instruments to assess disease and health-related changes.[197] Construct-specific subjective measures are also strongly recommended, including the Freezing of Gait questionnaire and Parkinson's Fatigue Scale.

Five core areas should be assessed: physical capacity, transfers, manual activities, balance, and gait. In addition, a clinician should also assess respiratory function and pain.[198] In the clinical setting, the exam should focus on impairments and functional activities. Highly recommended measures in the Body Structure and Function domain include MDS-UPDRS part 1 and the Montreal Cognitive Assessment (MOCA), while those in the Activity Limitation domain include 6-minute Walk Test, 10 m walk, mini-BESTest, Functional Gait Assessment (FGA), MDS-UPDRS part 2, five times sit-to-stand, and 9 Hole Peg Test. An integral component of the exam is a complete and thorough movement analysis during the tasks to generate links between impairments and activity limitation. Additionally, the time it takes to complete an activity must be measured. It is also valuable to address the effects of adding interfering stimuli (motor and cognitive) and complexity to a task to determine at which point a patient may begin having difficulties.[142,143]

Throughout all stages of the disease, a careful and comprehensive analysis of balance is imperative because a patient with Parkinson disease has a two to four times higher risk of hip fractures caused by falls compared to individuals without the disease.[199,200] The Activities-Specific Balance Confidence Scale (ABC) is highly recommended owing to its excellent reliability and validity in this population.[201,202] The ABC Scale, along with previous fall history and UPDRS motor score, were the most significant predictor of future falls.[203] It has become more evident that balance impairments and increased fall risk are present even in the early stages of the disease; decreased confidence in self-perceived balance is a known contributor for future fall risk.[204,205] Assessing challenges to balance such as tandem walking or standing on a compliant surface is important because this may be the first sign of balance impairment. Posturography is the most sensitive measure of postural instability, especially in the early stages of the disease (Hoehn and Yahr stages 1 and 2).[60] A clinically useful tool to assess dynamic balance is the functional reach test, which has been shown to be an effective, predictive tool in people with Parkinson disease as it is in the elderly, while the functional axial rotation (FAR) test has been shown to detect functional limitations in the early stages of the disease.[206,207] Evaluation of pain in an individual with Parkinson disease is important because this can have a detrimental effect on function and quality of life, although it is frequently underrecognized and often inadequately treated. While pain may come from different origins, pain of musculoskeletal origin is the most prevalent in people with Parkinson disease.[208,209] It is widely known that chronic pain can develop from, and lend itself to, avoidance of activities based on the fear of pain.[210] This further exacerbates decreased participation in functional activities and, ultimately, progression of disease-related symptoms.

An assessment of chest expansion and vital capacity should also be included because of their contribution to the complication of pneumonia. For this reason, when rigidity is assessed, the muscles of respiration, extremity, and trunk movement should be included. Active and passive range of movement, general strength, chest expansion, and vital capacity should also be measured on regular intervals. Clinicians should also be aware of swallow function, sleep-disordered breathing, and cough mechanism because these can also contribute to respiratory limitations.[211] Early recognition of contributors to respiratory limitations are imperative for timely interventions and, ultimately, improving quality of life and mortality. At present, a complete and easy-to-use form for evaluation does not exist for Parkinson disease.

General Prognosis, Treatment Principles, and Rationale

As with all treatment, the prognosis (functional goals, personal factors, and established time parameters) is based on the general goals related to the findings from the examination of each patient, the patient's expectations, and functional requirements. Parkinson disease must be understood as a degenerative disease when establishing the prognosis and treatment plan, initially emphasizing a recovery model of care, then evolving to a maintenance/compensatory approach. In general, goals include increasing movement and range of motion (ROM) in the entire trunk and extremities, improving endurance, chest expansion with emphasis on posture, balance reactions, and restoring or maintaining functional abilities. Increased movement may in fact modify the progression of the disease.[212,213] Nonpharmacological and nonsurgical interventions, especially physical therapy treatment, are essential at the beginning of the disease owing to potential complications associated with chronic medication use and surgical procedures.[214] Although levodopa decreases the bradykinesia, it alone will not be effective in increasing movement or improving balance; therefore aggressive intervention in the early stages is necessary.

Overall, physical rehabilitation is effective in the treatment of people with Parkinson disease and the results are greater when treatment is started early in the disease process. Although treatment initiated while the disease is still unilateral (Hoehn and Yahr stage 1) is more advantageous, it has been shown to be effective in Hoehn and Yahr stages 1 to 3.[215,216] The American Academy of Neurology recommends physical therapy in its practice parameters.[217] Animal studies have shown that exercise can induce neuroprotective and neurorepair changes in the brain. Neuroprotective changes can slow the disease progression by increasing DA generation and availability, while neurorepair changes slow motor deterioration and disability by improving the efficiency of available DA.[218–220] In the later stages of the disease, adaptive and compensatory approaches are utilized with increased reliance on undamaged systems, although increased angiogenesis and decreased brain damage marker expression in the striatum occur in response to exercise in animal studies.[221] In the clinical setting, therapists tend to see patients after motor symptoms appear, and thus patients are already in the neurorepair or adaptation window of the disease.

Basic principles for treatment of the person with Parkinson disease will depend on the areas of impairment and functional limitations revealed in the evaluation. Certain principles, however, are true for all stages of the disease. Interventions should incorporate neuroplasticity parameters addressing intensity, repetition, specificity, difficulty, and complexity of practice. Interventions should integrate goal-based activities for skill acquisition while also requiring cognitive engagement, which is essential for learning to occur.[222] Owing to diminished automatic movements from the loss of DA in the basal nuclei, increased

cognitive control and attentional strategies are indicated. Asking the patient to generate goals and activities of their interest encourages patient investment and consistency, while a collaborative clinician-patient relationship helps improves compliance. Patients should engage in moderate to vigorous intensity-based training because higher-intensity training has been shown to induce DA D2 receptor-binding potential; this pathway has been implicated in increasing inhibitory drive, leading to motor impairments caused by decreased DA.[223] Interventions should also address balance and an emphasis on increasing amplitude of movement because the DA-depleted state results in slower and smaller movements. Treatment should also involve strengthening, gait training, incorporating transitional movements (changes in directions and turns), and dual-tasking activities.

Variety is important to facilitate shifts in movement as well as in thought. To date, many rehabilitative techniques and exercises have demonstrated improvement in function for people with Parkinson disease, and numerous randomized clinical trials have proven the efficacy of the varied techniques. Programs that emphasize sensory-motor integration, agility, and motor learning demonstrate decreased progression of disease and improved motor function.[224–240] Programs that involve dual motor-cognitive tasks, complex sequences of movements, and force the participant to quickly change movements dependent on environmental conditions have resulted in improved performance on the Timed Up-and-Go Test, the UPDRS, the 10 m walk test, and a variety of balance tests. The words *big, fun,* and *novel* are good words to remember when planning treatment.

Although a majority of evidence supports interventions in the earlier stages of the disease (Hoehn and Yahr stages 1 to 3) and there is evidence of some disease modification in the later stages, as the disease progresses, goals may shift to more task-specific activities, assessment and training for assistive devices, addressing posture and positioning for respiratory and pain management, and caregiver training. Task-specific activities often include turning in bed, getting in/out of bed, rising from a chair, dressing, grooming and hygiene activities, and being aware of posture. At the later stages of the disease, breathing exercises and positioning will need to be a more prominent aspect of treatment. Throughout the course of the disease, large amplitude movements during all activities should be emphasized. Frequent conversations with the patient and caregivers regarding expectations, concerns, and caregiver training should also be ongoing throughout the provider's care.

Therapeutic programs and approaches. As previously stated, exercise itself is important for the person with Parkinson disease. There is a relationship between longevity and physical activity, with those who exercise having lower mortality rates.[241] A link has been demonstrated between a lack of exercise and development of Parkinsonian symptoms. Some evidence also indicates that exercise may alter the magnitude of free radicals and other compounds linked to aging and Parkinsonism. Given the evidence that physical activity can induce disease-modifying changes, especially in the earlier stages of the disease, it is strongly recommended to establish a consistent exercise routine as early as possible in the disease process.[225,242]

Individuals with Parkinson disease are strongly encouraged to achieve the World Health Organization's recommendations for physical activity. Intensity has been shown to be necessary for beneficial effects, so patients are encouraged to perform 3 days of moderate intensity activity and 2 days of vigorous intensity exercise per week, as well as at least 3 days of balance training and 2 days of muscle-strengthening exercises. For individuals who may be at a lower activity level, shorter bouts of exercise of at least 10 minutes should be encouraged to reach the recommended dosage. Clinicians are encouraged to gradually increase intensity when first introducing higher effort exercises with use of percentage of maximum heart rate and/or perceived exertion.[234,243]

Movement throughout a full ROM is crucial, especially early in the disease process, to prevent changes in the properties of muscle itself. Rigidity of some degree is present in up to 99% of people with Parkinson disease, with the contractile elements of flexors becoming shortened and extensors becoming lengthened, enhancing the development of the flexed posture that is traditionally present.[225] Rigidity can be the cause of, and further contribute to, the pain the patient may experience. For most patients, treatment proceeds better if rigidity is decreased early in the treatment session. Many relaxation techniques appear to be effective in reducing rigidity, including gentle, slow rocking, rotation of the extremities and trunk, and the use of yoga. Yoga is also beneficial to target spinal extensor strength and flexibility. Furthermore, because the proximal muscles are often more involved than the distal muscles, relaxation may be easier to achieve by following a distal-to-proximal progression. The inverted position may be used with care. Initially, this position facilitates some relaxation (increase in parasympathetic tone) and then increases trunk extension, which is important for the Parkinsonian patient. Once a decrease in rigidity has been achieved, movement must be initiated to use the newfound range in a functional way.

Implementation of aerobic exercise is essential in the management of a patient with Parkinson disease. The role of aerobic fitness itself may be a factor in reducing dysfunction, with studies showing that it may be necessary to promote neuroplasticity to help restore automatic movement.[244] Animal studies indicate that functional exercise decreased DA loss after a variety of lesion models.[125,215,216] As stated before, clinicians should emphasize increased intensity into their interventions to gain the aforementioned benefits. Animal research indicates that exercise and forced functional movements may protect the dopaminergic neurons, with earlier intervention having greater beneficial effects on the dopaminergic system.[215,216] Alberts and colleagues performed a classic study investigating the use of tandem bicycling, during which a person with Parkinson disease was required to pedal at a higher rate and intensity than their preferred rate. They found this forced exercise led to increased connectivity between cortico-subcortical regions that underlie automaticity on fMRI, and the pattern of activation was similar in patients who were on medication and those following forced exercise while off medication. Furthermore, a study investigating the effects of high-intensity, moderate-intensity, and a no exercise control group demonstrated that the high-intensity exercise group had significantly lower reductions in mobility scores at 6 months follow-up compared to the control group, while the moderate group did not experience a significant change.[245] High-intensity interval training is often utilized to help patients achieve the intensity and time necessary for neuroplastic changes to occur.

Aerobic exercise may also improve pulmonary function in patients with Parkinson disease because these functions appear to suffer from deficiencies in rapid force generation of the respiratory muscles, similar to limb musculature.[246] If patients practice regular physical exercise in conjunction with disease-specific exercises, the ill effects of inactivity will not potentiate the effects of the disease process itself. Although most patients with Parkinson disease can achieve an adequate exercise level, many patients have low fitness levels before the medical diagnosis.[120] Exercise, even once a week, can be effective in improving gait and balance in patients with Parkinson disease when practiced over several months.[198,220] Given these benefits, as well as known benefits of general aerobic exercise on brain and cardiopulmonary health, it is concluded that regular aerobic exercise is the single strategy with compelling evidence for slowing Parkinson disease progression.[247] Programs emphasizing sensory awareness of the size of movement have shown improvement in both speed of limb movement and gait parameters.[226,227,229] In Parkinson disease, for any given amplitude of movement, velocity of movement is reduced, with velocity decreasing as the amplitude of movement gets larger. Cues for large amplitude movements result in bigger and faster movements as opposed to cues for speed.[229] There are various programs that employ sensory awareness for amplitude of movement, such as PD SAFEx, LSVT BIG, and Parkinson's Wellness Recovery (PWR!). Sensory awareness programs have evolved to incorporate movements that specifically address the primary Parkinson disease movement deficits while integrating balance, coordination, and automaticity. Furthermore, patients are encouraged to perform these movements in different postures to challenge the body in functional positions. These programs have been shown to improve gait and function on the UPDRS.[227] These authors concluded that programs emphasizing increased sensory feedback and awareness, with emphasis on amplitude and effort, are the best behavioral strategy to decrease hypokinesia and bradykinesia while improving the function of people with Parkinson disease.

Treadmill training has been used in Parkinson disease exercise programs, with strong recommendations of its use to improve walking speed and stride length, improve balance, reduce fear of fall, and number of falls.[240,248,232] In addition to forward walking, multidirectional treadmill training (backward, left, and right sidestepping) at the patient's fastest tolerated speed in each direction improved spatiotemporal gait measures in all walking directions, balance performance, and gait kinematics.[249] The use of the treadmill with body-weight support increases safety and allows the therapist to control speed of movement, introduce perturbations, and challenge multidirectional walking. Studies have shown that cued treadmill training, such as visual cues to target stride length or auditory cues for gait speed, exhibits good results and carryover to the home.[250–251] Cognitive tasks and other dual tasks have also been added during treadmill training with good results.

Rhythmical exercise has been shown to decrease rigidity and bradykinesia and improve gait over time.[224,243,252–271] Ballroom dancing is a form of rhythmical therapy for patients with Parkinson disease that incorporates rotation, large amplitude and multidirectional movements, weight shifting and turning, speed variation, and coordination.[224,272] Given that dance requires high-level multitasking and progressive learning, it is both cognitively and physically challenging; the socialization aspect can help improve mood and adherence. While tango has been the mostly widely researched form of dance, other forms have also shown to have benefit. A program of tango versus waltz and foxtrot indicated that both groups improved on the UPDRS motor scale, Berg Balance Scale, 6 minute walk distance, and backward stride length, although the tango group had greater improvements.[227,236,239] The waltz and foxtrot, which are easier dances, may be beneficial for those at more advanced stages of the disease. Latin dance and other weight-bearing exercises demonstrated similar improvements in balance and especially initiation of gait.[224,259,271,273] Dance therapy also has beneficial effects on cognitive tasks, with improvements seen on the Brooks Spatial Test and Trail-Making Parts A and B.[274] Similar effects were seen in tai chi as a form of rhythmical therapy, which demands attention to movement and increases challenges to balance and control of movement. Tai chi has been shown to be effective in improving gait and balance parameters, as well as nonmotor function such as mood and overall quality of life.[233,275] There is growing evidence for the use of technologies in Parkinson disease rehabilitation. Virtual and augmented reality can be used to optimize motor learning in a safe environment, stimulating motor and cognitive processes while providing augmented feedback about performance and address repetition and task specificity. Although there is currently limited high-quality evidence, virtual reality interventions have greater effects on step and stride length compared to conventional therapy, and similar gains in balance, ADL function, Quality of Life (QOL), and cognitive function compared to conventional therapy.[276] Mirelman and colleagues demonstrated that an intensive treadmill program incorporating virtual reality obstacle negotiation significantly improved fall risk and fall rates 6 months after training compared to treadmill training without virtual reality.[277] For some with Parkinson disease, even in the early stages, games are too fast or too confusing; therefore the use of disease-specific exercise programs may be superior to commercial systems and could be used and enjoyed by those with Parkinson disease.[278] There is also growing research into biofeedback, in which a somatosensory cue is provided in real time to improve balance and weight shifting to minimize freezing of gait. Despite the limited research and evidence, technological advances and its use in rehabilitation for Parkinson disease is promising.

Physical activity and movement can increase quality of life by decreasing depression and improving mood and initiative.[258,279] Group classes can serve as an extra support system for patients with Parkinson disease and their spouses, providing both extrinsic and intrinsic motivation. Exercise programs should be designed to meet, and progress, a patient's current functional level. A carefully structured low-impact aerobics program appears to be beneficial to patients even with long-standing disease.[271] For example, individuals in Hoehn and Yahr stage 2.5 or 3 can begin with seated activities with upper-extremity exercises (Fig. 18.8A) and combination movements (see Fig. 18.8B) then progress to standing and marching activities that incorporate coordinated movements of arms and legs, balance, and trunk rotation (Fig. 18.9). All movements are performed to music similar to that used in aerobics classes in any gym or health club (Fig. 18.10). A cool-down period allows participants to practice fine motor coordination activities of the hands (Fig. 18.11). Many Parkinson disease associations also have audiotapes for exercises (e.g., United Parkinson Foundation).

Most studies have found that exercise under the guidance of a physical or occupational therapist or trained instructor is effective in reducing Parkinsonian symptoms.[226,240,268,269] There is long-standing evidence of the benefits of exercise, with improvements in gross and fine motor functions, as well as of general well-being[270]; however, it is necessary for continued, consistent participation for long-term carryover. The most successful exercise programs appear to be those that incorporate context-dependent responses and a varied environment (Box 18.1), although noncontext-dependent aerobic exercises are also effective (Box 18.2). Research has shown the importance of adjusting the response to the specific task and has also demonstrated the importance of practice for the Parkinsonian patient.[280,281] The principles of motor learning are of paramount importance in the treatment

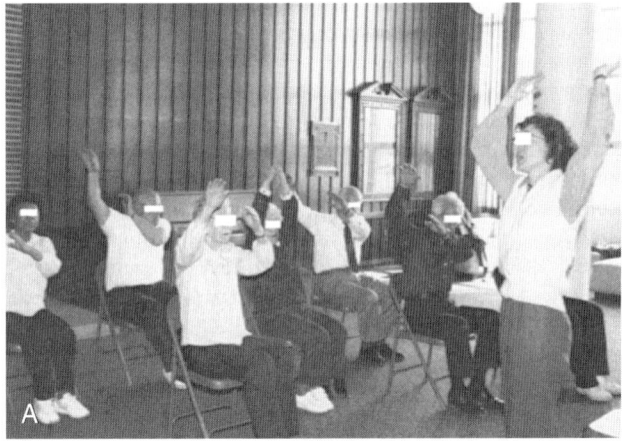

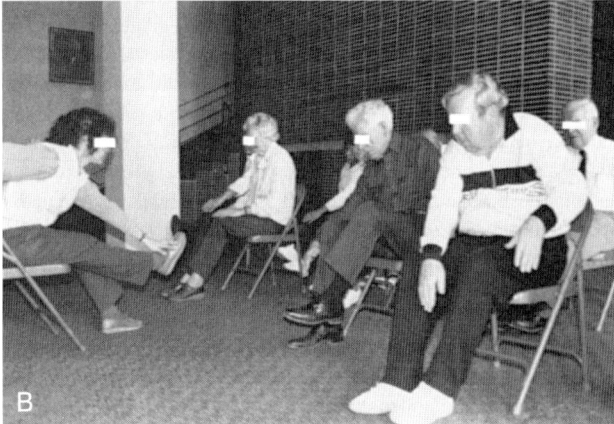

Fig. 18.8 Seated Aerobics or Warmup Exercises. **(A)** Patients are using bilateral upper-extremity patterns to facilitate trunk rotation. Instruction was to let the head follow the hands. **(B)** This exercise encourages trunk rotation, large movements, and coordination of the upper and lower extremities. Patients are to reach with the arms and touch the opposite foot. This coordination is difficult for those with Parkinson disease, and many patients initially could not move their arms and legs at the same time.

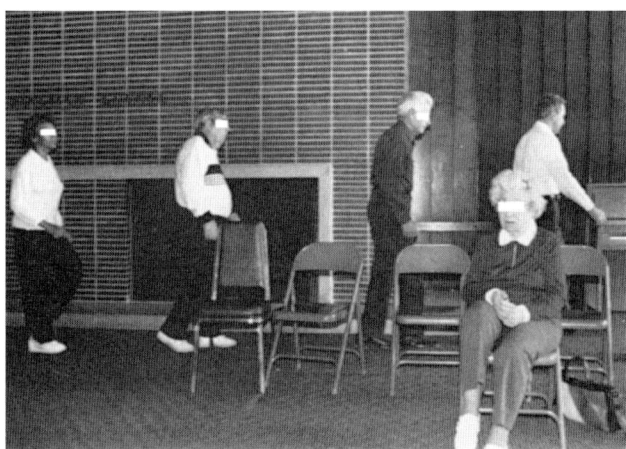

Fig. 18.9 Initial Warmup in Standing. Patients are to walk with their head up, with the back as straight as possible, and to take large steps. When the group began, walking was the major aerobic activity and was used to increase endurance and encourage movement. Nonambulatory patients march in place while seated.

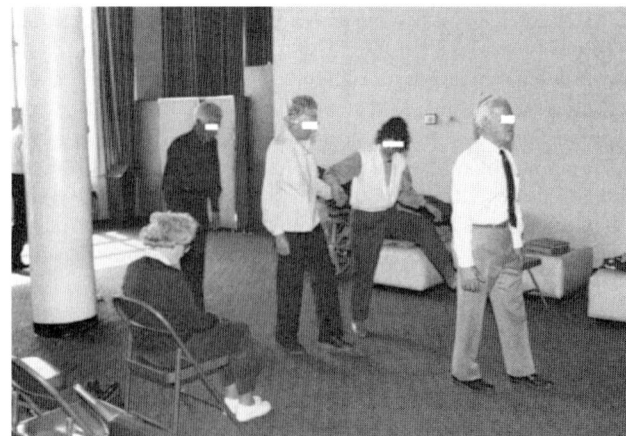

Fig. 18.10 Walking in a "Waltz Rhythm" (Slow, Quick, Quick) Emphasizes a Big Step for the Slow Step. Note lack of automatic arm swing. Also, note flexed posture of seated patient during rest period.

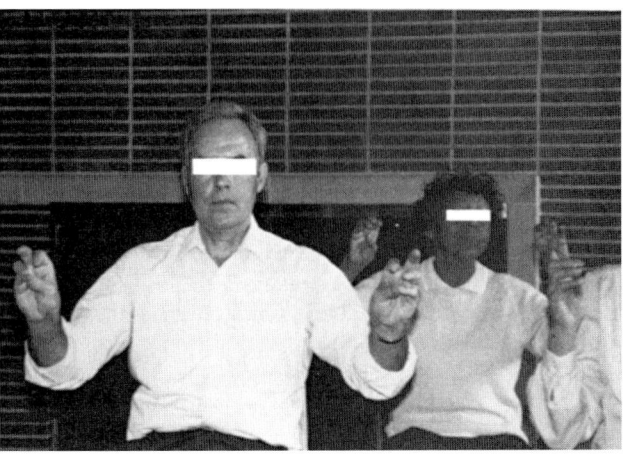

Fig. 18.11 Cool-Down Period Allows Time to Work on Fine Finger Movements. Thumb abduction with rounded fingers and various rhythms are used to increase coordination. Note "masked face" appearance.

BOX 18.1 Exercises That Promote Context-Dependent Responses

The following exercises promote context-dependent responses and are recommended for people with movement disorders:
1. Walking outdoors
2. Karate and other martial arts (Tai Chi and Qi-Gong specifically)
3. Dancing (all forms), particularly to music
4. Ball sports (various types)
5. Cross-country and downhill skiing
6. Well-structured, low-impact aerobics classes
7. Treadmill training with guidance of a movement specialist
   This list is a sample of activities; it should not be considered all inclusive.

Hackney ME, Lee HL, Battisto J, et al. Context-dependent neural activation: internally and externally guided rhythmic lower limb movement in individuals with and without neurodegenerative disease. *Front Neurol.* 2015;6:251.

BOX 18.2 Exercises That Promote Fitness and Increase Range of Motion But Not Context-Dependent Responses

The following exercises promote fitness and increase range of motion but not context-dependent responses and are recommended for people with movement disorders.
1. Treadmill walking without guidance or supervision
2. Stationary bicycle riding
3. Using strengthening machines and free weights (with low weights or low resistance)
4. Using step exercises and stair climbers
5. Using rowing machines
6. Swimming laps
   This list is a sample of activities; it should not be considered all inclusive.

program of these patients. Random practice may enable the patient to learn the correct schema by which to regulate the extent, speed, and direction of the movement and may also be important in facilitating the ability of the patient to shift attention and to learn to access "working memory." The Parkinsonian patient may benefit from visual instruction and mental rehearsal before performing the movement.[135,152]

In addition, the instructions used need to be pertinent to the task at hand.

Strengthening. Strengthening exercises have been promoted for patients with Parkinson disease because disuse contributes to decreased strength. Weakness occurs with initial and prolonged contraction. Deceased leg strength is associated with increased fall risk and gait velocity, and hip strength is specifically related to sit-to-stand performance in people with Parkinson disease.[282] Manual muscle testing may not reveal losses in strength; however, most successful exercise programs include functional strength training as part of the program. High-resistance eccentric exercises can produce muscle hypertrophy and may affect improvements in mobility.[283]

Functional strength training seems to be more effective than weightlifting for the goal of ADL improvement owing to task specificity.[154] An important part of any strengthening program is the trunk musculature. As extensors become weaker compared to flexors, spinal and hip extensors need to be strengthened, and flexibility likewise encouraged.[284] When implementing progressive strength training, the clinician should train effort. Large amplitude, high-velocity movements at mid-range to low resistance should be performed because bradykinesia contributes to reduced power generation at lighter loads, but not heavy loads.[285]

Use of cues for improving gait. As the disease progresses, intensive exercise programs may need to be revised or altered. By Hoehn and Yahr stage 2.5, gait disorders are the most common diagnosis for which the person with Parkinson disease will see a therapist. Owing to reduced internal control for timing and scaling of automatic and repetitive movements, external cues and attentional strategies are needed to compensate. Visual cues can be used for spatial awareness to increase amplitude of movement, while auditory or tactile cues can be utilized to improve timing and generate rhythm. As the disease progresses and attentional and executive functions become more impaired, external cues can be used to guide attention to the task.[234] The problems that cause the biggest ambulation limitation are freezing and small steps. Studies have demonstrated that the use of rhythmical exercise programs, a metronome, or carefully synthesized music improved gait characteristics, such as stride length and speed, with immediate and longer-lasting improvements.[271,286] A study by Nieuwboer and colleagues[251] used auditory, visual, or somatosensory cues during gait in the patient's home per patient preference. The cues were provided in a variety of conditions, including dual tasking, over uneven surfaces, and multidirectional walking. Cues were effective in improving step length, gait speed, and decreasing freezing, but no carryover effects were observed at 6 weeks. The frequency of cueing is patient specific and will be activity and context specific (i.e., cuing indoors may be slower than outdoors); however, in patients who experience freezing, auditory cueing frequencies should be below the patient's baseline frequency because higher may trigger freezing.[287] Furthermore, cueing may be more effective for those who do not have frequent freezing episodes owing to the disordered movement rhythmicity seen in freezers.[287]

Visual stimuli has been shown to be effective in initiating movement during freezing episodes in context-specific situations. These include the use of lines on the floor and stair climbing because stairs can provide visual stimulation. Martin[57] found that parallel lines were more facilitating than other lines, with the space between lines being important. There is also increasing use of visual cues incorporated into assistive devices, such as a Laser Cane or U-Step walker;[288] however, the use of visual stimuli has limited evidence of carryover. Morris and colleagues[144] have tried to increase carryover of visual stimuli by incorporating them with a visualization program. Patients practiced walking with lines until the steps were near normal in size, then progressed to visualizing the lines on the floor as they walked; their visualization program met with initial success. Increasing the magnitude of the step, weight shifting before stepping, or the amplitude of the movement appears to be the most important component for improvement in gait and a decrease in freezing, and can be accomplished using either cueing strategies, attentional strategies, or a combination of both.[144]

Gait rehabilitation must include walking in crowds, through doorways, and on different surfaces. Speed variations are important, as is walking with differing stride lengths, owing to varying context-dependent environmental demands. The principles of motor learning appear to be very helpful for facilitating carryover of the therapeutic effects; however, the individual with Parkinson disease can have difficulty dual tasking and may have to initially concentrate only on walking as the disease progresses to increase patient safety.[111,124,151]

Balance. Another problem for which therapy is indicated is impaired balance, especially because drug and surgical treatments are ineffective in remediating this problem. This problem will eventually affect all persons with Parkinson disease.[289] Fall risk earlier in the disease can be caused by proprioceptive impairments, increased trunk rigidity, and medication side effects, whereas fall risk later in the disease can be associated with increased sedentary behavior and immobility.[290] The patient should be instructed to practice balance exercises at the early stages of the disease. Equilibrium reactions in all planes of movement and under different conditions should be addressed. Techniques to increase dynamic balance control should be included, especially turning the body and turning the head. All three balance strategies need to be addressed and then practiced in a variety of environmental conditions. Postural instability is higher in freezers than nonfreezers, with more fear-of-falling avoidance behavior; people who improved balance also improved freezing of gait most.[291] The newer computerized games that target balance have provided a fun and therapeutic method for keeping interest in balance exercises.[124,133,134,139,140]

Dual task performance. Rarely will the patient with Parkinson disease state that he or she has difficulty performing two tasks at once; however, as dual tasking involves executive functioning, a patient with Parkinson disease will demonstrate mistakes with both mental and motor tasks when performed concurrently. This becomes quite apparent in very simple activities, such as requiring the patient to count backward and walk at the same time.[143,292] This impaired ability to perform dual tasking is associated with increased loss of balance and freezing of gait because people with Parkinson disease tend to prioritize a cognitive task at the cost of balance and posture.[293] One solution is to instruct the patient to attend to only one task at a time, while another is to have the patient practice doing two things at the same time and constantly alter activities in a random practice mode during treatment; both consecutive and integrated dual task training led to similar and sustained improvements in gait velocity without increasing fall risk.[294]

Activities of daily living. Transitional movements pose great problems for the patient, especially by Hoehn and Yahr stage 3. This is most likely because normal postural adjustments are no longer automatic and become a sequential task. Task specificity with repetition is helpful, and visualization of the task has demonstrated carryover. Some researchers report improvement in moving from a seated to a standing position after practicing techniques designed to increase forward weight shift.[295,296] Compensatory strategies to alter the environment may become necessary if the task becomes too difficult.

Bed mobility is an important consideration for patients with Parkinson disease. Rolling in bed and rising from the supine position become difficult and should be practiced; emphasis should be placed on appropriate technique, with cues for amplitude and effort during the transitional movements. A firm bed may make getting in and out

of bed easier. Most patients report that satin sheets with silk or satin pajamas make moving in bed far easier. Adjustable beds may be helpful as the disease progresses, but while sleeping the patient should lower their head as close to horizontal as possible.

Breathing exercises are crucial for the patient with Parkinson disease. As stated previously, the most common cause of death is pneumonia. Clinicians should address both inspiratory muscle training for pulmonary function, as well as expiratory muscle function for airway clearance and protection. Chest expansion may be included during functional activities. Other interventions include LSVT LOUD and expiratory muscle strength training, which integrates the sequencing and coordination of breath support with activities such as volume production.[297] With disease progression, specific breathing exercises may need to be incorporated, especially for patients who are no longer able to walk.

In addition to treatment in the clinical setting, patients with Parkinson disease should be given a home program that encourages moderate-to-vigorous, consistent exercise as part of the normal day. The clinician should guide and support the patient in selecting the most optimal type, intensity, and frequency of exercise to increase patient self-efficacy. This, along with periodic checks, may enhance compliance. Exercises should be graded to the individual's capability, and the therapist should keep in mind that learned skills such as various sports are sometimes less affected than automatic movements, perhaps because these skills may rely on cortical involvement.[14]

Fatigue is a frequent complaint of people with Parkinson disease. Although it has been correlated with disease progression, depression, and sleep disturbances, it also exists in up to 44% of those without depression or sleep difficulty.[298] This type of fatigue is over and above what is associated with the exertion of an exercise program and may be one reason people with Parkinson disease have difficulty exercising. The patient with Parkinson disease frequently experiences post-exercise fatigue. If a person is so tired after exercise that he or she cannot perform normal ADLs, exercise will not become a part of the patient's daily routine. Post-exercise fatigue is easily alleviated by a gradual and extended cooldown period.

Patients frequently ask about the timing of medication and exercise. For any form of exercise in Parkinson disease to be effective, movement must be possible, especially movement through the full arc of the joint. Therefore exercise should be performed during the "on" period of the medication cycle given the dopaminergic effect and ability to push intensity and amplitude; however, clinicians should also assess and work with patients during their "off" period. People with Parkinson disease feel their "off" time correlates more closely with quality of life and balance confidence; therefore providing strategies for safe mobility during these periods may help improve quality of life, functional mobility, and decrease falls.[299] "Off" times also affect nonmotor symptoms and mood, and assessment during these periods may show patients that they can do more than initially believed, thereby improving confidence. Patients are encouraged to be "in tune" with his or her own response and adjust medications and exercise to a schedule accordingly.

The therapist is also involved in the prescription of assistive devices. The use of ambulatory aids for patients with Parkinson disease is an area with no clear-cut guidelines, and assessment should be specific to each individual. Because coordination of upper and lower extremities is often difficult, the ability to use a cane or walker can be limited as learning to use the device can be seen as a dual task activity. Standard walkers sometimes increase the festinating gait and are not recommended for people with freezing owing to the close extrapersonal space and management of the walker over obstacles; as such, four-wheel walkers with pushdown brakes appear to work best for many patients.[300] A walker that is in the brake condition at the start and requires the patient to push on handles to walk may also be safer. For patients with a tendency to fall backward, an assistive device may be positioned behind them. Walking sticks or canes can be helpful for the person who is able to walk with a heel-toe gait pattern but lacks postural stability. The height of walker or cane should be adjusted carefully to promote trunk extension, while a walking stick (or two) is less likely to promote flexion than a cane. Patients with Parkinson disease may also benefit from assistive devices for eating or writing, such as weighted utensils or devices with extra-large handles for tremor management and improved manipulation, as well as tools for fine motor tasks, such as buttoning aid hooks for dressing. A survey by Mutch and colleagues[256] in Ireland found that nearly half of the patients responding used some type of assistive device. These devices included ones for walking, reaching, rising from bed, and performing ADLs.

As Parkinson disease progresses, the patient may experience impaired speech (hypophonia, impaired articulation, and speech rate), difficulty in chewing and swallowing, as well as decreased saliva management. Therapy for volume production and/or oral-motor control should be initiated to improve volume, respiration, intelligibility, and decrease risk of aspiration. A dietician consultation may be necessary to ensure adequate nutrition and may also be beneficial in guiding the patient's protein intake. A diet high in protein may reduce the responsiveness of the patient to DA replacement therapy, and regulating the amount and timing of protein ingestion can improve the efficacy of drug treatment in some patients.[143] The use of vitamins is a subject that appears on many websites for patients with Parkinson disease, and the patient should be reminded to consult with his or her physician when changing vitamins.

The resurgence of surgery as a treatment alternative in Parkinson disease, including stimulation of deep brain sites that may alter neuroplasticity, means that the therapist will face new and exciting challenges in treatment.[301] Intense physical therapy, especially incorporating complex motor skills, has been demonstrated to be effective in improving function after a subthalamic nucleus lesion in animal studies.[302] Therefore intense physical therapy after surgery should be performed to maximize benefits from all surgeries in Parkinson disease (as well as in Huntington disease and the dystonias).

Finally, therapeutic rehabilitation and exercise may modify but cannot halt or reverse the progression of this degenerative disease. The therapist should assist the patient and family in coping with the constraints of this disease, enhancing the patient's quality of life throughout its course.

Differences Between Parkinson Disease and Atypical Parkinsonisms: Theoretical and Practical Considerations

Several other neurodegenerative diseases are grouped together as "atypical Parkinsonisms" disorders. Patients with these syndromes usually have limited to no response to levodopa intervention and tend to progress more rapidly than Parkinson disease. The most common of these is progressive supranuclear palsy (PSP). Clinical features include progressive onset of symmetric symptoms, lack of tremor, bradykinesia, increased rigidity in the trunk and legs, frequent falls early in the disease, and pseudobulbar features (dysphagia, dysarthria, and emotional lability). They also present with vertical gaze palsy. These patients can be evaluated and treated in a manner similar to patients with Parkinson disease. Treatment is aimed at symptom management and relief, although within a decade the patient is typically immobile.

Multiple system atrophy (MSA) is the second most common atypical Parkinsonism that affects various areas of the CNS, with varying degrees of pyramidal, cerebellar, and autonomic dysfunction. The disease is characterized by symptoms including rigidity, bradykinesia, postural instability, ataxia, bladder dysfunction, and orthostatic hypotension. There are two main phenotypes: MSA-P, which presents with Parkinsonism-dominant features, or MSA-C, which presents with predominantly cerebellar features. Almost all patients will develop autonomic dysfunction, while those with MSA-P are more likely to have a greater functional decline. Cognitive impairments occur in some patients, including decreased executive function, loss of verbal memory, verbal fluency, and difficulty maintaining attention.[303] Assessment and treatment should be focused on addressing impairments and symptom management while maintaining/improving mobility.

The least common atypical Parkinsonism is corticobasal syndrome. As the name suggests, it involves cerebrocortical and basal nuclei dysfunction, characterized by asymmetric motor impairments, apraxia, myoclonus, postural tremor, speech and swallowing impairments, and predominantly upper limb dystonia. Cognitive deficits are not a predominant feature. In some cases, patients may experience "alien limb phenomenon." Interventions should be focused on symptom management.

Dementia with Lewy bodies is a progressive, neurodegenerative disease that shares symptoms of both Parkinson disease and Alzheimer disease caused by abnormal deposits of alpha-synuclein protein in multiple areas of the brain. One of the characteristic features is the appearance of cognitive impairments before motor symptoms. Progressive cognitive decline, confusion, changes in attention, and hallucinations or delusions are often seen. While the Parkinsonian features may be responsive to Parkinson disease medications, cognitive involvement may make rehabilitation and carryover difficulty, and treatment should be focused on symptom management.

Because these syndromes are rarer than Parkinson disease and far more variable, there are limited studies that have been undertaken regarding rehabilitation intervention efficacy. Accurate differential diagnosis is important in patient planning; thus a thorough evaluation by a neurologist is highly recommended.

Huntington Disease

Huntington disease (formerly *Huntington chorea*) is another degenerative disease of the basal nuclei resulting in hyperactivity in the basal nuclei circuitry.[304,305] This disease gets its name from the family of physicians who described its patterns of inheritance. Huntington disease is inherited as an autosomal dominant trait and affects approximately 6.5 per 100,000 people.[2] The defect is on the short arm of chromosome 4, and alters DNA so that there is an increase in the cytosine-adenine-guanine (CAG) sequence; in normal individuals there are 10 to 35 CAG triple repeats, but in the individual with Huntington disease there are 36 to 125 repeats.[305] The longer the length of the CAG triple repeats, the more likely an individual is to develop the disease. Greater than 40 CAG repeats will cause development of Huntington disease, and longer repeat lengths is correlated with earlier onset of the disease.[306] The CAG repeat is related to glutamine. The target protein affected by the polyglutamine expansion has been named *huntingtin*. Huntingtin combines with ubiquitin and induces intranuclear inclusions and interference with mitochondrial function. The defect is characterized by severe loss of the medium spiny neurons and preservation of the ACh aspiny neurons. There are decreases in choline acetyltransferase (CAT), ACh, the number of muscarinic ACh receptors, glutamic acid decarboxylase, and substance P. There is generally no decrease in DA, norepinephrine, or serotonin (5HT), although more recent studies with single-photon emission computed tomography (SPECT) indicate that DA does diminish significantly in the later stages of the disease.[307]

Huntington disease is usually manifested between 30 and 50 years old, although childhood forms appear rarely. Those younger than

20 years with the disease account for approximately 10% of all people with Huntington disease and experience a faster rate of progression of the disease. Death from this disease occurs approximately 15 to 25 years after the onset of symptoms, although as in Parkinson disease, the earliest symptom is not known.

A marker for the Huntington gene has been detected.[308] If the family pedigree is known and the chromosomes of the parents can be obtained, detection of which offspring have the faulty chromosome is possible pre-symptomatically. Of course, early detection of this disease involves ethical and practical issues. At present, although testing is available, it is not widely used. Furthermore, testing for Huntington disease is typically available only to those older than 18 years. Despite these problems, localization of the gene and the repeat is promising and offers hope for improved means of treatment.

Huntington disease affects neurons in the basal nuclei as well as the cerebral cortex, thalamus, and cerebellum. The movement disorders are presumed to be related to degeneration of the striatal neurons, specifically the enkephalinergic neurons, which results in excitation of the cortex via disinhibition of the thalamus, and resultant hyperkinetic, choreiform movements.[14] The cognitive and emotional symptoms are associated with cortical destruction.

Symptoms

Huntington disease is characterized by a triad of signs and symptoms involving movement, cognitive, and psychiatric disorders. Some of the signs and symptoms of Huntington disease are similar to those of Parkinson disease: abnormalities in postural reactions, trunk rotation, distribution of tone, extraneous movements, as well as a decrease in associated movements (e.g., arm swing). Individuals with Huntington disease, however, are at the other end of the spectrum; rather than a paucity of movement, they exhibit too much movement, which is evident in the extremities, trunk, and face. The extraneous movements are of the choreoathetoid type–involuntary, irregular isolated movements that may be jerky and arrhythmical as in chorea, to rhythmical and worm-like as in athetosis. The gait takes on an ataxic, dancing appearance (in fact, *chorea* means to dance in Greek), and fine movements become clumsy and slowed.[308,309] Usually, however, these movements occur in succession so that the entire picture is one of complex movement patterns. The "movement generator" aspects of the basal nuclei seem to be continuously active, as would fit the hypothesis of a disruption in the indirect pathway; however, as the disease progresses, the choreiform movements may give way to akinesia and rigidity. This is caused by the excitatory direct pathway of the basal nuclei becoming affected in the later stages of the disease, which inhibits thalamic activity and results in decreased activation of the cortex.

Disruptions in voluntary movement for the person with Huntington disease further reflect the role of the basal nuclei in movement. The person with Huntington disease, like the person with Parkinson disease, has difficulty responding to internal cues, as well as internal rhythms. Kinematic analysis of upper-extremity complex tasks demonstrates that the person with Huntington disease must rely on visual guidance in the termination of a movement. This has been interpreted to indicate impairment in the development and fine-tuning of an internal representation of the task.[310] Furthermore, these patients have increasing difficulty with more complex movements in the absence of advanced cues.[311,312] The lack of internal cuing in the person with Huntington disease has been linked to the increased variability of response seen in these patients.[313]

Gait patterns of the person with Huntington disease are in some ways similar to those of Parkinson disease. Gait velocity and stride length are decreased, with the decrease in velocity correlating with disease progression. Unlike the person with Parkinson disease, however, the person with Huntington disease has a decreased cadence as well.[309] The base of support is increased (again unlike the pattern seen in Parkinson disease). In addition, lateral sway is increased along with great variability in distal movements. Balance impairments are manifested as increased sway in static and dynamic standing, with delayed balance recovery reactions. A combination of disease severity, lower limb weakness, cognitive impairment, and executive dysfunction have been found to influence balance and mobility in people with Huntington disease.[314] The face is also affected in Huntington disease. Impaired voluntary eye movement is often the first sign of Huntington disease, with noted difficulty with initiation and control of saccadic eye movements and smooth pursuits. Speech, breathing, and swallowing lack normal control and coordination. Speech lacks rhythm, variability in volume control, and mistiming in breath control, as might be expected with decreased internal timing. Timing and coordination of the swallowing mechanism is also impaired and can lead to choking, aspiration, and weight loss. Studies suggest that a person with decreased body weight and a parental history of the disease is at greater risk of disease development and progression.[313,315,316]

The exact mechanisms for the production of choreoathetoid movements are unknown. Because these extraneous movements are part of a person's normal repertoire of movement patterns, they may be "released" at inappropriate times and without any modulation. A postmortem examination showed a decrease in GABA that was greater in the globus pallidus external segment than the internal segment, while the recent use of positron emission tomography (PET) scans demonstrates loss of ACh and GABA neurons.[317] A pattern may therefore be executed before it is necessary, and inappropriate portions of a movement pattern cannot be inhibited. Petajan[318] found motor unit activity indicative of bradykinesia. Recordings of single motor units in the muscles indicates that persons with Huntington disease have a loss of control evidenced by an inability to recruit single motor units.[318] As the efforts at control increased, these individuals demonstrated an overflow of motor unit activity that resulted in full choreiform movements. Those in the earlier stages of the disease demonstrated what the experimenters termed "microchorea," or small ballistic activations of motor units.[318] As in Parkinson disease, difficulty occurs in modulating motor neuron excitability. Yanagisawa[319] used surface Electromyography (EMG) recordings to classify involuntary muscle contractions in Huntington disease patients with varying movement disorders from chorea to rigidity. He found brief, reciprocal, irregular contractions in those patients with classic chorea, and tonic nonreciprocal contractions in those patients with rigidity. Presence of athetosis or dystonia was associated with slow, reciprocal contractions. During sustained contractions, EMG activity demonstrated brief, irregular cessation of activity in the choreic patients; thus patients with Huntington disease have interruption of normal motor function at rest and during sustained activity (e.g., stabilizing contractions).

In addition to the involvement of the motor systems, the individual with Huntington disease also shows signs of cognitive and behavioral disorders that become worse as the disease progresses. Cognitive impairments include difficulties in planning, memory impairments, poor initiation, impulsivity, lack of insight, perseveration, and severe deterioration in the ability to communicate (e.g., speech and writing). Psychiatric changes include depression, hostility, irritability, paranoia, apathy, and anxiety. Ideomotor apraxia and apraxia of speech can also occur, especially as the disease progresses.[320] Intellect decreases, with performance measures decreasing more rapidly than verbal levels. Neuropsychological tests are therefore part of the Unified Huntington's Disease Rating Scale (UHDRS).

	Engagement in occupation		Capacity to handle financial affairs		Capacity to manage domestic responsibility		Capacity to perform activities of daily living		Care can be provided at	
		Score		Score		Score		Score		Score
Stage 1	Usual level	3	Full	3	Full	2	Full	3	Home	2
Stage 2	Lower level	2	Requires slight help	2	Full	2	Full	3	Home	2
Stage 3	Marginal	1	Requires major help	1	Impaired	1	Mildly impaired	2	Home	2
Stage 4	Unable	0	Unable	0	Unable	0	Moderately impaired	1	Home or extended care facility	1
Stage 5	Unable	0	Unable	0	Unable	0	Severely impaired	0	Total care facility only	0

Fig. 18.12 Functional Stages of Huntington Disease. (Reprinted from Shoulson I, Fahn S. Huntington's disease: clinical care and evaluation. *Neurology.* 1979;29:2.)

Stages of Huntington Disease

Huntington disease is a progressive disorder. The initial motor symptoms are most often incoordination, clumsiness, or jerkiness. A classic test for eliciting choreiform movements in this early stage is a simple grip test. People with Huntington disease displays what is descriptively called the "milkmaid's sign"; alternating increases and decreases in the grip that are perhaps the equivalent of the electromyographic abnormalities seen during sustained contractions. Facial grimacing or the inability to perform complex facial movements also may be present very early. As mentioned, the patient with Huntington disease will initially exhibit hyperkinetic movements with deficits in gross and fine motor control, eventually progressing to a hypokinetic presentation and significant debility in the late stage.

In most cases the cognitive and psychological impairments of Huntington disease occur before the onset of the motor signs; cognitive impairments have been reported at least 15 years prior to when a motor diagnosis is given.[321] As the disease progresses, cognition will progress from difficulty with complex tasks to intellectual decline with impaired insight and dual tasking, ultimately progressing to global dementia in the late stages. In cases in which very subtle personality changes occur first, the diagnosis may be more difficult. Such persons may appear depressed, irritable, or forgetful, but can then develop apathy, perseveration, antisocial behavior, and experience delusions or hallucinations; the late stage is characterized by delirium. Early diagnosis may be important, and SPECT shows promise for early detection of the disease.[322]

With time, the combination of the motor, cognitive, and psychiatric problems cause the individual to lose all ability to work and perform ADLs. Eventually, this person can only be cared for in an extended care facility. By this time, the choreiform movements have given way to rigidity, and the patient is bedridden. Death is usually caused by infection, but suicide is also common. Fig. 18.12 shows the stages of Huntington disease according to Shoulson and Fahn.[323,324]

Pharmacological Considerations and Medical Management

Advances in the pharmacological management of Parkinson disease have led to a great deal of research in an effort to find appropriate drugs for the management of Huntington disease.[325–329] At present, however, no fully effective medication is available for this disease. Each symptom is treated with its own medication.

The symptoms of Huntington disease indicate an increase in dopaminergic effect. Owing to the decrease in GABA and ACh concentrations in the basal nuclei, drug therapy depends on drugs that are cholinergic or GABA-containing agonists and those that act as DA antagonists. To date, the DA antagonists have been more effective in ameliorating neurological symptoms and are often the first drug to be prescribed; however, these drugs have severe side effects, including depression, drowsiness, Parkinsonian symptoms, and tardive dyskinesia.[324] DA antagonists for chorea management have initially shown improved gait, balance, and transfers, and further research is warranted.[330]

In general, pharmacological treatment is not started until the choreiform movements interfere with function, as antichoreic drugs have side effects that may be worse than the chorea.[331] Tetrabenazine and deutetrabenazine are the only FDA-approved drugs for management of chorea in Huntington disease and act to deplete DA in the synapse, with deutetrabenazine requiring less frequent dosing and fewer side effects;[332] however, they can exacerbate depression and suicidal actions and are not indicated in people with unmanaged mood disorders. Second-generation antipsychotics (DA antagonists), such as olanzapine, risperidone, and tiapride, are becoming more commonly prescribed owing to their effects on chorea, as well as positive effects on sleep dysfunction, mood, and weight loss prevention, and especially if psychiatric symptoms are present.[333] Drugs such as choline, which would increase ACh concentrations, have produced only transient improvement.[180] Many efforts have been undertaken to find a GABA agonist that would reduce the symptoms of Huntington disease, but these have been unsuccessful so far.[331,334] A barrier to medications that increase GABA is that such a drug may cause inhibition throughout the brain, not just in the basal nuclei; thus the individual's level of alertness and ability to function might be reduced—something the person with Huntington disease can ill afford.[334] A drug trial is currently underway and has so far delivered promising results to reduce the levels of the huntingtin protein.[335,336] The cognitive and behavioral impairments interfere more with life tasks and quality of life than do the presence of movement disorders. Medications are usually prescribed as combinations of drugs to treat the specific emotional and psychological symptoms. Cortical degeneration is most certainly involved, but disruption of the heavy corticostriate projections may also be a factor in the progression of this disease. Although alterations in

DA have been implicated in psychiatric problems such as schizophrenia, the role of the basal nuclei in thought processes is, at best, little understood. In the words of Woody Guthrie, "There's just not no hope. Nor not no treatment known to cure me of my dizzy called Chorea."[337]

At present, the best hope for the person with Huntington disease lies in a better understanding of the genetic mechanisms causing destruction of the GABA-containing cells in the striatum and cortical destruction. In the meantime, correct and early diagnosis is important in providing the proper early intervention, which must include counseling.[338] To facilitate research into the causes as well as the treatment of the disease, the Commission for the Control of Huntington's Disease has set up several research centers, including a brain and tissue bank. Research has also begun on the use of tissue transplantation. As with Parkinson disease, the tissue does survive, but the results are even more preliminary than for Parkinsonism.

Examination of the Patient With Huntington Disease

The standard medical evaluation is the UHDRS.[339] This comprehensive evaluation examines cognitive function, motor function, behavioral, and functional ability. The physical or occupational therapy evaluation of a person with Huntington disease must be global, incorporate the different ICF domains, and include an assessment of the degree of functional ability. Initial assessment should occur as early in the disease as possible and be performed at regular intervals to optimize their progression through the disease. Patient-reported outcomes are integral to help prioritize and determine the efficacy of interventions. The SF-36 is recommended for generic assessment of health status and quality of life and is widely used in Huntington disease studies. The Huntington's Disease health-related Quality of Life questionnaire (HDQoL) is also suggested to assess disease-specific symptoms and their impact on quality of life throughout the course of the disease.[340]

The clinical exam of a patient with Huntington disease should emphasize impairments and functional abilities. Strength and ROM should be assessed, with particular attention paid to the ability to stabilize the trunk and proximal joints. Strength and ROM changes may not be evident in the early stages of the disease. As the disease progresses, the clinician should be aware that isolated strength tested may be confounded by cognitive impairments and motor impersistence; therefore functional strength assessments may be warranted. To reduce the effects of rigidity, ROM measurements become important as the disease progresses.

Assessment of chorea should include its presence in the extremities, trunk, and face. Clinicians should note how frequent the chorea occurs, its severity, and how it interferes with function; they should also make note of what may aggravate and ease the choreiform symptoms. A simple rating scale is the capacity to perform ADLs (see Fig. 18.12). A standardized ADL assessment with space to write how the patient performs these activities or why she or he cannot perform them would be helpful.

Fall risk and rate of falls is significantly higher in people with Huntington disease, warranting a thorough balance assessment, especially narrow base of support and dual tasking conditions. Patients with a falls history have higher chorea scores, increased bradykinesia, aggression, and cognitive impairments. When assessing balance, the clinician should also consider the impact of oculomotor impairments. Saccadic eye movement and smooth pursuit deficits may affect balance and walking, especially as oculomotor impairments occur early in the disease.

Gait analysis can include a timed walk test and cadence assessment; stride length can then be calculated. A subjective assessment of variability

and incoordination should also be made. In addition, posture and equilibrium reactions should be tested, with assessment of associated reactions. In assessing posture, care should be taken to observe the posture of the extremities in addition to the trunk, head, and neck. Dystonic posturing should be carefully noted, especially if the patient is taking medication. Any changes should be reported to the physician.

In the assessment of the patient with Huntington disease, the stage of psychological involvement and mental state must be reliably assessed during both evaluation and treatment. SPECT and other computer tomography scans may give some clues to the amount of cortical and basal nuclei degeneration, which can assist in determining possible cortical functioning. There does not seem to be a consensus in research or clinical practice for which measurements are most sensitive to change or best reflect function for the patient with Huntington disease.

General Treatment Goals and Rationale

As there is such wide variation of potential multisystem impairments that impact functional activity and participation within each stage of the disease, it is recommended to approach interventions with treatment-based classifications. Clinicians are encouraged to review the EHDN Physiotherapy Clinical guidelines classification and determine where the patient may fit. Using the classifications as a framework, appropriate evaluation measures and intervention strategies should be chosen. Maintenance of the optimal quality of life is the most important goal for treatment of persons with Huntington disease and their families, including maintenance of functional skills and adaptive equipment recommendations. Techniques that reduce tone may also reduce choreiform movements. Increasing stability of the core and proximal musculature helps maintain function, and respiratory function should be kept as high as possible. Examination results and patient/caregiver goals will ultimately guide treatment procedures.

Treatment Procedures

The Commission for the Control of Huntington's Disease[341] stated that these individuals are underserved by physical and occupational therapy. Peacock[342] surveyed physical therapists in one state. Of the 585 therapists who responded, only 15.5% had worked with at least one patient with Huntington disease, and 6.2% had worked with more than one patient; this confirmed the underutilization of physical and occupational therapy today. Hayden[337] and Peacock[342] suggest that therapy can improve quality of life for this population. A 2008 article by Busse and colleagues[343] demonstrated that there is still underutilization of therapy services. They also found that there are no routine outcome measurements for the stages of the disease, and they suggested that management of falls and decreased mobility could be a treatment goal of physical therapy interventions. Although animal models of Huntington disease exist, there have been few studies investigating possible movement interventions. In one animal study, even a little environmental enrichment improved the ability of Huntington mice on a rotarod test and slowed the progression of the disease.[344] The mice getting even more enrichment showed improvement on more behavioral tests as well as changes in the striatum. Several articles have been published examining physical and occupational therapy treatment techniques for holistic therapy and for treating specific problems.[345–347]

A study by Zinzi and colleagues[345] was a nonrandom pilot study that incorporated gait, balance, and transfer training. Strengthening of the extremities, trunk, and muscles of respiration as well as coordination and postural stability activities were included. The program was undertaken with occupational therapy to include cognitive, rehabilitation, and ADL training. Participants were engaged in an intensive inpatient program for 3 weeks for 8 hours per day, 5 days a week, and three times a year. The data indicate that there was significant improvement in motor function and in ADL performance and that these subjects did not show deterioration over the 3 years of the study—a positive outcome for a degenerative disease.

Treatment of the person with Huntington disease has some parallels with the treatment of athetoid cerebral palsy; however, these techniques must be adapted to the adult. Of critical importance are the techniques for improving coactivation and trunk stability. The use of the pivot-prone and withdrawal patterns of Rood is helpful, and their benefits may be increased with the use of Thera-Band. Neck co-contraction and trunk stability may improve, or at least oral functions may be maintained. In addition, the techniques of rhythmical stabilization in all positions as well as heavy work patterns of Rood should be helpful.[348] Movements practiced out of context may not, however, carry over into functional activities; thus practicing coactivation in functional patterns during treatment, if at all possible, is recommended. Whereas in Parkinson disease the emphasis is on large-amplitude movements, movements for the person with Huntington disease need to be of smaller amplitude and controlled.

The gait disorder of Huntington disease has been shown to respond to rhythmical auditory stimuli in one study.[349] The ability to respond decreases in those most severely involved, indicating that treatment in the later stages of the disease may not be amenable to rhythmical stimuli. Another finding of this study was that cadence was a larger problem than stride length, especially at normal and fast speeds (compare this with the findings in Parkinson disease). Interestingly, people with Huntington disease were able to modulate gait to a metronome but had more difficulty with musical cues even when the tempos were identical. Subjects with Huntington disease demonstrated short-term carryover of metronome auditory stimuli to gait without auditory stimuli. Although the long-term carryover was not studied, using a metronome in gait training may be helpful in patients with Huntington disease. A more recent study using a metronome to cue gait during single and dual-task gait activities found that participants with Huntington disease had difficulty synchronizing steps to a metronome in all conditions.[346]

In a controlled clinical trial published by Kloos and colleagues, participation in a video dance game (Dance Dance Revolution), for 25 minutes, two times per week for 6 weeks resulted in significant reduction in double support percentage for forward and backward walking. Additionally, those with less severe motor symptoms had reductions in heel-to-heel base of support during forward walking.[350]

Relaxation aids the reduction of extraneous movements. In the early stages of the disease, methods that require active participation of the patient, such as biofeedback and traditional relaxation exercises, may be included. As dementia becomes more apparent, more passive techniques such as slow rocking and neutral warmth must be used. These techniques are also helpful in reducing the choreiform movements of the mouth and tongue, which may prove useful for the dentist and those responsible for proper nutrition of the patient. In most cases of Huntington disease, the individual is quite thin (almost emaciated) and begins to age rapidly as the disease progresses. The extraneous movements, especially as they become more severe, increase metabolic demands, and nutrition, therefore becomes increasingly important. Attention therefore must be paid to head, neck, and oral-motor control. Increased pressure on the lips may aid in lip closure and facilitate swallowing. Special straws with a mouthpiece like a pacifier may be useful. A dietician should be consulted for assistance in teaching the family how to prepare balanced and appetizing meals and snacks that are still easy to swallow.

The degree of dementia influences treatment options. Conscious efforts to control extraneous movements will be more difficult as cognitive function decreases. New memories and new patterns of movements are more difficult to establish. The therapist must therefore use techniques that require subcortical control and must keep in mind that the patient can sometimes remember old, normal patterns of movement. An encouraging treatment method may be the use of imagery. Yágüez and colleagues[347] found that patients with Huntington disease could use imagery to compensate for impairments in a graphomotor design task.

Peacock's study[342] suggests that group programs including strength, flexibility, balance, coordination, and breathing exercises may be very successful, especially in the early stages of the disease, and this was confirmed in the study by Zinzi and colleagues.[345] No amount of physical or occupational therapy, however, can prevent neuronal cell loss. With Huntington disease being a progressive, degenerative disease, the patient's condition will get worse, although the Zinzi study suggested that the progression might be slowed with integrated therapy.[345] Eventually, goals must be aimed at preventing total immobility and assisting caretakers in transfer techniques and advising them in the use of adaptive equipment. One aspect of treatment that cannot be measured but is important in my view is the degree of hope offered just by the fact that a health professional is providing ongoing care. This may lessen the patient's degree of despair and depression and may help maintain quality of life.

Wilson Disease

Wilson disease, or hepatolenticular degeneration, is a disease caused by faulty copper metabolism. The toxic effects of copper lead to degeneration of the liver and the basal nuclei. Wilson disease, inherited as an autosomal recessive trait, affects a very small percentage of the population. If the disease is recognized and properly treated, the patient can expect function without restriction and a normal life-span.

Wilson disease is characterized by an increase in the amount of copper absorbed from the intestinal tract, a subsequent elevation in the amount of copper in the blood serum, and an increase in the amount of copper deposited in tissue.[351] Ceruloplasmin is concomitantly reduced. The increase in tissue copper may interfere with various enzyme systems of particular cells. The connection of copper with DA metabolism may account for the basal nuclei involvement.

Neuronal degeneration is present in the globus pallidus and putamen and, to a lesser extent, in the caudate nucleus. Atrophy may be present in the gray matter of the cortex and the dentate nucleus of the cerebellum.

Symptoms

The deposition of the excess copper in the cornea results in the classic diagnostic sign of Wilson disease, the Kayser-Fleischer ring: a brownish-green or brownish-red ring found in the sclerocorneal junction.

Several forms of Wilson disease have been classified based on signs and symptoms. One type entails only liver involvement and no neurological signs. A dystonic form is most common in those with an onset of the disease after the age of 20 years. The individual shows the same abnormal positioning of the limbs and trunk that characterizes the dystonia, rigidity, and bradykinesia seen in Parkinson disease. Associated reactions and facial expressions are absent. Festinating gait and flexed posture are present. Tremor of the hand, head, and body may be present.

If the onset of the disease occurs before age 20, the appearance of choreoathetoid movements of the face and upper extremities is usually present. The gait resembles that of the individual with Huntington disease. This early-onset form is accompanied by rapid deterioration.[352]

Common to all forms of Wilson disease that involve brain structures are difficulty in speaking and swallowing, incoordination, and personality changes. The personality changes are the first signs of the disease, especially emotional lability and impaired judgment. If the disease progresses, dementia and cirrhosis of the liver increase and motor function progressively decreases.

The postures and movement patterns seen in people with Wilson disease include dystonic movements involving twisting and rotation of limbs, with sustained contraction at the end of the movement.[16] As Wilson disease progresses, the classic abnormal posture of increased flexion occurs, along with rigidity that can progress to the inability to move if severe enough. Dystonia, like bradykinesia and choreoathetosis, belongs on a continuum of the extraneous movements present with basal nuclei involvement. Dysfunction of the cerebellum and intralaminar nuclei of the thalamus may also contribute to these impairments of posture and movement.[353] A peculiar aspect of dystonia is that it can be decreased with proprioceptive or tactile inputs.[14] As with other diseases of the basal nuclei, an imbalance or abnormal response in the neurotransmitters occurs in Wilson disease; however, the precise imbalance is not yet known.

Stages of the Disease

The first symptom of Wilson disease is usually a change in the individual's personality. When this becomes severe enough or when the movement disorder appears, a diagnosis can be made by the presence of the Kayser-Fleischer ring in the eye or by an analysis of copper metabolism. Because Wilson disease is now treatable by chemical means, the full progression of this disease is usually not seen. If left untreated, the dystonia becomes worse and the person becomes more rigid. In addition, muscle weakness can occur and progress, seizures may develop, and the dementia and personality disorder become worse.

Medical Management

Wilson disease is usually one of the first diseases to be ruled out when a patient manifests movement disorders and behavioral problems, especially in the younger patient. The signs and symptoms of Wilson disease are caused by an increased absorption of copper; thus the treatment consists of drugs that will inhibit this absorption. Concomitantly, copper intake in the diet is restricted; no nuts, chocolate, liver, shellfish, dried fruit, or mushrooms. Zinc salt, which blocks the absorption of copper in the stomach and has no side effects, is now the treatment of choice. Penicillamine and trientine increase urinary excretion of copper, but there are serious side effects to these drugs. If the copper imbalance is treated, the neurological signs do not progress.

Examination and Treatment Intervention

Wilson disease is fully managed medically and can be diagnosed early; hence it may not be of concern to the therapist. If the patient is referred for therapy, treatment techniques should be wholly based on symptoms. Examination is similar to that of the person with Parkinson or Huntington disease. It consists of describing the type of extraneous movement present, when it is present, and factors that influence the degree of dystonia. Ease of movement should also be assessed and may be timed as for the patient with Parkinson disease. In addition, functional mobility (transfers, floor transfer), range of movement, and strength should be evaluated, especially if the disease is progressing.

Treatment is then designed to alleviate the problems. Extraneous movements may be reduced by any technique that will reduce tone. Positioning is important. If bradykinesia is the major sign, then treatment would be similar to that used for people with Parkinson disease; if trunk stability is poor, the therapist proceeds as in Huntington disease. The patient with Wilson disease has knowledge of what normal movement feels like and usually has good cognitive abilities at the time treatment is started. As a result of the emotional lability, which is one

of the first symptoms in this disease, the treatment session should be well planned and quite structured.

Tardive Dyskinesia

Tardive dyskinesia is usually a drug-induced disorder and thus will be used to indicate the problems that can arise from drug intoxication. This section concentrates on the problems associated with drugs that affect DA metabolism and/or reuptake, including amphetamine, methamphetamine, haloperidol, and classes of drugs used in the treatment of psychotic disorders: the phenothiazines, butyrophenones, and thioxanthenes. As the use and misuse of drugs becomes more common, these types of disorders may become more frequent.

The use of phenothiazines (one of the neuroleptics) has become a very effective and common treatment for schizophrenia. This treatment protocol has enabled many schizophrenics to leave the mental institution. These drugs are DA antagonists and thus decrease the amount of DA in the brain. The exact site of the brain involved in schizophrenia itself is not within the scope of this chapter, but the neurological signs that occur will be discussed. As might be expected, they involve structures within the basal nuclei. Tardive dyskinesia is a gradual disease that occurs after long-term drug treatment. The most typical involvement is of the mouth, tongue, and muscles of mastication; thus tardive dyskinesia may be called *orofacial* or *buccolingualmasticatory* (BLM) dyskinesia.

Symptoms

Dyskinesia is defined as an inability to perform voluntary movement.[338] In practical terms, however, dyskinesia is usually a series of rhythmical extraneous movements. In tardive dyskinesia this typically begins with, or may be confined to, the region of the face. These extraneous movements may include choreoathetoid or dystonic movements. Because of abnormality in basal nuclei function, abnormalities in postural tone and postural adjustments are also present. Instead of the typical flexed posture of Parkinson disease, patients with tardive dyskinesia show extension of the trunk with increased lordosis and neck flexion.[354] This description of the disease is rather broad, but the problems of drug-induced movement disorders are varied. They may take the form of drug-induced Parkinson disease or dystonia. In tardive dyskinesia, akinesia and rigidity like that seen in Parkinsonism may exist simultaneously with the choreoathetoid-like movements. The key factor in tardive dyskinesia is its slow onset after the ingestion of neuroleptic medications.

Etiology

Although many people take neuroleptic medication, only a small percentage acquires tardive dyskinesia. Many factors may predispose an individual to movement disorders. One of these is age.[355] This might be expected because of the influence of aging processes on the concentration of DA. Gender may also be a factor. Women, and older women, are more at risk for tardive dyskinesia, perhaps because of decreased estrogen.[354] The absolute amount of neuroleptic ingested may also be a factor, but to date definitive studies have not been completed. So far, the length of time the individual takes medication does not appear to be a strong predisposing factor. As the biological abnormalities of schizophrenia become better understood, further understanding of the causes of tardive dyskinesia may also be elucidated. The development of tardive dyskinesia is hypothesized to be caused by supersensitivity.[338,356] With the use of drugs that deplete the brain of DA, the brain becomes more sensitive to it and, in fact, in humans the withdrawal of neuroleptics tends to heighten the disease; essentially, withdrawal of the DA antagonist means that far more DA is able to act on these already sensitive terminals.[338,356,357]

As a result of the effectiveness of long-term treatment for schizophrenia provided by neuroleptics, research into the underlying cause and therefore treatment of the major side effect, the motor disorders, has greatly increased;[358] however, as with Parkinson disease and Huntington disease, animal models are difficult to produce. Experimental evidence indicates that the basal nuclei are involved in movements about the face, especially the mouth, and buccolingual dyskinesia is the most frequently encountered symptom in tardive dyskinesia.[359,360] The response of basal nuclei neurons to sensory input shows increasing localization of response with age; the region about the mouth becomes increasingly sensitive.[359] Further research along these lines, both in normal animals and in those with lesions, may answer the question of what is happening at a neuronal level. This would facilitate pharmacological and therapeutic interventions.

Pharmacological and Medical Management

The most important treatment for tardive dyskinesia is prevention. Today, DA receptor agonists are prescribed only when other, newer medications are not effective. Tardive dyskinesia is often irreversible. The withdrawal of medication may, in fact, increase the movement disorders, or recovery may take even more time than that required for the onset of the disease. Strangely, sometimes the drug that caused the disease may be the drug that reduces the symptoms; that is, increasing the dose may lessen the movement disorder, and this might be expected if supersensitivity to DA is involved. Again, however, with time the increased dose will also cause a reappearance of the symptoms. The Movement Disorder Society recommends that the physician evaluate the schizophrenic patient at 3-month intervals to prevent the disease. (Refer to the list of websites at the end of this chapter.)

The use of other drugs in conjunction with the neuroleptics has been tried in various animal models of the disease. As might be expected, anticholinergic drugs (which would worsen an imbalance between DA and ACh) worsen the dyskinesia. Lithium has been successful in one animal model of dyskinesia.[338] Some neuroleptic drugs seem to have less effect on movement than others; however, the side effects of one such drug, chlorpromazine, are life-threatening. Reducing the buildup of phenylalanine is also indicated as a way to decrease occurrence of tardive dyskinesia. A medical food comprising branched-chain amino acids seems to reduce concentration of phenylalanine and was effective in reducing the movement disorder in one clinical trial. More research is needed into both the mechanisms of schizophrenia and the mechanisms for the production of the abnormal movements.

Evaluation and Treatment Interventions for Dyskinesia

The effectiveness of rehabilitation therapy intervention in drug-induced dyskinesia is not yet completely known; however, because the neuroleptics do provide an effective long-term treatment of schizophrenia, and because amphetamines and methamphetamine are being abused, therapists need to become aware of the problem and offer some assistance. Early drug holidays (time without use of drugs) may be of value in treatment of tardive dyskinesia, and therefore early awareness of incipient changes in motor function may be of value. Assessment of patients receiving drug therapy could perhaps begin before treatment and then at prescribed intervals. The knowledge that postural adjustments are abnormal in most basal nuclei diseases means that analysis of posture statically and in motion might provide early clues of development of movement disorders. The same would be true for balance reactions and changes in tone with changes in position. Once movement disorders appear, an assessment of when and where the extraneous movements occur is important.

General treatment is similar to that used in Huntington disease; oral treatment corresponds to that for the athetotic child with cerebral palsy. If a hyperreactivity to sensory stimulus exists, then oral desensitization may be of value.

Ameliorating the oral grimacing, of course, would be helpful for the schizophrenic person who is trying to return to society. The effectiveness of physical and occupational therapy treatment cannot be assessed until therapists become involved with these patients and record the effectiveness of their interventions. In cases in which the Parkinsonian-like symptoms are stronger than the dyskinetic movements, treatment would follow the plan for the individual with Parkinson disease. As yet, physical therapy for drug-induced dyskinesias is not mentioned on websites to the physician or the patient.

Other Considerations

Other drugs besides neuroleptics may also produce movement disorders. Amphetamine, for example, has been shown to cause long-term changes in brain function even with very small doses.[361–363] Adults who were hyperactive as children sometimes show a decrease in the readiness potential.[364] Further longitudinal research and research using PET scans and fMRI are underway to determine the role that medications used in treating hyperactive children, such as methylphenidate (Ritalin), might play in changing the architecture of the basal nuclei and causing movement disorders.[82] The problem of drug-induced movement disorders may become an ever-increasing one for the therapist.

In 1982, several young people were treated for rigidity and "catatonia" after the use of what they thought was heroin. Careful examination of these patients revealed that they had Parkinsonian-like symptoms.[36,103] The chemical responsible for the symptomatology was MPTP, a meperidine analog that was an impurity in the designer heroin. This discovery has enabled research in animals and clinical studies in humans and may enable better understanding of the pathogenesis and, in turn, of the treatment of the disease. One hypothesized cause of Parkinson disease implicated environmental toxins (because some herbicides such as paraquat resemble the chemical structure of MPTP) and the involvement of superoxide free radicals.[95,365,366] Epidemiological studies have shown that exposure to organophosphates is associated with an increased incidence of developing Parkinson disease.[367]

Methamphetamine use also induces movement disorders. The MRI of even infrequent users shows damage to the basal nuclei.[368,369] A child born to a mother using methamphetamine may also have movement disorders and delayed achievement of developmental milestones. Another recreational drug, cocaine has long been known to produce Parkinsonian movement disorders.[370]

Dystonia
General Information

Dystonia is a movement disorder characterized by sustained or intermittent muscle contractions causing abnormal, often repetitive movements, postures, or both. Dystonic movements are typically patterned, twisting, and may be tremulous. Dystonia is often initiated or worsened by voluntary action and associated with overflow muscle activation.[371] In 2013 it was proposed that classification of dystonias would fall into one of five classification systems.

- Focal. Only one body region is affected. Typical examples of focal forms are blepharospasm, oromandibular dystonia, laryngeal dystonia, and writer's cramp.
- Segmental. Two or more contiguous body regions are affected. Typical examples of segmental forms are cranial dystonia (blepharospasm with lower facial and jaw or tongue involvement) or bi-brachial dystonia.
- Multifocal. Two noncontiguous or more (contiguous or not) body regions are involved.
- Generalized. The trunk and at least two other sites are involved. Generalized forms with leg involvement are distinguished from those without leg involvement.

- Hemidystonia. More body regions restricted to one body side are involved. Typical examples of hemidystonia are caused by acquired brain lesions in the contralateral hemisphere.

In all cases of dystonia, excessive coactivation of agonists and antagonists occurs that interferes with the timing, execution, and loss of independent joint motions. Rarely are any abnormalities of muscle tone present, per se—that is, no increase in deep tendon reflexes or rigidity occurs. Muscle strength and ROM are usually within normal limits unless disuse leads to weakness or if Botox has been utilized as a treatment modality.

Generalized Dystonia

Symptoms. The person with generalized dystonia will begin a movement (such as walking) and will then experience a torsional contraction of the trunk; of the upper extremity, especially at the shoulder; and in the ankle, foot, and toes. These contractions may be so strong that further movement is impossible. Many patients experience pain as the muscles remain contracted for long periods of time.[372]

Etiology. The cause of generalized dystonia is predominantly genetic, involving the *DYT* gene.[373]

According to the Dystonia Medical Research Foundation, there may also be additional causes for generalized dystonia including birth injury, exposure to certain drugs, head injury, and infection.

Pharmacological and medical management. There are few treatments for generalized dystonia. DA agonists and L-dopa are sometimes effective.

Evaluation and treatment intervention. Evaluation of the person with generalized dystonia will be similar to the evaluation of the person with tardive dyskinesia or Huntington disease. Several ADLs should be examined. The way that dystonia interferes with these ADLs is of most importance for treatment. In addition to the full extent of the motoric abnormality, it is also important to test sensation, especially higher level sensory processing such as precise localization of touch, graphesthesia, and kinesthesia.

Movement therapy interventions are only now being developed for generalized dystonia. Overall, treatment similar to that in Huntington disease that emphasizes treating the symptoms may be beneficial. One successful program uses sensory integration and relearning techniques performed with attention.[374] Practice is a crucial element of treatment, and the patient must be willing to practice the sensory tasks many, many times throughout the day for benefit.

Other considerations. As with other extraneous movements associated with basal nuclei disorders, relaxation can reduce the muscle contraction; however, I have found that the time to incorporate relaxation is before the full-blown development of the muscle contraction—a difficult task. Therefore patients should practice relaxation on a regular basis. There is frequently a psychological aspect to focal dystonias that may necessitate intervention from a psychiatrist or psychologist.

Focal Dystonias

Spasmodic torticollis is the most common focal dystonia. The person with this disorder will have involuntary contractions of neck muscles that result in head turning or tipping and head extension and flexion movements that are often sustained for long periods of time. Other common sites of focal involvement are the vocal cords; the tongue and swallowing muscles; the facial muscles, especially around the eye; the hand; and the toes. Writer's cramp is a task-specific dystonia, unlike other focal dystonias. An interesting phenomenon of dystonia is the fact that many patients will develop a sensory or motor "trick" that will decrease the severity of the muscle contraction(s) and may even stop these movements.[372,375]

Symptoms. Symptoms of focal dystonia will depend on the site of involvement. For example, in the case of spasmodic torticollis, the symptom is pain and an inability to control a movement of the head to the side.

The signs and symptoms of focal hand dystonia are variable. The problem may initially manifest as an abnormality in the quality of sound produced by a musical instrument (e.g., a deterioration of vibration in a violinist),[376] increasing errors in task performance, unusual fatigue or sense of weakness, or involuntary or excessive movement of a single or multiple digits. Initially, the symptoms are subtle and virtually indistinguishable from the normal variations that may be seen in the execution experienced by all musicians studying technically demanding music or software engineers who spend excessive hours at the computer. Frequently, a person engaged in a profession with highly repetitive tasks who has minimal pain but vague motor control problems or somatosensory dysfunction is manifesting early signs of focal dystonia.[377] Although co-contraction of flexors and extensors can be observed while an individual with hand dystonia performs the target task, while at rest and during performance of nontarget tasks the hand appears to function normally. Some patients demonstrate a variety of subtle abnormalities such as reduced arm swing; loss of smooth, controlled grasping; a physiological tremor; hypermobility of interphalangeal joints; decreased ROM in some upper limb joints (e.g., shoulder abduction, external rotation, finger abduction, and forearm pronation); neurovascular entrapment; compression neuropathy; or poor posture.[378–383]

Etiology. The cause of focal dystonias is unknown and multifactorial. Frucht[379] observed that task-specific hand dystonia seemed to begin after motor skills had been acquired rather than during skill acquisition; thus focal hand dystonia in a musician is probably not a disorder of motor learning but a disruption of acquired, complex, motor programs. The data also suggested that peripheral environmental influences seem to play an important role in molding the dystonic phenotype. For example, the hand performing the more complex musical tasks (e.g., right hand in pianists and guitarists, left hand in violinists) seemed to be more predisposed to the development of dystonia. In addition, the dystonia usually began in one finger and spread to adjacent fingers, rarely skipping a finger. Furthermore, the ulnar side of the hand (fingers 4 and 5) was disproportionately affected, potentially because of the challenging ergonomics and technical stresses of the musical instrument required for this part of the hand in terms of gripping and activation of individual finger movements.[384]

Pharmacological and medical management. The most common medical treatment for focal dystonias is botulinum toxin. This toxin binds with the ACh receptors on the muscle and prevents the muscle from contracting. The injections are made under electromyographic guidance so that only those motor units involved in the production of the extraneous movements are paralyzed; however, the treatment does not cause permanent change, so the patient must repeat these injections every 3 to 4 months. Some people develop antibodies to the toxin, rendering it then ineffective.[385,386] Therefore medical management prevents the abnormal movement but is not a cure.

Evaluation and treatment. Overall, treatment of focal dystonia will depend on the joint or joints involved. The duration of the dystonia, the trigger, and the person's trick, if any, to relieve the dystonia must be noted. Tricks are sensory in nature and help relieve the pain often associated with the extreme movement. The Toronto Western Spasmodic Torticollis Rating Scale (TWSTRS) is one evaluation for the person with spasmodic torticollis.[387,388]

Several ADLs should be examined. For example, in hand dystonia, the person should be evaluated using the instrument producing the dystonia (i.e., the pen in writer's cramp) as well as other tools (e.g., a fork). In addition, there seems to be position dependence, so writing while prone may not evoke the dystonia despite severe inability to hold the pen at a desk.

In addition to the full extent of the motoric abnormality, sensation, especially higher-level sensations such as precise localization of touch, graphesthesia, and kinesthesia must be assessed. Byl and colleagues found changes in the sensory cortex after development of focal hand dystonia.[374,388–391] Recent evidence suggests that balance, particularly dynamic balance, should also be assessed in patients with torticollis.[392] These balance difficulties have not been relieved with botulinum toxin.

Movement therapy interventions are now being developed. One successful program uses sensory integration and relearning techniques performed with attention.[393] Practice is a crucial element of treatment, and the patient must be willing to practice the sensory tasks many times throughout the day for benefit. The patient practices cognitively demanding sensory discrimination tasks throughout the day and tries to use only tension-free movements.[388]

Treatment for the person with torticollis must include a relearning of midline before the person can begin to practice normal movement away from midline. The patient may find this relearning process easier after botulinum injection.

Other considerations. As with other extraneous movements associated with basal nuclei disorders, relaxation can reduce the muscle contraction; however, the time to incorporate relaxation is before the full-blown development of the muscle contraction—a difficult task. This task requires a shift in paradigm to a health and wellness model and prevention; therefore patients should practice relaxation on a regular basis. A psychological aspect to focal dystonias frequently necessitates intervention from a psychiatrist or psychologist.

METABOLIC DISEASES AFFECTING OTHER REGIONS OF THE BRAIN

All alterations of metabolism, if allowed to continue, will affect nervous system function. This includes alterations in sodium, water, sugar, and hormonal balance. Table 18.2 lists metabolic diseases that often have neurological sequelae. Proper treatment is usually medical management of the imbalance. Physical therapeutic intervention, if necessary, should address specific neurological symptoms.

Ingestion of, or exposure to, heavy metals may also lead to CNS disease. Table 18.3 describes the sequelae of these problems.

SUMMARY

This chapter has focused on the pathophysiology, evaluation, and treatment of genetic, hereditary, and metabolic diseases affecting adults. In all of these diseases the therapist or movement specialist is an important part of the rehabilitation team. Knowledge of the possible mechanisms involved in the production of varying movement disorders may make the appropriate evaluation and subsequent treatment more meaningful. Even with degenerative, progressive disorders the therapist plays an important role in maintaining quality of life, potentially improving movement and decreasing disability, and assists the patient and family in coping with the disease. The importance of documentation and publication of cases and larger controlled studies cannot be overstressed. Both will assist in the development of improved therapeutic

techniques and may help researchers in planning and interpreting appropriate experimental studies. Establishment of efficacy is the first step toward evidence-based practice and a critical link in the evolution of professionals who have been identified as movement specialists.

With the advent of the Internet, many websites have been created to focus on diseases and conditions mentioned in this chapter. In addition, the organization Patients Like Me has a website for both patients and care providers (www.patientslikeme.com). Sites such as this answer many questions for patients and provide information on making day-to-day life easier. Local and national support groups and foundations also provide information and support for the patient and caregiver. Most also have separate sections for health care providers.

TABLE 18.2   Neurological Complications of Metabolic Disorders

Metabolic Problem	Treatment	Neurological Complication
Decreased sodium (too much water)	Restriction of water intake	Muscle twitching, seizures, and coma
Increased sodium (too little water)	Slow rehydration	Cerebral edema, muscle rigidity, and decerebrate rigidity
Decreased potassium (hypokalemia), often caused by aldosteronism	Restoration of potassium levels after assessing primary cause	Changes in resting potential of neuron; hyperpolarization; muscle weakness and fatigue with eventual total paralysis
Magnesium imbalance	Improved diet, intravenous magnesium	Mental confusion, muscle twitching, myoclonus, tachycardia, hyperreflexia, extraneous movements, and seizures
Diabetes mellitus	Proper control of diabetes	Peripheral neuropathy, pseudotabes, possible seizures, and coma
Hypoglycemia	Treatment of primary cause; diet adjustment	Anoxia of the brain, seizures, confusion
Hyperthyroidism	Thyroid-blocking agents; intravenous fluids, hydrocortisone, and propranolol if patient is in thyroid crisis	Hyperkinesia, irritability, nervousness, emotional lability, and symmetrical peripheral neuropathy
Hypothyroidism	Thyroid supplement	Sluggishness, mental and motor retardation, muscle weakness, and sometimes muscle pain
Hypercalcemia	Treatment of primary cause, which is often hyperparathyroidism, vitamin D malignancy (therefore surgical removal)	Headache, weakness, fatigue, proximal neuropathy, rigidity, tremor, and disorientation
Hypocalcemia	Intravenous administration of calcium (possible medical emergency)	Hyperexcitability of the peripheral and central nervous systems, which can lead to tetany and convulsions

TABLE 18.3 Neurological Complications of Heavy Metal Poisoning

Type of Metal	Treatment	Neurological Complication
Lead Source: lead paint, industrial (fumes of molten lead)	Elimination of source, reduction of fluids, intravenous urea or mannitol, and use of chelating agents	Interstitial edema and hemorrhage (especially in cerebellum) in acute poisoning; all levels of central nervous system affected in chronic long-term poisoning In children: seizures, mental retardation, behavior problems, and hyperactivity In adults: spasticity, rigidity, dementia, and personality changes Peripheral neuropathy may occur in adults and children
Arsenic Source: paint and insecticides	Removal of source, gastric lavage, intravenous fluids, maintenance of electrolyte balance; penicillamine used in acute poisoning	Demyelination of peripheral nerves in all extremities
Manganese Source: industrial if manganese dust is not removed; symptoms appear 2–25 years after exposure	Levodopa	Neuronal loss in basal nuclei, substantia nigra, and cerebellum Initially psychiatric disturbances, including nervousness, irritability, and a tendency toward compulsive acts Later, muscular weakness and Parkinsonian symptoms
Mercury Rare, but may affect farmers and dental office workers	Penicillamine; function returns only with physical, occupational, and speech therapy	Loss of neurons, especially in cerebellum; also in cortex near calcarine fissure Alternating periods of confusion, drowsiness, and stupor with restlessness and excitability Ataxia, dysarthria, and visual deterioration

CASE STUDY 18.1 Patient With Parkinson Disease, Hoehn and Yahr Stage 1

Ms. T. is a 55-year-old woman who was diagnosed with Parkinson disease 1 year ago. The disease began in her left arm and leg when she noticed increasing stiffness and difficulty moving. She was initially seen in physical therapy 8 months ago for potential frozen shoulder, which did respond to traditional physical therapy. She complains of some instability in walking and has recently developed a slight resting tremor in the left hand. On initial evaluation she had full active and passive ROM in all extremities, neck, and trunk. There is a mild resting tremor present in the left hand. There is mild cogwheel rigidity in the left upper and lower extremities; there is some intermittent resistance to passive movement in the right upper extremity as well. Strength is grossly within normal limits throughout. Sensation is intact throughout. Equilibrium reactions are delayed, but the patient demonstrates an ankle strategy on a flat surface and a hip strategy when standing on the balance beam; there is no mixing of the synergies, and her balance responses are appropriate to the degree of displacement.

The patient is able to stand in the sharpened Romberg position for 30 seconds with eyes open and 20 seconds with eyes closed. She can stand on the right leg for 30 seconds with eyes open and 15 seconds with eyes closed; she can stand on the left leg for 15 seconds with eyes open and 10 seconds with eyes closed. When walking, she has a heel-toe sequence, shortened stride length, and normal stride width. There is no arm swing on the left and a diminished arm swing on the right. There is no trunk rotation and very slight trunk flexion throughout the gait cycle. Speed is within normal limits for a 25-foot walk. The patient is able to turn freely to complete Timed Up and Go in less than 10 seconds and cognitive Timed Up and Go (counting backward by 3s from 50) with correct accuracy, but her speed slowed to just more than 11 seconds, and her arm swing limitations were increased bilaterally. She recently began to experience a foot dystonia, which is worse with fatigue. It has interfered with her daily walking program and her tennis, an activity she enjoys with her husband twice a week. Her only medication is deprenyl.

This patient is in Hoehn and Yahr stage 1, with some beginning of bilateral symptoms and progression to stage 2. She is young, is employed full-time, and has been involved in regular exercise for the past 10 years. Her complaints are stiffness, slowed movements, and foot dystonia. Her symptoms are mild at present, and she has good balance in standing and walking; hence this patient should be encouraged to continue exercising regularly. She should try to maintain her tennis because this requires complex, sequential, context-dependent movements. Although tennis involves motor responses to external cues, it does necessitate rapid force generation and anticipatory movements. This should encourage continued motor learning. In addition, she should be encouraged to continue walking out of doors and practice alternating speed of walking. During her walks she has been instructed to exaggerate her arm swing and keep her hands open as she works to swing them contralaterally with each leg as she steps. Use of music at a cadence of 100–120 beats per minute was encouraged to set an external rhythm. The dystonia is more difficult to resolve. It may be tied to medication, and differing medication schemes are now being tried. She is also on a program of stretching and strengthening of the ankle as well as a sensory stimulation program for the feet. Foam between the toes has helped to decrease dystonia early in the day.

Ms. T. has also been informed about the importance of maintaining chest expansion and monitoring her breathing. This will be important as the disease progresses. She attends a support group to increase her awareness of the disease, new treatments, and support. As the disease progresses, she will need a home program appropriate for her symptoms. She should start considering exercise groups because the group setting can be very valuable for a patient with Parkinson disease at any disease stage. She will be seen by her physical therapist no less than every 6 months for reassessment and progression of her home program.

CASE STUDY 18.2   Patient With a Seven-Year History of Parkinson Disease, Hoehn and Yahr Stage 3

Mr. R. is a 68-year-old man with a 7-year history of Parkinson disease. He is currently in Hoehn and Yahr stage 3 of the disease. He falls two or three times a day, has difficulty eating, and has noticed weakness in his right hand. He would like to return to full activity including golf twice a week, swimming, and skiing. On evaluation he has moderate rigidity in all extremities; the right side is worse than the left. It is most marked in the right wrist, forearm, and hand. Shoulder flexion and abduction lack 15 degrees bilaterally. He has a 15-degree knee flexion contracture on the right; all other joints in the lower extremity have range within functional limits. Strength is grossly 4 to 4+/5 on manual muscle testing throughout, including grip strength. Sensation is within normal limits throughout. Sitting balance is good during static and dynamic activities.

The patient sits with a posterior pelvic tilt, rounded shoulders, and flexed neck. On rising to a standing position, he does move forward in the chair, which positions his feet under his knees. He does not lean forward as he stands and momentarily loses his balance backward on rising from a chair. Static standing and dynamic balance is fair. When pushed on the sternum, he takes 1 or 2 steps backward, even to a gentle push. When pushed from behind he takes several steps forward. He lost his balance and required assistance when trying to catch a large ball thrown to the side. His gait pattern is typical of a patient with Parkinson disease with shortened steps and flat foot contact bilaterally. He complains of festination and freezing, but neither are observed during the evaluation. He turns "en bloc," exhibiting no arm swing and no trunk rotation. He walks slowly and is unable to increase his speed measurably in a 25-foot walk. He is taking carbidopa-levodopa and deprenyl. He tried taking another D2 agonist but experienced hallucinations. He was able to ski until last winter. At that time, he found that he could not stand up once he fell, and sometimes he fell without realizing that he was falling. He stated that he "did not think it was safe to ski." He also no longer swims because he has difficulty breathing in the pool and coordinating his breathing with the strokes. He does not play golf because it takes him so long.

This patient was encouraged to continue to exercise and socialize while exercising. He was encouraged to resume golf at times when his course is less crowded. He was also encouraged to utilize a driving range so he can maintain his swing and add trunk rotation as part of his home program. In addition, he was given a home program consisting of activities to be performed in seated and standing positions that encourages trunk rotation and large movements and is coordinated with good breathing practices. He was given some balance exercises that challenge his equilibrium in a safe environment. His home program was monitored every 3 months because of the distance he must travel to come to the clinic. His wife was instructed to exercise with her husband and to exercise to music with him. He was referred to a speech pathologist for a swallowing evaluation and was given a therapeutic program for his speech and breathing. He is now able to play golf once a week; however, he is not yet ready to resume swimming or skiing. Future therapeutic interventions may include high-intensity exercise as his goals are significant for his disease level and he will need more aggressive treatment to reach these goals.

Websites

National Institute of Neurological Disorders and Stroke, National Institutes of Health

A comprehensive index of neurological disorders.

www.ninds.nih.gov/disorders/disorder_index.htm

International Parkinson and Movement Disorder Society

This organization is for professionals and patients and includes information regarding all movement disorders included in this chapter. Educational handouts for each movement disorder in this chapter may be found through this resource as well.

www.movementdisorders.org

The Parkinson's Disease Foundation

This website includes an exercise program for people with Parkinson disease.

www.pdf.org

The National Parkinson Foundation

News, medical information, events calendar, and more for people with Parkinson disease, families, and caregivers.

www.parkinson.org

American Physical Therapy Association Podcasts

www.moveforwardpt.com/radio

Huntington's Disease Society of America

Information, research, and help for people with Huntington disease, families, and caregivers.

www.hdsa.org

ACKNOWLEDGMENT

We would like to thank Marsha Melnick, PT, PhD, for her significant contributions to this chapter in the previous editions of the textbook.

REFERENCES

To enhance this text and add value for the reader, all references are included on the companion Evolve site that accompanies this textbook. This online service will, when available, provide a link for the reader to a Medline abstract for the article cited. There are 393 cited references and other general references for this chapter, with the majority of those articles being evidence-based citations.

19

Cerebellar Dysfunction*

Susanne M. Morton, Jennifer L. Keller, and Amy J. Bastian

OBJECTIVES

After reading this chapter the student or therapist will be able to:

1. Understand critical features of cerebellar anatomy and physiology and its role in motor control.
2. Describe the major movement deficits associated with damage to the human cerebellum.
3. Discuss important components of the physical therapy examination for patients with suspected cerebellar dysfunction.
4. Review the evidence for and against specific rehabilitation interventions targeting recovery of body functions, activities, and participation.
5. Discuss the factors involved in selecting recovery versus compensation approach in the physical therapy management of individuals with cerebellar dysfunctions.

KEY TERMS

ataxia
cerebellum
incoordination

motor learning
rehabilitation

OVERVIEW

The cerebellum is a highly unique brain structure, easily recognizable by its location on the dorsal surface of the brain stem and the distinct, dense folia, or foldings, of its cortex. For centuries, the cerebellum has been the object of intense investigation by scientists, in particular because of the extreme uniformity in the arrangement of neurons in the cerebellar cortex and the presence of very large Purkinje cells that have an extensive fanlike dendritic arbor. The human cerebellum contains more neurons than any other brain region, suggesting that whatever its role in behavior, it requires the integration of vast amounts of information and may perform rather complex computations. Researchers agree that the cerebellum plays a critical role in coordinating and adapting movements, although how it does so is still not fully understood. It is currently also clear that the cerebellum is connected to nonmotor regions of the brain, such as the prefrontal cortex, and therefore likely plays a role in cognitive and other nonmotor functions. Yet the most striking and debilitating effect of damage to the cerebellum is *ataxia*, which comes from the Greek and translates literally to mean "without order." We will focus on this hallmark feature of cerebellar damage, which is incoordination of movements without overt muscle weakness. In this chapter, we will review critical features of cerebellar anatomy and physiology that help to reveal its role in motor control, and we will describe the major movement deficits associated with damage to the human cerebellum. We will highlight the most valuable and unique components of the physical therapy examination for patients with suspected cerebellar dysfunction and review the evidence for and against specific rehabilitation interventions targeting recovery of body functions,

activities, and participation. Emphasis is placed on the importance of the physical therapist's judgment in determining whether a recovery or a compensation approach should be implemented.

Types of Cerebellar Damage

Cerebellar ataxia can result from damage to the cerebellum itself or the pathways to or from it. Damage can occur from a number of different causes, such as stroke, tumor, degenerative disease, trauma, or malformation. The etiology of cerebellar dysfunction is often an important consideration when determining a prognosis and developing a treatment plan. Other factors to consider include whether the cerebellar lesion is static or progressive, whether it involves only the cerebellum or multiple neural structures, and whether it was present at birth or acquired.

Cerebellar strokes are rarer than cerebral strokes but not entirely uncommon; they account for less than 5% of all strokes.[1] These strokes can involve any of the three arteries that supply the cerebellum: the superior cerebellar artery, anterior inferior cerebellar artery, and posterior inferior cerebellar artery. Depending on the territory supplied by the damaged vessel (Table 19.1), there are stereotyped patterns of cerebellar and extracerebellar motor dysfunction that results. However, there is certainly some variation in distributions from person to person. Stroke involving the superior cerebellar artery often leads to dysmetria of ipsilateral arm movements, unsteadiness in walking, dysarthric speech, and nystagmus.[1] Stroke involving the anterior inferior cerebellar artery often causes both cerebellar and extracerebellar signs (due to involvement of the pons) including dysmetria, vestibular signs, and facial sensory loss.[1] Finally, stroke involving the posterior inferior cerebellar artery is usually, in the long run, the most benign, although initially it often presents with vertigo, unsteadiness, walking ataxia, and nystagmus.[1] The best predictor of recovery from cerebellar stroke is

---

*Videos for this chapter are available at studentconsult.com.

TABLE 19.1 Territories of the Cerebellar Arteries[1,3]

Artery	Cerebellar Territory Supplied
SCA	• Superior/upper approximately one-half of the dorsal and upper approximately one-third of the ventral surface of the cerebellum except for the extreme lateral wing of the hemisphere • Portions of the vermis and nodulus • Substantial upper portions of the intermediate and lateral hemispheres • Portions of the deep cerebellar nuclei • Superior cerebellar peduncle
AICA	• Middle approximately 10%–30% of the ventral cerebellum, sometimes wrapping laterally to encompass a small portion of the most lateral aspects of the dorsal cerebellum • Flocculus • Small portions of the lateral hemisphere • Middle and inferior cerebellar peduncles
PICA	• Inferior/lower approximately one-half of the dorsal cerebellum and the inferior approximately one-fourth to one-third of the ventral cerebellum • Portions of the nodulus, vermis, intermediate, and lateral hemispheres • Portions of the deep cerebellar nuclei

Note: The cerebellar arteries also supply extracerebellar regions (i.e., portions of brain stem) not listed here.
AICA, Anterior inferior cerebellar artery; *PICA*, posterior inferior cerebellar artery; *SCA*, superior cerebellar artery.

TABLE 19.2 Selected Forms of Cerebellar Damage[5]

Acquired	Degenerative Nonhereditary
1. Stroke (infarct, hemorrhage)	1. Multiple system atrophy (MSA)
2. Tumor (primary brain tumor, metastatic disease)	2. Idiopathic late-onset cerebellar ataxia (ILOCA)
3. Structural (Chiari malformation, agenesis, hypoplasia, etc.)	
4. Toxicity (alcohol, heavy metals, drugs, solvents, etc.)	**Hereditary**
5. Immune mediated (multiple sclerosis, gluten ataxia, etc.)	1. Autosomal dominant disorders (episodic ataxias, spinocerebellar ataxias)
6. Trauma	2. Autosomal recessive disorders (Friedreich ataxia, early onset cerebellar ataxia, etc.)
7. Infection (cerebellitis, etc.)	3. X-linked disorders (mitochondrial disease, fragile X-associated tremor, etc.)
8. Endocrine (hypothyroidism)	

whether the deep cerebellar nuclei are involved: recovery is best when they are not damaged.[2]

Tumors in the posterior fossa (i.e., in or near cerebellum) do occur, although they are more common in children than adults. Depending on the type and location, tumors may be treatable with surgical resection, chemotherapy, radiation therapy, or some combination of these. Children with cerebellar tumors often have a good prognosis for recovery because many of the types of tumors most common in this population are benign and can be removed. Children also typically recover very well following cerebellar damage from tumor resection and show little signs of cerebellar ataxia. Tumors in adulthood often are due to a more aggressive form of cancer and therefore may have a poorer prognosis. Second to tumor type, damage of the deep cerebellar nuclei is an important factor that predicts recovery, even more so than age.[2]

Several neurodegenerative diseases can damage the cerebellum (Table 19.2). One of the more common types of degenerative diseases is a group of hereditary, autosomal dominant diseases referred to as the spinocerebellar ataxias (SCAs). Currently, there are 46 known distinct SCAs, which are named by numbers (e.g., SCA1, SCA2).[4] Depending on the genetic abnormality, they can cause either purely cerebellar damage or combined cerebellar and extracerebellar damage.[5,6] Most of the SCAs have onset in midlife and are slowly progressive, which means that children of an affected parent will likely not know if they are affected until adulthood. There are genetic tests for a subset of these diseases. Because onset of symptoms is delayed and there are no effective pharmacological treatments, genetic counseling is a must before families decide whether or not to have children undergo genetic testing. A related set of diseases are the hereditary episodic ataxias,[7] which are rare autosomal dominant diseases. As the name implies, patients with episodic ataxia will have periods of ataxia, lasting minutes to hours, brought on by exercise, stress, or excitement. Some of the episodic ataxias respond well to medications.[8]

Cerebellar damage can occur from other sources as well. In traumatic brain injury, damage of the cerebellum is almost always found in the presence of widespread brain damage and is seen as a predictor of poorer outcome.[9] The cerebellum is also particularly sensitive to toxins, including certain heavy metals and alcohol. Chronic alcoholism causes cerebellar atrophy preferentially involving the anterior superior vermis.[10,11] The inflammatory disorder multiple sclerosis also frequently produces lesions in the cerebellum. Finally, congenital brain abnormalities such as Chiari malformation damage the cerebellum by increased pressure and mechanical deformation. Recovery from cerebellar malformation is not understood; often these children have substantial damage to the brain stem or other neural structures, which may make therapy more challenging. A more comprehensive list of the variety of types of cerebellar damage is provided in Table 19.2.

Given the wide range of cerebellar disorders, it is useful for the clinician to categorize the damage as progressive or nonprogressive. Patients with progressive disorders, such as the SCAs, are likely to experience worsening ataxia and decreased mobility over time and will need periodic therapy over the life-span for optimal function. In contrast, those with nonprogressive disorders would not be expected to worsen and some may have the potential for substantial recovery. Note that when additional brain areas are involved, rehabilitation may be more challenging, theoretically because other compensatory brain mechanisms may be impaired. This type of information is vital for making an appropriate prognosis and developing a long-term plan of care for patients with cerebellar dysfunction.

CEREBELLAR ANATOMY AND PHYSIOLOGY

A brief review of specific anatomical and physiological features is critical to understanding the mechanisms by which the cerebellum helps to coordinate and adapt movement. Recall that most pathways

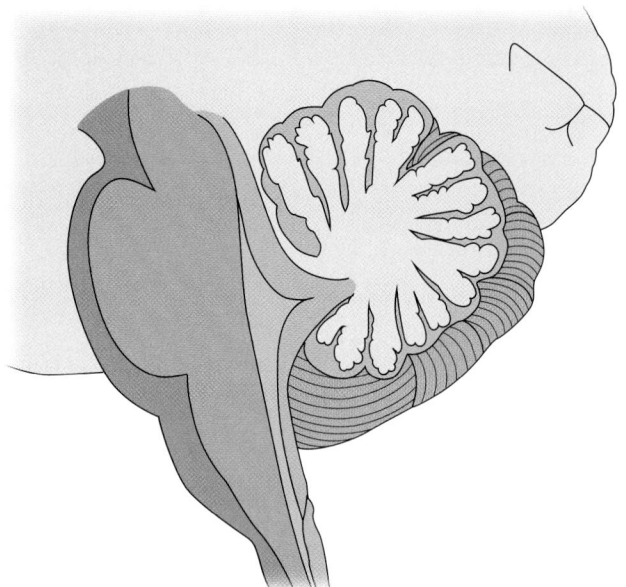

Fig. 19.1 The Cerebellum, Bisected Through the Midsagittal Plane.

between the cerebellum and spinal cord are uncrossed or double-crossed, whereas pathways between the cerebellum and cerebrum are crossed. Hence a lesion to one side of the cerebellum produces ataxia and related cerebellar deficits involving the same side of the body as the lesion. Also note that the cerebellum has relatively few direct projections to the spinal cord. Instead, it exerts a strong influence on movement through its projections to cerebral and brain stem motor structures, as described later.

Anatomical Divisions

The cerebellum is part of the hindbrain and is positioned on the dorsal surface of the brain stem at approximately the level of the pons (Fig. 19.1). It is connected to the brain stem by the superior, middle, and inferior cerebellar peduncles. The cerebellar peduncles contain all of the axons that transmit information to and from the cerebellum. The cerebellum can be anatomically divided into three lobes; the anterior, posterior, and flocculonodular lobes. The primary fissure divides the anterior and posterior lobes, and the posterolateral fissure divides the posterior and flocculonodular lobes (Fig. 19.2).

Looking at a sagittal slice through the cerebellum, distinct cellular regions can be visualized. The most superficial region is the cerebellar

cortex, which, unlike cerebral cortex, contains only three layers. The arrangement of cells within the cortex is strikingly uniform across all cerebellar lobes and plays a vital role in determining cerebellar function, which will be described later. Deep to the cerebellar cortex is the white matter layer, which contains the axons of Purkinje cells projecting out from cerebellar cortex and the axons of mossy and climbing fibers entering the cortex from other brain and spinal regions (see Fig. 19.1). The cerebellar nuclei are the output structures of the cerebellum, and they make up the deepest region. These are groups of neuronal cell bodies that receive information coming into the cerebellum from the periphery and also from the cerebellar cortex, via Purkinje cell axons. The deep nuclei are arranged in pairs, with one nucleus of each pair on each side of the cerebellum. Most medially are the fastigial nuclei, followed by the globose and emboliform nuclei and, most laterally, the broad dentate nuclei (see Fig. 19.2). The medial and lateral vestibular nuclei also receive inputs directly from the cerebellar flocculonodular lobe and are therefore sometimes considered an additional set of cerebellar output structures.

Functional Divisions and Their Afferent and Efferent Projections

Probably the most useful way of thinking about the anatomy of the cerebellum is to divide it into distinct functional longitudinal "zones."[12] Each cerebellar zone consists of a region of cerebellar cortex and its own pair of deep cerebellar nuclei. Each zone also has projections to and from distinct areas of the brain and spinal cord. Thus despite the regular arrangement of cells over the entire cerebellum, each functional longitudinal zone is uniquely positioned to control certain types of movement but not others.[12–14] See Table 19.3 for a summary.

The medial zone consists of the midline structure, the vermis, and the fastigial nuclei. This region of the cerebellum predominantly receives afferent information from the brain stem vestibular and reticular nuclei and the dorsal and ventral spinocerebellar pathways,[15–20] which convey important information regarding the current sensorimotor state of the trunk and limbs.[21–23] In turn its outputs, through the fastigial nuclei, are largely to reticular and vestibular nuclei, which will form part of the medial descending system (reticulospinal and vestibulospinal tracts), with some additional projections to the cerebral cortex via the thalamus.[24–26] The medial cerebellar zone is involved in the control of posture and muscle tone, upright stance, locomotion, and gaze and other eye movements.

The intermediate zone is made up of the intermediate hemispheres and the globose and emboliform nuclei. This region also receives inputs from the dorsal and ventral spinocerebellar pathways and brain stem reticular nuclei, as well as some projections from cerebral cortex

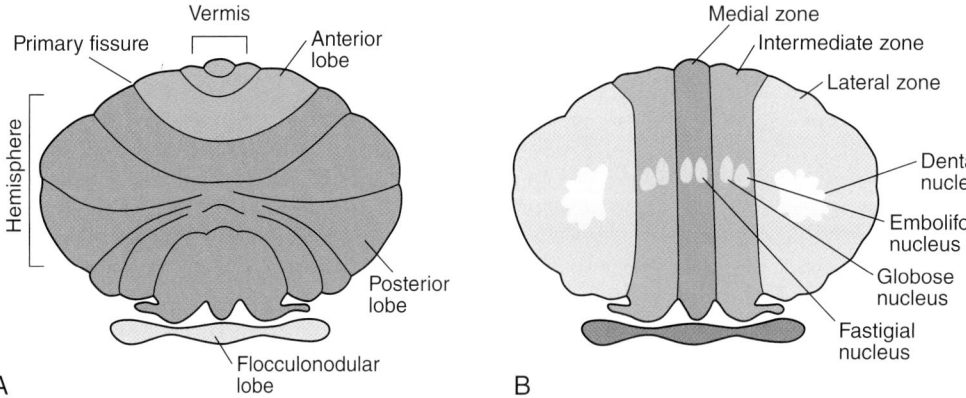

Fig. 19.2 The Cerebellum, Flattened, Showing Key Structures. **(A)** Different shading distinguishes the three lobes of the cerebellum. The cerebellar vermis and hemispheres are also shown. **(B)** Functional longitudinal cerebellar zones, distinguished by different shading, and the locations of the deep cerebellar nuclei within each zone.

TABLE 19.3 Functional Longitudinal Cerebellar Zones

Functional Zone	Alternate Name	Major Afferents	Major Efferents	Role in Movement	Clinical Signs If Damaged
Flocculonodular lobe Flocculonodular lobe; med and lat vestib nuclei	Vestibulocerebellum	• Vestib primary afferents • Vestib nuclei • Visual areas	• Med and lat vestib nuclei	• VOR • Gaze and eye movements • Posture and balance	• Nystagmus • Impaired VOR • Imbalance
Medial zone Vermis; fastigial nuclei	Spinocerebellum	• Vestib and retic nuclei • DSCT and VSCT	• Vestib and retic nuclei • Cerebrum	• Gaze and eye movements • Postural tone • Balance • Locomotion	• Oculomotor deficits • Hypotonia • Imbalance • Falls • Gait ataxia
Intermediate zone Intermediate hemispheres; globose and emboliform nuclei		• DSCT and VSCT • Retic nuclei • Cerebrum	• Cerebrum • Red nucleus	• Limb movements • Coordinate agonist-antagonist muscle pairs	• Imbalance • Gait ataxia • Tremor • Lack of check • Dysdiadochokinesia • Dysmetria
Lateral zone Lateral hemispheres; dentate nuclei	Cerebrocerebellum or Neocerebellum	• Cerebrum (wide range of areas: motor, pre-motor, prefrontal, so-matosensory, sensory association, visual, auditory cortices)	• Cerebrum (same areas as afferent projections) • Red nucleus	• Complex, multijoint voluntary limb move-ments • Visually guided movements • Motor planning • Sensorimotor error assessment	• Dysdiadochokinesia • Dysmetria • Dyssynergia • Decomposition

DSCT, Dorsal spinocerebellar tract; *Lat,* lateral; *Med,* medial; *Retic,* reticular; *Vestib,* vestibular; *VOR,* vestibuloocular reflex; *VSCT,* ventral spinocerebellar tract.

that arrive via the cerebropontocerebellar pathway.[13,15,16,27,28] Major projections from this cerebellar zone are to the cerebral cortex via the thalamus and to the red nucleus.[25,26,29] The intermediate zone is considered to be important in controlling coordination of agonist-antagonist muscle pairs during a variety of activities including walking and voluntary limb movements. The medial and intermediate zones of the cerebellum are collectively referred to as the spinocerebellum be-cause these are the only cerebellar regions that receive afferents from the spinal cord.

The largest region of the cerebellum is the lateral zone, which con-tains the two broad lateral hemispheres and their output structure, the dentate nuclei. Afferents to the lateral zone predominantly come from the cerebrum, from a wide variety of cortical areas including motor, premotor, and prefrontal cortices, parietal somatosensory and sensory association areas, and primary visual and auditory cortices.[27,28] Outputs from the dentate travel mostly back to large areas of the cere-brum (through the thalamus), to many of the same areas from which afferents arrived in the cerebellum. Again, these include vast regions of sensorimotor cortices.[29,30–35] Other efferent fibers project to the red nucleus in the brain stem. The lateral cerebellar zone plays a major role in control of complex, multijoint voluntary limb movements, particu-larly those involving visual guidance, and for the planning of complex movements and the assessment of movement errors. Because this re-gion of the cerebellum interacts predominantly with the cerebrum, it is also commonly called the cerebrocerebellum. It is also sometimes referred to as the neocerebellum because it is considered to have arisen fairly recently in the phylogenetic tree, being much more expansive in primates than in lower animals.[36]

The flocculonodular lobe can be considered a fourth zone of the cerebellum. It receives afferent projections directly from the vestibular primary afferents (semicircular canals and otoliths), as well as from vestibular nuclei and visual brain regions.[13,15,16,18,20] Outputs from the flocculonodular lobe project directly to the medial and lateral vestibular nuclei of the brain stem, without a synapse in a deep cerebellar nu-cleus.[14,24,37] For this reason, these vestibular nuclei are sometimes con-sidered an additional set of deep cerebellar nuclei. This cerebellar zone helps to control eye movements and balance. The well-known vestibu-loocular reflex (VOR), which provides gaze stabilization during head turning or walking, relies upon the cerebellum for proper function-ing.[38,39] Because of its critical ties to the vestibular system, the flocculo-nodular lobe is also known as the vestibulocerebellum (see Fig. 19.2).

Physiology of Cerebellar Neuronal Circuits

Within a longitudinal zone, thousands of microzones may exist,[13] each consisting of a highly organized group of connected cerebellar cortical neurons. A microcomplex is the name given to a neural circuit made up of a single microzone plus the other connected neurons with which it communicates directly. The following section provides a very brief overview of the circuits important for cerebellar function and reviews the flow of neuronal signals into and out of cerebellar microzones (Fig. 19.3).

Most afferent information enters the cerebellum through one of two pathways, the mossy fiber pathway or the climbing fiber pathway. Both have important actions on cerebellar Purkinje cells. The mossy fiber pathway affects "beams" or rows of Purkinje cells oriented along the cerebellar folia. Dense mossy fiber inputs arise from a wide variety

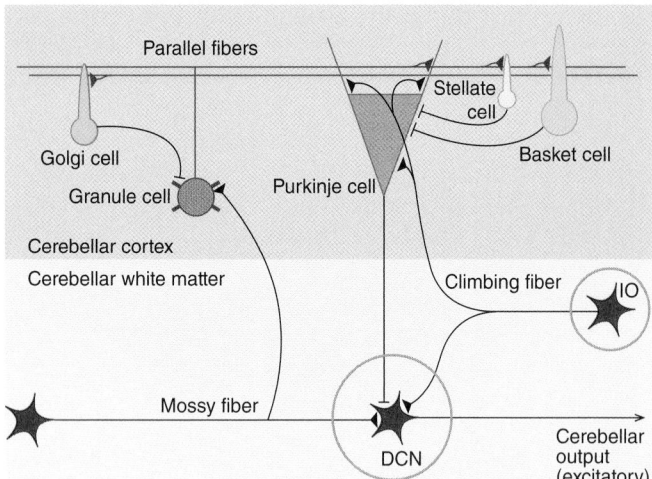

Fig. 19.3 Schematic of the Major Cell Types and Their Connections Within the Cerebellum. Excitatory synapses are indicated with a triangle; inhibitory synapses with a bar. *DCN,* Deep cerebellar nucleus; *IO,* inferior olive. (Adapted with permission from Elsevier, Ito M. Cerebellar circuitry as a neuronal machine. *Prog Neurobiol.* 2006;78(3-5):272-303.)

of regions, including cerebral cortex, several subcortical areas, the brain stem, and spinal cord. Mossy fibers enter the cerebellar cortex and synapse onto granule cells, whose axons ascend and branch into parallel fibers. Each parallel fiber extends long distances longitudinally and synapses onto many Purkinje cells all located along the same beam.[40] Each parallel fiber has a relatively weak effect on single Purkinje cells, but the mass effect of many thousands of parallel fiber contacts with Purkinje cells drives the Purkinje cells to fire at high rates.[41] In contrast, each climbing fiber arises exclusively from the inferior olive located in the brain stem and contacts only a few (approximately 1 to 10) Purkinje cells.[14,42,43] Each Purkinje cell receives information from only one climbing fiber, yet the climbing fiber's effect on the Purkinje cell is powerful, causing large complex spikes.

The Purkinje cell provides the output for the cerebellar cortex; each Purkinje cell axon projects to one of the deep cerebellar nuclei. The mossy fiber and climbing fiber pathways affect Purkinje cells differently and are thought to transmit different types of information. Mossy fibers are active at very high rates (generating action potentials at approximately 100 Hz) and are highly modulated by various sensory stimuli and motor activity. They have been speculated to relay information related to the direction, velocity, duration, or magnitude of movements or sensory stimuli.[44–47] However, climbing fibers are active at very low rates (approximately 1 to 4 Hz) and do not appear to be as strongly modulated by sensory stimuli or motor activity.[42,48,49] There is still some disagreement regarding what sort of information is encoded in the climbing fiber signals, but the frequency of discharge appears to be too low to transmit information pertaining to specific parameters of sensory or motor events. However, the role of the climbing fiber is clearly important because its firing produces large complex spikes in the Purkinje cells and can also powerfully affect subsequent Purkinje cell firing.[43,50] Therefore it is often considered to serve as a sort of "teaching" signal to Purkinje cells.

CEREBELLAR FUNCTION IN ADAPTING AND CONTROLLING MOVEMENT

The cytoarchitecture of the microzones is extremely stereotyped throughout the cerebellum, suggesting that it performs the same

overall function regardless of whether it is acting on circuits controlling standing balance, eye movements, or reaching and grasping, etc. So, what is the function of this cerebellar circuit? What aspect of motor control does it uniquely provide? Despite centuries of study, these questions have still not been answered completely. Although numerous theories of cerebellar function exist, here we limit the discussion to just a few that we view as particularly relevant.

Theories of Cerebellar Function

One general theory states that a primary function of the cerebellum is in coordinating multiple limb segments to generate smooth and fluid multijoint movements.[51–54] This "motor coordinator" theory has support from behavioral studies demonstrating that multijoint movements appear to be particularly impaired in patients with cerebellar lesions.[52] Multijoint movements are inherently more complex than single joint movements because they require control of mechanical interaction torques, those occurring at one segment but caused by movement of other linked segments.[55] This model suggests that the cerebellum predicts the mechanical interactions between segments based on a stored internal knowledge of limb dynamics and helps to generate the correct motor commands for appropriate multijoint movements.

A second popular theory is the timer hypothesis. This idea proposes that the cerebellum is the main site for the temporal representation of movements.[56,57] Supporters of this theory suggest that cerebellar output ultimately encodes the precise temporal sequence of muscle activation with such precision that when it is lesioned it produces obvious deficits in the spatial (e.g., movement direction and magnitude) as well as the temporal domain.[58] Other studies have shown that individuals with cerebellar damage also have impairments in perceiving time intervals, suggesting that this could be a more general cerebellar function.[59,60]

A third idea is that the cerebellum acts as an internal model to allow predictive control of movement. Sensory feedback is inadequate for movements that need to be both fast and accurate: it is too slow, and as a result, motor corrections would be issued too late. Instead, the brain generates motor commands based on an internal prediction of how the command would move the body. This "feedforward" control requires stored knowledge of the body's dynamics, the environment, and the object to be manipulated; it is learned from previous exposure. The neural representation of this knowledge is referred to as an internal model[61–64] because it provides the ability to reproduce the effects of motor actions in the brain. The internal model theory for cerebellar function states that the cerebellum serves as the site of an internal model for movement. Accordingly, the incoordination of movement associated with cerebellar damage is a consequence of a disrupted internal model, which disrupts nearly all aspects of feedforward motor control.[65] This idea is appealing because it could help to explain the wide variety of motor behaviors (e.g., reaching, standing balance, eye movements) and movement parameters (e.g., force, direction) that can be impaired following cerebellar damage. Likewise, human behavioral studies have recently pointed out that cerebellar damage is frequently associated with impaired feedforward control but relatively intact feedback mechanisms.[66,67]

A related theory originates from the seminal works of Marr,[68] Albus,[69] and Ito,[70] in which the cerebellum was theorized to be a sort of "learning machine." This theory was based on careful examination of the anatomy and physiology within cerebellar microcircuits and continues to provide the basis for many of the current theories of cerebellar function (i.e., those described above). Central to the idea of cerebellar involvement in learning was the discovery that Purkinje cell output can be radically altered by climbing fiber induction of long-term depression (LTD) of the parallel fiber–Purkinje cell synapse.[50] Hence climbing fiber inputs onto Purkinje cells can be viewed as providing a unique type of teaching or error signal to the cerebellum. More recently LTD, long-term potentiation (LTP), and nonsynaptic plasticity have all been shown to exist at numerous sites within the cerebellum, both in the cortex as well as the deep cerebellar nuclei.[71–74] Thus there are multiple avenues for activity-dependent plasticity to occur within the cerebellum over relatively short time scales. It is presumed that the plastic changes in cerebellar output are responsible for changing motor behavior during the process of learning new skills.

To summarize, although the precise mechanisms are still under debate, most researchers can agree upon a few central themes of cerebellar function. First, the cerebellum is an integral structure for the coordination of movements. Second, precisely timed interactions between neurons produce activity-dependent plasticity at a number of different sites within the cerebellum. Presumably, this plasticity plays a fundamental role in motor learning. Convergence of these two themes would seem to indicate that a major cerebellar function is to maintain optimal motor control through constant adaptive learning processes, so that movements are appropriately adjusted for varying environmental demands.

CLINICAL MANIFESTATIONS OF CEREBELLAR LESIONS

Ataxia is the primary sign of damage to the cerebellum or its input structures. Ataxia refers generally to uncoordinated or disordered movement, which, although most often associated with gait ("gait ataxia"), can also be used to describe uncoordinated arm or leg movements ("limb ataxia"). Ataxia is exacerbated by moving multiple joints together and by moving quickly. Because ataxia is a nonspecific term, it is important in both clinical and research settings to use more precise terminology to describe the specific aspects of motor performance that are impaired. Around the beginning of the 20th century, Joseph Babinski and Gordon Holmes were two of the earliest investigators to describe many of these specific features we now discuss here.[75–77]

Dysmetria

Dysmetria specifically refers to an impaired ability to properly scale movement distance. Movements are described as either hypermetric or hypometric, referring to overshooting or undershooting of targets, respectively. Many patients with cerebellar lesions will show both forms of dysmetria even during successive movements (Fig. 19.4).[51,52] Dysmetria can be seen in both proximal and distal joints and occurs during both single-joint and multijoint movements, although multijoint movements worsen dysmetria (Fig. 19.5).[52,78–80] Slow movements tend to produce hypometria, whereas fast movements almost always bring about hypermetria.[51] For this reason, it has been speculated that hypometria represents more of a voluntary compensation for hypermetria than a primary impairment from cerebellar damage. Sometimes large end point errors can be reduced to some degree with visual feedback, but even the corrective movements themselves are still abnormal.[81]

One proposed mechanism for dysmetria is an impaired ability to predict and account for the dynamics of the limbs. In particular, patients with cerebellar lesions have been demonstrated to have a specific deficit in the ability to account for interaction torques,[51,52] the rotational forces that act on a limb segment when another linked limb segment is in motion.[55] When the cerebellum is intact, the central nervous system is able to predict the effects of interactions torques and appropriately counter or exploit them so as to produce a smooth, straight, and accurate reach in a feedforward manner. When the cerebellum is damaged, an incorrect or absent accounting for interaction torques leads to an incorrect feedforward motor plan and subsequently,

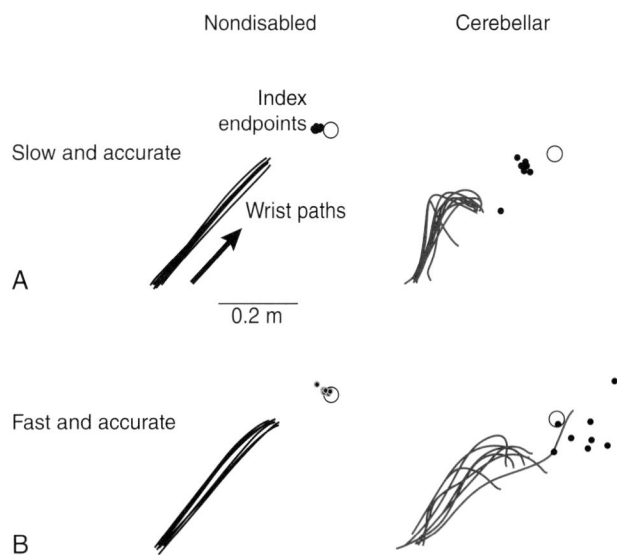

Fig. 19.4 Trajectories of the wrist *(solid lines)* and final end point positions of the tip of the index finger *(filled circles)* during **(A)** slow and accurate and **(B)** fast and accurate reaches from a typical nondisabled individual *(left)* and a subject with cerebellar damage *(right)*. The subject with cerebellar damage shows dysmetria and an abnormally curved wrist path. Note also the tendency for hypometria during slow movements and hypermetria during fast movements (the same control and cerebellar subjects are shown in [A] and [B]). Several reaches are overlaid for each subject. Arrow indicates the reach direction. Large open circles indicate the target locations. (Adapted with permission from the American Physiological Society, Bastian AJ, Martin TA, Keating JG, Thach WT. Cerebellar ataxia: abnormal control of interaction torques across multiple joints. *J Neurophysiol.* 1996;76[1]:492–509.)

an uncoordinated, overly curved and hypermetric or hypometric reach that requires feedback corrections to reach the target location.

Dyssynergia

Originally, Babinski[75] coined the term "asynergia" as a deficit in the coordination of movements of one body region or in one limb segment with movements of another. Currently, dyssynergia is used to describe impairment of multijoint movements, wherein movements of specific segments are not properly sequenced or of the proper range or direction, resulting in uncoordinated multijoint movement. As indicated earlier, it is nearly universally true that patients with significant cerebellar damage show greater impairments during multijoint movements than single-joint movements. However, it is not fully understood whether the reason for that is because the deficits of single-joint movements are compounded during a multijoint movement or because the cerebellum plays a special and unique role in multijoint control. Dyssynergia appears to be related to dysmetria and therefore is probably also related to a deficit in predicting limb dynamics.[51]

Dysdiadochokinesia

Dysdiadochokinesia specifically refers to a deficit in the coordination between agonist-antagonist muscle pairs elicited during voluntary rapid alternating movements.[82] It is typically tested during performance of simple, fast alternating movements such as forearm supination-pronation or hand or foot tapping. Characteristic deficits are excessive slowness along with inconsistency in the rate and range of the alternating movements, which worsen as the movement continues.[76] Dysdiadochokinesia appears to be caused by poor regulation of the timing of cessation of agonist and the initiation of antagonist muscle activity,[83,84]

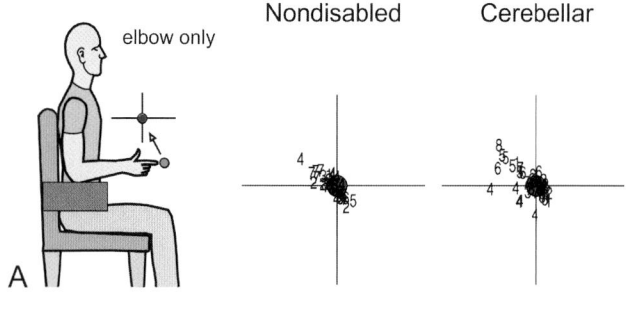

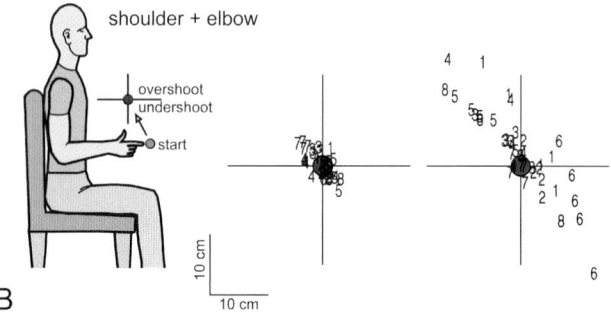

Fig. 19.5 Final end point positions of the tip of the index finger (numbers, each value corresponds to a different subject) during **(A)** single-joint (elbow only) and **(B)** multijoint (combined shoulder and elbow) reaches from nondisabled *(left)* and cerebellar *(right)* subjects. Cerebellar dysmetria (both hypometria and hypermetria) is greatly exacerbated during the multijoint reaching condition. Multiple reaches are shown for all subjects. *Arrow* indicates the reach direction. *Large open circles* indicate the target locations. (Adapted with permission from the American Physiological Society, Bastian AJ, Zackowski KM, Thach WT. Cerebellar ataxia: torque deficiency or torque mismatch between joints? *J Neurophysiol.* 2000;83[5]:3019–3030.)

which could be related to a deficit in predicting limb dynamics. Indeed, rapid reversals in movement are dynamically difficult to control.

Decomposition

Movement decomposition refers to the breaking down of a movement sequence or a multijoint movement into a series of separate movements, each simpler than the combined movement.[77] An example of this is the well-known finding that patients with cerebellar damage, when asked to reach to a target in front of and above the resting arm, will often flex the shoulder first and then, while holding the shoulder fixed, extend the elbow.[51] This approach is generally slower and will produce a more curved trajectory of the finger to the target compared with nondisabled individuals who would typically perform the shoulder flexion and elbow extension at the same time to produce a nearly straight-line finger trajectory. Most likely decomposition reflects a compensatory strategy for dealing with impaired multijoint movements than it does a primary sign of cerebellar damage.[51,85]

Lack of Check

Lack of check, sometimes also referred to as excessive "rebound," refers to the inability to rapidly and sufficiently halt movement of a body part after a strong isometric force, previously resisting movement of the body part, is suddenly released. Individuals without cerebellar damage can very quickly halt, or "check," this unintended movement. Individuals with cerebellar damage, on the other hand, are known to have considerable movement in the direction opposing the previous resistance, to the point that the unchecked movement risks upright balance and/or self-injury. This phenomenon is presumed to be caused by delayed cessation of agonist and/or delayed activation of the antagonist muscles.

Cerebellar Tremor

Despite being a very common neurological sign, tremor is poorly defined and not well understood. There are several different forms of tremor, many with different etiologies, only some of which are related to cerebellar dysfunction, so it is important to distinguish among them. Tremor associated with damage to the cerebellum is typically called action tremor, reflecting the fact that it is absent at rest and elicited during muscle activation, and importantly, distinguishing it from the resting tremor associated with Parkinson disease. Action tremor can be classified as postural or kinetic tremor.[86] Postural tremor occurs in muscles maintaining a static position against gravity (e.g., holding arms out in front of the body or standing in place), whereas kinetic tremor occurs in muscles producing an active voluntary movement. Therefore the movement oscillations are most visible in the same plane as the voluntary movement. Kinetic tremor typically occurs at relatively low frequencies (~2 to 5 Hz) and can be observed during simple non–target-directed movements such as forearm pronation and supination or foot tapping, or during targeted movements such as pointing during the finger-to-nose test. Intention tremor is a specific form of kinetic tremor, which occurs during the terminal portions of visually guided movements toward a target. It may actually represent the multiple corrective movements, driven by visual feedback, to reach the target. As such, intention tremor can be tested by repeating the test movement with eyes closed: if the tremor decreases substantially or disappears, it is intention tremor.[81]

Classic cerebellar tremor is kinetic tremor with intention tremor at movement termination. In general, cerebellar tremor is thought to be due to an insufficient ability to anticipate the effects of movement and excessive reliance on sensory feedback loops.[87] Cerebellar tremor is highly influenced by sensory conditions and has a strong mechanical component: it is significantly reduced during isometric conditions or when vision is removed. It also can be decreased in some patients by adding an inertial load to the limb,[88] although that strategy may also act to increase dysmetria.[89] There may also be a significant central component to cerebellar tremor, possibly related to influences from the thalamus or the inferior olive.[83,90]

Hypotonia

Hypotonia in patients with cerebellar damage was first described by Holmes.[77] It appears to arise from decreased excitatory drive to vestibulospinal and reticulospinal pathways, two major output pathways from the cerebellar vermis and flocculonodular lobe. The hypotonia usually presents as a decrease in the extensor tone necessary for holding the body upright against gravity. In cats, lesions to either the vestibular or fastigial nuclei cause this sort of postural hypotonia.[53,91–93] More recent observations in humans indicate that hypotonia is typically most problematic in cases of severe cerebellar hypoplasias affecting the vermis, such as Joubert syndrome,[94] or in adults during the acute stage of cerebellar injury only. In cases of adult-onset acute injury, hypotonia usually resolves naturally over time and patients recover normal passive muscle tone and normal reflexes quickly. Thus hypotonia typically presents minimal to no problems for physical function.[83]

Imbalance

Another cardinal sign of cerebellar damage is postural instability in both static and dynamic conditions. Specifically, patients with cerebellar damage usually show increased postural sway, either excessive or diminished postural responses to perturbations, poor control of equilibrium during voluntary movements of the head, arms, or legs, and sometimes abnormal oscillations of the trunk, called titubation.

Classically, cerebellar imbalance during stance was considered to be of a similar magnitude whether or not the eyes are open (i.e., little improvement noted with visual feedback[75,77] and a negative Romberg test). However, more recently, investigators using posturography measures have been able to distinguish several different categories of cerebellar imbalance during quiet standing, some of which do show improvement with visual stabilization.[95,96] For instance, patients with cerebellar damage relatively isolated to the anterior lobe typically show increased postural sway that is of a high velocity and low amplitude and occurs mainly in the anterior-posterior dimension. These individuals also tend to have associated postural tremor and increased intersegmental movements of the head, trunk, and legs and tend to improve when allowed visual information. On the other hand, localized damage to the vestibulocerebellum more often leads to increased postural sway that consists of low-frequency and high-amplitude movements without a preferred direction and without increased intersegmental movements. These individuals typically show no improvement with visual information. Patients with damage limited to the lateral cerebellum tend to have only slight or even no postural instability at all.[95–97]

Human cerebellar damage is also associated with hypermetric postural responses to surface displacements or during step initiation (i.e., dynamic instability).[98,99] Specifically, patients tend to produce larger than normal surface-reactive torque responses and exaggerated and prolonged muscle activity, thereby overshooting the initial posture during the return phase of the recovery from a perturbation (Fig. 19.6).

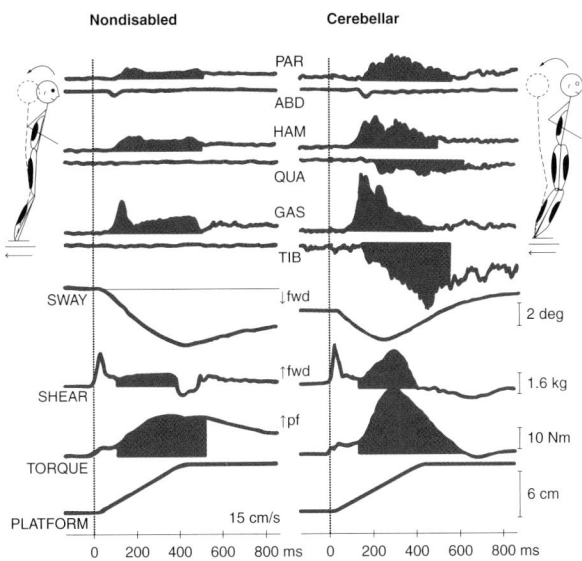

Fig. 19.6 Postural responses from nondisabled control and cerebellar groups (average of 10 trials from 10 subjects in each group) after backward platform translations of 15 cm/s for 6 cm. Traces show *(top to bottom)* electromyographic recordings from various postural muscle groups, postural sway, shear force, surface torque, and platform displacement. Filled areas indicate the first 400 ms of activation in the electromyographic traces and the active surface reactive forces in the shear force and torque traces. Postural responses of the cerebellar subjects are increased, with excessive and prolonged muscle activity (note especially the abnormal activation of flexor muscle groups), larger sway and greater torque production. *ABD*, Rectus abdominus; *fwd*, forward; *GAS*, gastrocnemius; *HAM*, biceps femoris; *PAR*, paraspinals; *pf*, plantarflexion; *QUA*, rectus femoris; *TIB*, tibialis anterior. (Adapted with permission from the American Physiological Society, Horak FB, Diener HC. Cerebellar control of postural scaling and central set in stance. *J Neurophysiol.* 1994;72[2]:479–493.)

Gait Ataxia

Probably the greatest complaint and the most obvious sign of cerebellar damage is gait ataxia. This abnormal pattern of walking is often described as a "drunken" gait because patients often stagger and lose balance as if intoxicated. Early work of Holmes showed that patients with cerebellar lesions have severe difficulty maintaining balance during walking, which often leads to falls, typically directed backward and toward the side of the lesion. Holmes reported specifically that walking is slowed, with steps that are short, irregular in timing, and unequal in length. The legs sometimes lift overly high during swing phase by excessive flexion at the hip and knee and then lower abruptly and with uncontrolled force. The trajectory of walking often veers erratically, and patients have difficulty with stops or turns, especially if performed quickly.[77]

Those initial reports have been confirmed numerous times; patients with cerebellar damage walk without the consistency in timing, length, and direction of steps typical of healthy adults.[79,100] In some cases, gait appears wide based. There is also increased variability in both the timing and movement excursion at the hip, knee, and ankle joints, and irregularities in the resulting path of the foot during swing. Coordination between joints of one leg and between legs (intralimb and interlimb coordination) is also abnormal.[79,100,101] As an example, the timing of peak flexion at one joint with respect to other joints' positions may be altered or inconsistent. Often decomposition is also observed between hip and knee, knee and ankle, and/or hip and ankle joints.[101,102]

A critical component of locomotor control is the requirement for stability and dynamic balance while maintaining forward propulsion. Thus imbalance, described earlier, is also a major contributor to many features of gait ataxia. In fact, it has been shown that patients with cerebellar damage and significant balance deficits also typically demonstrate nearly all the classic features of gait ataxia (i.e., reduced stride lengths, increased stride widths, reduced joint excursions, abnormal swing foot trajectories, increased variability in foot placement, and joint-joint decomposition). In contrast, patients with cerebellar damage and significant leg coordination deficits but minimal or no balance deficits typically have very few walking abnormalities (Fig. 19.7).[103,104] Therefore during typical conditions of level walking, balance deficits contribute much more strongly to cerebellar gait ataxia than do leg coordination deficits.

Oculomotor Deficits

Eye movements are often dramatically impaired following cerebellar damage. Saccades are often slowed and dysmetric (can be hypermetric or hypometric).[105] Smooth pursuit may be "choppy," referred to as saccadic pursuit, wherein the smooth tracking of a target is degraded into a series of shorter saccadic movements following behind the target.[106] The ability to cancel, or suppress, the VOR may be impaired or absent.[107] Finally, abnormal nystagmus may also be present. The nystagmus may occur during central gaze, or there may also be alternating nystagmus or rebound nystagmus. The most common form of nystagmus in cerebellar dysfunction is gaze-evoked nystagmus, indicating nystagmus elicited toward the end ranges of lateral and/or vertical gaze.[108,109]

Patients with significant oculomotor abnormalities may be referred to vestibular specialists, but these deficits should never be ignored. Impaired eye movements may have a significant negative impact on physical function. For example, impaired saccades can prevent a patient from reading and saccadic pursuit can exacerbate already poor visually guided limb movements.[110] Perhaps most devastating, deficits related to impaired oculomotor control and vestibular reflexes often worsen dynamic balance and walking abilities.

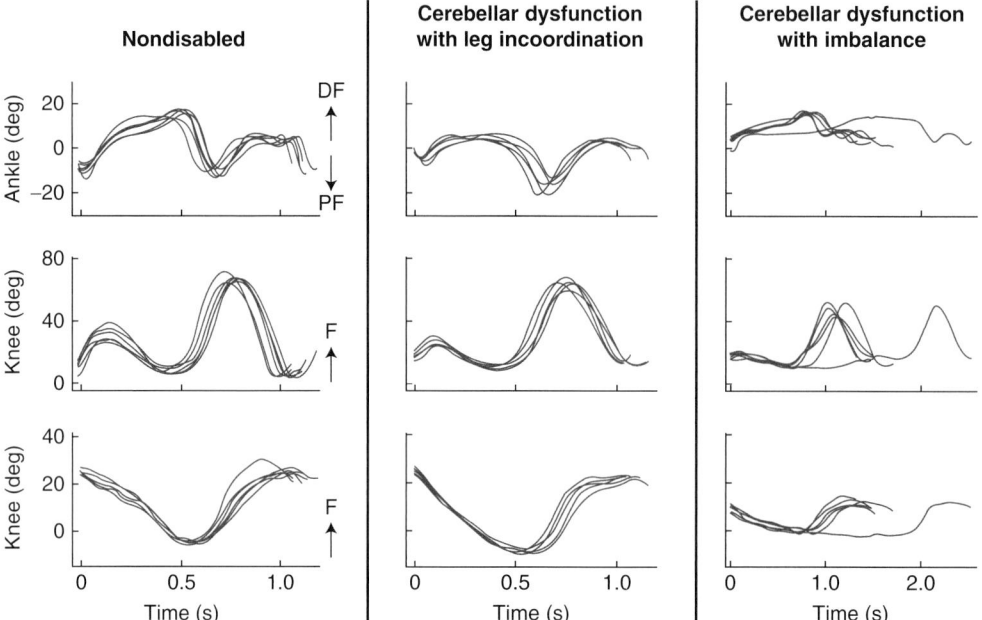

Fig. 19.7 Angular excursions at the ankle *(top row)*, knee *(middle)*, and hip *(bottom)* during fast walking from a typical nondisabled individual *(left column)*, a subject with cerebellar dysfunction who has significant leg incoordination but minimal imbalance *(middle)*, and a subject with cerebellar dysfunction who has significant imbalance but minimal leg incoordination *(right)*. Several strides (from initial contact to next initial contact) are overlaid for each subject. The patient with cerebellar imbalance *(shaded)* shows significant evidence of gait ataxia, including reduced joint excursions, excessive stride-to-stride variability, and abnormal timing between joints, whereas the patient with cerebellar leg incoordination and no imbalance shows no evidence of gait ataxia. *DF*, Dorsiflexion; *F*, flexion; *PF*, plantarflexion. (Adapted with permission from the American Physiological Society, Morton SM, Bastian AJ. Relative contributions of balance and voluntary leg-coordination deficits to cerebellar gait ataxia. *J Neurophysiol.* 2003;89[4]:1844–1856.)

Speech Impairments

Speech production may also be impaired when the cerebellum is damaged. Classically, the speech deficit associated with cerebellar damage is referred to as "scanning speech," although it may be more generally referred to as ataxic dysarthria. Similar to limb control deficits, the primary impairment of speech may be related to the planning and prediction of movements rather than in the execution of speech components directly.[111] Also like limb movements, most speech impairments appear to be attributable to alterations in timing and coordination.[112] The most consistent characteristics of ataxic dysarthria are impaired articulation (the correct pronouncement of speech sounds) and impaired prosody (the pattern of stress and intonation of certain syllables or words). Other common findings include slowed speech and either a lack of or excessive loudness variability.[111] Traditionally, speech impairments are treated primarily by speech and language pathologists.

Impaired Motor Learning

A critical problem associated with cerebellar damage is impaired motor learning. In humans, the cerebellum has been linked to learning of a wide variety of motor behaviors, including recovering balance after a perturbation,[98,99] learning new walking patterns,[66,102,113] adjusting voluntary limb movements,[67,114,115] and eye movements.[116,117] The type of learning that appears most reliant on the cerebellum is associative and procedural. Specifically, the cerebellum appears to be essential for learning to adjust a motor behavior through repeated practice of, or exposure to, the behavior and using error information from one trial to improve performance on subsequent trials. It is important to note

that cerebellum-dependent motor learning is driven by errors directly occurring during the movement, rather than other types of feedback, such as knowledge of results after the fact (e.g., hit or miss). Studies have suggested that the type of error that drives cerebellum-dependent learning is not the target error (i.e., "How far am I from the desired target?") but instead what has been referred to as a sensory prediction error (i.e., "How far am I from where I predicted I would be?").[115,118]

In the laboratory setting, cerebellar learning is most easily tested via motor adaptation, a form of motor learning that requires a modification of an already well-learned motor behavior for new environmental or physical demands (in contrast to learning of a completely novel skill). Adaptation is an error-driven learning process that is acquired on a time-scale of minutes or hours, as opposed to days or weeks.[119,120] It is an active process—movement adaptation takes trial-and-error practice of the task, where errors during one trial change movement on the subsequent trial. Storage of the adapted movement is shown by the presence of aftereffects when the new demand is removed. Specifically, aftereffects are movement errors in the opposite direction to the original errors during adaptation, and they provide strong evidence that the central nervous system adjusts the predictive control for body movements with practice.[64,121] Thus when the new demand is removed, a process of active "unlearning" or de-adaptation must occur to return the movement to its original form. An example of a locomotor adaptation is shown in Fig. 19.8. In this case a walking adaptation is induced by having subjects walk on a splitbelt treadmill, where one belt is moving at twice the speed of the other, forcing the two legs to walk at different speeds. Nondisabled subjects are able to rapidly restore appropriate step length symmetry after only a few minutes walking on the splitbelt treadmill. They also appear to store the newly learned set of (predictive) motor commands, demonstrated by large negative aftereffects (step length asymmetry in the reverse direction compared to early adaptation) when the treadmill belts are initially returned to a regular (nonsplit) pattern. In contrast, individuals with cerebellar damage typically show a slower rate of adaptation, a reduced magnitude of adaptation or no adaptation at all, and small or no aftereffects. See Fig. 19.8. All of these findings indicate a significant deficiency in the capability for motor adaptation in individuals with cerebellar damage. As indicated earlier, adaptation deficits have been demonstrated in this patient population with numerous behavioral tasks.[58,66,67,98,99,113-116]

Cerebellum-dependent adaptation is not the only form of motor learning, but it is an important one for rehabilitation several reasons. First, adaptation is a highly automatic process to rapidly adjust movements for new, predictable demands (e.g., adjusting the walking pattern for snow or sand; adjusting eye movements for glasses). Individuals with impaired cerebellar adaptive learning must use other means to handle new task demands, such as conscious control strategies. This is obviously inefficient and difficult, because it means that the individuals must think much more about their movements and cannot tolerate distractions. Adaptation is also important because when it is repeated many times, it can result in more permanent storage of a movement pattern that can be called on immediately (i.e., no error-based period of adaptation required). A clear example of this is the use of new bifocal glasses. Initially, there is an adaptation process to adjust eye movements when switching between the top and bottom lenses because eye movements have to be bigger for magnified objects. Yet with repeated adaptation, the brain eventually stores two calibrations, one for viewing through the top lens and one for the bottom, that can be switched between immediately. Thus adaptation can lead to a more permanent, learned calibration that is used in specific situations. Patients with cerebellar damage will not be able to make these short-term adaptations normally, and theoretically one would expect that they will not be able to form the more permanent calibrations with repeated adaptation.

Other forms of motor learning may not depend on the cerebellum and thus may be particularly useful for rehabilitation for patients with cerebellar lesions, although this has never been formally tested. One example is use-dependent motor learning, in which a person strengthens a movement pattern with repeated practice of that same pattern.[122] It is not clear what mechanisms subserve this form of learning, although a Hebbian-like process in the cerebral cortex seems likely (i.e., repeated use strengthens the synapses in the brain that are engaged). Another form of motor learning is reward or reinforcement learning. This may involve basal ganglia circuits to strengthen movements that are rewarded.[123] It has not been experimentally tested whether individuals with cerebellar damage can undergo either of these other forms of learning. Yet if they can, these learning mechanisms might provide important compensatory strategies for the loss of error-dependent adaptations.

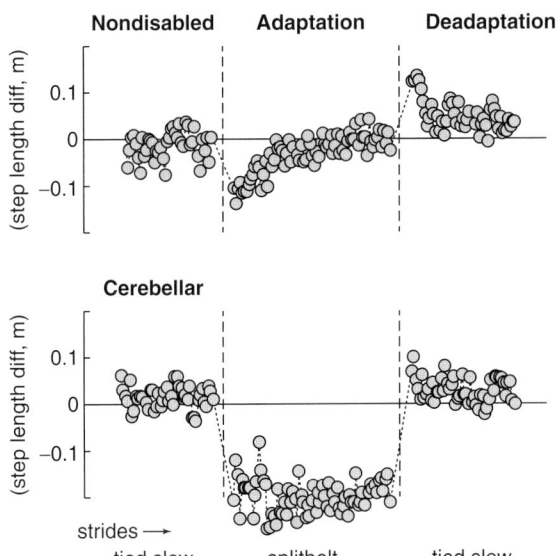

Fig. 19.8 Motor adaptation of step length symmetry during walking on a splitbelt treadmill from a nondisabled individual *(top)* and a subject with cerebellar damage *(bottom)*. Each data point represents the difference in step lengths between the legs (fast minus slow) for all strides during regular walking (belts tied, speed 0.5 m/s), splitbelt adaptation walking (fast belt speed 1.0 m/s; slow belt speed 0.5 m/s), and de-adaptation walking (belts tied, speed 0.5 m/s). Perfect symmetry between legs is represented by a step length difference value of 0. Note that the splitbelt condition perturbs step length symmetry initially in both subjects. The control subject rapidly adapts the walking pattern to restore appropriate step length symmetry while walking on split belts. The cerebellar subject does not adapt. Once the belts are returned to the tied condition, the control subject shows a large negative aftereffect (i.e., perturbed step length symmetry in the reverse direction), which again is rapidly adjusted to restore near-symmetric step lengths. The cerebellar subject shows a reduced aftereffect and no de-adaptation. (Adapted with permission from the Society for Neuroscience, Morton SM, Bastian AJ. Cerebellar contributions to locomotor adaptations during splitbelt treadmill walking. *J Neurosci.* 2006;26[36]:9107–9116.)

Nonmotor Impairments

Within the past 25 years, researchers have exposed a possible role of the cerebellum in a number of nonmotor, cognitive behaviors. Much of the early evidence for cerebellar involvement in nonmotor tasks came from functional imaging studies showing increased activation within the cerebellum during performance of certain tasks with a predominant cognitive component, such as language processing.[124,125] Speculation has since risen that the cerebellum may be involved in not only language, but also working memory,[126] learning nonmotor associations between objects,[127] and higher-order executive functions.[128] Loss of control over emotional behaviors[129] and certain neurodevelopmental and neuropsychiatric disorders have also been said to be linked to cerebellar damage.[130,131] However, interpretation of some investigations of the relationship between the cerebellum and cognition is limited in that it is sometimes difficult to separate the cognitive and motor components of a task, particularly in imaging studies in which subjects are instructed to perform some motor task to indicate a cognitive choice.[132,133] Nevertheless, anatomical studies have shown clearly that the cerebellum has connections to brain areas considered relatively purely cognitive in function, suggesting that a cognitive role for the cerebellum is likely.[134]

Clinical Signs by Functional Division

Because of the organizational structure of the cerebellum into functional longitudinal divisions, discreet areas are associated with specific signs and symptoms. Thus depending on the location and volume of cerebellar damage, patients may have just a few or nearly all of the clinical manifestations described earlier. Patients with damage to the flocculonodular lobe or midline zone typically present with some (although usually transient) loss of postural tone, impaired upright posture and balance, gait ataxia, and oculomotor deficits.[2,54] On the other hand, damage to the intermediate zone often results in action tremor, dysdiadochokinesia, and dysmetria of the limbs.[2,53] Finally, damage to the lateral zone commonly produces dyssynergia, dysmetria, and difficulty planning complex limb movements, especially those that are visually guided.[2,53]

Often, however, multiple longitudinal zones are affected at the same time. For instance, the arteries supplying the cerebellum each span more than one longitudinal zone, such that a stroke involving a single cerebellar artery would be likely to cause signs and symptoms associated with more than one zone (see Table 19.3). Degenerative disorders affecting the cerebellum also are typically pancerebellar, affecting large regions of the cerebellum. Hence these patients will also typically present with a wide variety of signs and symptoms. A careful and thorough clinical examination is therefore a requirement before a diagnosis for physical therapy can be made in patients with cerebellar damage.

MEDICAL MANAGEMENT OF CEREBELLAR DAMAGE

The greatest limitation in caring for patients with cerebellar damage is the lack of any curative treatment for most forms of cerebellar damage. Pharmacological agents have been used but with limited success. Often, patients with ataxia and degenerative forms of cerebellar damage may be prescribed vitamin E, coenzyme Q10, and/or its synthetic analogs, but the effectiveness of these drugs in minimizing symptoms or otherwise slowing or halting the disease is largely unsubstantiated.[135,136] Other drugs that may be used include acetazolamide, amantadine, 4-aminopyridine, and buspirone chlorhydrate,[8,137–139] but these also have questionable effectiveness. Studies of the effectiveness of medications for cerebellar ataxia have been significantly limited by inadequate sample sizes, inappropriate outcome measures, and/or limited follow-up. Given the unsatisfactory results from pharmacological interventions thus far, most patients with cerebellar ataxias must rely primarily or solely on physical rehabilitation approaches to restore or reduce the symptoms of their disease.

PHYSICAL THERAPY MANAGEMENT OF CEREBELLAR MOVEMENT DYSFUNCTION

As is the case with all brain lesions, there is nearly always some level of natural, or spontaneous, recovery following damage to the cerebellum. The extent of recovery depends on complex interactions among numerous factors including the source of damage, the severity, location and volume of damage, the presence or absence of damage to other brain regions, the presence or absence of other coexisting medical conditions, age, and other factors. Several studies have indicated that motor recovery from a first ever ischemic cerebellar stroke is generally excellent, with minimal to no residual deficits in up to 83% of individuals.[140–142] On the other hand, individuals with a degenerative cerebellar disorders tend to have progressively worsening clinical signs and symptoms.[143] One study has shown that people with damage to the deep nuclei do not recover as well as those with damage to only the cerebellar cortex and white matter.[2] Another consideration is the degree to which other brain regions are lesioned. Individuals with cerebellar stroke or tumor may also have damage of the brain stem. Patients with multiple sclerosis or head injury often also suffer from cerebral and spinal cord lesions. Moreover, the majority of the SCAs affect other neural structures well beyond the cerebellum; these are often the corticospinal tract, cerebral cortex, basal ganglia, and sometimes even the peripheral nervous system. In general, the presence of multiple lesion locations is associated with a poorer outcome, possibly because circuits that could otherwise serve in a compensatory role are also damaged.[144]

Physical Therapy Examination

A majority of the components of the physical therapy examination for patients with cerebellar dysfunction are the same as would be performed with any patient with a health condition that is primarily neurological in origin. Therefore we will discuss only the features that are unique or of critical importance for the patient with cerebellar pathology. As follows, we highlight just a few of these specific tests. Box 19.1 contains a

---

BOX 19.1 Typical Clinical Tests and Measures for the Physical Therapy Evaluation of Cerebellar Dysfunction

Tests of Impairments of Body Function or Structure

1. Muscle Tone

   Hypotonia Particularly involving postural extensor muscle groups. Can be assessed in supine, sitting, and/or standing.

2. Voluntary Movement Coordination

   *For all coordination tests, the following guidelines are recommended, when appropriate: (1) compare both sides; (2) repeat each test multiple times; (3) compare slow/preferred versus "fast as possible" speeds; (4) compare with and without vision.

   Finger-to-nose test: Vary the target (fingertip) locations. Require near-full excursion at elbow and shoulder. Observe for speed, dysmetria, dyssynergia, decomposition, kinetic tremor, intention tremor.

   Alternating forearm supination-pronation: Do not allow bracing of upper arm against trunk. Require elbow flexion/extension along with forearm movements. Observe for speed, dysmetria, dyssynergia, decomposition, dysdiadochokinesia, kinetic tremor.

   Hand/finger tapping: Observe for speed, dysmetria, dysdiadochokinesia, kinetic tremor.

   Drawing/handwriting sample: Compare with and without permitting bracing upper arm against trunk and/or forearm on writing surface. Observe for speed, dysmetria, dyssynergia, decomposition, kinetic tremor, intention tremor.

   Holding static position, arms outstretched: Patient holds position for several seconds. Observe for drift, postural tremor.

   Resisted movements: Compare different levels of resistance. Observe for lack of check (rebound). Note: ensure patient safety; rebound may be extreme and destabilizing and/or injurious in severe cases.

   Heel-to-knee test: Patient performs in supine to test full excursion at hip and prevent bracing of thigh/hip on support surface. Patient performs (a) repeated taps on knee with heel and (b) sliding the heel up and down the lower leg. Observe for speed, dysmetria, dyssynergia, decomposition, dysdiadochokinesia, kinetic tremor, intention tremor.

   Foot/toe tapping: Observe for speed, dysmetria, dysdiadochokinesia, kinetic tremor.

3. Static and Dynamic Balance

   Sitting balance: Patient performs with and without upper and lower extremity support or with and without trunk support (as skill level permits), with

BOX 19.1   Typical Clinical Tests and Measures for the Physical Therapy Evaluation of Cerebellar Dysfunction—cont'd

and without vision. Test for recovery from self-imposed (upper extremity or head movements) or external (gentle pushes by examiner) perturbations. Observe resting preferred posture, tremor, sway, ability, and effort required to maintain position, recovery from perturbations or other loss of balance. Inquire about vertigo, nausea, and subjective perception of stability.

Standing balance: Patient performs with and without upper and lower extremity support, with and without vision and with feet apart and together. Test for recovery from self-imposed (upper extremity or head movements) or external (gentle pushes by examiner) perturbations. Advanced testing: assume and maintain tandem stance and single limb stance. Observe resting preferred posture, natural foot position (base of support), tremor, sway, ability, and effort required to maintain position, recovery from perturbations or other loss of balance. Inquire about vertigo, nausea, and subjective perception of stability.

4. Oculomotor Performance

Smooth pursuit: In sitting, keeping the head still, patient follows pen tip or similar small object with eyes. Test in all movement planes and directions and through full range of motion. Vary speed. Observe for saccadic (choppy) pursuit.

Saccades: In sitting, keeping the head still and when verbally prompted, patient alternately fixes gaze on one of two pen tips, or a pen tip and the examiner's nose, or other small objects. Vary the target (pen tip) locations, testing a variety of end point locations, directions of movement, and

distances traveled, including full range of motion. Observe for dysmetria, particularly on initial trials.

Gaze-evoked nystagmus: In sitting, keeping the head still, patient maintains gaze in a variety of locations, including near end-ranges of lateral gaze. Observe for nystagmus, particularly toward the direction of gaze.

Tests of Activity Limitations

1. Bed Mobility

2. Transfers

3. Gait As skill level permits, patient performs natural, narrow, and tandem gait. Compare preferred versus fastest speed and with and without vision. Test for recovery from self-imposed (upper extremity or head movements) or external (gentle pushes by examiner) perturbations. Observe on inclines and declines, uneven surfaces, negotiating introduced obstacles. Observe walking while distracted (dual-task situation) and while holding an object with the upper extremity (e.g., hold a Styrofoam cup half-filled with water). Test turns and control through narrow areas such as a doorway. Observe for speed, irregularity of step height and distance, veering walking path, losses of balance, seeking out of upper extremity support surfaces/guarding, leg dyssynergia, decomposition (e.g., stiff knees, reduced ankle motion), widened base of support, truncal sway, kinetic tremor. Note distance tolerated and need for assistive devices and/or orthotics.

4. Stair Climbing

5. Activities of Daily Living (dressing, grooming, feeding, bathing, etc.)

---

more complete list. One important note is that many of the tests for cerebellar movement dysfunction are sensitive but not specific to cerebellar pathologies. That is, although they often will detect abnormalities in a patient with cerebellar damage, they are frequently also observed to be abnormal in patients with other, noncerebellar disorders of a neuromuscular origin. Therefore they should not be used to rule out cerebellar pathologies.

Tests of Impairments of Body Functions or Structures

At the level of body functions or structures, physical therapists use a variety of simple tests and measures to detect the typical movement impairments associated with cerebellar dysfunction. Many of these fall into the category of limb movement coordination tests. Particularly useful in the upper extremity are the finger-to-nose test, the alternating forearm supination-pronation test, and the hand or finger tapping test. The heel-to-knee test and foot or toe tapping test provide similar information for the lower extremity. Each of these tests informs the physical therapist about the presence and severity of many components of ataxia, including dysmetria, dyssynergia, dysdiadochokinesia, decomposition, and kinetic and/or intention tremor. Some general rules should be applied when performing and interpreting the findings from these clinical tests. First, it is usually important to perform the test on and compare both sides. Each test should be repeated multiple times with the same limb, as subsequent movements may look strikingly different (e.g., hypometric on some trials, hypermetric on others). Comparing slow or preferred to "fast as possible" speeds allows the clinician to determine the severity of the ataxia (generally worst with fastest movements) and how well the patient is able to compensate when allowed full use of feedback mechanisms (the degree to which the movement is improved when performed slowly). It is also generally useful to compare the same movements with and without vision, to determine whether or not visual feedback improves movement quality.

A final caution about the tests of voluntary movement coordination is that the examiner must carefully dissociate limb incoordination from deficits of balance and/or vision. For example, if the patient has difficulty maintaining quiet unsupported sitting, he or she will most likely demonstrate several abnormal movement patterns that resemble classic limb ataxia when asked to move the limbs (e.g., dyssynergia, dysmetria) if tested in this unsupported position. In this situation the examiner cannot distinguish whether the deficits observed are caused by a true incoordination of voluntary limb movements or because of an inability to maintain the trunk in a stable and upright position that provides the limb a stable base from which to generate movement. Thus to test coordination, the examiner must give the patient the necessary head and trunk support required for the limb movement task (e.g., test sitting in a high back chair with manual support at shoulders or perform in supine) if the patient is unable to provide this support by himself or herself. Similar confusion may arise if the patient has significant visual or other oculomotor impairments such as diplopia. Here, the patient would be likely to show apparent dysmetria during visually targeted movements, but it could not be determined whether it is caused by real limb ataxia or a visual impairment preventing the patient from accurately identifying the target location in space. This is not to say that it would not be beneficial to test limb coordination in positions or situations that also challenge balance and/or vision; only that during the initial examination of the patient, one should be careful to ensure an accurate determination of the source of the movement impairment.

Another major component of almost all physical therapy examinations of patients with cerebellar dysfunction is the posture and balance examination. Posture and balance should always be observed in both static and dynamic conditions and in both sitting and standing, as the patient's capabilities allow. The examination is performed the same as for patients with other neurological disorders, so it is not described in detail here (see Box 19.1 for suggested components to emphasize with patients with cerebellar dysfunction). Important considerations specific for patients with cerebellar dysfunction include careful monitoring for symptoms of nausea or vertigo (common in acute cerebellar stroke, may resolve quickly), observation for postural tremor or titubation and observation of the recovery from perturbations, and the presence of lack of check.

As described previously, because other areas of the nervous system are also frequently damaged along with the cerebellum, it may be appropriate to test for impairments of body functions or structures associated with pathology involving extracerebellar regions of the neuromuscular system. Most commonly, this involves testing of muscle strength, somatosensation (including cutaneous sensation and proprioception), reflexes, passive muscle tone, and observation for signs of other motor abnormalities such as spasticity, dystonia, abnormal synergies, chorea, bradykinesia, or resting tremor.

It is also important to examine the patient's initial level of endurance (fatigability), both in the cardiovascular and muscular systems. For the cardiovascular system, this can be approximated by recording the response to sustained aerobic exercise on one or more measurement scales (e.g., perceived exertion, heart rate, blood pressure, respiratory rate). For the muscular system, this can be approximated by recording the maximal number of repetitions of a specific set of muscle contractions or limb movements that can be tolerated before force output or range of motion is reduced. These types of measures can provide a gross gauge of the overall level of cardiovascular and musculoskeletal fitness of the patient. Because cerebellar dysfunction often leads to movements being much more effortful and often exaggerated, it is extremely important that the patient with cerebellar dysfunction obtain adequate endurance for safe participation in daily activities.

Tests of Activity Limitations

Tests of activity limitations should typically proceed similarly to the standard neurological examination. The observation of gait should be given particular attention because gait ataxia is considered one of the most sensitive signs of cerebellar damage and the inability to walk safely is a major participation limitation for most patients with motor disorders.[145] Box 19.1 provides suggested components of the gait analysis for patients with cerebellar dysfunction. In addition, it may be necessary to evaluate the activity limitations related to speech, visual, and/or oculomotor deficits common to cerebellar dysfunction. With careful interviewing, the patient may relay information about limitations in conversation and communication, reading, etc., that should be addressed in rehabilitation. The physical therapist may be the first health care professional to note these types of activity limitations and should refer the patient to the proper professional for additional services.

Documentation of the body function or structure impairments and activity limitations should include not only the level of assistance, if any, required to perform the skill (or for the voluntary limb coordination tests, the degree of impairment; e.g., none, mild, moderate, or severe), but also a detailed description of the deficits observed during the attempted movement (i.e., the movement quality). Specifically, the severity and frequency of the specific features of ataxia (e.g., decomposition, lack of check) should be reported when they accompany a given movement. Also useful is documentation of the time taken to perform certain tasks. For example, one might document performance of a functional reach and place task by a patient with cerebellar dysfunction in the following way: "The patient was able to perform five repetitions of a block stacking task with the right upper extremity in 9.4 seconds without significant drops or placement errors. Decomposition was observed between shoulder and elbow joints, and obvious intention

tremor was present during terminal block placement. When asked to repeat at a faster pace, the patient performed the same task in 6.0 seconds with one block dropped and two misplaced on the stack (dysmetria). Notable dyssynergia was also present."

Standardized Clinical Scales

There are two common standardized rating scales that quantify the severity of cerebellar ataxia. The more well-known is the International Cooperative Ataxia Rating Scale (ICARS).[112] This scale was first published in 1997 by the Ataxia Neuropharmacology Committee of the World Federation of Neurology in response to an established need for a universal scale to quantify ataxia in randomized clinical trials of pharmacological interventions for treating ataxia. The ICARS measures a patient's ability to perform 19 specific activities or movements using an ordinal scale. The activities are grouped into categories based on whether they relate to cerebellar dysfunction affecting (1) posture and gait, (2) limb movements, (3) speech, or (4) oculomotor performance. A subscore is tallied for each category, and a total score is obtained, ranging from 0 (no ataxia) to 100 (most severe ataxia). The ICARS has been found to be reliable in patients with cerebellar dysfunction and has established criterion-related and external validity.[146–149] More recently, it was shown that the ICARS is sensitive to increases in ataxia severity over 1 year in persons with chronic cerebellar degeneration.[143] The Scale for the Assessment and Rating of Ataxia (SARA) is a newer tool that was devised, at least in part, out of concern over the construct validity of the ICARS subscale structure.[150] The SARA is similar to the ICARS, in that it quantifies performance of specific movements or activities on an ordinal scale (many of the test activities are the same or similar to those in the ICARS), but it does not categorize individual test items by body part. The SARA has fewer test items (only eight) and can therefore be administered faster in the clinical setting. The SARA has been shown to be reliable and valid for patients with SCAs.[150] Either the ICARS or SARA scale may be useful for longitudinal tracking of disease progression in cerebellar degeneration or for quantifying improvement of ataxia in clinical trials. The scales are detailed in Appendices 19A and B.

Diagnosis, Prognosis, and Plan of Care

Patients with cerebellar dysfunction should be given a diagnosis for physical therapy that identifies the primary movement dysfunction and helps direct treatment interventions to return the patient to his or her desired level of activity and participation, if possible. Typically, determination of a diagnosis is based largely on both the results of the physical therapy examination and evaluation, as well as knowledge of the etiology of the disorder and the extent of the lesion. The prognosis for recovery likewise depends highly on the etiology and extent of the lesion. It is important to make a determination whether the impairments of body function or structure and activity limitations are expected to improve or expected not to improve or potentially to worsen over time (e.g., with disease progression). For impairments and activity limitations that are expected to improve, emphasis should be placed on recovery of those skills; for those expected not to improve or to worsen, emphasis should be placed on instruction and practice of compensatory strategies and general conditioning to minimize fatigue.

Physical Therapy Interventions for Patients With Cerebellar Dysfunction

The literature on the effectiveness of rehabilitation interventions for individuals with primary cerebellar damage is extremely limited: to date, there have been no randomized controlled clinical trials published, except for one small trial in patients with Friedreich ataxia.[151] Of the few studies on the effects of rehabilitation interventions in this patient population, all have been nonrandomized, noncontrolled small group[35,103,152–154] or case study[155–160] designs. The fact that there are so few studies available, each featuring different patient populations (e.g., post-stroke vs. postsurgical tumor resection vs. cerebellar degeneration) and different outcome measures, makes determining the most effective interventions difficult. Therefore we provide here a summary of the major themes that have arisen to date from these studies as well as some recent consensus reports.[161–165]

Gait and Balance Interventions

Many of the intervention studies for cerebellar ataxia emphasize stability and balance, especially during gait.[103,152–154,157,159] This likely is a reflection of the tight link between gait and balance[104] and the fact that gait ataxia is one of the most common and debilitating signs of cerebellar damage.[102] Common interventions include combinations of exercises targeting gaze, static stance, dynamic stance, gait, and complex gait activities.[103,157] Some examples of exercises in each of these categories are detailed in Box 19.2. Dynamic balance activities in sitting, kneeling, and quadruped have also been advocated.[103] Other interventions specific to the patient's individual impairments of body structure

or function should be implemented as necessary (e.g., stretching of short or tight ankle plantar flexors, exercises for the VOR).[103,157] Locomotor training over ground and on treadmills, and with and without body weight support, has also been used with some success in single case examples.[155,166] However, it is not clear how imbalance is corrected in the body weight support environment. With all gait and balance activities, it is critical that the exercise be sufficiently and increasingly challenging, so as to facilitate plasticity in the nervous system.[167,168] In mouse models, it has been suggested that trial-and-error practice is a requirement for regaining full motor recovery through cerebellar remyelination[169] and that motor training can ameliorate some symptoms of ataxia.[170]

Aerobic Exercise and Resistance Training

Integration of aerobic exercise and resistance training into the treatment plan is recommended for a majority of patients with cerebellar dysfunction, particularly if it is expected the patient will not regain his or her premorbid status. If full recovery is not attained, nearly all types of movements will be generally more effortful, requiring increased energy expenditure and demanding greater concentration. It is well

---

BOX 19.2 Common Gait and Balance Interventions for Patients With Cerebellar Dysfunction[103,157]

1. Gaze and Eye Movements
   a. Vestibuloocular reflex (VOR): (i) visually fixate on stationary target, slow head movements; (ii) visually fixate on target moving in opposite direction, slow head movements; (iii) VOR cancellation, visually fixate on target moving in same direction, slow head movements. Progression: increase and vary speed, perform eyes closed, add complexity to background.
   b. Saccades: active eyes alone and combined eye and head movements between two stationary targets. Progression: increase and vary speed.
2. Static Stance
   a. Feet together, arms across chest, eyes open and closed, with and without slow head movements. Progression: increase time with eyes closed, increase and vary speed of head movements.
   b. Stand on foam, feet apart, arms across chest, eyes closed briefly and intermittently. Progression: narrow base of support, increase time with eyes closed.
   c. Semitandem stance, arms across chest, eyes closed briefly and intermittently. Progression: narrow base to full tandem stance, increase time with eyes closed, perform semitandem stance on foam.
   d. Unilateral stance, arms across chest, eyes open. Progression: perform with intermittent, then longer periods with eyes closed, perform on foam.
3. Dynamic Stance
   a. March in place, arms across chest, eyes open and closed. Progression: increase time with eyes closed, add and incrementally increase pause time in unilateral stance, add head movements.
   b. Standing toe taps, forward/backward/side, alternating legs, arms across chest, eyes open and closed. Progression: increase step distance, increase time with eyes closed, add head movements.
   c. March in place on foam, arms across chest, eyes closed briefly and intermittently. Progression: increase time with eyes closed, add and incrementally increase pause time in unilateral stance.
   d. Standing 360-degree turn, rightward/leftward, arms across chest, eyes open and closed. Progression: tighten turns, increase speed.
   e. Standing reaches, feet apart and together, eyes open and closed. Progression: increase time with eyes closed, increase reach distance, vary directions, narrow base of support to feet together position.

   f. Standing bends and squats, feet apart and together, eyes open and closed. Progression: increase time with eyes closed, narrow base of support to feet together, reach to touch the floor.
   g. Transitions: standing to supine on floor and back up. Progression: transition in and out of all possible positions, with and without upper extremity support, eyes open and closed, including kneel, half-kneel, quadruped, side sit, squat, etc.
4. Gait
   a. Narrow base of support, arms at sides. Progression: increase gait speed.
   b. Normal base of support, arms at sides with periodic head movements. Progression: narrow base of support, increase and vary speed and frequency of head movements.
   c. Gait with wide turns, arms at sides. Progression: sharpen angle of the turn, increase gait speed, add head movements.
   d. Gait with eyes closed, arms at sides. Progression: add turns, add head movements, increase gait speed.
   e. Gait with perturbations: (i) self-imposed, e.g., large arm movements; (ii) external, e.g., pushes by therapist. Progression: increase speed and amplitude of perturbations, make external perturbations unexpected.
5. Complex Gait
   a. Sideways and backward gait, eyes open, arms at sides. Progression: narrow base of support, add head movements, perform with eyes closed, increase gait speed.
   b. Incline and decline gait, eyes open, arms at sides. Progression: narrow base of support, add head movements.
   c. Gait on foam, padded or other compliant surface, eyes open, arms at sides. Progression: narrow base of support, add turns, add head movements, perform with eyes closed.
   d. Semitandem gait, eyes open, arms at sides. Progression: narrow base to tandem gait, add head movements, perform with eyes closed.
   e. Gait while negotiating obstacles, eyes open, arms at sides, avoid/step onto/step over. Progression: increase obstacle number and size, vary obstacle placement.
   f. Gait while distracted, eyes open, arms at sides. Add cognitive task as a distracter; start with responding to simple yes/no questions, progress to difficult tasks (e.g., counting, performing two- or three-digit addition/subtraction).

known that repetitive fatiguing activity worsens postural control[171,172] and therefore may contribute to trips, falls, or other injuries.[173] Because imbalance is such a common outcome for patients with cerebellar dysfunction, incorporating both aerobic exercise to improve cardiovascular endurance and submaximal resistive exercise to improve muscle fatigue-resistance appears appropriate. Aerobic exercise activities might include walking, dance, recumbent or stationary cycling, rowing, arm ergometry, swimming and aquatic exercise, and many other possibilities.

Consider More Intensive, Longer Duration Interventions

Because the cerebellum is thought to be a primary site of motor learning and individuals with cerebellar damage often have motor learning deficits, it is a reasonable to consider whether these patients are capable of benefitting from any intervention that relies on trial-and-error motor practice.[103] It has been suggested that rehabilitation for patients with significant cerebellar dysfunction may take longer (more trials, more sessions) and might not ever be complete. The question remains unanswered thus far. Of course, cerebellum-dependent motor adaptation is only one of many motor learning mechanisms, so it is possible that other processes can be engaged during rehabilitation. In support of this idea, it now appears that at least partial "relearning" of more normal movement patterns is possible with selected cerebellar patient populations.[103,174] Notably, reported gains in the literature were made under conditions of very frequent (10 hours/week) or very long (6 months) training schedules. This could be a necessity for patients with health conditions in which motor learning is impaired. Much more research is needed to determine the full range of improvements possible, the minimal dosage of intervention required, and whether the benefits can be retained over the long-term in this difficult patient population. Fig. 19.9 shows improvements in SARA scores and self-selected walking speeds in a group of individuals with significant progressive ataxia, in response to an intensive rehabilitation program targeting balance and dynamic intersegmental control.

Compensatory Strategies

Compensation is a common component of the plan of care for patients with cerebellar dysfunction. Many patients begin using compensations unconsciously, whereas others need to be taught these strategies and when to use them. If the patient is not expected to recover "normal" movement patterns, compensation can enable the individual to regain a certain prior level of activity or societal participation despite an abnormal movement pattern. Instruction in compensation can also be valuable in situations when full recovery is expected, but the patient would benefit from the use of compensatory strategies for the short term, such as for safety purposes. One compensatory strategy that works well for patients with cerebellar dysfunction is the instruction to simply slow down movements. Recall that slower movements are less dyssynergic and less hypermetric.[51] Voluntarily reducing the number of segments moving at the same time (i.e., decomposition) also helps to reduce dyssynergia and dysmetria.[51,85] In some cases, reminding patients to use visual cues can also be helpful (e.g., use vertical markings of a doorway to maintain upright stability), although for certain types of cerebellar damage this is not effective.[95,96] For gait, deliberately widening stance can be helpful, both for maintaining balance and for preventing tripping over a foot. The use of assistive devices for gait should be considered on a case-by-case basis. For some patients, facilitating upper extremity support and increasing the base of support improves balance during gait. However, for others, the level of skill required to coordinate controlling the device with the movements of arms and legs is too difficult, and using the device actually worsens the instability. In general, patients with significant imbalance and limb ataxia but who are

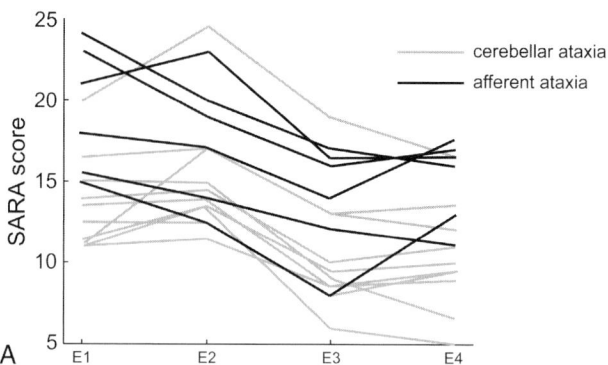

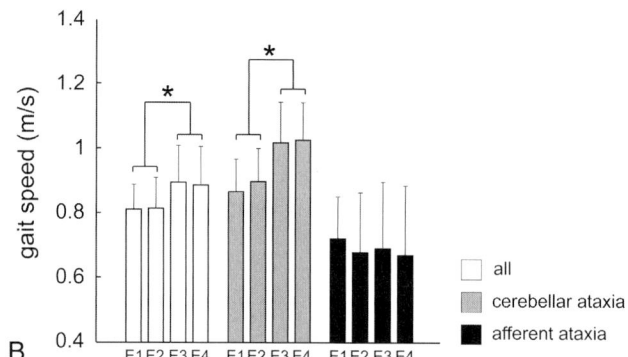

Fig. 19.9 Changes in **(A)** SARA score and **(B)** self-selected walking speed for a group of 16 individuals with progressive ataxia who completed 4 weeks of intensive (1 h/day × 3 days/week supervised training plus 1 h/day × 7 days/week independent home exercise) rehabilitation emphasizing balance. Measures were recorded at four time periods *(E1 to E4)*, corresponding to 8 weeks preintervention *(E1)*, immediately preintervention *(E2)*, immediately postintervention *(E3)*, and 8 weeks postintervention *(E4)*. Subjects were categorized as having either a predominant cerebellar ataxia (e.g., SCA 2, SCA 6, idiopathic cerebellar ataxia or another autosomal dominant cerebellar ataxia) or a predominant afferent ataxia (e.g., Friedreich ataxia or other significant somatosensory neuropathy). The group overall showed significant improvements in both measures (reduced SARA scores and increased walking speeds) after the 4 weeks of exercise and retained these improvements over a further 8 weeks. When broken down by ataxia category, subjects with a predominant cerebellar ataxia, but not the subjects with a predominant sensory ataxia, showed a significant improvement in walking speed. *SARA*, Scale for the Assessment and Rating of Ataxia. (Adapted with permission from the American Academy of Neurology, Ilg W, Synofzik M, Brötz D, Burkard S, Giese MA, Schöls L. Intensive coordinative training improves motor performance in degenerative cerebellar disease. *Neurology.* 2009;73[22]:1823–1830.)

ambulatory will often not be safe with any type of cane and instead require a wheeled walker and/or the physical assistance of a caretaker to walk. A final strategy is to remove or minimize distractions during effortful activities. Distraction (e.g., dividing attention between a motor and a cognitive task) can worsen ataxia.[175]

The Controversy of Weighting

Rehabilitation textbooks have traditionally supported the use of weights for adults and particularly children with cerebellar dysfunction and ataxia. Either the trunk may be weighted by having the patient wear a vest or pack that is weighted, increasing the load on the body axially,[176] or the limbs may be weighted individually[177,178] with simple wrist or ankle weights. Presumably this trend was based on the common finding, first noted by Holmes,[76] that patients with cerebellar dysfunction appear improved (move more smoothly and with reduced tremor) if they are asked to hold a heavy weight in the hand while moving the arm. Currently, it is known that cerebellar tremor is at least in part mechanical in nature, such that anything that adds inertia to the moving segment would reduce the amplitude of the tremor.[88] This most likely explains the improvement that has been reported. However, this apparent benefit would certainly not continue once the weight is removed, and a reduction in tremor does not indicate a normalization of any other parameters of movement. In fact, weighting of the extremities would seem a questionable choice, given the known difficulty of patients with cerebellar dysfunction to predict and account for limb dynamics or to account for interaction torques.[51,52] Addition of weights, particularly to the distal segments, would seem to only make this task more difficult. Evidence for this has been demonstrated in a study of patients with cerebellar ataxia in which it was shown that weighting the extremities worsens the amount of hypermetria during a simple wrist movement task.[89] Furthermore, more recent work showed that weighting the extremities especially exacerbates reaching errors during multijoint movements.[179]

One unintended consequence of weighting is that it tends to slow movements down. As described earlier, slower movements are less hypermetric and less dyssynergic than preferred-speed or fast movements. In early studies of weighting, speed was not monitored or controlled for, so a simple reduction in movement speed could account for the immediate apparent improvement described in some reports.[177,178] Therefore weighting may indeed provide a benefit to some patients with ataxia, but it is most likely an indirect one, related more so to decreased movement speed. Accordingly, the significant potential for negative consequences of weighting (i.e., worsened hypermetria, increased interaction torques, and the annoyance and physical awkwardness of weights, etc.) makes this intervention option seem inferior when compared with the simpler strategy of instructing the patient in voluntarily moving more slowly.[180] It is important to note that the analysis here relates specifically to ataxia of a cerebellar origin. The topic of axial or limb weighting for people with other forms of ataxia (e.g., sensory ataxia) is beyond the scope of this chapter and should be considered to be a different approach because the mechanism of movement incoordination is entirely different.

SUMMARY

The cerebellum is highly unique, in terms of its anatomy, physiology, and the movement-related consequences individuals suffer if it becomes damaged. Ataxia, or movement incoordination, is the major sign of cerebellar damage and can affect limb movements, eye movements, speech, balancing, and walking. Depending on which cerebellar functional longitudinal zone(s) is/are lesioned, one or more of these specific categories of movements will be impaired. Although the precise mechanisms are not yet fully understood, it is widely acknowledged that the cerebellum is integral for (a) coordination of movements, particularly fast, multijoint movements and (b) adapting movements to changes in body conditions or the environment and learning new movement patterns based on trial-and-error practice

(motor learning). Unfortunately, evidence for the effectiveness of rehabilitation interventions for individuals with primary cerebellar damage is extremely limited and incomplete. One critical factor in the evaluative process is the determination whether the body function or structure impairments and activity limitations are expected to improve or expected not to improve or even worsen in the case of progressive diseases. If expected to improve, emphasis should be placed on trial-and-error practice of increasingly challenging motor activities. Balance and gait skills may be highlighted. On the other hand, if recovery is not expected, instruction and practice of compensatory strategies and general conditioning may be effective in at least partially restoring prior participation levels.

ACKNOWLEDGMENTS

The authors are supported by the following grants: NIH P20GM103446 (SMM), NIH R01HD040289 (AJB), NIH R37 NS090610 (AJB).

REFERENCES

To enhance this text and add value for the reader, all references are included on the companion Evolve site that accompanies this textbook. This online service will, when available, provide a link for the reader to a Medline abstract for the article cited. There are 180 cited references and other general references for this chapter, with the majority of those articles being evidence-based citations.

International Cooperative Ataxia Rating Scale

I. POSTURE AND GAIT DISTURBANCES

1. **Walking capacities** (Observe walking 10 m, near a wall, including half-turn.)
   0 = Normal
   1 = Almost normal naturally but unable to walk with feet in tandem position
   2 = Walking without support but clearly abnormal and irregular
   3 = Walking without support but with considerable staggering; difficulties in half turn
   4 = Walking with autonomous support not possible; uses the episodic support of the wall
   5 = Walking only possible with one stick
   6 = Walking only possible with two special sticks or with a stroller
   7 = Walking only with accompanying person
   8 = Walking impossible, even with accompanying person (wheelchair)
   Score: _____

2. **Gait speed** (Observe only if subject scores <4 on preceding test; otherwise automatically score this test as "4.")
   0 = Normal
   1 = Slightly reduced
   2 = Markedly reduced
   3 = Extremely slow
   4 = Walking with autonomous support no longer possible
   Score: _____

3. **Standing capacities, eyes open** (Ask subject to stand on one foot; if impossible, ask to stand with feet in tandem; if impossible, ask to stand with feet together. For the natural position, ask subject to find a comfortable standing position.)
   0 = Normal; able to stand on one foot >10 s
   1 = Able to stand with feet together but no longer able to stand on one foot >10 s
   2 = Able to stand with feet together but no longer able to stand with feet in tandem position
   3 = No longer able to stand with feet together but able to stand in natural position without support, with no or moderate sway
   4 = Standing in natural position without support, with considerable sway and considerable corrections
   5 = Unable to stand in natural position without strong support of one arm
   6 = Unable to stand at all, even with strong support of two arms
   Score: _____

4. **Spread of feet in natural position without support, eyes open** (Ask subject to find a comfortable position, then measure the distance between medial malleoli.)
   0 = Normal (<10 cm)
   1 = Slightly enlarged (>10 cm)
   2 = Clearly enlarged (25–35 cm)
   3 = Severely enlarged (>35 cm)
   4 = Standing in natural position impossible
   Score: _____

5. **Body sway with feet together, eyes open**
   0 = Normal
   1 = Slight oscillations
   2 = Moderate oscillations (<10 cm at the level of head)
   3 = Severe oscillations (>10 cm at the level of head), threatening the upright position
   4 = Immediate falling
   Score: _____

6. **Body sway with feet together, eyes closed**
   0 = Normal
   1 = Slight oscillations
   2 = Moderate oscillations (<10 cm at the level of head)
   3 = Severe oscillations (>10 cm at the level of head), threatening the upright position
   4 = Immediate falling
   Score: _____

7. **Quality of sitting position** (on flat, hard surface, thighs together, arms folded)
   0 = Normal
   1 = With slight oscillations of the trunk
   2 = With moderate oscillations of the trunk and legs
   3 = With severe disequilibrium
   4 = Impossible
   Score: _____
   POSTURE AND GAIT SUBSCORE: _____ / 34

II. KINETIC FUNCTIONS

8. **Knee-tibia test: decomposition of movement and intention tremor** (Subject is in supine with head tilted to allow visual control. Ask subject to raise one leg in the air (to a height of ~40 cm) and place heel on opposite knee and then slide the heel down the anterior tibial surface of the resting leg toward the ankle. On reaching the ankle joint, the leg is again raised, and the action repeated. Repeat for at least three trials on each side.)
   0 = Normal
   1 = Heel lowering in continuous axis, but movement is decomposed in several phases (without real jerks) or abnormally slow
   2 = Heel lowering jerkily in the axis
   3 = Heel lowering jerkily with lateral movements
   4 = Heel lowering jerkily with extremely strong lateral movements or test impossible
   Score right: _____ Score left: _____

9. **Action tremor in the heel-to-knee test** (Same test as preceding one; visual control required. Observe action tremor of the heel when asked to hold the heel on the knee for a few seconds before sliding down the leg.)
   0 = No trouble
   1 = Tremor stopping immediately when the heel reaches the knee
   2 = Tremor stopping in <10 s after reaching the knee
   3 = Tremor continuing >10 s after reaching the knee

4 = Uninterrupted tremor or test impossible
Score right: _____ Score left: _____

10. **Finger-to-nose test: decomposition and dysmetria** (Subject sitting; visual control required. Start trials with hands resting on knees. Repeat for at least three trials on each side.)
   0 = No trouble
   1 = Oscillating movement without decomposition of the movement
   2 = Segmented movement in 2 phases and/or moderate dysmetria in reaching nose
   3 = Segmented movement in >2 phases and/or considerable dysmetria in reaching nose
   4 = Dysmetria preventing the patient from reaching nose
   Score right: _____ Score left: _____

11. **Finger-to-nose test: kinetic tremor of the finger** (Same test as preceding one. Observe movement tremor occurring during the ballistic phase of the movement.)
   0 = No trouble
   1 = Simple swerve of the movement
   2 = Mild tremor, estimated amplitude <10 cm
   3 = Moderate tremor, estimated amplitude 10–40 cm
   4 = Severe tremor, estimated amplitude >40 cm
   Score right: _____ Score left: _____

12. **Finger-finger test: action tremor and/or instability** (Subject sitting; under visual control. Ask subject to flex and abduct shoulders and then flex elbows so as to have both index fingers pointing at each other at midline. Subject is to maintain index finger positions for ~10 s, at distance of ~1 cm apart (not touching) and hands at the level of the thorax.)
   0 = Normal
   1 = Mild instability
   2 = Moderate oscillations of finger, estimated amplitude <10 cm
   3 = Considerable oscillations of finger, estimated amplitude 10–40 cm
   4 = Jerky movements, amplitude >40 cm
   Score right: _____ Score left: _____

13. **Pronation-supination alternating movements** (Subject sitting. Ask subject to raise the forearm vertically and alternate supinating and pronating the forearm on the lap, combining elbow flexion and extension with forearm supination and pronation.)
   0 = Normal
   1 = Slightly irregular and slowed
   2 = Clearly irregular and slowed, but without sway of the elbow
   3 = Extremely irregular and slowed movement, with sway of the elbow
   4 = Movement completely disorganized or impossible
   Score right: _____ Score left: _____

14. **Drawing of the Archimedes' spiral on a predrawn pattern** (Subject sitting at a table with a sheet of paper fixed in place. Ask subject to trace the spiral with a pen; no timing requirements.)
   0 = Normal
   1 = Impairment and decomposition, the line quitting the pattern slightly but without hypermetric swerve
   2 = Line completely out of the pattern with recrossings and/or hypermetric swerves
   3 = Major disturbance due to hypermetria and decomposition

4 = Drawing completely disorganized or impossible
Score: _____
LIMB KINETICS SUBSCORE: _____ / 52

III. SPEECH DISORDERS

15. **Dysarthria: fluency of speech** (Ask subject to repeat a standard sentence several times; e.g., "A mischievous spectacle is Czechoslovakia.")
   0 = Normal
   1 = Mild modification of fluency
   2 = Moderate modification of fluency
   3 = Considerably slow and dysarthric speech
   4 = No speech
   Score: _____

16. **Dysarthria: clarity of speech**
   0 = Normal
   1 = Suggestion of slurring
   2 = Definite slurring, most words understandable
   3 = Severe slurring, speech not understandable
   4 = No speech
   Score: _____
   DYSARTHRIA SUBSCORE: _____ /8

IV. OCULOMOTOR DISORDERS

17. **Gaze-evoked nystagmus** (Ask subject to look laterally at examiner's finger. Observe for nystagmus, mainly horizontal, but could be oblique, rotary or vertical.)
   0 = Normal
   1 = Transient
   2 = Persistent but moderate
   3 = Persistent and severe
   Score: _____

18. **Abnormalities of ocular pursuit** (Ask subject to follow the slow lateral movement of the examiner's finger.)
   0 = Normal
   1 = Slightly saccadic
   2 = Clearly saccadic
   Score: _____

19. **Dysmetria of the saccade** (Examiner's two fingers are placed, one in each temporal visual field of the subject whose eyes are in the primary position. Ask subject to shift eyes to look laterally at the finger, first on the right and then on the left. Average overshoot or undershoot of the two sides is then estimated.)
   0 = Absent
   1 = Bilateral clear overshoot or undershoot of the saccade
   Score: _____
   OCULOMOTOR SUBSCORE: _____ /6
   TOTAL ATAXIA SCORE (sum of four subscores): _____ /100

Adapted with permission from Elsevier, Trouillas P, Takayanagi T, Hallett M, et al. International cooperative ataxia rating scale for pharmacological assessment of the cerebellar syndrome. The ataxia neuropharmacology committee of the world federation of neurology. *J Neurol Sci.* 1997;145(2):205–211.

Scale for Assessment and Rating of Ataxia

1. Gait

Subject (a) walks at a safe distance parallel to a wall including a half-turn (turn around to face the opposite direction of gait) and (b) walks in tandem (heels to toes) without support.

0 Normal, no difficulties in walking, turning, or walking tandem (up to one misstep allowed)
1 Slight difficulties but only visible when walking 10 consecutive steps in tandem
2 Clearly abnormal, tandem walking >10 steps not possible
3 Considerable staggering, difficulties in half-turn, but walks without support
4 Marked staggering, intermittent support of the wall required
5 Severe staggering, permanent support of one stick or light support by one arm required
6 Walking >10 m only with strong support (two special sticks or stroller or accompanying person)
7 Walking <10 m only with strong support (two special sticks or stroller or accompanying person)
8 Unable to walk, even supported

Score: _____

2. Stance

Subject stands (a) in natural position, (b) with feet together in parallel (big toes touching each other) and (c) in tandem (both feet on one line, no space between heel and toe). Subject does not wear shoes, eyes are open. For each condition, three trials are allowed. Best trial is rated.

0 Normal, able to stand in tandem for >10 s
1 Able to stand with feet together without sway, but not in tandem for >10 s
2 Able to stand with feet together for >10 s but only with sway
3 Able to stand for >10 s without support in natural position but not with feet together
4 Able to stand for >10 s in natural position only with intermittent support
5 Able to stand >10 s in natural position only with constant support of one arm
6 Unable to stand for >10 s even with constant support of one arm

Score: _____

3. Sitting

Subject sits on an examination bed without support of feet, eyes open and arms outstretched to the front.

0 Normal, no difficulties sitting >10 s
1 Slight difficulties, intermittent sway
2 Constant sway but able to sit >10 s without support
3 Able to sit for >10 s only with intermittent support
4 Unable to sit for >10 s without continuous support

Score: _____

4. Speech disturbance

Speech is assessed during normal conversation.

0 Normal
1 Suggestion of speech disturbance
2 Impaired speech but easy to understand
3 Occasional words difficult to understand
4 Many words difficult to understand
5 Only single words understandable
6 Speech unintelligible/anarthria

Score: _____

5. Finger chase

Subject seated comfortably, feet and trunk supported if needed. Examiner sits in front of subject and performs five consecutive sudden and fast pointing movements in unpredictable directions in a frontal plane, at approximately 50% of subject's reach distance. Movements are approximately 30 cm in distance and occur approximately 1 reach every 2 s. Ask subject to follow the movements, pointing with his index finger, as fast and precisely as possible. Average performance of last 3 movements is rated. Rate separately for each side.

0 No dysmetria
1 Dysmetria, under/overshooting target <5 cm
2 Dysmetria, under/overshooting target <15 cm
3 Dysmetria, under/overshooting target >15 cm
4 Unable to perform 5 pointing movements

Score right: _____ Score left: _____ Mean score (R+L/2): _____

6. Nose-finger test

Subject seated comfortably, feet and trunk supported if needed. Ask subject to point repeatedly with his index finger from his nose to examiner's finger, which is in front at approximately 90% of subject's reach distance. Movements are performed at moderate speed. Average performance of movements is rated according to the amplitude of the kinetic tremor. Rate separately for each side.

0 No tremor
1 Tremor with an amplitude <2 cm
2 Tremor with an amplitude <5 cm
3 Tremor with an amplitude >5 cm
4 Unable to perform 5 pointing movements

Score right: _____ Score left: _____ Mean score (R+L/2): _____

7. Fast alternating hand movements

Subject seated comfortably, feet and trunk supported if needed. Ask subject to perform 10 cycles of repetitive alternation of pronation and supination of the forearm on his thigh as fast and as precise as possible. Demonstrate the movement at a speed of approximately 10 cycles in 7 s. Record times for movement execution. Rate separately for each side.

0 Normal, no irregularities, performs in <10 s
1 Slightly irregular but performs in <10 s

2 Clearly irregular, single movements difficult to distinguish or relevant interruptions but performs in <10 s

3 Very irregular, single movements difficult to distinguish or relevant interruptions, performs in >10 s

4 Unable to complete 10 cycles

Score right: _____ Score left: _____ Mean score (R+L/2): _____

8. Heel-shin slide

Subject in supine on examination bed without sight of his legs. Ask subject to lift one leg, point with the heel to the opposite knee, slide down along the shin to the ankle, and lay the leg back on the examination bed. The task is performed 3 times. The slide component of the movement should be performed within 1 s. If subject slides down without contact to shin in all three trials, rate as "4." Rate separately for each side.

0 Normal

1 Slightly abnormal, contact to shin maintained

2 Clearly abnormal, goes off shin ≤3 times during 3 cycles

3 Severely abnormal, goes off shin ≥4 times during 3 cycles

4 Unable to perform the task

Score right: _____ Score left: _____ Mean score (R+L/2): _____

TOTAL ATAXIA SCORE (sum of eight test scores): _____ /40

Adapted with permission from the American Academy of Neurology, Neurol (Schmitz-Hubsch et al. 2006).[150]

Balance Dysfunction*

Leslie K. Allison

OBJECTIVES

After reading this chapter the student or therapist will be able to:

1. Describe both central and peripheral sensory and motor components of the postural control system.
2. List common postural control system impairments and sensorimotor skill deficits found in patients with neurological problems.
3. List commonly used balance tests, and distinguish which are appropriate for patients at low, moderate, and high levels of function.
4. Differentiate how test results are used to identify postural control system impairments, sensorimotor skill deficits, and activity limitations that limit participation.
5. Analyze the interaction of individual, task, and environmental factors that affect balance.

6. Describe how to plan and progress balance exercise programs to increase the use of or compensation with available sensory inputs.
7. Describe how to plan and progress balance exercise programs to facilitate anticipatory postural adjustments to prevent balance loss and provoke automatic postural responses to regain balance after unexpected disturbances.
8. Describe how to plan and progress balance exercise programs to increase the control of center of gravity in upright postures and during gait.
9. Describe how to increase the difficulty level of balance exercise programs in order to promote the automaticity of postural control during functional activities.

KEY TERMS

activity limitation
anticipatory postural adjustments
automatic postural responses
balance
base of support
body structure and function impairments
center of gravity
impairment
limit of stability

motor learning stages
participation restriction
sensorimotor skills
sensory conflict
sensory environment
strategies
systems model or systems approach
volitional postural movements

No matter what the neurological diagnosis, a disease or injury that affects the nervous system is likely to compromise one or more of the postural control mechanisms. For example, patients with such diverse diagnoses as stroke, head trauma, spinal cord injury (SCI), peripheral neuropathy, multiple sclerosis (MS), Parkinson disease (PD), cerebellar dysfunction, cerebral palsy, and Guillain-Barré syndrome all experience postural control problems. One common thread among these different medical diagnoses is the presence of postural control system impairments and, consequently, sensorimotor skill deficits, including imbalance and abnormal gait. Patients with different medical diagnoses may have the same postural control system impairments, and patients with the same medical diagnosis may have different postural control system impairments, depending on which portions of the postural control system are involved.[1] To optimally understand and manage balance problems, assessment of each postural control system component and the interactive nature of the

components is important. The traditional medical "diagnostic" model does not provide this information and is not the most beneficial model for planning balance rehabilitation interventions. The medical diagnosis is relevant: knowing whether deficits are permanent or temporary, and whether recovery or progressive decline is expected is critical. This medical prognostic information will assist physical and occupational therapists in goal setting and intervention planning.

The International Classification of Functioning, Disability and Health (ICF) model described in Chapter 1 and illustrated in Fig. 20.1 describes the interactions of body function and structure problems (impairments) and activity limitations as seen in patients with neurological disease or injury, and how these functional activity limitations restrict an individual's ability to participate in life situations, thus decreasing quality of life. As valuable and beneficial as this model has been to rehabilitation practice, researchers and clinicians alike have had difficulty reaching a consensus about whether "imbalance" should be categorized as an impairment of body structure/function, or as an activity limitation. This is perhaps because the ICF categorizes some aspects of balance as impairments of body structure/function (e.g.,

---

*Videos for this chapter are available at studentconsult.com.

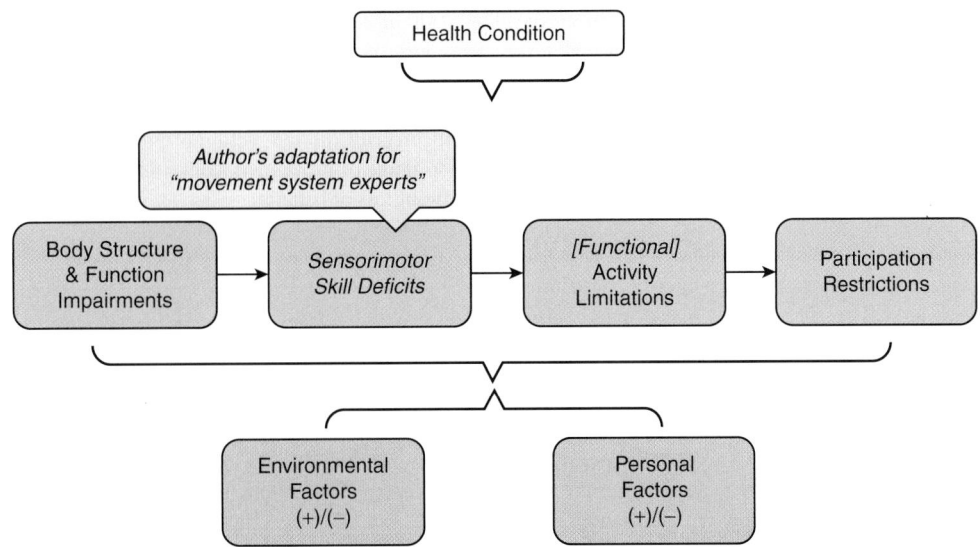

Fig. 20.1 An adapted version of the International Classification of Functioning, Disability and Health Model as conceptualized by the author. The addition of a Sensorimotor Skills category may increase the usefulness and applicability of the model for clinicians responsible for assessment and improvement of human movement.

"Involuntary movement reaction functions" including functions of postural reactions, righting reactions, body adjustment reactions, balance reactions, supporting reactions, defensive reactions) and other aspects of balance as activity limitations (e.g., "Mobility: Changing and maintaining body position," including sitting, maintaining a sitting position, standing, maintaining a standing position, shifting the body's center of gravity [COG]).[2] To align with the ICF model, in previous editions of this chapter, I have used the term "balance impairments" despite concerns that neither category offered an optimal fit. The ICF model was not developed or designed specifically for use by movement system professionals such as physical therapists (PTs), occupational therapists (OTs), or adaptive physical education teachers with expertise in normal and abnormal motor control, motor learning, and motor development. I believe it is useful to adapt the ICF model for our purposes by adding a "sensorimotor skills" category in between body "structure/function impairments" and (more functional) "activity limitations" (see Fig. 20.1). Sensorimotor skills (i.e., perceptual-motor skills) are learned, goal-directed movement abilities that require the interaction and integration of sensory inputs, perceptual processes, motor planning, and movement execution. When we consider *how* or *how well* a patient moves and are concerned with the quality of their movement or movement patterns not only their outcome, we are engaged in sensorimotor skill analysis. Balance and gait fit very well into this category.

Within this adapted ICF model, body structure/function impairments (e.g., sensory loss, leg weakness, slow reaction time) lead to sensorimotor skill deficits (e.g., imbalance, hemiplegic gait patterns, abnormal synergies in reaching), which in turn lead to real-life, functional activity limitations (e.g., requires minimum assistance for wheelchair transfers, moderate assistance for limited household ambulation with a straight cane), culminating in participation restrictions and decreased quality of life. Application of this adapted ICF model to patient-centered rehabilitation care includes the following assessment sequence: (1) identification of the patient's participation goals, (2) hypothesis generation about and evaluation of the functional activity limitations leading to participation restriction, (3) hypothesis generation about and evaluation of the sensorimotor skills leading to functional activity limitations, and (4) hypothesis generation about and evaluation of the body structure/function impairments

leading to sensorimotor skill deficits. For example, a patient may wish to participate in a tour of historical buildings but cannot perform stair-climbing without either two handrails or assistance (activity limitation). The therapist hypothesizes that the patient's dynamic balance is deficient and finds she cannot perform single-leg stance skills on either leg; further evaluation includes hypotheses and testing to reveal that she has weak hip extensors and abductors, and limited ankle dorsiflexion range of motion (ROM) bilaterally. Application of this adapted ICF model to the design of customized, individualized intervention programs thus requires that we *treat impairments*, *teach sensorimotor skills*, and *train functional activity abilities* if we wish to increase participation and improve quality of life. We cannot assume that doing one will automatically lead to another and should incorporate all three. For the patient described above, intervention would include treatment of impairments (e.g., closed-chain resistance exercises and ankle stretching), teaching dynamic balance skills (e.g., hands-free alternate toe touching on increasingly higher step stools, progressing to step ups/downs with dual-tasking), and training stair climbing (e.g., progressing to single or no handrail and counter-traffic).

Balance skill deficits negatively affect function, often reducing the individual's ability to participate fully in life.[3] These skill deficits often limit functional activity levels, produce abnormal compensatory motor behavior, and may require devices for support or assistance from another person. Falls can result when imbalance is severe, leading to secondary injuries. To avoid these consequences and advance the functional status of patients, therapists should understand both the demands that various environments and functional tasks place on postural control systems *and* the individual's impairments and skill deficits that may diminish the ability of those systems to respond adequately.

BALANCE

Definitions of Balance

Balance is a complex process involving the reception and integration of sensory inputs and the planning and execution of movement to achieve a goal requiring upright posture. It is the ability to control the COG over the base of support in a given sensory environment.[4,5] The COG is an imaginary point in space, calculated biomechanically from measured forces and moments, where the sum total of all the forces equals zero. In a person standing quietly the COG is located just forward of the spine at approximately the S2 level. With movement of the body and its segments, the location of the COG in space constantly changes. The base of support is the body surface that experiences pressure as a result of body weight and gravity; in standing it is the feet, and in sitting it includes the thighs and buttocks. The size of the base of support will affect the difficulty level of the balancing task. A broad base of support makes the task easier; a narrow base makes it more challenging. The COG can travel farther while still remaining over the base if the base is large. The "shape" of the base of support will alter the distance that the COG can move in certain directions.

Any given base of support places a limit on the distance a body can move without either falling (as the COG exceeds the base of support) or establishing a new base of support by reaching or stepping (to relocate the base of support under the COG). This perimeter is frequently referred to as the *limit of stability* or *stability limit*.[4,6] It is the farthest distance in any direction a person can lean (away from midline) without altering the original base of support by stepping, reaching, or falling.

Environmental Context

This biomechanical task of keeping the COG over the base of support is always accomplished within an environmental context, which is detected by the sensory systems. The sensory environment is the set of conditions that exist, or are perceived to exist, in the external world that may affect balance. Peripheral sensory receptors gather information about the environment, body position, and motion in relation to the environment, and body segment positions and motions in relation to the self. Central sensory structures process this information to perceive body orientation, position, and motion and to determine the opportunities and limitations present in the environment. This central sensory integration process also estimates where we will be in the immediate future, permitting APAs. Gravity is one environmental condition that must be dealt with to remain stable. It is a constant condition for everyone except astronauts in space. Surface and visual conditions, however, may vary significantly and may be stable or unstable. Unstable surface conditions might include the subway, a sandy beach, a gravel driveway, or an icy parking lot. Common unstable visual conditions are experienced on mass transit, in crowds, or on a boat. Rapid head movements may render even a stable visual environment unusable for postural cues, and darkness may preclude the use of vision. The more stable the environment, the lower the demand on the individual for balance control. Unstable (extrinsic) environments place greater demands on the (intrinsic) postural control systems.

Balance is also affected by an individual's intentions to achieve certain goals and the purposeful tasks that are undertaken. Volitional balance disturbances are self-initiated almost constantly, such as shifting from foot to foot, reaching for the telephone, or catching an object that is falling from a high shelf. Even reactions to involuntary balance disturbances, such as a slip or trip, are modified on the basis of the immediate task. A man carrying a bag of groceries who slips may drop the bag to reach with both hands and catch himself. If he is instead carrying his infant, he may reach with only one hand or even take the fall if by doing so he can protect the infant from harm. Often in real life we perform several tasks at once, such as carrying a laundry basket while walking or talking on a cellular phone while climbing a flight of stairs. When tasks are undertaken concurrently (dual-tasking or multi-tasking), attention must be divided between them, which may also affect balance abilities. This is especially true for individuals for whom balance skills are not automatic.

All of these variables—the location of the COG, the base of support, the limit of stability, the surface conditions, the visual environment, the intentions and task choices—are inconstant and produce changing demands on the systems that control balance. The integrity and interaction of postural control mechanisms allow a wide range of movement skills and real-life functions to be achieved without loss of balance.

HUMAN CONTROL OF BALANCE

Early studies of postural control mechanisms using selectively lesioned cats and primates focused on reflexive and reactive equilibrium responses that are relatively "hard-wired."[7] These valuable studies brought to light certain stereotypical motor responses to specific sensory stimuli, such as the crossed extension reflex or tonic neck reflexes. There is no doubt that these reflexive and reactive responses—for example, the vestibuloocular reflex (VOR) and protective extension reactions—are foundational to normal postural control. However, the postural control system encompasses much more than these subcortically driven components. Balance abilities are heavily influenced by higher-level neural circuitry and other systems (e.g., cognitive, musculoskeletal) as well.[6] In addition, the nervous system is influenced by and responsive to the demands placed on it by the tasks being accomplished and the environments in which those tasks are performed.[8–10] All of these facets are included in a systems approach to dynamic equilibrium.[11–13] Examination and intervention methods based on this systems model have consequently evolved.[12,14]

The Systems Approach

The systems model for dynamic equilibrium recognizes that balance is a result of interactions among the individual, the task(s) the individual is performing, and the environment in which the task(s) must be performed. These interactions are represented in Fig. 20.2. Within the individual, both sensory inputs and processing systems (left side of figure) and motor planning and execution systems (right side of figure) are critical. Both peripheral components (lower part of figure) and central components (upper part of figure) of the systems are involved in the cycle. The cycle is driven both by purposeful choices of the individual (tasks) and by demands placed on the individual by the environment. Successful function of the sensory systems allows recognition and estimation of body position and motion in relation to self and the world. The desired outcome from the motor systems is the generation of movement sufficient to maintain balance and perform the chosen, goal-directed task(s).

Peripheral Sensory Reception

The three primary peripheral sensory inputs contributing to postural control are the bilateral receptors of the somatosensory, visual, and vestibular systems.[5,11] Somatosensory receptors located in the joints, ligaments, muscles, and skin provide information about muscle length, stretch, tension, and contraction; pain, temperature, and pressure; and joint position. The feet, ankles, knees, hips, back, neck, and eye muscles all furnish useful information for balance maintenance. Somatosensation is the dominant sense for upright postural control and is responsible for triggering automatic postural responses (APRs) in almost all cases except a primary perturbation of the head. Somatosensory loss negatively affects balance. Loss of peripheral somatosensation occurs in patients with loss or disease of or injury to the peripheral sensory receptors or afferent sensory nerves. Examples include patients with diabetic neuropathy, peripheral vascular disease, spinal cord injury, MS, or amputation.

Dynamic Equilibrium

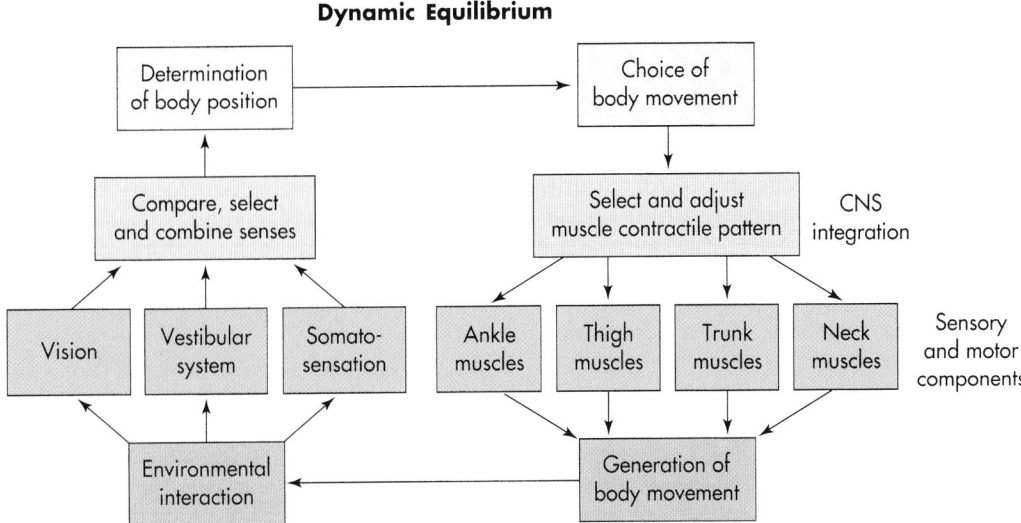

Fig. 20.2 The systems model of postural control illustrates the constant cycle that occurs simultaneously at many levels. *CNS*, Central nervous system. (Reprinted with permission from NeuroCom International, Clackamas, Ore.)

Visual receptors in the eyes support two functions. Central (foveal) vision allows environmental orientation, contributing to the perception of verticality and object motion, as well as identification of the hazards and opportunities presented by the environment.[11] For example, a kayaker may see rocks in a stream as a hazard to be avoided, whereas a hiker who wants to cross the stream may see the same rocks as a welcome opportunity. Peripheral (ambient) vision detects the motion of the self in relation to the environment, including head movements and postural sway. Peripheral vision is largely subconscious, whereas central visual inputs tend to receive more conscious recognition.[11] Both are normally used for postural control. Vision is critical for feedforward, or anticipatory, postural control in changing environments. This includes planning for functional movements such as reaching and grasping, and especially for successful navigation during gait. Vision loss also negatively affects balance. Loss of peripheral visual inputs occurs in patients with disease of or injury to the eyes or afferent cranial nerves. Examples include patients with cataracts, macular degeneration, glaucoma, or diabetic retinopathy.

The vestibular system provides the central nervous system (CNS) with information about the position and motion of the head. The position of the head in relation to gravity is detected through the otolith system. Horizontal and vertical accelerations, as in riding in a car or an elevator, are also detected by the otoliths.[15] Movements of the head are detected through the semicircular canals. Head movement stimulates both sets of semicircular canals, so that the vestibular nerve on one side becomes inhibited while the other becomes excited. The vestibular system provides sensory redundancy in the information obtained from each separate vestibular apparatus. If the peripheral vestibular system is damaged on one side, the information can be captured by the intact canals on the opposite side. The vestibular system is critical for balance because it uniquely identifies self-motion as different from motion in the environment. Vestibular loss also negatively affects balance. Loss of peripheral vestibular inputs occurs in patients with disease of or injury to the peripheral sensory receptors or afferent cranial nerves. Examples include patients with head injury involving temporal bone damage, acoustic neuroma, benign positional vertigo (BPV), or Meniere disease. For a comprehensive review of the vestibular system and vestibular disorders, see Chapter 21.

Orientation to the wider environment, primarily from vision, allows feedforward, or anticipatory, postural adjustments. Prior experience and high attentional capacity improve APAs significantly. Detection of head movement by the vestibular and cervical somatosensory systems and of body sway by somatosensory and peripheral visual systems provides feedback for APRs. Note that the better anticipatory abilities become, the fewer balance errors occur. Fewer balance errors means fewer losses of balance and a reduced need to produce rapid APRs.

Disease of or damage to any of the peripheral sensory receptors or afferent pathways impairs or removes the detection capabilities of the system rendering sensory information unavailable for use in postural control. Many patients with neurological diagnoses have peripheral sensory impairments.

Central Sensory Perception

The brain processes the environmentally available sensory information gathered by the peripheral receptors in varying degrees. This processing is usually referred to as *multisensory integration* or *sensory organization*.[5,11] Central sensory structures function first to compare available inputs between two sides and among three sensory systems. The somatosensory system alone is unable to distinguish surface tilts from body tilts. Also the visual system by itself cannot discriminate movement of the environment from movement of the body.[15] The vestibular system by itself cannot tell if head movement through space is produced by neck motion or trunk and hip motion. Therefore the brain needs information from all three senses to correctly distinguish self-motion from motion in the environment.

How are sensory inputs from separate senses combined to form perceptions of position and motion? To explain this, consider the example of the movement of turning your head quickly to one side to look over your shoulder. When the head turns to one side, firing will increase in one vestibular organ and decrease proportionally in the other. This is known as *push-pull function,* and the information from each side is considered to "match" reciprocally. With the same example, if the eyes are open while the head moves, the rate of the visual flow will be equal and the direction of the visual flow will be opposite to the rate and direction of information from the vestibular inputs. The muscles on one side of the neck will shorten and on the other side will stretch. The inputs from these three systems are congruent. If both sides and all three systems provide compatible inputs, the process of sensory organization is simplified.

When changes in the environment occur, the relative availability, accuracy, and usefulness of information from the three sensory systems may also change. Sensory organization also includes an adaptive process, called *multisensory reweighting,* that permits the CNS to prioritize the sources of sensory information when environmental conditions change.[16,17] Available, accurate, and useful information is "upweighted," whereas unavailable, inaccurate, or less-useful information is "downweighted." For example, in dark environments vision would be downweighted and somatosensory and vestibular information would be upweighted. This adaptive process is imperfect, however, and balance is not as well controlled when any sense must be downweighted as it is when all three senses are available and accurate. Individuals with peripheral sensory loss or central sensory processing deficits may have difficulty reweighting quickly and fully. This impairs their ability to adapt to, and remain stable in, changing environments.[18]

Sensory conflict can arise when information between sides or between systems is not synchronous. Sensory organization processing then becomes more complex because the brain must then recognize any discrepancies and select the correct inputs on which to base motor responses. The vestibular system may be used as an internal reference to determine accuracy of the other two senses when they conflict. For example, a driver stopped at a red light suddenly hits the brake when an adjacent vehicle begins to roll. Movement of the other car detected by the peripheral visual system is momentarily misperceived as self-motion. In this situation, the vestibular and somatosensory systems do not detect motion, but the forward visual flow is interpreted as backward motion. Because the brain failed to suppress the (mismatched) visual inputs, the braking response was generated. Note that "perception drives action," thus perceptual errors lead to movement errors.[19]

When the brain recognizes that the information coming from one sensory input is inaccurate or unavailable, as is the case when the perception of somatosensory information is diminished post-stroke, it must depend more on the remaining senses (in this case, vision and vestibular system) to determine position and motion in space. The brain then compares and uses information from senses it considers accurate for balance. An individual with the problem just described may compensate for the loss of somatosensory function by becoming visually dependent for balance during movement. If vision subsequently also becomes disrupted as this patient ages, his or her ability to orient in space will be further compromised. This will negatively affect balance and increase risk of falls.

Activities or environments that create sensory conflict or demand sensory resolution become more difficult to manage when the vestibular system is deficient or underused. These situations, such as going down stairs, riding escalators or elevators, walking on uneven ground, and making quick turns, are often avoided by patients with vestibular deficits. When sensory conflicts cannot be resolved rapidly, dizziness or motion sickness occurs.

Intrinsic central sensory processing impairments also can produce sensory conflict. An adult hemiplegic patient with pusher syndrome illustrates an inability to integrate visual, vestibular, and somatosensory inputs for midline and verticality orientation. Within a single system, discrepancies between the sides are also problematic. Unequal firing from opposite sides of the vestibular system, as in unilateral vestibular hypofunction, produces a mismatch that is subsequently interpreted as head rotation when head movement does not occur. This spinning sensation is known as *vertigo.*[15] Vertigo is resolved if the brain is able to adapt to the mismatch. For further information on vertigo, refer to Chapter 21.

Finally, the central processing mechanisms combine any available and accurate inputs to answer the questions, "What is my position and how am I moving now?" and "What will my position and motion be in the next moment?" This includes both an internal relation of the body segments to one another (e.g., head in relation to trunk, trunk in relation to feet) and an external relation of the body to the outside world (e.g., feet in relation to surface, arm in relation to handrail). CNS disease or trauma involving the parietal lobe may impair these processing mechanisms so that even available, accurate sensory inputs are not recognized or incorporated into determinations and estimations of current and future position and movement.[20,21] Impairments of central sensory processing may occur after stroke, head trauma, tumors, or aneurysms; with disease processes such as MS and Alzheimer disease; and with aging.

Central Motor Planning and Control

Whereas sensory processing allows the interaction of the individual and the environment, motor planning underlies the interaction of the individual and the task. Aside from reflexive activity such as breathing and blinking, most motor actions are voluntary and occur because some goal is to be achieved. That is not to say that reflexes occur separately from volitional movements; for example, the VOR is active concurrently with visual tracking activity, but most actions occur because of some purposeful intent.[15] These task intentions precede motor actions.[11,22] Wrist and hand movements vary depending on what is to be grasped (a cup vs. a doorknob); foot placement and trunk position vary depending on what is to be lifted (a heavy suitcase vs. a laundry basket). The initiation of volitional motor actions depends on intention, attention, and motivation.[11,23]

Once a task goal (Where do I want to be? What do I want to do?) has been chosen, the next step in motor planning is to determine how to best accomplish the goal given the many options that are potentially available. For example, when the task demands fine skills or accuracy, the dominant hand is preferred; when the task involves lifting a large or heavy object, both hands are preferred. In addition to which limbs, joints, and muscles will be used, motor planning also adjusts the timing, sequencing, and force modulation of muscle activity. This can be demonstrated in various reaching tasks. Reaching to remove a hot item from the oven will occur slowly, whereas reaching to put an arm through a sleeve will occur more quickly. Optimal motor plans are developed with knowledge of self (abilities and limitations), knowledge of task (characteristics of successful performance), and knowledge of the environment (risks and opportunities).[23]

The motor plan is generated in the cortex and refined in the basal ganglia, which responds to goal achievement with reward signals that increase motivation and the likelihood that the correct movement will be reproduced. Next, the motor plan must be transmitted to the peripheral motor system to be enacted. A copy of the intended movement plan is sent to the cerebellum during the transmission. When the movement begins, incoming sensory inputs (feedback) about the actual movements and performance outcome are compared with the intended movements and performance outcome. Movement errors (the difference between the intended and the actual movement) and performance errors (desired goal not achieved) are detected by the cerebellum and basal ganglia and transmitted to the cortex. Corrected motor plans are then formed in the cortex and transmitted for the next attempt to achieve the goal. This process of error detection and error correction is the foundation of motor learning.

Patients with CNS disorders often have central motor planning and control system problems. After a stroke, patients may have hypertonus and poor reciprocal inhibition; patients with head trauma may have difficulty initiating or ceasing movements; patients with PD exhibit bradykinesia; and those with cerebellar ataxia display force modulation problems.[24]

Peripheral Motor Execution

Movement is accomplished through the bilateral joints and muscles. Normal joint ROM, muscle strength and power, and muscle endurance of the feet, ankles, knees, hips, back, neck, and eyes must be present for the execution of the full range of movements needed for normal balance skills. Decreased ankle dorsiflexion ROM, for example, restricts the forward limits of stability. Strength deficits are a primary cause of movement abnormalities in both CNS and peripheral nervous system (PNS) disorders. In addition, weakness may be the result of force modulation deficits or disuse.[12] Balance is directly negatively affected by loss of muscle strength, power, and endurance. For example, weakness of the hip extensors and abductors will impede successful use of a hip strategy for upright trunk control. Low muscle power impedes the rapid generation of sufficient force to execute a successful APR. Initially adequate toe clearance may diminish with fatigue. Many patients with neurological issues also have stiffness and contractures as a result of persistent weakness or hypertonus. Restrictions in ROM, particularly extension, also limit balance skills.

The ability to achieve static postural alignment, although necessary for normal balance, is not sufficient to allow volitional functions. Adequate strength (to control body weight and any additional loads) through normal postural sway ranges is needed to permit dynamic balance activities such as reaching, leaning, and lifting. Postural control demands are increased during gait because the forces of momentum and the interaction between recruitment, timing, and velocity also must be regulated.[25] Traditionally considered orthopedic problems, deficits in muscle strength and power, ROM, posture, and endurance have a negative impact on balance skills. Attention must be given to these musculoskeletal system problems in examination of and intervention for patients with neurological diagnoses.

Influence of Other Systems

Balance skills are also influenced by other systems. Attention, cognition and judgment, and memory are critical for optimal balance skills and are often impaired in hemiplegic and head-injured patients, as well as those who have progressive neurological disorders such as MS and Alzheimer disease. Attentional deficits reduce awareness of environmental hazards and opportunities, interfering with anticipatory postural control.[13] When balance is threatened, an inability to allocate attention to the necessary task of balance versus a secondary, less necessary task increases the risk of falls. Cognitive problems such as distractibility, poor judgment, and slowed processing also increase the risk of falls. Memory loss may preclude recall of safety measures. Depression, emotional lability, agitation, or denial of impairments also can increase the risks for loss of balance. Fear of falling may lead to self-imposed participation restrictions that precipitate a downward spiral of more sedentary behaviors (leading to increased stiffness and weakness) and social isolation (leading to depression); all of these negatively affect balance and raise the risk of falls. In addition to having a direct impact on balance skills themselves, these cognitive and behavioral problems impede motor learning processes, which are crucial for the relearning of balance skills.

Constant Cyclic Nature

The systems model of postural control previously presented illustrates the constant cycle that simultaneously occurs at many levels. Attention and intention allow feedforward processing for active sensory search of the environment and motor planning, both of which are needed for anticipatory postural control. Movements are initiated and executed with resultant sensory experiences and error detection, or feedback. Successful movements are repeated and refined; unsuccessful ones are modified. The nature of this cycle presents the clinician with opportunities for intervention after the appropriate examination of sensory, motor, and cognitive functions. Through feedback and practice, balance skills can improve.[26]

Motor Components of Balance

Reflexes

Many levels of neuromuscular control must be functioning to produce normal postural movements. At the most basic level, reflexes and righting reactions support postural orientation. The VOR and the vestibulospinal reflex (VSR) contribute to orientation of the eyes, head, and body to self and environment.[11]

When motion of the head is identified by the semicircular canals, it triggers a response within the oculomotor system called the *vestibulo-ocular reflex (VOR)*. This causes the eyes to move in the opposite direction of the head but at the same speed. Stimulation of the otoliths drives the eyes to respond to linear head movement. Quick movements of the head will trigger the VOR.[27]

The VOR allows the coordination of eye and head movements. When the eyes are fixed on an object while the head is moving, the VOR supports gaze stabilization. Visuo-ocular responses often work concurrently with the VOR. They permit "smooth pursuit" when the head is fixed while the eyes move and visual tracking when both the eyes and the head move simultaneously.[11]

The VSR helps control movement and stabilize the body. Both the semicircular canals and the otoliths activate and modulate muscles of the neck, trunk, and extremities after head movement to maintain balance. The VSR permits stability of the body when the head moves and is important for the coordination of the trunk over the extremities in upright postures. Righting reactions support the orientation of the head in relation to the trunk and the head position relative to gravity and include labyrinthine head righting, optical head righting, and body-on-head righting.[11]

Automatic Postural Responses

At the next level, APRs operate to keep the COG over the base of support. They are a set of functionally organized, long-loop responses that act to keep the body in a state of equilibrium.[4,5] *Functionally organized* means that the responses, although stereotypical, are matched to the perturbing stimulus in direction and amplitude. If the stimulus is a push to the right, the response is a shift to the left, toward midline. The larger the stimulus, the greater the response. APRs always occur in response to an unexpected stimulus and are typically triggered by somatosensory inputs. Because they occur rapidly, in less than 250 ms, they are not under immediate volitional control.

Four stereotypical APRs have been described. Ankle strategy describes postural sway control from the ankles and feet. The head and hips travel in the same direction at the same time ("in-phase"), with the body moving as a unit over the feet (Fig. 20.3A). Muscle contractile patterns are from distal to proximal (i.e., gastrocnemius, hamstrings, paraspinals). This strategy is used when sway is small, slow, and near midline. It occurs when the surface is broad and stable enough to allow pressure against it to produce forces that can counteract sway to stabilize the body. Ankle strategy is typically used to control anterior-posterior sway, because most of the degrees of freedom at the ankle are in this direction.

Hip strategy involves postural sway control from the pelvis and trunk. The head and hips travel in opposite directions ("out-of-phase"),

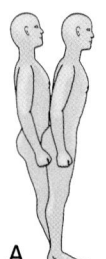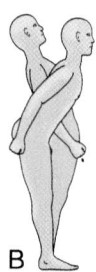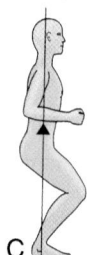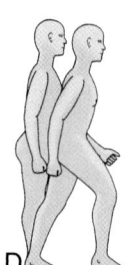

Fig. 20.3 Automatic Postural Responses. **(A)** Ankle strategy. **(B)** Hip strategy. **(C)** Suspensory strategy. **(D)** Stepping strategy. (From Hasson S. *Clinical Exercise Physiology.* St Louis: Mosby; 1994.)

with body segment movements counteracting one another (see Fig. 20.3*B*). Muscle contractile patterns are from proximal to distal (i.e., abdominals, quadriceps, tibialis anterior). This strategy is observed when sway is large, fast, and nearing the limit of stability or if the surface is too narrow or unstable to permit effective counterpressure of the feet against the surface. Hip strategy is used to control both anterior-posterior and medial-lateral sway. Hip strategy in the medial-lateral direction involves weight shifts from foot to foot; any patient with difficulty weight-shifting quickly and accurately will have difficulty with medial-lateral hip strategy.

Suspensory strategy involves a lowering of the COG toward the base of support by bilateral lower-extremity flexion, or a slight squatting motion (see Fig. 20.3*C*). By shortening the distance between the COG and the base of support, the task of controlling the COG is made easier. This strategy is often used when a combination of stability and mobility is required, as in windsurfing.

Stepping and reaching strategies involve steps with the feet or reaches with the arms in an attempt to reestablish a new base of support with the active limb(s) when the COG has exceeded the original base of support (see Fig. 20.3*D*). A successful stepping strategy (sufficiently large and fast) is the best way to avoid a fall after a slip or trip.

Misconceptions about these APR strategies are common. First, these strategies do not function in daily life as separately as they are described in the early research literature. In quiet standing, for example, frequency analysis of unperturbed postural sway in healthy adults reveals that both ankle and hip strategies occur in combination, simultaneously.[28] In perturbation studies, mixed use of strategies is often seen unless the perturbation is clearly below or above certain-sized thresholds. Second, these strategies occur in response to disturbances from all directions, not just in pure anterior-posterior or medial-lateral directions.[29] Third, although these strategies are stereotypical in humans, great individual variation in strategy selection and performance comes from other influential factors. For example, many people use stepping strategy for most perturbations unless specifically instructed not to step or unless the conditions do not permit a step. An anxious person may reach or step much sooner than a relaxed person with similar physical deficits. Last, all these strategies do *not* occur in sequence with every balance disturbance.[30,31] In other words, individuals normally do not try ankle strategy and wait until it fails before trying hip strategy, then wait until it fails before trying stepping strategy (although early learning in children may involve such exploration). Because these responses must occur extremely rapidly to prevent balance loss, such a sequential approach would be inefficient and ineffective. Instead, the normal adult response is the near-immediate emergence of the single strategy best suited to the particular perturbation, the limitations of the individual, and the conditions in the environment.

Abnormal use of APRs is often observed in individuals with neurological disorders. Patients with vestibular deficits typically rely on ankle strategy, which permits the head to remain aligned with the body and sustains congruence between vestibular and somatosensory inputs. Use of hip strategy may be modified or limited because when the head is moving in the opposite direction as the COG, vestibular and somatosensory inputs are not congruent. Activities that require use of hip strategy, such as standing in tandem or on one leg, can be a problem for patients with bilateral vestibular loss or an uncompensated vestibular lesion. However, some cases involve excessive use of hip strategy on a level surface (when an ankle strategy would suffice).[32] This may reflect abnormal integration of the somatosensory and vestibular information. If peripheral somatosensation is impaired, as in diabetic neuropathy, or central sensory weighting of somatosensory inputs is inadequate, hip strategy may dominate.

Patients with somatosensory loss, distal lower extremity weakness or hypertonus, restricted ankle ROM, and/or reduced limits of stability typically rely on hip strategy. This occurs because the patient cannot feel the surface or the feet well enough to modulate foot pressure against the surface, because the person cannot rapidly generate sufficient force against the surface with the ankle muscles, or because restricted ankle ROM prevents COG sway. The use of hip strategy is normal when the COG is at or near the limits of stability and a step is either not possible or not desired.

When the brain perceives that hip or ankle strategy will not be efficient enough to control the movement of the center of pressure, or if conditions and instructions permit a stepping response, stepping strategy may be preferred. Individuals who are fearful of falling often perceive even slight body sway as threatening instability. They may use stepping and reaching strategies exclusively whether or not these "rescue" strategies are actually necessary.

Anticipatory Postural Adjustments

APAs activate muscles in a manner similar to APRs, but they occur before the actual disturbance.[22] If a balance disturbance is predicted, the body will respond in advance by developing a "postural set" to counteract the coming forces. For example, if an individual lifts an empty suitcase thinking it is full and heavy, the anticipatory forces generated before the lift (to counter the anticipated weight) will cause excessive movement and brief instability. Failure to produce properly calibrated anticipatory adjustments increases the risk of sudden balance loss, creating the need to use rapid, reactive APRs to prevent a fall. For patients with deficits in reaction time or APRs, superior use of anticipatory postural control can help the patient avoid the unexpected perturbations that make APRs necessary.

In balance laboratories, APAs are studied using electromyography so that muscle activity before observable movement can be measured. In the clinic, problems with anticipatory adjustments may be observed when the patient fails to counteract a predicted disturbance, such as "don't let me push you backward," or fails to integrate postural control tasks during other activities; this can include the inability to step smoothly over an anticipated obstacle during gait or inability to maintain sitting balance when both arms are intentionally lifted overhead.

Patients with neurological disease or injury involving the cortex may have difficulty recognizing the need for and/or producing APAs. For example, individuals post-stroke or post–traumatic brain injury (TBI), or with MS, PD, or Alzheimer disease. Age-related white-matter changes in fall-prone older adults may also contribute to deficient APAs. Note that the motor learning needed to know when to generate and how to calibrate APAs requires practice and experience. Patients who are learning a novel task like a wheelchair "wheelie"—even patients without cortical involvement (e.g., individuals with SCI or Guillain-Barre)—need extensive repetition to be able to develop successful APAs for that task.

Volitional Postural Movements

Volitional postural movements are under conscious control. Weight shifts to allow an individual to reach the telephone or put the dishes in the dishwasher, for example, are self-initiated disturbances of the COG to accomplish a goal. Volitional postural movements can range from simple weight shifts to complex balance skills of skaters and gymnasts. They can occur after an external stimulus or be self-initiated. Volitional postural movements can occur quickly or slowly, depending on the goal at hand. The more complex or unfamiliar the task, the slower the response time. Use of a variety of movements that might successfully achieve a goal is possible. Volitional postural movements are strongly modified by prior experience and instruction. Automatic and anticipatory postural responses allow the continuous unconscious control of balance, whereas volitional postural movements permit conscious activity. This level of postural motor control is the most frequently tested and treated in clinical practice, but it is by no means sufficient by itself to produce normal balance.

CLINICAL ASSESSMENT OF BALANCE

Objectives of Testing

The patient interview should include determination of participation restrictions and the patient's goals. Then, when present, activity limitations need to be identified and measured. Functional scales (e.g., Functional Independence Measure) are typically used to determine the presence and severity of these limitations, not necessarily why those limitations exist. From these functional tests, decisions can be made about whether intervention is required and, if so, what tasks need to be practiced. If intervention is indicated, clinicians must make judgments about what should be included in the intervention plan. Further testing to identify and measure sensorimotor skills deficits and body structure/function impairments is then necessary to know what systems are involved. A comprehensive evaluation of balance includes functional activity abilities/limitations, sensorimotor skills, and postural control system impairment tests.[13]

No single quick-and-easy test of balance can adequately cover the many multidimensional aspects of balance, although many such tests have great value as screening tools. However, a comprehensive test battery, called the Balance Evaluation Systems Test (BESTest), based on the systems model has been developed that provides clinicians with a thorough examination covering the six major components of the postural control system (Fig. 20.4).[33] The BESTest takes more time to administer than, for example, a single-leg stance test, but results from the BESTest give the clinician a far more complete and accurate picture of the patient's balance deficits than any single-item test or screening test can. Armed with these results, the clinician can develop interventions specifically targeted to the deficient systems. For patients whose primary problems include imbalance, the clinician's investment of time to perform this comprehensive test battery yields a valuable outcome. Shorter versions of this test, the Mini-BESTest and the Brief-BESTest, have subsequently been published.[34,35] They take less time to administer but likewise provide a less complete picture of the patient's balance systems. Specifically, they do not include any items from the biomechanical constraints or stability limits categories. Even so, they are superior to single-item tests or screening tests that are not based on the systems model and do not identify balance system deficits that should be addressed in the intervention plan.

For some patients at lower functional levels, the BESTest may be too difficult. If this is the case, the Berg Balance Scale (BBS) is also an excellent test battery. Though not specifically designed to align with the systems model of dynamic equilibrium, the BBS contains 14 items

I. Biomechanical Constraints	1. Base of support	2. CoM alignment	3. Ankle strength and ROM	4. Hip/trunk lateral strength	5. Sit on floor and stand up		
II. Stability Limits/ Verticality	6. Sitting verticality (left and right) and lateral lean (left and right)	7. Functional reach forward	8. Functional reach lateral (left and right)				
III. Anticipatory Postural Adjustments	9. Sit-to-stand	10. Rise to toes	11. Stand on one leg (left and right)	12. Alternate stair touching	13. Standing arm raise		
IV. Postural Responses	14. In-place response, forward	15. In-place response, backward	16. Compensatory stepping correction, forward	17. Compensatory stepping correction, backward	18. Compensatory stepping correction, lateral (left and right)		
V. Sensory Orientation	19. Sensory integration on balance (modified CTSIB). A: Stance on firm surface EO; B: stance on firm surface EC; C: stance on foam EO, D: stance on foam EC		20. Incline, EC				
VI. Stability in Gait	21. Gait, level surface	22. Change in gait speed	23. Walk with head turns, horizontal	24. Walk with pivot turns	25. Step over obstacles	26. Timed "Get up & Go" Test	27. Timed "Get up & Go" Test with dual task

Fig. 20.4 Balance Evaluation Systems Test With Modifications of Both Long and Short Forms. Short form identified by 14 components shown in BOLD. *CoM,* Center of mass; *CTSIB,* Clinical Test of Sensory Integration on Balance; *EC,* eyes closed; *EO,* eyes open; *ROM,* range of motion. (Data from Horak FB, Wrisley DM, Frank J. The Balance Evaluation Systems Test (BESTest) to differentiate balance deficits. *Phys Ther.* 2009;89:484–498.)

that do challenge several different components of postural control. Selection of one of these two test batteries (based on patient ability level) to initiate a comprehensive balance evaluation is a valuable approach because results from these tests permit extensive hypothesis generation about what balance skills may be deficient and what postural control system impairments may be present.

No single, simple test for balance is possible because balance is such a complex sensorimotor process.[36] Many relatively simple balance tests exist, but not all tests are appropriate for all patients. Different tests may be needed to answer specific questions. For example, several good tests have been developed to determine the risk of falls in elderly people. These would be insufficient to discern whether an injured dancer can resume practice, or an injured roofer is ready to return to work. Clinicians should understand the advantages and limitations of different balance tests in order to be able to select appropriate evaluative tools.

In general, a balance test will not be useful unless it sufficiently challenges the postural control system being tested. Tests for stability ("static balance") are appropriate for patients who are having difficulty simply finding midline or holding still in sitting or standing. They are of much less value for patients with higher-level abilities. Conversely, single-leg stance tests or sensory tests with a foam surface may be far too difficult to perform for patients with lower-level abilities. Certain tests permit the use of arms and/or assistive devices, while others do not; clearly test choices are then limited for patients dependent on the use of upper extremities for balance.

A word of caution about interpreting test results is indicated. Most clinical tests rely on observations of motor behavior to arrive at some conclusion about what systems have problems and how they affect movement. Abnormal motor behavior has many causes, and clinicians should be careful before concluding that an observed behavior is caused by problems in a certain system. For example, the Romberg test is commonly assumed to test the use of vestibular inputs. Yet during the test, both somatosensory and vestibular inputs are (normally) used for balance control. If balance control is deficient, is the vestibular system necessarily the culprit? Could somatosensory system deficits also result in a poor test result? Or, alternatively, because the Romberg test is performed with feet together, what effect would hip weakness have on the ability to stand with a narrowed base of support? When using a test whose results may be altered by problems in more than one system, any relevant system should be evaluated. If multiple system deficits exist, and they often do in patients with neurological conditions, then use caution in making "commonly assumed" conclusions on the basis of clinical test results.

Because so many balance tests are available, several questions must be asked to determine whether a test is appropriate for use.[36] For what purpose and population was the test designed? Can that test be used legitimately for a different purpose or with a different population? Is it valid? Is it reliable, that is, repeatable by different examiners or by the same examiner multiple times? In what populations is it valid and reliable? What is the threshold (minimal detectable change [MDC]) for this test—that is, how large must true performance changes be before this test can detect them? Are normative data available for comparison? These questions are being investigated but have not yet been answered for many of the clinical balance tests commonly used by therapists with the many different neurological populations they treat. Some of the evidence already reported may be frustrating to clinicians. For example, the Timed Up-and-Go test (TUG) predicts falls in community-dwelling older adults but not in acute-care hospital populations.[37,38] For several balance tests such as the TUG, the BBS, and others, the cutoff scores used for accurate prediction of falls in patients with Parkinson disease are different from the cutoff scores used in older adults without Parkinson disease.[39] These examples make

it clear that clinicians must understand their patients and the characteristics of the various balance tests in order to select the most appropriate tests and interpret test results for each patient.

Types of Balance Tests

Balance tests can be grouped or classified by type. Different types of tests measure different facets of postural control (Table 20.1). Quiet standing (static) refers to tests in which the patient is standing and the movement goal is to hold still. Disturbances to balance, called *perturbations,* may or may not be applied. Active standing (dynamic) tests also position the patient standing, but the movement goal involves voluntary weight shifting. Transition tests require that the patient

TABLE 20.1   Types of Balance Tests

Type	Tests
Quiet standing (with or without perturbation)	Romberg Sharpened Romberg or tandem Romberg One-legged stance test (OLST) Timed stance battery Balance Error Scoring System (BESS) Postural sway via forceplate, accelerometry Nudge or push Push and Release Test Motor Control Test (MCT)
Active standing	Functional Reach Test (FRT) Multi-Directional Reach Test (MDFR) Limits of Stability (LOS) Star Excursion Balance Test (SEBT) and Y Balance Test
Sensory manipulation	Sensory Organization Test (SOT) Clinical Test of Sensory Interaction on Balance (CTSIB)
Active transitions and stepping	5-Times Sit-to-Stand Test (5XSTS) 30-s Chair Stand Test (CST) 4-Square Step Test (4SST)
Functional scales	Berg Balance Scale (BBS) Timed Up-and-Go Test (TUG) Tinetti Performance Oriented Mobility Assessment (POMA) (Balance subscale) Tinetti Performance Oriented Mobility Assessment (POMA) (Gait subscale) Gait Abnormality Rating Scale (GARS) Modified Dynamic Gait Index (mDGI) Functional Gait Assessment (FGA) Environmental Analysis of Mobility Questionnaire (EAMQ)
Combination test batteries	Balance Evaluation Systems Test (BESTest) Fregly-Graybiel Ataxia Test Battery High-level Mobility Assessment Test (HiMAT) Community Balance and Mobility Scale (CBM) Fugl-Meyer Sensorimotor Assessment of Balance Performance
Dual-task	Stops walking when talking (SWWT) Dual-Task TUG, Manual and Cognitive Multiple Tasks Test (MTT) Walking and Remembering Test (WART)
Balance confidence	Activities-Specific Balance Confidence Scale (ABC) Falls Efficacy Scale—International (FES-I) Survey of Activity and Fear of Falling in the Elderly (SAFFE) Fear of Falling Avoidance Behavior Questionnaire (FFABQ)

move from one point to another, but do not require walking; examples include items #1 Sit-to-Stand, and #4 Transfer in the BBS, and the 4-Square Step Test (4SST).[40] Sensory manipulation tests use altered surface and visual conditions to determine how well the CNS is using and reweighting sensory inputs for postural control. Functional balance, mobility, and gait scales involve the performance of whole-body movement tasks, such as Item #9 "Pick up object from floor" in the BBS, walking, and stepping over objects. A few test batteries offer a combination of the preceding tests. The BESTest is the most comprehensive test battery to date. Dual-task tests have been developed to examine the effect of concurrent activities and divided attention on balance and mobility performance. Tests of sitting balance in adults are being developed because patients with neurological problems often need sitting balance retraining in early stages of recovery. Examples include the Seated Functional Reach Test[41] (used to measure excursion in seated individuals with spinal cord injuries), Postural Assessment Scale for Stroke Patients[42] (PASS), Trunk Impairment Scale,[43] Kansas University Sitting Balance Scale,[44] Sitting Balance Assessment Tool[45] (SitBAT), Function in Sitting Test,[46] and Ottawa Sitting Scale.[47]

Quiet Standing

The classic Romberg test was originally developed to "examine the effect of posterior column disease upon upright stance."[48] The patient stands with feet parallel and together and then closes the eyes for 20 to 30 seconds. The examiner subjectively judges the amount of sway. Quantification of sway can be accomplished with a videotape, forceplate, or, more recently, accelerometer.[49,50] Excessive sway, loss of balance, or stepping during this test is abnormal. The sharpened Romberg,[48] also known as the *tandem Romberg*, requires the patient to stand with feet in a heel-to-toe position and arms folded across the chest, eyes closed for 60 seconds. Often four trials of this test are timed with a stopwatch, for a maximum score of 240 seconds.

One-legged stance tests (OLSTs) are commonly used.[48,51] Both legs must be alternately tested, and differences between sides are noted. The patient stands on both feet and places hands on the hips or crosses the arms over the chest, then picks up one leg and holds it with the hip in neutral and the knee flexed to 90 degrees. The lifted leg may *not* be pressed into the stance leg. This test is scored with a stopwatch. Five 30-second trials are performed for each leg (alternating legs), with a maximum possible score of 150 seconds per leg. Normal young subjects are able to stand for 30 seconds, but this may not be a reasonable expectation for frail older patients.[48]

In both the Romberg test and the OLST, problems in sensory organization processes can be observed. To determine how much of the stability is achieved through visual stabilization, each test can be repeated with eyes closed. The patient with visual dependency for balance will often have an immediate loss of balance when the eyes are closed. (Remember, visual dependency may be a sign of somatosensory or vestibular loss, or both.) As noted earlier, the patient with somatosensory or vestibular loss may have difficulty producing the hip strategy necessary to perform these tasks.

A battery of timed stance tests has been developed by Bohannon and Leary[52]; designed for acute care bedside use, it can be used in other settings as well. This set of tests varies the foot position (apart, together, tandem, and single leg) and the availability of visual information (eyes opened and closed) to produce eight different combinations. Maintenance of balance in each condition is timed for a maximum of 30 seconds; the assigned score is the total number of seconds that balance could be maintained. The best possible score on this test is 240 seconds. This test is reliable, valid, and sensitive to change over time.[52]

A related test is the Balance Error Scoring System, or BESS test, which was developed for use with athletes to screen for concussion effects.[53,54] The original BESS test involved three stance positions (double-leg stance with feet together, single-leg stance, tandem stance) on two surfaces (firm and foam), thus providing six conditions. The eyes are closed in all conditions. Each trial is 20 seconds in duration. The examiner observes and counts the number of balance errors that are made in each condition. The six observed errors include hands lifted off waist; opening eyes; step, stumble, or balance loss; moving a hip past 30 degrees of abduction; lifting the forefoot or heel; and remaining out of the test position for more than 5 seconds. If more than one error occurs at the same time, for example, opening eyes and hands off waist, only one error is counted. When measured in high-level young adults, the reliability of this test improved with the removal of the double-leg stance condition, which produced few to no errors in this high-functioning population, and the addition of three trials in each of the remaining four conditions. The modified BESS test thus includes only four conditions.[55] This test has not been investigated for use in traditional neurological rehabilitation populations but may be a valuable alternative for high-functioning young patients post-concussion or mild TBI.

Objective postural sway measures can be obtained by computerized force plates (Fig. 20.5) or wearable accelerometers (Fig. 20.6).[50,56–58] The patient is asked to adopt a standardized foot placement, if possible (this varies by manufacturer), and to stand quietly with arms at the sides or hands on the hips for 20 or 30 seconds. Sway with both eyes open and eyes closed is commonly measured. Graphic and numerical quantification is provided. Normative data may be provided. These more technical measures are able to detect more subtle problems and are more sensitive to change in performance after treatment than are rating scales or timed measures.

APRs are assessed by the patient's response to perturbations. It is imperative that clinicians include APR testing in their balance

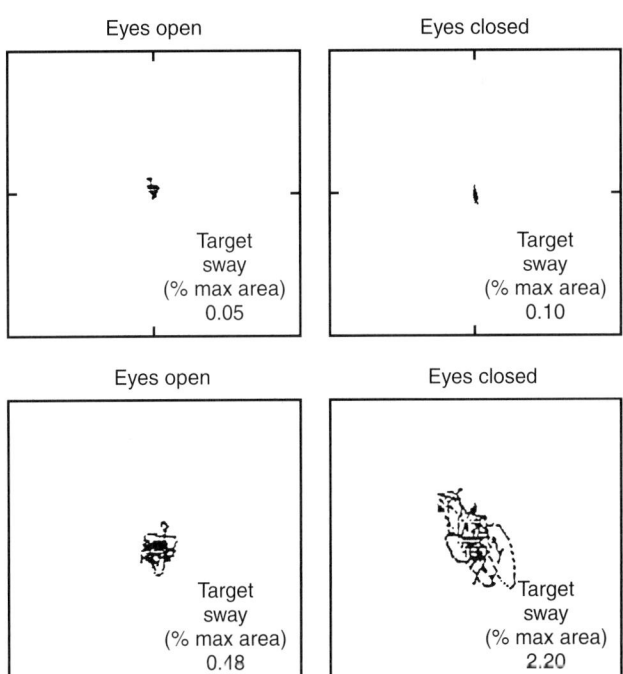

Fig. 20.5 Graphic and Numerical Postural Sway Measures Using a Computerized Force Plate System. *Top left,* Normal subject, eyes open. *Top right,* Healthy subject, eyes closed. *Bottom left,* Patient with Parkinson disease, eyes open. *Bottom right,* Patient with Parkinson disease, eyes closed. (Reprinted with permission from NeuroCom International, Clackamas, Ore.)

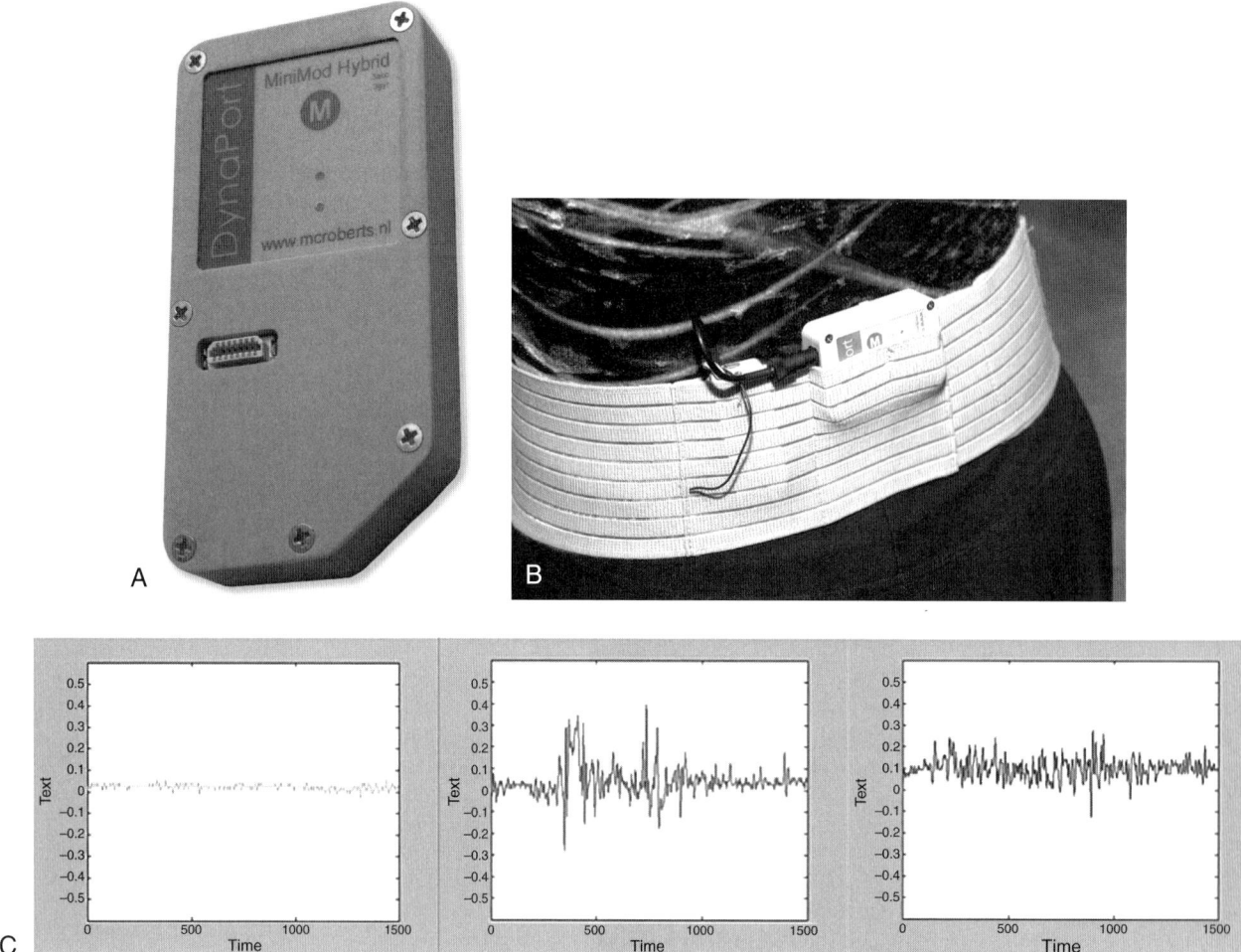

Fig. 20.6 **(A)** A wearable accelerometer for motion detection that can be used to measure postural sway and other physical motions. **(B)** The accelerometer worn in a belt at the L5 to S1 level. **(C)** Postural sway data recorded by the accelerometer. (Photographs courtesy McRoberts B, The Hague, The Netherlands.)

assessment because APRs are the motor responses necessary to prevent loss of balance and falls. The push-and-release test is a clinically useful method with a five-point ordinal rating scale.[33,59,60] Testing for ankle and hip strategies ("in-place" strategies) requires that the clinician (1) place his or her hands on the front or back of the patient's shoulders, (2) ask the patient to remain still and centered by resisting the pressure applied by the hands (producing isometric muscle activity), (3) watch for the toes or heels to begin to raise slightly (the clinician increases pressure until this occurs), then (4) suddenly release the push. Both forward and backward directions are tested. For safety, the clinician always stands where he or she can support the patient in case of balance loss. Testing for stepping strategy follows the same concept but is performed differently. Instead of keeping the patient's COG at midline, the patient leans his or her weight into the clinician's hands, shifting the COG away from midline toward the outer limit of stability before the release. The correct patient response is to step to reestablish a new base of support underneath the new position of the COG. Forward, backward, and both lateral directions are tested. When nudge or push tests are performed predictably (i.e., "Don't let me push you backward."), this is assessment of anticipatory postural control. When the release happens unpredictably (no cues, unpredictable timing), APRs can be assessed. Perturbations of different strengths from multiple directions should be given.

The Motor Control Test (MCT) is a computerized test of APRs that perturbs the patient through surface displacement (Fig. 20.7B).[4] The patient stands on a dynamic (movable) forceplate with feet parallel and arms at sides. The support surface rapidly translates (slides) forward or backward. This surface displacement results in a rapid shift in the relation between the COG and the base of support. The expected responses are directionally specific (to the direction of the stimulus) forces generated against the surface to bring the COG back to the center. Response latencies, strength, and symmetry are measured. Normative data are available. This test can be used to look for abnormal stepping strategies when failure to select hip strategy occurs. The MCT is the most standardized and reliable test of APRs but is less widely used because it requires computerized equipment.

Active Standing

Volitional control of the COG is evaluated by asking the patient to make voluntary movements that require weight shifting. The Functional Reach Test (FRT) was developed for home health use with older adults to determine risk of falls.[61] The patient stands near a wall with feet parallel. Attached to the wall at shoulder height is a yardstick. The patient is asked to make a fist and raise the arm nearest the wall to 90 degrees of shoulder flexion. The examiner notes the position of the fist on the yardstick. The patient is then asked to lean forward as far as

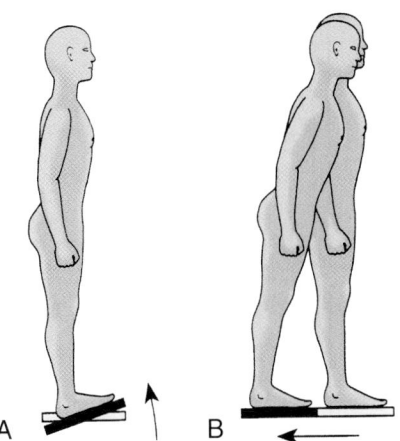

Fig. 20.7 Surface perturbations during **(A)** the adaptation test and **(B)** the motor control test using computerized dynamic posturography. Forceplate measures include latency and amount of response and adaptation of the response to repeated perturbations. (From Hasson S. *Clinical Exercise Physiology.* St Louis: Mosby; 1994.)

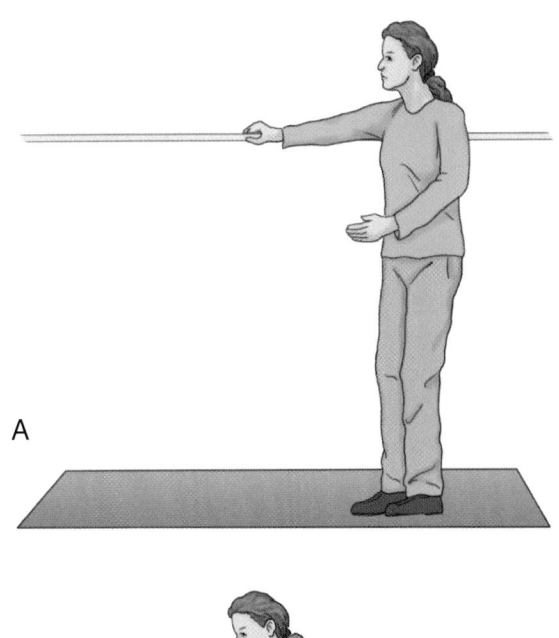

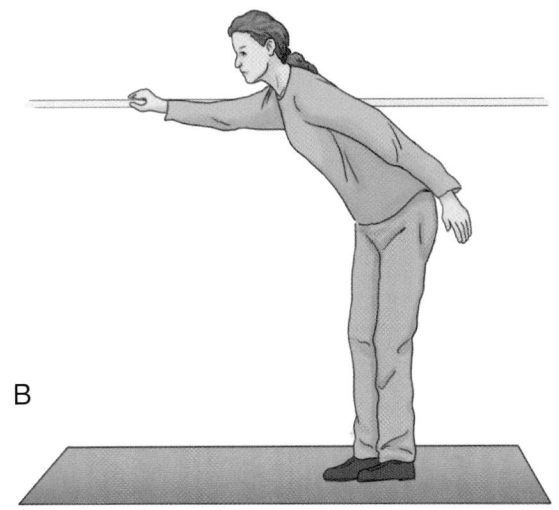

Fig. 20.8 During the Functional Reach Test, the patient is asked to reach forward as far as possible from a comfortable standing posture. The excursion of the arm from start to finish is measured by a yardstick affixed to the wall at shoulder height. **(A)** Functional reach, starting position. **(B)** Functional reach, ending position.

possible, and the examiner notes the end position of the fist on the yardstick (Fig. 20.8). Beginning position is subtracted from end position to obtain a change unit in inches. Three trials are performed. Normative data are available, and the test is reliable. However, the standard error of measurement for this test may be as high as 2 inches, meaning that a change in score of less than 2 inches cannot be attributed to clinical improvement because it may reflect only measurement error. Subsequent studies have not shown that this test is useful for fall prediction.[62–64] For these reasons the FRT is not recommended as a stand-alone test, rather it should be used in conjunction with other tests. Both the BBS and the BESTest include the FRT.

One serious limitation of the FRT is that it measures sway in only one direction (forward). An expansion of this test has been devised to measure sway in four directions.[65] The multidirectional functional reach test (MDFR) is conceptually equivalent but measures sway anteriorly, posteriorly, and laterally to both sides. This test should provide a more comprehensive picture of volitional COG control limitations. Validity and mean values have been established for community-dwelling older adults.[66] The BESTest includes the forward and lateral directions from the MDFR test.

The Limits of Stability test (LOS) uses a computerized forceplate to measure postural sway away from midline in eight directions.[56,67] Patients assume a standardized foot position and control a cursor on the computer monitor by shifting their weight. They are asked to move the cursor from midline to eight targets on the screen (Fig. 20.9). Measures include movement velocity, directional control (path sway), measures of excursion (length of the trajectory of the COG), and reaction time. This test should be performed once for familiarization, then a second time for scoring purposes. Second and subsequent tests are reliable and normative data are available.

A very challenging test used primarily in athletic populations is the Star Excursion Balance Test (SEBT) (Fig. 20.10).[68,69] The SEBT could be used, for example, in high level TBI patients who require more demanding test conditions. However, although there is evidence for the validity and reliability of this test in orthopedic populations, as yet this test has not been investigated for use in neurological populations. The SEBT is in concept a lower-extremity functional reach test, requiring single-leg stance on one leg and a reach with the other leg. The original SEBT included eight directions; currently the SEBT is

typically performed in three directions: center-forward, right-rear, and left-rear.[70] Three tape measures are taped to the floor, radiating out from the same center point. The two rear tape measures are at a 45-degree angle from the center line. The patient stands on one foot with the great toe on the center point, then reaches the maximum distance away from the center with the lifted foot. The distance is recorded by the examiner. This is done in all three directions, with the lifted leg having to cross behind the stance leg to reach to the opposite-side rear tape. Six practice trials in each direction are given before recording scores to eliminate a learning effect, although recent evidence suggests four practice trials may be sufficient.[71] Three scored trials in each direction are performed; both legs are tested.[72] A commercial version of this test, the Y Balance Test, is available and has the advantage of being portable.

Sensory Manipulation

Sensory inputs play a critical role in postural control, but few tests to measure their use to produce a balance performance outcome have

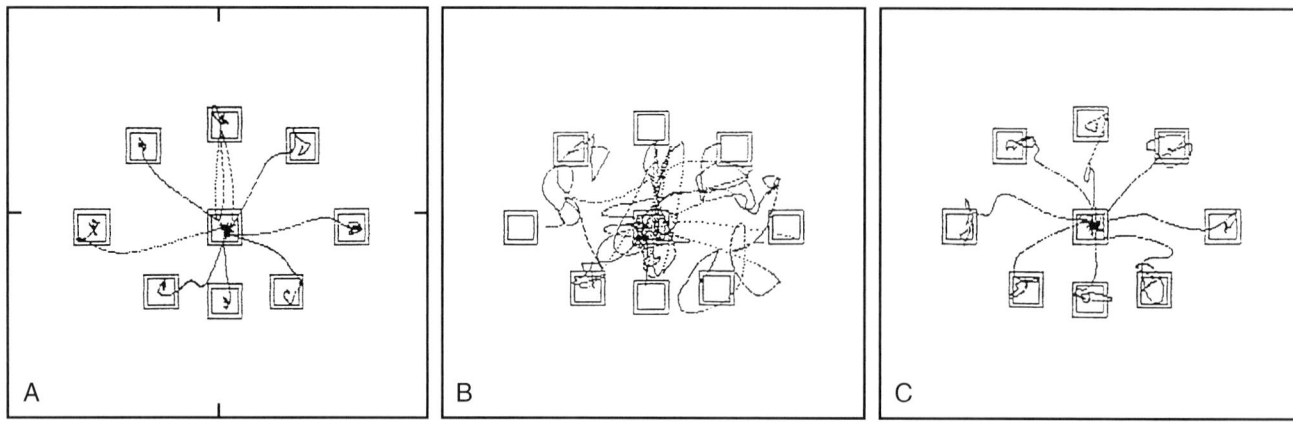

Fig. 20.9 Graphic postural sway measures from the limits of stability test using a computerized forceplate system (numerical measures not shown). Patients are asked to move away from and return to midline. **(A)** Subject with normal postural sway. **(B)** Hemiplegic patient on initial evaluation. **(C)** Hemiplegic patient on discharge evaluation. (Reprinted with permission from NeuroCom International, Clackamas, Ore.)

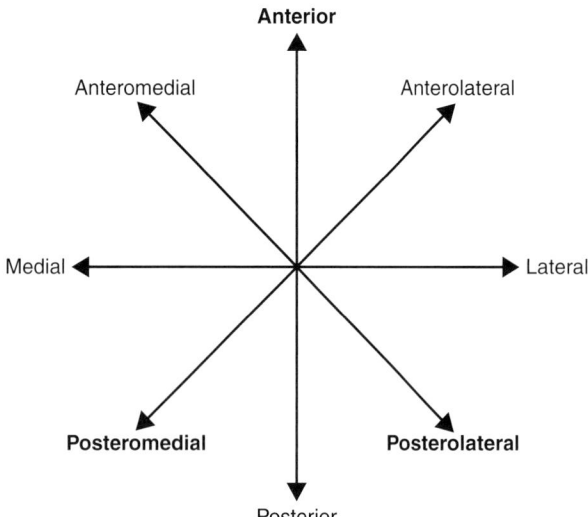

Fig. 20.10 The floor grid layout for the original Star Excursion Balance Test (SEBT) with eight directions. Bolded arrows in the anterior, posteromedial, and posterolateral directions indicate the three directions used in the modified SEBT. (From Brumitt J. Assessing athletic balance with the Star Excursion Balance Test. *NSCA Perform Train J.* 2008;7:6.)

Fig. 20.11 The Six Sensory Organization Test (SOT) Conditions. The SOT determines the relative reliance on visual, vestibular, and somatosensory inputs for postural control using computerized dynamic posturography. (From Hasson S. *Clinical Exercise Physiology.* St Louis: Mosby; 1994.)

been developed. The Sensory Organization Test (SOT) uses a computerized, movable forceplate and movable visual surround to alter the surface and visual environments systematically.[4,5] The patient stands on the forceplate with feet parallel and arms at the sides and is asked to stand quietly. Three 20-second trials under each of six sensory conditions are performed (Fig. 20.11). In conditions one, two, and three the support surface (forceplate) is fixed. During conditions four, five, and six the support surface is sway referenced to the sway of the patient. In other words, the movement of the surface is matched to the movement of the patient in a 1:1 ratio. This responsive surface movement maintains a near-constant ankle joint angle despite body sway, rendering the somatosensory information from the feet and ankles inaccurate for use in balance maintenance. Visual inputs are undisturbed in conditions one and four. Vision is absent (eyes are closed) in conditions two and five. The movable visual surround is sway referenced in

conditions three and six. This responsive visual surround movement maintains a near-constant distance between the eyes and the visual environment despite body sway, rendering visual inputs from the eyes inaccurate for balance maintenance in those two conditions.

Under condition one, all three senses (vision, vestibular sense, and somatosensory sense) are available and accurate. Body sway is measured by the forceplate; this initial measurement forms the baseline against which subsequent measures are compared (Fig. 20.12).

SENSORY ANALYSIS			
Ratio Name	Test Conditions	Ratio Pair	Significance
SOM Somatosensory	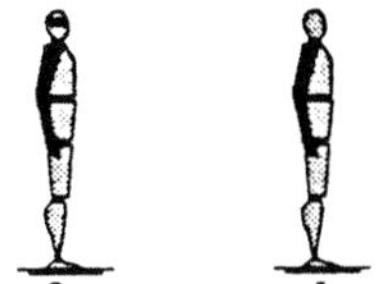 2 1	Condition 1 / Condition 2	Question: Does sway increase when visual cues are removed? Low scores: Patient makes poor use of somatosensory references.
VIS Visual	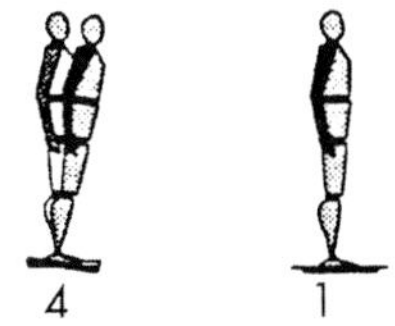 4 1	Condition 4 / Condition 1	Question: Does sway increase when somatosensory cues are inaccurate? Low scores: Patient makes poor use of visual references.
VEST Vestibular	5 1	Condition 5 / Condition 1	Question: Does sway increase when visual cues are removed and somatosensory cues are inaccurate? Low scores: Patient makes poor use of vestibular cues, or vestibular cues unavailable.
PREF Visual Preference	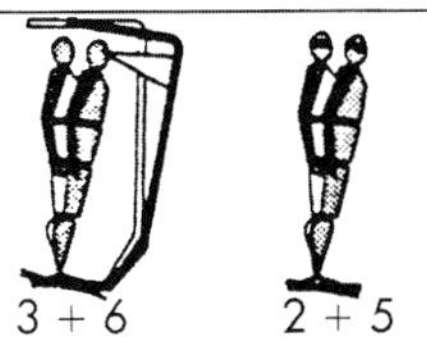 3 + 6 2 + 5	Condition 3 + 6 / Condition 2 + 5	Question: Do inaccurate visual cues result in increased sway compared to no visual cues? Low scores: Patient relies on visual cues even when they are inaccurate.

Fig. 20.12 Postural sway measures from each of the six sensory organization test conditions are compared, and the ratios are used to identify impairments in the use of sensory inputs for postural control. (From Jacobson GP, Newman CW, Kartush JM. *Handbook of Balance Function Testing.* St Louis: Mosby; 1993.)

Under condition two the eyes are closed, so only somatosensory and vestibular cues remain. In an individual with normal movement function, the somatosensory inputs will dominate in this condition. By comparing sway during condition two with sway during condition one, detection of how well the patient is using somatosensory inputs for balance control is possible. Patients with somatosensory loss from incomplete SCI, diabetes, or amputation have difficulty in condition two. Functional situations with inadequate lighting or unusable visual cues (e.g., busy carpeting) are similar to condition two.

Under condition four, the support surface is sway referenced (somatosensory cues are available but are inaccurate), so only visual and vestibular cues remain useful. In a normal patient the visual inputs will dominate in this condition. Comparing sway during condition four with sway during condition one indicates how well the patient is using visual inputs for balance control. Patients with visual loss caused by diabetes, cataracts, or field loss have difficulty in condition four. Functional situations that correlate with condition four include compliant surfaces (beach, soft ground, gravel driveway) and unstable surfaces (boat deck, slipping throw rug).

Under condition five, the eyes are closed (visual cues are absent) and the support surface is sway referenced (somatosensory cues are inaccurate), leaving the vestibular inputs as the only remaining sensory inputs that are both available and accurate. Comparison of sway during condition five with sway during condition one indicates how well the patient is using vestibular inputs for balance control. Patients with vestibular loss caused by head injury, MS, or acoustic neuroma may have difficulty with condition five. Many older patients with age-related vestibular loss also may be unstable in this condition. Functional situations in which these patients may be at risk for falls would have both inadequate lighting and compliant or unsteady surfaces (e.g., walking on a gravel driveway or thick carpet in the dark).

Under both conditions three and six, the visual surround is sway referenced (visual cues are available but inaccurate). By comparing sway during these two conditions with sway in the absence of vision (conditions two and five, with eyes closed), determining how well the patient can recognize and subsequently suppress inaccurate visual inputs when they conflict with somatosensory and vestibular cues is possible. Some patients with CNS lesions (e.g., head injury, stroke, tumor) may have difficulty with this condition. Patients who cannot recognize or ignore inaccurate visual cues cannot distinguish whether they are moving, or the environment is moving. If they perceive that they are moving (away from midline) when they are not, they may often actively generate postural responses to "right" themselves. These responses, invoked to bring the COG to midline, then result in movement away from the midline. The inaccurate perception leads to a self-initiated loss of balance. Functional situations that correlate with this test condition include public transportation, grocery and library aisles, and moving walkways.

The SOT is valid and reliable in the absence of motoric problems, which increase sway for reasons unrelated to sensory reception and perception. Normative data are available.

Visual conditions

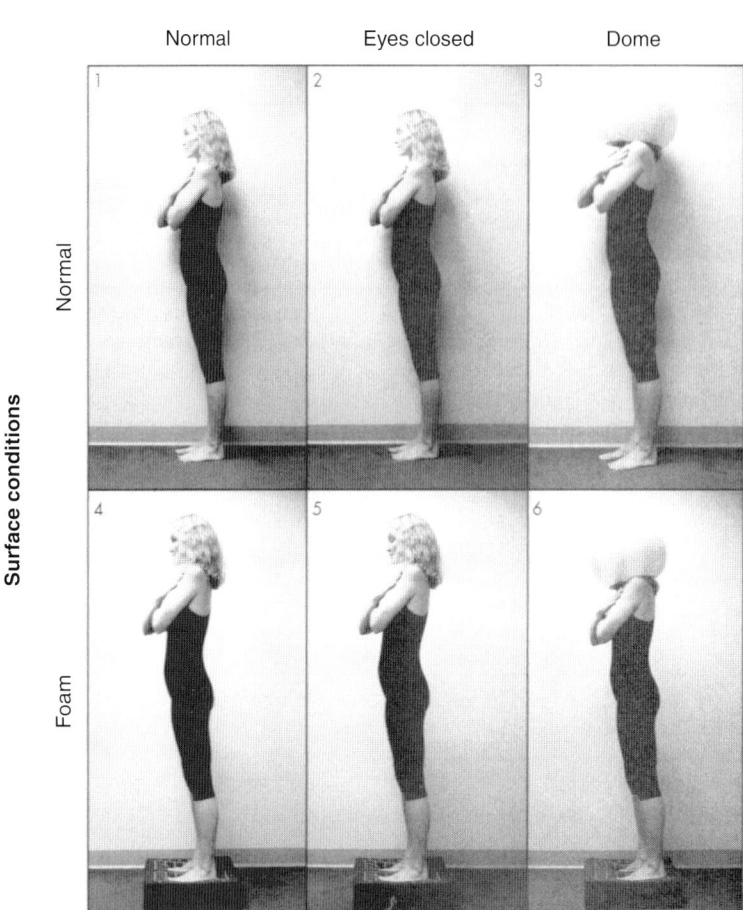

Fig. 20.13 The clinical test of sensory interactions on balance uses foam and a Japanese lantern to replicate the six sensory conditions. A stopwatch is used to time trials.

The Clinical Test of Sensory Interaction on Balance (CTSIB) is a clinical version of the SOT that does not use computerized force-plate technology.[73] The concept of the six conditions remains intact (Fig. 20.13). Instead of sway measures, the examiner uses a stopwatch and visual observation. A thick foam pad substitutes for the moving forceplate during conditions four, five, and six. In normal individuals and patients with peripheral vestibular lesions, measures with foam correlate to moving forceplate measures.[74] Originally, a modified Japanese lantern substituted for the moving visual surround in conditions three and six. Studies have not shown that measures using the Japanese lantern correlate with the moving visual surround measures. Most clinicians now perform the modified CTSIB with just four conditions, eyes open and closed on a firm surface and eyes open and closed on the foam surface. The patient is asked to stand with feet parallel and arms at the sides or hands on the hips. At least three and up to five 30-second trials of each condition are performed.[20] The watch is stopped if the patient steps, reaches, or falls during the 30 seconds. If the patient is very steady for 30 seconds on the first trial of a condition, some clinicians choose not to test the remaining trials in that condition and will give the patient a full score for that condition. A maximum score for five trials of each condition is 150 seconds. Individuals with normal movement abilities are able to stand without stepping, reaching, or exhibiting loss of balance for 30 seconds per trial per condition. It is normal for sway to increase slightly as the conditions increase

in difficulty. The CTSIB may not be a reliable measure in patients with hemiplegia or other conditions that involve motor deficits in, or abnormal response time through, the lower extremities and trunk.[75] The clinician can use the information regarding patient response in a variety of environmental conditions to determine intervention management strategies.[76]

Vestibular System Tests

Please refer to Chapter 21 for a thorough presentation of vestibular disorders and their management.

Active Transitions and Stepping

The ability to change the base of support without balance loss and then to reestablish COG stability over the new base of support is a balance-dependent skill critical for functional activities. The 5-Times Sit-to-Stand Test (5XSTS) and the 30-second Chair Stand Test (CST) are both quantifiable measures of the sit-to-stand skill often used to screen for leg weakness.[77,78] For both tests, the patient sits with arms crossed over chest in a stabilized standard height chair without arms. The starting position is seated slightly forward so that the patient is not resting against the back of the chair, with the feet underneath and slightly behind the knees. In the 5XSTS the patient is asked to stand up (all the way up to an erect stance) and sit all the way back down (weight transferred from feet to buttocks) 5 times; the clinician uses a

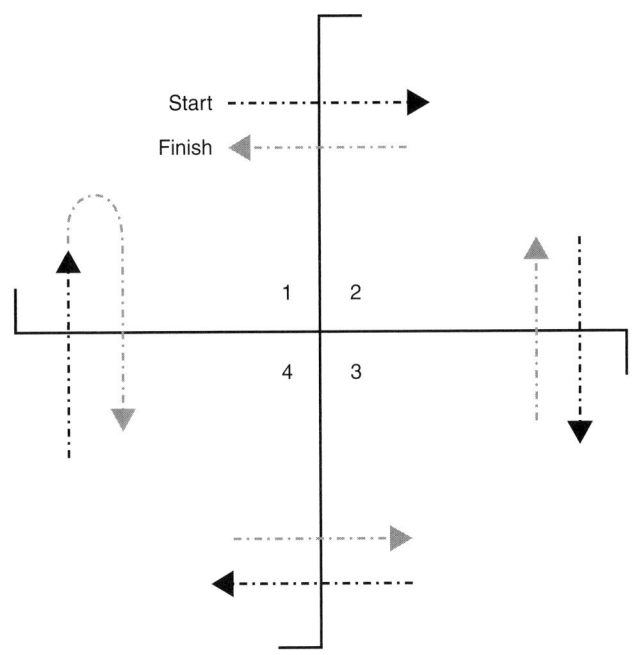

Start

Finish

1 2

4 3

Fig. 20.14 The Floor Grid for the Timed 4-Square Step Test. Arrows indicate the direction of the steps. (From Dite W, Temple VA. A clinical test of stepping and change of direction to identify multiple falling older adults. *Arch Phys Med Rehabil.* 2002;83:1568.)

stopwatch to time the performance beginning when the clinician says "Go" and ending when the patient is fully seated the fifth time. In the CST the instructions to the patient and their performance of full sit-to-stand motions are the same, but the clinician counts the number of times the patient can perform the motion in a 30-second timeframe. Rests are permitted but the timer continues to run, so rests should only be taken if needed. The longer duration of this test requires muscle endurance in addition to strength. Normative data and cutoff points for fall risk screening are available for both tests.

The 4-Square Step Test is a timed stepping test in a standardized, structured format in forward, backward, and lateral directions (Fig. 20.14).[40] A simple plus sign–shaped grid is laid out on the floor using four straight canes, dowel rods, or lengths of plastic piping. This creates four quadrants. The patient begins standing in the rear-left quadrant, steps forward over the first bar to stand with both feet in the front-left quadrant, steps rightward over the second bar to stand with both feet in the right-front quadrant, steps backward over the third bar to stand with both feet in the right-rear quadrant, steps leftward over the fourth bar to stand with both feet in the left-rear quadrant (starting location). The patient then reverses direction, going back through each quadrant in the same way until standing again with both feet in the rear-left quadrant. The outcome measure is the time it takes the patient to perform this task correctly, clearing each bar completely with each foot. This test has been used with older adults, individuals with vestibular disorders, and with patients post-stroke.[79,80]

Functional Scales

A comprehensive balance evaluation must include impairment-based tests of body systems, tests of balance skills, and activity-based functional measures. Functional scales help identify the activity limitations. By asking the patient to perform functional tasks that demand balance skills, the clinician can determine the presence of activity limitations that will affect the individual's ability to participate in life and identify

the tasks that the patient needs to practice. Three mobility scales and three gait scales focus on postural control; five of these were developed for the elderly population to determine risk of falls. Many clinicians are also using them to assess patients with neurological conditions, although their usefulness with neurological populations is less well-documented. Far fewer standardized tests for high-level balance skills have been developed; some clinicians adapt tests used by athletes, but these are often too difficult for many neurologically involved patients.

The BBS consists of 14 tasks that the patient is asked to perform.[81] The examiner rates the patient on each task by using an ordinal rating scale of 0 to 4, in which 0 is unable to perform and 4 is able to perform without difficulty. This test is highly reliable. It was originally designed for assessing risk of falls in older adults, and cutoff scores for fall risk vary depending on which of several studies is consulted.[82,83] Use of higher cutoff scores may erroneously identify nonfallers as fallers; use of lower cutoff scores may erroneously identify fallers as nonfallers. The BBS has also been used with patients after stroke.[84–87]

The original Get-Up-and-Go Test is made up of seven items and subjectively scored on an ordinal rating scale of 1 to 5, in which 1 is normal and 5 is severely abnormal.[88] This test has been modified by making it a timed measure to increase its objectivity and reliability, which is now high. The TUG test eliminates the "standing steady" segment and uses a stopwatch to time the performance.[89] Patients are asked to rise from a chair with arms, walk 3 meters as fast as they safely can, turn, walk back to the chair, and sit down. This test may be performed with an assistive device; however, the use of a device will alter the speed at which the task can be accomplished, and any retesting must be done with the same device to produce comparable results. Originally designed to assess frailty in older adults, the test is now more commonly used to assess fall risk in this population. Young adults typically perform this task in 5 to 7 seconds, healthy older adults in 7 to 9 seconds (low-risk), moderate-risk older adults in 10 to 12 seconds, and high-risk older adults in 13 seconds or more.[90,91] These cutoff scores are for older adults walking without assistive devices. Improvements in test performance that are not captured by the time score alone should also be documented; for example, if the patient can now perform the test without the use of chair arms to stand up, or without an assistive device.

The Tinetti Performance-Oriented Mobility Assessment—Balance subscale (POMA-Balance) is a list of nine items scored on scales of either 0 to 1 or 0 to 2, with the higher numbers reflecting better (more normal) performance.[92] The score value is specific to the item. The best possible score is 16, with a score of 10 or lower indicating a high risk of falls.[93] This test is appropriate for onetime use, for example at a health fair, but is not ideal for documenting progress over time due to the limited scoring range.

Most balance and mobility scales have been developed to assess risk of falls in older adults. Many share similar items. See Table 20.2 for a summary of scale items.

The Tinetti Performance-Oriented Mobility Assessment—Gait subscale (POMA-Gait) is a list of seven normal aspects of gait that are observed by the examiner as the patient walks at a self-selected pace and then at a rapid but safe pace.[92] Scoring scales are again either 0 to 1 or 0 to 2, and higher numbers indicate better performance. Score values are specific to the item being observed (Table 20.3). The best possible score is a 12; scores of 8 or below indicate a high risk of falls. When combined, the Tinetti POMA balance and gait scales offer a best possible score of 28, with scores of 19 or less indicating a high fall risk. Again, if the clinician will need to document change over time, the scoring range of this test renders it less able to detect that change.

TABLE 20.2   Balance and Mobility Scale Items

Activity	Berg Balance Scale	Dynamic Gait Index and Functional Gait Assessment	Timed Up-And-Go Test	Tinetti Balance Assessment
1. Sitting unsupported	√			√
2. Sitting to standing	√		√	√
3. Standing to sitting	√		√	√
4. Transfers	√			
5. Standing unsupported	√		√	√
6. Standing with eyes closed	√			√
7. Standing with feet together	√			
8. Tandem standing	√			
9. Standing on one leg	√			
10. Rotating trunk while standing	√			
11. Retrieving object from floor	√			
12. Turning 360 degrees	√			√
13. Stool stepping	√			
14. Reaching forward while standing	√			
15. Sternal nudge	√			√
16. Walking		√	√	
17. Abrupt stop		√		
18. Walking then turning		√	√	
19. Stepping over obstacle		√		
20. Stairs		√		
21. Walking at preferred and varied speeds		√		
22. Walking with horizontal and vertical head turns		√		
23. Stepping around obstacles		mDGI only		
24. Walk with narrow base of support		FGA only		
25. Walk with eyes closed		FGA only		
26. Walk backwards		FGA only		

TABLE 20.3   Gait Scale Items

Gait Activities	Tinetti Gait Scale	Gait Abnormality Rating Scale
1. Initiation (hesitancy)	√	√[b]
2. Step length	√	√[b]
3. Step height	√	√
4. Step symmetry	√	√
5. Step continuity	√	√[b]
6. Path deviation	√	√
7. Trunk	√	√
8. Walking-heel distance	√	
9. Staggering		√[b]
10. Heel strike		√[b]
11. Hip ROM[a]		√[b]
12. Knee ROM[a]		√
13. Elbow extension[a]		√
14. Shoulder extension[a]		√[b]
15. Shoulder abduction[a]		√
16. Arm-heel strike synchrony		√[b]
17. Forward head[a]		√
18. Shoulders held elevated[a]		√
19. Forward flexed trunk[a]		
20. Gait speed		√[b]

[a]During gait.
[b]Items that were retained for the Modified GARS.
ROM, Range of motion.

The original Gait Abnormality Rating Scale (GARS) is a list of 16 abnormal aspects of gait observed by the examiner as the patient walks at a self-selected pace (see Table 20.3).[94] These abnormalities are commonly seen in older adults who fall, who are fearful of falling, or both. The items are scored on a scale of 0 to 3, with lower numbers reflecting better (less abnormal) performance. The best possible score is 0. This gait scale provides some relative numerical indication of the quality of gait. A shorter, modified version of this test, the Modified GARS (GARS-M), has been developed. The GARS-M includes nine of the original items plus a gait velocity measure. It provides equivalent sensitivity and takes less time to perform.[95] These two gait scales were developed to assess risk of falls in older adults.

The Dynamic Gait Index (DGI) is a gait test specifically designed to look at postural control during gait.[13] It includes eight items requiring changes in gait speed, walking with horizontal and vertical head turning, whole-body turns during gait, stepping over and around obstacles, and stair ascent and descent. The presence of head motion and whole-body turns in this test may help identify patients with potential vestibular dysfunction.

Items on this test were originally scored with a focus on the gait pattern using a 4-point ordinal scale of 0 to 3, with 3 being normal performance and 0 indicating severe impairment. The best possible score on the original test is a 24, and scores of less than 19 points were associated with impairment of gait and fall risk. The reliability of this test is high.[83,96,97] The Modified DGI (mDGI) includes the same eight test items, but the scoring system has been changed by the original test developers to better capture multiple aspects of gait performance.[98]

Each item is now scored using a combination of gait pattern, time to complete the task, and level of assistance needed, on the same scale of 0 to 3. The maximum possible score for this test is also 24. The mDGI is a valid, reliable measure in persons with stroke, TBI, vestibular dysfunction, and gait abnormalities.[99]

A modified and slightly more difficult version of this test, the Functional Gait Assessment (FGA), has been developed specifically for use with patients with vestibular disorders.[100] The FGA has 10 items, seven of which are identical to the DGI. The FGA eliminates the "step around obstacles" item and adds three new items, gait with narrow base of support, gait with eyes closed, and backwards walking. The best possible score on the FGA is 30 points, and a score of 22 points or below can be used to classify fall risk and predict unexplained falls in community-dwelling older adults.[101] Normative data for community-dwelling older adults is available.[102]

The three gait tests listed previously are distinct from traditional gait tests because they focus on elements of postural control during gait. Two very important traditional gait measures that should be included in the assessment of balance and gait in older adults and patients with neurological disorders are gait speed and distance/endurance. Gait speed has been termed "the sixth vital sign" for older adults because of its strong association with level of dependence in activities of daily living (ADLs) and instrumental ADLs (IADLs), probability of hospitalization, risk of falls, eventual discharge location, and ambulation category.[103] Reliable and valid measures of gait speed and distance include the Six-meter and Ten-meter Walk tests for speed, and the Two-minute and Six-minute Walk tests for distance and endurance[104–107]

Patients whose balance and gait deficits negatively affect their ability to manage environmental demands on mobility are considered to have "mobility disability" and are likely to have limited community participation.[108,109] Eight environmental dimensions that together describe the demands placed on an individual for community mobility include distance, time/speed, ambient conditions (lighting, weather, etc.), physical load (carrying), terrain, attentional demands, postural transitions, and traffic level (density and need to accommodate others). To minimize mobility disability and maximize community participation, clinicians need to assess their patients' abilities in all of these eight dimensions (and where deficient, intervene to improve patient capacity in those dimensions). Most clinical measures of gait do not capture the level of complexity and challenge found in community mobility activities.[110] As yet, no standardized performance measure of these dimensions of community mobility has been developed, however, a self-report measure based on these eight dimensions is available and does correlate with directly observed performance. The Environmental Analysis of Mobility Questionnaire (EAMQ) has 41 questions about "trips away from home" that address how frequently the patient encounters various environmental demands, and how often the patient intentionally avoids those encounters.[111] Improved scores on the EAMQ may demonstrate increased capacity for community-level participation.

Combination Test Batteries

Because no single test can give a complete picture of a patient's balance abilities, individual test items are often combined to form a test battery. Several of the tests described earlier, such as the BBS and the Tinetti POMA, include a combination of multiple items and could be categorized as combination test batteries. Different items on a test may challenge different components of the postural control system to permit a more complete assessment of the patient's balance abilities.

The BESTest is an excellent comprehensive test battery based on the systems model of postural control (see Fig. 20.4).[33] It includes 36 items

grouped into six categories of balance "sub-systems" representing components of postural control: biomechanical constraints; stability limits/verticality; APAs; APRs; sensory orientation; and stability during gait. Within each category are individual test items and, in some cases, existing tests. For example, the sensory orientation category contains the individual item "Stand on incline with eyes closed" and the four-condition CTSIB discussed earlier. Each item is scored on a 0 to 3 scale, with a maximum score of 108. Although the BESTest takes approximately 30 minutes to administer, the information acquired helps to identify which underlying components of the postural control system are causing the observed balance problems. Armed with this critical information, the clinician can design a customized, individualized intervention program that targets the sources of imbalance in each patient.

Two shorter versions of this test have been developed. The Mini-BESTest (see Fig. 20.4)[34] includes 14 of the original 36 items in four of the original six categories. It has a compressed rating scale (0 to 2), a maximum score of 28, and takes approximately 15 minutes to administer. It does not include any items from the biomechanical constraints category or the stability limits/verticality category. This does not mean that these components need not be measured, however. Biomechanical constraints such as hip and ankle weakness, and constricted limits of stability, seriously negatively affect balance and should be tested in addition to administration of the Mini-BESTest. The compressed rating scale may reduce the ability of this test to reflect a patient's progress over time. The Brief-BESTest (see Fig. 20.4)[35] includes 6 of the original 36 items, one in each of the original 6 categories. Two of the 6 items are tested bilaterally, for a total of 8 scored items using a 0 to 3 scale, and a maximum score of 24. The Brief-BESTest takes the least time to administer and provides the highest sensitivity for discriminating fallers from nonfallers. Normative data for older adults is available for all three versions of the BESTtest.[112]

For patients with higher-level balance skills, more challenging test batteries are needed. The Fregly-Graybiel Ataxia Test Battery includes eight test items that the patient must perform (Fig. 20.15).[48] Standing trials in tandem stance both off and on a rail with eyes open and closed are timed. Timed single-leg stance trials also are performed for each leg. Walking 10 steps with eyes closed is included. Five trials of each task are given. Trials are stopped if the patient uncrosses the arms, opens the eyes (during eyes-closed trials), steps (during standing trials), or falls. Trials are judged on a pass-fail basis. This test battery is valid for use with patients who have peripheral vestibular dysfunction. Normative data are available from a normative database composed primarily of findings in young men. As noted earlier, patients must be at a high level motorically to perform these tasks. This test is a good choice for patients with higher-level abilities because it does provide more demanding balance tasks. Interpretations regarding a patient's use of sensory inputs when motor involvement is also present cannot be made with certainty.

The High-Level Mobility Assessment Tool[113] (Hi-MAT) is a balance-challenging mobility measure that was designed to quantify mobility outcomes after TBI. It includes a total of 11 items, 9 are timed (walk, walk backwards, walk on toes, walk over obstacle, run, skip, hop on affected leg, ascend/descend stairs), and 2 are distances measures (bound on affected leg/unaffected leg). Each of these interval measures is converted to an ordinal scale score (0 to 4 or 1 to 5 depending on item), and these are added together to obtain a total score. The maximum possible score is 54. For many young patients, tests designed for older adults are much too easy; this test was designed for young adults and is challenging.

The Community Balance and Mobility Scale[114] is likewise a balance-challenging mobility scale designed for young adults post-TBI. Despite the title, the test is performed in a clinical setting. It contains 13 items,

FREGLY TEST

	Trials				
Condition	1	2	3	4	5
1. Sharpened Romberg, EC (60 s; feet in tandem)					
2. Walk on Rail, EO (5 steps; best 3/5 trials)					
3. Stand on Rail, EO (3 trials; 60 s/trial)				x	x
4. Stand on Rail, EC (3 trials; 60 s/trial)				x	x
5. Stand on Right Leg, on Floor, EC (5 trials; 30 s/trial)					
6. Stand on Left Leg, on Floor, EC (5 trials; 30 s/trial)					
7. Walk on Floor, EC (3 trials; 10 steps each)				x	x
8. Stand sideways on rail (characterize sway)[a]					

[a]Added by the author to observe the movement strategy used by the individual.
EO, eyes open; EC, eyes closed.

Fig. 20.15 A combination of tasks (Romberg test, one-legged stance test, walking) and environments (eyes open, eyes closed, rail) are included in the Fregly-Graybiel Ataxia Test Battery. (From Newton R. Review of tests of standing balance abilities. *Brain Inj.* 1989;3:335.)

6 of which are assessed on or to both right and left sides. These items are unilateral stance, tandem stance, tandem pivot, lateral foot scooting, hopping, crouch walking, lateral dodging, waking and looking, walk-look-and-carry, run with controlled stop, forward-to-backward walking, descend stairs, and step-ups. A majority of items are graded using both movement performance quality combined with either time, distance, or quantity. Each item is scored on an ordinal scale of 0 to 5, and the maximum score is 96.

The Fugl-Meyer Sensorimotor Assessment of Balance Performance is a subset of the Fugl-Meyer Physical Performance Battery, which was designed for use with hemiplegic patients (Fig. 22.16).[20] Three sitting and four standing balance activities are listed. The items are scored on a 0 to 2 scale, with score values specific to each item. Higher scores indicate better performance; the maximum (best) score is 14. However, a patient could achieve this score of 14 and still not have normal balance.

Dual-Task Tests

In everyday life tasks, normal balance is largely unconscious and does not compete for attentional resources. In patients with balance disorders, however, the challenge of maintaining postural control during upright activities and gait is often sufficient to demand the use of attentional resources. The interaction of cognitive demands and postural control demands is examined in dual-task tests that add concurrent cognitive and motor tasks to gait tasks. At the simplest level are the walking while talking (WWT) and stops walking when talking (SWWT) tests.[115–118] In these tests the patient is asked to walk and while the patient is walking, the clinician asks the patient one or more questions and observes if the patient must stop walking to answer the question(s). If so, the test result is positive—that is, the patient must stop attending to the postural control demands of walking to reallocate attention to the cognitive task. These are gross measures, apt to identify only those with more severe attentional balance problems or to misidentify patients who prefer to chat and rest rather than keep walking. A more formalized dual-task test is the Multiple Tasks Test (MTT), which includes eight items involving gait plus other verbal cognitive and motor tasks such as carrying a tray and avoiding obstacles.[119,120] Two dual-task versions of the TUG have been developed. The TUG-Manual involves performing the TUG while carrying a cup nearly full of water. The TUG-Cognitive involves performing the TUG while subtracting backward from a randomly selected number or spelling words backward.[121] The Walking and Remembering Test (WART) requires the patient to remember a set of numbers or grocery list items that the tester speaks aloud while the patient walks as quickly as possible while trying not to step off of a narrow path.[122] Once the walk is completed, the patient must repeat the numbers/items in sequence. For all dual-task tests, performance of each single task is measured separately first. Then the dual-task performance is recorded. The difference for each of the two scores (physical and cognitive performance) between undivided attention and divided attention conditions is calculated. This is calculated as (dual-task score minus single-task score) divided by the single task score, then multiplied by 100 to provide a percentage score termed the "dual-task cost" or "dual-task effect." This calculation can be done once using the physical single- and dual-task scores (e.g., time in seconds for the TUG), and again using the cognitive single- and dual-task scores (e.g., number of shopping list items recalled for the WART).

Balance Confidence Tests

Reduced participation in functional activities may occur not only because balance impairments impede participation, but also when patients are anxious about falling. Fear of falling may lead individuals to avoid activities that they remain quite capable of doing.[123] In turn, prolonged self-restriction of activity leads to the many negative consequences of being sedentary—decreased ROM, weakness, low endurance, and so on—and thus ironically further impairs balance and increases fall risk.[124,125] As this worsening balance and increased risk is perceived by the patient, further activity restriction occurs, creating a self-perpetuating downward spiral leading to social isolation, anxiety, and depression.[126,127] It is just as important to address poor balance confidence as it is to address poor balance, for without sufficient balance confidence a patient will not participate in activities even if balance abilities permit him or her to do so. The patient will lose all the gains made in therapy if he or she does not remain active, and he or she will not be active if fearful of falling. Evidence-based group programs like "Stepping On" and "A Matter of Balance" are designed to educate and empower older adults[128,129]; participation in these programs decreases the fear of falling and increases willingness to engage in balance-challenging exercise programs like "Otago," "Tai Chi Moving for Better Balance," or "FallProof."[130–132]

The two most commonly used measures of balance confidence are the Activities-specific Balance Confidence Scale (ABC Scale) and the Falls Efficacy Scale (FES) or Falls Efficacy Scale—International (FES-I).[133,134,135] Both are questionnaires that are easy to administer.

FUGL-MEYER

Test	Scoring	Maximum Possible Score	Attained Score
1. Sit without support _____	0—Cannot maintain sitting without support 1—Can sit unsupported less than 5 min 2—Can sit longer than 5 min		
2. Parachute reaction, non-affected side _____	0—Does not abduct shoulder or extend elbow 1—Impaired reaction 2—Normal reaction		
3. Parachute reaction, affected side _____	Scoring is the same as for test 2		
4. Stand with support _____	0—Cannot stand 1—Stands with maximum support 2—Stands with minimum support for 1 min		
5. Stand without support _____	0—Cannot stand without support 1—Stands less than 1 min or sways 2—Stands with good balance more than 1 min		
6. Stand on unaffected side _____	0—Cannot be maintained longer than 1–2 s 1—Stands balanced 4–9 s 2—Stands balanced more than 10 s		
7. Stand on affected side _____	Scoring is the same as for test 6		
		Maximum Balance Score	/14

Fig. 20.16 The Fugl-Meyer sensorimotor assessment of balance performance includes both low-level and high-level tasks. (From DiFabio RP, Badke MB. Relationship of sensory organization to balance function in patients with hemiplegia. *Phys Ther.* 1990;70:20.)

The ABC Scale consists of 16 items that range in difficulty from "walk around the house" to "walk outside on icy sidewalks." Several of the items inquire about activities in public places, for example, parking lots and escalators. Patients are asked how confident they are that they could do each of the activities without losing their balance or becoming unsteady. Responses are given on a scale from 0 to 100 in increments of 10, with higher numbers indicating higher confidence. More recently a short version, the ABC-6, has been developed. It has 6 of the original 16 items and takes less time to administer yet retains good reliability and correlation with balance and fall risk measures.[136] The FES consists of 10 activity items that are less difficult than the items on the ABC Scale. Items on the FES include getting in and out of a chair and answering the door or a phone. All of the items refer to activities done in the home. Patients are asked how confident they are that they could do each of the activities without falling. Responses are given on a scale from 1 to 10, with lower numbers indicating higher confidence. The Modified FES (MFES) has 14 activity items and includes 2 activities done outside the home and 3 activities done in public spaces. It also takes into account whether or not an assistive device is used.[137] Scoring is identical to that of the original FES. The FES-I is a 16 activity-item questionnaire that includes 7 of the original 10 items from the FES and adds 9 more difficult items, 2 household and 7 community-based. Responses are given on a scale from 1 to 4, with lower numbers indicating higher confidence. There is also a Short FES-I with 7 items using the identical scoring system.[138]

A third measure of fear of falling is the Survey of Activities and Fear of Falling in the Elderly (SAFFE).[139] This measurement instrument is more involved than the ABC Scale or FES-I; however, it provides additional information specific to activity restriction that is valuable to the clinician. The SAFFE has 11 activity items that are similar in nature to the items on the other 2 scales, including community activities. This questionnaire asks if the patient actually does the activity or not. If he or she does the activity, the questionnaire asks how worried the patient is that he or she might fall during the activity, on a scale from 1 to 4. Lower numbers indicate increased worry. If the patient does not do the activity, the patient is asked whether the reason he or she does not do the activity is fear of falling, with degree of fear scored on the scale from 1 to 4, or whether the patient does not do the activity for reasons other than fear, and what those other reasons are. For each item, patients also indicate whether the frequency of doing the activity has increased, decreased, or remained the same. The SAFFE takes longer to administer than the ABC Scale or FES/MFES/FES-I/S-FES-I but provides explicit results about activity restriction not obtained from the other two scales. Improvement on this measure captures both reduction in fear and increase in participation.

The Fear of Falling Avoidance Behavior Questionnaire (FFABQ) is a recently developed instrument with a focus on activity avoidance versus fear.[140] It lists 14 different activities, ranging in difficulty from walking and preparing meals to going up and down stairs to engaging in recreational activities such as sports or traveling. Patients rate whether or not they agree with a statement that they avoid a specified activity on a 5-point scale from 0 (completely disagree) to 4 (completely agree). This questionnaire is reliable with scores that discriminate between previous fallers and nonfallers, and more versus less active individuals. The shift from an emphasis on fear or confidence as in the ABC and FES, to activity avoidance as in the SAFFE and FFABQ is an important and positive one for PTs and OTs. As the ICF health and disablement model describes, the goals are to increase activity and participation to achieve an improved quality of life for patients.

Tests Recommended by Expert Consensus or Systematic Review for Specific Populations

The sheer number of available balance tests has on one hand made it much easier for clinicians to use standardized measures with good to excellent psychometric properties, while on the other hand has resulted in a lack of standardization between clinical institutions and research sites. Consequently, though individual patient documentation may have improved, the ability to compare clinical outcomes and research findings has become more complicated. In response the American Physical Therapy Association Section on Research formed the Evaluation Database to Guide Effectiveness (EDGE) Task Force to produce recommended outcome measures including but not limited to balance. Subsequently the Academies of Neurologic Physical Therapy and Geriatric Physical Therapy (ANPT and AGPT, respectively) have convened clinician groups with shared expertise in various patient populations to produce recommendations about which outcome measures are best and ought to be used most consistently. See Table 20.4 to locate recommended balance tests for

neurological patients with stroke, PD, TBI, MS, and community-dwelling older adults undergoing fall-risk screening.

Considerations in the Selection of Balance Tests

To determine the type and level of challenge of the tests to be used during the examination, a thorough subjective history is critical. In describing the symptoms and the situations that cause imbalance or falls, the patient offers clues to possible deficits and thereby the measures that will help identify them.

Many of the functional balance scales previously reviewed were designed to determine whether balance is abnormal in elderly patients who have no medical diagnosis (i.e., as screening tools). Clinicians working with clearly diagnosed patients with neurological conditions often do not need such tools to establish that balance skills are

TABLE 20.4 Balance Outcome Measures: Evidence-Based Recommendations From Academies of Neurologic Physical Therapy and Geriatric Physical Therapy Evaluation Database to Guide Effectiveness Task Force Groups

Test	Core Set (All Neuro)	Stroke	PD	TBI	MS	Fall-Risk Screening
ABC	X	X	X	X	X	
BERG	X	X	X	X	X	X
FGA	X	X	X	X	X	
5XSTS	X	X	X	X	X	X
6-min Walk	X	X	X	X	X	
10 Meter Walk	X	X	X	X	X	
BESTest		X	X			
Chedoke-McMaster		X				
Fugl-Meyer		X				
PASS		X				
Rivermead		X			X	
STREAM		X				
Trunk Impairment Scale		X			X	
MDS-UPDRS P2			X			
FGA			X			
BESS				X		
CM&B				X		
HiMAT				X		
TUG					X	
TUG Cognitive					X	X
TUG Manual					X	
Timed 25' Walk					X	
[DGI] mDGI					X	
4SST					X	
Single-Leg Stance Time						X
Self-selected Walking Speed						X
FES-I						X

abnormal because the deficits are patently obvious. These screening tools can be useful, however, to identify disabilities, establish a baseline, monitor progress, and document outcomes.

Many clinical facilities have their own therapy evaluation forms that include a section on balance. Items and scoring are usually defined by the facility. They are not standardized across sites, as are published scales, and are rarely tested for measurement qualities such as validity and reliability. As rehabilitation professions evolve toward evidence-based practice, nonstandardized tests with unknown measurement quality are no longer acceptable. Clinicians should use standardized, objective, quantifiable, valid tests with high reliability, sensitivity, and specificity whenever possible. If a test will be used to document progress following intervention, it also needs to be responsive to change over time. A functional balance rating scale is important in the evaluation of patients with neurological impairment. To be responsive enough to measure changes in patients who clearly are not (and may never be) clinically normal, ordinal scales should have at least five, and perhaps seven, possible relative scores.

Following functional balance testing, additional impairment tests are necessary to assess the systems that may affect postural control to help identify and measure impairments (e.g., ROM, strength, sensation and sensory organization, motor planning and control). These types of measures should be sensitive, objective, and quantifiable. Unfortunately, some body system components do not have objective, quantifiable clinical measures (e.g., motor planning, coordination). In these cases, clinicians must continue to use subjective rating scales.

Other factors to include when deciding what tests to use are the time required to perform the test, the number of staff members who must be present, and the space and equipment needed. Clinicians must weigh the potential benefits of technological tools (e.g., computerized forceplates, accelerometers, isokinetics, motion analysis, electromyography) against their cost and practicality (i.e., their cost-effectiveness). The test must be suitable for the patient's level of functioning (physical and cognitive). Many head-injured patients, for example, cannot initially participate in traditional forms of testing because of cognitive limitations.

PROBLEM IDENTIFICATION, GOAL SETTING, AND TREATMENT PLANNING

Clinical Decision Making

Treatment of patients with neurological diagnoses is based on the particular set of impairments, skill deficits, and activity limitations possessed by each individual. Remediation of balance skill deficits similarly must be specific to the involved body systems and functional activity losses in each patient. Clinicians should generate an overall problem list for each patient; if imbalance is a listed problem, then a sublist of balance problems also can be developed (Fig. 20.17).

To direct and establish priorities for treatment, clinicians must review the problem list and ask themselves the following questions (Fig. 20.18): Which impairments are temporary and can be remediated? How much improvement can be expected? How soon will it occur? Which impairments are permanent or progressive and must be compensated for? What other body systems can be counted on to substitute? What external compensations may be needed?

For some patients with neurological impairments, knowing whether a problem is permanent or temporary is not possible, as in recovery from a stroke or head injury. In others with progressive diseases such as Parkinson disease or MS, the rate of decline is unknown and abilities may fluctuate. In these cases the clinician should consider the following issues: Would a consultation provide the required information? If so, referral is appropriate. Do any contraindications to treatment exist? What are the risks and benefits of providing versus withholding treatment? Is some amount of functional improvement possible? If no contraindications are present, the benefits outweigh the risks, and

EXAMPLE OF BALANCE PROBLEM LIST

General Problem List	Balance Problem List
1. Decreased strength (L) side	
2. Decreased ROM (L) shoulder	
3. Decreased endurance	
4. Impaired sensation (L) side	
5. Decreased balance	a. Decreased weight bearing on left (L) LE b. Unable to maintain midline orientation c. Extraneous sway with eyes closed d. Unable to stand on (L) LE e. Decreased limits of stability to 40/100% f. Unable to shift to (L) side g. Unable to establish stable base of support h. Unable to stand on unstable surface i. Unable to perform hip strategy
6. Increased tone (L) side	
7. Synergistic movement (L) side	
8. Min. assist transfers	
9. Mod. assist ambulation	

Fig. 20.17 An example of a balance-specific problem list (as a subset of a general problem list), which should be developed to guide balance rehabilitation treatments.

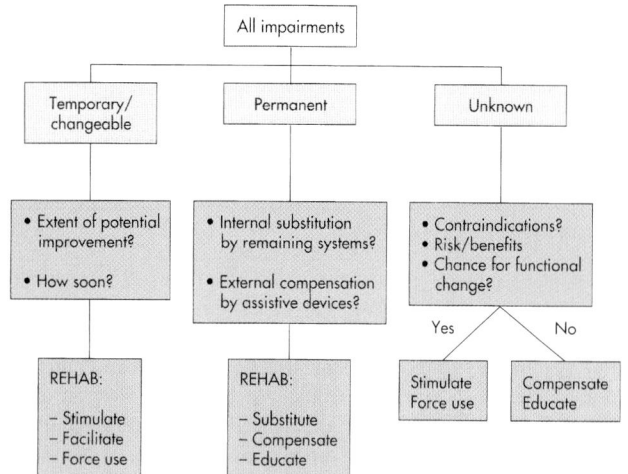

Fig. 20.18 A clinical decision making tree to illustrate the treatment-planning process in balance rehabilitation *(REHAB)*.

functional improvement is expected, then a trial of treatment may be given, even if knowing for certain whether the problem(s) will respond to the treatment is not possible. In these cases especially, a baseline must be established against which to measure any change. Change for the worse or no change after a reasonable trial period indicates that treatment should be altered or discontinued.

Using the Systems Model to Identify Postural Control Impairments

The systems approach is useful to develop a balance problem list because it can be applied to different diagnoses equally well and allows deficits in multiple systems to be recognized. Table 20.5 illustrates several examples of ways this framework is used to identify balance deficits in patients with different neurological diagnoses.

For each patient, problems affecting postural control should be described in objective, measurable terms whenever possible. For example, the term "impaired vision" is too vague; "four-line drop on eye chart" is more specific. "Poor use of visual inputs for balance control" is an interpretation; the objective result could be stated "Loss of balance after less than 15 seconds on 5/5 trials of standing on foam, eyes open." Documenting problems in this manner makes goal writing (and subsequent treatment planning) much easier.

Writing Goals on the Basis of Body Structure and Function Impairments, Balance Skill Deficits, and Activity Limitations

Goals also should be stated in objective and measurable terms so that their achievement can be judged. "Improved balance" is open to any interpretation, whereas "able to stand on right leg for 30 seconds on 3/3 trials" and "walks tandem entire length of balance beam without misstep 7/10 times" are measurable goals. These types of goals may be helpful to the clinician who understands the link between

TABLE 20.5	Examples of Medical Diagnoses and Related Impairments Affecting Balance		
Impairments From Systems Model	**Diabetic Patient With Stroke**	**Older Patient With Parkinson Disease**	**Patient With Incomplete Paraplegia**
Peripheral Sensory			
Vision	Retinopathy	Cataracts	
Vestibular		Hair cell loss	
Somatosensory	Peripheral neuropathy	Slowed transmission time	Complete loss below level of lesion
Central Sensory			
Vision	Hemianopia	Vision dominant	Needs superior use to compensate
Vestibular	Failure to use inputs		Needs superior use to compensate
Somatosensory	Failure to use inputs	Failure to use inputs; unaware of posture and small movements	
Strategy selection	Step dominant	Ankle dominant	Hip dominant
Perception of position in space	Midline shift with left neglect	Flexed posture; restricted limits of stability	Cannot detect relationship of body to feet/surface
Central Motor			
Timing	Increased reaction time	Bradykinesia	
Sequencing	Disordered	Co-contraction	
Force modulation	Spasticity, hypertonus, weakness	Hypokinesia, rigidity	Flaccid paralysis below level of lesion
Error correction	Use right side only	Loss of automaticity; must use intentional cortical attention	Relearning abilities and limitations of "new" body
Peripheral Motor			
Range of motion	Knee hyperextension	Bilateral ankle plantar flexor contractures	Hip flexion contractures
Strength	Decreased left side	Decreased bilateral extremities and trunk	Paralysis bilateral lower extremities and trunk
Endurance	Severely impaired	Moderately impaired	Mildly impaired

impairments, skill deficits, and functional activity limitations, but they may seem nonfunctional (and therefore unnecessary) to others who read them (e.g., case managers, third-party payers). From their standpoint, incorporating the functional task that will be positively affected by its achievement into the impairment goal is beneficial; for example, "able to stand on right leg for 10 seconds at a time so that stairs can be ascended and descended step-over-step without railing," or "walks tandem on balance beam to demonstrate ability to avoid falls using hip strategy." By describing the specific system problem (e.g., muscle power, joint range) or skill deficit (e.g., "unable to stand in on one leg") as it relates to function in the treatment objectives, clinicians force themselves to focus on functional outcomes and illustrate for others reading the documentation why these goals are meaningful. The need for and validity of the intervention are then more likely to be clearly perceived. At times, goal documentation requirements may specify that the goals be purely functional in nature. Writing goals without impairment components may meet the needs of the reviewer, but they will not help to direct clinical interventions to the specific components that need to be addressed in each individual patient. Documentation must meet reviewer requirements, but for one's own benefit, writing a separate set of goals with the dual impairment-function or skill deficit-function components will assist the clinician with planning and prioritizing treatment.

If a problem cannot be alleviated and requires compensation, the goal(s) should reflect this as well. For example, a patient with diabetes has progressive peripheral neuropathy with somatosensory loss and ineffective ankle strategy. If the patient's visual and vestibular sensory systems and proximal strength are relatively intact, however, then the goals might mention improved use of visual cues and successful substitution of hip and stepping strategies. Educational and environmental modification goals for safety also are appropriate in these situations.

Developing an Intervention Plan

Once the goals have been listed and priorities established, the intervention plan is developed. The most effective and efficient treatments focus first on those problems with the greatest impact on function and address more than one problem at a time. Teaching balance skills on an unstable surface contributes to the use of visual and vestibular inputs as well as to the use of hip strategy, increased lower-extremity

strength, and increased motor control (skill) on that type of surface. Gait training on an inclined treadmill with eyes closed or head movement increases the use of somatosensory and vestibular inputs, endurance, postural control, ROM, and lower-extremity strength. Creative clinicians develop comprehensive intervention plans with this type of multiple-problem approach to maximize the time available with patients.

The clinician must thoughtfully choose environments and tasks that together stimulate and challenge the appropriate postural control systems. To stimulate one sensory system, the other systems must be placed at a disadvantage to force reliance on the targeted system. The environment is then structured to put the other systems at a disadvantage (e.g., training with eyes closed or in the dark puts vision at a disadvantage and forces the use of somatosensory and vestibular inputs). If one side or limb is significantly more affected, such as in hemiplegia, then the other side must be disadvantaged to force reliance on the targeted side. Tasks are then selected to disadvantage the less affected side. For example, placing the less affected leg on a step or small ball makes it more difficult to use for balance and forces the transference of weight to the more affected leg. To achieve optimal function, however, all systems and all sides must be capable of working together, so *treatment* to improve postural control system impairments and *teaching* to improve balance skill deficits must be incorporated and interspersed with *training* functional tasks. For effective teaching of balance skills that results in carryover of improvements into real-life situations, training tasks should be varied enough to promote motor problem solving on the part of the patient.[141] For example, sitting balance and transfers should be taught using stable and unstable surfaces, with different heights and levels of firmness, with and without armrests and back supports, and using both right and left sides. This technique may improve the patient's abilities to perform safe sitting and transfers in new situations not previously practiced in therapy.[26]

Tables 20.6 and 20.7 illustrate the process of test choice, problem identification based on test results, goal setting based on impairments and disabilities, and treatment planning based on goals in three different types of patients. Note that only selected tests were performed for each patient. Goals were directly related to the problems that were identified by the tests, and treatment plans followed directly from the goals.

TABLE 20.6 Example of How Treatment Planning Flows From Test Results in an Older Adult Patient With Frequent Falls

Patient profile: 72-year-old woman
Diagnosis: Disequilibrium of aging, frequent falls
Course of examination and treatment: Cardiologist → neurologist → outpatient physical therapy

Test	Problems Identified	Goals Set	Treatment Plan
Peripheral sensory	Mildly decreased vibration sense bilateral lower extremity	Compensate for permanent sensory loss	Educate about safe surfaces and lighting
Somatosensory			Home safety evaluation
Vision	Acuity, cataracts		
	Depth perception		
SOT	Absent use of vestibular inputs 0/Decreased use of somatosensory inputs 60/Dependent on vision	Increase use of vestibular inputs to 30/increase use of somatosensory inputs to 75/100	Somatosensory and vestibular stimulation[a]
Static postural sway	Excessive sway—2 standard deviations outside normal range for age	Standing sway within normal limits for age	COG control training
Nudge or push test	No use of ankle or hip strategy Steps immediately	Survives 5/10 pushes with hip strategy	Hip strategy exercises[a]

Continued

TABLE 20.6 Example of How Treatment Planning Flows From Test Results in an Older Adult Patient With Frequent Falls—cont'd

Test	Problems Identified	Goals Set	Treatment Plan
LOS	No ankle strategy—uses hip strategy Sway to 45% LOS anterior, 35% LOS posterior Slow movement time	Uses ankle strategy to reach 40% LOS anterior and posterior Reaches 8/8 targets at 75% LOS using hip or ankle strategy within 4 s	COG control training
ROM	Neck extension 0–10 degrees Lumbar extension 1–15 degrees Hip extension 0–5 degrees	Spinal extension neck 0–20 degrees Lumbar extension 0–20 degrees Hip extension 0–10 degrees	ROM exercises*
Strength	Flexion 4/5 (B) Hip abduction 3+/5, extension 3/5 (B) Knee extension 4+/5, flexion 4/5 (R) Ankle dorsiflexion 3−/5 (L) Ankle dorsiflexion 2/5 (B) Ankle plantarflexion 3+/5	(B) Hip abduction and extension to greater than 4/5 (B) Ankle dorsiflexion and plantarflexion to 4−/5	Progressive resistive exercises, including bicycle*
Gait (GARS)	Score 35/48 Deviations Forward flexed trunk Double limb stance prolonged bilaterally Short step length	GARS scales 25/48 (I) Ambulation with walker in home, community	Gait training[a] 1—starts, stops, turns 2—treadmill 3—uneven surfaces, curbs, stairs, carpet, outdoors
Endurance	Fatigue after ambulating 60 ft	Ambulates more than 200 ft without stopping	Gait training as earlier
Tinetti balance scale	6/16 score	Tinetti balance score 10/16	Gait training as earlier
Tinetti gait scale	5/12 score Falls and catches self	Tinetti gait score 8/12	Gait training as earlier

[a]Also included in home exercise program.
LOS, Limit of stability; *(B)*, bilateral; *COG*, center of gravity; *GARS*, Gait Abnormality Rating Scale; *(I)*, independent; *(L)*, left; *(R)*, right; *ROM*, range of motion; *SOT*, Sensory Organization Test.
Reprinted with permission from NeuroCom International, Clackamas, Ore.

TABLE 20.7 An Example of How Treatment Planning Flows From Test Results in a Patient With Right Hemiparesis

Patient profile: 69-year-old woman
Diagnosis: Left cerebrovascular accident with right hemiparesis
Course of examination and treatment: Acute rehabilitation → home health → outpatient rehabilitation

Test	Problems Identified	Goals Set	Treatment Plan
Peripheral somatosensory		None	
SOT	Average overall stability 47/Absent use of vestibular inputs 0/100	Average stability 60/use of vestibular inputs 15/100	Vestibular stimulation with forced use and head movements
Postural sway			COG control training
Functional reach	Forward lean restricted to 5 inches	Able to reach forward 8 inches	
Static balance	Weight shift asymmetry to left in static standing and medial or lateral sway, 25% LOS to left of midline	Control of COG Stands midline	
Limit of stability	Forward weight shift restricted to 25% LOS	Forward LOS to 50% Right LOS to 50%	
Rhythmic weight shift	Extraneous sway off desired path	Extraneous sway scores by 50%	
OLST	Unable on right leg, 30 seconds on left leg	Stands on right leg, 10 seconds	COG control training
Nudge, push (motor strategy selection)	Switch from ankle to hip strategy noted but unable to withstand perturbation	Able to stand upright after mild perturbations 5/10 times Able to "catch" self by stepping or reaching 5/10 times	Hip and stepping strategy training
Range of motion	None		

TABLE 20.7   An Example of How Treatment Planning Flows From Test Results in a Patient With Right Hemiparesis—cont'd

Test	Problems Identified	Goals Set	Treatment Plan
Strength: right leg	4/5 Knee extension 3/5 Knee flexion 2/5 Ankle dorsiflexion 3/5 Ankle plantarflexion	RLE strength 5/5 Knee 4/5 Ankle	Progressive resistive exercises
Endurance	Standing tolerance less than 10 min	Able to stand unaided for 15 min	Standing tolerance tasks
Gait	Step length—RLE Step height—RLE Heel strike—RLE Toe-off—RLE	Symmetrical step height and length 5/10 times Heel strike RLE 5/10 times	Gait training on treadmill
Tinetti Gait Subscale	Unable to turn, reach, or bend without loss of balance Falls: Uneven surfaces Low lighting Head turning No community ambulation Requires cane Requires supervision for household ambulation	8/12 score No falls Gait independent without cane in household; with cane in community	Gait training on uneven surfaces, with head movements, with low lighting Safety education

COG, Center of gravity; *LOS,* limit of stability; *OLST,* one-legged stance test; *RLE,* right lower extremity; *SOT,* Sensory Organization Test. Reprinted with permission from NeuroCom International, Clackamas, Ore.

BALANCE RETRAINING TECHNIQUES

Motor Learning Concepts

Although covering the principles of motor learning is not within the scope of this chapter, the discussion of balance retraining methods is not possible without some consideration of several motor learning concepts that must be incorporated into treatment. The clinician must remember that successful treatments address the interaction of the individual, the task, and the environment (Fig. 20.19).[13,26]

Individual

Therapists should know their patients' impairments: sensory and motor, peripheral, and central. Whenever possible, therapists should know which impairments can be rehabilitated and which require compensation or substitution. Because of the nature of neurological insult, this includes an awareness of cognitive and perceptual impairments that may affect the ability to relearn old skills or develop new ones.

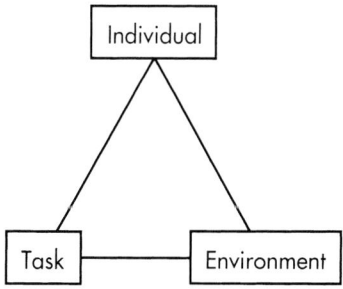

Fig. 20.19 Interactions of the individual, the environment, and the task are critical to postural control skills. Although they may be isolated in the mind of the clinician for assessment purposes, they are never isolated in the function of the patient.

Optimal learning of skilled movement requires that the patient have (1) knowledge of self (abilities and limitations), (2) knowledge of the environment (opportunities and risks), (3) knowledge of the task (critical components), (4) the ability to use those knowledge sets to solve motor problems, and (5) the ability to modify and adapt movements as the task and environment change. To the extent that a patient is missing these characteristics, the clinician should attempt to support his or her development or even supply them until they are present. Different types of patients vary with regard to which characteristics are likely to be missing. For example, a cognitively impaired, head-injured patient may lack awareness of self and environment, even though his or her physical abilities make modifying and adapting movements possible. Conversely, a quadriplegic patient may be aware of his or her limitations, the environment, and the task demands but may initially have limited experience to know how to solve a motor problem and limited physical ability to modify movements.

The clinician must also ask what motor learning stage the patient is in for different skills needed to successfully perform tasks. Skill acquisition is the first stage. The objective is for the patient to "get the idea of the movement" to begin to acquire the skill.[142] In this stage, errors are frequent and performance is inefficient and inconsistent. Within the nervous system only temporary changes are occurring. Skill refinement is the second stage. The goal is for the patient to improve the performance, reduce the number and size of the errors, and increase the consistency and efficiency of the movements. Skill retention is the final stage. The ability to perform the movements and achieve the functional goal has been accomplished, and the new objective is to retain the skill over time and transfer the skill to different settings. Retention and transfer are the hallmarks of true learning, in which some relatively permanent changes have occurred within the nervous system. A patient may have attained the skill retention phase for sitting balance tasks, be in the skill refinement stage for standing balance tasks, and be in the skill acquisition stage for locomotor balance tasks.

Therapists use practice and feedback to teach motor skills. Repetition is necessary to develop skill; feedback is necessary to detect and correct errors. During skill acquisition, frequent repetition of a movement or task and frequent feedback are beneficial to help the patient begin to be able to perform the desired movements and tasks. As soon as the patient progresses to the skill refinement stage (the clinician observes reduced errors and less variable performance), however, then practice should be varied and feedback briefly delayed. For example, the task of standing and reaching to one side to take an object from the therapist might initially be repeated to the same side and at the same height several times. Then the therapist should begin to vary the task demands gradually: reach farther or faster; take different objects of various weights, shapes, and sizes; and take the object from higher and lower heights and alternately reach to right and left sides. This variation introduces a problem-solving demand for the patient: modifications in timing, force, and sequencing are now necessary.

Feedback, which is especially helpful for those with sensory reception or perception problems, initially may contain information to assist the patient in detecting errors about the goal achievement (knowledge of results, such as "you stood up five times without using your hands") or about a movement error (knowledge of performance, "you did not straighten your knee enough last time").[143] Early feedback also may contain cues about what to do better next time, such as "straighten your knee before you shift weight onto that leg." If feedback is always provided by an external source, such as the therapist, a mirror, or a computer monitor, then the patient is not given the opportunity to develop internal error detection and error correction mechanisms and will not be as likely to retain or transfer the skill. By delaying the feedback and asking the patient to estimate or describe her or his own errors, and afterward providing the feedback, the therapist allows the patient to compare her or his own developing internal frame of reference with the correct external frame of reference. By asking patients to suggest what might be done to correct the errors, the therapist shifts the error correction process from the external source to the patients, supporting motor problem-solving processes. As patients progress to the skill retention level, variations should increase (including task and environmental demands) and feedback delays should be longer. The clinician must develop a sense of how to use practice variation and feedback delay therapeutically to progress patients through the stages of motor learning. Too much variation and too little feedback early on impede skill acquisition; insufficient variation and excessive feedback later on hamper skill retention and transfer.

Task

Functional rating scales performed as a part of the evaluation yield information about what tasks, or functional activities, are limited by the postural control system impairments and balance skill deficits. Bed mobility, sitting, sitting to standing, transfers, standing, walking, working, and sports participation may be affected. Repeating the problematic tasks over and over is one approach; however, analyzing the problematic tasks to determine what postural control demands are placed on the patient when undertaking those tasks is far more productive for the clinician. Does a task demand predominantly stability? Mobility? Both? For example, standing to take a photograph demands the ability to hold still; standing to move laundry from the washer to the dryer requires weight shifting; and standing to don a pair of pantyhose calls for both steadiness and movement. All three are standing dual-tasks, but each places different postural control demands on the patient. By using task analysis, the therapist may consciously select or design tasks to place specific demands on the patient such that the postural control systems that need improvement will be challenged to respond, and skills that need to improve will be practiced extensively.

Analysis of mobility tasks includes attention to timing, force, and duration of movements. Consider the different timing demands for weight shifting and reaching to catch an item falling from a shelf, take a hot casserole out of the oven, or open a door. Compare the different amounts of force necessary to pick up a heavy suitcase, pick up a baby from a crib, or replace a ceiling light bulb. The duration of a balance demand may be brief, as in recovering from a trip, or extended, as in walking across an icy parking lot. Clinicians should choose tasks that vary these parameters to prepare patients for activities with various mobility demands. Activities that incorporate changing head positions will further challenge the individual with vestibular insufficiency.

Therapists also need to consider whether the elements of the task are predictable or unpredictable. In other words, will the postural control demand be a voluntary movement (e.g., sweeping the porch), an APR (e.g., missing the last step on a flight of stairs), or an APA (e.g., preceding a lift)? Patients need to learn to respond in all three conditions, which are often combined. For instance, lifting is a voluntary movement. Predicting the load to be lifted leads to anticipatory postural preparation. Counteracting the destabilizing force of a greater-than-predicted load requires an APR. If during therapy the clinician says "don't let me push you" before nudging the patient, the demand is for APA. If the disturbance is provided without warning, the demand calls for APRs. If the clinician requests a lean to the right, that is a voluntary postural adjustment. Activities that demand all three types of balance control, either one at a time or in combination, should be included in balance retraining programs.

Environment

Just as tasks can be purposefully selected to promote improved postural control, environmental conditions also must be included in the design of the therapy plan to stimulate the necessary systems and challenge the deficient skills. Gravity cannot be manipulated by the clinician, but the patient needs to learn to counteract it at different speeds and from different positions, among other things. Familiarity with how gravity can aid movement, as in walking, is also important. The therapist can vary the surface conditions. They may be stable, even, and predictable (hospital hallway, sidewalk), unstable (boat, subway, gravel driveway), uneven (grass, curbs, stairs), or compliant (beach, padded carpeting). Visual conditions also may be manipulated. Visual cues may be available and accurate (daylight, fluorescent lighting), unavailable (darkness or poor lighting, or lack of environmental cues such as a busy carpet pattern on a stairway), unstable (moving crowd, public transportation), used for purposes other than balance (fixation on a ball in tennis), or dependent on head movements. Clinicians should help prepare their patients to function in the real world by training them to maintain balance under different combinations of surface and visual conditions. This includes situations in which cues from the environment agree—that is, visual, somatosensory, and vestibular inputs are all sending the same message, so to speak—as well as in sensory conflict environments where cues from one system may disagree with cues from the other sensory systems. Functional situations in which sensory conflicts may exist include elevators, escalators, people movers, airplanes, and subways. An emphasis on being able to adapt to changes in environmental conditions rapidly and effectively is important.

Intervention

Successful intervention for the individual with a balance disorder depends on the ability of the *clinician* to identify the components of the problem. The therapist must create a program that addresses several components at a time, not just for efficiency, but because these systems should be able to function together, and multiple skills must be simultaneously coordinated to perform functional activities in real-world environments. *Treatment* is oriented toward multiple impairments, with tasks and environments selected to best correct involved or facilitate compensatory systems. *Teaching* is focused on critical balance skills, with tasks and environments chosen to develop adaptive sensorimotor problem-solving abilities. *Training* is targeted to the patient's real-life functional activity limitations, with tasks and environments designed to replicate real-life situations as closely as possible.

The intervention must be matched to the level and combination of body system impairments and the degree of skill deficits. For example, tasks related to the different functions of the sensory systems should be identified and not treated as a single body system problem. The clinician should have a good idea of the level of stimulus during each exercise program so that the facilitation is as accurate as possible. Progression of the program follows the changes seen from one session to the next to promote carryover and retention of learning. The exercise progression integrates activities that reflect those changes. This usually involves more complex movement skills and more demanding tasks in a greater range of gradually more challenging environments.

Sensory Systems

In general, the less sensory information available, the more difficult the task of balancing. An intervention progression might therefore start with full sensory inputs (vision, somatosensory, and vestibular: 3/3) available in the environment and perhaps augmented feedback if intrinsic sensory channels are deficient, as with somatosensory loss or a vestibular disorder. Challenge is added by manipulating either visual or somatosensory inputs so that equilibrium must be maintained by using only two of three senses (vision and vestibular or somatosensory and vestibular). If both vision and somatosensory inputs are manipulated, then only the vestibular inputs are a reliable source of sensory information and balance is accomplished with only one of three senses.

Most patients with permanent or progressive vestibular or somatosensory losses naturally compensate and become visually dependent. In cases in which improving the use of somatosensory or vestibular inputs is necessary, the training of vision for stability can be counterproductive, teaching compensation versus improvement of normal function. On the other hand, visual retraining is entirely appropriate for the patient with severely compromised somatosensation that cannot be changed, as is common in persons with diabetes.

To stimulate the use of visual inputs, environments are designed to disadvantage somatosensation while providing reliable visual cues (stable visual field with landmarks). Somatosensation cannot be removed as can vision, but it can be destabilized by having the patient sit or stand on unstable surfaces (rocker board, biomechanical ankle platform system [BAPS] board, randomly moving platforms) or confused by having the patient sit or stand on compliant surfaces that give way to pressure, such as foam, "space boots," or responsively moving platforms.

To stimulate the use of somatosensory inputs, environments are designed to disadvantage vision while providing reliable somatosensory inputs (stable surfaces, level or inclined). Having the patient close the eyes or practice in low lighting or darkness removes or decreases visual inputs. For patients with an overreliance on visual input for balance, the somatosensory system needs to be facilitated while the visual system is disrupted. This can be accomplished by having the patient sit or stand on a stable surface while performing quick head turns. For the patient with self-limited head movement, the intervention may begin with head movement during quiet standing and progress to head movements during weight shifts and then walking. Eyes-closed standing and weight shifting also increase the use of somatosensation for balance. Optokinetic stimuli in the visual surround also stimulate use of somatosensory inputs.

To stimulate the use of vestibular inputs for adaptation of the CNS, environments are designed to disadvantage both vision and somatosensation while providing reliable vestibular cues (detectable head position). Practicing on unstable or compliant surfaces, with vision either absent (eyes closed), destabilized (eye movements or head movements), or confused (e.g., optokinetic stimulation) provides challenging combinations. Adding neck extension and rotation to place the vestibular organs at a disadvantaged angle can increase difficulty. Gaze stabilization with head turns while standing on an uneven surface or while walking creates a higher-level challenge. Quick movements of the head, head tilts, or forward bending trigger vestibular signals to add input to the system. Combining these types of activities can create progressively more complex challenges. Standing or weight shifting on foam with eyes closed, and head and eye movement while walking all require vestibular input for successful performance.

Additional vestibular challenge can be added by including activities that require quick changes of position in a superior or inferior direction, such as a lunge or going up and down stairs. Other exercises involving up-and-down body movements, such as sitting to standing, seated bouncing on a Swiss ball, and standing bouncing on a mini-trampoline, all with eyes closed to eliminate use of vision for stability, increase the demand on the vestibular system. To train the patient who is overreliant on vision to improve the use of vestibular inputs versus vision, activities such as watching a ball being tossed from hand to hand while walking, walking backward, or walking with eye movements can be used. Reading while walking requires the use of vision for reading so that it cannot be used for postural orientation, forcing the other sensory sources to be used for orientation.

Multisensory and Motor Control Dysfunction

Older patients often have dysfunction in all three sensory systems—that is, a multisensory balance disorder. Disease-related disruptions of the somatosensory or visual system (e.g., a peripheral neuropathy or cataracts) are combined with age-related declines in the vestibular system. In some cases therapy aimed at increasing vestibular function can have a significant impact on postural stability. If sensory loss is permanent or progressive, safe function may require the use of an assistive device.[144] Choosing an assistive device for these patients can be a challenge. An individual with cerebellar or visual-perceptual problems may have more difficulty using an assistive device, and thus it may be contraindicated. For these patients, careful assessment of safety and gait both with and without the device is demanded. A single cane often does not allow for compensation for changes in direction of an impending fall, and a standard aluminum walker does not provide support when changing directions because it must be lifted. The ideal walker has four rotating wheels and thus the ability to change direction without being lifted. This device greatly increases stability, and the patient usually describes a significant increase in confidence. Of course, the use of a walker also limits normal use of the upper extremities and trunk during gait and restricts the types of environments that can be negotiated. Making sure the patient stands erect in walking versus leaning forward into a permanent flexed position is important in order to retain and/or improve existing postural function.

Many patients with neurological conditions have temporary difficulty with head control early in their recovery, and others have chronic head control problems. Their ability to orient the vestibular organs, eyes, and neck proprioceptors properly is impaired, which negatively affects the ability to perceive internal and environmental cues that could assist in balance maintenance. Thus developing head control is very important. Patients with spasticity or contractures of the ankles and feet who cannot place their feet in full contact with the floor are at a biomechanical disadvantage and also have difficulty receiving somatosensory inputs that could support postural control processes. The more accurate and reliable sensory information there is available, the greater the chances that the sensoriperceptual processes that contribute to balance can fulfill their role. Intervention progressions should include attention to increasing the patient's ability to receive and process sensory information pertinent to balance control through oculomotor, head, and peripheral limb positioning and movement.

Control of the Center of Gravity

Effective control of the COG depends on accurate awareness of body position and motion in space and the relation between body parts (perception), as well as biomechanical and musculoskeletal systems (execution). Trunk and head control abilities are primary. For patients with paralysis or degenerative disease that limits the ability of arms and legs to assist with postural stability, head and trunk control may be the dominant means of balance. Both the head and neck and the trunk need to be able to achieve and hold a midline position, rotate around this midline axis, and move away from and return to the midline without loss of balance. The term *midline* here refers not to a line between right and left sides, but to a point at which the right and left and forward and backward components are centered in all planes—medial-lateral, anterior-posterior, rotary, and side bending (shortening and elongation on either side). Midline problems can certainly be caused by body system problems such as weakness, pain, or sensory deficits but can also be caused by perceptual problems (e.g., patients with "pusher syndrome" following stroke).

Sitting balance. In sitting, the pelvis and posterior thighs form the primary base of support, with additional stability provided by the feet in contact with the floor. The axis of anteroposterior movement rotates around the greater trochanter, and forward and backward leans are achieved through pelvic and trunk movement. Anterior pelvic tilt with upper trunk extension allows forward reaching and begins the sitting-to-standing transition. Lateral weight shifts with trunk elongation precede right and left reaching and scooting. Lateral weight shifts with trunk rotation permit cross-midline reaching and begin the sitting-to-supine progression. The use of arms to prop in sitting is an extension of the base of support.

Standing balance. In standing, the feet form the base of support. The axis of anteroposterior movement rotates around the medial malleolus. Mediolateral movement occurs with weight shifts from foot to foot. Weight shifts move the COG through space for reaching and lifting tasks as well as in preparation for stepping. Ankle strategy is most effective for forward and backward movement of the COG through the central range of the limits of stability on a stable surface. As the COG nears the sway boundary, hip strategy works to restrict its travel. If this fails, stepping or reaching strategies are used to reestablish a new base of support.

Balance during gait. During gait, the COG follows a sinusoidal path as forward progression of the body mass combines with alternating lateral weight shifts to the stance foot (Fig. 20.20).[25] Each step creates a new base of support. Assistive devices such as canes, walkers, and crutches extend the base of support and thus reduce the demands on the intrinsic balance control system. In sitting, standing, and walking, control of the COG involves the ability to establish a stable base of support and transfer weight over it. Treatment progressions for COG control then involve training to establish, maintain, and reduce the base of support and to produce automatic, anticipatory, and voluntary postural responses to restrict or produce weight shifts.

Early treatment progression for COG control may include "neurodevelopmental sequence activities" (e.g., prone on elbows, all fours, kneeling, right or left side sitting, half-kneeling), not for the purpose of "reflex

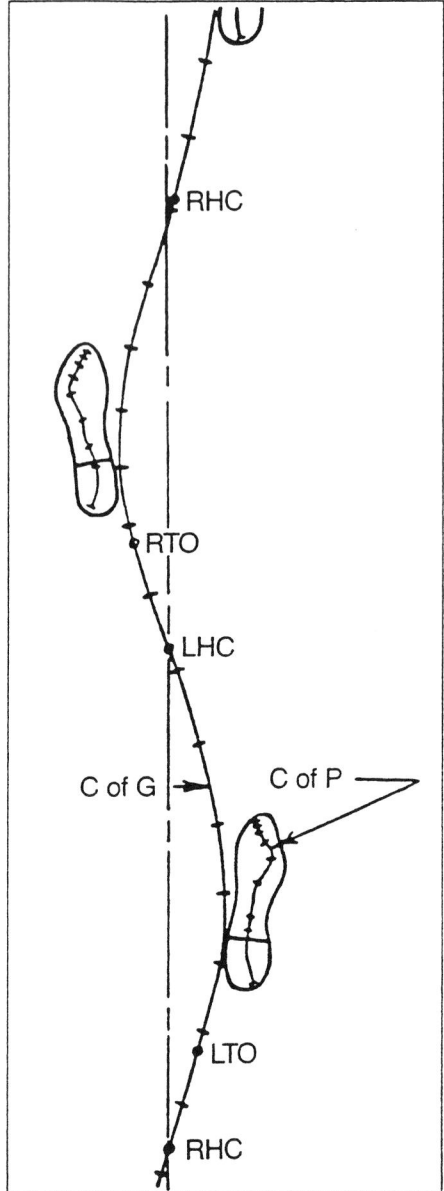

Fig. 20.20 The Trajectory of the Center of Gravity *(C of G)* and the Center of Pressure *(C of P)* During a Gait Cycle. *LHC,* Left heel contact; *LTO,* left toe-off; *RHC,* right heel contact; *RTO,* right toe-off. (From Palia AE, Winter DA, Frank JS, et al. Identification of age-related changes in the balance control system. In Duncan P, ed. *Balance: Proceedings of the APTA Forum.* Alexandria, VA: American Physical Therapy Association; 1990.)

development" in the traditional sense but because the task demands are to balance with progressively less surface contact (i.e., shrinking the base of support). Additional benefits include greater control, coordination, and generation of power of the neck, trunk, and axial muscles. It also is useful for simultaneously addressing impairments such as lower extremity extensor tone, trunk weakness and asymmetries, and head and neck extensor weakness. Note, however, that for adults these activities should be considered exercises to remediate impairments and improve skills, not as directly transferable to many adult functional tasks. Functionally, bed mobility and floor-to-stand transfers are related to these progressive position exercises and should be practiced concurrently in low- and high-level patients, respectively.

Sitting balance can be progressed by (1) removing upper-extremity support (hands on firm surface to movable surface [e.g., ball, bolster, rolling stool], one hand free and both hands free); (2) making the seating surface less stable (mat to bed to rocker board to Swiss ball); and (3) removing the use of one foot by crossing the leg, or of both feet by raising the height of the seat so the feet do not touch the floor. Tasks might include multidirectional weight shifts with the hands in contact with a bolster or ball that is pushed or pulled to and fro, reaching or passing objects, performing upper body tasks (grooming, dressing), managing socks and shoes, wheelchair armrests and footrests, and so forth.

Sitting to standing and transfer balance. Transitional movements such as sitting to standing and transfers involve large COG excursions over a stable base of support. For sitting to standing, the base of support must change from the seat to the feet. The feet begin to accept the weight first by downward pressure through the heels as the pelvis rolls anteriorly. The weight moves to the front of the feet as the trunk comes forward and the pelvis lifts from the surface, then backward toward midline as the trunk extends into standing. The COG stays near midline if both legs are participating equally, but it will often deviate to a preferred side during the transition in patients with hemiplegia. Training should include disadvantaging the preferred leg (perhaps by moving it a bit forward) to allow the more affected leg and foot to experience the weight transference. During transfers, a lateral weight shift is required in addition to the partial stand. The COG does not remain near midline; it instead moves forward to load the feet and then laterally toward the side of the transfer. Progression of balance skills in sitting to standing and transfer tasks may involve gradually lowering the height of the surface, removing armrests to preclude upper-extremity assistance, and transferring to surfaces of different heights and levels of firmness. Remember that velocity is a normal part of sitting-to-standing movements because the momentum is used to assist the weight transfer from seat to feet, so the clinician must allow some speed during this task. If the patient is unsteady on arising (cannot dampen or slow the speed in a controlled manner), working gradually from standing to sitting initially may be beneficial before progression to sitting to standing. Practice of sitting to standing with the eyes closed can be an effective way to train patients who are over-dependent on vision for balance. Without the use of vision for stability, integration of vestibular and somatosensory systems can be facilitated.

Standing balance. Standing balance tasks also can begin with finding midline and becoming stable there. Controlled mobility (volitional) should be encouraged as soon as possible, first on a stable surface with slow, small weight shifts. Challenge is added by increasing the distance traveled away from midline, moving toward restricted regions of the limits of stability, altering speed of sway, adding combined upper-extremity activities (e.g., dribbling a basketball, reaching), or adding resistance (manual, flexible bands). Narrowing the base of support (Romberg, tandem, single leg) makes control of the COG more demanding. Placing the feet in a diagonal stride position is more desirable for pregait weight shifting than is symmetrical double stance. Attention should be given to the stance (loading) leg with regard to pelvic protraction, hip and knee extension, and ankle dorsiflexion, with the tibia traveling forward over the foot. Focus on the swing (unloading) leg should include pelvic drop with knee flexion as the heel comes up and pressure through the ball of the foot and toes to load the opposite leg maximally. Standing balance exercises can be made more difficult by training on a less stable surface (carpet, foam, rocker board, BAPS board) and by adding combined head and eye movements or closing the eyes. The goals for dynamic sitting and standing balance exercises are to increase the size and symmetry of the limits of stability and improve the ability to transfer weight to different body segments

with control at different speeds and with varied amounts of force. To facilitate somatosensory and vestibular integration, these activities can be performed with decreased or distorted visual cues. Closing the eyes, turning the head quickly, turning the lights down low, or wearing sunglasses may decrease the use of vision for stabilization.

Strategy training. Training ankle, hip, and stepping strategies may begin in a voluntary manner but must progress to an automatic level of use to develop more normal balance and for real-life prevention of balance loss. Before strategy training, the clinician should be sure that the patient has the ability to develop the desired strategies. The observed dominance of other strategies is appropriately compensatory, not dysfunctional, if a missing strategy cannot be effectively executed. Patients use these strategies to prevent loss of balance, so the clinician must take care not to reduce reliance on an effective strategy but to add additional strategies to the repertoire.

Ankle strategy should be practiced on a firm, broad surface. Patients can be asked to sway slowly in anterior-posterior, right-left, and diagonal directions, first to and from midline, progressing to passing midline, and finally progressing to sway toward the periphery without return to midline. Head and pelvis should be traveling in the same direction at the same time. Patients can practice standing near a wall with a table in front of them, swaying forward to touch the table with the stomach (leading with the pelvis) and backward to touch the wall with the back of the head. Cues are given not to "bow" to the table and not to touch the wall with the buttocks. As soon as the patient is able to perform this protocol, functional meaning should be added with maneuvers such as forward or lateral reaching tasks, hands over head to take things off shelves, and leaning backward to rinse hair in the shower. To improve anticipatory and automatic ankle strategy use, add slight perturbations to the body or the surface when midline, progress to gentle perturbation when away from midline, and finally progress from predictable to unpredictable perturbations.

Hip strategy is practiced on either a narrow or an unstable surface, such as standing sideways on a balance beam, a two-by-four, a half-slice foam roller, foam, or a rocker board. The head and pelvis travel in opposite directions to counterbalance each other in a forward bow–backward bending motion for anterior-posterior sway. Rapid sway is requested in forward-backward, right-left, and diagonal directions. By using the wall and table setting previously mentioned, patients can be cued to how to touch the nose toward the table while simultaneously touching the wall with the buttocks. Lateral hip strategy can be trained similarly, with the patient standing sideways to the wall, touching the table with one hip and the wall with the opposite shoulder. Sway close to the edge of the patient's limit of stability should produce a shift from ankle to hip strategy, so to enhance the use of hip strategy the patient should practice sway control as far away from midline as possible without stepping. As soon as the patient demonstrates the ability to perform this strategy, it should be incorporated into functional tasks such as low reaching (e.g., trunk of car, laundry dryer). To promote anticipatory and automatic use of hip strategy, the patient is in midline and given moderate, rapid perturbations to the body or the surface such that ankle strategy will be insufficient to counteract the force. Then the size of the disturbance is increased, and the patient is positioned away from midline when the perturbation is given so that righting to midline is appropriate. The shift should be made from predictable ("don't let me make you step or fall") to unpredictable perturbations.

Stepping strategy can be practiced first from atop a step, curb, or balance beam. Both legs should be included in training because real-life situations such as a slip or trip often preclude the use of one limb and demand the use of the other. It may be necessary to fix one foot in position to prevent stepping by the less affected leg in order to allow a stepping response on the more affected leg to emerge (a forced-use paradigm). Progress is made by stepping on a level surface and then to stepping up onto a step or curb or over progressively larger obstacles (appliance cord, shoe, phone book). All directions should be practiced, including lateral and diagonal perturbations, if safe recovery from real-life unexpected balance losses is to be learned. Large, rapid perturbations are given such that ankle and hip strategies will be inadequate and stepping or reaching is demanded. Again, progress should be made from predictable to unpredictable disturbances. For any APR—ankle, hip, stepping, protective reaching—to be effective in real life, successful demonstration of the response to *unexpected* perturbations is imperative.

Many patients, especially those who are fearful of falling, are dependent on the use of hands for stability. Therapeutic balance retraining activities should provide the maximal level of challenge that can be managed without the need for upper-extremity support. If the patient physically needs to hold on, then the activity is at too high a level and should be modified. Otherwise, what is being taught is a "hand strategy" that will not be useful if the patient experiences loss of balance when nothing firmly fixed is available to grasp for stability. Extremely anxious patients may initially benefit from training with an overhead harness system that will permit hands-free motion but provide tangible reassurance that a fall will be prevented if balance loss occurs. In this case, treatment progression would include weaning the patient off the use of the harness. If the only harness available is on a body-weight support treadmill or gait system, move the balance retraining to that harness. The treadmill does not need to be moving.

Gait training. The initial focus for controlling the COG during gait is a stable base of support that can be continually reestablished quickly and reliably through stepping. Unlike standing balance in which the base is stable and the COG moves over it, during locomotion the base is moving and the COG moves to stay over the base. Achieving a symmetrical, smoothly oscillating COG movement is the objective, with the forces of gravity and momentum being exploited.

The training is begun first in the forward direction but also includes backward and sideways directions (sidestepping, braiding, or carioca) to increase postural control demands. Challenge can be added by narrowing the base of support (tandem) or reducing the foot-surface contact (walk on toes or heels). Training to integrate postural control with locomotor skills is best accomplished not through continuous, steady-pace walking, but by starting, stopping, turning, bending, varying the speed, and avoiding or stepping over obstacles. Difficulty is added by increasing the abruptness, frequency, and unpredictability of these types of tasks and by adding tasks such as carrying or reading while walking. Altered surface conditions (carpets, ramps, curbs, stairs, grass, gravel) or reduced lighting conditions also heighten the challenge. Head and eye movements while walking should be

added as the patient improves. Walking quickly while reading signs on the wall or room numbers, for example, or looking toward and away from the therapist while walking makes vision more difficult to use for stability. Walking in crowds or in busy, cluttered environments is also challenging. Locomotion training on the treadmill reduces some abnormal asymmetries and increases control of gait with increased extension of the trailing limb.[145] Again, gait training specifically for balance enhancement should occur without holding onto fixed surfaces with the hands, for example, parallel bars or the side rails of the treadmill. This is because the nervous system needs to learn to solve the balance problem using the legs and trunk, not the hands.

Patients with somatosensory loss in the feet should use a cane or walker. They may not need the device for biomechanical support, but they do need to obtain as much information about the surface as possible. Through use of a cane or walker, preserved somatosensation in the hands can detect surface information that is important for balance control, and biomechanical support is available if needed in case of balance loss.

Other Considerations
Treatment Tools

Therapists use both high-technological and low-technological equipment in the remediation of balance deficits; each has advantages and disadvantages. High-technological options include accelerometers with motion biofeedback, forceplate systems with postural sway biofeedback, electromyographic biofeedback, optokinetic visual stimulation (from visual surround or moving lights), videotaping, and treadmills with biofeedback. Options for the evaluation and treatment of balance and gait deficits are expanded with the addition of advanced technology such as forceplate measures of postural sway and pressure mat measures of gait, giving the therapist a more quantitative and sensitive measurement than visual observation or timed measures. Most high-technological systems provide computer-generated reports with charts and graphs quickly. For training, overhead harness systems allow safe, hands-free practice, and computerized sway feedback supports motor learning (Figs. 20.21–20.24). Computerized systems allow advanced monitoring of progress and biofeedback, which supports motor learning. Fig. 20.21 is an example of technology in which force plates measure pressure-generated signals (center of force [COF]). The systems shown use height and COF data to calculate the COG, which is used to measure postural sway. The COG icon may be displayed on the monitor screen for feedback to the individual if desired. Fig. 20.22 is an example of how surface motion provides both biomechanical and somatosensory challenges. Balance measurement characteristics vary; some systems measure the motion of the

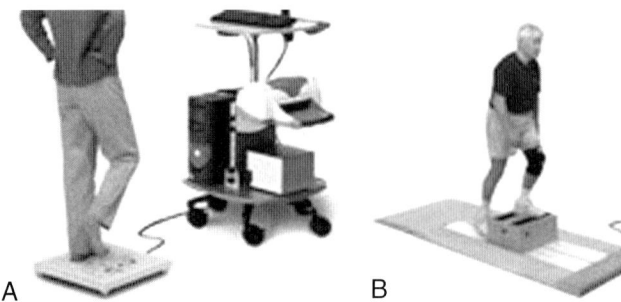

A   B

Fig. 20.21 Advanced Technology to Support Balance and Gait Retraining. The forceplates shown here are static, or fixed when in use. They are portable. The patient using these systems may be given static balance exercises ("Hold still"), or dynamic balance exercises ("Move with control"). These systems provide visual feedback options, which may be given during or after the balance exercise task, or not at all. **(A)** Bertec Portable Essential. **(B)** Bertec Portable Functional. (Courtesy Bertec, Inc.)

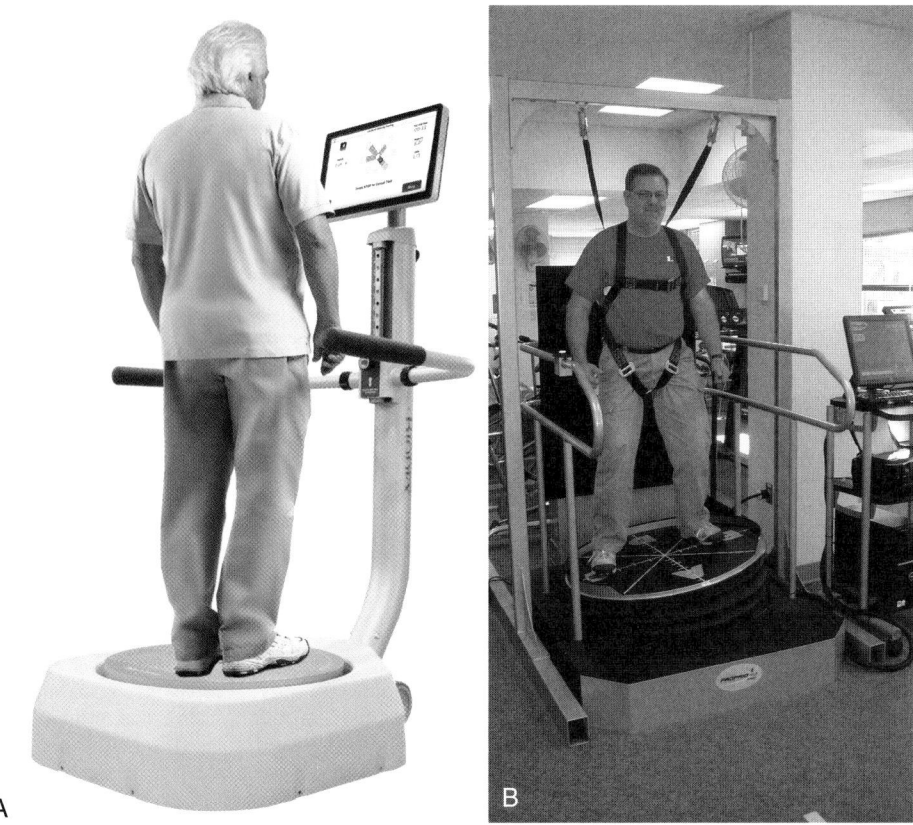

A   B

Fig. 20.22 Advanced Technology to Support Balance and Gait Retraining. Other systems provide surfaces that can be made unstable **(A)** or made to move **(B)**. The surface motion provides both biomechanical and somatosensory challenges. Amplitude and velocity capacity also vary from system to system. Both systems shown here provide omnidirectional motion. **(A)** Biodex Balance System SD measures the motion of the surface, **(B)** Proprio Reactive Balance System uses motion sensors on the body placed at the level of the center of gravity. (**A,** Photo courtesy of Biodex Medical Systems, Inc. **B,** Courtesy Perry Dynamics, Decatur, IL.)

surface (see Fig. 20.22*A*), whereas others use motion sensors on the body placed at the level of the COG (see Fig. 20.22*B*). Other systems provide the ability to generate visual motion. Fig. 20.23*A* shows a system with a three-sided booth with unidirectional motion combined with a movable forceplate with unidirectional motion. Both visual and somatosensory inputs can be manipulated for testing (e.g., SOT) and training. Omnidirectional visual motion (see Fig. 20.23*B*) can be produced by rotating display systems that are used in a dark room.

The ability to challenge balance during gait training is improved if the patient is secure in an overhead harness system as seen in Fig. 20.24*A* and *C*. These systems allow hands-free training as soon as possible to increase reliance on the lower extremity and trunk reactions critical for balance recovery strategies. Rapid and recordable measurement of gait characteristics (e.g., velocity, step length, step width) is possible with instrumented systems. Some systems are made for overground walking (see Fig. 20.24*B*) and are portable. Other systems are incorporated into treadmills and provide feedback during gait training. All motorized systems provide the ability to manipulate the environment easily and efficiently and to graduate tasks and environmental challenges safely. Drawbacks to high-technological equipment include cost, space requirements, and operator training requirements.

Low-technological options include mirrors, soft foam pads, hard foam rollers, rocker boards, BAPS boards, tilt boards, Swiss balls, minitrampolines, balance beams, and wedges or incline boards. All these items are accessible (low cost, easy to obtain), portable, and easy to use.

The main drawbacks for low technological equipment are that it does not provide novel feedback, objective scoring, or graphic recording, and clinicians must be skilled and creative in the use of such equipment in order to provide appropriate gradation of task difficulty and environmental conditions.

Safety Education and Environmental Modifications

Remediation of balance deficits is not always possible, but the clinician is always responsible for ensuring the safety of each patient. When permanent deficits exist, the patient and the family should be taught in what environments the patient is at risk (e.g., a patient with vestibular loss on a gravel driveway at night), what tasks are unsafe (e.g., ladder climbing, changing ceiling light bulbs), how the patient can compensate (e.g., use a cane at night or in crowds), and what changes in the home or workplace are needed (e.g., night lights, stair stripes, raised toilet seats). Clinicians can ask the patient (or family) to problem solve risky situations: "What would the patient do?" Home evaluations should be followed by a list of recommended safety modifications. Falls are frightening and dangerous, so clinicians should do their utmost to prevent them. If falls are likely, patients and families should be taught what to do if a fall occurs and, once the patient is on the floor, how to perform floor-to-standing or floor-to-furniture transfers. Home monitoring services such as Lifeline may be indicated if the patient lives alone and is prone to falling. Hip protectors will not prevent falls but do significantly reduce the risk of hip fracture.

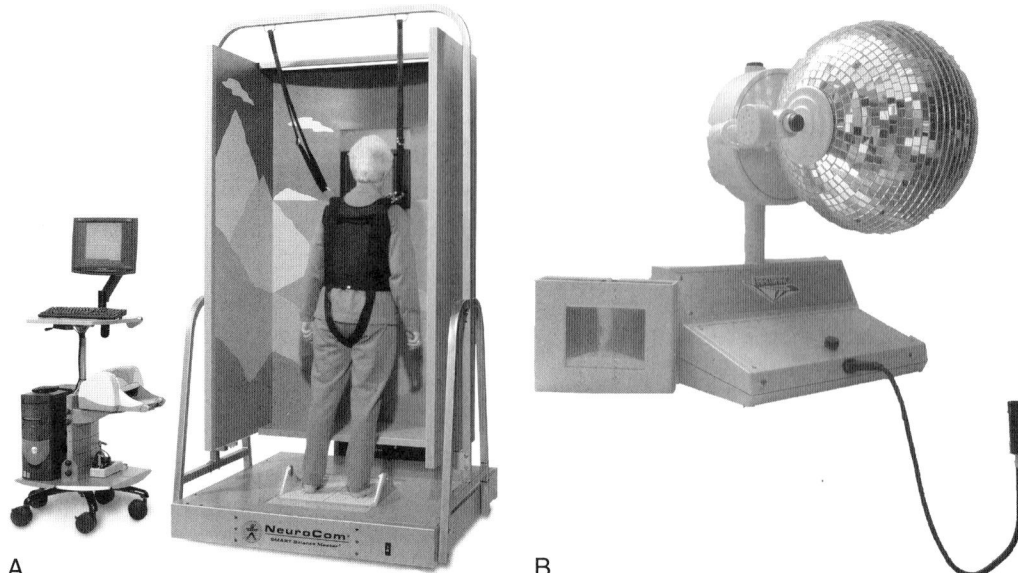

Fig. 20.23 Advanced Technology to Support Balance and Gait. (A) The Bertec Computerized Dynamic Posturography system allows the manipulation of somatosensory and visual inputs via surface motion (unidirectional anterior/posterior) and visual screen motion (omnidirectional or optokinetic), respectively. Evaluation components include the Sensory Organization Test, Motor Control Test and Adaptation Test; intervention components include progressive multisensory integration training. (B) The Bertec Vision Trainer system, used in conjunction with a static forceplate, offers dual task/concurrent task balance training exercises incorporating visual, cognitive, and upper extremity motion task demands. (Courtesy Bertec, Inc.)

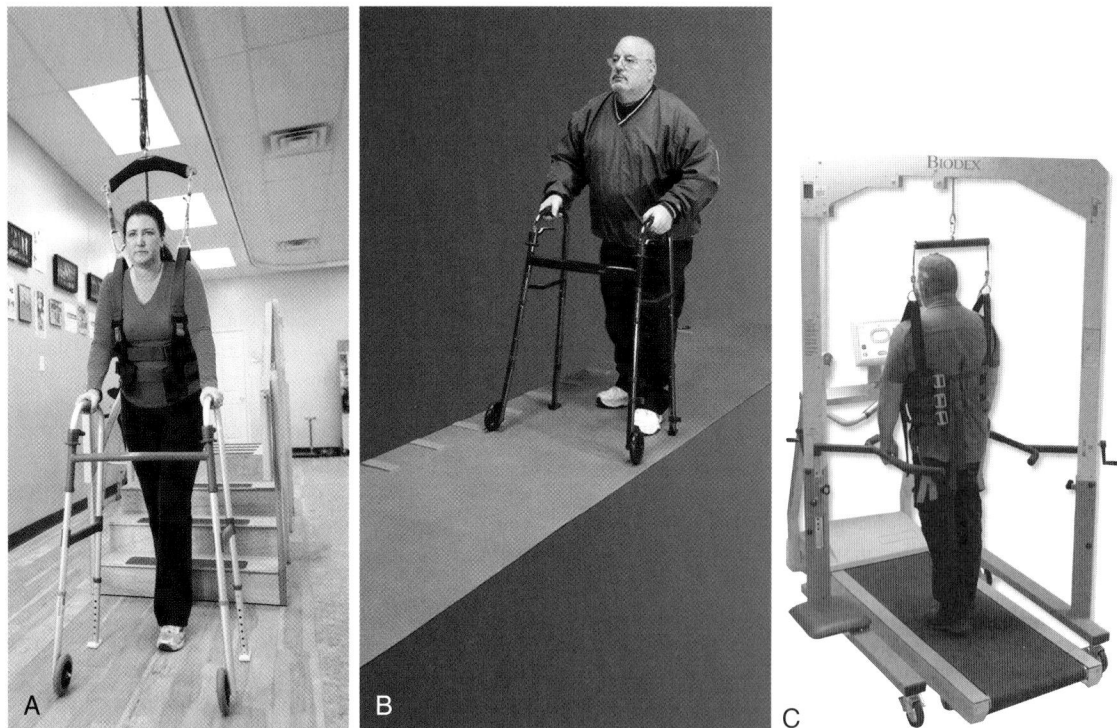

Fig. 20.24 Advanced Technology to Support Balance and Gait Retraining. High technology used to challenge gait. The ability to challenge balance during gait training is improved if the patient is secure in an overhead harness system. These systems allow hands-free training to increase reliance on the lower extremities and trunk reactions critical for balance recovery strategies. Rapid and recordable measurement of gait characteristics is possible with instrumental systems. (A) Biodex FreeStep SAS uses an overhead harness system to challenge balance during gait. (B) GAITRite Portable Walkway System challenges gait during overground walking. (C) Biodex Gait Trainer 3 with Unweighting System is another example of how to challenge balance during gait training. (A and C, Photos courtesy of Biodex Medical Systems, Inc. B, Courtesy CIR Systems, Havertown PA.)

Home Programs

Strengthening, stretching, posture, and endurance exercises can all be performed safely at home so that time in the clinic can be spent on balance-challenge exercises requiring supervision. Improvements in strength, ROM, posture, and endurance support improvements in balance. Many balance exercises can and should be performed at home if safety and adherence can be ensured; however, *unstable patients should always be supervised.* Standing balance tasks can be completed in a corner or near a countertop so that in case of balance loss the patient can use the hands (reaching strategy) to prevent a fall if other APR strategies are inadequate. However, balance exercises should not be routinely done while holding onto countertops, furniture, or other surfaces. If the patient needs to use her or his hands to perform the balance task, the task is too difficult and should be modified so that it can be safely performed without needing to hang on to a stable object. The community setting is ideal for postural control gait training. Grocery or library aisles, public transportation, elevators, escalators, grass, sandboxes or beaches, ramps, trails, hills, and varied environmental conditions in general provide both challenge and functional relevance.

Concurrent Tasks

Normal balance is largely subconscious. One objective in balance retraining is to force the nervous system to solve postural control problems at the automatic, subconscious level. A great deal of practice and dual-task training are necessary to accomplish this; the conscious brain is focused on accomplishing some other goal(s) and thus balance control must be achieved at a less conscious level. Alternative tasks can be physical in nature, such as carrying a tray or dribbling a basketball, or cognitive, such as conversing or solving verbal or math problems, or a combination of physical and cognitive demands.

This objective is not universal. Patients with permanent or progressive deficits in automatic motor processing, particularly those with advanced Parkinson disease, lose automaticity. They must learn to produce motor actions volitionally, with attention and intention, unless there are external sensory cues to drive the motor system.

Fall Prevention

Patient safety is always paramount; for any patient with balance deficits the risk of falls is increased and must be addressed in every clinical management program. In older adults, even those without documented neurological conditions, falls are prevalent and may lead to severe injury (including head trauma) and death. Fall risk is even greater and is especially high in persons with stroke and Parkinson disease. Fall prevention is a critical primary objective for clinicians serving patients with neurological conditions who have impaired balance and gait.

Fall risk factors are categorized as intrinsic, relating to the individual, and extrinsic, relating to the environment. Intrinsic risk factors include but are not limited to medical conditions (e.g., stroke, Parkinson disease); medications; impaired balance and gait; somatosensory, visual, or vestibular sensory loss; central processing problems; slow reaction time and other central motor deficits; lower-extremity weakness and decreased ROM; cognitive deficits; depression; urinary urgency or incontinence; and footwear. Extrinsic risk factors are hazards in the environment, such as inadequate lighting or excessive glare; slippery or cluttered surfaces; lack of handrails or grab bars; attention distracters; and timing demands (e.g., hurrying to answer the phone). The more risk factors present, the greater the likelihood of falls. Most falls in community-dwelling older adults are trips and slips and occur because of a combination of intrinsic and extrinsic risk factors. For example, a patient with hemiplegia who has limited ability to rapidly and maximally dorsiflex the ankle who encounters a trip hazard such as a rumpled doormat may not be able to clear the obstacle by lifting the hemiplegic leg and foot quickly. If the number and/or severity of intrinsic risk factors is great, falls may occur without any provoking extrinsic hazard.

Additional factors influence fall risk levels. The location of the patient may have an effect on fall risk. While in an institutional setting, the physical environment may be safer and the level of supervision and assistance higher, thus lowering risk. Yet if the surroundings are unfamiliar or confusing to the patient, the patient does not remember to call for assistance before getting up, or the environment holds barriers such as bedrails, wheelchair footrests, and so on that must be dealt with when hurrying to the bathroom, then an institutional setting may pose increased risk. The amount of supervision or assistance the patient receives may alter risk level. Confused or forgetful patients in facilities with high staff-to-patient ratios or who have family or caregiver supervision most of the time will have lower risk than those in facilities or homes where supervision and assistance are sparse. Lastly, the relative dependence-independence level of the patient, both physical and cognitive, affects risk level. Very dependent patients who cannot get up by themselves, and very independent patients with high-level balance and gait skills, are both at lower risk than patients in the middle of that spectrum. Patients who have sufficient ability to get up out of the bed or chair, and perhaps to walk, but who have impaired balance and gait skills and poor judgment or memory are at a much higher risk level.

A separate but equally important risk to consider is the risk of injury from a fall. Injury risk also depends on both intrinsic and extrinsic factors. Patients with low bone mineral density (BMD), low body mass, and impaired protective responses (APRs, especially reaching or protective extension) are more likely to be injured. Falls that occur from a greater height onto a harder surface are more apt to result in injury. An overweight patient with adequate BMD who, while in her yard gardening, stumbles and falls to the grassy ground from standing height with both arms out to break her fall would have a lower risk of injury. A thin patient with osteoporosis who, while at the store shopping, stumbles off a curb and falls to the concrete parking lot without getting her arms out in time to protect her would have a higher risk of injury.

Clinicians should consider fall risk and injury risk factors as they carry out their assessments and evaluation. This would begin with the chart review or history taking; as problems are noted, the clinician should be "red-flagging" those that are risk factors for falls. For example, you might note that the patient is on more than six prescription medications; polypharmacy is a risk factor for falls. You also note that one of the medications is a drug to remediate bone loss, and further inquiry reveals that the patient does have a diagnosis of osteoporosis, a risk factor for injury. During your own therapy assessment, you find substantial lower-extremity weakness, balance impairments, and gait limitations requiring the use of an assistive device, all major risk factors for falls. One of the identified balance impairments includes deficient APRs, a risk factor for injury. Later, during a team meeting to discuss the new patient, you learn from the OT that the home safety survey completed by the patient's spouse indicates numerous safety hazards, extrinsic risk factors for falls and perhaps injury. For fall prevention and injury prevention purposes, a list of all fall and injury risk factors pertaining to that patient should be generated for use in intervention planning.

The aim of intervention for fall prevention is to eliminate or minimize risk factors, with emphasis on four risk factors that appear to be more influential than others (in community-dwelling older adults). These four interventions are exercise, medication management, home safety modification, and vision management. The single best intervention for fall prevention is exercise—specifically, individualized exercises that target balance, gait with balance challenges, and leg strength. The challenge level of the balance and gait exercises should be high in relation to the patient's abilities. The balance and gait training program must be of high intensity and frequency and of long duration. For a reduction in fall rates in community-dwelling older adults, a minimum of 50 hours of exercise delivered over at least 2 months but not more than 6 months, is required.[146] For more neurologically involved patients, the overall amount of practice would likely need to be greater. Gains that are made during therapy will not be maintained unless exercise or physical activity that includes balance challenge is continued after therapy. Patients should be intentionally transitioned from therapy to a community-based balance exercise or physical activity program as an integral part of their discharge plan. Clinicians may consider doing their last therapy session or two at the community-based program to support the patient through the transition and increase the probability of follow-through. It is critical for patients to persist with physical activity to maintain or even further lower their fall risk level.

The second area of intervention is medication management. This requires a team approach and tactful, professional communication with the patient's physician(s). The goal is to have the patient take as few medications as possible, in the smallest doses possible, and to eliminate or when necessary replace certain drugs that are known to raise the risk of falls substantially (e.g., benzodiazepines). (Refer to Chapter 36 for a discussion of the impact of drug therapy on patients undergoing neurological rehabilitation.) Clinicians must understand that medication management for fall prevention is a difficult balancing act for the physician. For example, antidepressants and sleeping pills raise the risk of falls. Yet depression and sleep disorders are serious conditions with many negative effects, and depression, inattention, and fatigue are all risk factors for falls. Both the condition and its treatment increase risk! Patients on blood-thinning medication who are at risk for falls are also at risk for serious bleeding problems should a fall occur; the physician, patient, and family or caregiver should all be alerted to this risk. Medication management guidance for fall prevention directed to physicians is available from the American Geriatrics Society.

Home safety modification is an effective intervention for those who are already at high risk for falls. Ideally an in-person home safety evaluation is performed by a trained professional, usually a physical or occupational therapist. If this is not possible, a home safety survey may be completed by a reliable source (patient, family member, or caregiver). The clinician and patient or their responsible decision makers should then have a frank discussion about recommended home safety modifications. The clinician should convey what is recommended and why, highlighting the benefits. However, factors such as time, expense, and personal preference also influence patient and family decisions. Identification of barriers to safety modification implementation is helpful and may lead to solutions that permit initial resistance to be overcome.

Vision management is critical for any patient with visual deficits. (Refer to Chapter 28 for a discussion of disorders of vision and visual-perceptual dysfunction.) These visual impairments might be at the peripheral level, such as macular degeneration, or the central level, such as homonymous hemianopsia. Occupational therapy is recommended for a visual-perceptual evaluation and potentially for low-vision rehabilitation, if needed. Vision professionals (ophthalmologists, developmental optometrists), preferably those with specialization in neurological populations if indicated (e.g., TBI, cerebrovascular accident [CVA], MS), should also be involved. Objectives include maximizing vision for the patient and including visual support within the home safety modification plan, if needed.

Footwear assessment is important. Walking indoors barefoot or in socks is associated with increased fall risk. The footwear most highly associated with hip fractures is slippers. Shoes and slippers that do not provide adequate foot support, or that have slick soles, are unsafe and not recommended. Footwear lacking a secure back (flip-flops, mules, or sling-backs), high-heeled shoes, and platforms are poor choices for patients at risk for falls. Running shoes with very thick, cushioned soles and a heavy tread are also not ideal. The optimal shoes for fall risk reduction are well fitted with thin, hard soles. Shoes with a tread sole and a tread beveled heel are more stable on wet or slippery surfaces.[147] Just as with home safety modifications, factors such as expense, habit, and personal preference may create obstacles to patient adoption of suggested footwear changes. These obstacles should be recognized, respected, and addressed directly with professional communication strategies designed to facilitate positive behavior change.

Clinicians should assume that patients at risk for falls will fall when they are discharged home. Though clinicians work to ensure this will not happen, they also prepare for the possibility that it will. Patients who are able must be taught how to get up from the floor independently, with and without furniture if the latter is possible. If patients cannot get up from the floor by themselves, then family members or caregivers should be taught how to assist patients to get up from the floor. This may be as simple an act as bringing a chair close to the patient so the patient can use the chair to get up independently. Patients at risk for falls who will be home alone for extended periods of time would benefit from a wearable home alerting system. If such a system is cost-prohibitive, the patient should develop the habit of carrying a cell phone at all times. For patients without cell phones, a landline phone should be left on the floor or a chair seat so that it is within reach from the floor should a fall occur. Older patients with osteoporosis should consider wearing hip protectors. Hip protectors do not reduce the risk of falls but when properly fitted and worn may reduce the risk of hip fracture. Adoption of and adherence to wearing hip protector apparel is typically low and requires commitment and effort.

The combined aim of balance retraining and fall prevention is to assist the patient to become as active as is safely possible. With improved balance and gait skills, the patient achieves higher levels of function and physical activity. With attention to and emphasis on fall prevention, safety is maintained, injury is prevented, and the opportunity for improved quality of life is preserved.

CONCLUSION

Many patients who once thought their quality of life was permanently diminished and their ability to participate in meaningful activities had been taken away now show tremendous improvement in postural control system components, balance and gait skills, and functional abilities. The effectiveness of therapists working with these patients depends on their understanding the breadth and depth of the clinical problems, the use of standardized outcome tests that show measurable change, and the design and implementation of interventions that treat impairments, teach balance skills, and train functional activities. The importance of active patient participation cannot be overemphasized when discussing motor control and motor learning principles needed to optimize positive changes in balance disorders. Balance problems dramatically affect an individual's function, participation, and quality of life, and the role occupational and physical therapists play in providing appropriate interventions has established efficacy in practice.

CASE STUDY 22.1 Andy

Andy is a 27-year-old man who sustained a severe closed-head injury in a skiing accident. He was hospitalized for 2 months and resided at a long-term care facility for 6 months before cranial surgery for removal of bilateral subdural hygromas and revision of a ventriculoperitoneal shunt. After surgery he demonstrated marked improvement and was transferred to a rehabilitation unit. His initial physical therapy assessment revealed the following impairments, which had a negative effect on postural control:

1. Oculomotor deficits (difficulty tracking to the right and upward)
2. Disorientation
3. Delayed and slow motor responses
4. Bilateral ankle plantarflexion contractures (1–10 degrees left, 1–15 degrees right); limited right shoulder flexion (0–100 degrees) and external rotation (0–20 degrees)
5. Hypotonic trunk (right, moderate; left, mild), hypertonic (extensor) lower extremities (right, moderate; left, mild), hypertonic right upper extremity (mild)
6. Fair head control
7. Poor trunk control with right scapular atrophy, shortened right side, strength 3−/5
8. Left upper and lower extremity movement isolated and coordinated but slow, strength 4/5 at shoulder, 4+/5 elbow, wrist, hand, 4/5 hip and knee, 3+/5 ankle, able to place and hold for weight bearing
9. Right upper extremity rests and moves in synergistic pattern but can move out of synergy with request or demonstration; strength 3−/5 at shoulder and 4−/5 distally; coordination is poor; can place and hold for weight bearing if cued but not spontaneously
10. Right lower extremity moves in flexor-extensor pattern, grossly 3+/5 in hip and knee flexion, 20°ā hip extension, 3+/5 knee extension, no isolated ankle movement, cannot place or hold for weight bearing

Functional activity and balance skill tests found the following activity limitations:

1. Minimum assist supine-to-sit
2. Sitting balance, poor
3. Moderate assist sit-to-stand
4. Standing balance, unable
5. Moderate assist transfers
6. Nonambulatory

Body system impairment goals were the following:

1. Increase ROM to within normal limits throughout
2. Increase trunk tone to normal and strength to 4+/5
3. Decrease right-sided tone to normal
4. Increase spontaneous use, isolated movement, and strength (4+/5) in right extremities
5. Able to place and bear weight on right lower extremity

Short-term functional and skill goals were the following:

1. Independent in all bed mobility
2. Independent in wheelchair transfers
3. Good static and fair dynamic sitting balance
4. Contact guard sit-to-stand
5. Minimal assist static standing balance

Note: Ambulation goals were temporarily deferred because of the ankle contractures and balance deficits.

Early treatments included the following:

1. Standing frame activities for head control, visual tracking, trunk control, reduced lower-extremity extensor tone, and heel cord stretching with ultrasound
2. Neurodevelopmental sequence activities for head and trunk control; trunk strengthening; decreased lower-extremity extensor tone; balance on all fours, heel-sitting, kneeling
3. Supine to and from sitting, especially over the right arm
4. Sitting balance with upper-extremity functional tasks (e.g., putting glasses on and taking them off, taking shirt off and putting it on, wiping nose with tissue), with focus on right visual tracking, right trunk elongation, and incorporation of right lower-extremity ground pressure for stability
5. Transfer training with incorporation of right upper extremity to push up, reach and grasp, and right lower-extremity placing and weight bearing

As soon as Andy's ankle dorsiflexion ROM was near neutral on the right (was then 0 to 5 degrees on the left), neurodevelopmental activities were phased out and standing balance and pregait activities in the parallel bars were initiated with moderate assistance. He rapidly progressed to minimal-assistance gait in the parallel bars but with significant scissoring of the lower extremities. Gait outside the bars was begun with a quad cane on the left, but Andy was not able to organize the sequence for cane use and did not use the cane when loss of balance occurred, so use of the cane was discontinued. Gait without an assistive device required moderate assistance from the therapist for balance. A line drawn on the floor provided a visual cue to remind him to keep his feet apart; when walking without this cue, approximately 25% of his steps were close or crossed.

At discharge 2 months after admission, Andy had good visual tracking; normal ROM with the exception of right lower-extremity dorsiflexion, which was limited to 0 to 5 degrees; normal tone in the left extremities; mildly increased tone in the right extremities with slight extensor patterning in the leg; good head and trunk control; and strength grossly 4+/5 throughout. Functionally, he was independent in bed mobility, wheelchair mobility, and activities requiring sitting balance such as grooming and dressing. He required supervision for safety in transfers and standing activities and minimal to moderate assistance for indoor ambulation without an assistive device depending on his fatigue level.

CASE STUDY 22.2 Doris

Doris is a 73-year-old woman with a long history of Parkinson disease who had fallen 4 times within the 6 months before referral to physical therapy. As a result of her most recent fall during which she hit her head, Doris had ear pounding, lightheadedness, and headaches. After referral to an otolaryngologist, she was diagnosed with unspecified peripheral vestibular dysfunction and referred to outpatient therapy. Her therapist found that Doris reported increased lightheadedness and dizziness with anterior-posterior head movements, rolling in bed, sit-to-stand, and the Hallpike-Dix maneuver (worse to the right). Multiple impairments that could be contributing to her instability and falls, as well as symptoms related to the vestibular disorder, were also noted. Doris had mildly decreased

ROM in her left ankle, shoulders, and neck; mild left-sided weakness and lack of coordination; marked bilateral upper-extremity tremor; and moderately forward-flexed posture.

She could not perform an ankle strategy at all and continually used hip strategy; she also used stepping strategy frequently with the least shift or sway. Static postural sway tests indicated that Doris had excessive sway when attempting to stand still and that she kept her COG slightly posterior and to the right of midline. Sway increased tenfold with eyes closed, indicating poor use of somatosensory inputs for postural control. Doris could not perform repeated weight shifts in either anterior-posterior or medial-lateral directions. Her limits

Continued

CASE STUDY 22.2 Doris—cont'd

of stability were severely restricted to less than half of normal sway range anteriorly, and her movement time was slow.

Functional testing revealed that Doris had several disabilities. She had to use a walker or have manual assistance to ambulate and could negotiate level surfaces only. Without her walker or handhold assistance, Doris could stand for less than 30 seconds and take a maximum of 10 steps. For community ambulation, Doris needed minimum assistance with her walker and could go only short distances. She also required minimum assistance with bathing and household tasks.

Doris participated in therapy twice a week for 6 weeks and also performed a home exercise program daily. Her treatment plan included vestibular exercises for the dizziness and balance retraining exercises for instability and falls. The vestibular exercises she was given were designed to provoke her symptoms repeatedly and included head turning in supine and sitting (progressed to standing), rolling in bed, rocking in a rocking chair, and sit-to-stand practice. As her dizziness subsided, her home program was modified to increase the number and rate of head movements. To improve her use of somatosensory and vestibular inputs, Doris also practiced standing on a firm surface with eyes closed (with family supervision). In the clinic, Doris did stretching, strengthening, and postural extension exercises to address her musculoskeletal limitations. For

increased use of somatosensory and vestibular inputs, she practiced standing and weight shifts with optokinetic stimulation. By using postural sway biofeedback, she practiced achieving the midline position, controlled anterior and left-sided weight shifts at progressively faster speeds, and ankle strategy. Gait training included starts, stops, turns, and obstacle avoidance and progressed to community ambulation tasks such as curbs and ramps. As her endurance improved, she also did gait training on the treadmill to increase the gait speed, stride length, hip strength, and use of vestibular inputs.

Despite her multiple problems, Doris was able to reduce the severity of her impairments and consequently improve her functional level. Her dizziness resolved completely. Although she still had excess sway during static standing, she was able to achieve and hold a midline position, and her sway with eyes closed reduced by more than half. Doris could shift her weight in both anterior-posterior and medial-lateral directions at moderate speeds by using ankle strategy without stepping. Her limits of stability were expanded from 35% to 80% of normal, and she was able to shift her weight much more quickly. Functionally, she could stand without the walker for 8 minutes and walk independently indoors on level surfaces without the walker for short distances. She was independent in community ambulation with the walker. At a 3-month follow-up visit, Doris reported that she had experienced no more falls.

ACKNOWLEDGMENT

I wish to extend my gratitude to Darcy Umphred, PT, PhD, FAPTA, and Rolando Lazaro, PT, PhD, DPT, for the opportunity to share my passion for balance rehabilitation through this chapter. I thank Kenda Fuller, PT, NCS, for her insightful contributions to this chapter revision.

REFERENCES

To enhance this text and add value for the reader, all references are included on the companion Evolve site that accompanies this textbook. This online service will, when available, provide a link for the reader to a Medline abstract for the article cited. There are 147 cited references and other general references for this chapter, with the majority of those articles being evidence-based citations.

Vestibular Dysfunction*

Kenda Fuller

OVERVIEW: THE ROLE OF THE VESTIBULAR SYSTEM

The vestibular system is critical for postural control because it uniquely identifies self-motion of the head as different from motion in the environment. The vestibular system is a mechanical system that creates neural output to create this sense. Fig. 21.1 shows the components of the vestibular mechanism as it sits with the cochlea, the organ of hearing. The vestibular system detects the direct pull of gravity to identify head position during balance activities and maintains vertical alignment of the eyes. This contributes to the head righting or labyrinthine response and activates the ocular tilt triggered by lateral head bend as seen in Fig. 21.2. Horizontal and vertical accelerations, such as riding in a car or an elevator, are detected by the vestibular otolith mechanism depicted in Fig. 21.3. The otolith structures provide this input during head movement by identifying the degree and direction of deflection of the hair cells projecting into the macula of the saccule in the vertical plane and macula of the utricle in the horizontal plane. It is the mass of the otoconia that sits on top of the macula and creates the mechanical pull on the hair cells when the head accelerates or tilts. The vestibular system calibrates the speed of head movement or degree of tilt in relation to the input from the nerve cells that project from the otoliths.

The vestibular spinal reflex (VSR) creates the response from the otolithic structures of the vestibular mechanism to the muscles to provide postural control through the activation of the vestibulospinal tracts. The medial vestibulospinal tract (MVST) descends only to the axial cervical musculature. The coordination of head movements and the integration of head and eye movements are activated through the

medical tracts. The lateral vestibulospinal tract (LVST) descends to the muscles of the trunk, providing orientation for body position in space to support upright balance activities and gait. Together these tracts provide efficient head righting. Activation will cause ipsilateral increased tone in extensors with reciprocal inhibition of reciprocal inhibition of flexors. Someone with an acute vestibular disorder that affects the VSR will often increase weight shift to the side of the lesion. It is important to remember that vestibular nuclei are connected to other sensory and motor systems involved with balance. The connection to the cerebral cortex is associated with spatial orientation. Both top down and bottom up referencing (see later) are used to create the necessary integration for balance. The inferior vestibular nuclei connect to the reticular activating system, which is the cause for the nausea and anxiety often associated with disruption within the vestibular system.

Angular and linear acceleration of the head are detected through the semicircular canals that are part of the labyrinth on each side. When the head moves or changes position, there is movement of endolymph fluid within the canal that moves in the opposite direction of the head movement. The ampulla, which appears as a bump in the canal, houses the cupula containing a group of hair cells; the kinocilia are the longer hair cells, and the stereocilia are shorter hair cells. The hair cells are deflected as the endolymph pressure increases or decreases, reflecting the speed and direction of the head motion. When the stereocilia move toward the kinocilium, the canal is excited, and when the pressure moves the kinocilium toward the stereocilia, the canal is inhibited. In the posterior canal and anterior canal the stereocilia are closest to the otolith, whereas in the horizontal canal the kinocilium is closest to the otolith. This relationship will determine the how the nervous system will react to changes in head position and rotation of the canal. The canals are aligned to provide information about head position and angular acceleration in all planes of movement. For example, the posterior canal

---

*Videos for this chapter are available at studentconsult.com.

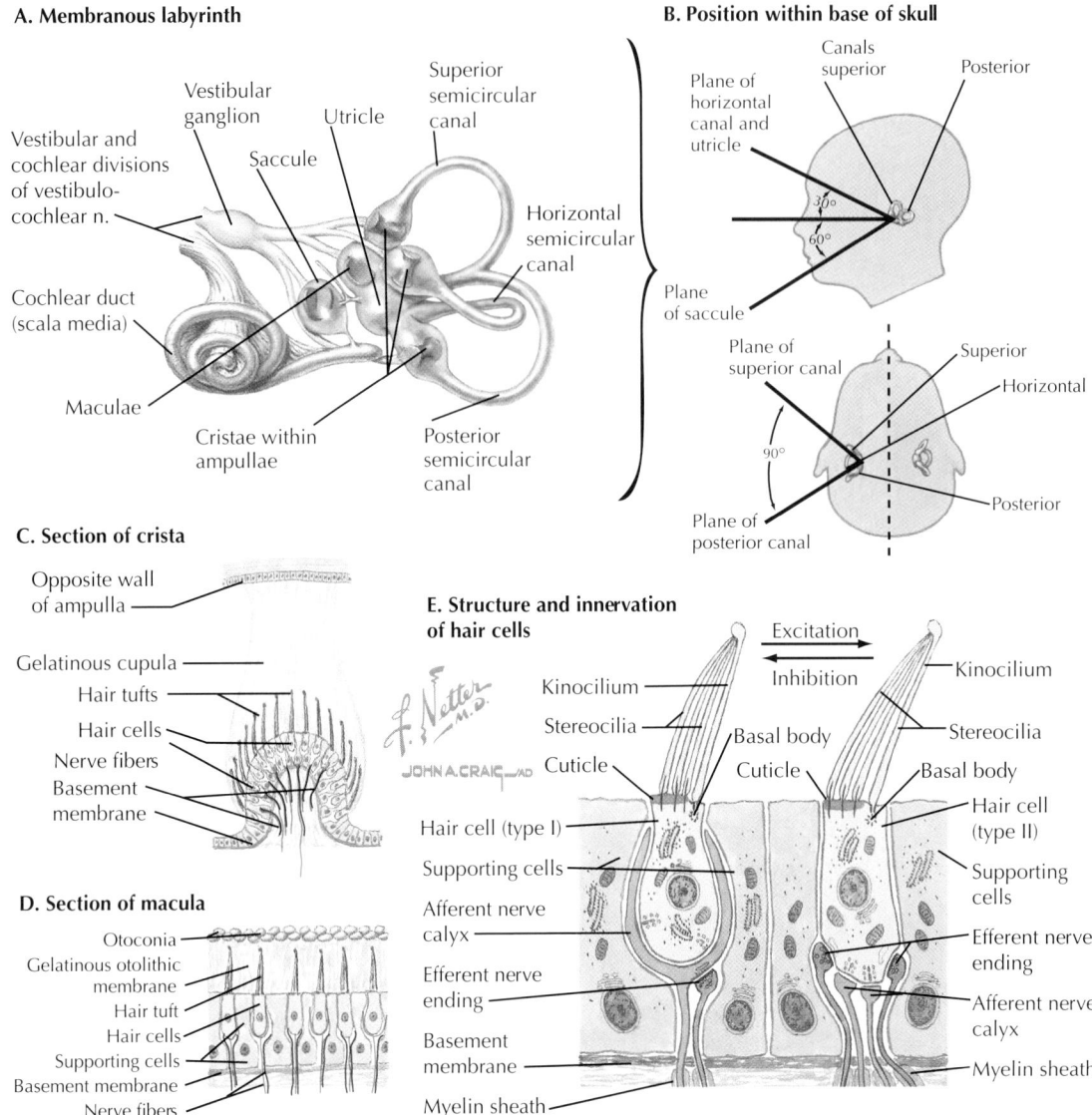

Fig. 21.1 Components of the Vestibular System and Cochlea With Distribution of Neural Connections.
(A) Membranous labyrinth refers to the structure of the vestibular and cochlear mechanism. **(B)** Plane of reference for the canals and otliths. **(C)** Cross section of the ampulla within the semicircular canal. **(D)** Cross section of the macula of the otoliths. **(E)** The structure and activation pattern of the nerves within the semicircular canals and otliths. (From Felten DL, O'Banion K, Maida M. Sensory Systems. In: *Netter's Atlas of Neuroscience*; 3rd ed. Elsevier; 2016.)

on one side is in relative alignment with the anterior canal on the opposite side. This allows for redundant information to be provided by the canals through a push–pull relationship.

To maintain a stable gaze during head movement, the eyes respond through the vestibulo-ocular reflex (VOR). This is achieved as the excitation signal is activated as described previously in the direction of head turn. For example, in a right head turn, the movement of the fluid in the semicircular canal is in the opposite direction, or toward the left. The endolymph presses the kinocilium of the right horizontal canal toward the otolith (excitation), and the endolymph in the left horizontal canal pulls the kinocilium away from the otolith (inhibition). The excitation moves through the vestibular nerve to the level of the oculomotor nuclei activating the medial rectus muscle of the ipsilateral eye and the lateral rectus of the contralateral eye. This pulls the eye in the opposite direction as the head turn. At the same time, the medial rectus of the contralateral eye is inhibited

along with the lateral rectus of the ipsilateral eye, which allows the eyes to move without resistance. In a properly functioning system, the eyes move at the same time and at a speed exactly opposite the head, providing a gain of 1:1 (eye movement speed reflects head movement speed). The relationship between eye movement and head movement can be seen in Fig. 21.4.

When the signals from the labyrinth mechanisms are not equal and opposite, usually when there is damage to one side anywhere along the pathway, nystagmus results. Nystagmus is nonvoluntary, rhythmic oscillation of the eyes, with movement in one direction clearly faster than movement in the other direction. Nystagmus reflects the abnormal VOR response when the system is not calibrated. The eye movements represent the slow drift of the eye with a fast catch up saccade returning the eye to the original position. This is due to the unopposed neural activity in the intact vestibular pathways. The slow phase represents the vestibular insult, and the fast phase is the central reset.

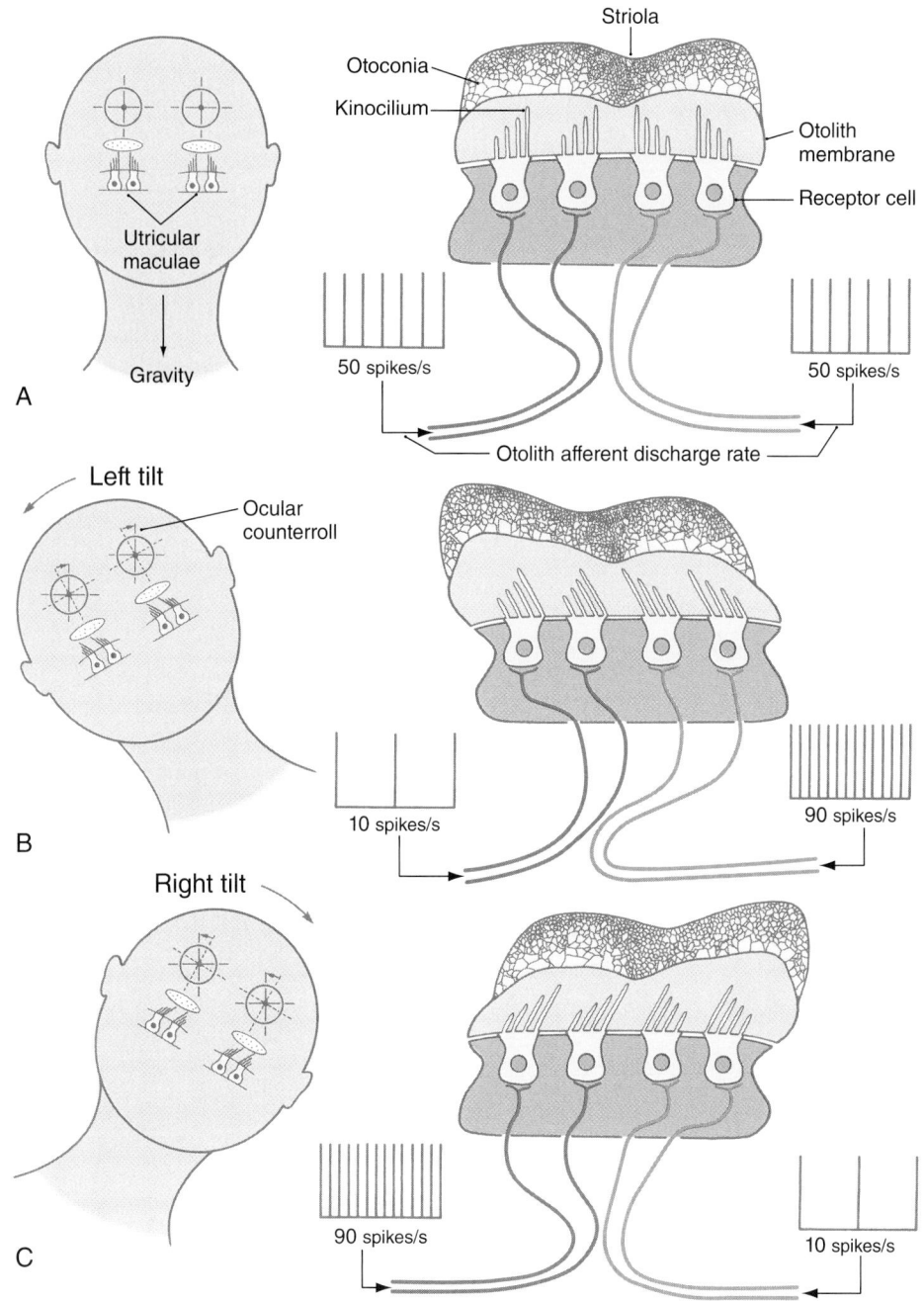

Fig. 21.2 Patterns of excitation and inhibition for the left utricle and saccule when the head is upright **(A)**, tilted with the left ear 30 degrees down **(B)**, and tilted with the right ear 30 degrees down **(C)**. The utricle is seen from above and the saccule from the left side. (From Haines DE. *Fundamental Neuroscience for Basic and Clinical Applications*. 3rd ed. Philadelphia: Churchill Livingstone; 2006.)

Nystagmus is labeled by the fast phase. In a patient with a peripheral vestibular disorder, horizontal nystagmus will intensify with the gaze toward the fast phase; this is known as Alexander's Law. Disruption of the vestibular system resulting in nystagmus causes an immediate sensation of blurriness of vision or the sense the room is moving, known as vertigo. Vertigo is a specific type of dizziness that reflects the vestibular system involvement. Vertigo can cause imbalance as it disrupts the visual reference for head position.

Abnormal eye movements can also reflect the vestibular system function as it passes through the cerebellum, where the Purkinje cells provide inhibitory control of the vestibular nuclei. The flocculonodular lobe and medial zone of the cerebellum will affect postural control

and eye movements. For example, dysfunction in the flocculus will cause abnormal smooth pursuits, abnormal VOR suppression, and nystagmus patterns, which include downbeat, gaze-evoked, and rebound. Central positioning and periodic alternating nystagmus (PAN) patterns are seen in nodulus lesions. Saccadic movement, or the ability to move the eyes quickly between targets, is controlled in the vermis so a lesion can cause hypometric eye movements. Disruption of function in the fastigial nucleus can cause hypermetric eye motion. The cerebellum also has a role in motor skill adaptation and error correction. Disease processes, such as multiple sclerosis, which can progress to disruption of cerebellar pathways, can cause nystagmus and loss of postural control. Strokes that affect the cerebellum can cause

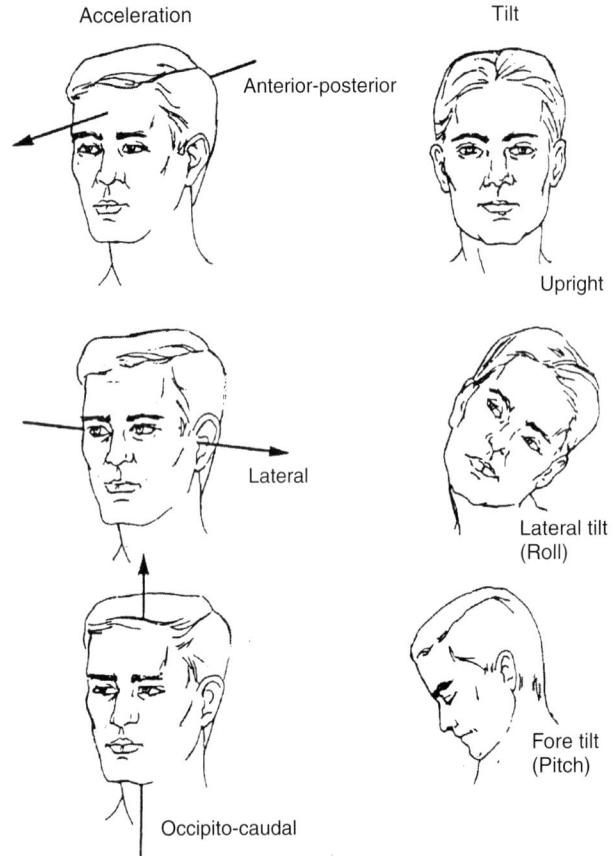

Fig. 21.3 The Otoliths Register Linear Acceleration and Static Tilt of the Head. (From Hain TC, Ramaswany TS, Hillman MA. Anatomy and physiology of the normal vestibular system. In: Herdman SJ, editor. *Vestibular Rehabilitation*. 3rd ed. Philadelphia: FA Davis; 2007.)

persistent dizziness as well as imbalance, even when the vestibular testing is normal and there is no concomitant hemiplegia.

The hippocampus is linked to the functionality of the vestibular system and contains "place cells" that create an inner map of our environment. These cells work together with connections in the entorhinal and thalamic areas to assist us in way finding, or spatial orientation. These cells become dysfunctional with peripheral vestibular lesions. The evolutionary gravity sensing function of the otoliths may be connected to both spatial and cognitive functions. There is a further connection to the striatal component of the basal ganglia, which has an additional impact on both spatial orientation and cognition.[1] This may be the reason that diseases affecting the basal ganglia, such as Parkinson disease, have components that may overlap. There appears to be a connection to vestibular dysfunction related to atrophy of the hippocampus and changes in the posterior parietal–temporal, medial temporal, and cingulate regions seen in people with Alzheimer disease, mostly in the subset known to have spatial disorders that lead to wandering.[2]

The vestibular projections to the cortex pass through other parts of the brain. The thalamus works as part of the sensory relay system. It has a connection with the vestibular cortex and the reticular formation, so it affects arousal and conscious awareness of the body to provide the determination of self-movement compared to environmental movement as described in the opening paragraph. Vestibular connections to the cortex provide spatial orientation and perceived

vertical. The roles of the vestibular cortical areas, such as the parieto-insular vestibular cortex, are the focus of research directed toward changing firing patterns in the brain to address concerns as mal de debarquement noted later in this chapter. The connections to the autonomic nervous system, such as the locus coeruleus, amygdala, and parabrachial nucleus, provide the link to symptoms of stress and panic, activation of the fight or flight response, emotional memories, and the malaise that includes nausea. This is another area of active research (see Fig. 21.5).[3]

It is very important to remember that the vestibular system never works in complete isolation; it is always integrated with the somatosensory system or the visual system. Vestibular rehabilitation as an intervention is always dependent on sensory integration. The vestibular and somatosensory systems preferentially operate at different velocities of postural sway because of differences in sensory thresholds and sensitivities. It is believed that misinterpretation of multisensory inputs during postural sway may underlie the imbalance associated with either vestibular or somatosensory impairments. The term "sensory reweighting switch" describes the unconscious shift from a surface reference using somatosensory input to a gravitational reference that relies on the vestibular system information. This can be described as a switch from a "body on support" to a "body in space" orientation.

Top Down Postural Control

Vestibular inputs are critical to determine whether the body is moving on a fixed surface or if the surface is moving.[4] The perception of verticality used to orient to gravity, when the support surface is perceived to be unstable, is provided by the vestibular system. Vestibular inputs are used to recognize the changes in angle of the support surface.[5,6] The vestibular system provides a top-down reference for the head and trunk stability in line with gravity, while the leg segment is coordinated to maintain surface reference. It is important to remember that at the same time the vestibular system is activated in this moving surface condition, the somatosensory system is still providing feedback about the relationship to the surface.[7] Resulting patterns of muscle activation reflect vestibular and somatosensory integration to maintain continuous upright postural control.

Studies performed on rotating surfaces demonstrate how the use of vestibular, visual, and somatosensory reference differs under conditions that mimic environmental situations. At very slow speeds, somatosensory reference is the primary reference used. As a surface rotates greater than 6 degrees of tilt and increases velocity (range of 2 to 8 degrees per second) there is more focus of the sensory systems away from the somatosensory reference toward the vestibular and visual references. Correct visual information can compensate for loss of vestibular information. However, when the eyes are closed, individuals with vestibular deficits will typically lose balance as the surface tilts at 4 degrees per second. Patients with missing or mal-adapted vestibular function lack the awareness of angle changes and demonstrate abnormal firing patterns in the muscles of the lower leg, aligning their bodies with respect to the surface instead of gravity, which is described as active postural destabilization. Instead of changing the ankle angle to adjust to the tilt, the torque around the ankle remains locked with excessive reference to the surface. The head and trunk follow the direction of the surface tilt.[8] This concept can be seen in Fig. 21.6. As the surface tilt angle exceeds 8 degrees, the individual who cannot activate gravitational reference or adjust the ankle angle will be unable to maintain balance without visual input.[4,9] When the surface is uneven, compliant, or narrow, the vestibular system will provide adequate information on head position, even if vision is occluded.

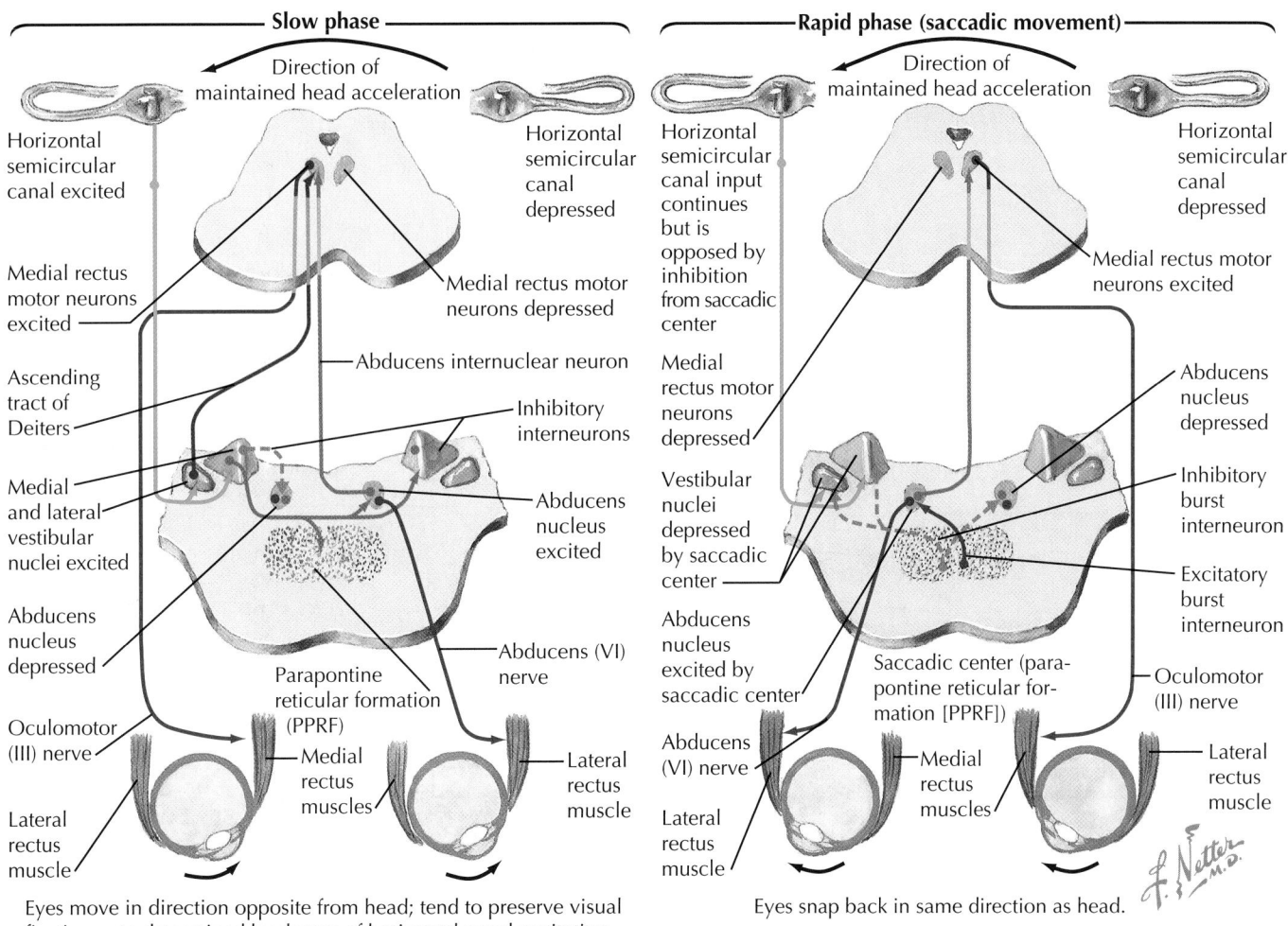

Slow phase

Direction of maintained head acceleration

Horizontal semicircular canal excited

Horizontal semicircular canal depressed

Medial rectus motor neurons excited

Medial rectus motor neurons depressed

Abducens internuclear neuron

Ascending tract of Deiters

Inhibitory interneurons

Medial and lateral vestibular nuclei excited

Abducens nucleus excited

Abducens nucleus depressed

Abducens (VI) nerve

Parapontine reticular formation (PPRF)

Oculomotor (III) nerve

Medial rectus muscles

Lateral rectus muscle

Lateral rectus muscle

Eyes move in direction opposite from head; tend to preserve visual fixation; rate determined by degree of horizontal canal excitation.

Rapid phase (saccadic movement)

Direction of maintained head acceleration

Horizontal semicircular canal input continues but is opposed by inhibition from saccadic center

Horizontal semicircular canal depressed

Medial rectus motor neurons excited

Medial rectus motor neurons depressed

Abducens nucleus depressed

Vestibular nuclei depressed by saccadic center

Inhibitory burst interneuron

Excitatory burst interneuron

Abducens nucleus excited by saccadic center

Saccadic center (parapontine reticular formation [PPRF])

Oculomotor (III) nerve

Abducens (VI) nerve

Medial rectus muscles

Lateral rectus muscle

Lateral rectus muscle

Eyes snap back in same direction as head.

Fig. 21.4 Vestibuloocular Reflex. When the head is turned to the right, inertia causes the fluid in the horizontal semicircular canals to lag behind the head movement. This bends the cupula in the right semicircular canal in a direction that increases firing in the right vestibular nerve. The cupula in the left semicircular canal bends in a direction that decreases the tonic activity in the left vestibular nerve. Neurons whose activity level increases with this movement are indicated in solid lines. Neurons whose activity level decreases are indicated in dotted lines. For simplicity, the connections of the left vestibular nuclei are not shown. Via connections between the vestibular nuclei and the nuclei of cranial nerves III and VI, both eyes move in the direction opposite to the head turn. (From Felten DL, O'Banion K, Maida M. Sensory Systems. In: *Netter's Atlas of Neuroscience*; 3rd ed. Elsevier; 2016.)

Bottom Up Reference for Postural Control

As stated previously, the somatosensory system can determine the orientation of the head compared to the surface tilt through cutaneous, proprioceptive, pressure, and stretch receptors of the muscles and joints, primarily related to pressure through the balls of the feet.

The somatosensory system is necessary to interpret vestibular information.[7] It contributes significantly to balance when the surface is stable or moving slowly (at less than 4 degrees per second). At the other end of the spectrum, in very fast oscillations, the muscle spindles provide stabilizing information that can contribute to head and trunk stability. Patients with vestibular deficits typically rely primarily on their ankle strategy during typical activities by keeping the head aligned with the body. This can be seen in a patient who demonstrates rotation "en bloc"; the head will stay aligned with the body while turning. This can be seen in Fig. 21.7 during a lateral tilt where the trunk will follow the direction of the platform.

The vestibulospinal system also activates the neck muscles in response to head motion. When the vestibular system function is missing or inaccurate, there is abnormal muscle activation in the muscles of the neck.[7] This is usually seen as excessive co-contraction of both flexors and extensors. Abnormal firing of the sternocleidomastoid (SCM) with restriction of rotation of the head is often seen in both acute and chronic settings. The suboccipital muscles can develop a pattern of overuse that can contribute to headache. See cervical spine function and dysfunction in concussion in Chapter 23.

Having even the slightest touch reference, so that the somatosensory system can orient the trunk through upper extremity joint position sense, is another way to substitute somatosensation for vestibular reference.[10] The position of the head and trunk can be determined by this touch even when the vestibular system function lacks normal function and the eyes are closed. Because the arm stabilizes the trunk more than the legs do, reaching for a stable surface is a common way

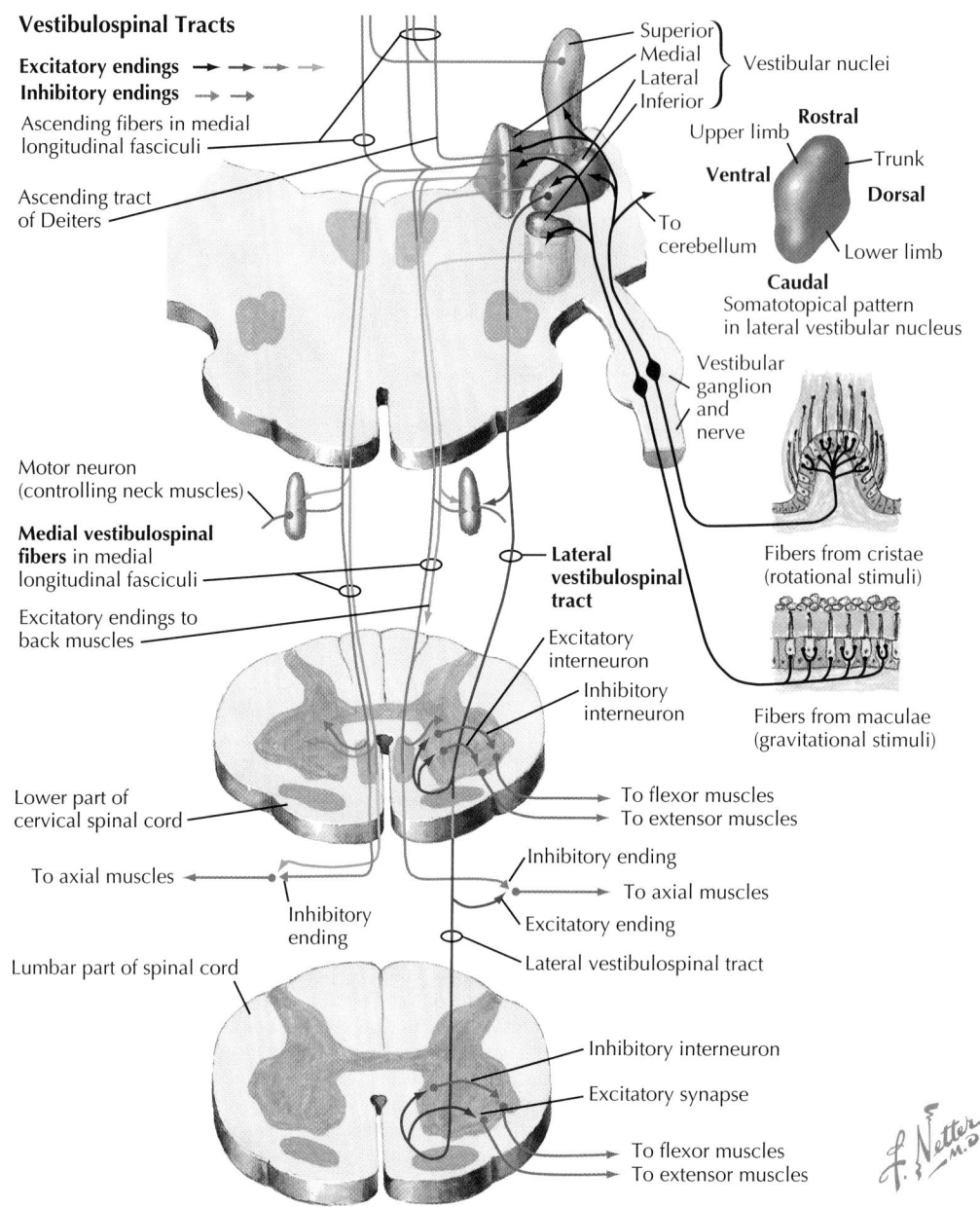

Fig. 21.5 Potential Location of Lesions That May Affect the Vestibular System. (From Felten DL, O'Banion K, Maida M. Sensory Systems. In: *Netter's Atlas of Neuroscience*; 3rd ed. Elsevier; 2016.)

to maintain balance when challenged. The therapist must recognize when the patient is using this touch reference to substitute for gravity orientation.

When the brain is not able to use somatosensation to identify the relationship between appropriate body segments and the surface, the patient often will report feeling lightheaded or has the sense of floating. When somatosensory inputs from the neck are reduced, absent, or distorted, it affects the stability and mobility of the individual spinal segments. Co-contraction of the SCM, levator scapulae, upper trapezius, and superficial neck extensors may indicate abnormal sensory feedback, altered afferents, and recruitment patterns, which are ineffective. Nociception from cervical segments can create "noise" in the postural control system contributing to dysmetric postural responses and nausea. Impaired cervical afferents will cause changes in cadence and length of stride when neck motion is introduced to gait. This should be considered in planning interventions for patients who are sent for vestibular rehabilitation.[11,12]

Visual Reference for Postural Control

Orientation of the head in space is possible through predictive control of vision. A stable environment provides visual vertical and horizontal references for balance. Recognizing self-movement as it relates to visual movement can be disrupted momentarily in a normal individual experiencing unexpected movement in the peripheral visual environment. This is a common sensation noticed when the car next to you rolls backward, and you press the brake, thinking that you are rolling forward. Vestibular system function is necessary for a comparison of self-motion to motion in the environment. For example, when you are walking and someone is walking toward you, your visual system will detect that the person is getting closer; however, you cannot determine

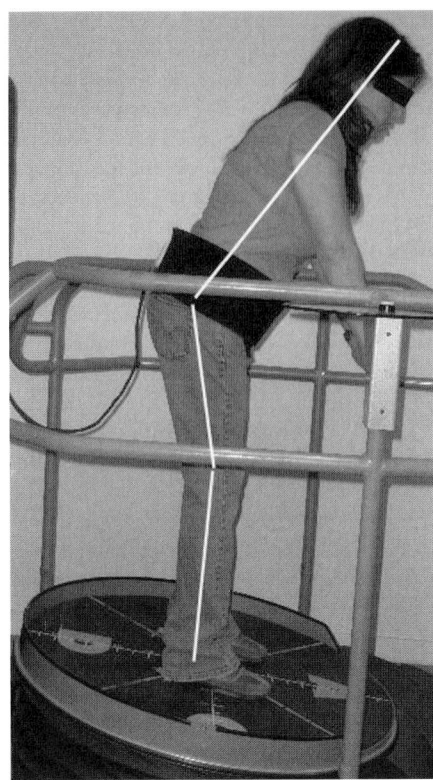

Fig. 21.6 In anterior tilt of the platform, the head and trunk follow the reference of the platform rather than maintaining a gravity-neutral position. This is reported as surface reference. (Courtesy Perry Dynamics, Decatur, IL.)

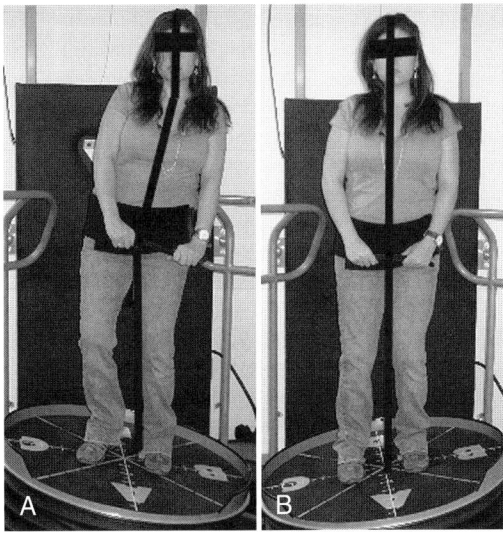

Fig. 21.7 **(A)** The patient references her trunk to the platform, shifting weight downhill to the downhill leg. **(B)** The patient has referenced her trunk and head to gravity, resulting in improved postural control. (Courtesy Perry Dynamics, Decatur, IL.)

how fast the other person is moving unless your vestibular system is able to independently recognize your own speed to calibrate the relative movement in the visual field. This is why driving can be challenging; it is hard to determine the distances and speeds of other cars when the vestibular system is not providing accurate information about self-movement.

Visual disorders can independently disrupt balance, cause the sensation of dizziness, and limit the function. Information from both smooth pursuits and saccades are integrated with the vestibular system information to help interpret the relationship of the body to the environment. Accurate evaluation of the visual system is critical in differential diagnosis. A clue that the visual system is causing dizziness can be discovered when the patient reports less dizziness with eyes closed than when the eyes are open. Disorders of convergence are common in the vestibular-deficient patient and can cause delay in the process of adaptation.

If there is a visual–vestibular mismatch, the patient will complain of motion sickness or visual motion sensitivity. These individuals will have dizziness when there is movement in the visual environment, especially if there is a pattern to it, as when driving on a wooded mountain highway or in the presence of optokinetic stimulation. The brain is unable to use the visual reference to determine body motion, speed, or upright position. In this visual environment, it is the vestibular system that provides the correct reference. If the visual–vestibular integration is faulty in these circumstances, the result is dizziness often with nausea. The oscillopsia associated with acute VOR disruption or with bilateral loss gives the patient a sensation that the room is moving around them, or bouncing as they walk. Oscillopsia as a result of visual system disorders is less common and is usually evaluated and treated by a specialist in vision.

A normal visual response called physiological diplopia (double vision) can contribute to visual discomfort in patients with vestibular dysfunction. See Box 21.1. When a person looks at an object close to them (within 6 to 12 inches), there is an apparent doubling of the objects in the peripheral field of view. Because this is normal, the awareness of the double vision is typically extinguished and not perceived. Patients with uncompensated vestibular systems, who rely excessively on visual reference, can become sensitive to this physiological diplopia as it destabilizes the visual field. This can cause a sense of visual motion hypersensitivity during daily activity as they attempt to look at near objects. When there is sensitivity to this apparent movement, it is difficult for the patient to distinguish this when there is movement in the visual field. Optokinetic stimulus, or movement in the visual field, especially if it is in a pattern, will cause dizziness and loss of balance. Visual motion sensitivity can be measured and tracked via the Visual Vertigo Analogue Scale or the Pediatric Visually Induced Dizziness Questionnaire.[13]

Abnormal responses in neck muscle activity associated with eye motion have implications for control of posture and movement. The smooth pursuit neck torsion test (SPNT) is used to delineate abnormal cervical afferent influences on oculomotor function from vestibular influences. There is considerable evidence to support the importance of cervical afferent dysfunction in the development of dizziness especially with visual disturbances during head movement following neck trauma, especially in those with persistent pain. This should become an essential part of the routine assessment and management of those with traumatic neck pain, including those with concomitant injuries

> **BOX 21.1 Physiological Double Vision**
> - Everything in front of and behind the central focal point is perceived as double
> - The closer the focal point, the more distance appears to be between the *perceived* double images
> - As the central focal point moves in space, the background image appears to move

BOX 21.2   **Smooth Pursuit Neck Torsion Test**

Test: Smooth pursuits tested in the head-neutral position, and then compared with the head rotated right and left
Findings: Compare gain in three head positions
Considerations: Shows relationship to cervical pain, proprioception, and oculomotor control

such as concussion, vestibular system damage, and visual pathology or deficits.[14] Testing of SPNT is described in Box 21.2.

GAIT DYSFUNCTION

Chapter 20 on Balance describes automatic postural responses and describes balance testing in detail. It is important to understand the role of the vestibular system in movement disorders related to balance. These consequences can have an impact on the gait patterns related to vestibular dysfunction.

Vestibular system losses can result in motor responses that are larger than necessary for the task, which can predispose a patient to falling. This can be seen in the gait cycle when the body center of mass moves faster and farther than the individual can control. This movement appears similar to that of the patient with cerebellar dysfunction, and indeed may represent the loss of vestibular input to the Purkinje cells in the cerebellum that would normally modulate vestibular pathways.[7,15] The gait pattern reflected by vestibular dysfunction, or lack of integration, often involves flat-foot gait with minimal heel strike and abnormal foot placement requiring larger than normal trunk adjustment. To control the position of the trunk, the base of support is widened. Speed of gait is another indication of vestibular function from the perspective that patients with bilateral loss or uncompensated vestibular loss demonstrate a slower self-selected speed. Typically, there is increased double limb stance time and decreased stability at heel strike.[16] Vestibular control of position for the upper body and head appears to be separated from the lower body in gait in a similar pattern as noted during perturbed stance. Head and trunk stability normally remain constant throughout the phases of gait, and vestibular inputs appear to be most critical during initiation of gait, toe off, and heel strike. Vestibular information contributes to the planned foot trajectory and placement of the foot to prevent disequilibrium. It is interesting to note that during steady state gait—and even more so with running—vestibular contribution appears to diminish in importance. This may be because movement in running is highly automatic and the trajectory remains steady.[17]

When the vestibular system does not accurately inform the patient about the speed and direction of head movement, visual cues are used to determine movement speed and direction of gait in relation to nonmoving objects. However, in environments with a lot of motion, or when someone approaches in the opposite direction, determining speed and direction of self-movement becomes more difficult. Patients often report dizziness and imbalance in a crowd. Walking with head turns becomes even more challenging as the vestibular system is activated and the somatosensory and visual systems are disadvantaged. Head turns included in the Functional Gait Assessment provide a way to identify this impairment. Because head movement can cause visual disturbances and dizziness, the patient with a vestibular disorder will significantly limit head movement while walking. When visual cues are used predominantly for balance, the patient will try to keep the body in line with vertical and horizontal visual targets. This will decrease the

small, natural movements typically made during the gait cycle. A change in visual environments can trigger imbalance in the patient with visual dependency. Walking into a darkened room, especially if the surface is uneven (e.g., in a theater where the surface is sloping), can often trigger a fall or stumble. Patients with permanent vestibular loss should be educated about these potentially high-risk environments and taught compensatory strategies to ensure safe mobility. Patients with potentially recoverable vestibular function should be trained to walk with eye and head movements, trunk rotation, and arm swing.

Vestibular contributions to stability during transitions from sit-to-stand, initiation of gait, and abnormal foot placement can be identified during standard tests such as the Timed Up and Go, the Tinetti, and Dynamic Gait Index. Scores are adversely affected when vestibular system functions are diminished. The Functional Gait Assessment has been developed specifically for use in patients with vestibular disorders (see Table 20.1 in Balance chapter).[18]

RECOVERY OF FUNCTION: ADAPTATION VERSUS SUBSTITUTION

During most daily functions, the vestibular system creates little awareness or sensation that it has been activated. When it is stimulated beyond the typical level (e.g., during a fast spin or when a roller coaster suddenly drops), it creates a strong sensation of uneasiness or dizziness. This is often accompanied by nausea, sweating, and feeling out of control. Often the balance system is also affected for a short time, causing an unsteady gait. The dizziness that occurs in the normal individual when the vestibular system is overstimulated can mimic the feeling of dizziness that occurs when the brain encounters sudden changes or losses of input from the vestibular system.

Acute disorders of the vestibular system can cause devastating lack of visual stability, loss of balance, and inaccurate sense of movement. As stated previously, there is an initial loss of trunk and gaze stability with vestibular dysfunction. Central nervous system (CNS) adaptation is critical to recovery of function.[19] During recovery, the visual or somatosensory systems may be used excessively to counteract the loss of information from the vestibular system.

In the patient with an acute unilateral vestibular disorder, the brain identifies this abnormal state, recognizing that the perceived motion from the visual system is not congruent with the feedback provided by the somatosensory system. If there is stable visual input available, the brain will begin to use the stable visual input to assist the CNS recalibration. There is usually adequate central adaptation to stop the spontaneous nystagmus in a lighted environment within 3 days.[20] The spontaneous nystagmus may continue to be active in a dark room, and even for weeks after the insult there may still be a sensation that the head is rotating when the eyes are closed.

CNS adaptation represents the highest level of recovery in the patient with a vestibular dysfunction, and therefore as much adaptation as possible should be facilitated to improve functional outcomes.[21,22] Although some patients with vestibular lesions appear to be well-compensated, they often require increased attention to perform daily activities. This increased demand for attention appears to extend beyond postural control and may be associated with sensory integration resolving multiple sensory signals for spatial orientation.[23] Vestibular adaptation programs should challenge the patient at the limit of his or her ability. Patients often choose to do the easiest exercise and avoid the more difficult exercises if they are not educated about the need to trigger the symptoms. Conversely, if the challenge is too far above the ability of the patient, the CNS will fail to adapt. Comorbid dysfunction can also affect functional recovery, especially if it affects the visual or somatosensory inputs. Disorders that effect the autonomic nervous system can significantly impede recovery. Trauma, either physical or psychological, can cause maladaptive responses that are inconsistent with typical recovery. Conditions such as concussion and persistent postural-perception dizziness (PPPD) are prime examples of this concept and are discussed later in the chapter.[24]

Clinicians are exposed to patients at many different levels of adaptation in clinical settings. It is critical to understand the level of adaptation and potential for recovery for each patient. For example, tests such as video nystagmography (VNG) will identify an existing impairment; the level of physiological adaptation is identified by nystagmus in room light or tests such as the head impulse test. Functional adaptation is determined through activities such as dynamic visual acuity (DVA), loss of balance during gait with head turns, tandem gait, and walk with sudden stops. Dependency patterns are identified by observing the change in status when vision or somatosensation is removed, for example, by using the sensory organization test, namely Clinical Test of Sensory Organization and Balance, or moving platforms. Functional scales (e.g., the Functional Gait Index) can help the knowledgeable clinician identify which impairments may be having the greatest impact on the activity limitation of the patient. Successful intervention is achieved by accurate analysis of both the missing and available components of the system—facilitating adaptation, avoiding excessive sensory substitution, and determining appropriate compensatory strategies when necessary. Home exercise programs must be created to optimize the recovery process while keeping the patient safe. The patient should clearly understand the purpose for each exercise and the progression to higher-level activities. Guided home-based vestibular rehabilitation programs will likely become more widely used with enhanced education and increased adherence.[25]

IMPORTANCE OF TAKING THE HISTORY

The term "dizziness or dysequilibrium" can mean something different to each person who describes the experience. For the therapist, this description is the first opportunity to begin the differential diagnosis to determine the appropriate impairments to focus on during the evaluation process. The onset or circumstance that created the dizziness can give a clue to the cause. In patients with long-term dizziness, it is important to determine the most recent concern, or the reason that brought the patient in for this evaluation. The intensity of symptoms and what makes them better or worse can guide both the evaluation and intervention. A true spin, or vertigo, indicates an asymmetry of neural activity from the vestibular system that occurred rapidly. This most often represents a lesion below the pons or cerebellum, such as vestibular neuritis, or a disruption of blood flow in the basilar or vertebral artery. Lightheadedness can indicate problems with maintaining postural tension of blood pressure, lesions deeper into the CNS that likely involve somatosensation, peripheral somatosensory loss such as diabetic neuropathy, or the inaccurate somatosensory input after whiplash or concussion. When dizziness is accompanied by dysphagia, dysarthria, diplopia, and dysmetria, this can be a red flag for brain stem lesions or those that may involve the cerebellar or cerebral cortex.

Dizziness can be reported as panic, heart palpitations, tingling in the face or hands, or feeling out of touch with the environment. This may be associated with PPPD or may be the phenomenon of posttraumatic stress. Autonomic nervous system dysregulation can cause dizziness that can be orthostasis, exercise induced, and related to other factors such headache and gastrointestinal symptoms. In these cases, the underlying disorder needs to be diagnosed and managed properly as noted later in the chapter.

The temporal course of the symptoms can assist diagnosis. Slow onset of dizziness especially with progressive imbalance can indicate a mass effect, perhaps an acoustic schwannoma or infratentorial meningioma. Determining the timing of the symptoms when there is a sudden onset can determine the cause. When it is described in seconds, one might think first of benign paroxysmal positional vertigo (BPPV), but when it is hours or days, a migraine or Meniere disease is suspected. A report of continuous dizziness with exacerbations will lead toward a diagnosis of possible fistula, perhaps superior canal dehiscence, mal de debarquement, or other causes of inhibited adaptation. Provocation with head motion gives additional clues to the diagnosis. Motion-provoked symptoms may indicate inadequate adaptation. Head position dizziness can be related to BPPV if symptoms are brief, or central dysfunction if symptoms persist. Maladapted patients can describe constant and vague symptoms. Comorbid complaints of hearing loss, tinnitus, and fullness in the ear are indications of conditions that involve the cochlea. These conditions will be described in detail at the end of this chapter.

DETERMINING THE ADAPTATION STATUS THROUGH EXAMINATION THAT GUIDES INTERVENTION

There are many known ways to identify acute vestibular lesions. To determine the level of adaptation using visual cues, look for nystagmus in room light with the patient looking at a stable object. Nystagmus from peripheral vestibular lesions is easily inhibited with visual fixation. Nystagmus caused by central lesions of the brain stem or cerebellum is not inhibited with visual fixation. Blocking visual fixation to look for spontaneous nystagmus is achieved with the use of infrared goggles or Frenzel lenses.

Videonystagmography (VNG) captures eye movements related to vestibular dysfunction using video goggles or electrodes surrounding the orbit (electronystagmography). Oculomotor testing is included in this test to determine the status of saccades and smooth pursuits as well as eye speed and optokinetic response. It is critical to determine the baseline oculomotor functions because, as noted previously, this can be an independent cause of dizziness. Nystagmus patterns are determined to be spontaneous, positional, with head motion, or during the Dix Hallpike positioning. The vestibular component of the VNG is the caloric test, the use of warm and cold air to manipulate the fluid in the horizontal canal to isolate the ear and indicate the relative function on one side compared to the other. Central disorders will produce nystagmus patterns that are different than those related to a peripheral lesion. The caloric portion of this test is reported as a relative percentage of reduced vestibular response in the affected ear.

Vestibular-evoked myogenic potentials (VEMP) is based on the principle that the saccule of the otolith is sensitive to sound and responds in a similar fashion to clicking sounds as it does to tilt. A click produced in the ear stimulates the saccule that in turn inhibits the synchronous discharges of muscles in the SCM on the same side. It is thought that this reflex allowed the head to turn toward the sound of a predator. Abnormal hearing can interfere with the ability to perform the test as will dysfunction in the SCM muscle.

The rate of firing or tone of the SCM is inhibited during the recorded sounds, and this change is captured using surface electromyography (SEMG). Surface electromyography the response in one ear can be compared to the response on the other side in the same person. VEMPs are abnormal when they are very asymmetrical such that one side is more than two times as large as the other, low in amplitude, or absent. An abnormal VEMP can represent an ipsilateral lesion in the saccule, the inferior vestibular nerve, the lateral vestibular nucleus, or the MVST. The inferior component of the vestibular nerve can be preserved in a neuritis, and the VEMP can be normal even with loss of superior innervation of the horizontal canal. Intervention in this case would be determined with enhanced use of head righting and the adaptation of VOR.

Subjective visual vertical (SVV) is used to test the degree of ocular torsion present in unilateral lesions. The SVV is tested in absolute darkness or an environment that prevents visual reference to the vertical. The patient is asked to orient a rod to gravity, and the degree of off-axis tilt represents the torsion of the eye, or skew deviation, which is common in acute unilateral lesions.[26] When looking at skew it is important to realize that the vestibular system skew is a nonparalytic ocular misalignment due to utricle-ocular motor pathway asymmetry. This should not be confused with a paralytic skew that represents a nerve palsy or intranuclear ophthalmoplegia (INO). This can be tested with a Maddox rod, or the Cover-Uncover and Alternate Cover tests can help determine a con-concomitant or nonconcomitant dysfunction. Medullary and medial longitudinal fasciculus lesions need to be ruled out as well when a skew is identified.

Sensation of Motion at Rest

The tonic firing of the vestibular system, when the head is in a neutral nonmoving state, is symmetrical, at approximately 90 spikes per second recorded in the canal and otolithic systems. When there is disruption of signal from only one side of the vestibular pathway, it will change the relative input into the CNS resulting in a perception of the head rotating even if the head is not actually moving.

To determine the degree to which the patient has adapted using somatosensory cues, ask them to sit still on a stable surface with eyes closed. If there is a sensation of motion, the somatosensory system and vestibular system are still out of synch. If the sensation is that of rotation, it is likely that the CNS has not adapted to the unequal signals caused by vestibular system lesion.

Enhanced input through stable joint surfaces can facilitate the CNS recalibration early in the adaptation process. This appears to be most effective through mechanical pressure through the top of the head or as shown in Fig. 21.8 with the use of weights on the shoulders to increase the vertical reference of the spine in a neutral position with vision occluded. In the very acute patient, this may need to be started in the supine position. This allows the vestibular system to calibrate using somatosensory input as a reference. This activity, known as settling, is a good way to allow the patient to manage symptoms when they have been exacerbated by activity. Using the weight or pressure for several minutes at a time can control symptoms. The use of settling is reduced as the system adapts during movement—the final goal of the intervention. If the use of weights increases the sensation of movement with a report of being lightheaded, the clinician should suspect abnormal central sensory weighting of somatosensory inputs. Slow progressive introduction of weights may be necessary to achieve decreased sensation of movement. Closer examination of the musculoskeletal system may be necessary. Joint position sense and neck torsion smooth pursuits should be examined and treated as well. It is a critical first step in the rehabilitation process to achieve accurate CNS recalibration with the head at rest before initiating intervention that requires movement of the head.

Gaze Stability

The ability to hold the eyes fixed on a target while the head is moving is known as gaze stabilization and is a manifestation of the VOR. The gain of an intact VOR is should be equal to one (1:1) as stated previously, which means movement of the eyes is equal to the movement of

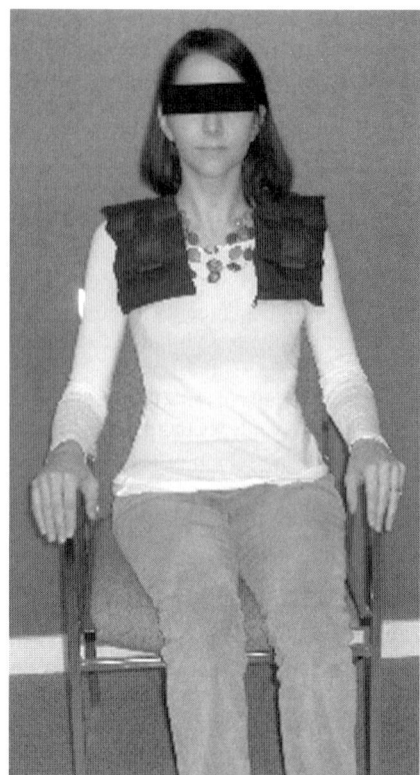

Fig. 21.8 The use of 5-pound weights on each shoulder to increase the somatosensory reference allows the vestibular system to recalibrate to the body reference. Eyes are closed so that the head position is not referenced by vision.

the head.[27] To test the accuracy of the vestibular system gain, the head is rotated and/or moved up and down at a rate of 2 Hz to 4 Hz. This is the rate the head moves during typical daily tasks increasing with sports activity. When an individual is unable to achieve similar clarity of vision at rest and at 2 Hz, you would expect that the VOR is not sufficiently calibrated.[28]

Head Impulse Testing Paradigm

In the presence of vestibular system dysfunction, when the head is passively rotated or tilted while a patient is looking at a fixed target, there are saccadic eye movements required to move the eye back to the target, as the gain falls below the 1:1 ratio. The eye moves in the same direction as the head; hence, a saccade is required to move the eye back in the opposite direction where the target remains. This can be tested manually as the clinician asks the patient to fixate on a target and then grasps the patient's head performing a fast passive horizontal or vertical head thrust, observing the eyes during the thrusts. A normal VOR will allow the patient to maintain the eyes on the target. If there is a refixation saccade, it indicates abnormal gain of the VOR. This refixation saccade can be recorded electronically with a video head impulse test using the head impulse testing paradigm (HIMP) protocol, so that catch-up saccades can be identified and measured. This is an indicator of vestibular loss.

Suppression Head Impulse Testing Paradigm

The suppression of the VOR is a way to identify the remaining function in an individual with partial loss of vestibular function. It is a way to determine the level of adaptation using a quick head turn as indicated in the HIMP, but the target moves with the head so that the VOR must be suppressed. There is a reversal of saccades in this test, with smaller and later saccades in the same direction as the head movement. The parameters for the suppression head impulse testing paradigm (SHIMP) testing can be integrated into video head impulse testing and may be more useful for the therapist to have an idea of the level of function that remains in the vestibular system.[29] This can be especially useful in conditions that cause bilateral vestibular loss but may have sparing of anterior canal function such as ototoxicity and progressive Meniere disease.

Rotary Chair Testing

In this test the patient is rotated in a sitting position while eye movements are measured. It is used to confirm the degree of bilateral loss and determine whether there is adaptation after a unilateral lesion by testing the gain of the system during these full body rotations. Lesions of the central VOR patterns can lead to changes in the gain of rotation-induced nystagmus. Cerebellar dysfunction will result in abnormal amplitudes.

Dynamic Visual Acuity

DVA can be tested with manual head turns using a Snellen chart, with the patient reading the smallest line that is possible when the head is still, then the therapist passively rotates the head at 2 Hz and the patient attempts to read the same line.[30] When acuity drops more than three lines, the patient will be unable to maintain visual acuity during typical daily activity. Quantified DVA can be recorded as the logarithm of minimal angle of resolution (LogMAR). As seen in Fig. 21.9 this can be tested and quantified by use of equipment such as inVision (NeuroCom Int.). Gaze stability also can be quantified using the same equipment, but the measure is one of function, reporting the head speed that can be obtained while maintaining gaze stability. This is a good way to clarify the amount of deceleration that is necessary for the patient to maintain proper vision.

In the clinical examination, the VOR is reported as abnormal only if there is loss of gaze stability that leads to blurring of target object with head movement at 2 Hz to 3 Hz.

If the vestibular ocular reflex is not functioning efficiently and it does not drive the eyes to the correct position for a stable gaze, the result is known as vestibular driven oscillopsia, causing visual targets to appear to move as the head moves. This disorder has significant

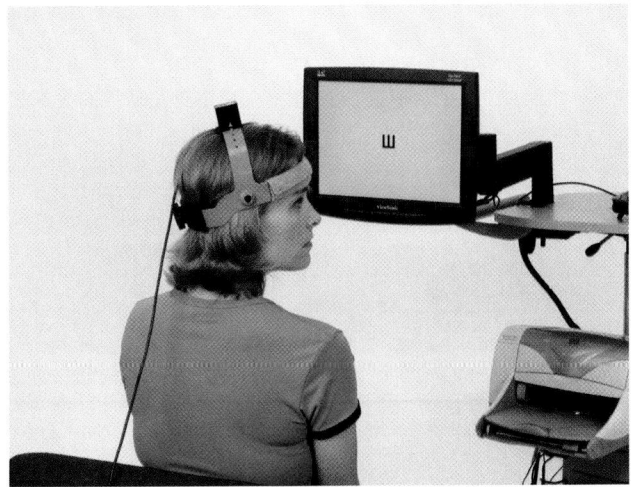

Fig. 21.9 Quantified Dynamic Visual Acuity Is Possible With Systems Such as in Vision. (Courtesy NeuroCom International, Clackamas, OR.)

functional implications: the individual will try to limit the head motions that cause gaze instability, walk with increased base of support to enhance somatosensation, and increase the use of hand holds or use wall walking (touching the wall to stay upright while walking). Gait speeds slow while trunk and head remain locked in relation to each other during turns. This can often be observed during the initial evaluation.

VOR adaptation requires movement of images on the retina, or retinal slip. Therefore intervention begins with head movement at the speed that allows stable vision.[27,31] Adaptation of the VOR is accomplished by having the patient move the head while trying to maintain gaze stabilization, keeping a stationary object in clear focus.[32] As the system adapts, the speed of head movement increases, with the goal of achieving head movement at 2 Hz without the object blurring. Initially, the patient can focus on the thumb or a business card held at arm's length. The activity is progressed to a higher level of difficulty by adding background visual stimulus such as a television set or a visually complex environment. Gaze stabilization with head turns while standing on an uneven surface or while walking creates a higher-level challenge. Many patients have avoided head movement, so simply turning the head may initially trigger dizziness. As stated previously, dizziness with head motion should not be confused with abnormal VOR; in VOR dysfunction, the visual image blurs as the head moves.[28]

Vestibulo-Ocular Reflex Cancelation (VOR Cancel)

VOR cancel reflects the ability to synchronize simultaneous eye and head movements in the same direction; it is associated with the ability of the brain to suppress the VOR. This function allows an individual to track an object while moving the head at the same speed. Testing is reported as normal if the eye can remain in the center of the orbit as the head and eyes track an object as it moves across the visual field. If the central integration capabilities are abnormal, the patient will not be able to override the reflex activity and cannot keep the eye and head moving at the same rate in the same direction. The clinician must also be aware that the peripheral visual field will appear to move in the opposite direction to the head movement during these testing procedures. This normal visual phenomenon can cause dizziness in the patient with visual dependence or visual motion sensitivity.

Head Motion Dizziness

The quality of somatosensation in the spine and muscles of the upper body can contribute to dizziness with head motion. The vestibular nuclei have the job of integrating somatosensory information on its way to the cortex. There must be adequate input from both the somatosensory and vestibular systems to distinguish between head on body or body on head movement. Impaired somatosensation, pain, and guarding of movement will disrupt the accuracy of calibration related to head movement. The patient who has an abnormal VOR will be constantly decelerating his head movement to less than 2 Hz to try to prevent blurred vision. That unconscious deceleration by the muscles in the neck can cause stiffness and decrease the sensitivity of the somatosensory mechanisms in the neck and shoulders. Dizziness with head movement can persist even after the VOR has recalibrated if the somatosensory system continues to send abnormal signals from the muscles of the neck. Most often this is described as a lightheaded sensation rather than the spinning sensation that is associated with vestibular dysfunction.

Abnormalities of head motion related to the quality of somatosensation known as head motion–provoked dizziness can be tested by holding the head upright and still, in gravity-neutral position while the patient rotates back and forth in a chair, known as body rotation under a stable head (BRUSH). This should be done with the eyes closed to eliminate the use of visual cues. The movement may illicit dizziness if the somatosensory system is impaired. If the patient has been relying on somatosensation as a primary reference for head position, there may be co-contraction of the cervical muscles to keep the head aligned to the trunk to provide head position reference. This will feel like resistance to the motion, often reported as neck stiffness. To eliminate the co-contracted pattern this movement should be initiated by teaching a family member to gently hold the head in place while the patient rotates the chair side to side. Using a mirror for feedback about head position while rotating the body in a chair also can be effective but relies on visual cues.

Rotation of 360 degrees in a chair at 1 Hz to 3 Hz allows the head to move at the same speed as the body and isolate the vestibular system response to rotation of the head. This should be done with the eyes closed to eliminate visual feedback. Movement at this speed will cause an increase in dizziness even in a normal system, reflecting the velocity storage mechanism of the vestibular system. In an intact vestibular system, dizziness should resolve in less than 10 seconds once the rotation has stopped. If the dizziness persists for greater than 15 seconds, it represents abnormal vestibular calibration. This can be used as a home exercise to enhance recalibration. The patient sits in a swivel chair, rotating around three times at a speed that is tolerable but increases vertigo, then stops moving, keeping his and her eyes closed, and counts to see how long it takes for the dizziness to stop. Calibration is achieved when the dizziness lasts less than 10 seconds. This can increase normal head motion without dizziness during typical activities and can reduce the fear of increasing symptoms.

Sensory Substitution for Postural Control

When, as noted several times previously, critical information from one system is absent or inaccurate, the CNS will begin to rely more heavily on the other systems for necessary reference. While this is used initially to provide stability during the recalibration process, it can limit adaptation over the course of recovery. Visual or somatosensory dependency patterns develop when the patient persistently makes use of either or both of those systems in preference to vestibular references when the most efficient reference for the environmental condition would be the vestibular system. This can persist as evidence that an individual has not achieved complete adaptation of vestibular function. On testing there was an average of only 50% use of vestibular system weighting (trunk in gravity neutral) resulting in trunk sway in reference to the surface tilt, when tested on a rotating (tilting) surface. Individuals with normal functioning systems showed 100% reliance on gravity by the time the surface made the 6-degree rotation and the individuals showed minimal head and trunk sway following the surface tilt.[7]

Dependency patterns are typically observed in an individual who does not recover satisfactory adaptation and integration of the sensory systems required for normal balance responses in a variety of environmental conditions. Clinically, these substitution patterns often present as hyperreliance on vision or somatosensory cues even when the vestibular system may have adequate potential for recovery.[33,34] When given standard vestibular rehabilitation, these patients often do not recover a full return to activity and are left with activity and participation limitations, or complain of symptoms that have a negative impact on their lives.

Visual Dependency

Patients may experience discomfort when their eyes are closed or may find it impossible to walk down an incline in a visually challenging environment without the need to hold on to a railing. Patients with visual dependency often report excessive fatigue after activity because

of the strain of using vision for postural stability. When these patients are in situations with excessive visual stimulation, reports of dizziness increase. The subtle eye movements associated with viewing a computer monitor cause more fatigue for the individual with vestibular disorder when they display visual dependency. These individuals also often avoid crowds as in a mall, grocery store, or airport. Attending religious services, which are often characterized by low lighting, visual stimulation, and the need to stand with eyes closed or read a hymnal while singing, can create challenges to the vestibular system and can reduce an individual's participation.

Destabilization can occur when the peripheral visual references appear to move as a component of physiological diplopia. When the eyes are tracking something moving in the central gaze field, the background or peripheral visual field will appear to move in the opposite direction. During diagonal smooth pursuit tracking, for example, the patient with visual dependence will orient the head and trunk to the perceived movement in the room creating postural adjustment patterns as if the room is tilting. The patient is pulled off balance when they align themselves with the apparent visual motion. This can also be tested when a patient is standing on a compliant surface or on a single leg, tracking a target moving in a figure of eight. Head and trunk sway match the apparent visual field movement instead of actual gravity vertical in the patient who is visually dependent. This test can be used in a clinical battery to determine degree of visual dependence to compensate for missing the gravity reference. Patients can be taught to perform this and other activities at home to increase the use of the vestibular system function as seen in Fig. 21.10. Tossing a ball in the air and following it with the eyes while standing on a compliant surface, or while walking, will allow for balance without visual fixation as seen in Fig. 21.11.

Walking backwards while tossing the ball increases the challenge. Increased efficiency of vestibular weighting can improve the ability to accomplish activities of daily living and improve balance confidence.[35]

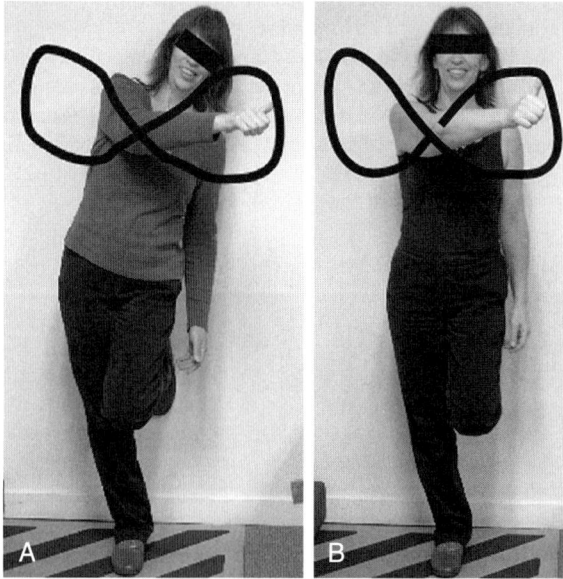

Fig. 21.10 When the visual reference is dominant for the head position, the position of the head changes to match the tilted peripheral visual reference that results from the eye following the thumb in a figure-of-eight. **(A)** The head tilts off-center as the perception of the visual field tilts. **(B)** If the vestibular system is dominant, suppression of the apparent shift in the visual field allows the head to stay in alignment over the base of support. (Courtesy Ray Hedenberg, IRB Solutions, Silverthorne, CO.)

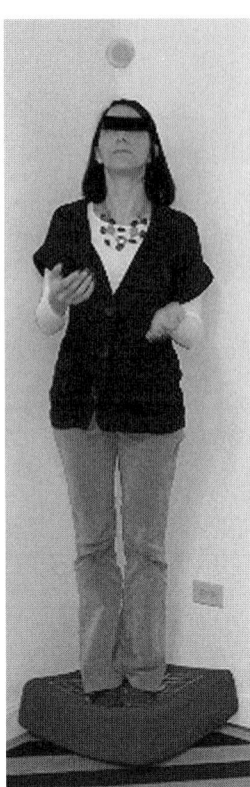

Fig. 21.11 Keeping the gaze directed at the moving ball while standing on a compliant surface eliminates the primary use of visual targets to stabilize the head and is an effective way to shift reference from visual to vestibular. (Courtesy Ray Hedenberg, IRB Solutions, Silverthorne, CO.)

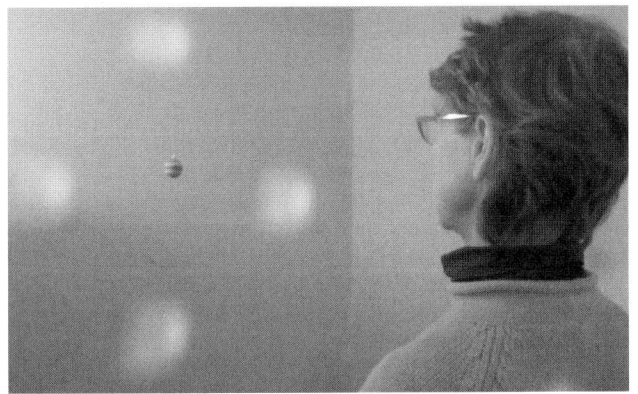

Fig. 21.12 Projecting Peripheral Movement Activates the Optokinetic Response. Individuals with visual dependence for balance, or visual motion hypersensitivity, are not able to adequately achieve gaze stability of the central object or will lose balance as they match head position to the peripheral reference. In the patient with maladapted responses, this stimulus can cause significant nausea and other abnormal autonomic nervous system responses.

Elimination of visual dependence is a therapeutic goal with these patients. The optokinetic stimulus, which provides full field stimulus in a clinical setting as seen in Fig. 21.12, can be used to stimulate the use of vestibular references and decrease the visual dependence that leads to visual hypersensitivities. For the visually sensitive, this can start with the patient sitting and progress to standing on a compliant surface, or walking.

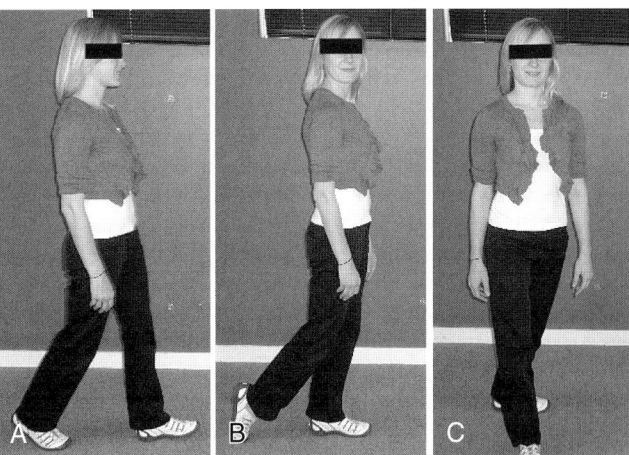

Fig. 21.13 The "Spot Turn" for the Patient With Bilateral Vestibular Loss. (A) When the patient is ready to turn, the front foot is planted to provide somatosensory reference. (B) Once the foot is planted, the head is turned. (C) Visual reference on a nonmoving target is maintained while the body turns under a stable head. (Courtesy Ray Hedenberg, IRB Solutions, Silverthorne, CO.)

Somatosensory Dependency

To increase somatosensory input, patients with a vestibular disorder often put the whole foot down at once to get better input on the position of the body relative to the ground. The normal heel-toe weight progression over the ball of the foot is diminished. The use of touch through the upper extremities increases, especially during turning or reaching. Allowing a patient to touch a stable surface during balance training should be quickly eliminated from intervention to avoid dependence on surface reference when attempting to activate the vestibular system. Walking on uneven surfaces can be a challenge if the patient is primarily reliant on somatosensory input. Balance training on compliant foam, unsteady or perturbed surfaces, with eyes closed will facilitate use of vestibular input. Adding optokinetic stimulus, head turns, and other visual challenges will further facilitate adaptation. Gait training on progressively less-stable surfaces is appropriate for patients who need to reduce dependence on somatosensory cues and improve visual–vestibular interaction. Walking backwards on a treadmill with the trunk gently supported can be a good task to improve balance in gait. Patients often have difficulty reaching the foot backwards as they have become dependent on the foot forward to determine head position. Standing with a ball supported against a corner and reaching one foot backward at a time is a way to work on trunk control for balance.

Permanent bilateral vestibular loss requires the substitution of somatosensation and vision to orient to the environment. A cane or walking stick can increase the use of somatosensation and allow more time to prepare for the next step, thereby increasing confidence in gait. Control of turns can be achieved by the use of double limb support while the head is turning, performing a rapid saccade to find a stable visual target, and then completion of the turn with a fixed gaze on the target as the body turns as shown in Fig. 21.13. This process can become second nature and be performed on a regular basis to increase stability during daily tasks.[36] Driving can be trained in a safe manner by controlling head turns and visual references.[37]

Head-Righting Responses

The otolithic labyrinthine reflex, commonly reported as head righting, is developed early in life. As stated earlier, it provides input to maintain eyes in horizontal and nose vertical by identification of the pull of gravity by the vestibular system. Ocular skew and abnormal subjective visual vertical testing reflect this dysfunction. Another way this phenomenon can be tested is by observing the head-righting response while a patient has his or her vision blocked while sitting on a tilt board. The tilt starts at the pelvis; this should trigger the head-righting response to keep the head in the gravity neutral upright position. In the patient with vestibular dysfunction causing abnormal gravity reference, co-contraction of the neck muscles occurs to lock the head into position with the trunk. The head stays in alignment to the trunk and orients to the surface tilt, which causes imbalance. Because the lateral head-righting response is absent, the patient will often institute a parachute reaction with the arms out to the side to support the trunk. In addition, you will also see an attempt to increase the base of support through the legs and feet. Often there is a startle response activated, which is further evidence of somatosensory responses. This is evidenced in higher-level activities that require gravity reference, such as a tandem walk in visually stimulating environments or with vision occluded. The narrow stance of tandem will limit the contribution of surface reference in the lateral plane, and the patient must take a step out to control the excessive lateral tilt of the trunk and head. Normal and abnormal responses are seen in Fig. 21.14. It is the vestibular inputs that should drive the appropriate lateral head righting and resulting postural strategies that are required in these conditions. Observation of the alignment of the head during a tandem walk or single leg stance is critical in patients with vestibular deficits. Training should always include feedback on head position.

Head turns during balance tasks will decrease the ability to substitute somatosensory input. Activities that require quick changes of position in a superior or inferior direction, such as a lunge or going up and down stairs, can be difficult when the otoliths are damaged. Good program components for otolith stimulation are activities involving up-and-down body movements. Examples include sit-to-stand and seated bouncing on a Swiss ball—with eyes closed to eliminate the use of vision for stability. The use of the hip strategy may be modified or limited in the vestibular-deficient patient because when the head is moving in the opposite direction as the center of gravity (COG), vestibular and somatosensory inputs are not congruent.[38] Standing on a narrow surface such as a 2×4 piece of wood should activate a hip strategy. The clinician can identify functional deficits as the patient locks the ankles at 90 degrees and the entire body tilts forward or backward causing the 2×4 to tilt. Often the patient will avoid using an appropriate stepping strategy as well and falls without recovery. As an exercise this is performed in the corner so that the walls will catch the patient and the patient has room to perform a backward step. In this exercise, a stepping strategy is preferable to reaching out to the wall.

As stated previously, the vestibular system provides a top-down point of reference that the somatosensory system uses to prevent the head and trunk from aligning with surface changes. Perturbations in the form of oscillating surfaces provide a mechanism to activate the gravity receptors, and feedback about the alignment of the trunk to gravity neutral can help to discourage surface dependence when it should not be the dominant reference.[39] Certain positions or movements of the head during upright activities can affect balance even if just one part of the vestibular system has abnormal function. If the otoliths are damaged or hypersensitive, a voluntary lateral tilt of the head when standing with the eyes closed can cause destabilization. Training strategies with head tilts will improve stability.

Central Maladaptation

There can be many conditions that create inadequate sensory reference for the adaptation process to occur. The problem may be that the competent information from the periphery is not processed correctly at the

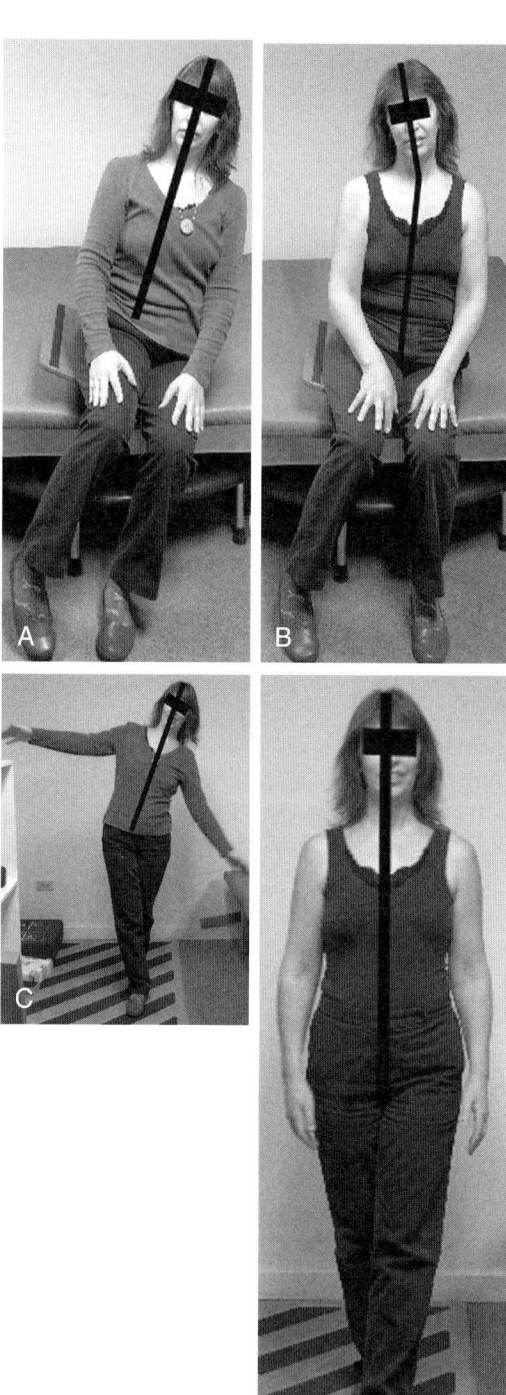

Fig. 21.14 (A) When a surface reference is used in preference to a vestibular cue, the head remains in alignment with the surface. **(B)** As the patient is able to regain vestibular function and gravity reference, the head remains in alignment with gravity, as a head-righting response. **(C)** Lack of head-righting responses can cause excessive use of upper-extremity activity to try to reference to the surface, with bottom-up firing patterns; hip strategy is activated but inefficient. Abnormal reference patterns result in loss of balance in a tandem stance with eyes closed. **(D)** When the vestibular reference is restored, the head remains over the feet, so balance is restored. This is why it is important to observe the angle of the head during examination of a tandem stance or gait. (Courtesy Ray Hedenberg, IRB Solutions, Silverthorne, CO.)

CNS level. The vestibular, visual, and somatosensory systems may test normal, but the individual is not able to use them adequately for functional activity. The peripheral information also can be so disrupted that the CNS is not able to adapt; this can be the case in concussion wherein the visual, somatosensory, and vestibular systems may all be damaged to some degree. When the vestibular information fluctuates, as in the case of Meniere disease, migraine dehiscence, or fistula, the adaptation process cannot stay effective over time. Autonomic nervous system disorders are common contributors to maladaptation. Postural orthostatic tachycardia syndrome (POTS), dysautonomia, and autoimmune ear disease fall into this category and will be discussed later. The mechanisms that underlie chronic pain in terms of sensitization of either the peripheral nervous system or CNS may have a parallel construct to chronic dizziness. This concept is under investigation and may help identify the hypersensitivity to stimulus that is often a part of this disorder.[40,41]

Hypersensitivity patterns can create intolerance of typical environmental conditions that include apparent visual motion, ground vibrations, or conflict between sensory references. As described previously in visual sensitivity, many patients will avoid provoking environments, such as airports or malls, often wear dark glasses when inside, and self-limit their driving. Box 21.3 presents environmental conditions that may drive hypersensitivities.

These patients often report abnormal sensations with the head at rest with eyes closed, such as "flickers, explosions, or racing," which do not reflect vestibular or somatosensory deficits. They will often demonstrate fear or avoidance behaviors during the testing process. Often they will perform better on the tests of balance that are harder to perform, such as eyes closed on foam, especially when distracted by a concurrent mental task. This can be misinterpreted as malingering. Visual motion hypersensitivity during oculomotor testing is common, and excessive startle is often seen during tests of head righting as noted previously.[42]

Visual motion hypersensitivity is a hallmark of PPPD (see later) and other disorders that affect the autonomic nervous system. These patients typically have not been able to return to previous function despite time and therapies, and generally under-perform in life roles. Routine vestibular rehabilitation is usually not successful unless sensitivities are identified early in the intervention process so that the correct referrals can be made.[43] A patient in this category may become identified only when several other treatment regimens fail. Based on the status of normal vestibular testing the patient has often been told that there is nothing wrong and thus the problem is in their heads. Indeed, this category of patient often has an overlapping psychological disorder that should be treated concomitantly.

Anxiety, depression, posttraumatic stress, and a history of physical or verbal abuse are common comorbidities that will affect intervention and outcome. Management of these patients should include focus on self-regulation, which can include referral to someone to assist with the identification and treatment of psychological or psychiatric components. Successful outcomes with interventions are possible; however, the process may take longer because the central modulation of sensory input is compromised, and therefore adaptation will occur in smaller increments.[44] Most types of central dysfunction will negatively affect the recovery rate. Patients with persistent dizziness had significantly more anxiety and depression, which correlated with a higher emotional subscale of the Dizziness Handicap Inventory.[45] The patient with maladaptation will often have more difficulty with relationships and may create more demands on the health care system, families, or caregivers. Activities such as scheduling appointments, attendance for sessions, and compliance with home programs are often compromised and can cause frustration for the clinician. It is critical for the clinician to have a proper understanding of the behavioral aspect of intervention to avoid burnout with these patients. Mindfulness training for both the clinician and the patient can have a positive impact on interventions and follow through.

Head Position Dizziness

Sometimes just changing the position of the head, such as when bending forward or looking up, can cause dizziness. BPPV is the most common form of head position dizziness in adults. The onset is sudden and often severe.

In this condition, otoconia from the utricle floats into the semicircular canal. The canals are designed to respond to fluid movement that accompanies head motion as described previously. Think of the otoconia in the endolymph as steel balls in corn syrup. The otoconia drifts through the fluid in the canal as the head moves into a gravity-dependent position. This causes a drag on the endolymph, which pulls on the cupula, causing excessive deflection of the hair cells. The increased firing of the hair cells creates a sensation of rotation of the head. Fig. 21.14 shows how the falling otoconia activates the cupula. The VOR is stimulated in response to the abnormal message that the head is rotating quickly. The eyes are activated to respond to the perceived movement, and as the VOR is attempting to establish the appropriate gain of the system, there is nystagmus. As soon as the head stops moving, otoconia come to rest at the lowest point in the canal, the pressure on the hair cell is relieved, and the nystagmus subsides. This takes about 20 to 60 seconds. There is no nystagmus until the head is moved into another gravity-dependent position causing the otoconia to roll once again through the canal.[46]

By looking at experimentally induced canalithiasis using the principles of mechanics of the falling otoconia the clinician can identify the nature of the nystagmus, and this can help determine the likely cause. The otoconia will typically fall to the lowest portion of the canal in relationship to the head position. Depending on the exact head position, the otoconia will fall through the center of the canal, creating a strong nystagmus, or it may roll along the wall of the canal, moving slower and causing less drag on the cupula, thereby resulting in a smaller amplitude nystagmus. The timing of the fall, or sedimentation, is dependent on how many of the otoconia have stuck together, which determines the canalith size. A single large canalith will fall faster and create more drag than several smaller canaliths falling at the same time in the canal.[47] Due to the architecture of the canals in relation to the otoliths, the otoconia can appear on either side of the cupula appearing in the short arm or the long arm of the canal. The otoconia will either push or pull the hair cells depending on the head position, and this will determine the nystagmus pattern. Identification of the

---

BOX 21.3 Environmental Conditions That May Cause Visual Motion Hypersensitivities

Grocery stores—cans and boxes appear to be moving backward when one walks down an aisle

Airports with moving sidewalks

Malls with open walkways and glass elevators

Disco lights

Escalators, if the "down" and "up" escalators are side by side

Department stores, especially during holidays or when displays are moving

Large "box" stores where the ceiling is unusually high

Large-format TV and movies, especially IMAX or 3D

Walking outside when the wind blows the tree limbs

Driving in rain or snow with windshield wipers active

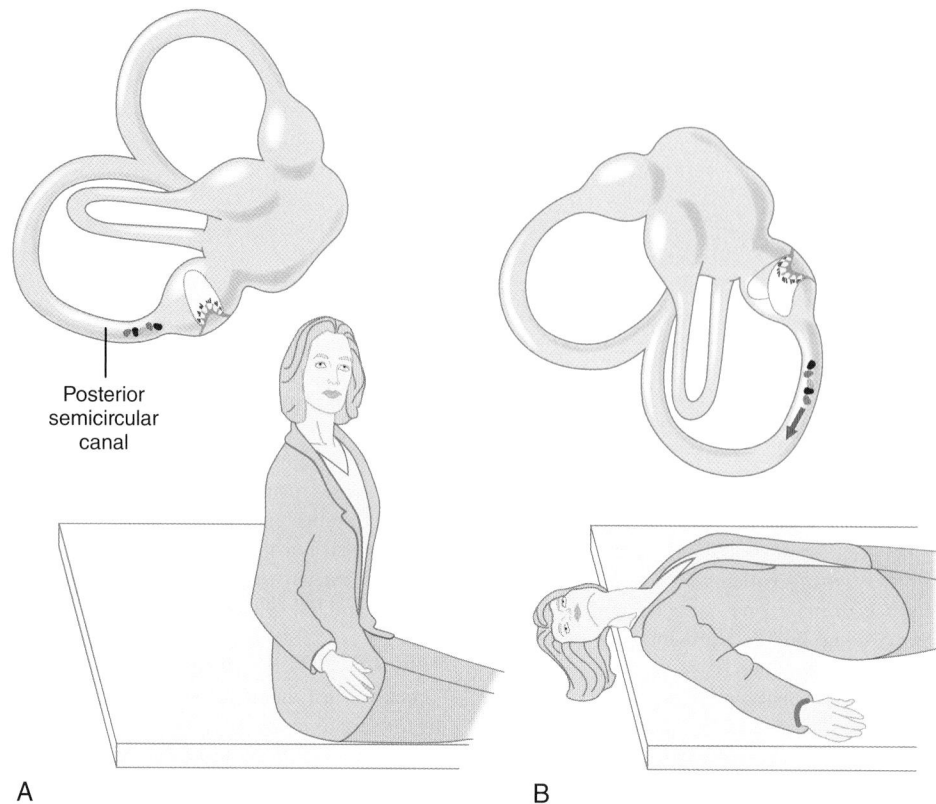

A   B

Posterior
semicircular
canal

Fig. 21.15 **The Hallpike-Dix Maneuver. (A)** Starting position with head rotated toward the side to be tested. **(B)** Lowering the patient's head backward and to the side allows debris in the posterior canal to fall to its lowest position, activating the canal and causing eye movements and vertigo. (From Lundy-Ekman L. *Neuroscience: Fundamentals for Rehabilitation.* 3rd ed. Philadelphia: Saunders; 2007.)

nystagmus pattern with respect to the involved canal is key to determining the appropriate intervention as each canal will create its unique nystagmus pattern.

Cupulolithiasis occurs when the otoconia is adhered to the cupula, which causes a direct pull on the hair cells and is not dependent on the drag of the endolymph. This changes the nature of the nystagmus pattern, with immediate onset and longer duration before there is accommodation to the stimulus. The otoconia can adhere to either side of the cupula, depending on which part of the canal it entered. The nystagmus pattern will reflect the direction of pressure on the cupula and the resulting bend of the kinocilium.

Positional testing is indicated when a patient describes episodic vertigo or other symptoms such as dizziness, nausea, or imbalance.[48]

Vertical Canals

The Dix-Hallpike maneuver is the gold standard test to establish the diagnosis of posterior and anterior BPPV.[49] With posterior or anterior canal BPPV, the patient typically experiences symptoms with bending forward, looking up, and rolling in bed. These movements place the vertical canals in the plane of gravity, causing loose debris (otoconia) to shift and stimulate the cupula.[50]

To perform the Dix Hallpike test, the patient is brought from long sitting to supine position with the head turned 45 degrees to one side and the neck extended 20 degrees. The examiner holds the head in this position for 20 to 30 seconds while monitoring for symptoms of vertigo and observing the eyes for nystagmus.[38] A positive response for posterior canal BPPV is torsional upbeating nystagmus with a latency of 3 to 15 seconds. The intensity of the nystagmus increases

before decreasing until it completely resolves, typically fatiguing in less than 60 seconds.[51]

When the Dix-Hallpike test indicates BPPV, specific and highly effective procedures can be performed in the clinical setting to remediate the disorder.[52] Canalith repositioning is a series of passive movements designed to move the otoconia through the canal and back into the otolith. During the Epley maneuver for posterior or anterior canal BPPV, the patient is first brought down into the extended and rotated position that causes the nystagmus and vertigo (the positive Hallpike-Dix position). The head is held in that position until the symptoms fade completely or for 60 to 90 seconds. The head is maintained in extension and then slowly rotated toward the unaffected side and kept in that position for an additional 1 to 2 minutes to allow movement of the otoconia through the canal. The patient then rolls to side-lying position with the head turned to a 45-degree position relative to the ground and is kept in the position for another 1 to 2 minutes. This position often produces more vertigo and nystagmus as the otoconia continue to move through the canal. The head is then tipped toward the chest, and the patient is assisted into the sitting position. The stages of the Epley maneuver are shown in Fig. 21.16.

An alternate maneuver for posterior canal BPPV is the Semont liberatory maneuver. The patient quickly moves from sitting on the edge of a table to lying on the affected side with the head turned up. This position is held for at least 20 seconds after nystagmus has resolved. The patient then moves quickly through the sitting position to lying on the unaffected side with the head facing up. This nose down position is held for 60 seconds or longer. The patient then moves back

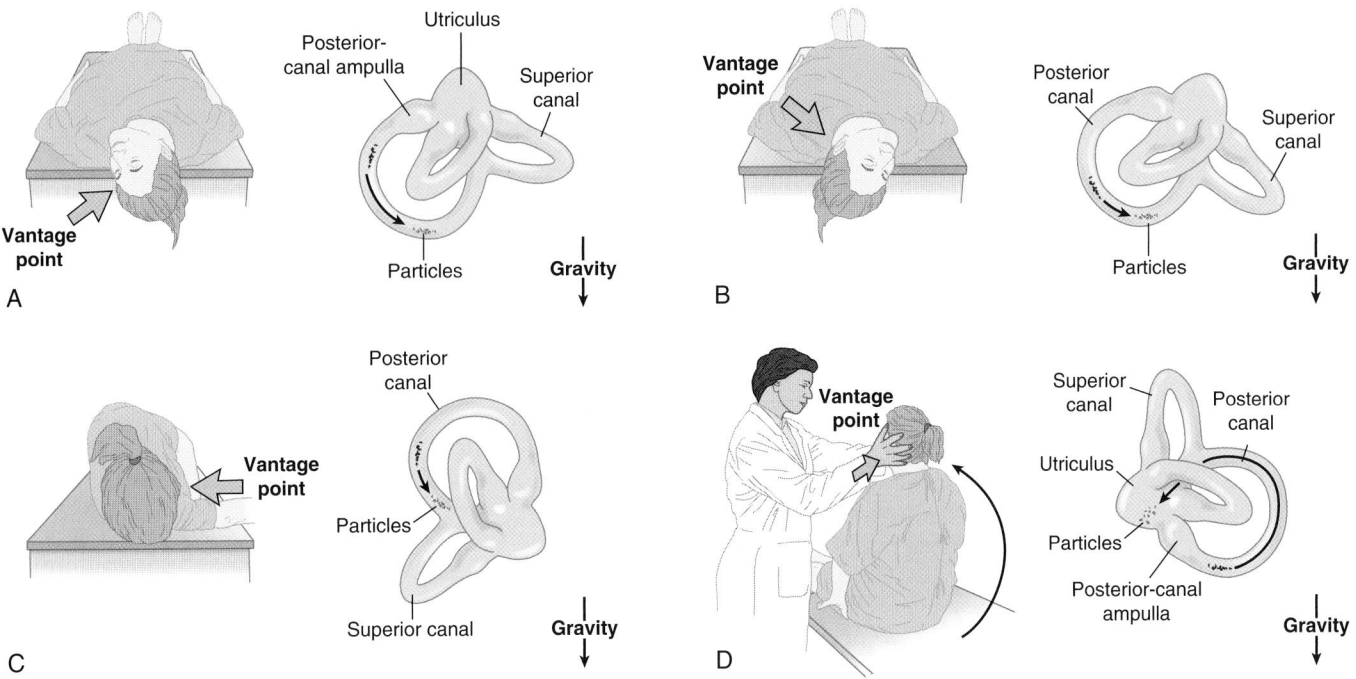

Fig. 21.16 Epley maneuver: Canalith repositioning maneuver for the patient with posterior canal benign positional vertigo (BPPV). The figure represents the procedure for right-side BPPV. The movement of particles through the canal is shown in each position.

to sitting.[53] Some recent clinical recommendations for the Semont maneuver are to maintain an extension angle of head and neck at 110 degrees in the nose up position and 220 degrees in the nose down position. A velocity of 135 degrees per second, which should take 0.66 seconds for the nose up, and 1.33 seconds to move to the nose down position should be achieved during the movement. It is recommended that resting time between movements should be at least 45 seconds. If the patient requires slower movement, there should be more resting time between movements (up to 60 seconds).[54,55]

Horizontal Canals

When otoconia are present within the horizontal canal, the patient will experience vertigo with rolling in either direction, especially when the head is elevated on a pillow, and may have vertigo with bending forward. Horizontal canal BPPV is usually associated with autonomic symptoms such as lightheadedness, nausea, and vomiting. The supine horizontal roll test[51] is the most commonly used test to determine the presence of horizontal canal BPPV. During the roll test, the patient lies in supine with the head held in 30 degrees flexion to keep the horizontal canal perpendicular to the ground. The head is then turned 90 degrees to one side while the eyes are observed for nystagmus. The head is returned to neutral and then rotated 90 degrees to the other side. A positive response is horizontal nystagmus that changes direction when head position is changed (e.g., right beating with the head turned right and left beating with the head turned left) and is stronger on one side than the other. The nystagmus can be either geotrophic or apogeotrophic. In geotrophic horizontal canal BPPV, the more intense nystagmus beats toward the affected ear (toward the ground) when the patient is lying on the affected side. This suggests the otoconia are located in the long or posterior arm of the horizontal canal. In the apogeotrophic type, the more intense nystagmus beats away from the affected ear (away from the ground) when the patient is lying on the affected side.

Apogeotrophic nystagmus indicates the otoconia is adhered to the ampulla on either the utricular or canal side (cupulolithiasis) or is located in the short arm or in the anterior portion of the long arm of the horizontal canal (canalithiasis).

The posterior arm of the canal opens to the otolith, which allows the otoconia to be moved back into place. It is the goal of repositioning maneuvers to shift the otoconia toward the otolith. When the otoconia is in the anterior portion of the horizontal canal, it must be moved into the posterior portion of the canal to be removed from the canal.

Identification of the involved side is critical to treating horizontal canal BPPV. The bow and lean tests can be performed in addition to the horizontal roll test to provided increased certainty about the side of involvement. The bow test is performed by having the patient bend the head forward by 90 to 120 degrees in sitting position, while the lean test is performed by having the patient lean the head backward by 45 to 60 degrees or by having the patient lie supine with the head supported on a pillow.[54] The direction of nystagmus is noted.[56] In geotrophic BPPV, nystagmus will beat toward the affected ear in the bow test and away from the affected ear in the lean test. In apogeotrophic BPPV, the reverse is true with nystagmus beating away from the affected ear in the bow test and toward the affected ear in the lean test.

For horizontal canal BPPV, several canalith repositioning maneuvers are effective. During the barbecue roll, the patient lies in supine, and the head or full body is turned toward the affected ear. The head is then turned away from the affected ear before turning the head down toward the ground. Traditionally, the maneuver was performed by turning the patient a full 360 degrees before returning to sitting with the head tucked. However, some recommend finishing the roll by having the patient sit up from the nose down position. Each position is held for 15 to 30 seconds.[57]

An alternate maneuver for horizontal canal repositioning is the Gufoni maneuver, during which the patient moves from sitting to lying on the unaffected side for 30 seconds. The head is then rotated quickly down 45 to 60 degrees and is held for 1 to 2 minutes. The patient then sits up with the head rotated toward the unaffected side. This moves the otoconia, which is in the posterior portion of the canal, toward the otolith.[58] The Gufoni maneuver is modified for apogeotrophic BPPV to have the patient lying on the affected side. This moves the otoconia from the anterior toward the posterior portion of the canal to gain access to the otolith.[59] A final treatment that can be used in conjunction with the barbecue roll or the Gufoni maneuver is forced prolonged positioning during which the patient lies on the unaffected side (for geotrophic BPPV) or the affected side (for apogeotrophic BPPV) for the entire night. Again, the goal is to move the otoconia to and through the posterior portion of the canal to the otolith.[57]

Traditionally, the patient was instructed to follow specific instructions for 24 hours following canalith repositioning to prevent displacement of the otoconia back into the treated canal.[60] These instructions included sleeping with the head elevated to at least 30 degrees and avoiding head movement.[61] More recent studies suggest there is insufficient evidence to support the recommendation of these restrictions following canalith repositioning for posterior canal BPPV.[62] However, some patients, such as those with frequent reoccurrence of BPPV, may still benefit from these restrictions.

Because BPPV is the most common cause of dizziness and should not require a hospital stay, emergency room personal are being training to identify, rule out other causes, and provide the appropriate repositioning procedures.[63]

When BPPV is not found to be the cause, position-provoked dizziness may alternatively be related to canal sensitivity, a light or heavy cupula (see later), or abnormal firing through the brain stem or cerebellum as described previously. In this case, exercises may be done to increase the patient's tolerance to the provocation. For example, rolling on a bed or spinning in a chair can help the adaptation process when it involves the horizontal canal. In cases of maladaptation creating sensitivity of head position, moving gradually into the position of discomfort while minimizing input from the other sensory systems can be successful. In addition to exercise sessions, incorporating the provoking positions into daily activities is important.

FEEDBACK

Biofeedback is used to improve adaptation to vestibular disorders. Feedback regarding the correct postural responses remains the task of the therapist in the training paradigm. Visual feedback about the head and trunk movement versus total movement on a perturbed surface can provide the patient with knowledge of the abnormal pattern and

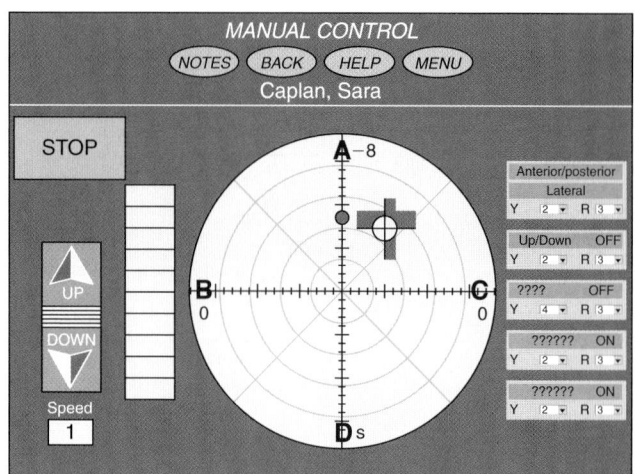

Fig. 21.17 Feedback regarding the position of the trunk in relation to the center of the platform, as well as feedback regarding the amount of trunk flexion, extension, and rotation, can be provided to the patient during the perturbations. The patient can also receive summary feedback after sessions performed with the eyes closed. (Proprio 5000, Perry Dynamics, Decauter, IL.)

give clues of correct postural responses as seen in Fig. 21.17. Feedback has been used to supplement the center of pressure reference for the control of weight shifting using vision to supplement vestibular integration to somatosensory inputs. When visual feedback is provided, it is important to consider the patient's level of visual sensitivity and recognize the need for modified feedback. Audio feedback has been used in the patient with vestibular system loss to provide information about sway when surface and visual reference is lacking. Vibrotactile feedback using accelerometer or gyroscopic information can assist the alignment of body position and movement. This has been successful on many levels, and the modes of input are becoming less intrusive to those who wear them.

ACKNOWLEDGMENT

Chelsea Van Zytveld assisted in this chapter with a focus on head position dizziness. Thanks to Leslie Allison for years of working on the integration of the vestibular system into the larger concepts of balance and function. It has been wonderful to work with Rolando Lazaro who is bringing forward the wisdom and wonder that Darcy Umphred shared with all of us over the years. Thanks to my many patients who have taught me the importance of knowing how to help.

CASE STUDY 21.1   Mr. Hu

At the initial visit, Mr. Hu reported dizziness that started approximately 12 years ago with vertigo that woke him up in the night. He was unable to get out of bed for 2 days following that episode. He reported that this has happened about four times in the past 10 years, with the most recent episode about 5 years ago. He reported that his balance has not felt normal for years. His vestibular testing (VNG) showed a 48% reduced vestibular response on his right side with a suspected viral etiology. He scored 50/100 on the Dizziness Handicap Inventory (moderate impairment). He had difficulty at work at the botanical gardens with both visual discomfort and pain when lifting. He had difficulty when he had to walk across the gardens.

He reported a comorbidity of neck pain with radiation to the hand, which has been progressive. His orthopedic surgeon has recommended surgery.

Patient's reported problem list:

1. Head motion provoked dizziness primarily with horizontal head turns and when looking up.
2. Visual motion hypersensitivity creating dizziness and discomfort with computers, fluorescent lights, loud and crowded restaurants, and similar environments.
3. Increased anxiety.
4. Hyperventilation with exertion.

CASE STUDY 21.1   Mr. Hu—cont'd

Examination Highlights

- Sensation of motion at rest with eyes closed reported as a tilting sensation. Increased sense of being lightheaded with 5-pound weights on shoulders.
- Normal oculomotor exam. Visual motion hypersensitivity with oculomotor testing.
- Vestibulo-ocular reflex testing normal with one line drop on dynamic visual acuity. Dizziness reported during testing.
- Increased dizziness with body rotation under stable head. Excessive stiffness and guarding of his cervical paraspinals.
- Head on body orientation during sitting side tilts, inefficient head righting, strong startle and parachute responses.
- Positive smooth pursuit neck torsion test on right.
- Increased sway during standing with eyes closed on firm surface. Increased sway but no loss of balance on foam. Loss of balance on foam with eyes closed head turns.
- Excessive sway with evidence of strong visual dependence and surface reference during standing perturbations.
- Positive Dix Hallpike test with torsional up-beating nystagmus about 20 seconds duration, indicating probable right posterior canal BPPV.

Progression of Intervention in First Month

The Epley maneuver was performed 2× with the resolution of nystagmus. This remained resolved in subsequent visits, so a balance program was initiated. This started with work to integrate the somatosensory system and vestibular with eyes closed. He was given 2-pound weights to put on his shoulders when sitting with his eyes closed. He was given sequential numbering activities to perform during sitting with weights, which was progressed to 5 pounds. Standing activities began with weights on shoulders, eyes closed. Small fast perturbations were initiated with eyes closed to facilitate the use of somatosensation for balance. Slower deeper tilts were used with eyes closed to facilitate vestibular response. Feedback was provided to maintain the trunk in a gravity neutral position. The cervical spine was addressed with soft tissue work to decrease stiffness along with the use of laser light and targets to improve the efficiency of kinesthesia in the neck. Sitting tilts were performed to activate normal head righting starting with manual feedback for the gravity neutral head position.

Progression of Intervention

In the following months, Mr. Hu was able report no sensation of tilt with eyes closed with 5-pound weights on each shoulder; however, he had increased anxiety when his eyes were closed. He showed improved head righting and could stand on perturbed surfaces during both fast and slow speed, but again had increased guard when his eyes were closed. His exercises were progressed to stand on a single leg with eyes closed and with visual pursuits. He stood on foam tracking a ball toss and would do this while walking as well. He worked to activate hip and stepping strategies while standing on a 2×4. His balance was improved in testing. Functional gait assessment improved from 20/30 to 28/30. Improvements were seen in walking with head turn and tilt, tandem gait, backward walking, step over obstacle, and stair climbing. He was given optokinetic stimulus in the clinic while standing on both a firm surface and on foam with follow-up computerized optokinetic flow exercises performed at home, which he had downloaded from various internet sites.

His kinesthesia continued to be abnormal, and it was felt that this was associated with the extensive pain and movement disorder related to his cervical spine.

Of concern, he continued to complain of the same vague dizziness that had plagued him for years, and with further questioning, he reported that this would fluctuate daily and persisted despite his improved balance. He continued to experience hyperventilation with exertion. His neck surgery was approaching, and he was reporting increasing anxiety and dizziness. During the session that was designed to begin to work on self-regulation through modulation of the autonomic nervous system, he became extremely fearful and agitated when asked to lie quietly in a dark room and begin controlled breathing. During this session, he reported that his father, who was in his home country, has Alzheimer disease and was doing poorly. His father had also had episodes of dizziness during his lifetime, and the patient had connected his own experience of dizziness to the probable onset of Alzheimer disease. This was likely related to his high levels of anxiety surrounding the dizziness. His orthopedic surgeon told him that his dizziness might be worse during recovery, so Mr. Hu wanted to postpone the surgery.

The patient was educated to gain the understanding that his father may have also been having bouts of BPPV or other vestibular events in his life, but this was not the direct cause of his Alzheimer disease. Imbalance is a part of Alzheimer disease, but it is not the primary precursor. As the patient began to understand this his agitation decreased.

In the weeks before surgery, his sessions were devoted to continued work on self-regulation and control of his ANS response. He was able to participate in the sessions without fear and was referred to a physical therapist dual trained as a psychotherapist as well, who specializes in trauma work.

His cervical spine surgery was performed as scheduled. The rehabilitation for that surgery was incorporated into continued work with kinesthesia, progressing to performing during both sitting and standing perturbations. As his cervical kinesthesia improved, he was able to tolerate increasing optokinetic challenges. With significantly increased tolerance to required activities, he was able to return to workand the.

It has been 3 years since this patient's initial visit. He has had occasional return of BPPV and will have increased dizziness when he is over stressed. He continues to work on improvement of cervical function with integration of balance tasks. He benefits from clinical intervention when he has episodes of head position dizziness. His anxiety will increase when he is dizzy but is not disabling as it had been in the past. He reports that he will be forever grateful for the understanding of his problem within this context and feels like he "got his life back."

Summary

This case highlights the need to understand how a vestibular event can trigger PPPD and the need for comprehensive history taking. Although the BPPV brought him into therapy at this time, the reduced vestibular response was likely related to the report of dizziness that occurred 12 years ago. He did not have full adaptation without therapy at that time, which led to anxiety and persistent symptoms. Intervention targeted to the ANS can have a positive impact. In the patient with maladapted sensory system integration, the visual, somatosensory, and vestibular systems should be modulated throughout the program. Improvement in one area often leads to increased capacity for other sensory systems to integrate. Research may someday uncover a link to the vestibular system and dementia, as noted earlier in this text. At the same time, there may be more options for intervention and prevention.

Common Vestibular Disorders

BENIGN PAROXYSMAL POSITIONAL VERTIGO

This is the most common cause for head position dizziness with vertigo as its primary symptom. It is a common sequela of concussion, viral labyrinthitis, hydrops, and vascular occlusion in the distribution that feeds the inner ear. The mechanism and intervention of benign paroxysmal positional vertigo (BPPV) are described in the *Head Position Dizziness* section. Any of the six semicircular canals can collect the loose otoconia. The posterior canal is most common because of its relationship to the otoliths when the person is in the recumbent position. The horizontal canal, while less common, can have more intense symptoms. This dizziness seems more persistent and more easily triggered with the typical head movements of daily life.

Despite the use of the term *benign,* the symptoms related to positional vertigo are intense and can cause significant disability. There is often a strong sense of falling or spinning out of control, even when the individual is lying on a bed. Before the individual is aware of the mechanism, the symptoms seem uncontrollable and the person will avoid head movement. Spontaneous remissions are common, and many current patients will describe an earlier episode that resolved without intervention. Recurrent episodes may reflect an underlying disorder such as hydrops or migraine-induced ischemia. Infections or inflammations may occur months or years before the onset; it is believed that the otoconia may loosen as the nerve degenerates. Adverse life events are reported to trigger an episode, especially in those individuals with an underlying disorder.[61] It is critical to rule out other conditions that can cause head position dizziness. (Common causes are described in Box 21.4.)

> ### BOX 21.4 Alternative Causes of Head Position Dizziness and Nature of Dizziness
>
> *Unilateral vestibular dysfunction:* Dizziness when changing head position while supine
> *Vestibular migraine:* Episodic dizziness that can usually be related to specific triggers
> *Cerebellar nodulus:* Nystagmus is downbeat without torsion, fatigue, or habituation
> *Vertebral artery compression:* Nystagmus with extreme rotation or extension of neck
> *Central vestibular pathways:* Nystagmus without dizziness, usually unidirectional
> *Geriatric supine nystagmus:* Vertical nystagmus when supine
> *Perilymph fistula:* Episodic dizziness after trauma increases with Valsalva or head hanging
> *Superior canal dehiscence:* Dizziness with loud noises or change of head position
> *Hypermobile stapes:* Unstable at oval window; allows fluid pressure changes that cause dizziness with head positions
> *Head extension:* Otoliths outside of functional range, causing dizziness
> *Orthostatic intolerance:* Dizziness when bending or quickly standing from sitting; never when lying

There is often some imbalance reported that may take some time to improve after the dizziness has resolved. Evaluation of underlying vestibular function and sensory integration should be done for patients with BPPV.

INFECTION

Acute unilateral vestibulopathy affects the vestibular nerve directly or associated with the labyrinths. Most often the infection is viral in nature and is known as neuronitis or neuritis. It can also be due to bacterial infection from a variety of causes, either as a primary infection or secondary to bacterial meningitis or encephalitis. Vestibular neuritis can be partial, affecting the superior afferents from the horizontal and anterior semicircular canals primarily along with the utricle. This can leave the saccule function intact so that the head motion concerns are greater than the imbalance.

The infection often is preceded by a systemic illness or an upper respiratory tract infection, but it can be an isolated infection affecting the nerve or labyrinths. Initial impairment may include ocular tilt, skew deviation, or lateropulsion as described previously. Recovery reflects central adaptation to loss of input on one side of the vestibular system. Herpes virus infection can result in a condition known as Ramsay Hunt syndrome. It is often seen along with unilateral facial weakness as the facial nerve is also affected by the infection. The patient is usually treated with antiviral medications. In Ramsey Hunt syndrome, the symptoms follow the typical pattern of acute vestibular and hearing loss, but these are not as profound as the facial weakness.

The adaptation mechanisms described previously are typically successful. In patients with less than a 40% loss, adaptation is achieved with typical vestibular rehabilitation strategies to facilitate adaptation. When there is 40% to 70% unilateral loss, the adaptation will take longer, and it is more likely that dependency patterns will develop, so the clinician should look for these patterns and isolate challenges to the vestibular system to avoid dependency. When the loss is greater than 70% and the nerve does not heal, the patient may have a much harder time with the adaptation process and may need to be trained on substitution strategies. Even a moderate vestibular loss can trigger symptoms of hypersensitivity when the adaptation process is prolonged or incomplete.

ENDOLYMPHATIC HYDROPS

Increased fluid pressure within the labyrinth, known broadly as hydrops, will cause vertigo. The increased size of the endolymphatic cavity can be imaged with magnetic resonance imaging (MRI).[64] The pressure may increase within the canal because the fluid cannot move out of the system through the endolymphatic sac, which normally provides drainage of excess fluid. This is usually a unilateral problem. As the fluid pressure increases on the cupula, the hair cells are activated as if there was quick head movement and results in the sensation of spinning with the vestibulo-ocular reflex activated.

Ménière disease is a type of hydrops that occurs intermittently with spontaneous vertigo. There is often concurrent low-frequency loss of hearing related to the fluid pressure in the cochlea. The episode can last from just a few minutes to a day but is usually between 2 and 4 hours in duration. A low-salt diet is usually the first line of defense. The use of diuretics can control the fluid changes and decrease the number and intensity of symptoms. In some cases, steroid injections are administered.

In the early course the person has normal balance and hearing when not in an episode. However, there appears to be a gradual degradation of the vestibular system over time, resulting in symptoms associated with chronic unilateral vestibular loss associated with progressive hearing loss. These patients often have a diffuse dizziness and complain of imbalance between episodes. Intervention is targeted at the adaptation of the abnormal vestibular responses, and this can improve symptoms, although it cannot remedy the disease itself. Tinnitus[65] may persist beyond hearing loss, and often this is one of the biggest complaints. If episodes persist, a Minette device can be helpful, or the ear function can be ablated via gentamicin injections or shunt surgeries.[66] Box 21.5 gives the criteria for the diagnosis of Ménière disease.

Traumatic hydrops can be the result of a blow to the head during a fall or a whiplash injury. The mechanism is not fully understood, but it may be related to damage of the endolymphatic sac during the trauma, resulting in inflammation or scarring that limits the regulation of fluid in the sac. Patients often appear drunk during an episode; therefore they may limit social interactions or driving for fear of an attack. Drop attacks can develop over time, and in some individuals an attack can include the "crisis of Tumarkin," resulting in feeling as if they are thrown to the ground without a sensation of dizziness. Intratympanic gentamicin can be used to manage the drop attacks.[67] However, there is a sudden unilateral vestibular loss associated with gentamicin. Progressive introduction of gentamicin can be considered along with prehab for those who are appropriate for the procedure but do not want to experience the severe symptoms of sudden loss of function.[68]

PERILYMPH FISTULA

Fistula, or an abnormal communication of the inner and middle ear, can occur at the round or oval windows. This may be related to congenital temporal bone deformity or trauma through the middle ear by surgery, blasts, head injury, or even sneezing. The Valsalva maneuver or tragal pressure can trigger an intense sensation of dizziness and cause abnormal lateral weight shift because of the increased pressure in the system. Loud sounds can trigger the same responses and is described as the Tulio phenomenon. Daily activity can produce an almost persistent sense of dizziness that is relieved by recumbent positions with minimal head movement. Typical vestibular testing is nondiagnostic,

but the use of pressure in the ear may assist this diagnosis. Vestibular rehabilitation for adaptation fails because the system has a persistent fluctuating nature. Successful surgical repair of the fistula produces the stability needed to resume rehabilitation efforts.

SUPERIOR SEMICIRCULAR CANAL DEHISCENCE SYNDROME

Dehiscence or thinning of the bone overlying the superior (anterior) semicircular canal creates a "third mobile window," and the effect of change in pressure of the canals appears to mimic the fistula. Loud noise or pressure can cause disequilibrium, vertigo, and oscillopsia. Surgical repair usually produces good results.

VESTIBULAR MIGRAINE

The aura or even the primary symptom of migraine may be dizziness. Diagnosis of vestibular variant of migraine is based on the episodic nature with the specific reports of one or more of the following: spontaneous vertigo, visual motion hypersensitivity, sensation of disrupted spatial orientation, head motion dizziness often with nausea, and occasional head position dizziness without evidence of BPPV. Recognition of triggers, history of migraine, and combination of dizziness with the other typical prodromes of migraine, including photophobia, nausea, and vestibulo-cochlear symptoms of tinnitus as well as sensitivity to sound can help identify migraine.[68] Symptoms are moderate or severe intensity. Duration of acute episodes is limited to a window of between 5 minutes and 72 hours.[69] Younger to middle-aged females are affected the most, often with a history of motion sickness or a family history of migraine.[70–72] Box 21.6 describes the criteria to determine vestibular migraine.

BOX 21.6 Vestibular Symptoms Associated With Vestibular Migraine as Defined by the Barany Society's Classification

A. At least five episodes with vestibular symptoms of moderate or severe intensity lasting 5 min to 72 h
B. Current or previous history of migraine with or without aura according to the International Classification of Headache Disorders (ICHD)
C. One or more migraine features with at least 50% of the vestibular episodes
  - headache with at least two of the following characteristics: one sided location, pulsating quality, moderate or severe pain intensity, aggravation by routine physical activity
  - visual aura
  - photophobia (visually induced vertigo, triggered by a complex or large moving visual stimulus)
  - phonophobia
  - spontaneous vertigo including:
    - internal vertigo or a false sensation of self movement
    - external vertigo, a false sensation that the visual surround is spinning or flowing
  - positional vertigo, occurring after a change of head position
  - head motion induced vertigo, occurring during head motion (can be accompanied by nausea)
D. Not better accounted for by another vestibular or ICHD diagnosis

Modified from Lempert T, Olesen J, Furman J, et al. Vestibular migraine: diagnostic criteria consensus document of the Barany society and the International Headache Society. *J Vestib Res.* 2012;22:167–172.

BOX 21.5 Definite Ménière Disease

A. Two or more spontaneous episodes of vertigo, each lasting 20 min to 12 h
B. Audiometrically documented low to medium frequency hearing loss in the affected ear on at least one occasion before, during, or after one of the episodes of vertigo
C. Fluctuating aural symptoms (hearing, tinnitus, or fullness) in the affected ear
D. Not better accounted for by another vestibular diagnosis

Diagnosis criteria from the International Classification of Vestibular Disorders

BOX 21.7 Factors to Consider for Return to Play and Learn, Which May Represent Vestibular Involvement

1. Report of sensation of motion at rest with vision occluded
2. Abnormal oculomotor findings
3. Visual dependence or visual motion hypersensitivity
4. Somatosensory dependence or hypersensitivity
5. Head-motion-provoked dizziness
6. Loss of gaze stability with head motion
7. Abnormal smooth pursuit neck torsion test
8. Headache and/or neck pain
9. Abnormal head-righting response
10. Abnormal exertion test and excessive fatigue

The pathophysiology follows that of migraine headache in which there are multiple levels of dysfunction from gene defects that drive familial autosomal disorders and an inherited migraine threshold, brain stem activity that can trigger vascular responses of dilation or restriction, serotonin platelet activity, and spreading neuronal depression. Afferent vestibular and pain information in pre-parabrachial and pre-thalamic pathways have consequences on cortical mechanisms influencing perception, interoception, and affect. There are remarkable parallel neurochemical phenotypes for the inner ear and trigeminal ganglion cells, and these afferent channels appear to converge in shared central pathways for vestibular and nociceptive information processing. These pathways share the expression of receptors targeted by anti-migraine drugs[73] It can be difficult to distinguish vestibular migraine (VM) from Ménière disease in its early stages. VEMPs may provide a way to help discriminate between these two vestibular disorders.[74,75] The criteria to determine VM is described in Box 21.7.

Patients with vestibular migraines have increased anxiety compared to migraines without vertigo.[76,77] The autonomic nervous system plays a major role in all migraines and can be related to dysregulation in the activity of the parasympathetic–sympathetic branches. Interventions targeting control of the autonomic nervous system (ANS) through mindfulness meditation can help normalize related phenomenon such as heart rate variablility.[78]

Rehabilitation is indicated when avoidance of activity has changed the sensory integration, or when multiple episodes have influenced the system toward dependency or hypersensitivity patterns.[79] Visual sensitivity can be addressed in the patient with vestibular migraine, but the exposure must be introduced slowly and for brief episodes.

VASCULAR DISORDERS

Ischemia or bleeds in the areas of the vestibular system (brain stem, cerebellum, parietal-insular cortex) can cause dizziness and imbalance. The anterior inferior cerebellar artery feeds the peripheral vestibular system and the lower two-thirds of the pons and the ventrolateral cerebellum. The posterior inferior cerebellar artery feeds the dorsolateral medulla and posterior inferior cerebellum. Vertebral basilar artery insufficiency syndrome and lateral medullary syndrome (Wallenberg syndrome) present with dizziness and nystagmus, but will have associated brain stem findings. Ischemia is usually seen in individuals older than 50 years, but it can also be associated with bleeding disorders such as leukemia. Bleeds near the brain stem can be seen in younger individuals associated with recreational drug use. Migraine headache can cause intermittent dizziness from the compromise of blood flow in the

areas of the vestibular system. See chapters on cerebellar disorders and hemiplegia. Identification of direction changing gaze evoked nystagmus and presence of skew deviation can be used to assist early diagnosis of stroke. Oculomotor findings are used to assist in diagnosis.[80]

NEOPLASIA

This can compromise vestibular function when it occurs near any part of the vestibular system. Vestibular schwannoma (commonly, but mistakenly, known as acoustic neuroma) can cause damage as it slowly grows on the sheath of the vestibular nerve. Because the tumor grows slowly, the system may have adapted to the gradual compression of the nerve so dizziness is not the primary complaint. Hearing loss is the most typical phenomenon, and sometimes when it is excised, the patient will develop dizziness and imbalance due to acute swelling around the tumor, or damage inflicted by surgical techniques. The schwannoma can grow into the pontocerebellar angle and cause symptoms typically associated with cerebellar lesions. Meningiomas (encapsulated tumors found most often deep in the brain) growing near the temporal lobe can cause pressure on the vestibular mechanism.

OTOTOXICITY

Aminoglycosides and antibiotics used in cases of massive or systemic infection can be ototoxic (causing damage to the vestibular hair cells). Although a small percentage of users experience this adverse effect, it can affect both sides of the bilateral vestibular apparatus and cause significant disability. Often the patient does not begin to experience the symptoms until the medication has been used for more than a week.

TRAUMATIC BRAIN INJURY AND CONCUSSION

A brain injury, either considered moderate/severe or mild (concussion), can affect the vestibular system in several ways. It can cause direct damage to the vestibular end organ (in the temporal bone), cause BPPV, and, in many cases, disruption of the integration of the vestibular nuclei (in the brain stem) and cerebellum. Comorbid visual dysfunction often results from damage to brain stem areas such as the pontine gaze centers or central damage in the medial longitudinal fasciculus, or from direct damage to the third, fourth, or sixth cranial nerves. The oculomotor system should be carefully examined for efficiency of saccades, pursuits, and convergence. Initial training of oculomotor function should start with minimal background visual stimulus. If the oculomotor system is functioning normally, but the testing makes the patient dizzy, interventions to reduce visual sensitivity should be initiated.[81]

Recognition of the connections between the cervical spine and eye movement is also critical in the early stages of recovery. Excessive co-contraction in the neck and upper back may represent disrupted signals between the eye muscles and the cervical musculature. Neck torsion smooth pursuits should be tested when there is dizziness and neck pain. If the VSR is not providing appropriate signals to the cervical musculature, the small intrinsic cervical muscles that fire in response may be overpowered by the extrinsic stabilizers of the neck and shoulders. Often overactivity is noted in the sternocleidomastoid, levator scapulae, and upper trapezius. This will affect the ability to perform head-righting tasks and can lead to tension-type headaches. This is further explained in the Cervical Spine Function and Dysfunction in Chapter 23. Excessive surface reference during balance and gait can lead to lack of confidence in mobility and increase energy costs.[82]

The autonomic nervous system function is negatively affected post brain injury and may represent the prolonged recovery and symptoms that interfere with daily tasks. Conditions related to ANS dysfunction are prevalent post traumatic brain injury (TBI; see below in Autonomic Nervous System Dysregulation) and may lead to postconcussive symptoms of anxiety and depression. Preexisting issues may be exacerbated after TBI and should be evaluated and addressed concurrently by a professional who is familiar with brain injury.[83]

These multiple impairments are responsible for the central maladaptation pattern seen in brain injury that leads to hypersensitivities and avoidance of environmental stimulus. Intervention should be directed toward physiological function and symptom control. Increased recovery times may be related to the lack of precision in the examination and poor choice of interventions. Traditional vestibular rehabilitation that depends on intact visual and somatosensory integration for adaptation has limited success for the individual with brain injury. As new understanding of the factors related to maladaptation arise, there will likely be a way to achieve better outcomes in rehabilitation.[84,85]

Box 21.7 describes the basic criteria to consider during return to play decisions. (See Chapter 23 for more information on the vestibular system testing and vestibular rehabilitation for the concussed individual.)[86]

METABOLIC DISORDERS

Vertigo and dizziness are often reported with metabolic disorders such as diabetes. Autoimmune diseases such as rheumatoid arthritis, lupus, and human immunodeficiency syndrome infection can also cause symptoms when the disease process damages components of the vestibular system. Management of the underlying disorder is essential to create as much stability in the system as possible for adaptation to occur.

AUTOIMMUNE EAR DISEASE

Autoimmune ear disease (AIED) appears most commonly in females between 20 and 50 years of age. A rapidly progressive, often fluctuating, bilateral sensorineural hearing loss (SNHL) occurs over a period of weeks to months. The progression of hearing loss is often too rapid to be diagnosed as presbycusis and too slow to conclude a diagnosis of sudden SNHL and is likely to be bilateral. Imbalance, ataxia, motion intolerance, and episodic vertigo are often present. Systemic autoimmune diseases coexist in about one-third of patients such as systemic lupus erythematosus, rheumatoid arthritis, Sjögren syndrome, myasthenia gravis, Hashimoto disease, Cogan syndrome, sarcoidosis, colitis, and polychondritis. There is strong evidence that immune mechanisms are involved in the pathogenesis of inner ear damage, together with viral infection, trauma, vascular damage, and genetic factors. Steroid responsiveness is high, and with prompt treatment hearing loss may be reversible.[87]

AUTONOMIC NERVOUS SYSTEM DYSREGULATION

Dizziness, vertigo, nausea, and instability can be attributed to dysautonomia. A larger constellation of symptoms is often present, and symptoms are typically elicited in orthostatic postures, during exertion or postprandial. Additional signs of dysautonomia may be orthostatic intolerance, POTS, presyncope or syncope, headaches, fatigue, lightheadedness, tremulousness, blurry vision, reduced mental clarity, changes in bowel and bladder function, gastrointestinal motility issues, altered sleep, and body temperature dysregulation. Diagnostic testing

for assessment of the ANS function includes multiple studies as there are many subtypes of dysautonomia that fall along a spectrum of severity, some of which involve hereditary disorders, autoimmune diseases, and metabolic disorders.[88] Adrenergic function is examined through heart rate and blood pressure responses during passive head-up tilt table testing (TTT) and Valsalva maneuver studies as well as variation in plasma norepinephrine measures in supine and standing positions. Sudomotor function testing involves a combined quantitative sudomotor axon reflex test (QSART) and thermoregulatory sweat test (TST), and cardiovagal response is evaluated by heart rate variability (HRV) during deep breathing and Valsalva maneuver studies.

Increased evidence has steadily emerged regarding the involvement of peripheral and central vestibular pathways in ANS regulation[89] when hemostasis is disrupted by viral, infectious, allergic and immunological, or traumatic stressors. Vestibular contributions exist throughout the afferent and efferent pathways from the brain stem to the thalamus and include neurotransmitters and antibody receptors that influence orthostatic tolerance and blood pressure modulation.[90] Improved functional mapping of the central vestibular system and specific vestibular and ANS testing promote obtaining a differential diagnosis for what historically involved complex management of a very broad and evasive symptoms of dizziness.[91] For example, in a prospective study of patients with chronic dizziness lasting longer than 6 months, a significant number of participants who tested positively for the presence of dysautonomia also demonstrated alterations in smooth pursuits and otolithic function testing.[92] Additionally, a lesser portion of subjects classified as having vestibular migraine, psychogenic dizziness, or unspecified chronic dizziness had abnormal findings on sympathetic and cardiovagal autonomic function testing. Larger volumes of research have been conducted following traumatic brain injury and concussion to describe a transient dysautonomia, which often coexists with vestibular and oculomotor dysfunction as well as migraine patterns, as discussed in the (Chapter 23). Proper diagnosis of the etiology of symptoms related to dizziness is imperative as medical management for regulation of autonomic dysfunction, such as plasma volume expansion, may contrast from specific vestibular syndromes that indicate the use of diuretic therapy, such as Ménière disease.

MAL DE DEBARQUEMENT (DISEMBARKMENT SYNDROME)

This is a phenomenon described as "sickness of landing." The symptom of continued rocking, or the sensation that one has just gotten off a boat, is the hallmark of this phenomenon. It usually occurs after a long boat ride or airplane ride, often when there is turbulence. The vestibular system seems to be activated to a high degree, then is unable to calibrate back to normal in reference to the somatosensory input available.[93] In addition to the oscillating sensation there are complaints of fatigue, mental clouding, visual motion intolerance, anxiety, tinnitus, and headaches. The sensation is greater when the patient is at rest, and movement is actually preferable to standing or sitting. The sensation nulls or is reduced when reexposed to passive motion. Many patients describe relief of symptoms when they are riding in a car. The system typically remains maladapted, and the condition can persist over months and years, causing significant disability and frustration. Rehabilitation is directed toward recalibration of the somatosensory and vestibular systems with a focus on the somatosensory input activities. Traditional vestibular rehabilitation is not helpful with this population. The use of transcranial stimulation may give some insight into the condition as well as some potential intervention. The assumption that the brain is made up of oscillators and Mal de Debarquement occurs after exposure to oscillation (passive movement of the boat) is the basis of this approach.[94] It appears that the neural activity in the brain in the individuals who develop Mal de Debarquement is different than the control population in studies performed. The hypothesis of introducing oscillation through TMS may be able to uncouple the abnormal functional connectivity associated with Mal de Debarquement. Ongoing research is targeted toward the most appropriate area of the brain to stimulate.[95]

PERSISTENT POSTURAL-PERCEPTUAL DIZZINESS

Persistent postural-perceptual dizziness (PPPD or 3PD) is a syndrome that unifies key features of what was known as chronic subjective dizziness, phobic postural vertigo, and related disorders. It describes a common chronic dysfunction of the vestibular system and brain that produces persistent dizziness, nonspinning vertigo, and/or unsteadiness. The disorder constitutes a long-term maladaptation to a neuro-otological, medical, or psychological event that triggered vestibular symptoms, such as vestibular neuritis or BPPV, and is believed to be a specific complication to healing following an inner ear crisis. The phenomenon appears to negatively affect normal adaptation and therefore creates a more conscious effort into maintaining control of posture.

The increased burden of abnormal self-monitoring results in the common occurrence of dissociation and fatigue resulting from mental overload. The cycle of fear and avoidance can give rise to secondary phobic disorders such as agoraphobia.

Symptoms of PPPD include hypersensitivity to visual motion environment with an intolerance of apparent visual motion in the environment. Strong visual patterns can trigger symptoms, and there can be discomfort in moving surrounds such as crowds, grocery stores, airports, and theaters. Misleading vertical reference cues can cause both dizziness and imbalance. Tasks that require specific eye/hand coordination can become difficult. There can be intolerance to head and body movement often associated with changes of visual focus, such as moving from a text book to a projected screen, which is typical of current classroom activity. These patients will also avoid anything that would normally trigger dizziness, which usually involves head turns or quick movements. This can cause neck stiffness as they avoid movement. Patients often develop secondary functional gait disorder, anxiety, avoidance behavior, and severe disability.

There is interest in the possibility of inherited vulnerabilities in sensory processing that may underlie the processing disorder. Brain imaging shows some distinct areas of decreased functional connectivity during functional MRI.[96] Early neuroimaging studies suggest that there may be an additional pathophysiological mechanism underlying PPPD, perhaps a deficiency in cortical processes that supports locomotion and spatial orientation. Activity and connectivity appear to be greater in visual versus vestibular regions of the cortex, in keeping with physiological data on visual dependence. Activity and connectivity between key cortical regions that process space/motion

---

BOX 21.8 Cardinal Symptoms of Persistent Postural Perception Dizziness

1. Symptoms present for 3 months or more
2. Symptom must be present for prolonged periods on most days but will wax and wane in intensity
3. Dizziness triggered by visual motion or visually complex environments
4. Hypersensitivity to any passive motion
5. Generalized head motion dizziness that is not reported as vertigo
6. Symptoms cause significant distress or functional impairment
7. Symptoms are not better attributed to another disease or disorder
8. Persistent postural perception dizziness may coexist with other diseases or disorders. Evidence of another active illness does not necessarily exclude this diagnosis but may indicate the presence of a comorbid condition

Symptoms according to AA51.53 Persistent Postural-Perceptual Dizziness

---

information, such as the posterior insula and hippocampus, are decreased. Threat responses modulated in the anterior cingulate cortex are reduced. The abnormal functionality in the cortical networks may fail to suppress the bottom-up influences of instinctive threat on postural control and spatial orientation, leading to the sustained use of high guard balance strategies. This understanding may lead to new intervention strategies.[97]

PPPD has also been documented in association with migraine, concussion, primary anxiety, panic attacks, dysautonomia, or an acute medical crisis that disturbs postural stability orthostasis or syncope. (See section on autonomic nervous system disorders.) Increased levels of distress measured using the Hospital Anxiety and Depression Scale or the Generalized Anxiety Disorders Scale in patients with chronic symptoms suggest that the emotional status of the patients may contribute to prolongation of dizziness symptoms from the acute phase. Medical management[45] includes the use of low-dose selective serotonin reuptake inhibitor/serotonin norepinephrine reuptake inhibitor medications.[98] Therapy should include visual/optokinetic, motion desensitization, and recalibration of the somatosensory reference. Management of the autonomic phenomenon through interventions that decrease the fight or flight response can increase tolerance to the adaptation process and can be critical as noted previously. While diagnostic tests and conventional imaging usually remain negative, patients with PPPD present in a characteristic way that fits with positive diagnostic criteria.[99] Box 21.8 describes the characteristics associated with the diagnosis of PPPD.

REFERENCES

To enhance this text and add value for the reader, all references are included on the companion Evolve site that accompanies this textbook. This online service will, when available, provide a link for the reader to a Medline abstract for the article cited. There are 99 cited references and other general references for this chapter, with the majority of those articles being evidence-based citations.

22

Traumatic Brain Injury*

Doris Chong and Sheri Kiami

OBJECTIVES

After reading this chapter the student or therapist will be able to:

1. Describe the epidemiology, pathophysiology, and mechanisms of injury of moderate to severe traumatic brain injury.
2. Describe common clinical changes after traumatic brain injury.
3. Describe common medical interventions for traumatic brain injury.
4. Plan and select appropriate physical therapy examination techniques and tests and measures for people with traumatic brain injury using the Hypothesis-Oriented Algorithm for Clinicians (HOAC) II and International Classification of Functioning, Disability and Health (ICF) framework.
5. Develop a comprehensive plan of care with appropriate physical therapy interventions for people with moderate to severe traumatic brain injury using the ICF framework.
6. Describe prognosis and outcomes for people with moderate to severe traumatic brain injury using evidence-based prognostic indicators.

KEY TERMS

axonal injury
brain injury
contusions

hematomas
hemorrhages
ischemia

SECTION I—OVERVIEW OF TRAUMATIC BRAIN INJURY

Traumatic brain injury (TBI) is defined as a blow or jolt to the head or a penetrating head injury that disrupts the function of the brain. Not all blows or jolts to the head result in a TBI. The severity of such an injury may range from mild—a brief change in mental status or consciousness—to severe—an extended period of unconsciousness or amnesia after the injury. www.cdc.gov/traumaticbraininjury/get_the_facts.html. A TBI can result in short- or long-term problems with independent function.[1]

Epidemiology of Traumatic Brain Injury

TBI is a global health issue and is affecting around 10 million people in the world each year.[2] The Centers for Disease Control and Prevention (CDC) estimated in 2010 (www.braintrauma.org/faq) that approximately 1.7 million Americans sustain a TBI every year.[3] More than 2.5 million emergency department (ED) visits in the United States are related to TBI.[4] Of these, falls constituted the most frequent visits (45%), followed by motor vehicle accidents (43%), and violence (6%).[5] The admission diagnoses include concussion, skull fracture, cerebral laceration and contusions, and different types of hematoma/hemorrhages. The most prevalent age groups include 0 to 4 years old,

15 to 19 years old, and those who are older than 75 years of age.[1] Males (around 64%) are more likely to sustain a TBI than females.[5] The TBI-related hospital admission costs in 2010 were $21.4 billion.[4]

The incidence of TBI is 506.4 per 100,000 population, with around 43% of those hospitalized experiencing long-term activity limitation.[6] It is estimated that 3.2 million to 5.3 million people are living with TBI-related disabilities.[7] The estimated lifetime cost for each individual with severe brain injury exceeds $4 million. Annual costs for all TBIs in the United States exceed $60 billion. It is thought that the incidence and costs related to TBI have been underestimated due to gaps in capturing data in certain populations, for example sports-related injuries, or for those who do not seek medical advice after an injury. The actual burden of care is estimated to be much higher than the reported data and figures.

Mechanisms of Injury

There are four main types of injury, as follows:

1. Those from external forces hitting the head or the head hitting hard enough to cause brain movement. Injuries include those with skull fracture and those without skull fracture (closed head injuries). Direct blows to the head can cause coup injuries (at the site of impact) and contrecoup injuries (distant from the site of impact).
2. Severe acceleration and deceleration of the head, which can cause TBI without the head hitting an object. An example is shaken baby syndrome.
3. Blast injuries mainly affecting military personnel.

---

*Videos for this chapter are available at studentconsult.com.

4. Penetrating objects causing direct cellular and vascular damage. Injuries to the face and neck can cause brain injury by disrupting the blood supply to the brain.[8]

Pathophysiology of Injury

Acceleration, deceleration, rotational forces, and penetrating objects cause tissue laceration, compression, tension, shearing, or a combination, resulting in primary injury.

Primary Damage

- **Contusions.** A bruise or bleeding on the brain and lacerations can occur with or without skull fractures. Either an object hits the head, neck, or face, or the head hits an object. Damage can be to any area of the brain. Occipital blows are more likely to produce contusions than are frontal or lateral blows. Areas in which the cranial vault is irregular, such as on the anterior poles, undersurface of the temporal lobes, and undersurface of the frontal lobes, are commonly injured. Lacerations of blood vessels within the brain itself or of blood vessels that feed the brain from the neck or face reduce the flow of blood carrying oxygen to the brain. Contusions and lacerations can also injure the cranial nerves. The most commonly injured are the optic, vestibulocochlear, oculomotor, abducens, and facial nerves. Lacerations of the dura or in the arachnoid space may cause cerebrospinal fluid to discharge from the nose (cerebrospinal fluid rhinorrhea discharge increases with neck flexion, coughing, or straining).[9]
- **Epidural hematomas or hemorrhages.** These occur mostly in adults when tearing of meningeal vessels results in blood collecting between the skull and dura. Skull fracture is present in the majority of cases. This is accompanied by intervals of lucidity and can result in death unless treated early.
- **Subdural hematomas.** These occur with acceleration-deceleration injuries when bridging veins to the superior sagittal sinus are torn. Blood accumulates in the subdural space. Symptoms include weakness and lethargy. Symptoms such as weakness and lethargy that come on acutely are life-threatening. Symptoms caused by slow bleeding may not be present for several weeks.
- **Diffuse axonal injuries.** Also known as diffuse injuries, these are among the most common types of primary lesions in persons with brain trauma.[10,11] Brain tissues that differ in structure or weight experience unequal acceleration, deceleration, or rotation of tissues during rapid head movement or during impact, causing diffuse axonal injury and changes in chemical processing. Severing of the axons may be severe enough to result in coma. In milder forms, more spotty lesions are seen, including deficits such as memory loss, concentration difficulties, decreased attention span, headaches, sleep disturbances, and seizures. Damage often involves the corpus callosum, basal ganglia, brain stem, and cerebellum.[10,11]
- **Penetrating injuries.** These usually happen with objects with high velocities, such as bullets or shrapnel from explosives, and can cause additional damage remote from the areas of impact as a result of shock waves. Foreign objects such as sticks and sharp toys cause low-velocity injuries, directly damaging the tissues they contact.
- **Blast injuries.** These occur when a solid or liquid material explodes, turning into a gas. The expanding gases form a high-pressure wave, called an overpressure wave, that travels at supersonic speed. Pressure then drops, creating a relative vacuum or a blast underpressure wave that results in a reversal of air flow. This

is then followed by a second overpressure wave. Blast-related injury can occur through several mechanisms. The primary blast wave generates extreme pressure changes that can cause stress and shear injuries. For example, rupture of the tympanic membranes is very common after blast injury, and lung and gastrointestinal injuries also occur. The exact mechanism of injury to the brain is unknown, with speculation about both axonal shearing and shearing of vasculature.[12,13]

Secondary Damage or Insult

Secondary injuries are mainly caused by a lack of oxygen in the highly oxygen-demanding and dependent brain. Secondary problems may result from the following:

- **Increased intracranial pressure** (ICP) resulting from swelling or intracranial hematoma. Swelling of the brain causes distortion because the brain is held in the skull, a rigid, unyielding structure. The resultant increased ICP can lead to herniation of parts of the brain. The most often seen herniations include cingulate herniation under the falx cerebri, uncus herniation, central (or transtentorial) herniation, and herniation of the brain stem through the foramen magnum.[14] Acute hydrocephalus occurs when blood accumulates in the ventricular system, expanding the size of the ventricles and causing increased pressure on brain tissue being compressed between the skull and the fluid-filled ventricles. The increased pressure can then result in changes in Pco_2, which is harmful to nervous tissue. Increased ICP has been correlated with poorer outcomes and higher mortality rates.[15]
- **Cerebral hypoxia or ischemia** occurs when blood vessels are ruptured or compressed. Hypoxia can occur from a lack of blood to the brain or from lack of oxygen in the blood as a result of airway obstruction or chest injuries.
- **Intracranial hemorrhage** causes hypoxia to tissues fed by the hemorrhaging blood vessels and adds pressure and distortion to brain tissue. Metabolic products from damaged cells and blood bathe the brain. Cell death occurs within minutes after injury from ischemia, edema, necrosis, and the toxic effects of blood on neural tissues.
- **Electrolyte and acid-base imbalance.** Secondary cell death occurs either by swelling and then bursting of the cellular membrane (necrosis), or by destruction from within the cell through changes in the deoxyribonucleic acid (DNA)—apoptosis. Cell death can occur days, weeks, or months after injury.[16]
- **Infections.** Infections may arise from open wounds (e.g., penetrating injuries) or from prolonged invasive monitoring (e.g., ICP monitoring). If infection is present in brain tissue, it may cause swelling and cell death.
- **Seizures from pressure or scarring.** Seizures are most common immediately after injury, and 6 months to 2 years after injury. Seizure activity can cause additional brain damage owing to high oxygen and glucose requirements.

Clinical Features of Traumatic Brain Injury
Disorders of Consciousness

Disorders of consciousness (DOCs) is a collective term describing conditions where consciousness or arousal have been affected by brain damage. The damage can be of direct insult to structures and systems regulating arousal and awareness, or of indirect damage to systematic neural connections of the brain.[17] The main DOCs are coma, vegetative state (VS), and minimally conscious state (MCS). Some clinicians and scientists include locked-in syndrome as a DOC, while some perceive it as a differential diagnosis. A brief description of the various disorders under this broad spectrum is provided below.

- **Coma.** *Coma* is defined as a complete paralysis of cerebral function or a state of unresponsiveness. The eyes are closed and there is no response to painful stimuli. There are no obvious sleep-wake cycles.[17] Oculomotor and pupillary signs are valuable in assisting with the diagnosis, localizing brain stem damage, and determining the depth of coma.[18] In coma, brain stem responses may include grimacing to pain, which is frequently associated with a flexor or localizing motor response, loss of hearing or balance, abnormal palate and tongue movements, loss of language, and loss or distortion of taste.

- **Vegetative State.** This state is characterized by a wakeful, reduced responsiveness with no evident cerebral cortical function. The difference between coma and VS is that there are intermittent periods of wakefulness in VS.[17] VS can result from diffuse cerebral hypoxia or from severe, diffuse white matter impact damage. The brain stem is usually relatively intact. Patients may track with their eyes and show minimal spontaneous yet involuntary motor activities, but they do not speak, nor do they respond to verbal stimulation.[19] When VS lasts for over 1 month after TBI, the term persistent vegetative state (PVS) may be applied, though some now advocate for the term chronic VS due to the fact that brain injury is a dynamic rather than static process. Functional magnetic resonance imaging (fMRI) was recently used to test patients who were diagnosed with PVS. Five of 54 patients diagnosed with PVS demonstrated "willful, neuroanatomically specific blood-oxygenated–level–dependent responses when told to visualize one of two tasks."[20] The diagnosis of PVS indicates lack of cortical function, and fMRI may be useful in this diagnosis in the future. Recovery of consciousness, if it occurs, includes a gradual return of orientation and recent memory.[18] The duration of each of these stages is variable and can be prolonged. Improvement can stop at any point.

- **Minimally Conscious State.** In MCS, consciousness is severely altered but there are signs demonstrating self or environmental awareness.[17] Patients will have to be able to demonstrate motor response in a reproducible manner. That is, for a diagnosis of MCS a person must be able to follow simple one-step commands inconsistently and may even demonstrate some verbal responses to stimuli. Smooth pursuit may be present. MCS is often viewed as a transitional state signifying improvement of consciousness. The previous terminology for this state includes obtundity. It describes the condition of a person who sleeps a great deal and who, when aroused, exhibits reduced alertness, disinterest in the environment, and slow responses to stimulation.

- **Posttraumatic Confusion or Clouding of Consciousness.** In this state the person is awake most of the time, but is confused, easily distractible, with faulty memory, and with slowed but consistent responses to stimuli. Functional communication emerges in this state and is a clinical sign of improvement.

Autonomic Nervous System Changes

Changes in the autonomic nervous system (ANS) after TBI are not uncommon. Hilz and colleagues[21] found that in persons with mild TBI, cardiovascular regulation shifts from parasympathetic activities to sympathetic activities at rest and there is a decrease in orthostatic responses. The dysfunctions are thought to be due to the close connections between the frontal cortex and various ANS functions.[22] Because the ANS is a system that functions without voluntary control and it regulates multiple systems in the body, autonomic dysfunctions can

---

> ### BOX 22.1 Possible Autonomic Nervous System Symptoms Resulting From Brain Injury
>
> - Variabilities in heart rate (e.g., tachycardia) and respiratory rates
> - Irritable bowel syndrome
> - Temperature elevations
> - Blood pressure changes
> - Excessive sweating, salivation, tearing, and sebum secretion
> - Dilated pupils
> - Vomiting
> - Anxiety, panic disorder, and posttraumatic stress disorder

cause system-wide abnormalities and increase mortality.[22] It is recently reported that autonomic dysfunction at rest and in standing are more prominent in persons with moderate to severe TBI and dysfunctions can be prolonged after TBI.[21] Box 22.1 lists possible ANS symptoms resulting from brain injury.

Motor, Sensory, Perceptual, and Functional Changes

Motor impairments are common after TBI yet understudied in humans due to the overwhelming focus on consciousness and cognitive changes. A cohort study showed that during the inpatient rehabilitation phase, 20% or more of patients had paresis in upper extremity (UE) and/or lower extremity (LE), 30% or more had incoordination, and between 13% and 27% had gait and balance problems.[23] Dizziness and disequilibrium were reported in 30% to 65% of people with TBI.[24] Although dystonia appears not to be a significant issue in people post-TBI,[23] spasticity could develop as soon as one week after the injury.[25] It is still not well understood why these changes occur, but animal studies point towards imbalance between excitation and inhibition neuronal signals after brain injury. In particular, the imbalance favors excitation causing sensory deficits, which in turn causes cognitive and motor deficits in TBI.[26] Box 22.2 lists common motor changes and provides symptoms of sensory and perceptive involvement.

Cognitive, Personality, and Behavioral Changes

Cognitive and behavioral sequelae can result from generalized or focal brain injuries. For example, emotional changes may be seen with lesions in the orbitofrontal areas. Septal area lesions result in rage and overall irritability. Pseudobulbar injuries can result in emotional lability of involuntary laughing or crying not associated with feelings of emotions. Memory impairment, a very common finding after TBI, is an aftermath of generalized lesions.

Amnesia is a term that describes memory impairment. Posttraumatic amnesia (PTA) is defined as "the time lapse between the accident and the point at which the functions concerned with memory are judged to have been restored."[27] Two types of PTA are frequently associated with brain injury: retrograde and anterograde. Retrograde amnesia is a deficit in memory retrieval with inability to recall events that occurred prior to the injury.[28] Anterograde amnesia refers to the inability to form new memories after the injury, and it is often more impaired in declarative tasks as compared to procedural.[28] The duration of PTA is considered a clinical indicator of the severity of the injury; it may guide clinical management decisions, and it is also one of the prognostic indicators in TBI.[27,28]

The patient's inability to develop new memories can be quite challenging for the rehabilitation team and for the patient because memory is an important component of learning.[29] There are two types of memory: declarative and procedural. Memory in which the patient

BOX 22.2 Motor, Sensory, Perceptual, and Functional Changes Resulting From Brain Injury

Motor changes may Include any or all of the following:
- Paralysis or paresis such as monoplegia or hemiplegia
- Cranial nerve injury resulting in paralysis of eye muscles, facial paralysis, vestibular and vestibuloocular reflex abnormalities, slurred speech (dysarthria), swallowing abnormalities (dysphagia), and paralysis of the tongue muscles
- Poor coordination of movement
- Abnormal reflexes
- Abnormal muscle tone: flaccidity, spasticity, or rigidity. (The terms *decorticate rigidity* and *decerebrate rigidity* are often used to denote abnormal posturing. *Decerebrate rigidity* denotes extension in all four limbs. *Decorticate posturing* includes flexion of the upper extremities and extension of the legs.)
- Combinations of asymmetrical cerebellar and pyramidal signs and of bilateral pyramidal and extrapyramidal signs have all been reported[15]
- Loss of selective motor control
- Poor balance
- Loss of bowel or bladder control

Sensory and perceptual may include any or all of the following:
- Hypersensitivity to light or noise
- Loss of hearing or sight
- Visual field changes
- Numbness and tingling (peripheral nerves are often injured)
- Loss of somatosensory functions
- Dizziness or vertigo
- Visuospatial abnormalities
- Agnosia
- Apraxia

BOX 22.3 Cognitive, Personality, and Behavioral Changes Resulting From Brain Injury

Cognitive changes might include any or all of the following:
- Temporary or permanent disorders of intellectual function
- Memory loss
- Shortened attention span
- Concentration problems
- Confusion
- Changes in motivation
- Difficulty sustaining attention
- Executive function loss
- Reduced problem-solving skills
- Lack of initiative
- Loss of reasoning
- Poor abstract thinking
- Shortened attention span

Behavioral changes could include the following[31]:
- Agitation
- Aggression
- Irritability
- Substance abuse
- Behavior with legal consequences
- Apathy
- Depression
- Anxiety
- Posttraumatic stress disorder
- Obsessive-compulsive disorder
- Psychosis
- Suicidal ideation and attempts
- Suicide

can recall facts and events of a previous experience is declarative memory. Explicit learning, a conscious verbal learning, is based on declarative memory. However, many patients who cannot reproduce memories through conscious recollection do have the ability to learn new motor skills. Implicit learning, a noncognitive type of learning in which patients can show changes in performance after prior experience, is based on procedural memory. Patients can show the ability to change motor, perceptual, or cognitive behaviors with practice or training but may lack declarative memory. Another type of short-term memory that is often compromised after TBI is working memory, which is crucial for processing everyday life information. An example of working memory is the ability to remember the steps of a recipe during cooking. Quality of life is thought to be affected when working memory is impaired.[30]

Behavioral changes can be present even without cognitive and physical deficits. A recent systematic review[31] grouped behavioral changes after TBI into four categories: (1) Disruptive behaviors by excess, for example agitation, aggression, irritability, drug addiction, and behaviors with legal consequences; (2) disruptive behaviors by default, such as apathy and decreased goal-oriented behaviors; (3) affect disorders, including depression, anxiety, and post-traumatic stress disorder (PTSD); and (4) suicidal attempts and suicide. Even though the extent and types of behavioral changes depend upon the severity of injury, all of these behaviors (except for substance abuse) have higher prevalence rates among persons who have sustained a TBI than the general population. The social consequences of inappropriate behavior can be disastrous and interfere with achieving therapy goals.

Box 22.3 lists common cognitive and behavioral changes resulting from brain injury.

Other Complications

A list of the complications that may accompany brain injury would be limitless. In addition to any concomitant injuries, some of the diagnostic, monitoring, and therapeutic procedures themselves carry hazards as does prolonged bed rest. Catheters, nasogastric tubes, and tracheotomies can cause iatrogenic injuries. Infections, contractures, skin breakdown, thrombophlebitis, pulmonary problems, heterotopic ossification (HO), and surgical complications are but a few of the risks. Posttraumatic epilepsy is also a possible sequela. Depression occurs frequently after brain injury and appears to be the most prevalent mental disorder post-TBI.[32] It appears that a combination of neuroanatomical, neurochemical, and psychosocial factors is responsible for the onset and maintenance of the depression.[32] Depression post-TBI often negatively impacts outcomes related to productivity and quality of life.

Locked-in syndrome may be grouped differently from DOCs. In this syndrome the patient cannot move any part of the body except the eyes but cognition remains intact and the person is conscious.[33] Communication disorders are also common complications after TBI and may include expressive and receptive aphasia, dysarthria, loss in reading comprehension and social communication, and many others.

BOX 22.4 Glasgow Coma Scale

Eye Opening (E)	
Spontaneous	4
To speech	3
To pain	2
Nil	1
Best Motor Response (M)	
Obeys	6
Localizes	5
Withdraws	4
Abnormal flexion	3
Extensor response	2
Nil	1
Verbal Response (V)	
Oriented	5
Confused conversation	4
Inappropriate words	3
Incomprehensible sounds	2
Nil	1
Coma Score (E + M + V) =	3–15

From Jennett B, Teasdale G. *Management of Head Injuries.* Philadelphia: FA Davis; 1981.

Types and Classifications of Traumatic Brain Injury

Severity of TBI is categorized as mild, moderate, or severe based on specific measurements on scales such as the Glasgow Coma Scale (GCS) (Box 22.4), duration of loss of consciousness, and duration of PTA. See Table 22.1 for details. In addition, the Brain Injury Association of America[34] provides qualitative descriptions according to the severity of injury. For mild TBI, there is usually a brief to no loss of consciousness and there may be vomiting, dizziness, lethargy, and memory loss. For moderate TBI, unconsciousness can last up to 24 hours. There are signs of trauma, contusions, and/or bleeding on neuroimaging. For people with severe TBI, coma persists for more than 24 hours, there are no obvious sleep/wake cycles, and there are signs of trauma on neuroimaging.

Another scale that is commonly used to classify levels of TBI is the Rancho Los Amigos Levels of Cognitive Functioning Scale (LOCF).[35] The scale measure levels of consciousness, cognition, and behavior post-TBI and is often used as an outcome measure for these impairments as patients progress through various stages of TBI. Briefly, there are eight levels describing persons' responses and behaviors, namely no response (LOCF I), generalized response (LOCF II), localized response (LOCF III), confused-agitated (LOCF IV), confused-inappropriate (LOCF V), confused-appropriate (LOCF VI), automatic-appropriate (LOCF VII), and purposeful-appropriate (LOCF VIII). See Appendix 22.A for detailed descriptions of typical behaviors observed in each level.

TABLE 22.1 Severity of Traumatic Brain Injury

Measurement	Mild	Moderate	Severe
Glasgow Coma Scale	13–15	9–12	3–8
Loss of consciousness	<30 min	30 min–24 h	>24 h
Posttraumatic amnesia	0–1 day	>1 to ≤7 days	>7 days

SECTION II—MEDICAL MANAGEMENT OF TRAUMATIC BRAIN INJURY

Initial Care and Acute Management

For persons with severe TBI, medical management begins at the prehospital phase where the person is monitored for oxygenation, blood pressure, cognitive function (using the GCS), pupillary function, and signs of brain stem herniation. Transport to a trauma center with CT scanning, neurosurgical evaluation, and ICP monitoring is the goal to monitor and minimize secondary injuries.[3] A determination of GCS score is performed either at the prehospital stage or in the ED to test the function of the brain stem and the cerebrum through eye, motor, and verbal responses.[36] It provides a measure of the level of consciousness and an idea of injury severity. Scores range from 3 to 15, with lower scores associated with lower levels of function. Scores from 13 to 15 indicate a mild brain injury, 9 to 12 a moderate brain injury, and 8 or less a severe injury.

On admission to the ED, a neurosurgeon usually assumes initial and primary responsibility for the person. The first priority in acute care is resuscitation and prevention of secondary insult. The Brain Trauma Foundation[34] recommends the following guidelines for severe TBI management in the acute phase: airway control and ventilation to optimize oxygenation, monitoring and maintenance of cerebral perfusion pressure (CPP) and blood pressure, monitoring and management of ICP, fluid management, hyperosmolar therapy, sedation, and prophylaxis of infections, deep vein thrombosis (DVT), seizures, and hypothermia.[3,9,27,37] The details of the guidelines can be found at www.braintrauma.org.

In addition to the traditional neuroimaging such as CT, magnetic resonance imaging (MRI), and positron emission technology (PET) scan for monitoring of neurological functions, advanced multimodal neuromonitoring is recommended to improve outcomes of TBI. These include jugular venous oxygen saturation ($SjvO_2$), focal brain tissue oxygen tension ($PbrO_2$), cerebral microdialysis, and continuous electroencephalography (EEG). For patients who are candidates for decompressive craniectomy due to elevated ICP, a large frontotemporoparietal approach is recommended versus a small one as it has been found to have better neurological outcomes.[37]

Common Neurosurgical Interventions

Decompressive craniectomy, as mentioned above, is a procedure where a large portion of the skull is removed to allow the brain to swell. This procedure is used when ICP is elevated over 25 mm Hg for 1 to 12 hours despite other medical interventions.[3] The goal is to prevent brain stem herniation and maintain CPP for brain tissue viability.

External ventricular drain (EVD) is another frequently used neurosurgical procedure to control elevated ICP. Usually a catheter is inserted through the skull into the anterior horn of one of the lateral ventricles to drain cerebrospinal fluid. The catheter is also connected to an external transducer for constant ICP monitoring. The amount of fluid drained from the ventricle needs to be precise and, oftentimes, a few milliliters of drained fluid results in a decrease in ICP. Although EVD may increase the risk of infection, there is strong evidence proving its effectiveness in immediate reduction of ICP.[38]

Persons with epidural hematomas often undergo craniotomies with blood evacuation to relieve pressure within the cranium. Subdural injuries are frequently treated by removing the blood through bur holes.

Common Pharmacological Interventions

Medications are chosen according to symptoms to be treated.

Medications That Decrease Intracranial Pressure

Osmotic agents such as mannitol are used to pull fluid from brain tissue back into the blood system, thus lowering ICP. Use of mannitol is recommended for patients who have perfusion problems,[35] and the evidence is strong for the effectiveness of mannitol to reduce ICP.[38] Propofol, a barbiturate (sedative), may reduce the need for ICP treatment. Sedative treatment may be reduced as well if it is used together with morphine.[38] Propofol is recommended only if ICP cannot be controlled by other means because it may potentially reduce CPP.[39,40] Hypertonic saline is another osmotherapy to control ICP, although the best solution and administration has yet to be determined. The Brain Trauma Foundation in 2016 recommended a stepladder approach using mannitol or hypertonic saline, together with other procedures for best control of elevated ICP.[37] Corticosteroids are commonly used in the acute phase to stabilize brain injury; however, it has been shown that mortality may be increased by methylprednisone, and it should be avoided.[38] See Chapter 36 for additional information.

Medications That Control Blood Pressure and Cerebral Perfusion Pressure

Blood pressure control is important in patients with brain injury. CPP[41] or adequate blood pressure to maintain cerebral blood flow against increased ICP is calculated by subtracting the ICP from the mean arterial pressure. If fluid management cannot maintain adequate blood pressure, then vasopressor medications such as phenylephrine (Neo-Synephrine) are used to constrict peripheral vessels but not the vessels of the brain. Norepinephrine is also shown to support CPP in a consistent and predictive manner.[37] The Brain Trauma Foundation recommended to maintain the systolic blood pressure at ≥100 mm Hg for persons aged between 50 and 69 and ≥110 mm Hg for persons aged between 15 and 49 or those over the age of 70.[42] In general, CPP should be maintained between 60 and 70 mm Hg for positive outcomes.

Medications That Decrease Intracranial Bleeding

Intracranial bleeding is common after TBI, and it can cause permanent disability and even death. Therefore controlling intracranial bleeding is usually a goal in the acute management of TBI. Hemostatic drugs work by increasing coagulation. Antifibrinolytic medications, including lysin analogues and plasmin inhibitors, work by reducing fibrinolysis and increasing clot stability.[40] Although some studies have shown effectiveness, systematic reviews fail to show reliable evidence on their effects for reducing mortality and morbidity.[40]

Medications to Control Seizure

Seizure is a common complication after TBI, and its presence may have an adverse effect on ICP; therefore anticonvulsants are routinely used in acute TBI as a preventative measure. Examples of anticonvulsants include phenytoin, sodium valproate, levetiracetam, and carbamazepine. Recent systematic review and the Brain Trauma Foundation guidelines recommended that an anticonvulsant should be routinely administered within the first week of acute TBI.[40,42] The effectiveness for late seizure prevention remains inconclusive.

Medications for Prevention of Brain Cell Death

Hypothermia is frequently used in acute severe TBI because of its possible neuroprotective effect. Although it does not appear to change the mortality rate, it is associated with improved functional outcome on the Glasgow Outcome Scale (GOS) (Box 22.5).[43] Progesterone is a hormone that has been shown to reduce cerebral edema and neuronal loss in acute TBI; however, further research is still needed to support its use in medical management of TBI.[40]

> ### BOX 22.5 Functional Outcomes on Glasgow Outcome Scale
>
> **Vegetative State**
> A persistent state characterized by reduced responsiveness associated with wakefulness. The patient may exhibit eye opening, sucking, yawning, and localized motor responses.
>
> **Severe Disability**
> An outcome characterized by consciousness, but the patient has 24-h dependence because of cognitive, behavioral, or physical disabilities, including dysarthria and dysphasia.
>
> **Moderate Disability**
> An outcome characterized by independence in activities of daily living and in home and community activities but with disability. Patients in this category may have memory or personality changes, hemiparesis, dysphagia, ataxia, acquired epilepsy, or major cranial nerve deficits.
>
> **Good Recovery**
> Patient able to reintegrate into normal social life and able to return to work. There may be mild persisting sequelae.

Modified from Jennett B, Bond M. Assessment of outcome after severe brain damage: a practical scale. *Lancet.* 1975;1:480.

Medications for Prevention of Infections

Antibiotics may be used after TBI due to risk of infection from injuries, wounds, or invasive monitoring. It is recommended that antibiotics be delivered for 1 to 2 weeks for persons sustaining penetrating injuries.[37] However, the evidence on the use of antibiotics in other forms of TBI is unclear and may even lead to an increased rate of infection.

Medications That Affect Behavioral and Cognitive Functions (also see Chapter 36)

Medications to treat behavioral or cognitive dysfunction are difficult to standardize. A recent systematic review suggested the following medications for various behavioral dysfunctions after TBI.[44] There is some evidence to use carbamazepine (Tegretol) and valproate as a first line treatment for agitation and aggression. Propranolol (Inderal) can also help to improve aggression. For persons with depressive symptoms, selective serotonin reuptake inhibitors (SSRIs) are recommended. Confusion and other neuropsychotic symptoms have been treated using neuroleptic medications; however, there is no evidence of their efficacy.

For patients with attention deficits, monoaminergic agonists such as amantadine or methylphenidate may increase information processing, aid functional recovery, and prevent permanent functional loss in some patients, but the evidence remains inconclusive.[40,45] In a recent systematic review, amantadine is recommended for people with DOC to improve arousal.[46]

Medications That Affect Motor Functions (see Chapter 36)

Medications also may be prescribed for motor abnormalities involving increases in tone. Oral medications for treating spasticity include baclofen, diazepam, dantrolene sodium, and tizanidine.[25] They can be used alone or in combination depending on the severity of spasticity. Baclofen works at the CNS level and may cause drowsiness. Baclofen can also be delivered intrathecally where the side effect is less. Dantrolene sodium works directly at the muscle level and therefore is less likely to cause cognitive disturbances but more likely to cause generalized weakness.[47] Botulinum toxin type A (Botox) is commonly used to treat focal muscle hypertonicity, such as the finger flexors, biceps, or gastrocnemius. Diazepam (Valium) initially was the drug most commonly administered for spasticity or high tone. However, diazepam also promotes drowsiness and decreased responsiveness and can increase muscle weakness and ataxia.[48] Regardless of the medication used, it is recommended that medications be combined with complementary therapies, such as transcranial magnetic stimulation (TMS) and therapeutic exercise, in order to achieve greater benefits of tone reduction medications and improve functional outcomes.[25]

Regenerative Medicine and Management of Traumatic Brain Injury

Regenerative medicine is an interprofessional field of research and clinical practice for the repair, replacement, or regeneration of cells, tissues, and/or organs in order to restore function lost due to disease or damage.[49] Recent advances in stem cell and tissue engineering technology have led to a rapid proliferation of research, though limitations exist, including the survival and appropriate differentiation of implanted cells. Studies on the combined effects of regenerative approaches and physical rehabilitation following stroke and TBI, referred to as regenerative rehabilitation, are very promising and show greater recovery than either approach used in isolation in animal model studies.[50-53] Several clinical trials are underway to explore the impact of regenerative rehabilitation in stroke and TBI, as well as muscular conditions such as muscular dystrophy.[49] Scientists in this field are encouraged by positive results to date, and predict that with further advances in the stem cell and tissue technologies and rigorous interprofessional research, regenerative medicine has the potential to become the standard of care in the treatment of many neuromuscular and other health conditions.[49]

SECTION III—REHABILITATION MANAGEMENT OF TRAUMATIC BRAIN INJURY

Terminology and Structure for Patient Management

The World Health Organization (WHO), in the International Classification of Functioning, Disability and Health (ICF),[54] has developed a common terminology that is used in this chapter. Definitions are as follows (see also Chapter 1):

- *Body functions* are physiological functions of body systems (including psychological functions).
- *Body structures* are anatomical parts of the body such as organs, limbs, and their components.
- *Impairments* are problems in body function or structure such as a significant deviation or loss.
- *Activity* is the execution of a task or action by an individual.
- *Participation* is involvement in a life situation.
- *Activity limitations* are difficulties an individual may have in executing activities.
- *Participation restrictions* are problems an individual may experience in involvement in life situations.
- *Environmental factors* make up the physical, social, and attitudinal environment in which people live and conduct their lives.

The American Physical Therapy Association (APTA) has published levels of patient management leading to optimal outcomes.[55] The Association's Guide to Physical Therapist Practice, which uses examination, evaluation, diagnosis, prognosis, intervention, and outcomes as its basis, will be followed in this chapter. Although this is the terminology used by physical therapists, its application and integration into the

profession of occupational therapy should be simultaneously acknowledged. The method used in this chapter for gathering the guide information is based on the Hypothesis-Oriented Algorithm for Clinicians (HOAC) II model.[56] See Box 22.6 for an overview of this method, and see the text that follows for details of how to perform these procedures.

Examination

Data are collected from referral information, from the medical record, via observation, and from the patient or family interview. A history is taken and should include information regarding the mechanism of injury, initial GCS score, extent and time since onset of injury, patient's age, and duration of PTA. This information will be used to help establish a prognosis. Other information about education, family support, and living circumstances will also help with the prognosis and discharge planning. Complications, as well as coexisting diseases, are reviewed with the patient in order to discuss a thorough plan of care and determine appropriate referrals. Included under examination are systems review and tests and measures. Systems review is considered a screening of major systems that helps therapists to identify areas of focus during selective tests and measures. Therapists use information collected in examination to identify service needs.

Examination should lead to an understanding of the underlying causes of the activity limitations and participation restrictions and should be the basis of the intervention program. Patients usually present their chief complaints as activity limitations, for example, "I can no longer walk very far." Once activity limitations have been determined, a task analysis can be completed by having the patient demonstrate the problem—in this case, walking. The therapist will develop a hypothesis as to why the observed deviation from typical performance is present. Tests and measures and standardized outcome measures will be chosen on the basis of the therapist's knowledge of their importance in the task being performed and recommendations from peer-reviewed resources, such as the Academy of Neurologic Physical Therapy,[57] to confirm the hypothesis and to establish baseline measurements. For example, in a patient who drags the foot

---

BOX 22.6 Development of Intervention Approaches Based on HOAC II Model

1. Collect initial data.
2. Have patient and family identify patient problems with activity and participation limitations.
3. Develop an initial set of hypotheses based on a task analysis of identified activity limitations; choose and apply examinations to test those hypotheses.
4. Reassess hypotheses in light of examination findings and confirm or deny. Repeat first three steps if denied.
5. Develop list of non–patient-identified problems, including anticipated problems (such as skin breakdown when sensation is impaired).
6. Choose and apply appropriate outcome measures to monitor progress that address the impairments or activity limitations.
7. Develop an evaluation and diagnosis identifying why the problems exist or are likely to occur in the future.
8. Establish a prognosis and set goals with time frames for achievement.
9. Develop interventions that most effectively ameliorate the problems based on current literature or best practice.
10. Reexamine using outcome measures to determine progress.

HOAC, Hypothesis-Oriented Algorithm for Clinicians. From Rothstein JM, Echternach JL, Riddle DL. The hypothesis-oriented algorithm for clinicians II (HOAC II): a guide for patient management. *Phys Ther.* 2003;83:455–470.

in initial swing, the patient might lack 45 degrees of full passive knee flexion, but this is not critical in the task of walking. However, being able to dorsiflex the foot at initial swing is important. Therefore testing of both the ability to dorsiflex with the leg in the extended position and the speed at which the patient can perform this task would be appropriate. The tests and measures should be chosen on the basis of the hypothesis that the therapist generates from the task analysis. Details of task analysis and examinations of impairments, activity limitations, and participation restrictions will be provided in later sections of this chapter.

The Academy of Neurologic Physical Therapy Outcome measures recommendations, and Evidence Database to Guide Effectiveness (EDGE) Task Force developed recommendations for outcome measures for selected clinical conditions (e.g., stroke, TBI) based on vigorous evaluations of available measures.[58] The recommendations of outcome measures are classified according to settings and practices. Physical therapists should choose outcome measures from the recommendations for TBI when possible.[57] For example, gait outcome can be measured using the 6 minute walk test or 10 m walk test in the inpatient or outpatient setting, or the High-Level Mobility Assessment Tool (HiMAT) if the patient is high-functioning and seen in an outpatient setting. Recommended outcome measures by settings/practices are presented in Tables 22.2 to 22.4. For various components of examination, see Box 22.7.

Evaluation

Evaluation identifies the needs that can be managed by the therapist; serves to delineate those factors that influence or restrict the choice of therapeutic approaches; and states which components are most critical for the identified activity limitations. Evaluation provides a qualitative means of determining why a need is present. It includes considerations of subjective findings, objective findings, and environmental/contextual and personal factors (as illustrated in the ICF model). Thus the evaluation determines goals and intervention. The purpose of the evaluation is to determine what prevents the patient from performing in a functional, acceptable manner as identified by the patient, the therapist, and society.

Diagnosis

Diagnosis takes into consideration the integrated evaluation findings and classifies the problems into diagnostic categories. These diagnostic categories define the primary dysfunctions of an individual and in turn enable the therapist to formulate appropriate intervention. The diagnostic process involves discernment of what the individual desires to achieve and the capacity of the individual at the moment. Additional information from other healthcare professionals may need to be sought during the diagnostic process. Likewise, the therapist may need to share information with other healthcare professionals if the diagnostic process reveals problems outside of the therapist's scope of practice. The ultimate goal of diagnosis for the therapist is to verify the needs of the individual and act accordingly.

Prognosis and Outcomes

Prognosis is the determination of the optimal level of functional improvement and the time required to reach that optimal level. In addition to the highest functional level the individual is capable to obtain, the therapist needs to consider the individual's habitual level of function in order to identify a realistic and reasonable prognosis. This is important to manage expectations of the individual and the therapist and is crucial to motivate the individual during intervention. Prognosis often includes short- and long-term goals that are specific to improve functions along with duration and frequency of intervention to achieve those goals.

On the other hand, outcomes are the actual results of intervention and are chosen to measure all levels of dysfunction from impairment through participation limitation to determine effectiveness of the intervention strategies and whether or not the patient has met rehabilitation goals. Again, outcomes should ideally follow the recommendations listed above by TBI EDGE Taskforce.[57] An example of the process is presented in Box 22.8.

TABLE 22.2 Academy of Neurologic Physical Therapy Outcome Measures Recommendation for Traumatic Brain Injury—Acute Care[58]

General	Moderate to severely dependent	Mildly dependent to independent in ambulation
• Agitated Behavior Scale • Coma Recovery Scale—Revised • Moss Attention Rating Scale • Rancho Levels of Cognitive Functioning	• Functional Assessment Measure • Functional Independence Measure	• 6 min walk test • 10 m walk test • Balance Error Scoring System • Community Mobility and Balance Scale • Functional Assessment Measure • High-Level Mobility Assessment Tool

From The Academy of Neurologic Physical Therapy.

TABLE 22.3 Academy of Neurologic Physical Therapy Outcome Measures Recommendation for Traumatic Brain Injury—Inpatient and Outpatient Rehabilitation[58]

Inpatient Only	Outpatient Only	Both In- and Outpatient
• Coma Recovery Scale—revised (highly recommended) • Moss Attention Rating Scale (highly recommended) • Agitated Behavioral Scale • Barthel index • Cog-Log and O(rientation)-Log • Disorders of Consciousness Scale • Functional independence measure	• High-level mobility assessment tool (highly recommended) • Action research arm test • Apathy Evaluation Scale • Balance Error Scoring Scale • Community integration questionnaire • Dizziness handicap inventory • Global fatigue index • Sydney Psychological Reintegration Scale	• 6 min walk test • 10 m walk test • Berg balance scale • Community Balance And Mobility Scale • Disability Rating Scale • Functional assessment measure • Patient health questionnaire • Quality of life after brain injury • Rancho levels of cognitive function

From The Academy of Neurologic Physical Therapy.

TABLE 22.4 Academy of Neurologic Physical Therapy Outcome Measures Recommendation for Traumatic Brain Injury—Research[58]

Body Structure/Function	Activity	Participation
• Agitated Behavior Scale • Apathy Evaluation Scale • Awareness Questionnaire • Coma Recovery Scale—Revised • Disorders of Consciousness Scale • Dizziness Handicap Inventory • Functional Status Exam • Glasgow Coma Scale • Glasgow Coma Scale—Extended • Global Fatigue Index • Modified Ashworth Scale • Montreal Cognitive Assessment • Moss Attention Rating Scale • Motivation for TBI Rehabilitation • Neurologic Outcome Scale—TBI Orientation Log • Patient Health Questionnaire • Rancho Levels of Cognitive Function	• 2 min walk test • 6 min walk test • 10 m walk test • Action Research Arm Test • Activity Measure Post Acute Care • Balance Error Scoring System • Barthel Index • Berg Balance Scale • Community Mobility and Balance Scale • Functional Independence Measure • Functional Assessment Measure • Functional Gait Assessment • Functional Reach • High-Level Mobility Assessment Tool • Sensory Organization Test • Walking and Remembering Test • Wolf Motor Function Test	• Activity-specific Balance Confidence Scale • Assessment of Life Habits • Canadian Occupational Performance Measure • Community Integration Questionnaire • Craig Handicap Assessment and Reporting Techniques-SF • Craig Hospital Inventory of Environmental Factors—long and short forms • Disability Rating Scale • EuroQOL • Impact on Participation and Autonomy • Mayo-Portland Adaptability Inventory-4 • NeuroQOL • Participation Assessment with Recombined Tools-Objective • Quality of Life After Brain Injury • Satisfaction with Life Scale • SF-36 • Sydney Psychosocial Reintegration Scale • WHO Quality of Life-BREF

TBI, Traumatic brain injury.

BOX 22.7 Examination Framework SPECIFIC for TBI

I. History: injury, age, PTA, GCS score, job, home environment, educational level, previous injuries, etc.
II. Patient and family data: patient and family perception of the limitations, goals, personal factors, socioeconomic factors relating to participation limitations
III. Other health care team member evaluations
IV. Screens
  A. Systems review to emphasize precautions during intervention and to identify any "red flags" that will require referrals.
    1. Circulatory and respiratory
    2. Integumentary
    3. Musculoskeletal
    4. Autonomic nervous system—bowel, bladder
    5. Cognitive
    6. Language
    7. Emotional
V. Assess activity limitations (perform task analyses) of patient-identified problems
VI. Formation of underlying impairments (hypotheses) from the task analyses
VII. Choose specific tests and measures and recommended outcome measures to test underlying impairments or confirm the hypotheses; these might include:
  A. Sensory
    1. Somatosensory
    2. Vestibular
    3. Visual
    4. Hearing
  B. Integrated, perceptual
  C. Motor
    1. Muscle strength
    2. Muscle flexibility
    3. Response speed
    4. Tone
    5. Movement speed
    6. Endurance and fatigue
    7. Complex impairments
      • Basic motor patterns available
      • Modification of motor patterns possible
      • Anticipatory and adaptive responses
      • Variability of performance
  D. Autonomic nervous system
  E. Cognitive
  F. Language
  G. Emotional

GCS, Glasgow Coma Scale; *PTA*, posttraumatic amnesia.

Examination for People With Traumatic Brain Injury
Task Analysis of Activity Limitations

Often the physical therapist begins the examination at the activity limitation level. This involves observing those functions that the patient or family identifies as problematic. Activity limitations in patients with TBI may include loss of mobility in bed, coming to sit, sitting to standing; impaired static and dynamic balance; loss of household and community ambulation and stair negotiation; loss of running, jumping, and kicking skills; poor reach and grasp; loss of activities of daily living (ADLs) such as dressing, toileting, and feeding; and loss of instrumental ADLs such as shopping and driving. The physical or occupational

BOX 22.8   Case Example of Examination, Evaluation, and Prognosis for a Patient With Traumatic Brain Injury

Examination

A patient comes to your clinic reporting that he falls several times a week during walking and would like to improve his balance. He is 21 years old and suffered a moderate traumatic brain injury (TBI) 6 weeks ago. He had a Glasgow Coma Scale (GCS) score of 11 initially and 1.5 days of posttraumatic amnesia (PTA). He was at ABC Rehabilitation Center for 5 weeks and was discharged home last week. He lives with his parents in a single-story house. He is in his third year of college studying geology. His systems review demonstrates slight decreased vital capacity of 3.8 L (4.6 L would be normal), but no abnormalities in the musculoskeletal systems or integumentary system. His cognitive functions are within normal limits according to neuropsychological testing, except for memory deficits.

Task Analysis

You observe this patient during walking and note that he has decreased knee flexion in preswing and decreased dorsiflexion throughout swing phase, with the toe intermittently catching on the carpet when you have him speed up his walking. He also has decreased dorsiflexion at initial contact and in terminal stance.

Testing of Impairments

Because of the decreased dorsiflexion in terminal stance (which is passive), you hypothesize that the decreased dorsiflexion is secondary to gastrocnemius-soleus muscle tightness rather than anterior tibialis weakness. You test the range of motion (ROM) at the ankle, and it is within functional limits. You now develop a second hypothesis that there is increased tone in the gastrocnemius-soleus. On an Ashworth test, the patient scores a level 3 for the gastrocnemius-soleus. Because the patient does not get adequate plantarflexion at preswing (neutral vs. 15 degrees for typical adults), you also hypothesize that the patient is unable to generate plantarflexion fast enough in preswing to achieve the normal 15 degrees of plantarflexion. Testing by having the patient plantar flex rapidly in standing shows that it takes a full 3 seconds (s) to achieve 15 degrees of plantarflexion—much too long to be used in walking.

Outcome Measures for Activity Limitations

The patient is in an outpatient setting and appears to be high functioning. The high-level mobility assessment tool (HiMAT), 6 min walk test, 10 m walk test for gait speed, and various balance scales appear to be appropriate.

Evaluation

The patient is experiencing multiple weekly falls secondary to toe drag at initial swing when walking at speeds over 1.17 m/s. The toe drag comes from decreased dorsiflexion and decreased knee flexion at initial swing because of inadequate plantarflexion. Testing demonstrated both increased gastrocnemius-soleus tone (Ashworth level 3) and decreased ability to generate adequate plantarflexion to achieve the normal 40 degrees of knee flexion during preswing.

Prognosis and Outcomes

The patient has a good prognosis. He is early postinjury, is young, and has good family support and a high education level. There is no history of previous TBI. The patient started rehabilitation immediately and in a center specialized for people with TBI. His PTA was short.

loss of balance in the extension phase, a hypothesis may be poor timing of the gastrocnemius firing. Both of these hypotheses are based on the task analysis but also on the literature, which defines the importance of trunk momentum to initiate seat-off and timing of gastrocnemius firing during the end of the sitting-to-standing activity to maintain balance.

Examining activity limitations requires knowledge of typical movement patterns and task performance among persons without neuromuscular disorders of about the same age as the patient. Tasks that are described in the literature for typical performance include rolling, rolling to sit, sitting, sitting to standing, standing to sitting, standing balance, walking, hopping, jumping, kicking, running, reaching and grasping, throwing, batting, and golfing. The form is a bit messy and we have decided to remove it from the chapter.

Assessing Underlying Impairments

Once the task has been analyzed, the impairments leading to poor performance of the task are identified. Breaking motion down to its most basic components may be helpful, but two caveats are necessary. First, improvement in abnormal components may not lead to improvement in activity limitations. Some critical impairments will have more influences on an activity than will others. For example, Perry and colleagues[60] showed that for normal walking velocity to be attained, although cadence and stride length are important, a strength level of $3+/5$ is a critical component in the ankle muscles. Deficiencies of timing, strength, or sequencing can contribute to poor hand function, but sensory deficits at the hand level may be the critical impairment related to poor manipulation skills. In addition, impairments in the circulatory, respiratory, integumentary, and musculoskeletal systems can account for activity limitation in the patient with TBI (Fig. 22.1). Relative contributions of the impairments to the activity limitation or participation limitation are addressed by the therapist's task analyses, hypothesis, subsequent evaluation, and diagnosis,[61] which will determine the focus of the intervention program.

The second caveat is treating the individual impairments will not necessarily result in the patient learning a skill. Skills result from an organization of many motor functions together and require whole task practice. Conversely, not having a critical component, such as arm strength, may be the one factor preventing a person from learning to perform a skill (e.g., enough force cannot be generated to throw a ball 5 feet in the air to hit a basket). Commonly seen impairments after TBI are reviewed below along with recommended measures.

Impaired consciousness and cognition. As previously mentioned, changes in consciousness are common in the acute phase of TBI. The duration of this change varies depending on the extent of the injury and recovery. Physical therapists often include measures of consciousness to capture changes in this impairment, as consciousness commonly depicts different stages of interventions. Recommended outcome measures for consciousness include Coma Recovery Scale-Revised, LOCF, and GCS.[57]

Cognitive impairments are also common after TBI and may affect overall disability more significantly than physical impairments.[62] It was reported that cognitive impairment was the primary contributor to activity limitation in most patients with TBI who scored at moderate to severe levels on the GOS.[63] The spectrum of cognitive dysfunctions include, but are not limited to, impaired attention, frustration, lack of spontaneity, easily distractible, impaired executive functions, inappropriate affects, altered memory, slowed information processing, and impaired judgment. Traditionally, neuropsychologists, speech pathologists, and occupational therapists all perform testing of cognitive function. Depending on the profession and types of cognitive impairment,

therapist performs a task analysis of the impaired function by comparing the patient's performance of the task with typical task performance. For example, the therapist would observe the patient performing the sitting-to-standing activity, observing that there is inadequate forward trunk momentum in the preextension phase.[59] A reasonable hypothesis may be that the patient is fearful of falling forward. If the problem is

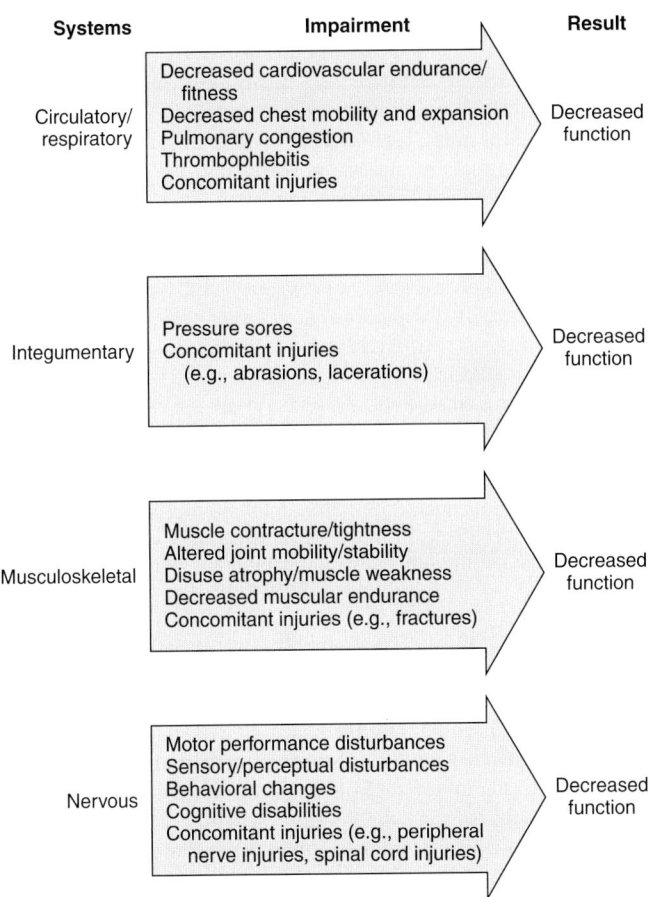

Systems	Impairment	Result
Circulatory/ respiratory	Decreased cardiovascular endurance/ fitness; Decreased chest mobility and expansion; Pulmonary congestion; Thrombophlebitis; Concomitant injuries	Decreased function
Integumentary	Pressure sores; Concomitant injuries (e.g., abrasions, lacerations)	Decreased function
Musculoskeletal	Muscle contracture/tightness; Altered joint mobility/stability; Disuse atrophy/muscle weakness; Decreased muscular endurance; Concomitant injuries (e.g., fractures)	Decreased function
Nervous	Motor performance disturbances; Sensory/perceptual disturbances; Behavioral changes; Cognitive disabilities; Concomitant injuries (e.g., peripheral nerve injuries, spinal cord injuries)	Decreased function

Fig. 22.1 Therapists develop intervention strategies to deal with functional deficits that may result from a variety of problems occurring primarily in one or more of the body systems depicted.

various cognitive tests are employed, and it is beyond the scope of this chapter to introduce all of these cognitive tests and batteries. For physical therapists, the TBI EDGE Task Force highly recommended a physical therapy examination to include the Coma Recovery Scale-Revised or Moss Attention Rating Scale in inpatient settings for moderate to severe TBI.[57] The LOCF (see Appendix 22.A) is also a commonly used measure by physical therapists to record changes of cognitive functions as the patient progresses through various stages of consciousness. The Montreal Cognitive Assessment (MoCA) is a recommended test that has memory testing embedded within it. Refer to Box 22.2 to 22.4 for the full recommendation list by setting and practice.

Autonomic dysfunctions. As mentioned earlier, changes in the ANS after TBI may cause system-wide issues due to the broad spectrum of body functions regulated by the ANS. These functions can directly or indirectly affect the rehabilitation process, and therefore it is important for therapists to measure these functions from time to time. These measures surround vital sign measurements, for example heart rate, respiratory rate, blood pressure, etc. Since orthostatic challenge is reported,[21] therapists should monitor appropriate vital signs in various patient positions, especially when persons are symptomatic. Sophisticated measurements of ANS functions are usually performed by physicians, for example, using electrocardiographic marker to track sympathetic and parasympathetic activities, measuring pupillary light reflex, measuring arterial pulse wave, and measuring eyeball pressure.[22]

Impaired strength or force production. Evidence consistently shows that strength and force production are common impairments in both the UEs and LEs after TBI. When strength control or force gradations are significantly impaired at initial admission (about 25% of patients), research has shown improvements with near to full resolution at a 2-year follow-up, with only 12% impairment remaining in the UEs and 7% in the LEs.[23] Low power production is also thought to be the major contributor to impaired mobility.[64]

In the case of upper motor neuron lesions, weakness can be a major problem. The number of motor neurons activated, and the type of motor neurons and muscle fibers recruited, affect force. Motor neurons in the motor cortex can be deficient, leading to disordered and reduced recruitment. Individuals with brain damage show early atrophy and loss of motor units, as well as motor units that fatigue easily.[65,66] Disuse, cast immobilization, joint dysfunction, improper nutrition, medications, and aging can cause differential weakness with altered morphological, biochemical, and physiological characteristics within the muscle.[67] Electromyography (EMG) studies by numerous investigators[68,69] suggest that reduced activity alters motor unit properties, discharge frequency, and recruitment patterns. Performance problems are reflected in the inability to generate force in different directions and against different loads, as well as in problems sustaining force output.[14]

Changes in muscle length affect strength. In patients who have had a cerebrovascular accident (CVA), shortened muscles tend to be strong in short ranges and lengthened muscles are strongest in lengthened ranges but weak in shorter positions compared with the strength-length curves of normal muscles.[70]

Strength may be examined functionally—for example, by seeing if the patient has enough strength to lift the arm overhead, out to the side, and up to the mouth, or is able to go from sitting to standing. In some cases, such as those in which the patient is unable to perform balance reactions or has been on extended bed rest, testing individual muscles may be important. Traditional manual muscle testing (MMT) with force transducers or strength testing with isokinetic testing[71] throughout the range provides good strength information. The level of testing chosen should be consistent with the deficit and the therapist's knowledge of its importance in contributing to the activity limitation.

Muscle endurance refers to the ability of a muscle to produce the same level of contraction over time. The subjective feeling of effort and weakness after fatiguing exercise may be related to the need to recruit more motor units and to increase the mean firing frequency of the motor units to maintain constant force output.[72] EMG with medium-frequency analysis can test this type of fatigue. Fatigue can also be assessed by measurement of maximal voluntary force, maximal voluntary shortening velocity, or power.[72] Decreased force production, prolonged time to relaxation of muscle fibers, and recruitment of additional muscles during an activity are characteristic of fatigue.[73] Although repeated muscle testing can pick up decreased strength in specific muscles, in most instances overwork fatigue is first noted by an altered pattern of movement of body segments during activity.

Impaired muscle length and joint range of motion. Flexibility at the muscle and joint level is critical for normal posture and movement. Muscle atrophy occurs rapidly,[65] and changes in muscle fiber type and function can be seen as early as 3 days. Viscoelastic properties change with paralysis so that the muscle feels stiffer.[74,75]

The examination should determine the contribution of muscle tone, joint structure, and tissue factors in limiting flexibility. Active and passive motion should be compared because stiffness (not contracture) often prevents normal function. For example, active dorsiflexion is often limited in patients who have full passive ankle range of motion (ROM) because stiffness begins at neutral. The functional result is foot drop or toe catch in the early part of the swing phase of gait because the anterior tibialis muscle cannot generate adequate force production to overcome the stiffness in the gastrocnemius and soleus. This restriction also may limit forward movement of the tibia over the foot during the stance phase of gait, resulting in hip retraction or an apparent balance loss. Knee hyperextension also can result from lack of forward motion of the tibia. Flexibility measurements are done with goniometers, motion analysis systems, tape measures, inclinometers, photographs, or electronic devices. Taking both passive and active measurements is critical in identifying intervention approaches.

Abnormal muscle tone and reflexes. In the motor learning theories of today, many of the behaviors and resulting motor patterns after brain injury are seen as attempts by the CNS to compensate for loss. For example, spasticity may be the result of an attempt to compensate for the patient's inability to increase force. When the amplitude of a contraction cannot be increased because of the injury, the CNS may increase the length of time the muscle fires or may recruit muscles not normally used in a particular pattern of movement; both are characteristics seen in spasticity.

Whatever the cause of increased tone, the therapist can evaluate tone at two levels: is it interfering with function, and, if so, can it be changed? Spasticity is not a single problem.[66–69,74,76–80] Spasticity can have any or all of the following characteristics:

- Changes in response to stretch
- Decreased ability to produce appropriate force for a specific task
- Increased latency of activation
- Inability to rapidly turn off muscles
- Loss of reciprocal inhibition between spastic muscles and their antagonists
- Changes in the intrinsic properties of the muscle fibers
- Inability to generate enough antagonist power to overcome spastic muscles

Examination begins with identifying whether there is increased or decreased muscle tension at rest. If it is increased, is the tension at the muscle level (stiffness or sarcomere involvement) or the neurological level? Muscle stiffness resulting from tissue changes is common in the patient with brain injury. If there is increased tone during movement, EMG may be beneficial to determine the nature of the tone. Is it a problem of co-contraction of agonist and antagonist at a joint? Is it a problem of prolonged contraction? Or is it poor sequencing, either temporally or spatially, of other muscles involved in the movement?

Spatial sequencing of movement involves the contraction of a preset group of muscles. Temporal sequencing involves the contraction of muscles in a fixed sequence. EMG and video analysis provide additional depth of information regarding the sequence and timing of movement patterns. For example, is the normal temporal sequencing in the distal-to-proximal manner present in the UE during a reaching task? In a balance reaction, are the ankle, hip, and back extensors (spatial sequencing) all contracting in response to a forward perturbation?

The most commonly used tool in examination of tone is the Ashworth Scale or Modified Ashworth Scale (MAS) (Box 22.9).[81] The Tardieu Scale[82] is similar, but testing is done at three different velocities and may provide a clearer picture of what is caused by tone versus muscle shortening. Testing of deep tendon reflexes identifies problems with stretch reflexes, and surface EMG (sEMG) can determine the presence of co-contraction, prolonged contraction, sequence and timing problems, and increased latencies.

Impaired coordination. Ataxia was one of the most common findings among military personnel who had sustained TBI,[23] with 32% of patients showing ataxia initially and 14% at the 2-year follow-up. There are many subcategories of ataxia, including dysmetria, dyssynergia, rebound phenomenon, dysdiadochokinesia, and intention tremor.

BOX 22.9 Modified Ashworth Scale

Grade	Description
0+	No increase in muscle tone
1+	Slight increase in muscle tone, manifested by a catch and release or by minimal resistance at the end of the range of motion (ROM) when the affected part(s) is moved in flexion or extension
1+	Slight increase in muscle tone, manifested by a catch, followed by minimal resistance throughout the remainder (less than half) of the ROM
2	More marked increase in muscle tone through most of the ROM, but affected part(s) easily moved
3	Considerable increase in muscle tone, passive movement difficult
4	Affected part(s) rigid in flexion or extension

Reprinted from Bohannon R, Smith M. Interrater reliability of a Modified Ashworth Scale of muscle spasticity. *Phys Ther.* 1987;67:207, with permission of the American Physical Therapy Association.

Many clinical tests to assess coordination impairments are available. Common tests include finger-nose-finger test for UE coordination, and heel to shin/heel slides for the LEs.

Impaired sensory function. Sensory functions are often impaired after a moderate to severe TBI. Problems in the sensory system are often reflected in the motor system, creating distorted movement through faulty information in the feedforward or feedback processes.

Two broad categories of sensations can be defined on the basis of the type of information: primary sensation and cortical, or integrative, sensation. This arbitrary division is useful functionally, but it is not anatomically based. Primary sensation includes exteroception and proprioception. The exteroceptors of smell, sight, and hearing are sometimes referred to as teloreceptors. Vision, hearing, olfaction, gustation, pain, touch, temperature, proprioception, and kinesthesia are commonly affected primary sensations. Sensation cannot be clinically tested without patient participation.

- **Proprioception.** Deficits associated with poor balance included a high number of subjects with discriminative touch deficits in one study,[83] an impairment related to poor UE function. Traditional examinations of proprioception include the ability to distinguish motion and motion direction at each joint. Some patients who cannot distinguish direction or movement still function well. They may have proprioceptive function at the unconscious level (e.g., cerebellar) while not perceiving the input at the parietal level (conscious level).

  Testing is performed by having the patient close his or her eyes; then the therapist places a joint in a specific position (e.g., flexed, extended) and asks the patient to name/identify the position either verbally or with the uninvolved limb. Asking the patient to close the eyes and identify when the therapist passively moves a joint while the patient indicates specific direction of movement can test joint movement sense, or kinesthesia, especially for those with multilimb involvement. Very small joint movements of about 1 degree are within the discrimination level of typical individuals.

- **Light touch.** Light touch is tested with a brush for localization and quality of sensation. For more definitive light-touch discrimination, especially on the hands and feet to determine peripheral neuropathies, a monofilament test[84] can be used.

- **Two-point discrimination.** Two-point discrimination can be tested with instruments specifically designed to measure how far apart two separate spots of contact need to be to identify them as distinct. For patients who are thought to be ignoring stimuli on one side, testing at the same time bilaterally is first performed, and then each limb is retested separately. Patients who extinguish stimuli will respond that they feel only one stimulus when both limbs are tested simultaneously but will perceive the stimulus just fine when each limb is tested separately. This is called the bilateral extinction test.
- **Stereognosis.** Stereognosis, the ability to identify objects placed in the hand without visual assistance, may be critical to normal hand use. The therapist places multiple common and culturally appropriate objects, such as pens, coins, and safety pins, in the hand and asks the patient to identify the objects while the eyes are closed.

Impaired vision and visual perception. Vision is critical in recovery of many motor functions because it is responsible for much of the feedforward, or anticipatory, control of movement and the initial development of a movement pattern. For example, balance can be maintained through the visual system by modifying synergies before surface change occurs. Feedback through the peripheral field via the movement of the visual array on the retina can also trigger balance responses. Campbell[83] found problems with visual functions in most patients with mild to moderate TBI; these problems involved poor visual acuity (48%) and problems with vergence (85%), which can cause blurring and doubling of vision, and smooth pursuit (63%), which can cause a "jumping" of the visual image.

Some patients are able to use their hands for grasp and release, in spite of severe somatosensory deficits, when they are able to use vision to guide the motion. Many of the standard movement tests should be performed with and without vision.

General visual functions can be screened by the physical or occupational therapist as follows:

1. Tracking is assessed by use of an H pattern of movement of the object being tracked with the eyes and not with head movement. The examiner observes any nystagmus or refixation saccades. Eye muscle paralysis can be observed during tracking if the patient cannot move the eye(s) laterally, up, down, or medially.
2. Focus, or accommodation, can be checked by observing constriction and dilation of the pupil. Constriction occurs as an object is moved toward the nose, and dilation as the object is moved away from the nose.
3. Binocular vision is controlled through feedback from blurred or doubled vision. This reflex signals whether the eyes and fovea are focused on a single point or target, as the images in both eyes fall on the same retinal points. A "cover test" can screen for binocular vision. The patient stares at an object at about 18 inches from the nose. The therapist covers one eye. If there is movement to adjust the remaining uncovered eye back to the object, both retinas may not be focusing on the same point. Observing whether light reflections fall on exactly the same place on both pupils is useful in evaluating binocular eye focus. Vergence testing can also be an indicator of binocular visual functions.
4. Visual fields can be grossly tested by having the patient look forward at a point (observer sits in front of the patient to be sure the patient remains focused straight ahead). The patient indicates when he or she first sees an object coming into the peripheral field from behind, or the "spotter" notes when the patient looks toward the object.
5. Vergence is tested by having the patient observe an object or pen tip as it is brought from about 20 inches away. The patient is told to follow the object with his or her eyes. The object is moved at a moderate speed toward the bridge of the nose, and the patient

reports when the object becomes blurred or doubles. When typical convergence is present, there will be no blurring or doubling until the object is 2 inches away or closer, and when the object is moved back out, the patient will report the object as single within 4 inches.
6. Visual interactions with the vestibular system are assessed through the vestibuloocular reflex (VOR). This reflex allows people to maintain a fixed gaze on a target as the head moves. The object should not appear to blur, move, or double during head motion at various speeds.
7. Perceptual tests that evaluate how visual information is used include visual memory tests, cancellation tests, and figure-ground tests.
8. Visual acuity is tested using a Snellen eye chart. Poor acuity can affect balance responses. Neuro-optometrists and neuro-ophthalmologists are appropriate referrals for patients needing in-depth visual workups, especially when visual perception is involved. See Chapter 28 for additional information on vision and visual testing.

Deficits in the vestibular system. The vestibular system monitors the position of the head in space and helps distinguish if the body or the visual surrounding is moving. It also provides a vertical reference to gravity to maintain the head upright. Vertigo, dizziness, eye-head incoordination, and postural and balance complications occur as a result of problems in the vestibular-cerebellar systems. Details of vestibular rehabilitation are described further, and readers are encouraged to see Chapter 21 for more information.

Vestibular deficits are common after TBI with an estimated 30% to 65% of people affected.[85] Patients with mild or moderate TBI have a high rate (23.8% to 81%) of complaints of dizziness.[86,87] In many cases dizziness is a sign of vestibular dysfunction and may prolong recovery from TBI.[23,87] TBI-related vestibular disorders can be central or peripheral, for example benign paroxysmal positional vertigo (BPPV), central vertigo, or perilymphatic fistula. Testing of the vestibular system should be conducted according to the patient's complaints of symptoms. A comprehensive history and vestibular examination are instrumental for accurate diagnosis, targeted interventions, and promoting recovery.

In general, a vestibular system examination should include assessment of the oculomotor system (e.g., smooth pursuit, saccades, vergence), assessment of VOR function (e.g., head thrust test), and position test (e.g., Dix-Hallpike) according to the patient's complaints.[87] For example, symptoms occurring only with specific head movements can be an indicator of problems in the semicircular canals, which points toward the diagnosis of BPPV. Dizziness with head tilts might indicate problems in the otolithic system and VOR tests should be conducted. Other advanced evaluation tools, such as electronystagmography, may be used when symptoms and complaints are more complex. Since postural instability is also a common manifestation in patients with vestibular disorders, outcome measures on balance and/or sensory organization are common tests to be included, which will be discussed in the following section on Assessing Activity Limitations. See Chapter 20 and 21 for additional information on balance and vestibular testing.

Impaired cardiovascular endurance (deconditioning). For persons after TBI, peaked aerobic capacity is found to be lowered by 25% to 35% compare to matched sedentary group.[88] In addition, the ventilatory anaerobic threshold (submaximal exercise response correlated with cardiovascular fitness) after TBI is also found to be below the demand of many everyday activities.[89] It is therefore imperative to investigate cardiovascular endurance in people with TBI. Mossberg and colleagues[90] in their review paper stated that maximal graded exercise tests using leg cycle ergometry and treadmill are both reliable for persons after TBI, though treadmill is preferred over cycle ergometry due to its functional nature. Submaximal tests are good alternatives when equipment and time are concerns. The 6 minute walk test is a recommended choice by both Mossberg and colleagues[91] and the TBI EDGE Task Force.[57]

Fatigue, which is separate from impaired endurance, may result from increased energy requirements resulting from less efficient motor patterns or from more CNS activity. Fatigue is a common complaint after TBI[92] and is associated with insomnia.[93] Testing for fatigue is challenging because it is multifactorial. The Global Fatigue Index is recommended for physical therapists to assess fatigue in outpatient settings.[57]

Impaired communication. Primary damage to the language and communication centers in the brain sustained during the accident or injury, alone or in combination with cognitive, motor and sensory impairments, often result in impaired communication following a TBI. Various communication disorders after TBI are reported in the literature (e.g., aphasia, dysarthria, social communication,[94] reading comprehension[95]). Although it is not within the scope of practice for physical therapists to formally assess and treat communication disorders, it is a domain included in many commonly used measures by physical therapists, for example the MoCA. Physical therapists need to be aware of the deficits and modify communication strategies during rehabilitation intervention. The speech and language therapist typically assesses and treats communication disorders, and makes recommendations for interprofessional team members regarding augmented or alternative communication strategies.

Emotional and behavioral problems. Examining behavioral changes after TBI is important because they are major sequelae of the injury. These changes include impulsiveness, disinhibition, anger, lack of initiative, and apathy, among others. Because the effect of behavioral changes is multidimensional, it is thought that all health care professionals play a role in evaluating behavioral issues in persons post-TBI.[96] It is, however, still best for neuropsychologists or neuropsychiatrists to administer neurobehavioral tests as special training is required.[96] Some measures are appropriate for physical therapists to administer, namely the Agitated Behavior Scale, Apathy Evaluation Scale, and LOCF.[57]

Assessing Activity Limitations

Activity in the ICF model is defined as the execution of tasks or an action with a functional purpose. Examples of activities include bed mobility (e.g., rolling), transfer, balance, ambulation, wheelchair mobility, running, bathing, grooming, toileting, and dressing. When assessing these activities, it is important to evaluate both the quality of movements, as well as the quantitative components (e.g., speed of movement, distance). Physical therapists should pay attention to the following quality of movements when assessing a task:

- Is the patient able to use the basic motor patterns for the task in a functional manner?
- Is the patient able to modify and then accomplish the task?
- Is there good interlimb coordination as demonstrated by coordinated two-handed activities, good timing between limbs in walking, and jumping?
- Does the patient appear to have the ability to coordinate motions (decrease the degrees of freedom), or are they limited by too few degrees of freedom?
- Does the patient respond correctly to environmental changes or stimuli such as stepping over or around objects or being able to walk on different terrain?

- When motor patterns are used, are they appropriate for the stimulus? For example, is the ankle strategy used for standing on a firm surface and when stopping walking?
- Are automatic movement patterns present (e.g., balance synergies, walking, and running)? Are volitional or voluntary movements present?
- Can the patient accomplish the same task in several ways? Can the patient adapt to different task demands?

The following subsections reviewed the commonly seen activity limitations after TBI and recommended outcome measures in this ICF domain.

Basic functional mobility. Functional mobility usually includes bed mobility, transfer (sit to/from stand and transfer to/from different surfaces), basic locomotion, and basic ADLs. After a TBI, approximately 40% of patients experience limited functional mobility[97] due to physical and cognitive impairments, resulting in need for personal assistance.[98] Assessing functional mobility is therefore imperative, especially during the early phase of rehabilitation. Recommended outcome measures for assessing basic functional mobility include Functional Independence Measure (FIM), Functional Assessment Measure (FAM), and Barthel Index.[57] More than one functional mobility type is usually included in the measure to capture a comprehensive picture of the person's mobility and functional level. These measures are often administered in acute or inpatient rehabilitation settings when patients require more assistance in mobility and improvement in this area is more substantial.

Sitting balance. Brown and colleagues[99] found sitting balance to be impaired in 52% of the patients with TBI at initial examination in their review. Testing usually includes static sitting without arm support and dynamic sitting with the patient reaching in multiple directions or ability to resist perturbations. These are not standardized tests but are commonly used clinical tests to assess sitting balance.

Standing balance. Standing balance after TBI is usually affected in mild, moderate, and severe injuries, with 82% of patients exhibiting standing balance deficits. Deficits include both motor strategy problems and appropriate use and integration of somatosensory, visual, and vestibular information. Newton[100] reported that patients with moderate and severe TBI showed significantly impaired reaction times to perturbation in standing. Although they could grade their responses to the perturbations appropriately, the responses were often asymmetrical.

The TBI EDGE Task Force recommended various outcome measures for assessing standing balance in patients with TBI.[57] Depending on the patient's functional level and settings where therapy occurs, different measures should be selected. For example, the Berg Balance Scale and Community Balance and Mobility Scale are recommended for both inpatient and outpatient rehabilitation settings. The Balance Error Scoring System is recommended for outpatient rehabilitation settings where the patient is tested on the types of standing balance error in double leg stance, single leg stance, and tandem stance on firm and foam surfaces. Sensory Organization Test is also a recommended test and is an appropriate choice for the patient with vestibular symptoms.[87]

Gait and dual-task gait ability. The motor impairments of TBI often result in spatiotemporal gait deficits, including a decrease in velocity, asymmetry of step lengths, increased double limb support time, reduced step length, and increased mediolateral sway.[101,102] Tandem gait (ataxia) is also prominent post-TBI and can remain at 2-year follow-up.[23] For individuals with ataxia after TBI, it was found that they have reduced interjoint coordination during gait, and this coordination further deteriorated during more complex walking situations such as narrow base of support or when carrying an object.[103]

Impaired gait mobility is also perceived as a contributor to falls in post-TBI.[104] It is obvious that gait abnormalities after TBI can pose a significant limitation in everyday activity and warrant detailed measurement.

There is a wide range of gait outcome measures. Similar to other impairments and activity limitations, selection of appropriate gait outcome measures is based upon patients' functional level and settings where therapy takes place. For acute care and inpatient rehabilitation settings, gait assessment is oftentimes included in generic functional mobility measures such as FIM and FAM.[57] Together with these outcome measures, a qualitative gait description through task analysis should be done in order to identify underlying impairments.

For individuals with basic ambulatory function, more robust gait outcome measures are recommended and include the 6 minute walk test, 10 m walk test, HiMAT, and Functional Gait Assessment.[57]

Another type of gait outcome measure that should be included for high-functioning patients with TBI is gait ability during dual-task situations. Dual tasking is a common daily function (e.g., walking while attending to a conversation) and entails performing one cognitive and one motor task at the same time. Since motor and cognitive impairments are major sequelae of TBI, it is expected that dual-task abilities are even more compromised. In fact for persons post-TBI, despite well recovery of motor gait ability, reaction time during dual-task gait activity is significantly longer compared to age-matched group.[105] The TBI EDGE Task Force recommended the Walking and Remembering Test to assess dual-task gait ability in persons post-TBI.[57] In addition, the modified Walking and Remembering Test and Timed Up and Go-Cognitive together with the Walking and Remembering Test have been shown to be reliable and feasible for persons in inpatient rehabilitation settings.[106] Physical therapists are encouraged to include dual-task measures when appropriate because they may be more indicative of functional outcomes.

Upper extremity function. UE function includes tasks that require reaching, grasping, pinching, etc. and can be affected after TBI. Clinical presentations for upper limb dysfunction after TBI may be similar to those with hemiplegia or hemiparesis—for example, impaired timing and reduced accuracy of reaching and grasping.[107] The Action Research Arm Test and Wolf Motor Function Test are recommended outcome measures specifically for assessment of upper limb function.[57] There are also generic outcome measures that assess activities requiring upper limb functions. An example being FIM where grooming is included as a test item and is a task where upper limb function is highly indicative.

Assessing Participation Restrictions

Participation restrictions refer to limitations an individual experiences in his or her life roles. As such, each individual's participation restrictions after TBI can be very different and limitless. Examples include inability to drive, restriction in work duties, inability to participate in school activities, or restriction in carrying out the role as a parent. While the focus of rehabilitation programs for TBI is on improving motor and cognitive outcomes at the impairment and activity limitation levels, measuring participation is equally important as it affects the patient's quality of life after an injury. The ultimate goal for rehabilitation is for patients to resume participations at preinjury level, such as returning to work or school.[108] A recent Cochrane review[109] included several indicators as primary and secondary outcomes when investigating effectiveness of cognitive rehabilitation programs. These outcome indicators include return to work, independence in ADL, community integration, and quality of life. Most of these outcomes are in the participation category of the ICF model, implying the ultimate long-term goal of effective rehabilitation is to improve patients' functioning in society, and hence assessment in this area should be included.

Some common participation measures are introduced for inclusion in the examination process. The ultimate choice depends upon the patient's role and meaningful function in the society in which they live. From the physical therapy perspective, the TBI EDGE Task Force recommends to include outcome measures on community integration and quality of life in outpatient settings.[57] These measures include Disability Rating Scale, Quality of Life after Brain Injury, Community Integration Questionnaire, and Sydney Psychosocial Reintegration Scale. Usually, participation restriction measures are administered in outpatient or community clinical settings because this is the time when patients and family/caregivers focus on long-term life plans. Specific participation measures associated with certain impairments can also be included. For example, if balance and falling is an issue after TBI, therapists could include the Activity-specific Balance Confidence Scale to assess the impact of balance on daily life.

Interventions for People With Traumatic Brain Injury

Roles and Responsibilities of the Interprofessional Rehabilitation Team

TBI results in a myriad of physical, psychological, behavioral, and cognitive impairments. Comprehensive rehabilitation requires an interprofessional team approach due to the complex clinical presentation following a moderate to severe TBI. Research has shown that medical management, in addition to early onset and continuous rehabilitation, is most effective when delivered in a specialized neurotrauma/brain injury unit by an interdisciplinary health care team.[110,111]

As most people who have experienced a moderate to severe TBI have cognitive impairments and reduced ability to learn, consistency and repetition of management strategies is required to optimize effectiveness. This requires regular, ongoing communication among interprofessional team members, including the patient, family, and friends involved in their care. Each member of the interprofessional team will focus their plan of care on interventions within their primary scope of practice. However, all providers will need to carefully consider other aspects of the injury and incorporate recommendations for managing impairments outside their scope of practice into their plan of care to optimize patient outcomes. For example, PT's should incorporate strategies for managing communication impairments, memory loss, reduced orientation, as well as behavior modification, into their interventions in order to be effective. See Table 22.5 for a list of interprofessional health care team members and their primary role in caring for people with TBI.

Physical Therapy Interventions Through the Care Continuum

The continuum of care and common practice settings for persons with moderate to severe TBI are presented in Fig. 22.2. As each person and brain injury is unique, the settings required for optimal care, and length of time spent in each, will differ. The focus of rehabilitation will vary depending upon the practice setting, severity of the brain injury, the person's level of consciousness, physical functioning, and personal goals. However, there are general physical therapy management goals that are prioritized among the settings. Regardless of practice setting or patient acuity, physical therapists should work with the interprofessional team to prevent secondary complications, including pneumonia, pressure sores, adaptive shortening of soft tissue, disuse atrophy, heterotropic ossification (HO), joint contractures, and deep vein thrombosis (DVT) through aggressive bronchopulmonary hygiene, positioning schedules, tone management techniques, pressure relieving mattresses, cushions and splints, and daily ROM and stretching programs. Physical therapists working with individuals with head injury should also receive competency training on the medical monitoring and treatment devices commonly used in the neurological intensive

TABLE 22.5 Interprofessional Team and Roles/Responsibilities in Care of Persons With Traumatic Brain Injury

Discipline	Roles and Responsibilities
Social Worker/Case Manager	Coordination of care and discharge planning with team, family, and insurance company
Neuropsychologist/Neuropsychiatrist	Evaluate and treat cognitive, emotional, and behavioral issues due to CNS disorders
Neuro-optometrist/Ophthalmologist	Diagnose and treat visual disorders due to CNS injury
Neurologist/Neurosurgeon	Physicians specializing in diagnosis and treatment of nervous system disorders
Physiatrist	Physicians specializing in physical medicine and rehabilitation; often coordinates care during the rehabilitation process
Pharmacist	Experts in medications and drug interactions; prepare medication as ordered by prescribers
Nurse	Maintain and/or restore health of all body systems; administer medications ordered by prescribers
Occupational Therapist	Focus on improving activities of daily living such as feeding, bathing, grooming, driving, etc.; address cognitive, visual, and social skill impairments
Physical Therapist	Movement specialists; focus on improving functional mobility by addressing the movement system and movement dysfunction
Speech and Language Pathologist	Focus on improving ability to speak, swallow, and communicate orally, through writing or augmented communication devices
Recreational Therapist	Focus on improving self-esteem, social skills, motor skills, coordination, endurance, cognitive skills, and leisure skills

Brain Injury Association of America. *CNS,* Central nervous system.

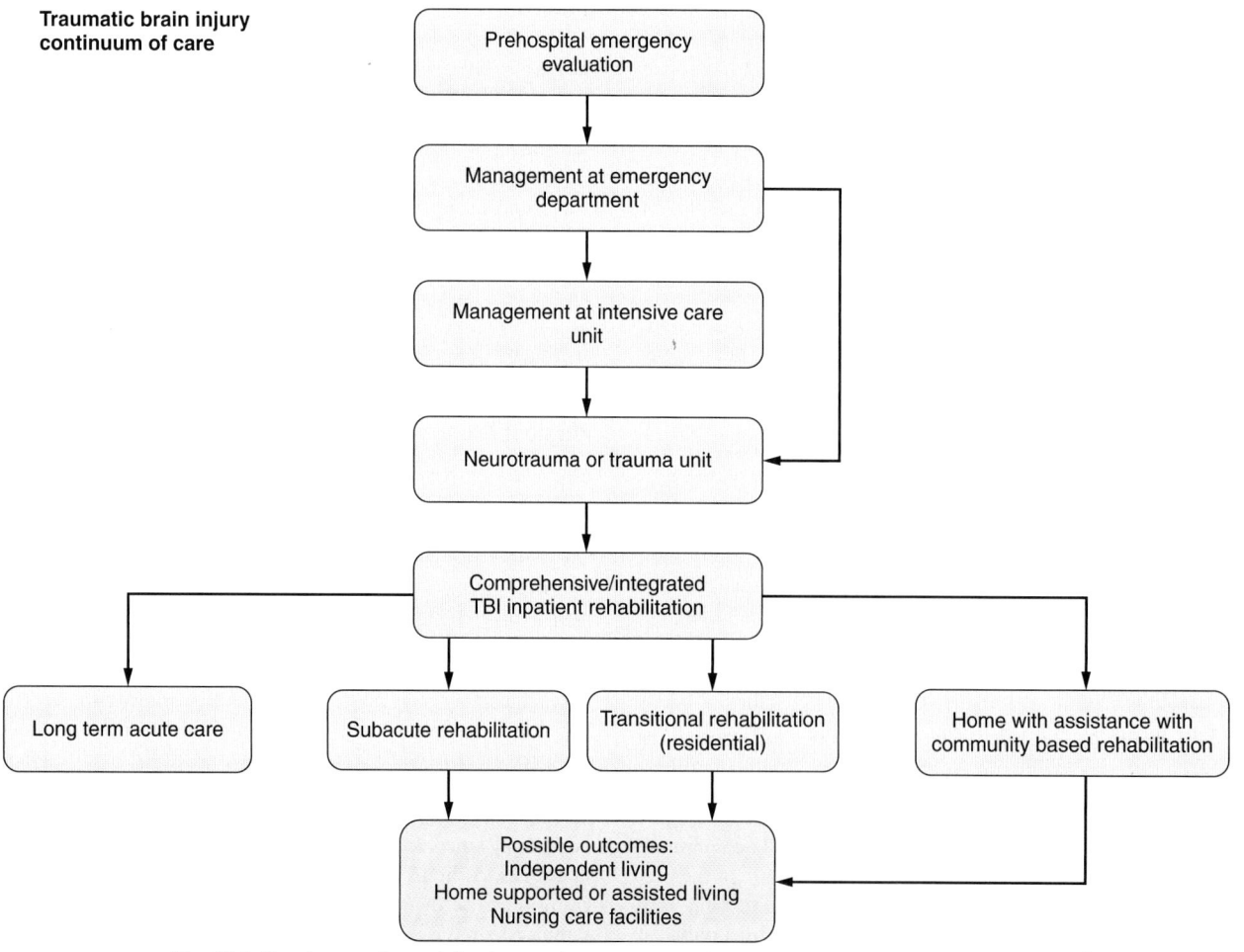

Fig. 22.2 Continuum of care following moderate to severe brain injury. *TBI,* Traumatic brain injury.

care unit (ICU) and acute care settings. Precautions for all of the devices must be observed, and therapists should closely monitor all lab values and vital signs throughout physical therapy sessions to maintain patient safety and prevent complications.

Within the ED, neurological ICU, and/or trauma center, the primary focus of all care is on preservation of life and neural tissue, and prevention of secondary complications. In these acute stages of a moderate to severe TBI while the person is in the ICU or trauma center, physical therapy interventions that should be prioritized are early mobility, and improving level of arousal and awareness for people with DOC. Early mobilization is well supported in the literature to improve long-term outcomes and reduce costs of care and has been shown to be safe for people in the neurological ICU.[112–114]

Once the person is transferred to a step-down unit or is in a neurological acute care unit and level of arousal is improved, the priorities shift towards increasing mobility and improving meaningful interactions with the environment. In acute or subacute rehabilitation, priorities are on maximizing safety and independence with functional mobility, performance of ADLs, and appropriate interactions with others and the environment. For persons who remain in a lower level of consciousness such as coma or VS, discharge is often to a long-term care facility due to payor issues and eligibility requirements for rehabilitation facilities. Unfortunately, signs of emerging from VS and progressing to MCS and beyond are often missed in this setting, and people do not receive regular or intensive physical therapy as they are not capable of making consistent progress early in recovery. Further, the time it takes for physical recovery from DOC is often much longer than the short length of stay, which is predetermined by insurance companies in the United States, currently.[17] It has been demonstrated that a specialized early treatment program for people with DOC can lead to over half of participants' progress to a level of consciousness that makes them eligible for admission to a mainstream inpatient rehabilitation facility.[115] Therefore a paradigm shift is needed in the clinical management for persons with trauma-related DOC.

The post-rehab goals for a person with moderate to severe TBI will depend on residual deficits and level of function; however, the focus is typically on participation in society and community reintegration, including return to school/work/family responsibilities and independent function. Despite advances in medical care and rehabilitation interventions, most people experience chronic effects of brain injury, including residual functional deficits, emotional problems, and cognitive impairments. Evidence now suggests that TBI may also lead to chronic brain injury (CBI), a degenerative process that can progress over a person's life-span and result in Alzheimer disease, as well as progressive motor deficits.[116,117] Thus long-term, individualized care plans with lifelong supports are needed to manage chronic effects of brain injury whether they are static or progressive.[118] Many clinicians now advocate for periodic therapy, sometimes referred to as a "dental model of care," for persons with CBI and other neuromuscular conditions such as Parkinson disease, multiple sclerosis, cerebral palsy, and others. The goal of periodic therapy is to improve overall health, physical function, and participation in life roles through self-management with an emphasis on healthy behaviors, including exercise, proper nutrition, and avoidance of substances like nicotine and alcohol.[119]

Interventions for Disorders of Consciousness (Levels of Cognitive Functioning I–III)

Consciousness comprises the domains of arousal, or level of alertness, and awareness to both self and environmental factors. As stated in the clinical features section of this chapter, DOCs are common after a TBI and may also be experienced by persons diagnosed with a stroke, brain tumor, infectious process, alcohol overdose, or poisoning.[119] The primary focus of management for people with DOC is on prevention of secondary complications and restoration of cognitive-behavioral functions.[17] The DOC state corresponds to LOCF I–III.

Standards of care for clinical management for DOC are lacking, and there is a dearth of evidence-based interventions shown to improve outcomes for this population despite many recent advances in understanding the neuropathophysiology, standardization of terminology, and improving accuracy of diagnosis.[120] The logistical and ethical issues related to placebo-controlled studies constrain this type of research.[121] However, clinicians are reminded that a tenant of evidence-based medicine is the integration of clinical expertise with best available external evidence, thus past clinical experience should be utilized in decision making for the management of persons with DOC.[122] Further, clinicians are obligated to provide reasonable treatments within their scope of care regardless of the state of the published literature.[120] Lastly, the considerable data on long-term outcomes (which will be discussed at the end of this chapter) shows that the majority of people emerge from DOC following head trauma, providing justification for physical therapy interventions and other rehabilitation measures.

The physical therapy plan of care for people with DOC should include interventions previously mentioned for limiting common secondary complications, including contractures, thrombo-embolic disease, HO, pulmonary infections, and pressure sores. Additionally, diligent management of spasticity is recommended to prevent contractures, limit need for costly tendon release surgeries, improve positioning and comfort, and promote readiness for active therapy such as transfers and standing balance, which would be precluded if there were plantarflexion contractures. Effectively managed hypertonia can also decrease the effort and time required to provide all other routine care and possibly reduce caregiver burnout.[115,123] It has been demonstrated that frequency of physical therapy influences spasticity in a positive manner, and that persons with DOC who receive four sessions of therapy per week have less spasticity and fewer contractures than persons who receive less therapy.[123] Interventions, including prolonged stretch, prolonged positioning with splints and/or serial casts, modalities such as heat and cold, and weight bearing have all been shown to reduce spasticity. If conservative measures fail to address the hypertonicity, communication with team members, including the neurologists and physiatrist, are indicated for further medical management, which may include phenol or Botox injections, oral medications, or intrathecal pump delivery of Baclofen.

Restorative treatments within a physical therapist's scope of practice include increasing level of arousal to promote normal sleep-wake cycles.[120] There are two primary types of interventions used in neurorehabilitation to increase arousal level: upright positioning and sensory stimulation. Placing a person with head injury in an upright position has been shown to increase responsiveness and behaviors.[124] People post brain injury who are diagnosed with VS or MCS are most responsive in standing, but also more responsive sitting in a wheelchair compared to lying supine.[125] This is widely believed to be due to increased activation of the reticular formation, the central core of nuclei that run through the brain stem and are responsible for maintaining consciousness.[126] Sound clinical reasoning with careful consideration of factors such as medical stability and comorbidities, level of consciousness, activity orders, precautions (spine, weight bearing, craniectomy, aspiration, behavior, seizure, etc.), and availability of equipment and personnel should be used to determine the safest method of mobilizing a person and achieving upright positioning. For persons who are in a coma and/or medically unstable, a hospital bed that moves into a reverse Trendelenburg position or converts to a chair may

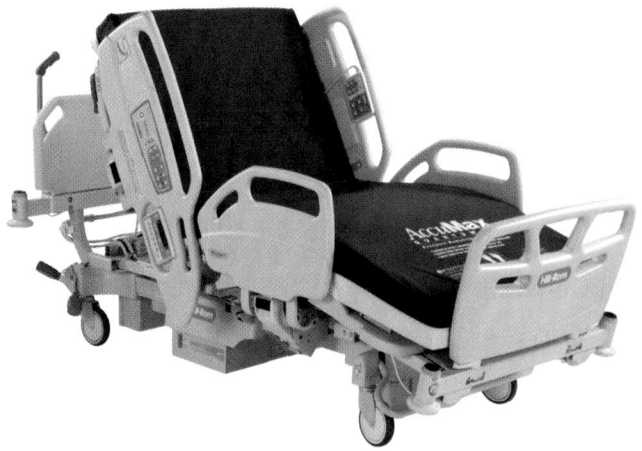

Fig. 22.3 Hospital bed converts to chair for upright positioning to improve level of arousal.

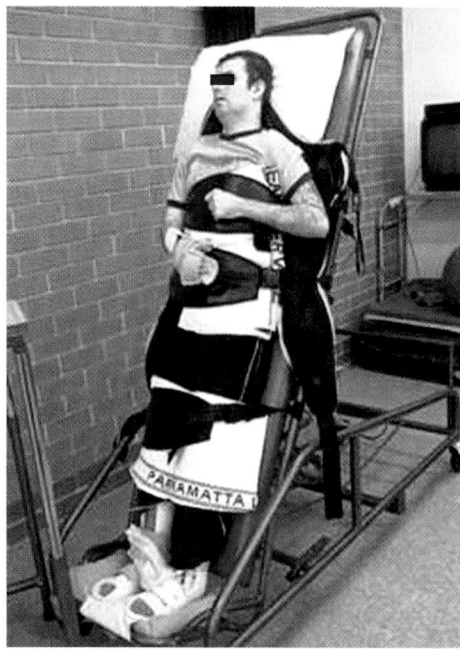

Fig. 22.4 Use of tilt table to promote arousal, increase weight bearing through lower extremities, and improve cardiovascular tolerance to position changes.

be most appropriate to initiate upright positioning if available (Fig. 22.3).

Use of a tilt table (Fig. 22.4) to gradually increase upright posture and position is also used for this patient population due to the fact that safety can be maintained even when the patient is unable to follow commands or actively participate in the treatment. The person can be transferred via a slide board or with bed sheets from hospital bed to the tilt table, then safely strapped to the table with harnesses and belts before moving the person to an upright position, which limits risk of a fall. Additional benefits of using a tilt table include early weight-bearing to promote circulation and prevent DVT, redistribution of pressure points on skin, improve renal function, improve ankle ROM, decrease spasticity in the LE, improve respiration, preserve bone density, reduce orthostasis, and improve cardiovascular response to

position changes after prolonged bedrest.[127] Rolling and transferring the person to sitting position on the edge of the bed is another option; however, this method requires participation of several clinicians to prevent a fall for a person with DOC as total assist will be required for maintaining sitting balance. Transfer of a person from bed to a recliner or wheelchair via active, dependent transfers or using a mechanical lift are also indicated. Activity orders should be specified in the medical record prior to mobilizing the person, and ranges of acceptable vital signs, including ICP for mobility, should be checked as well. Abdominal binders and compression stockings may be beneficial for improving venous return, limiting orthostasis, and improving tolerance to upright position during early mobilization procedures.

Many people with TBI have concomitant internal injuries, orthopedic injuries, including fractures and subluxations, as well as soft tissue damage such as skin tears, lacerations, and muscle contusions. Therefore with mobilization and other interventions, therapists should observe persons for signs and symptoms of pain such as grimacing, agitation, withdrawal responses, and/or increased heart rate, blood pressure, and ICP. If any of these symptoms are noted during physical therapy, the therapist should discontinue the treatment and try to return the person to a comfortable state. The findings should be documented and reported to the interprofessional team, and a plan of care should be implemented to premedicate the person before treatment for comfort and safety. For people in MCS, aggressive pain management protocols are encouraged because subjective awareness of pain is intact but ability to communicate is often limited.[128–130] Additionally, therapists must carefully observe patients for sign and symptoms of seizure activity at all times as this is a common complication following TBI. Most people will be prescribed antiseizure medications prophylactically; however, seizures may still occur, and therapists must respond in an appropriate manner to maintain patient safety. Medical personnel and nursing should be alerted immediately, sharp objects should be removed from the immediate area, and the person's head should be supported with a pillow.

Sensorimotor stimulation has historically been the primary nonpharmacological treatment intervention used for rehabilitation of persons with DOC.[120] A study published in 1990 by Mitchell and colleagues found that a rigorous program of olfactory, visual, tactile, auditory, and gustatory stimuli provided by trained family members for 1 to 2 hours per day for 7 to 12 days shortened the time it took to follow commands and execute purposeful movements among people with severe TBI.[131] A Cochrane review published in 2002 did not find any evidence to support multisensory interventions; however, this was due to poor study quality, variable study designs, and lack of consistent outcome measures used in the reviewed articles.[132] More recently, an early interprofessional rehabilitation program for people with DOC consisting of a minimum of 90 minutes of therapy per day, mean length of stay 39.1 days and standard deviation of 29.4 days, resulted in improved levels of consciousness for most participants and only a 13% discharge rate to long-term care facilities.[115] Despite the lack of rigorous research studies to support the practice, sensory stimulation is routinely used in the treatment of persons with DOC with the purpose of increasing the level of arousal.

Examples of commonly used sensory stimuli are listed in Table 22.6. Noxious stimuli, including deep pressure or pin prick to the nail beds or palmar surfaces of the hands and feet, as well as sternal rub, may be used initially for nonresponsive people with DOC. Loud, brisk auditory stimulation introduced via dropping a book on the floor, clapping, or banging on an object may also be used in an attempt to induce an alerting, startle response. Education that includes thorough explanations of physiological rationales and potential benefits of these interventions should be provided as family members

TABLE 22.6 Types of Sensory Stimuli to Increase Awareness and Arousal Levels

Mode	Examples
Auditory	• Conversation, voice of family members • Reading books, magazines • Sounds, e.g., ringing bell, hand clapping • Play music
Tactile	• Light touch, massage • Temperature (hot/cold) • Brushing or stroking • Pressure, e.g., inflate a sphygmomanometer cuff or air sleeve • Noxious: sternal rub, deep nail bed pressure, pin prick
Visual	• Colored papers • Pen light, room lights • Daylight • Faces of the patient's family, friends, pet, etc. • Pictures of the patient's family, friends, pet, etc.
Olfactory	• Perfume • Vinegar • Orange • Lemon • Coffee
Gustatory	• Oral swabs • Lollipop • Popsicle • Providing oral hygiene care
Kinesthetic	• Any change of position, e.g., rolling, supine to sit • Vestibular, head turns if not contraindicated, rolling • Passive range of motion

present may perceive them as torturous or distressing if not well understood, and especially if the family believes there is little potential for meaningful recovery.[133]

Many other types of sensory stimulation, including visual, vestibular, kinesthetic, sensory, and gustatory, may be introduced to increase levels of arousal (see Table 22.6). Whenever the therapist is using sensory stimuli to promote arousal, it is recommended that the stimuli be presented in a graded manner to achieve an optimal level of arousal while maintaining sensory integration. If too many are introduced, or they are too intense, the person may become overloaded and overwhelmed. They may become agitated or shut down and not respond to any further stimulation. Thus it is best to start with one type of stimulation at a time, then gradually add additional forms, and/or increase the intensity of the stimuli, until arousal is achieved. People in lower levels of consciousness may need repeated presentation of stimuli to maintain a state of wakefulness, but often only remain awake for short periods of time and need frequent periods of rest. Therapists should document patient response to types and intensity of stimuli and avoid forms and intensities that agitate the person, as well as communicate these findings to interprofessional team members for consistency and efficiency. As people emerge and move to higher levels of consciousness, they may respond differently to stimuli, and any changes in response should also be documented and communicated with team members.

For persons in and emerging from MCS, physical therapy goals should focus on increasing the level of awareness of self and the environment. Persons in this stage of recovery may respond to stimuli and

demonstrate purposeful behaviors, albeit inconsistently. Nonetheless, therapists should encourage purposeful responses, eye and/or head tracking of familiar visual and auditory stimuli, and activities such as reaching, grasping, and placing objects. As learning will be compromised due to the brain damage and anterograde amnesia, activities should be familiar to increase the automaticity and motivation to participate. Sessions should be stimulating but not overstimulating. Delayed processing is also present, so allow adequate time for the person to respond to cues before attempting another trial or repeating cues. Therapists should carefully consider environmental factors such as temperature, lighting, and ambient noise and attempt to control these factors to keep the person as alert as possible for as long as possible but without overstimulating them. Treatment may need to be performed in a closed environment free of external distractions to promote participation.

Physical Therapy Considerations for Persons With Levels of Cognitive Functioning IV-VI

For persons emerging from DOC, or those who present in LOCF IV-VI immediately following their injury, the focus of rehabilitation is on motor recovery, and improving safety and independence with functional mobility. Motor learning principles, as well as the neurophysiological principle of neuroplasticity, should be applied throughout interventions for persons recovering from a TBI. Refer to Chapter 3 for more information on this topic.

Motor learning strategies specific to the TBI population and those with impaired awareness include use of implicit memory tasks in therapy. Several studies have demonstrated impairments in explicit memory tasks with preservation of implicit tasks, including priming and procedural learning following TBI.[134,135] Thus it is recommended that rehabilitation professionals utilize implicit-memory tasks, including priming and procedural learning, for interventions as this type of learning does not rely upon conscious awareness. Persons in LOCF IV through VI often benefit from use of priming, or fostering learning through prior exposure to the stimuli, and procedural tasks, such as riding a bike. These tasks are more automatic, and automaticity may be augmented by use of familiar and desirable items and objects. For example, a therapist may hand a basketball to a person who played on their high school team before the injury, then place a hoop in front of them to encourage them to place or throw the ball. This seemingly simple task provides an internal perturbation for sitting or standing balance, promotes trunk stabilization and motor coordination, is a functional strengthening task for the UEs, and may even improve activity tolerance if repeated multiple times. Therefore the therapist can simultaneously address several impairments of body structure and function commonly present in persons with TBI through this procedural task.

Therapists are encouraged to consider environmental factors and ensure context specificity whenever possible. If the person in the above example is not responding in the desired manner when in their hospital room, a more appropriate motor response of throwing the basketball may be elicited if taken to a gym or basketball court. Similarly, if the goal of the therapy session is to improve performance of an ADL such as brushing one's teeth, the individual should be brought to the bathroom, placed in front of the sink and mirror, then handed a toothbrush and tube of toothpaste. Therapists need to carefully consider the individual's premorbid preferred activities and hobbies, life roles, and impairments to develop and structure individualized physical therapy interventions that promote implicit learning.

An additional consideration for persons in LOCF IV-VI is the need for behavior modification strategies to be utilized during therapy sessions. Some examples of behaviors commonly observed for person recovering from a head injury, and examples of management strategies, are listed in Table 22.7. This list is not exhaustive, and therapists are highly encouraged to work with interprofessional team members to develop strategies that are then used consistently by all team members, visiting family members, and friends. Consistency is critical for success due to impaired learning and cognition. Simple cues and strategies often work best. For example, a simple verbal response such as "that is inappropriate," or "that is not safe," will be most helpful to extinguish unwanted behaviors such as swearing, hitting, or inappropriate sexual touching. Positive reinforcement plans are also encouraged. One example of this may be if the person does not exhibit an unwanted behavior throughout the entire therapy session, they

TABLE 22.7 **Sample Behaviors and Suggested Interventions**

Behaviors	Interventions
Agitation • Removing restraints/tubes • Crawling/getting out of bed • Mood swings • Screaming, crying, restlessness • Pacing, wandering	• One-to-one supervision • Remove restraints if order in place to do so • Redirection to tasks • Reduce stimulation (turn off TV, dim lights, check needs for bathroom or pain, limit visitors, keep door closed, etc.) • Education on importance of tubes, IVs, lines, etc. • Do not argue or yell, and stay calm • Consistent response by all team members to undesired behaviors
Aggression • Verbal (increase in voice volume and tone, swearing, name calling) • Physical (hitting, kicking, biting, choking, hair pulling, object throwing, etc.) • Demanding unreasonable requests (e.g., demanding to leave or go home)	• Remove breakable or sharp objects from reach • Keep safe distance from patient • Do not respond with physical force or restrain person unless for their safety • Reduce stimulation (turn off TV, dim lights, check needs for bathroom or pain, limit visitors, keep door closed, etc.) • Minimize safety risks: lower bed, lock brakes • Do not argue or yell, stay calm • Give patient breaks from activity/stimulation
Noncompliance • Refuse to take meds • Refuse to participate in therapy	• Identify motivators and use positive reinforcement • Education regarding purpose of interventions • Give patient some control and/or choices • Involve family who induce cooperation • Set goals with person • Behavioral contract-avoid punitive measures
Impulsivity • Quick verbal response without awareness of consequences • Quick physical action without safety awareness	• Verbalize or rehearse steps prior to starting a task or activity • Provide verbal cues for safety throughout task performance • Safe environment (use of assistive device, grab-bars, handrails, etc.) • Review consequences of unsafe movements or behaviors • Utilize bed alarm or door alarm if ordered • Restraints if ordered and all other interventions have failed
Confusion/Disorientation • Where am I? • What time is it? • Not recognizing staff members • Hallucinations or delusions	• Provide frequent orientation • Utilize same staff members (nurses and therapists) • Utilize consistent therapy schedule • Use bed alarm or door alarm if ordered • Give simple explanations prior to activity • Limit change and be consistent
Inappropriate Sexual Behavior • Inappropriate comments • Masturbation • Grabbing or groping staff	• Provide education that inappropriate sexual behavior is not allowed • Keep distance from patient • Utilize same sex staff if effective and able to do so • Involve family members to minimize inappropriate behavior if effective • Consistent verbal cues among the interprofessional team, e.g, "that is not appropriate"
Fatigue • Poor endurance or tolerance for therapy/activity • Frequent rests or desires to go back to bed • Always sleeping or requesting to skip treatment	• Identify cause of fatigue if possible (medication, depression, poor sleep/wake cycle, restlessness at night, etc.) • Use frequent rest breaks during and between therapy sessions • Minimize time in bed during the day to promote sleep at night • Education regarding need for breaks and cause of fatigue
Denial • Low insight into deficits • Unrealistic about abilities and outcomes	• Set up experiences with patient that bring out the deficit for patient's own observation (within safe limits) • Review deficit areas/outcomes with patient • Gradually prepare patient for outcomes and highlight progress • Provide support for acceptance of deficits/outcomes, social worker involvement

receive a reward such as watching a TV show, playing a game, going outside to the garden, etc. When possible, the reward should be predetermined and chosen by the patient, and delivered as soon as the goal is achieved, to increase motivation. Allowing personal choices in types or sequencing of activities may also be helpful with improving motivation to participate and limit unwanted behaviors. If you have to address a therapy goal that is less desirable to the patient, you could tell them that it is critical to do those interventions and provide a rationale but let them choose a desired activity to do next. Punitive measures such as isolating the person, not allowing them to eat dessert, etc. should not be used for behavior modification as these may be considered neglectful or abusive and are often less effective.

Communication and processing issues common after TBI may also impact the provision of therapy. Therapists working with persons in LOCF IV-VI may need to allow increased time for processing commands and use multimodal cues, including visual, verbal, and/or tactile, depending upon which systems are intact. Augmented communication devices may be beneficial, and the physical therapist should work closely with the speech and language pathologist to determine which systems are most effective.

Dosing factors, including timing and intensity of therapy, are also important factors to consider. Several published studies on timing and intensity of therapy for people with moderate to severe head injury report better outcomes, including less time to achieve independence with functional tasks, shorter hospital stays, and faster improvement in level of consciousness, with early and more intense therapy.[115,135–137] A recently published meta-analysis concluded that early provision of rehabilitation in the trauma center and more intense therapy in rehabilitation facilities promote improved functional recovery among people with moderate to severe TBI.[138] Unfortunately, many people with TBI do not engage in the number of repetitions of activities required for neuroplastic changes during therapy sessions.[139] This may be due to service delivery models that limit number of hours in therapy per day and require provision of therapy in a one-to-one manner. Further, persons with TBI are often limited in their attention span and activity tolerance, which may prevent active participation in highly intense therapy sessions. To address this problem and increase number of repetitions, alternative service delivery models such as group sessions and robotic assisted therapy have been suggested Kimberley and colleagues[139] Frequent, short duration rest breaks or split sessions, such as 30 minutes in the morning and 30 minutes in the afternoon rather than 60 consecutive minutes, may also allow more repetitions needed for improved recovery following TBI.

Interventions to Improve Motor Performance and Physical Function After Traumatic Brain Injury

Motor deficits commonly seen after a TBI include loss of selective or isolated control, weakness, impaired force production, altered tone, poor timing and sequencing, and loss of coordination. Physical therapy approaches to improving motor performance and improving function are similar to those used for persons with other neurological insults such as stroke, cerebellar lesions, and brain tumor, while incorporating the above considerations for changes in mood, cognition, personality, communication, and others. Refer to Chapter 24 for specific interventions aimed at improving motor function for hemiplegia, as these are currently the same as those recommended for persons with TBI.

Traditional approaches such as Bobath, neurodevelopmental treatment (NDT), and proprioceptive neuromuscular facilitation (PNF) are often blended by contemporary therapists into general neuromuscular reeducation and functional task-oriented retraining approaches. Constraint-induced movement therapy (CIMT) is also commonly

used to improve UE function and ADL performance for people post-TBI even though the research on this intervention has primarily used subjects who are post-stroke. Compared to stroke, there is limited research on outcomes for specific types of rehabilitation interventions for people post-TBI. Many published studies include subjects with hemiplegia due to both stroke and TBI; however, they are not a homogenous group, as people post-TBI often have extrapyramidal disorders from more extensive CNS damage. As a result, rehabilitation practices for persons with TBI are highly variable.[140]

Regardless of the limitations in research and variable nature of interventions, considerable evidence exists that supports the fact that persons with TBI make functional gains in rehabilitation.[141,142] Therapists should therefore engage persons post-TBI in intense, repetitive, task-oriented training to promote recovery of function and optimal motor performance with all functional mobility tasks, including rolling, transferring supine to/from sitting, sit to/from stand, bed to/from wheelchair, wheelchair mobility, ambulation, and stair mobility. Additional contemporary neurorehabilitation approaches for persons with TBI, areas of physical rehabilitation that are critical to address for this population, as well as emerging treatment interventions for TBI will be discussed in more detail below.

Treadmill training. Improvement of walking ability is often a priority for people who have had a TBI, and repetitive, intensive, task-oriented practice is required for recovery. The use of treadmill training, with or without body-weight support and robotic assist, has become common practice in rehabilitation of gait. The use of body weight supported treadmill training (BWSTT) has several potential benefits, including that it may allow a greater number of steps per therapy session than overground walking, and therapists have hands free to facilitate appropriate motor patterns (Fig. 22.5). However, it may require multiple staff members to facilitate the trunk and each limb. It may also allow earlier gait training and weight bearing for persons who have not recovered sufficient postural control to commence overground training safely. However, treadmill training as a gait intervention post-TBI has been shown to be no better than overground training.[143] Moreover, there is a lack of high-quality studies to support any gait interventions for people with TBI and higher-quality studies with standardized treatment approaches are needed in this area.

Robotic-assisted treadmill training (RATT) has grown in popularity recently as it can decrease the physical burden of gait training on the therapists and allow persons to take more steps per day than overground training, but the systems are quite expensive and not widely available in rehabilitation facilities. Studies on the use of RATT are also limited. Recent studies with small sample sizes found that people with chronic TBI benefit equally from RATT and manually assisted treadmill training to increase gait velocity, endurance, and mobility domain Stroke Impact Scale scores, but the RATT group showed greater improvements in symmetry of step length.[101,144]

Some participants reported skin irritation from the robotic assist. More high-quality research is needed to guide physical therapist practice in gait training for people with TBI. Factors that need to be considered in clinical decision making on use of these devices at this time, in addition to patient safety, which is always paramount, are availability and cost of equipment, as well as staff availability and training.

Virtual reality. Virtual reality (VR) involves the use of a 3-dimensional, computer-generated environment in which a person is immersed and is able to interact with or manipulate the objects in the virtual setting, thereby creating a safe and controlled milieu for therapy sessions (Fig. 22.6).[145] VR has been reported to increase motivation and compliance, especially among pediatric populations, which promotes

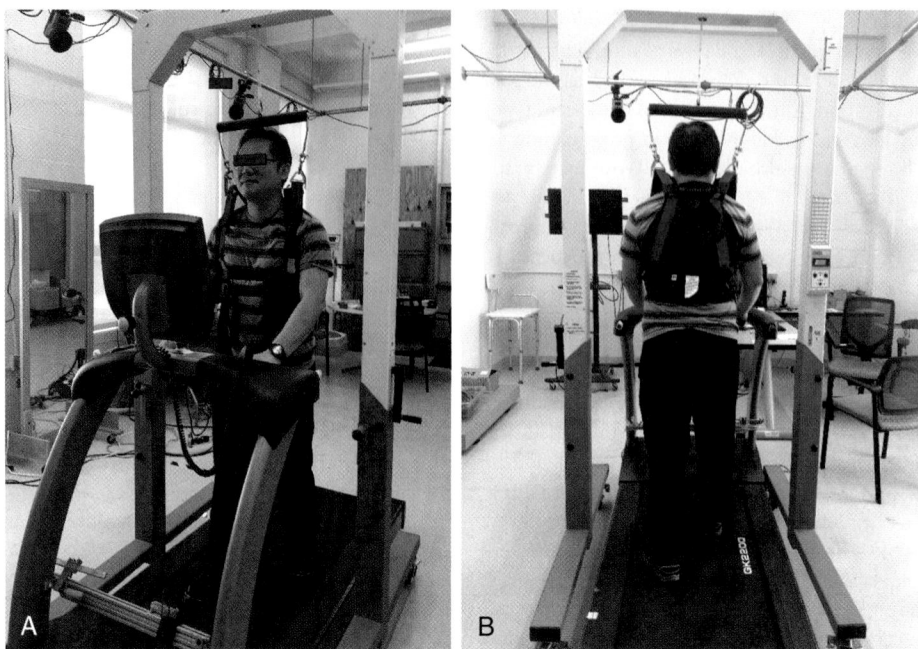

Fig. 22.5 Body Weight Support Treadmill Training. **(A)** Front view. **(B)** Back view.

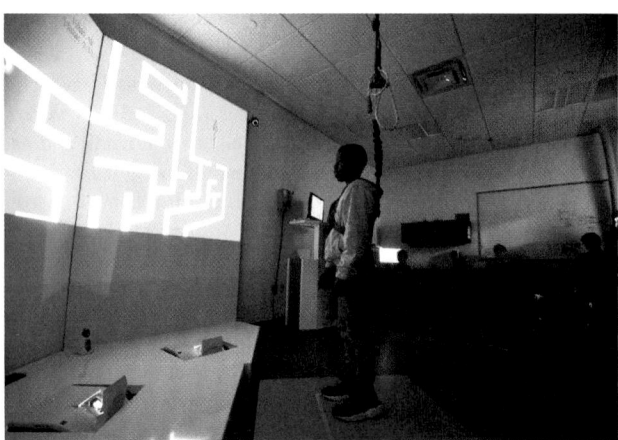

Fig. 22.6 Virtual Reality.

neuroplasticity and recovery through increased repetitions of activities. The recent decrease in cost for systems, as well as the emergence of commercially available serious games that create interactive, virtual environments, has resulted in an increased use of this technology in neurorehabilitation and for home-based programs. Research on VR in stroke rehabilitation is more robust than for TBI, and clinical practice guidelines now include using VR to address spatial, visual, verbal, mobility, and upper limb impairments post-stroke.[146] Recently published literature reviews agree that there is emerging evidence to support VR in rehabilitation for people post-TBI; however, the strength of existing evidence is limited by research design and methodology as most studies are case studies or noncontrolled trials with low numbers of participants.[145,147,148] There is a need for large, randomized controlled studies to demonstrate cost-effectiveness and efficacy.

Reported benefits of VR for adults and children post-TBI in studies included in these reviews include improved gait kinematics, motor coordination, cognition, memory, attention, balance, dual-task function, and

visual vertigo symptoms.[145,147,148] Further, it has been shown that VR can be an effective pain distractor and have an analgesic effect for persons during physical therapy sessions in inpatient treatment centers.[148] In available studies that include control groups, it is important to note that VR and conventional therapy groups typically have similar outcomes indicating that while VR may be more enjoyable and increase compliance for some persons, similar results may be achieved with traditional therapies.[145,147,149]

Interventions to improve vestibular function. Dizziness and balance issues can be a source of long-term disability following a head injury, and presence of dizziness after TBI is a risk factor for a longer recovery.[85,87] Unfortunately, these symptoms are often overlooked and undertreated in rehabilitation. Brain injuries have potential to damage all of the structures involved in visual-vestibular function, thus it is possible to have peripheral, central, or mixed vestibular pathology following a head injury.[85,150] Damage to the inner ear from the force of impact or blast may rupture the bony or membranous labyrinth or produce a hemorrhage that can result in BPPV, traumatic hydrops, or perilymphatic fistula. Contusions, hemorrhage, and axonal damage, involving the vestibulocochlear nerve, brain stem, cerebellum, or cerebral hemispheres, may produce central vestibular pathology. These may be compounded by the frequent presence of neck injuries and cervicogenic dizziness, as well as high rates of psychiatric conditions after TBI, including anxiety, which is also associated with dizziness.[85,150] While there is limited research on this issue and nearly all published literature to date focuses on persons who have sustained mild TBI or concussion, the VOR may be impaired in brain injuries of any severity, yet VOR testing is not routinely performed during assessments.[87] Thus visual-vestibular examination should be included in the physical therapy evaluation of all persons post-TBI, as stated in the Examination section earlier in the chapter. This will allow for an accurate differential diagnosis that can guide appropriate clinical management. Readers can refer to the chapter on Vestibular Disorders for details of examination and treatment procedures.

An interprofessional approach to management of vestibular symptoms, and balance and dizziness problems, is required for people post-TBI due to the complex nature of the clinical presentation, multitude of systems commonly involved, and the wide-ranging effects of most moderate to severe brain injuries. A neuro-ophthalmologist can assist in diagnosing a nervous system pathology that affects vision and eye movement. Occupational therapists are specially trained to treat visual and perceptual deficits, as well as improve function. Neuropsychologists and psychiatrists are experts in diagnosing and treating the psychological disorders common after TBI, which may exacerbate visual-vestibular dysfunction and dizziness.

Interventions to improve endurance and benefits of aerobic exercise. The physical, cognitive, and psychological sequelae of TBI often lead to reduced physical activity and a sedentary lifestyle, which results in reduced cardiorespiratory fitness and endurance. It also increases risk of developing secondary health conditions, including hypertension, coronary artery disease, osteoporosis, type II diabetes, and obesity.[90,151] Physical activity following TBI has been shown to improve neuroplasticity and promote recovery, as well as lower risk of secondary health complications associated with inactivity. Furthermore, it has been shown to have a positive impact on sleep, mood, and cognition, which are also frequently impaired after TBI.[90,152–155]

The physiological mechanisms related to brain injury, exercise, and recovery have been well documented in animal model studies, and more recently in research involving human subjects and advanced neuroimaging modalities and lab tests.[151] In brain injured animals and humans, activity-based rehabilitation induces neurogenesis and angiogenesis. Exercise also increases the production of molecules such as brain-derived neurotrophic factor (BDNF), a protein vital to neuroplasticity and essential to cognition, as well as insulin-like growth factor-1 (IGF-1), a growth factor that mediates exercise-induced neurogenesis and angiogenesis and upregulates BDNF during exercise.[156,157] Studies have also shown that regular exercise and activity increases levels of these molecules in healthy older adults who were previously sedentary, and that neuroplastic changes also occurred in subjects in the parahippocampal region and medial temporal gyrus, which are areas of the brain involved in learning and memory.[158] These effects have not been demonstrated yet in people who are recovering from a head injury; however, the neuroprotective effects of regular exercise prior to TBI have been and will be discussed further in the prognosis and outcomes section of this chapter.[159,160]

Experimental data supports the use of aerobic exercise in the clinical management of people who have sustained a head injury as it has been shown to promote neuroplasticity, speed recovery of physical functioning, and improve cognition, mood, and sleep. Dosing factors and timing must be carefully considered. Exercise that is introduced in acute stages, when there is inflammation, excess glutamate, and glucose metabolic depression in the brain, has been associated with decreased performance on learning tasks and cognition, and does not lead to an increase in BDNF levels in animal model studies.[152] As metabolic depression may last anywhere from days to weeks, therapists are cautioned to avoid implementing aerobic training when brain tissue is metabolically compromised, in order to prevent further loss of function and reduced neuroplastic potential.[152,161] Studies regarding the intensity of exercise required for optimizing recovery after TBI are lacking in the literature. Thus further research is required in human subjects to determine optimal time for commencing exercise programs, as well as appropriate intensity of exercise, post-TBI.

Modes of exercise should be chosen based on the patient's personal preferences and safety considerations. If the activity is safe and enjoyable, the person is more likely to engage in it on a regular, long-term basis. Typical activities for aerobic conditioning such as stationary bicycle, recumbent bicycle, walking on a treadmill or overground at a faster speed, jogging, upper body ergometry, and swimming may be

appropriate, and other interventions such as VR and serious games can also be used if parameters are intense and the person participates for longer periods of time. Therapists working with people in chronic stages of TBI across practice settings are encouraged to educate patients on the multiple health benefits of aerobic exercise programs and encourage regular participation in exercise for optimal health status.

Interventions to improve dual-task performance. As mentioned earlier in the chapter, impairments in attention, executive function, and working memory are common following TBI and contribute to reduced ability to engage in tasks regarding divided attention, or the ability to complete two tasks simultaneously.[106,162] Deficits in dual task, such as reduced gait speed and postural stability, have been correlated with restricted participation in life roles such as school and work, and affect social interactions.[105,163–165] Attentional deficits are one of the most commonly reported problems following moderate to severe TBI. Assessing and treating single-task gait will not necessarily translate into real-world environments requiring divided attention such as walking down busy city streets and safely navigating crosswalks, or remembering items to purchase while shopping in busy grocery stores.[166] Further, it has been shown that people who have had a TBI exhibit difficulty with dual task while walking even if they have normal gait speed.[105,165] Therefore it is essential to assess and treat dual-task performance for persons with TBI to promote participation in life roles and social functioning.

An international team of clinicians and researchers with expertise in TBI and cognition, known as INCOG (International Cognitive working group), recently published their recommendations for rehabilitation of attention.[167] They reported a lack of research in the area of interventions aimed at improving attention following TBI, yet concluded that there is moderate support for including dual-task training in rehabilitation when each task is trained singly then simultaneously, and that gains should only be expected on the specific tasks trained or very similar ones. Specificity of training principles need to be applied to dual-task interventions, and one cannot assume that skills will be generalized to environments or types of dual tasks that are not included in interventions. Therapists should therefore determine which dual-task skills are required of the individual patient based on their life roles and environmental conditions, and train them in these specific domains for optimal outcomes.

Emerging technology for the rehabilitation of moderate to severe traumatic brain injury. There are many emerging technologies currently being used and further investigated for neurorehabilitation, including robotics, VR, and noninvasive brain stimulation (NBS) techniques, including transcranial direct current stimulation (tDCS) and TMS (Fig. 22.7). Within this chapter, recent findings on NBS for persons with TBI will be explored.

Studies involving NBS for persons with a history of TBI are limited, yet promising. There is a strong theoretical basis for their use following TBI to modulate cortical activity and limit inflammation in acute stages, then enhance reorganization of neural networks for recovery.[168] Animal model studies have demonstrated that TMS is capable of reducing secondary damage in TBI by modulating glutamatergic and GABAergic processes, and reversing biomarkers associated with oxidative stress and apoptosis.[168,169] Additionally, tDCS and TMS have been shown to promote neuroplasticity and improve motor function in people with chronic stroke.[170–174] When combined with physical therapy interventions to promote motor relearning, effects of NBS could be further enhanced. Indeed, studies on the combined effects of NBS for priming and/or consolidating are yielding positive results.[175,176] While further studies with people post-TBI need to be conducted, the positive effects on motor recovery in those with brain injury from stroke are overwhelmingly favorable. One factor that may limit utility in people post-TBI compared to those post-stroke is the higher

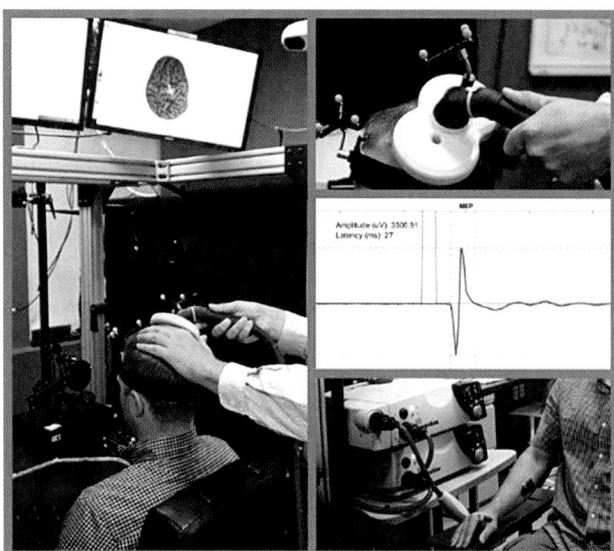

Fig. 22.7 Transcranial Magnetic Stimulation.

risk of seizure with brain stimulation after TBI; however, protocols and parameters that could make it safer to use in this population are being investigated.[177] Several low-level studies also support the use of NBS to improve cognition, attention, and depression following TBI.[178,179] Lastly, there is also low-level evidence to support use of NBS to increase the level of arousal among some people with DOC, especially those in MCS.[180,181]

SECTION IV—PROGNOSIS AND OUTCOMES AFTER TRAUMATIC BRAIN INJURY

Prognostic Models and Indicators

Predicting outcomes of TBI is challenging due to the complex clinical features of the condition. TBI is a heterogeneous condition, and each individual's presentation and clinical course is different.[182] Other confounding factors include the number of variables that are included in the prediction as it varies according to the model used, the possible effects of intervention strategies and bias in treatment on the basis of predictions, validity of prediction models (which include the percentage of error in prediction and generalizability), and the definition of positive outcomes. Understanding these problems is imperative because the therapist can provide persuasive suggestions regarding the type and intensity of rehabilitative care after injury.

Two models for predicting outcomes of TBI have been developed based on the largest population data, and they have been widely used in recent decades—the Corticosteroid Randomization After Significant Head injury (CRASH)[183] and the International Mission for Prognosis and Analysis of Clinical Trials (IMPACT) in TBI.[184] The CRASH trial was based on 10,008 persons with TBI and was validated externally on 8509 persons. Two models were developed from the CRASH trial, where the basic model included demographic and clinical variables only, while the CT model included CT results in addition to the basic model. The predictors are age, GCS, pupil reactivity, and the presence of extracranial injury. CT scan predictors include obliteration of the third ventricle or basal cisterns, midline shift, nonevacuated hematoma, petechial hemorrhages, and subarachnoid bleeding. The models predict death at 14 days, and death and disability at 6 months after the injury. Overall, the models possess excellent discrimination

and are simple enough to be used in different geographical regions for outcome predictions.

The IMPACT trial[184] is similar to the CRASH trial in that it uses admission variables to predict outcomes at 6 months after injury. The strongest predictors that this model identified are age, motor score, pupillary reactivity, and CT scan results. Again, the model discriminates persons with good and poor outcomes especially when CT scan results are included. Although both models are widely used and are relatively simple to administer, criticisms on these models include lack of consideration of secondary insults and persons' responses to treatment.[185]

In fact, there are more predictor models than the above two mentioned. Lingsma and colleagues[186] did an extensive review and identified 27 prognostic models for TBI in the literature. After reviewing the models, they listed several factors that are strong prognostic predictors for TBI. These factors include age, clinical severity, secondary insults, abnormalities on CT scan, and laboratory variables. The factors will be briefly described below with other evidence.

Age

Among all patient characteristics such as genotype, demographic factors, socioeconomic status, and education and medical history, age is a strong predictor of outcomes for TBI, with older age associated with poorer outcomes.[183–187] It was also found that increasing age is correlated with increased mortality.[185] The threshold depends on the individual studied population and may vary between 30 and 60 years of age.

Clinical Severity

It is well known that lower GCS, which indicates more severe injury, is associated with poorer outcomes.[183–187] In addition, clinical severity of TBI may need to be evaluated together with injury types. It was found that if TBI is milder, the coexistence of an extracranial injury may lead to higher morbidity and early mortality. Lingsma and colleagues[186] suggested that for persons with less severe injuries, health care professionals should pay more attention to the eye and verbal components of GCS as they may provide more relevant information than the motor component. Whereas for persons with more severe TBI, the motor component may be more indicative. Nonetheless, GCS should be conducted at regular intervals for better prediction of outcomes. It was found that a 1-point drop in GCS led to an increase of mortality rate by 19%.[185]

For persons under sedation or who are paralyzed, using pupillary reflex should be a better prognostic indicator compared to GCS.[183,184,186] Junior and colleagues[185] found that anisocoria (asymmetrical pupils) is associated with 38% of mortality in their studied population. Therapists should pay attention to this point as a number of persons in the acute phase are under these conditions.

Abnormalities on Computed Tomography Scan

For characteristics on CT scan, the strongest predictors of poor outcomes are the presence of subarachnoid hemorrhage and the obliteration of the basal cisterns.[183,184] Lingsma and colleagues[186] added that consideration of location of subarachnoid hemorrhage is also an important factor and should be included in any prediction model. Lesions in the brain stem do appear to cause poorer outcomes on the GOS than other lesions.[188] Junior and colleagues[185] reported similar findings that any category of Marshall classification of head injury based on CT scan, except for level I (no visible pathology), is associated with increased mortality rate.

Secondary Insults

Secondary insults such as hypoxia or hypotension (e.g., below 90 mm Hg) after TBI are shown to have adverse effects on clinical outcomes.[186,189] Literature in this area is sparse compared to other predictors and warrant more research.

Biomarkers

In the past few decades as more people survive moderate to severe TBI, a plethora of research has focused on biomarkers and genetic variations that may influence recovery.[190–193] There is a great deal of variability in the rate and extent of recovery, even among survivors of the same age who have experienced similar injury types and severity. A better understanding of the influence that biomarkers and genetic variation have on recovery has the potential to foster development of novel, targeted interventions for TBI. The research to date, however, has not been conclusive, and several limitations exist, including the complex pathophysiology of TBI and focus on a single marker of cell damage or gene that fails to account for the interrelationship of many factors in the nervous system.[194] Nonetheless, it is apparent that biochemical markers of brain damage and genetic factors influence neuroplasticity and outcomes after TBI. Some of the most frequently studied factors will be discussed further here.

Several different biomarkers have been studied in relation to TBI pathology and recovery, as well as in many other neurological conditions, including stroke, Alzheimer disease, and Parkinson disease. BDNF is one of the most commonly studied biomarkers. BDNF is widely distributed throughout the brain and is vital to the growth and differentiation of neurons, maintaining neuronal health, activity-dependent neuroplasticity, and memory formation.[190,195,196] Following brain injury, BDNF is believed to have a role in reducing secondary cellular damage through its neuroprotective effects and aid in the process of recovery through structural neuroplastic changes.[160,197] Animal and human studies have demonstrated changes in BDNF levels and gene expression in the acute phase of TBI, and the changes may be proportional to the severity of injury.[190,193] The serum BDNF levels measured on day of injury have also been shown to have predictive value for severity of injury and 6-month outcomes, as well as mortality when examined along with age.[193,198] Further, serum BDNF levels measured on the day of injury have been able to accurately discriminate TBI from nontrauma controls even in the absence of findings on CT scan, making it a good prospect for diagnosing mild TBI and guiding appropriate clinical management for concussion.[193] Future research on biomarkers will likely contribute to the knowledge of the highly complex pathophysiology of TBI and improve ability to accurately diagnose and treat TBI.

Genetic Factors

Similarly, the study of genetic polymorphisms and gene expression hold promise for improving treatment and promoting recovery after brain injury. While research to date is inconclusive, it is widely accepted that polymorphisms lead to variability in outcomes among TBI survivors.[194] That is, genetic factors influence the brain's susceptibility to injury and influence repair and regeneration.[199] There are many inconsistencies in research findings on this topic however, as gene expression is incredibly complex and interdependent on a confluence of personal, demographic, and environmental factors.[191] Much of the research on genetic polymorphisms have focused on BDNF and apolipoprotein E (APOE). Many studies have shown that the Val66Met polymorphism of BDNF and APOE-4 allele are associated with poorer outcomes following TBI and stroke.[200–203] However, a recent systematic review found incongruous results about the influence of APOE-4 allele on recovery after TBI, with stronger evidence of its negative consequence on recovery among people with severe TBI compared to moderate and mild brain injuries.[192] Large scale, multicenter genomic studies are currently being conducted and will hopefully shed more

light on this promising new approach to TBI management and allow for better functional, psychological, social, and cognitive outcomes following TBI.

Laboratory Values

For laboratory values, in general, high glucose concentration indicates poorer prognosis, but this laboratory value needs to be considered with other predictors. Subsequent persistent high glucose concentration and coagulopathy may cause poorer outcomes and higher mortality.[186]

Duration of Coma and Posttraumatic Amnesia

Duration of coma and PTA are well-known factors predicting outcomes after TBI. Shorter duration of coma[189] and PTA are strong predictors of better outcomes as measured by FIM[182,204]; and when PTA is combined with age, sitting balance, and limb strength at admission, prediction of outcome is high.[205] When comparing individual factors (e.g., age, employment status) and injury-related factors (e.g., duration of coma), PTA is the only injury-related factor that is equally predictive as individual factors.[206] It was found that when PTA lasted less than 4 weeks, a severe activity limitation was unlikely; however, if longer than 8 weeks, a good recovery was unlikely when measured by GOS.[207] As such, duration of PTA can be used as a functional prognostic indicator for therapists when setting goals and intervention strategies in rehabilitation.

Outcomes After Traumatic Brain Injury

Long-term impairments, activity limitations, and participation restrictions after TBI commonly exist due to the wide array of health issues this condition brings, be it physical or cognitive-behavioral. According to the Traumatic Brain Injury Model Systems National Data and Statistical Center, around 30% of persons with moderate to severe TBI worsen in their conditions within 5 years post-injury, around 26% of them stayed home, and around 22% of them died.[208] These persons are likely to die from seizures, accidental drug poisoning, infections, and pneumonia.[208] Overall, around 57% of persons who are still living have moderate to severe disability.

From an impairment level, emotional and cognitive impairments, for example memory problems, attention deficits, irritability, slowness, anxiety, and depression, were most common in people with severe TBI.[182] Depending on the cohort study, these emotional and cognitive problems may present in around 30% to 90% of persons with severe TBI even after 3 to 4 years of injury.[209,210] Motor impairment is less commonly reported but may be present in around 25% of persons.[210] Other somatic complaints were also reported, such as fatigue, headaches, and pain.[210] Communication and language impairments exist in around 15% to 25% of persons with mild to moderate TBI, and these impairments were found to correlate with quality of life and participation in work and leisure activities.[211]

With regards to activity limitations, balance, locomotion, and ADL limitations were reported in the literature. Balance complaints were reported in over 40% of persons with severe TBI 4 years post.[210] About 70% of persons with severe TBI still needed walking aids after a mean of 8 months of rehabilitation.[212] About 33% of persons needed help for daily activities[208] and 40% needed help for mobility-related ADLs.[210]

Most studies on long-term outcomes in TBI investigated areas in the participation level, such as quality of life, return to work, and/or community integration. Despite persistent cognitive and motor impairments post-TBI, persons were able to show improvements in time productivity and community integration with standard TBI programs or cognitive rehabilitation programs.[108] Return to work has been shown in around 20% to 36% of persons with TBI.[210,213,214] National Data and Statistical Center Traumatic Brain Injury Model Systems reported that 55% of persons are unemployed at 5 years post-injury.[208] Factors related to unemployment included low initial GCS score, low GOS score at discharge, low GOS-extended score at 1 year, long length of stay in ICU, longer time for following instructions, low Dysexecutive Questionnaire Revised score, transportation issues, residual cognitive impairments, and depression.[213,214]

Quality of life in all domains (social, physical, and emotional) post-TBI has been shown to be affected despite the severity of conditions, though persons with severe TBI improved the least, especially in mental

health aspect.[215] The predictors for lower quality of life after TBI included being female, older age, having comorbidities, and a more severe injury.[215] National Data and Statistical Center Traumatic Brain Injury Model Systems reported that 29% of persons are unsatisfied with life at 5 years post-injury.[208] With greater understanding of optimal medical management, effects of various rehabilitation protocols, and the long-term consequences of TBI, it is likely that medical guidelines, policies, and innovative rehabilitation programs will be developed that improve outcomes and meet the needs of this population.

CASE STUDY 22.1   Mrs. E.K.

Examination

History

Mrs. E.K. is a 60-year-old woman who sustained a brain injury in a fall 1 year ago. Injury was to the cerebellum and brain stem, resulting in left-sided involvement and incoordination. Currently she reports falling approximately two times per month. She complains of feeling tired constantly and not having enough energy to even accomplish her housework. She lives with her husband and 29-year-old son in a two-story house 1.5 h from a large western city. Her son is an alcoholic and is unemployed. Patient OR Mrs. EK's goals include being able to sew again and to return to square dance at her club.

Task Analysis of Activity Limitations

Gait (With Use of the Observation Gait Analysis Based on the Rancho System)

Mrs. E.K. has significantly decreased trunk rotation during right leg swing and a right pelvic drop in left leg stance. Left hip flexion during swing phase is reduced, and the leg circumducts. The left knee has limited flexion, and the foot has excessive plantarflexion. In stance phase on the left, she lacks hip extension during midstance and late stance, and initial contact is made with the foot flat. The left arm is held tightly against her chest with the elbow in flexion and the forearm in full supination. When she is asked to put her left arm to her side during ambulation, the arm swings uncontrolled in large arcs, actually hitting her in the chest. Gait speed is 0.8 m/s as measured by the 10 m walk test. Cadence is 73 steps per minute with a 0.8-m stride length.

Testing of Underlying Impairments for Gait Limitation

- Strength (manual muscle testing): 2+/5 left hip flexor and ankle dorsiflexors.
- Range of motion testing: Left rectus femoris reduced length with 100 degrees knee flexion test in prone. The gastrocnemius-soleus is shortened permitting dorsiflexion to neutral only.
- Tone: Modified Ashworth Scale (MAS) of 3 for left quadriceps and gastrocnemius-soleus.
- Balance testing: no ankle strategy on left, only combined hip-ankle strategy to all perturbations. There is a proximal-to-distal balance response during small perturbations.
- Proprioception is impaired when Mrs. E.K. is asked to note small changes in flexion and extension of the great toe and ankle; within normal limits for knee and hip.
- Motor patterns are poor in trunk. There is no trunk rotation during walking, and anticipatory responses are poor as measured by rapid forward reaching resulting in forward balance loss in standing.
- Vestibular function: underuse of vestibular system during sensory integration of balance as tested by the Clinical Test of Sensory Interaction on Balance (CTSIB). She also has a positive Head Thrust test indicating impaired vestibuloocular reflex (VOR) function, and a positive VOR cancellation test and positive convergence, indicative of a central vestibular disorder.

Outcome Measures for Activity Limitations (Gait, Balance and Upper Extremity Function)

- For measuring gait speed, the 10 m walk test was chosen, and it was 0.8 m/s on evaluation. Because Mrs. E.K. has two falls per month and her traumatic brain injury involved the cerebellum, it is imperative to test her balance stressing the vestibulocerebellar system and when out in the community. The Community Balance and Mobility Scale appears to be appropriate for her level as she is ambulatory and living in the community. She scored 45 out of 96 on the scale, indicating she may be at risk for community integration.
- For her upper extremity (UE) function, the Action Research Arm Test was chosen as it includes fine hand motor tasks mimicking sewing. She scored 43 out of 57.
- Since Mrs. E.K. also reports a lack of energy, the Global Fatigue Index and 6-min walk test could be included.

Upper Extremity Activity Limitation

Sewing (Large 4-Inch Needle With Yarn Rhrough 1-Inch Square Holes in Plastic Grid)

Mrs. E.K. hits the hole with the needle in one of three attempts. The left hand does not work in a distal-to-proximal manner. The scapula and shoulder initiate the reach rather than the hand, and moderate dysmetria is present, resulting in overshooting or undershooting of the target. The hand remains excessively supinated throughout the task. Fine motion of the fingers is within normal limits.

Hypothesis of Underlying Impairment for Sewing Limitation

Unable to perform sewing task because of poor timing and coordination of the scapula and shoulder muscles producing a sequentially uncoordinated movement pattern.

Testing of Underlying Impairments for Sewing Limitation

- Timing of movements: surface EMG—Poor sequencing and timing of movement of the scapular muscles with hand and wrist motion. Tremor of high frequency in the scapular stabilizers, especially in the external rotators at rest and with movement. There are lower-frequency tremors of larger amplitude in the wrist flexors and extensors during voluntary motion. Co-contraction of the biceps occurs with all shoulder and hand motions.
- Coordination: Finger-nose-finger test takes 10 s for 10 repetitions for right upper extremity, 20 s for left upper extremity. Amplitudes of movement are far too large for tasks but are repeated with each trial without modification.

Hypothesized Underlying Impairment for Gait Limitation

Gait is impaired in kinematics and speed as a result of poor force production in the left hip flexor and ankle dorsiflexors complicated by quadriceps and gastrocnemius spasticity. Slowed gait is also present because of poor trunk rotation during arm-fixed gait and instability when the arm is not fixed to her chest. Reduced muscle length of quadriceps and gastrocnemius-soleus may also contribute to the poor movement patterns, and there may be a disruption of the normal temporal sequencing of muscle firing in stance on the left. Ataxic gait qualities such as variable left foot placement are consistent with damage to the cerebellum and may be exacerbated by proprioceptive impairments. Mrs. E.K. may have anticipatory postural adjustment issues because gait is not compensated during the arm movements.

Outcome Measures for Participation Restriction
* In terms of participation restriction, Mrs. E.K.'s goals were to resume her social events (sewing and dance club). The Community Integration Questionnaire was administered, and she scored 20 out of 29.
* Quality of Life after Brain Injury could be added as a supplementary measure.

Evaluation and Diagnosis
UE is not being used functionally secondary to impaired coordination with poor sequencing and timing of muscle firing. Mrs. E.K. also exhibits impaired motor control of the left UE. The arm is held in co-contraction during walking and other activities to decrease the instability in balance caused by large movements of the entire arm. Impaired gait, slow gait velocity, and reduced balance are the result of impaired proprioception L foot and ankle, decreased strength in left hip flexors and ankle dorsiflexors, spasticity, and reduced muscle length of left quadriceps and gastrocnemius. Underuse of the vestibular system also contributed to poor balance during community mobility. Due to the above impairments and activity limitations, participation in community events is limited, and quality of life is reduced.

Interventions
Mrs. E.K. was referred to a psychologist, as it was suspected that fatigue was related to depression and she had a flat affect. She was diagnosed with depression. Mrs. E.K.'s physician then prescribed an antidepressant medication, which was not highly effective. She was later referred for repetitive transcranial magnetic stimulation (TMS) treatment sessions over several weeks, which improved her subjective complaints of fatigue and depression. Aerobic exercise was prescribed to improve endurance as well as symptoms of depression and fatigue.

Because Mrs. E.K. lived 70 miles from the treatment clinic, much of her treatment consisted of a home program. She was seen in the clinic once every 3 weeks, for 3 months, and then once a month for a year.

The initial home program focused on the basic impairments of improving quadriceps and gastrocnemius-soleus muscle length and reducing spasticity with a regular stretching program for these muscle groups. Strengthening exercises for her hip flexors and ankle dorsiflexors were prescribed and progressed accordingly. Exercises included sitting arom hip flexion and ankle dorsiflexion, standing marching, side stepping and walking on her heels while holding kitchen counter for support, sitting-to-standing repetitions with the knees bent past 100 degrees, keeping the heels on the floor.

Mrs. E.K. walked on a treadmill starting at 1.8 miles/h for 20 min, 3 days/week. Over a few months' time, she progressed to a walking speed of 3.2 miles/h for 30 min, 4–5 days/week, and she was starting to take walks with her husband outdoors. Lower-extremity (LE) interventions included improving coordination, balance, and vestibular function. Standing exercises with dim lights progressed to eyes closed while on variable surfaces such as a mat then foam were conducted in the clinic. Part-task activities for gait, including swing of left LE to target encouraging heel strike, were progressed to whole task walking over solid ground with occasional verbal cues for heel strike on the left side. Ankle strategies were promoted through rapid walking while the patient's husband told her to stop abruptly and the patient tried not to take a step after being

told to stop. She also stood 6 inches from the wall and kept the upper body rigid while she swayed back and forth around the ankle joints. This was progressed to doing the same activity with eyes closed. External perturbations were also applied by the therapist to her lower then upper trunk with increasing amplitudes to tolerance in the anterior-posterior directions to promote ankle strategies.

sEMG was used in standing to increase the force of contraction of the anterior tibialis. As the amplitude of arm motion decreased with use, Mrs. E.K. was able to walk with her hands clasped behind her back and worked on trunk rotation coordinated with gait. When this was accomplished, she was able to allow her arm to hang freely at her side and had improved natural trunk rotation in gait. Mrs. E.K. practiced line dancing with her husband, using an introduction videotape on line dancing. This activity provided higher-level balance challenges and provided enjoyment.

Virtual reality was used in the outpatient sessions to improve UE use for functional activities such as drinking from a cup, accurately placing kitchen items in drawers and on shelves. Biofeedback was also used to decrease the co-contraction of the biceps during functional activities of the arm. Blocked then eventually random practice of UE activities was utilized. To reestablish some control of amplitude of movement in the left arm, gross motor activities of the hand were done with the elbow stabilized on the support surface and a wrist splint to limit the degrees of freedom; for example, drawing large circles with a pen and pulling long pieces of yarn through some large holes. She also used her left forearm to stabilize paper while writing, finally progressing to using the hand only for stabilization. Fine motor tasks of the hand were also performed, including sewing with yarn on a mat with large, 1-inch squares, molding clay, and playing the organ. These activities were first performed with the elbow stabilized and a wrist splint, then with the elbow not stabilized, and finally without the wrist splint.

Vestibular rehabilitation exercises were used in the clinic, instruction provided for home exercise program (HEP), and were progressed accordingly on subsequent visits. These included VOR × 1 in sitting at slow speeds, for 1 min periods and plain background. VOR × 1 exercises were progressed to standing, faster speeds for up to 3 min and full (checkerboard) background for the visual target over a 2-month period. She was encouraged to repeat these exercises 3 times a day and reported compliance. She was also prescribed vergence exercises, or "pencil push-ups," and gaze substitution exercises, which were added to her HEP after 1 month. In the clinic she was challenged with higher level activities to improve vestibular function with dynamic activities. She participated in obstacle courses requiring walking on variable surfaces, direction changes, head turns to targets, and eventually dual task of counting forward and backward by 3's while in the obstacle course.

Outcomes
At discharge, Mrs. E.K. had improved patterns of motion in the left LE. An articulated ankle-foot orthosis was used for long walks or when she was fatigued. She walked with 90 steps per minute with a 1.2-m stride length. Spasticity of her gastrocsoleus was 2 on the MAS. Hip flexion improved to 20 degrees in midswing, but dorsiflexion was still limited to 5 degrees. She performed within normal limits on the CTSIB. Her gait speed had improved to 1.1m/s, and her Community Balance and Mobility score improved by 20%.

UE testing showed 100% accuracy in putting the needle through the 1-inch squares. She was able to sew and use the left arm for most activities, although a mild intention tremor persisted. She scored close to normal in the Action Research Arm Test. She reported attending the square dance once every 3 months. Medication, aerobic exercise, and TMS treatment had controlled her depression, and her fatigue was resolved.

Continued

CASE STUDY 22.2 C.H.

Examination

History

C.H., a 21-year-old woman, was in an automobile accident and sustained a severe brain injury and fractures of the left scapula, left radius, right ankle (fused), and jaw. She developed heterotopic ossification (HO) in the right elbow. C.H. was in a coma and vegetative state for 1 month and minimally conscious state for another 2 months. Her Glasgow Coma Scale score was 8 at 2 h after the accident. She had 8 days of posttraumatic amnesia. Her Rancho Los Amigos Level of Cognitive Function (LOCF) score was a V (confused, inappropriate) at 2.5 months. She is now at 5 months postinjury, and her LOCF is a VII (automatic, appropriate).

Expressive language is minimal with severe expressive aphasia and dysarthria. C.H. is able to follow two-step commands consistently and is able to nod her head "yes" or "no" appropriately. Her behavior is impaired, and she continuously tries to hug and kiss her boyfriend when he is present. She is easily frustrated by challenging tasks, and becomes extremely agitated and self-injurious, scratching herself to the point of bleeding.

Her memory and overall cognition are impaired, as noted by her score of 19/30 on the Montreal Cognitive Assessment (MoCA).

Mobility is by manual wheelchair. C.H. is independent in transfers. She can roll and come to sitting independently, but she needs moderate assistance to come to standing, minimal assistance for standing with feet shoulder width apart, and maximal assistance to ambulate. She is unable to perform self-care such as personal grooming, hygiene, and dressing or to do household chores. She has impaired posture with severe forward flexed head; however, she is able to extend her neck when asked to do so.

C.H. is a junior in college majoring in elementary school teaching. She worked part time in a clothing store prior to the accident, where she had to wait on customers, put out stock, and ring up purchases. She lives at home with her mother in a single-story house. Dancing and cooking were her hobbies.

C.H.'s goals include use of the left arm to put on makeup and dance with her boyfriend. Her mother, who is a psychologist, would like her daughter to hold her head upright, be able to walk again, and have better balance.

Review of Systems

- *Musculoskeletal system:* C.H. had HO in the right elbow; it was surgically removed 1 month ago with range of motion (ROM) 25–110 degrees. Scapular and clavicle fractures are healed. Left gastrocnemius is shortened, and she is only able to reach neutral dorsiflexion. Left shoulder has active flexion to 20 degrees but can hold at 90 degrees. Left elbow ROM is 20–135 degrees. Strength testing shows weakness in the left shoulder rotator cuff, lower trapezius, and deltoid with rapid fatigue by third repetition of movements.
- *Cardiopulmonary system:* She demonstrated poor endurance. Resting heart rate was 85 beats per minute (bpm) and 130 bpm after 5 min of standing balance and UE exercise. There was a 10-mm Hg increase in blood pressure of 115/65 to 125/72 after 5 min of examination. Vital capacity is documented as low normal (3 L).
- *Integumentary system:* Unremarkable. No pressure sores since her injury. Incision healed over right elbow.
- *Cognitive and behavioral system:* C.H. became easily frustrated, and on each occasion she scratched her left forearm with her right hand for approximately 30 s. C.H. was referred to a neuropsychologist for assistance with reducing frustration and self-injurious behaviors.

Task Analysis of Activity Limitations

Limited Reach and Grasp with Left Hand

C.H. is right handed. As her goal was to be able to put on her own makeup again, performance of this task was analyzed on evaluation. C.H. was asked to pick up an eyeliner pencil, switch it to her right hand, and apply the eyeliner to her

eyelids. Her neck was flexed with her chin resting on her chest. There was no anticipatory hand shaping before initiating the reach on the left. Reach component was with forward trunk lean, 20 degrees of left shoulder flexion, and elbow remaining at 90 degrees. She picked up the pencil with inferior lateral pinch and excessive grip force. She was able to switch the pencil to the right hand but had difficulty applying it to her eyelids.

Motor patterns appeared intact except in the cervical area, where her head was not held upright to maintain level eyes, and the left arm, in which there was a proximal-to-distal pattern of movement. C. H. was unable to modify the motor patterns in the left elbow, and intralimb joint coordination was poor.

Anticipatory responses were absent in reach and grasp; there was no hand shaping before the reach was initiated, and fingers were held wide open even as she approached the pencil. C.H. was able to reach and grasp and bend in many different ways with the right arm and was limited only by elbow ROM. The left arm was maintained in an adducted, internal rotation pattern with the elbow flexed at 90 degrees on the left. She also appeared limited in the degrees of freedom available at the forearm and hand.

Hypothesized Underlying Impairments for Upper Extremity Dysfunction

Disuse weakness and limited ROM in the left deltoid and rotator cuff group was present, likely due to immobilization after scapular fracture and prolonged bed rest. There was increased tone at the elbow and wrist on the left, likely to be contributing to impaired reaching. Problems with force production and gradation of force were the result of poor somatosensory function in the left hand. Loss of ROM in the right elbow from postoperative swelling after HO removal restricted movements of this limb. C.H. was unable to maintain her head in upright likely due to visual and proprioceptive deficits, and possibly altered perception of verticality. She may have had lack of head-righting reflexes, and overstretch weakness of the neck extensor muscles as well.

Impaired Standing Balance

C.H. stood in static standing, feet shoulder width apart with contact guard assist (CTG). There was hip flexion of 20 degrees with forward trunk lean, and she had asymmetrical weight bearing with greater weight on R LE. Upper trunk was rotated 20 degrees to the left, and she had a 15-degree upper-trunk left lean. Her chin was resting on her chest. She exhibited anterior-posterior sway in standing with no loss of balance after 30 s; sway increased moderately with eyes closed. Feet-together stance caused loss of balance in 15 s and in 10 s with eyes closed. When asked to reach rapidly forward, she fell forward and needed maximal assistance to recover her balance. She demonstrated a hip strategy with small perturbations to the trunk, and she continued to flex at the hips and knees with larger perturbations, again requiring assistance to recover her balance. When asked to take a step with the right foot in response to a perturbation, C.H. did not shift the weight to the left and required maximum assistance for balance recovery.

Hypothesized Underlying Impairment for Impaired Standing Balance

Forward lean may be caused by impaired vertical perception (seen with lack of head righting with and without vision) from visual, proprioceptive, and possibly vestibular dysfunction. There is overuse fatigue of hip extensors for maintaining continuous contraction whenever C.H. is upright. Trunk rotation may be secondary to increased tone in trunk, UE (scapular retraction), and LE. Balance losses were secondary to lack of anticipatory responses when reaching forward and for weight shift before right-foot stepping. The losses of balance with perturbation were secondary to a lack of stepping strategy and use of a mixed strategy for all standing conditions. Weakness of the gastrocnemius resulted in the premature use of the hip strategy.

CASE STUDY 22.2 C.H.—cont'd

Testing of Impairments of Body Structure and Function for Upper Extremity Dysfunction

- Strength: Manual muscle testing (MMT)—neck extensors: 3−/5. Left arm—not able to actively abduct shoulder but able to actively hold if placed at 90 degrees. Shoulder flexion and external rotation, elbow flexion and extension—3/5 (but range was limited). Wrist extension—2+/5 (half range) and flexion 3+/5.
- Grip strength: Poor on use of a dynamometer. C.H. could not regulate her force output; she either gripped with full grip or used minimal force when asked to change her grip from minimal, 1 pound per square inch (psi) to 5 psi to 8 psi to 12 psi.
- Passive ROM—Left shoulder limited to 100 degrees of flexion and abduction, 45 degrees of external rotation. Right elbow ROM—20–90 degrees in flexion and extension and 10 degrees in supination.
- Tone: Modified Ashworth Scale (MAS)—Left arm, 3 in biceps, triceps, and wrist flexors, 2 in the finger flexors, otherwise 0 or 1 throughout.
- Sensation: Proprioception and kinesthesia were impaired for left UE and hand. Stereognosis—identified 4 of 10 objects placed in the left hand.
- Visual-perceptual: C.H. complained of diplopia and identified a pen as vertical when in a left 10-degree tilt.

Testing of Underlying Impairments of Body Structure and Function for Limited Standing Balance

- Strength: MMT: 3/5 strength in left leg except 2+/5 in the left hip extensor and gastrocnemius.
- Tone: MAS 3 in the left quadriceps and gastrocnemius. The left lumbar extensors exhibited hypertonicity and forward bending elicited an extensor spasm.
- Muscle endurance: Poor in trunk and LE muscles; there was a reduction in amount of resistance tolerated after approximately five repetitions with isolated muscle testing of the quadriceps, hip extensors, back extensors, and cervical extensor muscles.
- Sensation: Proprioception was decreased (needs larger movement for accuracy) in the left ankle, knee, and hip.
- Visual testing: C.H. had a left hemianopsia. No nystagmus was present. (Vision and vestibular systems are also addressed under the activity limitation.) Left tilt off vertical 15 degrees in standing with eyes open and with eyes closed.
- Vestibular testing: C.H. complained of double vision and objects "jumping" with moderate and fast head motion with trying to maintain eye fixation on a pen tip. C. H. had increased sway during this test (in sitting). Unable to maintain balance for CTSIB testing.
- Verticality: Unable to hold head up consistently; no head righting reflexes to tilts. Did not right lower body to floor in standing. No change with eyes closed.
- *Balance synergies* to large and small perturbations: sEMG—appeared intact, in the right LE, but ankle strategy is absent in the left. Small perturbations to upper trunk are responded to with synergies showing a proximal-to-distal firing beginning in the trunk flexors and extensors. Amplitude of muscle contraction at the gastrocnemius was small even for large perturbations, less than 25% of her maximal contraction. Gastrocnemius reaction times were 400 ms to perturbation on sEMG.
- *Anticipatory responses* were generally absent in the left LE and trunk during stepping. C.H. fell to the right each time she tried to raise her right leg. There was no anticipatory shift of weight to the left. sEMG showed no left gastrocnemius firing before rapid forward reaching.
- Cognitive deficits: Attention span was about 2 min during therapy. Moss Attention Rating Scale score was 65/100, and she scored 19/30 on the MoCA.

Outcome Measures for Activity Limitations

- C.H. was in an inpatient rehabilitation setting, and she required assistance for her general mobility and activities of daily living (ADLs), thus the Functional Independence Measure is an appropriate outcome measure to use. Her score was 79/126 on admission.

- Since she requires maximum assistance with ambulation, it is not appropriate to include a gait outcome measure. Instead, the Berg Balance Scale is appropriate for her level, and it is also a recommended outcome measure for traumatic brain injury (TBI). She scored 25 out of 56, indicating high fall risk.
- For UE function, the Nine-Hole Peg Test was done, and she scored 1 min. She scored 1/5 in the Frenchay Arm Test.

Outcome Measures for Participation Restriction

The Quality of Life after Brain Injury is a recommended measure for persons post-TBI in the inpatient rehabilitation setting. However, since C.H. still exhibited abnormal behaviors such as anger, frustration, and self-destructive responses, it was not appropriate to conduct the test. As a result of her behaviors, she is restricted with participating in social activities with friends. Her impaired balance, as well as reach and grasp with the left hand, restricts her from performing her job in a clothing store. Cognitive impairments limit her ability to return to college at this time.

Evaluation and Diagnosis and Prognosis

Poor force control, timing and sequencing, lack of wrist and finger proprioception, co-contraction of the biceps and triceps, and poor anticipatory hand shaping during reach and grasp resulted in nonuse of the left UE. Contributing to the lack of use of the hand was poor strength in the scapular stabilizers due to a scapular fracture that was immobilized and prolonged bed rest from disorders of consciousness (DOC) for 3 months. Lack of adequate elbow ROM from HO and postoperative swelling in the right elbow prevented independent grooming, personal hygiene such as teeth brushing, and applying makeup when combined with deficits in the left hand.

C.H. was unable to stand or walk without moderate to maximum assistance because of a lack of appropriate balance responses to perturbations, lack of anticipatory responses to movements of her center of gravity, and impaired vertical orientation. Poor left gastrocnemius strength contributed to lack of an ankle strategy. Standing posture is with a forward lean owing to poor perception of vertical. The forward lean overstretched the back and hip extensors, and perhaps the gastrocnemius, which were weak from prolonged bed rest during the time when C.H. was in DOC.

C.H. has problems perceiving the vertical position in sitting and standing because of visual, vestibular, and proprioceptive impairments. Head righting is absent owing to loss of visual and proprioceptive head righting, as well as overstretch weakness of the cervical extensors. She has poor muscular endurance from prolonged bed rest. Her poor attention span and cognitive status likely contributed to all her activity limitations.

Prognosis

- *Long-term goals:* In 4 months C.H. will be independent in all self-care activities and ADLs using the left hand as an assist. C.H. will be able to participate in activities without exhibiting self-injurious behaviors 100% of the time. She will be able to stand with UE support with MI. C.H. will have fair + standing static and dynamic balance.
- *Short-term goals:* Improved force production and timing of left gastrocnemius using functional electrical stimulation (FES) daily for 15 min on a home exercise program and electromyography (EMG) biofeedback 3 × weekly for 2 weeks in rehab. Improved force gradation for grasp so C.H. can grasp and release a paper cup filled with water and not deform the cup or spill the water in 2 weeks.

The prognosis for meeting the above goals is good because C.H. is young, has a supportive family (sister and mother), and showed focal lesions on brain magnetic resonance imaging rather than diffuse injury. Return to college and work will be dependent upon cognitive recovery and progress with occupational therapy (OT), speech and language pathologist (SLP), and psychologists. Team will work with neuropsychologist to develop and implement a behavioral modification plan to improve emotional responses and limit self-injurious behaviors.

Interventions

Initial goals included addressing impairments that did not allow higher levels of functioning. These were improvements in neck and hip strength, gastrocnemius

Continued

CASE STUDY 22.2   C.H.—cont'd

strength and length, visual skills, particularly in tracking of objects into the left visual field, and perception of verticality.

Development of proper head control was a priority. FES was applied to the posterior cervical muscles (5:1 duty cycle and frequency at 35 pulses per second [pps]) for strengthening and upright head position. A sterno-occipital-mandibular immobilization support was worn intermittently to prevent further stretch weakness, then was weaned to a Philadelphia collar. Visual focus on a doorframe was used to encourage visual control of head and body position for improved alignment. Complex neck activities to encourage basic synergy use and modification included seated activities in which C.H. wore a "hat" with a flat top from which she tried to prevent an object from falling off (first flat stable objects and later more rounded objects). This exercise was performed first on a firm, flat surface and progressed to sitting on an exercise ball. The ball promoted automatic neck muscle motor patterns in which the body moves and the head is kept upright and still. To make the activity at the automatic level, C.H. did side-to-side leans while sitting on the ball, looking in a mirror to monitor head verticality, and then doing the activity without visual proprioception.

Upper extremities: Traditional basic left UE strengthening exercises included the use of Thera-Band. Functional activities that required scapular use such as emptying the dishwasher with the left hand were assigned homework. Bilateral hand use was encouraged early on. After C.H. could accomplish this, then only left-hand use was allowed; a 1-lb wrist weight was added, which was gradually increased to 3 lb.

PROM program for UE was implemented with nursing, family, OT, and PT daily, and she made slow gains with bilateral UE ROM. C.H. worked on picking up and manipulating objects of different sizes and shapes, throwing balls at targets, and doing two-handed carrying with a laundry basket, and quick release of the basket. She sorted different-sized objects by retrieving them from a bucket that also contained marble-sized balls with her vision occluded to force the development of stereognosis.

C.H. enjoyed cooking, so tasks were used in therapy that involved elbow extension, such as rolling out cookie dough. Exercises such as washing the dishes with hands in soapy water for proprioceptive feedback and practice of slip grip for enhancement of feedback through the fingertips were used. Setting the table with plastic dishes using the left hand helped improve functional use of the UE.

Bimanual UE tasks were added to her treatment plan. C.H. hooked a small rug. When able, she began two-handed typing. Two of her most motivating activities were applying makeup and inserting contact lenses.

Visual treatment used exercises that required visual fixation at different points in space and at different distances using letters and objects, while moving the head left and right with the goal of seeing only one image. These exercises advanced to include moving objects and head moving with a fixed object and progressed to both the object and head moving while a single image was maintained. Finally, full body movement with eyes fixed on a moving object was accomplished. Vergence exercises were worked on, first using a ball with an "X" marked on it on a string, swinging the ball toward and away from her. She did five swings at a time and wrote down how many times the X stayed single. The ball was swung side to side, and C.H. had to point at it with her finger for left visual field loss.

Standing balance exercises focused on developing anticipatory responses via throwing a gym ball and reaching activities. She also worked on kicking a ball to a goal with the right foot. Exercises to promote ankle strategy included gentle "tug-of-war" with a dowel, and Wii balance board games to improve gastrocnemius firing and timing.

After C.H. was able to stand and weight shift without support, small-angle, slow random tilts on a tilt board were used to promote both vertical upright and vestibular responses for balance. To promote vertical trunk control and anticipatory responses, C.H. practiced taking a full step forward with each foot. C.H. had a penlight attached by velcro to a belt she wore on her waist. The goal was to keep the light, aimed at a wall target in front of her, from moving more than 2 inches side to side. This was also facilitated by moving the parallel bars extremely close together (about 1 inch from each hip) and asking C.H. not to touch the bars with either hip as she practiced stepping.

Tone was modified with rhythmic rotation and aggressive passive range of motion (prom) with prolonged stretch, as well as deep pressure on tendons of spastic muscles. Biofeedback to teach decreased co-contraction during activities such as reaching and lifting improve motor performance of her UE.

C.H. used a Nustep bike and upper body ergometer to improve cardiovascular fitness and activity tolerance. The goal C.H. had when first starting therapy was "to dance with my boyfriend." To encourage functional use of postural and balance motor patterns, dancing was used. She started first with slow dancing with her boyfriend. Gradually she was able to dance to faster music without being held, by using trunk and arm motion and a sidestepping motion. Finally, forward-backward movements and turning and bending were added. In addition, C.H. agreed to model in the Brain Injury Association fashion show that was scheduled for 6 months later, which provided motivation to walk independently.

C.H. did not adhere to Home Exercise Program (HEP) despite maximal encouragement, reward programs, and education regarding benefits. A behavioral modification program was established so that she was given control to stop activities that were too stressful for her. She participated in a volunteer program with farm animals two or three times a week on a fixed schedule to establish personal responsibility and provide a positive learning environment. A program of rewards and withholding of rewards was established to extinguish self-destructive behavior. Verbal feedback was provided when immature behavior was exhibited. C.H. kept a diary of duties and accomplishments to help with memory and reinforce successes.

Motor learning was enhanced by using a program of blocked feedback to start, with only three trials before feedback was given. The number of trials increased to about 10, and then she progressed to random feedback, as C.H. was able to tolerate higher frustration levels. She began doing her own self-assessment of her performance after about 2 months of therapy for each of her activities.

Outcomes

C.H. reached the goals of independent standing static and dynamic balance in 6 weeks. She had vertical upright trunk and head posture but still needed the collar support intermittently for her neck. The left arm had good assistive and gross independent use. Tone in the left arm and left quadriceps was at a level 2 MAS at 6 weeks; however, the trunk tone was still interfering with standing posture and left side rotation remained, although at only about 50% of the initial rotation. Her attention had improved and scored 77/100 on Moss Attention Rating Scale. C.H. was independent in all grooming and with most other ADLs, except showering. The Functional Independence Measure score was 110/126, 10 m walk test revealed a gait speed of 1.2 m/s, Frenchay Arm Test scored 5/5, and Nine-Hole Peg Test 18 s. C.H. had no episodes of scratching herself and much higher tolerance for more difficult tasks. She continued to have some atypical behaviors, but the work at the farm helped her to assess her own deficits better. She made new friends, participated in social activities, and walked in the fashion show fundraiser for the Brain Injury Association after discharge.

REFERENCES

To enhance this text and add value for the reader, all references are included on the companion Evolve site that accompanies this textbook. This online service will, when available, provide a link for the reader to a Medline abstract for the article cited. There are 215 cited references and other general references for this chapter, with the majority of those articles being evidence-based citations.

Family Guide to the Rancho Los Amigos Levels of Cognitive Functioning

Cognition refers to a person's thinking and memory skills. Cognitive skills include paying attention, being aware of one's surroundings, organizing, planning, following through on decisions, solving problems, using judgment, reasoning, and being aware of problems. Memory skills include the ability to remember things before and after the brain injury. Because of the damage caused by a brain injury, some or all of these skills will be changed.

The Rancho Los Amigos Levels of Cognitive Functioning is an evaluation tool used by the rehabilitation team. The eight levels describe the patterns or stages of recovery typically seen after a brain injury. This helps the team understand and focus on the person's abilities and design an appropriate treatment program. Each person will progress at his or her own rate, depending on the severity of the brain damage, the location of the injury in the brain, and the length of time since the brain injury. Some individuals will pass through each of the eight levels, whereas others may progress to a certain level and fail to change to the next higher level. It is important to remember that each person is an individual and there are many factors that need to be considered when assigning a level of cognition. There are a range of abilities within each of the levels, and your family member may exhibit some or all of the behaviors listed below.

COGNITIVE LEVEL I

No Response

A person at this level will:
- Does not respond to sounds, sights, touch, or movement.

COGNITIVE LEVEL II

Generalized Response

A person at this level will:
- Begin to respond to sounds, sights, touch, or movement.
- Respond slowly, inconsistently, or after a delay.
- Respond in the same way to what he hears, sees, or feels. Responses may include chewing, sweating, breathing faster, moaning, moving, and/or developing increased blood pressure.

COGNITIVE LEVEL III

Localized Response

A person at this level will:
- Be awake on and off during the day.
- Make more movements than before.
- React more specifically to what he or she sees, hears, or feels. For example, he or she may turn toward a sound, withdraw from pain, and attempt to watch a person move around the room.
- React slowly and inconsistently.
- Begin to recognize family and friends.

- Follow some simple directions such as "Look at me" or "Squeeze my hand."
- Begin to respond inconsistently to simple questions with "yes" and "no" head nods or shakes.

What family and friends can do at Cognitive Levels I, II, and III:
- Explain to the individual what you are about to do. For example, "I'm going to move your leg."
- Talk in a normal tone of voice.
- Keep comments and questions short and simple. For example, instead of "Can you turn your head toward me?" say, "Look at me."
- Tell the person who you are, where he or she is, why he or she is in the hospital, and what day it is.
- Limit the number of visitors to two or three people at a time.
- Keep the room calm and quiet.
- Bring in favorite belongings and pictures of family members and close friends.
- Allow the person extra time to respond, but don't expect responses to be correct. Sometimes the person may not respond at all.
- Give the person rest periods. He or she will tire easily.
- Engage the person in familiar activities, such as listening to favorite music, talking about the family and friends, reading out loud to the individual, watching TV, combing his or her hair, putting on lotion.
- The person may understand parts of what you are saying. Therefore be careful what you say in front of the individual.

COGNITIVE LEVEL IV

Confused and Agitated

A person at this level may:
- Be very confused and frightened.
- Not understand what he or she feels or what is happening around him or her.
- Overreact to what is seen, heard, or felt by hitting, screaming, using abusive language, or thrashing about. This is because of the confusion.
- Be restrained to prevent injury.
- Be highly focused on basic needs—that is, eating, relieving pain, going back to bed, going to the bathroom, or going home.
- May not understand that people are trying to help.
- Not pay attention or be able to concentrate for a few seconds.
- Have difficulty following directions.
- Recognize family and friends some of the time.
- With help, be able to do simple routine activities such as feeding himself or herself, dressing, or talking.

What family and friends can do at Cognitive Level IV:
- Tell the person where he or she is and reassure the person that he or she is safe.
- Bring in family pictures and personal items from home to make the individual feel more comfortable.
- Allow the person as much movement as is safe.

- Take the person for rides in the wheelchair, with permission from nursing.
- Experiment to find familiar activities that are calming to him or her, such as listening to music or eating.
- Do not force the person to do things. Instead, listen to what he or she wants to do and follow this lead, within safety limits.
- You may need to give breaks and change activities frequently because the person often becomes distracted, restless, or agitated.
- Keep the room quiet and calm. For example, turn off the TV and radio, don't talk too much, and use a calm voice.
- Limit the number of visitors to two or three people at a time.

COGNITIVE LEVEL V

Confused and Inappropriate

A person at this level may:
- Be able to pay attention for only a few minutes.
- Be confused and have difficulty making sense of things outside himself or herself.
- Not know the date, where he or she is, or why he or she is in the hospital.
- Not be able to start or complete everyday activities, such as brushing the teeth, even when physically able. Step-by-step instructions may be needed.
- Become overloaded and restless when tired or when there are too many people around.
- Have a very poor memory (the person will remember past events from before the accident better than the daily routine or information the individual has been told since the injury).
- Try to fill in gaps in memory by making things up (confabulation).
- Get stuck on an idea or activity (perseveration) and need help switching to the next part of the activity.
- Focus on basic needs such as eating, relieving pain, going back to bed, going to the bathroom, or going home.
  What family and friends can do at Cognitive Level V:
- Repeat things as needed. Don't assume that the person will remember what you say.
- Tell the individual the day, date, name and location of the hospital, and why he or she is in the hospital when you first arrive and before you leave.
- Keep comments and questions short and simple.
- Help the person organize and get started on an activity.
- Bring in family pictures and personal items from home.
- Limit the number of visitors to two or three at a time.
- Give frequent rest periods when he or she has problems paying attention.

COGNITIVE LEVEL VI

Confused and Appropriate

A person at this level may:
- Be somewhat confused because of memory and thinking problems; he or she will remember the main points from a conversation but forget and confuse the details. For example, the person may remember having had visitors in the morning but forget what they talked about.
- Follow a schedule with some assistance but become confused by changes in the routine.
- Know the month and year, unless there is a severe memory problem.
- Pay attention for about 30 min but have trouble concentrating when it is noisy or when the activity involves many steps. For example, at an intersection, the person may be unable to step off the curb, watch for cars, watch the traffic light, walk, and talk at the same time.
- Brush teeth, get dressed, feed himself or herself, and so on, with help.
- Know when he or she needs to use the bathroom.
- Do or say things too fast, without thinking first.
- Know that he or she is hospitalized because of an injury but will not understand all of the problems he or she is having.
- Be more aware of physical problems than thinking problems.
- Associate his or her problems with being in the hospital and think that he or she will be fine once at home.
  What family and friends can do at Cognitive Level VI:
- Repeat things as needed. Discuss things that have happened during the day to help the individual improve his or her memory.
- If needed, help the person with starting and continuing activities.
- Encourage the individual to participate in all therapies. He or she will not fully understand the extent of the problems and the benefits of therapy.

COGNITIVE LEVEL VII

Automatic and Appropriate

A person at this level may:
- Follow a set schedule.
- Be able to do routine self-care without help, if physically able. For example, he or she can dress or feed himself independently.
- Have problems in new situations and may become frustrated or act without thinking first.
- Have problems planning, starting, and following through with activities.
- Have trouble paying attention in distracting or stressful situations—for example, family gatherings, work, school, church, or sports events.
- Not realize how the thinking and memory problems may affect future plans and goals; therefore the person may expect to return to previous lifestyle or work.
- Continue to need supervision because of decreased safety awareness and judgment. He or she still does not fully understand the impact of the physical or thinking problems.
- Think more slowly in stressful situations.
- Be inflexible or rigid and may seem stubborn. However, these behaviors are related to the brain injury.
- Be able to talk about doing something but will have problems actually doing it.

COGNITIVE LEVEL VIII

Purposeful and Appropriate

A person at this level may:
- Realize that he or she has a problem in thinking and memory.
- Begin to compensate for the problems.
- Be more flexible and less rigid in thinking—for example, the person may be able to come up with several solutions to a problem.
- Be ready for driving or job training evaluation.
- Be able to learn new things at a slower rate.
- Still become overloaded with difficult, stressful, or emergency situations.
- Show poor judgment in new situations and may require assistance.
- Need some guidance to make decisions.
- Have thinking problems that may not be noticeable to people who did not know the person before the injury.

What family and friends can do at Cognitive Levels VII and VIII:

- Treat the person as an adult by providing guidance and assistance in decision making. His or her opinions should be respected.
- Talk with the individual as an adult. There is no need to try to use simple words or sentences.
- Be careful when joking or using slang, because the individual may misunderstand the meaning. Also, be careful about teasing.
- Help the individual in familiar activities so he or she can see some of the problems in thinking, problem solving, and memory. Talk to the person about these problems without criticizing. Reassure him or her that the problems are because of the brain injury.
- Strongly encourage the individual to continue with therapy to increase thinking, memory, and physical abilities. He or she may feel completely normal. However, he or she is still making progress and may possibly benefit from continued treatment.
- Be sure to check with the physician on the individual's restrictions concerning driving, working, and other activities. Do not just rely on the individual for information, because he or she may feel ready to go back to the previous lifestyle.
- Discourage the individual from drinking or using drugs, because of medical complications.
- Encourage the individual to use note-taking as a way to help with the remaining memory problems.
- Encourage the person to carry out self-care as independently as possible.
- Discuss what kinds of situations make the person angry and what he or she can do in these situations.
- Talk with the person about his or her feelings.
- Learning to live with a brain injury can be difficult, and it may take a long time for the individual and family to adjust. The social worker and/or psychologist will provide the family and friends with information regarding counseling, resources, and/or support organizations.

LEVEL IX—PURPOSEFUL, APPROPRIATE: STAND-BY ASSISTANCE ON REQUEST

- Independently shifts back and forth between tasks and completes them accurately for at least 2 consecutive hours.
- Uses assistive memory devices to recall daily schedule, make "to do" lists, and record critical information for later use with assistance when requested.
- Initiates and carries out steps to complete familiar personal, household, work, and leisure tasks independently and unfamiliar personal, household, work, and leisure tasks with assistance when requested.
- Is aware of and acknowledges impairments and disabilities when they interfere with task completion and takes appropriate corrective action but requires standby assistance to anticipate a problem before it occurs and take action to avoid it.
- Is able to think about consequences of decisions or actions with assistance when requested.
- Accurately estimates abilities but requires standby assistance to adjust to task demands.
- Acknowledges others' needs and feelings and responds appropriately with standby assistance.
- Depression may continue.
- May be easily irritable.
- May have low frustration tolerance.
- Able to self-monitor appropriateness of social interaction with standby assistance.

LEVEL X—PURPOSEFUL, APPROPRIATE: MODIFIED INDEPENDENT

- Able to handle multiple tasks simultaneously in all environments but may require periodic breaks.
- Able to independently procure, create, and maintain own assistive memory devices.
- Independently initiates and carries out steps to complete familiar and unfamiliar personal, household, community, work, and leisure tasks but may require more than usual amount of time and/or compensatory strategies to complete them.
- Anticipates impact of impairments and disabilities on ability to complete daily living tasks and takes action to avoid problems before they occur but may require more than usual amount of time and/or compensatory strategies.
- Able to independently think about consequences of decisions or actions but may require more than usual amount of time and/or compensatory strategies to select the appropriate decision or action.
- Accurately estimates abilities and independently adjusts to task demands.
- Able to recognize the needs and feelings of others and automatically respond in appropriate manner.
- Periodic episodes of depression may occur.
- Irritability and low frustration tolerance when sick, fatigued, and/or under emotional stress. Social interaction behavior is consistently appropriate.

Copyright 1990, Los Amigos Research and Educational Institute (LAREI).

23

Concussion*

Brian M. Moore
Nicole Miranda (Tests and Measures in Acute Concussion, Headaches, and Management of Cervical Spine Dysfunction), Heather Campbell (Management of Cervical Spine Dysfunction), and Lisa D'Angelo (Cognitive/Neuropsychological Dysfunction, Cognitive Assessment, and Rehabilitation)

OBJECTIVES

After reading this chapter the reader will be able to:

1. Define concussion/mild traumatic brain injury (mTBI), sports-related concussion (SRC), postconcussive syndrome (PCS), and persistent postconcussion symptoms (PPCS).
2. Describe the epidemiology, pathophysiology, and the economic/personal costs associated with concussion.
3. Describe screening tools and medical tests used to diagnose the acute concussion and the medical management for individuals following a concussion.
4. Discuss considerations for cognitive and physical rest and recommendations for return to play (RTP) and return to school/learn for student-athletes following an SRC.

5. Describe the prognosis and outcomes for patients with persistent symptoms following an SRC considering pediatric/youth, adolescent, and adult athletes.
6. Describe the epidemiology, prognosis, and return to meaningful activities (e.g., work) for individuals following concussion including young adults, older adults, and military personnel.
7. Describe the clinical examination and evaluation for a rehabilitation specialist for individuals with PPCS and describe interventions for individuals with a slow recovery using a targeted approach to match intervention to a specific clinical profile.

KEY TERMS

cognitive rehabilitation
mild traumatic brain injury (mTBI)

return to learn/play
sports-related concussion (SRC)

INTRODUCTION

Concussion is one of the most common neurological conditions in the world, with at least 3 million cases each year in the United States alone.[1,2] Concussion may cause a variety of impairments that can impact an individual's ability to return to meaningful activities such as an athlete returning to sport, a student returning to school, a civilian returning to work, or a service member returning to duty. Due to the frequency of concussions, which some reports estimate to occur every 7 seconds in the United States, and the detrimental effect concussion can have on function, the Centers for Disease Control and Prevention (CDC) has labeled concussion a major public health issue[3] that is accompanied by considerable personal and social economic costs. The annual economic burden associated with concussion has been estimated to be $16.7 billion USD, with an estimated direct cost of $35,000 to $45,000 USD per patient.[4,5]

Concussion, also referred to as mild traumatic brain injury (mTBI), has been defined by the International Consensus Conference

of the Concussion in Sport Group (CISG) as a complex pathophysiological process affecting the brain, induced by biomechanical forces[6] that can cause sudden deceleration and rotation forces to the brain.[7] It is unclear and debatable whether concussion results in structural damage (e.g., microvascular hemorrhage) or functional injury characterized by transient metabolic damage.[8] What is clear is that concussion may cause a variety of short-lived neurological signs and symptoms that, in most cases, resolve spontaneously.[6] However, in a minority of concussive events, symptoms will evolve and persist over a number of days or weeks leading to a slow, prolonged recovery.[3,6,9]

Once termed the "silent epidemic,"[10] concussion has moved to the forefront of the public's consciousness in recent years. Perhaps the catalyst to the public's interest in the United States were reports that developed surrounding the potential long-term consequences of concussion in professional American football players. Since that time, several educational initiatives[11] have been developed to increase the public's awareness of the critical nature of concussion, how to recognize a concussion, and what action to take if a concussion is identified. By January 2014, laws had been established in all 50 states mandating

*Videos for this chapter are available at studentconsult.com.

school districts to develop information and policies related to concussion in children and adolescents. And if Twitter can be used as a measurement tool to gauge change in public awareness, the number of tweets related to traumatic brain injury increased twofold over a 6-year period, from 2010 to 2016.[12,13] These examples may point to increased public awareness of concussion; yet, unfortunately, there continues to be disheartening evidence, both empirical and anecdotal, which suggests continued mismanagement in the care of patients who sustain a concussion.

Although concussion research has increased in the last 25 years, in rehabilitation, there is still much that is not well understood.[3,14] Because of the challenges that exist in returning individuals to their life activities, it is imperative that medical professionals and rehabilitation specialists understand the risks, functional and medical consequences, level of evidence, current recommendations for management, and effective preventions programs to inform local, state, and federal policies.

This chapter was developed to review all stages of care following a concussion with an emphasis on topics for the rehabilitation specialist providing services to children, young adults, and older adults. The chapter was developed with an emphasis on sports-related concussion (SRC) as this is the well-developed area of research related to concussion. One substantial contribution to the literature comes from the CISG, which has provided recommendations from a formal consensus process in 2001 (Vienna), 2004 (Prague), 2008 (Zurich), 2012 (Zurich), and 2016, its last updated consensus statement in Berlin. For the most recent consensus statement,[6] specific clinical questions related to management of SRC were developed and a formal systematic review was completed by committee members and authors of the CISG to answer each of these clinical questions. The reports from the systematic reviews provided the basis for the updated recommendations. Throughout the chapter, the CISG will be used interchangeably with "international consensus." While the bulk of published evidence is found in the SRC and service member populations, the recommendations for evaluation and management of concussion injuries may be applied to individuals of all ages who sustain a concussion following falls, violence/abuse, motor vehicle collisions, and recreational or work-related trauma.

An important point of clarification for the reader regarding terms used in this chapter: although there are some texts that use the terms concussion and mTBI to refer to the same condition and others that use the terms to refer to different injuries,[6] the terms concussion and mTBI will be used interchangeably in this chapter to refer to the same health condition. Table 23.1 provides definitions of common terms used in concussion literature. The reader may find it useful to become familiar with the terms and consider how the definitions differ, depending on the organization or consensus body providing the definition.

TABLE 23.1 Definitions of Common Terms Used in Concussion-Related Literature and Care

Concussion

International Consensus: A complex pathophysiological process affecting the brain, induced by biomechanical forces[6]

American Academy of Neurology: A clinical syndrome of biomechanically induced alteration of brain function, typically affecting memory and orientation, which may involve loss of consciousness[15]

Cantu Grading Scale[16]:

  Grade 1: posttraumatic amnesia <30 min and no loss of consciousness

  Grade 2: loss of consciousness <5 min or amnesia 30 min to 24 h

  Grade 3: loss of consciousness >5 min or amnesia >24 h

Mild Traumatic Brain Injury (mTBI)

International Consensus: Physiological disruption of brain function resulting from traumatic force transmitted to the head[17]

WHO-ICD-10: Head injury resulting in a score of 13–15 on the Glasgow Coma Scale, without other factors such as acute substance abuse, other focal or systemic injuries, coexisting medical conditions, or penetrating craniocerebral injury. The patient must endorse one of the following: confusion or disorientation, loss of consciousness of <30 min, posttraumatic amnesia of <24 h, or transient neurological abnormalities.[18]

Term used to categorize the severity of a traumatic brain injury (mild, moderate, and severe) based on the Glasgow Coma Scale score of 13–15 and limited posttraumatic amnesia. The term may include concussion, but may also include small intracranial hematomas or skull fractures.[5,19]

American Congress of Rehabilitation Medicine: A traumatically induced physiological disruption of brain function including (1) any period of loss of consciousness; (2) any loss of memory for events immediately before or after the accident; (3) any alteration in mental state at the time of the accident (e.g., feeling dazed, disoriented, or confused); and (4) focal neurological deficits that may or may not be transient but where the severity of the injury does not exceed the following: loss of consciousness of 30 min, Glasgow Coma Scale of 13–15, and posttraumatic amnesia of 24 h.

Postconcussive Syndrome

WHO-ICD-10: A head injury usually sufficient to result in loss of consciousness after which at least 3 of 8 common symptoms arise within 4 weeks. The symptoms include headache, dizziness, fatigue, irritability, sleep problems, concentration problems, memory problems, and/or problems tolerating stress/emotionality/alcohol.[21,22]

American Psychiatric Association (DSM-IV): Diagnosis provided if the following criteria are met: (1) A history of head trauma that has caused significant cerebral concussion, the manifestation of which includes loss of consciousness, posttraumatic amnesia, and less commonly, posttraumatic onset of seizures; (2) evidence from neuropsychological testing or quantified cognitive assessment of difficulty in attraction or memory; (3) three (or more) of the following occur shortly after the trauma and last at least 3 months: fatigue, sleep disturbance, headache, vertigo or dizziness, irritability or aggression on little or no provocation, anxiety or depression, changes in personality. Note: Diagnosis supported when symptoms in criteria (2) or (3) have onset following head trauma or worsening of preexisting symptoms, which causes significant impairment in social or occupational functioning or decline from previous level of functioning.[21,23]

Continued

TABLE 23.1 Definitions of Common Terms Used in Concussion-Related Literature and Care—cont'd

Persistent Postconcussion Symptoms (PPCS)

International Consensus: A constellation of nonspecific posttraumatic symptoms that may be linked to coexisting and/or confounding factors that reflects failure of normal clinical recovery where symptoms persist beyond expected time frames of more than 10–14 days in adults and >4 weeks in children. Persistent symptoms do not reflect a single pathophysiological entity and do not necessarily reflect ongoing physiological injury to the brain.[6]

Sports-Related Concussion (SRC)

International Consensus: A traumatic brain injury induced by biomechanical forces. Several common features that may be utilized in clinically defining the nature of a concussive head injury include[6]:

A direct blow to the head, face, neck, or elsewhere on the body with an impulsive force transmitted to the head

A rapid onset of short-lived impairment of neurological function that resolves spontaneously. However, in some cases, signs and symptoms evolve over a number of minutes to hours

Neuropathological changes, but the acute clinical signs and symptoms largely reflect a functional disturbance rather than a structural injury and, as such, no abnormality is seen on standard structural neuroimaging studies

A range of clinical signs and symptoms that may or may not involve loss of consciousness.

Clinical Recovery

International Consensus: A resolution of postconcussion-related symptoms and a return to clinically normal balance and cognitive functioning that leads to a return to normal activities, including school, work, and sport, after injury[6]

Physiological Recovery

International Consensus: Time of recovery that may outlast the time for clinical recovery for which there is no modality (e.g., neuroimaging, biomarkers) that can define a single 'physiological time window' for recovery following a concussion[6]

Second Impact Syndrome

A rare, often critical condition that arises when an individual, typically an athlete, sustains a second head injury before symptoms associated with an initial head injury have fully cleared. The second injury, it is believed, results in catastrophic brain swelling and can lead to death.[24,25,26]

Complicated mTBI

Mild traumatic brain injury that results in a visible trauma-related intracranial abnormality on structural neuroimaging (e.g., hemorrhage, contusion, or edema) such as a CT scan or MRI.[27]

International consensus: consensus statements, definitions, and recommendations provided by the 2017 Concussion in Sport Group international conference held in Berlin; *WHO-ICD-10, World Health Organization International Classification of Diseases,* 10th edition; *DSM-IV, Diagnostic and Statistical Manual of Mental Disorders,* 4th edition. (Note: the definitions provided for the WHO-ICD-10 and DSM-IV are abbreviated definitions. Complete definitions can be found on the respective websites for the World Health Organization and American Psychiatric Association.

CT, Computed tomography scan; *MRI,* magnetic resonance imaging; *mTBI,* mild traumatic brain injury.

Epidemiology

The most recent population data estimates 2.5 million traumatic brain injury–related emergency department (ED) visits, hospitalizations, and deaths each year in the United States.[28] According to the Nationwide ED Sample, the rate of mTBI in ED visits was 807 per 100,000 visits in 2012,[28] with the highest rates of mTBI requiring medical attention occurring in 0- to 4-year-olds, followed by male 15- to 24-year-olds, and females 65 years and older. The lowest rates were found for 45- to 64-year-olds.[28] Across all age groups, males were found to have a higher rate of mTBI ED visits compared with females, except among those patients aged 65 years and older.[28] Among all patients diagnosed with mTBI, falls were found to be the most common external cause of injury.[28]

In the United States, estimates of 1.6 to 3.8 million athletes sustain an SRC each year, a statistic that includes those for which no medical attention is sought.[31] With nearly 8 million participants annually, high school athletes make up the single largest athletic cohort in the country who may be susceptible to head injuries.[32] The National High School Sports-Related Injury Surveillance Study[33] showed that concussion moved from the fourth most

commonly reported category of injury in 2005–06 (9% of all sports-related injuries) to the most commonly reported injury category in 2016–17, accounting for 24.8% of all sports-related injuries.[33] The National Athletic Treatment, Injury and Outcomes Network (NATION) study that used a convenience sample of 147 high schools drawn from 26 states to compile data on 31 sports[34] found a total of 2004 SRCs across 3 academic years (2011–2014), leading to an overall SRC rate of 3.89 per 10,000 athletic exposures (defined as one student participating in one athletic practice or competition). High school football had the highest overall SRC rate, followed by boys' lacrosse and girls' soccer (Table 23.2). For all sports, the rate of SRC was higher during competition compared with practice.[34] Nearly 3% of all SRCs were reported to be recurrent concussions[34]; however, recurrent concussions, specifically in the high school athlete population, have been reported to account for 11% of all SRCs.[35]

During the 2009–10 to 2013–14 academic years, it was estimated that SRCs constituted 6.2% of all injuries that occurred during participation in collegiate athletics.[37] Wasserman and colleagues reported a total of 1670 SRCs in schools participating in the National Collegiate

TABLE 23.2 Concussion Counts and Rates Among Collegiate and High School Athletes

Sport	NUMBER OF CONCUSSIONS		CONCUSSION RATE/10,000 ATHLETIC EXPOSURES[c] (95% CONFIDENCE INTERVAL)		
	Competitions	Practices	Competitions	Practices	Overall
High School Athletes[a]					
Boys' football	409	611	19.87 (17.95, 21.80)	6.78 (6.24, 7.31)	9.21 (8.64, 9.78)
Boys' lacrosse	74	37	17.51 (13.52, 21.49)	2.97 (2.01, 3.93)	6.65 (5.41, 7.89)
Boys' soccer	60	23	11.33 (8.46, 14.20)	1.48 (0.87, 2.08)	3.98 (3.12, 4.83)
Boys' wrestling	45	92	10.21 (7.23, 13.20)	4.75 (3.78, 5.72)	5.76 (4.80, 6.73)
Boys' basketball	45	47	4.93 (3.49, 6.36)	1.72 (1.23, 2.21)	2.52 (2.01, 3.04)
Girls' soccer	66	40	17.16 (13.02, 21.30)	2.96 (2.04, 3.88)	6.11 (4.94, 7.27)
Girls' lacrosse	30	26	11.75 (7.55, 15.95)	3.44 (2.12, 4.76)	5.54 (4.09, 6.99)
Girls' basketball	81	47	10.52 (8.23, 12.82)	2.22 (1.59, 2.86)	4.44 (3.67, 5.20)
Girls' field hockey	39	27	9.83 (6.74, 12.91)	2.47 (1.54, 3.40)	4.42 (3.36, 5.49)
Girls' softball	24	26	6.33 (3.80, 8.86)	2.54 (1.57, 3.52)	3.57 (2.58, 4.56)
Girls' gymnastics	2	6	5.27 (0.00, 12.58)	2.28 (0.45, 4.10)	2.65 (0.81, 4.49)
Girls' volleyball	28	46	3.67 (2.31, 5.03)	2.09 (1.49, 2.69)	2.50 (1.93, 3.06)
Collegiate Athletes[b]					
Men's wrestling	46	40	55.46 (39.43, 71.48)	5.68 (3.92, 7.44)	10.92 (8.62, 13.23)
Men's football	262	341	30.07 (26.43, 33.71)	4.20 (3.75, 4.64)	6.71 (6.17, 7.24)
Men's ice hockey	170	54	24.89 (21.14, 28.63)	2.51 (1.84, 3.18)	7.91 (6.87, 8.95)
Men's soccer	33	22	9.69 (6.39, 13.00)	1.75 (1.02, 2.48)	3.44 (2.53, 4.35)
Men's lacrosse	25	26	9.31 (5.66, 12.96)	1.95 (1.20, 2.69)	3.18 (2.31, 4.05)
Men's basketball	26	58	5.60 (3.45, 7.75)	3.42 (2.54, 4.31)	3.89 (3.06, 4.72)
Women's ice hockey	60	25	20.10 (15.01, 25.18)	3.00 (1.82, 4.17)	7.50 (5.91, 9.10)
Women's soccer	101	35	19.38 (15.60, 23.16)	2.14 (1.43, 2.85)	6.31 (5.25, 7.37)
Women's lacrosse	27	28	13.08 (8.15, 18.02)	3.30 (2.08, 4.52)	5.21 (3.84, 6.59)
Women's field hockey	10	5	11.10 (4.22, 17.99)	1.77 (0.22, 3.32)	4.02 (1.99, 6.06)
Women's basketball	50	66	10.92 (7.89, 13.95)	4.43 (3.36, 5.50)	5.95 (4.87, 7.04)
Women's volleyball	26	30	5.75 (3.54, 7.96)	2.69 (1.73, 3.69)	3.57 (2.64, 4.51)
Women's softball	36	17	5.61 (3.77, 7.44)	1.75 (0.92, 2.58)	3.28 (2.40, 4.17)
Women's gymnastics	2	10	4.83 (0.00, 11.52)	2.43 (0.92, 3.93)	2.65 (1.15, 4.14)

[a]Statistics from the National Athletic Treatment, Injury and Outcomes Network (NATION), 2011–12 through 2013–14 academic years.[34]
[b]Statistics from the National Collegiate Athletic Association (NCAA) Injury Surveillance Program (ISP) in collegiate athletes from 2009–2010 through 2013–2014 academic years.[36]
[c]Athletic Exposures = One athlete participating in one sanctioned practice or competition.
Note: Table comprises the sports with the *highest rate of concussion during competitions*. The table does not report all sports included in the NATION[34] or NCAA ISP[36] studies.
Adapted from O'Connor KL, Baker MM, Dalton SL, Dompier TP, Broglio SP, Kerr ZY. Epidemiology of sport-related concussions in high school athletes: National Athletic Treatment, Injury and Outcomes Network (NATION), 2011–2012 through 2013–2014. *J Athl Train.* 2017;52(3):175–185 and Wasserman EB, Kerr ZY, Zuckerman SL, Covassin T. Epidemiology of sports-related concussions in National Collegiate Athletic Association athletes from 2009–2010 to 2013–2014: symptom prevalence, symptom resolution time, and return-to-play time. *Am J Sports Med.* 2016;44(1):226–233.

Athletic Association (NCAA) Injury Surveillance Program (ISP), leading to a yearly national estimate of 10,560 SRCs in collegiate sports.[36] Although football contributed the greatest number of SRCs (36.1%), followed by men's ice hockey (13.4%) and women's soccer (8.1%), of the 25 collegiate sports investigated in the NCAA ISP, men's wrestling and men's and women's ice hockey were found to have the highest overall concussion rates (see Table 23.2).[36,37] Similar to high school athletes, a higher rate of concussions occurred during competition compared with practice, with an injury rate of 14.59 and 2.57 per 10,000 athletic exposures, respectively.[36] Nearly 1 in every 11 SRCs that occurred were reported to be recurrent concussions.[36] Overall, most concussions were related to player contact; however, other mechanisms, such as contact with the playing surface and equipment such as sticks and balls, have been described.[37]

It is well documented that females are at greater risk of experiencing an SRC compared with males participating in high school and collegiate sports.[34,37–39] In high school athletics, the rate of SRCs has been found to be 56% higher in girls than in boys,[34] and the disparity in SRC incidence between girls and boys has been reported to be twice as high when considering contact sports alone.[35] Some researchers have suggested that structural and physiological differences in cervical spine morphology, strength, and dynamic stability[37,40,41] account for sex differences in the incidence of SRCs; however, given the evidence that female athletes are more likely than male athletes to report a concussion,[42,43] it is unlikely that potential structural and physiological differences solely explain the biological sex gap in SRC incidence.

Pathophysiology

The basic neurobiology of concussion has been described as a neurometabolic cascade of events that does not always result in cell death, but will lead to a functional injury where cells undergo a significant energy crisis. This process, referred to as the *bioenergetic crisis*, is characterized by a mismatch between energy supply and demand.[44]

Neurons have a relatively high consumption of oxygen and depend almost exclusively on oxidative phosphorylation for energy production. Mechanical deformation of neurons, termed *mechanoporation*, caused by an acceleration/deceleration force quickly leads to two mechanisms of dysfunction: failure of energy-dependent ion transport pumps and release of large quantities of glutamate. Failure of the energy-dependent ion pumps allows charged ions to move across their electrical and concentration gradients, leading to an efflux of potassium and an influx of calcium and sodium. Excessive concentrations of calcium and sodium within the cell causes degradation of cytoskeletal proteins and cytotoxic edema as water follows positively charged ions into the cell. The ionic flux leads to an energy crisis as a considerable amount of the cell's energy reserve is spent attempting to restore ionic homeostasis by pumping calcium and water out of the cell. A direct consequence of the excessive calcium influx is release of excessive glutamate, a potent excitatory molecule, into the extracellular space. Glutamate then binds to *N*-methyl-D-aspartate (NMDA) receptors on neighboring neurons leading to calcium influx and release of more glutamate into the extracellular space. This process, referred to as *excitotoxicity*, leads to a self-perpetuating, deleterious cycle of hyperexcitability and cellular instability.

Another contribution to the energy crisis is an initial decrease in cerebral blood flow, which creates a mismatch between energy supply and demand (increased glucose metabolism to support increased neural activity) in the initial stages of concussion.[44] Functionally, the cell is then vulnerable to subsequent injury,[44] meaning the cell has less energy reserve or resources to address a subsequent stress, be it a second biomechanical stress (e.g., second impact syndrome) or a functional stress such as an increased cognitive or physical load. This point is important for medical professionals who consider return to play protocols in acute concussion as the impaired metabolic state can extend for weeks to months.[44–46]

Cytoskeletal and axonal alteration due to axonal stretch can interfere with axonal transport, leading to impaired synaptic transmission and in severe cases result in retraction and degeneration of the synapse.[44] This process, referred to as *axonal disconnection*, can be a transient event and in some cases may recover, but due to the poor regenerative capacity of the central nervous system, such stretching may lead to permanent axonal damage.[47,48]

Recent studies suggest that inflammatory changes are also triggered by mTBI[44] and cause functional disruption of neural activity.

Cytokines, cystokines, and immune-mediated responses may play in important role in neuroinflammation after injury.[49] Immunoassay of plasma cytokines, chemokines, epinephrine, and norepinephrine in individuals following brain trauma has revealed a relationship between systemic inflammation and autonomic nervous system dysregulation with an acute hyperadrenergic state.[50] A preliminary study of rugby players who have sustained concussion injuries indicates that genetic influences may trigger a postinflammatory brain syndrome (PIBS) that is congruent with prolonged symptoms after injury.[51]

It appears there is little to no cell death associated with mTBI; however, the impact of subsequent head injury or potential detrimental structural and physiological degeneration that occurs over time is unclear. In longitudinal studies of mTBI using rodent models, there is evidence of cortical and subcortical atrophy and depletion of dopaminergic neurons in subcortical nuclei[44]; however, the degree to which the changes occur in humans or how they relate to impaired cognitive, physical, and emotional function following a concussion in humans has not been determined at this time.

Persistent Symptoms/Prolonged Recovery

Injuries that seem mild initially can occasionally cause a constellation of somatic, cognitive, emotional, and behavioral symptoms.[52] In most cases, the majority of individuals will have a complete functional recovery and return to their life activities without the burden of these sequelae.[6,53] But a "miserable minority,"[54] approximately 10% to 33% of patients, will experience an incomplete recovery, and their symptoms often persist for months or even years after the initial injury.[52,55–58] Using these numbers, an estimated 200,000 to 600,000 individuals every year in the United States are likely to experience persistent symptoms after a head injury. With few longitudinal studies, there is limited information related to time periods that persistent symptoms may last; however, for concussions in general, the prevalence of persistent symptoms at 1 year following the injury is estimated to be 5%.[59]

As one may expect, differences have been found across age groups for patients who continue to endorse persistent symptoms following a concussion. For SRCs, higher rates of persistent symptoms have been reported following concussion in cohorts of high school athletes compared with collegiate and professional athletes. Using American football as an example, 17% to 30% of high school athletes have persistent symptoms greater than 21 days following injury,[60,61] and 10% to 15% of collegiate athletes have symptoms beyond 10 days,[62] while it is uncommon for professional athletes to experience persistent symptoms beyond 7 days.[63]

Although a small number of patients may have symptoms that persist for 1 year, several reports from specialty concussion clinics in rehabilitation have described children and adults who present for treatment with continued symptoms that have persisted for 2 to 5 years following injury,[64–66] which may represent up to 20% of the patients with mTBI who are referred for care in these specialty clinics.[64]

Several terms have been used to characterize symptoms following a concussion, such as postconcussion syndrome (PCS), persistent postconcussion syndrome,[59] persistent postconcussion symptoms (PPCS), prolonged recovery,[67] protracted recovery,[68,69] or slow-to-recover (see Table 23.1).[70] Importantly, there is continued controversy related to the time period used to classify individuals into one of these categories and what the underlying cause of the continued symptom complaint may be. Barlow and colleagues and Yeates and colleagues showed individuals who endorse somatic, cognitive, emotional, and/or behavioral symptoms following a biomechanical force to the head recover differently than those who endorse similar symptoms following an injury to the body without sustaining a hit to the head.[21,71] Barlow and colleagues conducted one of the largest prospective, population-based studies comparing symptom complaints of children (aged 0 to 18 years) after mTBI (as defined by the American Congress of Rehabilitation Medicine) to children who presented to the ED with an extracranial injury (ECI). Three months after injury, 11% of children were symptomatic in the mTBI group compared with 0.5% in the ECI group. Between group differences were even larger when considering children and adolescents between the ages of 6 and 18, where 13.7% of the mTBI group were symptomatic 3 months following the injury compared with only 1% of the ECI group.[21]

For simplicity, but not to suggest consensus in the literature related to proper classification of such individuals, we will use the term PPCS to refer to adults who continue to be symptomatic 10 to 14 days following injury and children (aged 0 to 18 years) who continue to be symptomatic 28 to 30 days following injury.[6] Risk factors and outcomes associated with PPCS and treatment options for different clinical profiles will be reviewed in later sections.

EXAMINATION OF THE ACUTE CONCUSSION

Given that a concussion is broadly defined as a complex pathophysiological process affecting the brain, induced by biomechanical forces, there are challenges for physicians to diagnose a concussion. The primary challenge is the absence of a valid and reliable diagnostic test or battery of diagnostic tests that can be used to diagnose concussion. In addition, signs and symptoms of concussion can mimic other health conditions, and the evolving nature of the clinical presentation can present a challenge to medical professionals as signs and symptoms, such as headache or change in mental status that may not appear immediately or may emerge minutes to hours later either when an individual is at rest or undergoes cognitive or physical exertion.[72] In relation to SRC, time constraints or pressures from coaches and parents can also pose challenges to diagnose the acute concussion.

For these reasons, during sporting events, it is recommended that licensed medical personnel, which may include a sideline physician and at least one athletic trainer, should use the Recognize, Remove, and Evaluate (Reevaluate) framework in the medical management of the acute concussion.[6,9,72] In short, where concussion is suspected (Recognize), the athlete must be removed (Remove) from participation in the sport to undergo an assessment (Evaluate) by a physician or other licensed medical professional. The sideline evaluation should be composed of multimodal testing that includes, at least, an evaluation of symptom complaint, mental status, cognitive performance, and motor control (Table 23.3).[6,72] It is important to note that standard orientation questions (e.g., time, place, person, and situation) are unreliable in sport situations; therefore more comprehensive mental status and cognitive testing is recommended.[6]

Recognize

Parents, coaches, spectators, and most importantly licensed medical professionals must understand that the brain can undergo a neurometabolic crisis without the head coming in contact with an object or the brain coming in contact with the inside of the skull.[6,9,72] The only requirement for a concussive event is the presence of a large enough acceleration/deceleration force, which can result from a direct blow to the head, or a blow to the body, that subsequently causes a whiplash movement of the head and neck.[72] Importantly, the injury does not require loss of consciousness, loss of memory, or the presence of apparent neurological decline.[6,72] Suspected diagnosis of SRC can include one or more of the following clinical domains[6]:

- Symptoms: somatic (e.g., headache), cognitive (e.g., feeling like in a fog), and/or emotional symptoms (e.g., lability)

TABLE 23.3 Tests and Measures Used for Preinjury Baseline Assessment and Sideline Examination for Acute Concussion

Preinjury/Preparticipation Baseline Evaluation

Full Neurological Examination

Clinical History

Past Medical History: previous number of concussions, recovery from previous concussions, prior history of migraine headaches, prior history of mental health problems/mood disorders, attention and learning disorders, sleep disorders and/or disorders

Family History: mood disorders, learning disability, ADHD, migraine headaches

Tests and Measures

Mental status, cranial nerves, reflexes, sensorimotor systems, gait, balance and coordination assessment

Cognitive Tests

Standardized Assessment of Concussion (SAC)[73,74]

Immediate Post-Concussion Assessment and Cognitive Testing (ImPACT)[75]

Axon Sports Computerized Cognitive Assessment Tool (CCAT)[76]

Physical Tests

Reaction time test: "Stick drop" test[77]

Oculomotor assessment: King-Devick test for visual tracking[78]

Balance assessment: Balance Error Scoring System[79,80]

Cervical Spine Joint Position Sense Error[81]

Sideline Examination

Cognitive Tests

SCAT5 or Child SCAT5[6]

Standardized Assessment of Concussion (SAC)[73,74]

Immediate Post-Concussion Assessment and Cognitive Testing (ImPACT)[75]

Axon Sports Computerized Cognitive Assessment Tool (CCAT)[76]

Physical Tests

Reaction time test: "Stick drop" test[77]

Oculomotor assessment: King-Devick test for visual tracking[78] or Vestibular/Ocular Motor Screening[82]

Balance assessment: Balance Error Scoring System[79,80]

Symptom Assessment

Postconcussion Symptom Inventory (PCSI)[83]

Post Concussion Symptom Scale[84] (PCSS)

Rivermead Postconcussive Symptom Questionnaire (RPQ)[85]

Health and Behavior Inventory[86]

Graded Symptom Checklist[87]

Mood/Anxiety Assessment

Center for Epidemiologic Studies Depression Scale (CES-D)[88]

ADHD, Attention-deficit hyperactivity disorder.

- Physical signs (e.g., loss of consciousness, amnesia, neurological deficit)
- Balance impairment (e.g., gait unsteadiness)
- Behavioral changes (e.g., irritability)
- Cognitive impairment (e.g., slowed attention speed)

Given the circumstances that may provide sufficient force to cause a functional injury, combined with the fact that such signs and symptoms can be observed or reported following physical exertion in a nonconcussed athlete,[58,89,90] it can be difficult for the medical professional to make the correct choice to Recognize and Remove in every case. It is therefore strongly recommended that the medical professional always error on the side of caution.[6,9] Once a concussion is suspected, the athlete should be removed from participation in the sport, and the athlete will not return to participation: (1) within the same day, and (2) until an evaluation by a licensed medical professional (Evaluate) has been completed.

Remove

There is overwhelming agreement across position statements and consensus reports that an athlete who is suspected of sustaining a concussion should not return to participation within the same day.[6,72,15] In fact, this recommendation is mandated by law in all 50 states in the United States with regard to children and adolescent concussions.[72] Athletes are removed from participation in sports, especially contact sports, to remove the risk of impact during a time when the brain is vulnerable to damage from an initial injury. The time period of this vulnerable state is unclear, as it has been shown to last up to 5 days in rodent models,[91] but it is not known how this time frame translates to human populations. Therefore it is important to note, the medical professional is not withdrawing the athlete from physical activity in general, although there is evidence that vigorous exercise during this vulnerable period of brain recovery can lead to delayed recovery in rodent models of mTBI[92]; instead, the athlete is removed from participation at the time of suspected concussion to reduce the risk of another mechanical force occurring on an already injured brain during the acute neurometabolic crisis, an event known as the rare but potentially dangerous second impact syndrome.[24,25]

If a concussion is suspected, medical personnel must address first aid issues including an assessment of the "ABCs" (airway, breathing, circulation). If any of these are compromised, or if there is prolonged loss of consciousness, seizure, suspicion, or evidence of cervical spine instability or a rapidly deteriorating level of consciousness, emergency medical services should be activated immediately.[6,72]

Evaluate

In the majority of cases the athlete is able to leave the playing area independently or with assistance from medical personnel and should be escorted to a safe, isolated environment[72] for a sideline evaluation. The objective of the sideline evaluation is to provide a rapid screening for a suspected SRC that may rule out the need for urgent referral to emergency services to address critical medical conditions (e.g., hemorrhage, elevated intracranial pressure, cervical spine instability).

The sideline evaluation should be composed of tests and measures that assess the functional system domains known to be affected by concussion, and at a minimum should include a neurocognitive, motor control, and symptom complaint assessment,[6,9,15] which could be accomplished by using the Sport Concussion Assessment Tool 5 (SCAT5) or Standardized Assessment of Concussion (SAC), combined with a physical test and a self-report checklist for symptom complaints (see Table 23.3). The following section describes the tests and measures that should be used in the sideline evaluation. The National Institute of Neurological Disorders and Stroke (NINDS) has supported the collaboration of basic science researchers, clinician-researchers, and clinicians to develop a recommendation for Common Data Elements (CDE) to be used in the assessment of individuals following SRC during the acute (less than 3 days), subacute (3 days to 3 months), and chronic (greater than or equal to 3 months) phases of recovery following

concussion.[93] Recommendations from the NINDS CDE can be obtained at https://www.commondataelements.ninds.nih.gov/SRC.aspx#tab=Data_Standards.

Neurocognitive Assessment

The SCAT5 was designed to provide an organized framework for performing a neurological sports concussion assessment[72,94] and currently represents the most well-established and rigorously developed instrument available for sideline assessment.[6] The SCAT5 is the most recent version of a comprehensive concussion assessment agreed upon by international consensus.[6] There is a brief version created for a sideline assessment, which takes 15 to 20 minutes to complete, and a more complete "off-field" evaluation designed to be completed in the clinic as a follow-up (Reevaluate) after the time of injury. The SCAT5 is most useful in differentiating concussed from nonconcussed athletes immediately after injury, as its utility appears to decrease significantly 3 to 5 days after injury.[6] The SCAT5 is designed for athletes 13 years and older, and the Child SCAT5 should be used for children 12 years and younger. Each test may be freely copied and distributed to individuals, teams, groups, and organizations to use; however, it is important to emphasize that the tools should be used and results should be interpreted by licensed medical professionals. Each tool can be found at the British Journal of Sports Medicine website: SCAT5: http://dx.doi.org/10.1136/bjsports-2017-097506SCAT5, Child SCAT5: http://dx.doi.org/10.1136/bjsports-2017-097492childscat5.

The Standardized Assessment of Concussion (SAC) is an instrument designed for rapid assessment (5 minutes) immediately following a suspected concussion consisting of four neurocognitive domains: orientation, immediate memory, concentration, and delayed recall.[72] The total score ranges from 0 to 30, with lower scores indicating more severe cognitive impairment. The assessment has poor test-retest reliability with an intraclass correlation coefficient (ICC) value of 0.39 with 95% confidence intervals of 0.36 to 0.42.[95] Similar to the SCAT5, the diagnostic utility of the SAC diminishes over time, as the ability to distinguish concussed from nonconcussed athletes decreases after 2 days.[89]

The Immediate Post-Concussion Assessment Tool (ImPACT) is a 25-minute test that assesses different neurocognitive domains such as attention span, working memory, sustained and selective attention time, visual processing speed, nonverbal problem solving, and reaction time.[95,84] The components of the ImPACT have fair-to-good test-retest reliability, ranging from ICC values of 0.47 for ImPACT reaction time to 0.72 for ImPACT visual motor speed.[95] The sensitivity (Sn) of the ImPACT has been found to be 81.9% and the specificity (Sp) to be 89.4% to rule in or rule out a concussion, respectively.[96] This product must be purchased, and the cost differs depending on the organization purchasing the rights to perform the test.

Oculomotor Assessment

The King-Devick concussion screening test. The King-Devick test requires patients to rapidly read single-digit numbers from a series of three cards, with cards uniquely arranged and spaced for progressively more challenging reading tasks with each successive card. Patients can be asked to read each card in right-left or up-down direction as fast as possible without making an error, as a means to evaluate saccadic eye movements. The time to complete each card is measured and the number of errors are calculated. The best time (fastest) of two trials without errors is used as the timed value for the test.[97] Worsening of time and/or errors identified during testing have been associated with concussive injury.[78,98,99] The King-Devick test has been found to have excellent test-retest reliability with ICC values of 0.96[98] and 0.97.[97] The King-Devick test can be administered in less than 2 minutes.

TABLE 23.4 Tool Used to Monitor Symptom Complaint During the Vestibular/Ocular Motor Screening Assessment

Vestibular/Ocular Motor Test:	Headache 0–10	Dizziness 0–10	Nausea 0–10	Fogginess 0–10	Other
Smooth pursuits					
Saccades—horizontal					
Saccades—vertical					
Convergence					Near point distance in cm: Measure 1: _____ Measure 2: _____ Measure 3: _____
VOR—horizontal					
VOR—vertical					
Visual motion sensitivity					

VOR, Vestibulo-ocular reflex.
Adapted from Mucha A, Collins MW, Elbin RJ, et al. A brief Vestibular/Ocular Motor Screening (VOMS) assessment to evaluate concussions: preliminary findings. *Am J Sports Med.* 2014;42(10):2479–2486.

Vestibular/Ocular Motor Screening

The vestibular/ocular motor screening (VOMS) assessment was created in part due to the absence of a brief, comprehensive clinical bedside assessment that could be used to evaluate vestibulo-ocular and ocular motor eye movements, as common tests completed at the time of injury such as the King-Devick, SCAT5, or Balance Error Scoring System (BESS) do not include comprehensive assessments of the vestibulo-ocular and ocular motor systems.[82] The VOMS tool measures symptom provocation after each assessment of smooth pursuit, horizontal and vertical saccades, near point convergence (NPC), horizontal and vertical vestibulo-ocular reflex (VOR), and visual motion sensitivity. Near point of convergence (NPC) testing is assessed based on the average measurement of three trials of NPC distance. Before the assessment, patients are instructed to rate symptoms of headache, dizziness, nausea, and fogginess on a scale ranging from 0, meaning *no symptoms at present*, to 10, meaning *severe symptoms at present*.[100] After each assessment, patients are asked to reevaluate their symptoms, paying specific attention to how their symptoms may have changed (Table 23.4).[82] The VOMS tool has demonstrated strong internal consistency and significant correlation with the Post Concussion Symptom Scale (PCSS). The VOMS can potentially differentiate children who sustain an SRC within 14 days as they were found to score significantly higher on all VOMS items, compared with healthy controls.[82,100] Specifically, an NPC distance of greater than or equal to 5 cm increases the probability of a concussion by at least 34% (positive likelihood ratio [LR+] = 5.8).

Elbin and colleagues[101] evaluated prospective changes in the VOMS at three time points (baseline, 1 to 7 days, and 8 to 14 days following SRC) in 83 high school athletes aged 14 to 18 years and found the total and change from baseline scores revealed significant impairment at 1 to 7 days with return to baseline levels by 8 to 14 days. The authors concluded that the interpretation of the VOMS cutoff values should be compared with baseline values (e.g., preparticipation scores), as there is a higher probability of a false-positive if the total score is assessed in isolation. In fact, up to 35% of high school athletes[101] and 11% of collegiate athletes[102] report total symptom scores above the clinical cutoffs on the VOMS at preparticipation assessments.

Balance Assessment

Balance error scoring system. The Balance Error Scoring System (BESS) is a clinical balance assessment of postural stability, which is a component of the SCAT5 and can be completed within 5 minutes.[79,103,104] The BESS was designed to evaluate steady-state balance for clinicians without instrumented laboratory equipment. The BESS has been validated in children, adolescents, and adults with concussion, and has compared favorably to laboratory-based posturography tools such as the sensory organization test (SOT).[104] The BESS consists of three stances: double-leg stance (hands on hips and feet together), single-leg stance (standing on the nondominant leg with hands on hips), and a tandem stance (nondominant foot behind the dominant foot) in a heel-to-toe fashion.[79] The six testing conditions are shown in Fig. 23.1. The stances are performed on a firm surface and on a foam surface with the eyes closed, with errors counted during each 20-second trial. An error is defined as any one of the following: opening eyes, lifting hands off hips, stepping, stumbling or falling out of position, lifting forefoot or heel, abducting the hip by more than 30 degrees, or failing to return to the test position in more than 5 seconds.[79] Multiple errors that are committed simultaneously are counted as a single error. The maximum number of errors in each trial is 10, and the maximum number of errors in total is 60.[103]

The BESS has high sensitivity (94%), when combined with a brief neurocognitive examination and symptom report, to detect individuals with concussion.[105] However, the sensitivity of the BESS declines rapidly in the days postinjury.[89,105] Test-retest reliability has been found to be moderate in children aged 9 to 18 years and young adults,[79] with large ranges of intrarater (ICC values of 0.60 to 0.92) and interrater (ICC values of 0.57 to 0.85) reliability depending on the age and mechanism of injury.[79] Scores can be compared with normative data for community-dwelling adults,[106] which may not be appropriate for comparison of performance in the child and adolescent populations. For this reason, Alsalaheen and colleagues[107] described percentile scores for the 6 testing conditions of the BESS in 91 high school students (mean age 15.6 years), which can be used to gauge age-normed performance on each of the conditions for the test. Findings from Alsalaheen and colleagues were consistent with previous studies showing the average number of errors accumulated in high school and

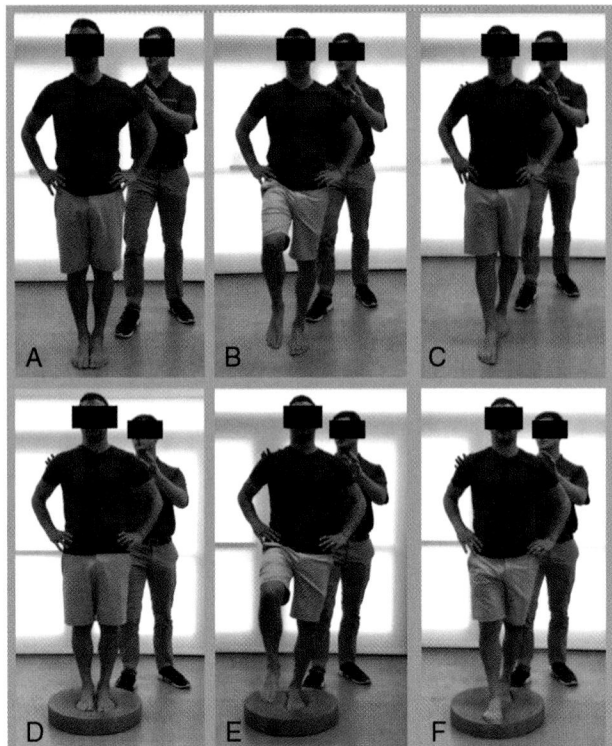

Fig. 23.1 Six Conditions of the Balance Error Scoring System to Assess Balance Performance in Acute Concussion. Stances used in Balance Error Scoring System: **(A)** double-leg stance; **(B)** single-leg stance (standing on the nondominant limb); **(C)** tandem stance; **(D)** double-leg stance with foam; **(E)** single leg on foam; and **(F)** tandem stance on foam. (Adapted from Bell, 2011.[79])

collegiate athletes without history of concussion ranges from 12 to 13 errors.[107] Therefore there is evidence to support the use of the BESS test, in combination with cognitive and symptom scales, as a diagnostic measure early following concussion or as a screening tool to compare a patient's performance to age-match norms for adolescents and adults. However, psychometric properties of the test do not support its use as an outcome measure, as it is not responsive to change in performance over time, nor has it been validated for use in the subacute and chronic stages of recovery following concussion.

Symptom Complaint

Postconcussion symptom inventory. The Postconcussion Symptom Inventory (PCSI) is a standardized self-report questionnaire that allows an individual to provide an overall rating of symptoms following concussion.[93] The scale covers six domains: affective, amnesia, cognitive, fatigue, physical, and sleep. The PCSI was modified from the original Postconcussion Scale[108] for appropriate use in children. The PCSI has three forms for children of different ages; the PCSI-SR5 (https://www.commondataelements.ninds.nih.gov/ReportViewer.aspx?/nindscdereports/rptNOC&rs:Command=Render&rc:Parameters=false&crfID=F2351) for ages 5 to 7 years; the PCSI-SR8 (https://www.commondataelements.ninds.nih.gov/ReportViewer.aspx?/nindscdereports/rptNOC&rs:Command=Render&rc:Parameters=false&crfID=F2355) for ages 8 to 12 years; and the PCSI-SR13 (https://www.commondataelements.ninds.nih.gov/

ReportViewer.aspx?/nindscdereports/rptNOC&rs:Command=Render&rc:Parameters=false&crfID=F2354) for children aged 13 to 18 years.[83] The tool has been found to have fair-to-good to excellent reliability with ICC values of 0.65 to 0.89 over a 2-week testing period for the four patient-centered questionnaires.[83] A questionnaire has also been developed for parents to report observations of symptom complaints in their children aged 5 to 18 years (PCSI-P; https://www.commondataelements.ninds.nih.gov/ReportViewer.aspx?/nindscdereports/rptNOC&rs:Command=Render&rc:Parameters=false&crfID=F1978). Interestingly, for individuals following concussion, parent-child concordance was low to moderate for individual symptom but moderate to strong for the subscales and the total score of the PCSI.[83] Test-retest reliability of the parent administered test has not been reported, and no information related to the responsiveness to change in the measure has been established.

Post concussion symptom scale. The PCSS is a portion of the SCAT5 that allows the patient to identify symptoms they are experiencing and attempts to quantify the severity of each symptom (Fig. 23.2).[6] The PCSS requires the patient to rate the severity of 22 different symptoms of concussion on a 0 to 6 scale, with higher scores indicating greater severity of symptoms. Patients can be assigned a symptom severity score from 0 to 132.

In the subacute and chronic stages of recovery, the scale has been validated for individuals with PPCS, though there are no cutoff values reported to rule in/out the condition. Instead, there are established norms for males and females, which the rehabilitation specialist could use to quantify symptom severity.[84] The scale can also be used as an outcome measure to monitor within subject changes in the number and intensity of symptom complaints over time. The PCSS was found to have a standard error of measurement (SEM) value of 5.3 points for high school and collegiate males and females who have sustained a concussion.[84]

Rivermead post-concussion symptoms questionnaire. The Rivermead Post-Concussion Symptoms Questionnaire (RPQ) is a 16-item self-report questionnaire in which patients rate the severity of cognitive, emotional, and physical symptoms in comparison with how the patient perceived they were functioning prior to their injury.[85] Items in the RPQ can be divided into two subcategories: the RPQ-3 and the RPQ-13. The RPQ-3 is associated with common sequela of postconcussive symptoms (e.g., headaches, dizziness, nausea and/or vomiting) that often occur early following the injury (score range 0 to 12). The RPQ-13 is associated with having a greater impact on individuals' participation, psychosocial functioning, and lifestyle (score range 0 to 52).[109] For both subcategories, a higher score indicates a more impaired condition. The RPQ has been shown to be a valid measure of outcome, particularly after a mild to moderate head injury.[110]

Health and behavior inventory. The Health and Behavior Inventory (HBI) is a 50-item self-report questionnaire, which requires parents and children to rate the frequency of somatic, cognitive, emotional, and behavioral symptoms over the past week on a four-point scale, ranging from "never" to "often."[111] Significant parent-child agreement at the item level and on composite symptom dimensions have been reported,[112] revealing two underlying dimensions of the HBI—cognitive and somatic symptoms.[111,113]

Graded symptom checklist. The Graded Symptom Checklist (GSC) is a 17-item self-rated survey of postconcussive symptoms, where patients score each item on a Likert scale of 0, indicating no symptoms to 6 indicating severe symptoms.[90] The total score ranges from 0 to 102, with lower scores reflecting a lower symptom burden. The tool is estimated to take 2 to 3 minutes to complete.

How do you feel?
"You should score yourself on the following symptoms, based on how you feel now."

	None	Mild		Moderate		Severe	
Headache	0	1	2	3	4	5	6
"Pressure in head"	0	1	2	3	4	5	6
Neck Pain	0	1	2	3	4	5	6
Nausea or vomiting	0	1	2	3	4	5	6
Dizziness	0	1	2	3	4	5	6
Blurred vision	0	1	2	3	4	5	6
Balance problems	0	1	2	3	4	5	6
Sensitivity to light	0	1	2	3	4	5	6
Sensitivity to noise	0	1	2	3	4	5	6
Feeling slowed down	0	1	2	3	4	5	6
Feeling like "in a fog"	0	1	2	3	4	5	6
"Don't feel right"	0	1	2	3	4	5	6
Difficulty concentrating	0	1	2	3	4	5	6
Difficulty remembering	0	1	2	3	4	5	6
Fatigue or low energy	0	1	2	3	4	5	6
Confusion	0	1	2	3	4	5	6
Drowsiness	0	1	2	3	4	5	6
Trouble falling asleep	0	1	2	3	4	5	6
More emotional	0	1	2	3	4	5	6
Irritability	0	1	2	3	4	5	6
Sadness	0	1	2	3	4	5	6
Nervous or anxious	0	1	2	3	4	5	6

Total number of symptoms (maximum possible 22)
Symptom severity score (maximum possible 132)

A

Circle one for each listed	None	Rarely	Sometimes	Often
I have trouble paying attention	0	1	2	3
I get distracted easily	0	1	2	3
I have a hard time concentrating	0	1	2	3
I have problems remembering what people tell me	0	1	2	3
I have problems following directions	0	1	2	3
I daydream too much	0	1	2	3
I get confused	0	1	2	3
I forget things	0	1	2	3
I have problems finishing things	0	1	2	3
I have trouble figuring things out	0	1	2	3
It's hard for me to learn new things	0	1	2	3
I have headaches	0	1	2	3
I feel dizzy	0	1	2	3
I feel like the room is spinning	0	1	2	3
I feel like I'm going to faint	0	1	2	3
Things are blurry when I look at them	0	1	2	3
I see double/two of things	0	1	2	3
I feel sick to my stomach	0	1	2	3
I get tired a lot	0	1	2	3
I get tired easily	0	1	2	3

B

Fig. 23.2 **(A)** Postconcussion symptom scale within SCAT5. **(B)** Postconcussion symptom score checklist recommended for children, kindergarten to sixth grade. (A, Modified from McCrory P, Meeuwisse WH, Aubry M, et al. Consensus statement on concussion in sport: the 5th International Conference on Concussion in Sport held in Belin, October 2016. *Br J Sports Med.* 2017;51:838–847. B, Modified from McCrory P, Meeuwisse WH, Aubry M, et al. Consensus statement on concussion in sport: the 4th International Conference on Concussion in Sport held in Zurich, November 2012. *Br J Sports Med.* 2013;47[5]:250–258.)

The sideline evaluation does not need to resemble the full, comprehensive neurological evaluation performed in the clinic by a physician with experience in the examination of individuals with brain injury (Reevaluate) or the complete evaluation used as the preparticipation baseline assessment (both of which may use neuropsychological testing). Although there is debate for the need of the preparticipation assessment across all youth, high school, and collegiate sports, it is recommended that all athletes participating in contact or collision sports undergo a baseline assessment.[9,15,72] It is true that the degree of cognitive, physical, emotional, and/or behavioral change that may occur in the athlete following a concussion can be assessed more accurately when compared with information obtained from a preparticipation assessment, the results of the sideline assessment can be interpreted without a preinjury baseline assessment.[6] Further consideration should be taken when comparing postinjury findings to preinjury baseline assessments as a recent analysis of the test-retest reliability for many tests and measures used in the baseline assessment have poor to fair test-retest reliability with a 1- and 2-year test interval.[95]

Reevaluate

It is beyond the scope of this chapter to describe the clinical interview and physical examination performed by a physician for a patient presenting with symptoms following a concussion. For a full discussion, the reader is directed to the following reviews: Matuszak and colleagues[114]; Ellis and colleagues[115]; McKeag and colleagues[116]; Kutcher and Giza.[72]

There is a strong recommendation that the reevaluation include neuropsychological testing (pencil and paper or computerized), which may be administered without a licensed Neuropsychologist or Speech-Language Pathologist (SLP), but requires the knowledge base and skill set of a Neuropsychologist or SLP to interpret the results of the neuropsychological tests.[72] For the majority of patients, a neurological screening examination will reveal no abnormalities[17,115]; however, any focal neurological deficits or severe neck pain presenting with malalignment or radicular symptoms should indicate imaging of the appropriate body area.[114,115] The objective of the follow-up clinical evaluation, performed by a neurologist or sports medicine physician who is experienced in the examination and treatment of athletes following a concussion, is to determine the diagnosis of concussion, inform medical management, and to determine recommendations for return to play/sport and return to school/learn.

Determination of Diagnosis of Concussion

As mentioned previously, no single test or battery of tests has the absolute sensitivity and specificity to diagnose a concussion; therefore concussion is a clinical diagnosis and requires the judgment of a physician. For this reason, a classification system has been proposed, which is based on the level of certainty for diagnosis of concussion being possible, probable, or definite.[72] The physician should consider if the mechanism of injury and the signs and symptoms follow a reasonable pattern and time course of concussion. The natural course of concussion being early symptom provocation within the first 1 to 2 days of injury improves gradually over time, given that no introduction to exacerbating activities occurs in that time.[17,72] Therefore an athlete who was unresponsive for ten seconds following a head-to-head collision in a soccer match who presents 36 hours later with headache, dizziness, and difficulty concentrating while reading would have a reasonable mechanism of injury (witnessed head-to-head collision) combined with a decline in mental status (loss of consciousness) to meet the criteria for a diagnosis of definite concussion. However, in the case of the athlete with a prior medical history of migraine who presents to the physician with complaints of headache, dizziness, and nausea exacerbated by physical exertion, which began 2 weeks

following a cross-country event where the athlete states she "may have hit her head," concussion is not the most likely cause of the clinical presentation given the absence of a reasonable mechanism of injury, the extensive delay in symptom provocation, and the symptoms that mimic a known comorbidity of migraine. The female cross-country athlete would likely be diagnosed with possible concussion, and the medical management of whether to treat as though this female athlete has a concussion would be the physician's discretion.

Medical Management

Some postconcussion injury symptoms may be addressed in the early stages with pharmacological therapies. Following concussion, pharmacological agents can be prescribed to treat headache, sleep disturbances, nausea, mood disorders, and cognitive deficits (e.g., attentional deficits), as they are indicated for nonconcussed patients.[72] Table 23.5 provides examples of commonly prescribed medications and side effects to manage postconcussion symptoms. It is important to note there is limited evidence demonstrating efficacy of such medications to address symptoms following concussion, and to date, there is still no FDA-approved pharmacological treatment for SRC.[3,14] Expert opinion suggests that medications should be tapered and then limited 2 to 10 days following the concussion, and then stopped by 2 weeks postinjury.[72] In the case of PPCS, pharmacological interventions should be combined with active rehabilitation programs and lifestyle management for optimal treatment.[3]

The final outcome of the reevaluation by a physician is to determine return to play/sport and return to school/learn recommendations. Given the absence of a direct method for measuring the pathophysiology of the injury to determine when the neurometabolic cascade has recovered (i.e., physiological recovery), once the patient is asymptomatic, he/she

TABLE 23.5 Commonly Prescribed Medications for Postconcussion Symptoms

Medication	Classification	Side Effects
Migraine Headache		
Aspirin	NSAID	Gastritis, gastrointestinal bleeding, peptic ulcer disease, rebound headache
Acetaminophen	Analgesic	Gastritis, gastrointestinal bleeding, peptic ulcer disease, rebound headache
Triptans	Serotonin 1B/1D-receptor agonists	Dizziness, fatigue, headache, numbness or tingling
Sleep Disturbances		
Trazodone	SSRI	Headache, nausea, vomiting, diarrhea, constipation
Melatonin	Hormone	Drowsiness, headache, nausea, depression
Amitriptyline	TCAs	Nausea, vomiting, drowsiness, weakness, headache
Mood Disorders (Depression)		
Sertraline (Zoloft)	SSRI	Nausea, diarrhea, constipation, vomiting, sleep disturbances, dizziness, fatigue, headache
Citalopram (Celexa)	SSRI	Nausea, diarrhea, constipation, vomiting, stomach pain, heartburn, decreased appetite, weight loss
Escitalopram (Lexapro)	SSRI	Nausea, diarrhea, constipation, change in sex drive, drowsiness, increased sweating, dizziness
Fluoxetine (Prozac)	SSRI	Nervousness, anxiety, sleep disturbances, nausea, diarrhea, weakness, loss of appetite, weight loss
Cognitive Deficits		
Amantadine	Neurostimulant	Diarrhea, constipation, nausea, orthostatic hypotension, increased irritability
Methylphenidate (Ritalin)	Neurostimulant	Elevated heart rate and blood pressure
Donepezil	Acetylcholinesterase inhibitor	Nausea, vomiting, diarrhea, loss of appetite, weight loss, urinary issues

NSAID, Nonsteroidal antiinflammatory drug; *SSRI,* selective serotonin reuptake inhibitor; *TCA,* tricyclic antidepressant.

should engage in routine activity and begin the process of graduated exertion.[6] For information related to rest and activity guidelines following concussion, see "Recommendations for Return to Play and Return to School/Learn." A critical point related to return to play that licensed medical providers must consider is that student-athletes must be asymptomatic prior to beginning a graduated return to activity, and should not be taking any pharmacological agents that may mask or modify symptom provocation when the decision to return to full participation is determined.[6]

Risk Reduction/Prevention of Sports-Related Concussion

Perhaps no other topic related to concussion has engrossed the general public more than how to reduce the risk for SRC, especially in children. Many organizations have disseminated information to school personnel, parents, coaches, athletes, and clinicians related to prevention of SRC. The most well-known program is the CDC's "Head Up to Schools: Know Your Concussion ABC's." As a result of the high incidence of concussion and the limited knowledge of the long-term consequences associated with concussion (e.g., chronic traumatic encephalopathy [CTE], dementia, mental health disorders), there has been misinformation related to what types of actions and/or policies are effective in reducing the risk of concussion. Table 23.6 provides a list of factors and characteristics associated with concussion risk.

It is well documented that a history of prior concussions is a strong risk factor for subsequent concussion.[6] Guskiewicz and colleagues found a dose-response relationship between the number of prior concussions and the likelihood of sustaining a future concussion, where collegiate football players with a history of three or more previous concussions were three times more likely to sustain a concussive injury than those without a history of concussion.[120] It is difficult to determine if these individuals have a decreased threshold/increased vulnerability due to never achieving a full physiological recovery, or if the phenomenon could be explained by "history repeating itself," as these individuals continue to put themselves in high-risk situations that increase the likelihood of sustaining a sufficient blow to the body/head. Still, this explains the importance of obtaining information related to the number of previous concussions in a medical evaluation (preparticipation baseline assessment or reevaluation), as the athlete can be identified as high-risk for concussion, which should impact future decisions made by the medical team. Identification of high-risk athletes can also be an opportunity for education to the athlete related to SRC prevention. The strongest and most consistent evidence leading to decreased incidence of SRC has been the adoption of policy to eliminate body checking in ice hockey for youth under the age of 13.[6] Other strategies used with the objective to reduce risk for SRC, such as helmets in American football and soccer or use of mouthguards, have not provided clear results in decreasing the risk for SRC.[6] Perhaps most surprising is the evidence that policy changes for fair play rules in youth ice hockey, tackle training without helmets and shoulder pads in youth American football, and tackle technique training in professional rugby do not lead to a reduction in SRC risk.[6] There is also insufficient evidence to determine whether age or level of competition (e.g., youth, collegiate, amateur, professional) increases the risk of SRC[15]; however, the argument could be made for continued attention toward reducing risk of SRC in children due to the potential added vulnerability of the developing brain at this age.

Potential Long-Term Effects Associated With Sports-Related Concussion

There is evidence that some former athletes in contact and collision sports experience depression and cognitive deficits later in life.[121] In addition to impaired clinical findings, there is evidence from advanced neuroimaging and electrophysiological studies of changes in brain function, activation patterns, and white matter fiber tracts in athletes with PPCS months and years following injury.[58] Perhaps more concerning, such structural and physiological changes have been identified even when the athlete has achieved clinical recovery (e.g.,

TABLE 23.6　Factors and Characteristics Associated With Concussion Risk

Variables Associated With Risk for Concussion
Prior history of concussion[6]
Female sex[15,34]
Body checking in ice hockey[6,15]
Type of sport
　Male
　　American football[15]
　　Rugby[15]
　Female
　　Soccer[15]
Use of protective headgear/helmet (decreased risk)
　Skiing/snowboarding[6]
　Rugby[15]

Variables Associated With Risk for Slow Recovery/Persistent Postconcussion Symptoms
[a]Prior history of concussion[15,117,118]
[a]Preinjury mental health problems (prior personal or family psychiatric history), particularly depression[6,117]
[a]Initial symptom severity[6,118]
[a]Younger age: adolescent[6,15,115,117]
Female sex[117,119]
Prior history of migraine headaches[15,119] or development of migraine headaches[6,115,118]
Prior history of multiple concussions[6]

[a]Indicates independent significant association with poor outcome, slow recovery, and/or persistent postconcussion symptoms.

asymptomatic at rest and with cognitive and physical exertion) and returned to play.[58] For example, Gosselin and colleagues[122] found a reduction in amplitude and increased latency in auditory evoked potentials in 20 symptomatic and asymptomatic athletes compared with 10 control athletes. Interestingly, the asymptomatic athletes had a similar electrophysiological profile to that of the symptomatic athletes, suggesting continued physiological impairment in athletes who were determined to be clinically recovered. At this time, it is unclear how to interpret these findings as abnormal brain activation patterns and white matter tract findings are not specific to concussion injury, and, due to a lack of methodologically sound, longitudinal investigations, the impact of structural and functional changes in neuroimaging studies on an individual's function across his or her life-span is unknown.

Due to the current level of discourse related to the association between neurodegenerative disease (e.g., Alzheimer disease and CTE) and concussion, it is worth discussing the state of evidence for the causal relationship between these two conditions. The most extensive review related to long-term effects of SRC was completed by Manley and colleagues,[121] who reviewed 47 studies that investigated neuroimaging, clinical, and neuropathology outcomes in athletes who sustained a concussion. The authors concluded there is emerging evidence that some retired athletes have mild cognitive impairment, neuroimaging abnormalities, and differences in brain metabolism disproportionate to their age, and there is an association between cognitive and psychological deficits and a history of multiple concussions in former athletes. However, the authors emphasize that *the majority* of former athletes report functioning at a similar level to the general public and are not at increased risk for death by suicide. Further, former high school American football players do not appear to be at increased risk for neurodegenerative diseases later in life. Finally, in terms of the link between CTE and repeated neurotrauma, there is consensus that a cause-and-effect relationship has not been established between neurodegenerative disorders and SRCs or exposure to contact sports; thus the implication that repeated concussion causes CTE remains undetermined.[6,121]

Retirement From Sports

For a select number of athletes, it may be important for medical professionals to discuss retirement from continued participation in sports-related activities, especially those with increased risk of concussion in contact or collision sports. At the foundation of this decision is consideration of the potential risks of prolonged or permanent neurological effects weighed against the positive aspects of continued participation in the sport, which may include the athlete's personal athletic goals (e.g., future aspirations of participation at a professional level), financial incentives (e.g., scholarship or athletics as a career), and/or the individual's identity as an athlete.[123] Unfortunately, the decision for retirement depends on many factors, for which there is limited supportive evidence to be used for guidance as there is uncertainty related to the long-term effects of repeated concussion.[121]

Kutcher and Giza[72] provide three scenarios that medical professionals should consider in the decision to recommend retirement from contact sports: (1) evidence of a clear lowering of a threshold for injury, meaning that over time, less force is required for an athlete to acquire postconcussion symptoms; (2) cases where the clinical syndrome is more severe than the average presentation and may last for several weeks, which outweighs the benefits of playing the sport; and (3) cases where an athlete demonstrates objective signs of declining or persistently impaired brain function (e.g., neuropsychological testing and/or diminished academic/work performance) without a plausible explanation other than exposure to impact forces (e.g., depression,

migraine headache). In addition to the considerations provided by Kutcher and Giza, medical professionals may use the Columbia SRC Retirement Algorithm proposed by Davis-Hayes and colleagues[123] to determine when a *discussion* related to retirement from sport may be indicated versus circumstances where a *recommendation* for retirement from sport should be provided to an athlete. For example, medical professionals should provide a recommendation for retirement where there is evidence of structural abnormality on routine neuroimaging (e.g., frontotemporal contusions or gliosis). Conversely, in cases where the cumulative effects of repeated concussions lead to relative contraindications for continued exposure, retirement from sports or recommendations for a replacement activity with reduced risk for contact or collisions[123] may be warranted. Symptoms or neurological signs persisting greater than 3 months, persistent cognitive impairment, diminished academic performance or social engagement, and evidence of a decreased threshold to trigger postconcussion symptoms may be useful criteria to suggest altered activities to prevent further injury.

CONSIDERATIONS FOR REST AND RETURN TO PLAY/LEARN FOLLOWING SRC

The rationale for rest draws from findings that functional injury and physiological dysfunction due to a neurometabolic crisis[44] may worsen in the presence of increased physical[124] and cognitive[125] load, suggesting the existence of a vulnerable period where the brain may be susceptible to further dysfunction or injury.[44,126,127] This has been shown in mice that exhibited impaired cognitive function when subjected to a second concussive brain injury within 3 or 5 days of the initial injury, but those subjected to a second injury at a later time (day 7 postinjury) showed normal cognitive function.[91] Similarly, Griesbach and colleagues found rats with an mTBI exposed to exercise within the first week of injury had impaired cognitive performance (learning acquisition and memory) compared with rats with delayed exposure to exercise 14 to 20 days after injury.[92] Likewise in humans, Majerske and colleagues reported that strenuous physical and cognitive exertion in acute concussion leads to poorer neurocognitive outcomes in adolescent athletes following an SRC.[128] Such findings suggest that rest following concussion may be necessary to (1) reduce the potential for a repeat concussion (e.g., second impact syndrome) while the brain may be still vulnerable from the initial concussion[44,120] and (2) facilitate recovery by preventing excessive physiological demands (e.g., physical exertion) that may hinder restoration of normal neurotransmission and neurometabolic function.[129,130]

Although rest has been considered a cornerstone of best practice[5,6,129,131–133] and is widely prescribed in the care of individuals who have sustained a concussion,[130] it has not been well defined. The term "rest" is quite broad when one considers the range of tasks children and adults engage in during daily activities. When a physician or medical professional provides instructions for rest, does she mean complete withdrawal from all recreational, social, academic, and work-related activities? Only some of those activities? Or is it the intensity of the activities that matters most? Perhaps not surprisingly, there are variations in what might qualify as rest. Thomas and colleagues[131] recommended 5 days of what the authors defined as "strict rest," which consisted of rest at home (specifically, no school, work, or physical activity) for which participants were provided excuses for missed days of school and work. Buckley and colleagues[134] provided a more detailed list of what constituted physical and cognitive rest. For 40 consecutive hours, student-athletes were instructed not to attend any classes, team meetings, or study hall, and not to perform any academic work. Participants were provided medical documentation for class absence, and coaches were informed of the restrictions for team activities. Further, to decrease cognitive load, participants were to refrain from excessive television, computer, or other electronics usage, and to limit text messaging, although no operational definitions of what constituted excessive or how much time to limit activities were provided. Finally, to encourage physical rest, student-athletes were withheld from all athletic activities, personal exercise, and instructed to rest in a quiet environment throughout the day.[134] Moser and colleagues[135] provided parents and adolescent athletes with a more exhaustive list of cognitive and physical activities to avoid, which included attending school, taking tests or notes, doing homework, performing general household chores, driving, taking trips outside of the home, visually watching TV, playing video games, using a computer or phone, reading, playing a musical instrument, engaging in aerobic exercise, or lifting weights. Participants were advised to avoid activities that might produce a sweat or exacerbate symptoms but were encouraged to engage in light exertion activities such as listening to an audiobook, relaxing music, or low-volume TV, folding laundry, setting the table, taking a slow walk outside, sleeping, and visiting with family members in the home. The examples of these three studies[131,134,135] show the variability in protocols for rest. Perhaps not surprisingly, there were mixed results in terms of persistent burden of symptoms, return to play/school, and performance on standardized physical and cognitive tests found across these three studies. Moser and colleagues[135] reported benefits following 1 week of restricted activity, whereas Thomas and colleagues and Buckley and colleagues found worse outcomes associated with rest.[131,134]

There is also variation related to the optimal amount of time an individual should rest following a concussion. There is agreement across international consensus, practice guidelines, and position statements[6,9,136,137] that an athlete should rest until asymptomatic. Using this recommendation, some medical professionals instruct athletes to spend several days in a darkened room (a type of rest referred to as "cocoon therapy")[138] or recommend prolonged rest where physical and cognitive activities are discouraged for weeks, months, or even longer, especially in children.[130] Although it may be advantageous in a minority of cases to recommend an extended period of rest in children,[6,132] there is convincing evidence emerging in the literature that shows rest, especially strict rest (e.g., withdrawal from all activities), and prolonged withdrawal from physical and cognitive activity during recovery of the acute concussion are associated with increased symptom burden[131,134] and delayed recovery.[128,131] The detrimental effects of prolonged rest and activity withdrawal are thought to occur, in part, because of anxiety formed by a patient's expectations of a lengthy recovery, physical deconditioning that can mimic postconcussive symptoms such as sleep disturbances and fatigue, and psychological complications arising from an inability to cope with reduced participation in life activities.[129,130] To this last point, one must consider the importance of self-identity, autonomy, and social engagement through recreational, sport, school, and work-related activities in adolescents. Current concussion management involves withdrawal from these activities, and an unintended consequence may be that missing social interactions and falling behind academically may contribute to an exacerbation of physical and emotional symptoms in some individuals.[130,131] This may help explain why it seems that adolescents are at greatest risk for experiencing PPCS, leading to a protracted recovery. Therefore medical professionals must be observant of this phenomenon for all individuals, but especially for adolescents, who may require additional encouragement of the likely positive outcome following concussion and potentially a referral for psychological or counselling services.

What Is the Evidence for Physical and Cognitive Activity in Acute Concussion?

Conversely, there is evidence that rather than strict rest, engaging in moderate levels of physical and cognitive activity can be beneficial for decreasing the burden of postconcussion symptoms,[139] promoting earlier return to baseline performance on standardized neuropsychological and physical assessments,[128] earlier return to play/sport,[140] and earlier return to school/work.[140] Majerske and colleagues[128] performed a retrospective chart review and found that individuals who engaged in moderate levels of exertion (slow jogging and sports practice) demonstrated better outcomes on neuropsychological testing compared with individuals with the least (no school or exercise) or greatest (full school and competition participation) level of activity. Lawrence and colleagues[140] reviewed charts of adolescents (aged 15 to 20 years) who engaged in either self-initiated or physician-prescribed physical activity within 14 days of an SRC. Although each athlete was symptomatic at the time of initiating aerobic exercise, the authors reported a shorter time to initiation of aerobic exercise (e.g., earlier physical activity) was associated with faster full return to sport and school/work-related activities.[140] Grool and colleagues[139] conducted a large prospective study investigating the association between participation in physical activity within 7 days and PPCS in children aged 5 to 18 years. Participants who met the criteria for concussion as defined by the CISG[17] completed surveys (via internet or phone) related to current level of physical activity and symptom complaint (using the PCSI). Among 2413 participants, 69.5% participated in some form of physical activity within 7 days following concussion, primarily with light aerobic exercise, which was associated with lower risk of symptom complaint at 28 days compared with no physical activity. The proportion of participants with PPCS at 28 days was 28.7% compared with 40.1% for those engaging in early physical activity versus no activity, respectively.[139] Therefore it appears that moderate physical and mental activity during the acute phase of recovery may be beneficial.

What Criteria Should Be Used to Determine Recovery?

Similar to diagnostic testing, at this time there is no single test or biomarker that can be used to determine prognosis for recovery following concussion.[5,44] Here, it is important to distinguish two types of recovery: clinical recovery and physiological recovery. Clinical recovery is the proxy that medical professionals (typically a neurologist, sports medicine physician, or rehabilitation medicine physician) use to determine an individual is able to perform all previous life activities without presence or exacerbation of baseline symptoms. The operational definition of clinical recovery provided by the CISG[6] encompasses a *resolution* of postconcussion-related symptoms and a *return to clinically normal* balance and cognitive functioning, which results in a return to normal activities, including school, work, and sport. However, using clinical recovery as the benchmark for return to activities, it is unclear to what extent there is continued physiological dysfunction (e.g., impaired metabolic activity, abnormal synaptic and neurotransmission, impaired cerebral blood flow, inflammation), as neurobiological recovery might extend beyond clinical recovery in some individuals. Results from neuroimaging studies[44,141–144] suggest that physiological recovery time may outlast the time to clinical recovery.[6] However, many of the neuroimaging techniques used to identify such dysfunction are not available in most medical clinics and are not used as a standard of care for individuals following concussion. Further, abnormalities found on neuroimaging studies are not specific to injury following concussion. Still, advanced neuroimaging and fluid biomarkers continue to be investigated for use in identifying physiological recovery.

At this time, fluid biomarkers to identify concussion injury are in development and are critical to the ability to diagnose and determine prognosis for recovery. On February 14, 2018, the FDA released approval for TBI Endpoints Development (TED) and TRACK TBI to study ubiquitin carboxyl-terminal hydrolase L1 (UCH-L1) and glial fibrillary acidic protein (GFAP), which are proteins released from the brain into the blood after brain injury.[145] A multicenter prospective study of 1947 adult blood samples showed that the Banyan Brain Trauma Indicator, a blood test that measures the presence of UCH-LI and GFAP, was able to predict intracranial lesions that would not appear on standard imaging (e.g., computed tomography).[147] Many other neuroimaging techniques and biomarkers for impaired neuroplasticity, inflammatory processes, and autoimmune antibodies are being investigated to better understand factors associated with comorbidities and prolonged recovery. For a discussion on neuroimaging and fluid biomarker research in concussion, the reader is referred to the following reviews: Makdissi and colleagues,[58] Kevin and colleagues,[148] Dambinova and colleagues,[149] and Schmidt and colleagues.[46]

The physician must rely on behavioral measures as a proxy for recovery; therefore at this time, recovery is synonymous with clinical recovery because the full physiological recovery process remains unclear. For this reason, clinical recovery constitutes waiting until the patient is asymptomatic and has returned to baseline on cognitive and physically based performance measures,[6,9,150] before initiating a graduated return-to-play (RTP) strategy.[5]

Recommendations for Return to Play and Return to School/Learn

Statements generated from international consensus, position statements, practice guidelines, and reviews related to RTP (also referred to as return to sport[6] and return to activity) can be found in Box 23.1.

Recommendations for Return to Play

International consensus makes the following recommendations for RTP progression[6]:

1. An athlete diagnosed with a concussion should not be allowed to return to practice/competition the same day.[6] This recommendation is made to reduce the potential for a repeat concussion and decrease the risk for the rare but dangerous second impact syndrome.[24,44,120]

2. After a brief period of initial rest (24 to 48 hours), symptom-limited activity can begin while staying below a cognitive and physical exacerbation threshold[6] (see stage 1 in Table 23.7). As there is no single test (or combination of tests) that can be used to determine physiological recovery, the clinician must use clinical recovery (ability to perform activity without symptom exacerbation) as a guide. Therefore the patient should be encouraged to engage in light-to-moderate-intensity, symptom-limiting physical and mental activities in order to avoid the detrimental effects of full withdrawal from activity[129,131,134] that may delay recovery[128,131] and potentially facilitate recovery.[128,139]

BOX 23.1 Recommendations From International Consensus, Position Statements, and Practice Guideline for Return to Play and Return to School/Learn

Considerations for Return to Play and Return to School/Learn

Return to Play

- Management of concussions include no same-day RTP[a] and prescribed physical and cognitive rest until asymptomatic.[3,5,6,9,137]
- Although most individuals follow a rapid course of recovery over several days to week following injury, concussions may involve varying lengths of recovery.[3,5,6,9]
- In the presence of continued symptom complaint following concussion, verbal or written education should be provided for reassurance that a good recovery is expected.[9,130]
- There is limited empirical evidence for the effectiveness of prescribed physical and cognitive rest.[3,6]
- Prescribed physical and cognitive rest may not be an effective strategy for all patients following concussion.[3]
- Strict brain rest (e.g., stimulus deprivation, "cocoon" therapy) is not indicated and may have detrimental effects on patients following concussion.[3,5,130,151]
- There is limited empirical evidence that physical and mental activity may be beneficial in acute concussion.[3]
- Return to school protocol should be prioritized over a return to sport strategy, so that the student-athlete should return to school with academic accommodations (if necessary) prior to advancing with return to sport progression.[6]
- Graduated activity strategy/progression should be used to guide a clinician's decision making for RTP.[b]
- Existing RTP progressions require validation as this approach has not been substantiated with prospective, randomized controlled comparative-effectiveness trials.[133]

Return to School/Learn

- When initiating return to cognitive (school-related) activities, there is a strong recommendation for academic accommodations,[3,5,6,152] which may include the following areas: attendance,[151] curriculum,[137,150,151,153] environmental modifications,[151,153] and activity modifications.[137,150,151,153]
- Concussions may involve varying lengths of recovery, with adolescents at greatest risk for protracted recovery. It may therefore be advantageous, in a minority of cases, to recommend an extended period of rest in children.[6,151]
- If symptomatic within first 72 h, the student should refrain from attending school and participation in all academic activities, to support cognitive rest and facilitate recovery.[5] A more conservative approach that children, symptomatic or asymptomatic, should stay away from school for 1 week has been recommended.[151]
- If symptomatic after 72 h postinjury, the student should refrain from attending academic activities for 1 full week.[5]
- After 2 weeks postinjury, the student should start attending school (nonphysical activities) with accommodations, even if he/she is still experiencing symptoms, to prevent psychological complications.[5,151]
- If reintegration into school is ineffective or unproductive at 4 weeks (symptoms persist or worsen), consider (1) greater academic accommodations, (2) move student's courses to audit status, or (3) consider whether student should continue in program for that term/semester.[5]

[a]References 3, 5, 6, 9, 15, 72, 137.
[b]References 3, 5, 6, 9, 137, 150.
RTP, Return to play.

TABLE 23.7   International Consensus for Graduated Return to Sport Strategy and Return to Participation Protocol

Stage of Rehabilitation	Functional Exercise	Objective of Each Stage
No activity	Complete physical rest	Recovery
Light cardiovascular activity	Stationary bike, walking, swimming, light skating	Increased HR and CBF
Sport-specific activity	Interval training, conditioning drills, running or skating drills, ball work sprints, etc.	Fluctuation in HR adding cognitive function to activity, adding movement
Noncontact practice	Complex training drills, noncontact team practices	Increased cognitive load, assess coordination and processing speed
Full-contact practice	Participation in normal training activities—only with medical clearance	Assess functional skills, assess for recurrence of symptoms by applying smaller magnitude of forces, ensuring self-confidence, and readiness to play
RTP	Full participation in game play	

CBF, Cerebral blood flow; *HR*, heart rate; *RTP*, return to play.
Adapted from McCrory P, Meeuwisse W, Johnston K, et al. consensus statement on concussion in sports, 3rd International Conference on Concussion in Sport held in Zurich, November 2008. *Clin J Sport Med.* 2009;19(3):185–200.

3. Once concussion-related symptoms have resolved, the athlete should continue to proceed to the next level (see stage 2, Table 23.7) if he/she meets all the criteria (e.g., activity, heart rate, duration of exercise) without a recurrence of concussion-related symptoms.[6] At this stage, the medical professional, including the rehabilitation specialist, may use a subsymptom exercise tolerance test[154] (Fig. 23.3) to guide exercise recommendations.

4. In general, each step should take 24 hours, so that athletes would take a minimum of 1 week to proceed through the full rehabilitation protocol once they are asymptomatic at rest.[6] If any concussion-related symptoms occur during the stepwise approach, the athlete should drop back to the previous asymptomatic level and attempt to progress again after being free of concussion-related symptoms for a further 24-hour period at the lower level.[6]

5. The time frame for RTP may vary with player age, history, and level of sport; therefore management must be individualized.[6]

6. For RTS, athletes should be symptom free, but also should not be taking any pharmacological agents that may mask or modify the symptoms of concussion at the time of returning the athlete to full participation in sport.[5,6]

Recommendations for Return to School/Learn

Statements generated from international consensus, position statements, practice guidelines, and reviews related to return to school/learn can be found in Box 23.1. Similar to RTP, providing cognitive rest and academic accommodations are two foundational components of return to school/learn protocols.[5,6,151] Removal from school-related activities until students are asymptomatic, followed by a graduated return to school-related activities (e.g., reading/writing, studying, homework), as the student can complete the tasks at a tolerable level has been recommended.[5,6] When returning to school-related activities, it has been reported that as many as 73% of students have academic difficulty,[155] which may substantiate the recommendation for instituting academic accommodations that may include the following: extension of assignment deadlines, rest periods during the school day, postponement or staggering of tests, reduced workload, and/or accommodation for light or noise sensitivity.[153] Such findings likely explain reports that student-athletes who sustain a concussion receive more academic accommodations and take longer to return to school compared with their student-athlete counterparts who sustain musculoskeletal injuries to other body parts.[156]

Although consensus and position statements recommend immediate withdrawal from school-related activities for 48 hours,[6] 72 hours,[5] and up to 2 weeks[5,151] following injury, the level of evidence supporting such recommendations is limited[128,157] (primarily based on prospective observational or retrospective reviews), as to date there are no multicenter randomized controlled trials (RCTs) validating the recommendations. In fact, there is evidence from a randomized control trial in children aged 11 to 22 years, which showed withdrawal from mental activity in acute concussion led to poorer outcome.[131] Thomas and colleagues[131]

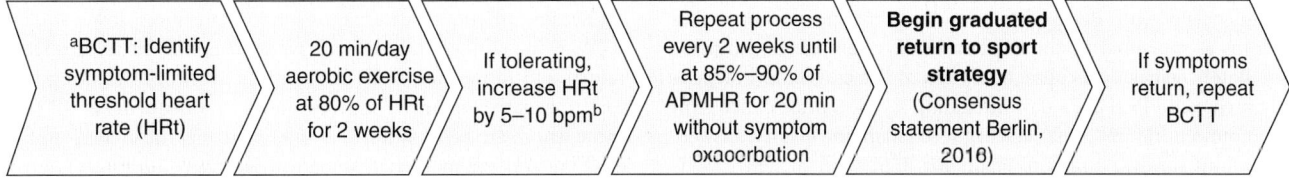

| aBCTT: Identify symptom-limited threshold heart rate (HRt) | 20 min/day aerobic exercise at 80% of HRt for 2 weeks | If tolerating, increase HRt by 5–10 bpm[b] | Repeat process every 2 weeks until at 85%–90% of APMHR for 20 min without symptom oxaocrbation | **Begin graduated return to sport strategy** (Consensus statement Berlin, 2016) | If symptoms return, repeat BCTT |

Fig. 23.3 Exercise Prescription Guided by Results of a Subsymptom Exercise Tolerance Test. Use of a subsymptom exercise tolerance test, Buffalo Concussion Treadmill Test *(BCTT)*, and exercise prescription for return to activity for individuals with exercise intolerance following concussion, as described in Leddy and Willer.[154] *APMHR*, Age-predicted maximum heart rate; *bpm*, beats per minute; *CISG*, concussion in Sport Group; *HR*, heart rate; *HRt,* heart rate achieved at symptom-exacerbation determined by stopping criteria. aAfter 3 weeks of persistent symptoms; b5 bpm for nonathletes, 10 bpm for athletes.

found a longer time to symptom resolution for students instructed to rest at home (e.g., no school-related work or physical activity) for 5 days compared with students who were provided instructions to rest for 24 to 48 hours prior to engaging in mental and physical activities below an exacerbation threshold. Evaluation of patient adherence in this study showed the physician's instructions did not significantly alter the amount of physical activity between groups, but did lead to a decreased amount of time spent performing mental activities in the strict rest group, which, in practice, suggests a detrimental effect on burden of symptoms due to withdrawal from cognitive activities alone (as physical activity levels were similar between groups). Again, withdrawal from social engagement with school-related activities and falling behind academically may contribute to an exacerbation of symptoms in some children.[130,131] In summary, similar to guidelines for RTP, return to school/learn recommendations lack strong evidence to support statements (see Box 23.1). This should emphasize the importance of a balanced approach between cognitive and physical rest with activity that should be modified to account for the age, severity of initial symptom complaints, and premorbid health conditions that may impact length of recovery.

PROGNOSIS AND OUTCOMES FOLLOWING CONCUSSION

Prognosis and Outcomes Following Sports-Related Concussion

There is a critical need to determine demographic characteristics and clinically relevant factors that are associated with clinical recovery prior to injury, at the time of injury, and postinjury. Such information would be useful for decision making for medical and rehabilitation approaches. For example, demographic and preinjury characteristics could be used by medical professionals to identify athletes who are at high risk for developing PPCS during preparticipation screenings and ensure careful monitoring and appropriately timed referrals for pharmacological and/or rehabilitation therapies in the event of a concussion. In addition, knowledge of variables at the time of injury and following the injury that contribute to a protracted recovery could impact clinical decision making for medical professionals on the field and in the clinic to better utilize resources for those at highest risk for protracted recovery, to promote successful and timely return to play and return to learn strategies.

The Predicting and Preventing Postconcussive Problems in Pediatrics (5Ps) study[119] was designed to develop and validate a clinical risk score in order to stratify PPCS risk after acute concussion in children and youth. Zemek and colleagues[119] completed a multicenter cohort study from 9 pediatric EDs within the Pediatric Emergency Research Canada network, where children aged 5 to 18 years underwent a comprehensive evaluation in the ED and completed electronic surveys at 7, 14, and 28 days following a diagnosis of concussion.[17] Out of 47 risk factors associated with PPCS (defined as 3 or more new or worsening symptoms as measured by the PCSI at 28 days compared with prior injury state), Zemek and colleagues[119] found 9 factors that independently predicted PPCS at 28 days, including age, sex, prior concussion and symptom duration, physician-diagnosed migraine history, answering questions slowly, number of errors for BESS tandem stance position, headache, sensitivity to noise, and fatigue. Depending on the PPCS risk score, the group was able to establish a probability of developing PPCS at 28 days. Although the clinical utility of the PPCS risk score needs to be established, the use of such a stratification system has the potential to individualize concussion care and lead to the identification

of children who are at risk for developing PPCS during the acute stage of recovery following a concussion.

A systematic review completed as a part of the CISG conference[6] synthesized the evidence regarding predictors of clinical recovery following concussion.[117] In general, Iverson and colleagues reported that the literature is mixed with positive and negative findings related to predictive factors of clinical recovery, because many of the included studies were found to use different criteria to establish clinical recovery, which made it difficult to provide definitive conclusions.[117] Still, Iverson and colleagues[117] reported that preinjury mental health problems (prior personal or family psychological history), especially depression, and prior concussions appear to be risk factors for PPCS. Importantly, adolescent years might be a particularly vulnerable time for experiencing persistent symptoms, with greater risk for girls than boys.[6,15,115,117]

It is also worth noting the variables that were not found to be associated with increased risk for protracted recovery or the development of PPCS, such as complaint of dizziness, initial severity of cognitive deficits, or development of oculomotor dysfunction, and individuals with prior cognitive and learning disabilities, and individuals with prior cognitive and learning disabilities (e.g., attention deficit hyperactivity disorder). There were also inconsistent findings related to "Red Flags" and memory assessment (e.g., loss of consciousness and posttraumatic amnesia) at the time of injury leading to PPCS.

A list of factors associated with increased risk for PPCS (continued symptoms beyond 14 days in adults and 28 days in children) is provided in Table 23.6.

Prognosis and Outcome Following Non–Sports-Related Concussion in Adults

To date, most studies evaluating outcomes for individuals following concussion have been directed almost exclusively toward clinical recovery after SRC. However, young and older adults sustain mTBI due to falls, motor vehicle accidents, physical assault, and participation in recreational activities. Similar to student-athletes, the majority of adults who sustain a concussion will resume normal activities within 10 to 14 days; however, a minority of these individuals will endorse PPCS and experience a slow return to participation in meaningful activities,[55] perhaps the most important of which is return to work (RTW).

Following concussion, perhaps due to instructions provided by a physician, but more than likely due to postconcussion symptoms, many patients will miss work for a period of time. Absence from work can lead to lost or reduced income, psychological stress due to pressures placed on family relationships, and secondary physical and mental health conditions due to prolonged withdrawal from typical activities (e.g., deconditioning and psychological distress). All of these factors can add to normal work-related, household, and financial stressors already present in most adult's lives.[158]

Because of various external or internal pressures, some adults will RTW while still symptomatic,[159] which can lead to an unsuccessful return and more time away from productive work, resulting in profound negative financial and emotional consequences.[160] Even for those whom are asymptomatic, it is possible that the increased physical or cognitive load may cause somatic, cognitive, emotional, and/or behavioral impairments. Despite these well-known complications that can create barriers for successful RTW, there is a paucity of literature related to RTW following mTBI.

The International Collaboration on mTBI Prognosis group completed a systematic review of the literature from 2001 to 2012 to update the previous World Health Organization Collaborating Centre Task Force on mTBI findings on RTW in 2004.[161] The group reported most workers returned to work within 3 to 6 months[162]; however, RTW rates varied widely based on the time from injury and the geographic area of the investigation. For example, as many as 84%[163] and as little as 41%[164] of individuals were found to RTW 1 week following mTBI, while other investigations reported a range of 25% to 100% of individuals returning to work 1 month postinjury.[160] Wäljas and colleagues[160] followed a group of 109 patients with an average age of 37.4 years, 76% of whom were working full time, 5.6% working part time, with the remaining patients being students, who were diagnosed with an mTBI at a University Hospital ED in Finland, and found the vast majority of the group (91.7%) returned to work within 2 months. Due to the repeated measure design of the study, the following RTW rates were reported; 46.8% RTW at 1 week, 59.6% RTW at 2 weeks, 70.6% RTW at 1 month, 91.7% RTW at 2 months, and 97.2% RTW at 1 year following mTBI.[160]

One major limitation of studies investigating RTW following mTBI is considering whether the patient achieves a full return to preinjury work-related activities. Two studies have somewhat disparate findings for full RTW rates at 6 months following injury, where 41.7% of individuals presenting to an outpatient concussion clinic[165] and 76% of individuals presenting to an ED[166] were reported to have a full RTW 6 months postinjury.

Perhaps it is obvious that work disability includes time off from work and sick leave, but it also incorporates reduced productivity or working with functional limitations.[162,167] However, few studies have evaluated RTW as a continuum based on a RTW hierarchy considering reduced workload, a change in roles/responsibilities, or lower productivity due to functional impairments such as cognitive deficits or symptom provocation.[66,159,165,168] Evaluating RTW as a dichotomy (employed vs. unemployed) rather than a hierarchy can lead to a drastic underestimation of disability an individual may experience when attempting to fully return to preinjury work. In 79 patients recruited from concussion specialty clinics in Vancouver, Canada, Silverberg and colleagues[165] reported that although 58.2% (46) of patients returned to any level of work, only 41.7% of patients fully returned to their preinjury work responsibilities at 6 months following injury. Importantly, at 6 months, 1 in 4 patients who had returned to work were still on modified duties, working reduced hours, or receiving accommodations, or took a different, less demanding job. Further, nearly 50% of patients who fully returned to work continued to report multiple somatic, cognitive, and emotional symptoms.[165]

A secondary objective of the study by Wäljas and colleagues[160] was to examine factors that influence RTW status in individuals who are slow to recover following mTBI. Wäljas and colleagues[160] concluded appearance of the following combination of factors within the first 4 weeks following mTBI strongly predicted RTW status: age, multiple bodily injuries, intracranial abnormalities on CT scan the day of injury, and fatigue ratings. Consistent with other studies, the authors reported that injury severity variables (e.g., duration of unconsciousness, Glasgow Coma Scale score, and duration of posttraumatic amnesia) were not associated with length of time to RTW.[160,169]

Based primarily on the Veteran's Affairs/Department of Defense (VA/DoD) Clinical Practice Guideline for Management of Concussion/mTBI, Marshall and colleagues provided the following recommendations for RTW following a concussion[5]:

- In some cases, vocational modifications are required and may include:
  - Modification of the length of the workday
  - Gradual work reentry (e.g., starting at 2 days/week and expanding to 3 days/week)
  - Additional time for task completion
  - Change of job
  - Environment modifications (e.g., quieter work environment)
- Individuals who continue to experience persistent impairments following mTBI or those who have not successfully resumed preinjury work duties following injury should be referred for an in-depth vocational evaluation by clinical specialists and teams (e.g., occupational therapist, vocational rehabilitation counsellor, occupational medicine physician, neuropsychologist, SLP) with expertise in assessing and treating mTBI.
- A referral to a structured program that promotes community integration (e.g., volunteer work) may also be considered for individuals with PPCS that impede return to preinjury participation in a customary role.

Prognosis and Outcomes Following Mild Traumatic Brain Injury in Military Personnel

Advances in the types of weapons used in warfare over the last 25 years have led to changes in the types of injuries inflicted on military personnel in combat. As a result, mTBI has been referred to as the "signature" injury of the two most recent US military operations in Afghanistan and Iraq,[170–172] where 15% to 22% of deployed US military service members sustained an mTBI.[172,173] Although service members may sustain an mTBI from falls, motor vehicle accidents, blunt head trauma, or recreational activities, blast-induced mTBI are the most concerning, not only because of the high frequency at which they occur (accounting for 78% to 80% of all injuries sustained in combat),[174] but also the limited understanding of how blast-induced mTBI differentially impacts outcome in service members.

Similar to SRC and non-SRC in the civilian population, blast-induced mTBI can lead to somatic, cognitive, behavioral, and emotional symptoms. One key difference is the increased risk for severe psychological effects that impact recovery from mTBI in military personnel.[175,176] It has been estimated that as many as 44% of deployed US military return from combat with posttraumatic stress, depression, and/or anxiety.[177] This is problematic, as it is clear from the literature in mTBI that psychological problems negatively impact recovery and may lead to slow recovery in service members, resulting in delayed return to duty (RTD) following injury. Although many reports have concluded most service members with combat related mTBI recover within 7 days, Kennedy and colleagues[176] evaluated rates of RTD in 377 US service members who sustained a concussion (52% with a loss of consciousness) while serving in Afghanistan and found 51.1% experienced an average RTD 7.6 days (range 0 to 13 days) following injury, whereas 48.9% experienced a delayed average RTD 24.4 days (range 14 to 51 days) following mTBI. The findings showed that in comparison to the recovery times for SRC, recovery time appears to be far greater in blast-induced mTBI.[176]

Just as it is important to ensure that athletes are asymptomatic with physical and mental exertion prior to RTP in order to decrease the risk of secondary injury (musculoskeletal injuries[178,179] as well as second impact syndrome), it is important that service members be able to perform a combat role effectively before RTD. Perhaps, because of the serious nature of responsibilities, full recovery is even more important for service members because RTD too soon has the potential to lead to catastrophic consequences.[176] The VA/DoD clinical practice guideline[180] for RTD recommends that all service members exposed to a potentially concussive event should be screened using the Military Acute Concussion Evaluation (MACE), a clinical assessment tool that was developed to assess the subjective symptom report, cognitive performance, and the neurological status (via a gross neurological screen) at the point of injury by a field medical provider. The cognitive performance section is based on the SAC,[73] and the neurological screen involves an assessment of visual, speech, and motor capacity. Regardless of the results, service members are required to rest for at least 24 hours[180]; however, beyond the initial rest period, there seems to be discrepancies in RTD strategy, as some studies require full symptom resolution at rest and during an aerobic exertional test, as well as neuropsychological testing (Automated Neuropsychological Assessment Metric [ANAM] results that are consistent with predeployment testing[176]). Conversely, the VA/DoD clinical practice guideline provides a strong recommendation not to use neuropsychological tests such as the ANAM or the ImPACT within the first 30 days of concussion to guide decision making.[180]

Mac Donald and colleagues[175] compared outcomes from 50 active-duty US military who sustained a blast-induced concussion to 44 combat-deployed control service members at 1 year and 5 years to investigate the long-term consequences of blast-induced mTBI. At 5 years postinjury, service members who sustained a blast-induced mTBI fared worse than their nonconcussed counterparts on global outcome measures (Glasgow Outcome Scale and Quality of Life After Brain Injury), reported greater headache impairment, and had significantly more mental health issues, including posttraumatic stress, depression, anxiety, and disrupted sleep. Further, Mac Donald and colleagues[175] reported that a number of service members with blast-induced mTBI continued to experience a worsening of symptom severity from 1-year to 5-year follow-up, which points to the need for effective treatments in this group of individuals. At this time, the VA/DoD clinical practice guideline[180] emphasizes that active and pharmacological therapy protocols should use a targeted approach to address delayed recovery and PPCS after blast-induced mTBI that matches the therapy to the clinical presentation and symptom complaint rather than the mechanism of injury. For information related to active therapy for service members with slow recovery following blast-induced concussion, the reader is directed to Morris & Gottshall.[23]

CLINICAL EXAMINATION FOR PERSISTENT POSTCONCUSSION SYMPTOMS

Concussion can produce a constellation of signs and symptoms that evolve over time, which reflect physical, cognitive, and emotional dysfunction.[5,23,154,181] Therefore the examination used by the rehabilitation specialist for the individual with PPCS should be comprehensive so as to consider all potential motor, sensory, cognitive, and psychological systems that may contribute to a patient's symptoms and functional limitations. Ideally, the examination should lead the therapist to identify the underlying impairments of functional systems that contribute to a patient's activity and participation restrictions, movement dysfunction, and/or symptom provocation.

Several frameworks have been proposed for the examination of the individual with PPCS.[68,70,115,182] Although some authors have proposed minor variations, most approaches are composed of similar components, which include:
- Description and documentation of baseline symptom complaint(s)
- Assessment of cognitive dysfunction
- Assessment of orthostatic tolerance and dysautonomia
- Assessment of exercise tolerance via a subsymptom exercise tolerance test
- Examination of the vestibular and oculomotor systems
- Assessment of the musculoskeletal and sensorimotor components of the cervical spine
- Appropriate screening and identification of comorbid conditions such as headaches, affective disorders, and sleep disturbance

A template describing the components of a comprehensive examination that may be performed by a rehabilitation specialist is provided in Table 23.8.

Symptom Complaint

A high prevalence of complaints of headache (83%), dizziness (65%), and confusion (57%) is reported by athletes following SRC.[14] Other common symptoms endorsed by patients who have sustained a concussion include nausea, intermittent vomiting, disturbances of balance or gait, tinnitus, photophobia, phonophobia, difficulty focusing, slowed speech, lightheadedness or fogginess, extreme fatigue, and other impairments in cognitive processing and memory.[44,115,186,187] Following concussion, 10% to 33% of patients will continue to endorse symptoms, which may persist for months or even years.[52,55–58] Although the time course of recovery that characterizes PPCS continues to be debated and has changed over time,[5,17,188,189] PPCS should be considered if symptoms continue for longer than 10 to 14 days for adults and more than 28 days for children.[6]

Special consideration should be taken for clinicians providing care to children and adolescents with persistent symptoms following concussion. Often children and adolescents do not have the insight or vocabulary to identify or articulate the symptoms they are experiencing.[115] It is recommended that clinicians working with this population, especially children, phrase interview questions in contexts that are appropriate to the child's life, such as inquiring about the child's experience for specific activities such as going to the grocery store, walking up the stairs, playing video games, and riding in the car, and will often illicit confirmatory evidence that those activities make the child feel anxious, foggy, or "not right."[115] Also, it is important to consider the method of obtaining symptom complaints can influence the number and severity of the symptoms reported,[190,191] and on average, even healthy children and young adults will endorse concussion symptoms listed on common symptom complaint assessments.[192] The Pediatric Visually Induced Dizziness (PVID) Questionnaire is an example of a

---

TABLE 23.8 Comprehensive Physical Therapist Examination for an Individual With Persistent Postconcussion Symptoms

I. History/Structured Interview
   Nature of injury, time since injury, initial symptoms, current symptoms, nature and behavior of symptoms, irritability status, previous treatments received, prior medical workup, previous ocular disorders (congenital)
   Past medical history: previous psychological history, previous concussions and recovery from previous concussions, comorbid or premorbid conditions (autoimmune conditions, heritable disorders of connective tissue, chronic fatigue, fibromyalgia, autonomic dysfunctions including POTS, pregnancy/breastfeeding)

II. Systems Review (in Accordance With Systems Review Described in Guide to PT Practice, APTA 1999)
   Cardiovascular/pulmonary system
   Integumentary system
   Musculoskeletal system
   Neuromuscular system
   Communication
   Affect: Screen for presence of anxiety and/or depression
   Cognition
   Learning style/educational needs

III. Patient's Goals

TABLE 23.8 Comprehensive Physical Therapist Examination for an Individual With Persistent Postconcussion Symptoms—cont'd

IV. Examination

A. **Self-Report Measures**

Symptom Complaint Scales (PCSI, PCSS, RPQ)

Health and Behavior Inventory (HBI)

Pain Rating Scale (visual analogue scale, McGill Pain Questionnaire)

B. **Subsymptom Exercise Tolerance Test**

Treadmill (BCTT) or cycle ergometer exercise test

C. **Vestibular System Assessment**

i. Self-report tests/measures

Dizziness Handicap Inventory (DHI)

Activities-specific Balance Confidence scale (ABC)

ii. Performance/clinical measures

Sensation of motion at rest

Positional testing (Dix-Hallpike, side-lying test, supine roll test)

VOR assessment (head thrust test, cDVA/GST)

Head tilt for otolithic assessment

Self-Motion Sensitivity (Motion Sensitivity Quotient[183])

Visual Motion Sensitivity (Pediatric Visually Induced Dizziness Questionnaire)[184]

Gait and Balance assessment (FGA, DGI, SOT, mCTSIB, Push-and-Release test)

D. **Oculomotor System Assessment**

Visual fixation

Ocular motility—H-test

Smooth pursuit and saccades

Vergence

E. **Cervical Spine Assessment (musculoskeletal and sensorimotor components)**

i. Self-report tests/measures (Neck Disability Index)

ii. Safety tests

a. Ligament integrity test

b. Vertebral basilar artery insufficiency test

iii. Performance/Clinical measures

a. Musculoskeletal evaluation (AROM, flexibility, PAVIM, strength, endurance)

b. Special tests (Spurling's, CFRT, Head lift, CCFT, neurodynamics)

c. Cervical proprioception (Joint Position Error test)[185]

e. Cervical influence on oculomotor control (SPNT)

f. Craniovertebral muscle recruitment with eye motion

g. Head righting response

h. Cervicothoracic extension (motion, motor control, strength, endurance)

i. Shoulder girdle screening

j. Respiratory pattern and thoracic cage motion

AROM, Active range of motion; *BCTT,* Buffalo Concussion Treadmill Test; *CCFT,* Craniocervical flexion test; *cDVA,* computerized dynamic visual acuity; *CFRT,* cervical flexion rotation test; *DGI,* Dynamic Gait Index; *FGA,* Functional Gait Assessment; *GST,* gaze stabilization test; *mCTSIB,* modified clinical test for sensory integration in balance; *PAVIM,* passive accessory intervertebral motion (PROM); *PCSI,* Postconcussion Symptom Inventory; *PCSS,* Post Concussion Symptom Scale; *POTS,* postural orthostatic tachycardia syndrome; *RPQ,* Rivermead Post-Concussion Questionnaire; *SOT,* sensory organization test; *SPNT,* smooth pursuit neck torsion test; *VAS,* visual analog scale; *VOR,* vestibulo-ocular reflex.

tool that has been developed and validated alongside the Pediatric Vestibular Symptom Questionnaire (PVSQ) to assess visually induced dizziness (ViD) in children aged 6 to 17 years.[184] The PVID shows utility in identifying and quantifying symptoms of ViD related to concussion, migraine, and other vestibular conditions—an important consideration in the assessment of children and adolescents, as they have been found to rely on the visual system as the predominant system for balance and to resolve sensory conflict until multisensory processing reaches maturation, even in the absence of injury.[193]

Tests and Measures to Evaluate Persistent Postconcussion Symptom Complaint

The NINDS CDE[93] recommends that symptom complaints of patients with PPCS be monitored using the PCSI, PCSS, RPQ, and the HBI. Information related to these self-reported symptom complaint questionnaires has been provided earlier in the chapter. A review of the decision making process of the rehabilitation specialist as it relates to symptom complaint is discussed here.

Clinicians are advised not to use the results from either the PCSI, PCSS, RPQ, or the HBI alone to direct their care. Symptoms can be nonspecific and can mimic symptoms associated with chronic pain, depression, and anxiety disorders[5]; therefore symptom complaints alone cannot be used to identify underlying impairments of functional systems that may cause common symptom complaints following concussion.[58,90,194] For example, a symptom complaint of a headache could be due to visual problems or cervical spine dysfunction, or could be related to prior history of migraines. Similarly, a symptom complaint of dizziness could be caused by orthostatic hypotension, vestibulo-ocular problems, or anxiety associated with the inability to return to sports, school, or social activities. Further, symptom complaints endorsed by individuals following a concussion are commonly reported among nonconcussed individuals.[58,89,90] For athletes specifically, the accuracy of symptom report from adolescents recovering from SRC has been questioned, as athletes may not disclose concussive signs and symptoms as they may intentionally withhold reporting them or, conversely, they may be motivated to inflate or continue reporting symptoms despite injury resolution as a means to leave a sport.[89,195,196] Therefore symptom complaints alone are not sensitive to either diagnose concussion or to identify underlying causes of dysfunction.

For this reason, the clinical examination should be made up of tests and measures that can provide the clinician with objective data about potential impairments of physical or psychological systems, or personal circumstances that may contribute to the reported symptoms. This point cannot be emphasized enough: the rehabilitation specialist should structure the examination to identify underlying impairments in functional systems and activity limitations so that interventions can be matched to the findings of the physical examination. In our experience, clinicians who rely on symptom complaint to guide decision making do not have successful outcomes in the management of concussion-related functional deficits.

Cognitive/Neuropsychological Dysfunction

As discussed previously, there is evidence that concussion may lead to neurocognitive dysfunction secondary to axonal shearing, secondary neuronal death, altered cerebral blood flow, and dysregulated biochemical function.[44,197] In most clinical cases, there are no obvious initial neuroimaging results that identify this damage or dysfunction.[198] However, the pattern of neurocognitive deficits is relatively consistent when evaluated clinically and behaviorally. Although the research debate continues on the existence of a constellation of neurocognitive deficits, the primary deficits reported by researchers, patients, and clinicians include attention, memory, executive functions, word retrieval, and social skills/pragmatics.[199–201]

Attention. Attention skills are critical for all cognitive function.[202–204] Attention domains have been identified and described in a variety of ways and with various names, but generally relate to sustaining attention, selective attention, alternating attention, and divided attention.[205] Sustained attention is the ability to maintain focus on a task, or for a period of time (i.e., completing a written task or listening to a phone conversation). Selective attention is the ability to attend to a task with distractions such as auditory, tactile, or visual stimuli (i.e., holding a conversation in a busy environment). Alternating attention is the ability to switch focus from one task to the next and back again (i.e., driving a car and watching the traffic in front, behind, while managing the controls). Divided attention is the ability to do one or more tasks at the same time (i.e., taking notes in class and scrolling through social media).[206]

Those with PPCS generally report these areas as the most frustrating deficits. The complaints typically focus on noise and feeling overstimulated while attempting to complete daily tasks.[207] Most individuals with PPCS report that they are able to generally sustain attention, but not for the length of time as they were able to premorbidly. In addition, any tasks that require alternating and divided attention result in significant fatigue, frustration, and sometimes lability. Frequently, the reduced abilities in sustained, selective, alternating, and divided attention are not evident to the person with PPCS until they return to their work or school responsibilities. Patients will sometimes attempt to ameliorate these deficits with sunglasses, noise-cancelling headphones, dimming lights, and reducing/controlling the amount of tasks.[208]

Memory. Memory is a broad category of cognition that is integral to daily and independent function, and learning throughout the lifespan. Memory domains include immediate memory, working memory, delayed memory, episodic memory (daily recall of a person's experience), prospective memory, semantic memory (i.e., vocabulary, general knowledge), procedural (i.e., recall of an overlearned motor task such as brushing teeth, riding a bike), and long-term/personal memory.[209] Memory abilities are closely aligned with attention domains: if a patient is unable to attend to information, it will be difficult to store and recall the information.[210] Processes involved in memory include attention, encoding (preparing information to store), storage, and recall. In general, the longer the information is stored and retrieved, the more stable in memory storage (i.e., name, address, family members are units of information that are easily recalled and automatic).[211] Memory can be visual, auditory, olfactory, and tactile. Memory systems are closely connected with attention and emotional areas of the brain.[212]

Memory is also one of the most common cognitive deficits reported by those with PPCS. Procedural, long-term, and personal memory units are not typically reported areas of concern. Semantic memory will be discussed further in relation to word retrieval. More recent memory that has not had extensive retrieval and recall over time are the areas those with PPCS identify as deficit areas: immediate, delayed, episodic,[213] working,[214] and prospective memory.[215] Common complaints include being unable to recall conversations, planned events, information just read, when or if medication was taken, and other daily interactions and new information. Most with PPCS indicate that when visual or auditory distractions are present, recall of new information is further impaired.

Executive functions. Executive functions are cognitive abilities that support personality, attention, flexibility, problem solving,

reasoning, awareness, and social skills/pragmatics.[216] These abilities are frequently impacted in those with PPCS.[217] These areas are also critical in daily human interaction, and may be conscious or subconsciously managed. For the most part, these abilities are not taught, but are learned through experience or subconsciously.[218] For example, awareness of self allows a person to interpret another person's reaction and change their own behavior in response. Flexibility supports a person's ability to make a choice, realize that it was not an appropriate choice, and change the plan or choice.

Executive function complaints with PPCS may not be as obvious to the patient. However, they may be identified by the family and significant others. Changes in mood and emotional control are reported: lability with anger, sadness, and laughter at inappropriate times or not consistent with premorbid status.[219] Inability to manage schedules, make adjustments with change, identify alternate solutions, and predict outcomes are demonstrated. Social skills/pragmatics differences are also experienced: inappropriate comments, difficulty with humor and sarcasm, and "personality changes" (i.e., those around the patient report that they are changed in some way). These deficits are further impaired by the lack of awareness and social repair abilities.

Word retrieval. Word retrieval refers to the ability of generating and producing the desired word. This ability is related to overall vocabulary level, speed of processing, and the expressive language system. Aphasia is the inability to express or comprehend language, typically after a cerebrovascular accident (CVA), TBI, or other neurological injury. Those with TBI sometimes present with various levels of aphasia, although their semantic memory system appears to be relatively preserved.[220] In PPCS, patients experience and report inconsistent difficulty in word retrieval that is significantly increased from premorbid levels. Speed of word retrieval is also significantly reduced from premorbid function.[200] This impairment can dramatically impact daily life.

Social language/pragmatic skills. Social language (i.e., pragmatic skills) are the skills used throughout interactions in daily life. They are skills that are generally not taught, but rather learned through experience or subconsciously.[221] Pragmatic skills include, but are not limited to, eye gaze, voice modulation, body language, topic maintenance, turn taking, appropriate behavior related to setting, emotional control, and overall Theory of Mind behaviors and abilities (i.e., consciously or subconsciously thinking about what others are thinking and adjusting behavior related to that perception).[222] Pragmatic skills significantly impact human communication. Notably, when they are appropriate, these skills go relatively unnoticed. When they are impaired, or deviant in some way, they are perceived and responded to sometimes in ways that are not overt and may be subconscious at some level (i.e., when a person is too close physically for the situation at hand, the other person will respond physically by moving away; when a person does something unexpected in a situation, the others in the interaction will make a judgment, consciously or subconsciously, and indicate their disapproval in a subtle or not subtle way).

Those with PPCS may experience subtle changes in their social language/pragmatic skills (SLPS).[223] As stated previously, due to the impaired executive function system, the patient may not be aware of these differences, although family and friends may notice. The frequent comment from family members usually is that the patient is "changed" or "different." Impairments frequently include difficulty with topic maintenance, inappropriate behavior for the setting, inability to use or understand humor or sarcasm, difficulty with social repair skills, perseveration on topics, and emotional control.[224] SLPS are sometimes confounded with personality. With typical lack of obvious physical impairment or injury, an added caveat is that those who do not know the patient may respond to impaired SLPS in a way that may socially isolate the patient, in that they assume the impaired behavior is by choice.

Cognitive/Neuropsychological Assessment

Two disciplines take the lead in cognitive/neuropsychological assessment. In some settings, specifically sports rehabilitation and/or concussion clinics, the two disciplines work together in the assessment process. Typically, however, neuropsychologists focus solely on assessment and counseling/support for the trauma and adjustment. In general, neuropsychological evaluations involve in-depth testing on all cognitive-communication domains, as well as intelligence testing, emotional adjustment, and visual-motor skills. This testing is usually completed many months or even years after the injury, and is typically part of vocational assessment, legal cases relating to the injury, and RTW and school. Notably, there is not always a neuropsychologist in every clinic or therapy setting, and their services may be cost-prohibitive.[225] Furthermore, as their focus is on assessment and support, neuropsychologists rarely provide direct cognitive-communication rehabilitation.

SLPs play a pivotal role in concussion management because of their expertise in the assessment, diagnosis, and treatment of persons with cognitive-linguistic disorders associated with traumatic brain injury.[226] SLPs are typically part of the clinical rehabilitation environments. The Scope of Practice for SLPs includes assessment and treatment for all areas of communication and cognition.[227] SLPs who work in medical and outpatient clinic settings specialize in the neurological population.

Cognitive-communication assessment should always be dynamic in nature and should be as functionally valid as possible. Artificial clinical environments with unfamiliar clinicians may not be as functional or ecological as real-life experiences. Therefore interviews with the patient and family and observations may also provide meaningful information. Several concussion symptom scales include parent or family ratings as well.[112]

Many tests are able to target cognitive-communication deficits in PPCS, and a partial list for all age ranges follows (Table 23.9). Some tests have specific subtests that target areas most critical in PPCS evaluation, and those are noted. In addition, intake interview questions are part of the interpretation of testing results. Prior level of function (PLF), including level of education, work experience, learning history including strengths and weaknesses, social history and

TABLE 23.9   Tests for Assessment of Persistent Postconcussion Symptoms Cognitive-Communication Function

Test	Standardization Age Range	Measures
California Verbal Learning Test–Children's Version California Verbal Learning Test (CVLT-2)	5–16:11 16–89	Memory for list learning, new information with repetition and semantic association, verbal learning and memory (differentiates encoding and retrieval) from retrieval skills
Comprehensive Assessment of Spoken Language–2 (CASL-2)	3–21:11	Supralinguistic skills: use of language in which meaning not directly available from the surface lexical and syntactic, pragmatics, and abstract language Pragmatic language: knowledge of language that is appropriate across different situational contexts and ability to modify language according to the social situation
Controlled Oral Word Association Test (COWA)	16–70	Semantic and phonetic verbal fluency
Clinical Evaluation of Language Fundamentals–5 (CELF-5)	5–21	Language memory for sentences and paragraph details/inferences, pragmatics checklist/profile Metalinguistics test for higher level language
Behavior Rating Inventory of Executive Function (BRIEF)–SR Behavior Rating Inventory of Executive Function (BRIEF)–A	11–18 18–90	Rating scales with indexes for behavior regulation, emotion regulation, and cognitive regulation
Developmental Neuropsychological Assessment, 2nd Edition (NEPSY-II)	3–16	Attention, memory, new learning, theory of mind
Rey Auditory Verbal Learning Test (RAVLT)	5–18	Immediate recall of words presented auditorily
Wisconsin Card Sorting Test (WCST)	7–89	Executive functions, mental flexibility
Test of Everyday Attention for Children (TEA-C) Test of Everyday Attention (TEA)	5–15 18–80	Attention: sustained, selective, alternating, divided
Elementary Test of Problem Solving–Elementary 3 (TOPS-E3) Adolescent Test of Problem Solving (TOPS-2 A)	6–15:11	Problem solving, perseveration, and abstract thinking: critical thinking based on students' language strategies, logic, and experiences, making inferences, determining solutions, interpreting perspectives, insights
Student Functional Assessment of Verbal Reasoning Executive Strategies (S-FAVRES) Functional Assessment of Verbal Reasoning Executive Strategies (FAVRES)	12–19 17–89	Evaluates aspects of complex comprehension (sarcasm, humor, intent, gist or central theme) discourse, social communication, verbal reasoning, problem solving, meta-cognition, executive functions

Continued

TABLE 23.9   Tests for Assessment of Persistent Postconcussion Symptoms Cognitive-Communication Function—cont'd

Test	Standardization Age Range	Measures
Repeatable Battery for Neuropsychological Assessment	12–89:11	Immediate memory, language, attention, visuospatial memory, and constructional abilities
The Word Test–3 Elementary	6–11:11	Word retrieval/expressive vocabulary (associations, synonyms, semantic absurdities, antonyms, definitions, and flexible word use)
The Word Test–2 Adolescent	12–17	
Pediatric Test of Brain Injury (PTBI)	6–16	Story recall, naming, immediate and delayed memory, verbal fluency, complex language comprehension, semantic associations
Boston Naming Test–2	18–79	Word retrieval/naming
Wide Range Assessment of Memory and Learning (WRAML-2)	5–90	Multiple tests for verbal and visual memory, immediate and delayed
Rivermead Behavioral Memory Test–Child (RBMT-C)	5–11:11	Verbal, visual memory immediate and delayed
Rivermead Behavioral Memory Test–3	16–96	
Test of Adolescent/Adult Word Finding (TAWF)	12–80	Word finding for nouns and verbs, sentence completion, description naming, and category naming
Test of Auditory Processing–4 (TAPS-4)	5–21	Four subtests for auditory memory, and three for auditory comprehension, inferences
Woodcock-Johnson Psychoeducational Battery: Tests of Cognitive Ability–3	2–90+	General intellectual ability and specific cognitive abilities: working memory, processing speed, cognitive efficiency
Ross Information Processing Assessment–P (RIPAP)	5–12	Immediate memory, recent memory
RIPA–2 (RIPA-2)	15–90	Temporal orientation (recent memory and remote memory) orientation, recall of general information, problem solving and abstract reasoning, organization auditory processing and retention
Expressive Vocabulary Test–2	2–90	Expressive vocabulary and word retrieval
Cognitive-Linguistic Quick Test-Plus (CLQT+)	18–89:11	Attention, memory, executive function, visuospatial skills, language[228–258]

support, as well as prior injuries, are important clinical evidence to use in when interpreting assessment results. The medical history of the injury and any prior therapy and testing should also be shared.

Standardized testing is critical in the assessment of PPCS. A study out of the military identified several tests in a battery that were comprehensive in evaluating the specific target areas in mild TBI(mTBI). Parrish and colleagues at the Naval Medical Center in San Diego[259] developed a standardized battery, including the Woodcock-Johnson III Tests of Cognitive Abilities (WJ-III),[260] the Attention Process Training Test (APT),[261] and the Functional Assessment of Verbal Reasoning and Executive Strategies (FAVRES; MacDonald, 2005).[262] In addition, for informal assessment, they developed a questionnaire about symptoms/concerns and observed SLPS in conversations with familiar and unfamiliar partners. Results of their evaluation of their assessment battery indicated that it was sensitive to the concerns and symptoms of their mTBI population. The Miami University Concussion Management Program utilized several different tests with the same goals in mind: Hopkins Verbal Learning Test,[263] Trail Making Tests A and B,[264] Controlled Oral Word Association Test,[228] Digit Span from the Wechsler Memory Scale (WMS), Grooved[265] Pegboard Test (GPT[266]), and the Post-Concussion Symptom Scale (PCSS[84]). In addition, they include the ImPACT computerized test, since they include that as baseline testing for all athletes at their university.

For TBI assessment, many studies recommend a combination of standardized and nonstandardized assessments to assess functional abilities.[268,269] An important aspect is the inclusion of nonstandardized and "informal" assessments, as the testing conditions themselves may

scaffold cognitive-communication skills that TBI patients have in the real world.[270] According to Coelho and colleagues,[271] the use of language within social contexts, communication competence, is best evaluated outside of the clinical setting in conversation, rather than in structured interviews in the clinic setting. Overall, cognitive-communication/neuropsychological assessment should provide the patient and the clinician with a clear picture of deficit areas, strengths, and the understanding of how these areas relate to the patient's life and goals.

Exercise Intolerance

Concussion can lead to physiological dysfunction, including neurometabolic challenges, altered cerebral blood flow, and/or autonomic dysfunction.[127,154,272] Patients with concussion have been found to have higher resting heart rates,[273] and there is evidence from imaging studies of abnormal cerebral blood flow volume and distribution in humans both acutely after concussion[274] and in those with PPCS.[275] Such cellular and physiological alterations lead to a mismatch between energy supply and demand that is thought to be a major contributing factor to exercise intolerance and prolonged recovery following concussion.

As mentioned previously, international consensus guidelines provide a strong recommendation for a period of rest (1 to 2 days), followed by a graduated return to activity (see Table 23.7). However, the clinician and patient with PPCS are often stuck in a gray area, questioning: What is the optimal amount of rest? When should exercise begin? And how can the exercise progress safely? For this reason, John Leddy's group at SUNY Buffalo developed a subsymptom exercise tolerance test, the Buffalo Concussion Treadmill Test (BCTT), to identify individuals with exercise intolerance following a concussion and provide clinicians with a tool for guidance in exercise prescription related to return to activity.

Assessment of Exercise Intolerance: Subsymptom Exercise Tolerance Test

The BCTT[154] has been shown to be a safe[276,277] and reliable[278] measure, which can be useful for identifying levels of exercise tolerance in patients following SRC, quantifying the clinical severity of the concussion, and developing exercise prescription for patients with PPCS.[115,154] Using a standardized Balke protocol, patients perform an incremental treadmill exercise test (Fig. 23.4) that is terminated upon provocation of new symptoms, elevation of symptoms beyond established criteria, or maximum exertion is achieved. The starting speed is set to 3.2 to 3.6 mph. During the first minute, the treadmill is set at a 0% incline. After 1 minute, the incline is increased by 1% grade and then by 1% grade each minute thereafter while maintaining the same speed until the patient can no longer continue, whether because of symptom exacerbation or fatigue. Rating of perceived exertion (RPE, using the Borg Rating scale) and symptoms, using a 1- to 10-point visual analog scale (VAS), are assessed every minute. Blood pressure (with an automated or manual cuff) and heart rate (HR) are measured every 2 minutes. For the most accurate information, it has been recommended that a heart rate monitor be worn across the chest during the test[277] (HR, by Polar HR monitor, Model #FIT N2965; Kempele, Finland).

The predetermined stopping criteria consists of either exacerbation of symptoms, or voluntary exhaustion (RPE of 18 to 20). Symptom exacerbation is defined as a greater than or equal to 3 point change from that day's overall pretreadmill resting symptom score on the VAS, where a point is given for each increase in a symptom (e.g., headache) or the appearance of a new symptom (e.g., dizziness).[154] The heart rate at which this event occurs is referred to as the threshold heart rate (HRt) and should be documented, as this threshold will be used as a reference for exercise prescription.[277]

The test should be deferred for individuals with significant pretest resting symptoms of greater than or equal to seven on the VAS or those with a history indicating increased risk for cardiopulmonary disease as defined by the American College of Sports Medicine.[154] A complete list of absolute and relative contraindications for exercise testing can be reviewed in Leddy and colleagues.[154] Special considerations should be established for transient dysautonomia, which has been identified in some cases of concussion, and has been described as the prolonged physiological response in individuals with exercise and activity intolerance.[279–281] There is a lack of consensus among medical professionals on the routine assessment of dysautonomia following mTBI in the acute phase postinjury. Evidence regarding heart rate variability testing is conflicting, and data is limited to within 2 weeks postinjury.[282] Autonomic function testing is not readily available, though the passive tilt table test is recommended for the diagnosis of postural orthostatic tachycardia syndrome (POTS) with well-established heart rate criteria in the presence of orthostatic symptoms.[283,284] In the absence of access to autonomic function testing or as a screening tool, an active standing test can be performed to compare the supine resting heart rate (obtained after 10 minutes of quiet rest) to the heart rate after 10 minutes of quiet standing. Sustained tachycardia may be an indication of dysautonomia as cerebral hypoperfusion may cause lightheadedness, blurry vision, or cognitive dysfunction brought on in upright postures or during exertion. Identification of signs consistent with dysautonomia or

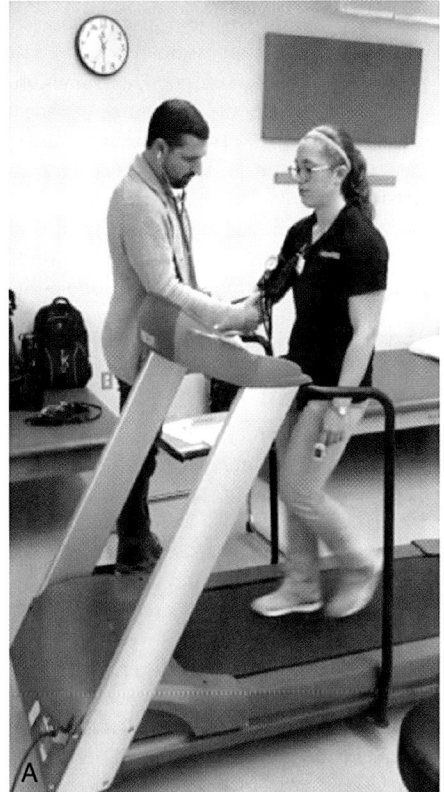
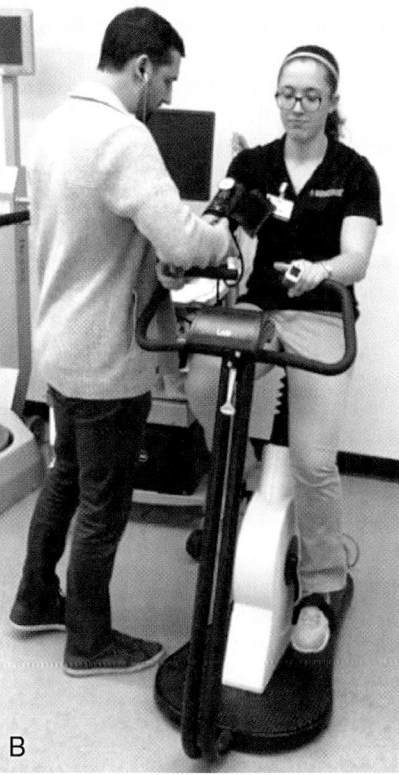

Fig. 23.4 (A) Subsymptom exercise tolerance test (Buffalo Concussion Treadmill Test) using a treadmill and **(B)** subsymptom exercise tolerance test using a bicycle, while medical professional monitors heart rate, blood pressure, rate of perceived exertion (Borg exertion scale), and a visual analog scale for symptom provocation

POTS requires consultation for medical management to improve response to vestibular neurorehabilitation. For those individuals with apparent dysautonomia or who meet diagnostic criteria for POTS, medical management and recumbent exercise may need to precede upright exertion testing.[285,286]

The safety of the test has been established for adult and adolescent patients aged 15 to 53 years with persistent symptoms at 3 weeks or more postinjury who attended a sports medicine clinic.[115,276] Because of a lack of evidence indicating the BCTT was safe to conduct during the acute phase of concussion recovery, Leddy and colleagues assessed the safety and potential predictive value of the BCTT in adolescents performed within 1 to 9 days following concussion.[277] Assessment of exercise tolerance using the BCTT a median of 4 days after injury did not significantly affect symptom reporting in the short-term (within 24 hours), did not delay recovery, nor did it increase symptoms in the long term (14 days postinjury). In addition, Leddy and colleagues[277] found exercise intolerance within the first week after concussion (as indicated by the HRt) strongly predicted recovery after concussion injury. Adolescents with a HRt below 135 bpm were approximately 45 times more likely to have a prolonged recovery (odds ratio = 44.75) than adolescents with a HRt above or equal to 135 bpm. The authors suggested academic and athletic teams use this cutoff with caution, as the study was not powered to determine sensitivity, specificity, or the positive predictive value associated with this cutoff. Still, the findings make a significant contribution to the utility of the BCTT, which has already been established as a useful guide for exercise prescription and return to play decision making.[17,154,188] Although it appears additional studies to establish the optimal modes and protocols for various populations are required to validate the BCTT as a diagnostic and prognostic biomarker,[287] the test's clinical utility and ability to predict prolonged recovery is promising.

Due to the common symptom complaint of dizziness, a stationary bicycle (see Fig. 23.4) can be used in place of a treadmill in order to reduce the magnitude of head excursion while walking or running on a treadmill[288] and to minimize conflicting sensory stimulation.[289] *Supplementary videos are available to provide examples of subsymptom exacerbation exercise tests using a treadmill and stationary bicycle. These videos can be found in the online resources for this text.*

A comprehensive examination of impairments that contribute to exacerbation of symptoms and decrease of function should be completed before the exertional assessment is started. When the examination identifies that there is a sensation of motion at rest, for example, that sensation will cause a decrease in the tolerance level when head motion is increased, as when walking on the treadmill. As intervention targeting sensation of motion at rest decreases this phenomenon, there will be more tolerance to most activity. This is further incorporated into activities that demand head turning, such as when turning the head to interact with the tester. If the somatosensory system is providing abnormal reference through the spine and weight-bearing joints, this can impact the sensation of stability when walking on a moving surface. Modifications and intervention for the visual system should be addressed as soon as possible so that the dizziness triggered by visual or visual/vestibular dysfunction can be reduced prior to testing. Other sensorimotor system changes, described as follows, will create exercise intolerance and should be addressed in an intervention regime prior to exertion.

Vestibular System Impairment

Function of the vestibular system relies on accurate information from the peripheral vestibular apparatus (sensory receptors and afferent pathways) and integration of the information by subcortical nuclei for appropriate motor output through the vestibulo-ocular and vestibulo-spinal reflexes, in order to provide gaze stability and postural control, respectively. Therefore damage to the peripheral or central vestibular structures can result in a cluster of signs, such as impaired gaze stability, gait, and balance, and symptoms including vertigo, dizziness, motion sensitivity, and/or imbalance.[115,187,290] Recent studies mapping the vestibular system through diffusion tensor imaging (DTI) and functional magnetic resonance imaging (fMRI) demonstrate the extensive network of interhemispheric and decussating relays between the vestibular nuclei and the parieto-insular vestibular cortex that could be affected by prolonged neurometabolic changes that may impact the integrity of vestibular reflexes and compensatory strategies.[291]

To perform efficiently the vestibular system information must be compared with the information provided by the visual and somatosensory systems to create the appropriate motor response. Central adaptation for vestibular dysfunction depends on intact references from these systems, or sensory integration. Concussion, in which dysfunction appears in more than one of the sensory systems, significantly challenges the adaptation process and leads to persistence of symptoms when compared with a person with primarily vestibular deficits. This is why an endorsement of dizziness during acute concussion has been shown to be a marker of poorer prognosis for athletes following an SRC.[61] Dizziness after concussion may be attributable to a variety of conditions. This point is critical, as "dizziness" is a nonspecific term that includes diffuse symptoms of disorientation and lightheadedness that may represent the somatosensory dysfunction. Early symptoms of vertigo (spinning) reflect unequal signals through the vestibular structures that can also affect balance problems[292] due to dysfunction of any combination of the peripheral vestibular system, central vestibular pathways, or comorbid conditions, including labyrinthopathy, vestibular migraine, autonomic nervous system dysfunction, or anxiety. Also, symptoms consistent with persistent postural-perceptual dizziness (PPPD) are common after concussion. For this reason, a comprehensive and thoughtful clinical interview, examination, and evaluation should be completed to identify the source of the symptom complaint,[181] and modifications of traditional vestibular rehabilitation strategies are often required to accommodate the visual and somatosensory deficits.

Common impairments and examination procedures observed in this patient population as they relate to the vestibular system are discussed in this section, which include positional vertigo, impaired dynamic gaze stabilization, ocular motor deficits, motion sensitivity, and balance and gait impairment.

Positional Vertigo

Benign paroxysmal positional vertigo (BPPV) following traumatic brain injury accounts for 8.5% to 20% of all cases of BPPV.[293] Therefore it is important that patients with symptoms of BPPV be screened with the Dix-Hallpike and side-lying tests to evaluate for potential BPPV of semicircular canals.[5,115,294–296] Treatment of BPPV for individuals with PPCS should follow the same clinical reasoning as nonconcussed patients who present with signs and symptoms suggestive of BPPV. Ahn and colleagues[293] reviewed medical records of 192 consecutive patients with positional vertigo to determine if there were clinical differences between BPPV after TBI and idiopathic BPPV. Of the 32 patients with BPPV following TBI, the majority (75%) had posterior semicircular canal BPPV, while the remaining patients had BPPV of the horizontal semicircular canal, which is consistent with prevalence of canalith involvement in idiopathic BPPV. Although recurrence rates were similar between the two groups, patients with BPPV following TBI required more treatment sessions than individuals with idiopathic

BPPV to lead to full resolution.[293] Posttraumatic hydrops may account for the need for increased intervention and may need to be addressed with use of diuretic in combination with the repositioning. Procedures for canalith repositioning maneuvers have been described in sufficient detail previously. Damage in the central structures can cause head position dizziness. When there is purely vertical nystagmus noted in supine head hanging that does not fatigue within 1 minute, it likely is of a central nature. For a review of this content, the reader is referred to Chapters 20 and 21.

Impaired Dynamic Gaze Stabilization

The VOR produces eye movements equal and opposite to head movements for the purpose of visual stability when the head is in motion. Proper function of the VOR requires intact peripheral and central vestibular pathways, which consist of the vestibular nuclei, cerebellum, thalamus, cerebral cortex, and the projections that connect subcortical and cortical areas to the ocular motor system to provide dynamic gaze stability. The forces that cause a concussion can disrupt the neurons that control the VOR,[187,297,298] causing blurred or unstable vision, difficulty focusing during head motion. This may lead to complaints of vertigo, nausea, and fogginess, or discomfort in busy environments (e.g., visual motion sensitivity).[100,115] There is evidence that symptom complaints suggestive of pathology to the vestibular system are associated with prolonged recovery[100]; it is therefore important that the rehabilitation specialist select reliable and valid measures that provide objective information related to the degree of involvement of the vestibulo-ocular system for patients following a concussion.

Dynamic gaze stabilization assessment. As measures used to evaluate the vestibulo-ocular system have been described previously in Chapters 20 and 21, special considerations of tests and measures (including their relevance as assessment tools and outcome measures for individuals with impaired dynamic gaze stabilization following a concussion) are discussed here.

The dynamic visual acuity (DVA) test and the gaze stabilization test (GST) are two functional measurements used for assessment of the VOR in individuals with vestibular disorders. The DVA can be assessed using a manual bedside test or a computerized version; however, reliability and validity studies support the use of the computerized DVA (cDVA) test[299–301] when available. Reliability and responsiveness of the cDVA and GST have been established for individuals with vestibular dysfunction. Due to the incidence of concussion in high school and collegiate sports, Kaufman and colleagues[302] investigated the psychometrics associated with the cDVA for high school and collegiate athletes as the required head speeds for athletic performance must be greater than the demands of regular daily activities. Test-retest reliability for the cDVA was found to be good in the yaw plane and fair-to-good in the pitch plane, with ICC values of 0.77 and 0.72, respectively. The minimal detectable change was found to be 0.16 logMAR and 0.21 logMAR in the yaw and pitch plane motions, respectively.[302] Findings show that even at high head speeds of 150 to 200 degrees per second (deg/s), which is considerably faster than the head velocity used for individuals with vestibular dysfunction (80 to 120 deg/s), the cDVA may be reliably used as an outcome measure to show change over time.

It is important to note that clinical examination tests used to assess the vestibular system may lead to general symptom provocation, which may not be sensitive to a specific vestibular impairment.[181] For example, symptom provocation during the VOR test as performed in the VOMS test is not equivalent to reduced VOR gain. Reduction of VOR gain can be detected using a head thrust test or with use of a functional assessment of the VOR, such as the cDVAT or GST. The symptom

provocation alone during one of these tests does not equate to dysfunction of the VOR. In this way, negative findings on tests used to evaluate the function of the VOR (head thrust test, cDVAT, GST), but with symptom provocation while performing head motion with visual fixation, should be recorded as such and addressed with interventions addressing *head motion provoked dizziness*, which may be related to vestibular-somatosensory maladaptation (see section on cervical spine) and does not necessitate the strict prescription of VOR exercises for patients with peripheral vestibular hypofunction, as described in Chapters 20 and 21. VOR retraining can increase symptoms in the presence of visual sensitivity, somatosensory impairments in the cervical spine, or stiffness caused by attempting to decelerate the head to avoid dizziness. These impairments should be addressed in the intervention before initiating dynamic gaze stability exercises.

Murray and colleagues[303] performed a systematic review of the literature to determine if specific outcome measures could be identified within vestibular rehabilitation treatment paradigms. Ten articles met the study inclusion criteria, including two RCT, two prospective cohort studies, one retrospective study, and five case studies. Three of the ten studies included children and/or adolescents; the remaining seven studies included young/older adults or military personnel. Interestingly, although 9 of the 10 included studies reported the incorporation of gaze stabilization or adaptation exercises, only two studies measured gaze stabilization using the DVA test. Schneider and colleagues[304] used the bedside DVA test, while Gottshall and colleagues[305] used the cDVA and GST. Although the symptom complaint of dizziness is not specific to impaired dynamic gaze stabilization, it is important to mention that self-report measures such as the Dizziness Handicap Inventory (DHI), the Vertigo Symptom Scale, and the dizziness analogue scale have been used in studies providing vestibular rehabilitation to patients with PPCS.[303]

Ocular Motor Impairment

The objective of the visual motor system, or the ocular motor system, is to direct the gaze to visual targets so that light waves land centrally over the fovea of the retina for best visual acuity. Eye movements can be driven voluntarily by motor control centers at the level of the cerebral cortex (frontal, occipital, and temporal eye fields) or reflexively by centers located in the brain stem (midbrain and paramedian pontine reticular formation, and vestibulocerebellum). The ocular motor system uses four primary eye movements to achieve its goals: saccades, smooth pursuit, vergence, and the VOR. This section reviews saccades, smooth pursuit, and vergence eye movements.

Saccades are rapid movements of the eyes that are used during voluntary searching movements from one target to another. Smooth pursuit eye movements are used to track moving objects or maintain the gaze on a moving target. Although the origin of voluntary movements for saccades and smooth pursuit eye movements originate in different areas of the cerebral cortex, the frontal eye fields or temporal eye fields, respectively, each system shares a final common pathway of cranial nerve nuclei to cause contraction of the extraocular muscles for horizontal (originating from paramedian pontine reticular formation) and vertical (originating from midbrain reticular formation) movements of the eyes.

Vergence eye movements require that the eyes move toward the midline (convergence) or away from the midline (divergence) of the visual field. Therefore vergence is used while maintaining fixation on a visual target as it moves from the far visual field to the near visual field or vice versa. Such eye movements are controlled reflexively by control centers at the level of the brain stem and cerebellum.

Ocular motor impairments are common after concussions, as oculomotor control can be compromised through axonal injury or blunt trauma to the ocular motor systems. Injury to the cerebral cortex can directly impact volitional saccades and smooth pursuit movements and damage to subcortical nuclei, and white matter structures may disrupt reflexive vergence eye movements resulting in convergence or divergence insufficiency. However, damage to the ocular motor system following concussion may not be isolated to central nervous system structures, as damage to cranial nerves (specifically oculomotor, trochlear, and abducens nerves) may occur following concussion leading to selective impairment to the extraocular muscles. Such injuries have the potential to cause indirect and direct limitations in daily functioning, including symptom provocation, cognitive deficits, impaired reading, and poor academic performance.

Similar to dysfunction of other functional systems, the symptoms associated with impairment to the ocular motor system are varied, nondescript, and are not sensitive to diagnose concussion. Symptoms may include blurred vision, diplopia, eye strain, difficulty in reading, dizziness, headaches, ocular pain, and poor concentration. In children and adolescents, guided questions may be necessary to obtain information related to ocular motor deficits, such as difficulty losing their spot or skipping words when reading, difficulty copying notes off the board at school, or feeling "outside of" or "one step behind" themselves.[100,115] In addition, children may endorse feelings of intense anxiety or overwhelming nausea when working on a computer for long periods or when inside a grocery store.

Ocular Motor Assessment

It is important to consider that examination tests used to detect the presence of BPPV, motion sensitivity, and vestibulo-ocular deficits can be some of the more provocative tests used in the evaluation of the patient following a concussion. Therefore tests used to assess the ocular motor system should be performed prior to the examination of positional vertigo, motion sensitivity, or the vestibulo-ocular system. In this way, the performance by the patient for the visual examination may not be influenced by the presence (or increased presence) of symptoms, such as dizziness and headache. This gives the clinician the opportunity to identify the degree of impairment to the static ocular motor system, prior to evaluating the more demanding task of gaze stability during head movement.

The rehabilitation specialist should begin with observation for ocular malalignment using the cover-uncover test that can help reveal esophorias and exophorias and an evaluation of the cardinal plane movements for ocular motility using the H-test, which should be completed under monocular and binocular conditions. A comprehensive oculomotor examination includes tests of fixation, saccadic, smooth pursuit, and NPC eye movements. Further, testing for fixation, saccadic, and smooth pursuit eye movements should be performed under monocular and binocular viewing conditions.

For visual fixation, the patient is instructed to look at a target (blunt end of a pen or pencil) at a 40 cm viewing distance. The clinician should evaluate the ability of the patient to maintain a steady fixation on the target for 10 seconds. An abnormal result would include ocular drift or gaze instability.

Saccadic eye movements are tested by asking the patient to look back and forth between two horizontal or two vertical targets separated by 20 cm at a 40 cm viewing distance. Eye movements should be evaluated in the horizontal, vertical, and oblique planes for accuracy, speed, and response to stimulus for no more than five repetitions in each direction. In healthy individuals, the target can be reached with a single eye movement or with one small corrective saccade. It is important to have discrete targets to observe so that the clinician can definitively determine if the patient consistently overshoots or undershoots the target position.

Smooth pursuit is tested by asking the patient to track, with the eyes, an object moving in the central 20 degrees of the visual field at a 40 cm viewing distance while the head is stationary. Smooth pursuit is abnormal if, during tracking, the eye movements are disrupted or interrupted by saccades. It is important to note that use of the VOMS in the acute screening of concussion involves testing smooth pursuits by tracking an object moving in the horizontal and vertical directions for two repetitions each. In the evaluation of PPCS, reduced ability to perform smooth pursuits, as evidenced by catch-up saccadic movements, may be detected with fatigue by increasing the number of repetitions or by tracking a more complex motion such an H or figure-eight pattern.

NPC measures the ability to view a near target without diplopia and is tested under binocular conditions with the patient wearing appropriate lenses necessary for near vision. The patient is asked to track a pen that is held in the vertical position at the midline of the visual field, as it is moved toward the nose from a 60 cm viewing distance to the point at which the object blurs or becomes double (NPC). From that position, the pen is moved back toward the 60 cm viewing distance and the patient is then asked to report when the object becomes a single, fused target again (divergence). The clinician should document the distance at which the patient is no longer able to maintain a single, clear perception of the target during the test for convergence and the distance at which the patient regains the perception of a single target for the test of divergence. Normal NPC values are within 5 cm. If there is visual dependence or visual motion sensitivity, performing convergence testing may trigger dizziness as the images in the peripheral visual field appear to move as the target moves closer. It is important to make sure that the normal physiological diplopia associated with this testing is not interpreted by the patient as double vision.

Motion Sensitivity

The topics of visual (e.g., environment) and self-motion sensitivity have been discussed in Chapters 20 and 21, as it relates to patients with vestibular dysfunction. Sensitivity to visual and self-motion are thought to be caused by impairment of primary sensory systems or the integration of sensory information by multisensory processing in the higher order cortical areas of the occipitoparietal and occipitoparietal-temporal areas.[184,291,306] The global neurometabolic and neural transmission injury caused by concussion can lead to dysfunction throughout cortical and subcortical areas that process information related to orientation to the environment and perception of self-motion.

Following concussion, children and adults have shown impaired postural responses and have reported exacerbation of concussion-related symptoms when exposed to visual motion[82,289,307] that can persist for months following injury.[184,307,308] Special consideration should be taken for adolescents, and adults with preexisting history of motion sensitivity may exhibit more prolonged vestibular dysfunction,[307] have a greater likelihood of experiencing posttraumatic migraine (PTM),[158] and, perhaps of more concern, may experience more symptoms of anxiety or mood disorders early in recovery.[307]

Brosseau-Lachaine and colleagues[307] found that objective perceptual impairment to simple and complex visual stimuli is present up to 3 months following injury in children and, interestingly, do not correlate with symptom complaints of dizziness and visual motion sensitivity endorsed by children on self-reported symptom complaint questionnaires. This points to the need for the rehabilitation specialist to use self-report measures as a supplement to objective measures of motion sensitivity in order to optimally target treatment to impaired functional systems. In addition to the assessment for visual and self-motion sensitivity already discussed for patients with vestibular dysfunction, Pavlou and colleagues[184] described the pediatric visually induced dizziness questionnaire (ViD), which has been shown to be a reliable and valid measure to assess for visual motion sensitivity specifically for children.

Sensation of motion at rest. As noted previously, when the sensory systems are not calibrated sufficiently, the brain is challenged to determine movement versus stability. If the vestibular system is the origin of the offset, there is a sensation of spinning. The CNS uses the visual system and somatosensory systems to assist in comparing movement to nonmovement. A persistent sense of spinning when the eyes are closed reveals poor adaptation through the vestibulospinal system. If the somatosensory system is off set, it limits the recalibration process, and a sense of being lightheaded may be prominent. (See section on cervical spine.) This can have significant functional implications and contribute to sense of disorientation. It is critical to determine stability in the perception of head motion during steady-state tasks before moving toward movement exercises. Interventions are included in Chapters 20 and 21 *(sensation of motion at rest)* and include settling, which is effective in controlling symptoms when they have been exacerbated.

Balance and Gait Impairment

Impaired postural control is also commonly reported following concussion.[14,65,290] This can be an issue especially for youth and adolescents with SRC, as returning to play with balance and gait impairments may lead to musculoskeletal injury.[178,179] While the mechanisms are not fully understood, it is reasonable to suspect forces that result in a concussion can disrupt the function of the vestibular system, especially with respect to integration of balance information between the vestibular nuclei, cerebellum, and the descending vestibulospinal tracts.[69,158,291] Such changes could result in impairment in the components of the balance system that the nervous system uses to maintain postural orientation and equilibrium[309,310] including, but not limited to, the inability to properly weight the three sensory systems (somatosensory, vestibular, and visual sensory systems), control graded and timed anticipatory postural adjustments, and provide adequate reactive postural responses. It is well documented that concussion can cause impairments under steady-state balance conditions, as well as during activities that require an individual to achieve or regain equilibrium under more dynamic conditions.[289,311,312] Following concussion, patients typically will use inappropriate righting reactions and have increased use of stepping and hip strategies for even the smallest losses of balance. This may be the result of dependency patterns (described later), which can extinguish the normal use of the *head righting reflex.* Testing of head righting is described in Chapters 2, 20 and 21. The contribution to abnormal head righting related to cervical spine dysfunction is described in the section on cervical spine.

It is the function of the vestibular system to maintain the trunk in a vertical position for balance on tilted or uneven surfaces when the visual system is not available. The somatosensory system can substitute at both slow and fast speeds, but there is a range in which the vestibular system must provide upright control. Horak and colleagues[313] determined that individuals with vestibular deficiency lost their balance in more than 90% of trials during the 4 deg/s tilt condition, but never fell during slower tilts (0.25 to 1 deg/s) and fell only very rarely during faster tilts (16 to 32 deg/s). If the somatosensory system is dominant, there is a loss of balance at the midrange speeds. The trunk and head follow the direction of the tilt beyond the point, at which the somatosensory system can provide adequate reference to remain upright. See Chapters 20 and 21 for further information on methods to isolate the vestibular system in this context.

Balance and Gait Assessment

Many of the same self-report measures, such as the Activities-specific Balance Confidence (ABC) scale and performance-based outcome measures such as the Modified Clinical Test for Sensory Integration in Balance (mCTSIB), SOT, BESS test, Timed Up and Go (TUG), Five Times Sit to Stand (FTSTS), Dynamic Gait Index (DGI), and Functional Gait Assessment (FGA), which have been described previously in Chapter 22, are useful for evaluation of balance impairment following a concussion. Body-worn sensors have also been shown to have clinical utility to monitor center-of-mass displacement in the assessment of balance impairment and function following concussion.[314,315]

It is important to consider that many of the performance-based balance assessments (mCTSIB, SOT, and BESS) primarily evaluate the contribution of the sensory systems (visual, vestibular, and somatosensory) to postural control. The nervous system uses many different components of the balance system to maintain, achieve, and recover postural orientation and equilibrium during daily activities[309,310]; therefore the rehabilitation specialist should select a battery of performance measures that evaluate all components of the balance system,[310,316] rather than restricting the assessment to the sensory systems. For this reason, the importance of a thorough examination cannot be overlooked as impairments in strength, flexibility, range of motion (ROM), coordination, muscle tone, and cognition can also impair postural stability.

Murray and colleagues[303] performed a systematic review of the literature to determine if specific outcome measures could be identified within vestibular rehabilitation treatment paradigms. The authors concluded that standardization and consensus on outcome measure usage is required for future studies to allow for comparisons across studies to perform meta-analyses. In terms of balance assessments, it was interesting that only four of the 10 studies included in the review used self-report balance measures, while 8 of the 10 studies used performance-based balance and gait measures, including DGI, FTSTS, SOT, BESS, FGA, TUG, High-Level Mobility Assessment Tool (HiMAT), and an instrumented mat for spatial-temporal variables of gait. As these measures have been described previously in Chapter 22, special considerations of the FGA have been highlighted here to report the appropriate use of each test for patients, with imbalance following a concussion. Importantly, recommendations from the NINDS CDE[93] suggest the BESS test should be used in acute concussion. Consistent with this recommendation, the test has not been validated for use in the subacute or chronic stages of recovery following concussion, and the psychometrics of the test do not support its use as an outcome measure, as it is not responsive to change in performance over time. Therefore the recommendation for motor control assessment from the NINDS CDE for individuals with PPCS includes the DGI and FGA.

Functional gait assessment. The FGA assesses postural stability during various walking tasks. It is a 10-item test that is scored on a 4-level ordinal scale (0 to 3). Aggregate scores range from 0 to 30, with lower scores indicating greater impairment. The FGA has demonstrated concurrent validity with other commonly used balance measures[317] and excellent intra- and interrater reliability. An important point to consider for the use of the FGA for individuals with concussion is a ceiling effect, which has been reported in a study of 180 adolescents, where 25% of participants reached the maximum score of 30 points.[107] In addition, there is limited evidence that a ceiling effect may also be a concern for the FGA when used with young and older adults with PPCS.[66] However, the components in the FGA such as head turns, quick stops, tandem, and backward gait can help identify impairments for those individuals in which vestibular deficits limit function.

Dependency Patterns

Central nervous system adaptation for vestibular disorders requires the use of vision and somatosensory references to recover function. As the vestibular system becomes more efficient, the need for substitution of the other systems should decrease. However, in the compromised CNS, this return to normal reliance on the vestibular system can be limited. Persistent overdependence on vision or somatosensory information can create inefficient strategies. The patient with visual dependence will rely on vision and will have abnormal increases in sway or instability when the eyes are closed. Instability can result in the presence of visual stimulation during pursuits and optokinetic stimulation. There is often a complaint of dizziness when the eyes are closed or when walking in the dark. Avoidance of activity where there is excessive visual stimulation is common. Somatosensory dependence is often seen as an overdependence on an ankle strategy for balance, even when a hip strategy would be more appropriate. This can be seen by examination using a compliant or narrow surface, or when tested on a tilting surface. Increased dependence on somatosensory input for postural stability can also be observed in attempts to reduce head motion by clenching to load the temporomandibular joint, extended neck posture to increase facet joint loading, or cocontraction of neck musculature. This concept is further defined in Chapters 20 and 21.

Cervical Spine Function and Dysfunction

The cervical spine has a unique role in supporting and orienting the head in space and to the trunk (or trunk to the head) to serve the sensory systems. Concussion is frequently, if not always, accompanied by cervical spine stress due to direct biomechanical attachment of the head and neck, and contributes to sensorimotor impairment. Symptoms of traumatic cervical injury, particularly whiplash-associated disorders (WADs), overlap with many of those associated with the clinical threshold for concussion. Overlapping symptoms from the SCAT and the Quebec Task Force (QTF) on Whiplash Associated Disorders[318] include headache, dizziness/unsteadiness, nausea/vomiting, ringing in the ears, memory problems, problems concentrating, and vision problems.[319] Cervical spine assessment is recommended as standard practice in the detailed clinical examination for concussed patients to aid in differential diagnosis and targeted management planning.[14,114,115,182] Surprisingly, Feddermann-Demont and colleagues[320] reviewed 46 prospective studies covering 3284 athletes and found no studies meeting their review criteria that reported on neck pain, despite being a frequent concomitant injury after a head trauma, contrary to current recommendations and research. Primary domains were neurocognitive testing, balance, and symptom complaint. Interestingly, the studies focused on the total number rather than type of symptoms, an unexpected emphasis since symptoms typically guide the diagnostic decision and therapeutic management. Finally, studies related to the non-SRC population were not examined or evaluated

for inclusion. The authors' recommendation for future research focus was to explore the less-studied domains of vestibular, ocular motor, visual, psychological, and cervical symptoms, including baseline test results.

Due to the number of sensory and motor pathways of the cervical spine that may be damaged following a concussion, it is critical that the physical therapist carefully identifies specific impairments in the context of any functional disruption. An impairment directed approach may lead to more efficient and effective management and intervention strategies with positive outcomes.

Movement, stability, and somatosensory components of the cervical spine. The neck is the most mobile portion of the human spine, houses all neural traffic between the body and brain, and encases 100% of the brain's life support. The articulations from the cranium to C2 (also referred to as upper cervical spine, subcranial spine, or craniovertebral region) provide one-third of the sagittal plane motion and nearly half the rotational (transverse plane) motion of the neck. Ligaments supply structural stability while joint morphology permits great motion, as seen in Table 23.10.

All ligaments, but particularly the facet capsules, are vascularized and innervated with nociceptors and mechanoreceptors. As in all synovial joints, facet mechanoreceptors respond to loading and tensile forces throughout their full ROM and stimulate firing from muscle spindles. Thus they are vital for stability[321] and motor control. Facet afferents have cell bodies in the Dorsal Root Ganglia (DRG), projecting to the deep laminae of the dorsal horn. Afferents from C2 and C3 DRG may converge upon other nociceptive afferents arising from the subnucleus caudalis of the trigeminal nerve, which extends into the spinal cord at least to the level of C3, creating the neural mechanism for pain referral from upper cervical structures to the face and cranium.[319,322]

Neck musculature can be classified in three groups: craniocervical, typical cervical (within the neck), and those that span both regions. The trapezius and levator scapulae attach the head to the shoulder girdle and thorax. Cervical musculature is arranged in two "sleeves": the deep intrinsic sleeve provides tonic activity, intersegmental stability, guidance, and coordination, which includes the subcranial group, multifidus, longus colli. Greater torque production for head-on body motion is produced by the phasic functioning of the superficial extrinsic sleeve,[323] which includes the splenius capitus and cervicis, scalene group, infra hyoid groups, and platysma. The sternocleidomastoid is a prime mover of the head on the body, with great leverage and no attachments in the cervical spine.

The intrinsic group of subcranial muscles are nearly a 60/40% mix of type I postural slow fatiguing and type II fast twitch (phasic)

TABLE 23.10 Cervical Spine Ligaments

Region	Ligament	Function
Intrinsic craniovertebral	Tectorial membrane	Prevents distraction of cranium from spine
	Alar-Odontoid (paired)	Limits side bending of cranium on C2
	Transverse ligament of the atlas	Limits forward nod of C1 on C2 and preserves the A-P dimension of spinal canal under foramen magnum
C2–S1 anterior and posterior vertebral bodies	Anterior and posterior longitudinal ligaments	Limit extension and flexion, respectively, invest in the outer layers of intervertebral discs from C2–C3 through L5–S1
C2–S1, lamina to lamina posterior border of the spinal canal	Ligamentum flavum (paired)	Elastic ligament forms anterior aspect of all facet capsules, limits excessive spine flexion, may assist in return from flexion
Cranium to cervicothoracic junction	Ligamentum nuchae	Limits excessive neck flexion, most superficial, thick, ropelike

fibers.[324] Thus the intrinsic group has both postural support and primary segmental movement roles. The subcranial musculature has an exceptionally rich density of muscle spindles with up to 240 spindles (γ) per gram of wet muscle weight, which is required for exquisite fine motor control. Such spindle densities are consistent with their important role in head/neck and eye coordination and segmental stability.[325] Twelve intrinsic subcranial muscles create a 360 degrees "rotator cuff" for the cranium on the neck, with direct neural connections to the cerebellum, vestibular nuclei, and oculomotor nuclei via the superior colliculus. In healthy subjects, deep cervical musculature may be facilitated with gaze direction but functions independently of neck rotation direction.[326]

Muscle spindles are important organs of proprioception, which can be considered the most important somatosensory component needed to integrate information from the visual and vestibular systems for normal movement and postural control.[327–329] As a group, mechanoreceptors in the neck help the nervous system distinguish between head motion accompanied by body center of mass, and head on body movements not accompanied by motion of the body center of mass.[330] Their disruption leads to sensorimotor changes with adverse effects on the feedback and feedforward mechanisms of motor control, as well as regulation of muscle stiffness needed for stability. Box 23.2 summarizes conditions that disturb muscle spindle function. Locally these conditions interfere with smooth and appropriately timed motor responses. Centrally, inaccurate afferents disturb sensory integration. The importance of anatomical structures in the cervical spine responsible for position sense cannot be overstated, as their integration within the CNS affects our ability to plan and execute effective purposeful movements.[321]

For a review of somatosensory neuroanatomy and function, the reader is directed to https://clinicalgate.com/the-somatosensory-system-i-tactile-discrimination-and-position-sense.

Through cerebellar, brain stem, midbrain, and cortical projections, neck afferents contribute to the integration and coordination of a trio of reflex pathways that help recruit deep neck muscles for stability during head and body movements. The tonic neck reflex (TNR) promotes extensor recruitment to stabilize the neck for head motion in response to gravity, the cervicocollic reflex (CCR) is activated by the body moving under the head, and the vestibulocollic reflex (VCR) helps stabilize during rapid head motions. The cervico-ocular reflex (COR) complements the VOR by contributing to gaze stabilization during object tracking at slow head speeds and when the body is moving under the head. An important distinction to consider is the COR and VOR are usually inversely active.

BOX 23.2   Conditions That Disturb Muscle Spindle Function

- **Pain** can alter reflex activity and the sensitivity of the gamma muscle spindle through chemosensitive type III and IV nociceptors, and centrally by somatosensory cortex reorganization.
- **Joint effusion** impairs proprioception by inhibiting skeletal muscle, even in the absence of pain.
- **Direct trauma** may result in loss of muscle tissue and mechanoreceptors.
- **Fatigue** alters the metabolic state, changes motor activation patterns and muscle spindle discharge, increases a sense of effort, and results in clumsiness and decreased fine motor control.
- **Ligamentous hypermobility and joint instability** evoke inconsistent and late mechanoreceptor firing, affecting the useful timing, tuning, and intensity of muscle spindle activation.
- **Psychological distress and anxiety** can upregulate sympathetic tone, increasing tonic firing.

Mechanisms of cervical injury in concussion events. Neck trauma includes whiplash, defined by the QTF as an acceleration-deceleration mechanism of energy transfer to the neck and head from indirect neck trauma, beyond the tissue's ability to dissipate.[318] Indirect transfer of rotational forces to the cranium may result in concussion injury during a whiplash effect. Cervical spine soft tissues are disrupted at much lower impact forces than those measured in typical football concussions.[331] Direct head impact is likely to create compression or tension forces within the cervical spine. Although any combination of forces can lead to injury, common examples include impact to the mid- or lower face, causing upper cervical extension/compression, lateral impact creating sudden side bending and rotation, posterior impact causing forced flexion, and vertex or crown impact creating compression. Indirect compression forces can be transferred to the cranium and upper cervical spine from a fall on the pelvis (e.g., falling off of a horse) or unexpectedly stepping into a hole with an extended leg. In blast-induced injuries, there is frequently a trauma component from being thrown into structures or the ground, or being struck by flying objects. Understanding the mechanism of injury may assist in directing assessments and interventions, although mechanism of injury is not a strong factor in prognosis of recovery.[332]

Morphological and functional changes in cervical spine structures have been identified after neck trauma injuries and in response to pain whether from trauma or nontraumatic etiology. These include transition of fiber types from slow fatiguing oxidative type I into fast fatiguing glycolytic type IIB fibers,[333] atrophy and fibrofatty infiltrate into both superficial and deep cervical musculature,[334] and mitochondrial changes. Endurance, strength, and power are adversely affected by any or all of those changes. Loss of muscle spindle density and quality impairs afferent quality and ultimately sensorimotor function. Cortical reorganization of motor strategies to avoid pain, and loss of endurance at low contractile loads is detrimental to cervical stability during prolonged static tasks such as desk work.[323,335] Damage to ligamentous and joint structures potentially causes pain, but also leads to impaired mechanics and deleterious tissue changes over time that compromise structural stability. The faster the intended movement task or pattern, the greater the impact of biomechanical constraints, with a more evident disruption of smooth motor control. Fig. 23.5 shows the interactions between peripheral and central cervical spine motor control.

Cervical Spine Assessment

As part of an overall assessment of the somatosensory system after concussion, the region of the cervical spine should also include temporomandibular, thoracic cage, and shoulder girdle function. Findings upon screening will direct a more detailed assessment. As noted in previous sections, contribution of any individual musculoskeletal finding needs to be considered in the global context of sensory integration and motor control. For the purpose of this chapter, the focus is cervical spine function. A hypothesis-driven approach will help prioritize assessment tool choices and lead to appropriate tailored interventions. Categories of cervical spine assessment are included in Box 23.4.

The interview with the patient should tease out red flag issues (Box 23.3), establish the time from injury, mechanism(s) of injury, nature and behavior of symptoms, status of irritability, and patient report on functional limitations and goals for recovery. The clinical interview is also an important screening tool for comorbid or contributing factors, and an opportunity to obtain information related to prior concussion history and recovery. Psychosocial contributions are particularly important in stratifying risk for chronicity in individuals with concussion and neck pain, particularly WAD.[336,337] Chronic conditions will be characterized by many adaptive—or maladaptive—changes in

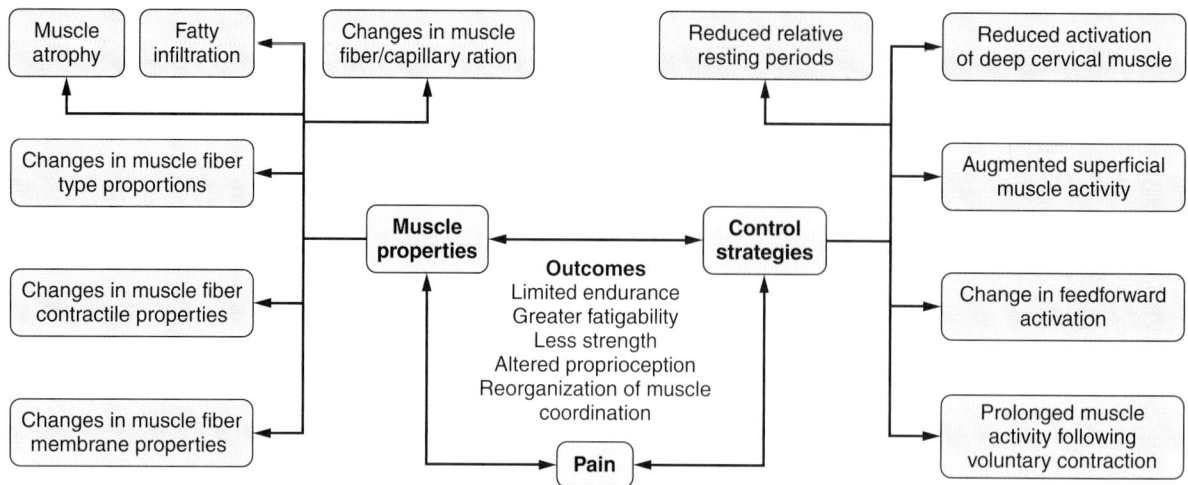

Fig. 23.5 Interrelationships between pain, altered control strategies, and peripheral changes of the cervical muscles. (Reproduced from Jull G, Sterling M, Falla D. *Whiplash, Headache, and Neck Pain.* St Louis: Churchill Livingstone; 2008:51, fig. 4.6.)

BOX 23.3   Red Flags for the Cervical Spine After Acute Concussion and Trauma

- Emergent referral: Risk and symptoms of myocardial infarction (risk factors, chest pain, nonmechanical arm pain, pallor, sweating, dyspnea, nausea, palpitations)
- Emergent referral: signs/symptoms of cervical artery dissection (see below)
- Neurological cord signs or cerebellar signs
- Rheumatoid conditions, heritable disorders of connective tissue (Ehlers-Danlos, Marfan), genetic conditions such as Down syndrome, oral contraceptive use, and pregnancy all are risks for hypermobility and craniocervical ligament injury.
- Congenital anomalies (canal stenosis, Klippel-Feil syndrome, os odontoideum)
- Diabetes mellitus II is a risk factor for delayed healing and excessive stiffness.
- Upper extremity motor or sensory loss (radiculopathy from spine segment disruption)
- Spinal accessory nerve (direct trauma, overstretch, asymmetry of the neckline, inability to shrug shoulders)
- Axillary nerve (>40 years. with shoulder dislocation, traction injury, shoulder abduction and flexion weakness, lack of sensation lateral aspect of upper arm)
- Long thoracic nerve (serratus anterior weakness with scapular winging)
- Endocrine changes—the thyroid may be injured in neck hyperextension.
- Vagus nerve dysfunction—cranial nerve X follows under the sternocleidomastoid muscle and can be overstretched during hyperextension with rotation.

Adapted from Boissonnault WG. *Primary Care for the Physical Therapist* (2nd ed.). St Louis: Elsevier Saunders; 2011:82.

BOX 23.4   Components of a Typical Cervical Spine Assessment

Components of a Typical Cervical Spine Assessment
- Interview: history of presenting complaint/medical history/nature and behavior of pain/pain and disability inventories/systems review/differential diagnosis begins
- Posture
- Active ROM
- Palpation
- Safety tests (ligaments, vertebral artery dependence)
- Spurling compression to rule out radiculopathy
  - If radiculopathy is suspected, neurological examination of the limb including sensation, vibration, reflexes, and strength.
  - If canal stenosis is known or suspected, neurological assessment of lower limbs, including cord signs.
- Passive accessory intervertebral joint motion
- Strength and endurance of neck and shoulder girdle musculature
- Shoulder girdle and thoracic spine screen
- Neural dynamic testing
- Functional assessment of movements or activities of concern to the patient
- Diagnosis, prognosis, plan, education

---

response to the initial injury, healing response, resilience, and contextual factors.[336]

Craniocervical ligament tests. Craniocervical ligament tests for signs of instability have moderate correlation to imaging findings and are more sensitive to degree of motion than imaging. Unfortunately, reliability and validity studies are scarce, and results are variable[338,339]; however, such tests are still recommended to identify patients who are not candidates for end-range subcranial treatments. Craniocervical ligament tests include the Sharp-Purser test for transverse ligament integrity, the alar-odontoid integrity test, and the tectorial membrane distraction test. Table 23.10 provides a summary of cervical spine ligaments and function. For details of strain tests for each ligament, the reader is directed to Aspinall.[340]

Vertebral artery dissection and vertebral basilar insufficiency. Craniocervical ROM is an important factor in treatment of cervicogenic headache (CGH), cervicogenic dizziness (CGD), and head righting responses (HRRs) after concussion. It is imperative that clinicians screen carefully for evidence of compromised vertebral basilar circulation, including history, risk, and symptoms suggesting potential artery dissection (Box 23.5).

The population occurrence of cervical artery dissection is 2.5 per 100,000 for internal carotid dissection, and 1 to 1.5 per 100,000 for vertebral artery dissection (VAD).[341] Cervical artery dissection is a

BOX 23.5 Signs and Symptoms of Vertebral Artery Dissection and Vertebral Basilar Insufficiency

The 5 Ds: dizziness, diplopia, dysarthria, dysphagia, drop attacks
Distress—feeling of impending doom
Nausea/vomiting
Presyncope/lightheadedness
Disorientation or anxiety
Tinnitus
Pallor, tremors, diaphoresis
Unexplained cranial nerve disturbances (facial paresthesia/anesthesia)
New headache and neck pain, unlike any other, moderate to severe
Cerebellar signs (finger to nose incoordination, limb or gait ataxia)
Unilateral limb weakness
Nasal speech pattern
Hiccups

significant cause of stroke in young people (<55 years), representing 20% of strokes affecting young people and 2.5% incidence of all strokes.[342] Traumatic dissection (TD) can be precipitated by head-neck motion, manipulation, violent coughing or sneezing, sudden deceleration, nonpenetrating head-neck injury, or direct arterial injury. Spontaneous dissection (SD) is associated with hereditary disorders of connective tissue (HDCT), such as Ehlers-Danlos or Marfan syndromes, cystic medial necrosis, polycystic kidney disease, osteogenesis imperfecta, and fibromuscular dysplasia.[342] Further risk factors include recent or current bacterial or viral infections, history of another arterial dissection (aortic, renal), or pregnancy.[343] Healthy arteries are not easily disrupted, suggesting that cases of dissection following minor trauma may carry some predisposition to arterial wall weakness. Kumar and colleagues[344] described a 16-year-old male wrestler who was injured in a forced "face plant" during a match. He was confused, slow to rise, and experienced nausea and vomiting in transport to hospital. His Glasgow Coma Scale score was 15 and initial CT scan was negative. He was diagnosed with a concussion but continued to develop neurological signs and experienced seizures. His presentation was misinterpreted, and he was not given anticoagulant therapy before developing a significant cerebellar infarct. The authors recommended that VAD should be suspected in any adolescent with advancing neurological signs, and that the threshold for ordering CTA or MRA should be lowered for males. For a comprehensive review of pathoanatomy, etiology, and current research, the reader is directed to Thomas.[341]

Clinical testing for vertebral basilar insufficiency (VBI) is intended to determine the safety of asking a patient to assume craniovertebral extension or rotation without signs of posterior ischemia. The test is for perfusion adequacy and not intended as a diagnostic test. Although possible, there is insufficient evidence to indicate that posterior circulation will be compromised in these positions; therefore a positive test (symptoms) is sensitive to ischemia, but a negative test does not rule out compromised posterior circulation.[345]

Somatosensory testing. For the assessments of individuals following concussion and neck trauma, the literature recommends several specific additions due to a preponderance of findings in the sensorimotor realm. The recommended order of screening and testing reflects a clearing of one component on to the next, a

reasonable order of physical movement, and an effort to minimize symptom aggravation.

Posture. Observe sitting and standing for comfort, symmetry, unusual alignment (e.g., subluxation of C1 to C2), head position relative to thoracic cage (forward head posture, FHP), and active support verses end-range support (resting in cervical extension to support the head).

Sensation of motion at rest (seated without support, eyes closed). This test assesses whether somatosensory references to stationary firm support surfaces are calibrated to vestibular references without visual inputs. Patients report feeling still or not. Recall that a hallmark of concussion is a global decrement in sensory integration. Observe for sway. CGD symptoms may include lightheadedness, imbalance, vertigo, or the sensation of floating. For a more detailed description, the reader is directed to Chapters 20 and 21.

Active range of motion (standing or seated, caution if patient complains of dizziness). Flexion, extension, side bending, and rotation are assessed overall and can be measured with a Cervical ROM device or inclinometers and compass. Gross restrictions or splinting (e.g., co-contraction that prevents motion) are signs for concern and may precipitate imaging. Note motions that reproduce symptoms—particularly headache or dizziness. Observe for symmetry and smooth execution. Observe for cervical movement progressing into the thoracic cage and screen shoulder girdle motion. Subcranial motion is observed separately, by asking the patient to nod "yes," nod "up," turn "no," and tilt "maybe" with just the face. Individuals with poor motor control, guarding, or restriction will have difficulty with such small localized motions.

Palpation (seated or supine). Examine for tone, guarding, muscle stiffness, edema, effusion of facets or sternoclavicular joints, myofascial trigger points. Palpate for tenderness or reactivity over the greater occipital nerve (GON), lesser occipital nerve (LON), and third occipital nerve (TON), which are also often reactive in CGH. A normal scalp is mobile and nontender, but after impact, or in cases of chronic headache, the scalp may be rigid due to stiffness in the occipitofrontalis or temporalis muscles. Subcranial stiffness and tenderness are common in CGH.

Passive accessory intervertebral motion (seated or supine). Each facet can be tested according to its biomechanical orientation. Normal synovial articulations have passive "give" or accessory motion due to capsular stretching. Range, discomfort, quality, effusion, or any other symptom provocation is recorded.

Of particular interest in patients following concussion are the atlanto-occipital joints (C1 to C2), where 40 to 45 degrees rotation from midline is normal and the concentration of mechanoreceptors is richest.

The cervical flexion rotation test (in supine). The cervical flexion rotation test (CFRT) is a validated method for measuring C1 to C2 rotation.[346] In supine, the head and neck are flexed toward the trunk to stabilize the midcervical joints and the head is rotated on the central axis right and left to end range, if tolerated. Capsular end range in the C1 to C2 articulation is soft and elastic, as the capsule permits so much motion. Less than 30 degrees is considered restricted. The test is not as useful in generally hypermobile people, those with a very thick chest, or when neck extensors are too stiff or painful to achieve sufficient flexion. An alternative is to cup the laminae and spinous process of C2 (using the thumb, webspace, and second and third fingers) to block motion below C1 to C2 and passively rotate the head (C1 turns with the cranium).

Joint position error test (seated, 90 cm from a wall). The joint position sense error test[347,348] (JPE or JPET) assesses the ability to relocate the head to a neutral position with vision occluded, or to relocate the trunk under a stable head to a neutral position.[185] Reacquiring a prescribed position can also be tested. A systematic review by de Vries and colleagues[349] looked at trials using JPE, and considered the possibility of vestibular effect. However, results were no different in patients with vestibular loss, indicating an increased weight on cervical proprioception for head repositioning. Deficits were consistently greater and of significance in subjects with neck pain compared with asymptomatic controls. Instrumented versions of testing are available. In the clinic, a small laser attached to a headband or hat brim suffices for an accurate depiction of head position. An error of 4.5 degrees (7 cm linear measurement) or greater is associated with poor proprioception and occurs more frequently in persons with neck pain of any etiology than in healthy asymptomatic individuals. A convenient calibrated color target is available for clinicians: http://www.skillworks.biz/Resources/Documents/JPE%20Target%20and%20Instructions.pdf. Due to printer differences in sizing, it is not suitable for research.

Hides and colleagues[81] included JPE testing in a preseason screening battery for 190 rugby football athletes to determine risk factors for head or neck injuries during the playing season. Previous SRC, a known risk factor for new concussion, was related to impaired or asymmetrical trunk muscle function and size, but not to vestibular, oculomotor, or cervical proprioceptive measures. Preseason cervical proprioception deficit was an independent risk factor with high specificity and sensitivity. Players who demonstrated 3 or more of 5 identified risk factors, including JPE, were 14 times more likely to have a head/neck injury than players with 2 or less risk factors. The study results were a strong endorsement for including JPE in preseason screening for contact sport athletes.

Kinesthetic sense. The assessment of kinesthetic sense is a variation on the JPE test, with an evaluation of coordination, motion accuracy, and time. The patient is asked to trace a figure or maze on the wall, where accuracy requires the patient to keep a head-mounted laser within 1 cm of the center line. The task can be timed and compared with the patient's future performance. Kristjansson and colleagues[350] demonstrated less accuracy in tracing computer-generated cursor patterns with the head in those with whiplash injuries and nontraumatic neck pain compared with healthy controls, with greater errors recorded in those who also complained of dizziness.

Smooth pursuit neck torsion test (performed seated or standing). The smooth pursuit neck torsion test (SPNT) assesses smooth pursuits while the body is maintained at 45-degrees rotation under a stable head to each side compared with performance in a neutral position.[351] Disturbances in oculomotor control during this test, seen as jerky pursuits or saccadic intrusions, are only seen in patients with complaints of neck pain, not in individuals with general CNS dysfunction or vestibular dysfunction. Therefore a positive test would suggest sensory impairment of afferent input from the cervical spine impacting the motor output of the COR.[352,353] In patients with whiplash injuries, the COR is augmented without the VOR being diminished, which may contribute to the sensory conflict reported as symptoms of dizziness and visual disturbances.[354,355] SPNT has been validated with electrooculography as a clinical method to detect oculomotor dysfunction induced by afferent inputs from rotation in the neck.[356]

Eye-head coordination, changes in neck recruitment and gaze in whiplash-associated disorder. Eye-head control is a complicated interaction among the cervically generated reflexes (CCR, COR), the VOR, optokinetic reflex, cortically generated saccades and pursuits, and cerebellar influences. Gaze stability during head/neck motion is impaired in persons with whiplash injuries, as are sequential coordinated movements of eyes and head, or head and eyes.[357] Patients report dizziness, unsteadiness, trouble reading and driving, with measured loss of visual field, blurry vision, photophobia, and disordered fusion. Treleaven and colleagues measured reduced ROM when turning the head during stable gaze. They also recorded reduced angular velocity of the head when gaze was offset 30 degrees then followed by head position, and subsequently reversed. Without electronic laboratory equipment, the rehabilitation professional can post targets for the patient to acquire visually, and with head position change. A head-mounted laser brings more precision to the task.

As a follow-up to their study of head/neck and eye motion in healthy subjects,[326] Bexander and Hodges recorded significant disruptions in the intricate coordination required for normal eye/head/neck control in subjects with chronic whiplash associated disorders.[358] By tracking muscular activity, eye motion, and slow head movement combinations, they discovered that superficial neck muscles (sternocleidomastoid) co-contract in both rotation directions in pain subjects; deep neck muscles showed a loss of independence from neck movement direction, reducing their fine motor control of segmental movement; and eye motions facilitated neck muscle responses far more than in asymptomatic controls activity. Their findings have implications for neck fatigue, chronic pain, and impaired eye-head/neck coordination. Muscle recruitment with eye motion can be palpated clinically and detected with surface EMG. Abnormal patterns may cause symptoms during rapid eye/head movement tests such as VOR and dynamic gaze stability, and should be screened for in advance.

Head righting response (seated). HHR develops in infancy and is driven by otolith inputs and the tonic labyrinthine reflex, which allows orientation of the head upright relative to gravitational force. The reader is directed to Chapters 2, 20, and 21 for more in-depth information. Although typically measured using the Functional Reach Test, it is the ability to maintain or recover an upright head position during eccentric trunk postures that is of interest. Instrumented measures using motion capture, such as with the PROPRIO Reactive Balance Systems (https://www.perrydynamics.com) can measure, record, and give the clinician visual feedback as to the patient's performance. A qualitative method of assessing HRR using observation is to perturb the seated patient at the shoulders, eyes closed. More challenging is to seat the patient on an unstable surface such as a tilt board or gym ball and observe the ability to maintain an upright head posture when perturbed. The HRR is also tested by observation in narrow based stance, single leg stance, or during gait. Following concussion, individuals have demonstrated increased medial-lateral displacement,[359,360] which may be a manifestation of impaired HRR. Biomechanical constraints in the cervical spine (restrictions, weakness, delayed speed of response, impaired proprioception) may disrupt a normal HRR despite an intact vestibular system. As concussion may cause global sensory system deficits, tests specific to the cervical spine may help elucidate its contributions to impaired head righting. Conversely, vestibular impairment of HRR may increase demand on neck function throughout the day and exacerbate symptoms.

Body rotation under a stable head. Walking and running require tolerance of rhythmic repeated trunk rotation under a head facing forward, as well as small amounts of subcranial side bending and sagittal plane motion described under HRR. When a patient is asked to swivel the body under a stable head, either seated or standing, the vestibular and auditory inputs are challenged to maintain dead-heading (straight on) by rotational torque in the neck. Individuals with increased dependence on neck somatosensation, poor proprioception, abnormal VCR or CCR, or musculoskeletal stiffness will have difficulty, particularly without visual input. The motion may also elicit complaints of dizziness. Although as yet this has not been published as a formal test, visual observation is sufficient to identify a deficit. Using a head-mounted laser aimed at a measured target during repeated body turns provides quantitative measures.

Strength and endurance tests. Strength and endurance at various percentages of maximum voluntary contraction (MVC) have been measured in healthy control and patients with neck pain. Deficits of endurance in the deep cervical flexors have been recorded across the spectrum of MVC in patients with neck pain and dysfunction, of both traumatic and nontraumatic origin.[335] Manual muscle testing can be performed at any level in the cervical spine, for gross or segmental control functions. The craniocervical flexion test (CCFT) captures the neuromotor control strategy of deep cervical flexors to sustain a prescribed level of contraction by flattening the cervical lordosis, measured using an air bladder device.[361] The cervical flexor endurance test (CFET), also referred to as the Head Lift Test, measures the time a subject can support the head in neck flexion one inch from the surface in a supine position.[362] The test ends when the subject is observed to lose chin tuck position and recruits more superficial flexors. Normal mean hold times are 39 seconds for males and 29 seconds for females. Neck extensor endurance is also reduced in adults and adolescents with neck pain of a variety of etiologies.[363] Tested in prone, a strap is used to stabilize the thoracic spine at T6. The head is supported off the table surface in a neutral position of the subcranial region and cervicothoracic junction. Unsupported hold is timed until the posture changes notably or the head drops more than 5 degrees. Adding a 2 kg weight suspended from the head by a wide strap reduces the hold time and is equally valid.[364]

Balance and gait. Tests of balance and gait represent multisensory system integration. Recommended assessments are described elsewhere in this chapter. It is important to observe all performance tests for neck guarding, changes in head-neck posture, and increased headache symptoms. Numerous authors have established gait parameter deficits in neck pain patients. Uthaikhup and colleagues demonstrated that patients with chronic neck pain produced shorter step lengths, slower gait speed with head pitches and turns, and slower "fast walk," which correlated to higher pain and perceived disability scores. In a cohort of older adults, after considering visual, vestibular, activity, lower extremity function, and health influences, Quek and colleagues ruled out all but neck pain and its detrimental influences on proprioception for gait disturbances and a twofold increased fall risk.[365]

By using pupillometry, Kahya and colleagues[366] demonstrated greater cognitive load during vision-occluded postural stability tests in normal healthy young adults. Although not yet tested in injured persons, the increased cognitive demand should be considered when testing acutely concussed individuals, as cerebral blood flow is reduced for 7 to 10 days.

Cervicogenic Dizziness

As a clinical diagnosis of exclusion, there is no single clinical test that identifies a patient's complaints of dizziness as generating from cervical structures. However, the collection of tests provided can implicate cervical contributions. A hypothesis-driven impairment-directed approach will lead the clinician to plan and prioritize patient education and intervention. As discussed earlier, concussion injuries impute global sensory system integration deficits, making specific identification much more difficult. A sensation of spinning in the head suggests a high cervical spine dysfunction. Dizziness or disequilibrium with trunk movements under a stable head, and oculomotor disturbances with neck torsion (SPNT), strongly suggest disturbed cervical afferents. Proprioceptive impairment (JPE) is consistently worse in neck-injury patients who complain of dizziness. Postural instability and gait disturbances may involve all subsystems, but specific testing may elucidate a particular contributor while ruling out others.

Cervicogenic Headache

The possible neural mechanisms for head pain that is generated by cervical structures are discussed above. It is important to differentiate cervical involvement, as CGH responds well to physical therapy intervention and contributes to multiple maladapted pain and motor behaviors when unresolved. Typical findings that alert the rehabilitation professional to primary cervical causes of head pain include unilateral pain, often episodic, worse with fatigue, which may be aggravated by neck motion; tender and tight suboccipital myofascial; trigger points referring to the head or face; restricted C1 to C2 rotation; sensitivity or tenderness over the GON, TON, or LON; JPE of 4.5 degrees or greater; strength and endurance deficits in deep cervical musculature; guarded neck behavior during activities that require head righting or rapid repeated motion; and reduced neck rotation range when stable gaze is required.[367]

Prognosis in Cervical Spine Dysfunction following Concussion

Stratifying persons by risk factors for protracted recovery can help identify those who may need more focused early intervention, as well as those who clearly will need multidisciplinary care. The statistics for chronic pain and disability in the WAD population have remained at 50% for the past 30 years of data collection, and the risk of PPCS has also been stable at up to 20%. This occurs despite research that recommends successful interventions. The heterogeneity of concussion and neck trauma injuries has not traditionally been captured, particularly in systematic reviews. The most frequently used outcome measures are pain and self-perceived disability, which may not represent meaningful participation in life. Newer studies featuring tailored interventions to identified problems, particularly considering sensorimotor function and sensory integration, demonstrate positive changes.

Risk factors associated with delayed recovery following WAD are described in Table 23.11.[337] Characteristics reported not to be useful for establishing prognosis include angular deformity of the neck (flattened lordosis or scoliosis), impact direction, seating position in the vehicle, awareness of impending collision, presence of a headrest, stationary or moving when hit, and older age.[368]

Not factored into the prognosis analyses, but potentially impactful, are conditions such as rheumatoid conditions (RA, ankylosing spondylitis, psoriatic arthritis), other autoimmune disorders, fibromyalgia, chronic fatigue syndrome, endocrine disorders, or autonomic dysfunctions, including POTS. Inflammatory markers are only recently being explored in concussion and are potentially significant for neck trauma injuries as well.

Mood and Psychological Disorders

A small but important proportion of patients present with mood or psychological disorders including anxiety, depression, and posttraumatic stress following a concussion. Importantly, a premorbid mood disorder diagnosis or the development of a mood disorder, such as

TABLE 23.11   Risk Factors Associated With Delayed Recovery Following Whiplash Injury

Construct	Recommended Tool	Useful Cut Score for Prognosis
High pain intensity	Numeric rating scale (0–10)	6 or greater
High self-reported disability	Neck Disability Index, original or shorter adaptations	>30%
High pain catastrophizing	Pain Catastrophizing Scale	20 or greater
High acute posttraumatic stress	Impact of Events Scale-Revised; here this scale is used to predict symptom chronicity, not to assess for posttraumatic stress disorder.	33 or greater
Cold hyperalgesia	Gold standard is the TSA-II NeuroSensory Analyzer (Medoc Ltd., Ramat Yishai, Israel), though cost may render it impractical for clinicians. Alternatives include the cold pressor task as a test of cold endurance (similar but not identical to cold pain threshold), use of an ice cube, or use of cold metal bars.	

Adapted from Table 6, Neck Pain Guidelines, Revised 2017.[337]

depression, following a concussion is a strong predictor of PPCS.[3,6,130,369,370] Considering long-term consequences of psychological disorders, specifically for athletes experiencing an SRC, a strong association has been reported between individuals with multiple concussions and affective disorders, particularly the development of depression.[121] Sandel and colleagues have described a pattern of symptoms and deficits that develop in some athletes, who may be classified by an anxiety and mood clinical profile where mental health or emotional disturbances become the primary concern for medical and rehabilitative management following concussion.[370] Sandel and colleagues[370] suggested that the anxiety and mood clinical profile is characterized by emotional disturbance such as experiencing anxiety, feelings of depression, apathy, hypervigilance of somatic complaints, panic, and/or sleep disturbances.

It is likely that a combination of physiological, psychosocial, and cultural factors may underlie the development of mood disorders following concussion. Preinjury risk factors such as personal or familial mental health history, female sex, and neurophysiological alterations, specifically in the emotional centers of the brain, may lead to changes in emotional responses of patients following concussion.[370] As mentioned earlier in the chapter, prior history of emotional instability,[370] a poor coping approach to lifestyle changes following injury,[129,130,370] and/or misguided clinical management such as prescribing unnecessarily long withdrawal from activities (physical, school-, or work-related) may exacerbate postconcussion symptoms, particularly anxiety or depression, and lead to prolonged recovery.[67,129,130] It is important to emphasize this latter point for adolescents following SRC as student-athletes who are removed from social, educational, and sporting activities for prolonged periods of time might develop, or cause an exacerbation of previous psychological problems, which can in turn disrupt social, recreational, and academic functioning, generating a vicious cycle leading to social and functional impairments.[67,130] It is well documented that diagnosed psychological distress or depressive disorders can impact cognitive function, even in patients who merely endorse symptoms of depression.[369]

For the assessment of mood and psychological disorders, a detailed history of previous psychological disorders, history of prior concussion(s), and response/recovery from previous concussion(s) are important to obtain, as each has been shown to increase the risk for development of emotional disturbance following concussion and contribute to prolonged recovery.[67] Medical professionals should document family history of mental health disorders (e.g., anxiety, major depressive disorder, posttraumatic stress, psychiatric disorders) and monitor current symptoms of emotional disturbance using general questions such as "Do your thoughts race when trying to sleep?,"[370] or "Are headaches brought on by stress?,"[370] or validated self-report

questionnaires, such as the Beck Depression Inventory II[371] or Beck Anxiety Inventory.[372] Medical professionals must acknowledge that elevated values on self-report questionnaires alone are not sufficient to diagnose patients with mood or psychological disorders. Symptoms caused by impairment of other functional symptoms may mimic or overlap with symptoms suggestive of emotional disturbances following concussion.[67,130,370] For example, sadness, excessive sleep, and fatigue may be clinical manifestations of chronic pain or injury to the cervical spine rather than symptoms of depression, just as endorsement of irritability, nervousness, and being more emotion may be related to impairment of the vestibular system rather than anxiety. Thus a detailed interview by a neuropsychologist or clinical psychologist with experience managing patients with brain injury may be required.

For the treatment of mood and psychological disorders following concussion, behavioral therapies, such as cognitive behavioral therapy, are recommended as an overall first-line treatment for anxiety and depression.[67,373] If emotional disturbances persist under conservative treatment, pharmacological therapies in conjunction with behavioral therapies are recommended.[67,370] Table 23.5 describes commonly prescribed pharmacological agents used to address mood and psychological disorders following concussion.

Headaches
Posttraumatic Headache

As previously mentioned, headache is the most common symptom reported after concussion injury and is referred to as posttraumatic headache (PTH) when there is a known traumatic event. The 3rd edition of the International Classification of Headache Disorders (ICHD-3) contains updated diagnostic criteria for primary and secondary headaches, as well as cranial neuralgias, facial pain, and other headaches.[374] PTH following mTBI is classified as a secondary headache attributed to trauma or injury to the head and/or neck,[374] as shown in Fig. 23.6. The diagnostic criteria require a 7-day temporal relationship between the date of injury and onset of headache symptoms. Secondary headaches attributed to trauma or injury to the head and neck are further differentiated into acute headaches lasting less than 3 months or persistent headaches lasting for more than 3 months from the date of onset of either a concussion or whiplash related injury. In some cases, where there is no known date of a traumatic event, but rather a potential for repeated minor events, the diagnosis is less precise. However, the diagnostic criteria for PTH is the same for children and adults.

The incidence of headache following head and neck injury has been reported in a variety of populations, typically investigated quarterly through the first year from the date of injury. In a retrospective study

5. Headache attributed to trauma or injury to the head and/or neck

5.1 Acute headache attributed to traumatic injury to the head
    5.1.1 Acute headache attributed to moderate or severe traumatic injury to the head
    5.1.2 Acute headache attributed to mild traumatic injury to the head
5.2 Persistent headache attributed to traumatic injury to the head
    5.2.1 Persistent headache attributed to moderate or severe traumatic injury to the head
    5.2.2 Persistent headache attributed to mild traumatic injury to the head
5.3 Acute headache attributed to whiplash
5.4 Persistent headache attributed to whiplash
5.5 Acute headache attributed to craniotomy
5.6 Persistent headache attributed to craniotomy

General comment

Primary or secondary headache or both? The general rules for attribution to another disorder apply to 5. *Headache attributed to trauma or injury to the head and/or neck.*

1. When a *new headache* occurs for the first time in close temporal relation to trauma or injury to the head and/or neck, it is coded as a secondary headache attributed to the trauma or injury. This remains true when the new headache has the characteristics of any of the primary headache disorders classified in Part One of ICHD-3.

2. When a *preexisting headache* with the characteristics of a primary headache disorder becomes *chronic* or is made *significantly worse* (usually meaning a two-fold or greater increase in frequency and/or severity) in close temporal relation to such trauma or injury, both the initial headache diagnosis and a diagnosis of 5. *Headache attributed to trauma or injury to the head and/or neck* (or one of its types or subtypes) should be given, provided that there is good evidence that the disorder can cause headache.

Fig. 23.6 Diagnostic Criteria for Posttraumatic Headache. From Headache Classification Committee of the International Headache Society (IHS) The International Classification of Headache Disorders, 3rd edition Cephalalgia 2018, Vol. 38(1) 1–211. DOI: 10.1177/0333102417738202

of 1953 pediatric patients aged 10 to 19 years who attended a hospital-based sports medicine clinic, headache was the most frequently identified symptom in 69.4% of participants following concussion.[375] At a medical university-based concussion clinic, 72% of 254 patients who were seen for concussion had PTH that was significantly related to symptoms severity scoring, which was reported using the SCAT3 even in those with non-SRC injuries.[376] In a population of active duty service members with PTH, who were evaluated retrospectively by a headache specialist postconcussion, more than 50% described more than one headache variant. Seventy-four percent of service members reported a continuous headache, which increased the odds of a medical discharge/retirement by 3.98 (95% Wald confidence interval 1.05 to 15.07).[377] There is some evidence that genetic predisposition may play a role in PTH, as athletes who carry the apolipoprotein (APOE) e4 allele are more likely to report headaches and have headaches of increased severity compared with those who do not carry the allele.[378]

The clinical manifestation of secondary headaches in PTH is most consistent with the presentation of primary headaches in the following frequency of occurrence: migraine, probable migraine, tension-type (TTH), and CGH. A prospective study of 212 adults in a level 1 trauma center following mTBI were evaluated for headache without inclusion of ICHD-3 classification available at the time, but instead assessed

headaches as primary migraine, TTH, cervicogenic, or another headache type.[379] Through the full year postinjury, 54% of subjects were found have new or worsened preinjury headache. For those who had headaches throughout the year, 49% were consistent with migraine or probable migraine, while 40% of people with headaches at 6 months presented with TTH profiles. In the case of head and neck trauma, the migraine and TTH are not considered primary because they are precipitated by a traumatic event within a 7-day window, but the clinical presentation and management is similar to that of primary headache and the classification criteria can be utilized to assess the headache behavior. Extensive details regarding headache pathology and implications for physical therapy can be found in Goodman and Fuller; the following sections provide an overview of headache topics specific to and commonly encountered during concussion recovery.[380]

Posttraumatic Migraine

PTM is a common headache type observed after concussion as reported in youth sports and recreation, high school, collegiate, and professional sports, and service member populations.[375,381,382] A familial history of migraine in a first degree relative has been found to increase the likelihood of having PTM in the first 2 weeks postconcussion by 2.6 times compared with those without a family history of migraine.[383] The presence of PTM is recognized as a poor prognostic factor in concussion recovery, as those with PTM have been shown to be seven times more likely to have prolonged recovery.[384] A preliminary study used brain network activation (BNA) to record electroencephalography (EEG) activity, which is known to detect the neurometabolic cascade of events that results in ionic changes following concussion, and evoked response potentials (ERP) during neurocognitive tasks in individuals postconcussion with and without PTM versus noninjured controls.[385] The results of this SRC study indicate there may be a future role for BNA analysis to investigate neurocognitive, vestibular, and oculomotor pathway involvement with PTM, and potentially to compare data pre- and postinjury in athletes.

Migraine headaches can occur with or without aura, and especially in children, migraine aura can occur without headache. The diagnostic criteria for different patterns of migraine headache are described in detail in the ICHD-3.[374] There are some important pediatric diagnoses to recognize as potential migraine precursors or variants, especially related to vestibular migraine (VM). Benign paroxysmal vertigo of childhood (BPVC) presents as spontaneous episodic vertigo or imbalance lasting seconds to minutes.[386] Children as young as 3 years of age diagnosed with BPVC were followed over a 15-year span into adulthood; 33% of those with PBVC developed migraine in young adulthood, which is nearly double the prevalence in the general population.[387] Benign paroxysmal torticollis of infancy (BPTI) is another vestibular disorder that can result in sudden onset head tilting, ataxia, dizziness, and signs of autonomic dysregulation.[388] BPTI has been associated with acquisition of BPVC in some children, and both disorders show an increased risk of developing VM through adolescence. Finally, abdominal migraine presents as recurrent periumbilical pain and discomfort, often in the absence of headache that lasts hours to days and significantly restricts participation in daily activities with overlay of dysautonomia symptoms such as nausea and pallor. Onset of abdominal migraine typically occurs between 3 and 10 years of age and is a poor prognostic indicator for the development of migraines later in life.[389,390]

Family history and developmental history are thus an important aspect of the patient interview after head and neck injuries that result in headache and dizziness. The use of a migraine diary or facilitated interview, as found in digital applications such as My Migraine Triggers, can be useful tools to track details of events and associated symptoms. Educating individuals to collect and present subjective and objective event data to medical providers can facilitate diagnosis of migraine headache, particularly when symptoms of dizziness, vertigo, and instability do not match other vestibular disorders and there is a known risk of head or neck injury. Common reported triggers for migraine headache may include stress, altered sleep, food exposures, dehydration, weather changes, hormone cycles, light, smoke or scented products/perfumes, exercise/exertion, or sexual activity.[391] Preexisting migraine history should be differentiated from altered migraine patterns that may occur following a novel injury.

Physical therapy following concussion involves complex sensory-motor processing of vestibular, oculomotor, cervical, and somatosensory neural pathways. Challenging any of these systems during an active migrainous event is counterproductive to therapeutic interventions aimed at neuroplasticity, habituation, and adaptation for recovery. The role of physical therapy in PTM involves recognition of migraine activity, referral for medical consultation if not already in place, and patient education to reduce any ongoing stimulating triggers that promote hyperexcitability and symptom burden. Efficacy of physical therapy assessment management of headache, dizziness, pain, and other symptoms between migraines is an area of ongoing investigation.[392]

Recognition of VM is of particular importance, due to the high incidence of both headache and dizziness following concussion.[158] Diagnostic criteria for VM has been developed from original studies that have resulted in a consensus between the International Headache Society and the International Bárány Society for Neurootology for the ICHD-3.[374,393–395] A person must have five episodes of vestibular symptoms lasting 5 to 72 hours with at least one of the following: headache (two of the four criteria: unilateral, pulsing, moderate to severe, aggravated by physical activity), photo and phonophobia, or visual aura. Much effort has been focused on use of imaging techniques to study the cortical and subcortical vestibular pathway activation during vestibular stimulation and as a diagnostic tool for vestibular dysfunction.[291,392,396] One particular study of individuals with VM found alterations in mediodorsal thalamic activation, correlated with the frequency of VM, compared with those with migraine without aura or healthy controls.[397] Future studies in advanced neuroimaging may help explain the role of vestibular and thalamic activation in the perception of pain and hypersensitivity patterns, such as motion perception, photophobia, and phonophobia. Successful medical management of VM requires proper recognition of symptoms to support effective use of prophylactic and/or abortive agents in both pediatric and adult populations.[398,399]

Tension-Type Headache

Tension-type headache (TTH) is another presentation of PTH found to occur after concussion and whiplash-associated disorders. According to the ICHD-3 diagnostic criteria, TTH can be differentiated into infrequent episodic, frequent episodic, or chronic based on the frequency of occurrence and duration of the headaches. All forms of TTH may or may not be associated with pericranial tenderness.[374] Primary TTH is described as bilateral pain and discomfort with a pressing or tightening sensation that is not exacerbated by physical activity or exertion, and most often does not include phonophobia or photophobia, nausea, or vomiting. While there is no current diagnostic test to differentially diagnose migraine and TTH, some imaging techniques show promising developments. An MRI and voxel-based morphometry (VBM) study of individuals diagnosed with episodic or chronic migraine or TTH were compared with health controls.[400] Reduction in gray matter volume found in the superior frontal gyrus and cerebellar regions appeared consistent with reduction in cognitive processing and in heightened pain due to reduced cerebellar inhibition of the trigeminal neuron activation in migraine compared with

TTH.[400] Further, changes in gray matter volume were found to have potential utility differentiating between headache types in veterans.[400]

A palpation examination and referred pain patterns may be hallmark clinical signs differentiating TTH from migraine activity, and headache diaries can be extremely helpful in deciphering symptom patterns. Patient questionnaires such as the Headache Disability Index (HDI), Headache Impact Test (HIT-6), and the Migraine Disability Index Assessment (MIDAS) are highly recommended to measure headache severity and to monitor change over time. The beginnings of a clinical prediction rule have been presented to differentiate between frequent episodic and chronic TTH through a correlation between pressure pain threshold testing and four strict criteria related to frequency and duration of headache, and bodily pain and vitality scores on the SF-36.[401] Subjects with less frequent and lower intensity headaches who met the prediction rule classification demonstrated generalized hyperalgesia and central sensitization with higher impact on quality of life, which may become a risk factor for development of chronic TTH and perhaps other generalized pain syndromes such as fibromyalgia.

Headache Attributed to Whiplash

Headache attributed to whiplash injury is classified as acute until persistence beyond 3 months from the date of injury, at which time it is deemed chronic.[374] This form of PTH is associated with a known whiplash associated injury that could include a concussive event. Whiplash injury is described as an unexpected acceleration/deceleration force of the head causing rapid flexion/extension of the neck at high or low speed. Keep in mind that few injuries occur in a pure head-on or rear-end fashion, in which case some rotational forces are present, causing diffuse axonal and diffuse vascular injuries to the brain and brain stem. Similar to other forms of PTH, the headache onset following whiplash injury must occur within 7 days of injury, and management follows that of other PTH headaches that mimic migraine, TTHs, or CGH if there has been injury to the cervical spine or soft tissues.

Cervicogenic Headache

By definition, a diagnosis of CGH can only be made if clinical or imaging evidence exists of a disorder or lesion related to the cervical spine or soft tissues that is known to cause headache.[374] Further diagnostic criteria from the ICHD-3 include all of the following: a temporal relationship between the cervical spine dysfunction and onset of headache pain, reduction of the headache in response to improvement in the cervical spine pathology, cervical ROM reduction causing headache exacerbation when provoked, and full resolution of headache with diagnostic blockage or a cervical structure or its nerve supply. See previous sections for a more detailed discussion of the diagnosis and management of cervical spine pathology.

Headache, Intracranial Hypotension, and Cerebral Spinal Fluid Leaks

There is an increasing awareness of headache associated with changes in cerebrospinal fluid (CSF) pressure after traumatic injury to the head and neck. However, the evidence for clear diagnostic workup of CSF leakage is limited in the published literature, and the diagnostic classification is restricted to headache related to low CSF pressure due to CSF fistula or spontaneous intracranial hypotension.[374] In individuals recovering from concussion and whiplash injuries, there is evidence that hereditary connective tissue disorders are a risk factor for CSF leak in the presence or absence of headache. Patients should therefore be screened for signs of hypermobility spectrum disorders, including Marfan's syndrome and Ehlers-Danlos syndrome.[402] The presence of headache or neurological symptoms, particularly with orthostatic positional changes, should be cause for referral for potential neuroimaging,[403] as altered CSF volume can occur in both the brain and spinal cord as a result of CSF leakage.[404]

Sleep Disturbances

Sleep is a critical function of human behavior; recent evidence support that sleep contributes to restoration of mental functions,[405] including learning and memory consolidation. Perhaps most importantly for rehabilitation following brain injury, sleep quantity and quality has been shown to be important for neural growth and plasticity,[406] and recent animal studies suggest sleep may even provide a neuroprotective role[407] in the presence of disease and injury to the nervous system.

Disrupted sleep is one of the most common complaints of patients who have experienced an mTBI. Interestingly, studies indicate greater subjective complaints and objective impairment in sleep experienced by patients with mTBI, compared with those with moderate and severe brain injury.[405,408,409] Following mTBI, sleep disturbances can persist for months following injury and may be the cause of, or lead to an exacerbation of, common postconcussion symptoms such as anxiety, headaches, fatigue, and irritability.[67,405,410] Further, sleep disturbances can cause impairments in cognitive function and physical performance, lead to diminished health-related quality of life, and are predictive of a prolonged recovery.[405,410,411] For these reasons, sleep disturbances should be an important consideration in the management of patients following mTBI.

The most common sleep disturbances that occur following mTBI include insomnia (difficulty falling asleep or staying asleep), hypersomnolence (daytime sleepiness), and circadian rhythm disorders (abnormalities of the timing of sleep).[67,405] Conservative management begins with emphasis on sleep hygiene, including regular bedtime and wake time, avoiding stimulants (e.g., caffeine) and heavy exercise late in the day, limiting technology use before bed, and avoiding spending time in bed awake.[412] However, in most cases, education for sleep hygiene will be insufficient, and a combination of rehabilitative strategies such as cognitive behavioral therapy and pharmacological agents are required for successful management of disrupted sleep in individuals following mTBI.[67] Table 23.5 describes commonly prescribed pharmacological agents used to address sleep disturbances. In general, there is limited evidence regarding medications to address sleep disorders in mTBI,[67] and the use of medications (over-the-counter and prescription) follow similar indications for patients with sleep disorders without brain injury, which include selective serotonin reuptake inhibitors (SSRIs), melatonin, and tricyclic antidepressants (TCAs) for insomnia, nonbenzodiazepine hypnotics or other neurostimulants to address hypersomnolence, and melatonin or regulated exposure to daylight/night (e.g., phototherapy) can be used in cases of circadian rhythm dysfunction.[67,405]

A critical component of the assessment related to a patient who endorses sleep disturbances following mTBI is consideration of other comorbid factors such as pain, psychiatric disorders (e.g., anxiety and depression), history of headaches, or fatigue. As mentioned previously, each of these disorders can be the cause of, or can be exacerbated in the presence of, sleep disturbance[405] and must be identified as a possible confounding factor leading to disrupted sleep. In addition, medical professionals should obtain information related to sleep history and current sleep patterns using self-report questionnaires that have been validated to assess sleep in patients with TBI, such as the Pittsburgh Sleep Quality Index[413] or the Epworth Sleepiness Scale.[414] The Pittsburgh Sleep Quality Index is composed of nine questions related to quality and patterns of sleep during the previous month. A cutoff score

of 8 has been established to identify patients with clinically significant insomnia following mTBI.[415] It is important that medical professionals consider that, similar to self-report measures of postconcussion symptoms, symptom complaint does not correspond well with objective sleep impairment. Several reports suggest an overestimation of sleep disruption on self-report measures of disrupted sleep in patients following mTBI.[416] Therefore in the presence of continued sleep disturbances, it is important that medical professionals consider referral to sleep specialists who have access to advanced clinical equipment to measure sleep, such as actigraphy and/or polysomnography, to better guide treatment approaches to address the underlying factors.

INTERVENTION

Education

The importance of education in providing care to individuals following a concussion cannot be emphasized enough. Education related to the patient's *current condition*, as well as discussing *expectations* about the patient's potential course of recovery, should not be overlooked by medical professionals, including the rehabilitation specialist. This aspect of care is critical for the individual at the time of injury, the patient who is in the acute stages of recovery following a concussion, and the patient who presents to the clinic with PPCS. Marshall and colleagues[5] published an updated clinical practice guideline in 2015 for concussion and persistent symptoms following concussion, as a synthesis of existing guidelines. The following recommendations related to education are supported by evidence of at least one randomized controlled trial, meta-analysis, or systematic review:

- Patients should be advised that they are likely to experience one or more symptoms as a consequence of the concussion/mTBI that may persist for a short period of time and that this is usually expected (normal course).[417]
- The patient should be advised that a full recovery of symptoms is seen in the majority of cases.[417]
- Education should be provided in printed material and combined with verbal review and consists of:
  - Symptoms and expected outcomes
  - Normalizing symptoms (education that current symptoms are expected and common after injury event)
  - Reassurance about expected positive recovery
  - Gradual return to activities and life roles
  - Techniques to manage stress

Active Training Intervention

Taken together, the findings from recent research indicate that active rehabilitation programs should be considered for management of individuals with concussion and PPCS. Across patient populations, the introduction of activity after concussion is potentially beneficial.[128,131,304,418]

A variety of treatment approaches have been described to assist the rehabilitation specialist in decision making to develop a training program, which includes models that use a classification system that match patients to a specific clinical profile,[115,381] an approach based on stage of recovery with a variation on international consensus for return to activity,[17,69] and a cognitive-behavioral approach with emphasis on self-efficacy and self-management in combination with active rehabilitation training designed for children and adolescents with PPCS.[70]

Given the subjective nature of a concussion diagnosis and the range of clinical signs and symptoms that can result after a concussion, there is consensus that rehabilitation strategies should be based on a targeted approach that matches interventions to a specific clinical profile.[14,115,419] Further, international consensus guidelines advocate for a multifaceted clinical approach for the assessment and treatment of concussion, which may include training of the cardiopulmonary and cardiovascular system, the vestibular and oculomotor system, and the musculoskeletal and sensorimotor systems of the cervical spine.[6,58,115,181,189,304] An example of such an approach has been proposed by Ellis and colleagues,[115] where results of an examination can lead the rehabilitation specialist to categorize a patient's presenting signs and symptoms into three clinical syndromes, defined as postconcussion disorders (PCD)—physiological PCD, vestibulo-ocular PCD, or cervicogenic PCD—which in turn provides targeted options for intervention.

It is important to consider that the current consensus of using a multifaceted approach has not yet been validated. Therefore despite these published models, there is little information to help guide clinicians on how to optimally match patients to specific interventions or in what order to address impairments, should the patient present with multiple needs.[181] Future research is needed to evaluate the efficacy and effectiveness of single as well as multidimensional active training programs, including cognitive/cognitive-behavioral, aerobic, cervical, vestibulo-ocular, vision, and postural control interventions for individuals following concussion.[181,420] Ultimately, a greater understanding of the optimal treatments, with consideration for the timing, dosage, and effects of multiple treatments, will inform best practice and potentially minimize health-related disability following concussion.[5,181]

The pharmacological therapies available for patients following concussion have already been discussed earlier in this chapter. For this reason, the reader is presented with evidence supporting the use of active rehabilitation strategies for individuals with slow recovery or PPCS following injury, which include cognitive rehabilitation, aerobic exercise, vestibular rehabilitation, vision therapy, management of cervical spine dysfunction, and multidisciplinary care.

Cognitive Rehabilitation

Cognitive rehabilitation is evidenced-based practice for the treatment of multiple neurological disorders, including TBI, right hemisphere CVA, neoplasms, and Parkinson disease.[421] Due to the heterogenic nature of TBI injuries, it is often difficult to initially assign a descriptor such as *mild* or *severe*: some of the most devastating injuries can present with mild deficits, while some of the most mildly appearing injuries can result in severe deficits). This is due to the fact that there are multiple variables affecting the injury: speed of impact, type of impact, premorbid functional levels, age, gender, drug or alcohol history, and prior injuries. Therefore though a person can be diagnosed with a concussion or a complex mild TBI versus a TBI, it is really a continuum, due to this injury heterogeneity. For the SLP, PPCS is not a different category of deficits, but rather on one side of the continuum of TBI, and as such, the treatment naturally connects to the evidence-based practice used in TBI cognitive rehabilitation. Notably, though there has been a paucity of research in PPCS cognitive rehabilitation, recent research has been robust in evaluating the outcome of cognitive rehabilitation for PPCS.[422]

The constellation of the cognitive-communication deficits reported by those with PPCS are similar to those with more severe injuries, although typically the PPCS patient is higher functioning and able to maintain independence (but may need support in some areas). As stated earlier, some tests or batteries may not identify the specific higher level cognitive-communication deficits.[259] This is consistent with rehabilitation efforts in this area, as well. Furthermore, as with assessment, rehabilitation therapy must be functional and ecologically valid for the PPCS patient's life and goals.

Results from assessment directly relate to development of therapy goals in all rehabilitation therapies. All cognitive-communication intervention/therapy is completed in a hierarchical approach, with cueing as needed, and with gradual fading or removal of cues.[423] Furthermore, in order to maximize outcomes, evidence-based practice recommendations include not only restorative practice (i.e., cognitive stimulation, practice in isolation), but also training on compensatory strategies, and practice in context or real-world situations.[424] A more recent approach in this area is the addition of Goal-Attainment Scaling (GAS).[425] This involves the patient and the therapist developing goals that relate specifically to the patient's life. A rating scale defines each level, with the patient describing and naming each level of the scale, and then as they move through therapy, the patient identifies where they are on the scale. This can be a very powerful tool, and a functional real-life connection of cognitive-communication skills and how we use them in life.

Cognitive-communication rehabilitation for PPCS generally addresses attention, memory, executive functions, social language/pragmatics, and word retrieval. Due to the heterogeneity of this population overall, it is possible that other specific deficits will be identified in assessment such as stuttering/dysfluency or writing; however, these are the primary areas that will be addressed in this chapter in relation to intervention.

Attention Training

Attention training can be completed for all domains of attention. Several programs have been developed to address sustained, selective, alternating, and divided attention, with one specifically for the mild TBI/concussion patient.[426] The starting point is identified through assessment results. Therapy usually involves starting where the patient is able to participate, and then gradually increasing in complexity, speed, and distractions. One example for divided attention from the APT program involves listening for two numbers presented slowly in an auditory list, while also crossing out numbers on a visual task.[427] Should the patient be able to complete at an 80% to 90% accuracy level, the next step will potentially be a list read more quickly, or more auditory or visual targets. An example of a selective attention task, without using a prepackaged therapy program, would be having the patient complete a checkbook balancing worksheet while an environmental noise tape or a TV program is on. Compensatory strategies may be identified, trained, practiced, and utilized, and ultimately gradually removed or diminished in usage (i.e., noise-cancelling headphones to complete sustained attention tasks, taking breaks frequently during tasks, working on one task at a time). The final goal for this therapy would be the patient being able to attend to tasks in their daily life with noise and distractions, as they were able to premorbidly.

Memory

Memory therapy for immediate, delayed, working memory similarly is based on the same hierarchical and cueing principles. Restorative practice and stimulation is also primary, as well as training on compensatory strategies, practicing use, and gradually incorporating them into real-life tasks.[428] Internal compensatory strategies may include visualization, repeating or reauditorization, association, mnemonics, and note-taking.[429] External strategies or aids may include smartphones, timers, visual schedules, dayplanners, and keeping items in the same location.[430] An example of a therapy activity for immediate memory could be listening to a factual paragraph, and the patient using strategies such as visualization, reauditorization, and association, then repeating or summarizing main points. The same task could be part of a delayed memory task with a timer set for a 20-minute delay, where the patient recalls the details or is asked detail questions. Cueing to support can also be involved. Prospective memory tasks can include scheduling tasks in the future, using compensatory strategies. This could start at minimal amounts of time up to future appointments, days and weeks ahead. Sohlberg and colleagues developed and evaluated the Prospective Memory Screening and Prospective Memory Training program, and this is one example of a program available in a hierarchical approach.[431]

Executive Functions

The ability to plan, organize, solve problems, be flexible in thought and generate multiple solutions, and reason through possible solutions are all used in daily life.[432] The best example in real life is creating and planning out chores with multiple units of information. (For example, say you need to go to the bank to get rolls of change for laundry, but they are only open until 4:00, and you do not get out of class until 4:30. And you need to get your laundry done by tonight since you need to have that shirt ready for your presentation in class in the morning. How are you going to get this done?) Executive functions also involve awareness of self, adjusting our behaviors to settings, and being able to see others' perspectives. Therapy for these behaviors and abilities can be more concrete for things like problem solving, or more abstract, as with role playing for awareness and perspective practice.[433] Compensatory strategy training can also be part of this hierarchy: taking notes, extra time, and breaking tasks down are just a few examples. Feedback from the therapist is also a powerful tool. An example of problem-solving/reasoning/planning could be the patient given and using a map, determining a route based on a few targeted stops. The next step in the hierarchy could be having the patient identify their daily chores from their life or home, and planning out the schedule and the tasks in the most appropriate order. Examples of perspective taking and awareness therapy activities could include role-playing, with videotaping of facial expressions, body language, and interactions, followed by guided review and feedback. A next step in this hierarchy could be a structured interaction with a planned script with another individual or the therapist, with videotaping and guided review and feedback. Much of this therapy is guided by identified deficits from assessment, as well as input from the family about premorbid executive function abilities, in addition to knowledge about cultural and personal strengths and weaknesses before the injury.

Word Retrieval

Word retrieval intervention involves stimulating the ability to generate specific words and training in the use of compensatory strategies. The inconsistency of word retrieval issues is very frustrating for the patient. Therapy can involve the production of specific words for description or in response to a question. This can be simple to complex in nature, and therapy is also hierarchical. For the PPCS patient, therapy usually focuses on this therapy process with the compensatory strategy training at the same time.[434] Strategies can include describing the word or concept (e.g., target word is *roller coaster*, and the patient describes a fast ride at an amusement park), gestures, and using semantically related words (e.g., "It's like a train").[435] These are the strategies that most people use in daily normal word retrieval issues. The PPCS patient may have to use these more consistently and automatically, and training in this will make it more automatic and reduce frustration. As reaction time or speed of processing is a related issue with word retrieval,[436] this extra time for processing used in compensatory strategy use can sometimes allow for the target word to be accessed.

Social Language/Pragmatic Skills

As stated previously, SLPS are highly correlated with executive functions and attention. They are also very abstract and sometimes subconscious in expression and perception. Therapy is driven by the weaknesses or deficits identified in observations, interviews, and rating scales by patient and family. Typically with the PPCS patient, the deficits are more subtle, and many in their inner circle may not even provide feedback to the patient since they feel as if they are being "rude" themselves by pointing it out. Therapy then involves identifying the issues, having the patient be able to identify (i.e., discriminate appropriate versus inappropriate behavior), providing specific training on target behaviors, and then practicing in structured situations through real-life scenarios.[434] An example would be perseveration on a topic and not recalling that the patient had shared that information multiple times prior. This could be identified via videotape review; the behavior could be negatively practiced (i.e., the patient can do it voluntarily), and then practiced using appropriate compensatory strategies or soliciting feedback (i.e., "Have I told you about my accident?"), and from there, the patient could practice being able to avoid the topic or getting back on the interaction topic. This would involve videotaping, practice, and role-playing, with eventual practice with structured and then unstructured real-life interactions. Cueing is a critical feature in SLPS therapy: the therapist must act as the frontal lobe external aid, and this cueing will eventually be faded.

Aerobic Exercise Training

It has been suggested that PPCS and exercise intolerance, which may be caused by persistent alterations in cerebral cellular metabolism, can be managed successfully with graduated, individualized aerobic exercise programs.[115,154,188] The use of subsymptom exacerbation exercise testing to assess for exercise intolerance of individuals following concussion has been discussed previously. Here the reader is presented with the prescription and progression of aerobic training and the evidence to support the use of graduated exercise training programs for the athlete and nonathlete of various age groups.

Schneider et al. completed a rigorous systematic review related to aerobic training for exercise tolerance as part of the CSG.[6] Authors concluded that closely monitored active rehabilitation programs involving controlled submaximal, subsymptom threshold exercise may be of benefit for adults and adolescents with PPCS.[189] Individuals with persistent symptoms at rest who experience an exacerbation of symptoms during the BCTT, or an equivalent subsymptom exacerbation exercise test, are considered to have exercise intolerance and should be prescribed aerobic conditioning at 60% to 80% of HRt obtained on the exercise test.[115,188,276,437] There is evidence showing superior outcomes in exercise tolerance and symptom complaints for individuals performing exercises at 60% to 80% HRt compared with those performing active training at 40% to 60% HRt achieved on a subsymptom exacerbation exercise test.[437]

Although the subsymptom exercise test has been deemed safe to perform acutely (3 to 7 days postinjury) and at 3 weeks postinjury for adolescents and young adults,[277] the exercise test and graduated exercise program has not been performed with children 10 years and younger; therefore clinicians should be cautious in the initiation of and prescription of graded exercise in children. As mentioned in Box 23.1, in the presence of persistent symptoms at rest and with cognitive load in children, it is important to establish academic accommodations and begin a structured return-to-learn program prior to return to activity, which can be safely initiated 4 weeks postinjury.[70]

Baker and colleagues[188] performed a study using a case series of 91 patients referred to a university clinic for treatment of persistent symptoms (individuals with more than 3 persistent symptoms at rest for a period of more than 3 weeks). Following a subsymptom exercise assessment (BCTT), 65 patients (71%) were found to have exercise intolerance, who were classified with physiological-postconcussive disorder (P-PCS). All patients were offered a graded exercise program; however, some declined to participate. More than two-thirds of the patients who completed the graded exercise program, whether or not the exercise prescription matched the patient clinical profile, returned to full function, on average 2 years following injury, while only 1 in 6 (16%) of the patients who declined to participate in the graded exercise reported return to full functioning. These findings show a potential benefit of graded aerobic training; however, the results should be interpreted cautiously, as there were differences between the two groups. The groups were not of equal size (65 patients were found to be classified as P-PCS compared with 26 patients without exercise intolerance), and follow-up for outcomes of return to function was completed by telephone, where 62% of the P-PCS group compared with 88% of patients without exercise intolerance were available for reporting their functional level.

Leddy and colleagues[276] performed a prospective cohort study with 12 participants (6 athletes and 6 nonathletes) with persistent postconcussive syndrome (diagnosis using WHO ICD-10 definition) and symptom exacerbation during the BCTT to show that controlled exercise is safe for individuals with PCS to perform and that graded exercise can improve PCS symptoms when compared with an individual's no-treatment baseline. After testing, athletes and nonathletes performed aerobic exercise for the same duration that they had achieved during the prior treadmill test, but at an intensity of 60% to 80% HRt once per day for 5 to 6 days per week. All of the participants reached age-predicted HR_{max} without symptom exacerbation within a range of 11 to 112 days. Although there was no difference in the amount of improvement between the two groups, athletes achieved maximum aerobic exertion (18 to 20 RPE) without symptom exacerbation in a shorter duration than nonathletes.

Leddy and colleagues[437] performed a quasi-experimental study to compare exercise capacity, symptoms, and fMRI activation patterns during a cognitive task in 10 athletes and nonathletes with PCS (using WHO ICD-10 definition). Ten athletes were assigned to an exercise treatment group ($n = 5$) or a placebo stretching group ($n = 5$), and were compared with a healthy control group ($n = 5$). Participants in the aerobic exercise group were instructed to perform a controlled, progressive aerobic exercise program at 60% to 80% HRt, attained on the BCTT for 20 minutes a day with a heart rate monitor for 6 days per week. All participants had an fMRI examination at baseline and again after approximately 12 weeks (range, 33 to 270 days). No adverse events were reported. A statistically significant increase in exercise heart rate was reported for the exercise group, while there was no significant change in exercise heart rate for the stretching group. The exercise group also experienced a statistically significant decrease in number of symptoms (measured by PCSS), whereas no change was observed in the stretching group. The fMRI results indicated that participants in the exercise group showed activation patterns that resembled those of healthy controls during the cognitive task, whereas the activation patterns for the stretching group continued to show impaired function.

Gagnon and colleagues[70] completed a case series of 16 children and adolescents (aged 10 to 17 years), which showed involvement in a controlled and closely monitored rehabilitation program initiated after 4 weeks of injury may be beneficial to children who are slow to recover following concussion. All participants showed improvements in aerobic activity duration tolerance and in symptoms, with a mean duration of 4.4 weeks in the program. In addition, Gagnon and colleagues[438] investigated outcomes in 10 adolescent athletes, between 14 and 18 years of age, who were referred consecutively to an aerobic and general coordination exercise program lasting a mean of 6.8 weeks (range, 3.6 to 26.2 weeks). Overall, a clinically meaningful decrease in postconcussion symptoms was found from initial assessment to the second assessment (Cohen's $d = 1.83$). In addition, moderate to large effect sizes were found for fatigue levels, depression scores, and performance on cognitive processing (Cohen's d ranging from 0.48 to 2.44).

In a randomized pilot study, Maerlender and colleagues[439] enrolled 33 college athletes who were removed from play due to concussion immediately into an exertion group (performed aerobic exercise on stationary bike for 20 minutes daily at a "mild to moderate level" measured by a 0 to 6 on RPE scale) or standard care group who were asked to engage in no systematic exertion other than normal activities for school. Median number of days to clinical recovery (measured by test scores on ImPACT and postride symptom complaint following bicycle exercise test) and number of athletes with prolonged recovery were no different between the two groups. The study findings provide emerging evidence that moderate physical activity may have a positive effect on time to recovery; however, the preliminary results should be interpreted with caution, because as a pilot study, it was not adequately powered to show between-group differences and the subsymptom exercise test protocol, nor if the RTP program was consistent with recommendations from international consensus guidelines.[17,154]

Chan and colleagues[440] randomized 19 adolescents aged 12 to 18 years with PPCS following an SRC into a treatment as a usual group (symptom management and RTP advice, return-to-school facilitation, and physiatrist consultation) and a treatment as a usual group plus an active rehabilitation program with subsymptom aerobic training, coordination exercises, visualization and imagery techniques, and a home exercise program for 6 weeks (mean, 3.4 sessions). The study corroborated with findings from previous studies[70,441] that an active rehabilitation program is safe to perform with adolescents with PPCS. In addition, a statistically significant treatment effect in symptom complaint as measured by the PCSS (Cohen's $d = .55$) was found for adolescents completing the treatment as usual plus active rehabilitation program.

Kurowski and colleagues[420] demonstrated the benefits of subsymptom exacerbation aerobic training in adolescents (mean age 15 years, range 14 to 17 years) with an average of approximately 2 months of persistent symptoms after concussion compared with adolescents randomized to a full-body stretching program. Medium to large effect sizes (Cohen's $d = 0.5–0.8$) were found between groups for the Postconcussion Symptom Inventory (PCSI) ratings of the parent/guardian and concussed adolescents, with a trend of greatest improvement found at 5 weeks of the 6-week-long aerobic training program. Interestingly, the study found a similar magnitude of effect size to that found in Chan and colleagues for aerobic exercise in adolescents.[440]

It is important to note, as mentioned previously, that a small population of individuals will experience prolonged signs of autonomic dysregulation and may have sustained exercise intolerance with poor ability to engage in aerobic exercise.[280] Symptoms of dizziness, particularly described as lightheadedness, nausea, heaviness of the extremities, tremulousness, reduced mental clarity, and generalized fatigue, can be signs of POTS, which is another syndrome whose clinical presentation mimics many symptoms of PPCS.[442,443] For those who have PPCS, it is suggested a monthly reassessment of orthostatic intolerance is prudent to rule out the development of POTS. Recumbent exercise training may be required as a mechanism to gradually build tolerance for upright aerobic training, and other comorbidities may further restrict participation in successful exercise training.[286] See Table 23.12 for levels of evidence to support the use of monitored, graduated aerobic exercise following concussion.

Vestibular Rehabilitation

Vestibular rehabilitation involves the use of a problem-oriented approach in which impairments are clearly identified in the examination to determine impact on activity limitations. Specific, targeted

TABLE 23.12 Levels of Evidence, as Described by the Center for Evidence Based Medicine,[444] to Support the Use of Monitored, Graduated Aerobic Exercise Training Following Concussion

	Acute Stage of Recovery (Training Initiated Within 14 Days Postinjury)	Persistent Postconcussion Symptoms (Training Initiated ≥ 3 Weeks Postinjury)
Children (<10 years)	NA/unknown	NA/unknown
Adolescents (10–18 years)	Level 2: Maerlender et al.[439] Level 4: Gall et al.[124]	Level 2: Chan et al.[440] Kurowski et al.[420] Level 4: Gagnon et al.[70] Gagnon et al.[438]
Young adults (18–55 years)	NA/unknown	Level 4: Baker et al.[188] Leddy et al.[276] Leddy et al.[437]
Older adults	NA/unknown	NA/unknown
Military personnel	NA/unknown	NA/unknown

interventions to decrease vertigo, lightheadedness, and disorientation should be introduced at the appropriate level. Balance exercises should be established focused on the impairment that is most likely to improve with the goal of avoiding the development of dependency patterns. The cervical spine should be examined to determine the contribution to both dizziness and pain. Posttraumatic headache is a common comorbidity and should be addressed early in the intervention. The concussed patient will likely have maladaptation issues, as there is potential damage to all three of the sensory systems involved, and there may be abnormal motor programs initiated that need to be corrected. The rehabilitation specialist should consider the following general guidelines related to vestibular rehabilitation in concussion:

- Determine the appropriate activity levels to avoid needless exacerbation of symptoms. Exercises that are likely to exacerbate symptoms should be saved for the end of a treatment session or home exercise program, and these should be carefully monitored for progression. The patient should be informed about which exercises are designed to decrease symptoms, and the ones that require the activation of vertigo for the recalibration process. Settling exercises should be provided to the patient to increase the ability to manage symptoms.
- When increasing one activity, reduce or keep other activities at the same level.
- Exercises should be introduced slowly to give the patient and therapist a chance to monitor responses. Remember that exercise for acute vestibular deficits are based on an intact visual and somatosensory system response, so they may be too aggressive for the concussed patient.
- Encourage rest that includes settling between activities (use the visual hygiene instructions provided later on in this chapter) and provide breaks during exercises to improve adherence and limit exacerbation of symptoms. For this reason, treatment sessions may be lengthened to allow sufficient time for active treatments to

promote recovery and decrease potential of worsening symptom provocation.
- Discuss medical management and refer when appropriate for control/resolution of headaches early in rehabilitation to increase exercise and activity tolerance.[290]
- Gradually include exercises with visual flow and complex visual stimuli.
  - Avoid complex environments initially (e.g., shopping malls, heavy traffic), followed by gradual exposure based on symptoms and tolerance.
  - Encourage the use of indoor and outdoor settings that patients typically encounter to promote reintegration into daily activities.

The trigger of symptoms can be aspects of the vestibular rehabilitation program as exercises are used to drive a change in the output of the vestibular system (VOR and VSR), which is in the business of providing stability in gaze and stability of the postural control system during daily activities, especially with head motion. However, specific considerations should be made for the concussed individuals compared with the patient who has intact vision and somatosensation available for the adaptation process.

Eye-Head Coordination Exercises

Impairments in eye-head coordination have been reported after brain injury[445] and may result from disruption in the VOR[446] or reflect increased symptoms with head and eye movement[447] (e.g., self-motion sensitivity). Eye-head coordination exercises involve movement of the head and/or eyes designed to enhance VOR adaptation. Oculomotor reeducation, if needed, should precede work on VOR and dynamic gaze stabilization exercises, which include eyes-open head movement.[445] The patient must be able to determine when the head is not moving when the eyes are closed. This can be achieved with settling exercises if necessary. It may also be appropriate to start performing eyes-closed head turns prior to starting eye-head coordination exercises to calibrate the somatosensory and vestibular systems if head motion is determined to contribute to symptoms. Body rotation under a stable head (BRUSH) can be performed in the clinic, as well as by caregivers, to decrease the stiffness in the cervical spine often associated with the habit of self-deceleration of head motion. This can be critical to allow normal speeds for VOR training.

Eye-head coordination exercises while standing, walking, and changing direction can be prescribed as an adjunct to adaptation exercises (e.g., VORx1) to incorporate the change in VOR gain into a functional activity. The direction of the head turn (yaw, pitch, roll plane motion), as well as the magnitude of the head turn, can be modified (head center to head right, head center to head left, head center head up, etc.), according to the determination of somatosensory sensitivity in the cervical spine. To active normal VOR, the head should be moved without stopping in the center. In all head turning activity, it is important that the patient does not stop at the end ROM to abnormally access somatosensory input. This should also be integrated into the frequency of the head motion, which can be modified by timing the head turns to the patient's steps as the patient walks. For instance, a clinician may ask a patient to turn their head to the left for three steps, then right for three steps, then back to the left for three steps, repeating this motion as they walk down a quiet, dimly lit corridor. As the patient progresses, the frequency of the head turns may be increased as the patient is asked to turn their head to the left for two steps, then right two steps, left two steps, and so on as they walk forward. In the advanced stage, head turns of 150 to 160 degrees can be made in the yaw or pitch plane every step as the patient walks forward. An important consideration is that rather than the clinician audibly instructing the patient when to turn the head, the patient can be encouraged to turn the head while counting the steps so that the movements can be anticipated and planned rather than unpredictable, as both types of perturbations are experienced during typical daily activities. In this way, the task could be considered in the divided attention paradigm.

Visual motion sensitivity can impact the performance of the eye-head coordination exercises and should be addressed concurrently. Use of activities that allow the patient to normalize responses to visual flow can be initiated early in the program. Visual pursuits, saccadic training, vergence, and VOR cancellation exercises are some examples. This can be started in supine or sitting, and progressed to standing on firm and compliant surfaces. Tossing a ball from hand to hand while tracking it can promote decrease in visual motion sensitivity and can be progressed through changes of surface and walking. Use of optokinetic stimulation can be integrated into the program.

Due to the limited guidance provided for vestibular rehabilitation exercise prescription and progression following concussion,

Alsalaheen and colleagues[445] reviewed home exercise programs designed by 8 physical therapists for 104 patients with persistent symptoms following a concussion that were referred to a tertiary clinic a mean of 58 days from injury. Exercises were categorized as eye-head coordination, sitting balance, standing static balance, standing dynamic balance, or ambulation exercises. Eye-head coordination exercises were the most commonly prescribed category, where 95% of patients received VORx1 viewing (88%) and VOR cancellation (64%) with common modifications to posture and the size of the base of support. Standing static balance exercises were prescribed in 88% of patients with common modifications of changing the surface, size of the base of support, direction of head movement, and visual input. Ambulation exercises were prescribed in 76% of patients with modifications to the size of the base of support and direction of head movement. Examples of prescription and progression of vestibular rehabilitation for individuals with PPCS are described in Table 23.13.

TABLE 23.13 Exercise Prescription and Progressions for Vestibular Rehabilitation Programs Published for Young Adults With Non–Sports-Related Concussion[448] and Children and Adults With Sports-Related Concussion and Non–Sports-Related Concussion[445]

Exercises	Kleffelgaard et al.[448]	Alsalaheen et al.[445]
Patient population/modality	Young adults, Non-SRC/Group-based VR program	Children and adults, SRC and Non-SRC
Adaptation/Gaze stability and eye-head coordination	VORx1: working most on far targets (2–3 m away) VORx2: target held in hand	Movement of head and/or eyes for the purpose of VOR gain adaptation, symptom habituation, or oculomotor re-education: VORx1, VOR cancellation, convergence VORx2
Habituation	Brandt-Daroff exercises, sitting or standing exercises with head tipped to knee, head turns, head pitches, standing whole-body turns, walking with head and body turns	Movement of head and/or eyes for VOR symptom habituation: VORx1, VOR cancellation, convergence VORx2
Oculomotor training	Substitution exercises for static gaze stability: active eye-then-head movement between 2 targets, remembered target	Convergence eye movement training
Balance	Circle training with different balance tasks: sitting on big ball/Airex mat, weight shifting, bouncing, turning head, standing on rocker boards, dual tasks	Seated, standing steady-state, standing dynamic balance exercises
Gait	Walking with head and body turns, start and stops, picking up objects from floor, catching/throwing beanbags, figure eight	Patient walks forward, backward, on stairs, with turns, skipping, jogging, and running
HEP	2–5 exercises, as appropriate + aerobic exercise program: 15–20 min of nonspecific activity (not guided by graded exercise test)	Participants were provided a HEP; however, no frequency or duration provided
Posture	Posture: sitting, standing, walking, jumping, running	Posture: sitting, standing, walking
Surface	Surface: level, mats, foam, Bosu balls, trampolines, wedges, wobble boards, obstacles, stairs	Surface: level, foam, uneven, obstacle, stairs, ramps
Base of support	Base of support: feet apart, feet together, semitandem, tandem, one foot	Base of support: feet-apart, feet-together, semi-tandem, tandem
Arm position	Arm position: away from body, close to body, crossed over chest, hands on hips, reaching, juggling	Arm position: close to body, away from body, reaching, carrying, juggling
Head movement	Head movement: still, nodding, rotating	Head movement direction: still, yaw, pitch, roll
Visual input	Visual input: eyes closed, eyes open, complex patterns, visually quiet environment, visually busy environment	Visual input: eyes closed, eyes open, complex visual patterns
Cognitive task	Cognitive task: secondary motor and cognitive tasks	Cognitive dual task: no examples provided
		Trunk position: upright, leaning, rotated
	Twice per week for 8 weeks (16 sessions)	Median 4 visits (range, 2–13)

HEP, Home exercise program; *SRC*, sports-related concussion; *VOR*, vestibulo-ocular reflex; *VORx1*, adaptation training strategy where the eyes match speed and distance of target (gain = 1); *VORx2*, adaptation training strategy for the VOR, gain = 2; *VR*, vestibular rehabilitation.

When considering the progression of exercises described by Alsalaheen and colleagues,[445] it is difficult to provide a clear recommendation due to the significant variability in the number of visits patients completed (7 to 181 days); however, it is worth noting that at initial evaluation the majority of patients were prescribed the VORx1 viewing exercise while standing with feet apart (43%), followed by standing with feet together (31%), and sitting (23%), demonstrating the modifications necessary to minimize potential symptom provocation. One interesting finding was that the VORx2 viewing exercise was prescribed less frequently (9%) than is typically prescribed for patients with unilateral vestibular hypofunction.[445] It is difficult to provide a definitive reason for the discrepancy in exercise prescription between the two groups. It may be due to the increased visual flow created by moving the head and the target in opposite directions. It may also suggest that patients become symptomatic with advanced adaptation exercises, and therefore the VORx2 viewing exercise should be reserved for the very late stages of return to play and after successful intervention for visual sensitivity when individuals are returning to intensive sport-specific activities that require precision of the VOR (e.g., dancing, skating, basketball) during repetitive, high velocity head turns. See Chapters 20 and 21 for more comprehensive information on the appropriate progression of intervention and exercise for sensory integration during eye-head movement exercises.

Balance Exercises

Prescription of balance exercises should follow the same guidelines related to sensory integration as eye-head coordination. They should be both specific to the impairments determined during examination and comprehensive enough to address all components of the balance system. In addition, modifications to steady state and dynamic balance exercises may need to be performed in a progression from seated to standing, then walking, changing direction, jogging, running, and athletic-specific movements if required for the patient's recreational/sports-related activities.

Effective use of hip strategy in both the anterior-posterior and lateral directions should be encouraged as soon as possible. Head-righting exercises and work on tilt surfaces are critical to avoid development of dependence pattern through the somatosensory system. Head righting can be initiated in sitting and progressed to tandem gait. These activities should be progressed to performance with eyes closed to avoid visual dependence. See Chapters 20 and 21 for a more complete description of the appropriate progression of exercise to facilitate normalization of balance.

Examples of balance prescription and progressions described in the literature are presented in Table 23.13.

Alsalaheen and colleagues[65] used a case series of 114 consecutive patients (67 children, 47 adults) to show that patients referred for vestibular rehabilitation after a concussion (median of 96 days postinjury; range 8–2566 days) may benefit from therapeutic interventions. Alsalaheen and colleagues[65] reported a significant treatment effect for self-report and performance-based measures for balance and gait impairment, including DGI, FGA, gait speed, and FTSTS. In addition, a significant interaction between treatment and age was found with children experiencing greater improvements in dizziness severity reports and balance performance.

The authors reported the group-based program, modified from a program developed at Oslo and Akershus University College for patients with chronic dizziness, is safe, feasible, and may be beneficial for individuals with targeted problems of dizziness and balance following concussion. Interestingly, one benefited from a prolonged vestibular rehabilitation period and might have continued to improve if provided an additional 4 to 8 weeks.[449] However, findings from Adams and colleagues[450] suggest that even long rehabilitation programs (up to

24 weeks) will not always lead to improved outcomes in this patient population. Evidence of potential "responders" and "nonresponders" to physical rehabilitation programs point to the need for more sensitive biomarkers to determine who and when individuals are likely to benefit from active rehabilitation strategies, if those individuals can be identified clinicians could potentially match patients to an effective treatment regimen at the ideal time for an optimal outcome. Future studies are needed to address these important questions in rehabilitation.

The highest quality of evidence to provide support for the use of vestibular rehabilitation has been reported by Schneider and colleagues[304] who performed an RCT comparing return to sport for 31 adolescents and young adults (mean age, 15; range, 12–30) receiving a combination of aerobic training, vestibular rehabilitation, and cervical spine physical therapy to a control group receiving aerobic training alone, one time a week for 8 weeks. At 8 weeks, a significantly higher proportion of patients who were treated with vestibular rehabilitation and cervical spine physical therapy (73% of the intervention group) were medically cleared to return to sport compared with just 7% of the control group. Although all individuals who were medically cleared reported feeling 100% and reported zero symptoms of headache and dizziness, it is unclear if this was at rest or if it was following the return to sport guidelines described by international consensus guidelines.[17] Another important limitation was the range of days from injury in the intervention group were within 30 days of injury while the control group was not—8 to 276 days compared with 31 to 142 days, respectively. Thus spontaneous recovery may have favored the vestibular rehabilitation and cervical spine physical therapy group.

Details related to the exercise prescription and progressions of the vestibular rehabilitation programs used in these studies[304,305,445,448] are provided in Table 23.13.

Reviews on vestibular rehabilitation following concussion have shown a paucity of strong evidence in support of vestibular rehabilitation for patients following concussion.[303,451] Evidence surrounding interventions to address vestibular impairment following concussion suggests that the potential benefits do outweigh the potential risks and vestibular rehabilitation may be most beneficial for a specific subset of patients with persistent symptoms following a concussion.[451] There is now a clear requirement for more high-quality RCTs for vestibular rehabilitation programs used to address vestibular impairment of patients following a concussion to determine the effectiveness of the treatment approach (Table 23.14).[303]

Vision Therapy

The most common oculomotor deficits that have been shown to be amenable to vision therapy include ocular misalignment, impaired visual fixation, versional dysfunction (saccadic and pursuit eye movements), and vergence ocular motility deficits.[100,453]

In the presence of visual fixation deficits, common treatment approaches are composed of rapidly changing focus on command and sustaining visual focus on targets for extended periods of time using attentional grids and near-far-vision focal shifting.[100] Basic scanning and searching exercises can be used in the presence of saccadic and smooth pursuit deficits, where the focus of the exercises should be on accuracy first and then building up to rapid saccadic eye movements or tracking tasks. For vergence ocular motility deficits, prisms may be used to accommodate motility deficits or to be used as a training tool, and far and near viewing (e.g., Brock string) can be performed as a restorative treatment option as well. Often these tasks involve the use of equipment that is only available through licensed optometrists and ophthalmologists, and there is evidence that the care of individuals with functional vision changes should be directed by qualified specialists

TABLE 23.14 Levels of Evidence, as Described by the Center for Evidence Based Medicine,[444] to Support the Use of Vestibular Rehabilitation Following Concussion

	Acute Stage of Recovery (Training Initiated Within 14 Days Postinjury)	Persistent Postconcussion Symptoms (Training Initiated ≥ 3 Weeks Postinjury)
Children (<10 years)	NA/unknown	Level 4: Alsalaheen et al.[65,a,c]
Adolescents (10–18 years)	NA/unknown	Level 2: Schneider et al.[304,a,b] Level 4: Alsalaheen et al.[65,a,c]
Young adults (18–55 years)	NA/unknown	Level 2: Schneider et al.[304,a,b] Level 4: Alsalaheen et al.[65,a,c] Kleffelgaard et al.[448,a,c]
Older adults	NA/unknown	Level 4: Alsalaheen et al.[65,a,c]
Military personnel	NA/unknown	Level 4: Hoffer et al.[381] Gottshall et al.[305,b] Carrick et al.[452]

[a]Improvements in symptom complaint of dizziness.
[b]Improvements addressing dynamic gaze stabilization.
[c]Improvements addressing self-report and/or performance related to balance and gait impairments.

such as a neuro-optometrist or ophthalmologist.[5,454] For this reason, underlying visual dysfunction should be given consideration for referral to specialists such as optometrists, ophthalmologist, neuro-optometrists, or occupational therapists, who specialize in vision therapy for individuals with brain injury.[100,290]

Special considerations should be incorporated for vision therapy in regards to patients with signs and symptoms consistent with impairment to the ocular motor system and visual perception following concussion. The rehabilitation specialist should provide:

- Instructions to the patient to "rest" eyes by looking at targets at a distance or by cupping hands around eyes to limit visual input
- Advice on the use of filter screens and glasses or printing on colored paper for visual comfort while reading
- Education to avoid/decrease exposure to light by dimming lights, using curtains, wearing sunglasses/filtered lenses, or wearing caps to shade the sun or indoor lighting

Overall, empirical evidence is limited for the effectiveness of vision therapy to address symptoms and functional deficits following concussion.[100] Preliminary evidence suggests that combined oculomotor therapies that target multiple impairments, including convergence and accommodative insufficiency and versional problems, may be effective in reducing symptoms and improving reading.[454,455]

Thiagarajan and colleagues[455] found oculomotor rehabilitation composed of versional (fixation, saccades, and smooth pursuit), vergence, and accommodation training two sessions per week for 6 weeks led to significant improvements in reading rate and was associated with improved subjectively based visual comfort and visual attention during reading in young adults (age range, 23 to 33 years) who were 1 year postinjury. Further, when oculomotor training was performed in conjunction with multiple therapies (vestibular, cognitive-behavioral therapy, speech therapy, and/or psychotherapy), Ciuffreda and colleagues[456] reported marked improvement in individuals' attentional state while reading under simple and complex environmental conditions for those with mTBI. However, given the small sample sizes, nonrandom group assignments, and inclusion of individuals with acquired and traumatic brain injury, findings from Thiagarajan and colleagues[455] and Ciuffreda and colleagues[456] need to be interpreted cautiously (Table 23.15).[100]

Management of Cervical Spine Dysfunction

Because of the heterogeneity of findings in people with neck dysfunction after concussion and whiplash injury, multimodal interventions based on identified impairments represent the most successful outcomes. Unfortunately, large-scale systematic reviews and meta-analyses present such inconsistent findings that it is difficult for clinicians to meaningfully synthesis research findings and draw informed conclusions.[457] The challenge remains to "provide the right intervention for the right person at the right time,"[457] which is a difficult approach to measure with conventional research methods.

Malmström and colleagues[458] used a clinical reasoning approach to assess and treat 22 patients with comorbid neck pain and dizziness, in whom vestibular dysfunction and trauma were ruled out. All improved whether acute or delayed care was rendered. Positive effects persisted at 6 and 24 months after treatment in 76% of subjects, suggesting that some may have required more specific maintenance strategies. As discussed in other sections, Schneider and colleagues[304] employed a multimodal treatment regimen addressing both vestibular and cervical findings. Cervical spine interventions included nonprovocative ROM exercises, stretching, postural education, manual therapy of cervical and thoracic spine regions, neuromotor retraining, and sensorimotor retraining. In order to control headache symptoms, cervical spine treatments preceded vestibular interventions. All participants in both the treatment and control groups had clinical findings suggesting cervical involvement, and 80% to 90% had clinical signs of vestibular dysfunction. The integrated approach resulted in student-athletes returning to play sooner than those not treated. Likewise, a case series of six pediatric athletes with PCS where multimodal assessments and care included cervical, aerobic activity, oculomotor, and postural control demonstrated successful return to activity.[68]

TABLE 23.15 Levels of Evidence, as Described by the Center for Evidence-Based Medicine,[444] to Support the Use of Vision Therapy

	Acute Stage of Recovery (Training Initiated Within 14 Days Postinjury)	Persistent Postconcussion Symptoms (Training Initiated ≥ 3 Weeks Postinjury)
Children (<10 years)	NA/unknown	NA/unknown
Adolescents (10–18 years)	NA/unknown	NA/unknown
Young adults (18–55 years)	NA/unknown	Level 4: Thiagarajan et al.[455,a,b]
Older adults	NA/unknown	NA/unknown
Military personnel	NA/unknown	NA/unknown

[a]Improvements in symptom complaint.
[b]Improvements in functional activities related to static gaze (i.e., reading, computer work).

Studies on the effects of neck treatment in the acute stage after concussion are few. Schneider and colleagues[459] identified a constellation of cervical impairments within 4 days of concussion in a cohort of elite youth ice hockey athletes that pointed toward appropriate treatment choices. A psychometrically sound battery of tests was used to explore cervical spine function, vestibulo-ocular function, dynamic balance, and divided attention tasks. Although individuals with persistent postconcussion often report issues in all categories, cervical spine dysfunction was most significant for this acute group. Impaired sensory integration was evident. Cervical tests included the CFET, cranial flexion rotation test, anterolateral neck strength, and joint position error.

Investigations of specific treatment approaches for individuals with traumatic neck injuries of greater than 3 months' duration have focused on proprioceptive retraining,[460] deep cervical muscle strength and endurance,[461,462] neuromotor retraining,[321,463] and manual therapy[464,465] interventions, including active mobilizations called sustained natural apophyseal glides (SNAGs). Shoulder girdle control also contributes to CGH treatment.[466] The methods of the recommended assessments outlined previously can not only identify impairments but be transitioned into interventions. Important principles to keep in mind for treating the cervical spine after concussion are:

1. Identify and prioritize impairments, and understand the known or theoretical mechanisms.
2. Group impairments into functional classifications, if possible, to maximize intervention effect.
3. Consider cognitive demands of multisensory processing after concussion.
4. Understand prognostic risk factors for chronicity, including psychosocial and contextual factors.
5. Invest the patient in the plan, provide appropriate images, and minimize written directions, as individuals with concussions may have difficulty following or remembering directions. Photos or videos captured on the patient's phone are very helpful.
6. Address basic impairments before advancing to complex activities.
7. Employ sound motor learning concepts to engender the most robust and lasting changes. In particular, consider appropriate feedback (both internal and external), high repetitions, attention, and salience to the patient.
8. Progress patients through sensory reweighting demands for enduring sensorimotor improvements. This also helps avoid developing excessive dependence on one sensory system.

The Neck Pain Clinical Practice Guidelines Revision 2017[337] promote four classifications of patients with neck pain: neck pain with mobility deficits, neck pain with movement coordination impairments, neck pain with headaches of cervical origin, and neck pain with radicular pain. Interventions with stringent levels of evidence are assigned by category with recommendations divided into acute, subacute, and chronic stages. The reader can appreciate that each of those categories can apply to concussed individuals with neck pain.

A selection of example interventions based on evaluative findings and test protocols follows:

- Repetitive nonaggravating small nods will encourage synovial joint healing and promote normal joint mechanoreception and motor recruitment in the highly problematic craniocervical region. Sucking the body of the tongue to the back of the hard palette encourages localized subcranial motion and reduces temporomandibular compression. Midcervical and cervico-thoracic movements may be localized by placing a hand, rolled towel, belt, or strap across the lower half of the target motion segment. Self-assisted localized facet and soft tissue mobility can be augmented with carefully placed belts or straps. Stretching exercises must not create excessive leverage across impaired articulations.
- Joint mobilization and manipulation in the cervical and upper thoracic regions where restrictions are identified are helpful in pain

reduction during the acute phase, but less so in the subacute and chronic phases. When supported by specific exercises for motion control, mobilization/manipulation can improve ROM.
- Cervical proprioception can be improved with progressive activities using the head-mounted laser, for head and trunk relocation activities as well as kinesthetic control such as tracing figures or mazes. More complex activities, including static and dynamic balance and gait, can incorporate proprioceptive tasks.
- Proprioception is also improved through strength and endurance training of deep cervical musculature. Beginning in the vertical position, the weight of the head may be increased as the trunk approaches horizontal. Limits must be set to ensure perfect form and control, just as in any skill development. Difficulty may increase through load, speed, and duration. For example, deep subcranial extensors may be challenged to meet their dual performance tasks of support and coordination in a four point kneel, head, and neck held in neutral, with nodding and turning added. The activity limit is reached when the two functions cannot both continue accurately.
- Eye-head coordination is described in detail in the vestibular intervention section. Serial eye-head motions should also be included, where gaze changes first, followed by head motion match, or gaze remains stable while head position changes with eyes following afterward. Slower speeds may help reset the COR. Additional tasks can be layered on, such as isometric head support in prone, four point kneel, side lying, or partial supine to challenge deep cervical musculature. "Foveal Glasses"[467] (only the pupil of each eye is exposed, with the remaining lens area taped over) are used to prevent eye drift during neck motion activities intended to strengthen the VOR cancellation, strengthen gaze stability, and improve cervical-visual coordination. Their effects are theoretical and untested. The clinician must decide if vision is the correct and desired feedback for the intended purpose.
- BRUSH movements may help normalize the CCR (eyes closed) and COR (eyes opened), reduce neck muscle guarding, and improve perception of head position relative to neck and body activity. Feedback may be visual, including use of a head-mounted laser for accuracy, somatosensory (rotating with a firm prop behind the head against a door frame), or auditory (ticking clock set straight ahead). Speed, repetitions, and duration constitute the dose, as well as choice of surface and body position.
- Head righting progression might include sitting or bouncing on an exercise ball, swinging hips and trunk from side to side under a stable head, or reaching into eccentric positions while maintaining a vertical head. On a firm seat, if ROM permits, the patient can tilt sideways until the elbow touches the sitting surface, alternating sides and maintaining a vertical head. This has the dual benefit of exercising the trunk. In standing, simple trunk side bending by sliding a hand down the leg can progress into more challenging stance positions and surfaces. Many yoga asanas are ideal for the challenge.
- Cervico-thoracic posture and mobility, respiratory patterns, and scapular carriage and control contribute to pain management and more efficient function (Table 23.16).

Multidisciplinary Care

Following concussion patients may experience symptoms and functional limitations caused by impairments of multiple systems, which can be best managed by practitioners across disciplines. For this reason, there is substantial, mostly anecdotal, support for multidisciplinary care for patients following a concussion.[58,118,181,303] Despite the number of reports advocating for the use of multidisciplinary care for the management of functional limitations following concussion, the recommendation is largely consensus based, as there is limited empirical evidence to demonstrate its superiority to isolated pharmacological or nonpharmacological (e.g., education, active intervention) treatments.

TABLE 23.16   Levels of Evidence, as Described by the Center for Evidence-Based Medicine,[444] to Support the Use of Management of the Musculoskeletal and Sensorimotor Deficits of the Cervical Spine Using Active Training Following Concussion

	Acute Stage of Recovery (Training Initiated Within 14 Days Postinjury)	Persistent Postconcussion Symptoms (Training Initiated ≥ 3 Weeks Postinjury)
Children (<10 years)	NA/unknown	NA/unknown
Adolescents (10–18 years)	NA/unknown	Level 2: Schneider et al.[304] Level 4: Hugentobler et al.[68]
Young adults (18–55 years)	NA/unknown	Level 2: Schneider et al.[304]
Older adults	NA/unknown	NA/unknown
Military personnel	NA/unknown	NA/unknown

Several large medical centers across the United States, Canada, and the United Kingdom have developed multidisciplinary Concussion Centers that incorporate teams dedicated to patient care and research from the acute stages through full recovery. For a detailed discussion related to the variety of disciplines that may be included in a comprehensive concussion center team and the roles of each team member, the reader is directed to the following reviews: Makdissi and colleagues,[58] Reynolds and colleagues,[182] and Ahmed and colleagues.[468]

Effective multidisciplinary care begins with a thorough assessment, which should start with a complete neurological examination ideally performed by an experienced sports medicine physician, neurologist, or neurosurgeon.[118] Results of a thorough examination by a medical physician specializing in brain injury can lead to referrals to different health care providers for specialized assessment and management of functional limitations that are within the rehabilitation specialist's scope of practice (see Ellis and colleagues[118] for review). This may include referral to a(n)

- or exercise physiologist physical therapist for a subsymptom exercise tolerance test and graduated aerobic exercise prescription;
- physical therapist for assessment and management of potential vestibular and cervical spine impairments;
- occupational therapist, optometrist, and/or ophthalmologist for visual deficits;
- psychiatrist or neuropsychologist to manage mood and psychological dysfunction;
- SLP or neuropsychologist for assessment and management of cognitive deficits;
- neurologist specializing in the management of headaches for migraine or migraine-like clinical presentation.

Schneider and colleagues[304] showed adolescents and young adults with PPCS, following an SRC who received a multimodal intervention of vestibular rehabilitation and management of cervical spine impairment performed by a physical therapist, were 3.91 (with 95% confidence interval of 1.34 to 11.34) times more likely to be medically cleared by 8 weeks, compared with a control group. The multimodal approach was completed by one physical therapist with 13 years of clinical experience and expertise in the area of vestibular rehabilitation and musculoskeletal physical therapy with treatments once per week that consisted of neuromotor retraining, manual therapy, and sensorimotor retraining exercises prior to initiating vestibular rehabilitative exercises.

Hugentobler and colleagues[68] carried out a case series including six adolescent athletes (age range 15 to 19 years) with postconcussion symptoms for a median of 80 days (range, 19 to 192 days) following injury. Although the study describes a problem-based assessment and treatment (similar to that described by Ellis and colleagues[115]) for physical therapists, including aerobic training, vestibular rehabilitation,

and management of the cervical spine, each patient received multidisciplinary care from rehabilitation specialists, including sports medicine, neuropsychology, psychiatry, physical therapy (vestibular rehabilitation and/or musculoskeletal physical therapy of the cervical spine), and headache specialist care, on average for 6.8 session over an average of 8.9 weeks. Outcomes suggest that a physical therapy program incorporating a multidisciplinary approach may help facilitate symptom reduction, improve self-management abilities, and safely enhance function in adolescents. In spite of improvements, only one of the six patients had returned to full preinjury activity levels at the time of their final physical therapy assessment; however, the majority (4/6) returned to preinjury levels and types of activity within 3 to 6 months. Similar findings for return to activity and RTW were reported by Moore and colleagues[66] in 14 young and older adults (median age = 43 years, range 18 to 72) with PPCS for a median of 107 days (range 14 to 992), who received multidisciplinary care, on average, for 19 sessions (range 12 to 27) over 24 weeks of treatment. The majority of patients did not return to preinjury work or physical activities until the 6-month assessment (86% and 57%, respectively) compared with the number of patients who returned to preinjury work and physical activities at the 3-month assessment (36% and 21%, respectively). In addition to aerobic exercise training, vestibular rehabilitation, and musculoskeletal cervical spine physical therapy, patients received vision therapy provided by an occupational therapist, cognitive therapy provided by a neuropsychologist, and psychology and vocational counseling, if appropriate.

Vikane and colleagues[469] randomized 150 participants with PPCS 2 months after an mTBI into an intervention group who received a multidisciplinary outpatient treatment program consisting of a specialist in rehabilitation medicine, a neuropsychologist, occupational therapist, social worker, and a nurse compared with a comparison group who received follow-up by a general practitioner. Intervention was performed once per week for 4 weeks, with a median of two sessions completed. The occupational therapist helped the patients with memory aids and structuring the day. Psychological distress or cognitive difficulties were followed-up by a neuropsychologist, who used cognitive behavioral treatment when appropriate. There was no difference on the primary outcome of *return to work* (defined as 5 consecutive weeks without absence), and there was no statistically significant difference in number of symptoms endorsed or severity of symptoms reported on the RPQ. Limitations of the study include potential differences in the type of nonpharmacological intervention provided, differences in scope of practice for rehabilitation services (study was completed in Norway), and most importantly, the severity of injuries in this sample population as 25% of the sample received a Glasgow Coma Scale score of 13 to 14 (75% were assigned a 15) and were hospitalized following injury. See Table 23.17 for a summary of levels of evidence to support multidisciplinary or multimodal care.

TABLE 23.17 Levels of Evidence, as Described by the Center for Evidence-Based Medicine,[444] to Support the Use of Multidisciplinary or Multimodal Care Following Concussion

	Acute Stage of Recovery (Training Initiated Within 14 Days Postinjury)	Persistent Postconcussion Symptoms (Training Initiated ≥ 3 Weeks Postinjury)
Children (<10 years)	NA/unknown	NA/unknown
Adolescents (10–18 years)	NA/unknown	Level 2: Schneider et al.[304] Vikane et al.[469] Level 4: Hogentobler et al.[68] Cordingley et al.[470] Grabowski et al.[471]
Young adults (18–55 years)	NA/unknown	Level 2: Schneider et al.[304] Vikane et al.[469] Level 4: Moore et al.[66] Ciuffreda et al.[456]
Older adults	NA/unknown	Level 2: Vikane et al.[469] Level 4: Moore et al.[66]
Military personnel	NA/unknown	Level 4: Janak et al.[472]

CASE STUDY 23.1

Ciara, a 17-year-old female, was a healthy adolescent, with no history of previously documented concussions or psychological disorders, sustained a high velocity direct ball-to-head contact injury during a soccer match. She was observed by coaching and athletic training staff to stagger and seemed disoriented as she ran the opposite direction of play once she arose from a downed position for 10 s following the hit. Due to the strong suspicion of a concussion because of her behavior following the injury, Ciara was pulled from the match and, as per mandated state laws to prevent a potentially life-threatening second impact syndrome, Ciara did not return to play.

During the on-the-field assessment using the Sport Concussion Assessment Tool 5 (SCAT5) testing, performed by the athletic trainer, Ciara endorsed headache, dizziness, and noise sensitivity with no evidence of impaired cognitive function. Results of the SCAT5 did not indicate the need for emergent care. The athletic trainer provided the recommendation for Ciara to not return to any sport or school-related activities until a full evaluation was completed by a Sports Medicine Physician. Her symptoms continued for the rest of the day and evening.

Acute Concussion

Follow-up examination by a Sports Medicine Physician 2 days following injury resulted in the following problem list:

- Posttraumatic headache described as dull, constant, and occipital in location, with some component of upper cervical discomfort
- Sleep disturbance of hypersomnolence (daytime sleepiness)
- Impaired cognitive function—specifically attention and memory
- Exercise intolerance as symptom exacerbation and abnormal heart rate response recorded during 4th minute of the subsymptom exercise tolerance test
- Endorsement of dizziness when rising from laying down or seated position
- Impaired balance as measured by the Balance Error Scoring System
- Slowed scanning right-to-left with multiple errors on King Devick test
  - eliminate

Education and Recommendations From Sports Medicine Physician

The nursing staff at the Concussion Center provided education to Ciara, through verbal report and physical pamphlets, indicating that it is common to experience a myriad of symptoms following a hit to the head, but in the majority of cases patients will return to prior functional activities without symptom provocation. Ciara was also

provided education for sleep hygiene with a discussion on regular bedtime and limiting technology use before bed. (Note: although not yet validated, the results of this examination indicate a score of 10 points on the PPCS risk categories reported by Zemek and colleagues,[119] with a 69% probability of developing PPCS.)

Recommendation for Return to Learn

As Ciara had already been kept from engaging in school for 2 days, the physician recommended partial return to school with accommodations. Communication with school counsellor and school nurse determined the following classroom accommodations:

- ½ day school for 2 weeks, but increase to full day of school if able
- Double time for homework and tests
- *Recommendation for return to play.*
- No engagement in vigorous physical due to failed subsymptom exercise tolerance test. Ciara was permitted to perform light activities such as daily chores, walking, and social activities.

Intervention (medical management): prescribed acetaminophen to manage continued headaches.

Reevaluation at 14 Days Following Injury

At 14 days following injury Ciara continued to be limited to ½ day of school, which resulted in an exacerbation of headaches, dizziness, and the development of new symptoms, including fatigue, "feeling like in a fog," and eye strain. She refrained from physical activity as instructed. Ciara was found to have exercise intolerance, as she had symptom exacerbation at 40% age-related heart rate maximum during the subsymptom exercise tolerance test. Ciara continued to be engaged in social activities, although she stated that this also caused an exacerbation of the previously listed symptoms. Further, Ciara was found to have continued sleep disturbances, cognitive dysfunction, and balance impairment.

Education and Recommendations From Sports Medicine Physician

Education was provided indicating that the majority of children and adolescents return to unrestricted school and sport-related activities within 28 days. Therefore Ciara was expected to continue to improve over time and, as able, she should increase the amount of time engaged in school-related activities.

Continued

CASE STUDY 23.1—cont'd

Recommendation for Return to Learn

No changes to the above listed recommendations for ½ day school and double time for homework and tests

Recommendation for Return to Play

Begin engaging in light jogging activities and individual soccer drills of low-to-moderate physical exertion below a symptom exacerbation level.

Reevaluation at 30 Days

At 30 days following injury, Ciara had returned to full days at school; however, she continued to report an exacerbation of nondebilitating headaches, dizziness, fatigue, and eye strain most days of the week. These symptoms were exacerbated during social engagement as well. She was able to engage in light aerobic exercise, but when she attempted to perform more intense soccer drills, she reported headaches and dizziness. Ciara was found to have exercise intolerance as she had symptom exacerbation at 80% age-related heart rate maximum during the subsymptom exercise tolerance test. Further, Ciara was found to have continued sleep disturbances, cognitive dysfunction, and balance impairment. In addition, screening for affective disorders indicated the presence of an anxiety disorder, potentially caused by her protracted recovery and inability to engage in school, social, and sport-related activities without an exacerbation of symptoms and unknown cause of the symptoms.

Patient met the classification for persistent postconcussion symptoms and was referred to the following health care providers (examination findings and interventions from a multidisciplinary team are provided):
- Referred to neurologist: headache management.
- Referral to sleep specialist for continued sleep disturbances
- Referral to psychologist for development of anxiety

- Referred to speech-language pathologist
  - Assessment findings
    - Impaired selective attention, alternating and divided attention per Test of Everyday Attention (TEA)
    - Impaired immediate memory, delayed memory on the Repeatable Battery for the Assessment of Neuropsychological Status (R-BANS) and the California Verbal Learning Test (CVLT-2)
  - Impaired executive functions per Functional Assessment of Verbal Reasoning and Executive Strategies
- Referred to Physical Therapist
  - Assessment findings
    - Oculomotor system
      - convergence insufficiency and slowed saccades
    - Vestibular system
      - Dynamic gaze stabilization
        - Impaired dynamic visual acuity testing
      - Motion sensitivity
        - Dizziness exacerbated by head turns in seated, standing, and walking activities
      - Balance assessment
        - Impaired vestibular functional test on sensory organization test
        - Unable to complete tandem walking with dual task
  - Cervical spine function
    - Musculoskeletal system
      - Reproduction of headaches with palpation of sub occipital musculature
      - Impaired active range of motion and passive accessory intervertebral motion for right rotation and extension in the mid to lower cervical spine
  - Sensorimotor system
    - Impaired cervical proprioception and head righting response

Examination and Intervention for Multidisciplinary Care Approach

Personnel	Examination Findings	Initial Intervention Provided
Neurologist	Posttraumatic headaches	Unclear whether posttraumatic headaches are posttraumatic migraine versus tension type headache. Conservative management through physical therapy as first-line management of headaches
Athletic trainer	Exercise intolerance on subsymptom exercise tolerance test: symptom exacerbation at 80% age-related heart rate maximum	Aerobic exercise at 70% heart rate maximum for 2 weeks prior to increasing to 80% heart rate maximum
Psychologist	Found to have posttraumatic anxiety and disrupted sleep	Cognitive behavioral therapy to begin addressing posttraumatic anxiety and sleep disturbances
Speech language pathologist	Impaired selective, alternating, divided attention. Impaired immediate memory, delayed memory. Impaired executive functions for identifying alternate solutions to problem, planning for task.	Cognitive-linguistic rehabilitation, with hierarchical approach and cueing, goal attainment scaling with patient goals for school
Physical therapist	Impaired dynamic visual acuity testing, motion sensitivity to self-motion, and dizziness exacerbated by head turns with seated, standing, and walking activities. Impaired vestibular contribution on sensory organization test and unable to complete tandem walking with dual task.	Dynamic gaze stabilization: VORx1 at a distance, seated Standing and walking with head turns Balance: tandem walking with EO/EC and with head turns
	Reproduction of headaches with palpation of suboccipital musculature. Impaired active range of motion and passive accessory intervertebral motion for right rotation and extension in the mid to lower cervical spine. Impaired cervical proprioception and head righting response.	Nonprovocative range-of-motion exercises, stretching and manual therapy for range of motion deficits. Sensory reweighting exercises for sensorimotor impairment.
Occupational therapist	Convergence insufficiency and slowed saccades	Convergence eye movement training (e.g., Brock string exercises). Basic scanning and searching exercises. Education on visual hygiene.

REFERENCES

To enhance this text and add value for the reader, all references are included on the companion Evolve site that accompanies this textbook. This online service will, when available, provide a link for the reader to a Medline abstract for the article cited. There are 472 cited references and other general references for this chapter, with the majority of those articles being evidence-based citations.

24

Movement Dysfunction Associated With Hemiplegia*

Susan D. Ryerson and Lauren F. Hurt

OBJECTIVES

After reading this chapter the student or therapist will be able to:
1. Identify the various types of neurovascular disease.
2. Identify the atypical patterns of movement in patients with residual hemiplegia.
3. Identify significant primary and secondary body system (impairments) that interfere with functional movement

patterns and limit ability to perform activities and participate in life.
4. Describe reeducation intervention strategies for improving functional activities in patients with hemiplegia.

KEY TERMS

aberrant movements
atypical movements
composite impairments
edema
evaluation of movement control
goal setting
hemiplegia

movement deficits
muscle activation deficits
orthoses
postural control
predictors of recovery
primary impairments
secondary impairments

shoulder pain
shoulder subluxation
standardized evaluations of function
trunk and arm linked movements
trunk and leg linked movements
trunk control
undesirable compensations

OVERVIEW

In this chapter, pathological conditions, body system problems (impairment), activity limitations, and intervention strategies for individuals with hemiplegia from stroke are reviewed. Although hemiplegia from neurovascular pathological conditions is the focus of the chapter, therapists can use this information and apply it to adults with hemiplegia caused by other central nervous system (CNS) pathological conditions, such as tumor, trauma, multiple sclerosis, and demyelinating diseases. Movement components and their relationship to functional performance are used as a basis for selection of therapy interventions.

Definition

Hemiplegia, a paralysis of one side of the body, is the classic sign of neurovascular disease of the brain. It is one of many manifestations of neurovascular disease, and it occurs with strokes involving the cerebral hemisphere or brain stem. A stroke, or cerebrovascular accident (CVA), results in a sudden, specific neurological deficit and occurs when a brain blood vessel is either occluded by a clot or bursts. It is the suddenness of this neurological deficit—occurring over seconds, minutes, hours, or a few days—that characterizes the disorder as vascular. Although the motor deficits of hemiplegia may be the most obvious sign of a CVA and a major concern of therapists, other symptoms are equally disabling, including sensory dysfunction, aphasia or dysarthria, and cognitive and behavioral impairments. CVAs can be classified according to location, size of lesion, pathological type—thrombosis, embolism, or hemorrhage—or according to temporal factors, such as completed stroke, stroke-in-evolution, or transient ischemic attacks (TIAs).

GENERAL MEDICAL ASSESSMENT

Epidemiology

In the United States, stroke is the fifth-ranking cause of death—nearly 133,000 people die each year—and is a leading cause of serious long-term disability.[1] The National Stroke Association estimates that 795,000 new or recurrent strokes occur each year: 610,000 are first attacks and 185,000 are recurrent attacks. The incidence of stroke rises rapidly with increasing age: two-thirds of all strokes occur in people older than the age of 65 years; and after the age of 55 years, the risk of stroke doubles every 10 years. With[1] the over-50-years age group growing rapidly, more people than ever are at risk. In the United States, the incidence of stroke is slightly greater in women than men. Stroke symptoms are more likely in blacks than whites, in those with lower income and educational status, and among people with fair to poor perceived health status. American Heart Association (AHA) projections demonstrate that from 2012 to 2030 there will be a 20.5% increase in stroke prevalence with the highest increase being in white Hispanic males.[1]

Cerebral infarction (thrombosis or embolism) is the most common form of stroke, accounting for 70% of all strokes. Hemorrhages account for another 20%, and 10% remain unspecified. Stroke is the largest single cause of neurological disability. Approximately 7.2 million

Americans have self-reported having a stroke and are dealing with impairments and disabilities from a stroke. Of these, 31% require assistance, 20% need help walking, 16% are in long-term care facilities, and 71% are vocationally impaired after 7 years. One study reported that 12% of subjects have complete functional arm recovery and 38% have some dexterity 6 months after stroke. In addition, loss of leg movement in the first week after stroke and no arm movement at 4 weeks are associated with poor outcomes at 6 months.[2]

The three most commonly recognized risk factors for cerebrovascular disease are hypertension, diabetes mellitus, and heart disease. Since the most important of these factors is hypertension, intensive blood pressure lowering is a critical factor in reducing stroke risk.[3] Because high blood pressure is the greatest risk factor for stroke, human characteristics and behaviors that increase blood pressure, including increased high serum cholesterol levels, obesity, diabetes mellitus, heavy alcohol consumption, cocaine use, and cigarette smoking, increase the risk of stroke. In addition, atrial fibrillation, an independent risk factor, increases the risk of stroke by 5 times.[4]

Ostfeld[5] noted that mortality rates for stroke declined, slowly at first (from 1900 to 1950) and then more quickly (from 1950 to 1970), with a sharp drop noted around 1974. From 1995 to 2005 the stroke death rate decreased by 30%. Experts have speculated that the greater use of hypertensive drugs in the 1960s and 1970s started this decline, and the creation of screening and treatment referral centers for high blood pressure may account for the continued marked decline.[4]

Outcome

The long-term follow-up on the Framingham Heart Study revealed that long-term stroke survivors, especially those with only one episode, have a good chance for full functional recovery.[6] For people left with severe neurological and functional deficits, studies have demonstrated that rehabilitation is effective and that it can improve functional ability.[7,8] It has been demonstrated that age is not a factor in determining the outcome of the rehabilitation process.[9] Currently it is thought that patients should be given an opportunity to participate in the rehabilitation process, regardless of age, unless it is medically contraindicated.

The prediction of ultimate functional outcome has been hampered by the heterogeneity of common stroke impairments and the diversity of commonly used predictors (medical items, income level, intelligence, functional level). Computed tomography (CT), magnetic resonance imaging, and regional cerebral blood flow studies are used to determine location and amount of insult for diagnosis, as predictors of functional recovery, and for research inclusion criteria.[2,10]

Pathoneurological and Pathophysiological Aspects
Classification

The pathological processes that result from a CVA can be divided into three groups—thrombotic changes, embolic changes, and hemorrhagic changes.

Thrombotic infarction. Atherosclerotic plaques and hypertension interact to produce cerebrovascular infarcts. These plaques form at branchings and curves of the arteries. Plaques usually form in front of the first major branching of the cerebral arteries. These lesions can be present for 30 years or more and may never become symptomatic. Intermittent blockage may proceed to permanent damage. The process by which a thrombus occludes an artery requires several hours and explains the division between stroke-in-evolution and completed stroke.[11]

TIAs are an indication of the presence of thrombotic disease and are the result of transient ischemia. Although the cause of TIAs has not been definitively established, cerebral vasospasm and transient systemic arterial hypotension are thought to be responsible factors.

Embolic infarction. The embolus that causes the stroke may come from the heart, from an internal carotid artery thrombosis, or from an

atheromatous plaque of the carotid sinus. It is usually a sign of cardiac disease. The branches of the middle cerebral artery are infarcted most commonly as a result of its direct continuation from the internal carotid artery. Collateral blood supply is not established with embolic infarctions because of the speed of obstruction formation, so there is less survival of tissue distal to the area of embolic infarct than with thrombotic infarct.[2]

Hemorrhage. The most common intracranial hemorrhages causing stroke are those resulting from hypertension, ruptured saccular aneurysm, and arteriovenous (AV) malformation. Massive hemorrhage frequently results from hypertensive cardiac-renal disease; bleeding into the brain tissue produces an oval or round mass that displaces midline structures. The exact mechanism of hemorrhage is not known. This mass of extravasated blood decreases in size over 6 to 8 months.

Saccular, or berry, aneurysms are thought to be the result of defects in the media and elastica that develop over years. This muscular defect plus overstretching of the internal elastic membrane from blood pressure causes the aneurysm to develop. Saccular aneurysms are found at branchings of major cerebral arteries, especially the anterior portion of the circle of Willis. Averaging 8 to 10 mm in diameter and variable in form, these aneurysms rupture at their dome. Saccular aneurysms are rare in childhood.

AV malformations are developmental abnormalities that result in a spaghetti-like mass of dilated AV fistulas varying in size from a few millimeters in diameter to huge masses located within the brain tissue. Some of these blood vessels have extremely thin, abnormally structured walls. Although the abnormality is present from birth, symptoms usually develop at ages 10 to 35 years. The hemorrhage of an AV malformation presents a pathological picture similar to that for the saccular aneurysm. The larger AV malformations frequently occur in the posterior half of the cerebral hemisphere.[12]

Clinical Findings

The focal neurological deficit resulting from a stroke, whether embolic, thrombotic, or hemorrhagic, is a reflection of the size and location of the lesion and the amount of collateral blood flow. Unilateral neurological deficits result from interruption of the carotid vascular system, and bilateral neurological deficits result from interruption of the vascular supply to the basilar system. Clinical syndromes resulting from occlusion or hemorrhage in the cerebral circulation vary from partial to complete. Signs of hemorrhage may be more variable as a result of the effect of extension to surrounding brain tissue and the possible rise in intracranial pressure (ICP). Table 24.1 summarizes the clinical symptoms and the anatomical structures involved according to specific arterial involvement.

The frequencies of the three types of cerebrovascular disease—thrombosis, embolism, and hemorrhage—vary according to whether they were taken from a clinical study or from an autopsy study, but they rank in the order presented in this section. The clinical symptoms and laboratory findings for each type are condensed in Table 24.2.

Medical Management and Pharmacological Considerations
Acute Medical Care

Evaluation. Assessment for severity of symptoms, time of onset, and differentiation of type of stroke as ischemic or hemorrhagic is critical in medical decision making. Speech difficulty and hemiparesis are the most common symptoms of an ischemic stroke. Facial weakness, arm or leg numbness, confusion, headache, and nonorthostatic dizziness may also occur. Severe and sudden headache is the

TABLE 24.1   Clinical Symptoms of Vascular Lesions

Affected Vessel	Clinical Symptoms	Structures Involved
Middle cerebral artery	Contralateral paralysis and sensory deficit	Somatic motor area
	Motor speech impairment	Broca area (dominant hemisphere)
	"Central" aphasia, anomia, jargon speech	Parieto-occipital cortex (dominant hemisphere)
	Unilateral neglect, apraxia, impaired ability to judge distance	Parietal lobe (nondominant hemisphere)
	Homonymous hemianopia	
	Loss of conjugate gaze to opposite side	Optic radiation deep to second temporal convolution
	Avoidance reaction of opposite limbs	Frontal controversial field
	Pure motor hemiplegia	Parietal lobe
	Limb—kinetic apraxia	Upper portion of posterior limb of internal capsule Premotor or parietal cortex
Anterior cerebral artery	Paralysis—lower extremity	Motor area-leg
	Paresis in opposite arm	Arm area of cortex
	Cortical sensory loss	Post central gyrus
	Urinary incontinence	Posteromedial aspect of superior frontal gyrus Medial surface of posterior frontal lobe
	Contralateral grasp reflex, sucking reflex	Uncertain
	Lack of spontaneity, motor inaction, echolalia	Uncertain
	Perseveration and amnesia	Supplemental motor area
Posterior cerebral artery		
Peripheral area	Homonymous hemianopia	Calcarine cortex or optic radiation
	Bilateral homonymous hemianopia, cortical blindness, inability to perceive objects not centrally located, ocular apraxia	Bilateral occipital lobe
	Memory defect	Inferomedial portions of temporal lobe
	Topographical disorientation	Nondominant calcarine and lingual gyri
Central area	Thalamic syndrome	Posteroventral nucleus of thalamus
	Weber syndrome	Cranial nerve III and cerebral peduncle
	Contralateral hemiplegia	Cerebral peduncle
	Paresis of vertical eye movements, sluggish pupillary response to light	Supranuclear fibers to cranial nerve III
	Contralateral ataxia or postural tremor	
Internal carotid artery	Variable signs according to degree and site of occlusion— middle cerebral, anterior cerebral, posterior cerebral territory	Uncertain
Basilar artery	Ataxia	Middle and superior cerebellar peduncle
Superior cerebellar artery	Dizziness, nausea, vomiting, horizontal nystagmus	Vestibular nucleus
	Horner syndrome on opposite side, decreased pain and thermal sensation	Descending sympathetic fibers Spinal thalamic tract
	Decreased touch, vibration, position sense of lower extremity greater than that of upper extremity	Medial lemniscus
	Nystagmus, vertigo, nausea, vomiting	Vestibular nerve
Anterior inferior cerebellar artery	Facial paralysis on same side	Cranial nerve VII
	Tinnitus	Auditory nerve, lower cochlear nucleus
	Ataxia	Middle cerebral peduncle
	Impaired facial sensation on same side	Fifth cranial nerve nucleus
	Decreased pain and thermal sensation on opposite side	Spinal thalamic tract

Continued

TABLE 24.1	Clinical Symptoms of Vascular Lesions—cont'd	
Affected Vessel	**Clinical Symptoms**	**Structures Involved**
Complete basilar syndrome	Bilateral long tract signs with cerebellar and cranial nerve abnormalities	
	Coma	
	Quadriplegia	
	Pseudobulbar palsy	
	Cranial nerve abnormalities	
Vertebral artery	Decreased pain and temperature on opposite side	Spinal thalamic tract
	Sensory loss from a tactile and proprioceptive	Medial lemniscus
	Hemiparesis of arm and leg	Pyramidal tract
	Facial pain and numbness on same side	Descending tract and fifth cranial nucleus
	Horner syndrome, ptosis, decreased sweating	Descending sympathetic tract
	Ataxia	Spinal cerebellar tract
	Paralysis of tongue	Cranial nerve XII
	Weakness of vocal cord, decreased gag	Cranial nerves IX and X
	Hiccups	Uncertain

Modified from Adams RD, Victor M. *Principles of Neurology.* New York: McGraw-Hill; 1981.

TABLE 24.2	Clinical Symptoms and Laboratory Findings for Neurovascular Disease	
Disease Type	**Clinical Picture**	**Laboratory Findings**
THROMBOSIS	*Extremely variable* Preceded by a prodromal episode Uneven progression Onset develops within minutes or hours or over days ("thrombus in evolution") 60% occur during sleep—patient awakens unaware of problem, rises, and falls to floor Usually no headache, but may occur in mild form Hypertension, diabetes, or vascular disease elsewhere in body	Cerebrospinal fluid pressure is normal Cerebrospinal fluid is clear Electroencephalogram: limited differential diagnostic value Skull radiographs not helpful Arteriography is definitive procedure; demonstrates site of collateral flow CT scan helpful in chronic state when cavitation has occurred
Transient ischemic attack (TIA)	Linked to atherosclerotic thrombosis Preceded or accompanied by stroke Occur by themselves Last 2–30 min A few attacks or hundreds are experienced Normal neurological examination findings between attacks If transient symptoms are present on awakening, may indicate future stroke	Usually none
EMBOLISM	*Extremely variable*	
Cardiac	Occurs extremely rapidly—seconds or minutes	Generally same as for thrombosis except for the following:
Noncardiac	There are no warnings	If embolism causes a large hemorrhagic infarct, cerebrospinal fluid will be bloody
Atherosclerosis Pulmonary thrombosis Fat, tumor, air	Branches of middle cerebral artery are involved most frequently; large embolus will block internal carotid artery or stem of middle cerebral artery If embolus is in basilar system, deep coma and total paralysis may result Often a manifestation of heart disease, including atrial fibrillation and myocardial infarction Headache As embolus passes through artery, patient may have neurological deficits that resolve as embolus breaks and passes into small artery supplying small or silent brain area	30% of embolic strokes produce small hemorrhagic infarct without bloody cerebrospinal fluid

TABLE 24.2 Clinical Symptoms and Laboratory Findings for Neurovascular Disease—cont'd		
Disease Type	**Clinical Picture**	**Laboratory Findings**
HEMORRHAGE		
Hypertensive hemorrhage	Severe headache	CT scan can detect hemorrhages larger than 1.5 cm in cerebral and cerebellar hemispheres; it is diagnostically superior to arteriography; it is especially helpful in diagnosing small hemorrhages that do not spill blood into cerebrospinal fluid; with massive hemorrhage and increased pressure, cerebrospinal fluid is grossly bloody; lumbar puncture is necessary when CT scan is not available
	Vomiting at onset	
	Blood pressure >170/90; usually from "essential" hypertension but can be from other types	
	Abrupt onset, usually during day, not in sleep	
	Gradually evolves over hours or days according to speed of bleeding	
	No recurrence of bleeding	Radiographs occasionally show midline shift (this is not true with infarction)
	Frequency in blacks with hypertensive hemorrhage is greater than frequency in whites	Electroencephalogram shows no typical pattern, but high voltage and slow waves are most common with hemorrhage
	Hemorrhaged blood absorbs slowly—rapid improvement of symptoms is not usual	Urinary changes may reflect renal disease
	If massive hemorrhage occurs, the individual may survive a few hours or days as a result of brain stem compression	
Ruptured saccular aneurysm	Asymptomatic before rupture	CT scan detects localized blood in hydrocephalus if present
	With rupture, blood spills under high pressure into subarachnoid space	Cerebrospinal fluid is extremely bloody
	Excruciating headache with loss of consciousness	Radiographs are usually negative
	Headache without loss of consciousness	Carotid and vertebral arteriography is performed only when diagnosis is certain
	Sudden loss of consciousness	
	Decerebrate rigidity with coma	
	If severe—persistent deep coma with respiratory arrest, circulatory collapse leading to death; death can occur within 5 min	
	If mild—consciousness regained within hours then confusion, amnesia, headache, stiff neck, drowsiness	
	Hemiplegia, paresis, homonymous hemianopia, or aphasia usually absent	

CT, Computed tomography; *TIA,* transient ischemic attack.
Modified from Adams RD, Victor M. *Principles of Neurology.* New York: McGraw-Hill; 1981.

most common symptom of a hemorrhagic stroke. Hemorrhagic strokes may also present with gradual development of reduced consciousness, vomiting, and hemiparesis. A neurological exam will help quantify the severity of symptoms by assessing mental status, focal weakness of the arm, leg and/or face, speech impairments, gait impairments, impaired eye movements, and visuospatial perceptual impairments. The National Institutes of Health Stroke Scale (NIHSS) is highly recommended due to its diagnostic and prognostic power of stroke severity. Additionally, imaging should be performed for differential diagnosis of other conditions as well as to differentiate the type of stroke as ischemic or hemorrhagic. Noncontrast head CT will help rule out hemorrhagic origin while an MRI is more sensitive for identifying ischemic stroke.[13] Other tests that may be performed include blood glucose, renal function, electrocardiogram (ECG), complete blood count, oxygen saturation, toxicology screen, blood alcohol level, and electroencephalography (EEG). Additionally, continuous cardiac monitoring is strongly recommended for a minimum of 24 hours.[13]

Ischemic stroke. Although infarcted tissue cannot at present be restored, medical management of the acute stroke from thrombosis or TIA is geared toward improving the cerebral circulation as quickly as possible to prevent ischemic tissue from becoming infarcted tissue. Cells that have 80% to 100% ischemia will die in a few minutes because they cannot produce energy, specifically adenosine triphosphate. This energy failure results in an activation of calcium, which

causes a chain reaction resulting in cell death. Around this area of infarction is a transitional area, the penumbra, where the blood flow is decreased 50% to 80%. Cells in the transitional area are not irreversibly damaged.[14,15]

An established pharmaceutical approach to acute ischemic stroke management is tissue plasminogen activator (t-PA) (see Chapter 36). t-PA must be given within 3 hours of symptom onset but is most effective if used within the first 90 to 180 minutes. It is absolutely contraindicated for hemorrhagic stroke. Permissive hypertension is often prescribed to assist with improving perfusion beyond the clot to limit the area of penumbra. Cerebral edema, if present, is managed pharmacologically during the first few days. Antiplatelet drugs such as aspirin are used to prevent clotting by decreasing platelet "stickiness" following TIA and/or within 24 to 48 hours following ischemic stroke.[13]

Endovascular surgical intervention may be indicated for ischemic stroke to remove/reduce the blood clot. Areas accessible to and suitable for surgery include the carotid sinus and the common carotid, innominate, and subclavian arteries. Although both surgery and anticoagulant therapy are used for TIAs, recently Ropper extensively reviewed the wide divergence of opinions.[12]

For individuals who have had a stroke yet recovered quickly and well, medical care focuses on prevention of recurrent stroke. Prevention usually includes maintaining blood pressure and blood flow, monitoring hypotensive agents (if given), and avoiding oversedation, especially for sleep, to prevent cerebral ischemia. Long-term anticoagulant therapy is effective in preventing embolic infarction in persons with cardiac problems such as atrial fibrillation, myocardial infarction, and valve prostheses.

Hemorrhagic stroke. Medical management to reduce ICP includes sedation, hyperosmolar agents, and hyperventilation. Surgical interventions including decompressive craniotomy and craniectomy are recommended only under extreme circumstances of rapid deterioration or if the ICP is not responding to other efforts. Following surgical intervention, medical management consists of lowering arterial blood pressures. Pharmaceutical management of hypertension for hemorrhagic stroke differs from that of ischemic stroke with an emphasis on reducing blood pressure as quickly as possible to reduce bleeding. Antiseizure medication may be used. Often a systemic anti-fibrinolysin is given to impede lysis of the clot at the site of rupture. Vasospasms are a common secondary condition following subarachnoid hemorrhage (SAH). Vasospasms result in secondary cerebral ischemia following the initial hemorrhage and result in increased morbidity and mortality. Nimodipine is considered a first-line drug to reduce the risk of vasospasm.[16]

Regardless of the type of the stroke, individuals who are comatose are managed by (1) treatment of shock; (2) maintenance of clear airway and oxygen flow; (3) measurement of arterial blood gases, blood analysis, CT, and spinal tap; and (4) control of seizures. Hypertensive hemorrhage is one of the most common vascular causes of coma.[17]

Recent studies indicate that 42% of patients who have sustained a stroke wait 24 hours before getting care, with the average being 13 hours.[15] The importance of community-wide programs to increase awareness of symptoms and effectiveness of emergency medical responses is immense in order to administer t-PA for best possible outcomes. The American Heart Association and the National Stroke Association are creating community campaigns to increase awareness of the medical emergency nature of stroke symptoms. These campaigns encourage people to call 911 immediately when any of the following warning signs, entitled BEFAST, occur:

Balance – trouble walking, dizziness, loss of balance or coordination

Eyes – trouble seeing with one or both eyes

Face – numbness or weakness of the face

Arm – numbness or weakness of the arm (or leg) especially on one side of the body.

Speech – confusion or trouble speaking and/or understanding

Time – call 911 immediately

Medical Management of Associated Problems

Spasticity. Research findings have refuted the earlier belief that spasticity is the cause of the atypical movement patterns in people with CNS dysfunction.[18,19] Spasticity, a reflex measured by velocity dependent stretch in the passive state, is an indication of damage to the CNS. The term "spasticity" is often used synonymously with hypertonicity, a resistance to passive stretch that is not velocity-dependent. Its treatment constitutes a major medical problem after stroke because patients complain about it and physicians continue to treat it aggressively. The pharmacological and surgical means are examined here, and therapy management is discussed later.

Two types of drugs are used to counter the effects of spasticity: centrally acting and peripherally acting agents. Centrally acting drugs, such as diazepam, have been used to depress the lateral reticular formation and thus its facilitatory action on the gamma motor neurons. This form of drug is used widely to treat spasticity, although the greatest disadvantage of centrally acting drugs is that they depress the entire CNS. Drowsiness and anxiety are common side effects.

Peripherally acting drugs are used to block a specific link in the gamma group. Procaine blocks selectively inhibit the small gamma motor fibers, resulting in a relaxation of intrafusal fibers. The effect of procaine blocks is transient. Intramuscular neurolysis with the injection of 5% to 7% phenol has been used to destroy the small intramuscular mixed nerve branches.[20] Phenol blocks relieve hypertonicity and improve function, especially when followed by an intensive course of therapy.[21] It can provide relief for 2 to 12 months, and the effects have been documented to last as long as 3 years.[20,21] Disadvantages of phenol use include its toxicity to tissue and the complications of pain that occasionally result.[22]

Botulinum toxin type A (Botox) is also used to decrease the effects of spasticity on functional movement in hemiplegia.[23–25] Local[26] injection of the toxin into spastic muscles produces selective weakness by interfering with the uptake of acetylcholine by the motor end plate. The effect of the toxin is temporary, depends on the amount injected, and is associated with minimal side effects. Repeat injections are recommended no sooner than 12 to 14 weeks to avoid antibody formation to the toxin. Researchers report positive functional results when botulinum toxin A injections are followed by intensive muscle reeducation and appropriate splinting.[26]

Dantrolene sodium is used to interrupt the excitation-contraction mechanism of skeletal muscles. Trials have shown that it has reduced spasticity in 60% to 80% of individuals while improving function in 40% of these patients. The side effects—drowsiness, weakness, and fatigue—can be decreased through titration of dosage. Serious side effects, including hepatotoxicity, precipitation of seizures, and lymphocytic lymphoma, have been reported when the drug has been used in high doses over a long time.[27]

Baclofen, in pill form, is used as a skeletal muscle relaxant to decrease spasticity. It can now be delivered intrathecally into the spinal cord with a pump that is surgically inserted into the body. It relieves spasticity with a small amount of medication (10 mg/20 mL, 10 mg/5 mL). Intrathecal baclofen has had dramatic results in cases of severe spasticity because it acts directly on the affected muscles instead of circulating in the blood. It is used for extremity spasticity that interferes with the ability to assume functional positions in patients with severe stroke, multiple sclerosis, head injury, and cerebral palsy.[28]

The surgical treatment of spasticity through tenotomy or neurectomy is considered when all other treatments fail, and it is used to correct deformity, especially of a hand or foot. A peripheral nerve block is often used as a diagnostic tool to evaluate the effect of surgical treatment. If anatomical or functional gains are made through a temporary nerve block, consideration is given to surgical release. The surgical treatment of spasticity does not necessarily result in increased movement control and, with the increased understanding of the causes of spasticity, does not seem appropriate in stroke.

Seizures. The highest risk for seizure after a stroke is immediately after the event; 57% of seizures occur in the first week and 88% occur within the first year.[29] Seizures after thrombotic and embolic stroke are usually of early onset, whereas seizures after hemorrhagic stroke are of late onset.[30] The management of seizures after stroke is usually with antiseizure medication. Commonly used drugs include phenytoin (Dilantin), carbamazepine (Tegretol), gabapentin (Neurontin), and divalproex (Depakote).[31] Side effects that interfere with movement therapy include drowsiness, ataxia, distractibility, and poor memory.

Respiratory involvement. Fatigue is a major problem for the person with hemiplegia. This fatigability, which interferes with everyday life processes and active rehabilitation, is attributed to respiratory insufficiency resulting from paralysis of one side of the thorax. Haas and colleagues[32] studied respiratory function in hemiplegia and found decreased lung volume and mechanical performance of the thorax to be significant factors, in addition to abnormal pulmonary diffusing capacity. Individuals with hemiplegia consume 50% more oxygen while walking slowly (regardless of the presence or absence of orthotic devices) than subjects without hemiplegia.[32] The decreased respiratory output and the increased oxygen demand that result from atypical movement patterns are responsible for early fatigue in persons with hemiplegia. Treatment objectives and techniques must reflect the understanding of this respiratory problem. For patients who walk at velocities greater than 0.48 m/s, a gain in walking capacity is associated with an increased peak Vo_2. Research exploring the role of exercise after stroke indicate that gains in respiratory fitness were associated with increased walking capacity. In clinical practice, therapists should remember to include standard respiratory measures and functions to evaluate the efficacy of treatment techniques.[33]

Stroke fatigue syndrome. Another potential cause of fatigue following stroke is Stroke Fatigue Syndrome or post-stroke fatigue. Although its etiology is not well understood, post-stroke fatigue is reported in 23% to 75% of Individuals following a stroke. It is known to reduce the quality of life and increase the risk of death in those who experience it. Research related to etiology and intervention for prevention and treatment is relatively new. Suspected mechanisms under current research include biological, psychosocial, and behavioral causes. Suggested interventions under recent and current investigation include pharmacological agents such as antidepressants and stimulants; psychological approaches including cognitive behavioral therapy and educational programming; and physical training including graded aerobic training. A recent systematic review indicated continued, high-quality research is needed to identify the most effective treatment intervention strategy.[34]

Cardiovascular health. In the chronic stage of recovery, Patients may have significant cardiovascular deconditioning with half the fitness levels of age-matched controls. This decrease in fitness affects the performance of daily activities and adds to these patients' morbidity and mortality risk. This decreased fitness results in part from decreased mobility of the leg, muscular atrophy, altered muscle physiology, increased muscular fat, and altered peripheral blood flow.[35,36]

Fractures. If the patient with hemiplegia has severe extremity or trunk weakness and relies heavily on the nonparetic extremities for function, poor balance and falls are possible. After a stroke the risk of hip fracture is greatest in the first year of recovery. Eighty percent of hip fractures occur on the paretic side and are the result of bone loss or falls.[37] In addition, other common fracture sites are the humerus and wrist.

Therapy intervention for a hip fracture with a hemiplegia is complicated by increased difficulty sustaining a symmetrical trunk posture over the fractured hip, decreased strength in the leg, pain, and spasticity. In addition to the loss of balance and protective mechanisms, the development of osteoporosis from disuse is a limiting factor for functional recovery after a fracture.[38]

Thrombophlebitis. Thrombophlebitis may occur in the acute and subacute stages of recovery and rehabilitation. Deep vein thrombosis is caused by altered blood flow, damage to the vessel wall, and changes in blood coagulation times. The vascular changes are aggravated by the inactivity and dependent postures of the weak extremities. Deep vein thrombosis is many times more common in the weaker leg.[39]

Complex regional pain syndrome. Formerly known as reflex sympathetic dystrophy, *complex regional pain syndrome* is a chronic pain condition affecting the paretic arm or leg. The extremity pain is reported as intense and burning and may be accompanied by swelling and redness. It leads to changes in bone and skin and, if left untreated, becomes debilitating. Medical treatment includes the use of chemical sympathetic blocks and oral or intramuscular corticosteroids. The use of blocks and corticosteroids often stops the burning pain. The length of time of the relief varies from patient to patient. Adverse reactions from blocks and corticosteroids occur about 20% of the time.[40,41]

Pain. The pharmacological management of joint pain after stroke (usually shoulder pain) includes the local injection of corticosteroids.

Sequential Stages of Recovery From Acute to Adaptive Phase
Evolution of Recovery Process

The evolution of the recovery process from onset to the return to community life can be divided into three stages—acute, active (rehabilitation), and adaptation to personal environment. The acute state involves the stroke-in-evolution, the completed stroke, or the TIA and the decision whether to hospitalize.

The stroke-in-evolution develops gradually with distinct demarcation of the damaged area over 6 to 24 hours. Thrombosis, the most common cause of stroke, results first in ischemia and finally in infarction. If ischemic tissue can be treated and saved before infarction occurs, the neurological damage may be reversible. Small hemorrhages also may become a stroke-in-evolution by effusing blood along nerve pathways and by attracting fluid.[42,43] A completed stroke has a sudden onset and produces distinct, nonprogressive symptoms and damage within minutes or hours. In contrast, the TIA has a brief duration of neurological deficit and spontaneous resolution with no residual signs. TIAs vary in number and duration.

The physician decides the extent of hospitalization. The trend to hospitalize is more common today than years ago.[44] However,[43] a mild stroke or TIA may produce minimal physical and mental symptoms, and the person may not even seek medical help. Cost-containment measures in hospitals and managed care have led to decreased lengths of stay and the development of critical pathway plans to deliver services more efficiently. The inpatient length of stay for acute stroke is currently around 5 days. After the inpatient stay, the patient follows one of four typical pathways: a return home with or without home care services, a rehabilitation hospital stroke unit stay, a subacute facility stay until able to tolerate a rehabilitation regimen, or to a long-term care facility for rehabilitation or maintenance care.

Once the stroke is completed, the clinical symptoms begin to decrease in severity. A person with a stroke caused by an embolic episode may have symptoms that reverse completely in a few days; more frequently, however, improvement occurs noticeably at first and then more slowly with varying degrees of functional recovery. The fatality rate is high within the first day but decreases substantially in the following months of recovery.[43] Evidence from efficacy studies of rehabilitation programs that aim at improving functional performance is limited. Studies by Bamford and colleagues indicate that early rehabilitation intervention reduces disability and improves compensatory strategies.[45]

The Framingham Heart Study has revealed that long-term stroke survivors have a good chance of returning to independent living. The greatest deficit in persons with hemiplegia who have recovered basic motor skills and who have returned home is in the psychosocial and environmental areas.[6]

Recovery of Motor Function

Recovery of motor function after a stroke was thought historically to be complete 3 to 6 months after onset. More recent research has shown that functional recovery from a stroke can continue for months or years.[46,47] Measuring recovery is difficult because the definition of "successful" or "complete" recovery varies greatly. Duncan reports that if recovery is defined at the disability level (Barthel score >90), 57% of stroke survivors have a complete recovery. However, if impairments are measured, less than 37% recover fully. If recovery is related to prior physical functioning, less than 25% are considered completely recovered.[48]

The initial functional gains after the stroke are attributed to reduction of cerebral edema, absorption of damaged tissue, and improved local vascular flow. However, these factors do not play a role in long-term functional recovery. The brain damage that results from a stroke is thought to be circumvented rather than "repaired" during the process of functional recovery. The CNS reacts to injury with a variety of potentially reparative morphological processes. Two mechanisms underlying functional recovery after stroke are collateral sprouting and the unmasking of neuropathways: regeneration and reorganization.[46] Research continues to provide important insights into the fundamental capabilities of the brain to respond to damage. Methods of intervention that use the environment and help the patient learn lead to long-term improved recovery.

The CNS has some predictable traits in response to injury. Twitchell, in his classic study, first documented the initial loss of voluntary function.[49] Although paralysis with flaccidity initially exists, there is seldom, if ever, total paralysis. He reported both an increase in deep tendon reflexes after 48 hours and the emergence of synergistic patterns of movement.[50] The synergistic movement patterns of the upper extremity and lower extremity have been described in detail by many.[51–53] Verbal description of a visual phenomenon often leads to differences in written and spoken communication, yet the visual array or behavioral patterns may be exactly the same.[54] Although it is stated that the leg recovers more quickly or better than the arm, a leg that is bound by an extensor synergy and that is as "rigid as a pillar" during gait has not recovered more quickly and has no better function than an arm that is flexed and held across the chest and that can only grasp in a gross pattern with no ability to manipulate or release.

Although studies continue to investigate the exact nature of the relationship between voluntary movement and spasticity, clinical evidence demonstrates that as voluntary function increases, the dependence on synergistic movement decreases.[19] With the knowledge that the CNS is capable of reacting to injury with a variety of morphological processes, we should no longer view the effect of a stroke as a fixed event. Because the brain immediately institutes neuromechanisms that reconstitute typical functions, therapy interventions should emphasize use of movement patterns on the affected side to maximize return and to help the patient achieve the highest level of function.

Predictors of Recovery

Research in motor recovery shows that although motor recovery may continue after 6 months, the functional status usually remains constant, and that 86% of the variance in 6-month recovery is predictable at 1 month.[55]

It would be useful to be able to predict recovery of functional activities both for intervention planning and to allow efficient utilization of post-stroke care. However, there are few multivariate models that take into account the various data points that must be taken into account: clinical, neurophysiological, and neuroimaging.[56,57]

Existing predictive studies that use clinical measures give us a general idea. In one study, although 58% of the patients regained independence in ADLs and 82% learned to walk, 30% to 60% of patients had no arm function.[58] Initial return of movement in the first 2 weeks is one indicator of the possibility of full arm recovery. However, failure to recover grip strength before 24 days was correlated with no recovery of arm function at 3 months.[57,58] In another study that used the modified Rankin scale as the outcome measure, half of the patients recovered within 18 months with the greatest amount of recovery present at the 6-month mark. Predictors of recovery in this group included stroke severity, no previous ischemic stroke, peripheral artery disease, or diabetes.[59]

As clinicians we can help minimize the problems in research methods by precisely formulating functional goals, stating movement components and significant impairments that interfere with functional performance, and following a model when making clinical decisions to postulate cause and effect during intervention.[60]

Classification of Atypical Movement Patterns

Although the *Guide to Physical Therapist Practice* groups patients with neurological dysfunction according to pathological condition, therapy intervention rarely is directed by the diagnosis of stroke and resultant hemiplegia.[60] The WHO classification system, the International Classification of Function (ICF-2), provides a model that allows us to consider multiple factors that impact our interventions: body function/structure, activity, and participation limitations as well as personal and environmental factors.[61,62]

Although the main focus of this chapter is the evaluation and treatment of activity limitations and impairments resulting from a loss of movement control, a stroke may result in damage to other systems that affect the patient's ability to perform functional skills. There may be deficiencies in sensory processing (vision, somesthetic sensation, and vestibular systems) and disorders of cognitive integration (arousal and attention, awareness of disability, memory, problem solving, and learning), which all have a large impact on functional retraining. Depression and, most important, problems of language and communication also affect the patient's ability to participate in a therapy program.

Impairments Contributing to Activity and Participation Limitations

Individuals with hemiplegia from stroke have movement problems—impairments—that lead to activity and participation limitations. These movement problems manifest themselves as loss of movement in the trunk and extremities, atypical patterns of movement, and involuntary nonpurposeful movements of the affected side that lead to compensatory functional strategies. These impairments interfere with normal functional movements and may lead to loss of independence in daily life.

Impairments are the signs, symptoms, and physical findings that relate to a specific disease pathology. Schenkman and Butler were among the first to apply a model of impairments to neurological physical therapy practice. Ryerson and Levit, using a similar format, specifically defined the impairment categories as primary, secondary, and composite (Box 24.1).[63,64]

Primary and secondary impairments. Primary impairments are a direct result of the brain damage and are present immediately. Secondary impairments develop over time and in body systems not originally affected by the brain lesion.

Composite impairments. Composite impairments are the combined effects of the primary and secondary impairments, stage of motor recovery, previous treatment, and behavioral factors.

The composite impairment category used in this chapter has three generalized movement patterns that create one model of classification: (1) movement deficits, (2) atypical movements, and (3) undesirable compensatory patterns.[63]

Movement deficits result from severe neurological weakness with either gradual, balanced return or no significant return. Functional movement patterns and levels of independence are based on the distribution and amount of return: trunk control greater than extremity control, extremity control greater than trunk control, distal extremity return greater than proximal extremity return or vice versa, and arm control greater than leg control or vice versa. These individuals do not have problems with hypertonicity but, when neurological weakness is severe, have long-term problems with the secondary impairments of muscle shortening and loss of joint range.

In the acute stage, the arm hangs by the side, the humerus is internally rotated, the elbow is extended, and the forearm is pronated. Inferior shoulder subluxation is common. The trunk is weak, the ribs flare, and spinal alignment is impaired: a convex lateral curve is seen

BOX 24.1   Impairments That Interfere With Functional Movement

Primary Impairments

Neurological weakness

Changes in muscle activation
- Initiation/cessation
- Difficulty sequencing patterns of muscle activity within an extremity
- Inappropriate timing of muscle activation
- Altered force production

Changes in sensation
- Touch
- Proprioception

Changes in muscle tone
- Hypotonicity
- Hypertonicity

Secondary Impairments

Changes in alignment and mobility

Changes in muscle and soft tissue length

Pain

Edema

Composite Impairments

Movement deficits

Atypical movements

Undesirable compensations

Modified from Ryerson S, Levit K. *Functional Movement Reeducation: A Contemporary Model for Stroke Rehabilitation.* New York: Churchill Livingstone; 1997.

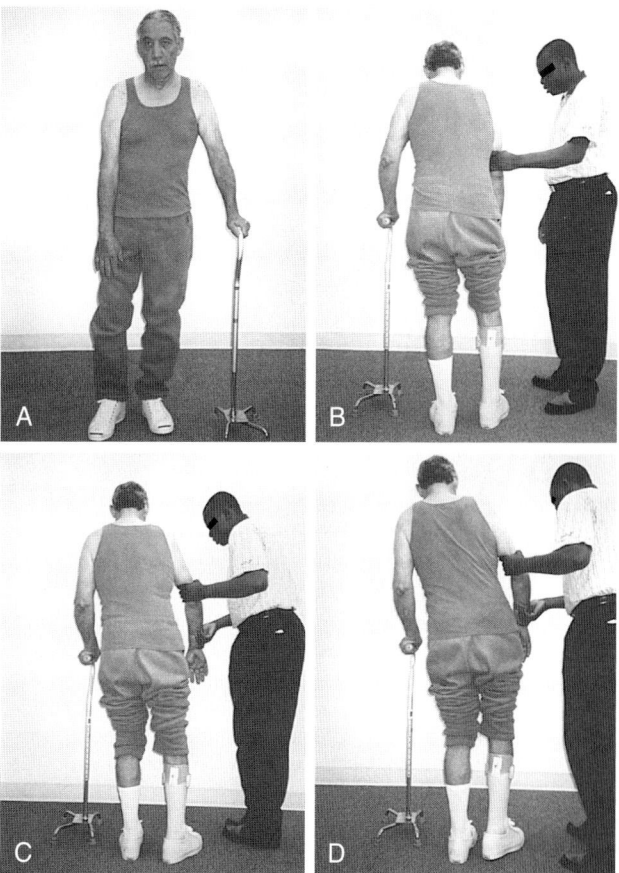

Fig. 24.1 **(A)** Patient with right hemiplegia. Movement deficit: neurological weakness (lack of initiation); patient was unable to move arm or leg in standing or sitting. **(B)** Patient uses cane and tries to shift to the right as he gets ready to step forward with the left leg. Note how the heavy weight of the right arm pulls the upper body into forward flexion and rotation left. **(C)** Patient prepares to step forward with the right leg. Note that his attendant has corrected his upper-body position. **(D)** Patient leans heavily onto cane (his upper body translates laterally to the left) to lessen weight on the right leg. He will accomplish the "step" by rotating his upper body to the left, a compensation for the loss of leg control in standing.

on the affected side. In standing, the patient has problems recruiting sufficient force production in the affected leg to counteract the downward pull of gravity. The pelvis lists downward, the hip and knee flex, and the ankle moves into plantarflexion. As the patient relearns to walk, the hip and knee may remain in flexion from weakness or the patient may compensate and push/lock the knee into extension.

A reliance on a cane for balance and the accompanying compensatory weight shift of the upper body onto a cane results in the use of pelvic elevation for swing initiation (Figs. 24.1 and 24.2).

Atypical movement patterns are found in patients with unbalanced muscle return and deficits of muscle activation not only in initiation/cessation, but also sequencing and timing. Atypical movements are movements that deviate from normal patterns of muscle coordination. They use patterns of muscle activation and sequences of joint movement that deviate from normal muscle synergies or biomechanical rules. Atypical movement patterns develop as a consequence of primary and secondary impairments. When motor recovery is incomplete, patients use the muscles that are available to produce movement. During attempts at functional activities, patients' movement patterns may occur with excessive effort and cocontraction (Fig. 24.3).

Undesirable compensatory patterns are patterns of function that may arise from either of the two previously described movement categories. Compensations are alternative movements or movement substitutions used to circumvent the challenge to the impaired side during daily activities. Although compensatory movements may be necessary and desirable to achieve the highest level of activity performance when there is no ability for recovery to occur, some may be more desirable than others. Undesirable compensatory patterns are noticeably one-sided; they rely on movements of the uninvolved arm and leg and are accompanied by asymmetrical postural trunk movements. They lead to unsafe patterns, or to secondary impairments, or

contribute to strategies that may have the potential to block or hinder future motor recovery. These undesirable compensatory patterns create "learned nonuse" of the affected arm and leg and foster asymmetrical postural patterns. Recent research findings indicate that limiting compensatory trunk movements may actually increase the performance of arm-reaching activities.[65]

Patients in the subacute to chronic phase of recovery who come into therapy with strongly established undesirable compensatory patterns do not respond quickly to any type of intervention. Although therapists may be tempted to train a one-sided pattern in early rehabilitation to quickly meet a stated goal, the long-term effects of learned nonuse of one side of the body include increased severity of secondary impairments and poor balance with an increased chance of falls (Fig. 24.4).

PHYSICAL THERAPY EVALUATION OF GENERAL NEUROLOGICAL FUNCTION

Evaluation is a process of collecting information to establish a baseline level of performance to plan interventions and to document progress. This section reviews mental status evaluation, communication, perception, cranial nerves, reflexes, and sensation.

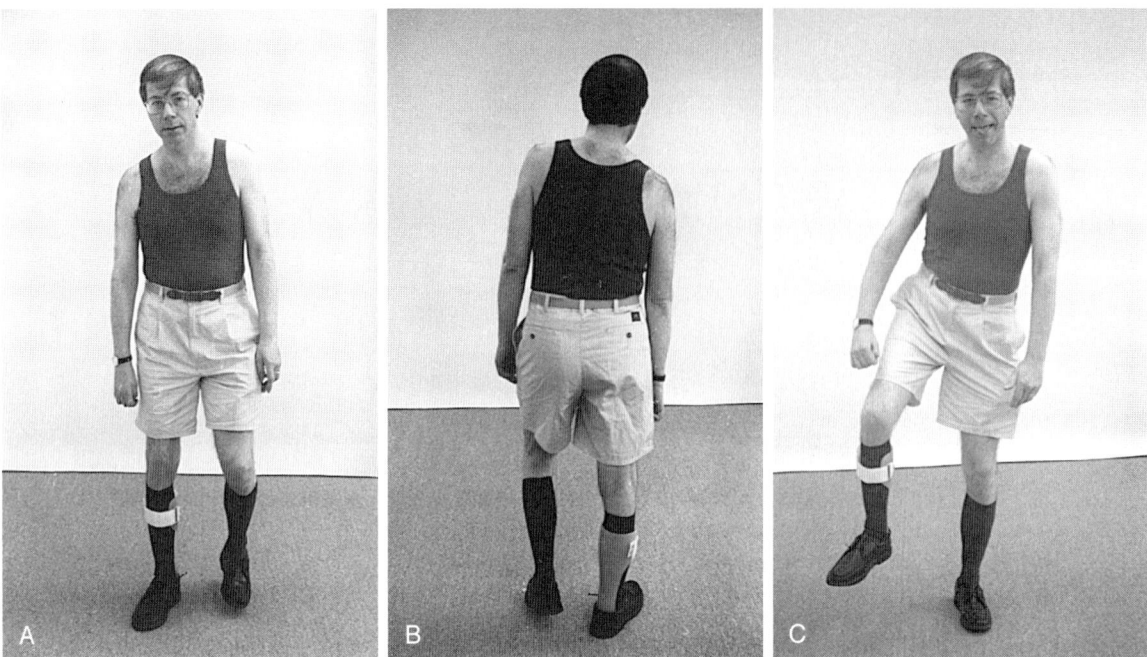

Fig. 24.2 (A) Individual with right hemiplegia. Movement deficit: Difficulty sequencing; patient is able to walk with a brace and does not need a cane. **(B)** During stance, his upper body moves laterally to the right and his right femur internally rotates as his knee hyperextends. **(C)** He has enough trunk control to stand and balance and sufficient leg control to lift the leg with knee flexion.

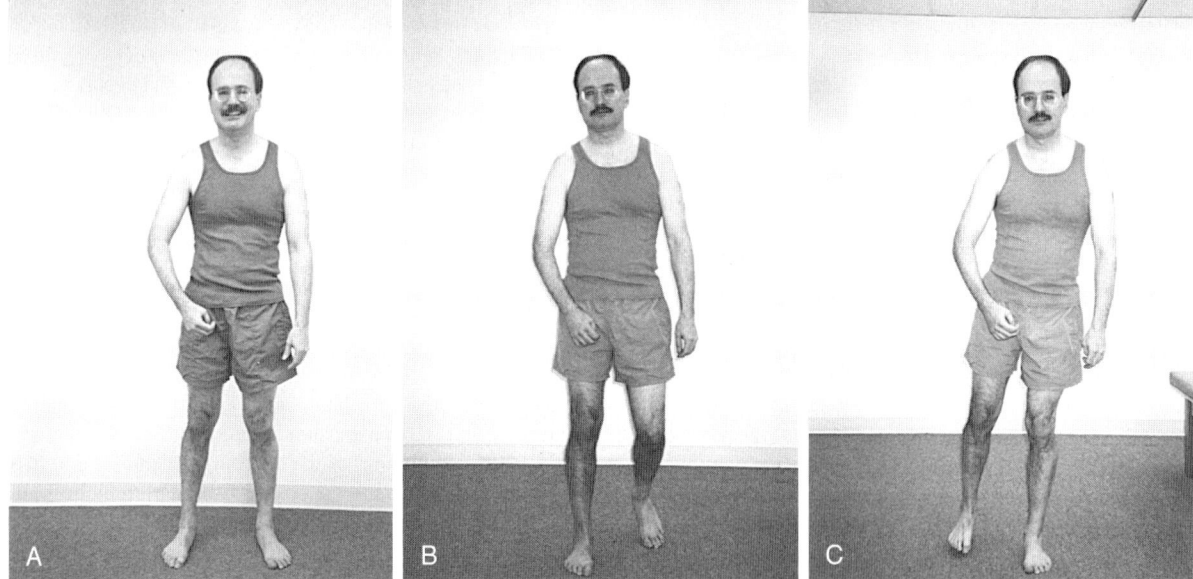

Fig. 24.3 (A) Individual with right hemiplegia. Movement deficit: atypical movement patterns—loss of initiation/cessation, timing, and sequencing. **(B and C)** Patient walking.

Mental Status Evaluation

The mental status evaluation requires arousal and alertness as prerequisites. If this is missing, the evaluation begins with an assessment of level of consciousness and then, when appropriate, considers the mental, affective, and emotional states.[66]

Levels of Consciousness

Consciousness consists of wakefulness and awareness. Wakefulness is identified by observing physical or electrophysiological evidence of arousal. Awareness requires reproducible and meaningful response to stimulus and/or evidence of comprehension of language. From these two components of consciousness, three levels of disordered consciousness have been defined, including coma, unresponsive wakefulness syndrome (UWS)—also known as vegetative state—and minimally conscious. When in a coma, a patient has no sleep-wake cycle and no response to stimulus. In UWS, a patient will have spontaneous eye opening, semiregular sleep-wake cycles, but no meaningful or reproducible response to stimulus. The patient has established wakefulness

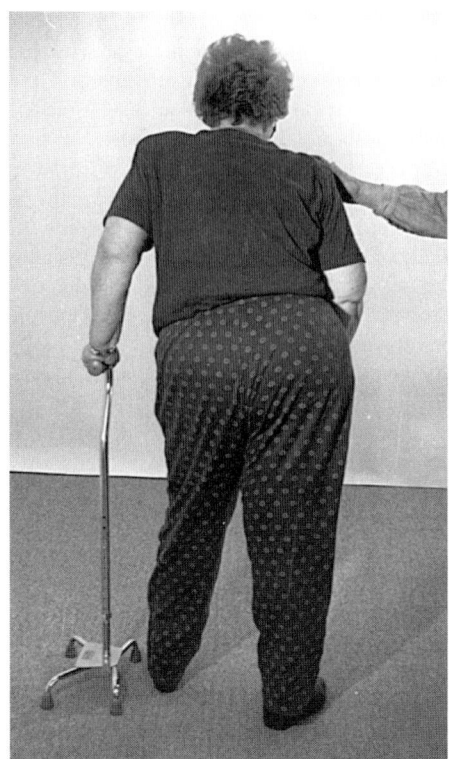

Fig. 24.4 Patient With Right Hemiplegia. Severe compensatory patterns. She walks with a quad cane and standby assistance. Pelvis rotates to the right, upper body rotates to the left, hip flexes, and knee hyperextends. There is strong lateral translation of upper body to the left (to the stable cane).

without awareness. In the minimally conscious state, a patient has established regular sleep-wake cycles and awareness as demonstrated by meaningful responses to visual, auditory, tactile, and/or noxious stimuli; however, the responses may be delayed and/or inconsistent. Further categorization of the minimally conscious state has been introduced based on higher versus lower levels of behavior response.[67]

Scales of varying types are used to measure the patient's level of consciousness, to assess the initial severity of brain damage, and to prognosticate recovery curves. The Glasgow Coma Scale, devised by Teasdale and Jennett in collaboration with Plum,[68] has been used for nontraumatic comas caused by stroke, head injury, and cardiac disease. This scale records motor responses to pain, verbal responses to auditory and visual clues, and eye opening. It assigns numerical values according to graded scales. Plum and Caronna[69] and Levy and colleagues[70] have also established criteria for correlating clinical signs of coma with prognosis.

The Coma Recovery Scale-Revised (CRS-R) is also a highly recommended, standardized clinical assessment of disordered consciousness. It consists of 23 hierarchically arranged categories with six subscales that evaluate level of arousal, auditory and language comprehension, expression, visuoperceptual ability, motor function, and communication. The lowest score on all subscales is 0 while the maximum score ranges from 2 to 6 depending on the subscale. Higher scores indicate higher levels of function.[71]

These descriptions of coma and related states are correlated with areas of suspected CNS damage but often leave a gap in the understanding of how the patient functions in life.[68] This gap was narrowed by the creation of a behavioral rating scale: The Levels of Cognitive Functioning Scale, developed at Rancho Los Amigos Hospital. This behavioral rating scale is not a test of cognitive ability but is an observational rating of the patient's ability to process and respond to information.[72]

Mental, Emotional, and Affective States

The history portion of the neurological evaluation leads to an assessment of the mental, emotional, and affective states. The patient's ability to describe the illness gives information on memory, orientation to time and place, the ability to express ideas, and judgment. If the examiner suspects a particular problem, a more thorough review is undertaken of the higher cortical function: serial subtraction, repetition of digits, and recall of objects or names. Patients with right hemiplegia may be cautious and disorganized in solving a given task, and patients with left hemiplegia tend to be fast and impulsive and seemingly unaware of the deficits present. These different response patterns stem from hemispheric involvement and prior hemispheric specialization.

Communication

A general evaluation of communication disorders is noted while taking the history. Cerebral disorder resulting from infarct or hemorrhage may produce aphasia—loss of production or comprehension of the spoken word, the written word, or both. Therapists should be familiar with expressive, receptive, and global aphasia and be prepared to modify their mode of communication to establish a good patient relationship.

Perception

Perceptual deficits in patients with hemiplegia are complex and intimately linked to the sensorimotor deficit. Sensory integration theory has begun to establish normative values and objective data for testing and documenting perceptual deficits in children. Currently, norms and testing procedures for adults have not been standardized, but perceptual deficits have been identified in patients with hemiplegia. Common perceptual deficits found in left and right brain damage are listed in Box 24.2.

Cranial Nerves

Thorough cranial nerve evaluation is necessary in hemiplegia because a deficit of a particular cranial nerve helps determine the exact size and location of the infarct or hemorrhage. In hemiplegia, it is imperative to check for visual field deficits, pupil signs, ocular movements, facial sensation and weakness, labyrinthine and auditory function, and laryngeal and pharyngeal function.

Tone

Tone, the resistance of muscles to passive movement, exists on a continuum from hypotonicity through normal to hypertonicity and finally, rigidity. Patients in the acute phase of hemiplegia exhibit, for varying periods of time, a lower-than-normal tonal state. The extremities feel like "dead weight" as the therapist moves them. As neuromuscular return slowly begins, the extremities may feel heavy, but some "following" of passive movement patterns is detected. At the further end, hypertonicity is defined as abnormal increase in resistance to passive movement and may be an indication of muscle shortening or the beginnings of joint contracture. Hypertonicity may be present without spasticity and vice versa (Box 24.3).

Postural tone refers to the overall state of tension in the body musculature. During the beginning of the 20th century, tone was thought of as postural reflexes. In the 1950s, the concept of tone was thought of as a state of light excitation or a state of preparedness.[73] Granit[74] later encouraged us to think of the relatedness of both these views. He believed that the same spinal organization is mobilized by the basal

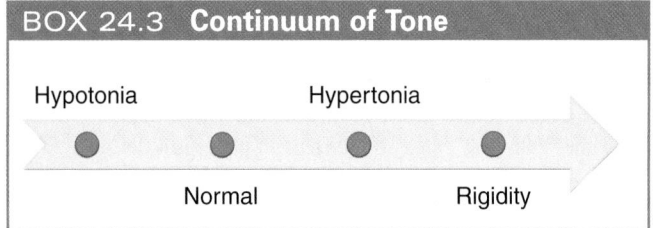
ganglia to produce both manifestations of tone: a state of preparedness and the postural reflexes.[74] Postural tone is tone that is "high" enough to keep the body from collapsing into gravity but "low" enough to allow the body to move against gravity. It is influenced by the input from the corticospinal tracts, the vestibular system, the α and γ systems, and peripheral-tactile and proprioceptive receptors.[75]

Reflexes and Spasticity

Standard areas of reflex testing include the triceps, biceps, quadriceps, and gastrocnemius muscles. According to Adams,[11] there are four plantar reflex responses: (1) avoidance–quick, (2) spinal flexion–slow, (3) Babinski–toe grasp, and (4) positive support.

Spasticity. Let's separate the definitions of spasticity and tone. Spasticity is a velocity-dependent reflex measured in the passive condition and is a sign of CNS injury. Spasticity, most likely, is the result of hyperexcitability of the medial rubrospinal tract.[76] Clinical characteristics of a muscle with spasticity include this increased velocity-dependent resistance to stretch, a clasp-knife phenomenon, and hyperactive tendon responses.

Spasticity versus hypertonicity. The terms hypertonicity and spasticity are often used interchangeably. This is incorrect. They are not the same construct. Spasticity is velocity-dependent, and hypertonicity is a resistance to passive stretch in a relaxed state and is NOT velocity-dependent (see Underlying Causes of Aberrant Movement).

Sensation

Traditional sensory testing is used to assess sensory deficits in the adult with hemiplegia: light touch, deep pressure, kinesthesia, proprioception, pain, temperature, graphesthesia, two-point discrimination, appreciation of texture and size, and vibration. A comparison of the differences in the two sides of the body and qualitative and quantitative measurements are important features of sensory testing. Sensory testing is difficult because it relies on the person's interpretation of the sensation, the patient's general awareness and suggestibility, and the person's ability to communicate a response to each test item.

The presence and quality of sensory loss must be considered during the process of reeducating motor control. Although Sherrington established the principle of interdependence of sensation and movement, current researchers have refined the concept and hypothesize that sensation modifies continuing movement by providing feed-forward information, feedback, and corollary discharge. They have provided evidence that sensation is not an absolute prerequisite for isolated movement[77]; however, impaired proprioception is a poor prognostic factor in recovery of functional movement.[78]

EVALUATION OF FUNCTIONAL MOVEMENT

Functional activities rely on the foundation of postural control and skilled extremity movement. These two elements are affected by primary impairments in the motor and sensory systems and secondary impairments in muscle and soft tissue that occur following a stroke. This section reviews normal components of postural control and skilled extremity movement and describes how the common primary and secondary impairments influence the performance of functional activities.

When evaluating functional activities, the therapist follows a pathway that includes the following: observation of the functional task, comparing what you observe with what you expect, generating hypotheses as to why differences are present, and finally assessing these hypotheses with assisted movement or objective tests and measures (see Objective Outcome Measures).

We assess the three phases of the movement pattern: *initiation*, which includes the body segment initiating the movement, the direction of movement, and the establishment of antigravity control; *transition or execution,* representing the point in the functional activity at which there is a switch in the muscle groups that provide antigravity control; and *completion/termination* of the activity, involving a final weight shift and the ability to maintain a steady state.[63] Assessing the

TABLE 24.3 **Upper-Body Initiated Weight Shift Pattern: Sitting**		
Direction of Movement	Spinal Pattern	Muscle Activity
Anterior movement—reach down to floor	Flexes	Eccentric extensor activity
Posterior—to sit back up	Extends	Concentric extensor activity
Lateral—reach sideways and down to right	Laterally flexes with concavity on right	Eccentric lateral activity on left
Lateral—comes back up to middle	Spine moves back to neutral	Concentric lateral activity on left

three phases of movement is performed with the concepts of both postural control and skilled extremity movement in mind.

Postural Control

Postural control allows the body to remain upright, to adjust to extremity movements, and to change and control body position for balance and function.[94–100] The postural control system has two major components: anticipatory and compensatory postural adjustments.[100–103]

Anticipatory Postural Adjustments

Anticipatory adjustments allow the coordinated linkage of trunk and extremity patterns before the activation of extremity movements: anticipatory postural adjustments (APAs) allow us to maintain our upright posture and balance in anticipation of a perturbation from an extremity or from the environment. Their presence minimizes changes in body alignment by correcting the effect of inertial forces on body segments. Clinically, we might say they link the trunk with the extremities. Researchers have identified altered anticipatory postural responses in people after stroke in both sitting and standing positions. The pattern or sequence of anticipatory responses post-stroke appears to be preserved, but the timing of the response is impaired; it may occur after a focal movement.[104]

Compensatory Postural Adjustments

Compensatory postural adjustments (CPAs) occur during activity when postural control is insufficient for the task. They occur after an unpredictable perturbation and serve to reorganize posture and regain balance.

Trunk Control

In a movement component model of postural control, trunk control forms the building blocks for anticipatory and compensatory adjustments.[105] Research in the field of postural control shows that the level of trunk control correlates with sitting balance and that extremity function correlates with trunk control.[106–108]

Levels of trunk control. Trunk control can be divided into levels of increasing complexity. The first level of trunk control is the ability to perform the basic movement components. Trunk control at this level provides a base that allows extremity movement to be combined and used for function. Retraining control of basic trunk movements in the three cardinal planes is a prerequisite for the coordination of trunk and extremity patterns for functional tasks.

Trunk movements in sitting are initiated from the upper trunk (head, C1 to T10) or the lower trunk (T11-pelvis) according to the demands of the task. In standing, functional trunk movements are initiated from the upper body (if the head or arm is initiating a task) or the lower body (if the leg is initiating a task). The two initiation patterns result in different spinal patterns, different types of muscular activity, and changes in the distribution of weight (Tables 24.3 and 24.4).[63]

The second level of trunk control allows the trunk to remain stable yet adapt to movement of the arms and legs.[104,109] There are three ways

this happens: the trunk remains stable during extremity movement around midline, during movements within extremity length, or during movements that extend the reach of the extremities. These coordinated movements can occur in supine, sitting, or standing positions as demonstrated in the following three examples.

1. Around midline: in sitting, the patient lifts up a leg to tie a shoe; the lower body initiates a posterior weight shift as the patient moves the lower extremity around midline.
2. Within arm's length: in sitting, the patient reaches a hand onto the edge of a table for support while the trunk remains active, yet stable.
3. Beyond arm's length: in sitting, the patient reaches down or sideways to the floor to pick up a shoe or cane. As the arm reaches down, the upper trunk initiates the anterior weight shift to extend the reach of the arm while the lower trunk provides stability and adjusts.
4. Beyond leg's length: in standing, the patient initiates a forward step with the right leg while the trunk and left leg follow the forward movement to extend the reach of the right leg to allow the foot to strike the ground.

The third level of trunk control allows stability and adaptability when the extremity receives or delivers impetus, for example, to push or pull an object. This highest level of trunk control allows for propulsive activities such as stair climbing, jumping, running, throwing, hitting, and rowing.

The model is summarized in Box 24.4.

Extremity Control

We use our extremities to perform a wide variety of tasks and functional movements. These functional movements of the extremities can be divided into two categories; movements in space and weight-bearing movements. Functional performance in the arm is more closely associated with the ability to move in space while functional performance in the leg occurs more evenly divided between movements in space and in weight bearing. Skilled extremity movements in space rely on well-timed and sequenced movements of proximal, mid, and distal joints to position the limb for function. Extremity movements in weight bearing are used to support body weight, to lift or move the body during transitional movements, and to stabilize objects for function. These weight-bearing patterns allow active, dynamic

TABLE 24.4 **Lower-Body Initiated Weight Shift Pattern: Sitting**		
Direction of Movement	Spinal Pattern	Muscle Activity
Posterior weight shift	Flexes	Concentric flexor activity
Anterior weight shift	Extends	Concentric extension activity
Lateral weight shift to right	Laterally flexes with concavity on right	Eccentric lateral activity on right Concentric lateral activity on left

---

BOX 24.4 Movement Component Control Model of Postural Control

Postural control
    Anticipatory postural adjustments
    Compensatory postural adjustments
Trunk control
    Level I: Basic movement components
        Upper-body and lower-body initiated movement
            Anterior/posterior; lateral; rotational
    Level II: Coordinated trunk and extremity patterns
        Trunk stabile in quiet sitting/standing
        Trunk stabile and adjusts to extremity movements
            *around midline
            *within extremity length
            *beyond extremity length
    Level III: Power production
        Trunk stabile and adjusts when extremity delivers/receives impetus

---

functional movement. Control of these skilled extremity movement patterns is altered post-stroke by both primary and secondary impairments. Patients who have had a severe stroke may have no visible movement in the extremities; the extremities display no resistance to passive movement and feel heavy. As strength and control in the muscles of the trunk and extremities increase, this hypotonicity lessens. If muscle activation deficits persist, the secondary impairments of poor joint alignment, muscle and soft tissue tightness, and eventually joint deformity or contracture will become predominant.

Objective Outcome Measures

During the initial interview the therapist and the patient together form a list of strengths and limitations and relate them to the patient's activity goals and personal and environmental needs. Objective baseline measurement is needed to follow recovery patterns and to document changes following rehabilitation interventions.

Objective Measures of Participation, Activity, Motor Function, Balance, Quality of Life

In 2018, the American Physical Therapy Association Stroke special interest group published outcome measure recommendations. The recommendations, known as StrokEDGE II, include outcome measures that are "highly recommended" as well as "recommended" based on their validity and reliability. They are divided into three groups: (1) core measures for all neurological disorders (6-minute Walk test, 10-Meter Walk test, Berg Balance Scale, Functional Gait Assessment, Activities-Specific Balance Confidence Scale, and 5 Times Sit-to-Stand), (2) post-stroke acute care (Orpington Prognostic Scale, Postural Assessment Scale for Stroke [PASS], and Stroke Rehabilitation Assessment of Movement [STREAM]) and, (3) post-stroke in/out patient rehabilitation (Fugl-Meyer Assessment, Functional Independence Measure, PASS, STREAM, and Stroke Impact Scale[79]). A Clinical Practice Guideline Task Force for stroke rehabilitation has additionally reviewed balance and gait measures and recommend the Functional Reach Test and the Timed-Up-and-Go (TUG).[80]

Descriptors of Gait Patterns

The evaluation of gait patterns includes the assessment of gait speed mentioned previously, including kinetic and kinematic descriptions of gait patterns to identify improvement in walking ability.[81,82] Gait speed assists with discharge planning in the acute and subacute phases of rehabilitation and is correlated with future health care utilization and functional decline.

Historically, gait deviations in persons with hemiplegia have been described according to their spatiotemporal and kinematic abnormalities and in terms of the loss of centrally programmed motor control mechanisms.[83,84] For example, Perry[84] described common problems of the hemiplegic person's gait in three phases: (1) loss of controlled movement into plantarflexion at heel strike, (2) loss of ankle movement from heel strike to midstance (resulting in loss of trunk balance and forward momentum for push-off), and (3) loss of the normal combination of movement patterns at the end of stance (hip extension, knee flexion, and ankle extension) and at the end of swing (hip flexion with knee extension and ankle flexion).

Knutsson and Richards[83] classified the motor control problems of the hemiplegic gait into three descriptive types. Type I is characterized by inappropriate activation of the calf muscles early in the gait cycle with corresponding low muscular activity in anterior compartment muscles. In the type I activation pattern, the calf musculature is activated before the center of gravity passes over the base of support. This thrusts the tibia backward instead of propelling the body forward in a push-off as normally occurs. The patient with hemiplegia compensates for the backward thrust of the tibia by anteriorly tilting the pelvis or flexing forward at the hip. Type II consists of an absence of or severe decrease in electromyographic activity in two or more muscle groups of the involved lower extremity. This pattern of markedly decreased muscular activity results in the adoption of compensatory mechanisms to gain stability. Type III activation patterns consist of abnormal coactivation of several limb muscles with normal or increased muscular activity levels in the muscle groups of the involved side. This type of pattern results in a disruption of the sequential flow of motor activity.

Mulroy classified post-stroke gait abnormalities of speed and weakness into four groups: fast walkers (44% of normal speed) with weakness in stance propulsion, moderate walkers (21% of normal speed) with greater weakness especially in hip and knee extensors leading to terminal stance abnormalities, and slow-flexed or slow-extended walkers (10% to 11% normal speed). Slow-flexed walkers have excessive hip and knee flexion in midstance while slow-extended walkers learn to use knee hyperextension to support body weight.[85]

A shift in conversation regarding hemiparetic gait pattern is occurring in the literature. To address the relationship between neural control, biomechanical constraints, and the variability of environmental constraints, Ivanenko described a module-based framework for human gait.[86] The modules describe the timing and activation profiles of groups of muscles during the phases of the gait cycle. Following stroke, as a result of damage to the cortex and the descending pathways, fewer modules are used.[87] Clark and colleagues identified four altered combinations of modular categories in the stroke population. They found people post-stroke merged these categories as the CNS's way of simplifying the task of walking: the altered ability to differentially activate muscle modules due to impaired motor initiation, cessation, and timing resulted in the "merging of module activation timing."[88]

They described the use of two modules as a low-complexity gait pattern, the use of three modules as a moderate-complexity gait pattern, and the use of four modules as a high-complexity gait pattern. These levels of complexity were correlated with functional mobility through measures of self-selected gait speed, fast gait speed, and step length asymmetry. A review of this modular-based framework was recently published.[89]

Evaluation of Movement Control

After the standardized testing has been performed, the therapist continues to a subjective evaluation of movement components to gather information to answer the question of "why" it is difficult for the patient to perform specific movements or tasks.

Patients who have sustained a stroke have difficulty moving the trunk and the arm and leg on the affected side because of the presence of primary motor impairments and secondary impairments.

In years past, weakness and paralysis after stroke were largely ignored because of a lingering focus on spasticity. Recent studies have shown that the inability of the muscle to produce force is, in fact, present and interferes with the ability to achieve functional performance.[90–92] Insufficient force production is present in 75% to 80% of patients after a stroke. There appears to be no difference in patients with left- or right-sided hemiplegia in terms of frequency or severity.[93]

When clinically assessing control of active movement patterns, the therapist observes, analyzes, and identifies the patient's functional patterns of posture and movement in the trunk and extremities and compares them to what is expected. Verbal directions or demonstrations may be necessary to help the patient understand what is desired. In this phase of the evaluation, the therapist should not physically assist the patient's movement but should be prepared to prevent loss of balance.

Assisted Movement

After the evaluation of movement during activity, therapists may use their hands while reevaluating the movements to gain additional information about the relationships between impairments. Whereas the use of handling must be judicious, handling is used during an assessment for the following purposes:

1. To correct alignment to gather additional information about strength, control, and orthopedic impairments (Fig. 24.5)
2. To limit degrees of freedom of one of the joints to assess relationships between intralimb segments
3. To assist the movement of a weak muscle
4. To block or stabilize a joint to assess the performance of a weaker muscle group or to limit the degrees of freedom of an intralimb segment (Fig. 24.6).[63]

Example.

Step 1. *Assessment of forward reach in sitting by patient with left hemiplegia.* Active movement patterns on left: patient initiates movement

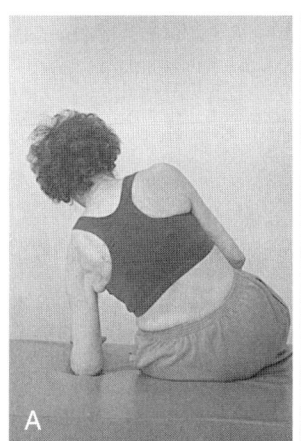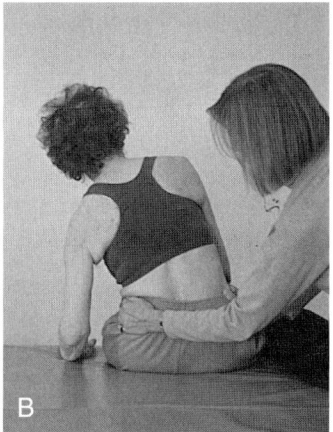

Fig. 24.5 (A) Patient with right hemiplegia trying to perform an upper-body–initiated lateral weight shift to the left. Note that the spine is straight and the right hip is off the surface. **(B)** Therapist uses her hands to correct and stabilize the lower trunk as the patient initiates the upper-body lateral movement to the left. The therapist gains information about trunk and hip control and secondary impairments of trunk muscle tightness. Note that the spine is beginning to curve as the patient uses eccentric activity of the right lateral musculature to control the movement. Active stretching of the right quadratus lumborum and latissimus occurs if tight muscles are present.

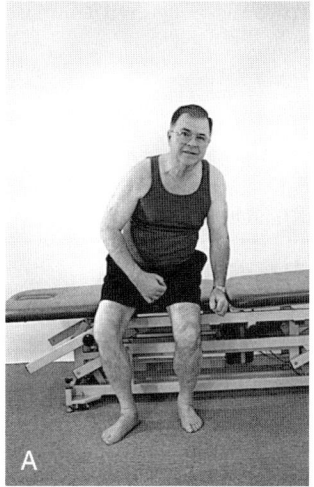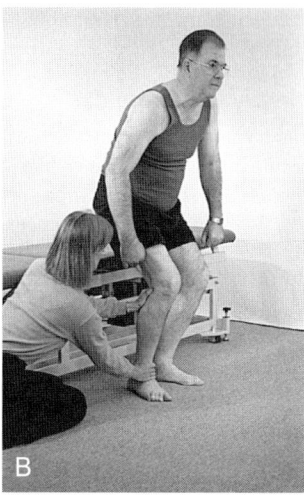

Fig. 24.6 (A) Patient with right hemiplegia moving from sitting to standing. Note the tendency to use the left leg more than the right, the left rotation of the upper body, and the position of the right arm. **(B)** Therapist uses her hands to stabilize the lower leg and to assist lower-leg movements as the patient initiates sit-to-stand. Note the change in upper-body position and the decrease in arm posturing.

proximally; shoulder flexes to 60 degrees, with internal humeral rotation; abducted, downwardly rotated scapula elevates during the movement; elbow flexes, forearm supinates to 10 degrees; wrist remains in flexion and radial deviation. Patient leans trunk forward to assist with task but cannot reach arm forward to place it on table.

Step 2. *Clinical judgment or hypothesis 1:* Weakness of scapula and humeral external rotators prevents antigravity use of elbow extensors during forward reach. Supination of forearm comes from strong proximal initiation and use of elbow flexors to lift arm. *Clinical judgment or hypothesis 2:* Forearm, wrist, and hand position prevent distal initiation and biases shoulder in internal rotation, thus blocking use of elbow extensors.

Step 3. *Test hypothesis 1:* Therapist uses her or his hands to externally rotate the humerus to neutral and asks patient to reach again. *Result:* Patient activates elbow extension halfway through range with shoulder forward flexion and places wrist and hand on table. *Clinical intervention implication:* Increased control of humeral external rotation and increased control of accompanying scapular pattern are important intervention goals to regain forward reach of arm. Retrain trunk, scapular, and humeral movement patterns, with emphasis on shoulder external rotation and scapular upward rotation. Assess secondary impairments of pectoral and rotator cuff tightness (rotator cuff is shortened if scapula is in an abducted position). *If result is unchanged, test hypothesis 2:* Therapist supports wrist and hand with wrist splint or with his or her hand and asks patient to reach again. *Result:* Patient activates elbow extension and places the wrist and hand on the table. *Clinical intervention implication:* Prevention or blocking of wrist flexion limits the degrees of freedom, changes the internal rotation moment on the distal portion of the lever arm, and allows use of existing elbow extensors. Use small wrist splint during independent practice or use object to assist or preset distal segment during practice.

DEVELOPING A PHYSICAL THERAPY ASSESSMENT

Following an evaluation of movement dysfunction, the physical therapist identifies the primary influencing factors to develop an effective treatment plan. The physical therapist considers the contributions of primary and secondary impairments.

Primary Impairments

Primary impairments are physical findings that are associated with a specific brain lesion. The primary impairments of stroke that relate to functional recovery of movement include neurological weakness, changes in muscle activation patterns, and changes in sensation.

Neurological Weakness

Weakness from stroke differs from generalized weakness and orthopedic weakness: it involves one entire side of the body and includes the trunk and extremities. After a stroke, the trunk, perhaps because of its bilateral cortical innervation, does not display the degree of weakness found in the extremities. As a result of differences in testing methods, position, and design, there is no consensus on the degree of trunk muscle weakness after a stroke: some research findings indicate a loss of lateral paretic-side trunk strength,[110,111] others report no significant difference in lateral trunk strength,[112,113] and others find slight weakness in the trunk extensors.[114,115] However, it is clear that weakness in the extremities interferes with functional use in either weight bearing or movement in space.[63,116]

Muscle Activation Deficits

Common muscle activation deficits include impaired initiation and cessation of the muscle, the inability to sequence muscles for selective extremity movement, and the inability to grade timing and force production.

Impaired initiation/cessation. Impaired initiation or cessation of muscle activity can take either of two forms: (1) an inability to turn a muscle on or off, or (2) improper initiation such as initiating a forward reach movement proximally instead of distally. The inability to turn a muscle on may be a result of the CNS damage or neurological weakness combined with altered alignment. The inability to turn a muscle off results in muscle overactivity and if combined with activity from neighboring muscles may result in cocontraction. Common examples of improper initiation are described below.

Example 1. The patient reaches forward to grasp an object and initiates the movement proximally with shoulder elevation (using the stronger proximal shoulder muscles) instead of initiating distally from the hand and forearm (due to weaker distal muscles).

Example 2. The patient initiates the swing phase of gait proximally (using stronger pelvic and hip muscles) instead of initiating distally from the ankle and foot.

Impaired sequencing. Impaired sequencing is inappropriate muscle selection or fixed patterns of muscle activity that do have a functional purpose. After a stroke, muscle sequencing patterns are related to the extent and area of insult. Abnormal sequences emerge as mass flexion or extension in the extremities. As the brain recovers, sequences become more complex and include the ability to combine patterns of flexion and extension. The level of ability to generate these sequences is assessed with the Fugl Meyer Assessment Scale.[117]

Inappropriate timing. During functional movements, muscles are activated in a particular sequence at a particular time to achieve a desired goal. Timing patterns that are too early, too late, or disorganized each contribute to loss of functional abilities.

Altered force production. Force production is the ability to move the body's mass. Altered force production, including difficulty producing sufficient force, or difficulty grading force, requires the therapist to consider a variety of possible contributing factors. These factors include the inability to turn a muscle on or off, inappropriate timing of muscle activation, neurological weakness, impaired trunk-limb coordination (the inability to keep the upper trunk aligned over the lower

trunk), abnormal sequencing of lower extremity flexors and extensors (the inability to combine flexor and extensor patterns), and/or incorrect joint alignment. Consider the task of sit-to-stand: a patient may have difficulty transitioning from a sitting to a standing position. A clinician must use observational skills to hypothesize which factor(s) are contributing to the difficulty of the task. If all factors have been addressed and the patient continues to have difficulty, the clinician may need to modify the environmental demands of the task to allow the patient to work within their force production ability.

Equilibrium and Protective Reactions

Equilibrium reactions help us to maintain or regain balance by keeping the center of gravity within the base of support. Equilibrium reactions are often referred to as the body's "first line of defense" against falling. They occur when the body has a chance of winning the battle against gravity. If equilibrium reactions cannot preserve balance, the second line of defense emerges: protective reactions. One of the best-known protective responses in the arm is the "parachute reaction." Protective responses in the leg in standing positions include hopping and stepping.

Equilibrium reactions are assessed while slowly moving either the limb or trunk away from the base of support. The amount of control in the trunk and supporting limb, the size of the base of support, and the available range of motion, as well as the evaluator's handling skills, affect the response (see Chapter 20). As the body moves outside the base of support, the extremities are recruited to help the postural system retain the body's balance. Once the control of the body is no longer sufficient to maintain balance, the extremities will respond in a protective fashion to prevent a fall.

Evaluation of Secondary Impairments

Secondary impairments occur as a consequence of the stroke or because of other medical and environmental influences, such as inactivity, falls, pneumonia, or phlebitis. As they develop, they influence one another and the primary impairments. Secondary impairments influence the patient's level of disability by contributing additional physical problems. There are four major categories of secondary impairments: changes in joint alignment and mobility, changes in muscle and soft tissue length, pain, and edema. During the chronic stage of rehabilitation, therapeutic interventions often focus on reducing secondary impairments to improve compensatory patterns of function, since the possibility of neurological recovery is lessened.

Changes in Joint Alignment

Weakness and activation deficits are the underlying causes of altered joint alignment in the acute recovery phase post-stroke. Included in this category are alterations in the normal resting alignment of bones (changes in spinal alignment) and changes in the normal mechanical relationships of joints (changes in glenohumeral alignment). Changes in resting posture arising from shortened muscles place the articular surface of joints in atypical positions, leading to changes in joint mechanics. In the foot, a shortened gastrocnemius muscle leads to a superior glide of the calcaneus and an equinovarus position. When the foot is placed into weight-bearing mode, the heel is not in contact with the ground and body weight is shifted to the mid or forefoot. This shift may result in additional changes of joint alignment in the foot. Changes continue in the subacute and chronic phase of recovery, especially with incomplete recovery of motor function.

Alignment changes develop quickly in the acute recovery phase, as in shoulder subluxation, when the pull of gravity and the weight of the paretic extremity exert traction on joints.

Shoulder subluxation. Shoulder subluxation occurs when any of the muscular and biomechanical factors contributing to glenohumeral joint stability are interrupted. In persons with hemiplegia, subluxation is related to a change in the angle of the glenoid fossa occurring because of muscle weakness. In the frontal plane the scapula is normally held at an angle of 40 degrees. When the slope of the glenoid fossa becomes less oblique (and more vertical), the humerus will "slide" down and out of the fossa.[118] Ryerson and Levit[119] first described three types of subluxation in patients with hemiplegia: inferior, anterior, and superior.

Inferior subluxation. The most common type of subluxation is an inferior subluxation. It occurs in patients with severe weakness and is present in the acute recovery stage. Weakness and the weight of a heavy arm result in downward rotation of the scapula. Downward rotation orients the glenoid fossa vertically, the unlocking mechanism of the capsule is lost, and the humerus subluxates inferiorly with internal rotation. With an inferior subluxation, the capsule is taut superiorly and vulnerable to stretch. Any downward distraction of the humerus will place an immediate stretch on the upper part of the capsule and the coracohumeral ligament, another superior structure. The rupture of this ligament is thought to be a contributor to shoulder pain.[120]

Anterior subluxation. Anterior subluxation occurs when the humeral head separates anteriorly from the glenoid fossa. Anterior shoulder subluxation occurs when the downwardly rotated scapula elevates, tilts forward on the rib cage, and the humerus hyperextends. An anterior subluxation places increased pressure on the proximal biceps tendon. This pressure on the tendon may lead to elbow flexion and forearm supination (actions of the biceps muscle). This subluxation is often found in patients with atypical patterns of return and trunk rotational asymmetries.[63]

Superior subluxation. A superior subluxation occurs when the humeral head lodges under the coracoid process in a position of internal rotation and slight abduction. The humeral head is "locked" in this position so that every movement of the humerus is accompanied by scapular movement. The scapular position in this subluxation is one of abduction, elevation, and neutral rotation. With a superior subluxation, the humerus abducts with elbow flexion. A superior subluxation occurs in patients with neurological weakness, unbalanced return, and cocontraction.

Subluxation itself is not painful but results in changes in muscle length–tension relationships, muscle shortening, and permanent stretch of the joint capsule. To correct a subluxation, the therapist corrects trunk, scapula, and humeral alignment before reeducating functional arm movement patterns.

Prevention of subluxation requires (1) proper assessment of secondary alignment problems (rib cage, scapular, humeral position), (2) early reeducation of trunk and arm linked patterns in sitting and standing, and (3) prevention of shoulder capsule stretch, including support and positioning as the patient sits, stands, and practices walking.

Changes in Muscle and Tissue Length

In the subacute or chronic recovery phase, continued loss of alignment leads to muscle shortening. Remember, this is a circular event: neurological weakness and/or muscle activation problems leads to altered joint alignment that leads to muscle and tissue shortening. Loss of alignment occurs early in recovery, whereas muscle and tissue shortening continue to occur over time. This muscle shortening (hypertonicity) is preventable through interventions that maintain range in key joints until motor control and activity levels increase. When evaluating muscle shortening, the therapist pays close attention to the functional consequences of two-joint muscle tightness.

Example. In sitting (hip and knee flexed), the patient may have ankle joint dorsiflexion range from 0 to 10 degrees; but in standing

(hip and knee extended), ankle joint dorsiflexion range may be significantly greater, for example, -20 degrees. This functional loss of ankle range due to two-joint muscle shortening causes significant problems for standing and walking. Loss of ankle joint range in standing may be the result of gastrocnemius and soleus shortening or two-joint muscles that influence the knee, such as tensor fasciae latae, or hamstring muscles. (Fig. 24.7).

Extremity muscles that cross multiple joints are the most common groups to shorten and limit joint range in hemiplegia. With prolonged changes in alignment and joint range, some two-joint muscle tendons may slip or shift.

Example. Long-standing wrist flexion may cause the ulnar wrist extensor to slip volarly and function as a wrist flexor. Similarly, a prolonged position of rearfoot equinovarus may lead to shifting of the anterior tibial muscle belly. As the muscle shifts, tension on the muscle belly results in increased foot supination.

Pain

In the patient with hemiplegia, arm pain can be caused by an imbalance of muscle activity, altered joint alignment, improper weight-bearing patterns, and muscle shortening; or it may be related to diminished or altered sensation. Although evidence-based approaches should be used to manage shoulder pain after stroke, systematic reviews show that there are few rigorous studies that can be used to guide treatment.[121]

The presence of pain in hemiplegia is devastating for the patient and makes movement reeducation difficult. Shoulder pain is the most frequent pain complaint after stroke.[122,123] Pain must be evaluated specifically and should not be allowed to occur during intervention; the "no pain, no gain" message that is sometimes used in orthopedic interventions should not be used in neurorehabilitation. Pain is an indicator that joint alignment or movements are incorrect. See Box 24.5 for questions helpful when identifying the cause and location of pain.

Joint pain. Joint pain is caused by poor shoulder joint mechanics during movement. Two common alignment problems are loss of scapular and humeral rhythm and insufficient humeral external rotation.[122,124,125] With a shoulder subluxation, the humeral head is not correctly seated in the glenoid fossa. At 60 to 90 degrees of forward flexion, impingement of the capsule may occur and the patient will report sharp pain on the superior aspect of the shoulder joint. The pain ceases when the arm is lowered. The subluxation and loss of scapulohumeral rhythm result from loss of trunk and arm movements or muscle tightness from either persistent arm posturing or weakness.

If the patient reports joint pain, the therapist should lower the humerus immediately, reestablish the mobility of the scapula, reseat the humerus if necessary, and maintain appropriate humeral rotation while moving the arm up again. Trunk movements in forearm weight bearing are used to teach a self-ranging practice routine that ensures scapulohumeral rhythm.

Muscle and tendon pain. When a shortened or posturing muscle is stretched too quickly or beyond available length, a strong "pulling" type of pain is often reported in the region of the muscle belly being stretched. If the amount of stretch is decreased a few degrees, the reported pain subsides.

If the inappropriate stretching is not stopped, muscle pain progresses to tendon pain. Proximal biceps tendonitis, distal biceps tendonitis radiating into the forearm, and wrist flexor tendonitis are most common. The usual cause of tendonitis is improper weight bearing, with an inactive trunk and "hanging" of the arm. The treatment of tendonitis is rest and modalities (i.e., heat, ultrasound, or electrical stimulation) or injection of corticosteroids. When movement

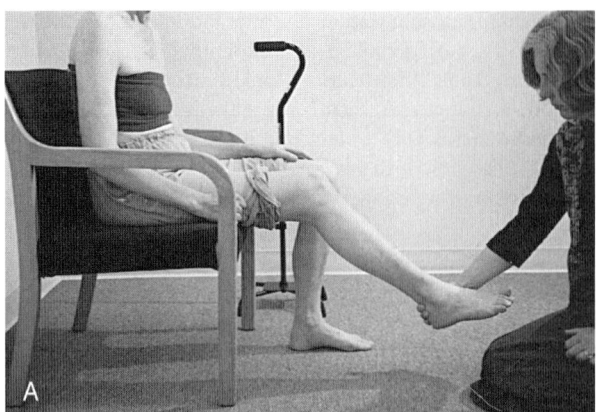

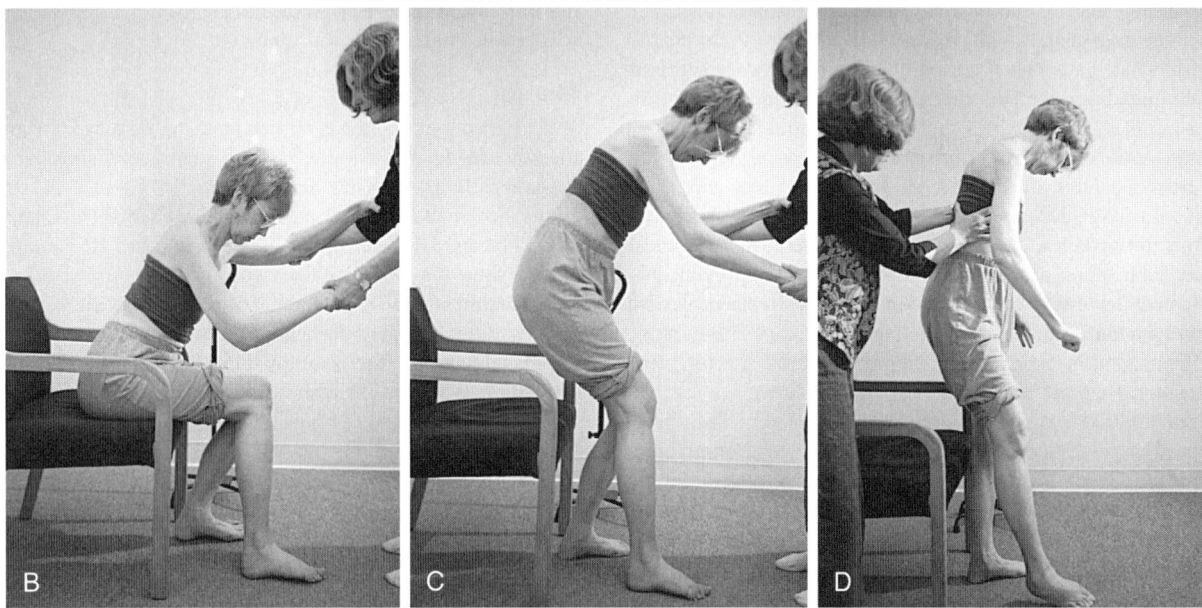

Fig. 24.7 (A) Patient with right hemiplegia with limited range in hamstring, tensor fasciae latae, and gastrocnemius and soleus muscles. **(B)** Patient has sufficient range at ankle to keep foot on the floor in sitting and as she initiates the rise to standing. **(C)** As she stands and reaches the limit of range of these two muscle groups, her body compensates. The pelvis rotates right, and the tight medial hamstring adducts and internally rotates the femur and pulls the knee into extension as its medial insertion becomes more anterior to the joint. **(D)** As the knee extends more, the calcaneus moves into equinus and varus. The foot supinates as a result of calcaneal varus and external tibial rotation from the tight tensor fasciae latae.

BOX 24.5 Questions for Subjective Evaluation of Pain

Location: Where is the pain? Pinpoint the location.

Type: What does it feel like?
- Sharp and stabbing
- Aching
- Dull
- Pulling
- Pins and needles

Occurrence: When does the pain occur?
- At rest
- During movement
  - Range-of-motion exercises
  - Weight-bearing exercises
  - A specific part of the movement

---

reeducation is restarted, it is important to avoid the "exercise" that caused the pain and to create a new intervention plan.

Complex regional pain syndrome: Shoulder-hand syndrome. One type of complex regional pain occurs in the shoulder and hand. It begins with tenderness and swelling of the hand and diffuse aching pain from altered sensitivity in the shoulder and entire arm.[125] This pain interferes with the reeducation of movement patterns and causes a general desire on the part of the patient to "protect" the arm by not moving it. Edema and limited shoulder, wrist, and finger range of motion soon occurs.

The second stage includes further loss of shoulder and hand range of motion, severe edema, and loss of skin elasticity. This is followed by the third stage, which includes demineralization of bone, severe soft tissue deformity, and joint contracture.[125,126]

Not every edematous hemiplegic hand leads to shoulder-hand complex regional pain syndrome. Hand edema results from an upper extremity that remains dependent and that does not move for long periods of time. It is essential to teach the person with hemiplegia how to properly care for the hand and to give the responsibility for the care of the hand and arm to the patient.

Ryerson and Levit[63] propose five intervention steps for severe or chronic shoulder pain: (1) eliminate pain from intervention or the home program, (2) desensitize the arm and hand to touch, (3) eliminate hand edema, (4) introduce pain-free arm movements by reestablishing scapular mobility, and (5) beginning with guided arm movements below 60 degrees, gradually increase the variety and complexity of arm movements.

Objective measures of pain. Two commonly used objective pain measurement scales are the Visual Analog Scale and the McGill Pain Questionnaire.[127,128] These scales focus on the intensity of pain and provide an objective measure of intervention effectiveness. For an in-depth discussion of the topic of pain management (see Chapter 30).

Edema

Edema in the hand and foot is another common secondary impairment that develops as a consequence of loss of movement control and hospitalization factors such as intravenous infiltrates and dependent limb positioning. Edema limits joint range and tissue mobility. The edematous fluid places the skin on stretch and acts as an interstitial "glue" that bonds the skin, fascial tissue, muscle tissue, and tendons. Hand edema is associated with the development of shoulder-hand syndrome. Foot edema is as common as hand edema, limits ankle joint dorsiflexion range, and is often ignored during intervention programs. Edema begins on the volar surface of the hand and foot, progresses dorsally, and then moves proximally across the wrist or ankle.

Edema interferes with the retraining of functional movement patterns by preventing the smooth glide of tissues. It must be eliminated before active reeducation begins. Edema has defined stages. When the involved tissue feels soft and fluid, the condition responds to retrograde massage and elevation. When the tissue is gelatinous and pitting, the edematous fluid cannot be physically expressed. At this stage, it begins to adhere to underlying tissues. The edema must be softened and liquefied through transtissue massage. The last stage of edema is characterized by hard, lumpy tissue that does not "pit" in response to manual pressure. This stage of edema requires gentle bilateral compression to break up the hard, solid areas into regions of softness. The soft regions then act as open spaces into which fluid released by massage of hard tissue is directed. The goal is to reverse the process of hardening—from hard, to pitting, to soft and fluid. In the pitting and hard stages, when the edematous tissue is not fluid, elevation, elastic gloves, bandaging, and retrograde massage are not effective. When edematous tissue is soft and fluid, active and active assistive extremity movement patterns produce muscular contractions that assist venous and lymphatic return of the fluid.[63]

Aberrant Extremity Movement

There is considerable debate in the academic and clinical therapy community over the clinical relevance of spasticity and the need to address it in treatment.[90,129] For years, spasticity, a velocity-dependent reflex measured in the passive condition and a sign of CNS injury, was thought to be a direct cause of atypical voluntary movement post-stroke. In the 1980s, scientists challenged this concept, and a new construct emerged that acknowledged the contribution of both neural and non-neural elements to the phenomenon of these atypical movement patterns. This newer concept helps explain why the stretch reflex or tendon tap response is an "epiphenomenon" and is not the cause of the "spastic movement problem."[18,130] Dietz[131] recommended that we assign different names to these two different phenomena of increased

tone: he suggested we reserve the term "spasticity" for the reflex and create a new term, "spastic movement disorder," to describe the extremity posturing that occurs during active movement. We suggest renaming Dietz's second category of spastic movement disorder *aberrant movements*. A knowledge of the underlying causes of aberrant movement is important for intervention planning. If we label aberrant extremity movement "spasticity," we may plan a treatment intervention that focuses on the aberrant movement itself instead of the underlying causes. For interventions to be successful, it is important to understand the situations in which this aberrant/atypical movement occurs.

Underlying Causes of Aberrant Movement

Ryerson and Levit along with Fisher have proposed several contributing factors. At least three different situations come to mind: (1) the patient's postural control ability is insufficient for the task, (2) altered biomechanical alignment results in increased tension on extremity muscles, and (3) voluntary activation of existing muscle sequences.[63,132] These situations are divided into three groups for ease of description, but, in reality, overlap may occur between groups.

Insufficient postural stability and trunk control. If postural control is insufficient for the functional task, extremity patterns of arm flexion or leg extension occur as a balance strategy; the body is recruiting activity in the limbs to help remain stable.

Example. If a patient has sufficient trunk control in sitting, the arm and leg display normal resting positions. However, during the rise to stand, the arm postures in flexion. The arm postures most obviously during the transition phase of the stand when the hips are off the surface and the center of gravity of the body is behind the feet, the new base of support.

Treatment of the increased tone, in this case, would not be directed at the arm. Rather, intervention would focus on increasing postural stability of the body, especially during the execution phase of the movement when the center of mass is behind the base of support. During this phase, trunk-limb coordination, lower-extremity sequencing, and sufficient force production are needed. As the trunk and leg gain more control, the arm posturing decreases (see Fig. 24.6).

Altered biomechanical alignment. A second cause of aberrant extremity movement, altered biomechanical alignment, may result in increasing tension and unwanted activity, especially in two-joint muscles.

Example 2A: Lower extremity. In sitting, tightness in the gastrocnemius muscle across the knee may not affect the ability to keep the heel on the floor. However, as the patient rising to stand and extends the knee, the limit of tightness in the gastrocnemius is reached, the distal end of the tendon shortens and the ankle plantar flexes. Gastrocnemius tightness pulls the calcaneus into equinovarus, resulting in foot supination (see Fig. 24.7).

However, after lengthening of the gastrocnemius across the ankle and knee in standing and correction of the calcaneal position, the patient can stand and keep the foot on the floor. Now, movement reeducation begins to restore the muscle activation control and strength needed to prevent this shortening from reoccurring.

Example 2B: Upper extremity. In anterior shoulder subluxation, the anterior movement of the humeral head increases tension on the biceps tendon proximally, resulting in increased elbow flexion. As the tension increases, the forearm may begin to supinate. With the knowledge that this altered alignment may be the underlying cause of the atypical movement, the therapist repositions the humeral head and scapula, the tension on the biceps is diminished, and the forearm slowly pronates and then the elbow extends.

For the atypical posturing to permanently stop, therapy interventions must help increase strength and muscle activation components to maintain active typical alignment.

Inappropriate voluntary muscle activation. This third underlying cause of aberrant movement occurs when the patient is actively using available patterns of return when trying to use the arm or leg. The patient uses the muscles in the only way he or she knows: patterns in synergy or combining synergies or with prolonged contraction. Historically, these patterns were labeled "spastic patterns." If we now think of these patterns as inappropriately initiated, sequenced, or timed, therapy intervention is directed at these underlying causes rather than at the symptoms (the aberrant movements). The aberrant movement of the extremity will change when the patient learns new activation patterns. Often, these are "learned" patterns and are difficult to change. Early reeducation should include training in these skills of more complicated sequencing, intensity, and duration of firing.

Conclusions

Hypertonicity is the increased resistance that you feel when you move a joint/muscle through its range during a state of relaxation. It may lead to contracture, but neither contracture nor hypertonicity are the cause of aberrant movement in patients post-stroke.

Using this new construct, inhibition techniques are inappropriate because they focus on the symptom, not on the underlying cause. Intervention techniques that focus on inhibition of extremity tone—maximal elongation, vibration, biofeedback, cold, or relaxation or static weight bearing—rarely result in a permanent change in the tone. The temporary decrease of clinical hypertonicity that occurs with any of these methods does not by itself directly lead to an increase in function.[133,134]

Motor Evaluation Forms

The foregoing information, once gathered, can be placed on an evaluation form in many ways. Every medical institution seems to have its own evaluation form and its own system of recording data. Active movement at the shoulder joint may be described in one institution in terms of percentages of synergistic stages, at another institution by a narrative of degrees and planes of movement, and at still another by functional outcomes of shoulder movement. At one hospital the documentation of pain may be descriptive, and at another it may be numerical. It is important to keep in mind the substance of the evaluative material, not the form in which it is described. A detailed motor evaluation form is necessary for the establishment of realistic goals and for subsequent treatment planning, but the specific form depends both on the needs of the specific clinical setting and on the clinician's choice.

Recognizing Needs

The information obtained from the total evaluation provides the basis for answers to the following questions:
- What activities are possible?
- What activities are not possible?
- How do the movement impairments and secondary impairments relate to activity performance?
- How do the environmental and personal considerations impact the ability to perform the activity?

By understanding the impairments and their relationship to activity limitations, the therapist can answer the following question: What significant movement components are missing? The answer to this question becomes a hypothesis for intervention planning. How the possible is accomplished and why the impossible exists provide logical suggestions for selection of intervention techniques.

If assistive devices are used, the following questions should be asked: Is the device always used? If not, when is it used? How is the device used? Could the device be used another way that would foster trunk symmetry and allow activity of the affected extremities?

Therapy intervention occurs at either the level of activity limitation or the level of movement-related primary and secondary impairments. The process of establishing goals and selecting activities for intervention begins with clinical decision making or problem solving.

CLINICAL DECISION MAKING AND PROBLEM SOLVING

Problem solving is a process of gathering and analyzing evaluation information from movement analysis, organizing and reflecting on this information to develop hypotheses for causal relationships between activity limitations and significant impairments, and establishing and prioritizing goals for therapeutic intervention. The problem-solving process is also used to hypothesize how the movement problems of the trunk, arm, and leg are interrelated and how these problems relate to the ability to perform tasks. Movement control deficits, secondary impairments, and compensatory movement patterns should be identified in relation to each significant activity limitation.

Analyzing Evaluation Material

The relationship between activity performance and primary and secondary impairments in people post-stroke, the basis for therapy intervention, is derived from clinical experience and judgment. Clinical reflection guides the evaluation process—what should be evaluated and how. As a result of the evaluation, the therapist has a list of functional skills that are difficult or impossible for the patient to perform and a list of primary and secondary impairments that relate to the attempted performance of that task. The therapist analyzes this information with the goal of identifying common impairments in categories of tasks: Which primary impairments are major impediments in each task analyzed? Are there secondary impairments that interfere with the patient's ability to perform specific critical movement components? What is the level of trunk-extremity control during task performance in each functional position evaluated? While analyzing the evaluation material, the therapist pays attention to all significant factors that limit performance of tasks, including environmental, cognitive, perceptual, and emotional barriers.

Common Combinations of Primary and Secondary Impairments

Therapists evaluating and planning interventions for people post-stroke need to identify both primary impairments of the motor and sensory systems along with the resulting secondary impairments of altered alignment and muscle length. Below are a few examples of common combinations of these impairment categories.

Acute Recovery

A patient after an acute stroke with left hemiplegia cannot perform morning daily care activities at the sink while sitting in a wheelchair, cannot transfer from bed to chair, and cannot rise to stand. Common primary impairments may include (1) neurological weakness of the left arm and leg, (2) inability to sequence forward arm movements, (3) an inability to coordinate trunk and lower-body movements to allow forward weight shifts in sitting and/or to perform transfers from bed to chair, and (4) impaired extremity sensation. Secondary impairments that begin to appear by the end of the acute recovery phase might include trunk asymmetries (lateral trunk flexion with a left spinal convexity, inferior shoulder subluxation, loss of extremity muscle length in the pectorals and gastrocnemius, and/or edema in the hand and foot).

During the acute recovery stage, weakness of the trunk on one side results in a flaring of the rib cage and lateral flexion of the spine with the *convexity on the affected side.* The appearance of a low shoulder contour on the affected side often is associated with trunk shortening (lateral flexion with the concavity). The heavy weight of the weak, hypotonic arm pulls the upper quadrant into *excessive forward flexion.* In this position, the scapula elevates and tips forward on a flexed, rotated thoracic spine (Fig. 24.8).

Inpatient/Subacute Recovery

In the inpatient rehabilitation phase of care, these primary impairments begin to improve. However, as the patient performs tasks that

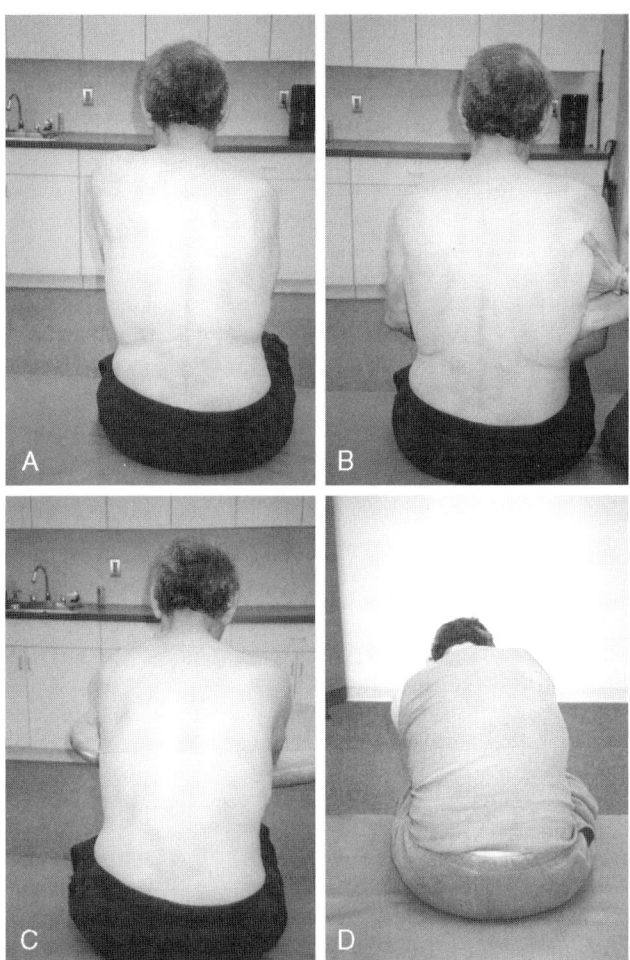

Fig. 24.8 (A) Patient with right hemiplegia. Contour of right shoulder appears lower and longer than on the left. Pelvis lists downward on the right. **(B)** Therapist lifts the patient's upper body up out of forward flexion and corrects the position of the glenohumeral joint. Note that the contour of the right shoulder is now higher and shorter than the left shoulder contour. The trunk is laterally flexed with the convexity on the right. These movement components, convexity of a lateral curve, high shoulder, and low pelvis, are compatible. **(C)** Patient's arms are supported symmetrically by a table. Note the convexity of the curve on the right and the low pelvis on the right. **(D)** Same patient moving forward and down with an upper-body anterior weight shift. This position allows the therapist to evaluate the position of the trunk. Note the tendency to avoid weight on the right hip. The trunk is laterally flexed with the convexity on the right, and the right shoulder is higher than the left shoulder.

exceed their level of postural control, aberrant movement in the arm or leg may increase as a strategy for maintaining balance. Secondary impairments of shoulder pain may increase, along with increasing instances and degrees of muscle tightness and altered alignment. These altered alignment patterns in the spine and girdles, as a result of muscle activation deficits and loss of trunk control, create an atypical starting position for functional movement.

If the patient relies heavily on the use of one-sided compensatory strategies (reliance on the nonaffected side with relative nonuse of the affected extremities) during sit-to-stand and walking, *lateral translation of the thoracic spine* may occur. This altered spinal alignment pattern also occurs when the patient relies heavily on a quad cane or hemiwalker. As the patient uses their arm to lean on and push down into this stable external assistive device (a "third leg"), the trunk translates laterally (from the hypermobile point of T10). This pattern creates a lower shoulder contour that may be mistaken for shortening of the affected side (see Fig. 24.4).

In standing, because the need for leg stability and movement control is much greater than in sitting, the trunk compensates to accommodate the demands of the leg. Often the upper body and lower body patterns are opposite one another (i.e., counterrotational). This counterrotational pattern is accompanied by a noticeable skin fold. However, the spinal asymmetry is rotational, not lateral (see Fig. 24.4).

Chronic Recovery

Another compensatory pattern, excessive spinal flexion throughout the spine, occurs in the chronic recovery stage especially with severe injury to the CNS. As patients with this asymmetry shift weight onto the stronger side, *spinal rotation toward the affected side occurs.* This pattern of spinal flexion and rotation to the affected side develops over time in patients who sit more than they stand or walk.

Distal and Proximal Relationships

Alignment problems in the distal extremity segments are related to loss of movement control and proximal alignment changes. Patterns in the distal arm and distal leg are strikingly similar. When the midjoint (elbow or knee) is extended, the proximal rotational alignment asymmetry translates down into the distal segment: into the hand or foot. Shoulder internal rotation translates across an extended elbow, resulting in forearm pronation (Fig. 24.9A). Similarly, when the knee is extended, hip internal rotation asymmetries translate across the knee and occur with tibial internal rotation and midfoot pronation. However, if the mid-joint is flexed, the proximal pattern no longer dictates distal asymmetries.

Example

A patient has an inferior shoulder subluxation resulting in humeral internal rotation. This tendency for internal rotation places tension on the biceps tendon, resulting in beginning elbow flexion and forearm supination. With unbalanced return and weakness of arm muscles, the emerging biceps activity predominates and reinforces a posturing pattern of shoulder internal rotation, elbow flexion with forearm supination (see Fig. 24.9B).

The weakness pattern of ankle plantarflexion and calcaneal equinovarus biases return in the anterior and posterior tibialis. During movements of the leg in space with hip and knee flexion, this distal supination pattern pulls the tibia into external rotation. To place the supinated foot on the ground, the patient compensates proximally by rotating the pelvis and femur, as a unit, toward the unaffected side. This incompatible tibial external rotation and femoral internal rotation may result in knee hyperextension.

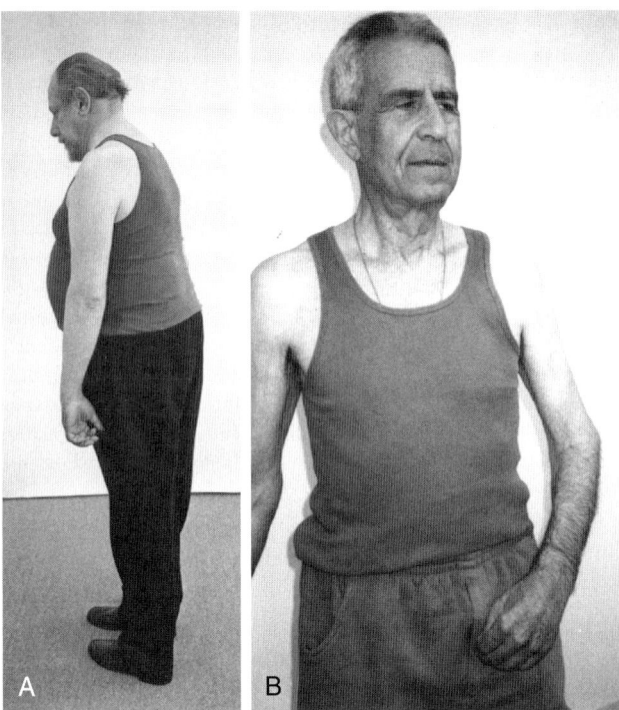

Fig. 24.9 **(A)** Patient with left hemiplegia and severe weakness. The left arm and hand are in shoulder internal rotation, elbow extension, and forearm pronation. The left wrist flexes, and the hand pronates and radially deviates on the wrist. **(B)** Patient with left hemiplegia with atypical movements. The left arm is positioned in shoulder internal rotation and elbow flexion. As the elbow flexes, the forearm begins to supinate on the internally rotated humerus. The wrist flexes and radially deviates with finger flexion.

Developing Hypotheses for Significant Impairments

The process of motor performance evaluation results in a list of activities and related impairments. However, not all these impairments directly relate to each activity limitation of the patient. The therapist, using clinical judgment, hypothesizes a causal relationship between frequently occurring impairments and activity limitation. These impairments, called *significant impairments,* are the ones that must be changed for measurable changes in movement and function to occur.[63] The other impairments are not forgotten but are reevaluated later as improvement begins and new activity goals are chosen. The significant impairments are often used as the focus of short- and long-term goals because they are the underlying building blocks of the selected activity goal. Because functional movement depends on the linkage of trunk and extremity movements, the therapist develops hypotheses between impairments in the extremities and specific levels of trunk control to set goals that result in improved activity performance. (See Chapters 3 and 7.)

Goal Setting

Once the therapist reviews the desired functional goal and identifies the underlying significant impairments, the intervention plan is created and discussed with the patient.

Functional Goals

Functional goals are based on the environment and personal needs of the patient and on the functional impairments that were identified by the therapist during the initial assessment. Functional goals should

represent a significant change in the patient's level of independence, be practical, and reflect improvement in a specific activity limitation. They state the desired function and the expected level of performance.[63]

Example. Patient will stand independently and safely while performing self-care activities at the bathroom sink.

Long-Term Goals

A long-term goal should reflect a major improvement in a primary or secondary impairment or an increase in level of performance of an existing skill. The time it takes to accomplish a long-term goal varies tremendously depending on the frequency of treatment and the length of time after stroke. Long-term goals may be stated in functional terms, but they usually reflect a change in a primary impairment: an increase in strength, movement control, or balance. The therapist may set many short-term goals to achieve one long-term goal.[63]

   Examples.
   Functional goal. Patient will be able to perform meal preparation activities in the kitchen safely (while standing).
   Long-term goals.
1. Patient will independently perform upper-body initiated movement (lateral and rotational) while standing, supporting hips against a kitchen counter.
2. Patient will safely stand near the kitchen counter and maintain balance during reach movements within and beyond arm's length.

Short-Term Goals

A realistic short-term goal should be achievable quickly and should be based on the result of the patient's response to handling during the evaluation of movement. Short-term goals should directly relate to the accomplishment of the long-term goal. Short-term goals are compiled from the list of relevant primary and secondary impairments. These goals are measurable but do not in and of themselves result in a functional change.[63]

When stated in terms of movement control rather than functional performance, these goals include the reestablishment of generalized movement patterns that link movement patterns of the trunk and extremities (Box 24.6).

Choosing Intervention Techniques

Once the problem-solving process of goal setting is finished, therapists can select specific intervention techniques and activities. Therapists have many techniques to choose from to meet their goals.

Controversy exists as to the means of increasing functional mobility and performance in patients who have had a stroke. One school of thought teaches compensatory patterns or hopes for some use of the affected side through task-specific practice without direct intervention for the neurological impairments. The other prevalent practice pattern is to increase functional movement patterns on the affected side to help achieve an activity goal by increasing control and strength of movement sequences of the trunk and limb through specific levels of reeducation.[63,135–137]

BOX 24.6 **Component Goals in Functional Training**

Component goal (power): Restore strength in trunk and extremity patterns (individual muscles, components, sequences)

Component goal (structure): Minimize or eliminate secondary impairments

Component goal (control): Reeducate patterns of control (sequencing and timing)

BOX 24.7   Reeducation Strategy for Intervention

Reeducating basic trunk movement components
Linking coordinated trunk and extremity patterns
- Weight bearing
- Movements in space

Preventing, minimizing, eliminating secondary impairments
Teaching appropriate compensations
Teaching independent practice routines

A combination of these two practices may be useful: impairment-based intervention strategies to reeducate movement, and task training strategies to foster desirable compensations—a functional reeducation strategy. This type of intervention includes activating trunk- and extremity-linked patterns of movement, minimizing or eliminating secondary impairments that interfere with regaining control, teaching appropriate compensations, and training the patient to practice functional movement patterns in the context of daily tasks (Box 24.7).[63,138] Research findings support a link between the trunk and upper extremity and the trunk and lower extremity during reaching activities.[139,140] One result of this research has been to design treatment interventions that restrain trunk movements during forward reach retraining to increase control of elbow extension movement in the paretic arm.[141,142]

For reeducation to be effective, therapists must allow the patient to initiate the active trunk and extremity pattern, must move from assisted practice to independent practice with the assistance of appropriately selected objects or verbal cues, and must teach the patient appropriately staged practice patterns. Studies based on the "learned nonuse" phenomenon demonstrate that when patients are encouraged to use the affected arm, movement and functional use, even if limited, are possible.[143,144]

Regardless of intervention type used, task-performance practice, or a reeducation strategy, there comes a time in the recovery process when therapists help the patient select practical compensatory strategies. Compensatory strategies are taught when the patient needs to function independently and cannot yet use the affected extremity because of insufficient recovery or the severity of damage. To be appropriate, the strategy should incorporate the use of the involved extremities and use appropriate trunk movement patterns to maximize future return of movement. Undesirable compensations are patterns that are so asymmetrical that they fail to incorporate available movements of the affected trunk and extremities (Fig. 24.10). Although there is a trend to stress task-based techniques, therapists in clinical settings use hands-on approaches to increase muscle strength and control and to decrease impairments that block the emergence of new functional patterns.[63] As research in movement science and recovery of movement increases, therapists must critically analyze research findings and judiciously integrate them with their clinical experience and judgment.

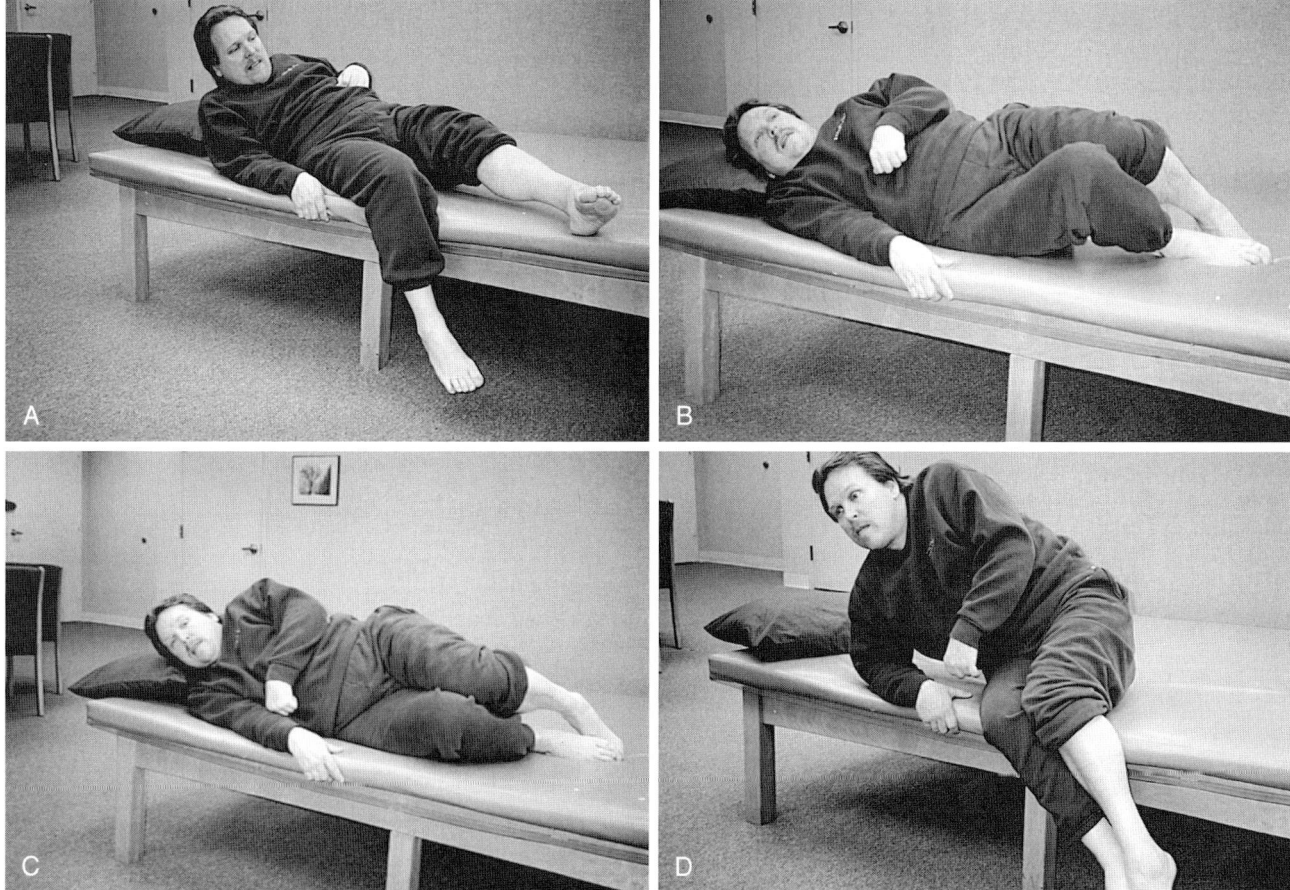

Fig. 24.10 (A) Patient with left hemiplegia using his right side to move to sitting and not incorporating movement of the left side—an undesirable compensation. **(B–D)** Patient moving to sitting while using as much control as possible on the left side to assist the movement to sitting.

INTERVENTION STRATEGIES FOR FUNCTIONAL RECOVERY

Functional mobility movement analysis, intervention techniques, and suggestions for task practice are documented in therapy literature.[145–147] In this section, representative mobility skills are selected in three functional positions: supine, sitting, and standing. For each task selected, the focus is on the basic trunk and extremity control patterns used, significant impairments in addition to weakness that make it difficult for the patient to perform the task, and observations from the clinic that relate to intervention and practice.

General Considerations

Weakness and loss of muscle activation control in the trunk and extremities results in ineffective and inefficient functional patterns in daily life. Interventions for extremity deficits include reeducation of movements in space, reeducation of weight-bearing movements, retraining appropriate initiation/cessation, sequencing of movement, and specific task practice. Most patient with hemiplegia regain enough control in the leg to stand and walk, but those same patients may not be able to use the arm for any purpose. Today the concept of "learned nonuse" may help therapists understand why this discrepancy between arm and leg recovery exists.

Distal reeducation is an important component of early reeducation that has been neglected by therapists because of a previous belief that proximal return comes before distal that has now been questioned.[148] Distal reeducation trains the patient to be able to initiate movements from the hand (foot), instead of the common proximal initiation patterns seen during attempted reach (stepping) (Fig. 24.11). Weight bearing on either the forearm or extended arm is used as a postural assist, may be used to reestablish scapulohumeral rhythm, to maintain range of motion in the arm, or to strengthen movement sequences in the arm (Fig. 24.12). The muscles of the arm are linked with trunk weight shifts during active weight bearing.[63] Table 24.5 presents the linked trunk and arm muscle activity during active weight bearing for one functional task.

The ability to support body weight on both legs for stability and movement control is similarly important. Movements of the trunk in sitting and standing occur with constant changes of muscle activity in the legs as part of the base of support, to adjust to demands of weight shifts, and to increase activity levels of leg muscles to initiate standing weight shifts. Loss of control of weight bearing on both legs or on one leg has an immediate effect on balance. Problems of weight-bearing control of the leg may exist as a result of insufficient force production, sequencing difficulty, or muscle shortening. When the leg cannot actively support body weight, undesirable asymmetrical compensations may result. A significant and often overlooked prerequisite for active

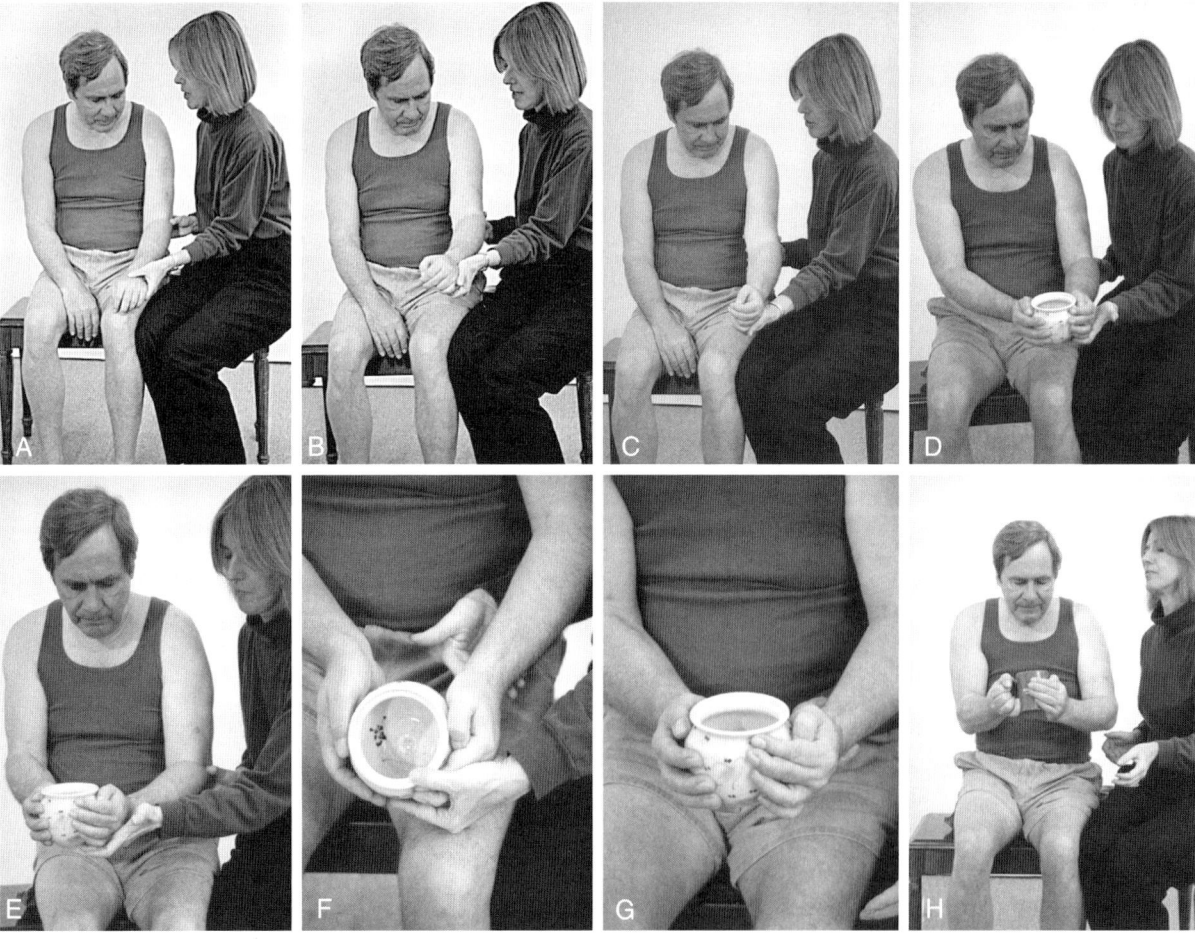

Fig. 24.11 **(A–C)** Patient with left hemiplegia. Therapist assists movements of forearm, wrist, and hand as patient practices increasing distal arm control. **(D–F)** Therapist introduces object and assists patient as he learns to control the object and the movement. **(G)** Independent practice. **(H)** Patient uses same movements with a similar object.

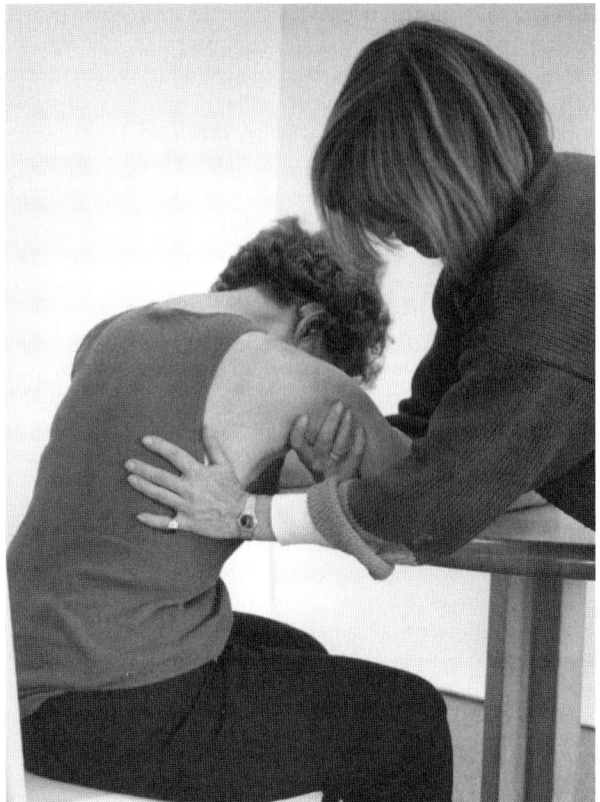

Fig. 24.12 Patient performs lower-body–initiated posterior movement during forearm weight bearing at a table. The therapist uses her hands to stabilize the humerus, and as the patient moves back, the therapist's left hand slowly stretches or releases tight tissue in the rotator cuff.

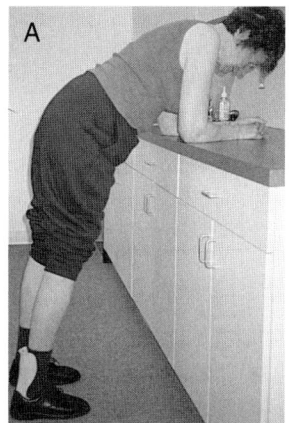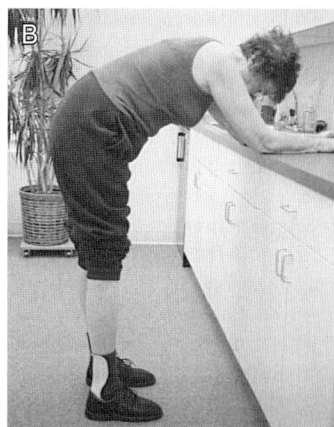

Fig. 24.13 **(A)** Patient with right hemiplegia practicing home program. During standing forearm weight bearing (providing upper-body stability), she initiates a lower-extremity forward-backward movement. As she moves her hips and lower leg forward, she thinks of keeping her knee straight and stretching her calf. **(B)** As she moves her hips backward, she may feel a stretch in the back of her thigh, on the lateral aspect of her trunk, or under her axilla.

TABLE 24.5 Trunk and Arm Coordinated Movements in Forearm Weight Bearing

Functional Task

Sit at a table with both forearms supported on the table. Keeping both arms on the table, move lower body back rounding spine, stop, then move body forward straightening spine.

	Anterior Weight ShiftLower Trunk Moves Forward	Posterior Weight Shift Lower Trunk Moves Back
Spine	Extends	Flexes
Scapula	Adducts and depresses	Abducts and elevates
Glenohumeral joint	Less flexion	More flexion
Elbow	Flexes	Extends

control of the lower body/leg in standing is a stable, aligned upper body. The use of forearm or extended-arm weight bearing in standing may provide external stability to the upper body while allowing the therapist to reeducate control lower extremity movements and provide environmental support when practicing at home (Fig. 24.13).

Supine
Rolling

Basic trunk movement patterns for rolling include (1) upper-trunk flexion and rotation initiation, (2) lower-trunk extension and rotation initiation, and (3) symmetrical (log-rolling) lateral flexion

initiation. These patterns link the trunk with either the arm or leg during the roll.

Trunk and extremity linked patterns. The *upper-trunk flexion rotation initiation pattern* links upper-trunk flexion rotation with arm reach across the body. Active assistive patterns, with the patient holding both hands together for a bilateral arm reach, are encouraged when strength is insufficient to lift the arm against gravity or, through therapist handling, when arm muscle weakness results in such a heavy feeling that the patient cannot control the extremity with the unaffected hand. If the therapist assists the arm, the goal of practice is for the patient to initiate the active antigravity trunk pattern.

A *lower-trunk extension rotation initiation pattern* is coordinated with either a leg-reach pattern or a flexed-leg "push" pattern. Active assistive patterns can be implemented through therapist handling to help train the sequencing or to grade the firing patterns of the leg when it is pushing into the bed. As the lower body moves from supine toward side lying, the upper body and arm follow the movement. The patient is encouraged to practice independently with a focus on the sequence. During independent practice, the therapist may provide verbal cues to help the patient with timing the movement of the upper body.

The *symmetrical lateral flexion initiation pattern* is known as "log rolling": in this pattern, the trunk does not rotate but is active in a coordinated fashion with the arm and leg on the same side; the arm and leg "reach or push" on the leading side. In rolling from supine to side lying, the trunk flexors initiate the antigravity movement, and when rolling from side lying to supine, the trunk flexors act as the antigravity movement control.

Impairments that interfere. Shoulder joint pain may occur when the patient rolls onto the affected side. Pain occurs if the shoulder is trapped under the trunk as the patient moves to side lying or when the humeral-scapular alignment causes the shoulder capsule to be impinged. If pain occurs during the roll, the therapist should teach the patient to stop, roll back a few degrees, adjust the position of the arm away from the trunk, and then continue the roll. Therapists should teach their patients how to avoid shoulder pain during all activities, especially during rolling or when lying on the more affected side.

In rehabilitative or outpatient care, muscle tightness in the latissimus, quadratus lumborum, biceps, or tensor fasciae latae may limit trunk rotation or trunk and extremity linked movements.

Clinical observations. Weakness in the extremities is a significant factor during rolling because the arm and the leg assist the trunk initiation patterns. Rotational patterns are difficult in the acute stage because they require an integration and sequencing of flexor and extensor muscle patterns. Symmetrical rolling may be the easiest independent pattern to train. Therapists should incorporate active assistive strategies and extremity strengthening in the early recovery period. Patients have an easier time rolling to the affected side because they use the strength of the unaffected side to initiate the roll. But they may not want to stay on that side because of shoulder pain, instability of the hip, or decreased sensation and the accompanying fear. The patient may prefer rolling to the unaffected side because it is easier to rest on, but initiating the movement is difficult because of loss of control on the affected, leading side.

The family is educated to understand the nature of the loss of movement and sensation and the effects of these losses on body awareness and early bed mobility. Family members are encouraged to sit with, visit, talk to, feed, and touch the person from the patient's affected side. They are instructed in simple movements such as rolling to promote symmetry, midline control, and activation of trunk and extremity muscles.

Feeding and Swallowing

Although detailed facilitation and inhibition of oral and neck muscle movement for feeding and articulated language are a specialty of speech pathologists, the movement therapist activates upper-body control to prepare for more automatic chew and swallow.

Basic trunk patterns to be reeducated include (1) lower-body anterior and posterior movement control to move toward a table and back into a chair and (2) upper-body anterior and posterior and lateral movement control to provide control for head and arm movements.

Impairments That Interfere

Oral problems include the following:
- Forward head, poor lip closure, loss of saliva and food
- Facial asymmetry during function greater than at rest
- Inability to swallow
- Inability to chew
- Inability to lateralize foods
- Inability to take liquids from cup or spoon
- Muscle weakness
  Central problems are as follows:
- Poor postural control
- Inability to feed self
  Compensations include the following:
- Use of gravity—head and neck extension
- Chewing on one side only
- Using the hand to place food in the mouth
- Using the hand to pull food from the cheek
- Using thicker food than liquids

Clinical Observations

Excessive drooling occurs with loss of head control and a decreased ability to automatically close the mouth and swallow if excessive extension is present. If the patient tries to extend the head from a flexed cervical spine position, the head may jut forward into a position of axial extension. As a result of the biomechanics of the forward head position, the jaw opens, automatic swallowing becomes difficult, and saliva runs out of the open mouth.

Drooling from one side of the mouth is annoying and embarrassing. The patient may not be able to maintain lip closure and, in addition, may not feel the saliva running out or may not identify a need to swallow.

In the majority of cases, swallowing problems are transient in persons with hemiplegia. After the initial insult, many patients exhibit a decreased gag reflex. In acute care settings, where liquid diets are often routinely given to persons with hemiplegia, education of hospital staff regarding the merits of using thicker foods should be considered. Thicker, chopped food is easier to swallow than soft food. Soft food is easier to swallow than liquids. Liquids with distinct taste or texture are easier to swallow than water.

Sitting

Function in sitting is based on the ability to maintain the trunk in an upright position, to automatically adjust the trunk when the arms or one leg moves around midline, and to follow movements of the arm and leg as they extend their reach. Control in sitting is also used to help change position, such as moving from sitting to standing, or lying down. The reestablishment of control in sitting for function is an important early goal in rehabilitation care.

Basic trunk movement patterns include the following:
1. Anterior, posterior, and lateral upper-trunk initiated movements. Upper-trunk movements are easier to retrain than lower-trunk movements because during upper-trunk movements the base of support (the lower trunk and thighs) remains on the surface.
2. Anterior and posterior lower-trunk initiated movements. With lower-trunk initiated movement, the upper trunk needs to be controlled and stable, yet adjust to and follow the movement of the lower trunk.
3. Lateral lower-trunk initiated movements. These movements are more difficult to reeducate than upper-trunk movements because as the movement begins, the base of support narrows.
4. Rotational movements. In sitting, upper-body rotational movements are easier to perform than lower-body rotational patterns for the reason noted previously.

Trunk and Arm Linked Patterns (Representative Examples)

Postural adjustments to arm movements around midline require the trunk to be upright, to be active, and to perform small adjustments. When the hand functions in front of the body, the trunk adjusts with small posterior weight shifts, whereas as the hand(s) move to function behind the body, the trunk adjusts with a small anterior weight shift.

The trunk moves with an arm to extend reach. If the reach is forward and down to the floor, as if to reach a shoe, the upper body initiates an anterior weight shift and the spine moves into flexion with control from eccentric contraction of the spinal extensors. If the reach is forward as if to grab an object on the front side of a table, the lower body initiates an anterior weight shift as the upper body remains stable and adjusts to the demands of the arm movement.

Trunk and Leg Linked Patterns (Representative Examples)

Small trunk adjustments occur with leg movements around midline. If the feet move back under the hips, the trunk adjusts with a small amount of anterior weight shift. When one foot is lifted up to slide into a slipper, the lower body adjusts with a small lateral weight shift. Upper-trunk stability allows lower-trunk initiated patterns when rising to stand. As the legs extend and the buttocks lift off the chair, trunk adjustments accompany the changing leg pattern to control trunk position over the legs.

Impairments That Interfere

Changes in alignment of the arm resulting from weakness and muscle shortening affect the position of the thoracic spine and rib cage. The weight of an extremely weak arm pulls the upper trunk into forward flexion.

Shoulder subluxation results in muscle shortening (biceps, pectorals, latissimus, subscapularis), alters the line of muscle pull, and interferes with scapulohumeral rhythm. Muscle shortening contributes to loss of upper-body alignment and interferes with reestablishing arm and trunk control.

Loss of trunk alignment as a result of extremity weakness and loss of trunk control creates an atypical starting position for movement and can become an undesirable compensation.

Clinical Observations

Alignment changes in the arm influence strength and control of the upper body. Therefore intervention techniques to restore alignment and control of the arm in relation to the upper trunk must be included in the list of short-term goals to achieve the functional goal of safe, independent task performance in sitting.

Active control of the pelvis in a neutral position is necessary for the reeducation of lower-body lateral and rotational weight shifts. Pelvic position influences leg position. If the pelvis is held in a posterior tilt, the leg initially tends to abduct; and if it is held in an anterior tilt, the leg initially adducts.

Patients with poor hip control do not regain functional trunk patterns while sitting until they can activate and strengthen hip muscles for stability during weight shifts. Loss of control in the hip results in a need to shift weight to the stronger side, thus creating pelvic and/or spinal asymmetry.

Lower-body–initiated lateral weight shift patterns are difficult to train because they require a narrowing of the base of support. Forearm weight-bearing movement patterns are used to increase the base of support to allow practice of these patterns that are needed for functional activities such as scooting, toileting, and lifting one leg off the surface.

Transfers

Transfers in the half-stand, pivot pattern require upper-body control over the lower body and combined trunk and leg control patterns. The squat, pivot position is trained when leg strength and control are weak and the goal is to train the patient to use the affected leg. Transfers are interim patterns that are trained before safe standing and stepping is possible.

The patient practices transfers to different objects (chair, bed, toilet) to either side. This promotes symmetry, encourages the use of the affected leg, and allows practice with varying environmental constraints. Transfers to the unaffected side have the advantage of being familiar to hospital staff because they are the "traditional" textbook way of transferring the person with hemiplegia. Nevertheless, transfers to the affected side need to be trained by therapists to allow function in either direction.

Sitting to Standing

Moving from sitting to standing is an important skill to retrain early after a stroke because it is used many times a day during functional activities. In a study investigating the relationship between sitting to standing and walking, Chou and colleagues[149] found that a critical component of sitting to standing was between leg vertical force displacement, the amount of weight transferred down into the floor. Those who had a maximal between-leg vertical force difference of less than 30% body weight between both legs displayed faster walking speeds and more typical gait parameters.

Two initiation patterns are commonly used, with or without the use of momentum, to train sitting-to-standing. A *lower-body initiated* anterior weight transfer occurs with a neutral spine as the shoulders move forward. Therapists should emphasize the forward weight shift

component of this pattern and hip flexion; the requirement of sitting to standing is a forward shift of the upper body and shoulders. Although individuals with a tendency for lumbar extension may have an anterior pelvic tilt as they shift forward, the anterior pelvic tilt is not as important a component as is a forward weight shift.

An *upper-body initiated* anterior weight transfer during sitting to standing requires control in spinal flexion. This pattern keeps body weight over the feet, the new base of support, but does not link the extension of the legs with the lower trunk. The demand on the trunk from liftoff to standing is greater than in the previous pattern because of the need to move the spine from flexion to upright neutral. In the previous pattern, the spine starts and remains in a neutral position through to standing. The upper-body initiated pattern is used in rehabilitation and extended care centers because it allows caregivers to keep weight firmly over the feet, thus allowing a safe, maximal-assistance transfer.

During transfer and sitting-to-standing training, techniques of directing manual pressure from the top of the knee through the tibia into the foot help the patient remember to keep weight on both feet and increase the dorsiflexion movement at the ankle. Full standing should not be attempted if loss of control in the leg results in nonuse. If the patient cannot activate leg muscles in a weight-bearing position in attempts to stand, the standing position will be precarious with undesirable trunk compensatory patterns.

Standing
Standing Control

Control in standing is a difficult early goal to achieve because not only is there a need for trunk and leg coordinated movements, but there is also a prerequisite need for upper-body (trunk and arm) control over the lower body. Control of basic movement patterns in standing is divided into upper-body–initiated control patterns and lower-extremity–initiated control patterns.[150]

Upper-body control in standing includes the ability to move the trunk and arm in all planes with appropriate lower-extremity responses, the ability to respond and adjust to weight transfer to each leg, and to provide postural stability for movements of each leg in space. As a prerequisite for reeducation of these movements, the upper body must have enough strength and control to provide stability and postural adjustments for movements of the lower extremity.

Basic trunk movements to be reeducated include the following:
1. Upper-body initiated anterior, posterior, lateral, and rotational patterns with critical corresponding adjustments in the leg (either hip, knee, or ankle strategies).
2. Control of the upper body over the lower trunk during lower-extremity–initiated weight-bearing movements.
3. Linked trunk and leg patterns during movements of the leg in space. These are easiest when the leg moves around midline and increase in difficulty as the leg moves within and beyond limb length and when movement in space increases in amplitude or speed.
4. Increased upper-body control to support power production for pushing, pulling, or lifting objects and increased upper- and lower-body control to support power production of the legs for activities such as stair climbing, hopping, jumping, and running.

Trunk and Arm Linked Patterns

Trunk and arm linked patterns include the following:
1. Upper-body initiated flexion movements that occur with forward and downward arm reach patterns
2. Upper-body initiated extension that occurs when the arm reaches up or up and back

3. Upper-body initiated lateral flexion when the arm reaches down and to one side
4. Upper-body flexion and rotation when the arm reaches down and to one side.
5. Upper-body extension and rotation when the arm reaches up and back to one side

Trunk and Leg Linked Patterns in Weight Bearing

Control of the upper and lower trunk during unilateral stance on either leg is one of the most difficult patterns to retrain. Control of the trunk in unilateral stance is linked with the need for abduction control on the stance leg. In patients with hemiplegia, the complicated control demands for leg and trunk control in standing combined with the presence of weakness and control problems result in loss of alignment in multiple joints and undesirable compensatory patterns.

Trunk and Leg Linked Patterns as the Leg Moves in Space

When the leg moves in space in small ranges, the adjusting movements of the upper body are small and occur as postural adjustments. The movement pattern of the femur and pelvis has a linked rhythm similar to that of scapulohumeral rhythm: the first 30 to 45 degrees of hip flexion occurs with no pelvic movements; from 45 to 90 degrees the pelvis flexes (posteriorly tilts) with the flexing hip; with continued hip flexion the upper trunk flexes. This pelvic-hip relationship occurs in the other planes of movement as well and is seen during the following functional movements:

1. Pelvic and lower trunk flexion occurs when the leg reaches forward and up; stepping up.
2. Pelvic and trunk extension occurs when the leg reaches back.
3. Pelvic elevation or depression with trunk lateral flexion occurs when the leg moves laterally.

Impairments That Interfere

In standing, loss of alignment in the upper body on the hemiplegic side may result in undesirable compensatory patterns that interfere with functional standing movements and balance. These patterns include (1) forward flexion of the upper trunk, (2) upper-body rotation toward the affected side, and (3) upper-body rotation away from the affected side.

Ankle range may decrease within a few days after stroke and needs to be minimized to allow early standing functions. Loss of ankle joint dorsiflexion range interferes with the ability of the body to recruit ankle strategies, and limited ankle joint dorsiflexion range often accompanies knee hyperextension in standing.

Loss of knee control during standing may result from loss of sufficient lower-extremity force production or low-level limb sequencing. Loss of knee control is also influenced by the position and movement control of the hip and ankle joints. Initially the knee flexes as more weight is shifted to the unaffected side, and the pelvis lists downward. If the pelvic position is not corrected (leveled) and the patient actively straightens the knee, a compensatory pelvic rotation (toward the affected side) may occur. Because of the instability of a weak, flexing leg, the patient may learn to "lock" the knee in hyperextension as a means of gaining stability (Fig. 24.14).

Clinical Observations

In the acute phase, therapists can help the patient practice standing with the hips and shoulders back against a wall to provide support for the trunk and pelvis while creating a safe situation for practicing active self-initiated leg weight-bearing movements. The patient can slide down the wall, activating eccentric control in the legs, and then slide back up, activating concentric control. By using the wall to assist the

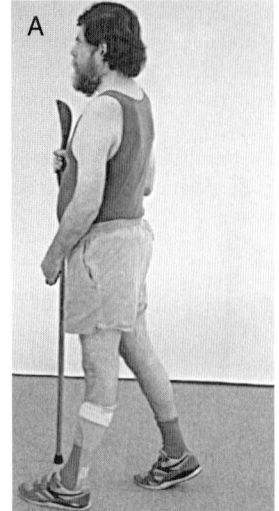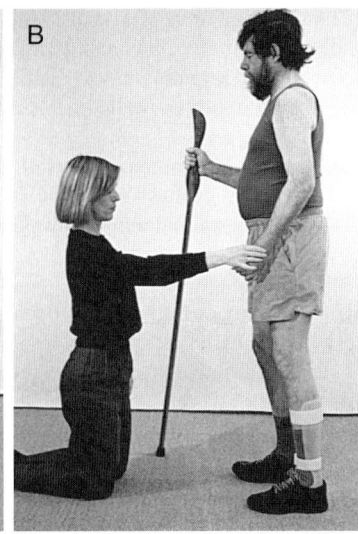

Fig. 24.14 **(A)** Patient with left hemiplegia with knee hyperextension wearing a lightweight prefabricated posterior leaf-spring brace that does not control his knee hyperextension. **(B)** A solid ankle brace with foot control that decreases knee hyperextension by providing distal stability.

stand, the therapist frees his or her hands to help correct leg alignment problems and lets the patient practice the initiation of movement early, independently, and safely.

The patient can practice controlled lateral weight transfer with appropriate trunk activity in this position. Whereas one study concluded that there is no relationship between lateral weight shift and walking, therapists should not conclude that unilateral weight acceptance is inappropriate functional training.[151] What may be more relevant than lateral weight transfer over the leg is learning to depress the foot into the floor, the vertical force, as it equalizes weight between the two legs.[152]

Upper-extremity forearm or extended-arm weight bearing provides upper-trunk stability for lower-extremity initiated practice. This practice pattern also allows a means of self-ranging for the ankle, knee, hip, and pelvis. This position is used not to inhibit tone in the extremities but to activate and strengthen the trunk and legs in linked patterns.

Walking

Independent, functional, and safe walking is difficult to retrain in the early phases of intervention because it requires control of the second level of the trunk: a stable yet adaptable trunk during extremity movement beyond limb length. Sufficient force production and appropriate timing in the leg is also needed to support body weight, to sequence complex patterns, and to control momentum and balance. Walking patterns in individuals who have experienced stroke are characterized by slow speed, uneven step and stride lengths, impaired balance with aberrant movement patterns in the arm and leg, and reliance on adaptive equipment.

In the current healthcare environment with the emphasis on limited therapy visits, therapists are confronted with major intervention dilemmas: Should they encourage the individual to walk without minimal prerequisites? Should they allow undesirable compensations although they predict future secondary problems? Should they use the benefits of the large health care systems to divide responsibility for continued gait training among therapy divisions (inpatient, rehabilitation, home care, outpatient)?

Prerequisites for functional, safe walking include the following:

- Upper-body control to support leg movements in unilateral stance and during swing
- Lower-trunk control to prevent atypical pelvic patterns
- Strength and control of the leg to initiate weight shifts
- Strength and control of the leg to move in space

Because gait is the most extensively studied, analyzed, and discussed in terms of intervention, this section describes the prerequisites for walking training and common impairments that interfere with walking.[153–155] Common impairments that interfere with walking are separated into three divisions of the walking cycle: (1) forward progression, (2) single- and double-limb support, and (3) swing.[156,157]

Impairments that interfere with functional walking are summarized in Box 24.8.

Research on and equipment for partial–body-weight supported treadmill walking training with or without robotic assistance have been ongoing.[158–162] In a 2004 review of randomized controlled studies, there was strong evidence for post-stroke treadmill training with or without body-weight support (Fig. 24.15).[163] Task specificity, speed, intensity, and symmetry of practice in this type of equipment were thought to contribute to improved overground walking performance.[158] However, a Cochrane review reported no statistically significant effect of treadmill training with or without body-weight support.[164] A 2011 randomized

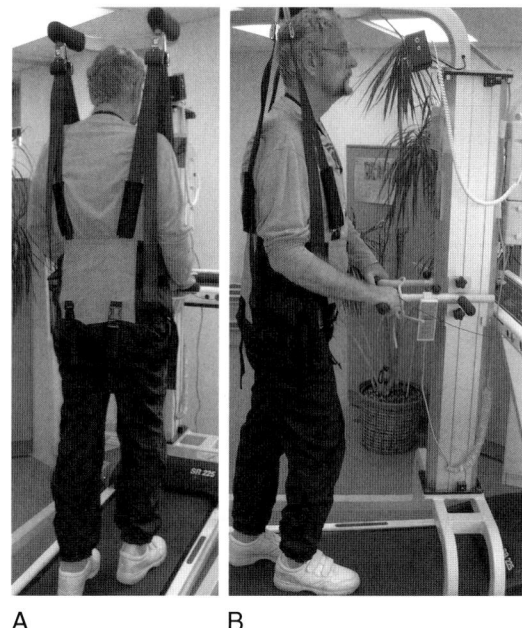

Fig. 24.15 (A and **B)** Patient with right hemiplegia walking on a treadmill with partial body-weight support.

controlled trial comparing body-weight–supported locomotor training with a therapist-supervised home progressive exercise and balance program reports improvements with both training methods.[165] Hershberg has extended that trial by developing an algorithm for clinical decision making in progressing either protocol based on patient presentation.[166] In the 2016 Clinical Practice Guideline, the authors point toward the potential impact body-weight support and robotic technologies may have; however, they state further clinical trials are needed to establish recommendations and protocols.[80]

Clinical Observations

If impaired sequencing in the lower extremity results in difficulty clearing the foot during stepping, compensatory strategies of hip hiking, circumduction, or posterior pelvic tilting arise. If allowed to persist, these atypical initiation strategies become difficult to retrain. Consider the post-stroke modular framework from Clark's study: intervention strategies should aim to improve muscle sequencing and timing to improve normal hip, knee, and ankle movements during swing phase.[88] Ferrante and Routson were able to demonstrate improved modular complexity and/or timing with the use of functional electrical stimulation and body-weight support treadmill training respectively.[167,168]

Additionally, consider minimal ankle and foot support during early walking as a means of preventing distal compensatory strategies and promoting distal initiation (Fig. 24.16). (See Chapter 32 for additional suggestions.)

Cardiovascular Health

A comprehensive physical therapy plan of care should include reducing the risk of recurrent stroke by addressing a patient's cardiovascular health through the prescription of physical activity and exercise. Physical activity and exercises have been shown to improve multiple aspects of stroke recovery including physical and psychosocial components; however, current research demonstrates underutilization and underprescription of cardiovascular rehabilitation programs.[169]

BOX 24.8   Summary of Significant Functional Impairments

Forward Progression—Heel Strike to Midstance

Impaired trunk control
- Altered alignment and control upper trunk over lower trunk
- Insufficient upper trunk control as leg initiates forward weight shift

Lack of proper initiation pattern
- Excessive forward trunk flexion
- Excessive lateral weight shift

Insufficient ankle joint dorsiflexion
- Muscle tightness
- Impaired muscle activation
- Edema

Inappropriate foot contact
- Weakness and altered muscle activation in foot and ankle muscles
- Muscle tightness

Single and Double Limb Support

Insufficient trunk control to maintain alignment over one leg
- Asymmetries during unilateral stance
- Loss of control of upper trunk over lower trunk

Altered lower-extremity control
- Hip instability
- Loss of knee control in unilateral stance
- Altered sequencing and timing of lower leg musculature

Loss of ability to transfer weight through foot
- Inability to maintain leg on floor behind body
- Loss of muscle length
- Weakness and inappropriate activation of leg muscles

Swing—Early and Late

Atypical leg muscle firing patterns
- Lack of distal initiation
- Inability to control trunk and lower-extremity sequencing patterns

Inability of the body to continue to move forward as leg swings

Aberrant foot movement

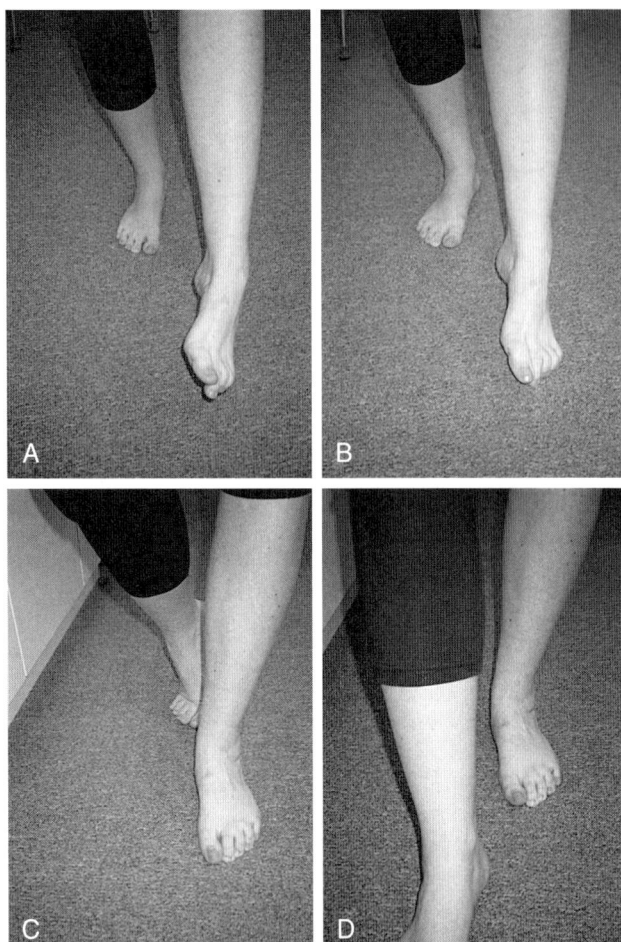

Fig. 24.16 (A and **B)** Patient with left hemiplegia. Supination of the foot during swing and during foot contact with ankle joint plantarflexion and calcaneal varus. **(C** and **D)** Compensatory pronation of the midfoot to allow the foot to contact the ground during stance.

Exercise counseling should aim to overcome identified barriers to participation in physical activity, including understanding of the benefits and feasibility of participation, access to resources, and limited knowledge on appropriate activities and intensity of activity.

Clinical Considerations

In the acute phase, early mobilization is recommended to abate orthostatic intolerance, limit edema, maintain joint mobility, and prevent deep vein thrombosis. Prior to initiating an exercise regimen in the outpatient setting, patients should undergo graded exercise testing. It is highly recommended initial graded testing be performed with ECG monitoring; however, if this is not feasible, an individualized training program should still be initiated. The current available data indicate a low risk of severe cardiovascular complications during submaximal graded exercise testing in stroke survivors when performed under appropriate guidelines including monitoring of heart rate, blood pressure response, O_2 saturation, subjective reporting of cardiac symptoms, and ratings of perceived exertion. The Bruce protocol and the modified Bruce protocol are appropriate graded tests for patients who are able to perform an ambulatory treadmill test. Other protocols are available for upright and recumbent cycle ergometers and upper extremity ergometers. It is recommended to discontinue a graded test when the patient has reached 70% age-predicted maximum heart rate

or greater than 250 mm Hg systolic or 115 mm Hg diastolic blood pressure to reduce the risk of adverse events.

Prescription of physical activity should be individualized to the patient based on their tolerance to activity, stage of stroke recovery, available social and environmental resources, activity preferences, and their unique impairments and limitations. Billinger and colleagues recommend exercise frequency to be three or more days per week for 20 to 60 minutes. They also support an interval training model including multiple sets of exercises (3 to 4× per day) for 10 to 15 minutes depending on the patient's capacity and exercise tolerance. Strength training is also recommended with higher repetitions (10 to 15 repetitions) and reduced loads performed 2 to 3 days per week. Exercises should focus on the torso and the major muscle groups of the upper and lower extremities.[170]

EQUIPMENT

Equipment for persons with CNS dysfunction can be thought of as supports or extra assists to allow better alignment, stabilization, or balance so that the patient can move and function more independently. Too much support or equipment may hinder the development of new movement control. Equipment should never be a substitute for treatment and should not be given without practice during treatment. One-handed equipment that is used as a compensation for trunk control is less successful than equipment that is used to compensate for loss of extremity function. Therapists should perform continuing assessments of the appropriateness of the equipment in relation to gains made in therapy.

Example

A "reacher" compensates for loss of trunk and limb linked control (reach beyond arm's length), but use of a reacher may prevent the development of this control, whereas an electric can opener designed for one-handed use substitutes for the ability to use the affected hand (when recovery is not possible).

Bedside Equipment

In acute and rehabilitation settings, pillows, blankets, or towels are used to position the patient in bed. With the patient in the supine position, the head pillow can be angled so that it slips under the shoulder and scapula to prevent loss of alignment: to prevent humeral hyperextension and internal rotation. A soft towel roll or pillow under the leg—greater trochanter or knee—maintains alignment of the leg in the first few days after a stroke. Once the patient begins to move to both sides in bed, the use of pillows for support is not necessary.

Wheelchairs

Wheelchairs must have a solid surface and, when possible, a supportive backrest. The soft leather seats and backs of transport chairs act as slings and allow the pelvis to posteriorly tilt and the spine to flex. Solid seats and backs allow the pelvis, trunk, and extremities to be more normally aligned. Wheelchairs specifically for patients with hemiplegia who are not expected to become household ambulators have lower seat heights and one-armed drive (two hand rims on one wheel). These adaptations make it easier for patients to propel the chair with the unaffected hand and foot.

Support for the hemiplegic arm when the patient is sitting in a wheelchair reduces the effect of the downward pull of gravity on the weak or paralyzed arm. Lapboards support both arms and provide symmetry for the upper body. However, in some health care settings, they are considered a form of restraint and cannot be used. The use of a pillow in the lap is another option for bilateral support of the arms.

Half-lapboards or arm troughs are used to support the arm. If an arm support is used, the patient should be taught how to protect the arm and hand while on the support.

Slings

Slings are used to support the glenohumeral joint to prevent capsular stretch, to temporarily maintain alignment that is gained in treatment, and to take some of the weight of the paralyzed arm off the upper trunk as the patient begins to learn to stand and walk. Capsular stretch accompanies shoulder subluxation, and it is difficult to reverse an existing subluxation once the capsule is stretched. Because subluxation is not inherently painful, a sling is not used to prevent pain. However, use of a sling can take the heavy weight of a weak arm off the trunk and may help break the cycle of shoulder pain.

Various reviews and comparisons of slings are available.[171–173] Shoulder subluxation is the result of loss of strength and control in the shoulder girdle and trunk, especially scapular upward rotation. There is no sling available that corrects a subluxation because no existing sling provides scapular upward rotation control. Slings act as an assist to "hold" a scapulohumeral position that has been restored in treatment.

The ideal shoulder sling helps maintain the normal angular alignment of the glenoid fossa, decreases the tendency of the humerus to internally rotate, takes some of the weight of the arm off the upper trunk, and allows the upper extremity freedom of movement. Therapists should not prescribe slings that cradle the arm in front of the body, prevent any movement, and in effect teach learned nonuse. The orthopedic-type *envelope arm sling* was used in the 1950s and 1960s is of this type. In the 1970s, influenced by Bobath,[101] sling use was thought to be undesirable. As more information about tone and movement became available, new slings were designed to allow the arm to be supported while movement was reeducated. Slings have different suspensions, provide different means of control for the arm, give differing "messages" to the arm and trunk, and have individual uses. Table 24.6, adapted from the work of Levit,[174] lists available slings and their characteristics.

Patients who come into therapy with a sling but who do not require one are weaned from a supportive sling into a less controlling one. Patients state that the *clavicle support* provides support during household tasks that require upper-body flexion, such as bed making or vacuuming. Patients who complain of "aching" in the arm at the end of the day may relieve this ache by using a support for a few hours around midday.

If the arm dangles or bangs against the body during active periods, the *shoulder saddle sling* can be adjusted to protect the arm from bruising. This sling is also helpful to patients with severe shoulder-hand pain because it allows full support of the arm and can be adjusted by the patient to allow the elbow to extend as the pain subsides. The *GivMohr sling* combines a humeral cuff with a hand support. *Humeral cuff slings* are the most practical from a functional standpoint because they do not restrict scapula, arm, or trunk position.

Canes

Canes are given to patients with hemiplegia to provide extra balance, not as a means to support body weight. Canes should be used after upper-body and lower-extremity initiated movements have been practiced.

If quad canes or hemiwalkers are used before trunk and leg activity is minimally established, they encourage lateral translation of the spine or counter rotation of the upper spine and pelvis. When patients shift off the weak leg onto the stable cane, the cane acts functionally as a third leg. This one-sided compensation encourages learned nonuse of the affected leg.

Single canes provide a balance assist. Often patients use the cane while walking outdoors or in crowded situations but not inside their homes. Reliance on a cane for walking eliminates the possibility of carrying objects and makes it difficult to perform one-handed tasks such as opening a door. Wrist loops allow the patient to use the unaffected hand without having to put the cane aside. Weighted cane tips, such as the AbleTripod[175] rubber cane tip, or the HurryCane[176] provide a bridge between quad canes and straight canes and allow a standard cane to remain upright.

Orthotics

Ankle-foot orthoses (AFOs) are used to allow foot clearance during walking, to ensure heel strike, to provide distal stability for early standing and walking in patients with severe weakness, to provide lateral lower-leg stability in patients who need an assist because of lateral hip weakness, and to control knee hyperextension caused by loss of ankle dorsiflexion control. Different design types provide different functions. Solid ankle bracing with plastic beyond the malleoli limits distal

TABLE 24.6 Examples of Slings and Their Characteristics

Basic Type	Supplier	Suspension	Message	Common Use
Clavicle support	DePuy (clavicle fracture sling with 1-inch soft foam axilla pad)	Figure-of-8 between scapulae Support under axilla	"Spine extend, scapula adduct"	Acute care Minimal support To wean out of other supports
Humeral cuff	Rolyan Hemi Arm Sling	Figure-of-8 between scapulae Velcro cuff support to humeral shaft	"Arm up"	Rehabilitative care
Unilateral shoulder orthosis	Bauerfeind Rolyan	Across body Elastic or spandex cuff support to humeral shaft	"Lift humerus up"	Rehabilitative care
Shoulder-saddle sling	Sammons	Saddle sits on top of shoulder Strap across body Forearm cuff—adjustable straps allow changes in elbow position	Maximal support of arm	To prevent "banging" of flaccid arm in active patients or during sports activities To provide support for painful arm
GivMohr sling	GivMohr	Figure-of-8 between scapulae Plastic cone in palm of hand	"Arm up"	To relieve weight of "heavy" flaccid arm

freedom but allows patients with severe weakness to practice gaining control of trunk and hip movements.

Polypropylene Orthotics

The use of polypropylene bracing to control foot posturing in adults began in the 1970s with information from pediatrics and podiatry. Foot control in a brace stops supination of the foot in swing and compensatory pronation of the foot in stance. This control is achieved through neutral rear foot positioning and long medial and lateral foot counters. Custom-made AFOs provide the best fit and control, but excellent prefabricated polypropylene braces are available through companies such as Orthomerica, or Wheaton Brace. These orthoses have long medial and lateral foot edges for control of foot posturing, come in multiple models and sizes, and can be ordered with regular or long foot plates or as blanks that can be self-trimmed (see Chapter 32).

Carbon Fiber Orthoses

Newer, lighter braces constructed from carbon fiber allow greater propulsive forces during late stance. The Phat brace, a custom fabricated energy-storing carbon fiber brace, allows exacting control of foot supination and pronation and with varying resistance strengths to replicate

the forces needed during walking (www.phatbraces.com). Techniques of Aquaplast fabrication have also created new possibilities for inexpensive, immediate, remoldable bracing for the foot and ankle.[177,178]

Wireless FES systems

Wireless Functional Electrical Stimulation (FES) foot-drop systems, the Bioness L300 and the WalkAide, are available for clinical use. These systems use low-level electrical activity to stimulate the nerves that lift the foot and are timed with walking stance and swing patterns.

Patients should be encouraged to spend time standing or walking short distances without the brace so that dependence is not established. Patients like to be able to walk to the bathroom at night without a brace. Orthopedic ankle and foot supports provide alternatives to plastic bracing. The MalleoLoc ankle support controls rear foot equinus and varus while allowing ankle and forefoot movement (Bauerfeind USA/AliMed). Patients with moderate supination posturing report a reassuring feeling of security with this support while walking short distances and during sports participation. This support, a substitute for the Aircast and Ace support, is a good choice for sports activities such as golfing, bicycling, jumping, and running.

Functions and limitations of commonly used braces are found in Table 24.7 and orthotic manufacturers in Appendix 24.A.

TABLE 24.7 Ankle-Foot Orthoses Used in Patients With Hemiplegia From Stroke			
Orthotic Design	**Function**	**Limitations**	**Patient Types (Categories)**
Solid ankle with foot control	Heel strike Distal stability Lateral hip stability Assists forward progression Assists knee control Stops foot posturing	No ankle mobility No toe break	Severe weakness in trunk and leg Need for distal stability
Modified solid ankle with foot control	Heel strike More distal mobility, less ankle control Stops foot posturing	Less knee control Reduced message of forward progression No control of knee	Increasing leg strength Increasing trunk and leg control
Posterior leaf spring	Toe clearance	No control of foot posturing	Good return of control in trunk and leg Need for minimal dorsiflexion assistance
Articulated ankle	Free dorsiflexion Heel strike if plantar stop used	Limited control of foot posturing Bulky at ankle	Normal ankle range—if range is limited, the movement of brace is translated into foot Functional needs; climb hills, stairs, move to and from ground
Supramalleolar foot orthoses in Aquaplast	Foot control Assist heel strike Used for weaning from AFOs Sports	No knee control Short shelf life of material	Increasing leg control Desire to begin increasing activity level
Foot orthoses	Balance small asymmetries of foot	No control of foot posturing No ankle or knee control	Persistent but minimal rear foot–forefoot asymmetries
Klenzak metal, double upright	Toe clearance Reminder of forward progression	No foot control Control of ankle and foot through shoe	Used before creation of polypropylene to provide heel strike and stop foot supination
Alternative Functional Electrical Stimulation Foot Drop Devices			
Bioness L300	Foot control Knee control assist Operates via heel pressure switch	Expensive Requires cognitive ability to don and adjust settings	
WalkAide	Foot control Operates via tibial tilt	Requires cognitive ability to don and adjust settings	

See Chapter 34 for additional suggestions.
AFOs, Ankle-foot orthoses.

Toe Curling/Clawing Aids

There are two patterns of toe posturing: toe clawing and toe curling. Toe clawing, metatarsal hyperextension with phalangeal flexion, is a result of altered alignment of the metatarsals and tarsals; and toe curling, metatarsal and phalangeal flexion, is a response to insufficient postural stability for the task: standing or walking.[63]

Toe curling and toe clawing interfere with comfort and may become painful. Problems of blistering on pads of the toes and on the top of the proximal interphalangeal joint are common in the later stages of recovery. Relief from pressure and pain on the toe pads (tips) comes with use of commercially available "hammertoe crest pads" or a "toe crutch" available from distributors[179] or from medical pharmacies.

Movable Surfaces

Movable surfaces such as gymnastic balls of varying sizes, large rolls, and adjustable stools with casters are used as environmental support for the trunk or extremities. Gymnastic balls provide symmetrical support to the rib cage when used in the hands-and-knees position and may be used to maintain spinal alignment or girdle muscle length. When spasticity was considered the major impairment in hemiplegia, therapists often placed patients prone over balls to "inhibit" tone. This is an inappropriate technique, considering advances in understanding of movement control and recovery.

Hand Splints

The practice of splinting the hemiplegic hand is controversial. Historically, the hand in patients with hemiplegia was splinted in a "resting" position of 15 degrees wrist flexion and a finger extension platform. After the introduction of neurophysiological approaches, splinting became "inhibitory" in design.[180–182] Now, with the understanding that spasticity is not the major problem, splinting the wrist and hand has undergone another change. A splint designed by Levit[183] as a neutral functional splint promotes functional retraining and hand use while minimizing secondary impairments. This splint, designed to hold the wrist and hand in a position of orthopedic neutral, helps maintain muscle length across the wrist and decreases aberrant movement that occurs with poor alignment or unbalanced muscle return. The splint promotes support of the wrist and hand to avoid the secondary impairments of muscle tightness, muscle shifting, and overstretching of weak wrist and finger muscles. This type of splinting has been reported to decrease hand edema and pain.[184]

Therapists custom-make the splints with the goals of supporting the wrist in neutral, preventing radial or ulnar deviation with long, high sides, and maintaining the palmar arches. The fingers are not incorporated into the splint but are left free to allow movement reeducation and practice. This functional splint is worn mainly during the day when aberrant arm movement may be greater and when support of critical joints decreases the degrees of freedom, thus allowing the emergence of active functional hand use.

Design Considerations

If joint range is limited, the therapist makes the splint to support available range. The splint can be revised as range increases. Alignment is corrected in three steps: (1) keeping the wrist in flexion, the lateral deviation is corrected by aligning the third metacarpal with the middle of the radius; (2) the carpal position is corrected (usually by gently lifting up from a low position under the radius); and (3) the hand is moved to wrist neutral (see *Functional Movement Reeducation*[63] for a step-by-step analysis). The warmed, soft splinting plastic captures this corrected position as it cools. The length of palmar support is decided by the therapist after assessment of degree and distribution of muscle return and muscle tightness patterns. The thumb is supported at its base in a neutral position, not one of abduction. As beginning grip returns, the thumb hole is widened to allow function.

A variety of neutral functional splints have been designed. The neutral wrist and thumb hole splinting design makes the splint hard to keep on the hand of patients with severe weakness. They sometimes find ulnar or radial trough splints or wide opponens splints easier to keep on.

As wrist extension control against gravity emerges, the therapist can fabricate a wide opponens splint to maintain the palmar arches as the patient begins practicing finger movements. The wide opponens splint supports the base of the hand and assists in maintaining carpal alignment. Patients can switch between the two splints as needed.

Patients with severe hand pain prefer a neutral wrist splint with a resting area for the thumb. This splint is fabricated with little or no correction initially but with gentle support for the wrist and palmar arches. As the pain decreases, this splint is modified to become the original neutral functional splint.

Although the move away from "inhibitory" splints and from night splinting to daytime functional splinting breaks many of the "rules" from the past, it is more compatible with concepts from research and clinical experts.

Recommended resources for practical solutions to one-handed functioning and devices that assist in independence are listed in Appendix 24.B at the end of this chapter.

PSYCHOSOCIAL ASPECTS AND ADJUSTMENTS

The suddenness of a stroke and the dramatic change in motor, sensory, visual, and perceptual performance and feedback may leave the person with hemiplegia confused, disoriented, angry, stressed, frustrated, and fearful.

Psychosocial issues may be more detrimental than any functional disability to long-term stroke survivors.[185] Decreased interest in social activity inside and outside the home and decreased interest in hobbies as a result of psychosocial disability hamper the hemiplegic individual's return to a normal social life.[186] Feelings of rejection and embarrassment may interfere with the hemiplegic person's interaction with people outside the home environment. Individuals with long-standing hemiplegia often become clinically depressed, with symptoms of loss of sleep and appetite, self-blame, and a hopeless outlook. The usual psychosocial adjustments to disability are compounded in persons with hemiplegia resulting from stroke by the issues associated with aging.

Family members and spouses may have difficulty assessing the capabilities of the hemiplegic person and may be overprotective. Overprotection among spouses may be a sign of affection and support or a sign of guilt.[187] Long-standing marriages do not tend to dissolve when one member has a stroke. However, previous marriage problems and personality traits may become exaggerated as a result of the presence of increased and changing demands and stresses that occur when the person returns home.

A comparison of occupational status of long-term stroke survivors in the United States and in Sweden reveals that 40% of the Swedes returned to a form of employment (including part-time work) but none of the US group returned to work.[188] The scarcity of part-time work and a shorter treatment period dictated by third-party payers in the United States may account for this discrepancy.

Age is a general predictor for return to employment, and younger people are more attractive to employers. Barriers to return to work for the person with hemiplegia include speech, perceptual, and cognitive deficits along with a need for psychosocial support. Architectural barriers also can create severe problems for hemiplegic patients with regard to both work and recreational activities. Stroke clubs, usually organized through hospitals, the National Stroke Association, or the American Heart Association, provide educational, social, and recreational support for the hemiplegic person and her or his spouse.

The impact of psychosocial disability and the need for its long-term treatment is great. Programs need to be established and continued for years to allow patients and their families to deal with the many problems that result from the stroke. Refer to Appendix 24.C for resources.

Sexuality

Most persons with hemiplegia experience a decline in sexuality through a decrease in frequency of sexual intercourse without a change in the level of pre-stroke sexual desire.[189] On return home, the person with hemiplegia faces uncertainty about sexual skills and the risk of failure. Sexual dysfunction that results from a stroke depends on the amount of cerebral damage and includes a decreased ability to achieve erection and ejaculation in men and decreased lubrication in women.[190,191] The sensory, motor, visual, and emotional disturbances of hemiplegia may cause awkwardness, but these disturbances can be overcome through the education of the spouse in alternate positioning and ways to provide appropriate sensory experiences. The normal factors of aging also interfere with the sexual performance of persons with hemiplegia. A person's pre-stroke sexual activity is a good indicator of post-stroke sexual activity. The closeness between partners achieved through a satisfactory sexual relationship can add to the quality of life after stroke (see Chapter 5).

SUMMARY

This chapter reviews the neuropathology of stroke, the evaluation of impairments that interfere with functional movement patterns, and intervention planning. Both evaluation of outcomes and evaluation of movement components are described. The chapter highlights significant impairments and provides clinical observations on critical areas of intervention. A detailed process of clinical problem solving helps the therapist organize and prioritize impairments to plan intervention programs that retrain movement components and train desirable compensatory patterns to help the patient gain the highest level of functional performance and independence in daily life. An example of the synthesis of this chapter's concepts and ideas can be found in Case Study 24.1.

CASE STUDY 24.1   History of Present Illness

Patient is a 61-year-old female who presents to outpatient physical therapy with right hemiparesis following hemorrhagic left anterior cerebral artery cerebrovascular accident. She began noticing right leg weakness resulting in a fall. Patient was admitted to inpatient rehab and participated in intensive therapy for 3 weeks. She currently reports difficulty with bed mobility, transfers, and ambulation. She arrives to therapy with a single-point cane and a Giv-Mohr sling provided by her inpatient therapy team.

Past Medical History: Hypertension

Medications: Lisinopril, Acetaminophen

Social History/Prior Level of Function: Patient is a retired FBI agent and now works in the executive offices of a department store. She also owns her own part-time baking business. She is currently not working due to medical status. She normally lives alone; however, she has been living with her brother to have assistance with activities of daily living (ADL) and independent ADLs. Patient's home is a multilevel home with two stairs with no rail to enter and bilateral rails for flight of stairs to second level.

Personal Goals: Patient wants to be more confident in walking, she is fearful of falling. Activities-Specific Balance Confidence Scale: 53%

Review of Systems

Integumentary: 3-mm wound on right lateral malleolus, no obvious signs of infection, normal granulation tissue.

Cardiopulmonary: At rest in supported sitting: blood pressure 140/80; heart rate: 70.

Mental Status/Communication/Preferred Learning Style: No cognitive or speech impairments. Patient demonstrates appropriate insight into deficits.

Objective Findings

Hypotonic Hemiparesis: Right-side affected.

Dominant Extremity: Right

Pain: No complaints of pain at this time.

Posture

  Unsupported sitting: asymmetrical weight bearing with reduced weight bearing on right pelvis, mild concavity to right, wearing Givmohr Sling. Right hip externally rotated with knee extended and foot contact to floor at lateral heel. Left lower extremity appropriately aligned for sitting posture with knee flexed approximately 90 degrees with complete foot contact to floor.

  Unsupported standing: weight bearing primarily through left lower extremity, mild left hip Trendelenburg.

Tone: Normal tone left hemi-body; Hypotonic right hemi-body

Sensation: Right side; light touch sensation impaired, proprioception severely impaired—tested at ankle and knee

Strength:

Motion	Left	Right
Hip flexion	5/5	3+/5
Knee extension	5/5	3+/5
Knee flexion	5/5	3+/5
Ankle DF	5/5	2+/5
Ankle PF	5/5	2/5

Objective Outcome Measures

Upright Motor Control Test:

  Hip Extension: 1
  Knee Extension: 1
  Ankle Extension: 1
  Hip flexion: 3
  Knee Flexion: 3
  Ankle Flexion: 1
  Score: 10/18

Trunk Impairment Scale:

  Static: 6/7
  Dynamic: 5/10
  Coordination: 2/6
  Score: 13/23

Balance: not formally tested; however, demonstrates balance impairments related to deficits in:

  Sensation/Sensory orientation
  Biomechanical constraints including impaired base of support, neuromuscular weakness
  Impaired trunk control as observed with Trunk Impairment Scale

Impaired anticipatory postural control related to impaired motor control of trunk and right hemi-body

Functional mobility: Patient is modified independent during sit-to-stand, from supine to and from long sitting requiring increased time to perform; modified independent with sit-to-from-stand with limited weight bearing on right LE, R knee extended with poor foot contact with ground, left lateral trunk lean and significant use of left UE to assist the stand.

Gait: With rigid Ankle-foot orthose and Givmohr sling: Patient ambulates with single point cane in L upper extremity with good coordination of cane use, step-to with intermittent step-through 3-point gait pattern.

Right Lower Extremity:

Initial Contact: forefoot/foot flat

Loading Response: limited knee flexion, increased ankle plantarflexion

Midstance: knee extension thrust, pelvis rotated right, left pelvis depressed, with insufficient anterior translation of the tibia

Terminal Stance: limited heel off, reduced knee flexion

Pre-Swing: reduced hip and knee flexion

Mid-Swing: mild circumduction with contralateral vaulting

Left Lower Extremity:

Initial contact: heel

Mid stance: vaulting to assist right foot clearance

Stride length: shortened length and duration (response to limited R stance time)

Assessment

Current impairments: Right hemiparesis: upper extremity > lower extremity, impaired trunk stability and motor control and impaired sensation resulting in limited functional strength and mobility. She will benefit from skilled care to improve functional strength and increase safety with transfers and ambulation to achieve modified independence with ADLs and IADLs. Patient's prognosis is limited by impaired sensation and limited activity tolerance. However, patient is relatively young and highly motivated with excellent social and family support. Her movement disorder is classified in the composite movement category with severe movement deficits.

Functional Limitation 1: Patient Is Unable to Perform Morning Self-Care at Bedside or Sitting in Wheelchair in Front of a Sink

Why?

Patient cannot perform anterior and posterior or lateral trunk movements in sitting without loss of balance and falling to left. Patient cannot feel right arm, and it hangs by side.

Evaluation

Primary Impairments

Neurological weakness in right arm and leg

Inability to initiate movements

Loss of postural control

Inability to coordinate trunk–limb movements

Decreased sense of touch in right arm, trunk, and right leg

Secondary Impairments

Loss of trunk alignment in sitting

Right shoulder subluxation

Muscle tightness—pectorals, latissimus, wrist flexors, ankle dorsiflexors

Loss of alignment of lower trunk and pelvis in sitting—spine laterally flexed, convexity on left, left pelvis lists downward

Loss of 10 degrees of right ankle joint dorsiflexion range

Functional Limitation 2: Patient Is Unable to Transfer From Bed to Chair Independently

Why?

Patient cannot control upper body while trying to activate bilateral leg activity when initiating transfers to either side. Right arm hangs by side with an inferior shoulder subluxation. Cannot lift right leg against gravity in sitting. Cannot depress left leg into surface. Tends to use left side exclusively during transfer with loss of balance. Patient uses left arm to support self at edge of bed.

Evaluation

Primary Impairments

Neurological weakness in upper trunk and right leg

Inability to coordinate trunk–leg patterns in weight bearing

Inability to sequence movement patterns in right in weight bearing

Secondary Impairments

Loss of upper-body alignment

Loss of right ankle joint dorsiflexion range

Functional Limitation 3: Patient Is Unable to Stand up From Chair Independently

Why?

Patient is unable to control upper body over lower trunk during lower-body–initiated transfers and sit-to-stand. Patient is unable to use right leg for support and movement during the transition of sit-to-stand. Patient is unable to keep weight (depress leg into floor) on right foot in standing.

Evaluation

Primary Impairments

Inability to control upper body over lower body, resulting in an inability to initiate lower trunk and leg movements

Inability to coordinate trunk–leg patterns in weight bearing

Impaired force production in right leg

Secondary Impairments

Loss of right ankle joint dorsiflexion range

Tightness in right gastrocnemius

Significant Impairments for Functions Evaluated

1. Loss of upper-body control during lower-body initiated movements, especially anterior-posterior plane
2. Shoulder subluxation contributes to loss of upper-body control
3. Loss of muscle activation control and neurological weakness of right arm and leg
4. Loss of ankle joint dorsiflexion range

Treatment Goals

Functional Goals

A. Perform morning self-care activities in wheelchair in bathroom independently
B. Transfer from chair to bed and back with contact guarding
C. Rise to standing with assistance of one person

Long-Term Movement Goals

A. Sit safely while performing tasks with right arm and leg around midline; that is, perform upper-body– and lower-body–initiated trunk movements in sitting independently
B. Increase upper-body control to prepare for independent, safe, lower-body–initiated movement patterns (extended-arm reach, sitting to standing, and standing balance)

Continued

CASE STUDY 24.1   **History of Present Illness—cont'd**

C. Increase leg strength and establish trunk and leg coordinated patterns in weight bearing (to allow transfers, rising to stand, and standing with minimal assistance to the upper body)

D. Establish a home or bedside program that the patient can perform independently

Long-Term Functional Goals (in 24 visits)

1. Patient will ambulate at self-selected gait speed >1.0 m/s with assistive device to achieve gait speed required for safe community ambulation
2. Pt will demonstrate demonstrate improved R Lower Extremity single limb stance time and stability for overall improved efficiency of gait.
3. Pt will report performing light home care activities including light cooking, light cleaning, and laundry with moderate assist to progress toward independent living
4. Pt will score greater than 85% on Activities Based Confidence Scale to demonstrate reduced fall risk and progress toward patient's goal.

Short-Term Movement Goals

A. Perform basic trunk movement patterns in sitting with contact guarding
B. Increase muscle activation control in upper body and shoulder girdle to decrease shoulder subluxation

C. Protect shoulder joint from excessive capsular stretch

D. Increase sequencing and force production in left arm: be able to lift arm up onto sink with unaffected arm, maintain sitting balance during morning ADL activities

E. Increase ankle joint dorsiflexion range in standing

F. Increase sequencing and force production in left leg and during trunk and leg linked patterns during lower-bodyinitiated transfers, during sit-to-stand, and in supported standing to allow lower-extremity assisted practice

Short-Term Functional Goals (in 10 visits)

1. Pt will demonstrate improved R Lower Extremity functional strength with increase in Upright Motor Control Test Score from 10/18 to 14/18 to improve R Lower Extremity stability in gait.
2. Pt will improve trunk impairment scale score from 13/23 to 20/23 to improve gait and functional mobility.
3. Pt will list at least three techniques to care for skin integrity.
4. Pt will perform sit-to-stand with bilateral upper extremity support, appropriate alignment and foot contact of R lower extremity to promote recovery of symmetrical use of lower limbs.

REFERENCES

To enhance this text and add value for the reader, all references are included on the companion Evolve site that accompanies this textbook. This online service will, when available, provide a link for the reader to a Medline abstract for the article cited. There are 191 cited references and other general references for this chapter, with the majority of those articles being evidence-based citations.

Product Manufacturers

Wheaton Brace Company
391 S. Schmale Road
Carol Stream, IL 60188
Orthomerica
505 31st Street
Newport Beach, CA 92663
AliMed
PO Box 9135
Dedham, MA 32703

Patterson Medical/Sammons Preston
1000 Remington Boulevard, Suite 210
Bolingbrook, IL 60440
Bioness, Inc
25103 Rye Canyon Loop
Valencia, CA 91355
WalkAide System
www.walkaide.com

Resources for One-Handed Adaptations

ONE-HANDED IN A TWO-HANDED WORLD

Tommye K. Mayer
Prince Gallison Press
PO Box 23
Boston, MA 02113

ADAPTIVE RESOURCES: A GUIDE TO PRODUCTS AND SERVICES

National Stroke Association
8480 E. Orchard Road
Englewood, CO 80111

Stroke Survivor Resources

INTERNET LINKS

National Stroke Association: www.stroke.org
American Stroke Association: www.strokeassociation.org
American Stroke Foundation: www.americanstroke.org
Stroke Survivor: www.strokesurvivor.com
Resource site: www.strokecenter.org
Stroke journal: stroke.ahajournal.org
Neurology stroke information: http://brainattacks.net
Useful stroke information: www.strokehelp.com

AUDIOVISUAL AND LITERARY RESOURCES

Films and Videotapes
Inner World of Aphasia, 35-minute film

American Journal of Nursing Film Library
267 W. 25th Street
New York, NY 10001

Candidate for Stroke, 35-minute film

American Heart Association

I Had a Stroke, 35-minute film

Filmmakers Library, Inc.
290 West End Avenue
New York, NY 10023

Living With Stroke

Rehabilitation Research and Training Center
The George Washington University
2300 I Street, NW, Suite 714
Washington, DC 20037

Books
Children

First One Foot, Then the Other, by Tomie dePaola. This book explores the feelings and fears of children about a relative who has had a stroke.

Adult

Berger PE. *How to Conquer the World with One Hand...and an Attitude* Merrifield, Virginia: Positive Power Publisher; 1999.
Bolte J. *Stroke of Insight: A Brain Scientist's Personal Journey.* Taylor; 2008.
Burkman K. *The Stroke Recovery Book: A Guide for Patients and Families.* 2010.
Levine PG. *Stronger After Stroke.* Demos Health; 2018.

25

Brain Tumors*

Corrie J. Stayner, Rachel M. Lopez, and Karla M. Tuzzolino

OBJECTIVES

After reading this chapter the student or therapist will be able to:
1. Identify the categories of primary brain tumors.
2. Recognize and interpret signs and symptoms of primary brain tumors specific to tumor location.
3. Recognize current diagnostic tests used to detect brain tumors.
4. Identity the types of medical and surgical management for brain tumors and how that management will affect functional movement.
5. Describe the side effects associated with the treatment of brain tumors and recognize their impact on therapeutic intervention.
6. Discuss the multiple considerations necessary to plan and execute an intervention program for the patient with a brain tumor.
7. Recognize the emotional and psychosocial impact of the disease process on the patient, the patient's support system, and the interdisciplinary team.

KEY TERMS

astrocytoma
biopsy
chemotherapy
Gamma Knife

glioblastoma
hospice care
Karnofsky performance status scale
meningioma

metastatic
radiation therapy
ventriculostomy

AN OVERVIEW OF BRAIN TUMORS

The rehabilitation clinician serves many different populations, including patients with brain tumors. Despite the prognosis for limited survival associated with primary brain tumors, these individuals have shown progress in the rehabilitation setting similar to that noted in patients with diagnoses of stroke or traumatic brain injury.[1] Advances in medical and surgical treatment for patients with cancer have resulted in improved survival rates and longer life expectancy, yet only incremental improvements for patients with brain tumors.[2] Progressive impairments, physical or cognitive or both, result from the disease process and require an interdisciplinary team approach to best facilitate the individual's participation in a meaningful lifestyle. In addition, clinicians must recognize the psychological and emotional needs of the individual given this diagnosis, and be sensitive and flexible in accommodating the patient's feelings. Improved quality of life, especially the opportunity to return home, remains the ultimate goal of the rehabilitation process.

The clinical presentation of patients with brain tumors mimics that of persons with other central nervous system (CNS) conditions. The location of the tumor or vascular accident determines the impairments the patient will exhibit. However, in the brain tumor patient, the burdensome effects of standard medical intervention and the aggressive nature of the disease course itself provide obstacles to therapeutic intervention. The patient's increased probability of eventual physical and functional deterioration provides a challenge to the clinician

attempting to formulate realistic goals and plan for future needs. Therefore a thorough knowledge of the tumor's natural history, the complications and side effects of treatment, and the neurological impairment the patient exhibits will assist the clinician in best developing a comprehensive, individualized plan of care.

Incidence and Etiology

The incidence of adult brain tumors is on the rise in the United States and has been for the past 3 decades,[3] with an estimated 86,970 new cases of primary benign or malignant brain and other CNS tumors anticipated for 2019.[4] It is estimated that 26,170 will be malignant and 60,800 will be nonmalignant.[2] For children aged 0–14, 3720 new cases of childhood primary and nonmalignant brain and other CNS tumors are expected in 2019.[4]

In the United States, brain tumors typically occur in two distinct categories of patients: (1) children aged 0 to 15 years and (2) adults in the fifth to seventh decades of life. In adults, white Americans have a higher incidence than black Americans, and in both pediatric and adult populations males are more frequently affected than females. A primary brain tumor is now the most common cause of cancer death in children and adolescents aged 0 to 19, and brain and other CNS tumors are the most common cancer site in children aged 0 to 14, with an annual average of 5.54 per 100,000.[2]

The frequently occurring meningioma, typically benign, accounts for 36.8% of all primary brain tumors. Glioblastoma, a malignant tumor, accounts for 14.9% of adult primary tumors and 47.1% of malignant primary brain tumors (Fig. 25.1).[2] The largest percentage

---

*Videos for this chapter are available at studentconsult.com.

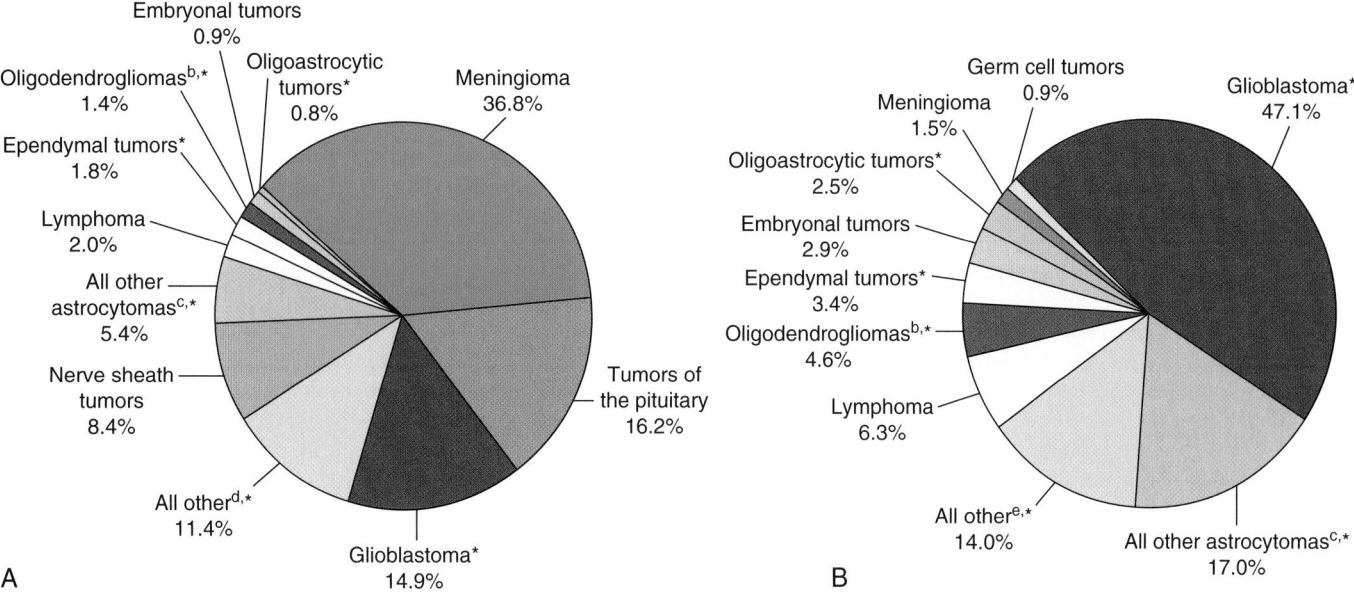

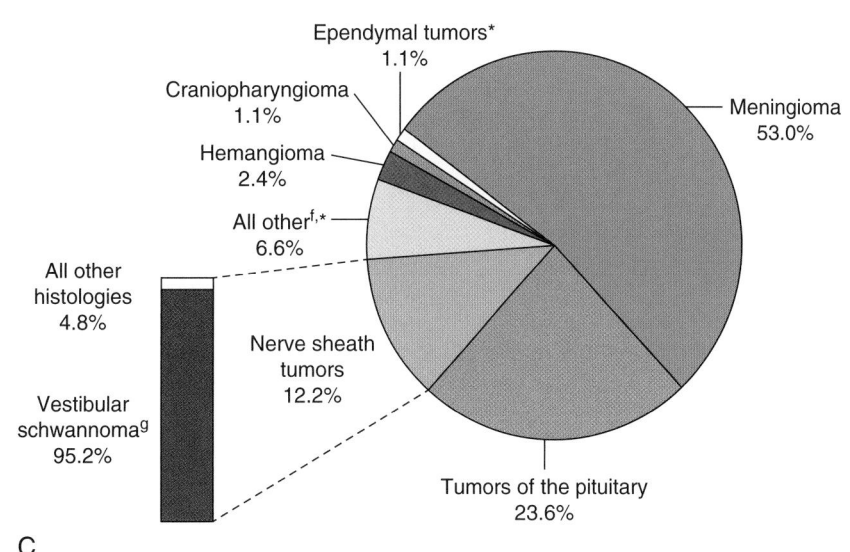

*All or some of this histology is included in the CBTRUS definition of gliomas, including ICD-O-3 histology codes 9380–9384, 9391–9460.
[a]Percentages may not add up to 100% due to rounding;
[b]Includes oligodendroglioma and anaplastic oligodendroglioma;
[c]Includes pilocytic astrocytoma, diffuse astrocytoma, anaplastic astrocytoma, and unique astrocytoma variants;
[d]Includes glioma malignant, NOS, choroid plexus tumors, other neuroepithelial tumors, neuronal and mixed neuronal-glial tumors, tumors of the pineal region, other tumors of cranial and spinal nerves, mesenchymal tumors, primary melanocytic lesions, other neoplasms related to the meninges, other hematopoietic neoplasms, hemangioma, neoplasm, unspecified, and all other;
[e]Include glioma malignant, NOS, choroid plexus tumors, other neuroepithelial tumors, neuronal and mixed neuronal-glial tumors, tumors of the pineal region, nerve sheath tumors, other tumors of cranial and spinal nerve, mesenchymal tumors, primary melanocytic lesions, other neoplasms related to the meninges, other hematopoietic neoplasms, hemangioma, neoplasm, unspecified, and all other;
[f]Includes unique astrocytoma variants, choroid plexus tumors, other neuroepithelial tumors, neuronal and mixed neuronal- glial tumors, tumors of the pineal region, embryonal tumors, other tumors of cranial and spinal nerves, mesenchymal tumors, primary melanocytic lesions, other neoplasms related to the meninges, other hematopoietic neoplasms, germ cell tumors, neoplasm, unspecified, and all other;
[g]ICD-O-3 histology code 9560.

Fig. 25.1 Distribution[h] of **(A)** all primary brain and other central nervous system (CNS) tumors by CBTRUS histology groupings and histology (N = 379,848), **(B)** malignant primary brain and other CNS tumors by CB-TRUS histology groupings and histology (N = 119,674), and **(C)** nonmalignant primary brain and other CNS tumors by CBTRUS histology groupings and histology (N = 260,174), CBTRUS statistical report: NPCR and SEER, 2010–2014. (From CBTRUS Statistical Report. Primary brain and other central nervous system tumors diagnosed in the United States in 2010–2014. *Neuro Oncol.* 2017;19[suppl 5]:v1–v88. doi:10.1093/neuonc/nox158; Neuro Oncol | © The Author(s) 2017. Published by Oxford University Press on behalf of the Society for Neuro-Oncology. All rights reserved. For permissions, please e-mail: journals.permissions@oup.com)

of childhood tumors, age 0 to 14 years (15.4%), are located in the frontal, temporal, parietal, and occipital lobes of the brain, 15.2% in the cerebellum, and 13.4% in the brain stem.[2]

The etiology of brain tumors remains unclear, and many environmental and behavioral risk factors have and are being investigated. The influence of cellular phones and occupational/industrial hazards has been researched; however, the results have been inconclusive.[5] Several hereditary CNS syndromes may be associated with increased risk of brain tumor; however, 95% of brain tumors are nonhereditary in nature.[6] Exposure to moderate to high doses of ionizing radiation (radiation generated by atomic bombs, computed tomography [CT] scans, x-rays, and therapeutic radiation) has shown an increased risk factor for primary brain and other CNS tumors.[3,7] Ionizing radiation, used therapeutically in high doses to treat tumors, has been found to have a causal relationship as well to the development of a second brain tumor.[3] A decreased risk for brain and other CNS tumors, specifically gliomas, has been linked to a history of allergy or other atopic disease, including eczema, psoriasis, and asthma.[3,8] Continued investigation into possible causal relationships is still ongoing and is essential if the incidence and mortality rates associated with brain tumors are to decrease.

Classification of Tumors

The World Health Organization (WHO) first published a universal classification system for CNS tumors in 1979, with its fourth edition published in 2007 and an update to the fourth edition in 2016.[9] This system grades tumors (grades I to IV) according to their microscopic (histologic) characteristics and has been accepted as the universal method for the classification of brain tumors. In the 2016 update, tumors are now classified by genetic molecular characteristics, in addition to the specific histology.[9] The hope is that by more specifically classifying tumors, treatment efficacy will improve.

Primary Brain Tumors

Primary tumors originate in the CNS, whereas metastatic or secondary tumors spread to the CNS from systemic cancer sites outside the brain.

Characteristics of the most common brain tumors are discussed in the following paragraphs, with information provided regarding age at onset, location, medical treatment, and prognosis.

Gliomas are primary tumors that arise from supportive tissues of the brain and are frequently located in the cerebral hemispheres. These tumors may also occur in the brain stem, optic nerve, and spinal cord. In children, the cerebellum is a primary location for gliomas.[10] Gliomas have four primary categories and are classified by their predominant cellular components: astrocytomas and oligodendrogliomas originate from glial cells, ependymomas from ependymal cells, and medulloblastomas from primitive cells.[11]

Astrocytomas are derived from astrocytes, which are star-shaped glial cells, and are the most common glial tumor in adults and children.[2] Astrocytomas vary in morphology and biological behavior, from those that are diffuse and infiltrate surrounding brain structures, to those that are circumscribed with a decreased likelihood of progression. In adults, the typical age of onset is after age 45, with the tumor frequently found in the frontal lobe. Most childhood astrocytomas occur in the cerebellum.[10,12]

Astrocytomas are further classified into four grades: pilocytic astrocytoma (grade I), which are well-differentiated, relatively benign low-grade tumors most common in children and young adults; diffuse astrocytoma (grade II), which are well-differentiated, low-grade tumors that grow slowly; anaplastic astrocytoma (grade III), which are high-grade tumors that typically have tentacle-like projections growing into the surrounding brain tissue and grow more rapidly; and glioblastoma (grade IV), which is the most aggressive of the astrocytoma tumors. The glioblastoma can be primary or evolve from a lower grade astrocytoma (secondary). The higher the grade, the worse the prognosis.[10,11]

Astrocytomas are typically treated with surgery, radiation therapy, and chemotherapy, depending on the grade, location of the tumor, age of the patient, and Karnofsky performance scale score (Table 25.1).[10,11,13] Typically, lower grade tumors are treated with surgery followed by radiation if necessary. Grade III tumors are treated with surgery, followed by radiation and possibly chemotherapy when needed. The

TABLE 25.1 Karnofsky Performance Status Scale

Condition	Performance Status (%)	Comments
A. Able to carry on normal activity and to work; no special care is needed	100	Normal; no complaints; no evidence of disease
	90	Able to carry on normal activity; minor signs or symptoms of disease
	80	Normal activity with effort; some signs or symptoms of disease
B. Unable to work; able to live at home, care for most personal needs; a varying degree of assistance is needed	70	Care of self; unable to carry on normal activity or to do active work
	60	Requires occasional assistance but is able to care for most of personal needs
	50	Requires considerable assistance and frequent medical care
C. Unable to care for self; requires equivalent of institutional or hospital care; disease may be progressing rapidly	40	Disabled; requires special care and assistance
	30	Severely disabled; hospitalization is indicated, although death not imminent
	20	Very sick; hospitalization necessary; active supportive treatment necessary
	10	Moribund; fatal processes progressing rapidly
	0	Dead

Adapted from Karnofsky DA, Burchenal JH. The clinical evaluation of chemotherapeutic agents in cancer. In Macleod C, eds. *Evaluation of Chemotherapeutic Agents.* New York: Columbia University Press; 1949.

lower grade tumors, pilocytic astrocytomas, carry a 5-year survival rate of 94%; however, patients with grade III astrocytomas have a 5-year survival rate of only 29.8%.[2]

Glioblastoma is the distinct name given to the highly malignant grade IV astrocytoma. These tumors grow rapidly, invade nearby tissue, and contain highly malignant cells. Glioblastomas are predominantly located in the deep white matter of the cerebral hemispheres, but may be found in the brain stem, cerebellum, or spinal cord. Fifty percent of these tumors are bilateral or occupy more than one lobe of a hemisphere.[11] Glioblastomas account for 14.9% of all primary brain tumors and 47.1% of all primary malignant brain tumors (see Fig. 25.1).[2] They are most common in older adults, with males having a 1.6:1 incidence rate over females. In children and adolescents (aged 0 to 19 years), only 3% of brain and other CNS tumors are glioblastomas.[2] The medical prognosis is poor for patients with glioblastoma: less than 40% survive more than 1 year and less than 5.5% survive 5 years.[2] Researchers have recently discovered that glioblastomas have four distinct genetic subtypes that respond differently to aggressive therapies, making treatment difficult and challenging.[9] These tumors are treated by surgical resection (only part of the tumor is typically resected), radiation therapy, stereotactic radiosurgery, and chemotherapy.[10,11]

Oligodendrogliomas are slow-growing but progressive tumors that typically develop over a period of several years. These tumors are most commonly located in the frontal and temporal lobes; however, they can be found anywhere in the cerebral hemisphere.[11] Seizures, headaches, and personality changes are the primary clinical manifestations of the tumor.[10] Oligodendrogliomas typically appear in the fourth to sixth decades of life, and the ratio of affected males to females is 2:1.[11] These patients have a 5-year survival rate of 81% and 10-year survival rate of 65%.[2] The 5-year survival rate decreases to 56% with anaplastic oligodendroglioma.[2] Treatment is dependent on symptoms and ranges from observation and seizure control with anticonvulsant drugs to surgical resection, radiation, and chemotherapy.[10,11]

Ependymomas are tumors arising from ependymal cells—cells that line the ventricles of the brain and central canal of the spinal cord.[10] These cells have glial and epithelial characteristics. Ependymomas grow into the ventricle or adjacent brain tissue. The most common site is the fourth ventricle (70% originate here), and they occur less frequently in the lateral and third ventricles.[11] Ependymomas are primarily treated with surgical resection followed by radiation therapy; however, chemotherapy is also used to treat tumor recurrence or when trying to delay radiation in young children.[10,11] Because of increased intracranial pressure (ICP), a shunt is commonly placed to improve survival. These tumors frequently recur, and prognosis is dependent on the success of resection, with a 5-year survival rate approaching 84%.[2]

Medulloblastomas are malignant embryonal tumors thought to arise from primitive neuroectodermal cells—specifically pluripotential stem cells that have been prevented from maturing to their normal growth-arrested state.[11] These tumors are typically located in the cerebellum.[10] Medulloblastomas typically grow into the fourth ventricle, blocking cerebrospinal fluid (CSF) flow, and cause hydrocephalus and ICP.[11] These tumors primarily occur in children or adults under the age of 45, accounting for 8% of childhood (0 to 14 years) brain tumors. The most common age of onset is 7 years old, with a prevalence in males over females.[2,11] An overall 5-year survival rate of 73% has been noted among adults and children, and the most common treatment is surgery followed by radiation and chemotherapy.[2,10,11]

Meningiomas are slow-growing tumors that primarily originate from cells located in the dura mater or arachnoid membrane, and account for 36.8% of reported brain tumors.[2,11] The incidence increases with age, with a more dramatic increase over age 65, and in females at a 2:1 ratio over males.[2,10,11] Often clinical symptoms are not manifested until the growing tumor compresses adjacent structures. Headache and weakness are the most common symptoms, followed by seizures, personality changes, and visual deficits.[10,11] If possible, tumors are treated with surgical resection. Recurring tumors are treated with surgery, radiation therapy, or stereotactic radiosurgery. Tumors in highly eloquent areas of the brain, however, may best be treated with serial scans to monitor for growth and compression of neural structures.[10,11] Patients with nonmalignant meningiomas (most meningiomas are not malignant) have a 10-year survival rate of 81.4% versus a 10-year survival rate of 57.4% with malignant meningiomas.[2]

Pituitary adenomas are benign epithelial tumors originating from the adenohypophysis of the pituitary gland and frequently encroach on the optic chiasm.[11] These tumors are characterized by hypersecretion or hyposecretion of hormones.[11] Age at onset spans all ages, but pituitary adenomas are rare before puberty, more common in older people, and more common in females than males, especially during child bearing years. These tumors are primarily treated by surgical resection, drug therapy, and radiation.[10,11] Prognosis is dependent on tumor size and cell type, with a 5-year survival rate of 96%.[2]

Schwannomas are encapsulated tumors composed of neoplastic Schwann cells that can arise on any cranial or spinal nerve.[11] A schwannoma on the eighth cranial nerve is called an *acoustic neuroma*. The tumors' location on the nerve produces otological, focal, or generalized neurological impairments. These tumors are often located in the internal auditory canal but may extend into the cerebellopontine angle.[11,12] Treatment typically involves surgical resection; however, stereotactic radiosurgery is increasing in popularity as an alternative method of treatment when the tumor is near vital nerves or blood vessels.[11] The prognosis for patients with these tumors is good, yet complications can result from treatment, including facial paralysis, deafness, and equilibrium impairments.[11] Deficits after surgery vary depending on the size and location of the tumor. A 10-year follow-up study looking at low dose linear accelerator stereotactic radiosurgery confirmed excellent tumor control and acceptable cranial neuropathy rates but a continual decrease in hearing preservation.[14]

Primary CNS lymphomas are rare tumors arising from cells in the lymphatic system, representing only 2% of primary brain tumors.[2] These lymphomas have a slightly higher incidence in men and peak in the sixth through eighth decades of life.[2] The tumor cells are similar in histology to systemic non-Hodgkin lymphoma cells, but it is uncertain how this tumor arises, as the CNS lacks lymphatic tissue.[11,15] The tumor may be solitary or multifocal, forming a poorly defined mass that may be difficult to distinguish from an astrocytoma.[11] Primary brain lymphomas appear primarily in the cerebral hemispheres, and the most common symptoms are behavioral and personality changes, confusion, dizziness, and focal cerebral signs, rather than headache and other signs of increased ICP.[10,11] Surgical resection is typically ineffective because of the deep location of these tumors. Radiation, chemotherapy, and steroids are the most common forms of treatment; however, the tumor recurs in 90% of individuals.[11] CNS lymphoma carries a poor prognosis, with only 33% of patients surviving longer than 5 years.[2]

Secondary Brain Tumors: Metastatic Brain Tumors

Metastatic brain tumors originate from malignancies outside of the CNS and spread to the brain, typically through the arterial circulation.[11] Approximately 25% of individuals with systemic cancer develop brain metastases, with approximately 80% of tumors in cerebral hemispheres and 20% in the posterior fossa.[11,15] One-third of brain metastases originate in the lung, followed by the breast, skin, gastrointestinal tract, and kidneys in order of frequency. Common clinical manifestations of metastatic brain tumors are similar to those of gliomas, including seizures, headache, focal weakness, mental and behavioral changes, ataxia, aphasia, and signs of increased ICP.[11]

Treatment for these tumors is tailored to the individual and dependent on the management of the systemic disease, the accessibility of the lesion, and the number of lesions.[11] Current treatment regimens include surgery and radiosurgery if the lesions are limited in number and accessible. Chemotherapy and whole brain radiation therapy (WBRT) may also be used. The average survival with treatment is approximately 6 months but varies widely and is affected by the extent of other systemic metastases. With some radiosensitive tumors, survival increases to 15% to 30% for 1 year and 5% to 10% for 2 years.[11]

Signs and Symptoms

The clinical manifestations of a brain tumor are dependent on the type and site of the tumor and rate of growth. These manifestations range from decreased speed in comprehension or minor personality changes to progressive hemiparesis or seizure.[16] Patients with brain tumors typically have headaches, seizures, nonspecific cognitive or personality changes, or focal neurological signs.[10,11] The presenting signs may be general, specific neurological symptoms, or a combination of both.

General Signs and Symptoms

General signs and symptoms of the presence of a brain tumor include headache, seizures, altered mental status, and papilledema. *Headache* is the presenting symptom in 50% of brain tumor cases; however, it is rarely the sole complaint or symptom in these patients.[10,16] It is important to identify the specific nature of the headaches, as certain features often indicate the presence of a brain tumor. These features include the following:

1. The headache interrupts sleep or is worse on waking and improves throughout the day.
2. The headache is elicited by postural changes, coughing, or exercise.
3. The headache of recent onset is more severe or a different type than usual.
4. The new onset of headache occurs in an older person.
5. The headache is associated with nausea and vomiting, papilledema, or focal neurological signs.[10,11,16]

Headaches can be caused by local tissue edema, distortion of blood vessels in the dura overlying the tumor, and increased ICP. The location of the headache is typically determined by the tumor's location. Tumors above the tentorium cause headaches on the same side as the tumor and the immediate surrounding area. Posterior fossa tumors cause headaches in the occipital lobe and ipsilateral retroauricular area. Increased ICP causes bi-frontal or bi-occipital headaches regardless of the tumor location.[10,11]

Seizures are a frequent symptom in patients with a brain tumor, and a first seizure during adulthood is suggestive of a brain tumor.[11,16] Seizure incidence and management is dependent on the tumor type, location, and at what point in the disease course the seizure presents.[16] Seizures may be solitary or occur frequently, preceding or following other symptoms.[11] More than 50% of patients with gliomas experience recurrent seizures, while only 11% of patients with brain metastases experience recurrent seizures.[16] Tumors can cause epilepsy, and the prognosis for complete seizure control in patients with tumor related epilepsy is poor.[16]

Altered mental status including cognitive and mental deficits are frequently seen in patients with brain tumors.[16] Cognitive changes range from decrease in concentration, memory, affect, personality, initiative, and abstract reasoning to severe cognitive deficits and confusion.[16] Subtle changes may be incorrectly attributed to worry, anxiety,

or depression.[11] Changes in mentation are common with frontal lobe tumors and in the presence of elevated ICP. Increased ICP causes drowsiness and decreased level of consciousness, which can progress to stupor or coma if edema is not immediately reduced.[11]

The incidence of *papilledema,* swelling of the optic nerve, is less frequent today because brain tumors are being diagnosed earlier with the use of sensitive imaging techniques. Papilledema is associated with symptoms of transient visual loss, especially with positional changes, and reflects evidence of ICP transmitted through the optic nerve sheath. Papilledema is more common in children than adults.[16]

Vomiting and dizziness are other less common symptoms associated with brain tumors located in the posterior fossa.[11,16] Vomiting can indicate a generally elevated ICP but can also occur due to pressure on the vomiting center (posterior fossa) with brain stem tumors. Projectile vomiting is usually seen in posterior fossa tumors in children but not adults.[16] Dizziness and/or positional vertigo can be a symptom of a tumor in the posterior fossa but also has other more common benign causes.[11]

Specific Signs and Symptoms

Certain clinical features are related to functional areas of the brain and thus have a specific localizing value in medically diagnosing a brain tumor. Therefore it is essential that clinicians be familiar with the lobes of the brain and their distinct functions to effectively manage the impairments resulting from the tumor (Fig. 25.2). These symptoms may vary among individuals and result in physical and cognitive deficits that range from mild to severe.

The *frontal lobe* is responsible for motor functioning, initiation of movement, and interpretation of emotion, including motor speech, motor praxis, attention, cognition, emotion, intelligence, judgment, motivation, and memory. Therefore frontal lobe tumors may result in movement disorders such as hemiparesis, seizures, aphasia, and gait difficulties, and cognitive impairments including personality changes such as disinhibition, irritability, impaired judgment, and lack of initiation. Initially, the tumor may be clinically silent; however, as the tumor grows, progressive symptoms develop based on the tumor's location in the frontal lobe.[16]

The *parietal lobe* processes complex sensory and perceptual information related to somesthetic sensation, spatial relations, body schema, and praxis. General symptoms of a parietal lobe tumor include contralateral sensory loss and hemiparesis, homonymous visual deficits or neglect, agnosias, apraxias, and visual-spatial disorders. If the dominant parietal lobe is involved, agraphesthesia, left-right confusion, and finger agnosia are typically present. With nondominant parietal lobe involvement, contralateral neglect and limited awareness of impairments is commonly found. Seizures with focal onset are often associated with tumors in the parietal lobe—particularly those in the region of the motor cortex.[16]

The *occipital lobe* is the primary processing area of visual information. Therefore lesions of the occipital lobe often result in dysfunction of eye movement and homonymous hemianopsia. If the parieto-occipital junction is involved, visual agnosia and agraphia are often present. Seizures are not common with occipital lobe tumors.[16]

The *temporal lobe* is responsible for auditory and limbic processing. If the lateral hemispheres are involved, auditory and perceptual changes may occur. When the medial aspects are affected, changes in cognitive integration, long-term memory, learning, and emotions may be seen. Anomia, agraphia, acalculia, and Wernicke aphasia (fluent, nonsensical speech) are specific to left temporal lobe lesions. Similar to the parietal lobe, seizures are common with temporal lobe tumors.[16]

The *cerebellum* is responsible for coordination and equilibrium. Midline cerebellar lesions can compromise CSF flow and produce

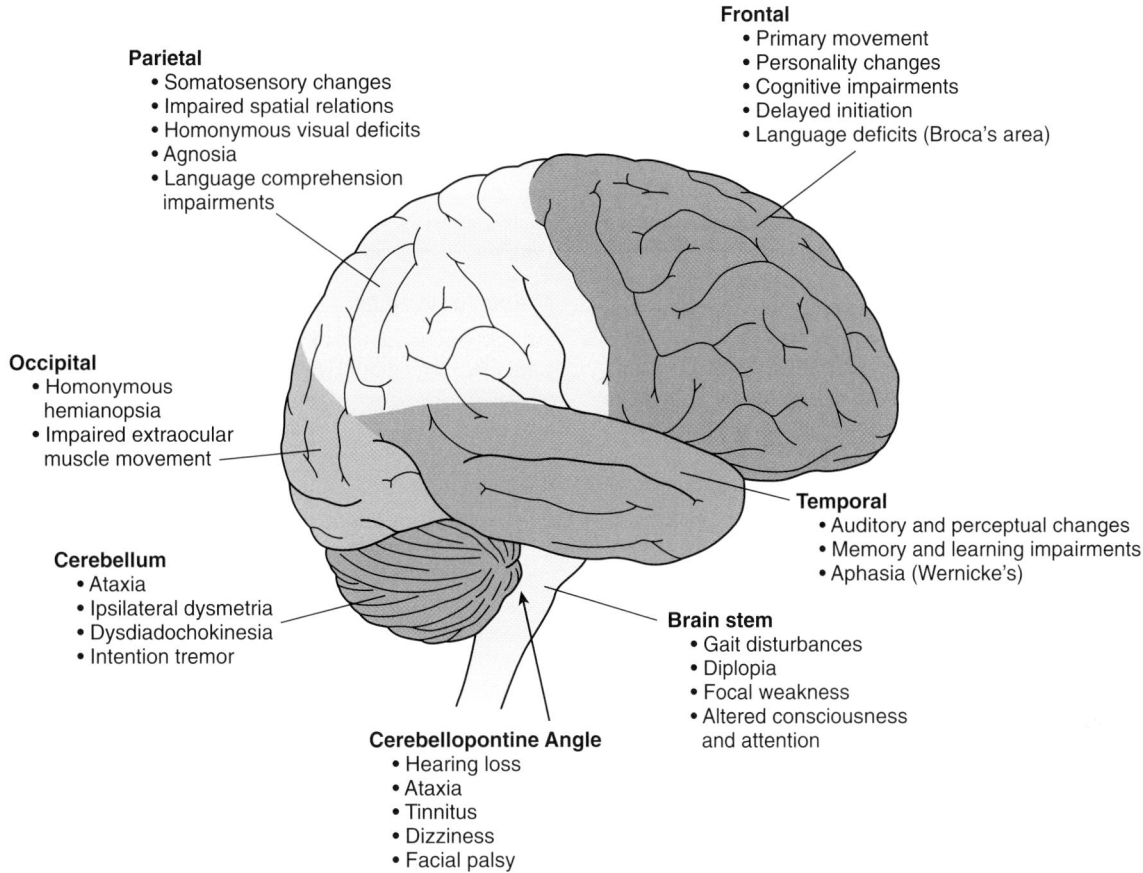

Parietal
- Somatosensory changes
- Impaired spatial relations
- Homonymous visual deficits
- Agnosia
- Language comprehension
  impairments

Frontal
- Primary movement
- Personality changes
- Cognitive impairments
- Delayed initiation
- Language deficits (Broca's area)

Occipital
- Homonymous
  hemianopsia
- Impaired extraocular
  muscle movement

Temporal
- Auditory and perceptual changes
- Memory and learning impairments
- Aphasia (Wernicke's)

Cerebellum
- Ataxia
- Ipsilateral dysmetria
- Dysdiadochokinesia
- Intention tremor

Brain stem
- Gait disturbances
- Diplopia
- Focal weakness
- Altered consciousness
  and attention

Cerebellopontine Angle
- Hearing loss
- Ataxia
- Tinnitus
- Dizziness
- Facial palsy

Fig. 25.2 Correlation between clinical symptoms and anatomical location of the tumor. (Used with permission from Barrow Neurological Institute.)

hydrocephalus, resulting in truncal ataxia. Lateral tumors are typically larger and are associated with limb ataxia (upper greater than lower extremity) and impaired coordination and nystagmus. Tumors invading the cerebellar pontine angle present with hearing loss, headache, ataxia, dizziness, and tinnitus. Facial palsy may occur due to cranial nerve compression, especially in the facial and acoustic nerves. If the cerebellar tumor infiltrates the meninges at the foramen magnum causing cerebellar tonsil herniation, sudden death may occur due to fourth ventricle obstruction and compression of the medulla.[16]

The *brain stem*, which communicates information to and from the cerebral cortex via fiber tracts, controls vital life functions. Even small tumors invading or compressing the brain stem can lead to death or devastating signs and symptoms. Within the brain stem, the reticular formation of the pons and medulla controls consciousness, sleep, and attention. If the reticular system is involved, symptoms of apnea, hypoventilation or hyperventilation, orthostatic hypotension, or syncope may occur. Symptoms of a brain stem tumor have an insidious onset and may include gait disturbances, diplopia, focal weakness, headache, vomiting, facial numbness and weakness, and personality changes. If the dorsal midbrain is involved, Parinaud syndrome, characterized by loss of upward gaze, pupillary areflexia to light, and loss of convergence, may be seen.[12,16]

The *pituitary gland* is an endocrine gland that secretes the hormones necessary to regulate the functions of the other endocrine glands in the body. The symptoms of pituitary tumors are caused by either a hypersecretion of hormones or the tumor compressing the gland itself, resulting in hormone hyposecretion (pituitary hypofunction). The symptoms that present are based on the specific hormone excess or deficiency, which can include headache, depression, vision loss, nausea and/or vomiting, behavior and cognitive changes, abnormal weight gain, abnormal growth in hands and feet, hair growth in women, amenorrhea, and impotence in men.[10,11]

Medical Diagnosis of Disease or Pathology

A clinical diagnosis is determined from the information that the physician gathers during a comprehensive evaluation. Information obtained while discussing the patient's medical history and the specific nature of the signs and symptoms is critical at the initial stages of the diagnostic process. Signs of an intracranial hemorrhage or infarction typically have an abrupt onset, whereas brain tumors usually have a more gradual onset and progressive symptoms.[17] The neurological examination may identify visual, cognitive, sensory, or motor impairments that may help identify the affected areas. However, sometimes symptoms may be subtle, depending on the tumor's location or if the brain has adapted to a low-grade glioma. In these cases, the patient may have a normal neurological exam in the presence of an underlying glioma.[18] After a thorough history and physical is performed, if the presence of a brain tumor is suspected, the next diagnostic step, tumor imaging, is warranted.[11]

In addition to imaging, specialized tests may be used to confirm the diagnosis and assess the structure and pathology of the brain tumor.[15,17] Advances in research and imaging techniques allow for earlier detection of brain tumors and more specialized treatment options. Conventional and advanced imaging in combination with biopsy and molecular diagnostics have revolutionized the diagnosis and management of brain tumors.[19]

Conventional Imaging

CT and magnetic resonance imaging (MRI) are the most common imaging modalities used to assess neurological deficits. Acutely, CT is a cost-effective method to quickly detect a hemorrhage; however, MRI is the modality of choice to evaluate a brain tumor. Conventional MRI provides exquisite anatomical details about tumor size and location, as well as surrounding intracranial structures. With MRI, different signal intensities differentiate normal brain from tumor and contrast enhancement sharpens the definition of a lesion. MRI enhanced with gadolinium can distinguish between tumor and edema.[11] Conventional MRI sequences with T1W, T2W, and fluid attenuated inversion recovery (FLAIR) are commonly used with cerebral malignancy.[20,21] Although conventional MRI can evaluate edema, hydrocephalus, and hemorrhage, it cannot reliably predict subtype or grade of glioma, and advanced imaging may be indicated to identify the pathophysiological characteristics of the tumor.[20]

Advanced Imaging

After the diagnosis has been confirmed, advanced imaging techniques are utilized to evaluate the cellular, hemodynamic, metabolic, and functional properties of the tumor have been shown to improve diagnostic, intraoperative, and postoperative management. Understanding pathophysiological properties such as microscopic tumor infiltration, microvascular characteristics, and early response changes is critical to the ongoing management of brain tumors. Advanced imaging improves the delineation of tumor margins and evaluates the extent of tumor invasion, including its relationship to eloquent cortical areas and major white-matter tracts. This advanced knowledge of the tumor has allowed for improvements in identifying optimal biopsy sites and making critical preoperative decisions, resulting in more effective treatment interventions.[17,20]

Diffusion-Weighted Imaging

Diffusion-weighted imaging (DWI) is a quantitative technique routinely used in research and clinical settings.[22] DWI utilizes MR to analyze the diffusion of water molecules in the extravascular extracellular space and determines an apparent diffusion calculation (ADC).[21] ADC can measure cellularity, cell density, and properties of the extracellular matrix. Restricted diffusion favors increased cellularity and therefore is a sign of tumor progression.[20] DWI has the capability of detecting tumor progression before it can be seen with contrast enhancement.[21]

Functional Magnetic Resonance Imaging

Functional MRI (fMRI) has become an important clinical tool in surgical planning by identifying eloquent areas of the cortex and their relationship to the tumor. When patients perform different tasks, fMRI can identify the different areas of the brain activated during the task. Research has shown that fMRI can be used for accurate mapping of motor, sensory, and language areas.[17,20] Identifying these critical areas preoperatively can ultimately improve a patient's quality of life by preserving these critical areas during surgery.[17]

Magnetic Resonance Spectroscopy

Magnetic resonance spectroscopy (MRS) is used in conjunction with other imaging techniques to assess the molecular content of brain tumors by using an imaging voxel.[17] Placement of the voxel in the center of the tumor ensures the sample contains only tumor cells. MRS has been shown to discriminate tumor recurrence from radiation necrosis.[23] Studies have identified Cho, a marker that identifies membrane turnover, which can identify the progression of low to high-grade malignant tumors.[24]

Perfusion Weighted Imaging

Perfusion weighted imaging (PWI) evaluates microvasculature and can indirectly measure the metabolic activity of a tumor. Tumors can initiate angiogenesis, developing blood vessels that are histologically disorganized, tortuous, and more permeable than normal. These pathological vessels lead to hemodynamic changes that can be identified with perfusion imaging. Newer methods of MR perfusion with arterial spin labeling are completely noninvasive and do not require contrast media.[21]

Molecular Imaging

Positron emission tomography (PET) and single-photon emission computed tomography (SPECT) are molecular imaging techniques that utilize radioactive compounds to study the metabolism and physiology of the brain tumor and the surrounding tissue. PET scans using radioactive markers to measure glucose metabolism can be useful in determining the grade of primary brain tumors and in differentiating tumor regrowth from radiation necrosis. PET with carbon 11 methionine tracer can differentiate between high- and low-grade tumors.[17] PET, along with MRS and magnetic resonance perfusion, are being explored as possible methods to distinguish tumor progression from treatment-related pseudoprogression.[18] SPECT evolved from PET and uses isotopes to assess cerebral blood flow and determine tumor location.[12] SPECT with Thallium-201 chloride can be used to stage gliomas and assess the tumor postoperatively; however, its anatomical resolution is limited.[11,25] PET and SPECT are not commonly used clinically due to high expense and limited availability, especially if other more cost-effective imaging modalities yield the same reliable diagnosis.[25]

Biopsy

Surgical biopsy is performed to obtain tumor tissue as part of tumor resection or as a separate diagnostic procedure.[10] Stereotactic biopsy is a computer-directed needle biopsy. When guided by advanced imaging tools, stereotactic biopsy yields the lowest surgical morbidity and highest degree of diagnostic information. This technique is frequently used with deep-seated tumors in functionally important or inaccessible areas of the brain in order to preserve function.

In the past, the biopsy site of a deep inoperable lesion was selected based on areas of solid enhancement on T1-weighted gadolinium-enhanced MRI or contrast-enhanced CT. However, sometimes a higher grade glioma would be misdiagnosed as a lower grade if necrotic tissue was centrally located and contained in the biopsy.[17] Newer modalities, MRS and PET imaging, highlight those areas of greatest metabolic activity, thereby improving diagnostic yield and minimizing sampling error.[17] PET with carbon 11 tracer can detect the most malignant areas of the tumor improving the accuracy of diagnosis.[25] Recently, a procedure in which a neuroendoscope simultaneously treats hydrocephalus while obtaining the biopsy (endoscopic tumor biopsy) has been successful with midline paraventricular gliomas.[26]

Molecular Diagnosis

As discussed earlier in the chapter, molecular and genetic characteristics of glial tumors are now being incorporated into tumor classification. Studies of the molecular pathology of gliomas have led to the discovery of molecular biomarkers that can be used to improve diagnosis, estimate prognosis, and determine treatment efficacy.[18] Researchers have discovered specific tumor mutations can be used as prognostic indicators and imaging can play a vital role in identifying these characteristics. Conventional MRI can identify enhancement, necrosis, and edema, which are associated with poor outcomes. Mutations specific to oligodendrogliomas and glioblastomas are also visible on MRI.[20] MR imaging with 5-ALA increases the concentration of intracellular iron by synthesizing heme in glioblastoma.[25]

Medical and Surgical Management

After diagnosis of a brain tumor has been confirmed, specific treatment must be selected. The ultimate goals of tumor management are to improve quality of life and extend survival, by preserving or improving body function and structures.[27] Treatment techniques are determined by histological type, location, grade, and size of tumor; age at onset; and medical history of the patient.[12,27] Four types of treatment are discussed: (1) traditional surgery, (2) chemotherapy, (3) radiation therapy, and (4) stereotactic radiosurgery.

Traditional Surgery

The primary goal of traditional surgery is maximal tumor resection with the least amount of damage to neural or supporting structures. Gross total resection is associated with longer survival rates and decreased neurological impairment.[28] Benign tumors, if accessible, are resected completely, whereas malignant tumors are typically partially resected secondary to location or size of the tumor.[27] The *purposes* of surgery in the management of brain tumors include the following:

1. Biopsy to establish a diagnosis
2. Partial resection to decrease the tumor mass to be treated by other methods
3. Complete resection of the tumor[29]

Biopsies are performed through open, needle, and stereotactic needle techniques. Open biopsies involve exposure of the tumor followed by removal of a sample through surgical excision. Needle biopsies involve insertion of a needle into the tumor through a hole in the skull and the excision of the tissue sample drawn through the needle. Stereotactic needle biopsies use computers and MRI or CT scanning equipment to assist in directing the needle into the tumor. This type of biopsy is useful for deep-seated or multiple brain lesions.[27]

Partial and *complete resections* are accomplished through craniotomy. Craniotomy involves removal of a portion of the skull and separation of the dura mater to expose the tumor. Stereotactic craniotomy uses technology to create computed three-dimensional pictures of the brain to guide the neurosurgeon during the procedure. CT scanning and MRI scanners are used to provide an evaluation of the tumor resection during the procedure.[29] Awake craniotomy allows for intraoperative brain mapping that helps identify and protect functional cortex, and in recent years has been used more frequently for most supratentorial tumors.[30]

Preoperative management. Before surgery, patients are evaluated for general surgical risks and the possibility of tumors in additional locations. Unless medically contraindicated, steroids are administered before surgery if brain edema is present or if extensive manipulation is anticipated during surgery. Anticonvulsant medications are also administered preoperatively to prevent seizures during or after surgery.[27]

Intraoperative management. During surgery, precautions are taken to prevent an increase in edema or ICP. Mannitol, a vasodiuretic to decrease ICP, is used to shrink the surrounding brain tissue, thus providing easier access to the tumor. Steroid use is continued and antibiotics are administered to prevent infection. Hyperventilation, with a carbon dioxide (CO_2) level of 25 mEq/L, is also used to reduce ICP.[27]

Postoperative management. Patients are observed in an intensive care unit for at least 24 hours for possible intracranial bleeding or seizures. Blood pressure is monitored continuously. After surgery, patients are at risk for developing deep vein thrombosis or pulmonary embolism, secondary to decreased muscle activity. Anticoagulants cannot be given, because these patients are at risk for intracranial bleeding. Therefore mechanical prophylaxis is used in an attempt to

prevent deep vein thrombosis. Steroids are tapered after surgery over 5 to 10 days. Antiepileptic medications are continued after surgery, with the length of time dependent on the presence of seizure activity before and after surgery.[27] The primary limitations of traditional surgery include the following:

1. Medical complications such as hematoma, hydrocephalus, infection, and infarction from the surgical procedure
2. Complications resulting from general anesthesia
3. Increased cost of the hospital stay and surgical procedure[27]

Chemotherapy

Chemotherapy is another treatment frequently used to manage brain tumors. It can be used independently or as an adjuvant to surgery or radiation. Chemotherapeutic drugs are not effective on all types of tumors. Some tumors are known to be resistant to certain drugs, and other treatment options must be pursued. Drugs can be given in combination to target all cell types present within the tumor. Because different drugs have different modes of action and side effects, combined drug therapy often proves to be one of the most effective treatments.[31] Chemotherapy can be administered in a number of different ways. Most agents are delivered intravenously through a peripheral intravenous line or through a catheter such as a peripherally inserted central catheter (PICC) or tunneled access central catheter (TACC). Other drugs are placed directly into the tumor bed or are given intramuscularly, orally, or by means of an implanted device.

Chemotherapy drugs impede cellular replication of the tumor cells, interfering with their ability to copy deoxyribonucleic acid (DNA) and reproduce. Once the replicating capability of the tumor cell has been disrupted, the cell dies. In this way, the tumor is prevented from growing and is destroyed at the cellular level.

Methotrexate is a highly toxic drug and is usually paired with an antidote drug, leucovorin, to reverse the side effects on normal cells.[31] Typically methotrexate is used to treat cancer outside of the CNS; however, it is the major chemotherapy drug used to treat CNS lymphoma.[11] The introduction of methotrexate has been found to increase the median survival for patients with primary CNS lymphoma, even those older than 60 years of age.[32]

Neurotoxic to surrounding tissue, methotrexate and cytarabine are drugs able to be introduced directly into the CSF through an intraventricular Ommaya reservoir.[33] The reservoir, implanted under the scalp, is filled by use of a syringe, and the medication is then circulated through the ventricles to the brain.[31] The drugs are routinely given in a clinic setting by a registered nurse certified in chemotherapy administration. A patient's chemotherapy schedule varies depending on the drug given. An on-off cycle is used to allow the patient time to recover from the drugs' harmful side effects.

One of the challenges in delivering cytotoxic drugs to the brain is the blood-brain barrier (BBB). The BBB is the brain's natural protective barrier against transmission of foreign substances from the blood into the brain.[31] One class of drugs that does penetrate the BBB is the *nitrosoureas*. These include BCNU (carmustine) and CCNU (lomustine), which are lipid soluble and cell cycle specific. These drugs are given in high doses and typically used to treat glioblastoma multiforme and anaplastic astrocytoma; however, often these high-grade tumors invade and destroy the BBB.

BCNU can also be administered in the form of wafers placed by the neurosurgeon directly into the brain tumor. An initial study for recurrent malignant gliomas found that patients' tumors responded to the treatment. This report was followed by an upfront study for glioblastoma.[34] The US Food and Drug Administration (FDA) granted approval for these wafers (Gliadel) for newly diagnosed high-grade glioma in 2002.[34]

Temozolomide is an orally available chemotherapeutic agent introduced in the 1990s for the treatment of malignant gliomas.[34] Initial results in treating recurrent anaplastic astrocytoma and glioblastoma were so successful that the drug was approved for the treatment of recurrent brain tumors by the FDA.[35] For recurrent tumors the drug is administered orally 5 days per month. Temozolomide was then tested for the upfront treatment of glioblastoma. This occurred in a multicenter study in which the drug was given daily as part of the initial treatment with radiation therapy, followed by five doses per month for maintenance treatment.[35] Survival increased substantially with this regimen, and as a result the FDA approved the use of temozolomide as part of first-line treatment of newly diagnosed high-grade glioma in 2005. The CATNON trial, just completed in 2017, demonstrated temozolomide chemotherapy was associated with significant survival benefits in patients with newly diagnosed anaplastic glioma.[36]

Another major breakthrough in chemotherapy for brain tumors was the finding that the antiangiogenesis monoclonal antibody Avastin (Bevacizumab) improved the progression-free survival and tumor images on MRIs of patients with glioblastoma.[37] The drug targets vascular endothelial growth factor (VEGF) and is administered intravenously. In 2017, the FDA granted full approval for the use of Avastin in the treatment of adults with recurrent glioblastoma. It is usually administered in combination with another chemotherapy agent such as irinotecan.[37]

Radiation Therapy

Radiation therapy can be used alone or in conjunction with surgery or chemotherapy to treat malignant brain tumors. It is typically chosen as a treatment option for tumors that are too large or inaccessible for surgical resection and to eradicate residual neoplastic cells after a surgical debulking. Radiotherapy consists of the delivery of high-powered photons, with energies in a much greater range than that of standard x-rays, as an external beam focused directly at the tumor site. The external beam is transmitted to the tumor through a linear accelerator or a cobalt machine that uses cobalt isotopes as the radiation source. External beam radiation is the most widely used form of radiation treatment.[38]

Conventional radiation therapy, as described previously, is fractionated into small doses delivered over a period of weeks. Often, if a large fraction is to be delivered, the dose is divided and given in multiple small doses; this is called *hyperfractionation*. The aim is to decrease the damage done to healthy surrounding tissue. Studies are investigating the use of a few high ablative doses of radiation known has hypofractionation radiotherapy. Preliminary findings suggest hypofractionation improves tumor growth control and may offer an increase in antitumor immune response as compared with hyperfractionation radiotherapy.[39,40]

Conformal radiation is the use of high-dose external beam radiation, produced by a linear accelerator, to precisely match or "conform" to the tumor shape. This method attempts to deliver a uniform amount of radiation to the tumor and minimize irradiation of healthy brain tissue.[41]

Radiosurgery involves relatively high-dose hypofractionated radiation beams directed at small tumor areas through the use of computer imaging.[41] This type of treatment includes the Gamma Knife, linear accelerators, and the Cyberknife, which are discussed later.

The radiation oncologist determines the dosage, frequency, and method of radiation delivery, depending on tumor type, location, growth rate, and other medical issues for each patient. A typical course of radiation therapy will last 6 weeks. Patients are irradiated for just 1 to 5 minutes, 5 days a week. The radiation is intended to destroy the malignant cells and preserve healthy ones; however, some rapidly

growing cells, such as skin tissue and mucosa, are killed, also producing the common side effects known to radiation.[38]

Radiation therapy has considerable limitations and disadvantages. There is an accepted maximum lifetime dosage of radiation that the brain and body can tolerate. As doses come close to this limit, the risk of radiation necrosis increases. Because the brains of young children are particularly vulnerable to radiation, other therapies, such as chemotherapy, are used until the developing brain is more tolerant of radiation. Metastatic lesions have invaded multiple organs or body systems; therefore a more systemic treatment such as chemotherapy is most effective for this type of brain cancer.[41]

Stereotactic Radiosurgery

Stereotactic radiosurgery is defined as delivery of a high dose of ionizing radiation, in a single fraction, to a small, precisely defined volume of tissue.[42,43] The high-energy accelerators involved improve the physical effect of radiation by allowing energy to travel more precisely in a straight line and penetrate deeper before dissipating. The goal is to arrest tumor growth by disrupting the tumor's DNA. This technique has been shown to be most beneficial for treating centrally located lesions less than 3 cm in size and for patients with increased surgical risk factors.[38] Advantages of stereotactic radiosurgery are as follows:
1. It is a noninvasive procedure using local anesthesia and sedation to place the stereotactic frame.
2. It avoids risks of general anesthesia and immediate postoperative risks such as bleeding, CSF leak, and infection.
3. It lowers treatment cost and shortens hospital stays.[42]

Stereotactic radiosurgery is used to treat benign, malignant, and metastatic tumors; vascular malformations; and functional disorders.[43] The primary modes of administration for stereotactic radiosurgery include the Gamma Knife, linear accelerators, and the Cyberknife.[42] The radiosurgery team consists of a neurosurgeon, radiation oncologist, medical physicist, oncology nurse, dosimetrist, and radiation therapist.

The Gamma Knife was first introduced in Sweden in 1968 and is now used worldwide at more than 300 sites (Fig. 25.3). The Gamma Knife uses 201 discrete sources of cobalt 60, which are focused precisely to one point in three-dimensional space within the cranium. The Gamma Knife is typically used for deeply embedded small tumors, often metastatic, that require precise delivery of radiation.[44,45]

MRI, CT scanning, or angiography is used to identify the exact location of the lesion to be treated after the stereotactic frame is placed on the patient's head. The stereotactic frame is then fixed to the machine and attached to a collimator helmet containing 201 holes

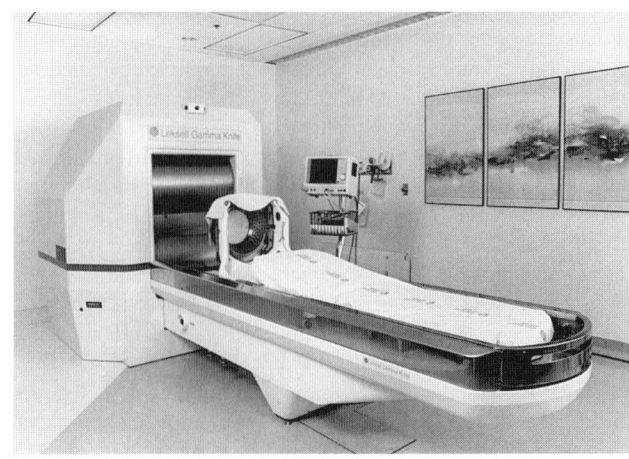

Fig. 25.3 The Leksell Gamma Knife.

for the radiation to pass through. The patient is then locked into position. The prescribed dose is given over 20 minutes to 2 hours. After treatment the frame is removed, the patient is observed and is frequently discharged after 24 hours. Return to previous activity typically occurs within a few days.[44,46]

With the Gamma Knife, the full dose of radiation is received only at the point where the 201 beams intersect, thereby giving only a minimal dose to uninvolved tissue when targeted accurately. Side effects are rare, but headache and nausea may occur. The primary limitations of the Gamma Knife are the limited brain volume that can be treated with one dose and the cost of the Gamma Knife machine.[27,44]

Linear accelerators used for conventional radiation can be modified for stereotactic radiosurgery. The brain lesion to be targeted is stereotactically placed in the center of the arc of rotation of the machine. A single, highly focused beam of radiation is delivered over multiple sweeps around the lesion. Linear accelerators can be used to treat larger tumors with precise shape while maintaining uniform dose. Because linear accelerators are used for conventional radiation, a quality check for beam accuracy is imperative before the machine is used for stereotactic radiosurgery.[12,27]

The *Cyberknife* uses a compact linear accelerator mounted on a robotic arm, with the robotic arm moving around the linear accelerator to multiple precalculated positions (Fig. 25.4). At each position, the accelerator fires a beam of radiation at the tumor or lesion. A high cumulative dose of radiation is achieved at the tumor or lesion at the convergence of the beams. This dose is typically strong enough to destroy the abnormal cells while minimizing the damaging effects of radiation to healthy surrounding tissue. The Cyberknife differs from other stereotactic radiosurgery because a linear accelerator is combined with an image guidance system. The robotic arm allows the Cyberknife to target difficult-to-reach areas of the body, as well as adjust quickly for changes in target location during treatment.[47,48]

These stereotactic radiosurgery techniques are widely used, due to the ability to precisely and accurately deliver a high dose of radiation to a target while sparing surrounding healthy tissue and minimizing the overall dose needed to ablate the tumor.[49] In recent years, studies have proven Gamma Knife to be a safe treatment modality for brain stem metastases.[50] A 2016 study looked at the use of stereotactic radiosurgery to the postoperative tumor bed after surgical resection.

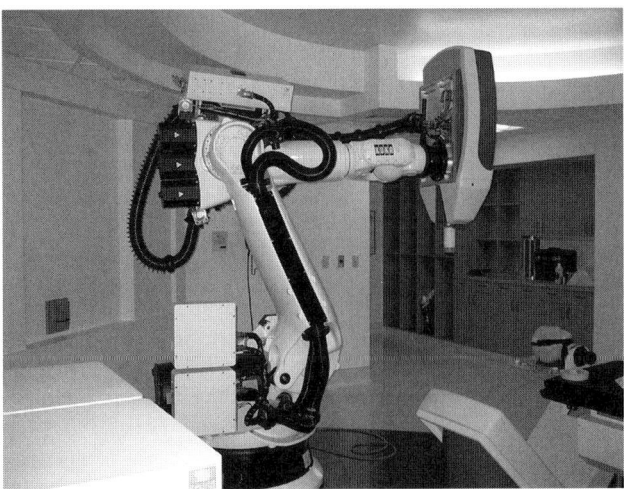

Fig. 25.4 The Cyberknife.

Results for local control and overall survival rate were comparable to WBRT.[51] Historically, microsurgical resection and radiosurgery have been utilized to treat acoustic neuromas, depending on the size and presence of brain stem compression. In these cases, stereotactic radiosurgery avoids the risk of an open procedure, has minimal side effects, and due to the overall decreased amount of radiation the cochlea receives, hearing is often preserved.[52]

Research suggests recurrent high-grade gliomas treated with stereotactic radiosurgery have median progression free survival and median overall survival estimates of 5.42 and 20.19 months, respectively. The combined rate of radiation necrosis was 5.9%.[53] The addition of radiosurgery at the time of recurrence after surgery and radiation has been found to aide in an increase in overall survival of patients with glioblastoma.[54]

The preferred treatment for *meningiomas* is surgical resection, if complete resection is possible. However, for meningiomas situated in the skull base, stereotactic radiosurgery is a good option, allowing for tumor control and preserved neurological function.[55] Cerebellopontine angle meningioma patients demonstrated a 98% progression free survival at 3 years and a low rate of adverse radiation effects.[56]

Research Trends

The standard of treatment for primary brain tumors has not changed much in the last two decades; most are still treated with surgical resection followed by chemotherapy and radiation. However, there are some promising new discoveries in the research and possible new treatment options and techniques on the horizon.

One such area of promise centers on inhibiting proteins responsible for the growth and division of glioblastomas by targeting glioma stem cells and glioblastoma stem cells (tumor precursor cells). Scientists from Massachusetts Institute of Technology (MIT) have identified the mechanism by which a specific protein, called PRMT5, drives glioblastoma tumor growth. By using PRMT5 inhibiting drugs to block this mechanism, glioblastoma growth was halted in mice. The finding indicates PRMT5 could be involved in a form of "gene splicing" that causes the tumor to grow out of control.[57] Another protein, oligodendrocyte transcription factor (OLIG 2), has been found to be a requirement for the proliferation of glioma stemlike cells. OLIG 2 is expressed in the CNS only; therefore it is a good target for highly targeted drug therapy. Ongoing research is being conducted to inhibit proliferation by targeting OLIG 2.[58]

The challenge of highly targeted drug therapy is getting through the BBB. Researchers are developing scaffolds for growing cell cultures, using polymers as carriers to transport drugs into the brain, and even using viruses. Preliminary studies have shown the Zika virus, devastating to the neural precursor cells in the developing fetus, seeks out and kills glioblastoma stem cells relative to normal neuronal cells.[59] Natural bioactive compounds, including retinoids and cannabis, have been shown to inhibit cell proliferation and migration in cultures of human glioblastoma.[60,61]

The FDA has begun Phase 0 advanced clinical trials, allowing new drugs to be entered into clinical trials with a smaller number of subjects much sooner. One such drug, AZD1775, was given to a recurrent glioblastoma patient prior to craniotomy resection to assess whether the drug had reached the tumor bed and was modulating as intended, thereby directing the course of further treatment.[62]

Tumor treating fields (TTF) is an FDA-approved antimitotic treatment modality that interferes with glioblastoma cell division and cellular assembly by delivering low-intensity, alternating electric fields to the tumor through transducer arrays applied on the shaved

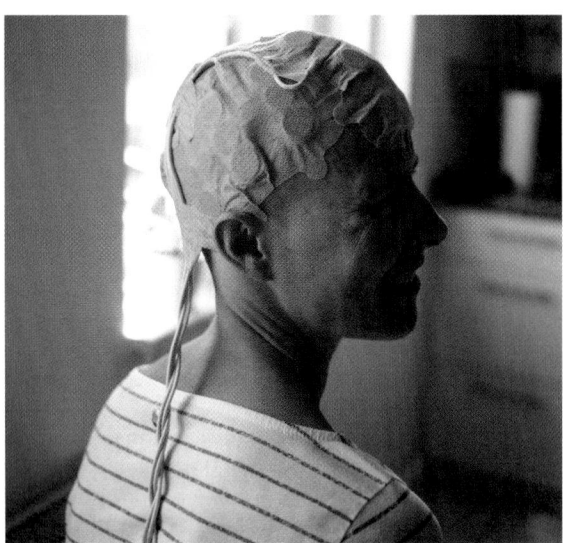

Fig. 25.5 Tumor Treating Fields (TTF) Device. Courtesy of Novocure.

scalp, connected to a portable device (Fig. 25.5). Studies completed using TTF and Temozolomide have resulted in both longer progression-free survival and median overall survival than with chemotherapy alone.[63]

REHABILITATION

Overview

Rehabilitation is a key component in the management of the patient with a brain tumor. With advances in technology and treatment intervention, survival rates of cancer patients with CNS involvement have improved over recent decades. Consequently, people are living longer with physical impairments resulting from the disease or its treatment, necessitating skilled therapeutic intervention.[64] The medical and psychological issues typically associated with cancer diagnosis are further complicated by loss of function and cognition specific to brain cancer. By preventing complications, maximizing function, and providing support, rehabilitation specialists ultimately improve the patient's quality of life.[13] Research has shown that the functional outcomes and discharge to home for individuals with brain tumors are comparable to those of individuals with stroke or traumatic brain injury.[65] The most effective rehabilitation plan is flexible, to allow for increasing impairment, and sensitive, to accommodate the highly emotional impact that accompanies the diagnosis of a primary brain tumor. The tumor's invasion is marked by complaints of pain and growing activity limitations. These functional consequences of the disease process are the target of the rehabilitation team. In addition to the side effects of therapeutic intervention, functional progress may be affected by cerebral edema, hydrocephalus, tumor regrowth, infection, and radiation necrosis. Compared with patients with other diagnoses, patients with brain tumors have a higher rate of unplanned transfers back to acute care, primarily due to infection.[66]

The management of a patient with a brain tumor is different from that of other CNS disorders, despite a similar clinical presentation. To establish an appropriate plan of care, the clinician must understand the nature of the specific tumor, consider the patient's fluctuating neurological status, and prepare for the likelihood of progressive decline. The preferred approach is holistic, addressing quality-of-life issues such as physical, psychosocial, and emotional needs,

incorporated into the systems model of motor control. Factors defining quality of life are unique to each individual, and therefore clinicians should identify and use these factors to construct a meaningful treatment program.[65] Individuals with advanced cancer who participated in exercise therapy have reported increased physical functioning, improved quality of life, and decreased fatigue.[67]

Evaluation, clinical analysis, intervention, discharge planning, and psychosocial issues specific to the management of the patient with a brain tumor are discussed in the following sections.

Evaluation

The evaluation process must include a comprehensive examination and assessment of all systems in order to establish an appropriate impairment diagnosis, problem list, prognosis, and plan of care. Before a neurological assessment is performed, a thorough review of the patient's medical history and an understanding of the medical diagnosis are necessary. The patient's occupation, support system, personal goals, and role in the family are important psychosocial factors that should be identified in the evaluation. These factors, along with a thorough functional and neurological examination, assist the clinician through the diagnostic process. This process includes identification of clinical problems, establishment of realistic and appropriate goals, selection of the most effective intervention, and discharge planning.

Although the neurological examination yields important information regarding strength, reflexes, sensation, vision, and cognition, it is important not to rely solely on its findings to determine an appropriate intervention. Because multiple systems interact to produce normal movement, it is difficult to examine isolated systems and apply the findings accurately to movement patterns. Therefore clinicians are encouraged to examine all systems through functional tasks to understand how the impaired neurological, musculoskeletal, and cognitive systems are affecting the patient's movement. During the evaluation process, the clinician notes systems that are functioning normally, identifies abnormal components of movement, and determines appropriate interventions to optimize motor recovery.[67] The progressive nature of the disease necessitates ongoing assessment followed by accommodating treatment intervention.

Goal Setting

The functional impairments and objective neurological findings provide the clinician with valuable information to establish goals and determine a treatment plan based on the patient's anticipated functional level. Despite the progressive nature of the disease, treatment goals should maximize the potential for function, introduce effective, task-oriented movement strategies, and offer multiple movement options.[64]

To set realistic and patient-oriented goals, it is important for the clinician to envision where the patient will be at discharge based on present level of function, prognosis, and disease course, while considering patient and caregiver personal goals. Appropriate goals range from comprehensive caregiver training to independent mobility with transition back to a work environment. Goals need to challenge the patient to attain an optimal level of function while also allowing for modifications due to disease progression. Patients who have the potential to return to work may require additional intervention from neuropsychology, vocational rehabilitation, or a multidisciplinary day program, depending on the nature of the job and the patient's specific deficits.

Because the rehabilitation potential for patients with brain tumors varies greatly, it is imperative that the patient, family members, rehabilitation team, and third-party payers understand and agree with the purpose of the patient's rehabilitation program. If a patient has a poor prognosis, the rehabilitation team can successfully train family members and order equipment within 1 week if the family understands the goals and the need to be present during treatment sessions. The patient's prognosis should be considered to make an ethical decision that ensures that time in rehabilitation does not compromise valuable time at home with family.[64]

Functional Assessment

Historically persons with primary malignant brain tumors have not been considered rehabilitation candidates because of the progressive nature of their disease. Physicians, health care providers, and third-party payers have questioned the efficacy of rehabilitation in this population because of poor prognoses and limited survival rates. However, advances in medical diagnosis and intervention are resulting in longer survival of people with multiple limitations that require rehabilitation. Functional assessment scales provide objective evidence that rehabilitation is effective and worthwhile for these patients.[64]

The functional assessment is a critical component in the development of the treatment intervention. It provides a method of analyzing deficits, compiling a problem list, developing a treatment plan, and measuring functional outcomes. The Functional Independence Measure (FIM) is a functional assessment tool used to measure degree of disability, regardless of underlying pathology, and burden of care to demonstrate functional outcomes of rehabilitation and assist clinicians with discharge planning.[67]

Functional outcome scales such as the FIM provide a means of documenting the patient's response to therapy intervention for clinicians, physicians, and third-party payers in the rehabilitation setting. Research using FIM data demonstrates efficacy for inpatient rehabilitation of brain tumor patients similar to that noted in those with traumatic brain injury or stroke when matched by age, sex, and functional status on admission.[64,68] In 2016, the Center for Medicare and Medicaid implemented a new functional outcome measure; however, these studies have not yet been published.[69]

Physicians use specific functional evaluation scales to measure the success of treatment. The Karnofsky performance scale, which rates patients' functional performance, is the tool most widely used in clinical research and treatment decisions (see Table 25.1). The patient receives a score from 0 to 100 based on independence or level of assistance required for normal activity. The scale is used in research to evaluate an individual's physical response to treatment.[13]

Side Effects and Considerations

Through advances in chemotherapy and radiation therapy, the ability to reduce tumor mass has greatly improved. Unfortunately, despite the often favorable long-term results of these treatments, the immediate effects create physical and psychological challenges for the patient and clinician. Patients who are receiving aggressive tumor treatment during the rehabilitation phase will probably experience a decline in neurological or hematological status. These declines often limit the individual's tolerance for treatment intervention and increase patient and caregiver feelings of depression and hopelessness. Clinicians have the opportunity to provide more than physical restorative services and should offer psychosocial support when possible to enhance successful rehabilitation.[67]

The side effects and special considerations that arise with this population range from physical to cognitive to psychosocial and emotional. The following paragraphs relate the spectrum of complications and side effects the patient may experience when undergoing medical treatment, and the impact these may have on therapeutic intervention.

Not everyone undergoing chemotherapy or radiation treatment will experience physical side effects; however, the possibilities include hair loss, fatigue, nausea, skin burns or irritation, difficulty eating or digesting food, anorexia, and dry, sore mouth.[67,70] The side effects are caused by the toxic effects the drugs have on healthy, rapidly dividing cells, including bone marrow cells, cells lining the mucosa, and hair cells.[70]

The toxic effect chemotherapy has on bone marrow impairs the patient's ability to produce red and white blood cells and platelets.[2] The patient may develop anemia, infection, or hemorrhage as a result of depressed hematological values.

The lining of the mouth, esophagus, and intestines may become inflamed and irritated and interfere with the ability to eat or digest food. The patient may experience nausea, vomiting, diarrhea, or constipation, any of which will impair mobility and energy for daily activities.[67]

Hair loss is a common side effect of brain radiation and chemotherapy. This requires an especially difficult adjustment for most people, because it causes a drastic change in appearance.[41]

Clinicians involved in the management of patients who are currently receiving radiation therapy or chemotherapy need to be mindful of these side effects when developing a plan of intervention. Fatigue, low blood count, and gastrointestinal complaints may limit a patient's ability to fully participate in the planned therapy session or may call for a modification in activity or environment.[71] Moreover, the clinician must use these factors to determine if the patient's health or safety would be jeopardized by therapeutic intervention at any particular time. In addition, the clinician must be flexible to determine the optimal time when intervention is most effective and does not interfere with medications or meals.

Together with the physical side effects mentioned previously, many patients with brain tumors have changes in cognition or personality as a result of the tumor's location. A patient with a frontal lobe tumor who was previously quiet and withdrawn may, over time, become loud and disinhibited as a result of tumor growth. Tumors that invade the speech-language area cause communication and comprehension difficulties that create challenges for the patient and clinician. The patient who has a left parietal tumor may be aphasic and not respond to verbal commands. In this case, the clinician must engage in alternate means of communication or provide therapeutic facilitation with tactile cues. An observant, critical analysis of the patient's physical deficits and impaired communication, comprehension, and feedback mechanisms is essential to select an effective, patient-specific intervention plan.

Because of the emotionally charged nature of the disease process, psychosocial and emotional issues frequently arise. Clinicians should be sensitive to fluctuations in temperament and mood that the diagnosis itself and subsequent treatment strategies create. Clinicians can offer psychosocial support and direct the patient and family to resources that may give direction and guidance during difficult transitions.

Intervention

The ultimate goal of rehabilitation is to achieve maximum restoration of function, within the limits imposed by the disease, in the patient's preferred environment. The clinician must recognize that the physical, cognitive, and emotional status of these individuals is inconsistent and changing as a result of the disease process or medical intervention. Treatment plans must be flexible to effectively manage fluctuations in the patient's presentation. A comprehensive rehabilitation plan is individualized to accommodate progressive changes in functional mobility and provides problem-solving experiences to prepare the patient and caregiver for these situations. The rehabilitation process typically begins in the intensive care unit and continues in the inpatient, outpatient, and home health settings.

In the intensive care unit, communication with nursing staff regarding the patient's present medical status and an understanding of ICP, hemodynamic values, and monitoring devices are crucial to determining tolerance for therapy intervention (Fig. 25.6). Mobilizing a patient with a ventriculostomy (a catheter placed in the third ventricle to drain CSF and to monitor ICP) is possible; however, nursing staff must close the drain before any positional change and should inform the clinician of appropriate treatment parameters. A patient's dependence on these monitoring devices does not prevent therapeutic intervention, but the critical status of these individuals must be considered. The monitoring equipment provides constant feedback that assists the clinician in assessing the patient's tolerance to activity and his or her ability to proceed with treatment.

As the patient becomes more medically stable, the clinician progresses mobility and prepares the patient for the next stage of rehabilitation. Despite the patient's upgraded medical status allowing for transfer to the rehabilitation setting, clinicians must continue to reassess functional and neurological status and alert physicians to any changes. Clinicians spend many hours with patients, and these daily interactions give them the opportunity to connect on a personal level and observe the patient in different settings. Intuitive therapists are often the first to notice physical, cognitive, and emotional changes. Communication to the physician of significant changes is imperative for appropriate follow-up procedures and referrals to provide optimal care.

In the inpatient rehabilitation setting, treatment focuses on optimizing functional capabilities to prepare the patient and family for discharge. Integrating the patient's personal goals and interests into therapeutic intervention invests the patient and family in the rehabilitation process. The incorporation of these quality-of-life issues encourages the pursuit of a meaningful lifestyle at discharge. If clinicians believe the patient's goals are unrealistic, gentle redirection is helpful to channel energy toward achievable goals. Goals for inpatient rehabilitation range from returning the patient to an independent lifestyle to training family members to be caregivers in the home environment.

The restoration of previous functional movement patterns is desired. The literature reports increasing evidence that the CNS has dynamic properties, including neural regeneration and collateral sprouting, which supports the concept of plasticity. Plasticity allows intact neural centers to recognize and assume functions of areas of the brain impaired or destroyed by the lesion or its medical management. The treatment focus may need to turn to compensatory strategies if the potential for motor recovery and learning is lacking. Once compensatory patterns are established, it is not clearly known whether recovery of normal movement will be achieved.[72,73] Compensatory techniques may be beneficial in increasing safety and efficiency with mobility and activities of daily living (ADLs), or in providing more independence for the patient. Increasing independence can assist in improving quality of life for the patient and may permit return to work or participation in previous recreational activity. For example, an avid golfer with right-sided hemiparesis and impaired standing balance can modify his clubs and return to the game at the wheelchair level.

The rehabilitation program should prepare the patient and caregivers for an efficient transition from the structured care setting to the home. Using motor learning principles (refer to Chapter 3) to teach functional mobility will best produce transfer of learning from a constant environment to an unpredictable home environment. Repetitious practice of specific parts of a skill in fixed surroundings, with physical and verbal guidance throughout the movement and frequent feedback during and after completion of the task, are beneficial in teaching acquisition of a specific movement or activity.[74,75] Recently, clinicians have incorporated more technology into treatments, including robotics to allow patients to perform high repetitions of movements with feedback mechanisms to promote motor learning. Studies have shown more accurate movement and positive affective responses of patients after ambulating with robotic-assisted gait training. Although research with robotics has focused on patients with spinal cord injury and stroke, the same principles can be applied to patients with brain tumors.[76–78]

Practicing the whole activity in a variable context, with irregular feedback and decreased physical and verbal guidance, expedites learning.[74] Learning results in the ability to execute a task in any setting. Community outings and home passes naturally provide an environment that facilitates learning. The clinician can measure retention and transfer of learning by the patient's performance in the community or at home. This information should be used to adjust the treatment plan and make recommendations for environmental modifications that minimize physical and cognitive demands on the patient. A patient whose individual treatment focus is transfers gains confidence when able to transfer from a wheelchair to a table chair in a crowded restaurant.

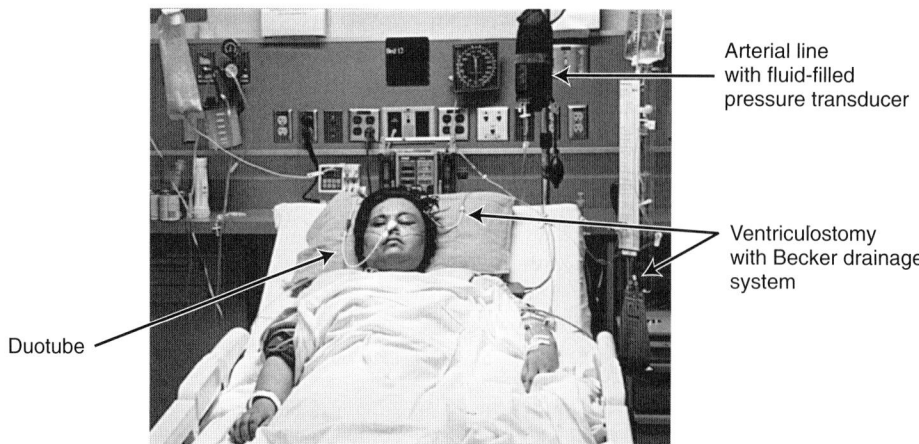

Arterial line
with fluid-filled
pressure transducer

Ventriculostomy
with Becker drainage
system

Duotube

Fig. 25.6 A Patient After a Partial Tumor Resection. Labels indicate the equipment commonly seen in the neurological intensive care unit.

An interdisciplinary team approach is used for community reentry to provide a meaningful experience for the patient. Recreational therapists play an integral part in identifying the individual's interests, reintegrating the patient into the community, and modifying leisure activities to meet physical abilities. Activities addressed in daily therapy sessions are practiced in the community, and feedback is provided to the appropriate clinician as well as the patient. Initial reentry into the community can be intimidating to the patient and may cause changes in the patient's behavior that will affect mobility performance. Therefore it is necessary for the clinician to be sensitive and recognize the issues the patient may be experiencing.

For caregiver training and education to be successful, a good rapport must be established among clinician, patient, and the family members or caregivers. Caregiver training includes mobility training and education regarding the effect the tumor may have on the patient's present and future mobility. Instruction should be given based on present level of function, but the probability of progressive decline should not be overlooked. An intuitive clinician should offer effective techniques and problem-solving to address potential obstacles created by the disease process. For example, when performing transfer training, the clinician may demonstrate a stand-pivot transfer but may also suggest a squat-pivot transfer if physical or cognitive changes mandate increased assistance by the caregiver.

Discharge Planning

Discharge planning is initiated early, continues throughout the rehabilitation process, and must allow for changes in the patient's functional status. On discharge from the rehabilitation setting, the patient will make the transition to one of the following settings: home, skilled nursing facility, or hospice. The transition to home is typically preferred by the patient, caregiver, and interdisciplinary rehabilitation team. If the patient cannot be physically or medically managed at home, then placement in a skilled nursing facility may be necessary. The patient may choose hospice care when medical treatment is no longer providing control of the tumor and the physical demands of the patient are not manageable by the caregivers. The case manager contacts insurance providers to determine coverage and, after conferring with the interdisciplinary team, gives the patient and family information regarding discharge options.

Patient and caregiver training and education constitute an integral part of discharge planning. Before discharge, the patient and caregiver should be instructed in functional mobility and ADLs, informed of equipment needs and vendor resources, and provided with community resources for support and education. During individual training, the clinician is able to provide feedback to the caregiver and patient to facilitate an easier transition to home. Documentation of caregiver education and training should be included in the progress and discharge notes.

Equipment necessary to assist the patient and family with mobility and ADLs is recommended by the appropriate clinician. When equipment is ordered, fluctuations in the patient's present status, as well as the probable progressive decline in function, are considered. If the patient is functioning without equipment at discharge, it is helpful to include resources of local charitable organizations and vendors for future equipment needs.

Prior to discharge, local and national resources specific to brain tumors should also be provided. These resources can be found on the internet or through communication with previous patients or health care professionals. Support groups provide the caregiver and the patient with an opportunity to share experiences and information, prevent isolation, foster hope, allow the patient and caregiver to discover coping skills, and offer emotional support.[79,80] National

BOX 25.1   National Organizations

NATIONAL BRAIN TUMOR SOCIETY
55 Chapel St., suite 200
Newton, MA 02458
617-924-9998
www.braintumor.org
AMERICAN BRAIN TUMOR ASSOCIATION
8550 W. Bryn Mawr Ave, suite 550
Chicago, IL 60631
(800) 886-2282
www.abta.org
e-mail: info@abta.org

organizations can provide educational information and support to patients (Box 25.1). These organizations can help the patient find local resources unfamiliar to the clinician.

PALLIATIVE CARE AND HOSPICE

As the disease process progresses, the patient and family often are faced with difficult decisions. When the prevalence of symptoms increase, and antitumor treatment is no longer effective, the end-of-life (EOL) phase has begun. During this phase, care is focused on reducing symptom burden while preserving quality of life, without inappropriate prolongation of life.[81] Both palliative care and hospice are resources that can provide support to patients and their families.

Palliative care provides for patients and families who are facing a life-threatening illness. The American Board of Medical Subspecialties has recognized palliative care since 2006. Palliative care is multidisciplinary care addressing the complex medical decisions necessary to identify patient and caregiver wishes regarding the prevention of suffering and EOL. The physical therapist focus is on mobility, caregiver training, and positioning to alleviate pain and promote comfort. Palliative care should be introduced early, soon after diagnosis, especially with a high-grade glioma. Due to the high likelihood of cognitive decline, possible seizures, and decreased consciousness as the disease progresses, sensitive EOL preferences and decisions need to be discussed early to ensure caregivers, if necessary, are aware and able to fulfill the patient's wishes.[81] Palliative care services may continue for a prolonged period of time until the illness is no longer deemed life threatening or the patient and family have decided to no longer seek curative treatment, choosing hospice.

Hospice always provides palliative care; however, patients choose hospice when they are no longer seeking curative therapy. Hospice refers to a type of care, not a place. Hospice care can be provided in the patient's home, in the hospital setting, in long-term care or nursing homes, or in freestanding hospice facilities. The hospice philosophy centers around the belief that we all have the right to die without pain and with dignity, and our loved ones are provided with the support they need to allow us to do so.[82] The dying patient experiences physical, psychological, social, and spiritual aspects of suffering. The hospice team is fully equipped and trained to support the primary caregiver (usually a family member) with a variety of services.

PSYCHOSOCIAL CARE

For many patients living extended lives with brain tumors, it is important to measure the efficacy of treatment not only in terms of functional outcome, but in terms of its effect on quality of life. *Health-related quality of life* (HRQOL) is a multidimensional concept that refers to an individual's functioning and well-being as measured by a personal perception of overall quality of life, including physical, emotional, spiritual, and intellectual functioning.[83] Despite advances, malignant brain tumors and metastases remain incurable. The treatment goal is to extend a patient's survival. Therefore in addition to overall survival, progression-free survival, and radiological response to treatment, HRQOL has become an important outcome measure. Recently, several self-reporting instruments to measure HRQOL specific for individuals with brain tumors have been developed.[84]

A strong supportive relationship with the patient and caregiver(s) is key to successful rehabilitation. This process begins with respecting the patient's unique experience and requires continual assessment of changing psychosocial needs. Many individuals with brain tumors experience higher levels of anxiety and depression, as well as feelings of loss, specifically loss of independence, loss of self, and loss of relationships.[85] Most people have a family, community, or belief system they identify with, and the acknowledgement and involvement of that bond should be part of their treatment.[86] The burden and strain on direct caregivers and family members can be devastating. The clinician must feel invested, demonstrate good communication skills, and exhibit self-confidence in the ability to discuss sensitive issues with the patient and family in order to develop a caring relationship. By active listening, the clinician can identify the patient's true concerns and feelings and assist the patient and family in coping with the cancer diagnosis. The clinician's consistent interaction with the patient can foster a supportive and safe environment in which the patient or caregiver feels comfortable sharing emotional and spiritual feelings. Once a trusting relationship has been established, the clinician's empathy can help decrease common feelings of isolation and helplessness and support the patient through the different stages of the disease.[86]

Hope is a key psychosocial need of the individual with cancer. It is an important coping strategy that can help patients with brain tumors face an uncertain and often fearful future. Clinicians working with brain tumor patients should see the preservation of hope as a therapeutic goal. A high level of hope for both the patient and family corresponds positively to a sense of well-being and good quality of life.[87] The clinician needs to maintain some degree of hope while remaining as realistic and honest as possible, focusing on short-term goals and functional improvements that are both achievable and meaningful to the patient.[87]

Psychological and social problems are not identified in 80% of physically ill persons, possibly owing to clinicians' personal behaviors or beliefs. Clinicians may find it easier to focus on the physical aspect of care to avoid becoming emotional or experiencing the patient's distress. Persons with cancer often experience feelings of powerlessness and isolation, which may be increased by distancing behaviors demonstrated by clinicians. Before offering support to patients, clinicians need to examine their own thoughts, feelings, and past experiences with death and dying. This awareness may prevent the clinician from internalizing the patient's grief, from protecting the patient and family members from the pain of grieving, and from allowing personal values to adversely influence their psychosocial support.[86] By recognizing that psychosocial care involves holistic healing, clinicians will be able to develop the best environment for interventions to improve multiple aspects of the patient's quality of life.[86]

SUMMARY

It is important for the clinician involved in the treatment of a patient with a brain tumor to anticipate the physical and cognitive deficits and the subsequent activity limitations that will develop as the patient deteriorates from the tumor progression or medical treatment. These limitations provide the foundation for treatment planning and goal setting. Improved quality of life is the goal of the rehabilitation process. This means restoring the patient to maximal functional capacity with the least amount of assistance from others. Regardless of the patient's life expectancy, the rehabilitation process should enable the patient to pursue a productive and meaningful life. Case Study 25.1 is an example of the complexity of the problems faced by an individual with a CNS tumor. These problems include both the medical condition and the functional activity limitations caused by the tumor and/or the medical management.

CASE STUDY 25.1 Medical Diagnosis: Metastatic Brain Tumor

Mr. S is a 66-year-old man diagnosed 13 years ago with melanoma, without lymph node involvement. He lived in Austria for 25 years, working in finance for the United Nations. Last July, he began to experience dizziness, mild weakness, and unsteadiness. He was diagnosed with a right frontal brain tumor and underwent a surgical resection (craniotomy) followed by WBRT in Austria. After surgery, he required a quad cane for ambulation; however, he was able to return to most activities of daily living (ADLs) except driving, due to his history of seizures. Prior to his initial diagnosis and surgery, he enjoyed playing squash, hiking, and "doing taxes."

Mr. S retired and returned to the United States in October to seek further cancer treatment and began taking Keytruda (pembrolizumab). In February, after progressive left hemiparesis, twitching, and numbness, diagnostic imaging revealed a large recurrent metastatic tumor in his right frontal lobe, causing cerebral edema and brain compression. He underwent a second craniotomy to resect this large tumor, situated directly adjacent to his primary motor strip. Postoperatively, he underwent CyberKnife radiosurgery to target five new areas of metastases. The following week, he was admitted to the neurorehabilitation unit to address his functional deficits due to impaired strength, coordination, balance, and motor planning.

Initially, he presented with impaired balance and motor planning impacting all ADLs and mobility. He required moderate assistance for bed mobility, maximal assistance for stand pivot transfers with a front-wheeled walker (FWW), and could ambulate only 5 feet with a FWW and maximal assistance, demonstrating shortened, inconsistent step length and left knee hyperextension during stance phase. After only a short week, his activity tolerance, high-level balance, and coordination significantly improved. He reached a functional level of modified independence for ADLs and ambulation on indoor, even surfaces using a four-wheeled walker. He required supervision in busy environments and on uneven surfaces due to impaired attention/concentration and intermittent decreased left-foot clearance with fatigue. At this point, Mr. S was discharged home with his brother and sister-in-law, after his family demonstrated safe proficiency, assisting him with all mobility tasks including ambulation, stair/curb negotiation, and car transfers. He continued to make slow but steady gains with physical and occupational therapy twice a week in the outpatient setting.

CASE STUDY 25.1   Medical Diagnosis: Metastatic Brain Tumor—cont'd

Mr. S returned to visit friends in Austria in June; however, he was forced to return home when his hemiparesis worsened. He had Gamma Knife Radiosurgery without significant improvement. Imaging revealed additional metastases and an increase in cerebral edema near the right frontal metastasis. This July he underwent his third craniotomy (this time a bifrontal craniotomy) to resect a right paramedian metastatic tumor. A few days after surgery, once again he returned to the neurorehabilitation unit.

It was a smooth transition back to rehab, as he was familiar with the process, the facility, and the staff; however, Mr. S's neurological deficits were significantly worse than at his previous admission. He required maximal assistance for bed mobility, maximal assistance of two for transfers, and moderate to maximal assistance for ADLs. He returned to rehab with a positive attitude, motivated to do his best despite the progression of his metastatic disease and his poor functional mobility. The therapists quickly positioned Mr. S. in a wheelchair and instructed him in wheelchair propulsion to provide him with some degree of independence; however, this task proved challenging due to his poor motor planning. The rehab team incorporated traditional treatment interventions with newer technology to allow him to perform movements that otherwise he was dependent or required maximal assistance to complete. For example, the occupational therapist utilized the Diego to perform active assisted arm exercises with a feedback monitor. With the assistance of the EKSO, the physical therapist was able to work with him on standing balance, weight shifting, and gait training. Assisted walking in the EKSO provided him with a sense of pride and accomplishment, as well as motivation to continue. As the weeks passed and Mr. S continued to need maximal assistance for mobility, it became clear that to maximize his independence and safety, he would need to discharge home at the wheelchair level. After many sessions of family training, ordering of adaptive equipment, and a wheelchair, he was discharged home with his family.

REFERENCES

To enhance this text and add value for the reader, all references are included on the companion Evolve site that accompanies this textbook. This online service will, when available, provide a link for the reader to a Medline abstract for the article cited. There are 87 cited references and other general references for this chapter, with the majority of those articles being evidence-based citations.

26

Inflammatory and Infectious Disorders of the Brain

Judith A. Dewane

OBJECTIVES

After reading this chapter the student or therapist will be able to:

1. Identify and comprehend the terminology for classifying different types of inflammatory and infectious disorders within the brain.
2. Discuss the range of neurological sequelae that occur.
3. Discuss the components of the comprehensive evaluation process and their interrelationships.
4. Structure the examination process to gather the information required to generate an appropriate plan of care.
5. Discuss the general goals of the intervention process.
6. Plan the interventions to meet the needs of the patient.

KEY TERMS

brain abscess
encephalitis
functional activities

hypertonicity
hypotonicity
intervention goals

meningitis
postural control

The diversity of neurological sequelae that may occur after an inflammatory disorder in the brain (brain abscess, encephalitis, or meningitis) provides a range of challenges to the rehabilitation team. The therapist must identify the problems underlying the individual's movement dysfunctions without the template of the cluster of "typical" problems available with some other neurological diagnoses. Each patient presents a combination of problems unique to that patient that requires the creative design of an intervention program. The following discussion of the therapeutic management of individuals recovering from an inflammatory disorder in the brain focuses on the process of designing an intervention plan to address the specific dysfunctions of the individual patient. Because the management of the clinical problems is built on an understanding of the underlying pathological condition and because therapists may not be as familiar with these disease processes, an overview of the inflammatory disorders of the brain is presented.

OVERVIEW OF INFLAMMATORY DISORDERS IN THE BRAIN

Categorization of Inflammatory Disorders

Inflammatory disorders of the brain can be categorized based on the anatomical location of the inflammatory process and the cause of the infection, which are as follows:

A. Brain abscess
B. Meningitis (leptomeningitis)
   1. Bacterial meningitis
   2. Aseptic meningitis (viral)
C. Encephalitis
   1. Acute viral
   2. Parainfectious encephalomyelitis

3. Acute toxic encephalopathy
4. Progressive viral encephalitis
5. "Slow virus" encephalitis

In most individuals, the defense mechanisms of the central nervous system (CNS) provide protection from infecting organisms. Compromises of the protective barriers can result in CNS infections as complications of common infections. The response of the CNS to the infection depends on several factors, including the type of organism, its route of entry, the CNS location of the infection, and the immunological competence of the individual. CNS infections occur with greater frequency and severity in individuals who are very young or elderly, immunodeficient, or antibody deficient.

The inflammatory process may be a localized, circumscribed collection of pus; may involve primarily the leptomeninges; may involve the brain substance; or may involve both the meninges and the brain substance. The infecting agents may be bacteria, viruses, prions, fungi, protozoa, or parasites. The most common agents producing meningitis are bacterial; the most common agents producing encephalitis are viral. However, bacterial encephalitis and viral meningitis also are disease entities. The following overview of the inflammatory processes within the brain is organized based on the anatomical location of the infection. More comprehensive discussions based on specific infecting organisms can be found in the references at the end of the chapter.[1] The site of the infection will determine the signs and symptoms of the CNS infections, whereas the infecting organism determines the prognosis, including the time course and severity of the problems.[2]

Brain Abscess

Brain abscesses occur when microorganisms reach brain tissue from a penetrating wound to the brain, by extension of local infection such as sinusitis or otitis, or by hematogenous spread from a distant site of infection. The route of infection influences the CNS region involved. The extension of a local infection tends to produce a solitary brain abscess in an adjacent lobe. Multiple abscesses may originate from the spread of microorganisms through the blood. The introduction of microorganisms by a penetrating trauma may result in an abscess soon after the trauma or several years later. As with the disorders presented in the subsequent discussions, circumstances that result in a compromised immune system (chronic corticosteroid or other immunosuppressive drug administration, administration of cytotoxic chemotherapeutic agents, or human immunodeficiency virus [HIV] infection) may predispose the individual to develop opportunistic infections.

The site and size of the abscess influence the initial symptoms. Evidence of increased intracranial pressure, a focal neurological deficit, and fever are described as the classic presenting triad.[3] However, the classic triad occurs in less than 50% of patients.[4] Most individuals experience an alteration of consciousness. In 47% of the cases, the frontal, parietal, or temporal lobe is involved.[4,5] Medical management of the abscess typically consists of antibiotic therapy (depending on the infecting agent and size and site of the abscess) and, often, surgical aspiration or excision. Bharucha and colleagues[3] describe neurological sequelae in 25% to 50% of the survivors, with 30% to 50% having persistent seizures, 15% to 30% having hemiparesis, and 10% to 20% having disorders of speech or language.

Meningitis

Meningitis (synonymous with leptomeningitis) denotes an infection spread through the cerebrospinal fluid (CSF) with the inflammatory process involving the pia and arachnoid maters, the subarachnoid space, and the adjacent superficial tissues of the brain and spinal cord. Pachymeningitis denotes an inflammatory process involving the dura mater. Meningitis can be caused by a wide variety of organisms, some of which cross the blood-brain barrier and the blood-CSF barrier. The CSF also can become contaminated by a wound that penetrates the meninges as a result of trauma or a medical procedure, such as implantation of a ventriculoperitoneal (VP) shunt. Once the organism compromises the blood-brain and blood-CSF barriers, the CSF provides an ideal medium for growth. All the body's typical major defense systems are essentially absent in the normal CSF. The blood-brain barrier may

impede the clearance of infecting organisms by leukocytes and interfere with the entry of pharmacological agents from the blood. The infecting organism is disseminated throughout the subarachnoid space as the contaminated CSF bathes the brain. Entry into the ventricles occurs either from the choroid plexuses or by reflux through the exit foramen of the fourth ventricle. The spread of the organism through the CSF circulation accounts for the differences in the variety and extent of the neurological sequelae that can result from meningitis.

Bacterial meningitis.

Clinical problems. The diagnostic categorization of meningitis depends on the infecting agent (e.g., *Haemophilus influenzae* meningitis, *Streptococcus pneumoniae* meningitis, and viral meningitis) and on the acute or chronic nature of the meningitis (acute, subacute, or chronic meningitis). The term *acute bacterial meningitis* denotes infections caused by aerobic bacteria (both gram-positive and gram-negative).[5,6] The most common infecting organism producing acute bacterial meningitis varies according to the age of the population. During the neonatal period and in the older adult, infections by gram-negative enterobacilli, especially *Escherichia coli,* and group B streptococci occur most frequently. Typical causative agents in children include *H. influenzae, Neisseria meningitidis,* and *S. pneumoniae.*[7] *S. pneumoniae, N. meningitidis,* and *H. influenzae* are the most common causes of community-acquired meningitis.[5,7,8] Individuals with a condition such as sickle cell anemia, alcoholism, or diabetes mellitus and individuals who are immunosuppressed are at increased risk.[1,9] Meningococci have been implicated in meningitis that strikes young children most often but can also infect adolescents and young adults. Freshman who live in dormitories are almost four times more likely to get meningitis when compared with other college students.

An example of an organism that uses a typical systemic route of bacterial infection is the *H. influenzae* organism—a member of the normal flora of the nose and throat. During an upper respiratory tract infection, the organism may gain entry to the blood. The route of transmission of the organism from the blood to the CSF is not well established.

The circulation of CSF spreads the infecting organism through the ventricular system and the subarachnoid spaces (Fig. 26.1). The pia and arachnoid maters become acutely inflamed, and as part of the

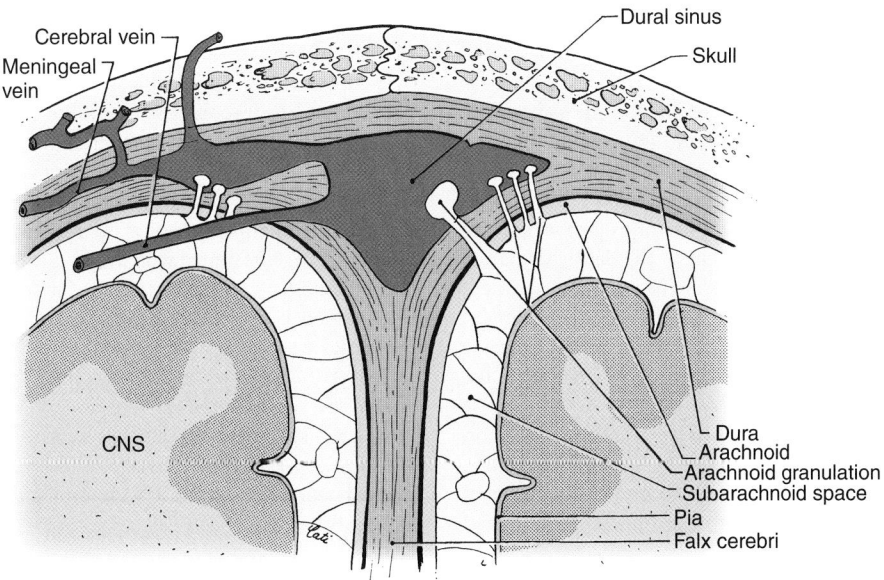

Fig. 26.1 The meninges, showing the layers of the dura, arachnoid, and pia mater and their relationship to the subarachnoid space and brain tissue. *CNS,* Central nervous system.

inflammatory response, a purulent exudate forms in the subarachnoid space. The exudate may undergo organization, resulting in an obstruction of the foramen of Monro, the aqueduct of Sylvius, or the exit foramen of the fourth ventricle. The supracortical subarachnoid spaces proximal to the arachnoid villi may be obliterated, resulting in a noncommunicating or obstructive hydrocephalus caused by the accumulation of CSF. As the CSF accumulates, the intracranial pressure rises. The increased intracranial pressure produces venous obstruction, precipitating a further increase in the intracranial pressure. The rise in the CSF pressure compromises the cerebral blood flow, which activates reflex mechanisms to counteract the decreased cerebral blood flow by raising the systemic blood pressure. An increased systemic blood pressure accompanies increased CSF pressure.

The mechanism producing the headaches that accompany increased intracranial pressure may be the stretching of the meninges and pain fibers associated with blood vessels. Vomiting may occur as a result of stimulation of the medullary emetic centers. Papilledema may occur as intracranial pressure increases.

Other routes of bacterial infection may involve a local spread as the result of an infection of the middle ear or mastoid air cells. Meningitis may occur as a complication of a skull fracture, which exposes CNS tissue to the external environment or to the nasal cavity. Fractures of the cribriform plate of the ethmoid bone producing CSF rhinorrhea provide another route for infection. Meningitis may be a further complication to the clinical problems of a traumatic head injury.

Clinical features of acute bacterial meningitis include fever, severe headache, altered consciousness, convulsions (particularly in children), and nuchal rigidity. Nuchal rigidity is indicative of an irritative lesion of the subarachnoid space. Signs of meningeal irritation are painful cervical flexion, the Kernig sign, the Brudzinski sign, and the jolt sign.[10] Cervical flexion is painful because it stretches the inflamed meninges, nerve roots, and spinal cord. The pain triggers a reflex spasm of the neck extensors to splint the area against further cervical flexion; however, cervical rotation and extension movements remain relatively free.

The *Kernig sign* refers to a test performed with the patient supine in which the thigh is flexed on the abdomen and the knee extended (Fig. 26.2A). Complaints of lumbar or posterior thigh pain indicate a positive test result.[10] This movement pulls on the sciatic nerve, which pulls on the covering of the spinal cord, causing pain in the presence of meningeal irritation. The same results are achieved with passive hip flexion with the knee remaining in extension. This is the same procedure described by Hoppenfeld[11] as the straight leg raising test for determining pathology of the sciatic nerve or tightness of the hamstrings. Passive hip flexion with knee extension can be painful because of meningeal irritation, spinal root impingement, sciatic nerve irritation, or hamstring tightness. The *Brudzinski sign* refers to the flexion of the hips and knees elicited when cervical flexion is performed (see Fig. 26.2B).[10] These signs will not be present in the deeply comatose patient who has decreased muscle tone and absence of muscle reflexes. The signs may also be absent in the infant or elderly patient. Finally, the jolt test, which has the patient turn his or her head from side to side quickly (two to three rotations per second), has a positive result if the maneuver worsens the patient's headache.[10]

The diagnosis of bacterial meningitis can be established based on blood cultures and a sample of CSF obtained by a lumbar puncture. CSF pressure is consistently elevated. The CSF sample in bacterial meningitis typically reveals an increased protein count and a decreased glucose level.

The type and severity of the sequelae of acute bacterial meningitis relate directly to the area affected, the extent of CNS infection, the age and general health of the individual, the level of consciousness at the

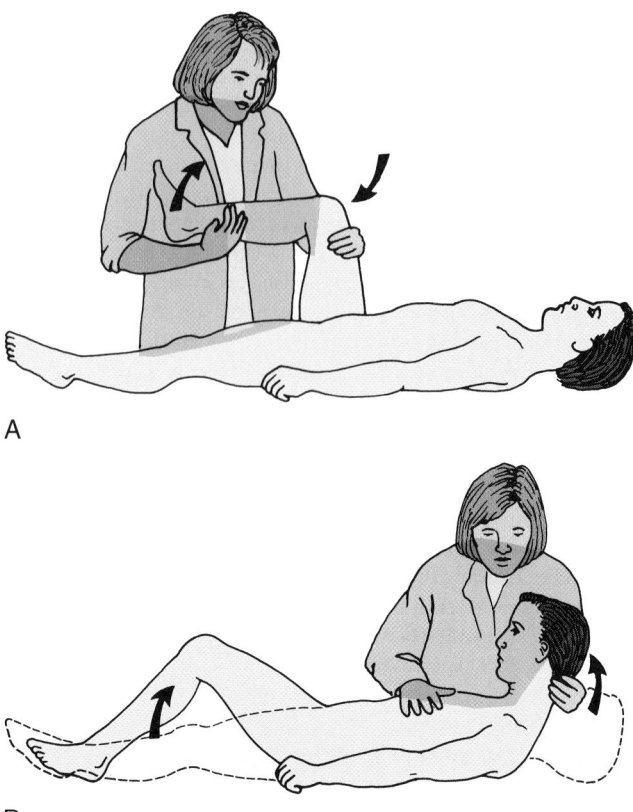

A

B

Fig. 26.2 **(A)** Kernig sign. **(B)** Brudzinski sign.

initiation of pharmacological therapy, and the pathological agent involved. Some of the common CNS complications include subdural effusions, altered levels of consciousness, seizures, involvement of the cranial nerves, and increased intracranial pressure.

Medical management. Medical management of bacterial meningitis consists of the initiation of the antimicrobial regimen appropriate to the infecting organism and procedures to manage the signs and symptoms of meningitis that have been described in the preceding paragraphs. Medical intervention strategies in both these areas change with the development of new pharmacological agents. Thus medical management can change within short periods. The reader is encouraged to always review recent literature for additional information on current aspects of the medical management of the patient with meningitis.

Prevention. Vaccination has significantly decreased the incidence of meningitis from *H. influenzae* type B in young children and infants. College freshmen who live in dormitories are four times more likely than other college students to develop meningococcus meningitis, and there is now a vaccine that has shown promise in reducing the outbreak rate.

Potential neurological sequelae. Even with optimal antimicrobial therapy, bacterial meningitis continues to have a finite mortality rate, which varies with the infecting organism, age of the individual, and time lapse to initiation of treatment, and has the potential for marked neurological morbidity. Neurological sequelae occur in 20% to 50% of the cases.[1,9] Bacterial meningitis is considered a medical emergency; delays in initiation of antibacterial therapy increase the risk of complications and permanent neurological dysfunction.[1,9]

Reports of the long-term outcome of individuals with bacterial meningitis indicate that up to 20% have long-term neurological sequelae.[1,5] The sequelae may be the result of the acute infectious pathological condition or subacute or chronic pathological changes. The acute infectious pathological condition could result in sequelae such as inflammatory or vascular involvement of the cranial nerves or thrombosis of the meningeal veins. Cranial nerve palsies, especially sensorineural hearing loss, are common complications. The risk of an acute ischemic stroke is greatest during the first 5 days.[9] Weeks to months after treatment, subacute or chronic pathological changes may develop, such as communicating hydrocephalus, which manifests as difficulties with gait, mental status changes, and incontinence.[10,12] Approximately 5% of the survivors will have weakness and spasticity.[6] Focal cerebral signs that may occur either early or late in the course of bacterial meningitis include hemiparesis, ataxia, seizures, cranial nerve palsies, and gaze preference.[1,13] Cognitive slowness has been found in 27% of patients after pneumococcal meningitis, even with good recovery as documented by a Glasgow Outcome Scale score of 5.[14]

Damage to the cerebral cortex can result in numerous expressions of dysfunction. Motor system dysfunction may be the observable expression of the damage within the CNS, but the location of the damage may include sensory and processing areas, as well as those areas typically categorized as belonging to the motor system. Perceptual deficits or regression in cognitive skills may present residual problems. Cranial nerve involvement is most frequently expressed as dysfunction of the eighth cranial nerve complex and produces auditory and vestibular deficits.

Aseptic meningitis. Aseptic meningitis refers to a nonpurulent inflammatory process confined to the meninges and choroid plexus, usually caused by contamination of the CSF with a viral agent, although other agents can trigger the reactions. The symptoms are similar to those of acute bacterial meningitis but typically are less severe. The individual may be irritable and lethargic and complain of a headache, but cerebral function remains normal unless unusual complications occur.[5,15] Aseptic meningitis of a viral origin usually causes a benign and relatively short course of illness.[16,17]

A variety of neurotropic viruses can produce aseptic (viral) meningitis. The enteroviruses (echoviruses and the Coxsackie viruses), herpesviruses, and HIV are the most common causes.[5,7,18] The primary nonviral causes of aseptic meningitis are Lyme *Borrelia* and *Leptospira*.[19] The diagnosis of this type of aseptic meningitis may be established by isolation of the infecting agent within the CSF or by other techniques. The glucose level of the CSF in bacterial meningitis is usually depressed; however, the glucose level in viral meningitis is normal.[2]

Treatment of aseptic meningitis consists of management of symptoms. The condition does not typically produce residual neurological sequelae, and full recovery is anticipated within a few days to a few weeks.

Encephalitis

Clinical problems. Encephalitis refers to a group of diseases characterized by inflammation of the parenchyma of the brain and its surrounding meninges. Although a variety of agents can produce encephalitis, the term usually denotes a viral invasion of the cells of the brain and spinal cord.

Different cell populations within the CNS vary in their susceptibility to infection by a specific virus. (For example, the viruses responsible for poliomyelitis have a selective affinity for the motor neurons of the brain stem and spinal cord. Viruses such as Coxsackie viruses and echoviruses typically infect meningeal cells to cause the benign viral meningitis discussed in the previous section.) In acute encephalitis, neurons that are vulnerable to the specific virus are invaded and undergo lysis. Viral encephalitis causes a syndrome of elevated temperature, headache, nuchal rigidity, vomiting, and general malaise (symptoms of aseptic or viral

meningitis), with the addition of evidence of more extensive cerebral damage such as coma, cranial nerve palsy, hemiplegia, involuntary movements, or ataxia. The difficulty in differentiating between acute viral meningitis and acute viral encephalitis is reflected in the use of the term *meningoencephalitis* in some cases.

The pathological condition includes destruction or damage to neurons and glial cells resulting from invasion of the cells by the virus, the presence of intranuclear inclusion bodies, edema, and inflammation of the brain and spinal cord. Perivascular cuffing by polymorphonuclear leukocytes and lymphocytes may occur, as well as angiitis of small blood vessels. Widespread destruction of the white matter by the inflammatory process and by thrombosis of the perforating vessels can occur. Increased intracranial pressure, which can result from the cerebral edema and vascular damage, presents the potential for a transtentorial herniation. The likelihood of residual impairment of neurological functions depends on the infecting viral agent. Patients with mumps meningoencephalitis have an excellent prognosis, whereas 20% to 60% of the individuals with herpes simplex encephalitis treated with acyclovir have some neurological sequelae.[20] Because of the slow recovery of injured brain tissue, even in patients who recover completely, return to normal function may take months.[21]

Plum and Posner[22] discuss viral encephalitis in terms of five pathological syndromes. Acute viral encephalitis is a primary or exclusively CNS infection. An example would be herpes simplex encephalitis, in which the virus shows a partiality for the gray matter of the temporal lobe, insula, cingulate gyrus, and inferior frontal lobe. Other examples are the mosquito-borne viruses, such as St. Louis encephalitis, California virus encephalitis, and most recently West Nile virus (WNV). While from 1999 to 2005 in the United States, the incidence of infection from the WNV increased from 62 cases to 3000 cases, the incidence has decreased in recent years to 2097 cases in 2017.[23] Currently all states have some level of WNV activity, and only two states are without human cases (Fig. 26.3). The majority (80%) of people infected by the WNV will be asymptomatic; of the remaining people infected, less than 1% will develop severe illness.[23] Risk of neuroinvasive disease from WNV is 40%; neuroinvasive disease involves meningitis, encephalitis, or poliomyelitis, with wide variety in clinical presentation (Fig. 26.4).[24] Parainfectious encephalomyelitis is associated with viral infections such as measles, mumps, or varicella. Acute toxic encephalopathy denotes encephalitis that occurs during the course of a systemic infection with a common virus. The clinical symptoms are produced by the cerebral edema in acute toxic encephalopathy, which results in increased intracranial pressure and the risk of transtentorial herniation. Reye syndrome is an example. Global neurological signs, such as hemiplegia and aphasia, are usually present, rather than focal signs. The clinical symptoms of the previous three syndromes may be similar. Specific diagnosis may be established only by biopsy or autopsy.

Progressive viral infections occur from common viruses invading susceptible individuals, such as those who are immunosuppressed or during the perinatal to early childhood period. Slow, progressive destruction of the CNS occurs, as in subacute sclerosing panencephalitis. The final category of encephalitis syndromes consists of "slow virus" infections by unconventional agents (the prion diseases) that produce progressive dementing diseases such as Creutzfeldt-Jakob disease and kuru.[25]

Medical management. The medical management of virally induced encephalitis has been, and with many infecting agents remains, primarily symptomatic. In some cases, intensive, aggressive care is necessary to sustain life. Pharmacological interventions are available to treat some viral infections, such as herpes encephalitis. The probability of neurological sequelae differs according to the infecting agent. Aggressive management of increased intracranial pressure is required

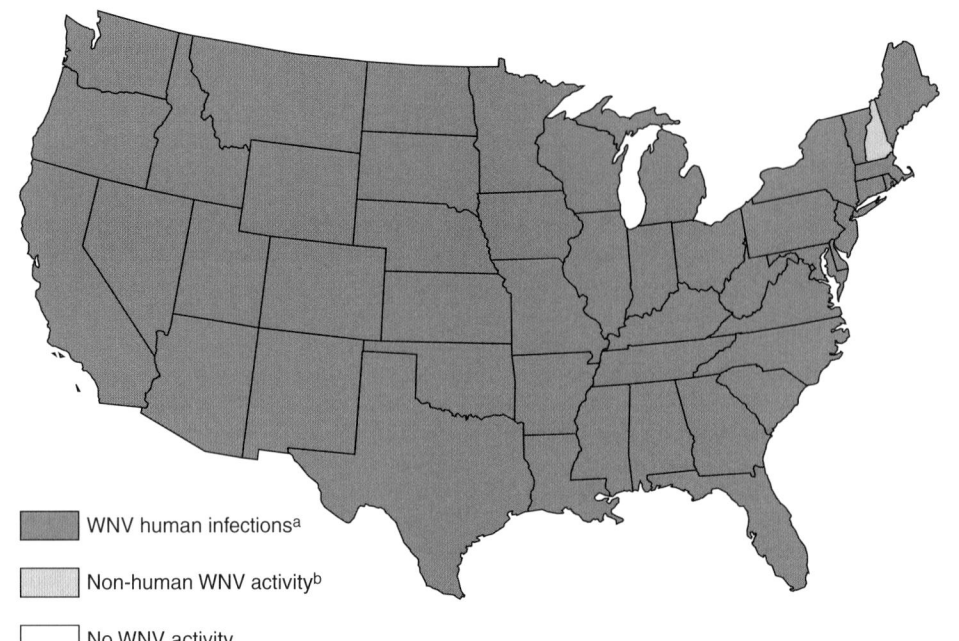

WNV human infections[a]

Non-human WNV activity[b]

No WNV activity

Fig. 26.3 West Nile virus *(WNV)* activity in the United States 2018. (From https://www.cdc.gov/westnile/statsmaps/preliminarymapsdata2018/activitybystate2018.html.)

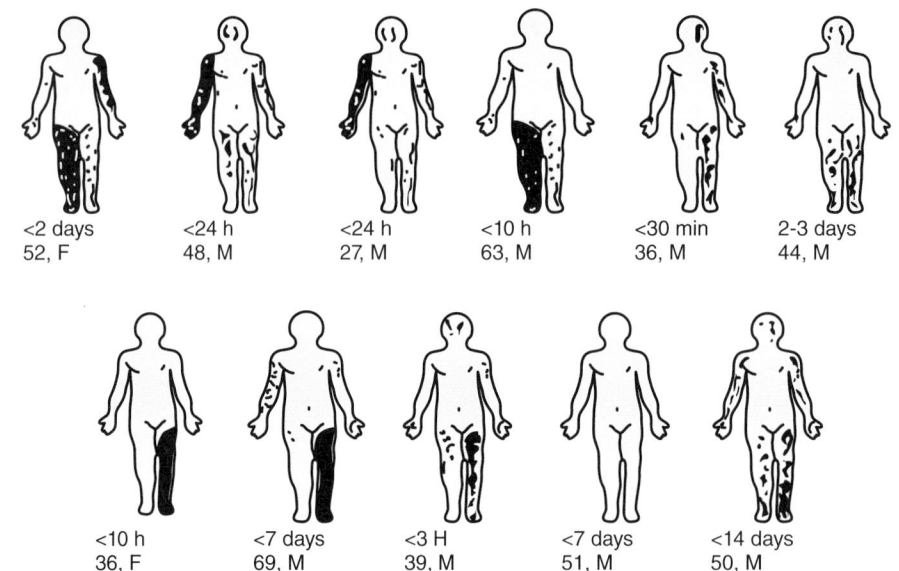

| <2 days | <24 h | <24 h | <10 h | <30 min | 2-3 days |
| 52, F | 48, M | 27, M | 63, M | 36, M | 44, M |

| <10 h | <7 days | <3 H | <7 days | <14 days |
| 36, F | 69, M | 39, M | 51, M | 50, M |

Fig. 26.4 Clinical Presentation of West Nile Virus. Weak limbs at the peak of paralysis are darkened. Degree of darkness corresponds to the severity of weakness. Duration of weakness and characteristics (age [years] and sex [*F*, female; *M*, male] are listed below each patient). (From Cao NJ, Ranganathan C, Kupsky WJ, Li J. Recovery and prognosticators of paralysis in West Nile virus infection. *J Neurol Sci.* 2005;236:73–80.)

because persistently elevated intracranial pressure is associated with poor outcome.[1,26] Further information concerning the clinical features, medical management, and potential for neurological sequelae of a specific type of encephalitis should be sought in the literature based on the infecting agent.

Clinical Picture of the Individual With Inflammatory Disorders of the Brain

An individual within the acute phase of meningitis or encephalitis or with residual neurological dysfunction from these disorders may demonstrate signs and symptoms similar to those of generalized brain trauma, tumor disorder, or other identified abnormal neurological state. The variability in the clinical picture is reflected in the inclusion of the category "infectious diseases that affect the central nervous system" in the *Guide to Physical Therapist Practice.*[27] It is therefore important for return to optimal function and return to quality life that the therapist understands the impairments of body functions and structures, the patient's activity limitations and participation restrictions, given the unique personal and environmental factors.

These concepts and selection of evaluation and intervention procedures are just as applicable for occupational therapists and other individuals working on movement dysfunction. In the acute phase the inflammatory process may result in impairments in arousal and attention that range from nonresponsiveness to agitation. The degree of agitation may range from mild to severe, depending on both the patient's unique CNS characteristics and the degree of inflammation. The agitated state may be the result of alterations in the processing of sensory input, with the consequence of inappropriate or augmented responses to sensory input. The patient may respond to a normal level of sound as though it were an unbearably loud noise. Low levels of artificial light may be perceived as extremely bright.

Perceptual and cognitive impairments may be present, resulting in a variety of functional limitations and disabilities. Patients may have distortions in their perception of events as well as memory problems. As their memory returns, accuracy of time and events may be distorted, leading to frustration and anxiety for both the patient and those family members and friends who are interacting within the environment.

In addition to alterations in mentation, the individual may demonstrate impaired affect, such as a hypersensitivity or exaggerated emotional response to seemingly normal interactions. For example, when upset about dropping a spoon on the floor, a patient may throw the tray across the table. When another individual was told his girlfriend would be a little late for her afternoon visit, the patient became extremely upset and stated his intent to kill himself because his girlfriend did not love him anymore.

Because of the variety of pathological problems after acute inflammation, the patient may have residual problems manifested as generalized or focal brain damage. The specifics of these impairments cannot be described as a typical clinical picture because they are extremely dependent on the individual patient. These variations require the therapist to conduct a thorough examination and evaluation process to develop an appropriate individualized intervention program. Although content from the *Guide to Physical Therapist Practice* has been incorporated into the discussion of the examination, evaluation, and intervention processes, the model presented provides a structure that can accommodate the specific disciplinary expertise of both occupational and physical therapists.

EXAMINATION AND EVALUATION PROCESS

Just as the medical intervention with patients who have an inflammatory disorder of the CNS is, to a large extent, symptomatic, so is the intervention by therapists. Designing an individualized intervention program based on the patient's problems requires a comprehensive initial and ongoing evaluation to define the impairments, functional limitations, and disabilities and to note changes in them. Although the discussion of examination procedures is separated from the discussion of intervention strategies, it must be recognized that the separation is artificial and does not reflect the image of practice. The evaluation process should be considered in relationship to both the long-term assessment of the individual's changes and the short-term within-session and between-session variations. For example, documentation of the level of consciousness of a patient on day one of intervention will provide a starting point for calculation of the distance spanned at the time of discharge. Perhaps more critical to the final outcome is determination of the level of consciousness before, during, and after a particular intervention technique to determine its impact on the individual's level of arousal and ability to interact with the environment. The evaluation process is a constant activity intertwined with intervention. The observations and data from the process are periodically recorded to establish the course of the disease process and the success of the therapeutic management of the patient.

Observation of Current Functional Status

The examination process should be conceptualized as a decision making tree that requires the therapist to determine actively which components are to be included in a detailed examination and which can be eliminated or deferred. The first step in this process is the observation of the patient's current functional status. If the patient is comatose and nonmobile, the focus of the initial session might be an assessment of the stability of physiological functions, level of consciousness, responses to sensory input, and joint mobility. If the patient is an outpatient with motor control deficits, the initial session might focus on defining motor abilities and components contributing to movement dysfunctions with a more superficial assessment of physiological functions and level of consciousness. The therapist must be alert to indications of the need for a more detailed evaluation of perceptual and cognitive function (e.g., the patient cannot follow two-step commands, indicating the need to assess cognitive skills).

Some of the components discussed in this process may be examination skills that are more typically possessed by other professions (e.g., assessment of emotional or psychological status). The inclusion of these items is not meant to suggest that the therapist must complete the formal testing. The items are included to indicate factors that will affect goal setting for the patient and that will have an impact on the intervention strategy. Although the therapist may not be the health care team member who has primary responsibility for evaluation of these areas, he or she should recognize these areas as potential contributors to movement dysfunctions.

Observation of the current functional status of the patient provides the therapist with an initial overview of his assets and deficits. This provides the framework into which the pieces of information from the evaluation of specific aspects of function can be fitted. The therapist must not allow assumptions made during the initial observation to bias later observations. The therapist might note that the patient is able to roll from the supine to the side-lying position to interact with visitors in the room. When the same activity is not repeated on the mat table in the treatment area, the therapist, knowing the patient has the motor skill to roll, might conclude that he is uncooperative or apraxic or has perceptual deficits. The therapist may have failed to consider that the difference between the two situations is the type of support surface or the presence or absence of side rails, which may have enabled the patient to roll in bed by pulling over to the side-lying position. It is characteristic of human observation skills that we tend to "see" what we expect to see. The therapist must attempt to observe behaviors and note potential explanations for deviations from normal without biasing the results of the subsequent observations.

The following discussion of the specific considerations within the examination process does not necessarily represent the temporal sequence to be used during the data collection process. As different items are discussed, suggestions for potential combinations of items will be made. The sequence of the process is best determined by the interaction of therapist and patient. Fig. 26.5 outlines the components that should be considered during the evaluation process and provides a synopsis of the following discussion.

The general philosophy in the evaluation of the patient with neurological deficits as a result of brain inflammation is a whole-part-whole approach. General observations of the patient's performance provide an overall description of the patient's abilities while indicating deficits in his or her performance. The cause(s) of the deficits (impairments) are explored to provide the pieces of data defining her or his performance. These pieces of data then are arranged within the framework provided by the general observation to define the whole of the

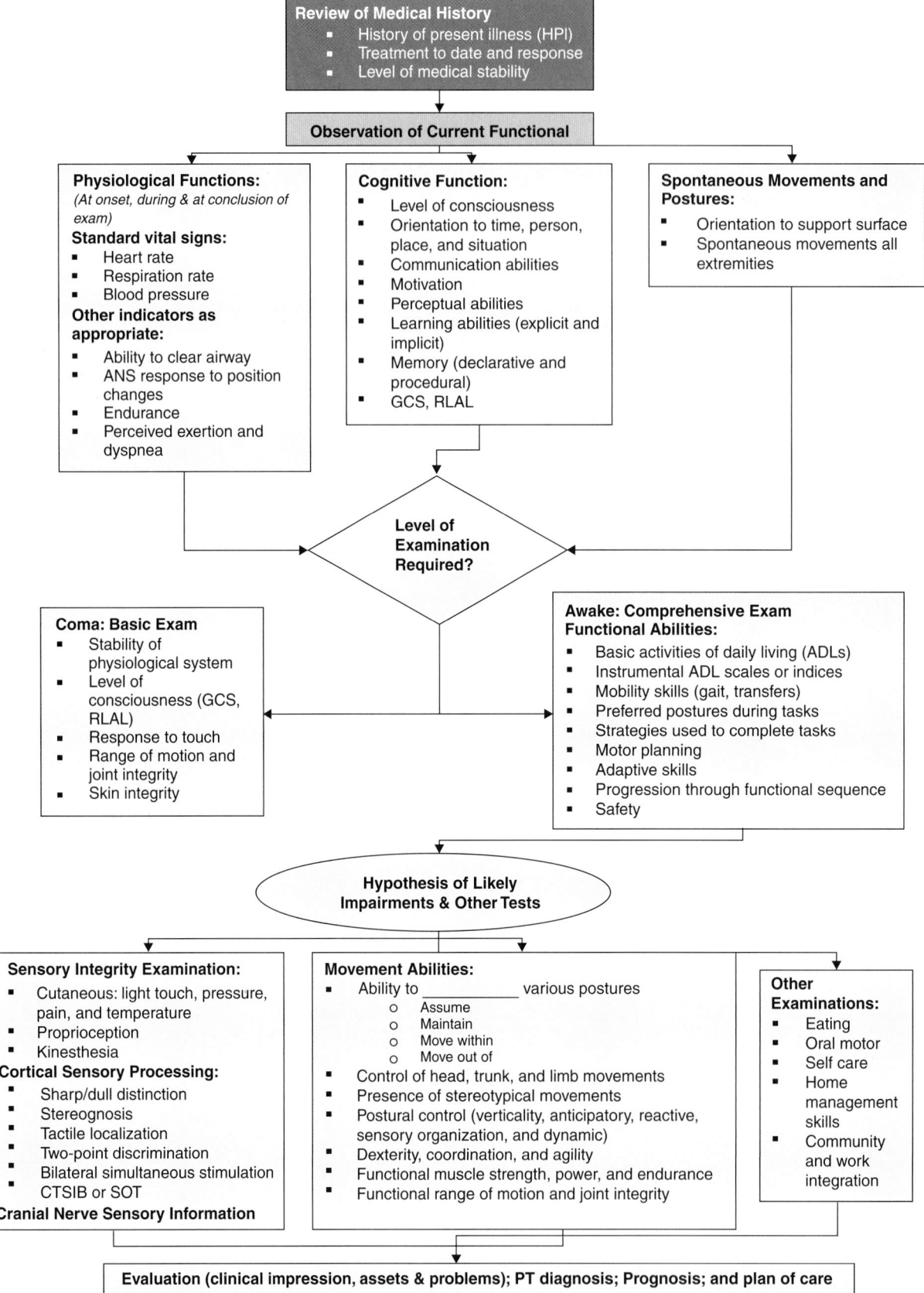

Review of Medical History
- History of present illness (HPI)
- Treatment to date and response
- Level of medical stability

Observation of Current Functional

Physiological Functions:
(At onset, during & at conclusion of exam)
Standard vital signs:
- Heart rate
- Respiration rate
- Blood pressure

Other indicators as appropriate:
- Ability to clear airway
- ANS response to position changes
- Endurance
- Perceived exertion and dyspnea

Cognitive Function:
- Level of consciousness
- Orientation to time, person, place, and situation
- Communication abilities
- Motivation
- Perceptual abilities
- Learning abilities (explicit and implicit)
- Memory (declarative and procedural)
- GCS, RLAL

Spontaneous Movements and Postures:
- Orientation to support surface
- Spontaneous movements all extremities

Level of Examination Required?

Coma: Basic Exam
- Stability of physiological system
- Level of consciousness (GCS, RLAL)
- Response to touch
- Range of motion and joint integrity
- Skin integrity

Awake: Comprehensive Exam Functional Abilities:
- Basic activities of daily living (ADLs)
- Instrumental ADL scales or indices
- Mobility skills (gait, transfers)
- Preferred postures during tasks
- Strategies used to complete tasks
- Motor planning
- Adaptive skills
- Progression through functional sequence
- Safety

Hypothesis of Likely Impairments & Other Tests

Sensory Integrity Examination:
- Cutaneous: light touch, pressure, pain, and temperature
- Proprioception
- Kinesthesia

Cortical Sensory Processing:
- Sharp/dull distinction
- Stereognosis
- Tactile localization
- Two-point discrimination
- Bilateral simultaneous stimulation
- CTSIB or SOT

Cranial Nerve Sensory Information

Movement Abilities:
- Ability to _____ various postures
  - Assume
  - Maintain
  - Move within
  - Move out of
- Control of head, trunk, and limb movements
- Presence of stereotypical movements
- Postural control (verticality, anticipatory, reactive, sensory organization, and dynamic)
- Dexterity, coordination, and agility
- Functional muscle strength, power, and endurance
- Functional range of motion and joint integrity

Other Examinations:
- Eating
- Oral motor
- Self care
- Home management skills
- Community and work integration

Evaluation (clinical impression, assets & problems); PT diagnosis; Prognosis; and plan of care

Fig. 26.5 Flow Chart of the Evaluation Process. *ANS,* Autonomic nervous system; *GCS,* Glasgow Coma Scale; *RLAL,* Rancho Los Amigos Level; *PT,* physical therapy.

patient's assets and deficits. As the whole picture is established (with the realization that it will be constantly adjusted), the process of goal-setting is initiated. These goals need to consider the patient's and family's desires. The process presented for refining evaluation data into an intervention plan is applicable whether the patient's neurological dysfunction is the result of a bacterial or viral infection, cerebrovascular accident, trauma, or other factors.

Evaluation of Physiological Responses to Therapeutic Activities

It is assumed that the therapist enters the initial interaction with a patient after reviewing the available background information. This may provide the therapist with information on the baseline status of the patient's vital physiological functions. Any control problems in these areas should be particularly noted. Until the therapist determines that the vital functions, such as rate of respiration, heart rate, and blood pressure, vary appropriately with the demands of the intervention process, these factors should be monitored. The monitoring process should include consideration of the baseline rate, rate during exercise, and time to return to baseline. The pattern of respiration and changes in that pattern also should be noted.

Other tests and measures of the status of ventilation, respiration, and circulation may be indicated in specific individuals. Individuals with limited mobility or motor control of the trunk or those with cranial nerve dysfunctions may demonstrate difficulty with functions such as moving secretions out of the airways. Inactivity during a prolonged recovery period may result in cardiovascular adaptations that compromise endurance and contribute to increases in the perceived exertion during activities.

Autonomic nervous system dysfunctions may be expressed as inappropriate accommodations to positional changes, such as orthostatic hypotension. Patients with depressed levels of consciousness may display temperature regulation dysfunctions. One mechanism for assessing the patient's ability to maintain a homeostatic temperature is to review the nursing notes. The events surrounding any periods of diaphoresis should be examined. If no causative factors have been identified, then interventions that involve thermal agents as discussed elsewhere in this text should be used judiciously.

Evaluation of Cognitive Status

Because the evaluation process encompasses the stages of recovery from the critical acute phase through discharge from therapy, a range of aspects are included under the evaluation of cognitive status. As indicated previously, the observation of current functional status will direct the therapist toward the appropriate component tests and measures.

Acute bacterial meningitis and various forms of viral encephalitis may result in changes in the patient's level of consciousness. *Consciousness* is a state of awareness of one's self and one's environment.[21] *Coma* can be defined as a state in which one does not open the eyes, obey commands, or utter recognizable words.[28] The individual does not respond to external stimuli or to internal needs. The term *vegetative state* is sometimes used to indicate the status of individuals who open their eyes and display a sleep-wake cycle but who do not obey commands or utter recognizable words. DeMeyer[29] presents a succinct description of the neuroanatomy of consciousness and the neurological examination of the unconscious patient. Plum and Posner[22] also provide extensive information in this area.

Several scales have been developed to provide objective guidelines to assess alterations in the state of consciousness. The Glasgow Coma Scale[28] assesses three independent items: eye opening, motor performance, and verbal performance. The scale yields a figure from 3 (lowest) to 15 (highest) that can be used to indicate changes in the individual's state of consciousness. The Rancho Los Amigos scale assesses level of consciousness and behavior.[28] The therapist can use assessment tools such as the Glasgow Coma Scale and the companion Glasgow Outcome Scale to determine if the intervention program has resulted in any recordable changes in the patient's level of consciousness. Ideally, the patient with decreased levels of consciousness will be monitored at consistent intervals to determine changes in status. Any carryover or delayed effects of the intervention could then be noted. The record of the patient's level of consciousness might also display a pattern of peak awareness at a particular point in the day. Scheduling an intervention session during the patient's peak awareness time may maximize the benefit of the therapy.

Performed in conjunction with the assessment of the patient's state of consciousness is the determination of the individual's orientation to person, time, place, and situation. Because the individual's level of orientation (documented as oriented times 4) is frequently recorded by multiple members of the rehabilitation team, the information in the medical chart may provide insights into fluctuations over the course of a day or a week.

Gross assessment of the individual's ability to communicate, both the expressive and receptive aspects of the process, is an important component of the examination. If a dysfunction is present in the patient's ability to communicate, the patient should be evaluated by an individual with expertise in this area so that strategies for dealing with the communication deficit can be developed. Evaluation of the movement abilities of the patient with communication deficits requires creative planning on the part of the therapist but usually can be accomplished if generalized movement tasks are used. With the patient who cannot comprehend a verbal command to roll, the therapist should use an alternate form of communication, such as manual cueing or guidance. The therapist could structure the situation to elicit the desired behavior by activities such as placing the patient in an uncomfortable position or positioning a desired object so that it can be reached only by rolling.

As the therapist progresses through the examination and intervention process, ongoing data collection should be occurring on factors that influence the motivation of the individual. Individuals with damage to certain areas within the frontal lobe will have difficulty with committing to long-term projects and may not be motivated to work during a therapy session by an explanation detailing the relationship of the current activity to the larger goal of returning home. In these situations, the therapist must create appropriate immediate rewards, such as a 2-minute rest break after completion of a specific movement task.

Deficits in cognition may be evident as problems in the area of explicit (declarative) or implicit (procedural) learning. Explicit learning is used in the acquisition of knowledge that is consciously recalled. This is information that can be verbalized in declarative sentences, such as the sequential listing of the steps in a movement sequence. Implicit or procedural learning is used in the process of acquiring movement sequences that are performed automatically without conscious attention to the performance. Procedural learning occurs through repetitions of the movement task (refer to Chapter 3). Because explicit and implicit learning use different neuroanatomical circuits, implicit learning can occur in individuals with deficits in the components underlying explicit learning (awareness, attention, higher-order cognitive processes) (refer to Chapter 3 for additional information regarding implicit and explicit learning).

The emotional and psychological aspects of the patient and the higher-order cognitive and retention skills of the patient should be evaluated informally by the therapist, with referral to appropriate professionals if dysfunction in these areas is suspected. A coordinated team approach is necessary for patients with emotional and psychological, cognitive, perceptual, or communication problems or a combination of these problems. A consistent strategy used by all team members eliminates the necessity on the part of the patient of trying to cope with different approaches by different people in an area in which she or he already has a deficit. The impact of cognitive deficits on the process of learning motor skills is further discussed in the next section on movement assessment. The assessment of the impact of perceptual dysfunctions is incorporated within the evaluation of sensory channels.

Examination of Functional Abilities

As indicated in the introduction to the evaluation of patients with inflammatory and infectious disorders of the brain, the examination process is not compartmentalized. As the therapist is examining the movement abilities of the individual through the format described in the previous section, he or she is also collecting information on the functional abilities of the individual. The components underlying the movement abilities of the patient can be examined within the framework of the basic or instrumental activities of daily living (ADLs), depending on the functional level of the person. The treatment setting and documentation requirements within that setting will determine whether the data on basic ADL and instrumental ADL skills are recorded with use of a formal scale or index or are gathered through an individualized process.

The introduction of specific tasks provides the therapist with the opportunity to observe the preferred posture used to accomplish the different tasks. The therapist should construct situations that require the individual to respond to unexpected occurrences to provide some insight into the person's ability to adapt to the unexpected. Throughout the process of examining a patient's movement abilities and functional abilities, the therapist is assessing the individual's awareness of safety considerations and judgment in attempting tasks.

The presence of motor planning dysfunctions can be noted as the patient attempts a movement sequence or a functional task. The therapist may have to cue the patient physically to initiate the sequence, which then flows smoothly. The therapist may observe that the patient has the correct components to a movement sequence, but that the sequence of the components is incorrect. Or the patient may demonstrate the ability to produce a movement sequence under one set of conditions but not another. Indications of these types of motor planning problems can be observed during the initial interactions with the patient. Similarly, the therapist also should be aware of indications of problems with dexterity, coordination, and agility, as well as with signs of cerebellar dysfunctions.

Another aspect of the evaluation process that can be integrated in the observations of movement abilities is identification of perceptual deficits. Aspects of the patient's motor performance can provide indications for detailed perceptual testing to classify the deficits. This testing should be conducted by the health care team member qualified in the area of perceptual testing. During the general evaluation procedures, the therapist can screen the patient for signs of perceptual deficits. Patients' abilities to cross their midlines with their upper extremities can be demonstrated in movement sequences, such as moving from the supine to the side-sitting to the sitting position (Fig. 26.6). The quality of the integration of information from the two sides of the body can be indicated by the symmetry or asymmetry of posture in positions that should be symmetrical. The therapist may suspect that the patient has a deficit in body awareness or body image by the poor quality of movement patterns that are within the motor capability of the individual. Spontaneous comments by the patient as to how he or she feels when moving ("my leg feels so heavy") also add to the thera-

pist's assessment of the patient's body image. Problems with verticality can be seen with the patient who lists to one side when in an upright posture. When the therapist corrects the list to a vertical posture, patients may express that they now feel that they are leaning to one side. Individuals who cannot appropriately relate their positions to the position of objects in their environments may have a figure-ground deficit or a problem with the concept of their position in space. When approaching stairs, these patients may fail to step up or may attempt to step up too soon. These examples should provide an indication of the observations that can indicate the need for detailed perceptual testing.

The preceding aspects of evaluation of movement abilities focused on facets of motor performance. Within this process the therapist should intertwine an appraisal of the individual's ability to learn motor tasks (or elements of the task). The therapist attempts to determine whether the patient can maintain a change in the ability to perform a movement throughout a therapy session and into the next session. The patient's ability to capture and integrate changes into the movement repertoire is fundamental to the success of the intervention program. The program can focus on the learning of movement sequences and the generalization of these sequences to movements within other contexts. Individuals with lowered levels of consciousness (typically Rancho Los Amigos Levels I to III) will be unable to learn or have difficulty learning and generalizing new motor skills. Therapy sessions may be more successful if the focus remains on the performance of motor tasks that were previously "overlearned" and automatic. Although the therapist may be able to manually guide the individual in coming to sit on the edge of the bed, until the individual demonstrates a higher level of processing, it may be unrealistic to expect that he or she will consistently reposition the legs without cueing before attempting the movement sequence. From looking at the "whole" of function, the therapist needs to determine the impairments that require further examination.

Evaluation of Sensory Channel Integrity and Processing

The examination process must include an assessment of the channels for sensory input. Knowledge gained in the assessment of the sensory systems will be used in the program-planning process to select the intervention strategies that have the highest probability of success. Although movements can be performed (and in some cases even learned) in the absence of typical sensory feedback, the presence of altered sensory function creates more challenges for both the patient/learner and the therapist/teacher. The therapist assesses both the patient's ability to perceive the sensory stimulus and the appropriateness of the response to the stimulus. Therefore it is important to determine if the sensory modality is intact, impaired, or absent, and if it is impaired, whether it hyperresponsive, hyporesponsive, or inconsistent. In addition, variations in the interpretation of sensory input may occur in some patients. Gentle tactile contact may be perceived by the person as a noxious input. Some individuals will have difficulty processing and discriminating information with high levels of one type of sensory input (e.g., the noisy clinic area) or with multiple simultaneous inputs (e.g., talking to the therapist while walking down a hallway with people moving toward the individual).

The therapist should develop a systematic approach to the initial cursory screen of the sensory systems. Deficits identified in the initial examination will provide structure for scheduling more comprehensive evaluation of deficits in specific systems. The therapist must also monitor changes in the status of physiological vital functions during sensory input, especially if the patient has a history of instability of heart rate, blood pressure, or rate of respiration.

Based on the information from the screen, the therapist will organize the components of the more detailed examination. Components to be considered include the integrity of the peripheral sensory

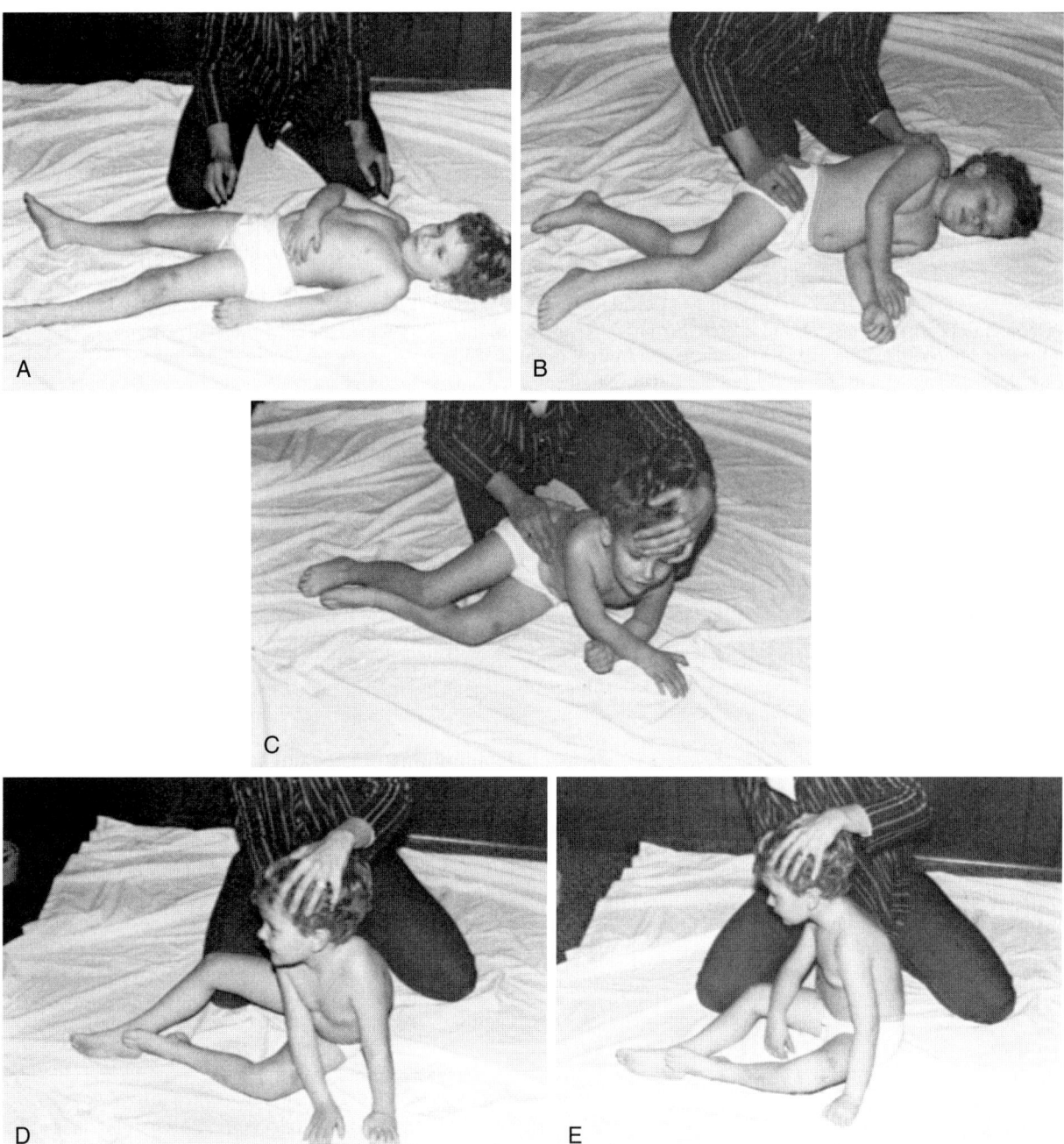

Fig. 26.6 Movement sequence from the supine to side-sitting to sitting positions. **(A)** Supine position. **(B)** Handling to side lying. **(C)** Handling toward side sitting; arm positions are important. **(D)** Side sitting; note propping patterns with arms. **(E)** Handling to symmetrical sitting.

circuits, the cortical level processing of the sensory information, the integrity of the cranial nerve sensory circuits, and the processing of multichannel input.

Cutaneous input has several aspects that must be assessed. Some of the inflammatory diseases of the brain may result in cutaneous distributions in which sensation is absent or diminished. These areas should be routinely evaluated for changes in distribution of level of sensation. Tests of light touch, pressure, and pain can be used if the patient can communicate reliably. In most cases, inclusion of assessment of differentiation of hot and cold will not add appreciably to the information needed for treatment planning unless thermal modalities are a consideration.

A gross assessment of the intactness of the touch system can be made in the noncommunicative patient by introducing a mildly aversive (not painful) stimulus, such as a light scratch, while monitoring the patient for changes in facial expression, posture, or tonus. The possibility of a spinal-level reflex response should be kept in mind when interpreting the results of such a gross assessment.

Assessment of the patient's response to proprioceptive input is incorporated within the assessment of the patient's movement abilities and is intertwined with the intervention process because a variety of intervention techniques are based on proprioceptive input. Evaluation of the proprioceptive channels can be conducted through assessment of the patient's static position sense and dynamic kinesthesis. These tests allow the therapist to make inferences concerning the patient's cognitive abilities to interpret proprioceptive information. Inherent in the successful completion of these tests is the necessity for the patient to be able to understand directions and to be able to communicate data to the therapist. Because information input, processing, and output are involved in these tests, failure to comply with the test instructions cannot be definitively attributed to dysfunction of the proprioceptive system. The therapist also should consider information obtained from watching the patient move before drawing a conclusion concerning the intactness of the proprioceptive channels. Some of the factors to consider include disregard of an extremity and variations in quality of performance between visually directed and nonvisually directed movements. Although tests of position sense and kinesthetics provide one aspect of the evaluation of the proprioceptive system, the therapist also must be involved constantly in assessing the patient's response to the intervention techniques that are part of the treatment plan. This again illustrates the intermingling of assessment and intervention. Intervention places a demand for movement on the patient. As the movement occurs, the therapist assesses the quality of the movement. If the quality is not appropriate, the therapist initiates intervention to improve the quality. If the technique does not produce the desired result, a second technique can be tried and the cyclical process continues.

In addition to determining the integrity of the peripheral sensory pathways and recognition of the input, it is important to assess the individual's ability to process more complex presentations of cutaneous input. Difficulties in the cortical-level processing of cutaneous stimuli are identified through tests of sharp and dull discrimination, stereognosis, tactile localization, texture recognition, two-point discrimination, and bilateral simultaneous stimulation.

Central processing and integration of sensory information as it affects postural control can be examined using the Clinical Test of Sensory Integration and Balance (CTSIB)[30] or with computerized dynamic posturography using the Sensory Organization Test (SOT). With both tests, the effectiveness of using vision or somatosensory or vestibular sensation at the appropriate time (sensory weighting) and changing from one sensory system to the other is examined.

Assessment of the integrity of the cranial nerve sensory channels is typically incorporated within the standard cranial nerve examination. Review of the physician's notes may provide sufficient information; however, the therapist may need to complete more specific tests before considering certain intervention techniques. Of specific note are vision and vestibular screening, both of which are discussed in detail elsewhere in this text. Simple visual system tests, such as identification of field deficits, assessment of tracking abilities, and a gross evaluation of visual acuity, can be performed quickly.

The complex functions of the vestibular system can be assessed through a variety of avenues such as the Ayres Post-Rotatory Nystagmus Test,[31,32] the SOT, and tests of the vestibular ocular reflex (head-thrust test, head-shaking test, and test of dynamic visual acuity [DVA]), and are discussed in detail elsewhere in this text. It is important to examine the vestibular influence in both postural control and gaze stability. The integrity of the connections underlying a vestibular-induced nystagmus response is assessed by physicians through the caloric test (warm and cold water or air introduced into the ear channel to induce nystagmus). The effect of rapid linear accelerations and decelerations can be evaluated as potential activating mechanisms increasing the level of consciousness or level of muscle activity. An example is the Dynamic Gait Index, a functional test that incorporates changes in speed and head movements during walking.[33] Slow, rhythmical reversals of linear movements may have a calming effect on the patient's behavior or level of muscle activation. Linear movements in all planes and diagonals should be explored.

During the evaluation of the patient as well as during intervention with the patient, the therapist must be aware of the potential to bombard him or her with sensory input and overload his or her ability to respond discriminatively to it. If the therapist detects that the patient has difficulty in responding appropriately to sensory input, as with a patient in a lowered state of consciousness or an agitated state, or demonstrating tactile defensiveness, sensory input should be used selectively during the initial examination or intervention sessions. If multiple sensory inputs are used, the positive or negative effects cannot be attributed to a specific input or necessarily to the series of inputs. Evaluation as well as intervention with sensory inputs should proceed in a controlled fashion. Inclusion of additional sensory modalities in the intervention plan should occur systematically.

The individual's response to multichannel sensory conflict input is typically assessed as a component of higher-level balance assessment and locomotor abilities. A more thorough discussion of sensory assessment is discussed elsewhere in the text. The therapist should apply these concepts during the evaluation of all motor tasks. Consider the following example: a patient who relies on visual input to supplement vestibular and somatosensory information is performing the task of sitting on the edge of the mat table. She remains relatively steady until someone walks directly toward her from across the clinic. This change in the environmental context of the performance requires her to assess whether she is moving toward the individual or the individual is moving toward her. Without reliable vestibular and somatosensory check points, the patient may activate a postural response to the incorrect assessment. As this example demonstrates, the evaluation of the sensory channels is intertwined with the evaluation of the person's movement abilities.

Examination of Movement Abilities

The initial assessment of the individual's movement abilities is conducted by observing as she or he moves through a sequence of functional postures. The therapist determines the functional postures to be examined for a specific patient, ranging from bed mobility activities (assessment of movement in prone and supine positions) through upright ambulation. The medical status of the individual, the extent of involvement, the intervention setting, and the age of the individual are considerations in determining the appropriate functional postures to be examined. The therapist gathers information on the movement abilities of the patient as he or she moves into, within, and out of the position.

The assessment focuses on both the quantity and quality of motor performance. The quantitative aspect of the movement assessment involves the number of different functional postures the individual can use. The quality of the movement abilities is assessed within the posture as well as in the process of moving between postures. For example, the therapist should assess the quality of the head, trunk, and extremity control demonstrated throughout the movement sequences. The use of stereotypical movement patterns should be noted because their presence may limit the adaptability of movements required to accomplish functional tasks. Other items relating to the patient's movement abilities are assessed during this process.

Indications of abnormal ranges of movement of all joints can be obtained. The range may show a limitation of movement or an indication of joint instability. Once the gross deviations are identified, these joints can be examined to determine the source of the problem: joint capsular, ligamentous, bony, skin, or muscular and fascial dysfunction. Conducting the gross assessment of range while the patient is moving eliminates the time spent in performing a joint-by-joint goniometric evaluation of articulations with normal excursions.

As the individual is moving (either independently or with the therapist assisting), an assessment of the distribution and fluctuations in muscle activity can be made and will provide information on functional muscle strength, power, and endurance. The timing, accuracy, and sequencing of muscle activation within the movement should be noted. The therapist can identify the postures that will be the most conducive to optimal motor performances and those that should be avoided. As the patient is moving through various postures, the function of specific musculature can be examined. Muscle groups should be examined with regard to their ability to function in both stability (distal segment fixed) and mobility (distal segment free) situations. Because numerous demands are being placed on each muscle group, therapists can assess the ability to perform isometric and isotonic (concentric and eccentric) contractions. Each different posture introduces a new set of variables; therefore the performance of a muscle group must be reexamined as each new movement pattern is performed.

The therapist can identify postural control in a variety of functional positions. Within each posture, the therapist must examine the control the patient displays over the posture. Because the assessment takes place as part of a dynamic sequence, the therapist can assess the patient's ability to assume the posture. If the posture cannot be achieved independently, the therapist assesses the factors interfering with achieving the position, the type of assistance necessary to facilitate assumption of the posture, and the effect of the various intervention techniques used to assist the patient in achieving the position. Once the patient is in the posture, her or his ability to maintain the posture is examined. Factors that interfere with the performance are noted. The patient's ability to move within the posture is identified. Movement demands placed on the patient should include aspects of both static and dynamic equilibrium. Static balance in the sitting position (such as on the side of the bed) could be demonstrated by the individual matching the strength of a force attempting to displace him backward and maintaining the position when the force is suddenly released.

The presence of dynamic balance of the upper torso in the sitting position could be demonstrated by the individual reacting to a quick sideways displacement force administered to the shoulder by activating the trunk lateral flexors to compensate for the displacement. Equally important is the individual's ability to demonstrate appropriate equilibrium responses to self-imposed perturbations. The absence of anticipatory control in standing could be demonstrated by having the patient do the rapid arm raise test with a 5-lb weight and noticing reactive stepping instead of doing a posterior weight shift in anticipation of the destabilizing force.

The final stage in examining the individual's movement abilities explores the individual's ability to move out of the posture. The patient should have the ability to move out of the posture to a lower-level posture and to a higher-level posture before mastery of the posture is considered to have been achieved.

Many aspects of the patient's performance are analyzed simultaneously. When the therapist assists the patient in moving to a new posture, an analysis of the influence of facilitation and inhibition techniques is being conducted. The individual's response to these handling techniques cues the therapist in projecting the patient's response to an intervention program. The therapist is constantly monitoring the patient for changes in physiological functions or changes in the level of consciousness. Anything that results in expressions of pain by the patient should be noted. Intervention programs should be a learning experience for patients. If they are attending to pain, they cannot attend to learning. The factor(s) producing the pain should be identified and measures instituted to eliminate the factor(s). If the factors producing the pain cannot be resolved, the intervention program should be designed to avoid triggering the pain.

In addition to looking at postural control in a variety of postures, it is also important to determine the type of postural control dysfunction, such as vertical orientation to the surface or to gravity as the situation dictates, anticipatory postural control, reactive postural control, sensory organization for postural control, and dynamic balance for gait.

DIAGNOSIS, PROGNOSIS, AND GOAL SETTING

Having collected data from the examination process, the first steps are to interpret the findings and integrate those findings with other information collected during the history to determine a diagnosis amenable to physical therapy management. Physical therapists identify the *impact of a condition on function at the level of the system (especially the movement system) and at the level of the whole person.*[27] This includes integrating specific problems (body functions [impairments], activity and participation limitations) and to interpret within the context of the individual and the environment. The individual factors will include her or his assets. Formulating an asset list focuses on the positive data elicited from the evaluation process and is critical for prognosing outcomes. Items on the asset list could be observations, such as the patient being able to assume the position of sitting on the side of the bed with setup assistance only, improved head control in this posture being facilitated by approximation, and controlled weight shifting being elicited by alternated tapping. The asset list provides a reference defining the postures and intervention techniques that are effective. This reference is used to develop the intervention goals and plan. Formulating and recording a problem list and an asset list can be completed relatively quickly as one gains familiarity with the process. Whereas novice therapists will benefit from generating a written asset list, experienced clinicians may formulate a mental asset list while completing the written evaluation format required by the facility. Just as the evaluation process is ongoing, so are the steps involved in goal setting. The asset and problem lists are redefined as the patient's status changes.

After assets and problems have been identified, the next step is to establish the expected outcomes from this episode of care. This is considered the prognosis. Ideally, the process of establishing the prognosis and setting the goals for a patient is a coordinated effort that involves all members of the health care team, including the patient (if feasible) and family. If the therapist is not functioning in a setting where involvement of many disciplines is viable, the therapist can progress through the goal-setting process in the context of his or her role in the patient's care.

These outcome statements represent the general objectives toward which the intervention process is oriented. They identify the end point of the intervention process and are the exit criteria for terminating the episode of care.

The *Guide to Physical Therapist Practice* views outcomes in relationship to "minimization of functional limitations, optimization of health status, prevention of disability, and optimization of patient/client satisfaction," whereas goals "relate to the remediation (to the extent possible) of impairments."[27] The breadth of acceptance of these definitions with the neurorehabilitation professions remains to be determined. These definitions at least give professionals a place to start communicating with consistency. The International Classification of Functioning, Disability and Health (ICF) model of the World Health Organization provides similar definitions, with the focus being patient centered.

Measurable, interim objectives should be established in relation to the outcome statements. To determine if the objective has been achieved, the objective should be measurable—either in terms of producing a numerical indicator of performance, such as time span, number of repetitions, distance covered, or accuracy of performance, or in terms of a precise description of the target motor behavior. The appropriate objective indicator must be carefully selected. Performing a movement more quickly may indicate that the individual is performing it with more normal control and therefore greater ease of movement, or it may indicate that the individual has become more skilled in using an abnormal pattern based on inappropriate muscle activation. If it is not appropriate to formulate the objective in terms of a numerical indicator, the objective can be formulated in terms of an observable behavior. The therapist can precisely describe body segment movements based on the component method of movement analysis presented by VanSant.[34,35] For example, the task of coming to standing from supine can be described in terms of the upper-extremity component, axial component, and lower-extremity component.[36] Formulation of an appropriate short-term objective could specify use of the upper extremities in a push-and-reach pattern during the task of coming to standing from supine. The interim objectives should be constructed so that observing the patient's behavior will allow the therapist to state whether the criteria of the short-term objective were achieved. Table 26.1 gives an example of some components of short-term objectives leading to mastery of functional activities in sitting.

The outcome statements define the patient's destination. The interim objectives define the mileposts. The therapist then uses the asset list to design the intervention program, which is the vehicle to get the patient to his or her destination. From the asset list, the therapist knows the intervention techniques that have the highest probability of success. Adopting this process simplifies the task of outlining the strategy for intervention.

As the therapist considers the appropriate outcomes and goals for the patient, a decision must be made as to whether the format of the intervention will focus on a "training" approach or a "motor learning" approach. During the assessment process, if the therapist concludes that the individual's level of cognitive function precludes the development of insight into movement errors (both the detection and correction of an incorrect performance) or the ability to retain the insight over time, then the therapist should delineate the outcomes and intervention plan to accommodate this limitation. The "training" approach requires more structure and repetition of activities within that structure. If it is more appropriate to design the intervention plan according to motor learning considerations, the therapist must consider the appropriate schedule and environmental context for the practice, the type and schedule for the feedback provided, and techniques to promote the generalization of the learning beyond the specific practice session.

General Goals for the Intervention Process

Whereas the goal-setting process described earlier results in specification of the outcomes, goals, and objectives for a specific patient, the general goals for the intervention process can be delineated to guide the process. As described in the overview of inflammatory disorders at the beginning of this chapter, the extent of the neurological sequelae may range from a single discrete problem to a devastating clinical picture composed of compromised functions in multiple areas. The goals for the intervention process address the problem areas that (1) jeopardize the efficiency and effectiveness of functional activities and (2) are the primary or secondary results of compromised neurological function. The listing of goals does not directly include consideration of secondary problems (such as decreases in joint range of motion [ROM], cardiovascular fitness, and endurance). The therapist should integrate these considerations in the overall assessment of the components of the movement problems.

The following goals are written as outcomes of the intervention process and not as goals for a specific patient. Because of the broad nature of the goals, other professions also will contribute to the attainment of the goals. The goals of the therapeutic intervention program for patients with inflammatory CNS disorders are as follows:

Goal 1: Postural control is optimized as demonstrated by the ability to maintain a position against gravity and the ability to automatically adjust before and continuously during movement.

Goal 2: Selective, voluntary movement patterns within functional activities are optimized.

Goal 3: Performance of functional activities is enhanced.

Goal 4: Integration of sensory information is fostered.

Goal 5: Cognitive status and psychosocial responses are optimized.

Each of these goals is discussed in conjunction with the general therapeutic intervention procedures that can be used to achieve the goal.

GENERAL THERAPEUTIC INTERVENTION PROCEDURES IN RELATION TO INTERVENTION GOALS

- *Postural control is optimized as demonstrated by the ability to maintain a position against gravity and the ability to adjust automatically before and continuously during movement.*

Because it is assumed that functional abilities are built on the base of the ability to control postures, the intervention goal of promoting optimal postural control underlies the ability to make selective, voluntary movement patterns (goal 2) and the performance of functional

TABLE 26.1   Examples of Short-Term Objectives Relating to Mastery of Functional Activities in Sitting

	Condition Variables[a]	Activity	Criteria
1. When sitting on a mat	a. Using the upper extremities for support	The patient will maintain the posture	For _____ seconds
2. When sitting on the edge of a mat table	b. Using one upper extremity for support c. Without using the upper extremities for support		
3. When sitting in a chair	d. With the therapist displacing the position of the: pelvis shoulders head lower extremities	The patient will make postural adjustments of the head and trunk	Appropriate to the degree of displacement
	e. Leaning forward and returning to erect sitting	The patient will bring the right foot to the left knee (as if to put on a shoe)	

[a]Therapist needs to consider all aspects of each variable (i.e., 1—a, b, c, d, e; 2—a, b, c, d, e; 3—a, b, c, d, e).
Outcome: The patient will master functional activities in sitting. Short-term objective: Select one phrase from each column.

activities (goal 3). Optimization of a postural set includes the concepts of decreasing muscle activity that is too high to allow performance of movement sequences, augmenting activation that is too low to support the accomplishment of a movement sequence, and fostering proper timing of the postural responses. Intervention techniques to achieve this goal demand that the therapist constantly monitor the patient's performance so that appropriate interventions are added when needed and continued only as long as they are needed.

Optimal postural control is defined by two elements. The patient should have the ability to maintain a vertical orientation with regard to gravity and should be able to maintain balance in the presence of both internal and external perturbations. Automatic adjustments in the postural set should occur in anticipation of and continuously during movements (internal perturbations). Both elements should be performed with minimal physical or cognitive effort on the part of the patient. Horak describes five components of normal postural control, including vertical orientation; anticipatory, reactive, sensory organization; and dynamic postural control for gait.[36] By looking at the subsets of postural control, interventions can be designed to specifically match the impairment (Table 26.2).

TABLE 26.2   Interventions for Postural Control Problems

Postural Control Problem	Possible Interventions
Malalignment and verticality problems	Augment sensory feedback: • Mirror • Static force plate • Flashlight on target • Videotape • Align without vision and check (knowledge of results) • Stepping with eyes closed
Limits of stability perception problems	Computerized feedback of actual versus possible Weight shifting exercise with feedback and targets (somatosensory, visual, both) Surface orientation exercises (static, ankle sway, hip strategies)
Anticipatory control problems	Hold on and slow down (lessen the need for anticipatory control—substitution) Mental rehearsal (weight shift, then move) Practice limb movements where balance must be controlled (start slow and get faster) • Interactions with the environment with a static base of support, such as reaching up in a cupboard, opening a door, opening a drawer, lifting a suitcase, lifting a bag of groceries, wearing a backpack • Interactions with the environment with a dynamic base of support (stepping up a step, kicking a ball, stepping over an object, stepping around an object, changing the pitch of the surface—inclines) Practice rapid limb movements where balance must be controlled (opening a door, opening a drawer, lifting a briefcase, lifting a bag of groceries, lifting a suitcase, wearing a backpack). Practice order: • Practice the anticipatory postural adjustment • Practice the focal action while supported • Combine the anticipatory postural adjustment with the focal action unsupported (slow to fast) • Practice varying similar tasks (predictable to unpredictable) Example: After the patient is doing better on a lifting task involving one object, he or she can work to be successful with several objects of different weights; first cognitively solve what must change for achievement of success in lifting one object versus another; then much repetition of alternating one object versus another; and eventually, work with a variety of objects in a varied pattern
Reactive postural control problems	Work to regain balance strategies (ankle, hip, and stepping) Remediate any biomechanical issues that affect use of balance strategies Begin with self-perturbation and progress to reacting to external perturbations Need to learn to match the magnitude and direction of perturbation Physioballs, T-stools, tilt boards, reaching, weight shifting
Sensory integration problems	If patient is overreliant on vision, be sure to help patient with another strategy before you take vision away Surface orientation exercises (tuning into somatosensory feedback) • Textured surface • Textured surface + visual tracking • Textured surface with vision occluded Enhancing use of vestibular system: • Compliant surface with stationary visual target • Compliant surface + visual tracking • Compliant surface with moving visual background • Changing surface + head turns • Changing surface + head turns + moving visual background • Obstacle course with varying sensory demands

Continued

TABLE 26.2 **Interventions for Postural Control Problems—cont'd**	
Postural Control Problem	**Possible Interventions**
Dynamic balance problems in gait	Alter the sensory contexts (e.g., resisted walking)
	Walking and reading signs right and left
	Carrying objects and looking at items carried
	Walking with quick stops (predictable distances and reactive)
	Practice falling without injury and getting up; practice slips and trips
	Walking and negotiating obstacles (around and over)
	• Practice both around and over obstacles
	• Larger steps, standing on one foot, changing directions
	• Practice stopping quickly with feet in target
	• Practice shorter steps, on a slippery surface; braiding
	Gesturing while walking

Verticality, or maintaining an upright posture, first requires the patient to recognize the desired alignment. Augmenting internal feedback mechanisms with the use of mirrors, force plates, or scales or even using a flashlight attached to the patient that shines on a target when he or she is vertical can be effective. Manual skills such as positioning the patient and using approximation to reinforce the position can be added to the treatment. Progression of intervention strategies can be done by having the patient maintain the posture and then begin to manipulate objects with the extremities. Research suggests that the CNS is organized around tasks and not movement patterns. Therefore as the patient learns to maintain a vertical orientation and moves in and out of the position, designing a task will likely give a better outcome. For example, Paul developed encephalitis, which left him with residual deficits in verticality. The simple task of keeping a book balanced on his head while sitting or walking gave him the type of feedback he needed without constant cues to "stand up straight" being the focus. Further progression involves teaching the patient to move to his limits of stability and find vertical again.

Anticipatory postural control involves the postural preset, which positions the trunk to allow skilled use of the extremities without loss of balance. It requires the patient to recognize the situation and the likely destabilizing force that will result, and posturally preset so destabilizing will not occur. The process requires memory and the ability to recognize the critical environmental and task cues. Interventions focus on practicing both the postural adjustment and the focal action before the two components are combined. Table 26.2 also has suggested interventions for reactive, sensory integrative, and dynamic balance in gait problems. Postural control is affected as well by biomechanical constraints, such as tonal abnormalities.

The patient's ability to demonstrate optimal postural control may be restricted by the presence of hypertonicity or hypotonicity in various muscle groups. These states may be relatively static or may fluctuate with the demands of a particular situation. Inappropriately high levels of muscle activity may be present in a stereotypical muscle distribution in the extremities, whereas the activity of the trunk musculature may be too low to support an antigravity posture. The therapist must design the interventions creatively to meet the shifting responses of the demands of a particular activity.

Being cognizant that spasticity is a reaction to initial peripheral instability, the therapist must select treatment that deals with the fact that as spasticity is modified, weakness or hypotonicity may be present. Inappropriately high levels of activity in a muscle group or groups may limit the patient's ability to demonstrate optimal postural control (and optimal selective movements as addressed in the second goal). The therapist can select intervention techniques that are mediated through

any of the sensory channels functional for that patient. The choice of which channel or combination of channels to use for the input is based on the therapist's initial and continuing evaluation of the patient's response to specific types of sensory input.

The therapist must address the hypertonicity influencing postural control as a generalized problem before demanding selective voluntary activation of specific muscle groups. Vestibular input that is slow and rhythmical may promote a generalized relaxation of skeletal muscle activity. In some patients, the trunk remains "stiff" in movement sequences in which a segmental response between the upper and lower trunk should occur. Repetitions of rhythmical movements in side-lying in which the therapist gently and progressively stretches the patient's pelvis in one direction around the body axis while moving the shoulder girdle in the opposite direction and then reverses the movement may effectively alter the biomechanical and neurological contributions to the stiffness (Fig. 26.7).

For some patients, changing the dynamics of a spastic extremity may permit the emergence of more optimal levels of postural control. The appropriately designed ankle-foot orthosis (AFO) may alter the individual's need to rigidly control the position of the pelvis to remain upright. Use of a soft webbing thumb loop to alter the resting position of the first metacarpal may change the overactivity of musculature throughout the upper extremity and allow appropriate adjustment of the shoulder girdle as part of postural responses.

If the patient is sufficiently alert that attending to and understanding directions is a possibility, the therapist should direct the person to focus on the effects of the movement responses rather than focusing attention on the movement of the body.[37] As the person begins to appreciate the consequences of what is transpiring, he or she should be

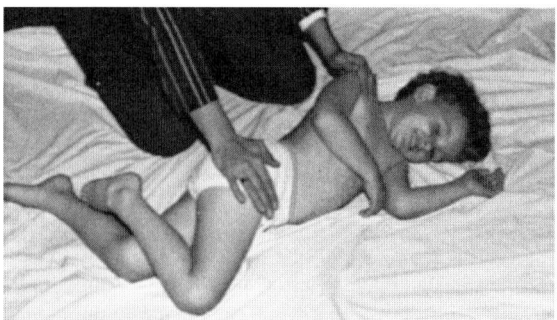

Fig. 26.7 Counterrotation of shoulder girdle backward (retraction) and the pelvis forward. Hand placement of therapist is important so that shoulder and hip movements can occur freely.

asked to assist in maintaining the changes that promote the more skillful movement response. Unless otherwise indicated by the patient's status, interventions must actively involve the individual in the process of planning, initiating, completing, and evaluating the movement. Although the therapist may manipulate the environment (internal and external) in which the response is made, the patient must be an active participant for learning to occur.

Although some patients will demonstrate a pattern of generalized overactivity of the postural muscles of the trunk, many will have difficulty generating sufficient activity in the appropriate groups to sustain a posture or to permit movement in the posture. With generalized hypotonia, temporary improvement in postural responses may occur by providing vestibular input that is characterized by rapid and irregular changes. The labyrinths should be stimulated by quick stops and starts with changes in direction. The program should include the introduction of movements in all planes. Approximation can be effective in developing appropriate postural activity from a state of either hypertonicity or hypotonicity. Empirically, it seems that more force is applied to increase than to decrease the postural response. Approximation appears to elicit a response in all the muscles surrounding a joint in preparation for responding to the demands on the erect posture or the demands of weight bearing. Approximation lends itself to combination with other proprioceptive techniques, such as quick stretch or tapping. Although the changes evoked by these techniques may be of short duration, the alterations can evoke movement components that would not otherwise occur and thereby provide the opportunity for the individual to learn from the movement. As the therapist applies various techniques in an attempt to elicit a specific response, the therapist must evaluate the desired response in relationship to the environmental context. If the patient is sitting on the edge of a mat table, the activity of the trunk musculature will vary depending on whether the feet are flat on the floor, the patient is engaged in an activity, the patient is leaning on one arm for support, or the patient is resting between activities. The patient who slouches in sitting when fatigued, bored, or overwhelmed by the sensory input may present a different clinical picture when the appropriate factors are altered.

• *Selective, voluntary movement patterns within functional activities are optimized.*

The concept of the influence of the environment on the quality of a movement response, discussed in relation to the first goal of the intervention process, is also incorporated in the second goal. High-quality, selective, voluntary movement patterns are sought within the framework of functional activities, rather than as isolated and abstract movements. Optimization of the selective movement patterns may require a decrease in the stereotypical linkages of certain muscle groups, an increase in the ability to selectively activate certain muscle groups, the development of the ability to execute the movement in different postures, or a number of other variations.

Performance of functional activities requires that the individual be capable of performing both mobility and stability patterns with the extremities. Mobility patterns are open kinetic chain movements in which the distal segment is free. These patterns are necessary for placing the extremities (e.g., swing phase of gait or reaching for a doorknob).

Patients who exhibit stereotypical posturing of the upper extremity with a restricted repertoire of available movement patterns require intervention to change the initial position of the extremity before movements are attempted. The influence of the spasticity that interferes with the repositioning of the extremity can be reduced by applying approximation through the long axis of the extremity. Preferably, the therapist's manual contacts for the application of the approximation force are on the weight-bearing surfaces of the hand. If

the flexed position of the wrist prohibits application of the force to the heel of the palm, the approximation can be applied gradually through the fisted hand. As the resistance to passive movement diminishes, the wrist can be moved toward the neutral position so that the therapist can apply the approximation through the heel of the palm (Fig. 26.8). The therapist is moving the extremity toward an alternative resting position so that a new movement sequence can be attempted. It is important to use an intervention technique, such as approximation, to reduce the level of spasticity before passive movement is attempted, so that a more appropriate position can be assumed without inappropriately stretching the spastic muscles.

The patient is asked to assist the therapist with the movement, with the person being cued to do so with a minimum of effort. Too often, patients attempt to make a selective movement through a massive effort and overactivation of the muscle groups, which compounds the underlying spasticity. Patients should be encouraged to make easy, effortless movements—those they are instructed to perform with reduced effort so that they can relearn selective activation of motor units rather than mass firing patterns. Working "harder" often creates additional impairments versus increasing normal functional movement responses. It is critical that the movements requested relate to a functional activity or skill. Research suggests that skilled movements require attention and therefore motivation. Shaping the activity to both interest the patient and afford some level of success is important.[33]

Electrical stimulation can be used as an adjunct to facilitate performance of a particular component of a mobility pattern. The wrist extension component of the proprioceptive neuromuscular facilitation (PNF) pattern of flexion, abduction, and external rotation can be reinforced by using a portable electrical stimulation unit with adjustable surge duration. The electrical stimulation elicits the correct movement so that the patient can learn from the feel of the correct pattern. Adjusting the practice schedule so that the pattern is performed with and without the electrical stimulation support of the movement avoids the potential problem of reliance on the device to produce the movement. Electromyographic biofeedback can be a useful adjunct to achieve activation of specific muscle groups or to guide the patient's attempts to reduce the level of activity of a muscle group.

Mobility patterns in the upper extremity have as their foundation the freedom of the scapula to adjust appropriately to the position of the humerus. The mobility of the scapula can be addressed through techniques that result in a general decrease in muscle activity and diagonal movement patterns of the scapula. The scapular stabilizers, such as the rhomboids, trapezius, and serratus anterior, must be capable of allowing appropriate adjustment of the scapula, as well as providing the fixation base on which humeral elevation can occur.

In stability patterns, the distal segment of the extremity is fixed (closed kinetic chain). These patterns are used in the weight-bearing components of the functional activities, such as the stance phase of gait or creeping. The components of the stability patterns are enhanced by proprioceptive input, such as approximation. During the performance of both stability and mobility patterns, the therapist should control the situation so that the patient learns the appropriate movement patterns and not those imposed on top of inappropriate muscle activation.

Performance of movement patterns should progress toward an ability to easily reverse the direction of the movement. This can be promoted by incorporating rhythmical movements within a posture or between postures as early as possible in the intervention sequence. The end point at which the reversal is required should vary. In preparation for mastering the movements required to move from supine to sitting on the edge of the mat table, the patient might be

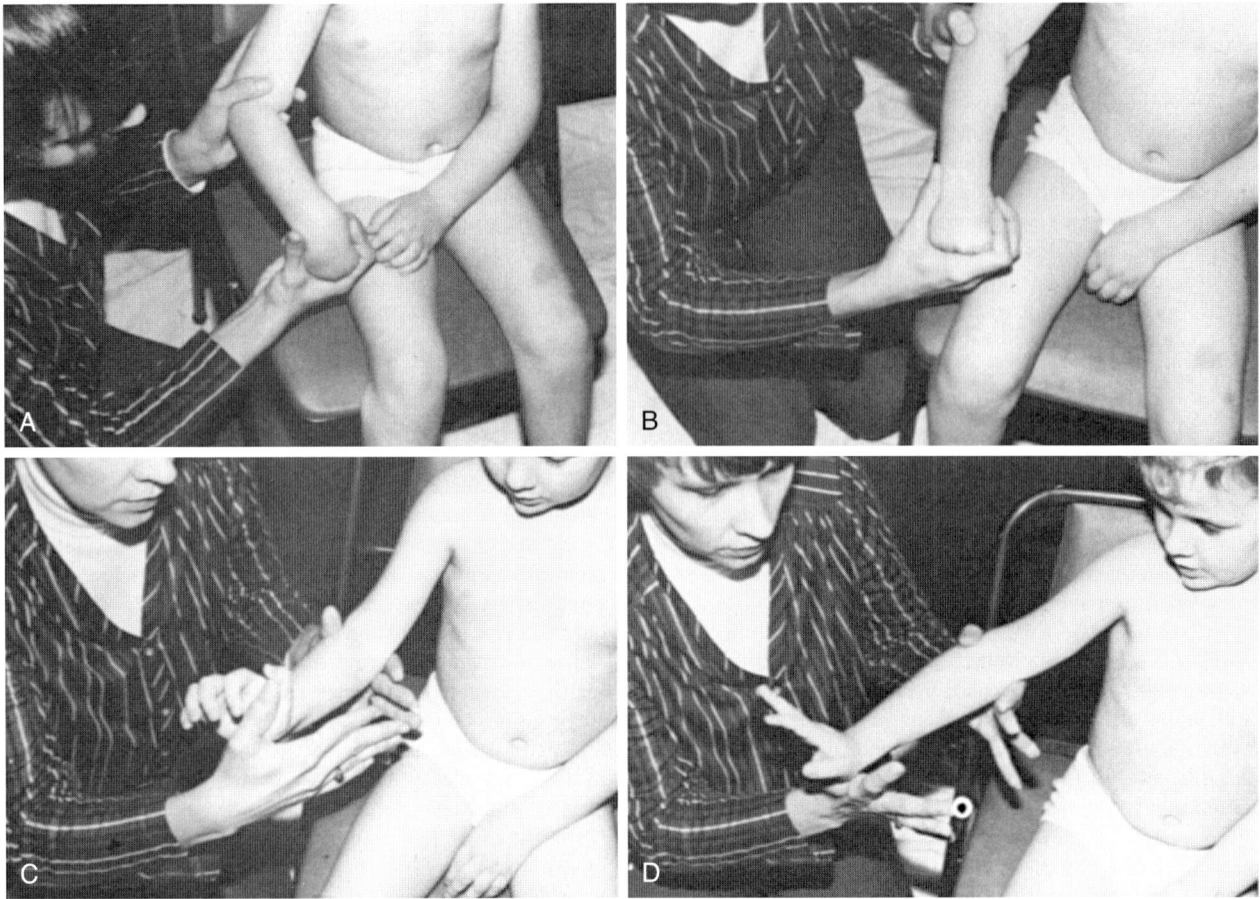

Fig. 26.8 Facilitating Opening of the Hand. (A) Fisted hand; stretch to the extensors and approximation through hand, wrist, and elbow is applied. **(B)** Approximation is continued; some resistance to the extensors may be applied. **(C)** Approximation is applied to thenar eminence to further facilitate extensor tone. **(D)** Full extension is achieved; approximation is maintained.

asked to move from the supine position to side sitting and back to supine; then the patient could move from the supine position to side-lying propped on one elbow (the halfway point in the overall movement), then reverse to supine. Incorporating reversal of movement patterns within the intervention program prepares the patient to deal with situations that mandate unexpected adjustments in the movement sequence.

Patients who demonstrate problems with the sequencing of movements, such as those with motor dyspraxia, frequently perform better if the movement is performed at a speed that is close to normal. Patients who had normal movement sequences before the brain infection seem to be able to trigger better movement responses at normal speeds than at slower speeds. The slower movement speeds appear to disrupt the typical flow of the movement. In working with patients with sequencing problems, all team members should provide the same, consistent sensory cues to elicit a movement pattern. For example, the therapist may establish a coupling of the verbal cue "roll" with a quick stretch to the ankle dorsiflexors to elicit a rolling pattern. These same cues can be used by other team members to assist the patient in changing positions in bed or in performing dressing activities. The consistency of cues may elicit a consistent response from the patient. Once the pattern is well established, the intervention program can be designed to reduce the cues progressing toward the ability of the patient to perform the activity in response to the demands of the situation rather than to externally imposed cues.

The flow of a movement pattern may be disrupted by problems categorized as incoordination. The origin of the coordination problems could be dysfunction of the visual-perceptual system (see Chapter 28) or vestibular system (see Chapter 21), dyspraxia (see Chapter 12), or dysfunction caused by cerebellar damage (see Chapter 19). If possible, the factors involved in producing a lack of coordination should be identified.

• *Performance of functional activities is enhanced.*

As the patient develops more appropriate postural control and the ability to perform selective movement patterns within functional activities, she or he is developing the basis to perform increasingly challenging functional activities. The movement patterns (and the postural control that underlies them) provide the building blocks for mastering an expanding variety of activities.

As the therapist designs the expansion of activities within the intervention program, the demands of each new functional activity and posture must be scrutinized. The patient's ability to meet these demands was examined in the evaluation process. The intervention strategy must focus on the quality of the patient's ability to assume a posture, maintain the posture, move within the posture (static and dynamic equilibrium responses to both self-generated and external perturbations), and move out of the posture. The therapist will change the sequence of this progression of activities to meet the needs of the patient. The patient may achieve independence in maintaining a posture while still requiring assistance in assuming the posture.

This progression should be grounded within the context of functionally relevant activities. Unless the individual has difficulty tolerating change, activities should be practiced within different environments to enhance generalization of learning. The creative therapist can design a variety of functionally relevant activities that require similar movement components.

With infants, the therapist may choose to use the developmental sequence as a general model for the functional activities progression. Progression through the developmental sequence should be viewed as a dynamic process so that the intervention incorporates movement both within and between postures. For individuals through the remainder of the life-span, the focus should be on the age-appropriate functional activities essential to the individual's daily life, such as bed mobility, sitting to standing, standing to sitting, ambulation, reaching, and manipulation.

Examples of handling techniques that can be adapted to enhance the individual's progression through the sequence of functional activities can be found in the works of Bobath,[38] Carr and Shepherd,[39,40] Duncan and Badke,[41] Levitt,[42] Ryerson and Levit,[43] Sullivan and Markos,[44] and Voss and colleagues,[45] as well as throughout this book. These authors can provide the therapist with ideas for ways to enhance the patient's performance within a specific activity.

- *Integration of sensory information is fostered.*

At the same time that the therapist addresses the previous intervention goals, the goal of fostering integration of sensory input must be considered. Unless the therapist has advanced knowledge of sensory integration theories, this goal may be secondary rather than primary; nevertheless, it cannot be ignored.

The potential for an exaggerated and inappropriate response to sensory input was discussed as part of the clinical picture. Before the therapist expects the patient to exhibit adaptive behavior to the potential bombardment of input from combinations of cutaneous, proprioceptive, auditory, and visual input, the therapist must assess the patient's ability to respond to multisensory inputs. The ability to respond adaptively progresses from a response to a single sensory system input, to a response to the input in the presence of multiple-system input, and then to an adaptive response based on inputs from two or more sources. The therapist must be sure that adding more sensory inputs augments an adaptive response rather than detracting from it. The patient may respond to handling techniques that provide proprioceptive and cutaneous cues but may demonstrate a deterioration of performance when auditory input is added. When verbal cues are added, the therapist should follow the philosophy that verbal commands should be concise, sparse, and appropriately timed.[46]

All sensory inputs should evoke the correct response on the part of the patient, rather than cause her or him to sift through the jumble of inputs to recognize the appropriate inputs to which a response should be made. At the highest level the patient will demonstrate cross-modal learning in which input from one sensory system will evoke a response based on input previously obtained through a different system. Recognition of a comb by touch is based on the precept of "combness," usually obtained initially by visual input. If the therapist recognizes the hierarchy in the process of integrating sensory input, intervention situations that require too high a level of performance from the patient can be avoided. The patient who can respond adaptively to input from only one source would not be expected to perform in a crowded treatment area that presents extraneous visual and auditory input. The therapist will also recognize the need to include in the intervention plan situations that involve the controlled introduction of sensory inputs so that the patient progresses toward the ability to deal with multiple inputs. Carr and Shepherd[40] discuss some general principles that can be used during

the training of motor tasks in the presence of somatosensory and perceptual-cognitive impairments.

Dysfunctions in perceptual integration are addressed as the patient moves through functional sequence activities. Although these movement activities would not provide the total program for an individual with a specific perceptual integration dysfunction, goals in this area can be addressed if the therapist is aware of indications of dysfunctions. The therapist must critically observe the performance of a movement sequence to identify substitute actions to compensate for problems such as inability to cross the midline. The therapist must then attempt to redesign the demands of the situation to elicit the desired behavior. The patient who moves from the supine to the side sitting to the long sitting positions without the upper extremities crossing the midline could be required to side sit to the left and transfer objects with the right hand from the left side of the body to the right side (Fig. 26.9). The therapist must determine whether the patient is truly crossing the midline or rotating the midline of the body to continue to avoid crossing it.

Therapists may be most aware of disturbances in the patient's ability to integrate sensory information into an appropriate response when this dysfunction disrupts balance. The ability to maintain and move in upright postures requires successful processing of information from the sensory triad of postural control: the visual, vestibular, and somatosensory systems. When one component is missing, unreliable, or discrepant with the other two, the person is at risk for loss of balance. During the ongoing evaluation process, the therapist gathers

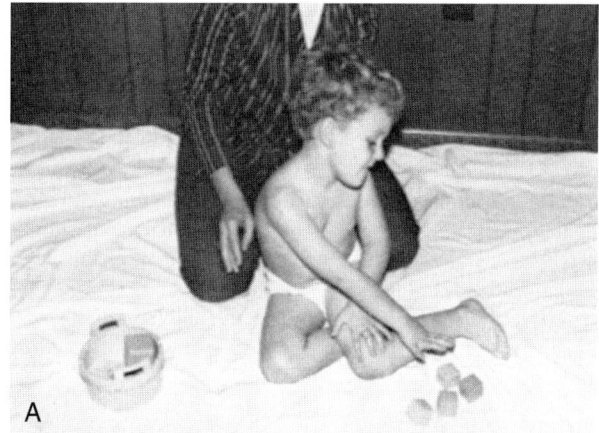

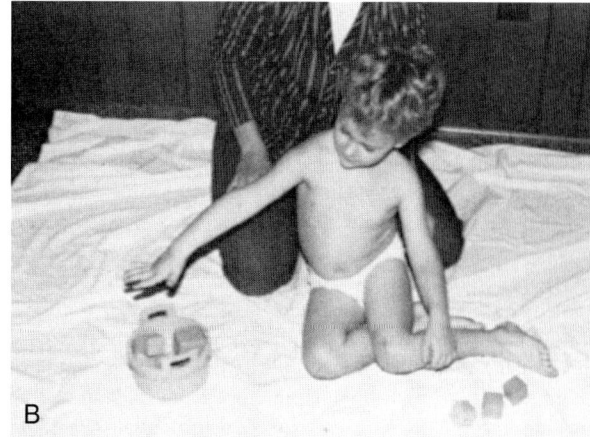

Fig. 26.9 Child crossing midline of body when transferring objects from left to right. **(A)** Beginning act on contralateral side. **(B)** Ending sequence by crossing midline and placing objects on ipsilateral side.

information on the integrity of each system and any evidence of central processing difficulties. Incorporated within the practice of activities to develop postural control, to promote selective movements with functional activities, and to develop mastery of increasingly difficult functional activities is the simultaneous practice of integrating sensory information so that a successful response can be generated.

Patients who are performing at higher levels can be challenged to maintain balance when one element of the sensory triad is missing (e.g., vision occluded) or altered (e.g., sitting, standing, or walking on a soft, compliant surface). Successful maintenance of balance outside the protective environment of the therapy clinic requires the ability to switch the primary information source to any one of the three systems. Walking in the dark requires the person to rely on vestibular and somatosensory input. Standing on a moving bus looking out a window requires resolution of the conflict between visual input (the external world is moving), vestibular input (you are moving), and somatosensory input (you are stationary). Movement experiences within the therapy program should foster practice of this sensory integration process (see Table 26.2).

• *Cognitive status and psychosocial responses are optimized.*

In addition to attending to the factors directly related to motor performance, the therapist also must attend to the patient's psychosocial and cognitive responses. Although the therapist does not have primary responsibility in this area, a goal of the intervention process should be to enhance the individual's psychosocial and cognitive responses.

Particularly in the agitated state that may be a component of the response to the inflammatory process, the patient may demonstrate exaggerated and inappropriate emotional responses to events. Dealing with these emotional fluctuations can become a major determinant in goal attainment in the other areas. Maintaining a positive, nonthreatening interaction allows the patient to use the therapist as a reference for judging the appropriateness of emotional responses.

If the patient's state of agitation is interfering with the intervention program, the therapist may alter the program to include techniques that have a calming effect. For example, the individual can be wrapped in a cotton sheet blanket and rocked in a slow, rhythmical, repetitive manner to decrease agitation. Auditory and visual input should be controlled to avoid overloading sensory processing mechanisms.

Earlier in this text, the psychosocial adjustment that occurs in the process of recovering from a neurological disability was discussed. The therapist must be aware of how the patient's regression in affective and cognitive domains affects the intervention process. The therapist should seek assistance from the health care team members responsible for intervention in these areas to deal with the patient constructively. The therapist must remember that both the family members and the

patient are in the process of adjusting to the patient's changed and, it is hoped, changing status. Family members may be an asset or a liability to the patient's recovery process. During the therapist's interactions with the family members in activities such as instructions in the patient's home program, the therapist should be prepared to deal with expressions of the individual's difficulty in adjusting to the situation. The therapist also should be prepared to assist family members in identifying appropriate sources to help them deal with their problems.

Changes in mentation, perception of events, and memory losses present challenges to both the patient and the therapist. Repetition in the recounting of past events may help reorder past knowledge. Use of brief verbal or visual cues may assist the patient in recalling safety instructions or the components of the exercise program. The therapist should try to generate a nonstressful environment when working on these deficits so that attention and recall are not overshadowed by emotional pressure. As the therapist works with the patient on an intervention program, situations arise that require problem solving to determine a way to accomplish a task. If the task is to accomplish an independent transfer from a wheelchair into a bathtub, decisions must be made concerning the sequence of movements. Therapists can approach this situation in two ways. They can instruct patients step-by-step in what to do, or they can involve patients to the extent possible in the process of deciding what to do. If the therapist instructs the patient step-by-step, the patient may master the task but may not be able to perform it under different conditions. If the therapist involves the patient in the decision making process, the patient may be learning not only how to accomplish the specific task, but also how to accomplish the task under varied conditions. The intervention process should lead to the ability to respond to the demands of a situation, and involvement of patients in the problem-solving process helps prepare them for independence. The therapist must structure the patient's role in decision making to the level of the patient's ability to participate so that the experience is not frustrating. Although the patient's participation may initially increase the time required to complete a task, it promotes skills that may lead more quickly to independence of function.

INTERACTION WITH OTHER PROFESSIONALS

The therapist needs to design an intervention program that is articulated with that of other members of the health care team. The recovery process of the patient should be facilitated by a care plan in which each team member reinforces the goals of the other team members. The care of the person must be a collaborative effort. Each patient deserves an intervention process that considers him or her as a whole person, not as a set of fragmented problems.

SUMMARY

This chapter has presented a brief discussion of the pathology and medical management of various inflammatory processes that affect the brain. The process of assessment, the role of assessment in designing an intervention program, the goals of the intervention process, and the means to meet those goals were presented to assist the reader in more effective management of patients with these diagnoses.

Although the problem-solving process presented in this chapter for assessment, prognosis, goal identification, and treatment planning is not limited to patients with inflammatory supraspinal disorders, its application in the presence of typical neurological sequelae has been described. When dealing with inflammatory disorders of the brain, the variability of neurological sequelae is examined based on the

anatomical location of the inflammatory process and the cause of the infection.

Although the neurological disorders discussed in this chapter are life threatening, many patients recover and return to their previous lifestyles. Patients will vary within the spectrum of minimal to severe involvement and from specific to generalized CNS dysfunction and will demonstrate a range of recovery after the acute distress, from little recovery to full recovery. Prognosis for recovery depends on the type of infecting organism and the extent of involvement. The therapist must remain flexible and willing to adjust every aspect of therapeutic intervention to meet the specific needs of each patient. Yet the therapist must also remember that learning requires active participation on the part of the patient.

CASE STUDY 26.1

A 74-year-old patient with cryptococcal *(Cryptococcus gattii)* meningitis was seen in the outpatient setting 1½ years after onset with residual complaints of constant dizziness, imbalance, and need for assistance with mobility tasks.

History of Present Illness

Patient manifested dementia and overt meningitis 1½ years prior. He was treated with liposomal amphotericin B + 5FC for 3 weeks and then put on fluconazole. He was transferred to a skilled nursing facility with dementia and need for significant assistance for all ADLs. His cognition and functional status continued to diminish over the next 3 months, when it was determined he had hydrocephalus, and a VP shunt was placed. This resulted in significant improvement in mentation and function, and he was discharged home with home care 3 months later.

Past Medical History

The past medical history included profound bilateral sensorineural hearing loss postmeningitis, chronic obstructive pulmonary disease (COPD), and possible Parkinson-like symptoms.

Summary of Key Findings

The patient was alert and oriented to person, place, time, and reason for referral. He had some short-term memory loss. He lived with his wife in a single-story home. He was walking with a two-wheeled walker with standby assistance as his primary mode of mobility. He had difficulty with steadiness during transfers and when turning. He complained of constant dizziness, which he described as a sense of movement and at times spins. All movements worsened the symptoms, and being still decreased the symptoms.

Vision screen was normal, but he complained of increased dizziness with eye movement. Vestibular ocular testing findings were abnormal; patient had a positive head-thrust test result bilaterally, and abnormal DVA with head movements at 2 Hz. Light touch and proprioception were intact for both legs. The accompanying table presents a summary of objective findings.

	FTSST	Strength	Berg	SOT	Ambulation	DVA (2 Hz)
Initial	18.73 s	LE 5/5, except hip extensor 4/5, and PF 2/5 bilaterally	38/56	28% (fell 9/18 trials—all sway referenced support)	Two-wheeled walker with SBA	20/200
1 month	15.12 s	Not tested	55/56	Not tested	Two-wheeled walker independent	20/125
2 months	Not tested	LE 5/5 except PF 4/5	Not tested	39% (fell 6/18 trials— conditions 5 and 6) Use of vision significantly improved from 0% to 55%	Single-point cane	20/80 horz
3 months	15 s	Not tested	55/56	Not tested	Single-point cane	20/63−2[a] at 2 Hz (horz); 20/80 (vert)
4 months	12.1	LE 5/5 with PF 4/5	Not tested	56% (fell 4/18 trials—first 2 attempts conditions 5 and 6)	No device on level surfaces, cane on uneven surfaces	20/50
5 months	51 s	Hip abductor 4/5 and ankle PF 2+/5	34/56	Fell conditions 3 and 4 of M-CTSIB in <5 s	Two-wheeled walker	20/100
10 months	16.9 s	LE 5/5 except PF only 2+/5	52/56	Only falls condition 4 of M-CTSIB	Single-point cane all surfaces	20/125

[a]The patient read the line with two errors.
DVA, Dynamic visual acuity test; *FTSST,* five-times-sit-to-stand test; *horz,* horizontal; *LE,* lower extremity; *M-CTSIB,* Modified Clinical Test of Sensory Interaction and Balance; *PF,* plantar flexors; *SBA,* standby assist; *SOT,* Sensory Organization Test; *vert,* vertical.

Physical Therapy Movement Diagnosis

The patient had an increased risk of falls, with significant balance impairment and gaze instability consistent with mixed peripheral (bilateral hypofunction) and central vestibular dysfunction postmeningitis (Physical Therapy Practice Patterns 5D and 5A). He also had lower-extremity weakness and reduced vertical orientation. His strengths included supportive family and excellent motivation.

Goals

1. Patient will be able to ambulate independently in his home without assistive device (4 months).
2. Patient will improve gaze stability to 20/80 with head movements at 2 Hz in either direction (4 months).

3. Patient will be independent and safe to negotiate a flight of stairs with rail (2 months).
4. Patient will be able to maintain standing with eyes open on foam surface >30 s (2 months).

Interventions

The patient lived 2 h from the clinic, so many of the interventions were through progressive home exercises. Patient was seen one or two times each month, and the program consisted of balance retraining, gaze stability exercises (vestibulo-ocular reflex [VOR] retraining beginning in sitting, plain background), lower-extremity strengthening, endurance activities, and gait training. Given the patient's hearing loss and memory deficits, teaching included demonstration, written instructions, and instruction of the patient's wife. The patient

Continued

CASE STUDY 26.1—cont'd

progressed steadily the first 4 months, then he began not feeling well. He complained of increased nausea and trouble eating and had a slow decline in mentation. At the 5-month visit, the patient's condition had declined significantly, and after discussion with the patient's physician, he underwent a series of tests that concluded the patient was having intermittent shunt malfunction. After the shunt revision, the patient did improve as noted at the 10-month follow-up visit.

Key Take Home Points
1. It is not unusual to have both cranial nerve and CNS involvement with meningitis.
2. Remember to monitor for signs of shunt malfunction, and the importance of educating the patient and family members concerning this.
3. Use standardized objective measures in case management.

ACKNOWLEDGMENT

I would like to thank Dr. Rebecca Porter, PhD, PT, for her contributions to the first four editions of this book. She not only has made a significant contribution through her publications and this chapter in the book but also is an inspiration to many of us within the profession of Physical Therapy.

REFERENCES

To enhance this text and add value for the reader, all references are included on the companion Evolve site that accompanies this textbook. This online service will, when available, provide a link for the reader to a Medline abstract for the article cited. There are 46 cited references and other general references for this chapter, with the majority of those articles being evidence-based citations.

27

Aging, Dementia, and Disorders of Cognition

*Mark David Basco, Edward James Gorgon, Ronald Barredo, Osa Jackson Schulte,
James Stephens, and Joyce Ann*

OBJECTIVES

After reading this chapter the student or therapist will be able to:
1. Define the basic terminology and discuss the prevalence of cognitive disturbances seen in older persons.
2. Describe normative changes in brain function with normal aging and their relevance to the diagnoses of delirium and dementias.
3. Discuss how symptoms are altered with normal aging (specifically related to the Arndt-Schulz principle, law of initial values, and habitual biorhythms) for an individual.
4. Describe normal sensory changes with aging and how they alter a person's overall ability to adapt to stress.
5. Describe how (and for what type of patient) to use the Mini-Mental State Examination as a part of the physical or occupational therapy examination.
6. Describe common sensory changes with dementia and implications for adapting physical or occupational therapy evaluation and intervention.
7. Discuss common changes in learning styles with aging and implications for adapting physical or occupational therapy intervention to enhance patients' ability to perform at their highest functional level.
8. Describe how environmental design and ergonomics can enhance patient performance in activities of daily living and instrumental activities of daily living.
9. Describe a strategy to evaluate a patient's emotional capacity to participate in a learning task and its clinical relevance to both occupational and physical therapy outcomes.
10. Describe criteria for delirium and reversible dementia and sample strategies for modifying evaluation and treatment procedures.
11. Discuss symptoms and disease progression in irreversible dementia.
12. Discuss the therapist's role on the treatment team in educating key caregivers and support personnel and sample training strategies.
13. Discuss treatment skills that are helpful in working with persons who have irreversible dementia.
14. Describe research activities and new findings that affect physical evaluation and treatment of the patient with dementia or delirium.

KEY TERMS

aging
Alzheimer's disease
caregiver training and support
dementia and delirium
function

physical and occupational therapy examination and intervention
problem solving
risk reduction and rehabilitation
therapeutic environment

THE STARTING POINT WITH OLDER PERSONS IN PHYSICAL OR OCCUPATIONAL THERAPY

Older persons can adapt to new physical problems. It is critical to use the processes of habilitation and rehabilitation to train caregivers (family, friends, or staff) to bring out the best functional performance in the older person. The health care staff, caregivers, family, and friends relating to the older person in a time of crisis need to prioritize creating a sense of safety, acceptance, and support based on the patient's preferences and habits. The specific actions in this process include the following:
1. Evaluate, document, and make available to the hands-on caregivers what the patient "likes"—his or her preferences and habits for all activities of daily living (ADLs) and instrumental activities of daily living (IADLs).
2. Train caregivers to create a care plan for daily living and nursing that builds in the patient's preferences to support his or her personal identity and self-image.
3. Create specific physical therapy or occupational therapy functional goals that build on and reinforce patient preferences with regard to mobility, eating, bathing, grooming, dressing, socialization, and so on. (Note: If caregivers change, training needs to be added and new goals may need to be developed because not all caregivers have the same capacity to relate to the patient.)
4. Train caregivers with the older person to use specific strategies to (a) enhance breathing, (b) increase bed mobility, (c) improve

balance in sitting and standing, (d) perform active range of motion (AROM) and active assisted range of motion (AAROM) for ADLs and IADLs, (e) achieve skeletal weight shift for ADLs and IADLs, (f) encourage head, neck, and spine to upright postural response during ADLs and IADLs, and (g) encourage walking and stair climbing safely and as able.

5. Screen for signs of reversible cognitive losses.

6. Provide adaptations and training for performance of ADLs when chronic cognitive problems exist.

7. Train caregivers and the older person in ways to adapt the ADLs and IADLs to maximize ability.

PARADIGM FOR AGING, THE BRAIN, AND LEARNING

Aging is a process that requires ongoing adaptation to and compensation for the losses that are imposed on human beings from the *outside* world and the internal physiological changes that occur with the passage of time, physical activities, emotional state, fatigue, digestive and elimination processes, and habitual rest-activity cycle. If a person's health is altered by illness or trauma, then he or she goes through an adaptive process. If too many changes happen too quickly, the brain is unable to create a functional adaptive response, and the individual must alter or simplify her or his life processes or face negative mental or physiological reactions. As human beings explore coping with unfamiliar experiences, they require more nurturing, rest, and physical contact that are perceived as empowering.

Human beings progress to adulthood through the millions of perceptions and choices that are recorded and responded to throughout the developmental years. With advancing age, there is a gradual decrease in the acuity of the kinesthetic and sensory information received. These changes can affect interactive learning for the older adult.[1–3] Active participation has a positive impact on recall and learning,[4] predictable events support recall,[5] and ordered events are easier to recall. Differentiations in the nervous system for human beings do not happen uniformly.[6,7] As a person grows, the result of this lack of uniformity is that some adults prefer to relate to the world visually, others aurally, and still others by touch or kinesthetically. Therefore people specialize with their sensory processing and, at the same time, become more vulnerable to issues of sensory adaptation and selection.[8]

The adult phase of central nervous system development will, for most people, involve a gradual narrowing of the focus in the development of new skills as well as increased repetition of certain activities. The tendency is to narrow down one's activities more and more to those in which a person excels or feels comfortable. Intuitive or practical people continue to pursue self-knowledge and explore ways to maximize their talents. By accident or through mentoring, these people discover that lifelong learning is the gift of life itself. Ongoing and ever-increasing self-awareness allows for enhanced adaptability at any age.

Indeed, the human brain has been found to be malleable and adaptable in old age, and even in the presence of various neurological insults. Neural growth has been observed in mature neurons,[9] hippocampal volume increases with physical activity, and myokines derived from muscle contraction have been found to modulate brain function.[10–15] Thus the presence or absence of physical experiences (e.g., human movement) and an enriching environment[16] provide powerful stimuli for brain activity.[17–19] The challenge for the rehabilitation professional is how to harness such potential and structure the therapeutic environment to attain an optimal outcome for the patient/client.

In this chapter, the paradigm for aging and lifelong learning presumes the following:

1. The central nervous system is viewed as the master system and the controller of other human systems (e.g., digestive, cardiovascular, muscular, and endocrine).

2. Capacity exists for ongoing learning (self-awareness), self-regulation, and adaptability throughout the life-span.

3. The whole (human being) is greater than the sum of its parts.

4. Language shapes reality and the experience and perceptions of life.

5. Enjoying a comfortable and easy pace for new learning is beneficial. Being able to learn new skills is important for adaptability and lifelong well-being.

6. The mind and body are not separate. Multiple chronic medical conditions, smoking, lack of physical mobility, and loss of muscle strength (among others) impact the mind, while a physically active lifestyle, healthy dietary intake, and lack of cardiovascular diseases mitigate the risks associated with an aging mind and body.[20–23]

7. Optimal aging begins in early adulthood. It is rooted in advocating for a healthy lifestyle, which reduces one's risk of acquiring debilitating mental and physical illness in later life.[24,25]

8. Personal variations in learning style and preferences for relating can be used to maximize adaptation in the presence of physical and cognitive decline.

9. The activation of the limbic system for "fight or flight" is normal, and the ability to release the limbic activation and return to a resting state once a crisis (real or imagined) is over becomes a critical skill for adapting as people grow older.[26]

10. The creation of environments that encourage safe exploration of new ideas and ways of self-expression can generate lifelong human growth and development.

FRAMEWORK FOR CLINICAL PROBLEM SOLVING

Therapists working with patients with cognitive impairments need to have received adequate advanced training in the assessment of communication skills and neurological functioning as well as gerontology so they can work with maximal efficacy and enjoy the clinical interactions with each patient. In the United States, there is a lack of adequately trained professionals to address the many health issues that accompany the rising number of older adults in the general population.[27] In 37 BC, the Roman poet Virgil wrote, "Age carries all things, even the mind, away."[28] Nearly 400 years ago, Shakespeare described the last stage of human life as "second childishness and mere oblivion, sans teeth, sans eyes, sans taste, sans everything."[29] This pessimistic view of the fate of older adults persists among health care workers today despite the fact that significant cognitive deficits affect only 9%[30] of older adults (people older than age 65 years) in the United States.[31,32] Clinicians therefore should not assume that older individuals have impaired cognitive functioning.[33]

Perhaps the most crucial concept for clinical problem solving is that the clinician must not assume that the current abilities reflect the true capacity of the person. When a patient is observed to have altered brain function, description of the extent and type of the distortion of intellectual capacity and determination of the time of onset (sudden or gradual) are necessary to enable a diagnosis and the provision of appropriate and effective treatment and care. The capacity to learn is a possibility, although the process of learning may be altered or different from that of unaffected older adults.[34–37] When age, illness, or medications create a temporary or permanent change in cognitive abilities, all functional training requires alteration to meet the unique cognitive abilities of the patient at the moment. For example, the son of a patient who needed physical and occupational therapy showed staff how to communicate with his mother so that she would not get scared. The therapist walked slowly into the room and greeted the patient by touching her softly on the cheek with the back of her hand. The patient looked up and smiled. The therapist smiled back and stroked the patient softly on the top of her head. The patient smiled again. The therapist kneeled down so that she was eye-to-eye with the patient sitting in the wheelchair. She took the patient's hand in her own hand and with her other hand slowly stroked the back of the patient's hand. The patient smiled again. The therapy session had begun. For this patient, words were actually confusing, so they were avoided.[38] The need for tactile nurturing input persists as people age.[39] Nurturing tactile input done at a pace that is pleasant for the patient can actually support a positive clinical outcome.[40]

Definition of Terms

Neurocognitive disorders, including dementia, arise from acquired changes in the brain, which lead to declines in the cognitive function of an individual.[41,42] They differ from mental retardation (developmental disability) in which changes arise early in life and baseline cognitive function do not necessarily decline. Though commonly associated with older adults, neurocognitive disorders in the younger population do occur, especially among individuals with human immunodeficiency virus (HIV) infection and traumatic brain injury.[41,42] In 2013, the American Psychiatric Association published the 5th edition of its Diagnostic and Statistical Manual (DSM-5) and incorporated concepts such as "dementia" and "mild cognitive impairment" into its revised classification system. Major neurocognitive disorder corresponds with dementia, while minor neurocognitive disorder is similar to mild cognitive impairment (Table 27.1).

Major neurocognitive disorders are differentiated from minor neurocognitive disorders in the (a) severity of cognitive decline from a previous level of performance and (b) interference with independence in everyday activities. Cognitive decline in one or more domains could be expressed by the patient or a reliable informant, and/or observed by a clinician. The severity of decline could then be classified as modest or substantial using standardized testing procedures or similar objective clinical evaluation tools.

- Modest cognitive decline: Test score between 1 and 2 standard deviations below the appropriate norm, or between 3rd and 16th percentile rank.
- Substantial cognitive decline: Test score below 2 standard deviations of the appropriate norm, or below 3rd percentile rank.

Cognitive decline in both Major and Minor Neurocognitive disorders could manifest in one or more of these domains: complex attention, executive function, learning and memory, language, perceptual-motor-visual perception praxis, and social cognition. Recognizing early signs of decline (red flags) in any of these domains is paramount in establishing a diagnosis and formulating a timely management plan.

Delirium differs from major and minor neurocognitive disorders in its *sudden and rapid onset*.[41,43] A person with delirium shows an acute disturbance in attention, environmental awareness, and cognition from baseline; changes in sleep-wake cycle and emotional states; and worsening of behavioral problems.[41,44–46] The patient is often less alert than normal and may be sleepy or obtunded; however, many are hypervigilant and may be extremely agitated and suspicious. Early identification of the symptoms as well as formal medical assessment and treatment are critical to ensure the return of a normal level of

TABLE 27.1 DSM-V Diagnostic Criteria for Major and Minor Neurocognitive Disorders

Diagnostic Criteria	Major Neurocognitive Disorder (Dementia)	Minor Neurocognitive Disorder (Mild Cognitive Impairment)
A	*Significant cognitive decline* in one or more cognitive domains, based on: 1. Concern about significant decline, expressed by individual or reliable informant, or observed by clinician 2. Substantial impairment, documented by objective cognitive assessment	*Modest cognitive decline* in one or more cognitive domains, based on: 1. Concern about mild decline, expressed by individual or reliable informant, or observed by clinician 2. Modest impairment, documented by objective cognitive assessment
B	Interference with independence in everyday activities	No interference with independence in everyday activities, although these activities may require more time and effort, accommodation, or compensatory strategies
C	Not exclusively during delirium	
D	Not better explained by another mental disorder, e.g., major depressive disorder, schizophrenia	
E	Specify one or more etiological subtypes, "due to" • Alzheimer's disease • Cerebrovascular disease (Vascular neurocognitive disorder) • Frontotemporal lobar degeneration (Frontotemporal neurocognitive disorder • Dementia with Lewy bodies (Neurocognitive disorder with Lewy bodies) • Parkinson disease • Huntington disease • Traumatic brain injury • HIV Infection • Prion Disease • Another medical condition • Multiple etiologies	

Adapted from American Psychiatric Association. *Diagnostic and Statistical Manual of Mental Disorders*. 5th ed. Arlington, VA: American Psychiatric Publishing; 2013.

TABLE 27.2 Key Characteristics in Depression, Delirium, and Dementia

	Delirium	Depression	Dementia
Onset	Acute (hours to days)	Acute or insidious	Insidious (months to years)
Course	Fluctuates hourly, lucid periods in a day, confusion usually worsens at night Commonly results from acute illness, medical emergency	Episodic; may be self-limiting, recurrent, or chronic	Chronic, slow progression Starts in mid-life, may take 20 years from onset of mild cognitive impairment to severe dementia
Duration	Days to months Usually reversible	Variable	Months to years Irreversible
Consciousness	Reduced, fluctuates	Clear	Clear in the early stages, progressively gets worse in the later stages
Hallucinations	Frequent, usually visual and/or auditory in nature	Variable, predominantly auditory	Often absent in early stages; may have visual hallucinations in the later stages
Delusions	Fleeting, poorly systematized	May have sustained, systematized delusions	Often absent
Poor attention	Variable	Variable	Present, progressive
Disorientation	Present	Variable	Progressively gets worse in the mid-late stages
Memory	Immediate and short-term memory impaired	Variable, may be minimally or selectively impaired	Gradually worsens with disease progression
Psychomotor	Variable, may be increased or reduced	Variable, may range from hypoactivity to hyperactivity in the case of agitation	Often normal
Speech	Often incoherent Slow or rapid	Normal	Initially coherent; speech impairment worsens in later stages
Thinking	Disorganized	Impoverished	Limited, executive functions deteriorate with disease progression
Affect	Variable	Depressed, presents with apathy and anhedonia	Variable, may present also present with anhedonia and apathy in later stages
Sleep/wake cycle	Disturbed; changes every hour	Disturbed; hypersomnia may be present during the day	Disturbed; day/night reversal

Adapted from Canada, Winnipeg Regional Health Authority, Occupational Therapy. "WRHA Occupational Therapy Cognition Toolkit FAQs." WRHA Occupational Therapy Cognition Toolkit FAQs, Winnipeg Regional Health Authority, Feb. 2013. Available at: www.wrha.mb.ca/professionals/cognition/files/Survey-07.pdf. Accessed December 24, 2018. Updated data from Downing LJ, Caprio TV, Lyness JM. Geriatric psychiatry review: differential diagnosis and treatment of the 3 D's—delirium, dementia, and depression. *Curr Psychiatry Rep.* 2013;15(6): 365. doi:10.1007/s11920-013-0365-4 and Reisberg, Barry, et al. "Staging Dementia." *Principles and Practice of Geriatric Psychiatry*, 3rd ed. Hoboken, NJ: John Wiley & Sons; 2011:162–166.

alertness and intellectual function and to prevent the development of secondary functional impairments.[43,47,48]

Psychiatric problems may be present before old age or may develop as a result of dementia and need to be assessed and treated along with the dementia. Depression, for example, can mimic dementia and may be hard to recognize given its atypical and subtle nature among older adults. Pain, weakness, headaches, agitation, fatigue, unexpected change in weight/appetite, chronic constipation, insomnia, hypersomnia, and irritability may be observed. Table 27.2 outlines the key characteristics of delirium, depression, and dementia.[49,50]

Epidemiology

Currently, 50 million people worldwide have dementia, with nearly 10 million new cases every year.[33,51] In the United States, 5.7 million Americans and one in ten people over the age of 65 years are estimated to have Alzheimer's disease (AD),[52] the most common cause of dementia.[33,51,52] By 2050, the number of people with AD is estimated to increase to 13.8 million in the United States and 132 million globally, if current trends continue and no cures or effective preventive

measures are found.[52] The percentage of adults aged 85 years and older with AD will increase from 2.1 million in 2018 (37% of all older adults) to 7 million (51% of all older adults) in 2050.[52] The prevalence of dementia rises from approximately 3% at ages 65 to 74 years to 17% at ages 75 to 84 years, and to 32% at age 85 years[52,53] or higher (Fig. 27.1). The increasing number of people older than the age of 85 will be paralleled by an increase in the incidence of dementia. Disorders causing cognitive deficits are expected to continue to be a growing public health problem for at least the next 50 years.

More than 70 conditions are known to cause dementia.[54] Secondary behavioral problems in the patient with dementia can be interpreted as a response to somatic, psychological, or existential stress. Because memory impairments, impairments of abstract thinking or judgment, or global cognitive impairments in an older adult may be symptoms of acute physical illness, the patient's physical, emotional, social, and cognitive status and physical, social, and caregiver environment need to be systematically evaluated.[54]

Gradual or sudden changes in intellectual capacity or memory function are not a normal part of the aging process. Any change,

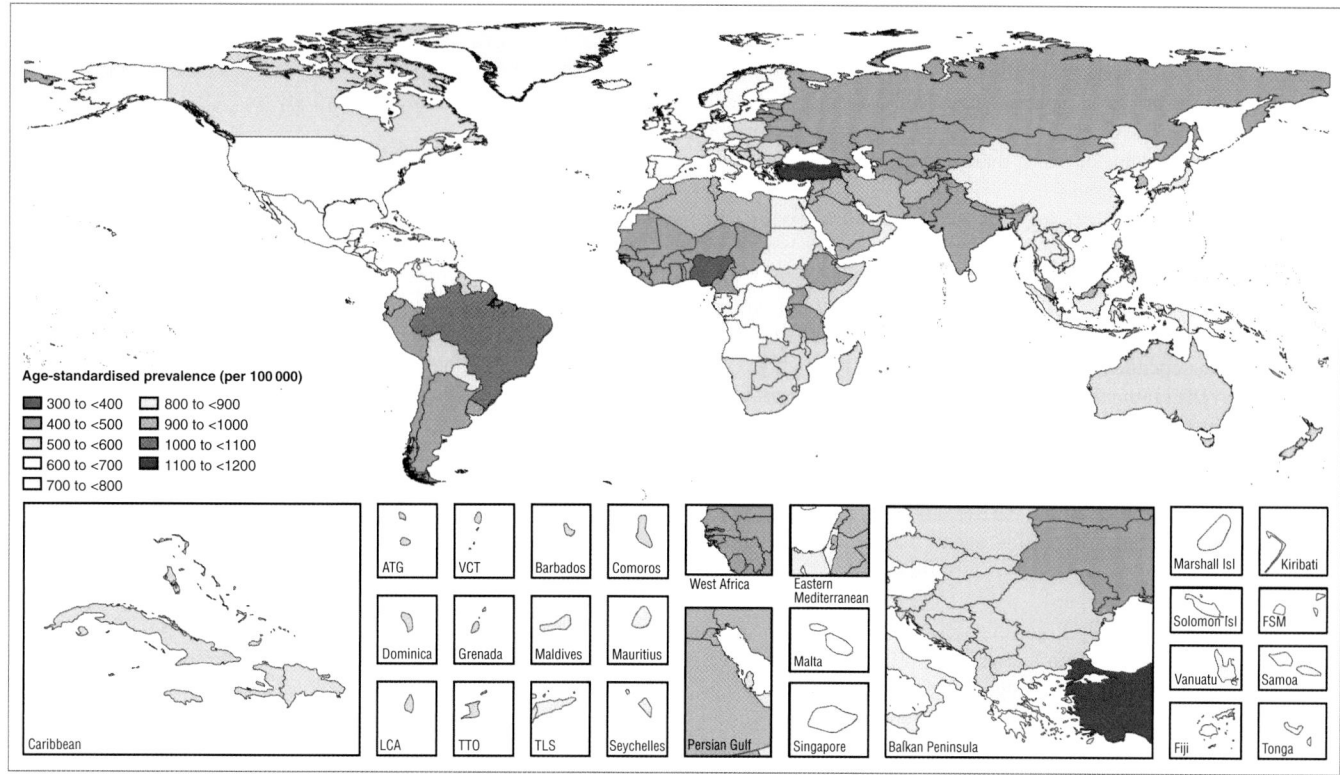

Fig. 27.1 Global age-standardized prevalence of Alzheimer's disease and other dementias by sex, 2016. (From GBD 2016 Dementia Collaborators. "Global, Regional, and National Burden of Alzheimer's Disease and Other Dementias, 1990–2016: a Systematic Analysis for the Global Burden of Disease Study 2016." The Lancet Neurology, vol. 18, no. 1, 26 Nov. 2018, pp. 88–106.)

whether it develops slowly over time or happens suddenly, should be diagnosed, and when possible, the underlying cause(s) of the delirium or dementia should be treated. Even if the cause of the dementia is untreatable, teaching the patient and significant others strategies to make the patient's ADLs and IADLs easier to manage is always possible.

Physical and occupational therapists are an important part of the comprehensive evaluation, treatment, and caregiver training for patients with delirium or dementia.[55–59] All treatment planning should occur as a part of a team effort in which the patient, the family or significant others, physician, nurses, social worker, physical therapist, and occupational therapist collaborate so that a consistent treatment plan and orientation are followed. Inclusion of the day-to-day caregivers is crucial for all training because they—more than anyone—need to know and use the adaptations for the patient's personal style of communication and how to facilitate functional movement for ADLs and IADLs.

PHYSIOLOGY OF AGING: RELEVANCE FOR SYMPTOMATOLOGY AND DIAGNOSIS OF DELIRIUM AND DEMENTIAS

The Normal Brain

The brain of a normal person at age 80 years shows several significant anatomical, physiological, and neurochemical changes when compared with the brain of a younger person. Brain weight decreases with advancing age.[60] Neuropathological changes, such as the deposition of senile plaques and neurofibrillary tangles, and multiple-domain cognitive decline do occur. However, such changes are not associated with

significant functional limitations in healthy older people. In contrast, older people with neurodegenerative conditions demonstrate tremendous neuronal loss and substantial declines in cognitive function.[61–63] Normal age-related changes vary from person to person in degree and severity and can include the following:

- Disturbance in the ability to register, retain, and recall certain recent experiences[33,64]
- Slowed rate of learning new material[36]
- Slowed motor performance on tasks that require speed[36,65]
- Difficulties with fine motor coordination and balance[66–72]

A motivated, upbeat older adult who is not undergoing emotional stress will show few negative changes in intellectual capacity and may actually demonstrate an increase in intellectual functioning over time.[29,73–75] Neuroplastic changes continue through old age and research has shown that specific parts of the brain can increase in volume, functional connectivity in the brain can improve, and cognitive performance can be enhanced if older persons are immersed in optimal experiences and exposed to enriched environments.[12,76–81]

Because many of the variables that need to be considered as part of the clinical evaluation of the rehabilitation potential of the person with dementia are affected by both aging and disease, therapists working with the older adult should be aware of these variables. The therapist explores ways to compensate for these changes; as a result, the patient will have a greater possibility of achieving her or his potential for self-care and contentment.

A slowing of the natural pace of movement is commonly noted in older adults. This slowdown is manifested in the brain as a slowing of resting electroencephalogram (EEG) rhythms (e.g., the mean frequency of the occipital rhythm is 10.3 Hz at the age of 60 years versus 8.7 Hz at the age of 80 years). The speed of nerve conduction in older adults can be 10% to 15% slower than in younger persons.[82–84] Because of these physiological changes, if the process and structure of evaluation and care of the healthy older adult emphasize speed of execution or timed activities, they will appear less capable than they really are. The therapist may need more time when working with persons older than 70 years than is generally required with younger individuals.

The brain is the most physiologically active organ in the body. The brain represents only 2% of the total body weight, yet it consumes up to 20% of the oxygen and 65% of the glucose available in the circulation in the entire body.[28] The minimal cardiovascular output required to deliver this is 0.75 L/min, which is equal to 20% of the total circulation (also dependent on body size). Because of the high level of nutrient use by the brain, it is one of the organs of the body most likely to be affected by any acute change in homeostasis. The homeostasis of the older adult brain is more vulnerable to disruption because of the normal age-related changes already discussed, as well as the increased permeability of the blood-brain barrier and increased sensitivity of neurons to the effects of outside agents such as drugs,[85] food, and allergens.

Arndt-Schulz Principle

The Arndt-Schulz principle summarizes the differences between the abilities of the younger brain and the aged brain to discriminate or respond to stimuli.[86] In older adults, a higher level or a longer period of stimulation is required before the threshold for initial physiological response is reached. Their physiological response is rarely as large, as visible, or as consistent as noted in younger individuals. The implication of the Arndt-Schulz principle for clinical problem solving is that the level of a stimulus (e.g., heat, cold, sound, light, or emotional input) needs to be adjusted to compensate for the altered physiology of the older adult patient. Optimal balance of the levels of sensory stimulation and emotional stimulation that is therapeutic for a young person may not be therapeutic for the older adult. The stimulus may be too low so it does not reach the threshold for generating a physiological response, or it may go beyond the safe therapeutic range for the older adult and become harmful. Therefore when an older adult patient does not respond to treatment or presents an unusual physical response, the clinician needs to ascertain whether the strength of the stimulus is too strong or too weak and whether modification of the stimulus is necessary because of factors associated with the aging process or the patient's cognitive deficits (e.g., he or she may be unable to accurately report the response because of a cognitive deficit). The older person with mild or moderate confusion needs small, slow clinical input and precise monitoring of the general response (heart rate, blood pressure, and respiration) as well as of the local response. This adjustment in approach is especially important for people with hearing impairment. Because the patient may not hear what is being spoken, the therapist may assume that the patient does not have the capability to comprehend what is being said.

Law of Initial Values

The law of initial values is both a physiological and a psychological principle stating that with a given intensity of stimulation, the degree of change produced tends to be greater when the initial value of that variable is low at the onset of stimulation. Therefore the higher the initial level of functioning, the smaller the change that can be produced.[87,88] The law of initial values, when defined and applied to younger individuals, presumes that homeostasis is a stable and consistent process. When the law is used to describe physiological and psychological responses in older adults, it cannot be presumed that homeostasis for any variable is predictable or consistent from one person to the next, or even within a 24-hour period for the same individual. For example, an older person with mild dementia may eat only sweets if left without companionship at a meal. As a result, after the meal, the individual may feel unsteady and afraid to walk back to the room.

Biorhythms

The brain has a biological clock that controls all physiological functions in a precise temporal course, whether daily (e.g., secretion of some hormones), monthly (e.g., menstruation), or during a certain period of the life cycle (e.g., ability to become pregnant)[89–91]. Before evaluating an older adult patient with dementia or a disturbance of intellectual functioning, assessment of the patient's premorbid biorhythm is helpful. What was his or her daily schedule of activities before the medical crisis? An assessment or time study can map such things as rest periods, activities and level of exertion, sleep or rest periods, mental stimulation, emotional stimulation, eating, and elimination cycles across a 24-hour period. The patient assessment must allow for and assess the current and past variability of individual biorhythms. These biorhythms should be clearly documented, and their stability should be evaluated and maintained as much as possible (critical if the patient will be going back to the family). Defining the peak times of day for awareness and intellectual capacity for each individual is necessary. For example, some patients are best able to participate in learning a new skill in the early morning, and some only in the late afternoon. If a woman has worked for 40 years as a night nurse, being primarily active from 11 p.m. to 7 a.m., she will most likely be alert and best able to participate in a rehabilitation program during those hours. In most cases the patient should be allowed to choose the best time for treatment. For patients whose dementia is too severe for them to make this determination, the staff can monitor the patient's behavior and choose a time for treatment when the person is most alert. For older adults with dementia, the time of assessment and treatment must be documented to maximize the person's rehabilitation potential.[92,93]

Cognitive Changes in Normal Aging

The idea that cognitive decline is a necessary part of aging is a myth. This belief has been debunked by research on crystallized and fluid intelligence.[94,95] Crystallized and fluid intelligence are components of general intelligence. Crystallized intelligence involves the ability to perceive relationships, engage in formal reasoning, and understand intellectual and cultural heritage. Crystallized intelligence can be affected by the environment and the attitude of the individual.[96] Crystallized intelligence can increase with self-directed learning and education as long as a person is alive. The measurement of crystallized intelligence is usually in the form of culture-specific items such as number facility, verbal comprehension, and general information.

Fluid intelligence, what has been called "native mental ability," is the product of the brain's information processing system. It includes attention and memory capacity and the speed of information processing used in thinking and acting.[97] It is not closely associated with acculturation. It is generally considered to be independent of instruction or environment and depends more on the genetic endowment of the individual.[4] The items used to test fluid intelligence include memory span, inductive reasoning, and figural relationships, all of which are presumed to be unresponsive to training. Because fluid intelligence involves those intellectual functions most affected by changes in neurophysiological status, it has been generally assumed to decline with age. Several studies have shown this to be untrue; one study noted that during middle age, scores on tests for fluid intelligence are similar to scores in midadolescence.[73,98] These changes, however, are primarily associated with processing speed, working memory, and executive function.[7,99]

Studies on the effects of cognitive changes in activities have shown that older people perform activities at a slower rate and use different areas of the brain in the process compared with younger people. Those additional areas of the brain used have mostly to do with monitoring and processing the ongoing activity.[8,100] Activities are therefore performed more in a feedback rather than a feedforward manner, which also requires more time. So, if older adults are given time to complete tasks, they usually do well.

Botwinick[101] described the classic pattern of changes in intelligence with aging. In the adult portion of the life-span, verbal abilities decline little, if at all, whereas psychomotor abilities decline earlier and to a greater extent (greater decline if the individual is not engaged in regular physical activity). The period between ages 55 and 70 years is a transition time, and some decreases in performance are noted on many cognitive tests. A substantial decline on laboratory tests of cognitive function is generally limited to those older than 75 years.[102] In these latter years, however, the decline in fluid intelligence is offset by the growth in crystallized intelligence for most people unless dementia is present (Fig. 27.2).[103] Although changes may be demonstrated in the laboratory, they may not be significant in the "real world," and the older adult may be as capable as the young of participating in rehabilitation training. For older adults to benefit maximally, however, they must control the pace of training because the tasks that are the most difficult for older adults are those that are fast paced, unusual, and complex.[104] All physical and occupational therapy treatments with older patients need to be structured to encourage the patient to set his or her own pace. The goal is to have a pace that allows ease of breathing and a comfortable, functional upright posture so that the person can enjoy the experience. Interventions should be predictable and progress by adding one new concept at a time.

Stress and Intellectual Capacity

Selye[75] defined stress as the nonspecific response of the body to any demand made on it. All human beings require a certain amount of stress to live and function effectively. When a stressor (stimulus) is applied, the body predictably goes through the three stages of response

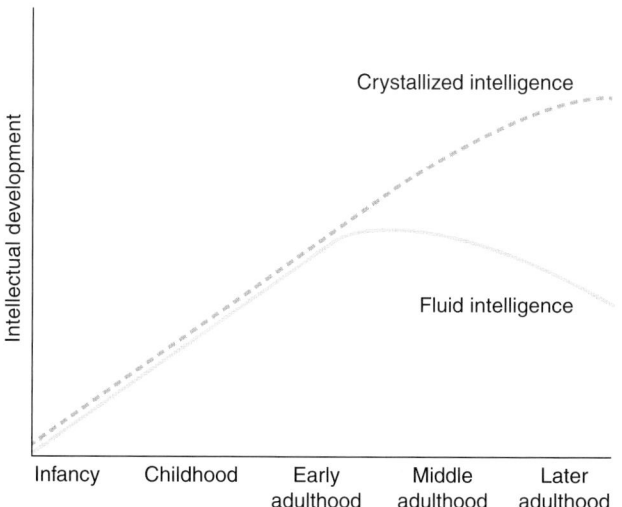

Fig. 27.2 Gains in crystallized intelligence throughout adulthood compensate for potential declines in fluid intelligence. (From Avers D, Williams A. "Cognition in the Aging Adult." Geriatric Physical Therapy, Elsevier Mosby, 2012, pp. 132–134.)

called the *general adaptation syndrome* (GAS). The first response is a general alarm reaction, a "fight-or-flight" response that mobilizes all senses in an effort to make a judgment about the response needed. The older person is at a disadvantage because collecting and processing accurate sensory data are decreased with normal aging owing to short-term memory loss. The sensory memory in an older person lasts less than 1 second.[36] The next stage involves judgment and the selective adaptation to the stressor. A decision is made regarding which action is needed, and all other bodily activities return to homeostasis. If the stimulus continues and goes beyond the therapeutic or functional level, then the body system or part will gradually experience physiological exhaustion. A person in physiological exhaustion is likely to manifest abnormal responses to any new stimulus.

When a person is under perceived stress (whether real or imagined), a predictable set of cognitive changes can occur such as preoccupation; forgetfulness; disorientation; confusion; low tolerance to ambiguity; errors in judgment in relation to work, distance, grammar, or mathematics; misidentification of people; inability to concentrate, solve problems, or plan; inattention to details or instructions; reduced creativity, fantasy, and perceptual field size; decreased initiative; decreased interest in usual activities, the future, or people; and irritability, impatience, anger, withdrawal, suspicion, depression, and crying. Differentiating whether the patient is having a stress reaction or has dementia is critical. If the changes occur with a sudden onset, they are probably related to a medical or pharmaceutical problem, which may be indicative of delirium and amenable to intervention.

With aging, the brain undergoes physiological changes that make the older people less physiologically efficient in her or his response to stressors. The general alarm reaction is poorly mobilized and takes longer to become activated (Arndt-Schulz principle). The stage of resistance should yield a series of responses that allows the body to economize in its response to stress. In persons of all ages who receive too many different stimuli and in older adults who experience normal levels of stimuli, the body becomes less efficient at turning off the general alarm response and replacing it with more appropriate and limited responses. When a person is overwhelmed by this type or level of stress, the individual may demonstrate mild global or specific cognitive impairments, especially mild short-term memory loss.[105]

The assessment of an older adult, with or without dementia, must include a determination of the type, number, and severity of the patient's current stressors. Positive life events (e.g., marriage or the birth of a grandchild) are also stressful life events. Scores that rate stressful life events can identify patients who are at greatest risk of physiological and emotional exhaustion.[106] Developed in the 1970s, the Holmes-Rahe Social Readjustment Rating Scale is still a commonly used life stress evaluation tool (see www.stresstips.com).[107] Older adults, with their numerous psychosocial problems and chronic and acute illnesses, are likely candidates for physiological and emotional exhaustion and the development of psychopathology. Thus the environment and process of rehabilitation need to be modified to counteract the effect of stress on the intellectual capacity of the older adult patient. Any action that modifies stress so that a deterioration of intellectual function is stopped or reversed is an efficient and cost-effective part of the total rehabilitation effort.

STRATEGIES FOR ASSESSING, PREVENTING, AND MINIMIZING DISTORTIONS IN INFORMATION PROCESSING

At the outset of the process of patient assessment, *it is important to identify whether the patient communicates best with verbal, written, or a combination of both strategies.* With an overview of the patient's cognitive capacity, the rehabilitation staff may be able to modify the process of evaluation to maximize the patient's performance (e.g., several 15-minute interactions spread over the 8-hour workday instead of an hour without rest; performing the assessment in the presence of a regular caregiver the patient trusts). A basic assessment of the patient's functional abilities (ADLs and IADLs) at a given moment to allow a comparison of cognitive capacity at other times in the 24-hour cycle provides the clinician a specific description of what aspects of intellectual function appear to be impaired and pinpoints those aspects of intellectual functioning that are still intact. Based on this approach, the rehabilitation evaluation can proceed in a language (perhaps the native language of childhood) and at a pace that are comfortable for the patient and at the time of day when the patient is most alert.

Screening Tests for Cognitive Impairment

The Mini-Mental State Examination (MMSE) provides a screening test for identifying unrecognized cognitive disorders in older adults. The MMSE assesses only cognition and can identify whether the patient is oriented; remembers (short term); and can read, write, calculate, and see and reproduce in drawing the relation of one object or figure to another. The MMSE may also be used in a serial fashion to quantify changes in a patient's cognitive status over time. All caregivers must be part of the team effort to get a real 24-hour picture of the cognitive capacities of the patient. This examination can be used as a springboard for planning how to carry out the traditional rehabilitation evaluation of a patient who has some intellectual dysfunction.[108,109]

The MMSE has been standardized for older adults living in the community, with scores correlating significantly with the Wechsler Adult Intelligence Scale and the Wechsler Memory Test. It has been found that when a cutoff score of 24 is used for the detection of dementia, the MMSE had a sensitivity of 87.6% and a specificity of 81.6%.[110] Several studies have noted that interviews with informants are highly consistent with older adults' scores on the MMSE.[111]

The entire examination grades cognitive performance on a scale from 0 to 30. A score of 24 or less usually indicates some degree of cognitive dysfunction, but some patients with dementia may score above 24 and some with depression or delirium may score significantly below 24. A low score on this examination can mean that the patient probably has dementia, delirium, mental retardation, amnestic syndrome, or aphasia. A low score on the MMSE can indicate the areas of specific cognitive impairment and gives the rehabilitation team data about how to best communicate with the patient. MMSE scores are also correlated with educational level, with scores dropping 10% to 20% for people with an eighth-grade education or less if older than 70 years.[112] A shortened version of the MMSE has been developed that uses only 12 of the 20 original variables.

The MMSE was freely available when it was first released in 1975, but its developers have since enforced copyright use restrictions[113,114] (USD 81 for 50 test forms, as of 2018).[115] Fortunately, a growing number of screening tools have been developed and could be used as possible alternatives to the MMSE.[114,116–118] Free educational versions of the MMSE are widely available on the Internet, including sites such as those maintained by Oxford Medical Education.[118a] In 2013, the Alzheimer's Association formed a workgroup to develop recommendations that would operationalize cognitive assessment in the primary care setting. As mandated in the Patient Protection and Affordable Care Act of 2010, Medicare beneficiaries can avail an Annual Wellness Visit (AWV), which includes the detection of any cognitive impairment by assessing an individual's cognitive function.[119] The assessment should be done using direct observation while taking into account

---

BOX 27.1   Brief Cognitive Impairment Screening Tools

Ascertain Dementia 8-item Informant Questionnaire (AD8)
Clock Drawing Test (CDT)
General Practitioner Assessment of Cognition (GPCOG)
Memory Impairment Screen (MIS)
Mini-Cog
Montreal Cognitive Assessment (MoCA)
Short Informant Questionnaire on Cognitive Decline in the Elderly (Short IQCODE)
Short Portable Mental Status Questionnaire (SPMSQ)
St. Louis University Mental Status (SLUMS)
Verbal Fluency
7-minute Screen (7MS)

From Cordell CB, Borson S, Boustani M, et al. Alzheimer's Association recommendations for operationalizing the detection of cognitive impairment during the Medicare annual wellness visit in a primary care setting." *Alzheimers Dement.* 2013;9(2):141–150. doi:https://doi.org/10.1016/j.jalz.2012.09.011; Lin JS, O'Connor E, Rossom RC, et al. Screening for cognitive impairment in older adults: a systematic review for the US Preventive Services Task Force. *Ann Intern Med.* 2013;159(9):601–612.

---

information obtained subjectively from the patient, the patient's care providers, family, friends, and others concerned. The workgroup identified the Memory Impairment Screen (MIS), General Practitioner Assessment of Cognition (GPCOG), and Mini-Cog as suitable brief cognitive assessment tools in primary care. All three tools require less than 5 minutes to administer, have been validated in a primary care setting, have good-to-excellent psychometric properties, and do not require permission or payment for copyrights when used in the clinical setting.[114] Clinicians may also select from a number of alternate tools in Box 27.1 and supplement the information with those obtained from a patient informant using the Ascertain Dementia 8-item Informant Questionnaire (AD8), GPCOG informant score, and short Informant Questionnaire on Cognitive Decline in the Elderly (Short IQCODE). Patients who present with any indication/s of cognitive impairment would need to be referred for further evaluation, as shown in Fig. 27.3.

The recent American Academy of Neurology guideline on mild cognitive impairment (MCI) recommends the assessment for MCI in cases wherein a patient and/or a close contact voices concern about memory or impaired cognition.[120] The guideline further emphasizes that clinicians not assume such concerns as a part of normal aging. Validated assessment tools should be used in the screening process, and if positive, more formal clinical assessment should follow. The guideline cautions against a premature diagnosis of dementia in the absence of functional impairments and detailed testing. Lastly, clinicians lacking experience and training in assessing cognitive impairments should refer patients suspected of having MCI to the appropriate specialist. A summary of the practice recommendations is outlined in Table 27.3.

Sensory and Perceptual Changes With Dementia

Patients with dementia may have specific problems that inhibit the integration of sensory input. Aphasias and disruption of association pathways may inhibit the patient's ability to integrate accurately perceived sensory information in a meaningful way. Patients with AD, multiinfarct dementia,[121] and alcoholic dementia may demonstrate disturbances in visual acuity, depth perception, color differentiation, and differentiation of figure from ground when compared with normal age-matched control adults and normal younger adults.

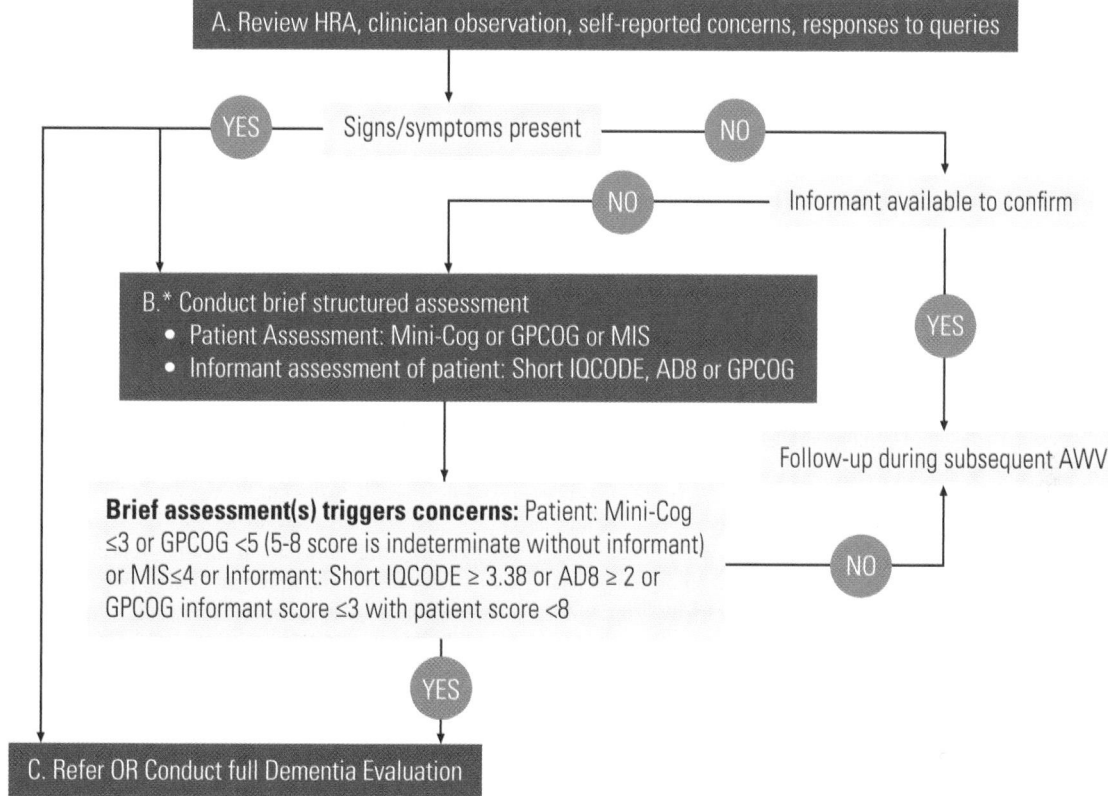

ALZHEIMER'S ASSOCIATION®

Medicare Annual Wellness Visit Algorithm for Assessment of Cognition

A. Review HRA, clinician observation, self-reported concerns, responses to queries

YES — Signs/symptoms present — NO

NO — Informant available to confirm

YES

B.* Conduct brief structured assessment
- Patient Assessment: Mini-Cog or GPCOG or MIS
- Informant assessment of patient: Short IQCODE, AD8 or GPCOG

Follow-up during subsequent AWV

Brief assessment(s) triggers concerns: Patient: Mini-Cog ≤3 or GPCOG <5 (5-8 score is indeterminate without informant) or MIS≤4 or Informant: Short IQCODE ≥ 3.38 or AD8 ≥ 2 or GPCOG informant score ≤3 with patient score <8

NO

YES

C. Refer OR Conduct full Dementia Evaluation

* No one tool is recognized as the best brief assessment to determine if a full dementia evaluation is needed. Some providers repeat patient assessment with an alternate tool (e.g., SLUMS, or MoCA) to confirm initial findings before referral or initiation of full dementia evaluation.

AD8 = Eight-item Informant Interview to Differentiate Aging and Dementia; **AWV =** Annual Wellness Visit; **GPCOG =** General Practitioner Assessment of Cognition; **HRA =** Health Risk Assessment; **MIS =** Memory Impairment Screen; **MMSE =** Mini Mental Status Exam; **MoCA =** Montreal Cognitive Assessment; **SLUMS =** St. Louis University Mental Status Exam; **Short IQCODE =** Short Informant Questionnaire on Cognitive Decline in the Elderly

Cordell CB, Borson S, Boustani M, Chodosh J, Reuben D, Verghese J, et al. Alzheimer's Association recommendations for operationalizing the detection of cognitive impairment during the Medicare Annual Wellness Visit in a primary care setting. *Alzheimers Dement.* 2013;9(2):141-150. Available at http://download.journals.elsevierhealth.com/pdfs/journals/1552-5260/PIIS1552526012025010.pdf.

800.272.3900 | alz.org®   alzheimer's ᪥ association®

Fig. 27.3 Alzheimer's Association Medicare Annual Wellness Visit Algorithm for Assessment of Cognition. (From Avers D, Williams A. "Cognition in the Aging Adult." Geriatric Physical Therapy, Elsevier Mosby, 2012, pp. 132–134. In the book this is Figure 8.2.)

TABLE 27.3   Practice Recommendations in the Assessment of Mild Cognitive Impairment

Recommendation	Grade
For patients for whom the patient or a close contact voices concern about memory or impaired cognition, clinicians should assess for MCI and not assume the concerns are related to normal aging	B
When performing a Medicare Annual Wellness Visit, clinicians should not rely on historical report of subjective memory concerns alone when assessing for cognitive impairment	B
For patients for whom screening or assessing for MCI is appropriate, clinicians should use validated assessment tools to assess for cognitive impairment	B
For patients who test positive for MCI, clinicians should perform a more formal clinical assessment for diagnosis of MCI	B
For patients with MCI, clinicians should assess for the presence of functional impairment related to cognition before giving a diagnosis of dementia	B
For patients suspected to have MCI, clinicians who lack the necessary experience should refer these patients to a specialist with experience in cognition	B
For patients diagnosed with MCI, clinicians should perform a medical evaluation for MCI risk factors that are potentially modifiable	B
For patients and families asking about biomarkers in MCI, clinicians should counsel that there are no accepted biomarkers available at this time	B
For patients diagnosed with MCI, clinicians should perform serial assessments over time to monitor for changes in cognitive status	B

MCI, Mild cognitive impairment.
From Petersen RC, Lopez O, Armstrong MJ. Practice guideline update summary: mild cognitive impairment: report of the Guideline Development, Dissemination, and Implementation Subcommittee of the American Academy of Neurology. *Neurology.* 2018;90(3):126–135; DOI:10.1212/WNL.0000000000004826

An assessment of specific sensory systems is necessary when a person demonstrates cognitive losses. The challenge in rehabilitation is to design a process and environment of care so that compensation and modification maximize the ability of the older adult with sensory deficits to adapt to most life situations. The example of visual deficits is a case in point. One of every two blind persons in the United States is older than 65 years (see www.afb.org/ and click on AFB senior site).[122] Techniques of environmental adaptation and special measures to organize care to help blind older adults have allowed many of them to live independently in the community.[123] However, many older adults with visual impairments are not blind. Some of the structural changes that result in mild to moderate deficits of vision include yellowing; uneven growth, striation, and thickening of the lens; increasing weakness of the muscles controlling the eye; alteration in the perception of color (especially fine distinctions in tone and brightness); and slower adaptation to light.[124] Modifications of the environment can include adequate effective lighting (including adequate intensity and controlling of reflection), dark and clear large-print, low-vision aids (e.g., magnifying glass), verbal orientation and escort by persons accompanying patients in a new environment, consistent furniture placement, explanation when changes occur, clear hallways, a systematic storage system for clothes and toilet articles, and the use of consistent contrasting colors to identify doors, windows, baseboards, and corners.[124–127]

Older Adult Learning Styles and Communication

Learning occurs throughout life.[104] In physical and occupational therapy, habilitation occurs when the patient learns new skills, and rehabilitation occurs when the person relearns old adaptive skills. As with intelligence, the learning process does not change abruptly when an individual reaches old age, but differences in performance have been reported. One challenge for rehabilitation therapy is to find ways to improve the efficiency of learning by the older person (Box 27.2).

Learning and performance are not the same. Poor performance on a learning task may mean that insufficient learning has occurred, that learning has not transferred to a new environment or task, or that

the performance does not accurately reflect the extent of learning achieved.[4] The key variables that affect a person's ability to participate in a learning task can include intelligence, learning skills acquired over the years, and flexibility of learning style. Noncognitive factors can also have a strong bearing on an individual's performance. The noncognitive factors include visual and auditory acuity, health status, motivation to learn, level of anxiety, the speed at which stimuli and learning is paced, and the meaningfulness to the individual of the items or tasks to be learned. Research has shown that learning styles change over the life-span and that people learn better when instructional approaches are matched to their learning style.[37] Therefore a rehabilitation assessment needs to include a review of the preferred learning style of the patient. This strategy is particularly important before discharging a patient from a rehabilitation program. The rationale is that a lack of progress may not reflect the patient's lack of capacity for rehabilitation but rather may reflect a dissonance between the patient's learning style and skills with the presentation of materials in the treatment program (e.g., verbal input has not been adapted to match the level or pace of comprehension of a person who may have a strong preference for visual learning and slower pace).

Interference

Interference can make the learning process less efficient in two major ways.[128] First, interference can result from a conflict between present knowledge and the new knowledge to be learned. Second, if the task to be learned has two or more components, secondary components may interfere with the learning of primary components. This situation is particularly true if secondary components overlap in time or use the same sensory modality.[97] Older adults have special difficulties if they must concentrate on intake, attention, and retrieval processes at the same time. Therefore the process and therapeutic environment of rehabilitation for the older adult patient must not be disturbed by background noise, other stimuli in the environment, or anxiety. When learning a new task, the older adult patient may require a quiet room with no stimuli other than that offered by the therapist. The need to rid the environment of distractions is particularly important when working with an older adult patient with dementia because this patient will have greater difficulty filtering out irrelevant sensory input compared with other patients without dementia.

Pacing

The pacing of therapeutic intervention is a significant variable in helping an older adult learn. Older adults (with or without dementia) perform best if they are given as much time as they need and when learning is self-paced.[101] The major drawback of a fast pace (as perceived by the patient) is that an older adult generally chooses not to participate rather than risk making a mistake. A lack of response by the patient is often interpreted as apathy, poor motivation, or "confusion."[129] Patient participation is increased when extra time to complete a rehabilitation task is offered. After the individual assessment, group work (where concepts can be presented, reviewed, and examined at leisure) also can be used to reduce the psychological pressure of faster paced one-on-one learning. The details of therapy must be planned carefully, including how questions are asked (this involves asking clear and precise questions in nonmedical language) and, most importantly, setting aside enough treatment time so the patient can respond at a manageable pace.

Organization

If data are organized in the brain as part of the learning process, the retrieval of these data becomes easier. Older persons are less likely than members of other age groups to organize data spontaneously to facilitate learning and later retrieval (memory) of that learning.[130] Older adults who are highly verbal show fewer weaknesses in the ability to organize stimuli. Older adults with poor verbal skills show significant improvement in data retrieval when strategies for data organization are provided by others (e.g., the therapist). In addition, organizing therapy by beginning with an overview of the entire lesson may be helpful as this presents a conceptual map of the learning experience. Older learners have difficulty following content because they cannot anticipate what will be taught and do not see the "whole picture" of what is being presented.[131] The use of purposeful organizing can help bridge the gap between what the older person knows and the new information or task to be learned. This is an example of how organization may influence the learning process.

Inefficient learning and, at times, an inability to learn occur in the older adult if material is presented in one way and the older person is expected to apply it in some other way. Instructions need to be provided in the format and context in which they are to be used. If possible, pieces of new data should be presented one at a time. A conscious transition needs to be made by the therapist from the patient's current frame of reference to the understanding of the new data, and the pace needs to be set by the patient.

Several other strategies exist for maximizing the efficiency of older adult learners based on awareness of normal age-related changes. Some of the more frequently used techniques are summarized in Box 27.2.

Communication

Therapists can begin by inquiring into what the reality of the patient looks like. The first goal should be to communicate with words, gestures, positioning, and so on, so that stimuli bring out functional responses in the patient.

The therapist needs to be sensitive to the entire communication—what is said and what is withheld. The patient with cognitive problems may not understand the content, but many patients still have the ability to sense and respond to the therapist's affective state at the moment. When beginning communication, be clear of all previous concerns and

---

BOX 27.2 Techniques for Maximizing the Efficiency of Older Adult Learners

1. Use mediators; the association of words, story, mnemonics, or visual inputs can help the person remember.
2. Choose learning activities that are meaningful for the patient.
3. Use concrete examples to make learning easier.
4. Provide a supportive learning environment to prevent stress, which can interfere with efficient learning.
5. Use supportive or neutral feedback and avoid feedback that is presented in a challenging tone.
6. Reward all responses, but reward correct responses more than incorrect responses. This can encourage older adults persons to decrease the number of errors by omission, which are often interpreted as apathy or lack of cooperation.
7. Use combinations of auditory and visual input to facilitate the learning process. This is effective only if the data presented are similar because variation between the two kinds of messages can result in interference and a decrease in the efficiency of learning.
8. Active learning is more effective. A patient who moves the involved body part while receiving verbal and visual input is likely to better master the new skill.
9. Design the learning situation so that successful completion of the task is likely. Older people are more likely to focus on errors, which increases anxiety and lowers self-esteem. Worst of all, with all the energy focused on the error, there is a strong chance of repeating the error.

---

bring no extraneous emotions into the interaction. Caregivers and therapists bring into the conversation the power of intention to create a therapeutic interaction and the choice to stay on task. Patients bring their own set of concerns at any particular moment. Knowing something about the patient's concerns helps the process.

Therapists and caregivers need to be self-aware. What is the therapist's favorite strategy for communication? What is the therapist's favorite sentence structure? Our habitual forms of presentation need to be assessed with regard to whether they are effective, because the patient needs to be the focus of attention. Honoring the communication habits of the patient is necessary if effective communication is to occur with a person with cognitive deficits. If the therapist chooses to speak to the patient as if there were no cognitive deficits, consistent results will not occur, and the patient may be upset or agitated. The patient could be approached as if he or she were a person from another culture that has its unique customs, norms, and ways of communication. The patient-therapist interaction becomes an inquiry in which success is measured by the achievement of functional outcomes that are needed and wanted (e.g., the patient transferring into bed and feeling safe).

Now the question becomes what is the specific process of interaction with which the patient appears to be most comfortable and feels safe? Every patient is different, and it may depend on the time of day or whether the patient is feeling tired or threatened. Persons commonly respond best to one particular style of communication and are predictably upset or agitated by another style. If a patient wants to joke around and be playful, this should be a cue to staff that this is a workable style of communication. Another patient smiles whenever the tone of the conversation is soft, nurturing, and tender, and if staff is willing, this is where ease of relating can occur. Other patients relate best to rules and need predictable structures and boundaries. They love to know what is coming next. Still another category is people who can relate and communicate when definite admiration and respect are built into the conversation or when patient and therapist can agree to disagree. Each patient with cognitive problems needs to have caregivers develop a chart of what works to create a sense of relatedness and ease in communication. A challenge here for caregivers is that the patient's abilities can change; guidelines for communication when new caregivers are introduced to the patient can also be helpful. Someone who is familiar and enjoys interacting with the patient should introduce new staff to the patient.

For people with cognitive disturbances, familiarity and rituals are keys to the ease of adaptability. The basis for rituals is well-organized documentation to which all caregivers have access and contribute on an ongoing basis. This information needs to be filtered and organized so that each shift can see what is working for the patient today. Even a nonverbal patient can relate effectively to bathing if a ritual exists regarding dressing and undressing (e.g., the socks always come off first). Another detail that requires staff or caregiver attention, evaluation, and adaptation in daily care is *ideational apraxia*. LeClerc and Wells[132] described this as "a condition in which an individual is unable to plan movement related to an object because he or she has lost the perception of the object's purpose." Consideration is especially important in relation to feeding, dressing, toileting, and bathing. The authors described a tool that can help caregivers assess ideational apraxia and problem-solving compensations to prevent unnecessary agitation or disability and take actions to preserve existing abilities. Savelkoul and colleagues[133] emphasized the importance of effective communication between staff and patients and the importance of routines for patient care to maximize functional behaviors for institutionalized older adults living in residential homes.

As a patient goes through gradual deterioration of cognitive status, as is common in AD, staff, family, and caregivers must be trained in nonverbal, positional, and manual cues and emotional communication techniques. Many patients come to a place in their lives with dementia when words are a source of confusion. Other strategies to communicate should then be used. Sign language is initially a possible tool until the associative functions begin to disappear. Accurate assessment needs to create adaptations in communication. It may be necessary to use hand-guided communication, in which the patient is led through a task or parts of a task to get his or her cooperation. At this stage of communication, ease and trust are the most important goals. It may take 5 minutes of tenderly holding a patient's hand before the patient is ready to walk to the dining room or bathroom. This strategy requires much patience on the part of caregivers. Positional communication can be used as well as simple touch. As patients begin to feel safe with their state of being, they will relax and choose to participate. At times, patients have unique needs, such as only wanting to be cared for by a female caregiver or a male caregiver. Honoring patient needs is critical because the cognitively impaired may not be able to learn or adapt to the demands of the staff member because of previous trauma (assault or incest, real or imagined).

As a way to summarize the considerations regarding communication with a person with cognitive impairment, therapists may find it useful to examine their own intentions from moment to moment. "What is my goal in this interaction?" "Who am I being at this moment?" The task may be important, and the "doing" of it may be critical. For the patient with cognitive disturbance, therapists must provide life-enhancing stimuli on the basis of the patient's perceptions. If in the zeal to "do," the patient is accidentally scared, intimidated, or bullied, the damage may not be able to be undone. The patient with cognitive impairment presents a unique challenge if a threat has been created, because reestablishing their trust is often difficult. Often, the patient may be afraid of the therapist and simply needs the therapist to leave the room for some time. The saving grace for many patients is that their short-term memory is poor so they may not remember the incident tomorrow. The problem with agitation occurs when other patients who are cognitively impaired in the area also get upset.

The solution to the crisis moment, when a breakdown in communication has occurred, is to redirect communication and the focus of the present moment effectively. For example, a staff member could purposely bump into a chair and knock it over, drop a cup of water or a book, start to sing, whistle loudly, or clap his or her hands. At that moment, a distraction is created. If the distraction works, then the patient's attention is pulled away from his or her old thought and focused to a new topic. At that moment, the staff needs to be intentional. The new focus needs to offer comfort or nurturing or a predictable sense of well-being (e.g., helping to clean up, eating some food, looking at a picture of a favorite thing, holding a favorite item, touching a favorite comfort object, hugging).

ENVIRONMENTAL CONSIDERATIONS

Hypothermia

The temperature of the living environment must be carefully controlled because older adult patients may not perceive that the environment is cold and may not experience shivering. Accidental hypothermia can develop in an older person even at temperatures of 60°F (15.5°C) to 65°F (18.3°C). Accidental hypothermia is a drop in the core body temperature to less than 95°F (35°C). Patients at risk for hypothermia are presented in Box 27.3.

The symptoms of hypothermia may include a bloated face, pale and waxy or pinkish skin color, trembling on one side of the body without shivering, irregular and slowed heartbeat, slurred speech, shallow and slow breathing, low blood pressure, drowsiness, and symptoms of delirium. The two principles of treatment of hypothermia are that the person will stay chilled unless the body temperature is slowly increased and that he or she should be evaluated by a physician, regardless of the apparent severity of the hypothermia.[4,134]

If a person continues to be at risk for hypothermia, specific measures can be taken to prevent subsequent distortions of cognitive status. First, the room temperature should be set to at least 70°F (21°C). Second, the person should wear adequate clothing; this may include long underwear and an undershirt. Adequate nutrition also may be a factor in preventing hypothermia.

Patients and their caregivers may attempt to save money by lowering room temperatures and thus inadvertently cause hypothermia. To prevent accidental hypothermia in institutions with central air conditioning, special accommodations for older adults, such as a special wing of the building or individual temperature controls in the rooms, are required.[134]

Transplantation Shock

Some older adults seem to function well in a familiar environment but become severely disoriented and unable to perform ADLs if taken out of their own homes. As a general rule, these persons have mild

---

BOX 27.3 Patients at High Risk for Hypothermia

Persons older than 65 years

Persons showing no signs of shivering or pale skin in response to cold

Persons taking medications containing a phenothiazine (to treat psychosis or nausea)

Persons with disorders of the hormone system, especially hypothyroidism

Persons with head injuries, strokes, Alzheimer's disease or other dementia, Parkinson disease, or other neurological conditions

Persons with severe arthritis

Persons with arteriosclerotic peripheral vascular disease, chronic ulceration, or amputation

symptoms of dementia that are not readily apparent when they remain in a structured, familiar, stable environment and maintain a consistent daily routine. When faced with the need to adapt to a new environment bombarded with multiple unfamiliar sensory stimuli, however, their limited brain capacity is unable to make sense of the large volume of new stimuli. If a patient was oriented before admission to an institution and then becomes disoriented, the patient's cognitive functioning will likely return to its baseline level of functioning on return to the familiar environment. Therefore all moves by a patient from one hospital room to another or from one institution to another, and all changes in a treatment regimen, need to be carefully planned. If a change is anticipated, the patient should be involved in the decision making. If the change is a permanent move, the patient needs to have a chance for one or two trial visits before the actual move. The patient needs to be informed of all changes well in advance, and this information needs to be given repeatedly to the patient with dementia. The precautions mentioned can help the patient relocate without creating transplantation shock and any related negative cognitive and emotional changes.

DELIRIUM AND REVERSIBLE DEMENTIA: EVALUATION AND TREATMENT

This section focuses on the patient's internal environment (physiological, psychological, spiritual, and pathological) and presumes that all unnecessary external environmental stressors have been removed.

Delirium and dementia have been previously defined (see Table 27.1) and differentiated (see Table 27.2). Delirium can manifest suddenly or over a period of hours or days. Delirium may occasionally be chronic, but this is relatively infrequent. Dementia usually has a much longer time of onset, although an acute onset can occur.

Diagnosis of the underlying cause of dementia or delirium is key to effective care. Although the diagnostic process is primarily at the level of pathology, the therapist can obtain information, as part of a team evaluation, which will help establish the underlying diagnosis. Historical information needs to be obtained regarding the following:

- The amount of time that has elapsed since the onset of symptoms
- The progression or lack of progression of symptoms
- Associated functional impairments and associated medical signs and symptoms
- Use of prescription drugs, over-the-counter medications, home remedies, illegal drugs, alcohol, caffeine, and nicotine
- Exposure to toxins at work or during recreation

Even in a patient with cognitive disturbances, this information can frequently be obtained and corroborated by obtaining a history from significant others.

The causes of delirium and reversible dementia are many. In older adults however, certain causes are more common than others (Box 27.4). Alcohol and drugs (prescribed, over-the-counter, or illegal medications and home remedies) are prime offenders (see Chapter 36). The delirium may be the result of intoxication, side effects, or withdrawal syndromes.[135] Benzodiazepines are among the most

---

BOX 27.4 Common Causes of Delirium and Reversible Dementia

Alcohol or Drug Abuse or Dependence
Intoxication
Toxicity
Side effects
Withdrawal

Cardiovascular or Pulmonary Conditions
Congestive heart failure
Cardiac arrhythmia
Hypertensive crisis
Hypoxia
Chronic obstructive pulmonary disease

Metabolic or Endocrine Conditions
Electrolyte disturbance (especially hyponatremia)
Hypercalcemia
Dehydration
Overhydration
Renal failure
Hypoglycemia
Diabetic ketoacidosis
Hypothyroidism
Hyperthyroidism
Malnutrition
Vitamin B_{12} or folate deficiency
Hepatic failure
Wernicke-Korsakoff syndrome
Cushing syndrome

Infection
Urinary tract infection
Pneumonia or acute bronchitis

Tuberculosis
Other acute infections

Neurological Conditions
Stroke
Head trauma
Mass lesion (e.g., tumor, hematoma)
Seizure

Pharmacological Causes
Benzodiazepines
Barbiturates and other sedative-hypnotics
Antidepressants
Neuroleptics
Antihistamines
Anticholinergics
Cardiac glycosides
Steroids
Antineoplastic drugs
Narcotics
Antiarrhythmics
Antihypertensives

Miscellaneous Causes
Sensory deprivation
Sensory overstimulation
Acute or chronic pain
Constipation or fecal impaction
Urinary retention

commonly prescribed offenders; even a low dose (2 mg) may cause demonstrable cognitive changes.[74] Other common drugs that cause delirium or reversible dementia are alcohol, oral narcotics, psychotropic medications, steroids, antineoplastic drugs, digoxin, anesthetic agents, antiparkinsonian drugs, and antihistamines. However, all drugs have the potential to cause significant cognitive problems in older adults.[136] These symptoms often resolve with discontinuation of the offending agent or treatment of the withdrawal syndrome. For some patients, a medication holiday of longer than 24 hours may be needed before a positive change in cognition can be noted.[93]

At times, the symptoms may be clearly correlated with the pharmacokinetic profiles of the medications taken by the patient. The dose or frequency of administration of medications can be a contributing factor to a delirious state.[137] Every member of the rehabilitation team needs to document the patient's ability to participate in learning tasks and the time of the assessment because timing of medication administration can affect functional performance. The rehabilitation team needs the input of a clinical pharmacologist who can help the team focus on concepts such as biological half-life, clearance, bioavailability of drugs, and the time course of drug concentration in plasma as a function of dose and frequency.

Several medical diseases are likely to cause symptoms of delirium. Urinary tract infections, more common in women, are the cause of delirium in 28%[138] of older adults patients. Fecal impaction is another common cause of acute cognitive change in older adults persons. Others are distended bladder caused by prostate enlargement or drug-induced urinary retention, dehydration, malnutrition, cardiovascular disorders,[134] metabolic disturbances (particularly undiagnosed diabetes mellitus),[28] endocrine diseases, renal diseases, hematological diseases, pneumonia or bronchitis,[134] and vitamin B_{12} deficiency.

Transient (and usually mild) cognitive deficits may be the result of a cerebrovascular accident (CVA). The cognitive deficits after a CVA are often reversible, although they may last for several months after the stroke. The rehabilitation team needs to evaluate and regularly reevaluate the patient's cognitive capacity and build a program of care around current abilities. A program of therapeutic intervention that allows the older person to work in a self-paced program for 1 to 3 months can yield good therapeutic results and prevent unnecessary secondary deconditioning until part or all of the patient's cognitive capacity returns.[139]

In older adults, depression shares some common characteristics with dementia, making diagnosis and management more complicated[134,140,141]. Depression can result in mild and subtle cognitive changes affecting immediate recall, attention, and the ability to perform basic ADLs. A history of depression has been implicated in increasing the risk for both all-cause dementia and AD. Together with memory and cognitive decline, depression has also been reported to precede dementia by 12 years.[140] Depression is a treatable disorder, and many patients with cognitive impairments show some improvement in their cognitive functioning if the depression is treated; however, the underlying cognitive problem does not resolve with treatment of the depression.[142] Because the presence of depression can interfere with the progress of rehabilitation through cognitive deficits or its effects on motivation, this disorder needs to be diagnosed early and accurately. The Geriatric Depression Scale (GDS), a 30-item yes-no questionnaire, screens for this disorder.[143] A shorter 15-item version is also available and has shown strong correlation (0.96) with the 30-item version.[144,145] Both long and short versions have been translated in multiple languages, and can be freely accessed in the authors' website (https://web.stanford.edu/~yesavage/GDS.html). The 15-item GDS is also available as a free mobile app in both Android and iPhone platforms. Scores >11 in the 30-item GDS, and >5 in the 15-item version indicate possible depression in older adults.[145–147]

The treatment of major depression generally involves pharmacotherapy, psychotherapy, and environmental manipulation, which can require support from the entire rehabilitation team.[148] In the treatment of a patient with depression, therapeutic techniques can promote a relaxation response, enhance upright posture, decrease anxiety level (e.g., through massage or heat), and help bring the patient to the point at which aerobic training is possible and can provide a beneficial effect. All aerobic training for older adults needs to begin with a stress test, modified as necessary to determine the patient's exercise target heart rate. The modification most commonly required is use of the upper extremities to achieve the training effect, because lower-extremity function may be limited, or use of major ADLs involving the upper extremities as the stress test or training program.

The causes of delirium are usually treatable, and if diagnosis and care are provided in a timely fashion, the patient can likely regain full command of his or her cognitive processes. When this does not happen, the patient probably had mild, irreversible dementia that remained hidden until the onset of an acute problem that uncovered the poor cognitive functioning. The length of time in an institution (hospital or nursing home) needs to be kept as short as possible to avoid learned dependency and learned helplessness,[148] which make a return to full cognitive functioning and independent living difficult.[141]

Therapy for older adults with delirium consists of treating the underlying causes of the cognitive changes. A close working relationship among all members of the rehabilitation team, including a geriatric psychiatric consultant, is necessary. Even before the cause of the disorder is elucidated, the patient should receive the same emotional and physical support as any patient with dementia. The therapist must adapt all activities to the extent and types of cognitive losses that are present. The patient needs to feel secure, live in an environment that has as few changes as possible, and have a consistent and stable schedule for activities.

IRREVERSIBLE DEMENTIA

The course of dementia is unique for each patient. The variation in clinical course occurs based on the cause of the underlying disease and superimposed biological and psychosocial factors, including medications, concurrent illness (including delirium), the nature of the social support system, and the patient's premorbid personality structure. The causes of irreversible dementia are summarized in Box 27.5.

Regardless of the cause of the dementia, the clinical course of these disorders has several commonalities.[98] Most of these diseases are progressive. Symptoms may be subtle early in the course of the illness, and the onset of disease is usually noted by the person with the disorder, family members, friends, or colleagues at work rather than by a physician. The signs of impairment of mental ability are typically memory loss, poor judgment, or incompetence at work. The patient can often succeed at hiding his or her symptoms for a while. The social consequences of the cognitive impairment usually bring the patient to the attention of health care professionals. In addition, the patient with dementia can manifest a variety of psychiatric symptoms, including mood disturbance, agitation, violent behavior, socially inappropriate behavior, delusions, hallucinations, catastrophic reactions, and perseveration.[109,149] The pattern of onset and the types of psychiatric symptoms are often directly related to the underlying pathological condition.

When a physician is finally consulted, the diagnostic process can begin. When a complete diagnostic evaluation—including history, physical examination, neurological examination, neuropsychological testing, and laboratory testing (Box 27.6)—is performed, an accurate

BOX 27.5   Common Causes of Irreversible Dementia

Degenerative Causes
Alzheimer's disease
Parkinson disease
Huntington disease
Pick disease
Fahr disease
Multiple sclerosis

Infectious Causes
Neurosyphilis (general paresis)
Tuberculosis
Acquired immunodeficiency syndrome (AIDS)
Creutzfeldt-Jakob disease

Vascular Causes
Multiinfarct dementia
Stroke
Binswanger dementia
Anoxia
Arteriovenous malformation

Other Causes
Normal-pressure hydrocephalus
Mixed dementia
Alcoholic dementia
Toxins
Head trauma
Mass lesions

BOX 27.6   Laboratory Evaluation for Delirium and Dementia

Complete blood count
Thyroid function tests
Vitamin B_{12} or folate levels
Urinalysis
Blood levels of drugs patient is taking
Urine drug screen
Electrocardiogram
Magnetic resonance imaging scan of head (computed tomographic scan if magnetic resonance imaging is contraindicated)
Automated chemistries (including electrolytes, glucose, renal function, hepatic function, protein and albumin, cholesterol, and triglycerides)
Blood alcohol level
Human immunodeficiency virus (HIV) titer
Chest radiograph

diagnosis can be made in approximately 90% of patients, although experienced geriatric psychiatrists can make an accurate diagnosis in more than 95% of patients.[150]

Once the diagnostic process is completed, treatment can be started. Medications can assist in reversing underlying causes in only a small percentage of cases. Currently, medications approved by the Food and Drug Administration only treat cognitive symptoms related to AD and are unable to stop AD progression (e.g., Donepezil, Rivastigmine, Galantamine, and Memantine).[151] Psychotropic drugs may reverse depression or the behavioral symptoms associated with dementia.[148,152,153] Medical management also involves the prevention and treatment of other medical conditions and side effects of the new interventions as they are added.

Medical management of dementia focuses on maximizing the patient's remaining functions and roles, rehabilitating some lost functions, and providing family education and support.[109] Training caregivers to adapt to the patient (e.g., modifications for getting the patient out of bed, bathing), simplifying the individual's living space, and referring relatives to family support services are some of the issues to be addressed.[154]

Alzheimer's Disease

The treatment of major neurocognitive disorder/dementia is a long-term process. Studies have found that the average duration of illness from first onset of symptoms to death is 8.1 years for AD, 6.7 years for multiinfarct dementia,[155] and 5.6 years for Pick disease.[152] Medical and nursing care can extend the life expectancy of patients with dementia for up to 20 years or more.

In 1907, Alois Alzheimer[156] described the case and neuropathology of a 54-year-old woman who developed morbid jealousy, which was followed by loss of memory, inability to read and understand, and death 4.5 years after onset of the illness. AD is now the sixth leading cause of death in the United States and the fifth leading cause of death in older adults.[157] In 2017, the total health care cost related to the management of patients with AD and other dementias was USD 259 billion.[158,159] In making the diagnosis of AD, all other causes of cognitive dysfunction must be ruled out. The disease can occur at any age, but the onset of the disease is almost always after the age of 65 years. The prevalence of the disease gradually increases to a rate of 20% in persons older than 85 years.[54]

AD can be clinically staged. The use of staging enables the family and health care team to plan ahead for the individual's needs. Staging helps the family prepare longitudinally for the process of interacting with the patient. It allows the treatment team to plan for appropriate levels of services as the individual's abilities decline. Finally, it allows the health care team to quantify change in functional and cognitive abilities over time, which helps assess the effectiveness of the patient's treatment plan and establish evidence-based practice. The use of staging requires an accurate description of the patient's behavior (without the use of jargon) as well as an assessment of the patient's mental state.

Traditionally, the symptoms of AD have been thought to progress in three overlapping stages.

Stage 1 lasts from 2 to 4 years and involves loss of functional skills or orientation, memory loss, and lack of spontaneity. The patient is often aware of the losses and is, in many cases, able to cover up the cognitive losses by talking around the issues. During this stage, the patient and family may need to deal with the issue of giving up a job, hobbies, or other types of meaningful activity because of the patient's inability to carry them out safely and independently. The patient begins to lose the ability to handle money and a personal budget, drive a car safely, and tell time. The family or significant others may have to come to terms with the question of whether the patient can live alone. Depression is common during this stage of the disorder.

Stage 2 is characterized by progressive memory loss and the presence of a variety of neurological symptoms such as aphasias, apraxia, wandering, repetitive movements and stereotypical behavior, increased or decreased appetite, constant movement, and a peculiar wide-based gait can manifest. Psychotic symptoms (especially paranoid delusions and hallucinations), agitation, violent behaviors, and uncontrollable screaming are common symptoms during this stage of the disorder.

In stage 3, the patient develops vegetative symptoms. The patient may become mute, stop eating, and become incontinent of bowel and bladder. Muscle twitches or jerks, spasms of the diaphragm, and an inability to walk generally occur. The patient may develop seizures, and

TABLE 27.4 Barthel Index

	With Help	Independent
1. Feeding (score as "with help" if food needs to be cut)	5	10
2. Moving from wheelchair to bed and return (including sitting up in bed)	5–10[a]	15
3. Personal toilet (wash face, comb hair, shave, clean teeth)	0[a]	5
4. Getting on and off toilet (handling clothes, wipe, flush)	5	10
5. Bathing self	0[a]	5
6. Walking on level surface (or if unable to walk, propel wheelchair)	10	15
7. Ascending and descending stairs	5	10
8. Dressing (includes tying shoes, fastening fasteners)	5	10
9. Controlling bowels	5	10
10. Controlling bladder	5	10

A patient scoring 100 is continent, feeds himself or herself, dresses, gets up and out of bed and chairs, bathes himself or herself, walks at least a block, and can ascend and descend stairs. This does not mean that he or she is able to live alone. The patient may not be able to cook, keep house, and meet the public but is able to get along without attendant care.

[a]A score of 0 is given in the activity when the patient cannot meet the criteria as defined (see Appendix 27.A).

Modified from Mahoney FI, Barthel DW. Functional evaluation: the Barthel index. *Md State Med J.* 1965;14:61.

TABLE 27.5 Physical Performance Outcome Measures for Older Adults With Alzheimer's Disease and Related Dementias

Performance Domain	Outcome Measures
Fitness	6-minute walk test (6MWT) 2-minute walk test (2MWT) 2-minute step test
Functional Mobility	30-sec chair stand test 5-time sit-to-stand test (FTSST) Timed up and go test (TUG) Performance Oriented Mobility Assessment (POMA) Functional Independence Measure (FIM) Short Physical Performance Battery (SPPB)
Gait	Short-distance fast-paced gait speed (m/s) Short-distance usual-paced gait speed (m/s) Quantitative gait analysis using instrumentation
Balance	Berg Balance Scale (BBS) Functional Reach Test Single-leg stance test Frailty and Injuries Cooperative Studies of Intervention Techniques-Subtest 4 (FICSIT-4) Instrumented postural sway Figure-of-8 walk test (F8W)
Strength	Isometric measures using handheld dynamometers for handgrip and lower extremity Dynamic measures using 1-RM test for lower extremity

From McGough EL, Lin SY, Belza B, et al. A scoping review of physical performance outcome measures used in exercise interventions for older adults with Alzheimer's disease and related dementias. *J Geriatr Phys Ther.* 2019;42(1):28–47. doi:10.1519/JPT.0000000000000159.

emotional responsiveness, if present, is at a primitive level. Eventually, the patient dies from the disease.

The MMSE also may be used as a staging tool. Scores of 26 or more are generally associated with minimal, if any, dementia; scores of 21 to 25 are associated with mild dementia, scores of 15 to 20 with moderate dementia, scores of 10 to 14 with severe dementia, and scores of 9 or less with profound dementia. The severity of most other symptoms correlates well with the MMSE score.

Selected Outcome Measures for Older Adults With Dementia

The Barthel Index (Table 27.4) is a profile scale that rates 10 self-care, continence, and mobility criteria.[160] The specific rating guidelines used in scoring are presented in Appendix 27.A. The advantage of the Barthel Index is its simplicity and usefulness in evaluating patients before, during, and after treatment. It is functionally oriented and may be best used when accompanied by a clinical evaluation.[161] The scale allows documentation of functional changes over time. It is useful when discussing with families the need for help for the patient who cannot manage self-care (ADLs and/or IADLs).

Aside from the Barthel Index, clinicians could also use physical performance outcome measures to capture changes in physical function related to the disease process and assess the effectiveness of exercise interventions in older adults with AD and other related dementias.[162] A 2019 scoping review categorized these outcome measures into five domains of physical performance as follows:

1. Fitness—Cardiorespiratory and muscle endurance to sustain effort that requires combined work capacities for cardiopulmonary, biomechanical, and neuromuscular function.

2. Functional Mobility—Ability to perform physical tasks needed for everyday mobility, including chair stands, stair climbing, transfers, and multicomponent movement patterns.

3. Gait—Spatial and temporal aspects of gait described with camera systems, electronic walkways, or inertial sensors for motion analysis.

4. Balance—Ability to maintain upright positioning during static and dynamic standing or postural sway measured with instrumentation during static standing.

5. Strength—Muscle capacity for maximum force generation.[162]

Table 27.5 outlines 20 physical performance outcome measures that were identified in the study. The outcome measures were found to be reliable and responsive for older adults with mild to moderate dementia, though none was found to be optimal for severe dementia.

STRATEGIES FOR TREATMENT AND CARE

Most older adults with decreased cognitive abilities live with family or friends and not in institutions. Because of this, the rehabilitation team needs to include the caregivers and the patient as much as possible in treatment planning. The goal of rehabilitation is to ensure that the patient remains safe, independent, and able to perform ADLs and

IADLs for as long as is reasonable. The planning to reach these goals is best done within the context of the patient's social support system.

The rehabilitation process begins while the diagnostic workup is still in progress. At this stage of treatment, the rehabilitation plan includes basic training for the patient in performing and adapting the ADLs. It also includes caregiver training and support for significant others so they can make needed environmental modifications to ensure the safety of the patient with dementia.

Once the diagnosis is established, treatment planning for long-term care at home or in an institution must be carefully made. No matter where the patient will be living, involvement of the caregivers and significant others is essential to maximizing functional outcomes. The emotional, physical, and financial resources of the patient and family or significant others who will be the caretakers must be ascertained. A review of the caregivers' willingness to perform basic tasks or make visits, their willingness to learn and teach the necessary skills, and the realistic need for respites must be determined.[163] Family training and orientation manuals[109] that deal with all the details of caring for a person with dementia are available (see www.alz.org). The same detailed orientation is needed for institutional staff who care for patients with dementia. The structure and process of care can help patients be maximally active in their self-care and prevent unnecessary anxiety and catastrophic reactions.

Supporting Families and Caregivers With Their Own Sense of Loss, Frustration, and Helplessness

Family, significant others, and caregivers go through their own coping and adaptive process as the patient experiences gradual or sudden cognitive disturbances.[164] These people have a history with the patient and have expectations about what the relationship and communication should be. As cognitive disturbance occurs, they experience a series of losses because the patient is no longer able to respond and interact as he or she has in the past. With progressive cognitive decline, family and friends experience ongoing losses because the patient is continually changing and is less able to relate. For many patients with cognitive disturbances, at the final stage all communication disappears, and the family is left with only nonverbal communication or no communication at all. Staff who work with a patient over a period of time also face their own personal reactions of loss, unfulfilled expectations, and a continual need to reassess how to relate effectively to the patient. The responsibility for creating a positive relationship falls on the people who are interacting with the patient. The family and caregivers themselves need training and ongoing support in learning how to nurture and maintain an ongoing relationship with the patient. This process of training and support requires that caregivers and family members be aware that they are in a healing process as they relate to the loss of the relationship that previously existed.[165]

Epstein: Stages of Healing for Caregivers

Epstein[166] provides a workable description of the stages of healing that occur when major trauma or loss occurs. Epstein defines *healing* as "putting right our wrong relation to our body, to other people and . . . to our own complicated minds, with their emotions and instincts at war with one another and not properly understood and accepted by what we call 'I' or 'me.' The process is one of reorganization, reintegration of things that have come apart."[166] When a patient experiences cognitive changes, the first stage of response by those who care for or love this person is suffering. Chaos exists during this traumatic time. For example, the patient suddenly cannot understand simple directions on how to operate the new electric cart and insists on getting the old one back. The family is upset, and arguments ensue. The family and patient together eventually get a medical workup and are told that

"Mom has some type of degenerative cognitive problem." They all experience a profound sense that "something is wrong." The response to helplessness for most human beings is to resist. The lesson of this stage is acceptance. When acceptance is present, then detachment from emotions is possible. With acceptance present, adaptation and compensation for losses are possible. In the example noted, this would mean that the family would return the new electric cart and have the old (familiar) model refurbished. The family would get training from the therapist in exactly what skills of interaction Mom does not have so that they can work to avoid creating situations in which she feels "stupid and helpless." When a cognitive loss is truly present, training in skills only creates frustration in the patient that may lead to anger and rage. The staff and family need to be trained to understand the exact nature of the losses and provide appropriate compensations in their oral communication and how they relate to the patient.

Stage 2 has been alluded to as a part of stage 1. Therapists, the family, and caregivers search for second opinions, see other types of physicians, and try alternative treatments to gain power over the sense of helplessness. The polarities and rhythms of this process define this stage. All persons involved, even the patient, eventually begin to note that the emotions of the interactions may actually be making things worse. Acceptance that no magic solution is available begins. Everyone involved looks with interest at the proposition, "What can I do to make *this* life—*this* person—cope more effectively and have a reasonable quality of life (regardless of my opinion about what cognitive loss means to me personally)?" The lesson at this stage is another level of acceptance.

The third stage invites an examination of the ways in which people are "stuck in a perspective." When overwhelming stimuli occur, people commonly resort to their favorite strategy from childhood. For some people, the favorite strategy is to withdraw, whereas for others it may be to eat to create a distraction, and for others it may be anger. The emotional and mental options created to adapt to a difficult situation are as varied as the human race itself. Human beings dwell in the desire to know why or how to fix something. The lesson of this stage is, again, another level of acceptance and insight about how involved individuals contribute to the problem by reactions at the moment.

Stage 4 begins the process of "reclaiming power." This is the stage at which people realize that the "script" (their internal dialogue) from the last three stages is not workable or even desirable. The anger is recognized, and it brings an awareness that this reaction is not helping. Recognition begins that resisting is also not working because the condition of the patient is not affected in a positive way by the emotional reaction on the part of the caregiver(s). The truth of the matter is that the first four stages of healing often cause family and caregivers to become part of the problem and not part of the solution. The problem is how to support the patient to heal and adapt to the cognitive changes, whether temporary or permanent. Family and caregivers need to bring their healing process to their own support system, which needs to be separate from the patient. When caregivers attempt to share their frustration, suffering, sadness, or anger with the patient, the patient is usually upset because he or she cannot comprehend what the details of the issue really are. The patient knows only that people are upset. This will cause the patient to be increasingly upset and agitated. The stages of healing in staff and family must be recognized and services created or referral to support groups made so the patient can interact with people who are able to adapt to his or her needs and not cause further upset.

Stage 5 is called "merging with the illusion" and represents the first step in being able to "relate to the facts in a powerful way" rather than resisting or trying to manipulate them. It is the step at which family and caregivers begin to integrate the facts into their view of the world. The adult son may say, "I hate the fact that my mom cannot live alone;

it makes me feel so helpless [or frustrated or angry or upset or inadequate]." Many health care providers get upset when cognitive losses occur in their loved ones. The cognitive loss seems to be a failure that they take personally.

Stage 6 begins with active steps to prepare for the resolution of the emotions connected with the process. Many people describe this stage as the time when they really admit that their parents are never going to be able to give them advice again, babysit, or travel alone. The healing comes in allowing people to notice the emotions that come with accepting these big changes in reality.

Stage 7 brings the actual physical or emotional discharge. The process can be expressed as laughter, crying, fever, the urge to be physically active, sneezing, coughing, and so on. Resolution is marked by a deep sense of peace and inner strength. The person will have gone through the six stages, and the release of emotions or movement results in a deep shift away from resistance. *Family and caregivers need to create their own healing experiences separate from or away from the patient with cognitive losses.* When therapists work with the patient with cognitive losses, they must create for the patient a world that works and is safe and respectful of his or her unique abilities. In most cases, the profound emotional and physical release that comes with resolution tends only to upset the patient.

At stage 8, affected individuals are emptied and the board has been wiped clean. In the space of nothingness is an opportunity for new possibilities for relating to the patient. *The relationship should not be based on the past but on moment-to-moment information that comes from the patient.* Therapists can now enjoy being with the patient and begin to feel gratitude. Family and caregivers begin to look for ways to make things work more easily.

Stage 9 is a time when the caregivers and family relate to the energy of the universe and begin to see the connections to all life around them. At this stage, involved individuals begin to see that they are also a part of the great flow of time and energy and that an opportunity for joy exists. The process of illness and dying becomes the focus of awe and a reason to connect with other people and appreciate other people because they are a part of the whole process of life.

Stage 10 is the time to connect with the creative force of the universe. The spiritual process is brought to the issue at hand. A sense of great wisdom and oneness with all creation is felt. *When working from this state of being, the caregiver has the unique capacity to speak or act to bring out the best in others.* In health care, some caregivers have the special gift of allowing themselves to step into the mental world of the other person and thereby create communication that will be heard and that can be acted on even by those with limited mental capacities. The most interesting thing is that the patients can often tell if a caregiver is in this unique state because they will come and sit next to the caregiver or want to hold hands. This state of ease and connection can be learned. A possible resource for exploring these skills is an organization called Landmark Education ([415] 981-8850; www.landmarkeducation.com), which provides programs and courses that examine how people listen, what bias they bring to the communication process, and specific speech strategies to bring out the best in others.

Epstein stage 11 is when people live day to day without being attached to the situation. Epstein notes that in this stage, "we communicate with ourselves and others through our wounds instead of from them." As healing progresses, caregivers become part of the solution in the care of the patient with cognitive losses. They know they can make a positive difference and take action to create what needs to be done. *They are able to sort out the facts of a situation from the first impression, which is often loaded with judgments and wishful thinking. As caregivers relate to the verifiable facts, they speak to the issues at hand with power and create positive outcomes in which "win-win" becomes the norm.*

In the last stage, caregivers bring their unique individuality to the service of the community. They become aware that the limits to what they can bring to the community are connected to the limits to their sense of wholeness. This insight sends them back to their earlier stages of healing to create further self-awareness and healing on other issues.

In-service training can offer a basic introduction to strategies for lifelong learning, healing, and self-awareness. "What works for me?" "What is the easiest way to learn new skills?" "What strategies enhance adaptability?" This type of learning is nonlinear and is the model a scientist uses to conduct an inquiry. Recently, more attention has been paid to managing stress and the role of spirituality in processing grief and loss among caregivers and family.[167–169]

Nonlinear Learning

Nonlinear learning begins with the posing of a question. Then data and information are collected, and additional questions are generated that are related to the first question. At some point an "Aha!" moment or insight occurs. A new relationship is suddenly made possible that was not possible before. Nonlinear learning is not about small gradual steps of progress but occurs similarly to how learning balance occurs when riding a bicycle—one minute balance is impossible, and the next is the breakthrough moment. Nonlinear training offers precise strategies that can enhance communication with someone who has cognitive deficits. Nonlinear learning is built on scientific communication that operates on the basis of verifiable facts at the present moment. Nonlinear learning invites each person to examine all strategies for communication to be sure that problems are not occurring as a result of misinterpretation of the facts. Communication can occur without verbal language, and fear does not need to be present. When a patient has cognitive deficits, the art and science of human interaction need to be precise so that caregivers do not speak in words that are not understandable to the patient. Which caregiver prejudgments are brought to the interaction with the patient needs to be understood: experiencing the stage of awe, sharing joy in the moment, or suffering because the person is "difficult"? The care and therapy provided to a person with cognitive disturbances need to be created based on the facts of the moment and carried out in a state of gratitude, vulnerability, and nurturing for the staff and the patient.

Role of the Clinician: Development of Interventions and Caregiver Training[170,171]

All people with cognitive losses should have access to caregivers who are trained to manage emotional responses in order to provide precise strategies for communication with those with dementia. A gracious and secure existence is possible even when cognition is diminished if the caregivers are committed to adapting the environment and its demands to match the capacity of the patient. The challenge for health care is designing training programs that truly prepare families and caregivers to be effective, empowering communicators. All caregivers need training to create this experience for a person with cognitive deficits.

As a part of the rehabilitation program, caregiver training for this group of patients needs to emphasize reassurance, hands-on interventions, and communication to allow treatment to proceed at a pace perceived as reasonable by the patient.[93] In the early and middle stages of all dementias, physical therapy intervention usually can prolong the ability to move with ease in ADLs and IADLs, and maintain the ability to participate in some social activities. This therapeutic outcome is extremely important for caregivers because deficits in the patient's ability to perform ADLs and IADLs often relate to the inability to physically perform these activities under supervision.[67] The ability to walk is lost late in most dementias, but gait and coordination disturbances

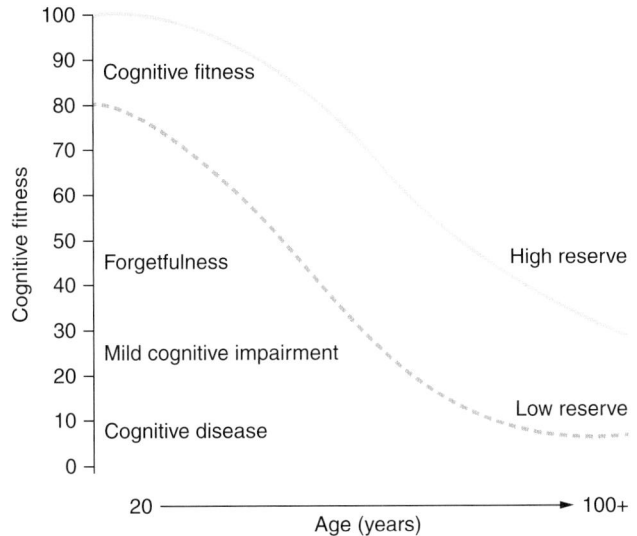

Fig. 27.4 Achieving and maintaining high cognitive fitness through exercise and physical activity in early to mid-adulthood may influence the onset and severity of cognitive impairment in later life.

are common and can benefit from physical therapy.[172–174] Therapeutic intervention to assist the patient and train the caregivers involves facilitation of ease of movement and motor planning and developing or refining environmental and cognitive cues to assist in carrying out complex tasks. Ultimately, caregivers require training in how to move, lift, and otherwise assist the patient.

Although not able to reverse the progressive cognitive decline, the exercise intervention that the physical therapist can develop may improve the level of function, confidence, vitality, and safety of the patient and ease the burden of care for the caregivers. Research has demonstrated an important role for exercise in maintaining physical activity[175–177]—contributing to general health, improving cognitive[178] reserve,[57] and slowing of cognitive decline,[179–182] as well as maintaining strength and aerobic conditioning[55,183] (Fig. 27.4). Guidelines for exercise prescription include aerobic, strength, balance, coordination, and flexibility activities determined by direct assessment, and suggestions for motivational and problem-solving strategies. The Seattle Protocols are an important contribution in this area.[184,185] Research shows that exercise not only increases strength, coordination, and aerobic capacity but also creates beneficial changes in brain plasticity.[81,186,187] Further studies need to be done to work out more clearly what types of exercise are beneficial in what ways and for which populations.[188]

Cognitive impairment is a key limiting factor in the performance of ADLs and IADLs as well as a limiting factor for participating in rehabilitation. Accurate assessment and training by the therapist help the caregiver provide only the help that is absolutely needed, with patients continuing to perform for themselves as many ADLs as possible. For example, when brushing the teeth, the patient needs to be able to remember the command to brush, must recognize the toothbrush, and must perform a complex but repetitive motor action. The patient may only need the help of someone placing the toothbrush in his or her hand and slowly guiding it to the mouth to be able to safely brush the teeth.

The accurate assessment of IADLs and ADLs is more reliable than medical diagnosis for predicting the amount of assistance and interaction a person will need in a nursing home (see Table 27.4, Table 27.5, and Appendix 27.A).[160] The first goal of rehabilitation for

patients with dementia is to create a supportive emotional and physical environment. The environment must actively work to compensate for the patient's cognitive and functional losses as they occur. The ultimate goal is to help patients feel they are capable so that they will continue to try to do those things for themselves that they can do safely, whether they remain in their home or live in an institution. Orientation and training of significant others are also important so that they feel comfortable allowing the patient to participate safely in activities and basic self-care tasks modified to their cognitive level.

The Alzheimer's Association ([800] 272-3900; www.alz.org) is a resource for professionals and caregivers of people with dementia. The goals of the association are the following:

- To support research related to the diagnosis, therapy, cause, and cure of AD and related disorders
- To aid in organizing family support groups; to educate and assist affected families
- To sponsor educational programs for professionals and laypersons on the topic of AD
- To advise government agencies of the needs of the affected families and to promote federal, state, and private support of research
- To offer help in any manner to patients and their caregivers to promote the well-being of all involved

The Alzheimer's Association promotes the provision of humane care to the patient with dementia or related disorders throughout the course of the illness. Other support groups have been tried in communities in which spouses have worked to develop ongoing respite care.[189]

As a member of the rehabilitation team, the physical or occupational therapist can conduct an inventory of services as a part of the annual review of the quality of care that is provided for a patient with dementia. Surveys of persons caring for patients with dementia listed the following services in their perceived order of importance[98,190]:

1. Availability of respite care services (i.e., short-term care provided by a third party to relieve the primary caregiver; a paid companion can come and stay at home for a few hours to several days giving caregivers a chance to go away and rest)[190a]
2. Assistance in locating people or organizations to provide patient care
3. Assistance in applying for government programs, such as Medicaid, disability insurance, and income support programs
4. Personal home care for the person with dementia to help with activities such as bathing, dressing, or feeding in the home
5. Support groups composed of others who are caring for people with dementia and other cognitive deficits
6. Special nursing home care programs only for people with dementia and other cognitive deficits while the caregiver is away
7. Adult day care providing supervision and activities away from the home
8. Visiting nurse services for care at home

In the home care category, information about the availability of services and government programs and various forms of respite care were also highly ranked in the survey. Overall, caregivers (family and friends) of the patient are often able and willing to provide care for the patient throughout the illness if appropriate professional consultation can help them cope with problematic situations and if adequate respite time is provided to the caregiver(s).

Not mentioned in this chapter is the need for psychological support for caregivers. The stress on caregivers is extreme, and symptoms of anxiety and depression are common. Because of the relative lack of counseling services for caregivers, however, the use of (and probable abuse of and dependence on) psychotropic medications by caregivers is high.[85,191] Because these medications may impair the cognitive functioning of caregivers, the risk of harm to the patient with dementia is also high.

EMERGING INTERVENTIONS AND FUTURE TRENDS ON THE ROLE OF REHABILITATION THERAPISTS IN DEMENTIA CARE

Most current research in delirium and dementia is focused on AD. Research is underway to explore possible causes of dementia, including work that examines the roles of neurotransmitters, structural brain changes, nutrition, viruses, drugs, immunological deficits, and heredity in the etiology of AD. Studies to increase the diagnostic accuracy of different forms of dementia, including making a distinction between cortical and subcortical dementia[190] or using *Diagnostic and Statistical Manual of Mental Disorders,* Fifth Edition (DSM-V) criteria[41] or neuropsychological criteria, are also underway. Newer diagnostic models of dementia, including that caused by stage II or III human immunodeficiency virus infection, are also being studied.[192,193] The recent discovery of lymphatic vessels in the dural venous sinuses offers a potential direct link between the human brain and the body's immune system, a connection which was previously believed to be nonexistent.[194,195] This development raises the possibility of the role the immune system plays in brain function and in the development of AD. In a separate study, increased levels of two human herpesviruses (HHV-6A and HHV-7) were observed in the brains of people with AD compared with normal controls.[196,197] The herpes virus genes were then found to interact with genes known to increase AD risk and those that modulate amyloid precursor protein processing. People with dementia who also have parkinsonian symptoms, delusions, and hallucinations have been reported to experience faster decline that those

who do not.[198] This research team found a relation between the presence of Lewy bodies (abnormal structures in the brain that contain a protein called *synuclein*) and parkinsonian symptoms; affected individuals had lower survival rates than those with either symptom present by itself.

Finding a cure for AD has been largely unsuccessful, with a failure rate of 99.6%.[199] The last time a drug was approved for AD was in 2003. In a review of the drug development pipeline, 63% of agents targeted disease modification, 23% have cognitive-enhancing effects, and 12% controlled neuropsychiatric symptoms.[200] Almost all were directed at patients with mild AD, severely limiting treatment options for patients already in the moderate to advanced stages. In the absence of a drug to halt or reverse the progression of AD, nonpharmacological strategies such as exercise, increasing physical activity, having a healthy/nutritious[201] diet, and improving sleep quality could play a role in preventing and/or delaying the onset of AD[202,203] (see Box 27.7). Results from a 44-year longitudinal population study in women suggest the importance of maintaining high cardiovascular fitness in midlife in reducing dementia risk and delaying its onset. In the said study, women who had high fitness (assessed by step-wise ergometer cycling) decreased their dementia risk by 88% compared to those with medium fitness, and those that developed dementia manifested it 11 years later than those with medium fitness.[24]

The most exciting area of research is dementia prevention by targeting known modifiable risk factors. Findings from the Singapore Longitudinal Ageing Study showed a 1.5- to 2-fold increased risk of developing MCI in those who had metabolic syndrome, diabetes mellitus, central obesity, and dyslipidemia; a fourfold increased risk of progressing from MCI to dementia in those with metabolic syndrome, and a twofold risk in those with diabetes mellitus.[204] Thus it is imperative to address these risk factors as early as possible to mitigate

---

BOX 27.7 **Highlights From the 2017 National Academies of Sciences, Engineering, and Medicine Report on the State of Knowledge Regarding Prevention of Cognitive Decline and Dementia**

The National Institute on Aging, in partnership with the National Academies of Sciences, Engineering, and Medicine, convened a committee to examine the current state of knowledge on the prevention of cognitive decline and dementia. Specifically, the Committee on Preventing Dementia and Cognitive Impairment was tasked to *evaluate the existing evidence on interventions for preventing cognitive decline and dementia, and based on this evidence, to recommend the appropriate content for inclusion in public health messages, as well as priorities for future prevention research.*

The Committee was not able to identify a specific intervention supported by conclusive evidence that would justify a widespread, assertive public health campaign for its adoption. However, **"encouraging but inconclusive evidence"** have been found for three classes of intervention:

1. Cognitive Training, interventions aimed at enhancing reasoning, memory, and speed of processing to delay or slow age-related cognitive decline
2. Blood Pressure Management in People with Hypertension, to prevent, delay or slow clinical Alzheimer's-type dementia
3. Increased Physical Activity, to delay or slow age-related cognitive decline

The report also highlights that these areas of study were the "highest priorities for research" for the National Institutes of Health and other interested organizations. Research is needed to elucidate the effectiveness of cognitive training, blood pressure management, and increased physical activity. In particular, it is important to *evaluate the comparative effectiveness of different forms of*

cognitive training interventions and determine which specific intervention elements are responsible for the observed positive and long-term impacts on cognitive performance; determine whether there are optimal blood pressure targets and approaches across different age ranges; and comparing the effects of different forms of physical activity such as aerobic and resistance training.

Aside from the above-mentioned interventions, the Committee also identified several that were currently supported by **insufficient evidence** from RCTs, but had promising findings derived from observational studies, knowledge of dementia risk factors, and/or strong argument for biological plausibility.

- New antidementia treatments that can delay onset of slow disease progression
- Diabetes Treatment
- Depression Treatment
- Dietary Interventions
- Lipid-lowering Treatment
- Sleep Quality Interventions
- Social Engagement Interventions
- Vitamin B12 plus Folic Acid Supplementation

Full report can be accessed online for free via http://nationalacademies.org/hmd/reports/2017/preventing-cognitive-decline-and-dementia-a-way-forward.aspx

National Academies of Sciences, Engineering, and Medicine. *Preventing Cognitive Decline and Dementia: A Way Forward.* Washington, DC: The National Academies Press; 2017. doi: https://doi.org/10.17226/24782.

cognitive impairment in later life. A landmark multiple-center randomized controlled trial, the Finnish Geriatric Intervention Study to Prevent Cognitive Impairment and Disability (FINGER),[20,205–209] has shown that a 2-year multiple-domain intervention consisting of nutritional guidance; exercise; cognitive training and social activity; and management of metabolic and vascular risk factors can prevent cognitive decline in older people from the general population who are at risk of dementia.[20,208] The success of the FINGER Trial helped establish the World Wide FINGERS (WW-FINGERS) initiative, an international collaborative effort to identify cost-effective preventative approaches for various at-risk groups that are accessible, feasible, and sustainable for different geographical, economic, and cultural settings.[209] As of the writing of this chapter in 2018, the US study to PrOtect through a lifestyle INTErvention to Reduce risk (US POINTER), a clinical trial modeled after the FINGER, has begun identifying its targeted 2500 participants aged 60 to 79 years. Aside from the US POINTER study, similar projects are being planned in China (Multimodal Intervention to delay dementia and disability in rural China/MIND-CHINA), Singapore (Singapore intervention study to prevent cognitive impairment and disability/SINGER), Australia (Maximising technology and methodology for internet prevention of cognitive decline: the Maintain Your Brain Trial/MYB trial), and Europe (Multimodal preventative trials for Alzheimer's Disease:towards multinational strategies/MIND-AD trial). These studies highlight the critical contribution of physical exercise in dementia prevention and rehabilitation therapists are strategically placed with the expertise to design and implement appropriate physical activity and exercise interventions. Findings from a 2×2 factorial randomized clinical trial in adults with cognitive impairment but no dementia showed that those who engaged in aerobic exercise had significant gains in executive function compared to those who were assigned in the Dietary Approaches to Stop Hypertension (DASH) diet group.[210] Adults who exercised and adhered to the DASH diet had the largest increase in executive function compared to controls. To further underscore the positive impact of exercise on cognitive function, the American Academy of Neurology now recommends exercise as part of the overall management plan for patients with diagnosed with MCI.[211] The guideline specifically states that, "*For patients diagnosed with MCI, clinicians should recommend regular exercise (twice/week) as part of an over-all approach to management*".

Various interventions have shown promise in improving cognitive and physical functions in people who already have dementia.[203] These interventions include the use of virtual reality or gaming technology like the Nintendo Wii for physical activity and exercise,[212,213] dance,[214,215] and the use of assistive technology to promote home safety[216]—all of which have been demonstrated to be feasible at various stages in the progression of dementia and are being further examined in research.

Research is also being funded to investigate the best ways to provide care and support in the home and in long-term residential settings.[54]

SUMMARY

Why some people stay lively and creative in their older years is not known; Michelangelo designed St. Peter's when he was nearly 90; Picasso painted at 90; and Arthur Rubenstein, Pablo Casals, and Martha Graham all worked creatively in their older years. What is clear is that lonely, isolated older people are much more likely to be confused and disoriented than their peers who remain actively involved with family and friends. Perhaps what is needed is to invite the world to explore rules of conduct in which older persons are honored and included.

In working with an older person with dementia or delirium, the therapist can do much to improve the quality of life for the patient, family, and caregivers.[109] A thorough listing of the details needed to develop an environment and process of care for older adults and people with cognitive deficits can be found in other texts (see www.alz.org/living_with_alzheimers.asp).[109,149]

Specific examples of modifications of physical and occupational therapy examination and treatment may include working in collaboration with the family, close friends, and other members of the rehabilitation team and developing a consultative relationship with key caregivers (professional and nonprofessional and all shifts of institutional staff) to encourage problem solving and patient participation in self-care. Another important modification includes the evaluation of each patient's communication abilities before the therapy assessment to adapt the assessment in such a way as to promote patient participation. Case study examples in the next section (refer to Case Studies 27.1 and 27.2) to provide clinical scenarios and corresponding physical and occupational therapy examination and treatment strategies.

CASE STUDY 27.1 The Complexity of Aging

The patient was a 78-year-old woman who had the following deficits on the MMSE: She was not aware of where she lived, the date, or the year; had poor short-term memory; could not spell the word "world" backward; and could not copy two overlapping pentagons. The patient was generally happy and enjoyed having someone sit with her. The patient had fractured her femur and, because of the location of the fracture site, a surgical procedure was performed to allow total weight bearing. The surgeon and the psychiatrist decided that partial weight bearing would not be a concept that the patient could understand. The physical therapist and assistant worked together with the family and caregivers in the nursing home to develop a plan of care. At the initial care conference, the main question was whether the patient should receive physical therapy. The family was fearful that the patient would fall again if she were taught how to walk. The focus of the conference was to educate the family and other staff regarding the importance of physical therapy so the patient could learn how to

participate in and eventually perform transfers from wheelchair to toilet as well as to bed. The decision was made to begin physical therapy, with the initial goal being to achieve all functional ADL transfers with standby physical assistance.

The patient was not interested in walking and was fearful of falling. The key change in physical therapy intervention was in the style of communication used to teach basic bed mobility and the components of transfer skills. Through the use of trial-and-error, it was determined that the patient responded best to a smile, verbal encouragement, hand signals, and gentle manual pressure to indicate the desired task to be performed. If the task was broken down and components were identified, the patient became frustrated and refused to participate. If the patient was invited by manual cues and verbal reassurance to stand up and sit on the bed, the patient would hesitate for up to 1 minute and then would attempt to perform the task. It became obvious that the patient needed at least 30 to 60 s of waiting time between when a verbal request was made and when

Continued

she was ready to act on the request. If additional time was not given, the patient appeared to become frustrated and would refuse to cooperate. A sign was placed over her bed with instructions for communication: smile, reassure, use your hands to guide her to perform the desired action, and wait 60 s; let her feel there is plenty of time.

A sliding board was introduced in therapy, and the patient enjoyed the idea. The board allowed transfers for all ADLs to involve no lifting for the staff. The patient would lean her head on the shoulder of the staff member while sitting and then she would assist in sliding across on the board. All transfers for ADLs using the sliding board were possible within five visits of physical therapy. A bed was located that was 17 inches high to facilitate bed-to-wheelchair transfers. The bed could be raised to assist the nursing aide in cleaning activities. The decision was made to leave the bed at 17 inches unless the nursing staff needed to perform special in-bed procedures with the patient. The wheelchair footrests were modified so that they formed a solid flat surface to allow the patient to rest in a natural position. The patient was only 5 feet 2 inches tall, and the standard wheelchair allowed her only to comfortably put both feet on one foot pedal and sit with her weight mostly on one buttock. A smaller wheelchair and the adapted footrest provided the patient with equal pressure on both sitting bones, and the patient began to sit at rest in a natural upright posture. The other goal of physical therapy was to teach the patient wheelchair mobility by using her hands to push the chair. Once the patient was given gloves for her hands (she did not like germs), she was willing to try to push the wheelchair. The patient was instructed in the physical therapy department during two visits. The patient was next seen by the therapist on the unit to allow the nurse's aide to become a part of the physical therapy instruction. The rationale was that the nurse's aide would need to help reinforce the skills and encourage the practice of wheelchair mobility skills as a part of daily activities. During the last visits, the physical therapist watched daytime, afternoon, and evening staff practice with the patient and addressed new situations that arose. All caregivers on three shifts were trained to ensure consistency of verbal and manual cuing for the patient.

Before discharge to restorative nursing, the patient's current level of functional abilities was documented by using an ADL chart that specified the task(s) and times of day when they were easiest, equipment needs, special positioning, clothing and other assistive devices, verbal cuing, and other communication requirements for each critical task that had been mastered in physical therapy. The cataloging of functional skills reminded the nurse's aide of the ingredients involved for the patient to successfully perform ADLs. The other advantage of the detailed discharge summary to the nursing staff was that new staff could use the document and, as needed, contact physical therapy for clarifications if the patient was suddenly unable to perform the tasks (a signal of possible medical or psychosocial problems).

Key Points
1. Common goals were identified and agreed upon among all team members and the patient's significant others.
2. Education was provided as needed to allow for consistency of verbal and manual cuing to the patient.
3. Physical therapy treatment began in a quiet, undisturbed area where the patient could concentrate. As mastery of a skill was achieved, the skill was practiced with supervision, and instruction of other staff was provided as needed.
4. Equipment and furniture were adjusted to help the patient perform tasks with minimal assistance.
5. Discharge from therapy involved providing nursing staff with a detailed description of functional abilities and the conditions required to help maximize patient participation, sense of safety, and control (as had already been reviewed with all aides working with the patient).
6. The physical therapist was designated as a resource person for nursing staff for simplifying functional tasks in patient care, problem solving, communication, and movement-related issues.

The patient was a 64-year-old man who, until 1 month ago, was working. He was forced to retire because he kept forgetting the natural sequences of his work tasks. For example, his partner would see him direct someone to wait for him in the waiting room and subsequently forget about that person. On the MMSE, he had difficulty with date and year and would try to redirect the question in an apparent attempt to cover up for the loss of short-term memory. He could not or would not spell the word "world" backward, and he poorly copied the overlapping hexagons (looked more like squares). He was a runner but now could not remember how to get home and, as a result, would pretend to be hurt and get someone to drive him there. The man reported feeling restless.

The patient, along with his wife and two sons, were seen by the team at a psychiatric clinic. The wife was very upset, and the family was asking for help. The role of therapy at this early stage of AD involved the following:
1. Functional assessment of basic ADLs and IADLs and home assessment.
2. Orientation of spouse and significant caregivers regarding the functional changes that could occur in the near future and how to compensate for current functional losses (e.g., patient had difficulty dressing in the morning and would become frustrated).
3. Orientation to the role of therapy in hands-on treatment related to techniques to help the patient relax. After initial evaluation, the team decided to teach caregivers massage techniques identified by the therapist as soothing and relaxing for the patient. (Note: The emphasis in hands-on intervention is to create slow, predictable, and nurturing contact that is perceived by the patient as soothing and relaxing.)

4. Orientation of caregivers to the use of manual contact and hand signals to communicate and reinforce the intention. Kinesthetic contact and the ability to follow kinesthetic cues can help the patient with ADL tasks at home. At this time, the kinesthetic cuing may not be critical for the patient, but the caregivers need to get in the habit of cuing the patient as a compensatory tool for future cognitive losses.
5. Orientation of caregivers to the benefits of a ritualized schedule of daily events for the patient and assistance in developing the daily schedule. The predictability of the ritual would help the patient feel safe and in control. The ritualizing would be especially helpful to address the frustrations with dressing in the morning.
6. Written information about local support groups, day treatment centers, and the availability of the rehabilitation team, including therapy for problem solving.
7. Participation in the evaluation of patient and family need for placement in a day treatment center or use of a home health aide. Supervision was needed for cooking (he would leave burners on), working in the woodshop (he would leave power tools running), and in self-care to ensure his safety. Supervision in the home was decided, with family members sharing the load. The idea of going to a new place was not positively received by the patient. (Note: The patient may function better in the environment where he or she has lived for a long time because of the familiarity with the details of the surroundings.)
8. The therapist participated in development of the home care plan and provided patient and family education during a home-health visit. The next contact

CASE STUDY 27.2 A Patient in the Early Stage of Alzheimer's Disease—cont'd

that the family made with therapy was 1 month later to address the patient's inability to settle down and go to sleep at night. A home visit was made to evaluate the bedtime ritual, the relaxation strategies being used, and communication with the physician about current medications taken. The patient disliked bathing and undressing for bed. After discussion with caregivers, the patient was allowed to go to bed in his clothes without bathing and undressing (bathing and undressing would be carried out in the morning when he was less tired). Relaxation massage was modified to involve the face, neck, hands, and feet, and the caregivers were instructed and practiced during two visits under the supervision of the therapist. A satisfactory bedtime ritual was developed, and home health care was workable for the patient and the caregivers.

The next request for therapy consultation came 4 months later when the wife and the daughter-in-law (who had been taking turns being the primary caregiver) both felt the need to hire and train an attendant-companion for the patient for 8 h a day. At this time, the patient preferred to be in the home, walk in the yard, or take long walks in the local park. The therapist, in cooperation with other team members, trained the patient regarding how to sequence for ease in ADL tasks; the use of kinesthetic cuing; how to facilitate ADLs, bathing, and dressing with a slow pace and ritualized format; and how to sequence the tasks and relaxation techniques to help the patient settle down and go to sleep. Foot massage was the only technique that the patient now allowed and appeared to enjoy. After three physical therapy visits over a 2-week period, the attendant was able to carry out home health care effectively for the patient.

The last request for help occurred when the family was concerned because the patient was trying to run away. The therapist made a home visit and found that the patient sat most of the day. The MMSE showed that he could not give his own first or last name and had no short-term memory. Based on the evaluation, the therapist proposed that the family or attendant go with the patient for a walk when the patient showed an interest in leaving the house. This strategy worked for a few months, but then the patient began to sit down on the sidewalk when he was tired. Another visit was made after a wheelchair was ordered to train the caregivers in use of the wheelchair and to orient the patient to the desired procedures and to reassure the patient. After this visit, the patient showed gradually less interest in leaving the home over the next few months until he eventually stayed in the house constantly. At this time, the patient also became incontinent of bowel and bladder. The patient refused to use the toilet, and the decision was made to seek nursing home placement.

Key Points

1. Physical (or occupational) therapy is a part of the team providing guidance and care for the patient and the family of the patient with AD and other dementias.
2. Evaluation of functional skills, communication related to functional skills, and home modifications to enhance patient participation in self-care can be continued as long as the caregivers request support and help problem solving.
3. Problem solving with caregivers and educating caregivers are the primary roles once the therapist has identified the intervention of choice to solve the key functional problems.
4. All therapy intervention needs to be coordinated with actions of others providing care for the patient (family, neighbors, and friends as well as other health care providers).

Modifications of treatment include the use of gentle, nonverbal neurological rehabilitation techniques (e.g., the Feldenkrais Method). The key is to acknowledge the now well-established research finding that nondeclarative learning and memory (procedural) are available long after declarative learning and memory (ability to consciously learn and remember facts and events) are lost for a person with AD. Motor ability is one of the last areas to be affected by AD.[217] Assisting a person with AD to edit procedural memory and increase walking safety is

therefore possible. The functional outcomes of this learning can include a decrease in abnormal muscle tone, enhanced sensory awareness and organization for the position of the eyes and head in space, an increase in the ease of movement, an increase in the ease of breathing, enhanced endurance, minimized anxiety, minimized resting muscle rigidity in the chest, and increased patient coordination. The therapist needs to modify the process of neurological facilitation by decreasing patient effort and adding extra cuing and more frequent breaks for integration of learning. Tasks may need to be simplified so that the patient can perform them, and the caregiver is trained to perform only those tasks that the patient cannot perform.

Each month, the therapist, treatment team, patient, and caregiver(s) need to identify safe physical activities that the patient can be encouraged to perform for recreation, relaxation, and overall fitness. The goal is to enhance the performance of simple ADL and IADL tasks (e.g., washing socks, setting the table), which can enhance patient self-esteem. In addition, the physical therapist, along with other members of the rehabilitation team and caregivers, needs to monitor the patient for new signs and symptoms of concurrent delirium or reversible dementia so that treatment can be initiated early and further deterioration can be prevented.

A hospital and nursing home patients' "Bill of Rights" defines the minimal quality of care required for any patient. The concepts presented apply to the care of patients with cognitive deficits no matter what the setting. The provision of considerate and respectful care for the patient with dementia or other cognitive deficits is possible and necessary. Well-planned and gentle care prevents unnecessary distortions in cognitive function brought on by feelings of fear or being rushed and thereby maximizes all remaining cognitive function. To use his or her remaining emotional and cognitive resources, the patient with cognitive deficits needs to live in an environment and experience a process of care that is modified to meet the special needs created by delirium or dementia.

AD is progressive and irreversible, but pharmacological therapies for cognitive impairment and nonpharmacological and pharmacological treatments for behavioral problems associated with dementia can enhance quality of life. Psychotherapeutic intervention with family members is often indicated, as nearly half of all caregivers become depressed. Health care delivery to these patients is fragmented and inadequate.[218]

Physical and occupational therapy are key resources for the creation of a therapeutic environment and for the effective and timely assessment and treatment of the patient with cognitive deficits. The goal of therapy is to create a process of care in which the patient feels safe and the caregivers are given training and support in problem solving to guide the patient to participate in self-care, ambulation, and recreation as long as it is safe and functionally possible.

Caregiver agreements can enhance the capacity of older people with dementia to participate in daily life—exploring the possibility of living a life with safety, dignity, and love. The following is a brief list of basic environmental supports for encouraging the activation of procedural memory:

1. I will ask my patient if he or she would like to pray or worship today, and I will make arrangements to meet those needs.
2. I will speak or communicate in a way that is functional and workable for the patient.
3. I will repeat what I hear and perceive back to the patient to ensure that I capture her or his perspective.
4. I will encourage natural participation by creating a pace that is pleasant for the patient.
5. I will close doors quietly.
6. I will not raise my voice or shout except in a real emergency.
7. I will talk to someone on staff when I get upset or take something personally so I can have peace with co-workers, creating a positive atmosphere in which the patients can live.

Continued

CASE STUDY 27.2   A Patient in the Early Stage of Alzheimer's Disease—cont'd

8. I will offer to warm up the patient's tea or coffee and make sure it is not so hot that it could cause a burn.

9. I will create only one choice at a time so the patient can understand and then choose yes or no.

10. I will know what "my" patient has eaten on my shift.

11. I will know my patients' timing for toileting so I can support their continence and dignity.

12. I will tell the patient I am going to touch him or her before I do so to avoid surprises.

13. I will walk (rolling or ambulating) with every one of my patients outdoors as often as possible or at least every 3 days to encourage good sleep and mental and physical stimulation.

14. I will sit and visit with each of my patients for 10 min (every shift).

15. I promise to listen with an open heart to the patients' perception of life at the moment.

16. I promise to close the blinds in every room at night (unless the patient requests otherwise) and open the blinds every morning to reinforce day-night orientation.

17. I will discover and use the "personal" get ready for bed routine for all patients so that they sleep well.

18. I promise to talk and walk at a pace that encourages a sense of safety for my patients.

19. I promise to be self-nurturing and come to work well rested and ready to share myself.

20. I promise to avoid confrontational actions and body language except in an emergency.

21. I promise to respect the unique ergonomics of each patient and adapt as needed.

22. I promise to offer to add support to explore ways to increase comfort.

23. I promise to notice how my patients relate so that no one agitates or bothers another.

24. I promise to be kind to myself, other staff, and my patients.

25. I promise to be of service and adapt to meet my patients' needs.

26. I promise to report problems (equipment, environment, relationships) to the person who can do something about them.

27. I promise not to gossip (talk about others in a way that leaves a negative impression and no resolution of the problem).

28. I promise to leave my workspace clean and restocked after I have taken care of the patient (or at least to leave a note to alert the next shift about what has not been done).

REFERENCES

To enhance this text and add value for the reader, all references are included on the companion Evolve site that accompanies this textbook. This online service will, when available, provide a link for the reader to a Medline abstract for the article cited. There are 219 cited references and other general references for this chapter, with the majority of those articles being evidence-based citations.

Rating Guidelines for Barthel Index

1. Feeding
   10 = Independent. The patient can feed himself or herself a meal when someone puts the food within reach. Patient must put on an assistive device, if needed, to cut up the food alone. The patient must accomplish this in a reasonable time.
   5 = Some help is necessary (with cutting up food, and so on, as listed above).

2. Moving from wheelchair to bed and return
   15 = Independent in all phases of this activity. Patient can safely approach the bed in the wheelchair, lock brakes, lift footrests, move safely to bed, lie down, come to a sitting position in the wheelchair if necessary to transfer back into it safely, and return to the wheelchair.
   10 = Either some minimal help is needed in some step of this activity or the patient needs to be reminded or supervised for safety in one or more parts of this activity.
   5 = Patient can come to a sitting position without the help of a second person but needs to be lifted out of bed, or he or she transfers only with a great deal of help.

3. Doing personal toileting
   5 = Patient can wash hands and face, comb hair, clean teeth, and shave. He may use any kind of razor but must put in blade or plug in razor without help as well as get it from drawer or cabinet. Female patients must put on own makeup.

4. Getting on and off toilet
   10 = Patient is able to get on and off toilet, fasten and unfasten clothes, prevent soiling of clothes, and use toilet paper without help. If a bedpan is necessary instead of a toilet, patient must be able to place it on a chair, empty it, and clean it.
   5 = Patient needs help because of imbalance or with handling clothes or using toilet paper.

5. Bathing self
   5 = Patient may use a bathtub or a shower or take a complete sponge bath. Patient must be able to do all the steps involved in whichever method is used without another person being present.

6. Walking on a level surface
   15 = Patient can walk at least 50 yards without help or supervision. Patient may wear braces or prostheses and use crutches, canes, or a walker (but not a rolling walker). Patient must be able to lock and unlock braces, if used; assume the standing position and sit down; get the necessary mechanical aids into position for use; and dispose of them when sitting. (Putting on and taking off braces is scored under dressing.)

   10 = Patient needs help or supervision in any of the above but can walk at least 50 yards with a little help.

6a. Propelling a wheelchair
   5 = Patient cannot ambulate but can propel a wheelchair independently. Must be able to go around corners, turn around, and maneuver the chair to a table, bed, toilet, and so on. Must be able to push a chair at least 50 yards. (Do not score this item if the patient gets a score for walking.)

7. Ascending and descending stairs
   10 = Patient is able to go up and down a flight of stairs safely without help or supervision. Patient may and should use handrails, canes, or crutches when needed. Must be able to carry canes or crutches when ascending or descending stairs.
   5 = Patient needs help with or supervision during any one of the above items.

8. Dressing and undressing
   10 = Patient is able to put on, remove, and fasten all clothing as well as tie shoelaces (unless adaptations are necessary). The activity includes putting on, removing, and fastening corset or braces when these are prescribed.
   5 = Patient needs help putting on and removing or fastening any clothing. Patient must do at least half the work. Patient must accomplish this in a reasonable time. Women need not be scored on use of a brassiere or girdle unless these are prescribed garments.

9. Continence of bowels
   10 = Patient is able to control bowels and have no accidents. Can use a suppository or take an enema when necessary.
   5 = Patient needs help in using a suppository or taking an enema or has occasional accidents.

10. Controlling bladder
    10 = Patient is able to control his or her bladder day and night. Patients who wear an external device and leg bag must put them on independently, clean and empty bag, and stay dry day and night.
    5 = Patient has occasional accidents or cannot wait for the bedpan or get to the toilet in time or needs help with an external device.

Modified from Mahoney FI, Barthel DW. Functional evaluation: the Barthel index. *Md State Med J.* 1965;14:63.

28

Disorders of Vision and Visual-Perceptual Dysfunction

Domenique Hendershot Embrey and Laurie Ruth Chaikin

OBJECTIVES

After reading this chapter the student or therapist will be able to:

1. Identify and analyze visual anatomy and physiology as they pertain to visual function.
2. Analyze the functional visual skills and how visual dysfunction may affect functional performance.
3. Identify the symptoms of visual dysfunction.
4. Develop the skill necessary to take a visual case history by use of behaviors and clinical observations.
5. Identify the difference between phoria and strabismus.

6. Identify and evaluate the difference between visual field loss and unilateral neglect.
7. Identify and differentiate various pediatric and age-related disease conditions that may affect vision.
8. Clearly differentiate nonoptical and optical assessment and intervention adaptations for patients with low vision.
9. Differentiate basic tools for vision screening.
10. Identify when and why to refer and the tools necessary to document that decision.

KEY TERMS

anatomy of the eye	refractive error	visual-perceptual dysfunction
eye diseases	strabismus	visual rehab
functional visual skills	treatment	visual screening

Vision is an integral part of development of perception. Some aspects of vision, such as pupillary function, are innate, but many other aspects are stimulated to develop by experience and interaction with the environment. Visual acuity itself has been demonstrated to rely on the presence of a clear image focused on the retina. If this does not occur, a "lazy eye," or amblyopia, will result. Depth perception develops as a result of precise eye alignment. This ability will be delayed, less precise, or absent if correction of eye misalignment is not done within the first 7 years of life. Research has demonstrated that, in fact, most visual skills such as acuity, binocular coordination, accommodation, ocular motilities, and depth perception are largely intact by age 6 months to 1 year.[1] Visual skill development parallels postural reflex integration and provides a foundation for perception.

Early in infancy visual input is associated with olfactory, tactile, vestibular, and proprioceptive sensations. The infant is driven to touch, taste, smell, and manipulate what he or she sees. Primitive postural reflexes such as the asymmetrical tonic neck reflex help provide visual regard and attention.

By combining the sensory input from vision, oral exploration, and tactile input, at some point the young child is able to look at an object and determine both the texture and the shape without having to touch or taste it. In adults, vision has moved to the top of the sensory hierarchy, providing full multisensory associations from sight alone. Even the visualized image of eating an apple can recreate the smell, sound of

crunching, taste, and feel of the experience; this occurs based on previous input provided to the brain by the senses.

Early visual impairment and later acquired impairment can affect the quality of the image presented to the brain and thus affect the learning process. In addition, damage to association centers involved with spatial perception, figure-ground, and directionality can interfere with learning and performance. Altered function may be the result of congenital and developmental disorders, birth trauma, physical trauma, or neurological or systemic diseases.

It is important therefore to isolate the primary visual processes of seeing from the secondary or associational processes of perceiving in the evaluation of perceptual disorders. The identification of a vision problem becomes part of the differential diagnosis of a perceptual deficit. Visual screening must be done before perceptual evaluation so that visual problems do not bias or contaminate the perceptual testing. It is just as important to eliminate vision as a contributing factor to a perceptual problem as it is to find a possible vision problem.

Our understanding of the ability to improve vision or recover visual function frequently needs to be updated as we apply new research and understanding of neuroplasticity. Principles of visual rehabilitation involve understanding how to provide visual feedback to the system in an optimal learning environment for the patient. The boundaries of improvement are slowly expanding as we refine this understanding.

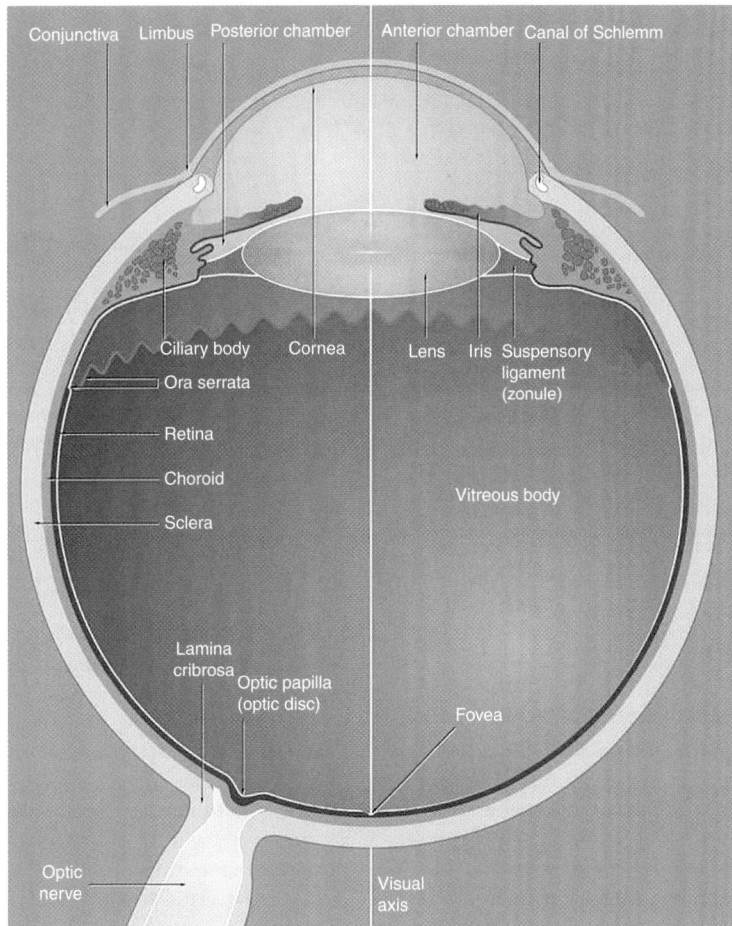

Fig. 28.1 Horizontal Section of the Eye. (From Young B. *Wheater's Functional Histology.* Elsevier: Philadelphia; 2014.)

ANATOMY OF THE EYE

An operational analogy of the eye as a camera may be useful up to a point in understanding the physical function of the structures. Once an image hits the retina and image enhancement begins, metaphors, however, must change to match our ever-changing comprehension of brain function. Using computer analogies such as microprocessing of feature detectors comes closer. Many aspects of how we see remain a mystery inside the "black box" of our brain.

Eye Chamber and Lens

Structures and function are discussed from anterior to posterior (Fig. 28.1). The first structure that light hits after it is reflected from an image is the cornea. (Technically, light first hits the tear layer, which has its own structure and rests on the corneal surface.) Corneal tissue is completely transparent. Light is refracted, or bent, to the greatest degree by the cornea because the light rays must pass through different media, which change in density, as in going from air to water.[2] The refraction of light can be observed by noting how a straw placed into a glass of water appears bent where it enters the water (Fig. 28.2).

Damage to the cornea from abrasions, burns, or congenital or disease-related processes can alter the spherical shape of the cornea and disturb the quality of the image that falls on the retina. In people diagnosed with keratoconus, the cornea slowly becomes steeper and more cone shaped, distorting the image and causing reduced vision.[3]

Radial keratotomy, a surgical procedure done in the 1980s to reduce nearsightedness by placing spoke like cuts in the cornea,

sometimes had the side effect of scarring the cornea and causing distorted vision. This surgery is no longer done, although you may see older patients who had this surgery. The newer surgeries such as laser-assisted in situ keratomileusis (LASIK) are far superior and more predictable in their reduction of refractive error (near-sightedness, farsightedness, or astigmatism) and induce virtually no scarring or distortion. In keratoconus the cornea slowly becomes steeper and more cone shaped, distorting the image and causing reduced vision.[3]

Iris

Behind the cornea is the iris, or colored portion, which consists of fibers that control the opening of the pupil, the dark circular opening in the center of the eye. The constriction and dilation of the pupil control the amount of light entering the eye in a similar fashion to the way the f-stop on a camera changes the size of the aperture to control the amount of light and the depth of field.[4] Under bright light conditions the opening constricts, and under dim light conditions it dilates, allowing light in to stimulate the photoreceptor cells of the retina. This constriction and dilation are under autonomic nervous system (ANS) control, with both sympathetic and parasympathetic components.[5] Under conditions of sympathetic stimulation (fight or flight), the pupils dilate, perhaps giving rise to the expression "eyes wide with fear." Under parasympathetic stimulation, the pupils constrict. The effect of drugs that stimulate the ANS can be observed.[6] For example, someone who has taken heroin will have pinpoint pupils.

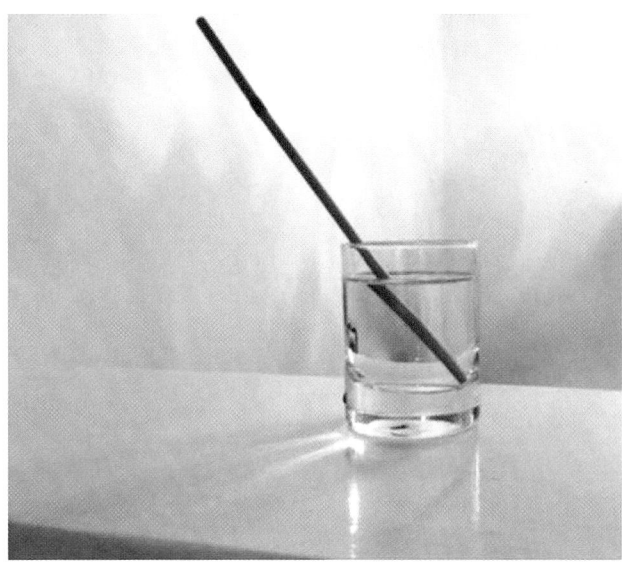

Fig. 28.2 Refraction: Bending of Light at Air-Water Interface. (From Khalili K. *Diagnostic Ultrasound*. Elsevier: Philadelphia; 2018.)

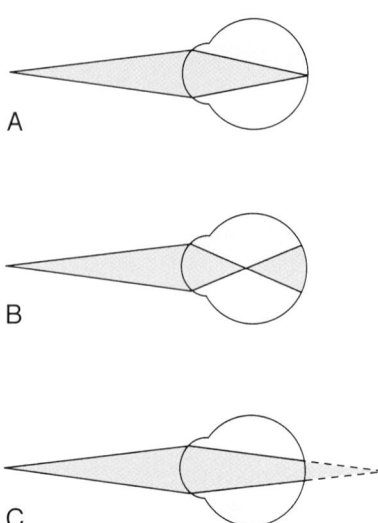

Fig. 28.4 Refractive Error. (A) Image focused on retina; no refractive error. (B) A nearsighted or myopic eye. (C) A farsighted or hyperopic eye.

Exercise 28.1: Observation of Pupillary Constriction and Dilation

Observe pupillary dilation and constriction on a willing subject (or on yourself in a mirror) by flashing a penlight at her or his pupil. Observe the decreased size of the pupil. Remove the light and watch the pupil dilate. Now go in a room with low natural light, observe the pupils, then walk into a room with bright overhead lighting. How do the pupils change? What does this tell you about the importance of lighting?

Lens

Behind the iris is the lens. The lens is involved in focusing, or accommodation. It is a biconvex, circular, semirigid, crystalline structure that fine-tunes the image on the retina. In a camera, the lens is represented by the external optical lens system. The ability to change the focus on the camera is achieved by turning the lens to change the distance of the lens from the film, which effectively increases or decreases the power of the lens, allowing near or distance objects to be seen more clearly. The same effect, a change in the power of the lens, is achieved in the eye by the action of tiny ciliary muscles, which act on suspensory ligaments, thereby changing the thickness and curvature of the lens. A thicker lens with a greater curvature produces higher power and the ability to see clearly at near distances. A thinner lens and flatter curvature produces less optical power, which is what is needed to allow distant objects to be clear (Fig. 28.3). The process of lens thickening and thinning is accommodation.[4,5]

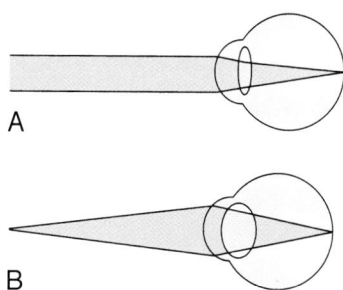

Fig. 28.3 Accommodation. (A) Looking far away. (B) Looking up close.

Ideally, the lens will bring an image into perfect focus so that it lands right on the fovea, the area of central vision. If the focused image falls in front of the retina, however, then a blurred circle will fall on the fovea (Fig. 28.4). In this case the lens is too thick, having too high an optical power. One simple remedy is to place a negative (concave) lens externally in front of the eye in glasses (or contact lenses) to reduce the power of the internal lens and allow the image to fall directly on the fovea. In presbyopia (old eyes), the flexibility of the lens fibers decreases and the lens becomes more rigid.[7] Accommodation gets weaker until the image can no longer be focused on the retina. Normal-sighted individuals first begin to notice these changes in their early forties. When this occurs, a plus (positive) lens (or bifocals, progressive lenses, bifocal or monovision contact lenses) may be worn to aid in reading.[4]

Other solutions to the problems of aging can be implemented during the time of cataract surgery, where a bifocal implant may be inserted, or monovision implant correction performed in each eye.

The lens can be affected by the age-related process of cataract development, in which the general clarity of vision is impaired from a loss of transparency of the crystalline lens. Incoming light tends to scatter inside the eye, causing glare problems. When vision is impaired to such a degree that it affects function, the lens may be removed surgically and replaced with a silicone implant placed just posterior to the iris.

Vitreous Chamber

The space behind the lens, which is filled with a gel-like substance, is called the *vitreous chamber*. As we age, the gel tends to liquefy, and some of the remnants of embryological development that were trapped are released to float freely. This can cause the very common perception of "floaters," the shadows cast by these particles onto the macular region. They can be disturbing but generally float out of view over time.[5]

Retina

The retina at the back of the eye is the photosensitive layer, like the film in a camera, receiving the pattern of light reflected from objects. The topography of the retina (Fig. 28.5) includes the optic disc, which is where the optic nerve exits and arteries and veins emerge and exit. This is also the blind spot because there are no photoreceptor cells on the disc. The macula is temporal to the optic disc and contains the fovea, providing central vision. The surrounding retina provides peripheral vision and defines a 180-degree half-sphere.[5]

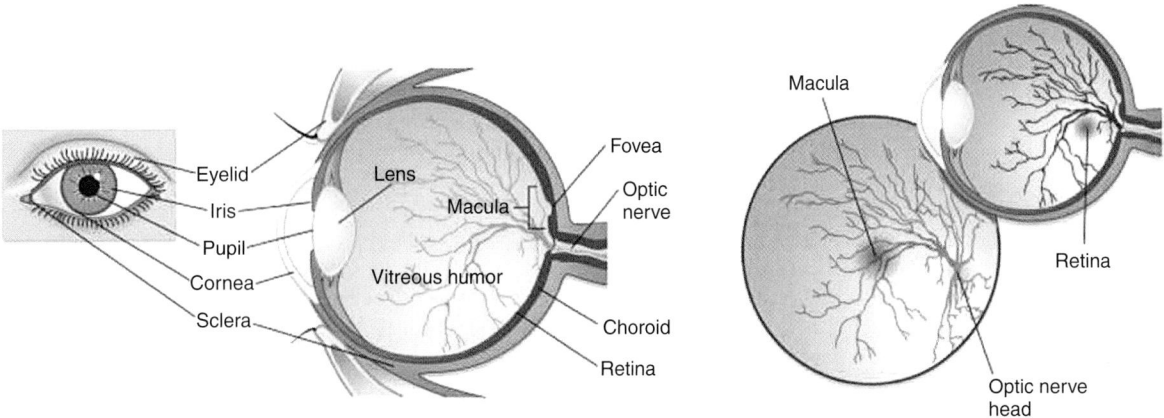

Fig. 28.5 Retinal Topography. (From Bhatia K. *Emergency Medicine.* Elsevier: Philadelphia; 2013.)

Exercise 28.2: Blind Spot

Your blind spot may be observed by doing the following: draw two dots 3 inches (7.5 cm) apart on a piece of paper. The dots can be ¼ inch (0.5 cm). Cover your left eye and look at the dot on the left. Starting at about 16 inches (40 cm), slowly bring the paper closer. Make sure you can see the two dots—one you are looking at directly and the other peripherally. At approximately 10 inches (25 cm) the dot on the right will disappear. This is your blind spot! Why can this exercise only be done monocularly (with one eye)?

Visual Pathway

The visual pathway begins with the photoreceptor cells, which begin a three-neuron chain exiting through the optic nerve. This chain consists of the rods and cones, which synapse with bipolar cells that synapse with ganglion cells (Fig. 28.6).[5,8]

There are two types of photoreceptor cells: rods and cones. The cone or rod shape is the dendrite of the cell. Variation in shape and slight variation in pigment give each one different sensitivities. The rod cell has greater sensitivity to dim light but less sensitivity to color,

whereas the cone cell has greater sensitivity to color and high-intensity light and less to reduced light conditions. The highest concentration of cone cells is in the fovea and macula, with decreasing concentration of cone cells and increasing concentration of rod cells moving concentrically away from the macula. The high degree of low-light sensitivity can be most appreciated in survival mode conditions such as being lost in the woods on a moonless night. By swinging the eyes side to side, one can maximize the image and keep the macula from interfering.

The phenomenon responsible for the high degree of neural representation of the foveal region and that accounts for the tremendous conscious awareness of the central view is called convergence.[5] At the periphery of the retina, the degree of convergence is great; many photoreceptor cells synapse on one ganglion cell, which accounts for poor acuity but high light sensitivity. The closer to the macula, the less the degree of convergence, until, finally, at the fovea there is no convergence. This means that one photoreceptor cell synapses with one bipolar cell and one ganglion cell.

The awareness of what is seen is directly related to the amount of convergence, which reflects the extent of neural representation. The 1:1

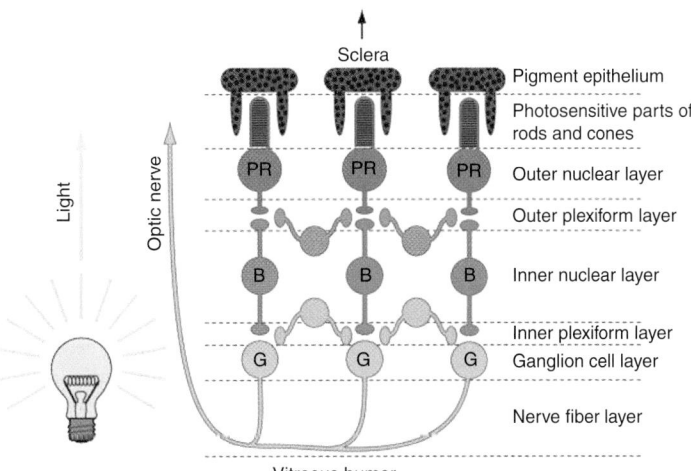

Fig. 28.6 The Connections Among Retinal Neurons and the Significance of Prominent Layers. The neurons shown are photoreceptors *(PR)*, horizontal cells *(H)*, bipolar cells *(B)*, amacrine cells *(A)*, and ganglion cells *(G)*. It has been suggested that ganglion cells dominated by bipolar cell inputs represent newer circuitry. The arrow indicates the direction of light as it passes through the retina to reach the photoreceptors. (From Vanderah T. *Nolte's Essentials of the Human Brain.* Elsevier: Philadelphia; 2019.)

correspondence between photoreceptor and ganglion cell at the fovea means that there is a high degree of neural representation of the foveal image in the brain. It is even greater than the neural representation of the lips, tongue, or hands.[9] This accounts for the primary awareness of what is in the foveal field and secondary awareness of the peripheral field. Conscious awareness of the environment is whatever is in the foveal field at the moment. But continuous information about the environment is flowing over the peripheral retina, usually subconsciously. Attention quickly shifts from foveal to nonfoveal stimulation when changes in light intensity or rapid movement are registered. This type of stimulus arouses attention immediately because it could have specific survival value. For example, a person is driving down the street and senses rapid motion off to the right. The foveae swing around immediately to identify a small red ball bouncing into the street. This information goes to the association areas, in which "small ball" is associated with "small child soon to follow." Frontal cortical centers are aroused, and a decision is made to initiate motor areas to take the foot off the accelerator and put it onto the brake, while simultaneously moving the wheel away from the ball and scanning for the object of concern—that is, the child.

Exercise 28.3: Peripheral Central Awareness

We have a unique ability to change our awareness by consciously shifting attention from our foveal or central awareness to our peripheral awareness. For example, as you read these words, become aware of the background surrounding the paper or screen; note colors, forms, and shapes; and continue to expand your awareness to include your clothes, the floor, walls, and ceiling if possible. You are consciously stimulating your primitive, phylogenetically older visual system. The ability to do this has considerable therapeutic value because a typical pattern of visual stress is associated with foveal concentration to the exclusion of peripheral information. The ability to expand the peripheral awareness at will is a skill that can help you to relax while you drive, can improve reading skills, and can be used in visual training techniques.

The moment light hits the retina, the photographic film model must be abandoned exchanged for the image processing or computerized image enhancement model. The primary visual pathway at the retinal level is a three-neuron chain. From back to front the first neuron is the photoreceptor cell, rods, or cones. They synapse with a bipolar cell, which in turn synapses with a ganglion cell. The axon of the ganglion cell exits by means of the optic nerve. Image enhancement occurs at the two junctions of the three–nerve-cell pathway. Lateral cells at the neural junctions have an inhibitory action on the primary three-neuron pathway, and through the inhibition of an impulse the image is modulated. For example, at the first junction between photoreceptor cell and bipolar cell, there are horizontal cells. These cells enhance the contrast between light and dark by inhibiting the firing of bipolar cells at the edge of an image. This makes the edge of the image appear darker than the central area, which increases the contrast and thereby increases attention-getting value. After all, it is by perceiving edges that we are able to maneuver around objects. In a similar manner, amacrine cells act at the second neural junction between bipolar and ganglion cells to enhance movement detection.[10]

This image enhancement process continues throughout the visual pathway. The process has been likened to the way in which a computer enhances a distorted picture of outer space received from a satellite. The first image may be unclear and fuzzy; by adjusting the settings to improve clarity the brain ultimately is able to obtain a clear perceived image. The image goes through a series of processing stations in the inner workings of the computer—much the same way that mapping software on your phone may initially give you an image of a grid, then

the area and finally the streets and roads that you need to take. The computer-generated, enhanced image shown on the screen is like the end product in the brain: the perceived image.

The visual pathway continues through the brain (Fig. 28.7). The ganglion cell axons exit the eyeball by means of the optic nerve, carrying the complete retinal picture in coded electrochemical patterns. From there the patterns project to different sites within the central nervous system (Fig. 28.8). Projections to the pretectum are important in pupillary reflexes; projections to the pretectal nuclei, the accessory optic nuclei, and the superior colliculus are all involved in eye movement functions.[5] The largest bundle, called the *optic tract*, projects to the lateral geniculate body in the hypothalamus, where additional image enhancement and processing occurs. The next group of axons continues to the primary visual cortex and from there to visual association areas.

At what point does the retinal image become a perception, and with what part of the brain does one see? Current theory regarding visual perception is the result of Nobel prize–winning research by Hubel and Wiesel in the 1960s called the *receptive field theory*.[11] This theory states that different neurons are feature detectors, defining objects in terms of movement, direction, orientation, color, depth, and acuity. Research in 1990 by Hubel and Livingstone[12] was able to locate a segregation of function at the level of the lateral geniculate body. They identified two types of cells, one type being larger and faster magno cells, which are apparently phylogenetically older and color-blind but that have a high-contrast sensitivity and are able to detect differences in contrast of 1% to 2%. They also have low spatial resolution (low acuity). They seem to operate globally and are responsible for perception of movement, depth perception from motion, perspective, parallax, stereopsis, shading, contour, and interocular rivalry. Through linking properties (objects having common movement or depth) emerges figure-ground perception. Much of this perception occurs in the middle temporal lobe.

The other type of cell, called the *parvo cell*, is smaller, slower, and color sensitive and has a smaller receptive field. These cells are less global and are primarily responsible for high-resolution form perception. Higher-level visual association occurs in the temporal-occipital region, where learning to identify objects by their appearance occurs. It appears that these two types of cells are functionally and structurally related to the two visual systems represented in retinal topography—the foveal (central) and peripheral visual systems.

Eye Movement System

The eye movement system consists of six pairs of eye muscles: the medial recti, lateral recti, superior and inferior recti, and superior and inferior obliques (see Fig. 28.8). Together they are controlled by cranial nerves III (oculomotor), IV (trochlear), and VI (abducens). The eye movement system has both reflex and voluntary components. Reflexive movements are coordinated through vestibular interconnections at a midbrain level. The vestibulo-ocular reflex (VOR) functions primarily to keep the image stabilized on the retina. Through connections between pairs of eye muscles and the semicircular canals, movement is analyzed as being either external movement of an object or movement of the head or body. From this information the VOR is able to direct the appropriate head or eye movement.[5]

Two types of eye movements are the result. Smooth, coordinated eye movements are called *pursuits*, and rapid localizations are called *saccades*. Voluntary control of both these motions indicates cortical control. Pursuits are used for continuously following moving targets, and they are stimulated by a foveal image. Saccades are stimulated by images from the peripheral system, where a detection of motion or change in light intensity results in a rapid saccadic eye movement to

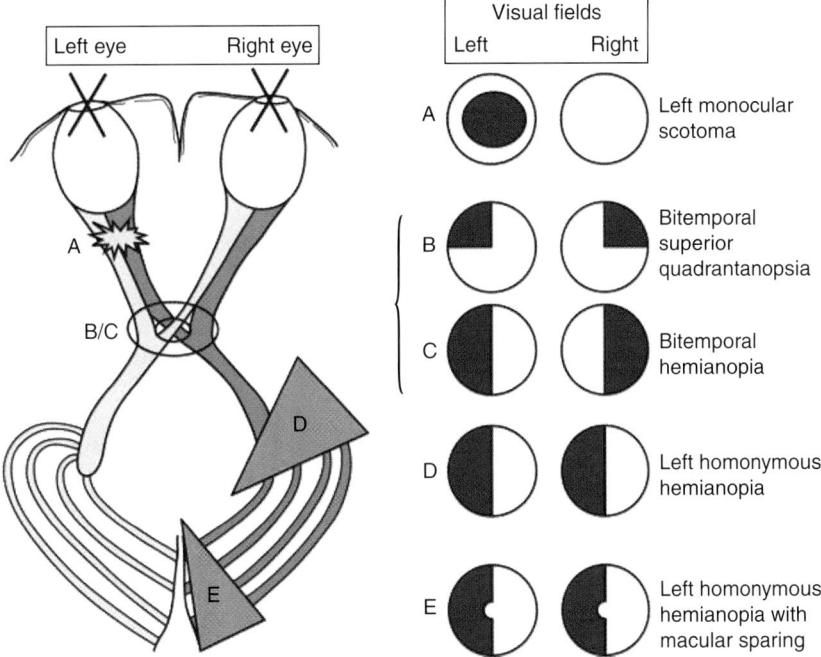

Fig. 28.7 Visual Field Disturbances at Various Points Along the Optic Pathway. (A) Lesions in the optic nerve could result in an ipsilateral scotoma (partial loss of vision or blind spot). **(B)** Lesions in the optic chiasm from below when small (small ring) can cause superior bitemporal quadrantanopsia (outer upper quadrant loss of vision) and **(C)** when large (larger ring) can result in bitemporal hemianopia (loss of vision in the outer half of both the right and left visual field). **(D)** Optic tract or lateral geniculate lesion can cause a contralateral homonymous hemianopia (blindness in the opposite half of both visual fields). **(E)** Lesion in the occipital lobe lesion can cause contralateral homonymous hemianopia (blindness in the corresponding half of each visual field) but with macular sparing. (From Kaufman DM. *Kaufman's Clinical Neurology for Psychiatrists.* Elsevier; 2017.)

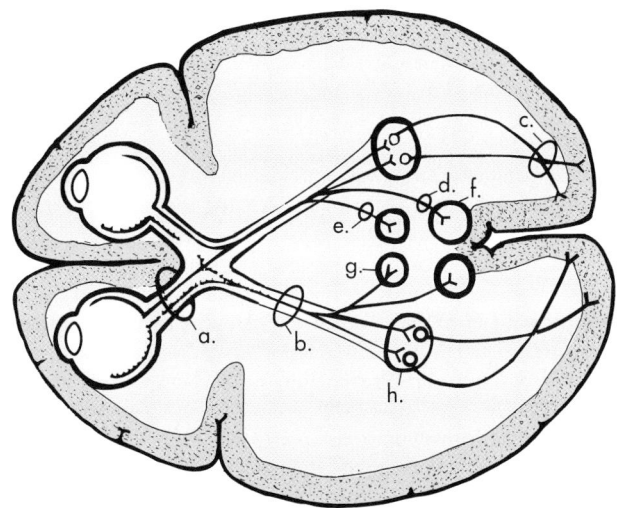

Fig. 28.8 Visual tract system: *a,* optic nerve; *b,* optic tract; *c,* geniculate-occipital radiators; *d,* retinocollicular radiation; *e,* radioprotector tracts; *f,* superior colliculus (midbrain); *g,* pretectal area (tegmentum); *h,* lateral geniculate.

bring the object into the foveal field. Either difficulties in the eye movement system or altered functioning of the vestibular system can affect the coordinated, efficient functioning of eye movement skills.

A third type of eye movement is specifically related to eye aiming ability. This is the coordinated movement of both eyes inward toward the nose, as in crossing the eyes, or outward along the midline, as when looking away in the distance. The inward movement is called *convergence*, and the outward movement is called *divergence*. The most important result of efficient vergence abilities is depth perception, or stereopsis. Small errors in aiming can dramatically affect stereopsis. Problems such as double vision, wandering eyes, and strabismus are discussed in greater depth in a later section.

Exercise 28.4: Pursuits, Saccades, Convergence

Pursuits. Take a pencil or pen and look at the pointed end. Follow a moving target such as a pencil point as you move it across your field of gaze, while keeping your head still. Continue to move it in different directions, vertically, horizontally, diagonally, and circularly, to stimulate all pairs of eye muscles. For a more challenging demonstration, find a fly and follow its flight path around the room. If you lose sight of it, note that the detection of the movement of the fly will signal your eye movement directly toward it.

Saccades. Hold two pencils about head width apart. Shift your eyes from pencil to pencil without moving your head. Note that your awareness is of the two pencils, not of the background between them. In general, perception occurs the moment the eyes are still, rather than while moving during saccades. For a more challenging exercise, move the pencil you are not looking at, then shift quickly to it; move the other pencil while looking at the one you just moved. In other words, you will pick up the location of the other pencil peripherally and direct your eyes to the foveal region. The size and degree of blur of the peripheral image will tell the brain where the image is and how far to move the eyes. This ability again is a result of the function of neural convergence, which is related to neural representation.

Convergence. Hold a pencil at arm's length along your midline. Slowly bring the pencil closer in toward you along your midline. Feel your eyes moving in (crossing). Try to bring the pencil to your nose, keeping the pencil visually single. (It is okay if you cannot.) Move the pencil away now, and your eyes are diverging.

FUNCTIONAL VISUAL SKILLS

Refractive Error

Before discussing binocular coordination and the individual visual skills, it is important to describe refractive errors and how they can affect binocular coordination. Three common types of refractive errors are myopia or nearsightedness, hyperopia or farsightedness, and astigmatism.[5,10]

The myopic eye is too long, or the cornea is too steep, so the focused image falls in front of the retina. It is easily corrected with a negative or minus lens, which optically moves the image back onto the retina.

The hyperopic eye is too short, or the cornea is too flat, such that the focused image falls behind the retina. A positive or plus lens optically moves the image onto the retina. A young hyperopic person will be able to use accommodation to bring the image focus back onto the retina, but because accommodation is finite, this can cause reading difficulties earlier than normal or can affect binocular coordination at near distances.

An eye will have astigmatism if it is not perfectly spherical. An aspherical eye will cause the image to be distorted, where part of the focused image will be in front of the retina and part on or in back. A person with astigmatism may see vertical lines clearly and horizontal lines as blurry, depending on the specific aspherical shape. A cylindrical type of lens is used to correct astigmatism. This lens corrects the distortion of the image so that it is placed right on the retina.

The following are examples of ways you may see different refractive errors documented in a chart and what it means functionally:

−5.50 DS (diopter sphere): myopia

+4.00 DS: hyperopia

+1.50 c⁻ − 1.50 × 180: astigmatism (Note: × stands for the axis of the cylinder correction.)

When significant refractive errors are uncorrected, they can reduce vision. Uncorrected refractive error also can interfere with binocular coordination. The symptoms are described in greater detail in the next section.

Binocular coordination is the end result of the efficient functioning of the visual skills (Box 28.1). The individual visual skills include accommodation, eye alignment or vergence, eye movements with normal vestibular coordination, stereopsis (depth perception), and peripheral and central coordination. During normal activities, all the skills are inseparable.

Accommodation

Accommodation is the ability to bring near objects into clear focus automatically and without strain. As demonstrated in Exercise 28.4, relaxation of accommodation allows distant objects to come into focus. The primary action is that of the ciliary muscles acting on the lens, and the primary system of control is the ANS, with sympathetic and parasympathetic components.[5]

Both accommodation and pupil size changes are reflexes that work in concert: as accommodation relaxes the pupil dilates and as accommodation increases the pupil constricts.[4] As a person focuses on a near object, the lenses thicken, allowing the near object to come into focus. At the same time the pupils constrict to increase depth of focus (just as in a camera). As a person looks into the distance, the lens gets flatter, relaxing accommodation, and the pupil dilates, decreasing the depth of field.

Accommodative ability is age dependent. A young child can focus on small objects just a few inches in front of the eyes. At about the age of 9 years, the accommodative ability slowly begins to decrease. By the mid-40s, the reserve focusing power diminishes to the point that near objects begin to blur. At this stage, reading material is pushed farther away until the arms are not long enough, and then reading glasses are needed. This is called *presbyopia* (old eyes) and, as stated earlier in this chapter, is caused by a loss of elasticity of the lens of the eye as part of aging.

Problems in accommodation may contribute to myopia, hyperopia, and presbyopia. Symptoms include blurriness at either near or far distance, depending on the age and the problem.

Accommodation is important mainly for up-close activities: reading, hygiene, dressing (specifically, closing fasteners), use of tools, typing, tabletop activities, and games.

Exercise 28.5: Accommodation

Accommodation cannot be directly observed, but it can be implied indirectly through observation of pupillary constriction while doing an accommodative task. Cover one eye. Hold a finger in front at about 10 inches (25 cm). Focus on the finger, making sure that the fingerprint is clear. Shift focus to a distant object. Continue shifting far to near and near to far while a partner observes the pupil. The partner should be able to observe pupillary constriction with near focus and dilation with far focus.

Vergence

Vergence includes convergence and divergence. It is the ability to smoothly and automatically bring the eyes together along the midline to singly observe objects that are near (convergence) or conversely to move the eyes outward for single vision of distant objects (divergence). Specific brain centers control convergence and divergence.

With regard to reflexes, vergence is associated with accommodation: convergence with accommodation, and divergence with relaxation of accommodation. The function of this reflex is to allow objects to be both single and clear, at either near or far positions. Vergence has both automatic and voluntary components. Most of the time it is not necessary to think about moving the eyes inward while looking at a close object; yet if asked to cross the eyes, most people can do this at will.

Problems can occur in vergence ability when the eye movement system is out of sync with accommodation or from damage to cranial nerves III, IV, or VI. Problems can be slight, in which there is merely a tendency for the eyes to converge in or out too far, or the eyes can be grossly out of convergence. Tendencies to underconverge or overconverge are called *phorias* and are not visible except by special testing in which they are elicited. An individual may be asymptomatic, but symptoms may occur under conditions of increased stress or fatigue, such as excessive reading or working at a computer terminal, or from drug side effects (prescription and recreational).

Some phorias may worsen to the extent that binocularity breaks down, at which point the individual becomes strabismic. There are two

---

BOX 28.1 **Binocular Coordination**

- Corrected refractive error
- Accommodation
- Eye alignment
- Stereopsis
- Central and peripheral coordination
- Efficient eye movement skills

main types of strabismus: esotropia and exotropia. An esotropia is an inward turning of the eye, and an exotropia is an outward turning. A third, less common type of strabismus is hypertropia, in which one eye aims upward relative to the other eye. Strabismus and dysfunctional phorias are discussed in greater detail in the next section.

Vergence ability is needed for singular binocular vision; thus it is basic to all activities. At near positions the patient may have difficulty finding objects; eye-hand coordination may be decreased, affecting self-care and hygiene tasks; and reading may be difficult. Distance tasks that may be affected include driving, sports, movies, communication, and, frequently, ambulation. Individuals with impaired vergence ability may also have difficulty focusing and may have decreased or no depth perception. Interpreting space can be quite difficult and confusing. If decreased vergence is a result of traumatic head injury or stroke, it may contribute to the patient's confusion, and he or she may not be able to identify or communicate the problem.

Exercise 28.6: Vergence

Hold a pencil in front of you at eye level at about 12 inches (30 cm). Look at the pencil. Look away into the distance. Looking at the pencil is convergence, and looking into the distance is divergence. As you converge and diverge slowly back and forth, note any changes you may feel: changes in how relaxed you feel, how focused or spaced out you feel, feelings of dreaminess, or nothing at all. Observe a partner's eyes as he or she shifts back and forth as well.

Pursuits and Saccades

Eye movement skills consist of pursuits and saccades. Pursuits are the smooth, coordinated movements of all eye muscles together, allowing accurate tracking of objects through space. Perception is continuous during pursuit movements. Saccades are rapid shifts of the eyes from object to object, allowing quick localization of movements observed in the periphery. The systems involved in eye movement skills are the oculomotor system with the VOR, in conjunction with coordination of the central and peripheral visual systems. The peripheral visual system is finely tuned for detecting changes in light levels and small movements.

Problems in pursuits or saccades can be the result of a dysfunction of any individual muscles, the VOR, or areas of the brain controlling pursuits or saccades.[13–15] Because the VOR helps stabilize the image on the retina and to differentiate image movement from eye movement, simple tracking can be more difficult. In addition, visual field loss, either central or peripheral, can dramatically affect localization ability. People with blind half- or quarter-fields can be observed to do searching eye movements rather than directly jumping to the object.

Activities affected include searching for objects; visually directed movement for fine motor tasks, gross movement, and ambulation tasks; eye-hand coordination; self-care; driving; and reading.

Memory also may be affected by an eye movement dysfunction. Research by Adler-Grinberg and Stark[16] and Noton and Stark[17] examined patterns of eye movements as subjects looked at a picture. Distinct eye movement patterns, called scan paths, became apparent. When the subject was asked to recall the picture, the same eye movement pattern was elicited as when the subject originally saw the picture. It would appear that a type of oculomotor praxis is involved in recall. Applying this idea to the clinical setting, if a patient has inaccurate eye movement with poor pursuits or excessive saccades, then perhaps the stored memory is less efficiently stored and consequently more difficult to reconstruct from memory. In addition, if a patient has a type of brain damage with generalized dyspraxia, the eye movement system could quite likely be affected and might be involved in the patient's perceptual dysfunction. Frequently, the treating occupational or physical therapist are the first to note a patient's dyspraxia, in which case a recommendation for a comprehensive eye exam is warranted.

Another more recent example of the relationship between eye movements and memory is the use of eye movement desensitization and reprocessing (EMDR) therapy to help individuals with posttraumatic stress disorder reintegrate traumatic experiences.[18] This technique is still being evaluated, but a systematic review by Wilson and colleagues[19] indicated good potential in the treatment of posttraumatic stress disorder. Although the exact mechanism is at this time unknown, the prevailing hypothesis is that the lateral eye movements elicit an orienting response, scanning the environment for further danger, and that this is an investigatory reflex associated with a relaxed physical state.[20]

SYMPTOMS OF VISUAL DYSFUNCTION

History

The identification of a visual problem begins with case history. It is important to get some idea of the patient's prior visual status or any history of eye injury, surgery, or diseases. Information can be elicited by direct questioning of the patient or family members or by clinical observation. Sample questions include the following:

- Are you having difficulty with seeing or with your eyes?
- Do you wear glasses? Contact lenses? For distance, near, bifocals, or monovision (one eye near, other distance)?
- Does your correction (glasses, contact lenses) work as well now as before the (stroke, accident, etc.)?
- Have you noticed any blurriness? Near or far?
- Do you ever see double? See two? See overlapping or shadow images?
- Do you ever find that when you reach for an object that you knock it over or your hand misses?
- Do letters jump around on the page after reading for a while?
- Are you experiencing any eyestrain or headaches? Where and when?
- Do you ever lose your place when reading?
- Are portions of a page or any objects missing?
- Do people or things suddenly appear from one side that you did not see approaching?
- Do you have difficulty concentrating on tasks?

Clinical observations of the patient performing various activities are a valuable source of problem identification. This situation varies considerably from the physician's observations in the more contrived environment of the examination room. Therapists in general are in an ideal position to observe patients in a variety of functional tasks that require near vision, far vision, spatial estimations, depth judgments, and oculomotor tasks. This situation varies considerably from the physician's observations in the more contrived environment of the examination room. In addition, the therapist's initial observations can be used in documenting difficulties within the therapy realm that may be amenable to visual remediation in terms that can be applied to reimbursement of therapy.

Clinical observations include the following:

- Head turn or tilt during near tasks, or postural adjustments to task
- Avoidance of near tasks
- One eye appears to go in, out, up, or down
- Vision shifts from eye to eye as indicated by head tilting
- Seems to look past observer
- Closes or covers one eye
- Squints
- Eyes appear red, puffy, or irritated or have a discharge (Notify nurses or physician of these observations.)
- Rubs eyes a lot
- Has difficulty maintaining eye contact (Be aware of cultural factors.)
- Spaces out, drifts off, daydreams

- During activity, neglects one side of body or space
- During movement, bumps into walls or objects (either walking or in a wheelchair)
- Appears to misjudge distance
- Underreaches or overreaches for objects
- Has difficulty finding things

Near Point Blur

Blurred vision up close is not a symptom that by itself is indicative of a problem in any one area. It could indicate farsightedness (hyperopia), astigmatism, or reduced accommodative ability (insufficiency). The patient may move objects or the head farther or closer, may complain of eyestrain or headaches, may squint, or may even avoid near activities as much as possible. The therapist might observe excessive blinking, and the patient may complain of glasses not working well.

Distance Blur

Distance blur could also have a number of different causes, including nearsightedness (myopia), a pathological problem (such as beginning cataracts or macular degeneration), or accommodative spasm. Most people have some experience with accommodative spasm. After spending long periods of time either studying or reading a novel and then glancing up at the wall across the room, it may be blurry and then clear up slowly. For some individuals, this spasm eventually develops into nearsightedness if the reading habits continue for a long time.

Patients with distance blur may make forward head movements and frequently squint in an attempt to see. They may not respond or orient quickly to auditory or visual stimuli beyond a certain radius. The therapist may also note excessive blinking and a withdrawn attitude because the patient cannot see well enough to interact with the environment.

Visual hygiene can be recommended to assist in the development of good visual habits. This should include attention to good lighting and posture, taking frequent breaks, and monitoring the state of clarity of an environmental cue such as a clock across the room.

Phoria and Strabismus

The next area of eye alignment problems can be divided into two types of problems: phoria and strabismus. A *phoria* can be defined as a natural positioning of the eyes in which there is a tendency to aim in front of or behind the point of focus. It may or may not be associated with symptoms. Fusion is intact, and depth perception may also be intact to some degree.

Everyone has a phoria, just as everyone has a posture. It may be within normal range, or, just as someone may have scoliosis, a high phoria may cause problems. The following phorias may cause problems:

- Esophoria: The eyes are postured in front of the point of focus.
- Exophoria: The eyes are postured in back of the point of focus.

Phoria is measured in units of prism diopters, which indicate the size of the prism needed to measure the eye position in or out from the straight-ahead position.[4]

Phorias tend to produce subtle symptoms. These include having difficulty concentrating, frontal or temporal headaches, sleepiness after reading, and stinging of the eyes after reading.

A strabismus, or tropia, is a visible turn of one eye, which may be constant, intermittent, or alternating between one eye and the other. The person may have double vision, or if the strabismus is long term, the person may suppress or "turn off" the vision in the wandering eye. Suppression is a neurological function that is an adaptation to the confusing situation of double images. In the developing brain the individual must choose (unconsciously) which eye is dominant, and the image is confirmed by motor and tactile inputs as being the

"real" image. The other fovea's image is then neurologically suppressed. The peripheral vision in the suppressing eye is still normal, and the eye still contributes to other aspects of vision such as orientation and locomotion.

The essential concept in understanding the difference between phoria and strabismus is that in strabismus fusion and depth perception are not present. Definitions of different types of strabismus are presented in Box 28.2. It is not a conclusive list; many other types and permutations are beyond the scope of this discussion. The intent here is to expose the therapist to different terms that may be used by the physician in diagnosing the type of strabismus.

In strabismus, one eye appears to go in, out, up, or down, and there is frequently an obvious inability to judge distances, especially if the strabismus is of recent onset (acquired). The patient may underreach or overreach for objects, cover or close one eye, complain of double vision, or exhibit a head tilt or turn during specific activities. He or she may appear to favor one eye, have difficulty reading, appear spaced out, or avoid near activities. In addition, especially if the patient sees double but is unable or unwilling to talk about it, she or he may be confused or disoriented.

Certain postures may facilitate fusion for some patients. The eye doctor will be able to determine which head position may be best. Frequently, many patients will automatically move around to the best position. At other times, however, head position will be used to avoid using one eye. Head and body position therefore are important aspects to consider.

Many convergence problems are amenable to vision therapy,[21–23] but some are not.[24] Whether a particular problem can be helped by vision therapy can be determined by an eye doctor, who can prescribe specific exercises.

Oculomotor Dysfunction

Oculomotor dysfunction is a very common sequela of neurological deficits, with an incidence as high as 90%, according to Ciufredda and colleagues.[25,26] Commonly the smooth pursuit system will be affected, such that the smooth movement is interrupted by a series of fixation stops and the movements appear jerky. Damage anywhere along the visual motor pathway may cause a variety of eye movement disorders. This includes injury to the pontine and mesencephalic reticular formation, oculomotor nucleus in the brain stem, caudate nucleus and substantia nigra, cerebellum, and vestibular nuclei.[25]

Patients with oculomotor disorders frequently also experience dizziness, nausea, and balance difficulties. Many times an eye movement will elicit dizziness and disorientation. It is thought that these symptoms are in part caused by a loss of integration of information coming from the two aspects of the visual system that process central vision (parvocellular pathway) and peripheral vision (magnocellular pathway).

As mentioned previously, detection of peripheral targets serves to direct an eye movement with a specific velocity and direction to bring the foveae in line for purposes of identification. Therapy for facilitating rehabilitation of eye movement disorders should be directed at using peripheral awareness with slow controlled eye movement toward the target. Once these movements are tolerated, head movement can be added, then slowly body movement.[27,28]

While doing any sort of tracking activity, the patient is encouraged to maintain peripheral awareness. This technique will help the patient keep her or his place. The oculomotor system is guided by the peripheral location of an object.

Visual Field Defects—Hemianopsia and Quadrantanopsia

Visual field loss may indicate damage that is prechiasmic, at the optic chiasm, postchiasmic, in the visual radiations of the thalamus, or in the visual cortex. The resultant visual field loss is characteristic (even diagnostic) in each case. The visual field loss pattern will generally reflect the location of the lesion. It could be bitemporal (outer half of each field), half-field loss (hemianopsia) with or without macular involvement, or quarter-field loss (see Fig. 28.7). Some symptoms of field loss are an inability to read or starting to read in the middle of the page, ignoring food on one-half of the plate, and difficulty orienting to stimuli in a specific area of space.

Hemianopsia is a loss of half of the visual field in each eye, and quadrantanopsia is loss of a quarter of the visual field in each eye. *Homonymous hemianopsia* refers to the inner or nasal half and the outer or temporal half of each eye being affected. The retina itself is intact, but a neurological lesion has interrupted the ability of the visual cortex to receive recognition of the image. Vision processing may be occurring at lower centers, such as the lateral geniculate body, but if signals are not being received by the cortex, then they are not recognized as "seen." In 1979, Zihl and von Cramon[29] published their findings that damaged visual fields could be trained by use of a light stimulus presented repeatedly at the border of the visual field defect. Balliet and co-workers[30] (when attempting to repeat the experiment, adding controls for oculomotor fixations) proposed that subjects were actually learning to make small compensatory eye movements rather than experiencing true improvements in the visual fields. In the 1980s and 1990s, a group of German researchers developed a computer-based field training system for researching the question of visual field

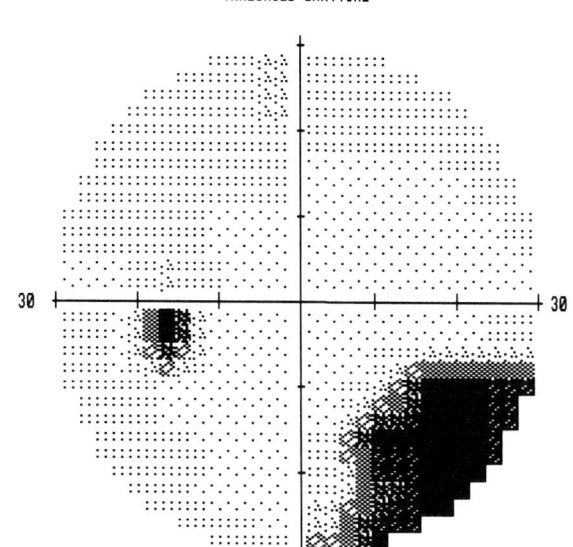

THRESHOLD GRAYTONE

Fig. 28.9 Visual Field Defect (Inferior Temporal) as Measured on Humphrey Visual Field Tester.

training. They found in their research that visual fields did expand on average by 5 degrees, with functional improvements noted by more than 80% of their patients (Fig. 28.9).[31-35] A company called NovaVision introduced the computer-based visual field restitution training program in the United States with good results (Appendix 28.A). This author has also noted documentable and functional improvements in visual fields, even when trained with less sophisticated methods.

Compensation training may also be required to allow the patient to resume activities such as reading. Compensation techniques include use of margin markers and reading with a card with a slit in it (typoscope) to isolate one line or a couple of lines at a time. Holding reading material vertically also can help. For those who do their reading using a computer, there are apps that can color code each line of a text to assist in maintaining visual attention. Changing font size or type can also help.

SUMMARY OF DISORDERS OF VISION

Table 28.1 summarizes primary visual deficits. Once a therapist or other specialist has eliminated the possibility of primary visual deficits, the clinician must assess whether the identified problem is resulting from central associative processing that is causing visual-perceptual dysfunction.

TABLE 28.1 Primary Visual Deficits Associated With Central Lesions, Functional Symptoms, Management, and Treatment

Visual Deficit	Functional Deficit	Management	Treatment
Decreased visual acuity (distance or near)	Decreased acuity for distance or near tasks (reading)	Provide best lens correction for distance and near vision	May not be correctable May be appropriate for low vision
Inconsistent accommodation	Inconsistent blurred near vision	Ensure appropriate lenses are worn for appropriate activities Determine whether bifocal is usable; if not, provide separate lenses for distance and near vision Enlarge target, control density, use contrast and task lighting	Accommodation training may be appropriate

Continued

TABLE 28.1   Primary Visual Deficits Associated With Central Lesions, Functional Symptoms, Management, and Treatment—cont'd

Visual Deficit	Functional Deficit	Management	Treatment
Cortical blindness	Marked decrease in visual acuity Severe blurring uncorrectable by lenses	Evaluated by vision specialist to determine areas and quality of residual vision Present targets of appropriate size and contrast in best area of visual field	Use headlamp to improve visual localization (i.e., functional use of residual vision) Multisensory input
Visual field deficits include homonymous hemianopsia, quadrantanopsia, scotoma, visual field constrictions	Blindness or decreased sensitivity in affected area of visual field	Be aware of normal field position in all meridians of gaze Ask patient to outline working area before beginning task Partial press-on Fresnel prism to facilitate compensation	Scanning training to facilitate compensation Training in use of prism NovaVision VF training
Pupillary reactions	Slow or absent pupillary responses	Sunglasses to control excessive brightness	
Loss of vertical gaze (external ophthalmoplegia)	Inability to move eyes up or down	Raise target or working area to foveal level Teach patient head movement to compensate	Prism glasses to allow objects below to be seen as directly in front
Conjugate gaze deviation	Inability to move or difficulty in moving eyes from fixed gaze position		
Lack of convergence	Diplopia or blurred vision for near tasks Decreased depth perception for near tasks	Convergence exercises prescribed by vision specialist	
Oculomotor nerve lesion (strabismus)	Intermittent or consistent diplopia in some or all meridians of gaze Loss of depth perception	Fresnel prism to fuse image in select cases Occlude deviant eye	Oculomotor and binocular exercises with prism use prescribed by vision specialist
Pathological (motor) nystagmus	Movement or blur of image during reading, near activities, decreased activities	Enlarge print or target to decrease blur Contact lens provides feedback, reduces movement, and increases acuity	Rigid gas-permeable contact lens prescribed by vision specialist
Poor fixations, saccades, or pursuits	Erratic scanning Unsteady fixation	Decrease density of material Isolate targets during evaluation and treatment Sensory integration activities Scanning training Use of kinesthetic and tactile systems to lead visual system (eye movements)	Oculomotor exercises prescribed by vision specialist

Copyright by Mary Jane Bouska, OTR/L, 1988. Modified by Laurie R. Chaikin, OD, OTR/L, FCOVD.

EYE DISEASES

Areas addressed in this section are common ocular and systemic diseases of the pediatric and geriatric populations, an introduction to low vision, and recommendations for adaptations of the treatment plan. If reduced vision (low vision) is a result of eye disease, the patient may be assisted by magnification aids. Also, the therapy treatment program may need to be altered to accommodate any special visual needs of the patient (lighting, working distance, inclusion of magnifiers, use of filters, and contrast-enhancing devices).

Pediatric Conditions

Retinopathy of Prematurity

The incidence of retinopathy of prematurity is increasing because of the improved survival of premature infants as a result of improved ventilation.[36] Immature retinal vessels are sensitive to high oxygen tension. The effect on the vessels is vasoconstriction, eventually leading to obliteration of the vessels. This creates a state of ischemia, which stimulates the growth of new blood vessels. These small, fragile vessels bleed easily, leading to fibrosis and traction on the retina. As a result of the traction, the macula gets stretched, interfering with the function of central vision.

The temporal vessels are most affected because they develop last. The degree of damage may be mild or severe, depending on the amount of prematurity.[7]

Retinoblastoma

Retinoblastoma is the most common malignant tumor in children.[1] The current incidence is 1 in 20,000 live births, a rate that has been increasing over the past 30 years, apparently owing to inheritance of a mutated gene.

The young child may have a strabismus resulting from impaired vision in the eye with the tumor. As the tumor grows, the pupil may appear milky white. If not detected early, the tumor will lead to loss of the eye; and if the tumor invades the brain, death will occur. Clearly, early detection is critical.

Mental Retardation

There are a higher number of visual problems in the mentally retarded populations.[1] These individuals have a higher incidence of refractive error (myopia, hyperopia, and astigmatism), strabismus, nystagmus, and optic atrophy than children with normal intelligence.

Cerebral Palsy

Therapists who work with children with cerebral palsy may have noticed a high incidence of vision problems. Many studies confirm these observations. A study by Scheinman[37] examining the incidence of visual problems in children with cerebral palsy and normal intelligence found the following incidences: strabismus in 69%, high phorias in 4%, accommodative dysfunction in 30%, and refractive errors in 63%.

Hydrocephalus

Various studies have found that the most common visual problem in children with hydrocephalus is strabismus, with an incidence of 30% to 55%. The strabismus may develop either from the hydrocephalus itself or from the shunting procedure.

Fetal Alcohol Syndrome

Children affected by fetal alcohol syndrome have several characteristic features and visual problems. They have a higher incidence of strabismus, myopia, astigmatism, and ptosis. These children frequently have some degree of mental retardation as well and are of small stature.

Conditions of Aging
Cataracts

The most common malady affecting vision in elderly persons is cataracts. General clarity of vision is impaired from a loss of transparency of the crystalline lens of the eye.

In the senile cataract, the lens slowly loses its ability to prevent oxidation from occurring, and liquefaction of the outer layers begins. The normally soluble proteins adhere together, causing light scatter.[3] Vision slowly declines as opacification and light scatter increase, until the lens must be removed.

Age-Related Macular Degeneration

Age-related macular degeneration (AMD) is the leading cause of blindness in the Western world and is the most important retinal disease of the aged (affecting 28% of the 75- to 85-year-old age group).[7]

Loss of central vision results from fluid that leaks up from the deeper layers of the retina, pushing the retina up and detaching it from the nourishing layer. New vessel growth and hemorrhage and atrophy further destroy central vision. There is much research going on regarding treatments for AMD. The most promising at this time is the use of bevacizumab (Avastin) or ranibizumab (Lucentis), which is injected into the eye; then the eye is treated with a laser. The drug targets the neovascular network of blood vessels, and the laser treatment obliterates the vessel network, sparing the photoreceptors.[38]

This condition has significant implications for independent functioning. Mobility tends to be less impaired because the peripheral visual system is still intact. All activities involving fine detail, such as reading, computer use, sewing, and cooking, are affected. Safety also can be affected.

Arteriosclerosis

In arteriosclerosis, vision may or may not be affected. There is a hardening of the retinal arteries, which may eventually lead to ischemia, with the areas of retina deprived of sufficient oxygen eventually dying.

Hypertension

Hypertension is usually accompanied by arteriosclerosis. There may be retinal bleeding and edema, which can affect central vision if the macula is involved.

Diabetes

Diabetes can affect the lens. In the diabetic "sugar cataract," sorbitol collects within the lens, causing an osmotic gradient of fluid into the lens, which leads to disruption of the lens matrix and loss of transparency. As the fluid increases and decreases within the lens, the patient's vision also can fluctuate, depending directly on the sugar level. This makes prescribing glasses during this time quite difficult. The cataract will need to be removed if vision is worse than 20/40.

The retinal effects include microvascular damage and the development of microaneurysms. Central vision may be reduced as a result of retinal ischemia. The ischemia leads to new blood vessel growth (neovascularization). These new vessels are weak, frequently leaking and causing hemorrhage. The hemorrhage leads to fibrosis, which puts traction on the retina, pulling it off and leading to retinal detachment and blindness. Laser treatment of the bleeding retinal vessels will stop the bleeding but also burns photoreceptors, creating blind spots. This result is far preferable to total retinal detachment and blindness.

Glaucoma

Glaucoma occurs in 7.2% of the 75- to 85-year-old age group.[7] It is generally caused by an increase in the intraocular pressure. This pressure interferes with the inflow and outflow of blood and nutrients at the optic disc. As it progresses, glaucoma can cause tunnel vision and, in some, complete blindness. Because of the type of vision loss affecting the periphery, mobility and safety are significantly impaired. Try walking around holding a paper towel tube to your eye while closing the other eye, and see what happens to your ability to maneuver around obstacles or find your destination.

A less common type of glaucoma is low-tension glaucoma, in which the internal eye pressures are essentially normal. The mechanism is not understood, and the disease is treated with eye drops to lower internal pressure, just like the other types of glaucoma.

In one type of glaucoma, called *open-angle glaucoma*, the outflow of aqueous humor is reduced, leading to increased intraocular pressure. There are no overt symptoms. In another type, closed-angle glaucoma, the outflow is blocked by the iris. Symptoms are a painful, red eye, which may be confused with conjunctivitis.

Corticosteroids used to treat many conditions in the elderly for long periods of time may have side effects in some people, such as glaucoma and cataracts.

Eye Muscle Dysfunctions

Eye muscle dysfunctions causing double vision may result from several disease conditions including thyroid disease (Graves disease and others), multiple sclerosis, myasthenia gravis, and tumors. The underlying condition must be diagnosed and treated.

Visual Field Loss

Visual field loss may be either central (macular degeneration, glaucoma, or retinal disease) or peripheral field loss from glaucoma, retinal damage, or stroke at any point in the visual pathway. This is potentially the most functionally disabling form of visual impairment (see Fig. 28.7).

Environmental Implications for Functional Performance
Lighting

Lighting conditions are important and vary depending on the nature of the condition. The person with presbyopia requires more light because the aging pupil gets smaller. The smaller pupil has the advantage of increasing the depth of focus, allowing the presbyope to see clearly over a wider range, but it has the disadvantage of eliminating more light from the eye. Thus providing a good source of direct lighting, especially on fine print, is helpful. Lighting for the low-vision patient is critical. Direct sources of low-glare light such as halogen seem to work best. This is, however, quite individual, in that some patients actually see better in lower-light conditions.

Glare

People who have problems with glare, such as those developing cataracts or other disease conditions, can be helped by several approaches. Incandescent or halogen lighting is preferred over fluorescent lighting. The use of a visor or wide-brimmed hat will reduce one source of glare, improving overall comfort. For some individuals who have trouble reading because of the glare coming off the white page, a black matte piece of cardboard with a horizontal slit in it (called a *typoscope*) can be used to reduce the surrounding glare and enhance reading. Various colored filters can be quite helpful; frequently a light amber color reduces glare while enhancing contrast. Other colors such as light green, plum, or yellow can be tried. The improvement noted is quite individual to the patient. Special photochromic, tinted antiglare lenses developed by Corning are available by prescription through the ophthalmologist or optometrist. An antireflective coating may also help. This is another area where adjusting the brightness on the computer screen or using an add-on to reduce glare can be quite helpful.

Low-Vision Aids

Many types of low-vision optical and nonoptical aids are available, usually by prescription by a low-vision specialist. Patients with damage to their central vision as in AMD or diabetic maculopathy and who still have some reduced central vision may be able to use various types of magnification aids.

Hand and stand magnifiers. One type is a stand magnifier, which is placed directly on the reading material and is useful for patients who have a tremor. Hand magnifiers are held in the hand and moved away from the page to the focal point of the lens, which may range from half an inch to 5 inches, depending on the amount of magnification. Some are equipped with their own internal illumination; others are equipped with halogen lighting systems.

Telescopes. Telescopes can be used for a number of different functions. To increase independence in orientation and mobility, a "spotting" telescope is held in the hand and looked through to identify approaching bus numbers, public transportation signs, stop or walk signs, or aisle signs. There are also telescopes that are worn on the head for hands-free usage or for viewing the computer screen. A telescope system can be attached to the patient's glasses frames. Special driving telescopes called *bioptic telescopes* are ground into the patient's glasses, angled in such a way as to allow viewing straight ahead and, with a tip of the head, viewing through the scope to read a sign. The best corrected visual acuity needs to be at least 20/100, but regulations vary from state to state. The greatest disadvantages of scopes are the small visual field and the additional training required to learn how to effectively use them.

The implantable telescope is an exciting new option available for patients with end-stage AMD. After careful evaluation the patient may be considered to be a good candidate for implantation. The tiny telescope is surgically implanted near the lens inside the eye. It has the benefits of having magnification immediately available for use for distance targets and reading; however, the peripheral vision in the implanted eye is significantly reduced. Similar to someone adjusting to monovision contact lenses, the patient with the implanted telescope learns to look through either the *telescopic eye or the other eye* (Fig. 28.10).[39–41]

Microscopes. Microscopes are high-powered reading glasses in which the magnification is created in the glasses rather than in the

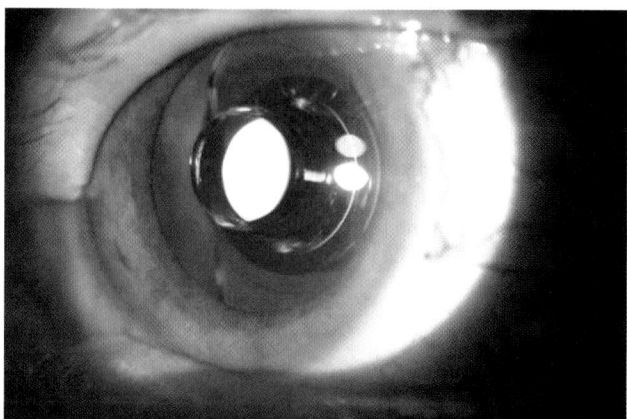

Fig. 28.10 Eye With Implanted 3× Telescope.

hand. The disadvantage of these is the close viewing distance, depending on the power. The viewing distance could be as close as 1.5 inches, creating discomfort in reading for many.

Electronic digital magnifiers. The best systems for severely impaired patients are the electronic digital magnifiers such as closed-circuit television (CCTV). The CCTV system consists of a camera housed in a device that can be directed at the object to be viewed. The scope of magnification is significantly larger, ranging from low power to 50×. Additional benefits include no distortion, like that caused by optical magnifiers, and a field of view limited only by the size of the screen. The housing for the camera may be in a stand, with a screen above, or portable, held in the hand or strapped to the head. Examples are the Merlin, Jordy, and MaxPort by Enhanced Vision Systems, and the portable digital magnifiers such as the Compact mini by Optelec.[42]

Nonoptical aids. Nonoptical aids include large-print materials, available at many libraries, typoscopes, mentioned earlier, and reading stands. Talking books are available for those for whom reading is an important hobby. New developments include text-to-speech synthesizers, screen reader software, computers that display large print or have large print/braille keyboards, large-print computers, and image intensifiers. Other simple aids are available such as lined paper with dark slightly raised lines, felt-tipped pens for writing, talking clocks, needle threaders, and many cooking and measuring aids. The website www.visionaware.org offers resources on this topic.

Visual field expansion. For patients with field losses, specially designed prism or mirror systems may be used. These frequently require training to get used to and are not useful for everyone. Compensation training also can be helpful, particularly in the use of eccentric viewing, or learning how to use a portion of the intact field by aiming the eye off center. The use of margin markers or reading slits and holding the book sideways so that the print is vertical are other helpful techniques.

Current research. Areas of research have included mounting a video camera onto spectacles and then transducing the visual information to electrodes implanted in visual cortical centers. In one study this system allowed a low-vision patient to see the large E (20/400) and detect large contours.[44,45] Recently a company called Second Sight Medical Products developed the Argus II, which includes implantation of a 60-electrode grid on the retina, which is used in conjunction with a video camera mounted on eyeglasses. A wireless microprocessor with battery pack is worn on the waist. Altogether the system enables rudimentary perception of shapes and forms, allowing improved mobility in patients whose vision has been impaired by retinal diseases such as retinitis pigmentosa.[46]

VISUAL SCREENING

Primary visual dysfunction must be differentiated from a visual-perceptual disorder so that appropriate treatment can be addressed for each problem. Gianutsos and colleagues[47] found that more than half the individuals in their study admitted for general head injury rehabilitation who were eligible for cognitive services had visual sensory impairments sufficient to warrant further evaluation. Visual screening can identify the need for referral for a complete eye examination. The results of the examination become part of the differential diagnosis regarding a perceptual dysfunction. Box 28.3 presents key elements in vision screening.

This section describes vision screening tools and adaptations for various populations. The following principles should be kept in mind:

- Acuities: Acuities should always be tested first because decreased acuities will bias other tests except for ocular motilities and the peripheral field test.
- Positioning: The body and head should be in good alignment or straightened with positioning devices, with the head in midline.
- Glasses: If the patient normally wears glasses, for either distance or near vision, the patient should be wearing glasses for tests for which spectacle correction is required. When in doubt, try it both ways, record the best response, and note whether glasses were worn.

Observations During Testing

The patient's response during the test can provide important qualitative information about his or her visual system, including postural changes (head forward or back, body forward or back, head tilts or rotation [turning to either side]), squinting, closing one eye, excessive blinking, rubbing, signs of strain or fatigue, and holding the breath. Patients should be encouraged to relax, breathe normally, and not squint.

Distance Acuities
Equipment

Needed to measure distance acuity are a distance acuity chart, an occluder, a 20-foot measure, and the patient's corrective lenses if worn for distance.

Setup

A distance chart is taped on a well-lighted wall at the patient's eye level, and a distance of 20 feet is measured from the chart.

Procedure

One of the patient's eyes is covered, and the patient is asked to read the smallest letters that he or she can see. Exposing one letter or line at a time can help if tracking or attention is a problem. The examiner should encourage the patient to guess and instruct the patient not to squint. The number of letters that were missed on the smallest line that the patient is able to see is noted. The procedure is repeated by covering the patient's other eye, and then both eyes are tested unoccluded.

Record

The smallest line the patient was able to read is recorded. If the patient missed any letters on that line, then the number of letters missed is subtracted. For example, if the patient read four letters correctly on the 20/30 line but missed the other two, then it is recorded as 20/30-2. The scores for the patient's right eye, left eye, and both eyes together are recorded.

If the patient is unable to see the top line at 20 feet, the patient is asked to move forward until able to identify the top letters. Then the distance and letter size (top line) are recorded. For example, if the patient had to move up to 4 feet to see the top line, then 4/100 is recorded. To calculate 20-foot equivalence, an equation is used where x equals the size of the letter (e.g., $4/100 = 20/x$); thus $4x = 2000$ and $2000/4 = 500$. The patient's vision is 20/500 (Box 28.4).

For patients whose attention is poor, the testing distance may need to be as close as 2 feet. Other testing stimuli can be used for children, such as the Broken Wheel Test* or the Lighthouse cards. Acuity in low-functioning patients or infants can be evaluated by use of preferential looking methods. Targets are usually high-contrast grating patterns of decreasing size. One such type is the Teller cards.

Implications

A patient who fails this test may require glasses or a change in the current prescription.

Near Acuities
Equipment

A near-point test card, an occluder, and the patient's corrective lenses, if normally worn for near vision, are needed.

Procedure

The procedure is the same as for distance acuity. The standard test distance is usually 16 inches (40 cm).

Record

The smallest line read is recorded.

Interpretation and Referral

A test result of 20/20 is considered normal, 20/40 is required for reading newspaper-sized print, and 20/100 is needed for large print. Referral to an optometrist or ophthalmologist should be made if vision is 20/40 or worse or if a difference of two lines exists between the two eyes. Neurological damage can affect the accommodative system. Sometimes it corrects itself spontaneously, but not always.

Visual retraining of the focusing system may be appropriate, depending on the patient's age. This can be determined by an optometrist familiar with vision therapy.

BOX 28.3 Key Elements in Vision Screening

1. Distance and near visual acuities
2. Oculomotilities (pursuits, saccades, and near point of convergence)
3. Measure of eye alignment to detect strabismus or high phoria
4. Measure of depth perception (stereopsis)
5. Measure of the visual fields

BOX 28.4 Interpretation or Referral

20/20 is considered normal.
20/40 is required by the Department of Motor Vehicles (DMV) in most states for full-time day and night driver's license, although requirements vary in different states.
20/80 is required by the DMV for daytime driver's license.
20/40 or worse indicates referral to an eye doctor.
20/200 corrected (with spectacle prescription) is considered legally blind.
A difference of two lines or more between the two eyes indicates referral to an eye doctor (e.g., right eye is 20/20, left eye is 20/30).

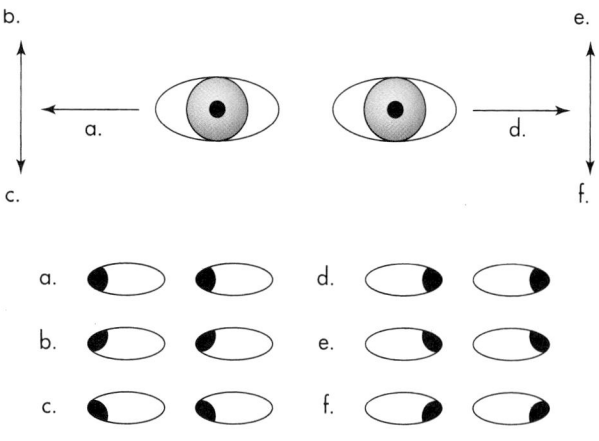

Then move from e→f, b→f, f→b, c→e to observe diagonal and midline pursuit patterns.

Fig. 28.11 Pursuit Patterns.

3		7	5			9			8
2	5			7		4		6	6
1			4		7		6		3
7		9		3		9			2
4	5				2			1	7
5			3		7		4		8
7	4		6	5					2
9		2			3		6		4
6	3	2		9					1
7				4		6	5		2
5		3	7			4			8
4			5		2			1	7
7	9	3			9				2
1			4			7		6	3
2		5		7			4		6
3	7		5			9			8

Fig. 28.12 Developmental Eye Movement Test.

Pursuits

Equipment

Any target that holds the patient's attention can be used, such as a pencil or small toy.

Setup

The patient is seated facing the screener.

Procedure

One pencil is held 16 to 20 inches in front of the patient, and the patient is asked to look directly at one part, such as the eraser, and to keep the head still, holding it if necessary. The pencil is moved around in the pattern shown in Fig. 28.11, which is designed to incorporate all directions of gaze. The examiner should observe for smooth following, noticing and recording jerks and jumps, where they occur, or if the eyes stop at a certain point. If one or both eyes stop tracking, the patient is encouraged to look at the pencil. If the patient is unable to do this, then the movement pattern is repeated with each eye separately and where the movement stops is recorded. Patients who have had a cerebrovascular accident (CVA) or head injury should be tested first monocularly (each eye separately).

Record

Results are rated as follows:
- Poor = Difficulty following target with any accuracy, jerky or jumpy, nystagmoid movements, incomplete range of motion
- Fair = Generally able to follow target but goes off target occasionally (1 to 2 times), with slight jerkiness
- Good = Eye movements smooth with no jerkiness

If one eye stops tracking at a certain point or if the patient reports double vision (diplopia) in certain directions, the examiner should record which eye or in which direction the problem is noticed (e.g., the right eye does not pass midline when moving from left to right, or diplopia is reported on upward right gaze). This specific information can be helpful to the ophthalmologist or optometrist.

Saccades

Equipment

Tracking pencils can be used, although a few saccadic tests are available. One is the King Devick Saccadic Test; the other is the

Developmental Eye Movement Test. These both require form perception (number reading) and may be difficult, depending on the patient's cognitive level.

Setup

The patient is seated facing the screener.

Procedure

A pencil is held in each hand about 17 to 20 inches from the patient, and the patient is told that he or she is going to be asked to look at one pencil while the other pencil is moved but not to look at it until told to do so. The patient is to move the eyes only, keeping the head still. While the patient looks at the first pencil, the other pencil is moved as the screener says "shift" or "look at this pencil." The screener then moves the other pencil, says "shift," then moves the pencil, says "shift," then moves the pencil, and so on, until a pattern of movement can be discerned.

This call-shift is repeated about 10 times, moving into different fields of gaze. The screener continues until the patient is seen to respond. The screener observes for overshooting or undershooting the target, for the ability to isolate the eyes from the head (hold head still), for controlled eye movement, and for ability to wait until the verbal command to look. It is important to observe for the patient's ability to shift to all fields of gaze. A lower level of testing would be to ask the patient to move the eyes from one target to the other as quickly as possible (Fig. 28.12).

Record

Results are rated as follows:
- Poor = Inability to control eyes with verbal command, consistent undershooting or overshooting, inability to isolate eyes from head
- Fair = Ability to maintain eyes on target with verbal command 50% of the time, with slight undershooting or overshooting, and ability to isolate eyes from head with verbal reminders
- Good = Ability to follow verbal commands 90% of the time, with no undershooting or overshooting, and complete eye from head isolation

Near Point of Convergence

Procedure

A pencil is introduced about 20 inches away from the patient's midline. The patient is asked whether the pencil looks single. If it is not, it is moved farther away. The patient is told that the pencil will be moved toward her or him and that it will be getting blurry but to keep watching it as far in as possible. When the pencil appears single, it is moved toward the nose at a moderately slow rate (but not too slow). The screener should watch the patient's eyes. As long as the patient's eyes are tracking the pencil, the pencil is kept moving toward the nose. At the point where one eye moves out, both eyes move out, or the eyes simply stop tracking, the distance of the pencil to the nose is measured. If the patient is wearing bifocals, it is important to make sure the patient is looking through the reading segment.

Record

The break point is the distance at which the eyes were observed to stop tracking the pencil. If the patient was able to track the pencil all the way to the nose, then record this fact.

Interpretation and Referral

A score of poor or fair on saccades or pursuits suggests the need for training. A near point of convergence with a break point of 5 inches or more is suggestive of convergence problems, and recommendations for referral should be made.

Implications

Difficulties with smooth pursuit, accurate saccades, or convergence can all present tracking difficulties for the patient. These difficulties can cause loss of place in reading, rereading of words or lines, skipping lines, and lower comprehension and concentration. Inaccurate eye movements also may affect visual memory.

An eye movement problem may be the result of direct damage to the eye muscles themselves (Fig. 28.13) or to the nerves controlling them, as in the case of a head injury. Damage to the vestibular center also may involve visual components. Neurons from cranial nerves III, IV, and VI synapse in the vestibular nuclei. Reflex control of eye movements occurs through the VOR and the optokinetic system.

Cover Tests
Purpose

There are two cover tests. The cover-uncover test is used to determine whether strabismus is present. The alternate cover test determines what type of phoria is present. The magnitude of the phoria generally determines the extent of the patient's symptoms.

Equipment

An occluder and a tracking pencil or a small, distinct target are needed.

Setup

The patient is seated facing the screener, who is also seated.

Procedure

A pencil is held approximately 16 inches in front of the patient, and the patient is asked to look directly at the target and to keep it in focus.

Near Cover Tests

Cover-uncover test. The movement of the uncovered eye is observed. The patient's right eye is covered, and the left eye is observed for movement in, out, upward, or downward. This is repeated a few times, allowing the eyes to be uncovered for about 2 seconds between trials. Then the left eye is covered to observe for movement in the right eye.

Alternate cover test. Eye movement is observed as the eye is uncovered. An occluder is held over the right eye for a few seconds while the patient looks at a near target. The occluder is moved from the right eye to the left eye while the right eye is observed for movement in, out, up, or down. After a few seconds, the occluder is moved back to the right eye, observing the left eye for movement. This is repeated back and forth several times until the screener is sure of what is seen.

Far Cover Tests

The preceding procedure is repeated with the patient looking at a distant target.

Interpretation and referral. Any visible eye movement seen during the cover-uncover test with good maintenance of fixation on the target indicates a strabismus. If there is no previous history of strabismus, referral is indicated. A large eye movement seen with the alternate cover test, along with the presence of symptoms such as eyestrain, headaches, or apparent difficulty in making spatial judgments, also indicates referral. In the clinic the therapist may notice that the patient has difficulty finding objects in a drawer, or that the patient appears cross-eyed or seems to be looking past the target. He or she may have difficulty with spatial judgments in reaching for objects or in mobility, especially with stairs or curbs.

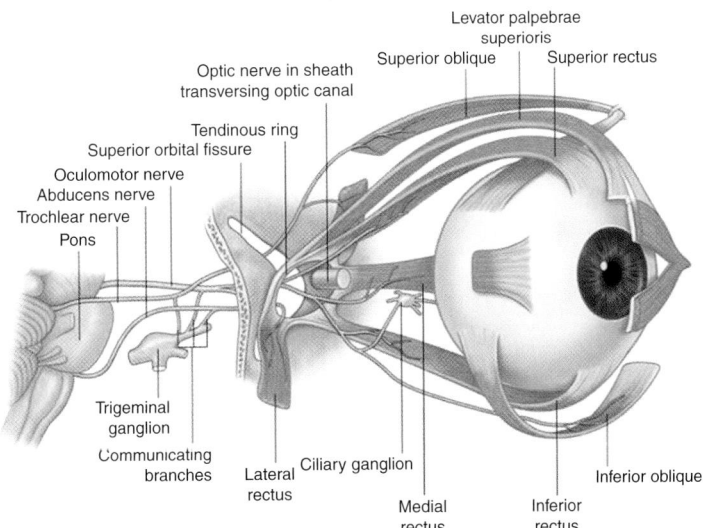

Fig. 28.13 Cranial Nerves III, IV, and VI. Oculomotor, trochlear, and abducens nerves and their innervation of the extraocular muscles. (From Tamhankar M. *Liu, Volpe and Galetta's Neuro-Ophthalmology.* Elsevier: Philadelphia; 2019.)

A visible eye movement may be part of a post-CVA patient's premorbid pattern. This should be determined by asking the patient or the family members before making a referral. Or the condition may be the result of neurological damage to cranial nerve III, IV, or VI from CVA, head injury, or cerebral palsy. Eye muscles are striated muscles, under voluntary control. Like other striated muscles that can be affected by neurological damage, they may recover spontaneously, they may not recover at all, or they may benefit from visual retraining. Many learning-disabled children with vestibular dysfunction have poor binocular skills. An ophthalmologist or optometrist specially trained in visual remediation can determine a patient's potential for vision therapy. Some published research has demonstrated the success of vision therapy for post-CVA patients.[48]

Stereopsis (Depth Perception)
Equipment
Any test that uses either Polaroid or red-green filters can test for stereopsis ability. Examples are the Titmus stereo fly, reindeer, and butterfly.

Procedure
The patient is asked to point to or say which test object appears closer. If the patient is able to grasp for the object in space, some stereo ability is present.

Record
The patient's response should be immediate. Long delays could indicate borderline ability.

Interpretation and Referral
If the patient fails this test, a referral to an ophthalmologist or optometrist is recommended. The patient must have best-corrected acuities for this test; otherwise, the results are invalid.

Implications
A deficit in depth perception can interfere with all activities involving spatial judgments—in particular, fine motor and eye-hand type activities in which judgments of relative depth are required (e.g., threading a needle, placing toothpaste on a toothbrush, and hammering). Although ambulation itself may not be affected, ambulation involving curbs or stairs will be affected.

Vision therapy training can be helpful for patients with problems in binocular coordination. Proper diagnosis and therapy prescription are essential.

Visual Field Screening
Equipment
An occluder or eyepatch is required, and a black dowel with a white pin on the end or just a wiggling finger can be used as a peripheral target.

Setup
The patient is seated facing the examiner.

Procedure
The patient holds the occluder over the left eye. The examiner explains that he or she is going to wiggle a finger out to the side and that the patient is to say "now" when he or she first detects the movement of the wiggling finger. The patient should look at the screener's nose the entire time and ignore any arm movement. The test is begun with the examiner's hand slightly behind the patient, about 16 inches away from the patient's head. The hand is brought forward slowly while a finger is wiggled. Different sections of the visual field are randomly tested in 45-degree intervals around the visual field. The left eye is then tested after the patient's right eye is occluded. Alternatively, if a dowel is used, it is slowly brought in from the side until the patient reports seeing the small pin at the end of the dowel.

These confrontation field tests are considered gross tests compared with a visual field perimeter test. Many patients cannot do the perimeter test because it requires a higher cognitive level. Confrontation fields will reveal a hemianopsia and a quadrantanopsia (quarter-field cut). For lower-functioning patients, the examiner can observe eye movements in the direction of the target to get a general idea of peripheral function once patients have seen it.

Record
The portion of field missing for each eye is noted.

Interpretation and Referral
If any hemianopsia or quadrantanopsia is noted, the patient is referred to an optometrist or an ophthalmologist.

Implications
A visual deficit has significant implication for the safe performance of many functional activities, including driving and mobility. Visually guided movement through space becomes impaired, as are efficient eye movements; if central field loss is present, reading and any other near activities are affected. The reader is referred to the discussion of assessment of unilateral inattention for differentiation between neglect and hemianopsia.

REFERRAL CONSIDERATIONS

The final outcome of the visual screening is referral to an optometrist or ophthalmologist, ideally to someone with an orientation toward visual rehabilitation. It is important not to make diagnostic statements but rather to indicate whether the patient passed or failed the vision screening. By law, only optometrists or ophthalmologists can diagnose visual conditions.

It is not always clear when to refer a patient or to whom. Many doctors do not test all areas of visual function. In general, behavioral or developmental optometrists have a functionally oriented philosophy quite similar to occupational therapy models of functional performance.

Recommended referral guidelines are shown in Box 28.5.

BOX 28.5   Referral Guidelines

1. Failure of either the distance or near acuity test (with glasses on). This could indicate an uncorrected refractive error, a disease process, or a neurological problem.
2. Failure of the oculomotility section only does not indicate referral because treatment of oculomotor dysfunction is currently within the scope of practice for rehabilitation. *Exception:* Failure of the pursuit test as a result of a reduced ocular range of motion in any direction of gaze, which indicates cranial nerve involvement.
3. Failure of the cover-uncover test indicates strabismus and is an indication for referral unless there is a history of an eye turn.
4. A large eye movement seen on the alternate cover test, along with apparent difficulties in stereopsis, such as spatial judgments, or symptoms, such as headaches, eyestrain, or difficulty with comprehension, constitutes an indication for referral.
5. Failure of the stereopsis test alone is an indication for referral if there is no history of an eye turn and if there is movement on either cover test.
6. Patients with quarter-field loss and half-field loss (hemianopsia) should be referred.

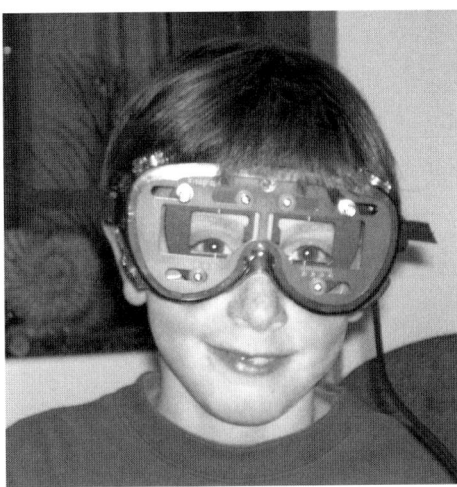

Fig. 28.14 The Visagraph (boy with goggles) measures eye movement while the subject is reading.

Rehabilitation Optometric Evaluation

Once the patient has been referred for evaluation, the eye doctor will evaluate any changes in the refractive error and the need for new correction to achieve the best possible vision. The eye alignment will be quantified, and determination will be made regarding whether there is an eye muscle paresis, which cranial nerve is involved, whether strabismus or phoria is present, and whether the eye deviation is better or worse in particular directions of gaze.

Oculomotilities will be evaluated grossly, and more specific tests may be done. One test is the Developmental Eye Movement Test (see Fig. 28.12). Another test is the Visagraph (Fig. 28.14). This instrument records eye movements while the patient is reading text. It will measure total reading rate, number of fixations and regressions per 100 words, span of recognition, and reading comprehension. The tool is excellent for in-depth evaluation and monitoring the progress of treatment over time.

Ocular health testing will include glaucoma testing, examination for cataracts, and retinal health evaluation. For visual field testing, either a screening field or a threshold visual field will be done on some type of automated perimeter such as the Humphrey Visual Field Analyzer or the Octopus. Threshold testing is done to determine the extent and depth of a defect, and it can help determine whether there is potential for visual field retraining. In Fig. 28.9 the black portions of the visual field are areas of absolute damage. The areas of white with small dots are intact visual fields. At the border of the damage area is a gray zone, which theoretically is amenable to training.[31–34]

The optometrist or ophthalmologist will deliver a report of the findings with recommendations for the treatment plan. Developing a professional relationship with an optometrist or ophthalmologist can be very beneficial for therapists who work in neurological rehabilitation.

Visual Intervention

Early intervention is recommended as soon as possible, when possible, to identify ways in which a vision problem may be interfering with other therapies.[48–51] Some treatments may be applied early on, as well. For example, if the patient has an eye muscle paresis, range-of-motion exercises for the involved muscle can prevent the development of a contracture of the unopposed muscle.

In cases in which the patient has double vision, a patching regimen can be instituted. One regimen is to alternate patching the eyes daily,

allowing some time to experience diplopia, so that the eyes may attempt to make a fusion response. The stimulus to fusion is double vision. If one eye is always patched, spontaneous recovery may be slowed. Another patching regimen is binasal taping, and another is to use partially opaque materials to allow peripheral vision in the occluded eye. The patching regimen should be prescribed by an optometrist or ophthalmologist.

In some cases of double vision, a temporary plastic (Fresnel) prism can be applied to the patient's glasses to reduce or eliminate the diplopia. This may significantly enhance the patient's functioning in other therapies, particularly when spatial judgments are being made (e.g., in fine motor tasks or ambulation).

Documentation

Vision problems should be documented in functional performance terms—that is, how the vision problem affects activities of daily living. Improvement can then be monitored according to function. This will also help in reimbursement. For example, a patient with an eye muscle dysfunction will have difficulty with spatial judgments such as placing toothpaste on a toothbrush, spearing objects, reaching for a cup handle, doing pegboard tasks, and using vision for balance.

THERAPEUTIC CONSIDERATIONS

Once a referral has been made, the patient has been seen, and the examination report has been received, what else can be done? How the dysfunction affects therapy can be considered, and some visual training, prescribed by the optometrist, can be initiated.

Accommodative Dysfunction

If the patient has an accommodative dysfunction, the treatment may be the prescription of glasses for reading or tabletop tasks or possibly near-far focusing exercises,[4] depending on the age of the patient. "Flipper bars" are special lenses that exercise the focusing system.[52]

If the patient needs glasses for near but cannot get them for some reason, the therapist can try moving the task farther away and increasing the lighting on the task.

Eye Alignment Dysfunction

If the patient has a problem in the eye alignment system, several factors should be considered. If the patient is able to fuse some of the time but loses fusion, seeing double when stressed or tired, then the most difficult tasks should be attempted when the patient is least fatigued. Otherwise, if the patient has constant double vision or the patient is seeing double at the time the therapist is working with her or him, patching may be prescribed by the ophthalmologist or optometrist. This will reduce the patient's confusion and increase attention to the task. For patients with acquired double vision, however, it is important to provide time without a patch so that the eyes will attempt to regain fusion. Wearing the patch constantly will discourage any attempts by the brain to overcome the double vision.

Visual Dysfunction and Balance Disorders

It is important to recognize the close interplay between the visual and the balance systems, including vestibular, proprioceptive, and tactile receptors, in maintaining balance. Altered visual input can affect perception of space, even with something as simple as getting a new pair of glasses. The nonneurologically impaired individual will eventually adapt and reset the coordination of information. Neurologically impaired patients can have much greater difficulty in resetting the coordination of sensory information from multiple systems, resulting in a feeling of sensory overload or being overwhelmed. Conversely, damage to areas of the brain that process vestibular or somatosensory information can create altered maps of space as well as affect the balance as the individual attempts to interact with the environment.

Therapy may be directed at both areas: improving balance by enhancing balance and proprioceptive mechanisms and/or by enhancing visual input through visual rehabilitation techniques. There has been recent research involving the strategic placement of small weights on the torso, which has had immediate and sometimes dramatic effects on balance.[53,54] Interestingly, these types of inputs to the torso can also affect visual processing (observations by BalanceWear vest developer Cindy Gibson-Horn, RPT, and Laurie Chaikin, OD, OTR/L, FCOVD). It is hypothesized that the mechanism for this change may be mediated by cerebellar-visual pathways.[55]

VISUAL-PERCEPTUAL DYSFUNCTION

This discussion of visual-perceptual disorders is divided into a number of categories: unilateral spatial inattention; cortical blindness, defective color perception, and visual agnosia; visual-spatial disorders; visual-constructive disorders; and visual analysis and synthesis disorders. Cortical blindness is a disorder of primary visual input; however, because its variations may influence perceptual interpretation, it is discussed here. All other disorders listed involve direct problems with the interpretation of visual stimuli. Although each of these terms represents symptoms recognized by many authors, the reader is reminded that there are no clear boundaries between one deficit and another or one system and another. Apraxia and body image disorders are not discussed under separate categories because they are not considered "visual"-perceptual disorders per se, although their presence may influence and complicate an already dysfunctional visual-perceptual system.

Problems of Unilateral Spatial Inattention
Identification of Clinical Problems

General category. In its purest form, unilateral spatial inattention is defined as a condition in which an individual with normal sensory and motor systems fails to orient toward, respond to, or report stimuli on the side contralateral to the cerebral lesion. Although this condition is not often seen in its pure form, inattention has been documented in persons who demonstrate no accompanying visual field defect (homonymous hemianopsia) or limb sensory or motor loss.[56] In most cases, however, unilateral spatial inattention is not seen alone but is associated with (although not caused by) accompanying sensory and motor defects such as homonymous hemianopsia and decreased tactile, proprioceptive, and stereognostic perception along with paresis or paralysis of the upper limb.[57]

It is easy to become confused by the numerous terms used in the literature, for example, *unilateral spatial agnosia, unilateral visual neglect, fixed hemianopsia, hemi-inattention,* and *hemi-imperception.* All terms describe the same deficit. Unilateral spatial inattention is used in this chapter because (1) in severe cases the syndrome most likely involves tactile and auditory as well as visual unawareness (i.e., a total spatial unawareness) and (2) the syndrome results in an involuntary lack of attention to stimuli contralateral to the lesion, whereas the term *neglect* implies a voluntary choice not to respond.

Unilateral spatial inattention occurs most frequently in individuals with a diagnosis of stroke (CVA), traumatic brain injury, or tumor. Most authors agree that unilateral spatial inattention occurs more often with right hemisphere than with left hemisphere lesions.[58-62] This frequency supports theories that the right hemisphere is dominant for visual-spatial organization. It is clear, however, that inattention may be present in individuals with left hemisphere lesions, but that the

inattention tends to resolve more quickly.[63] The clinician should remember that, although the chances are statistically lower, the patient with right hemiplegia may exhibit inattention to right stimuli.

Unilateral spatial inattention has been associated with lesions in both cortical and subcortical structures. It is most commonly seen in inferior parietal lobe lesions[61] but has also been observed in lesions in the inferior frontal cortex, the dorsolateral frontal lobe, the superior temporal gyrus, and the cingulate gyrus[64] and with basal ganglia, thalamic,[65] and putaminal hemorrhage.[66-68] Finally, lesions in the brain stem reticular formation have induced inattention in cats[67] and monkeys.[65]

Although a number of theories have been postulated regarding the mechanism underlying unilateral spatial inattention, no mechanism has been validly documented in human subjects. The one fact that is clear from all theoretical postulates is that inattention is a hemispheric deficit. LeDoux and Smylie[69] demonstrated this point effectively in an interesting case study of a right-sided lesion. During full visual exposure (bilateral hemispheric) of visual-perceptual slides, the affected individual made visual-spatial errors in left space. However, when the same slides were directed only to the right visual field (left hemisphere), performance improved substantially. It is as if the deficient hemisphere fails to receive or orient toward incoming information while the intact receiving hemisphere remains oblivious and goes about its own business. Treatment for inattention is problematic mainly because the mechanisms underlying unilateral spatial inattention are not clearly understood.

Theories on mechanisms underlying unilateral spatial inattention have attempted to explain it as an integrative associative defect as opposed to simply a problem of decreased sensory input. Theories include a unilateral attentional hypothesis, suggesting that inattention results from a disruption in the orienting response—that is, the corticolimbic hemisphere is underaroused during bilateral input, and therefore stimuli presented to that hemisphere are neglected.[61,64] Another theory is the oculomotor imbalance hypothesis, which suggests that individuals with inattention have a visual-spatial disorder worsened by oculomotor imbalance. The hypothesis suggests that the lesion disconnects the frontal eye fields in the damaged hemisphere from their sensory afferent nerves, resulting in an oculomotor imbalance deviating the gaze toward the lesion. This imbalance can be compensated for only momentarily by a voluntary effort to gaze toward the opposite hemispace (i.e., neglected space).[70]

Unilateral spatial inattention with homonymous hemianopsia. Inattention occurs more commonly with visual field defects and is generally better when the macular projections are not involved. Individuals with pure hemianopsia are aware of their visual loss and spontaneously learn to compensate by moving their eyes (foveae) toward the lost visual field to expand their visual space and thereby gather information right and left of midline. On visual examination, other individuals may demonstrate no visual field defect on unilateral stimulation; however, during bilateral stimulation they extinguish the target contralateral to the lesion. Other persons may perceive both targets simultaneously, yet when engaged in activity they may not respond to visual stimuli in one-half of the visual space contralateral to the lesion. These individuals are unaware of their inattention. Careful observation of their activity reveals few eye movements into the neglected space. The fovea does not appear to be directed to gather information in this space.

Unilateral visual, auditory, and tactile inattention. Inattention has been described as a multimodal sensory associative disorder involving not only visual but also tactile and auditory unawareness. Clinicians are well aware of the patient with left inattention who continues to direct the head and eyes toward the right throughout an entire conversation, although the therapist is standing on the patient's left side. When one conceptualizes unilateral spatial inattention as a dynamic decrease or loss of sensory information within one-half of the sensory-perceptual sphere (irrespective of hypothetical mechanism), the peculiar behaviors exhibited by these patients are more easily understood as a loss of input creating a loss of response.

Unilateral spatial inattention and body image. Body image is often disturbed in individuals with inattention. The defect in these persons is unusual because it affects only that half of the body that is contralateral to the lesion—for example, the left side of the body in right-sided lesions. There appears to be a lack of spatial orientation and attention for one-half of intrapersonal space. Those with severe inattention fail to recognize that their affected extremities are their own and function as though they are absent. They may fail to dress one-half of the body or attempt to navigate through a door oblivious to the fact that the affected arm may be caught on the doorknob or door frame. In severe cases, individuals may deny their hemiparesis, or they may deny that the extremity belongs to them. This phenomenon is called *anosognosia.*

Behavioral manifestations of unilateral spatial inattention. Persons with inattention orient all their activities toward their "attended" space. The head, eyes, and trunk are rotated toward the side of the lesion for much of the time, including during gait. Careful observation of eye movements (scanning saccades) during activities indicates that all or almost all scanning occurs on only one side of the midline within the attended space; the individual never spontaneously brings the eyes or head past midline into contralateral "unattended" space. Oculomotor examination always shows full extraocular movements and no apraxia for eye movements, thereby highlighting the difference between function and exam.

Inattention, like all other perceptual disorders, may occur on a scale from mild to severe. Mild cases of inattention may go unrecognized unless behavior is carefully observed. Scanning is symmetrical, except during tasks requiring increasingly complex perceptual and cognitive demands. Leicester and colleagues[71] believe that inattention occurs mainly when the individual has a general perceptual problem with the material—that is, some other problem with processing the task. This performance difficulty or stress brings on the additional inattention behavior; for example, neglect in matching auditory letter samples is more common in those with aphasia than in those with right hemisphere involvement without aphasia.

Independence in activities of daily living is often impossible because of inattention to both the intrapersonal and the extrapersonal environment. The individual may eat only half the food on their plate, dress only halfway, shave or apply makeup to only half of their face, brush their teeth only halfway, read only half a page, fill out only half a form, fail to locate items in the store if they are located in an unattended space, collide with obstacles or miss doorways on the unattended side, and, when walking or driving a wheelchair, veer toward the attended space rather than navigating in a straight line.

Assessment

Because most tests used to measure cognitive, language, perceptual, and motor skills require symmetrical visual, auditory, and tactile awareness, it is most important to rule out inattention early in the evaluation process of any patient with a central lesion. The two most common methods used to distinguish inattention from primary sensory deficits are double simultaneous stimulation testing and assessment of optokinetic nystagmus reflexes. Double simultaneous stimuli should be applied in three modalities: auditory, tactile, and visual. Initially, stimuli should be presented to the abnormal side. If primary sensation is impaired (e.g., a visual field loss), this evaluation cannot proceed because double simultaneous stimulation testing is invalid in that modality. If responsiveness is normal, however, bilateral simultaneous stimuli should be applied. Unilateral stimuli should be interspersed with bilateral stimuli to ensure valid responses. Lack of awareness (extinction) of stimuli contralateral to the lesion during bilateral stimulation should be noted. Patients with extinction in only one sensory system often do not demonstrate inattention behaviors; however, those with extinction in more than one modality (e.g., tactile and visual) often demonstrate these behaviors. If critical diagnosis of inattention is necessary, the patient may be referred for optokinetic nystagmus testing.

One of the best evaluation tools is a keen sense of observation. The position of the patient's head, eyes, and trunk should be observed at rest and during activity. Persistent deviation toward the lesion may indicate unilateral inattention. The individual should be asked to track a visual target from space ipsilateral to the lesion into contralateral space and maintain fixation there for 5 seconds. The therapist may ask the patient to quickly fixate on visual targets both right and left of midline on command. Problems with searching for targets in contralateral space should be noted. Some erratic oculomotor searching is normal when making saccades into a hemianoptic field, because saccades are centrally preprogrammed by peripheral input. Slow searching or failure to search should be considered indicative of inattention.

Asymmetries in performance should be noted during spatial tasks. Specific spatial tasks have been designed for detection of inattention, including the following:

- Cancellation tasks. The patient may be given a sheet of paper with horizontal lines of numbers or letters and asked to cross out all the 8s or As.
- Crossing-out tasks. In this standardized test, the patient is asked to cross out diagonal lines drawn at random on an unlined sheet of paper.
- Line-bisection tasks. The patient is asked to bisect a 4- to 8-inch line on a piece of paper placed at the midline.
- Drawing and copying tasks. The patient may be asked to draw or copy a house, clock, or flower or to fill in the numbers of a clock drawn by the examiner. For copying tasks, it is important that the copy be placed in the patient's attended space.

Patients with inattention demonstrate one or more of the following behaviors: failing to cancel figures or cross out lines in the unattended space; bisecting the line unequally, placing their mark toward the side of the midline ipsilateral to their lesion; placing their drawing toward the edge of the paper ipsilateral to their lesion rather than in the middle of the page; drawing only the right or left half of the house, flower, or clock; crowding all the numbers of the clock into the right or left half of the clock; or completing numbers on only one-half of the clock (Fig. 28.15), and demonstrating differences in reaction time.[72] When interpreting performance, the examiner is looking specifically for asymmetries in performance. Patients with inattention often have other visual-perceptual deficits that result in faulty performance on these tasks; however, these deficits are always symmetrical—that is, evident in any space to which the individual attends.

Asymmetries in performance should be carefully observed during functional activities such as eating, filling out a form, reading, dressing, and maneuvering through the environment. The therapist may note unawareness of doorways and hallways in the unattended space; turns may be made only toward one direction. As a result, these patients lose their way in the hospital or even in the therapy clinic. This behavior should be distinguished from a topographical perceptual deficit in which the individual cannot integrate or remember spatial concepts well enough to find his or her way without getting lost. The Behavioral Inattention Test has recently been published as a standardized measure of functional inattention.[73]

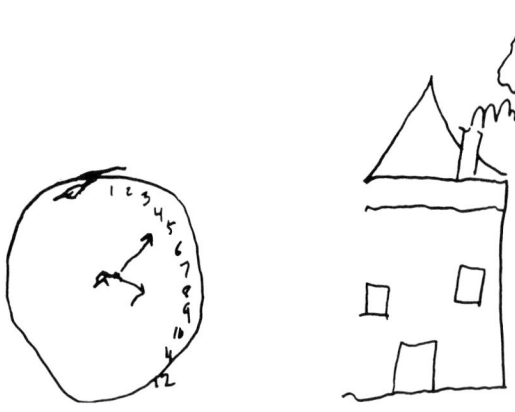

Fig. 28.15 Drawings of a clock and house by a patient with a right hemisphere parietal lobe tumor. Note the left unilateral spatial inattention in the drawings.

Finally, various studies have shown that inattention may occur during testing that requires visual processing and therefore may invalidate test results.[58,74,75] Unresponsiveness to figures on one side of the page during visual, perceptual, cognitive, or language assessments may be subtle but must be documented to rule out the influence of inattention on raw score—that is, if the patient did not see the entire test display for an item, that test item is invalid. Responses to figures on the right half and left half of the test page should be counted. If the frequency of answers is noticeably less on one-half of the page than would normally be expected, inattention may have occurred during testing. This may be used as additional evidence of inattention; but more important, this factor should be accounted for when computing the test score. Only those test items in which the correct answer was located in the attended space should be scored—that is, only those items in which the correct answer was right of midline in a patient with left inattention should be scored.

Interventions

As previously stated, the mechanisms underlying unilateral spatial inattention are not well understood; however, recent research has uncovered a strong correlation between nonspatial aspects of attention called *tonic* and *phasic attention* and spatial aspects of neglect. Tonic attention is intrinsic arousal that fluctuates on the order of hours to minutes and contributes to sustained attention and preparation for more complex cognitive tasks. Phasic attention is a rapid change in attention in response to a sudden and brief event and is related to orienting responses and selective attention.[76] This research has postulated that nonspatial attention mechanisms affect spatial and nonspatial behavior. Some highly successful training protocols using these attentional mechanisms have been developed, and the researchers have been able to demonstrate improved responses with carryover in the environment (see Appendix 28.A). They also demonstrated that this remediation approach was more effective than just scanning strategies. A number of studies have investigated the remediation of unilateral spatial inattention. They have attempted to (1) define effective remediation techniques and (2) measure changes in trained tasks and generalization to untrained tasks—that is, determine whether inattention training in one task carries over to other unrelated tasks such as activities of daily living. Treatment techniques used in all these studies resulted in less inattention during trained tasks.[59,77,78] An overview of these studies suggests that training may decrease inattention, although extent of change and generalization to other tasks may vary widely. Discrepancies in these results may be related to neurological variables in the various patient samples, severity of inattention, sample size, or tasks measured. A discussion of general principles of remediation follows.

Efforts should be made to increase the patient's cognitive awareness of the inattention. The individual should be made keenly aware of what a peripheral visual field loss is and how it is affecting her or his view of the world. The person with normal visual fields but with visual extinction should be treated the same as the individual with an actual visual field loss, because the visual experience is similar. Pictures of the visual field deficit may be drawn for illustration. Actual performance examples in the environment should be pointed out to the patient to demonstrate the biased field of view.

Visual scanning should be emphasized. Initially, the patient should be made aware of how eye and eye-head movements may be used to compensate for the deficit. The individual should be trained to make progressively larger and quicker pursuits and saccades and longer fixations into the unattended space. Training may be accomplished with interesting targets held by the therapist—for example, targets secured to the tips of pencils, such as changeable letters, colored lights, or bright small objects. Pursuit or tracking movements of the target leading the eye from attended into unattended space should be stressed first, followed by saccades into the unattended space. Initially the patient may be allowed to move the head during scanning exercises; however, eye movements without head movements should be the major goal. Individuals with inattention often move the head into the unattended space while the eye remains fixed on a target in the attended space (i.e., the visual field remains the same). The patient should be taught to independently carry out a daily right-left scanning program with targets appropriately positioned by the therapist. Eventually these targets can be moved farther into the unattended space.

Increased awareness and scanning abilities should be incorporated in increasingly complex visual-perceptual and visual-motor tasks. Because inattention often increases as task complexity increases, the therapist must select and structure tasks carefully. Examples of simple yet specific scanning tasks might include surveying a room repetitively, rolling toward and touching objects right and left of midline, assembling objects from pieces strewn on a table or the floor, completing an obstacle course, or selecting letters from a page of large print.

Scanning should be stressed during functional activities, for example, dressing, shaving, or moving through the environment. The patient may be taught to constantly monitor the influence of inattention on functional performance—for example, "When something doesn't make sense, look into the unattended space and it usually will."

Diller[79] has designed a number of specific training techniques to decrease inattention during reading and paper and pencil tasks. With a little creativity, these techniques may be applied to other activities. For example, when the patient is reading, a visual marker is placed on the extreme edge of the page in unattended space. The individual is instructed not to begin reading until he or she sees the visual marker. The marker is used to "anchor" the patient's vision. As inattention decreases, the anchor is faded. Each line may also be numbered and the numbers used to anchor scanning horizontally and vertically. To control impulsiveness, which often accompanies inattention, patients are taught to slow down or pace their performance by incorporating techniques, such as reciting the words aloud. Underlining and looping letters or words can also be used as a method to slow down impulsive scanning (Fig. 28.16). Finally, the density of stimuli is reduced; decreased density appears to decrease inattention in these tasks.

To stimulate tactile awareness in patients with tactile extinction, Anderson and Choy[80] suggest stimulating the affected arm as the individual watches. A rough cloth, vibrator, or the therapist's or patient's hand may be used. Eventually, this activity may be done before

				0	(1)	2	4	5	6	7	8	9	10							
1.	(1)	2	3	5	4	9	7	8	0	6	3	2	10	(1)	2	3	5	4	9	7	1
2.	3	4	9	6	7	10	8	(1)	2	5	0	6	4	9	6	7	10	8	2	8	2
3.	8	0	6	2	(1)	3	5	4	7	9	10	(1)	8	0	6	2	(1)	3	5	7	3
4.	5	7	3	9	6	(1)	2	8	4	10	0	3	5	5	7	3	6	(1)	2	5	4
5.	6	5	(1)	4	2	3	8	10	9	7	9	0	6	5	(1)	4	2	3	8	9	5
6.	4	8	10	0	7	6	9	1	3	2	5	6	3	4	8	10	0	7	6	9	6
7.	9	6	5	3	8	4	2	0	10	1	7	2	4	9	6	5	3	8	2	4	7

Fig. 28.16 Underlining During Visual Discrimination Tasks Helps Control Eye Movements (Scanning).

activities that require spontaneous symmetrical scanning, such as dressing or walking through an obstacle course.

During the early phases of treatment, when inattention is still moderate to severe, the patient should be approached from the attended space during treatment for inattention or other deficits such as apraxia, balance, or speech. This ensures that the individual comprehends and views all demonstrations and treatment instructions. Subsequently, as orientation and scanning improve, activities should be moved progressively into the unattended space and the therapist should be positioned in the unattended space during treatment. In the final stages of treatment, the patient should be able to symmetrically scan, regardless of the therapist's position (i.e., the therapist should vary position).

To enhance the integration of scanning behavior during functional tasks such as gait and dressing, the patient should be reminded of scanning principles and carried through a series of scanning exercises before initiation of the activity. If inattention reappears during the activity, the therapist should stop and assist the patient in becoming reoriented before the activity is resumed. Inattention results in confusion, and confusion increases inattention. As will be pointed out repeatedly in the following pages, the therapist must control the perceptual environment continuously so that the patient is able to sequence bits of information together meaningfully to learn or relearn.

Problems of Cortical Blindness, Color Imperception, and Visual Agnosia

Identification of Clinical Problems

Cortical blindness. Cortical blindness is considered a primary sensory disorder as opposed to a secondary associative disorder. It is discussed here, however, because of the many variations of this lesion that may result in problems with interpretation of visual stimuli. Cortical blindness, also known as *central blindness*, is a total or almost total loss of vision resulting from bilateral cerebral destruction of the visual projection cortex (area 17). Similar destruction limited to one hemisphere results in hemianopsia.[56] The lesion may be ischemic, neoplastic, degenerative, or traumatic. The patient may perceive the defect as a "blurring" of vision or as a marked decrease in visual acuity or may be unaware of the complete nature of the disability and even deny it, blaming the problem on eyeglasses that are too weak or a room that is too dark.

Color imperception. Color perception may be impaired in the patient with brain damage. This symptom is usually associated with right hemisphere or bilateral lesions.[81] This deficit is different from

color agnosia, in which there is a problem with naming colors correctly. Patients with defective color perception may see colors as "muddy" or "impure" in hue, or the color of a small target may fade into the background, decreasing the ability to differentiate it from the background.[62,82] Total loss of color monochromatism is rare, but it can occur.

Visual agnosia. A lesion circumscribed to the visual associative areas (areas 18 and 19) results in a number of unique visual disorders that are categorized as some form of visual agnosia. Lesions are usually bilateral with combined parietooccipital, occipitotemporal, and callosal lesions. Visual agnosia is defined as a failure to recognize visual stimuli (e.g., objects, faces, letters), although visual-sensory processing, language, and general intellectual functions are preserved at sufficiently high levels.[83] It also has been described as perception without meaning; perception apparently occurs, but the percept seems "disconnected" from previously associated meaning. In this pure form, visual agnosia is a relatively rare syndrome, and there is controversy as to whether it is simply an extension of primary visual sensory deficits (variations of cortical blindness) or whether it should be considered as a separate neuropsychological entity.

Three types of agnosia have been recognized: visual, tactile, and auditory. Agnosia is most often modality specific; that is, the individual who cannot recognize the object visually will usually give an immediate and accurate response when touching or hearing the object in use. In visual agnosia, then, poor recognition is limited to the visual sphere.

Visual agnosia is divided into a number of types: visual object agnosia, simultanagnosia, facial agnosia, and color agnosia. These deficits may be seen in isolation or in various combinations, depending on the size and location of the lesion.

Visual object agnosia. During evaluation for the presence of visual object agnosia, the individual is presented with a number of common objects (e.g., key, comb, brush) and asked to name them. The evaluator may assume that the object is recognized if the patient (1) names, describes, or demonstrates the use of the object; or (2) selects it from among a group of objects as it is named by the examiner. If the person recognizes (describes or demonstrates) but is unable to name the object, failure is most likely a result of an anomia rather than an agnosic defect. Individuals with real visual agnosia have no concept of what the object is.[83]

Simultanagnosia. Along the same vein are visual disorders that constrict or "narrow" the visual field during active perceptual analysis (i.e., when perceptions are tested separately, the visual field is within normal limits). Simultanagnosia is a disorder in which the person actually perceives only one element of an object or picture at a time and is unable to absorb the whole. As the individual concentrates on the visual environment, there is an extreme reduction of visual span. The problem is functionally similar to tubular vision. The narrowing of the functional perceptual field decreases the ability to simultaneously deal with two or more stimuli. It appears as if the person has bilateral visual inattention with macular sparing, although perimetric testing reveals full visual fields. A typical example is the individual whose visual attention is focused on the tip of a cigarette held between the lips and fails to perceive a match flame offered several inches away.[84]

Facial agnosia. Another special type of agnosia that has been documented is failure to recognize familiar faces. The disorder is also known as *prosopagnosia.* The individual is able to recognize a face as a face but is unable to connect the face and differences in faces with people he or she knows. This person is unable to recognize family members, friends, and hospital staff by face. One must be careful not to confuse this with generalized dementia. There may be categorical recognition problems with items involving special visual experience—for example, recognition of cars, types of trees, or emblems. Facial agnosia is usually seen in combination with a number of other deficits, including spatial disorientation, defective color perception, loss of topographical memory, constructional apraxia, and a left upper quadrant visual field loss. These other symptoms are most likely not causative but rather a result of the similar neurological location of these functions.[85]

Color agnosia. Finally, the individual may have difficulty recognizing names of colors, that is, an inability to name colors that are shown or to point to the color named by the examiner.[86] This defect is considered agnosic (as opposed to a defect in color perception) because the patient is able to recognize all colors in the Ishihara Color Plates[87] and is also able to sort colors by hue. The determining factor here appears to be a problem with visual-verbal association. Color agnosia is most common in patients with left hemisphere lesions and is often accompanied by the syndrome of alexia without agraphia.[83]

Assessment

Cortical blindness and variations of it should be thoroughly assessed by the vision specialist. Assessment for agnosia must be preceded by a thorough assessment for visual acuity problems, visual field deficits, and unilateral visual inattention because these primary visual sensory and scanning deficits are often mistaken for agnosic performance. Next, basic color perception should be measured by use of the Ishihara Color Plates[87] and color-sorting or color-matching tasks. Individuals with defective color perception will have difficulty with some visual-perceptual tasks because contextual cues related to color and shading are unavailable to them. Agnosia is a valid diagnosis only if (1) the aforementioned primary visual skills are intact and (2) language skills are intact (i.e., there should be no word-finding difficulty in spontaneous speech).

Although there are no standardized tests for agnosia, commonly used assessment methods have been included. The presence of simultanagnosia is determined by keen observation of performance that indicates perception limited to single elements within objects—for example, describing only the wheel of a bicycle or, within the environment, describing only one part of a room or an activity.

Object agnosia is tested for by placing common real objects (e.g., comb, key, penny, spoon) in front of the patient and asking the patient to name or point to the item chosen by the examiner. In pointing and naming tasks, the therapist must be sure that the patient is fixating on the appropriate target. The response is considered normal if the object is named correctly or described or its functional use demonstrated. Abnormal responses will be confabulatory or perseverative, with the individual often giving the name of a previous or similar object. Responses may also be completely bizarre and unrelated. The examiner may also present objects at an unusual angle. Abnormal responses will show lack of recognition or rotation of the head or body to try to view the object in the "straight on" position. The diagnosis of visual object agnosia is further confirmed if the individual can identify the object by touch or by hearing it in use, both of which should be attempted with vision occluded.

Color agnosia is evaluated by having the patient name a color and point to colors named by the examiner. Facial agnosia is evaluated by presenting the individual with photographs of famous world figures, actors, politicians, and family members.[62]

Interventions

There are no reliable studies regarding treatment of cortical blindness, color imperception, or visual agnosia. Treatment principles presented here are based on the experience of Bouska and Biddle[74] and Bouska and Kwatny.[58] If cortical blindness or simultanagnosia is suspected, the therapist must first attempt to increase the patient's knowledge of foveal versus peripheral vision, that is, where the patient is fixating. A small headlamp attached to the patient's forehead may be used under conditions of subdued lighting. The headlamp should not be used in a completely darkened room because the patient needs to use normal spatial cues from the environment. The movement of the projected light in the environment and kinesthetic input from the neck receptors augment knowledge of where the eye is fixed. To carry out this task, the patient must learn to position the eyes in midline of the head. The individual is asked to move the light (i.e., head and eyes) to locate and discriminate fairly large, bright stimuli placed on a plain background (e.g., yellow block on a brown table). As acuity and localization skills improve, stimuli and background should be made smaller and more complex (e.g., paper clip on a printed background or letters printed at different locations on a large page). The patient should be encouraged to accurately point to or manipulate targets once located with the light or to keep the light on a target as he or she slowly moves the target with one hand. Thus the kinesthetic input from the limb can augment visual localization abilities.[77] In patients with color imperception, treatment should initially involve materials and tasks with sharp color contrasts with minimal detail and should progress to less contrast (more hues) with more detail.

If the assessment has revealed a narrowing of the perceptual field, treatment should be aimed at progressively increasing the perception of large, bright, peripheral targets. For example, the patient may be asked to fixate on a centrally placed target while another bright target is brought in slowly from or uncovered in the periphery.[88,89] The individual is encouraged to maintain fixation on the central target while remaining alert for the presence of another target somewhere in the periphery. As the patient improves, targets should be smaller, multiple, and exposed for briefer periods. Peripheral targets should always have bright surfaces that reflect light because the peripheral receptors in the retina are mainly rods (light as opposed to color receptors). Another powerful variation of this technique is to involve hand use in peripheral location of objects. For example, the patient senses the presence of a peripheral object then reaches with the hand to pinpoint location, then shifts the eyes to identify it. This can further help differentiate between central and peripheral vision.

The treatment of patients with object agnosia should progress according to the abilities that return first in spontaneous recovery from agnosia. Common real objects should be used before line drawings in treatment. Presentations should be given "straight on," rather than at an angle or rotated. The patient should be asked to point to objects named by the examiner before being asked to name them. Manipulation of the object with simultaneous visual input should be attempted. This may help recognition, or it may simply confuse the patient; each case is unique. In general, tactile input with or without simultaneous visual input should be encouraged as a compensation method, although it may not be helpful during treatment sessions.

Color and facial agnosia may be approached by simply drilling the individual with regard to two or three names of colors or names of faces of people important to her or him. The patient may be assisted with picking out or memorizing cues for associating names with faces.[62]

Problems of Visual-Spatial Disorders
Identification of Clinical Problems

Individuals with brain lesions, particularly in the right posterior parietal and occipital areas, may have difficulties with tasks that require a normal concept of space.[56] Disorders of this nature have been termed *visual-spatial disorders*, *spatial disorientation*, *visual-spatial agnosia*, *spatial relations syndrome*, and numerous other names. Visual-spatial abilities are complexly interwoven within the performance of many perceptual and cognitive activities, such as dressing, building a design, reading, calculating, walking through an aisle, and playing tennis. An attempt is made here, however, to discuss spatial disorders in their purest form—that is, basic disorders—before dealing with visual-constructive disorders and disorders of analysis and synthesis. Constructional tasks require spatial planning, a type of planning that involves the building up and breaking down of objects in two and three dimensions. Constructional apraxia is viewed as a particular type of spatial-perceptual disorder and therefore is discussed separately under visual-constructive disorders and disorders of analysis and synthesis. Similarly, although perceptual skills such as figure-ground, form constancy, complex visual discrimination, and figure closure involve spatial concepts, tasks involving these skills often require the intellectual operations of synthesis and deduction. They, too, are discussed in the section dealing with analysis and synthesis.

All visual-spatial disabilities involve some problem with the apprehension of the spatial relationships between or within objects. Benton[90] has categorized them as the following disabilities:

1. Inability to localize objects in space, to estimate their size, and to judge their distance from the observer. The patient may be unable to accurately touch an object in space or indicate the position of the object (e.g., above, below, in front of, or behind). Relative localization may be impaired so that the individual may be unable to tell which object is closest. There may be difficulty determining which of two objects is larger or which line is longer. Holmes[91] reported cases of gross disorder in spatial orientation revealed through walking; affected individuals, even after seeing objects correctly, ran into them. In another example, a man intending to go toward his bed would invariably set out in the wrong direction. Difficulty in estimating distances may also extend to judgments of distances of perceived sounds and lead to overly slow and cautious gait or fear of venturing into public areas.
2. Impaired memory for the location of objects or places. An example is not being able to recall the position of a target previously viewed or the arrangement of furniture in a room. Individuals with this difficulty often lose things because they have no spatial memory to rely on for recall.
3. Inability to trace a path or follow a route from one place to another. Persons without this ability, known as *topographical orientation*, have difficulty understanding and remembering relationships of

places to one another, so they may have difficulty finding their way in a space, as in locating the therapy clinic in a hospital or locating the housewares department in a store previously familiar to them. Normally functioning individuals often have mild signs of topographical disorientation. Everyone is familiar with the disoriented feeling of not knowing how to get out of a large department store or losing a sense of direction in a familiar city. Many of the topographical errors made by patients result from unilateral spatial inattention. For example, someone with left inattention may make only right turns. Topographical disorientation, however, may be seen in a person with no signs of unilateral inattention. This individual will demonstrate route-finding difficulties at certain points and will apparently randomly choose a direction.
4. Problems with reading and counting. These high-level tasks require directional control of eye movements and organized scanning abilities. Eye movements (saccades) during reading bring a new region of the text on the fovea, the part of the retina where visual acuity is the greatest and clear detail can be obtained from the stimulus. During reading, the line of print that falls on the retina may be divided into three regions: the foveal region, the parafoveal region, and the peripheral region. The foveal region subtends about 1 to 2 degrees of visual angle around the reader's fixation point, the parafoveal region subtends about 10 degrees of visual angle around the reader's fixation point, and the peripheral region includes everything on the page beyond the parafoveal region. Parafoveal and peripheral vision contribute spatial information that is used to guide the reader's eye.[92] Visual-spatial disorders appear to interfere to varying degrees with the spatial schema of a page of type or numbers and the dynamic organizational scanning that must take place to gather information appropriately. Patients with unilateral spatial inattention will miss words or numbers located on one-half of the page. Other spatial problems unrelated to unilateral inattention include skipping individual words within a line or part of a line, skipping lines, repeating lines, "blocking" or having the inability to change direction of fixation, particularly at the end of a line, and generally losing the place on the total page. Performance usually deteriorates progressively as the individual continues to read. Eventually such persons cannot make sense of what they read, or if counting they complain of being lost or confused. This type of reading or counting disorder has nothing to do with recognition or interpretation of letters or numbers or their spatial configuration; rather, it represents a problem with dynamic sequential visual-spatial exploration during cognitive processing.

Other visual-spatial problems may include loss of depth perception, problems with body schema, and defective judgment of line orientation. There may also be difficulties with discrimination of right and left. Although unilateral spatial inattention is considered a visual-spatial disorder by many, it has been discussed separately in this chapter to increase clarity. Problems with judging line orientation (slant) or unilateral spatial inattention often interfere with a patient's spatial ability to tell time with a standard watch or clock. Perception of the vertical may also be considered a visual-spatial skill. Verticality perception is the interpretation of internal and external cues to maintain body balance. This maintenance is a complex neuromuscular process involving visual, proprioceptive, and vestibular systems. Patients with right lesions, particularly in the parieto-occipital region, have more difficulty perceiving verticality than those with left lesions. This may affect posture and ambulation.[93]

Assessment

The patient should be asked to accurately touch a number of targets in all parts of the visual field while fixating on a central point. Mislocation should be noted as well as the part of the visual field in which it occurred. Mislocalization within the central field is infrequent; however, defective localization of stimuli on one or both extramacular fields is more frequently seen.[56] The patient should be asked to determine which of a number of small cube blocks (placed perpendicularly in front of the patient) is closest, which is farthest, and which is in the middle. Differences in binocular (stereoscopic) and monocular viewing should be measured in this and other tasks. Impairment in both of these types of depth perception and subsequent inaccuracy in judging distances have been described in individuals with brain injury.[90]

With regard to memory for the location of objects or places, patients should be asked to describe the position of objects in their room from memory. They may also be asked to duplicate from memory the position of two or more targets (on a table or piece of paper) that have been presented for a 5-second period. As the number of targets increases, individuals with short-term memory for spatial localization will begin to make errors in spatial placement. Visual memory per se should be ruled out as a conflicting variable.

Topographical sense is assessed by asking patients to describe a floor plan of the arrangement of rooms in their house or to describe familiar geographical constellations, such as routes, arrangement of streets, or public buildings. After therapy, these persons may also be asked to find their way back to their rooms after being shown the route several times. Failure suggests a topographical orientation problem. Finally, such a patient may be asked to locate states or cities on a large map of the United States. In all of these procedures, the examiner must be sure to separate unilateral spatial inattention errors from topographical errors.

The influence of spatial dysfunction on reading and counting written material may be measured simply by asking the patient to read a page of regular newsprint. The examiner should observe performance carefully and document type and frequency of errors. If errors occur, eye movements should be observed to gather additional information. Pages of scanning material (letters or numbers) often give additional information on spatial planning during reading. These are pages of print in which the size and density of the print are controlled. Scanning behavior may be demonstrated by asking the patient to circle specific letters. Switching direction in the middle of a line, skipping letters or lines, perseveration, or any other abnormal performance behavior should be noted. Benton Judgment of Line Orientation Test[94] may be used to document problems with directional orientation of lines. If there is no indication of apraxia, the patient may simply be given a ruler and asked to match it to the directional orientation of the examiner's ruler.

Interventions

Treatment for visual-spatial deficits should follow basic developmental considerations, progressing from simple to more complex tasks. As with children, if the evaluation suggests disorders in body scheme, tactile or vestibular input, or right-left discrimination, these should be dealt with first.

Patients who do not know where they are in space need to internalize a spatial understanding before they can make judgments regarding the space around them. In gross motor spatial training, patients can be asked to roll and reach toward various targets. Supine, prone, sitting, and standing, with vision occluded, patients should try to localize tactile stimuli (various body locations touched by the therapist) and auditory stimuli (e.g., snapping fingers or ringing a bell) presented above, below, behind, in front of, and to the right and left of their bodies. The individual should state where the stimulus is and then point, roll, crawl, or walk toward it; this verbal, kinesthetic, and vestibular input augments spatial learning. In the occupational therapy kitchen,

the patient, once oriented to the room, may be asked to retrieve one type of object (e.g., cup) from "the top cupboard above your head," from "the bottom cupboard below your waist," from "the table behind you," or from "the drawer on your right (or left)." These patients may also place objects in various positions within a room. They should then stand in the middle of the room, close their eyes, and from memory visualize, verbalize, and point to where the objects are in relation to themselves. Having localized them, the patients should then walk through the space and retrieve the objects in sequence. Functional carryover should always be emphasized, such as having individuals remember through visualization where they put their glasses in the living room before they begin searching. Visualization is defined as the internal "seeing" of something that is not present at that moment: a vision without a visual input or internal visual imagery.[95] Visualization (spatial and other) is part of all perceptual tasks and may be used effectively as a treatment strategy. As previously discussed, a small feedback light placed in the middle of the patient's forehead can help teach spatial localization through eye-hand movements.

More complex spatial skills may be taught by asking patients to "partition" space and then localize within it. An excellent activity is one in which patients use a yardstick to divide a blackboard into four or more equal parts and then number each section.

Objects may be presented to patients, who must select the largest, the farthest away, or the one placed at an angle; they may be asked to place various objects in certain relationships to one another. As shape, size, and angle begin to "make sense" to these individuals, form boards, simple puzzles, and parquetry blocks may be added to training.

Topographical abilities should improve as patients begin to better conceptualize space; however, they may be trained directly. The therapist may help such patients organize a basic floor plan of the hospital room and the furniture within it while looking at the room. They may then be asked to do this from memory. Activities can progress to drawing plans or larger areas with a number of rooms. These patients should first "navigate" tactually through the area with a finger. Eventually, they should walk or wheel through the route themselves, visualizing and repeating the route until spatial concepts are learned. Imaginary routes also may be taken through maps of cities, states, or countries.

Organized visual-spatial exploration (eye movements) during reading or other scanning and cancellation tasks may be taught. Number and letter scanning sheets may be used for such training. Initially the size of numbers and the spaces between numbers should be large; this places less stress on visual acuity while training scanning. Before beginning, patients should orient themselves to the page spatially by numbering the right and left edges of each line. These numbers are used as additional spatial localization cues if needed during the scanning task.[46] Patients should then be asked to circle a specific number (or numbers) whenever it occurs. To control erratic or impulsive eye movements, they should be instructed to use a pencil to underline each line and then loop the selected letter as it comes into view (see Fig. 28.16). They may also be asked to read each letter. Underlining allows the kinesthetic and tactile receptors of the arm to control eye movements; verbalization allows the language and auditory systems to influence eye movements. Visual-spatial exploration exercises should progress to large-print magazines, books, or newspapers. The *New York Times* and *Reader's Digest* are both available in large print. In all training activities, it is most important that before the activity begins the patients fully comprehend the total space in which they will work. It is equally important that they reorient themselves at any point where errors occur. Those who lose their place during reading will eventually lose it again if the therapist simply points to where they should be. Chances are better that they will not lose their place again if they reorient themselves to the page spatially when an error occurs.

Problems of Visual-Constructive Disorders
Identification of Clinical Problems

Patients with lesions in either the right or left hemisphere may have problems when trying to "construct." Lesions in the parietal, temporal, occipital, and frontal lobes have been documented in individuals with visual-constructive disorders.[56,96] The normal ability to construct, also known as *visual-constructive ability* and *constructional praxis,* involves any type of performance in which parts are put together to form a single entity. Examples include assembling blocks to form a design, assembling a puzzle, making a dress, setting a table, and simply drawing four lines to form a square (graphic skills). The skill implies a high level of dynamic, organized, visual-perceptual processing in which the spatial relations are perceived and sequenced well enough among and within the component parts to direct higher-level processing to sequence the perceptual-motor actions so that eventually parts are synthesized into a desired whole. Visual-constructive ability may be compromised if any part of this process is disturbed.

Typical tasks used to measure this ability include building in a vertical direction, building in a horizontal direction, three-dimensional block construction from a model or a picture of a model, and copying line drawings such as of houses, flowers, and geometric designs.[85]

Patients with visual-constructive deficits, especially those with right lesions, often also have visual-spatial deficits. These individuals may rotate the position of a part erroneously, place it in the wrong position, space it too far from another part, be oblivious to perspective or a third dimension, or simply be unable to complete more than two or three steps before becoming entirely confused. This is usually evidence of breakdown because of faulty or inadequate spatial information.

Other patients, usually those with left lesions, have an "executional" or apraxic problem; they seem to have difficulty initiating and conducting the planned sequence of movements necessary to construct the whole. The problem seems to be in planning, arranging, building, or drawing rather than in spatial concepts. This deficit in its purest form is known as *constructional apraxia.* Constructional apraxia lies clinically outside the category of most other varieties of apraxia and is considered a special kind of "perceptual" apraxia. It occurs frequently in aphasic individuals; therefore the underlying mechanisms of aphasia and constructional apraxia may be related.[97]

Assessment

Constructional abilities are generally measured through tasks that require (1) copying line drawings of, for example, a house, clock face, flower, or geometric design (drawing may also be done without copying); (2) copying two-dimensional matchstick designs; (3) building block designs by copying or from a model; or (4) assembling puzzles. Table 28.2 lists common tests. The more complex the picture or design to be copied, the more complex are the constructional tasks. The following are examples of drawing and block construction deficits:

1. Patients may crowd the drawing or design on one side of the page or in one corner of the page or available space on the working surface, usually a result of the influence of unilateral spatial inattention.
2. Lines in drawings may be wavy or broken, too long or too short.
3. One line may not meet another accurately, or lines may transect one another; in block designs, parts may not be neatly placed but rather may have small gaps.
4. There may be "overdrawing" of angles or parts of the figure because of graphic perseveration (scribble), spatial indecision, or problems with executive planning.
5. Patients may superimpose their copy on the model or superimpose one of their drawings on top of another. In block design construction, they may become confused between the model and their

TABLE 28.2 Common Tests Used to Assess Visuoconstructive Skills

Test	Standardization
Drawing pictures or shapes with or without an example to copy	Not standardized
Reproducing matchstick designs	Not standardized
Assembling puzzles	Not standardized
Bender Visual Motor Gestalt Test	Standardized for children only
Kohs Blocks Test	Standardized for adults
WAIS Block Design Test	Standardized for adults
Benton's Three-Dimensional Constructional Praxis Test	Standardized for adults

reproduction and use part of the model to complete their design. This has been termed the "closing-in" phenomenon, a failure to distinguish between model and reproduction.[56]

6. Parts of the drawing or design may be reversed. Horizontal reversals are more common than vertical reversals.

A note might be appropriate here regarding dressing apraxia. This problem occurs most frequently with right hemisphere damage. It is considered a "perceptual" apraxia rather than a motor apraxia because the inability to dress is believed to result from body scheme, spatial, and visual-constructive deficits rather than difficulty in motor execution. Persons with dressing apraxia cannot correctly orient their clothes to their body. They often put clothes on backward or inside out. Failure to dress one side of the body is also often noted and is directly related to unilateral spatial inattention.

Interventions

It must be remembered that both visual-constructive and visual analysis synthesis skills are often used almost simultaneously during task performance. Thus treatment should not separate the two types of skills but rather should be a precise interrelationship of activities that require finer and finer levels of each facility. For example, arranging an office filing system is both an analytical-synthesis and a visual-constructive task. The individual must first analyze overall needs and translate them into an imagined visual-spatial plan (preliminary synthesis of the whole) that will help organization. Then the organizer begins to use the hands to categorize (segment visual space). This building is a visual-constructive task. Intermittently during building, new ideas of the whole surface, and visual-constructive tasks change in response to a "better idea" (final synthesis of the whole). Task performance, except for tasks that are rote, usually follows similar perceptual processes. Treatment therefore must be integral. Visual-constructive skills, however, may be emphasized more than visual analysis and synthesis skills or vice versa.

As previously mentioned, visual-constructive disorders are thought to result from different underlying problems in different individuals (e.g., visual-spatial disorders in persons with right hemisphere lesions and executive, planning, or synthetic disorders in those with left hemisphere lesions). There are few reliable studies on treatment strategies for visual-constructive disorders. One possible treatment strategy is known as *saturational cuing.*[98] This method involves presenting controlled verbal instruction on task analysis and sequence and presenting cues on spatial boundaries (cuing is also response related).

If there are problems with planning and sequencing of steps necessary to accomplish a visual-constructive task, the therapist should begin with simple tasks that require only three or four steps, such as positioning one place setting at a table. The patient should discuss the plan and sequence of steps before initiating the activity, while looking at the parts to be used, such as silverware, plate, and glass. These steps may even be written down for additional input. The patient should be helped to reorient the plan at any point during task breakdown. Eventually, tasks should increase in complexity (e.g., setting a table for five), and the patient should be encouraged to function more independently. Another technique often used by clinicians is known as backward chaining. This involves presenting a partially completed task and asking the patient to complete the final steps, for example, placing the knife and glass on a partially completed place setting. The perceptual cues of the task already begun appear to stimulate constructional abilities. As the patient progresses, he or she should complete more steps.

Intervention for problems with spatial planning during visual-constructive tasks should begin with the simple spatial exercises discussed previously. If problems still exist, the individual may be asked to draw around shapes (blocks) one by one. These shapes should first have been placed in a simple two-dimensional design. The patient is then asked to rebuild the design with the shapes alone. Therapy should progress from horizontal to vertical to oblique designs, from two-dimensional to three-dimensional designs, and from tasks with common objects to tasks involving abstract designs. For example, spatial problems with drawing, such as placing windows in a house or numbers on a clock face, are usually a result of an underlying spatial disorder. The patient should use a ruler or protractor to segment the space and plan placement before drawing. Dot-to-dot tasks may be designed that actually lead and sequence the drawing into a spatial whole. Simple puzzles also may be used to increase visual-spatial abilities during visual-constructive tasks. Finally, if task breakdown results from impulsive visual or motor behavior, these symptoms should be dealt with before further visual-constructive treatment continues.

Examples of visual-constructive tasks that may be designed for therapeutic use include the following:
- Setting a table for one to five people
- Wrapping a gift
- Assembling a piece of woodwork, a toy, a tool, a motor
- Changing a tire on a car
- Organizing a shelf in a library or a kitchen
- Organizing a filing system or cabinet
- Putting pieces of a sewing pattern together
- Addressing an envelope
- Rearranging furniture according to a preset plan
- Assembling a craft according to a preset plan
- Drawing from memory or copy
- Copying two-dimensional block designs
- Copying three-dimensional designs with oblique components

The key to effective visual-constructive learning, however, is not the task itself but rather how carefully the therapist organizes it and monitors performance. Patients with visual-constructive disorders are often visually or motorically impulsive; they often move or draw parts before analysis has taken place. Once a part is placed inappropriately, it begins to confuse the whole visual-perceptual process. This confusion increases anxiety and contributes to further breakdown in analysis and synthesis. Treatment should be directed at the underlying causes of task breakdown if these can be determined.

Problems of Visual Analysis and Synthesis Disorders
Identification of Clinical Problems
This separate discussion of visual analysis and synthesis is arbitrary. There is never any clear demarcation among the processes of visual-spatial orientation, visual construction, and visual analysis and synthesis. Analysis of likes and differences, relationships of parts to one another, and reasoning and deduction occur simultaneously with more basic spatial and constructive percepts. The final visual concept of a task (e.g.,

what a place setting on a table should look like) is necessary before the task is begun. Similarly, synthesis of one part of a task may be necessary before synthesis of the entire task can occur. For example, the person who is setting a table for four people must be able to conceptualize one place setting before conceptualizing the table with four place settings. Those points during perceptual processing when there is a colligation or blending of discrete impressions into a single perception are known as *synthesis*. This final stage of coordination and interpretation of sensory data is thought to be deficient in many individuals with perceptual problems. Deficits may be present with either left or right hemisphere damage but are more common and more severe with right lesions.[62,99]

Visual-perceptual skills considered to be analytical and synthetic in nature include making fine visual discriminations, particularly in complex configurations; separating figure from background in complex configurations (figure-ground); achieving recognition on the basis of incomplete information (figure closure); and synthesizing disparate elements into a meaningful entity, as, for example, conceptualizing parts of a task into a whole.[5]

Assessment
Many tests have been designed to measure the capacity for analysis and synthesis. Test items include complex figures in which small parts of a figure differ from another figure. The patient is asked to select the one that is different. Studies have shown that basic discrimination of single attributes of a stimulus such as length, contour, or brightness is intact in many patients.[100–102] The problem appears when these individuals are asked to discriminate between more complex configurations with subtle differences. Tests also measure figure-ground ability; the patient must select the embedded figure from the background. Functional examples of this problem are the inability of a patient to find her or his glasses if they are lying on a figured background, to find a white shirt on a white bedspread, and to find his or her wheelchair locks. Figure closure is measured by asking the patient to complete an incomplete figure, such as part of the outline of a common shape. Finally, synthesis of parts into a whole, also known as *visual organization*, is measured by asking the patient to conceptualize and organize the whole picture by, for example, looking at separate segments of the picture (e.g., cup or key) that have been divided and placed in unusual positions. This type of synthesis is necessary for high-level constructional tasks. Table 28.3 outlines examples of tests used to evaluate visual analysis and synthesis.

Interventions
Intervention for deficits in visual analysis and synthesis should follow developmental considerations described in the children's section. Visual discrimination tasks should begin with simple figures and obvious differences in complex figures. Color, size, texture, lighting, and verbal direction may help the patient "cue in" on subtle differences among objects or figures. The therapist should determine the threshold at which the patient is capable of discriminating differences and vary the dimension, contrast, and functional activity at this level. For

TABLE 28.3 Common Tests Used to Assess Visual Analysis and Synthesis

Test	Use
Hooper Visual Organization Test	Standardized for adults
Motor-Free Visual Perception Test	Standardized for adults
Raven's Progressive Matrices	Standardized for adults
Embedded Figure Test	Standardized for adults
Southern California Figure-Ground Test	Standardized for children only

example, if the individual cannot select a can of vegetables from a kitchen shelf stocked with cans of similar size, the therapist may simply change the task to fit that person's level of visual discrimination by removing some of the cans (decreasing the density of the display), replacing some of the cans with boxes of food (increasing the spatial contrast), moving the can to be selected forward or to one edge of the display (decreasing figure-ground difficulty), removing the label from the can (increasing the light and color contrast), or giving cues regarding what to search for (verbal direction). This example is described not as a method of compensation but rather as an approach to be used therapeutically in slowly building the patient's visual discrimination abilities. Eventually, high-level visual discrimination skills should be incorporated within tasks requiring three or more steps, such as selecting a can of vegetables, opening the can (which involves selecting the can opener from the utensil drawer), and emptying the vegetables into a specific bowl (which involves selecting the bowl from among other bowls). Visual discrimination and figure-ground skills may appear normal until the patient is required to do multiple-step activities, is given time constraints, or becomes anxious or confused. Tabletop games that require high levels of visual discrimination along with cognitive strategies may be therapeutic and motivating. Examples include *Monopoly* and card games such as solitaire. Matching and sorting tasks also may be helpful in enhancing visual discrimination. Examples include matching picture cards and sorting laundry, tools, silverware, or files.

Drawings of figures with subtle differences also may be used for therapy. The patient should be encouraged to point to, verbalize, or outline the subtle differences in two or more pictures; this enhances visual attention to detail. If the individual cannot select the discrepant detail(s) among three or more figures, the problem most likely results from an inability to select one feature and compare it with elements in the other figures. This is a fairly high-level skill that requires selective attention and analysis with internal visualization while the individual is still viewing the complete figures. This type of patient should practice feature detection and then begin systematic comparisons of similarities and differences between two figures, eventually progressing to three or more figures. The therapist may number or outline similar areas of each figure to help the patient (1) direct attention to similar areas of all figures and (2) sequence comparisons appropriately. The patient should verbalize, draw, or write details concerning similarities and differences in individual aspects of the figures. This enhances visual analysis and also informs the therapist about how the individual is selecting and comparing features. Eventually, speed should be stressed, the highest level being presentation of tachistoscopic designs.

Visual organization may be emphasized by presenting the patient with activities that have multiple parts that must be sequenced together into a whole. Activities involving this type of synthesis are discussed in the preceding section on treatment of visual-constructive disorders. Figure closure may be emphasized by presenting parts of figures or objects (e.g., half a plate covered by a towel) and asking the patient for identification. Figure-closure task difficulty may be increased by placing many objects on a table, some of which partially occlude others. Identification of objects in such a task requires figure closure simultaneous with figure-ground abilities.

Visual analysis and synthesis deficits reflect a disruption in cognitive function with specific regard to visual-perceptual features. The affected patient may function normally when analytical tasks require another system, for example, language. In others with generalized brain damage (e.g., traumatic head injury and senile dementia), general cognitive analysis and synthesis may be at fault rather than visual analysis. Because most cognitive performance requires visual processing, however, increased ability to analyze and synthesize visual-perceptual material often generalizes to an increase in cognitive function.

PERCEPTUAL RETRAINING WITH COMPUTERS

Numerous computer programs have been developed for rehabilitation of brain damage symptoms, including those affecting cognition (e.g., attention, sequencing, or memory) and perception. Because the computer is so highly visual, it becomes an obvious tool for treatment of visual-perceptual dysfunction. Treatment with computers has been named *computer-assisted therapy*. There is a growing interest in development of and research into programs for rehabilitation, for the prevention of Alzheimer's, and in normal healthy aging adults. The largest treatment study of 487 subjects was able to demonstrate statistically significant improvements in memory and attention by using a plasticity-based adaptive training program.[103] A number of other studies are in progress. Advantages of computer-assisted therapy include control and flexibility of perceptual variables during treatment (e.g., number, size, speed), immediate feedback regarding performance, automatic control for learning (e.g., items are repeated if incorrect to facilitate learning), and being motivational. Visual-perceptual training with computers, if used, should be viewed as one part of a patient's treatment program. One should always remember that the computer, monitor, and keyboard are just that: they do not require the many perceptual, vestibular, and motor responses typical of daily performance (e.g., scanning requirements may be bilateral, but they are not global and associated with head movement). A patient's total program may include computer-assisted therapy as an additional tool; however, it should never be substituted for more significant training within the multidimensional environment. Some computer programs for visual-perceptual training are listed in Box 28.6.

BOX 28.6 Computer Programs for Visual-Perceptual Training

HTS Home Therapy Systems
  homevisiontherapy.com
Visual Perceptual Diagnostic Testing and Training Programs
  H. Greenberg and C. Chamoff
  Educational Electronic Techniques
  1886 Wantagh Avenue
  Wantagh, NY 11793
Captain's Log MindPower Builder
  J. Sandford and R. Browne
  Computability Corporation
  https://www.braintrain.com/captains-log/captains-log-mindpower-builder/
    101 Route 46 East
  Pine Brook, NJ 07058
Cognitive Rehabilitation Therapy System
  http://www.psychological-software.com/psscogrehab.html
  Psychological Software Services
  P.O. Box 29205
  Indianapolis, IN 46229
Life Science Associates Programs
  Available at AbleData
  https://abledata.acl.gov/organizations/life-science-associates
  1 Fenemore Road
  Bayport, NY 11705 (Diagnosis and Training)
  Brain HQ
Posit Science
  https://m.brainhq.com
  1 Montgomery Street, Suite 700
  San Francisco, CA 94104
  (866) 599-6463
Online Brain Training
  http://www.lumosity.com

SUMMARY OF VISUAL-PERCEPTUAL DYSFUNCTION

Careful organized evaluation should delineate deficits well enough to result in a visual-perceptual function profile for each patient, including both primary and associative visual skills. Patients rarely come with isolated visual-perceptual deficits; more often, they exhibit a combination of visual-perceptual deficits usually interrelated with motor, language, and cognitive dysfunctions. For example, a visual-perceptual function profile may reveal strabismus, left unilateral visual inattention, visual-spatial deficits, visual-constructive deficits, and problems with visual analysis and synthesis, all affecting daily function. Treatment should be organized to progressively build skills, emphasizing one component more than another. The goal of treatment is eventual generalization of improvements in individual skills to spontaneous high-level function.

The presentation of information in this chapter is an attempt to use isolated and mechanistic terms to define a system that is extremely subtle, integrated, and complex. The reader is reminded that much of the normal and abnormal perceptual system has not been well defined. Preliminary studies cited throughout this chapter, however, suggest that disorders may be responsive to management and treatment. Research is needed to standardize evaluation procedures well enough to further define deficits and to investigate the effectiveness of various treatment approaches with various patient populations.

REFERENCES

To enhance this text and add value for the reader, all references are included on the companion Evolve site that accompanies this textbook. This online service will, when available, provide a link for the reader to a Medline abstract for the article cited. There are 103 cited references and other general references for this chapter, with the majority of those articles being evidence-based citations.

Bernell/USO, 4016 North Home Street, Mishiwaka, IN 46545; (800) 348-2225

CCTVs: Enhanced Vision Systems, 5882 Machine Drive, Huntington Beach, CA 92649, Tel: 888-811-3161, www.enhancedvision.com

Complete Visual Screening Kit: Laurie R. Chaikin, OD, OTR/L, FCOVD; 420 F Cola Ballena, Alameda, CA 94501; Laurie.chaikin@gmail.com

Teller Cards: Vistech Consultants, 4162 Little York Road, Dayton, OH 45414-2566

HELPFUL WEBSITES

American Optometric Association, Position Statement on Optometric Vision Therapy (includes excellent reference list): www.aoa.org/Documents/optometrists/vision-therapy-reimbursement-packet.pdf

Annotated reference list: www.visiontherapy.org/vision-therapy/vision-therapy-studies.html

College of Optometrists in Vision Development: www.covd.org

Computerized home vision therapy system: www.homevisiontherapy.com

Enhanced Vision systems for closed circuit TVs: www.enhancedvision.com

Neuro-Optometric Rehabilitation Association: www.nora.cc

Optometric Extension Program Foundation: www.oepf.org

Parents Active for Vision Education: www.pave-eye.com/~vision

Vision Therapy Information and Referrals

NovaVision: www.novavision.com/Home.html

Information on the Visual Field Restitution Training System.

Optometrists Network: www.optometrists.org

Optometrists Network: All About 3D: www.vision3D.com

The Vision Help Network: Hyperlink:>www.visionhelp.com

Full Circle Cognitive Rehabilitation has unilateral inattention training programs via computer and the internet. Please see http://mytrainedbrain.com/. The developer Tom Van Vleet can be reached through his website email address at tomvanvleet@gmail.com or by phone at (925) 580-2806.

Motion Therapeutics: www.motiontherapeutics.com. For information on the Balance-Based Torso-Weighting vest, email Cindy Gibson-Horn, RPT, at cindy@motiontherapeutics.com.

VisionCare Ophthalmic Technologies: www.visioncareinc.net

Information on the implantable telescope for macular degeneration.

29

Cardiovascular and Pulmonary System Health in Populations With Neurological Disorders

Marilyn Mackay-Lyons and Emily Nguyen

OBJECTIVES

After reading this chapter the student or therapist will be able to:

1. Explain the physiological principles related to cardiovascular responses to exercise testing.
2. Describe the factors that contribute to the deconditioned state in adults with neurological disorders.
3. Explain the adaptive responses to aerobic training in populations with neurological disorders and the factors underlying these responses.
4. Discuss general guidelines for designing exercise programs to improve cardiovascular health and fitness.

KEY TERMS

aerobic training	deconditioning	rating of perceived exertion
cardiovascular fitness	exercise tolerance	

The cardiovascular and pulmonary health of individuals with residual movement dysfunction after a neurological insult has become a topic of great interest in neurorehabilitation. In traditional practice, the state of the neuromuscular system preoccupied the attention of clinicians in the quest to optimize neurological recovery. Most interventions were based on strategies to improve the capacity of that system—an approach that has met with limited success in terms of restoring functional independence. It is now clear that recovery cannot be explained solely on the basis of improved neuromuscular function—three decades ago Roth and colleagues[1] determined that less than one-third of the variance in functional limitations after a stroke can be explained by the extent of neurological impairment. Nevertheless, the current approach to neurorehabilitation is somewhat perplexing. Evidence has accumulated indicating that many people with neurological disabilities are woefully deconditioned. There has been widespread acknowledgement of the central role that aerobic exercise plays in improving cardiopulmonary health and fitness. Furthermore, application of the principles of exercise physiology in cardiac rehabilitation has been widely endorsed. Yet neurorehabilitation clinicians have been observed to practice without full knowledge of their patients' cardiac status or without monitoring heart rate (HR) and blood pressure (BP).[2,3] Moreover, there is evidence to suggest that patients with neurological insults have not been challenged enough in therapy to induce the metabolic stress needed to enhance their cardiopulmonary fitness.[4-6] A troubling explanation offered for these observations is that clinicians lack either an understanding or an appreciation of the basic physiological principles of exercise.[7,8]

Fortunately, attention has turned to the introduction of interventions that encompass the neuromuscular, cardiovascular, and pulmonary systems and promote a more holistic approach to neurorehabilitation. The challenge of improving cardiopulmonary health and fitness in these populations is not trivial. For individuals with chronic conditions, fitness is affected by a host of interacting influences such as the location and extent of the lesion, the presence of comorbidities (particularly cardiovascular disease), and the premorbid activity level. To complicate matters further, testing and training protocols for individuals with compromised motor and postural control need to be tailored to ensure safety and effectiveness.

This chapter begins with an overview of basic physiological principles related to cardiovascular responses to exercise testing, much of the evidence for which was derived several decades ago. A summary of the evidence of cardiopulmonary fitness levels in adults and children with neurological disabilities is followed by a description of factors that contribute to the deconditioned state. Possible mechanisms responsible for reduced exercise capacity are then reviewed. Adaptive responses to aerobic training in patients with neurological conditions are examined, as are factors underlying these responses. The chapter closes with a summary of guidelines for the design of exercise programs that can be used to improve cardiopulmonary health and fitness. Appendix 29.A at the end of this chapter clearly identifies the meanings of the abbreviations used throughout the chapter.

PHYSIOLOGICAL RESPONSES TO EXERCISE

At rest the human body consumes roughly 3.5 mL of oxygen (O_2) per kilogram per minute, or 1 metabolic equivalent (MET).[9] In the resting state, skeletal muscle activity accounts for less than 20% of the body's total energy expenditure; the brain, making up only 2% of body weight, also consumes 20% of the available O_2.[10] Activities at rest, such as breathing and contracting of the heart, can be sustained indefinitely because the power demands of these activities are met by the rate of energy turnover. In other words, these activities occur well below the *critical power* of the muscles, defined as the maximal rate of work that can be endured indefinitely.[11] Any physical activity beyond the resting state requires more O_2; the increase is dependent on the intensity of the effort involved. The rise in metabolism relies on O_2 transport by the pulmonary and circulatory systems and O_2 usage by the active skeletal, cardiac, and respiratory muscles to convert chemical potential energy to mechanical energy.[12] The components of the O_2 transport system are outlined in Fig. 29.1.

Selective distribution of the increased blood flow to regions with heightened metabolic demands—the working muscles—is largely a result of local vasodilation mediated mainly by metabolites acting on the vascular smooth muscle (e.g., carbon dioxide [CO_2], hydrogen ions [H^+], nitric oxide, potassium ions, adenosine) and vasoconstriction in

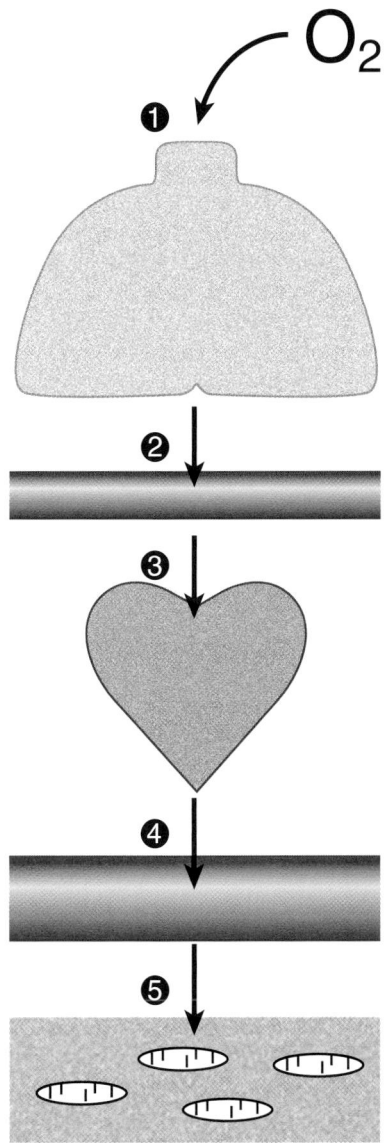

Fig. 29.1 Diagrammatic Representations of the Components of the O_2 Transport System. *(1)* During inspiration O_2 from the air is delivered to the alveolar gas space by the process of respiration. *(2)* O_2 diffuses across the blood-gas barrier into the pulmonary capillary blood, where almost all of the O_2 is bound to hemoglobin. *(3)* The heart acts as a pump, and *(4)* the vascular system acts as the plumbing to transport O_2 to the various tissues, including the exercising muscle, *(5)* where it diffuses from the red blood cells into the mitochondria within the myocytes. Reduced conductance of any component impairs O_2 transport, whereas improved conductance of any component augments O_2 transport.

tissues with low metabolic demands.[13] Blood flow to other vascular beds (e.g., renal and splanchnic bed) either is unchanged or decreases through active vasoconstriction resulting primarily from increased sympathetic discharge.[13] Cerebral autoregulation maintains regional and total cerebral blood flow and normal tissue oxygenation over a wide range of BPs[14]; thus cerebral blood flow and O_2 delivery during exercise either remain stable[15,16] or increase slightly.[17,18] As exercise intensity increases, systolic BP (SBP) increases markedly, whereas diastolic BP (DBP) either remains unchanged or lowers slightly, resulting in a moderate increase in mean arterial pressure.[19]

Extraction of O_2 from the muscle capillary blood to mitochondria is dependent on an adequate O_2-diffusion gradient. During a progressive increase in workload, the arterial hemoglobin saturation and arterial O_2 content remain relatively constant, whereas the venous O_2 content decreases substantially as a result of increased O_2 extraction in the active muscles.[20] As the metabolic rate rises, the minute ventilation (i.e., respiratory rate multiplied by the tidal volume) increases to remove CO_2 and to regulate pH balance of the active muscles. At low-intensity exercise, ventilation (mainly tidal volume) increases in a linear manner relative to the volume of O_2 use (Vo_2) and CO_2 production (Vco_2). Above the critical power, the energy demand of the muscle exceeds the capacity of the aerobic process to supply energy for muscle contraction; the additional energy is supplied by the anaerobic glycolytic system.[20]

During more intense exercise, ventilation is extremely variable among individuals; the respiratory rate usually increases without a substantial change in tidal volume.[19] The point at which the rate of glycolysis exceeds that of oxidative phosphorylation is called the *anaerobic threshold* (which approximates the ventilatory threshold or lactate threshold).[19] Pyruvic acid is converted to lactic acid, which completely dissociates to lactate and H^+, resulting in a rise in blood lactate levels and a fall in intramuscular pH. Exercise-induced muscular fatigue is caused by the exponential accumulation of lactate and a drop in intramuscular pH, with negative effects on the actin-myosin turnover rate, enzyme activities, and excitation-contraction coupling.

Maximal oxygen consumption (Vo_2max) is defined as the highest O_2 intake an individual can attain during physical work.[19] The Fick equation describes the relationship between cardiovascular function and Vo_2max:

$$Vo_2\,max = Q\,max \times a\text{-}vO_2 diffmax$$

where $Qmax$ is the maximal cardiac output and a-vO_2diffmax is the maximal arteriovenous O_2 difference. Given that $Qmax$ equals the product of maximal HR (HRmax) and maximal stroke volume (SVmax),

$$Vo_2\,max = HR\,max\ SV\,max \times a\text{-}vO_2 diffmax$$

Thus Vo_2max reflects both O_2 transport to the tissues and O_2 usage by the tissues. Increases in Vo_2 during exercise are caused by increases in both cardiac output and a-vO_2diff, with HR and stroke volume (SV) increasing progressively over the lower third of the workload range. Thereafter HR continues to increase while SV remains essentially constant,[21,22] resulting, at maximal effort, in a cardiac output three to six times greater than baseline levels. An increase in SV (50% over resting volume) is caused by enhanced myocardial contractility and increased venous return resulting from compression of the veins by contracting muscles and reduced intrathoracic pressure.[23] At low-intensity exercise, the increase in HR is mainly a result of decreased vagal tone, but as exercise intensifies, sympathetic stimulation and circulating catecholamines play a greater role, yielding, at maximal workloads, a rise in HR 200% to 300% above the resting level.[24]

MEASUREMENT OF CARDIOPULMONARY FITNESS

Exercise (aerobic) capacity is the principal determinant of the ability to sustain the power requirements of repetitive physical activity. Vo_2max is generally accepted as the definitive index of exercise capacity and cardiopulmonary fitness.[25] Vo_2max is a relatively stable measurement; variability of repeated measures of Vo_2max has been reported to be 2% to 4%[26] or 0.2 L/min.[27] Accurate determination of Vo_2max requires (1) adequate duration and work intensity by at least 50% of total muscle mass, (2) independence from motivation or skill of the subject, and (3) controlled environmental conditions. Also, because test performance is sensitive to time of day, the time of repeat testing should be consistent.

Before any fitness test, a 3- to 5-minute warm-up of slow treadmill walking on a level grade or unloaded pedaling that raises the metabolic rate twofold (i.e., 2 METs) above resting should be performed.[28] A proper warm-up prevents excessive local muscle fatigue from occurring before Vo_2max has been attained.[29] Furthermore, a 3- to 5-minute cool-down should follow test completion to aid in venous return to prevent blood pooling in the peripheral vasculature and a subsequent drop in DBP. The intensity of exercise can be increased in a continuous progressive manner (i.e., step or ramp protocol) or, less commonly, in a discontinuous progressive manner (i.e., subject rests between stages). Throughout testing, continuous monitoring of the electrocardiogram and periodic monitoring of BP are essential. The optimal duration of a graded exercise test is 8 to 12 minutes, with testing terminated when the subject can no longer generate the required power, is limited by symptoms, or is unable to continue safely.[30] Variables of interest during exercise testing include Vo_2max expressed in absolute terms (liters of O_2 per minute) or relative to body mass (milliliters of O_2 per kilogram of body weight per minute), MET level, percent of predicted HRmax, respiratory exchange ratio (RER; ratio of Vo_2 to CO_2), peak power, minute ventilation, tidal volume, respiratory rate, and rating of perceived exertion (RPE) according to the Borg scale.[31] Because there is considerable variability in HRmax among healthy individuals, the percent of predicted HRmax attained is not a robust indicator of exercise capacity.[32] Similarly, because both total exercise time and peak exercise intensity (or power attained; i.e., peak treadmill speed and grade or peak power on bike) are dependent on the test protocol, neither is a reliable measure of exercise capacity.[33,34] In addition, noninvasive estimation of the anaerobic threshold by identifying the point of nonlinear increases in minute ventilation and Vco_2 can be highly subjective and thus unreliable.[35]

The principal marker of exercise capacity is attainment of a plateau in Vo_2, beyond which there is a change of less than 100 mL/min, with further increases in workload dependent solely on anaerobic metabolism.[30] In cases in which a Vo_2 plateau is not observed (typically in deconditioned or elderly individuals or in patients with heart disease), the preferred term for the value obtained is *peak Vo_2* (Vo_2peak).[36] Criteria for attainment of Vo_2peak include achieving the age-predicted HRmax, RER in excess of 1.15, minute ventilation greater than the predicted maximal voluntary ventilation, tidal volume greater than 90% of the inspiratory capacity, and obvious patient exhaustion.[29]

Testing Modality

The modality of testing (e.g., treadmill walking, cycling, stepping, arm cranking) can affect Vo_2max values. The treadmill has the greatest potential to recruit sufficient muscle mass to elicit a maximal metabolic response, particularly in deconditioned individuals.[37] Bike ergometry yields 85% to 90%, and arm ergometry 70%, of the Vo_2max achieved with a treadmill.[37] Ideally the mode of exercise should be consistent with the patient's typical activity. Thus the treadmill is often preferred because the pattern of muscle activation during treadmill walking is similar to that for most mobility tasks. In patients with neuromuscular conditions, however, impaired balance and motor control often preclude the use of standard treadmill testing protocols. To resolve this limitation, we devised and validated an exercise protocol using a body-weight support system to permit safe and valid testing of Vo_2max early after stroke.[38] For subjects with paraplegia, tests with wheelchair treadmills are more functionally relevant than those using arm ergometry.

PREDICTING MAXIMAL OXYGEN CONSUMPTION WITH USE OF SUBMAXIMAL EXERCISE TESTS

Although submaximal tests do not measure the systemic response, they are inexpensive to administer and have a low risk of adverse events. The essentially linear relationship between Vo_2 and HR permits the estimation of Vo_2max from HR measurements taken during submaximal exercise. For example, for people without physical disability the HR increases approximately 50 beats per uptake of 1 L of O_2, independent of sex and body size.[39] For unfit individuals and patients with cardiac impairment, the increases in HR are greater per liter, except for patients taking β-blockers, who demonstrate blunting of the HR response throughout exercise. The Åstrand-Ryhming nomogram has been used to predict Vo_2max from submaximal HR.[40] The HR-Vo_2 relationship is independent of the exercise protocol. However, HR, unlike Vo_2max, is markedly affected by many stresses (e.g., dehydration, changes in body temperature, acute starvation), resulting in substantial error and inaccurate Vo_2max estimations.[37] In fact, discrepancies between estimated and measured Vo_2max in individuals with low exercise capacity can be as high as 25%.[41]

FITNESS LEVELS IN POPULATIONS WITH NEUROLOGICAL DISORDERS

Documentation of exercise capacity in populations with neurological disorders has been hindered by the lack of testing protocols that can safely and effectively accommodate the motor and balance disturbances common to these populations. Not surprisingly, the evidence to date suggests that most individuals with neurological disabilities are significantly deconditioned. Variability results from a multitude of factors, including differences in testing protocols, as discussed in the previous section, and differences in subject characteristics; these points are discussed in the following section.

Impact of Low Fitness Levels on Health of People With Neurological Disorders

People with high fitness levels use only a small fraction of the *physiological fitness reserve*[42] of the cardiovascular, respiratory, and neuromuscular systems to respond to the metabolic challenge of activities of daily living (ADLs).[43,44] Thus small declines in exercise capacity may not be noticeable in carrying out ADLS. In contrast, relatively minor reductions in capacity can substantially influence performance of ADLs by deconditioned individuals. Light instrumental ADLs require approximately 10.5 mL of oxygen per kilogram per minute (3 METs), whereas more strenuous activities have metabolic costs of about 17.5 mL/kg per minute (5 METs).[45] Cress and Meyer[46] reported that the Vo_2peak of 20 mL/kg per minute is needed for older adults to meet the physiological demands of independent living. It is evident that many people living with neurological disabilities (particularly stroke, tetraplegia, and postpoliomyelitis syndrome) do not have the level of fitness required for the more strenuous ADLs and independent living. Moreover, relative exercise capacities (expressed as a percentage of normative values) are of concern, given that Vo_2peak values less than 84% of normal are considered pathological.[47]

For individuals with neurological disabilities, the minimum Vo_2 requirements for ADLs are actually greater than the previously mentioned levels because of the increased energy requirements resulting from gross motor inefficiencies and other related factors.[48–50] In other words, the percentage of Vo_2peak required for activity at a fixed submaximal workload (termed *fractional utilization*) is increased. When the anaerobic threshold is exceeded prematurely and lactate accumulation is accelerated, accomplishment of low-intensity ADLs is unsustainable for extended periods and achievement of mid- to upper-intensity ADLs is virtually impossible. Moreover, the combination of poor exercise capacity and elevated energy demands results in diminished reserves to support other activities. For example, in the case of people with postpoliomyelitis syndrome, the energy costs of walking are about 40% higher than for healthy peers and are highly correlated with lower-extremity muscle strength.[51] Thus in the calculation of fractional utilization for walking, the numerator (Vo_2 during walking) is increased and the denominator (Vo_2peak) is decreased, increasing fractional utilization substantially.

Of the neurological populations, people post-stroke are the largest consumer group in need of rehabilitation services. This group also has received the most attention in the literature with regard to functional capacity. Exercise capacities documented in this population are consistently low—with a reported range of 8.3 mL/kg per minute in the subacute period[52] to 22.0 mL/kg per minute in the chronic period.[53] As much as 75% to 88% of Vo_2peak (almost twice that of the healthy control subjects) is required to perform household chores,[54] and one and a half to three times the Vo_2 levels of nondisabled people are needed to walk on level ground.[48,55,56] Not surprisingly, as many as 70% of patients complain of fatigue after stroke,[57] with poor energy levels rated as the area of greatest personal concern in comparison to mobility limitations, pain, emotional reactions, sleep disturbances, and social isolation.[58]

In addition to contributing to reduced ADL performance and increased fatigability, low fitness levels are associated with higher mortality. Exercise capacity has been reported to be an independent predictor of mortality in persons with coronary artery disease (CAD), a comorbidity prevalent in some populations of people with neurological conditions.[59,60] Those with a Vo_2peak <21 mL/kg per minute are classified as the high-mortality group and with greater than 35 mL/kg per minute as the excellent-survival group.[61] Thus determining an individual's Vo_2peak is of clinical value. Individuals who are being encouraged, or are internally motivated, to perform beyond their capacity and beyond the capabilities of the interaction of multiple systems are in a high-risk category. Conversely, individuals who are undermotivated or depressed and are performing below their capacity can be trained to self-monitor, which empowers them to reach goals that are safe and have the potential to improve the quality of their lives.

Factors Affecting Fitness Levels in People With Neurological Disorders

To identify appropriate measures to improve fitness levels in people with neurological disorders, the myriad factors at play that contribute to the deconditioned state must be considered. A useful conceptual framework to discuss the interaction of these factors is the International Classification of Functioning, Disability and Health (ICF)[62] (see Chapter 1). The ICF uses a biopsychosocial approach to organize factors related to the health conditions into two components: (1) personal and environmental contextual factors and (2) functioning and disability, which further subdivided into components of body functions and structures, activity, and participation (Fig. 29.2).

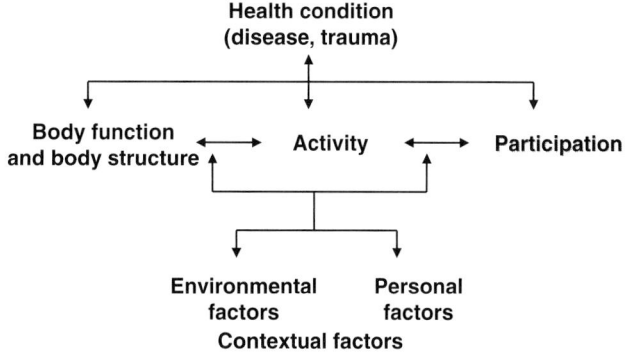

Fig. 29.2 Interaction of the Various Components of the International Classification of Functioning, Disability and Health (ICF). The ICF is a conceptual framework that uses a biopsychosocial approach to organize factors related to health condition into two components: (1) personal and environmental contextual factors and (2) functioning and disability, which are further subdivided into components of body functions and structures, activity, and participation.

Through application of the ICF framework, the complexity of interacting influences on cardiovascular and pulmonary health and fitness becomes more understandable.

Personal and Environmental Contextual Factors

For both able-bodied and disabled people, personal contextual factors contributing to individual differences in exercise capacity include age, sex, race, and lifestyle habits.

Age

A decline in Vo_2max of approximately 1% per year (0.4 to 0.5 mL/kg per minute per year) occurs from 25 to 75 years of age.[63] In accordance with the Fick equation, a reduction in Vo_2max is caused by reductions in both O_2 transporting (i.e., Qmax) and O_2 utilization capacity (i.e., a-vO_2diffmax) associated with cardiac, respiratory, and muscular changes. Decreased Qmax is the result of increasing myocardial stiffness and decreased left ventricular contractility, manifested by reductions in both ejection fraction and HRmax—hallmarks of cardiovascular aging.[64] In fact, the reduction in HRmax, which decreases 6 to 10 beats per minute (bpm) per decade, is responsible for much of the age-associated decline in Qmax.[65] Older adults also have a smaller SVmax,[65] and BP and systemic vascular resistance are higher during maximal exercise in older versus young adults.[66]

With advancing age, reduced elastic recoil of the lung and calcification and stiffening of the cartilaginous articulations of the ribs restrict compliance of the lungs, thus limiting increases in minute ventilation during exercise.[67] Age-related decline in oxidative capacity of the working muscles and hence decreased a-vO_2diff during peak exercise[68] have been attributed to alterations in mitochondrial structure and distribution, oxidative enzyme activity,[69] and skeletal muscle microcirculation, as well as sarcopenia resulting from a reduced number and size of fibers, particularly type II fibers.[70] Nevertheless, despite loss of aerobic capacity with aging, people without chronic health conditions retain adequate reserves for daily activities. However, for aging individuals with a neurological impairment, the decrease in aerobic capacity with age can further reduce their reserves and thus threaten living an independent lifestyle. In fact, age is a significant independent predictor of recurrent stroke.[71] Particularly disadvantaged are people with cerebral palsy (CP) or other developmental disabilities as a result of an incomplete development of their musculoskeletal and cardiorespiratory systems at the time of the neurological event, which accelerates the aging process.[72] In the case of people with Down syndrome, however, Baynard and colleagues[73] found that age-related changes in exercise capacity did not follow the typical pattern of decline after the age of 16 years. Older people with spinal cord injury (SCI) are at an increased risk for cardiac and respiratory complications.[74]

Sex

The absolute and relative Vo_2max of women is typically about 77% of that of men, after adjustment for body weight and activity level.[75] However, no significant gender differences have been reported in the percentage of exercise-induced improvement in Vo_2max of older adults.[76] Although older men and women generally exhibit similar responses to maximal exercise, older women tend to have lower SBP during maximal exercise.[66]

Race

Little attention has been paid to the differences in exercise capacity among racial groups; however, in one study no differences were found between 66 black and 52 white stroke survivors in the level of physical deconditioning post-stroke.[77]

Lifestyle Factors

Smoking is one factor that has been shown to impair exercise capacity in the general population.[78] Smoking causes increases in HR, myocardial contractility, and myocardial oxygen demand, which can lead to atherosclerosis and acute cardiovascular events.[79] In the stroke population, smoking doubles the risk of death (equivalent of about a 7-year reduction in life-span) compared with that of nonsmokers and ex-smokers.[80]

The relationship between cardiovascular disease and diet has attracted international attention.[81] Indeed, obesity increases the risk of cardiovascular risk factors such as impaired glucose tolerance and type 2 diabetes, hypertension, and dyslipidemia.[82] Abdominal obesity not only increases the risk of atherosclerotic disease but also the risk of primary ischemic stroke.[83,84] In addition, when compared with corresponding normal-weight populations, overweight youth with SCI and spina bifida (SB) have lower cardiovascular fitness.[85]

The lifestyle factor that has received the most attention in the literature is sedentary behavior. The evidence of the link between physical activity and cardiopulmonary health and fitness is irrefutable.[78,86–88] In fact, in the stroke population, prestroke physical activity has been found to decrease stroke severity as well as to result in better long-term rehabilitation outcomes.[89] Cardiovascular alterations resulting from physical inactivity (i.e., reduced Vo_2max and Qmax) parallel, in many ways, the changes that occur with aging; in fact, sedentary lifestyles explain a significant proportion of these age-related declines. If physical activity levels and body composition remain constant over time, the expected rate of loss in aerobic power associated with senescence is reduced by almost 50%.[70] Nonetheless, people with chronic health conditions often rate poorly in terms of daily physical activity, in part because of underlying physical impairments (e.g., paralysis, pain). For example, people with SCI have been reported to spend as little as 2% of their walking time participating in leisure physical activity,[90] making them among the most sedentary members of society.[91] Some people with multiple sclerosis (MS) avoid physical activity to prevent elevated body temperature and minimize symptoms of fatigue.[92,93] Inactivity can lead to increased cardiovascular risk factors such as hypertension and dyslipidemia, as seen in youth with chronic disabilities (including CP and SCI).[94] Bernhardt and colleagues[6] found

that after a stroke, patients spend more than 50% of their time resting in bed. Short periods of bed rest cause rapid decreases in aerobic capacity—a 15% reduction in healthy, middle-aged men after 10 days of recumbency[95] and a 28% reduction in healthy young subjects after 3 weeks.[96] Inactivity-induced reductions in Vo_2peak have been attributed to both central changes (decreased SV from impaired myocardial function and increased venous pooling) and peripheral changes characteristic of aerobically inefficient muscle fibers (decreases in oxidative enzyme concentrations, mitochondria, and capillary density).[24]

Environmental Factors

Significant associations have been found between physical activity and physical environmental factors such as accessibility, esthetic attributes, and opportunities for activity within the general public.[97] However, the influence of such factors on cardiovascular and pulmonary fitness of people with neurological disabilities has garnered little attention in the literature.[98]

Health Condition

Exercise capacity reflects both systemic capacity and the health of the component systems. Thus differences in Vo_2peak among individuals with neurological disabilities are a result of not only the contextual factors discussed previously but also pathological conditions involving the neuromuscular, cardiovascular, and pulmonary systems.

Neuromuscular System

For most individuals with neurological conditions, the existence of neuromuscular impairments confounds interpretation of Vo_2peak testing. When people with an intact nervous system are tested, normal biomechanical efficiency is assumed; an impaired nervous system increases the complexity of physiological responses. Both primary effects of upper motor neuron damage (e.g., paralysis, incoordination, spasticity, sensory-perceptual disorders, balance disturbances) and secondary "peripheral" changes in skeletal muscle (e.g., gross muscular atrophy[99] and changes in muscle fiber composition[100]) affect the response to exercise. As a result, people with neurological disabilities manifest not only metabolic but also biomechanical deficiencies, both of which contribute to reduction in functional capacity. Consequently, the decline in exercise capacity is greater than expected (e.g., in people with postpoliomyelitis syndrome, deterioration in Vo_2peak over a 3- to 5-year period was 12% greater than the predicted decline[101]).

Paresis reduces the pool of motor units available for recruitment during physical work, thereby reducing the metabolically active tissue and lowering the oxidative potential.[102] In the case of stroke, on average about 50% of the normal number of motor units are functioning,[103] and a strong relationship between muscle mass and Vo_2peak has been reported.[104] In addition, along with altered joint kinematics and decreased postural reactions,[105] children with CP exhibit high levels of co-contraction (simultaneous contraction of agonist and antagonist muscle groups), which may prematurely induce skeletal muscle fatigue, further increasing the energy expenditure of walking and decreasing Vo_2peak.[105] Thus when compared with able-bodied individuals, children with CP experience greater levels of fatigue at slower walking speeds.[105] For people with postpoliomyelitis syndrome, muscle weakness of the lower extremities is strongly associated with energy expenditure of walking.[51] In fact, when compared with healthy age- and sex-matched subjects, the energy cost of walking is found to be significantly higher (40%) for people with postpoliomyelitis syndrome.[51]

Altered fiber composition and recruitment patterns of paretic muscle may also contribute to poor fitness.[106] Skeletal muscles are composed of fibers that express different myosin heavy chain (MHC) isoforms. Slow (type I) MHC isoform fibers have higher oxidative function, are more fatigue resistant, and are more sensitive to insulin-mediated glucose uptake; fast (type II) MHC fibers are recruited for more powerful movements, are more reliant on anaerobic or glycolytic means of energy production, fatigue rapidly, and are less sensitive to the action of insulin. Although relatively equal proportions of slow and fast MHC isoforms are found in the vastus lateralis of healthy individuals,[102] elevated proportions of the fast, more fatigable fibers that are less glucose sensitive have been found in the paretic leg of people after a stroke.[107] Hence it is likely that reduced insulin sensitivity and increased use of the anaerobic processes during dynamic exercise at the level of the muscle contribute to reductions in $\dot{V}o_2$peak. Furthermore, alterations in the structure of mitochondria[102] and reduced activity of oxidative enzymes (e.g., succinate dehydrogenase)[108] may contribute to the reduced oxidative capacity of paretic muscles.

Cardiovascular System

Cardiovascular comorbidities, prevalent in populations with neurological disorders, contribute to metabolic inefficiency. In fact, cardiovascular complications are leading causes of death in persons with stroke,[109] MS,[110] and SCI.[111] As many as 75% of patients who have had a stroke are hypertensive,[112] and the same proportion of patients have underlying cardiovascular dysfunction.[113] In fact, most persons who have had a stroke have atherosclerotic lesions throughout their vascular system,[114] and a high correlation has been reported between the number and degree of stenotic lesions in the coronary and carotid arteries.[115] The high prevalence of CAD in this population should not be surprising because stroke and cardiac disease share similar predisposing factors (e.g., older age, hypertension, diabetes mellitus, cigarette smoking, sedentary lifestyle, and hyperlipidemia) and pathogenic mechanisms (e.g., atherosclerosis).[116]

Metabolic syndrome is a usual construct in identifying patients at high risk for future vascular events (e.g., a second stroke, myocardial infarction).[117] *Metabolic syndrome* refers to a constellation of markers of metabolic abnormalities (i.e., hypertension, abdominal obesity, abnormal lipid profile) that interact to accelerate the progression of atherosclerosis and increase the risk of development of cardiovascular or cerebrovascular disease.[118] The prevalence of metabolic syndrome in neurological populations is high. A retrospective study reported that about 61% of 200 patients in stroke rehabilitation met the criteria for the syndrome.[119]

Factors that elevate HR for a given $\dot{V}o_2$, such as CAD, result in attainment of a peak HR (HRpeak) at a $\dot{V}o_2$peak below that predicted for that individual. Cardiac dysfunction contributes to a lower aerobic capacity through two principal mechanisms: ischemia-induced reductions in ejection fraction and SV with exercise[120] and chronotropic incompetence—the inability to increase HR in proportion to the metabolic demands of exercise.[23] For persons who can attain HRmax within 15 bpm of the predicted maximum, limitations in exercise capacity probably do not have cardiovascular causes.

Impaired peripheral blood flow also contributes to reduced cardiovascular fitness. Inadequate blood flow to the periphery impairs O_2 transport and limits energy production in the working muscles, thereby compromising the ability to sustain physical activity. Both resting blood flow and postischemic reactive hyperemic blood flow have been found to be lower (approximately 36% less) in the paretic leg of people post-stroke.[121,122] In addition, despite near-normal (above 0.90) mean ankle brachial index values, arterial diameter has been found to be reduced post-stroke.[121] Potential mechanisms responsible for reduced blood flow on the hemiparetic side include altered autonomic function,[123] enhanced sensitivity to endogenous vasoconstrictor agents,[124] and altered histochemical and morphological features of

the vascular network itself.[125] However, the relative contribution of each of these factors is unknown. In addition, local metabolic mediators associated with changes in muscle fiber composition in the paretic limb (previously discussed) may contribute to impaired limb blood flow.[102]

Trauma to the spinal cord may disrupt the autonomic reflexes and sympathetic vasomotor outflow required for normal cardiovascular responses to exercise.[126] As a result, reduced venous return and cardiac output (referred to as *circulatory hypokinesis*) impair delivery of O_2 and nutrients to and removal of metabolites from working muscles, intensifying muscle fatigue.[127] For people with paraplegia, an exaggerated HR response may occur during exercise in order to compensate for reduced SV. However, adrenergic dysfunction associated with lesions above the T1 sympathetic outflow prevent this compensatory mechanism,[128] thereby increasing the risk of cardiovascular disease.

Pulmonary System

Typically, in able-bodied individuals, the pulmonary system does not limit cardiopulmonary fitness because the lungs of people without chronic health conditions have a large reserve.[129] Nevertheless, at maximal workloads as much as 10% of $\dot{V}o_2$max is needed to support the mechanical work of the diaphragm, accessory inspiratory muscles, and abdominal muscles.[120] In contrast, people with neurological impairments may have limited O_2 availability for exercise as a result of pathological conditions involving the pulmonary system, either as a direct complication of a neuromuscular condition (e.g., muscle weakness, impaired breathing mechanics) or as a result of cardiovascular dysfunction, comorbidities (e.g., chronic obstructive pulmonary disease), or lifestyle factors (e.g., physical inactivity, smoking habits).[130,131] These impairments can reduce the *ventilatory reserve*, defined as the difference between the maximal available ventilation and the ventilation measured at the end of exercise.[132]

As previously mentioned, minute ventilation is closely associated with $\dot{V}co_2$ during exercise. At peak exercise, a ratio of minute ventilation to $\dot{V}co_2$ above between 35[133] and 40[134] indicates an abnormal ventilatory response. Neu and colleagues[135] reported an 87% incidence of obstructive pulmonary dysfunction in patients with Parkinson disease, despite the finding that $\dot{V}o_2$peak levels in this patient group tend to be in the normal range.[136,137] For children with CP, reduced exercise capacity may be partly caused by respiratory muscle spasticity resulting in reduced breathing efficiency.[138] In the case of stroke, pulmonary function is usually affected to only a modest extent, notwithstanding acute respiratory complications (e.g., pulmonary embolism, aspiration pneumonia).[130,139] Impaired respiration may be attributed to cardiovascular dysfunction or lifestyle factors (e.g., physical inactivity, high incidence of smoking) or a direct result of the stroke, particularly brain stem stroke. The overwhelming fatigue felt by some persons after a stroke may be partly caused by respiratory insufficiency as manifested by low pulmonary diffusing capacity, decreased lung volumes, and ventilation-perfusion mismatching.[140] Impaired breathing mechanics with restricted and paradoxical chest wall excursion and depressed diaphragmatic excursion have been also reported.[130,141] Expiratory dysfunction appears to be related to the extent of motor impairment (e.g., abdominal muscle weakness), whereas inspiratory limitations appear to be related to the gradual development of rib cage contracture.[142]

To summarize, a host of interacting factors are associated with abnormally low cardiopulmonary fitness in people with neurological disorders. Neuromuscular and respiratory dysfunctions are often superimposed on an already-compromised state as a result of comorbid cardiovascular disease and premorbid health- and lifestyle-related declines. Paresis and the subsequent reduction in lean muscle mass, changes in the muscle fiber phenotype, and increased reliance on anaerobic processes for energy production result in high metabolic costs of moving paretic limbs. As a consequence, cardiac reserves available for meaningful activity-level functions are limited, which in turn has a negative impact on participation-level functions. Collectively, impairments in the neuromuscular, cardiovascular, and pulmonary systems converge to promote a sedentary lifestyle and reduced health-related quality of life, which in turn leads to further inactivity and further reductions in cardiopulmonary fitness. The contribution of skeletal system impairments to this downward spiral has received little attention. Pang and colleagues[143] studied the relationship between bone health and physical fitness in patients who had had a stroke and found a significant correlation between paretic femur bone mineral density and Vo_2max. They concluded that further study is needed to determine the clinical implications of this finding.

ADAPTIVE RESPONSES TO AEROBIC TRAINING IN POPULATIONS WITH NEUROLOGICAL DISORDERS

It is well documented that healthy young and old individuals who begin participating in regular activity, even after years of inactivity, can enjoy greater health and fitness than those who remain sedentary. Training studies involving people with neurological disability, although limited in number and sample size and, in some cases, lacking a control group, provide evidence of cardiopulmonary adaptations to physical work. For example, for adolescents with chronic disabilities (including CP, SB, and SCI)[94] and younger children with CP,[144-146] cardiovascular fitness training is found to produce positive results on aerobic capacity and fitness. There is also strong evidence supporting the benefits of aerobic training in people with stroke of mild to moderate severity.[147] Exercise training has been found to improve the physical capacity of people with SCI.[148,149] In the case of people with traumatic brain injury, evidence regarding the effects of exercise training has been inconclusive.[150] Unlike nondisabled populations, in neurological populations, cardiovascular adaptations in response to aerobic training enhance metabolic efficiency, and neuromuscular adaptations in response to strength and gait training improve mechanical efficiency. The result is improved functional capacity with lowered energy costs of ADLs, enhanced fatigue resistance, and increased exercise tolerance (Fig. 29.3).

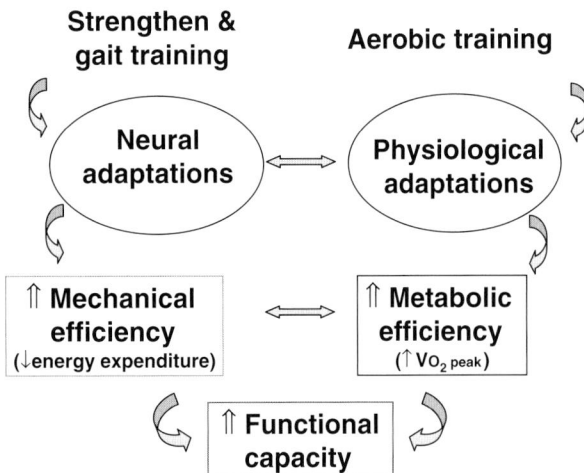

Fig. 29.3 Interaction of Influences That Enhance Functional Capacity. Neurorehabilitation interventions result in neural and physiological adaptations that in turn increase mechanical and metabolic efficiencies and ultimately improve functional capacity.

The magnitude of change in Vo_2peak in training studies involving neurological populations (mean gain of approximately 20%) is comparable to the improvements[151,152] reported for healthy, sedentary adults and participants in cardiac rehabilitation.[153,154] Substantial intersubject variability in results is attributable to many factors, including differences in neurological condition, severity, and time after insult, as well as variations in intensity of training, mode of exercise, and level of compliance with the exercise regimen. Within studies, considerable individual differences have been noted, of which only a small portion have been attributed to recognized covariates such as initial fitness status and measurement error. The most rapid improvements in exercise capacity are seen in previously sedentary people,[155] and similarly, the highest overall gains occur in individuals with the lowest initial values of Vo_2peak.[156] Age and sex have not been shown to have a substantial effect on exercise trainability.[157]

The dramatic increases in exercise capacity reported in some of the studies (e.g., improvements of 30%[158] to 94%[52]) may not be possible for most people with neurological disabilities. Yet the subtle gains realized in other studies (e.g., 8%,[159] 11%,[160] 15%[161]) may yield meaningful dividends by extending the time in which muscle contraction can be sustained through oxidative processes, thus elevating the lactate threshold. Enhanced functional capacity could spell the difference between being dependent and independent. In other words, interventions that result in even small changes in aerobic capacity may be of practical significance for people with neurological disorders.

Mechanism of Improved Exercise Capacity in Neurological Disorders

It remains unclear whether training-induced increases in Vo_2peak in people with neurological disorders result from central mechanisms or peripheral mechanisms. In nondisabled individuals both peripheral and central adaptations occur; and in those with CAD and an intact nervous system, central[162,163] and peripheral[163,164] adaptations have been variably reported. In accordance with the Fick equation, central adaptations rely on improved SV because HRmax remains unchanged with training. Enhanced myocardial contractility, together with decreased vasoconstriction in the nonworking muscles and improved venous return, account for the higher Qmax without a concomitant increase in mean arterial pressure.[165,166] There is preliminary evidence that exercise training can improve ejection fraction,[167] coronary blood flow,[168,169] and possibly blood hemoglobin content.[170]

Peripheral adaptations in the exercising muscle tissue include increases in capillary density,[171,172] size and number of mitochondria,[173] myoglobin levels, Krebs cycle enzymes (e.g., succinate dehydrogenase), and respiratory chain enzymes (e.g., cytochrome oxidase).[24] As a consequence of these skeletal muscle adaptations, a-vO_2diff, and hence Vo_2peak, increase.[63]

The possibility of "spontaneous" increases in exercise capacity during neurological recovery should not be overlooked. There have been early reports of non–exercise-induced positive adaptations after myocardial infarction.[174,175] In our lab we documented a significant increase (13%) in Vo_2peak over the course of a stroke rehabilitation program that lacked an aerobic training component.[176] Haisma and colleagues[177] reported that patients with tetraplegia and paraplegia demonstrated improvements in Vo_2peak of 17% and 23%, respectively, over the course of inpatient SCI rehabilitation; however, the extent and mode of aerobic training were not indicated. The authors speculated that the improved capacity could be, in part, a result of natural recovery and recuperation from trauma and complications.[177] Dressendorfer and colleagues[178] hypothesized that the metabolic demands of unregulated daily activities after myocardial infarction may have an insidious training effect. In support of this notion, a review of the threshold exercise intensity to improve cardiorespiratory fitness indicated that for deconditioned participants an effective training intensity is lower than previously reported.[179]

Additional Benefits of Aerobic Training

In addition to increased exercise capacity, other benefits of endurance training realized by healthy people appear to be attainable for individuals with neuromuscular disabilities. However, direct evidence of the impact on ICF-related domains remains limited, discussed as follows.

Cardiopulmonary Function

Decreases in HR at a fixed submaximal workload after training have been attributed to increases in total blood volume[180] and vagal activity and to concomitant reductions in sympathetic-adrenergic drive and resting HR (HRrest).[181,182] However, according to Wilmore and colleagues,[180] the decrease in HRrest is of minimal physiological significance. Reductions in SBP at fixed submaximal workloads,[183] resting SBP,[184] and resting DBP[28,185] have been demonstrated in individuals after stroke. Related to this finding, training can also reduce the rate-pressure product (product of HR and SBP) at submaximal loads,[65] which reflects improvement in cardiac efficiency.[186] After a 4-week single-limb exercise training program with the hemiparetic limb, Billinger and colleagues[121] reported significant improvements in femoral artery blood flow and diameter compared with the non-hemiparetic limb post-stroke. The authors reasoned that in order to maintain homeostasis, the diameter increased to adjust for the coupling of increases in metabolic demand and improved blood flow.[121]

In patients with CAD, training has resulted in decreased ST segment depression (a marker of myocardial ischemia) during submaximal exercise performed at the same baseline rate pressure product,[162] thus raising the anginal threshold and extending the time that submaximal tasks can be performed without triggering myocardial ischemia. Cardiovascular and muscle adaptations also lower minute ventilation at a given submaximal workload, intimating improved ventilatory efficiency.[187] After training, Vo_2 at a given submaximal workload is usually modestly reduced[188] because the increased a-vO_2diff in trained muscles is offset by reduced blood flow to the working muscles and a less pronounced decrease in blood flow to the nonexercising muscles resulting from depressed sympathetic reflex activity.[165] As a result of improved pulmonary function resulting from targeted expiratory[189] and inspiratory[190] muscle training in people with MS, it may be possible for members of this population to increase exercise tolerance. In fact, cardiorespiratory training improves respiratory function, Vo_2peak, and working capacity and reduces fatigue in people with MS.[191] Similarly, there is strong evidence that within stroke populations exercise training increases Vo_2peak[159,183,192–196] and reduces fatigue.[197,198]

Cardiovascular Risk Factor Reduction

Although limited physical activity is an independent predictor of risk of stroke,[199,200] the capacity of exercise to confer the same protective benefits against stroke recurrence is unknown. It is clear that endurance exercise training lowers resting BP in both young and older hypertensive adults.[201] Training is also associated with lower fasting and glucose stimulated plasma insulin levels and with improved glucose tolerance (if initially impaired), insulin sensitivity,[202] and glycemic control in patients with type 2 diabetes.[203] Aerobic training in individuals post-stroke has been demonstrated to reduce insulin resistance[203a] and increase glucose tolerance.[204] Evidence also suggests that stroke populations achieve similar training-induced improvements in lipid profile,[205–207] as previously documented for participants in cardiac

rehabilitation.[208] Patients with MS showed reductions in triglyceride and very-low-density lipoprotein levels after a 15-week training program.[209] Similarly, an 8-week training program for individuals early after SCI led to improved lipid profiles, with more pronounced changes in response to high-intensity training.[210] However, the previously mentioned improvements in vascular risk factors may be a result of training-induced reductions in body fat stores.[211] The potential for training to reduce intraabdominal fat is particularly significant because it is the body fat depot that is associated with aging and is most closely associated with other cardiovascular disease risk factors.[212] Because of the positive effects on glucose homeostasis, lipid lipoprotein profiles, and cardiovascular fitness, exercise training has been found to be effective in reducing the risk of cardiovascular disease and comorbidities (e.g., type 2 diabetes, hypertension, obesity) in people with SCI.[149] Stroke survivors participating in a 10-week cardiac rehabilitation program obtained greater improvements in cardiac risk score compared to those in usual care,[213] due, in part, to changes in systemic and cerebrovascular hemodynamics,[121] including improves endogenous fibrinolysis profiles[214] and decreased arterial stiffness.[215,216]

Impairments in Body Structure and Function

Benefits of training to impairments in body structure and function of people with neurological disabilities, other than improved endurance and exercise tolerance, are gradually being documented. In patients who have had a stroke, training studies have noted increases in balance,[193,217] walking speed,[218,219] and paretic lower-extremity muscle strength.[220,221] A 15-week aerobic training program for patients with MS resulted not only in improvement in exercise capacity but also in upper- and lower-extremity strength.[209] In people with Parkinson disease, aerobic exercise has immediate beneficial effects in improving motor action, balance, and gait.[222,223] Children with CP have shown improved gross motor function after participating in an 8-month circuit-training program.[224]

An exercise training program designed to improve ambulatory efficiency of patients with traumatic brain injury failed to reduce energy costs of walking despite a 15% improvement in Vo_2peak.[225] In contrast, two studies reported mean reductions in energy costs of walking of 30%[54] and 23% after stroke rehabilitation (although not specifically aerobic exercise),[56] and a pilot study reported a 32% reduction in the energy cost of walking in individuals with incomplete SCI after a 12-week program of body weight supported treadmill training (BWSTT).[226] The task specific nature of BWSTT is also had beneficial outcomes for individuals with improved disability scores and muscular strength and decreased fatigability.[227] Macko and colleagues[42] interpreted gains observed in ambulatory workload capacity as a reflection of both improved exercise capacity and greater gross motor efficiency. The investigative team postulated that the repetitive, stereotypic training may induce these adaptations by stimulating central neuromotor plasticity involving cerebellum-midbrain circuits.[228]

In the past 2 decades the possible role that dynamic exercise may play in enhancing cognitive function has become a focus of research. In fact, in older adult populations without known cognitive impairment and in cardiac populations, there is evidence supporting the benefit of exercise training on improving cognition.[229–231] In stroke populations aerobic training has been shown to improve global cognitive ability,[219] attention and visual spatial ability,[232] and implicit memory and information processing speed.[233,234] Similar effects on cognition have been demonstrated in populations with Parkinson disease.[235,236]

Neeper and colleagues[237] observed upregulation of brain-derived neurotrophic factor (BDNF) in the cerebral cortex of rats housed in an environment with free access to a running wheel. Since then, other researchers have demonstrated increased BDNF production and synaptic plasticity in rodent models engaged in voluntary running.[238-240] Gordon and co-workers[241] drew on the findings from these animal studies to postulate that the improved cognitive function of individuals with traumatic brain injury who exercised regularly may be attributable to exercise-induced increases in BDNF or other growth factors. A 2017 systematic review and meta-analysis concluded that aerobic training can increase levels of BDNF in people with a neurological disorder when compared to usual care or no therapy.[242]

Emotional Well-Being

Increased exercise capacity has been shown to improve mental well-being (reductions in anxiety and depression) in cardiac patients.[243,244] There is moderate evidence regarding the effect of exercise training on improving mood in patients with MS.[245,246] Limited evidence exists to support the relationship between aerobic exercise and emotional well-being post-stroke—a population with an increased risk for depression.[247] High levels of physical disability, cognitive impairment, and severity of stroke have been found to be predictors of post-stroke depression.[247] Nevertheless, a several aerobic training studies have reported outcomes of reduced depressive symptoms,[213,248-251] improved psychosocial health, perceived health and well-being,[182] and reduced mental health distress[197,251,252] in patients post-stroke. In the Parkinson population, demonstrated benefits of aerobic training include improved mood and sleep.[235,236] Preliminary evidence of exercise-induced reductions in general fatigue (which is associated with emotional well-being) have been reported in people postpoliomyelitis,[252] post-stroke,[253] MS,[227,245,254,255] and Guillain-Barré syndrome.[256]

Activity, Participation, and Quality of Life

Exercise-induced changes in activity, participation, and quality of life for people with neurological disabilities have been reported in the literature. However, whereas small improvements in Vo$_2$peak can have a substantial impact on the ability to perform daily activities, particularly in individuals with limited cardiac or ventilatory reserves, there is less documentation of these benefits in people with neurological disorders. Turner and colleagues[257] reported better physical and mental health, as well as social functioning, in veterans with MS who exercised (only 26% of the 2996 veterans engaged in physical activity). In patients with SCI, exercise and gait training were shown to have a positive impact on work, social life, family, and leisure participation.[258] In stroke survivors, exercise-elicited gains have been observed in balance, gait speed,[193,220] walking tolerance,[193,194] and enhanced performance satisfaction regarding ADLs.[259]

The positive impact of exercise training on quality of life has been demonstrated in people with MS,[209,227,244,257,260,261] CP,[224,262] stroke, Parkinson disease,[263] and postpoliomyelitis.[252] However, evidence on the effects of cardiovascular exercise on quality of life after stroke remains inconclusive.[147,218,259,264,265]

Aerobic Exercise Prescription to Optimize Fitness of People With Neurological Disabilities
Safety and Screening

In general terms, the risks imposed by lack of exercise are far greater than those imposed by exercise. Nevertheless, it is of paramount importance to recognize that symptomatic and asymptomatic cardiovascular disease, and related comorbidities such as diabetes, are much more prevalent in patients with many neurological conditions than in the general population. Because there is limited evidence regarding safety of aerobic exercise for people with neurological disorders, best clinical judgment should be used in aerobic exercise prescription. Thorough

review of the health records of potential participants is critical to identify problems that may preclude safe participation in aerobic training programs. Cardiac screening is recommended, with an exercise stress test for people with a known cardiovascular condition that may be provoked by exercise at the intended training intensity. Table 29.1 provides a compilation of contraindications to testing and training.[28,266] Before implementing an exercise program without preliminary exercise testing, the following should be considered: (1) Careful screening for possible contraindications must be conducted. (2) Motor function, mobility, balance, swallowing, and communication (ability to follow instructions and ability to express pain or distress) should be evaluated. (3) Training must be done under the close surveillance of trained personnel. (4) A period of continuous electrocardiography and telemetry at the initiation of training is recommended. (5) Monitoring of BP, HR,

TABLE 29.1 Contraindications to Exercise Testing and Aerobic Training

Signs and Symptoms	Contraindications
Myocardial infarction	Acute myocardial infarction
Angina	Unstable angina (not controlled with medication/intervention)
Cardiac arrhythmias	Uncontrolled cardiac arrhythmias causing symptoms or hemodynamic compromise
Resting ST segment displacement	>1 mm displacement in more than one lead
Heart failure	Uncontrolled symptomatic heart failure
Aortic stenosis	Symptomatic severe aortic stenosis
Large vessel intracranial stenosis	Severe stenosis
Aortic dissection	Acute aortic dissection
Endocarditis	Active endocarditis
Myocarditis/pericarditis	Suspected or known acute myocarditis or pericarditis
Hypertension	Resting SBP >200 mm Hg or resting DBP >110 mm Hg
Pulmonary embolus or infarction	Acute pulmonary embolus or pulmonary infarction
Metabolic diseases	Uncontrolled diabetes, thyrotoxicosis, or myxedema
Acute systemic infection	Accompanied by fever, body aches, or swollen lymph glands
Impaired cognitive function	Only if unable to understand risks associated with exercise and/or express pain or distress presenting a safety concern
Dysphasia	Inability to understand risks associated with exercise and/or to express pain or distress
Emotional distress/psychosis	Significant emotional distress
Dizziness	Severe motion-induced dizziness/vertigo
Arthritis	Severe pain on weight bearing or exercise
Seizures	Uncontrolled seizure disorder

and signs of exercise intolerance is essential. For subjects with pulmonary comorbidities such as chronic obstructive pulmonary disease, O_2 saturation levels should be monitored, with saturation levels less than 85% as the criterion to terminate exercise.[267]

In the past, clinicians were apprehensive about the possibility that the overload necessary to achieve an aerobic training effect could aggravate spasticity in patients with neurological disorders; however, such concerns have not been substantiated.[147,268,269] In fact, there is evidence from studies of cats[270] and humans with SCI[271] that treadmill training may, in fact, reduce spasticity by improving stretch reflex modulation.

Another concern raised regarding the implementation of aerobic training in neurological disorders is the potential for eliciting excessive fatigue. For people with MS, increased fatigue levels have been reported after high-intensity exercise[271]; however, exercising at an appropriate intensity actually yields benefits without aggravating fatigue.[246,272,273] Dawes and colleagues[274] found that early after traumatic brain injury, increasing the workload during cycling exercises did not elicit a disproportionate increase in energy cost in most of the patients with spasticity.

The issue of when it is safe to initiate exercise training with neurological populations is of ongoing interest. Most training studies on such populations have involved patients with chronic neurological impairments; however, the optimal time to introduce training is unknown. Macko and colleagues[275] expressed caution about training in the acute post-stroke period, speculating that abnormal cardiovascular responses to exercise (e.g., hypotension, arrhythmia) may impede perfusion of ischemic brain tissue during the period when cerebral autoregulation is most often impaired. Nevertheless, no adverse events have been reported in exercise training studies of people either early post-stroke[52,276,277] or in subacute stages post-stroke.[278,279]

Training Environment

High-risk individuals, such as patients in the early stages of neurological recovery or with cardiac comorbidities, should be trained in a setting with quick access to emergency medical equipment and trained personnel. An adverse event protocol should be posted and rehearsed. Lower-risk individuals, after appropriate screening to ensure an appropriate response to exercise, can be trained in supervised community[280] or home-based[193] aerobic exercise programs. A study of people with postpoliomyelitis reported reductions in fatigue and improvements in quality of life when patients were trained in either a hospital or home setting.[252] Similar gains in outcomes were achieved for people post-traumatic brain injury trained in an unsupervised home-based program versus a supervised facility-based exercise program.[281] Telehealth is being explored as a strategy to help deliver aerobic training remotely, particularly in rural areas.[282,283]

Regardless of the setting, certain safeguards are required. Because thermal dysregulation is common in patients with neurological disability, particularly MS[284] and SCI,[285] the ambient temperature should be carefully controlled and fans, spray bottles, towels, and a water cooler are recommended. Hydration before and during exercise and rehydration after exercise should be monitored by use of a water bottle with volumetric indicators. The exercise area should be wheelchair accessible, free of obstacles and blunt objects, and sufficiently large to permit safe transfer to and from exercise equipment.

Preparation of Participants

Participants should be advised to avoid eating 2 hours before training and to empty bowel and bladder before training, when possible, especially for patients with SCI above T6 who are at risk of autonomic dysreflexia. Comfortable clothing and supportive footwear, appropriate

for dynamic exercise, prepare the participant both physically and psychologically for training.

Scheduling of Sessions

Many patients with neurological involvement report a decline in energy levels in the afternoon. If fatigability is a concern, training should be scheduled for morning hours, when circadian body temperature is at its lowest. For certain patient groups, including people with Parkinson disease, training should be coordinated with the timing of medication to optimize performance.

Duration of Program

A meaningful increase in aerobic capacity (i.e., >10% improvement) of individuals without neurological impairment is unlikely to occur in less than 4 weeks.[286] The minimal exposure required for people with neurological disabilities has not been fully investigated. The available literature suggests a minimum of 8 weeks of aerobic training is required in patients post-stroke. In an overview of exercise studies, Ivey and colleagues[287] noted that program durations ranging from 8 weeks to 6 months elicited improved cardiorespiratory fitness and function in stroke survivors; however, because a plateau in Vo_2peak gains was not achieved at 6 months, program durations longer than 6 months may produce even more benefits. Nonetheless, da Cunha and colleagues[52] reported a mean improvement of 35% in Vo_2peak after 2 to 3 weeks of treadmill ergometry in people early post-stroke. Regardless of the minimum, participation in training must be sustained indefinitely to prevent return to the deconditioned state measured at the beginning of the program. Therefore a maintenance program should be followed after termination of formal training sessions.

Frequency and Duration of Sessions

To elicit a training effect, three to five sessions of aerobic exercise per week for a minimum of 20 minutes per session are required, although fitness can improve with twice-weekly sessions.[28] For those with low fitness levels or who are very deconditioned (which would include the majority of patients with neurological involvement) training may be initiated with 5-minute exercise "bouts" with rest periods between bouts. Two additional 5-minute periods are required for warm-up and cool-down; hence the minimal time required to complete a training session is 30 minutes. Incrementally increasing the duration to a target of 40 to 60 minutes of aerobic training is recommended. However, the greater the intensity of exercise, the shorter the duration needed to achieve improvement in cardiopulmonary fitness; conversely, low-intensity exercise can be compensated for by longer duration.[288] In addition, the accumulation of 10- to 15-minute periods of activity throughout the day can yield similar physiological improvements, provided that the total volume of training is comparable.[289]

Mode of Training

To induce central adaptations, training must incorporate large muscle mass activities that require elevated levels of Vo_2. Treadmill or overground walking is a preferred mode because of its task-specific, functional relevance; however, extensive motor disability may preclude this approach. Suitable alternatives include the cycle ergometer with toe clips and heel straps, recumbent ergometer, arm-leg ergometer, wheelchair ergometer, and stepping machine and swimming. Indeed, water-based exercise post-stroke has shown positive effects on cardiovascular fitness and coping with life after stroke.[195,290,291] Although arm ergometry activates a smaller portion of total muscle mass, its effectiveness in the aerobic training of patients with quadriplegia has been demonstrated.[160,292]

Innovative approaches have been introduced to overcome limitations to exercise training imposed by upper motor neuron damage. For example, body-weight–supported treadmill training provides external support while walking to facilitate lower limb advancement while reducing the risk of falls.[293] Robotic-assisted gait training has been shown to improve Vo_2peak[294,295] and walking capacity,[296,297] as well as reduce energy costs of walking.[298] A combination of electric stimulation of lower-extremity muscles and voluntary upper-extremity rowing has been applied to augment the muscle activation of patients after SCI.[160,292,299] Immersive virtual reality has been used to engage people after traumatic brain injury,[300–302] with Grealy and colleagues[298] postulating that interaction between the training apparatus and participant might enhance attention to the task of exercising and increase the potential of structural changes in the brain.

A continuous, interval, or circuit training regimen may be used. Typically, training studies involving patients with neurological disabilities have used short bouts of exercise with a gradual transition to continuous training. However, it has been recommended that if continuous training results in either a lack of improvement or a plateau in response, interval training should be instituted.[151]

Music, if properly selected, can be helpful in pacing the repetitive, alternating movements characteristic of aerobic exercise such as walking or cycling. With close matching of the cadence of music and alternating movements, music can potentiate muscle activation.[303] For example, McIntosh and colleagues[304] reported that music facilitated the gait pattern of people with Parkinson disease.

Muscle Strengthening

Traditionally, aerobic training programs emphasized dynamic exercise. However, the addition of resistance training improves outcome,[151] including greater improvements in Vo_2peak, walking endurance, and lipid profile in people with type 2 diabetes.[305] Improved fitness outcomes have also been reported in people post-stroke,[269] despite controversy about the benefits versus risk of resistance training of the paretic upper limb, particularly in the shoulder region. To offset this concern, a meta-analysis by Harris and Eng[306] found no reported adverse affects after upper-limb strength training post-stroke. In addition, in the SCI population, increases not only in fitness level but also decreases in shoulder pain were observed after circuit training involving resistance exercises and arm cranking.[307]

The order of performing aerobic versus resistance exercise does not appear to affect the extent of gain in exercise capacity.[308] Strength training decreases the cardiac demands of daily tasks while simultaneously increasing the endurance capacity to sustain these submaximal activities.[309] Muscle strengthening of key muscle groups (e.g., triceps, biceps, abdominals, hip and knee flexors and extensors, hip abductors, ankle dorsiflexors, and plantar flexors) is recommended 2 to 3 days per week, beginning with one set of 8 to 12 repetitions.[151]

Intensity of Training

Determining an appropriate intensity is the most challenging aspect of exercise prescription. The cardiovascular system responds to overload; hence, the metabolic load must be sufficient to provoke central and peripheral adaptations. However, excessive stress imposed on the heart and contracting skeletal muscles can evoke abnormal clinical signs or symptoms. The initial exercise intensity and progression must be individualized using the participant's HR or Vo_2peak data (Table 29.2). The RPE can serve as a valid proxy to more physiological measures[31]; to initiate training, ratings of 11 ("fairly light") to 13 ("somewhat hard") on the RPE scale of 6 to 20 are often recommended with progression to 12-16 on the Borg (6 to 20) category scale or 4-6 on the Borg (0 to 10) scale.[28] Despite considerable inter-individual variation in RPE, the ratings have been shown to correlate well with exercise intensity,[310] even in patients taking β-blockers.[311] When exercise intensity is being

TABLE 29.2 Formulae Used to Determine Threshold Intensity for Exercise Training

Formula	Comments
Karvonen method: HRrest + x% of heart rate reserve unfit (HRR), where HHR = predicted HRmax[a] − HRrest	Training intensities of 40%–85% HHR are recommended,[28] but for patients intensities of 30% HHR can be effective.[361]
x% of predicted HRmax = 220 − Age, where predicted	Deconditioned individuals can benefit from intensities as low as 55%–64% of predicted HRmax.[28]
HRmax = 220 − Age OR = 206.9 − (0.67 × age)[362]; if on β-blockers, predicted HRmax = 164 − 0.7 × Age[319]	
HRrest + x beats	The recommended intensity after myocardial infarction is HRrest + 20 beats and after cardiac surgery is HRrest + 30 beats.[28]
x% of Vo_2peak	Deconditioned individuals can benefit from intensities as low as 40%–50% of Vo_2peak.[28]

[a]*HRmax*, Maximal heart rate.

established, other variables (e.g., anginal symptoms, arrhythmias) should also be considered. Continuous monitoring of HR and periodic monitoring of BP and RPE will ensure that an appropriate intensity is sustained during training.

In addition to the RPE, another proxy measure of intensity is the talk test, in which the participant's intensity is regulated by whether he or she can sing (in which case intensity should be increased) or whether he or she is unable to talk (in which case intensity should be decreased). In general, the appropriate training intensity is at or near the ventilatory threshold, which is the point at which a participant can speak comfortably[312] or hear his or her breath.[313] The counting talk test (CTT) was introduced as another proxy measure; it measures how high the participant can count aloud without taking a second breath (e.g., "one, one thousand; two, one thousand…").[314] The percentage of resting CTT has been reported to be strongly correlated with the percentage of HR reserve, Vo_2 reserve, and RPE, with moderate intensity coinciding with 50% of CTT.[267] Validity of RPE has established in studies of people with MS,[315] SCI population,[316] and subacute stroke (at moderate but not high intensities).[317] However, Bae and colleagues[318] found that, for people in the chronic poststage period, HR reserve was a better guide of exercise guide than RPE (6 to 20 scale).

The American College of Sports Medicine guidelines recommend light to moderate-intensity physical activities to optimize *cardiopulmonary health*.[289] In fact, a meta-analysis revealed that for very unfit patients (which would include many people with chronic neurological conditions), the initial intensity can be much lower than previously recommended.[179] However, the only consistent beneficial cardiovascular response to low levels of training is reduction in BP in older hypertensive adults. To reduce cardiovascular risk factors and increase *cardiopulmonary fitness*, moderate- or high-intensity exercise appears to be necessary.[212] For people post-stroke, Billinger v[199] recommended intensities of 40% to 70% of Vo_2peak or heart rate reserve (HRR), 50% to 80% of maximal HR, or an RPE (6 to 20 scale) of 11 to 14. The exercise intensity recommendations for people with MS are similar: 40% to 70% of Vo_2peak or HRR, 40% to 60% of HRR, 60% to 80% of maximal

TABLE 29.3	Guidelines for Determining the Initial Intensity of Training of People Post-Stroke		
	Low Intensity	**Moderate Intensity**	**High Intensity**
Intensity %HRR	Minimum target HR = HRrest + <40% HRR	Minimum target HR = HRrest + 40%–60% HRR	Minimum target HR = HRrest + >60% HRR
Intensity RPE	RPE_{0-10} <4 or RPE_{6-20} <10	E_{0-10} of 4–5 or RPE_{6-20} 11–13	RPE_{0-10} ≥6 or RPE_{6-20} ≥14
Cardiac signs	Mild-moderate abnormalities on ECG ± BP ± HR responses	Borderline abnormalities on ECG ± BP ± HR responses	Normal ECG ± BP ± HR responses
Fitness level	Vo_2peak <40% predicted	Vo_2peak 40%–60% predicted	Vo_2peak >60% predicted
Motor control	Chedoke-McMaster stage of leg: 1 or 2	Chedoke-McMaster stage of leg: 3 or 4	Chedoke-McMaster stage of leg: >4

BP, Blood pressure; *ECG*, electrocardiogram; *HR*, heart rate; *HRR*, heart rate reserve; *RPE*, rating of perceived exertion.

HR, or an RPE (6 to 20 scale) of 11 to 13.[246] For people with CP, Verschuren and colleagues[144] recommended intensities of 50% to 65% of Vo_2peak, 40% to 80% of HRR, or 60% to 95% of maximal HR. Nevertheless, light to moderate-intensity physical activity programs may prove adequate to reduce the rate of age-associated deterioration in a variety of physiological functions, and in the long run may improve both quantity and quality of life.[212,235,263]

For many people with neurological involvement, determination of an appropriate intensity of exercise for the individual person is confounded not only by cardiac status but also by the extent of neurological impairment. We have derived guidelines for determining the initial intensity of treadmill training for people after stroke, based on baseline cardiac signs, prescription of β-adrenergic blockade therapy,[319] fitness level, and motor control of the involved lower extremity (i.e., Chedoke-McMaster stage of recovery of the leg)[320] (Table 29.3).

There is growing evidence to suggest that high-intensity training may be more effective than moderate or low intensities in increasing aerobic capacity, walking speed, and endurance in individuals post-stroke.[279,321–326] High-intensity interval training (HIIT, >80% to 85% HRR) has been shown to induce neuroplastic, cardiovascular, and functional improvements in people who are in subacute or chronic stages of stroke.[322,327] HIIT has the advantage of reducing overall training time, but requires careful screening for orthopedic and cardiovascular conditions, including exercise stress testing.[322,328] While the optimal parameters of HIIT remain unknown, Boyne and colleagues[317] outlined three types of HIIT protocols: (1) short-interval, with short high-intensity bursts (15 to 30 seconds at 100% to 120% Vo_2peak) and a 1:1 recovery time; (2) low-volume, with small bursts of the highest neuromuscular intensity possible (10 to 30 seconds, up to 60 seconds) followed by a small burst of active recovery (1:4 or 1:12); and (3) long-interval, with high-intensity bursts (3 to 4 minutes at submaximal workload of 80% to 90% Vo_2peak) at 1:1 or 4:3 of active recovery.

Progression of Training Program

Exercise progression must be individualized because people with neurological disabilities have a wide range of functional capacities. Progression usually occurs over a 3- to 6-month period from an initial conditioning phase to a training phase and then to a maintenance phase. In general, the first goal of training is to reach a target frequency (i.e., a minimum of 3 days/week), then duration (minimum of 20 minutes), and finally an appropriate intensity (40% to 60% of HR reserve, or 11 to 13 on the Borg scale). Gradual progression of frequency, duration, and intensity is needed in order to minimize muscle soreness, fatigue, and injury. Careful monitoring of BP, HR, and rating of perceived exertion is necessary to assess the participant's response to

increased exercise demands. Subsequently, exercise duration should be increased at tolerated, often in increments of 5 to 10 minutes every 1 to 2 weeks for the first 4 to 6 weeks, with a goal of achieving 20 to 30 minutes of continuous exercise before increasing the intensity.[28] Training intensity should be increased by 5% to 10% HRR every 1 to 4 weeks, depending on individual health status, fitness, training responses, and exercise goals. Gradual increases in the percentage of HRR can be achieved by systematically manipulating training parameters such as speed, revolutions per minute, incline, and extent of balance support. Patients with higher baseline fitness levels can be progressed more rapidly than those with lower initial capacities.

Laboratory Outcome Measures

Laboratory tests are useful not only to identify limitations in exercise capacity and establish exercise training protocols but also to evaluate the effectiveness of a training program. The principal indicator of a training effect is attainment of a higher Vo_2peak than was achieved in the pretrained state. The greatest increments tend to occur in individuals with the lowest initial Vo_2peak.[156] Ideally, Vo_2peak should be measured directly because indirect methods of predicting exercise capacity are more variable and prone to error. However, because Vo_2peak testing requires special equipment and trained personnel, clinicians often resort to clinical measures of functional capacity.

Clinical Outcome Measures

Six-minute walk test. The distance walked in 6 minutes is sometimes used as a clinical surrogate for Vo_2peak testing. However, the systemic response to the 6-Minute Walk Test (6MWT) is less than that of an incremental test using a treadmill cycle[329] or cycle ergometer.[330,331] Subjects tend to walk at a constant speed, achieve a Vo_2 steady-state condition after the first few minutes of exercise, and, with practice, walk at a pace approaching critical power.[328,332] Pang and colleagues[333] found a low correlation ($r = 0.40$) between 6MWT distance and Vo_2 in patients after stroke, concluding that the 6MWT alone should not be used as an indication of cardiopulmonary fitness after stroke. The same laboratory recommended that, to enhance the usefulness of the 6MWT, BP and HR should be recorded at initiation and termination of the test.[334] Various reference equations are available to compute the percent of predicted total distance walked in the 6MWT. For example, for men, Distance (m) = (7.57 × Height [cm]) – (5.02 × Age [years]) – (1.76 × Weight [kg]) – 309; for women, Distance (m) = (2.11 × Height [cm]) – (5.78 × Age [years]) – (2.29 × Weight [kg]) + 667.[335]

Shuttle walk test. The shuttle walk test is a standardized incremental test during which walking is initiated at an audio-guided set pace for a prescribed length of time.[336] Walking speed is increased at each stage until the subject can no longer maintain the required pace. Peak systemic responses have been reported to be consistent with those achieved during a progressive cycle test.[331] A variation of this test, the endurance shuttle walk test, involves walking as far as possible at a constant speed determined in a previously performed progressive walk test.[337]

Adherence to Program

The benefits of training are lost unless exposure to some form of training stimulus is maintained; therefore sustained behavioral change must be an important goal in any exercise program. A decrease in mobility or inactivity can lead to rapid loss of cardiovascular and pulmonary fitness. For example, a 25% reduction in maximum oxygen uptake has been observed in nondisabled young adults after 3 weeks of bed rest.[96] In secondary prevention of stroke, behavioral modifications may be as beneficial as antihypertensive and cholesterol-lowering agents.[80] Yet establishing and maintaining a regular fitness regimen in patients with neurological impairments pose challenges. In one study, 39% of 691 patients did not engage in the exercise program created by their physical therapist.[338] In addition, a majority of people post-stroke surveyed reported that they were not ready to incorporate exercise into their lifestyle.[213,339]

Some individuals are reluctant to engage in exercise owing to the fear of increasing their symptoms. Indeed, people with Parkinson disease avoid exercise out of fear they will increase their already high levels of fatigue.[340] Similarly, people with MS avoid exercising to avert increases in their level of fatigue and body temperature.[92] Furthermore, the frequency of MS-related symptoms has been found to be significantly and inversely related to physical activity.[341] It has been shown that less than 30% of 2995 people with MS reported engaging in any form of exercise,[257] with one study revealing an overall adherence rate of 65%.[342] Morris and Williams[343] reported that many individual factors (e.g., sex, level of disability), social factors, and environmental factors (e.g., access to facilities, travel) influence the level of engagement in exercise and physical activity in people with mixed disabilities. In addition, numerous psychological, cognitive, and emotional factors have been identified as potential mediators of engagement in physical activity (e.g., self-efficacy, attitude, competence, intention, knowledge of health and exercise benefits, motivation, readiness to change, and the value of exercise benefits).[344]

The role that self-efficacy (i.e., confidence in ability to execute a task) plays as a psychological predictor of level of engagement in physical activity and exercise has become a topic of growing interest, particularly in the stroke literature.[345–347] French and colleagues[348] demonstrated that self-efficacy after stroke mediates the relationships between performance-based measures of walking and real-world walking and participation. Interventions to enhance self-efficacy and participation include counseling and information,[349–351] behavioral change techniques (e.g., goal setting, barrier identification, self-monitoring),[347] self-management programs,[352,353] social support and education,[354] and motivational counseling through videotapes.[355] Snook and colleagues[341] reported that self-efficacy was significantly and moderately correlated with physical activity in people with MS.

A better understanding of theoretical frameworks of behavior change (see overviews[28,356]) would be helpful for neurorehabilitation clinicians to increase participant engagement. Garner and Page[339] exposed community-based, chronic stroke survivors to a theoretically based intervention using the transtheoretical model with five stages of change (i.e., precontemplation, contemplation, preparation, action, and maintenance). In another stroke study a score of readiness to change behavior based on the transtheoretical model was used to assess in patients undergoing secondary stroke prevention.[357] The authors found that the prevention program, which consisted of conventional rehabilitation plus additional advice, motivational interviewing, and telephone support, improved exercise frequency, and increased consumption of fruits and vegetables when compared with the control group receiving conventional rehabilitation.[357] Several other behavioral theories (i.e., social cognitive theory, theory of reasoned action, theory of planned behavior, health belief model, protection motivation theory, and self-determination theory) may also be useful in facilitating long-term engagement.[358] The American College of Sports Medicine[28] acknowledged that assessing the participants' self-motivation and readiness for change can provide important information toward adapting the exercise program to meet the specific needs of the participants.

In the cardiac rehabilitation literature, Piepoli and colleagues[359] recommended that in order for an individual to pursue and engage in an exercise program, both physiological and psychosocial changes are needed. Progression from promotion of physical activity within the patient's current domestic, occupational, and leisure settings to participating in vigorous and structured exercise programs is recommended.[359] In a literature review of cardiac rehabilitation, evidence supported the use of educational sessions, spousal and family involvement, flexible and convenient scheduling of sessions, ongoing positive reinforcement and enjoyment (e.g., motivational letters, pamphlets, conversations), and self-management aids (e.g., self-report diets, activity logs, individualized goal setting).[360] Other strategies to enhance long-term exercise adherence include gradually progressing the exercise intensity, establishing regularity of training sessions, minimizing the risk of muscular soreness, and exercising in groups. Training sessions should be scheduled at a convenient time and in an accessible location, and if feasible, assistance with transportation and childcare should be offered. With the established emphasis on patient-centered care, it is consistent to have the patient identify individual goals and time frames to achieve these goals. Incorporating physical activity within everyday life will help promote cardiovascular and pulmonary fitness as a life activity and not solely an exercise program conducted within a medical environment or rehabilitation setting.

Aerobic training alone is not sufficient to optimize the health and fitness of people with neurological disabilities. Education and counseling regarding daily physical activity, nutrition, energy conservation techniques, smoking cessation, and coping strategies are essential.

CONCLUSION

Several conclusions can be made based on available evidence. Neuromuscular, cardiovascular, and pulmonary impairments associated with most neurological conditions interact with contextual factors and the health condition itself to adversely affect exercise capacity and cardiovascular fitness. Aerobic training is now unequivocally regarded as an effective intervention to reduce the functional decline associated with the deconditioned state. Research, albeit limited, suggests that although patients with neurological impairments generally manifest poor cardiopulmonary fitness, they have the capacity to respond to exercise training in essentially the same manner as individuals without impairments. Trainability is evidenced by their ability to increase exercise capacity or Vo_2peak in response to the metabolic stress imposed by aerobic exercise. Although not abundant, research findings also suggest that involvement in aerobic exercise can also improve walking capacity and reduce risk factors for secondary complications. On the basis of the positive results of training studies, more aggressive training programs are now being introduced into neurorehabilitation, with the goals of interrupting the cycle of debilitation and enhancing neurological recovery. There is an obvious need for further, properly controlled research to examine the impact of aerobic training on all domains of function and quality of life, of neurological populations. Also, a more personalized approach to both screening and prescription protocols for aerobic training needs to be developed to optimize safety, effectiveness, and resource allocation. Patients with neurological insults clearly have compounding system variables that interact when they trying to perform any movement. A clinician who is assisting individuals to regain functional control over movement to improve their quality of life cannot afford to ignore the cardiovascular and pulmonary system regardless of the medical diagnosis.

REFERENCES

To enhance this text and add value for the reader, all references are included on the companion Evolve site that accompanies this textbook. This online service will, when available, provide a link for the reader to a Medline abstract for the article cited. There are 362 cited references and other general references for this chapter, with the majority of those articles being evidence-based citations.

29.A APPENDIX

Abbreviations Commonly Used When Discussing Cardiovascular and Pulmonary Problems and Their Effect on Function

6MWT: 6-Minute Walk Test

ADL: activities of daily living

a-vO_2diff: arteriovenous oxygen difference

a-vO_2diffmax: maximal arteriovenous oxygen difference

BP: blood pressure

CAD: coronary artery disease

CO_2: carbon dioxide

CP: cerebral palsy

DBP: diastolic blood pressure

ECG: electrocardiogram

H^+: hydrogen ion

HR: heart rate

HRmax: maximal heart rate

HRpeak: peak heart rate

HRR: heart rate reserve

HRrest: resting heart rate

ICF: International Classification of Functioning, Disability and Health

MET: metabolic equivalent

O_2: oxygen

Q: cardiac output

Qmax: maximal cardiac output

RER: respiratory exchange ratio

RERpeak: peak respiratory exchange ratio

RPE: rate of perceived exertion

SPB: systolic blood pressure

SV: stroke volume

SVmax: maximal stroke volume

Vco_2: carbon dioxide production per minute

Vo_2: oxygen consumption per minute

V$o_2$max: maximal oxygen consumption per minute

V$o_2$peak: peak oxygen consumption per minute

30

Pain Management

Annie Burke-Doe

OBJECTIVES

After reading this chapter the student or therapist will be able to:
1. Understand the definition of pain
2. Describe the pain pathways.
3. Describe how pain is modulated within the nervous system.
4. Identify the causes of acute and chronic pain.
5. List the signs and symptoms of central nervous system, autonomic nervous system, and peripheral pain and give an example of each.
6. Perform a comprehensive pain evaluation, including taking a pain history, measuring pain intensity, measuring pain character, and examining the patient.
7. Design a comprehensive pain management program that addresses the objective and subjective aspects of the pain experience.

KEY TERMS

ANS pain: complex regional pain syndrome
acute pain
behavioral manipulations: exercise, operant conditioning, hypnosis, biofeedback
chronic pain
CNS pain: thalamic pain

cognitive strategies: relaxation exercises, body scanning, humor
nociceptor
pain intensity measurements: visual analog scale (VAS), simple descriptive pain scale (SDPS), pain estimate, faces pain scale
pain localization tools: pain drawing

pain modulation: gate control theory, neurotransmitters, neuromodulators
pain pathway
pain quality measurements: McGill Pain Questionnaire (MPQ), pediatric verbal descriptor scale, caregiver checklists
point stimulation

More than 25 million adults suffer daily from pain; over 10 million report high levels of pain most days, and 8 million have pain severe enough to interfere with their lives.[1] Acute and chronic pain have a profound impact on all aspects of an individual's life. Pain influences relationships with family members, friends, co-workers, and health care providers. It affects the ability to fulfill responsibilities, to work, and to participate in social activities. Perhaps more than any other factor, the presence of chronic pain and the response to it determine the overall quality of an individual's life.

Acute pain is one of the most common reasons for patients to seek treatment at an emergency department.[2,3] Acute pain is defined as "pain of recent onset and probable limited duration." It usually has an "identifiable temporal and causal relationship to injury or disease."[4] Mounting evidence that tissue injury often results in changes to nervous system function has provided a new understanding of mechanisms that explain how acute pain can often lead to chronic pain.[5,6] The Centers for Disease Control and Prevention (CDC) estimate that chronic pain affects approximately 50 million US adults, and high-impact chronic pain (i.e., interfering with work or life most days or every day) affects approximately 20 million US adults.[7] Higher prevalence of both chronic pain and high-impact chronic pain are reported among women, older adults, previously not currently employed adults, adults living in poverty, adults with public health insurance, and rural residents.[7]

Studies of pain medicine education in medical and health care curriculums show that many medical schools have gaps between recommended pain curricula and documented educational content.[2,8] Additionally, pain education in medical schools internationally did not adequately respond to societal needs in terms of the prevalence and public impact of inadequately managed pain.[9] The result is inadequate or inappropriate care of individuals who report having pain.

The use of the biopsychosocial model of pain treatment as a framework for understanding the relationship among biological (e.g., disease-specific, neurological, immunological, genetic), psychological (e.g., mood/affect, cognition, resilience), and social (e.g., discrimination, cultural influences, social support) mechanisms has been identified as the model of choice to determine the variability in the experience of pain for both populations and individuals.[10] In terms of application of the biopsychosocial model of pain treatment, the clinician must understand that chronic pain is a biopsychosocial condition that often requires integrated, multimodal, and interdisciplinary treatment, all components of which should be evidence-based.[11]

The World Health Organization's International Classification of Functioning, Disability and Health (ICF) considers determinants of health and disability from the perspective of the biopsychosocial model.[12] The ICF model is utilized in the management of pain and includes[13-17] impairments (problems with body structure or function), activities (the execution of a task or action by an individual), activity limitations (difficulties an individual may have in executing activities), participation (involvement in a life situation), and participation restrictions (problems experienced in life situation or social role involvement). The ability to identify appropriate rehabilitation approaches to improve activity and participation depends on the clinician's ability to identify different impairments that cause pain, or the resulting impairments and activity and participation problems caused by pain through validated performance-based measures.

This chapter deals with the complex issue of acute and chronic pain management. In the first section, an overview of the anatomy and physiology of pain is presented. In the second section, examination and evaluation of pain are explained. In the third section, a number of treatment interventions are suggested. Finally, case studies are presented to guide clinicians through the problem-solving process for designing pain management programs.

DEFINING PAIN

The International Association for the Study of Pain (IASP) defines pain as "an unpleasant sensory and emotional experience associated with actual or potential tissue damage or described in such terms as damage."[18] The primary purpose of pain is to protect the body. It occurs whenever there is tissue damage, and it causes the individual to react to remove the painful stimulus. Pain is also a sensation with more than one dimension. To the individual, pain is both an objective and a subjective experience. The objective dimension is the physiological tissue damage causing the pain. The subjective dimensions include the following[19]:

- A perceptual component: the patient's awareness of the location, quality, intensity, and duration of the pain stimulus
- An affective component: the psychological factors surrounding the patient's pain experience, including the patient's personality and emotional state
- A cognitive component: what the patient knows and believes about the pain resulting from his or her cultural background and past pain experiences (both personal pain experiences and those of others)
- A behavioral component: how the patient expresses the pain to others through communication and behavior

All these components taken together constitute the patient's pain experience. Thus all must be addressed for a successful pain management program. When the subjective components of the pain experience are ignored, it is entirely possible that the patient's underlying tissue damage may be corrected without her or his pain perception being cured.

In addition, recognizing that pain is more than simply a physical injury or disease process helps clinicians explain some of the inconsistencies observed in patients with chronic pain. Why is a patient's pain report out of proportion to the magnitude and duration of the injury? Why is pain intolerable to one person and merely uncomfortable to another? And why is pain tolerable in one instance but overwhelming to the same individual when experienced at a different time?

The answers lie in the interconnectedness of the nervous system and the fact that pain transmission involves several higher centers. To select the most appropriate intervention, it is important for clinicians to have at least a general idea of the pain pathways. An overview of pain anatomy and physiology is discussed next.

PAIN ANATOMY

Pain arises from the stimulation of specialized peripheral free nerve endings called *nociceptors*. Injurious stimulation to the skin, muscle, joint, viscera, or tissue can trigger these peripheral terminals, whose cell bodies are in the dorsal root ganglia and trigeminal ganglia. The density of nociceptors varies between as well as within these tissues. Nociceptors are extremely heterogeneous, differing in the neurotransmitters they contain, the receptors and ion channels they express, their speed of conduction, their response properties to noxious stimuli, and their capacity to be sensitized during inflammation, injury, and disease.[20]

Nociceptors found in interstitial tissues become excited with extreme mechanical, thermal, and chemical stimulation,[21] whereas nociceptors found in vessel walls become excited with these stimuli plus marked constriction and dilation of the vessels.[22] These receptors respond directly to some noxious stimuli and indirectly to others by means of one or more chemicals (histamine, potassium, bradykinin) released from cells in the traumatized tissues.[23]

Thermal nociceptors are triggered by intense hot or cold temperatures (>45°C or <5°C). They have fibers that are of small diameter and thinly myelinated with moderately fast conduction signals of 5 to 30 m/s. Mechanical nociceptors are triggered by intense pressures applied to the skin, such as a pinch. They also have thinly myelinated, moderately conducting fibers with speeds of 5 to 30 m/s.

Polymodal nociceptors are triggered by more than one sensory modality (mechanical, chemical, or thermal). These nociceptors have small-diameter, nonmyelinated fibers that conduct more slowly, generally at velocities less than 1.0 m/s (see Table 30.1). Stimulation of these receptors causes sensations of diffuse burning or aching pain. The difference in the fibers' size and myelination determines the speed at which impulses will travel to the brain.

These three types of nociceptors are broadly distributed in the skin and tissues and may work together. One example would be hitting one's shin against a table: a sharp "first pain" is felt immediately, followed later by a more prolonged aching, sometimes burning, "second pain."[23] The fast, sharp pain is transmitted by A delta fibers that carry information from thermal and mechanical nociceptors. The slow, dull pain is transmitted by C fibers that are activated by polymodal nociceptors.

Nociceptive input travels on A delta and C fibers into the dorsal horn of the spinal cord, where the gray matter is laminated and organized by cytological features. The first-order A delta and C fibers synapse with second-order neurons in lamina I (marginal layer), II (the substantia gelatinosa [SG]), and V. The second-order neurons do one of three things. A small number synapse with motor neurons, causing reflex movements (e.g., withdrawing the hand from a hot object). Others synapse with autonomic fibers, causing responses such as changes in heart rate and blood pressure and localized vasodilation, piloerection, and sweating. Most, however, travel a multisynaptic route to the higher centers by means of the ascending tracts.[21,24]

There are four major classes of neurons[25] responding to pain in the dorsal horn: low-threshold nociceptive-specific neurons designated class I; wide dynamic range (WDR) neurons designated class II; high-threshold nociceptive neurons designated class III; and a fourth, non-responder group of neurons that develop spontaneous activity with exposure to

TABLE 30.1	Nociceptors			
Receptor Type	**Stimulus to Fire**	**Diameter/Myelination**	**Speed**	
Thermal nociceptors	Intense hot or cold temperatures (>45°C or <5°C)	Small diameter and thinly myelinated	Moderately fast conduction signals of 5 to 30 m/s	
Mechanical nociceptors	Intense pressures applied to the skin, such as a pinch	Small diameter and thinly myelinated	Moderately conducting fibers with speeds of 5 to 30 m/s	
Polymodal nociceptors	More than one sensory modality (mechanical, chemical, or thermal)	Small-diameter, nonmyelinated fibers	Conduct more slowly, generally at velocities less than 1.0 m/s	Diffuse burning or aching pain

endogenous inflammatory cytokines, designated class IV. Nociceptive-specific neurons are most abundant in superficial lamina; their receptor fields are discrete and vary from one to several square centimeters.[26] WDR neurons, in contrast, respond to a wide range of stimuli from A delta, A beta, and C fibers in a graded manner (i.e., the rate of firing escalates with increasing intensity of stimulation), can be found in all lamina, and are the most prevalent cells in the dorsal horn.[26] Because of their unique response to innocuous or nociceptive input, as well as their larger receptor field, WDR neurons play an important role in the central sensitization and the plasticity of the spinal cord.[26]

Nociceptive input crosses at the cord level to the anterolateral quadrant of the ascending contralateral spinothalamic tract (Fig. 30.1). The axons of the anterolateral quadrant are arranged so that the sacral segments are most lateral, with the lumbar segments more medial and the cervical segments most central. This arrangement may be important clinically in that symptoms may be provoked according to dermatomal maps to some degree.[27] Pain dermatomes overlap to several adjacent dorsal roots, so boundaries can be less distinct, requiring the clinician to distinguish the pain and dysfunction.

The anterolateral tract is divided into three ascending pathways: the spinothalamic, spinoreticular, and spinomesencephalic. The spinothalamic tract conveys information about painful and thermal stimulation (location and intensity) directly to the ventral posterior lateral nucleus of the thalamus, as well as sending collaterals off at the brain stem to join the spinoreticular tract. Axons within the spinoreticular tract synapse on neurons of the reticular formation of the medulla and pons, which relay information to the intralaminar and posterior nuclei of the thalamus and to other structures in the diencephalon, such as the hypothalamus (emotional response to pain).

Axons in the spinomesencephalic tract relay information to the mesencephalic reticular formation and periaqueductal gray matter by way of the spinoparabrachial tract. It then projects to the limbic system, which is involved with the affective component of pain (central modulation of pain).

The thalamus processes and relays information to several higher centers.[22] Each projection serves a specific purpose. Axons of the spinothalamic tract project information to both the lateral and medial nuclear groups of the thalamus. The lateral nuclear group of the thalamus is where information about the location of an injury is thought to be mediated.[23] Injury to the spinothalamic tract and the lateral nuclear group of the thalamus causes central neuropathic pain, which is discussed in further detail later.

Projections from the spinoreticular tract to the medial nuclear group of the thalamus are concerned with processing information about nociception, and they also activate nonspecific arousal systems. These pathways project from the thalamus to the basal ganglia and many cortical areas.

Projections to the postcentral gyrus (sensory cortex) are responsible for pain perception. It is from this projection that pain can be localized and characterized. Projections from the thalamus to the frontal lobes and limbic system are concerned with pain interpretation. It is from all these projections that an individual perceives pain as hurting. Projections from the thalamus, as well as from the limbic system and sensory cortical areas, to the temporal lobes are responsible for pain memory; and projections from the thalamus to the hypothalamus are responsible for the autonomic response to pain.

PAIN TRANSMISSION

Ascending transmission of pain impulses is mediated by the action of the chemical excitatory neurotransmitter glutamate (A delta and C fibers) and tachykinins such as substance P (C fibers). Glutamate and neuropeptides have distinct actions on postsynaptic neurons, but they act together to regulate the firing properties postsynaptically.[23]

Tachykinins' activity is thought to prolong the action of glutamate, as levels are increased in persistent pain conditions.[26] The substrates of nociception that exist at the spinal level are complex in that more than 30 different neurotransmitters acting on more than 50 different receptors have been identified in the spinal cord and associated with some pain-related phenomenon.[28] Modulation of these substrates will assist in the effectiveness of therapeutic interventions and will be discussed next.

PAIN MODULATION

Nociceptive transmission is modulated at several points along the neural pathway by both ascending and descending systems.

The Gate Control Theory

The SG contains an ascending gating mechanism to block nociceptive impulses from leaving the dorsal horn of the spinal cord. The first-order neurons for both nociceptive and non-nociceptive information synapse with second-order neurons in the SG. The second-order neurons for both types of information project to specialized neurons named *T-cells* (transmission cells) in lamina V. For pain transmission to occur, T-cells must be stimulated while the SG is inhibited. The input from A delta and C fibers stimulates the T-cells and inhibits the SG (Fig. 30.2). Therefore A delta and C fiber input opens the gate, allowing pain transmission to the higher centers. On the other hand, when the SG and T-cells are both stimulated, the T-cells are inhibited, and the gate is closed to pain transmission. The input from non-nociceptive A beta fibers carrying information from pressoreceptors and mechanoreceptors stimulates both the T-cells and the SG. Therefore A beta fiber input closes the gate, blocking pain transmission.[27]

One example that illustrates the gate control theory is the use of transcutaneous electrical nerve stimulation (TENS) in an area that overlaps the injury. It works to reduce pain by activation of large-diameter A beta fibers that "closes the gate," thereby preventing pain transmission to the higher centers of the brain. This is also why shaking (vibrating) your hand after hitting your thumb with a hammer temporarily relieves pain.

Descending Pain Modulation System

There are at least two descending pain modulation systems. One involves the action of neurotransmitters, including serotonin, dopamine, norepinephrine, and substance P. High concentrations of brain serotonin and L-dopa (a precursor of dopamine)[29] have been found to inhibit nociception, whereas norepinephrine appears to enhance nociception.[30–33] The spinal mediators of descending nociceptive inhibitory influences include serotonin, norepinephrine, and acetylcholine (ACh). This may be relevant to the action of antidepressants in relieving pain in the absence of depression. Substance P is thought to be the neurotransmitter for neurons transmitting chronic pain.[34]

The second descending modulating system is mediated by neuromodulators—chemicals capable of directly affecting pain transmission. The neuromodulators include enkephalin and β-endorphin, which are referred to as *endogenous opiates* because they have morphine-like actions and are found in areas of the central nervous system (CNS) that correspond to opiate-binding sites. Endogenous opiates are believed to modulate pain by inhibiting the release of substance P. They have been shown to have a profound effect on nociception and mood.[35–37] Their levels in the brain and spinal cord rise in response to emotional stress, causing an increase in the pain threshold and providing a possible reason that acute stress decreases acute pain.[38,39]

Although serotonin is not classified as an endogenous opiate, it exerts a profound effect on analgesia and enhances analgesic drug potency. High concentrations of serotonin lead to decreased pain by inhibiting transmission of nociceptive information within the dorsal

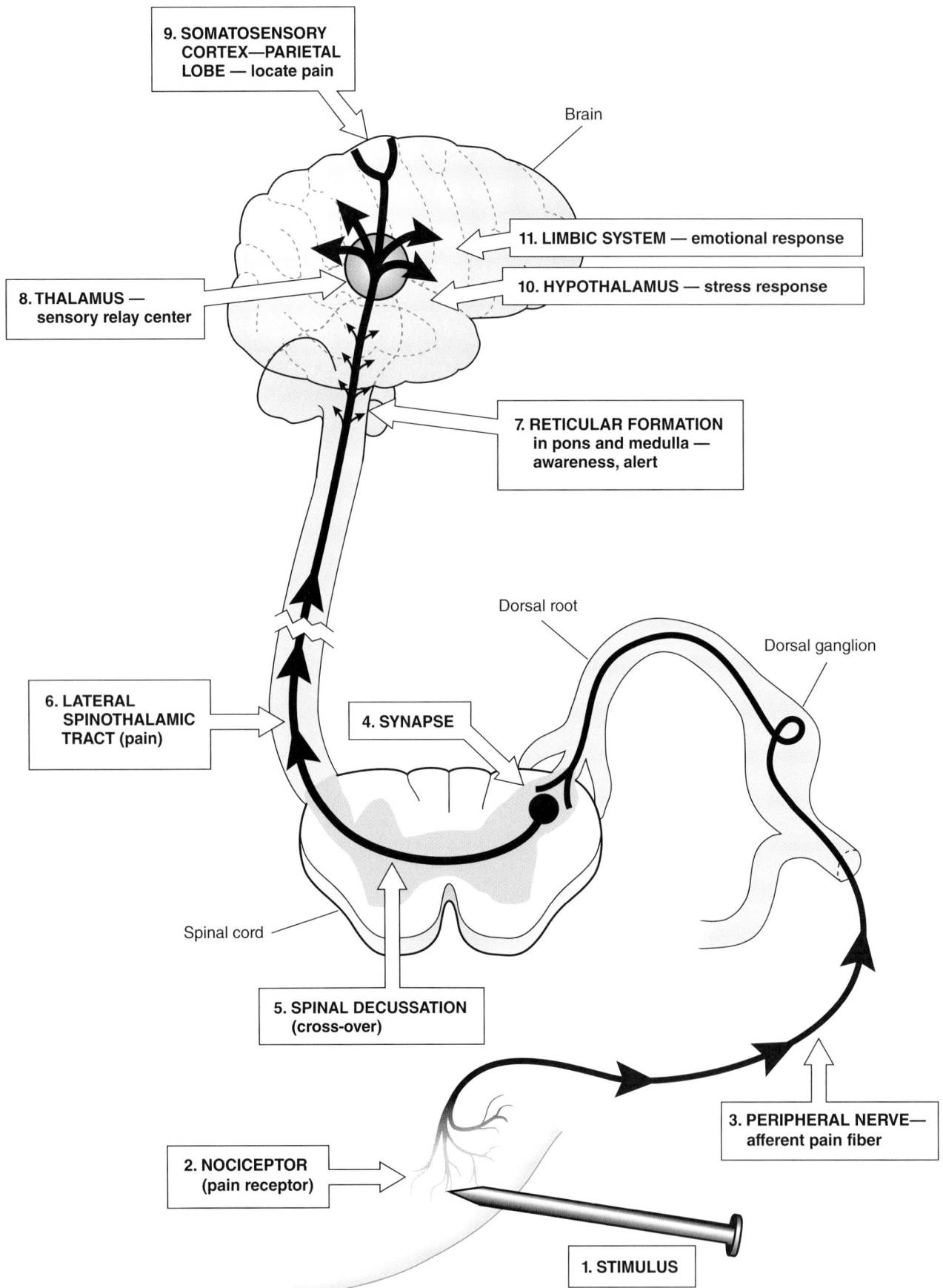

Fig. 30.1 Pain Pathway. (From Gould BE. *Pathophysiology for the Health Professions.* 2nd ed. Philadelphia: WB Saunders; 2002.)

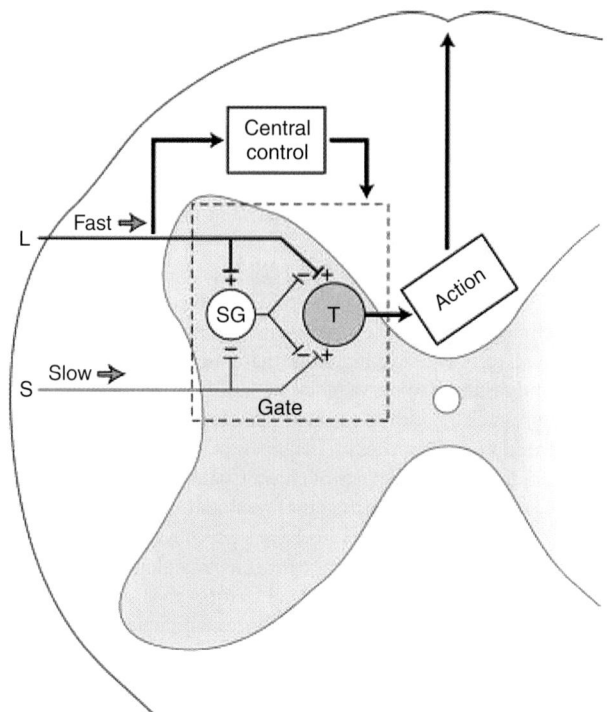

Fig. 30.2 Schematic Representation of Spinal Structures Involved in the Gate Control Theory of Pain Transmission. Afferent input by means of both large- and small-diameter fibers is theorized to influence the transmission cell *(T)* directly and through small internuncial neurons located within the substantia gelatinosa *(SG)*. (From Nolan MF. Anatomic and physiologic organization of neural structures involved in pain transmission, modulation, and perception. In: Echternach JL, ed. *Pain.* New York: Churchill Livingstone.)

horn,[40,41] whereas low concentrations result in depression, sleep disturbances, and increased pain.

The success of several therapeutic modalities, including noxious counterirritation (e.g., brief intense TENS or acupressure) and diversion (including hypnosis), is attributed to raising the level of endogenous opiates in the body.[39]

CATEGORIZING PAIN

Pain is grouped into several categories: acute, chronic, referred, central neuropathic, autonomic, and peripheral.

Acute pain is the normal predicted physiological response and serves as a warning. It alerts the individual that tissues are exposed to damaging or potentially damaging noxious stimuli. Acute pain is localized, occurs in proportion to the intensity of the stimuli, and lasts only as long as the stimuli or the tissue damage exists (1 to 6 months).[42] Although acute pain is associated with anxiety and increased autonomic activity (increased muscle tone, heart rate, and blood pressure),[43] it is usually relieved by interventions directed at correcting the injury. The pain experience is usually limited to the individual.[44]

Chronic pain is usually referred to as *intractable pain* if it persists for 6 or more months. It is defined as pain that continues after the stimulus has been removed or the tissue damage heals. Physiologically, chronic pain is believed to result from hypersensitization of the pain receptors and enlargement of the receptor field in response to the localized inflammation that follows tissue damage.[45] Chronic pain is poorly localized, has an ill-defined time of onset, and is strongly associated with the subjective components outlined previously. It does not respond well to

interventions directed solely at correcting the injury. Chronic pain patients frequently report other symptoms, such as depression, difficulty sleeping, poor mental and physical function, and fatigue. The effects of the pain experience extend beyond the individual and affect the family, the workplace, and the social sphere of the individual.[44]

Referred pain is felt at a point other than its origin. Pain can be referred from an internal organ, a joint, a trigger point, or a peripheral nerve to a remote musculoskeletal structure. Referred pain usually follows a specific pattern. For example, cardiac pain is frequently referred to the left arm or jaw; the referral pattern for trigger points is exact enough to be used as a diagnostic tool and is often used by physicians to diagnose pathology. Referred pain is the result of a convergence of the primary afferent neurons from deep structures and muscles to secondary neurons that also have a cutaneous receptive field.[46,47]

Although it is now recognized that all neuropathic pain results in abnormal activity within the CNS,[48] pain initiated or caused by a primary lesion or dysfunction of the CNS[49] is referred to as *central neuropathic pain.* The involvement of the nervous system can be at many levels: nerves, nerve roots, and central pain pathways in the spinal cord and brain. In this circumstance, there is permanent damage to the nervous system (usually a peripheral nerve) and likely anatomical reorganization of spinal terminations of surviving axons or ectopic activity from a neuroma that contributes paroxysmal, persistent input to the spinal cord.[50] In addition to anatomical reorganization in the spinal cord, there could be some reorganization in the rostroventral medulla (RVM) as well, but more likely there is prolonged input to the RVM that sustains facilitatory influences that descend to the spinal cord. Less appreciated, descending facilitatory influences on spinal sensory processing could also be important to maintenance of chronic pain conditions, particularly those that persist in the absence of obvious tissue pathology.[50]

Central neuropathic pain is medically diagnosed by its defining neurological signs and symptoms; it is verified with neuroimaging tests that identify a CNS lesion and rule out other causes. It is important that the therapist be able to localize the level and differentiate between central and peripheral pain. Central neuropathic pain can be caused by vascular insult; traumatic, neoplastic, and demyelinating diseases; and surgery (including vascular compromise during surgery). Central neuropathic pain is distinct from nociceptive pain (nonneuronal tissue damage).

The onset of central neuropathic pain is usually delayed after the occurrence of the initial episode that results in damage to the CNS; onset of pain may occur during the phase of recovery from neurological deficits.[51] Pain originating from a cerebrovascular incident and spinal cord injury usually begins weeks or months after the insult, whereas pain originating from tumors may take years to begin.[48]

Individuals with central neuropathic pain may have difficulty describing their pain and report burning, aching, pricking, squeezing, or cutting pain after cutaneous stimulation, movement, heat, cold, or vibration. A normally non-noxious stimulus, such as moving clothing across skin, becomes agonizing. In some cases, pain begins spontaneously.[52] Pain intensity varies, but it does seem to be associated to some degree with the location of the lesion.[48] Allodynia (pain from normally non-noxious stimuli) and dysesthesia are common, and one of the characteristic features of central neuropathic pain is that the clinical symptoms persist long after the stimulus has been removed.

Central neuropathic pain is topographical. The site of the lesion determines the location of the symptoms. The pain may involve half the body, an entire extremity, or a small portion of one extremity.[48] It is frequently migratory. Thalamic pain is the classic example of central neuropathic pain.

Central neuropathic pain is difficult to treat. Surgery is not helpful for most individuals with central neuropathic pain, and medications have not been effective in permanently relieving the symptoms.[21]

Therefore the treatment of patients with central neuropathic pain stresses coping strategies and prevention of loss of activity and participation. The ideal management of a chronic pain patient is by a multidisciplinary approach, including disciplines such as internal medicine, neurology, anesthesia, nursing, psychology, pharmacy, rehabilitation medicine, physical therapy, occupational therapy, and others. The limitation of this approach is that access to such a wide range of specialists is often available only at large medical centers and special pain clinics, which restricts access to a limited number of patients.

Under normal conditions there is a fine balance between the parasympathetic and sympathetic branches of the autonomic nervous system (ANS). Parasympathetic activity maintains homeostasis, whereas sympathetic activity functions to make "fight-or-flight" changes in response to stress. Stimulation of the autonomic efferent fibers is not normally painful. However, the balance between afferent input and the descending sympathetic nervous system (SNS) is disrupted when there is injury, resulting in exaggerated and prolonged sympathetic activity, allodynia, and hyperalgesia (increased response to normally painful stimuli)—hence, autonomic pain.

Allodynia is a product of the phenomenon of central sensitization.[53] After injury, new axons sprout from the sympathetic efferent neurons. These fire spontaneously and, because they synapse on the cell bodies of the primary afferent neurons, cause them to fire as well. In addition, the dorsal horn neurons themselves become more excitable. They show an enlargement in their receptive field and become more sensitive to mechanical, thermal, and chemical stimulation. The result is an increase in the neuronal barrage into the CNS and the perception of pain with usually nonpainful stimuli.[23]

Complex regional pain syndrome (CRPS) is an example of pain that arises from abnormal activity within the ANS.[54] CRPS has been classified into two distinct types[49]: CRPS type I (formerly *reflex sympathetic dystrophy*) follows mild trauma without nerve injury, and CRPS type II (formerly *causalgia*) follows trauma with nerve injury. CRPS type I generally begins within the month after the injury, whereas CRPS type II can occur any time after the injury.[55]

The main features of CRPS type I are constant burning pain that fluctuates in intensity and increases with movement, constant stimulation, or stress. There are also allodynia and hyperalgesia, edema, abnormal sweating, abnormal blood flow and trophic changes in the area of pain, and impaired motor function. CRPS type I is relieved by blocking the SNS, indicating that the pain is sympathetically maintained.[55]

CRPS type II occurs in the region of a limb innervated by an injured nerve. The nerves most commonly involved in CRPS type II are the median, sciatic, tibial, and ulnar; involvement of the radial nerve is rare. Pain is described as spontaneous, constant, and burning and is exacerbated by light touch, stress, temperature change, movement, visual and auditory stimuli, and emotional disturbances. Allodynia and hyperalgesia are common and may involve the distribution of more than one peripheral nerve. As with CRPS type I, edema, abnormal sweating, abnormal blood flow, trophic changes, and impaired motor function occur. The symptoms spread proximally and can involve other areas of the body. Evidence also points to sympathetic involvement in CRPS type II.[55]

The treatment of CRPS is complex and must be carefully coordinated among members of an interdisciplinary team including the neurologist (medications), psychologist (behavior), anesthesiologist (injections), and therapist (functional recovery). The therapist provides the core treatment to improve function. Therapists need to pay close attention to the following aspects of the disorder: (1) the degree of motor abnormalities, including restricted active range of motion (ROM), abnormal posturing, spasm, tremor, and dystonia; (2) true passive range restriction; (3) hyperesthesia and allodynia; (4) swelling and vasomotor changes; and (5) evidence of osteoporosis by radiograph.[56] Please refer to Case Study 30.1 for interventions for patients with CRPS.

Peripheral pain results from noxious irritation of the nociceptors. The character of peripheral pain depends on the location and intensity of the noxious stimulation, as well as which fibers carry the information into the dorsal gray matter. As noted previously, information carried on A delta fibers is sharp and well localized, begins rapidly, and lasts only if the stimulus is present, whereas information carried on C fibers is dull and diffuse, has a delayed onset, and lasts longer than the duration of the stimulus. The treatment of peripheral pain is covered in detail in Chapter 16.

The management of central versus peripheral pain is determined by the type of pain—acute or chronic—and the clinical features present, including clinical localization; time of onset; laboratory study localization; response to analgesics, including narcotics; response to antidepressants; and response to nerve block or neurectomy.[51] Differentiation among features will drive the treatment plan, but because some peripheral and central forms can coexist, diagnosis may be difficult.

The multidimensional aspects of chronic pain make it important to evaluate the causes as well as the emotional and cognitive sequelae.[57] Persistent pain is now considered to have a psychogenic component.[58] The longer an individual has pain, the more a psychological component may become dominant. Many emotional factors can strongly influence pain, such as pain thresholds, past experiences with pain, coping styles, and social roles. The emotional experience that we perceive with pain reflects the interaction of higher brain centers and subcortical regions, such as the amygdala and cingulate gyrus (limbic system).[59] Positron emission tomography of patients with chronic neuropathic pain demonstrates a shift of acute pain activity in the sensory cortex to regions such as the anterior cingulate gyrus.[60] Understanding the physical limitations imposed by chronic pain is an area that therapists commonly assess; it is the mind-body connection that is often less articulated by the patient and more difficult for the practitioner.

Treatment of chronic pain should include a patient-centered approach, given the unique manifestations that occur in an individual's response to pain. Patient-centered models, such as the biopsychosocial and ICF model, provide a framework that embraces a multidisciplinary team approach practiced in pain clinics. In such models, chronic pain has been noted to include psychological factors such as feelings of fear, anxiety, and depression,[61] which are known to have the ability to modulate and exacerbate the physical pain experience.[62] For example, a patient with chronic pain who has the fear that movement will increase pain may alter his activity, causing muscular shortening, spasms, and a spiraling course of more pain and disability. The focus in treating patients with chronic pain should be on improving functional physical activity, decreasing peripheral nociception and central facilitation, and providing cognitive and behavioral strategies to help in resuming normal activities.

EXAMINATION OF THE PATIENT WITH PAIN

The examination of a patient with pain can be challenging because the therapist must frequently weed through the individual's emotions, behaviors, and secondary gains to identify the source of the symptoms. Many patients are not referred to therapy until they have participated in weeks, months, or even years of failed interventions, and their expectations and patience are at low levels. They often approach therapy anticipating more instructions, more frustration, and more pain. Despite these obstacles, therapists must strive to complete pain evaluations that include evidence-based measurable, reproducible information that identifies the source of pain and provides direction toward treatment that is both beneficial and cost-effective and that assists in establishing attainable goals. The time allotted for the examination may be dependent on the type of practice setting; many therapists send a comprehensive questionnaire to the patient or ask the patient to arrive early to complete important paperwork. It is essential to develop a trusting relationship, ensuring that the patient feels that the therapist has listened to his or her concerns and has acknowledged his or her fears, and will participate in a plan for improving his or her physical, mental, and functional abilities.

Pain History

Every evaluation of a patient with pain should begin with a comprehensive pain history. It is important to have a standardized format to decrease chances of missing important information and to minimize having the patient "lead the interview." The following alphabetical mnemonic device may prove helpful (OPQRST):

- Observation: Observation of the patient from the moment of entry until (and sometimes beyond) the moment of exit from the clinic. By observing the patient outside of the evaluation, the therapist can assess the patient's movement. The patient's nervous system will accurately express itself to the therapist, especially when the patient is asked to focus attention on a topic other than pain and the patient is not aware that movement is being observed.
- Origin and onset: Date and circumstances of the onset of pain. How did the pain start? Gradually or suddenly? Was there a precipitating injury? If so, what was the mechanism of injury? If not, can the patient correlate the onset to a activity or posture?
- Position: Location of the pain. Have the patient demonstrate where the pain is located rather than relying on description alone. In addition to being more accurate, demonstration allows another observation of the patient's ability and willingness to move. Patients can also be asked to draw their symptoms on a schematic, such as the pain drawing, which is described later.
- Pattern: Pattern of the pain. Is the pain constant or periodic? Does it travel or radiate? Which activities and postures increase or decrease the pain? Does medication or time of day have any effect on the pain? Have there been any recent changes in the pattern? Does the patient believe that the pain is improving, worsening, or remaining the same?
- Quality: Characteristics of the pain. Does the patient use adjectives indicating mechanical (pressing, bursting, stabbing), chemical (burning), neural (numb, "pins and needles"), or vascular (throbbing) origin? Two tools for describing pain character are described later.
- Quantity: Intensity of the pain. How has the pain intensity changed since the onset? Several methods that allow for monitoring change in pain intensity are presented later.
- Radiation: Characteristics of pain radiation. Does the pain radiate? What causes the pain to radiate? Can the radiation be reversed? How?
- Signs and symptoms: Functional and psychological components of the pain. Has the pain resulted in any functional limitations? Has it caused any changes in the patient's ability to participate in life, including employment and recreational activities? Does the patient's personality contribute to the pain, or has the pain caused changes in the patient's emotional stability? Does the patient benefit from the pain? How? It may be necessary to interview the patient's significant others or family members for an accurate picture.
- Treatment: Previous and current medical and therapeutic treatment and its effectiveness, including medications, home remedies, and recommendations for movement activities. It is also important to determine the patient's attitude and expectations concerning therapy in addition to obtaining a treatment history.
- Visceral symptoms: Physical symptoms of visceral origin that can accompany and be responsible for the pain (Box 30.1). Visceral causes of pain require referral to the patient's physician for further investigation before the initiation of treatment by a therapist.

Pain Outcome Measurement

Outcome measures have become well established in pain research. Because of the variability in outcome measures across clinical trials

---

BOX 30.1 Viscerogenic Back Pain

General Signs and Symptoms
- Pain does not increase with spinal stresses or strains.
- Pain is not relieved with rest.
- Visceral symptoms accompany back pain.

Gastrointestinal Tract Signs and Symptoms
- Pain is accompanied by altered bowel habits.
- Pain is related to eating.
- Peptic pain is relieved with vomiting.

Kidney Signs and Symptoms
- Increased pain with diuresis indicates hydronephrosis.

Pelvic Signs and Symptoms
- Low back pain associated with vaginal bleeding or discharge.

Prostate Signs and Symptoms
- Low back discomfort associated with micturition.

Lung Signs And Symptoms
- Posterior thoracic pain associated with respiration in chronic obstructive pulmonary disease.

Vascular Signs and Symptoms
- Deep, boring, pulsating low back pain associated with a palpable abdominal aortic aneurysm.
- Back pain with or without calf pain after walking and relieved with standing still; possibly impaired lower extremity pulses and trophic skin changes associated with occlusive disease of the internal iliac artery or its branches.

Modified from Klineberg E, Mazanec D, Orr D, et al. Masquerade: medical causes of back pain. *Cleve Clin J Med,* 2007 Dec;74(12):905-13.

---

hinders evaluation of efficacy and effectiveness of treatments, the Initiative on Methods, Measurement, and Pain Assessment in Clinical Trials (IMMPACT) has recommended that six core outcome domains should be considered when designing chronic pain clinical trials. These six core outcome domains were (1) pain; (2) physical functioning; (3) emotional functioning; (4) participant ratings of improvement and satisfaction with treatment; (5) symptoms and adverse events; and (6) participant disposition (e.g., adherence to the treatment regimen and reasons for premature withdrawal from the trial).[63] These domains can assist in determination of outcome measures appropriate in clinical practice. Pain measurement tools are designed to provide information about the intensity, location, physical function, and character of a patient's symptoms at the time of the evaluation. This information can then be merged with the pain history, the disease or pathology history, and the physical findings to identify the cause of the pain. The disease or pathology management and its pain measurement will be the responsibility of the physician, whereas the movement limitations caused by the pain are the responsibility of the therapist. A number of pain measurement tools are available. These tools are used by professionals whose focus is pathology, as well as professionals whose responsibility is helping the patient to regain functional activities and life participation. The applications and limitations of several are discussed.

Patient reported outcomes have been utilized in the treatment of pain. The National Institute of Health funds the Patient-Reported Outcomes Measurement Information System (PROMIS),[64] which provides psychometrically sound and validated patient-reported outcome measures free of charge that can be used in a wide range of chronic conditions. PROMIS is comprised of calibrated item banks to measure diverse health concepts such as pain, physical function, and depression; these are

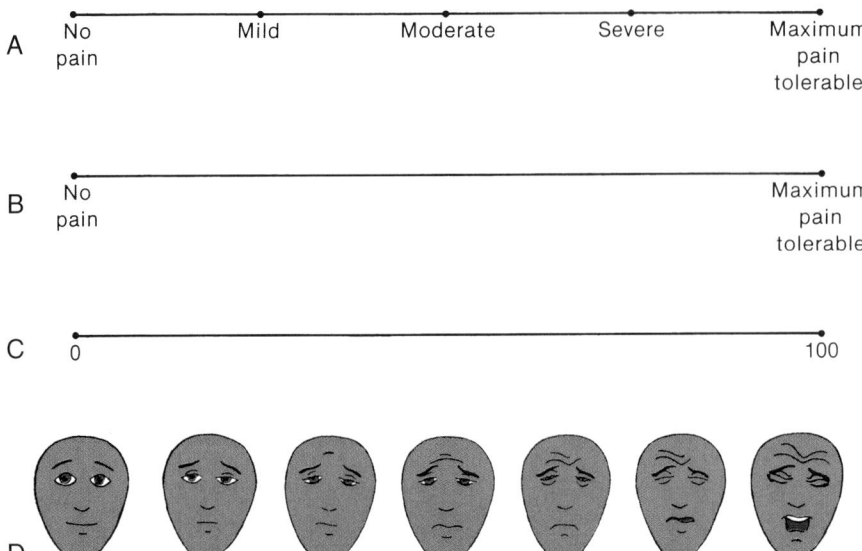

Fig. 30.3 Rating Scales for Measuring Pain Intensity. **(A)** Simple descriptive pain scale (SDPS). **(B)** Visual analog scale (VAS). **(C)** Pain estimate. **(D)** Faces pain scale. (D Reprinted from Bieri D, Reeve DA, Champion GD, et al. The faces pain scale for the self-assessment of the severity of pain experienced by children: development, initial validation, and preliminary investigation for the ratio scale properties. *Pain*. 1990;41:139–150, with permission from Elsevier Science.)

presented for each domain as individual items and/or instruments of various lengths. In addition, PROMIS includes several collections of items, termed profiles, which measure multiple domains. For example, the PROMIS-29 profile assesses seven domains, each with four questions; depression, anxiety, physical function, pain interference, fatigue, sleep disturbance, and ability to participate in social roles and activities. There is also an additional numeric pain intensity 0 to 10 rating scale (NPRS).

Measuring Pain Intensity

Research has shown that pain memory does not provide an accurate measure of pain intensity.[65]

Pain intensity rating tools are scales that have the patient rate the current level of pain by marking a continuum or assigning a numerical value to the pain intensity (Fig. 30.3).

Each of the first three tools described here has been found to be reliable over time when used to measure pain that is present at the time of the rating. In general, however, patients who are depressed or anxious tend to report higher levels of pain and patients who are not depressed or anxious tend to report lower levels of pain on all three of these scales.[66]

Visual analog scale. With the visual analog scale (VAS), the patient rates the pain on a continuum that begins with "no pain" and ends with "maximum pain tolerable." This tool provides an infinite number of points between the extremes, making it sensitive to small changes in pain intensity. However, it has not been found reliable for individuals who have impaired abstract thinking skills[67] and may be unable to translate their pain intensity into a corresponding point on a line.

Simple descriptive pain scale. With a simple descriptive pain scale (SDPS), the patient rates the pain on a continuum that is subdivided using descriptors that gradually increase in intensity. Sample descriptors are "no pain," "mild pain," "moderate pain," "severe pain," and "maximum pain tolerable." This tool is more useful than the VAS for patients with impaired abstract thinking because it is easier for them to identify with the pain descriptors than with the line found in the VAS. However, patients have been found to favor the points corresponding to each descriptor rather than points between, resulting in a less sensitive tool than the VAS.[68]

Pain estimate. With a pain estimate, the patient assigns a numerical rating to the pain, staying within defined limits (most commonly between 0 and 100, where 0 represents no pain and 100 represents maximum pain tolerable). Because it provides a numerical range of scores, this tool is valuable for statistical analysis purposes. However, whereas some patients find assigning a numerical rating to their pain intensity easy, patients with impaired abstract thinking may have difficulty similar to that encountered with the VAS.

Faces pain scale. With the Faces Pain Scale, the patient selects one of seven schematic faces representing gradually increasing pain intensities. The scale begins with a face representing no pain and ends with a face representing the most pain possible. This tool is designed for use with young children who do not have the ability to use any of the three previous tools. The Faces Pain Scale has been found to be valid across cultural lines[69] and to have a strong correlation with other pain measures.[68] It is simple to use, does not require verbal skills, and requires little instruction. It has been used successfully with children as young as age 3 and with individuals who are limited in verbal expression.

Localizing Pain Symptoms

Pain drawings. The patient is asked to draw his or her symptoms on a schematic of the human body using a provided list of symbols (Fig. 30.4). The result is a diagram describing the nature and location of the patient's pain, which can be compared with the patient's verbal report. In addition to providing a database, the pain drawing has been found to be useful in identifying individuals who have a heavy psychological or emotional component to their pain, making it helpful also in identifying patients who would benefit from further psychological evaluation.[70]

Describing Pain Quality

McGill pain questionnaire. One of the most popular scales to rate pain quality is the McGill Pain Questionnaire (MPQ), which includes 20 categories of descriptive words covering the sensory (numbers 1 to 10), affective (numbers 11 to 15), and evaluative (number 16) properties of pain (Fig. 30.5). Sensory properties are measured using temporal,

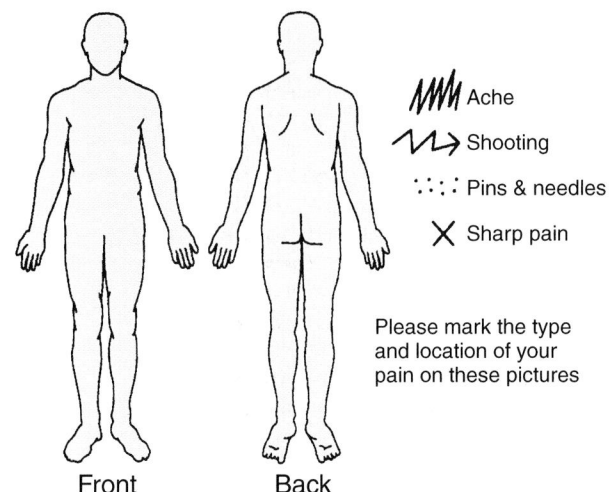

MMM Ache

Shooting

Pins & needles

✕ Sharp pain

Please mark the type
and location of your
pain on these pictures

Front   Back

Fig. 30.4 Pain Drawing for Describing the Nature and Location of a Patient's Pain Symptoms. (From Cameron MH, ed. *Physical Agents in Rehabilitation.* Philadelphia: WB Saunders; 1999.)

thermal, spatial, and pressure descriptors. Affective properties are measured using fear, tension, and autonomic descriptors. Evaluative properties are measured using pain experience descriptors.[71] Each word has a numerical value based on its position within its category.

The patient is instructed to "select the word in each category that best describes the pain you have now. If there is no word in the category that describes the pain, skip the category. If there is more than one word that describes the pain, select the word that best describes the pain."[71]

The MPQ can provide the following types of information[71]:
- A pain-rating index based on the sum of the values of all the words selected
- A pain-rating index based on the sum of the values of all the words in a given category
- The total number of words chosen

The MPQ has been studied extensively and found valid for adults with acute and chronic pain as well as for those with a variety of specific pathological states.[72–74] It provides clues into the specific cause of pain because it describes the patient's symptoms.

However, the MPQ does pose some disadvantages. It is time-consuming, requiring more time to complete than any of the previously

---

What Does Your Pain Feel Like?

Some of the words below describe your present pain. Circle ONLY those words that best describe it. Leave out any category that is not suitable. Use only a single word in each appropriate category–the one that applies best.

1	2	3	4
Flickering	Jumping	Pricking	Sharp
Quivering	Flashing	Boring	Cutting
Pulsing	Shooting	Drilling	Lacerating
Throbbing		Stabbing	
Beating		Lancinating	
Pounding			

5	6	7	8
Pinching	Tugging	Hot	Tingling
Pressing	Pulling	Burning	Itchy
Gnawing	Wrenching	Scalding	Smarting
Cramping		Searing	Stinging
Crushing			

9	10	11	12
Dull	Tender	Tiring	Sickening
Sore	Taut	Exhausting	Suffocating
Hurting	Rasping		
Aching	Splitting		
Heavy			

13	14	15	16
Fearful	Punishing	Wretched	Annoying
Frightful	Grueling	Blinding	Troublesome
Terrifying	Cruel		Miserable
	Vicious		Intense
	Killing		Unbearable

17	18	19	20
Spreading	Tight	Cool	Nagging
Radiating	Numb	Cold	Nauseating
Penetrating	Drawing	Freezing	Agonizing
Piercing	Squeezing		Dreadful
	Tearing		Torturing

Fig. 30.5 The McGill Pain Questionnaire Used to Rate Pain Quality. (Reprinted from Melzack R. The McGill Pain Questionnaire: major properties and scoring methods. *Pain.* 1975;1:277, with permission from Elsevier Science.)

TABLE 30.2   Pediatric Verbal Descriptor Scale

Dimension	Word	Dimension	Word	Dimension	Word	Dimension	Word
A	Annoying Bad Horrible Miserable Terrible Uncomfortable	S	Biting Cutting Like a pin Like a sharp knife Pinlike Sharp Stabbing	S	Itching Like a scratch Like a sting Scratching Stinging	A	Crying Frightening Screaming Terrifying
E	Aching Hurting Like an ache Like a hurt Sore	S	Blistering Burning Hot	S	Shocking Shooting Splitting	A	Dizzy Sickening Suffocating
S	Beating Hitting Pounding Punching Throbbing	S	Cramping Crushing Like a pinch Pinching Pressure	S	Numb Stiff Swollen Tight	E	Never goes away Uncontrollable
A	Awful Deadly Dying Killing						

A, Affective; *E*, evaluative; *S*, sensory.
Reprinted from Wilkie DJ, Holzemer WL, Tesler MD, et al. Measuring pain quality: validity and reliability of children's and adolescents' pain language. *Pain.* 1990;41:151–159, with permission from Elsevier Science.

described rating scales. Thus it is not appropriate for quick estimates of pain after treatment. Patients, especially children, are frequently unfamiliar with some of the descriptors and ask the evaluator to assist by defining words. However, reliability and validity of this test are based on examiner objectivity, and care must be taken to avoid the introduction of evaluator bias by helping the patient to select appropriate descriptors.[71] This issue can be dealt with by telling the patient, "If you do not recognize a word, it probably does not apply to you."

Pediatric verbal descriptor scale. Because a child's description of pain is limited by a smaller vocabulary, Wilkie and associates[75] have developed a verbal descriptor scale specifically for use with children (Table 30.2). Their list includes 56 words commonly used by children aged 8 to 17 to describe their pain experience. The word list is divided into the four categories found in the MPQ. The evaluators' research has shown the list to be useful for children with a variety of diagnoses because it is relatively free of gender, ethnic, and developmental bias.

Caregiver checklist. Patients who are unable to communicate verbally because of neurological disabilities may be unable to use any of the just-described pain measurement scales. However, because of pain associated with their medical conditions, extensive and repeated surgery, and behavioral oddities that might limit pain expression, these individuals are at high risk for having their pain go unrecognized. McGrath and colleagues[76] have attempted to develop and categorize a checklist of demonstrated pain behaviors identified by caregivers of severely handicapped individuals. Although their list did not pass validity criteria, the researchers propose that clinicians develop a patient-specific checklist that could be used to gauge changes in the patient's pain from the information gained during the caregiver interview portion of the evaluation of nonverbal handicapped patients.

In addition to qualifying and quantifying the patient's pain, pain measurement tools have an additional value. They can be used to identify inconsistencies between a patient's pain report and the clinician's objective findings. For example, a patient with normal objective findings would not be expected to give a high pain report or draw symptoms over the entire pain drawing. Conversely, a patient with a multitude of objective findings within the severe range would be expected to provide a high pain rating. In addition, as objective symptoms subside, it is expected that the patient will report a similar decline on the rating scales. Inconsistencies between the patient's pain descriptions and the therapist's findings should serve to alert the clinician that the patient might require cognitive or affective intervention in addition to physical treatment.

PSYCHOSOCIAL ASSESSMENT

Psychosocial factors are key variables in the comprehensive assessment of chronic pain. Davidson and colleagues[77] determined seven factors using a "prototypical" pain assessment battery that included pain and disability, pain description, affective distress, support, positive coping strategies, negative coping strategies, and activity. Depression is commonly experienced in patients with chronic pain.[78] Screening for depression should be part of the clinical exam, and available evidence suggests that two specific questions from the Primary Care Evaluation of Mental Disorders patient questionnaire can be used in physical therapy settings.[79] The questions suggested for use are (1) "During the past month, have you often been bothered by feeling down, depressed, or hopeless?" and (2) "During the past month, have you often been bothered by little interest or pleasure in doing things?" The patient responds to the questions with "yes" or "no," and the number of "yes" items are totaled, giving a potential range of 0 to 2. If a patient responds "no" to both questions, depression is highly unlikely, with a –LR of 0.07. Answering "yes" to 1 or both questions should raise suspicion of depressive symptoms.[79] Irving and Squire[80] described two key individual personality features that affect pain: catastrophizing and health-related anxiety. Persons who catastrophically misinterpret innocuous bodily sensations, including pain, are likely to become fearful of pain, which results in pain-related fear. Pain-related fear is associated with avoidance of movement and physical activity, which directly affects recovery of function. Pain-related fear is also associated with increased pain levels and an exacerbated painful experience. Three validated tools to screen for these features include the Fear-Avoidance Beliefs Questionnaire (FABQ)[81], Pain Catastrophizing Scale (PCS), and the Tampa Scale of Kinesophobia (TKS).[82]

EXAMINATION OF THE PATIENT

The clinical examination should begin the moment the patient enters the door. Patients frequently change posture and affect when they are being formally evaluated, and it is important to gain an accurate view of pain behavior during spontaneous activities to assess the validity of complaints. The following should be included in the examination:
- Observation of gait and movement patterns, including the use of assistive devices.
- Notation of body type and anomalies.
- Examination of sitting and standing posture, including both the normal posture and that assumed because of the pain. (Observe the patient during activities, if possible, to differentiate movement patterns altered by intent vs. automatic adjustments.)
- Inspection of the skin for pliability, trophic changes, scar tissue, and other abnormalities.
- Palpation of the soft tissue structures to identify changes in temperature, swelling, tenderness, and areas of discomfort.
- Palpation of the anatomical structures to determine end feel—the sensation felt at the end of the available movement.[83]
  - Bone to bone: hard normal, for example, at the end range of elbow extension.
  - Spasm: muscular resistance abnormal.
  - Capsular feel: rubbery normal at the extreme of full ROM; abnormal when encountered before the end of ROM.
  - Springy block: rebound abnormal.
  - Tissue approximation: soft tissue normal at the extremes of full passive flexion.
  - Empty feel: no physiological resistance, but patient resists movement because of pain.
- Examination of ROM: active ROM testing is performed to assess the patient's willingness to move and to identify any limitations or painful areas; passive ROM testing is used to further refine the observations.[83]
  - When active and passive movements are painful and restricted in the same direction and the pain appears at the limit of motion, the problem is most likely arthrogenic.
  - When active and passive movements are painful or restricted in opposite directions, the problem is most likely muscular.
  - When there is relative restriction of passive movement in the capsular pattern, the problem may be arthritic in nature.
  - When there is no restriction of passive movement, but the patient cannot perform the movement actively, the muscle may not be functioning, either from intrinsic problems within the muscle or interruption in the neural pathway (central or peripheral).
- Examination of muscle strength[83]:
  - When the movement is strong and painful, there is a minor lesion in the muscle or tendon.
  - When the movement is weak and increases the pain, there is a major lesion that needs to be identified with further testing.
  - When the movement is weak but does not increase the pain, there is the possibility of either complete rupture of the muscle or tendon or a neurological disorder.

- When all resisted movements are painful, the pain may be organic, or the patient may be emotionally hypersensitive.
- When movement is strong and painless, the test results are normal.
- Assessment of bilateral neurological function:
  - Reflexes: peripheral lesions tend to diminish deep tendon reflexes (DTRs). CNS lesions tend to intensify DTRs and testing frequently elicits a clonic reaction.[84] Note any asymmetries in response.
  - Sensation: test light touch, sharp (noxious) touch, and vibration. Pressure on a nerve usually affects conduction on the large, myelinated fibers first. Therefore vibration is the first sensation to be diminished. Where there is decreased perception of touch and noxious stimuli, the lesion is more severe.[85] Note any asymmetries in response.
  - Allodynia and hyperalgesia: delineate areas of allodynia and hyperalgesia to touch, hot, and cold. Exact descriptions of these areas, along with areas of decreased perception of vibration, will provide information concerning A beta versus C fiber involvement in the production of pain.[85]
  - Stretch and pressure tests to nerve trunks.

It is not always possible to complete a pain evaluation in one session. Patients may not be able to tolerate all the required activities at one time, or there may be enough inconsistencies for the therapist to want a second appointment to refocus on specific tests. However, with the limitations on number of visits common with managed care, the therapist may feel pressured to identify a cause for the patient's pain in the initial visit. This is not necessary. It is far better to take more than one visit and be accurate than to take only one visit and develop a treatment plan that is not appropriate for the patient's needs.

REHABILITATION MANAGEMENT OF THE PATIENT WITH PAIN

There are three broad avenues of intervention for pain management: physical interventions, cognitive strategies, and behavioral manipulations.[86] Each avenue addresses a different aspect of the pain experience, and each requires a different level of participation from the patient.

Physical interventions are directed at the patient's body with the goal of healing the tissue injury. Examples include medication, surgery, and the therapy modalities. Physical interventions are of use most frequently with acute pain or recurrent pain resulting from reinjury. Physical interventions are often passive and, for the most part, soothing. When used long term, they promote dependence on the clinician. Therefore it is best to use them as a short-term adjunct in the overall treatment program.

Cognitive strategies are directed at the patient's thoughts with the goal of changing the patient's pain paradigms. Cognitive strategies include body scanning and reinterpretation of self-statements. Cognitive strategies are self-initiated and performed independently; therefore they encourage personal responsibility and independence.

Behavioral manipulations involve a behavioral change on the part of the patient to bring about the desired response. They include exercise, biofeedback, hypnosis, relaxation exercises, and operant conditioning. There is usually a brief learning period until the patient becomes proficient with these techniques; however, once learned, behavioral manipulations can be initiated and performed independently. Behavioral manipulations also encourage personal responsibility and independence.

A brief review of the benefits, indications, contraindications, and precautions for many of the interventions provided by therapists should provide an overview of the complexity of pain management.

The purpose of this section is to provide guidance in the selection of one treatment option over another so that intervention will be based on sound physiological principles. Readers who wish to explore an intervention in greater depth are directed to the references listed at the end of this chapter.

Physical Interventions

Thermotherapy

The physiological effects of heat depend on the method of application, the depth of penetration, and the rate and magnitude of temperature change. In the use of thermotherapy to control pain, several mechanisms have been established. Muscle spasm decreases as a result of decreased activity in gamma motor efferents, decreased excitability of muscle spindles, and increased activity of Golgi tendon organs.[87,88] This modality will often decrease peripheral pain. Ischemic pain is relieved by the influx of oxygen-rich blood into the dilated vessels, and muscle tension pain is decreased by interruption of the pain-spasm cycle. In addition, the pain threshold itself rises through gating at the spinal cord level.[89,90]

Several textbooks[91–95] on physical agents and rehabilitation discuss the physiological effects, precautions, contraindications, and method of application for these modalities. The reader is advised to refer to the textbooks for details.

Superficial heat can be applied by conduction, convection, or radiation. Conductive heating involves the exchange of heat down a temperature gradient by two objects that are in contact. The depth of penetration with conductive heating is usually 1 cm or less.[96] Moist heat packs and paraffin are examples of therapeutic conductive heating. Convective heating involves heat transfer through the flow of hot fluid. Therapeutic convective heating takes place during hydrotherapy and Fluidotherapy (Encore Medical Corporation, Austin, Texas). Molecules with a temperature greater than absolute zero are in an excited state and emit energy, thus creating radiant heat. Objects that are warmed by the energy are heated by radiation. Therapeutic radiant heat is applied with infrared or ultraviolet light. Because of the contraindications of ultraviolet light, this type of radiant heat is seldom used by therapists today in rehabilitation settings.

Patients can be taught how and when to apply superficial heat independently. Once they have demonstrated independence, responsibility for the application of superficial heat should be transferred to the patient or her or his caregiver.

The deeper tissues can be heated using conversion, the alteration of one form of energy into another. Examples of heating by conversion include use of shortwave diathermy or ultrasound.

During shortwave diathermy, the patient is placed into an oscillating magnetic field. The systemic ions create friction as they attempt to line up with the continuously reversing current, resulting in an increase in tissue temperature deep within the body. Shortwave diathermy is contraindicated for patients with metal implants because of the potential for the implant to become hot and burn the surrounding tissues. It is also contraindicated for patients with cardiac pacemakers because of the pacemaker's metal components and because the electromagnetic radiation may interfere with the pacemaker's operation. Shortwave diathermy should not be used for patients with cancer or multiple sclerosis or who are pregnant, and it should not be used over the eyes, the reproductive organs, or growing epiphyses. Female therapists should avoid prolonged exposure to shortwave diathermy because some research has demonstrated a possible negative effect on pregnancy outcome and fetal development.[97]

Ultrasound is another modality that heats deep tissues by conversion. As its name implies, ultrasound consists of sound waves delivered at a frequency too high to be perceived by human hearing. Sound

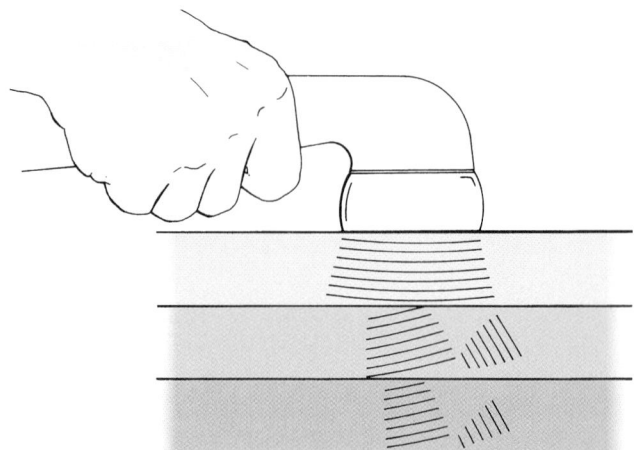

Fig. 30.6 The longitudinal wave of ultrasound is refracted at tissue interfaces where it encounters tissues of differing acoustical resistance. When the wave changes direction, energy is transferred to the tissues, resulting in the production of heat.

waves are repeatedly refracted as they encounter tissues of differing acoustical resistance while traveling through the skin toward the bone (Fig. 30.6). Tissues with high collagen content (tendon, ligament, fascia, and joint capsule) are heated more efficiently than tissues with low collagen content (fat, muscle). The extent of the temperature increase is related to the dose of ultrasound energy delivered. As the dose of ultrasound energy is increased by increasing the treatment duration or intensity, more energy is available to the tissues and the heating effect increases.[31] Moreover, the higher the frequency of ultrasound delivered, the more superficial the effect. Ultrasound delivered at 1 MHz heats tissues at depths to 5 cm, whereas ultrasound delivered at 3 MHz heats tissues in the upper 2 cm.[98]

The thermal effects of ultrasound can be used to increase tissue extensibility, cellular metabolic processes, and circulation; to decrease pain and muscle spasm; and to change nerve conduction velocity. The number of impulses traveling along the nerve decreases at low doses but begins to rise slowly beginning at 1.9 W/cm^2. Sounding of C fibers yields pain relief distal to the point of application, whereas sounding of large-diameter A fibers brings relief of spasm by changing gamma fiber activity, making the muscle fibers less sensitive to stretch.[99] Because it is impossible to treat C or A fibers selectively, ultrasound provides both pain relief and relief from muscle spasm, making it effective in the treatment of peripheral neuropathies, neuroma, and muscle spasm associated with musculoskeletal pathology, including sprains, strains, and contusions.[100]

In addition to thermal effects, ultrasound has nonthermal effects that come from the mechanical effects of the ultrasound wave on the tissues. Ultrasound causes cavitation, the development and growth of gas-filled bubbles, in the tissues. Ultrasound also causes tissue fluid to move or stream. The movement of fluid around the gas bubbles formed by cavitation is called microstreaming, and the movement of fluid within the ultrasound delivery area is called acoustic streaming. The nonthermal effects of ultrasound include accelerating metabolic processes, enzyme activity, and the rate of ion exchange, as well as increasing cell membrane permeability and the rate and volume of diffusion across cell membranes. These effects are thought to explain the role of ultrasound in enhancing the healing of soft tissue and bone.[101–103] The nonthermal effects of ultrasound can be achieved without raising tissue temperature by applying ultrasound in the pulsed mode.

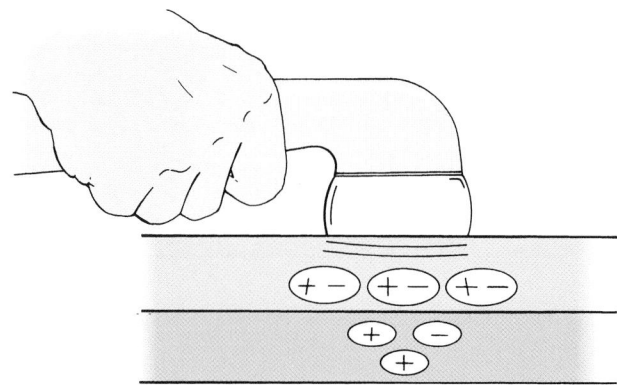

Fig. 30.7 Phonophoresis. Molecules of a substance are driven into the tissues by the ultrasound wavefront. They are not free for use by the body until they are broken down into chemical ions.

Phonophoresis is the use of ultrasound to deliver pain-relieving chemicals to the tissues. Chemicals are delivered to the cells by the ultrasound wave, where they are broken down into ions and taken up into the cells (Fig. 30.7). Common pain-relieving chemicals that can be administered with phonophoresis include 5% lidocaine ointment (Xylocaine) for acute conditions in which immediate pain relief is the primary goal, and 10% hydrocortisone cream or ointment for conditions in which pain is the result of inflammation.[104]

After phonophoresis, measurable quantities of these molecules have been found at tissue depths of up to 2 inches.[105] The contraindication to use of any chemical during phonophoresis is having an allergy to that chemical. Patients should be questioned about any adverse reactions to dental local anesthesia (lidocaine) or aspirin.

Cryotherapy

The physiological effects of cold make it superior to heat for acute pain from inflammatory conditions, for the period immediately after tissue trauma, and for treating muscle spasm and abnormal tone. Peripheral nerve conduction velocity in both large myelinated and small unmyelinated fibers decreases 2.4 m per degree centigrade of cooling. As a result, pain perception and muscle contractility diminish.[106] Peripheral receptors become less excitable.[106] Muscle spindle responsiveness to stretch decreases; as a result, muscle spasm diminishes.[99]

Local blood flow initially decreases, local edema decreases, the inflammatory response decreases, and hemorrhage is minimized. However, cold application for longer than 15 minutes results in increased local blood flow. Known as the "hunting response," this protective mechanism brings core temperature blood to the surface and prevents tissue injury resulting from prolonged cooling.[96] Cellular metabolic activities slow. The oxygen requirements of the cell decrease.[106]

As with heat, several precautions must be taken when using cold as a therapeutic modality. Cryotherapy is contraindicated in individuals with Raynaud phenomenon or cold allergy. Cryotherapy should not be used in individuals with rheumatic disease who, with the application of cold, have increased joint pain and stiffness. Cryotherapy should be used with caution in young, frail, or elderly individuals and those with peripheral vascular disease, circulatory pathological processes, or sensory loss.[107]

Cryotherapy is applied in three ways. Convective cooling involves movement of air over the skin (fanning) and is rarely used therapeutically. Evaporative cooling results when a substance applied to the skin uses thermal energy to evaporate, thereby lowering surface temperature. Most commonly, this substance is a vapocoolant spray. Conductive cooling uses local application of cold via ice packs, ice massage, or immersion. Cooling is accomplished as heat from the higher-temperature object is transferred to the colder object down a temperature gradient. Conductive cooling is the most commonly used form of therapeutic cold application.

Because muscles, tendons, and joints respond differently, the best method of cold application depends on which tissues are causing the pain.[108] Acute injuries are best treated with cryotherapy along with rest, compression, and elevation (RICE). Muscle spasm is decreased with cold packs and stretching. Trigger points, irritable foci within muscles, are best treated with vapocoolant spray, deep friction massage, and stretching. Tendinitis responds well to ice massage and exercise. Cold packs are often the only source of pain relief in acute disc pathology. The inflamed joints of rheumatoid arthritis frequently respond to cold packs or ice massage with decreased inflammation, increased function, and long-lasting pain relief.[107,109]

Patients and caregivers can be taught how and when to perform cryotherapy independently. Once they have demonstrated their proficiency, responsibility for the use of cryotherapy should be transferred to the patient or the patient's caregiver.

Transcutaneous Electrical Nerve Stimulation

TENS is the use of electricity to control the perception of pain. It appears that at a high rate TENS selectively stimulates the low-threshold, large-diameter A beta fibers, resulting in presynaptic inhibition within the dorsal horns,[110] either directly through the gating mechanism or indirectly through stimulation of the tonic descending pain-inhibiting pathways.[111] Research has shown that the neurons in the brain stem fire in synchrony with the TENS stimulation frequency,[112] and although the significance of this is not known at this time, it does indicate that the action of high-rate TENS is not limited to the dorsal columns. TENS delivered at a low rate is thought to facilitate elevation of the level of endogenous opiates in the CNS.[113]

Stimulation frequencies of 1 to 250 pulses per second (pps) decrease pain. Frequencies of 50 to 100 pps have proven most effective for sensory-level (high-rate) TENS, and frequencies of 2 to 3 pps are most effective for motor-level (low-rate) TENS.[41] Stimulation at exactly 2 pps causes an increase in the pain threshold.[64] As the frequency is decreased, more time is needed before the onset of relief, but the effects are more long-lasting.[114] Pulse width duration determines which nerves are stimulated. Sensory nerves are stimulated at widths of 20 to 100 ms, and motor nerves at 100 to 600 ms.[115]

There is a variety of modes of TENS delivery. Each mode relieves pain through a specific physiological mechanism and is therefore most beneficial for a specific type of pain.

When TENS impulses are generated at a high rate (greater than or equal to 50 pps) with a relatively short duration, the stimulation is referred to as *sensory-level* or *conventional* or *high-rate TENS*. Sensory-level TENS produces mild to moderate paresthesia without muscle contraction throughout the treatment area. Sensory-level TENS is thought to control pain through the gating mechanism in the spinal cord. The onset of relief is fast (seconds to 15 minutes)[41] because the gate is closed at the onset of stimulation. The duration of relief after stimulation stops is short-lived (at best up to a few hours). Sensory-level TENS has been found to be beneficial for acute pain syndromes and for some deep, aching chronic pain syndromes. (Refer to Chapter 31.)

Stimulation using high-rate and long-duration impulses is called *brief-intense TENS*. Brief-intense TENS decreases the conduction velocity of A delta and C fibers, producing a peripheral blockade to transmission.[41] Brief-intense TENS is useful in the clinical setting for short-term anesthesia during wound debridement, suture removal, friction massage, joint mobilization, or other painful procedures.

When the impulses are generated at a low rate (less than or equal to 20 pps) and have a relatively long duration (100 to 300 μs), the stimulation is referred to as *motor-level* or *acupuncture-like* or *low-rate TENS*. Motor-level TENS produces strong muscle contractions in the treatment area with or without the perception of paresthesia. Motor-level TENS is associated with deployment of endogenous opiates within the CNS. The onset of relief is delayed 20 to 30 minutes, presumably the time it takes to deploy the opiates. Relief frequently lasts hours or days after treatment. Because motor nerves are not stimulated in isolation, sensory fibers are also excited, causing the gating mechanism to come into play.[115] Motor-level TENS has been found to be beneficial for chronic pain syndromes and when sensory-level TENS has not been successful.

Modulating TENS parameters is one way to avoid the negative aspects of each of the treatment modes. Rate modulation is most commonly used to avoid neural accommodation during TENS. By setting the initial pulse rate so that, even with the programmed decrement, it will remain within the treatment range, there will be continuous variation in the stimulus, and neural accommodation will be avoided.

Width modulation is most commonly used with motor-level TENS. By setting the initial pulse duration so that, even with the programmed decrement, the impulses are able to recruit the desired motor units, there will be a continuous variation in perceived strength of the muscle contraction, rendering motor-level TENS more tolerable.

Stimulation in which the impulses are generated in pulse trains is called *burst TENS*. Burst TENS is another form of TENS modulation. The stimulator generates low-rate carrier impulses, each of which contains a series of high-rate pulses. Because burst TENS is a combination of high-rate and low-rate TENS, it provides the benefits of each. The low-rate carrier impulse stimulates endorphin release, and the high-rate pulse trains provide an overlay of paresthesia. The advantage to burst TENS is that muscle contractions occur at a lower, more comfortable amplitude, and accommodation does not occur. Burst TENS is beneficial whenever motor-level TENS cannot be tolerated and sensory-level TENS is ineffective because of neural accommodation.[116]

TENS, like all electrical stimulation, is contraindicated for patients with pacemakers, in the low back and pelvic regions of pregnant women, and over areas with thrombus. TENS should be used with caution for patients who have decreased sensation in the area being stimulated and for patients who have difficulty with understanding or expression. TENS electrodes should not be placed over areas of skin irritation, the eyes, or the carotid sinuses. It also should not be used in the immediate area of an operating diathermy unit.

TENS appears to be of greatest benefit for acute conditions with focal pain, chronic pain syndromes, postoperative incision pain, and during delivery. It has been found least effective with psychogenic pain[117] and pain of central origin.[118] For additional information on TENS, see Chapter 33.

Patients and caregivers can be taught how and when to apply TENS independently. Once they have demonstrated independence, responsibility for the use of TENS can be transferred to the patient or to the caregiver.

Iontophoresis

Iontophoresis is a process in which chemical ions are driven through the skin by a small electrical current. Ionizable compounds are placed on the skin under an electrode that, when polarized by a direct (galvanic) current, repels the ion of like charge into the tissues. Once subcutaneous, the ions are free to combine with the physiological ions, resulting in a physiological effect dependent on the characteristics of the ion (Fig. 30.8). Ionizable substances that are known to be effective analgesics include the following[119]:

- Five-percent lidocaine ointment (Xylocaine) administered under the positive electrode for an immediate, although short-lived,

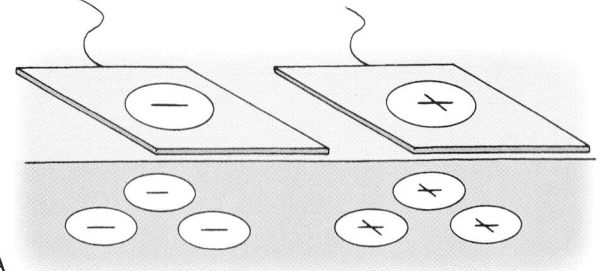
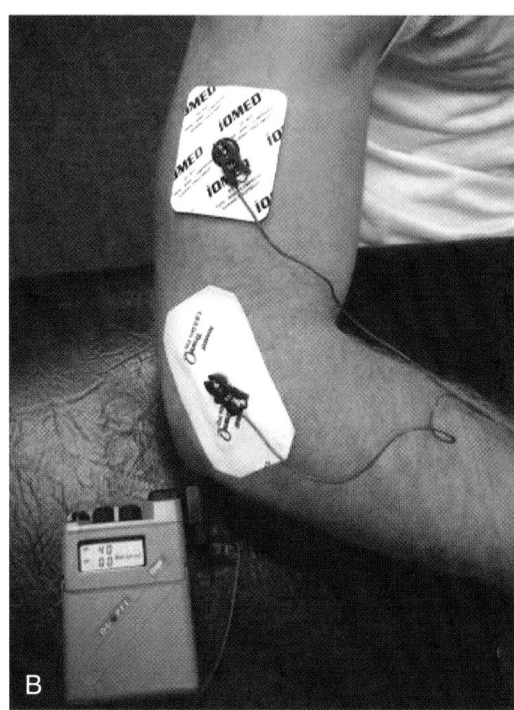

Fig. 30.8 Iontophoresis. (A) Chemical ions are driven into the tissues by a small electrical current. Once subcutaneous, they are immediately free to take part in chemical reactions within the body. **(B)** Iontophoresis treatment.

decrease in pain. Iontophoresis with lidocaine is recommended before ROM exercises, stretching, and joint mobilization and when immediate relief of acute pain (as in bursitis) is the object of treatment.

- One-percent to 10% hydrocortisone and dexamethasone administered under the positive electrode for relief of inflammatory pain in conditions such as arthritis, bursitis, or entrapment syndromes. Iontophoresis with hydrocortisone has a delayed onset but a prolonged effect, and it frequently eliminates the underlying cause of pain.
- Two-percent magnesium (from Epsom salts) administered under the positive electrode for relief of pain from muscle spasm or localized ischemia. High levels of extracellular magnesium inhibit muscle contraction, including the smooth muscle found in the walls of the vessels, leading to localized vasodilation.
- Iodine (from Iodex ointment [Lee Pharmaceuticals, South El Monte, California]) administered under the negative pole for relief of pain caused by adhesions or scar tissue. Iodine "softens" fibrotic, sclerotic tissue, thereby increasing tissue pliability.
- Salicylate (from Iodex with Methyl Salicylate [Lee Pharmaceuticals] or Gordogesic Creme [Gordon Laboratories, Upper Darby, Pennsylvania]) administered under the negative pole for relief of pain from inflammation. Salicylate is effective for arthritic joint inflammation, myalgia, and entrapment syndromes.

- Two-percent acetic acid administered under the negative pole to dissolve calcium deposits.
- Two-percent lithium chloride or lithium carbonate administered under the positive pole to dissolve gouty tophi. In both acetic acid and lithium iontophoresis, the insoluble radicals in the deposits are replaced by soluble chemical radicals so the deposits can be broken down through natural processes.

The contraindication to the use of any ion is an allergy to that ion. Because most patients will not have had iontophoresis previously, it is important to inquire about experiences that might indicate an allergy. For example, intolerance to shellfish may be the result of an allergy to iodine, and a poor reaction to dental local anesthesia may indicate a problem with lidocaine. Moreover, because iontophoresis involves the application of direct current, the likelihood of polar reactions under each electrode is greater than with electrical stimulations using alternating current (for example, TENS), and therefore the risk for skin burns is greater.

Massage

Massage has been recognized as a remedy for pain for at least 3000 years. Evidence of its beneficial effects first appeared in ancient Chinese literature, and then in the writings of the Hindus, Persians, Egyptians, and Greeks. Hippocrates advocated massage for sprains and dislocations as well as for constipation.[120]

Massage decreases pain through both direct and indirect means. Massage movements increase circulation through mechanical compression of the tissues, resulting in reflex relaxation of muscle tissue and direct relief from ischemic pain. Massage also indirectly stimulates A delta and A beta fibers, causing activation of the gating mechanism and the descending pain-modulating system.[44]

Massage movements are classified by pressure and the part of the hand that is used.[121] The two massage movements that may cause a decrease in pain include stroking (effleurage) and compression (kneading or pétrissage). Stroking involves running the entire hand over large portions of the body. Stroking causes muscle relaxation and elimination of muscle spasm or improved circulation depending on the depth and force of the strokes. Compression is applied with intermittent pressure using lifting, rolling, or pressing movements meant to stretch shortened tissues, loosen adhesions, and assist with circulation.

Massage is useful in any condition in which pain relief will follow the reduction of swelling or the mobilization of the tissues. These include arthritis, bursitis, neuritis, fibrositis, low back pain, hemiplegia, paraplegia, quadriplegia, and joint sprains, strains, and contusions. Massage is contraindicated over infected areas, diseased skin, and thrombophlebitic regions.

Patients or caregivers can be taught how and when to perform massage. Once they have demonstrated independence in the appropriate technique, responsibility for the performance of massage should be given to the patient or caregiver.

A specialized massage technique is lymphatic massage, which consists of light-pressure rhythmic strokes to encourage organizational flow of the lymphatic system. This type of massage can be beneficial with patients who have peripheral swelling with or without pain. A popular form of lymph massage called *manual lymphatic drainage* (MLD) is used after surgical procedures to reduce swelling (for example, mastectomy for breast cancer). Evidence-based studies show conflicting results regarding the efficacy of this technique, and more research needs to be done to validate it.[122–124]

Myofascial Release

Myofascial release (MFR) techniques are used to release the built-in imbalances and restrictions within the fascia and to reintegrate the fascial mechanism. The therapist palpates the various tissue layers,

beginning with the most superficial and working systematically toward the deepest, looking for movement restrictions and asymmetry. Areas of altered structure and function are then "normalized" through the systematic application of pressure and stretching applied in specific directions to bring about decreased myofascial tension, myofascial lengthening, and myofascial softening,[125] thereby restoring pain-free motion in normal patterns of movement. MFR is useful in treating musculoskeletal injuries, chronic pain, headaches, and adhesions or adherent scars.[126] MFR has been shown to be effective in the treatment of chronic prostatitis (CP) and chronic pelvic pain syndrome (CPPS) in conjunction with paradoxical relaxation therapy (PRT).[127] More research is needed to provide evidence regarding the efficacy of MFR in pain control.

MFR is contraindicated over areas with infection, diseased skin, thromboembolus, cellulitis, osteomyelitis, and open wounds. In addition, it should not be used with patients who have osteoporosis, advanced degenerative changes, acute circulatory conditions, acute joint pathology, advanced diabetes, obstructive edema, or hypersensitive skin.[126] (See Chapter 39 for more in-depth information regarding MFR.)

Joint Mobilization

Joint mobilization consists of passive oscillations that restore normal accessory movements.[128] In addition, the rhythmical repetition of the motions provides pain relief through the spinal gating mechanism.[129] Grades I and II oscillations are performed to maintain joint mobility and for pain relief, making them the choice for subacute conditions in which pain and potential loss of motion are the primary considerations. Grades III and IV oscillations are performed to increase joint mobility and are indicated for chronic conditions in which regaining lost motion is the goal. Grade V thrusts are performed to regain full joint mobility and have been recommended based on strong evidence for acute and chronic patients with low back pain.[13,128]

Joint mobilization is contraindicated with rheumatoid arthritis, bone disease, advanced osteoporosis, and pregnancy (pelvic mobilization), as well as in the presence of malignancy, vascular disease, or infection in the area to be mobilized.[64]

Light Therapy

Light therapy is described by Bot and Bouter[130] as a light source that generates extremely pure infrared light of a single wavelength. When applied to the skin, infrared laser light produces no sensation, and it does not burn the skin. Because of the low absorption, it is hypothesized that the energy can penetrate deeply into the tissues, where it is assumed to have a biostimulative effect.[92,130,131] It has been suggested that laser therapy may act by stimulating ligament repair,[132,133] producing antiinflammatory effects,[134] increasing production of endogenous opioids,[135] reducing swelling,[136] and influencing nerve conduction velocity.[137] To promote wound healing and manage pain, rehabilitation centers use lasers with power outputs less than 500 mW at a power density of 50 mW/cm^2 and wavelengths ranging from 600 to 1500 nm.[92] Contraindications to light therapy include exposing photosensitive areas, hemorrhagic areas, any area that has undergone 4 to 6 months of radiation treatment,[131] neoplastic lesions, and unclosed fontanelles in children; the abdomen of pregnant women; areas over the heart, the vagus nerve, or sympathetic innervations routes to the heart of cardiac patients; or, locally, endocrine glands.[92,131,138,139] In addition, exposure to the cornea of the eye is contraindicated, so protective eye equipment should be worn by the patient and the therapist. Caution should be used for areas with compromised somatosensation, the epiphyseal plates in children, the gonads, and infected areas and with patients displaying fever, epilepsy, or mental confusion.[92,131,138]

Therapeutic Touch

A description of therapeutic touch can be found in Chapter 39. Therapeutic touch has been effective in treating painful conditions resulting from anxiety and tension. In a report by Keller and Bzdek, 90% of individuals treated with therapeutic touch experienced tension headache relief, and 70% had continued relief for more than 4 hours; only 37% of the placebo group expressed sustained relief.[140] A meta-analysis and systematic review on therapeutic touch revealed that the available studies have varying approaches and protocols on therapeutic touch, subject selection, and description. Although most of these studies confirm the efficacy of the technique, several studies also have demonstrated negative or mixed results.[141] Therapeutic touch and other approaches are being more widely accepted; however, the therapist must continue to be diligent in using outcome studies to substantiate the use of any complementary therapy. (See Chapter 39 for additional information.)

Point Stimulation

Refer to Chapter 39 for an in-depth discussion of point stimulation. It is interesting to note that acupuncture points frequently correspond in location to trigger points, which are tight, elevated bands of tissue that are extremely sensitive when palpated and have a characteristic pattern of radiation of remote regions of the body. Trigger points appear to be areas of "focal irritability" that are myofascial in origin and are usually the site of small aggregations of nerve fibers that produce continuous afferent input when stimulated.

Needling therapies include trigger point injections (anesthetics, corticosteroids, Botox) and trigger point dry needling. Needling therapies are used in myofascial pain conditions. Trigger point injections are usually restricted to medical doctors and their professional support staff.[142] Trigger point dry needling consists of superficial and deep dry needling, and the exact mechanism of pain relief is not known. It is thought that needling and injections may trigger changes in the end plate cholinesterase and ACh receptors,[142] may involve central pain mechanisms, and may activate enkephalinergic, serotonergic, and noradrenergic inhibitory systems in association with A delta fibers through segmental inhibition.[142] Acupressure (i.e., finger pressure applied to acupuncture or trigger points) is thought to decrease their sensitivity through the same mechanism. The therapist applies deep pressure in a circular motion to each point for 1 to 5 minutes, until the sensitivity subsides. Pressure must be applied directly to each point for the treatment to be effective. Acupressure can be accompanied by a vapocoolant spray to provide additional sensory stimulation.

Sensitive points also can be stimulated using electricity. A point locator is used to identify points along the appropriate meridians that are sensitive to stimulation or more conductive to electricity. Each is then stimulated at the patient's level of pain tolerance for 30 to 45 seconds. The points farthest from the site of pain are treated first.

Points that are most sensitive to stimulation are beneficial sites for TENS electrode placement. When point stimulation alone does not provide enough pain relief, TENS can be used between sessions for continuous stimulation for more prolonged relief. (See Chapter 39 for additional information on electrical acupuncture.)

Cognitive Strategies, Including Cognitive Behavioral Therapy

The extent to which an individual perceives and expresses pain is a result of his or her emotional state, expectations, personality, and cognitive view. Each individual feels and responds to pain differently. Melzack and Wall[129] identified the following three nonphysical components of pain that interact and determine how an individual will respond to pain:

- The individual's sensory and discriminative interpretation of the pain

- The individual's motivation and attitudes relating to the pain
- The individual's cognitive and evaluative thoughts and beliefs concerning the pain experience

Cognitive strategies are part of a holistic approach to health that looks at the total person and the interaction among the three components of body, mind, and spirit. Cognitive strategies recognize that the mind is not separate from the body, accept that there is a mental component to pain, and use the inner resources of the mind to influence the pain experience.

Cognitive strategies work in two ways. First, they activate the descending cortical modulating systems, and second, they teach the individual to control, rather than be controlled by, the pain. Used in conjunction with other modalities necessary for physical relief, these approaches can play a significant role in long-term pain management and should not be overlooked in seeking a viable pain management alternative.

As mentioned previously, current research has given the medical community a much deeper understanding of chronic pain. Many new intervention approaches have been developed based on these new theories, and physical rehabilitation clinicians play a significant role in these new interventions. Of particular importance is the increasing role of clinicians in using cognitive behavioral therapy (CBT) in the management of individuals with chronic pain.[143] CBT for pain management involves the integration of cognitive, affective, and behavioral factors into the case conceptualization and treatment.[143] It is thought that a person's beliefs about pain are associated with various functional outcomes[144,145] and that changes in patients' beliefs about pain are related to changes in functioning.[146,147] Techniques potentially used may include coping skills, education and rationale about the course of an illness, relaxation, imagery, goal setting, pacing, distraction, and cognitive restructuring as well as homework assignments. A thorough discussion of this approach as it applies to physical rehabilitation is beyond the scope of this text. The work of Butler and Moseley provides clinicians a great resource on how to better explain pain to patients and patients, as well as how to use the most current evidence on pain science and chronic pain management in treating individuals with chronic pain.[148,149]

Relaxation Exercises

People who are in pain experience stress. Chronic stress can trigger increased pain. Both pain and stress cause an increase in SNS activity, including increased muscle tension. Relaxation exercises can bring about muscle relaxation and a generalized parasympathetic response.[150] Benson[151] has named this effect the *relaxation response* and reports that it is accompanied by an increase in alpha brain waves.

Relaxation reduces ischemic pain by normalizing blood flow to the muscles by making way for more oxygen to be delivered to the tissues. In addition, relaxation reduces muscle tension, resulting in an interruption in the pain-spasm cycle.[152]

Relaxation exercises all have two elements in common: a single focus and a passive attitude toward intruding thoughts and distractions. The end product of relaxation is a lowered arousal of the SNS and a lessening of the symptoms caused by or worsened by stress.[153]

Deep relaxation can be achieved through progressive relaxation and attention-diversion exercises. Progressive relaxation involves alternately tensing and relaxing the muscles until, eventually, the entire body is relaxed. This activity teaches the individual how to recognize and relieve muscle tension within the body.

Attention diversion is an active process in which the individual directs her or his attention to non-noxious events or stimuli in the immediate environment to achieve distraction from the pain. Attention diversion is categorized as passive or active. Passive attention diversion includes meditation and involves concentrating on a visual or auditory stimulus rather than the painful sensation, whereas active attention diversion involves active participation in a task (e.g., serial subtraction).

Meditation involves quieting the mind and focusing the attention on a thought, word, phrase, object, or movement. The individual becomes more alert to the constant stream of conversation taking place within the mind. Meditation calms the body through the relaxation response and keeps the attention focused in the present moment. Individuals in Eastern cultures have traditionally focused on a mantra, a word with spiritual meaning; however, there are no rules for where to focus the attention. The word or object should bring the individual a sense of peace and should allow the attention to be pleasantly directed toward the immediate moment.

Imagery is another form of attention diversion. During imagery the individual uses his or her imagination to produce images with pain-weakening potential. This can take two forms. In one, the individual imagines experiences that are inconsistent with the pain (e.g., imagining rolling in snow to alleviate burning pain). In the other, the individual imagines experiences that modify specific features of the pain experience (e.g., imagining that the pain is the result of a sports injury or that the sensation is "numbness" rather than pain).

Attention diversion works by activating the relaxation response and by diverting the individual's attention from the pain. However, attention diversion also has been found to activate the higher brain centers and may have an inhibitory effect on pain through the spinal gating mechanisms.[54,86] Lautenbacher and colleagues[154] found that individuals who used attention diversion for pain management reported decreased intensity and unpleasantness of their pain.

Patients can be taught to perform relaxation exercises independently and should be encouraged to perform them regularly because the benefits of these exercises are gained through regular practice.

Body Scanning

Patients with chronic pain frequently become one with their suffering; they do not view themselves as individuals with pain, but rather as painful individuals. Body scanning is a technique that endeavors to separate the individual from the pain.[155]

During body scanning, the patient is taught to achieve a meditative state, and then to focus attention on each body area, one area at a time. The patient is instructed to breathe into and out from each area, relaxing more deeply with each exhalation. When the area is completely relaxed, the patient "lets go" of the region and dwells in the stillness for a few breaths before continuing. Painful areas are scanned in an identical manner as nonpainful areas. The patient notes, but does not judge, changes in sensation, thoughts, and emotions during scanning of each area.

Individuals who practice this technique report new levels of insight and understanding concerning their pain experience. They separate the pain experience into the following three parts[155]:

- An awareness of the pain sensation and their thoughts and feelings about it
- An awareness of a separation between the pain sensation and their thoughts and feelings about it
- An awareness of a separation between themselves and their pain, because they are able to examine objectively the sensation and their thoughts and feelings about it

Once patients have accepted that they are not their pain or their reaction to the pain, they can determine how much influence and control pain will have in their lives.

Studies of chronic pain patients at the Stress Reduction Clinic at the University of Massachusetts Medical Center revealed that 72% of patients who used body scanning along with traditional medical interventions experienced at least a 33% reduction on their McGill-Melzack Pain Rating Index score.[155] In addition, at the end of an 8-week training period, the individuals perceived their bodies in a more positive light, experienced an increase in positive mood states, and reported major improvements in anxiety, depression, hostility, and the tendency to be overly occupied with their bodily sensations.

Humor

Ever since Cousins[156] reported in his book *Anatomy of an Illness* that he used humor to manage pain and enhance sleep during his illness, the role of humor in healing has been well studied. Humor has been found beneficial for both acute and chronic pain management.[111,157]

Laughter increases blood oxygen content by increasing ventilation. It helps to exercise the heart muscle by speeding up the heart rate and enhancing arterial and venous circulation, resulting in more oxygen and nutrients being delivered to the tissues.[158] Laughter decreases serum cortisol levels (cortisol levels increase with stress and are thought to have a negative effect on the immune response)[159,160] and increases the concentration of circulating antibodies.[158] As little as 10 minutes of belly laughter a day has been found to decrease the erythrocyte sedimentation rate and provide 2 hours of pain-free sleep.[159] Finally, laughter releases energy and emotional tension and is followed by generalized muscle relaxation.[158,161]

Therapeutic humor can be used to provide distraction from pain and as a coping mechanism to decrease the anxiety and tension associated with chronic pain. The muscle-relaxing effect can be used to interrupt the pain-spasm cycle.

Therapeutic humor should not be used with individuals who do poorly with humor. This includes individuals who despise or misunderstand humor, individuals who find joy threatening or guilt-inducing, and narcoleptic individuals who become cataleptic with laughter.[162]

Very few patients will benefit from all these cognitive strategies, and it may take some trial and error to find the appropriate cognitive strategy for an individual patient. Some patients will have no difficulty learning and practicing cognitive strategies, whereas others will not be able to perform any of these techniques independently. It may be beneficial to provide the patient with an individualized relaxation tape or to have the patient repeat coping affirmations over and over throughout the day. The success of cognitive strategies is dependent on applying the appropriate strategy to the appropriate patient and fine-tuning the strategy so that it matches the patient's needs.

In conclusion, it is important to reemphasize that all individuals with chronic pain have some degree of emotional or cognitive involvement, or both, in their pain experience. Many patients will live with pain regardless of the treatment they receive. Therefore it is imperative for health care practitioners to address the emotional and cognitive components of each patient's pain to allow her or him to function at the highest level and as comfortably as possible and to find joy in each day.

General Conditioning Through Exercise

Deconditioning is a major source of disability with chronic pain. Pain causes an intolerance for activity, which in turn leads to physiological and pathological changes in the organ systems. Exercise improves overall functional performance by improving ROM, muscle strength, neuromuscular control, coordination, and aerobic capacity, as well as offering higher self-esteem.

All three types of exercise are beneficial for pain management. ROM and stretching exercises restore normal joint mobility and correct muscle tightness. The joints are held in normal alignment and are subjected to normal stresses during movement. ROM and stretching exercises are indicated where there is decreased mobility.

Strengthening exercises increase muscle strength and cardiovascular endurance. When performed with high intensity for a short duration, strengthening exercises result in increased muscle mass, improved neuromuscular control, and improved coordination. When performed at low intensity for a long duration, they increase the aerobic capacity of the muscles.

Aerobic exercises improve cardiovascular fitness. More oxygen is supplied to the tissues because there is an increase in the number and size of capillaries and a decrease in the diffusion distance between the capillaries and the muscles. The tissues use oxygen more efficiently, and the individual has a higher energy level.

All exercise has an analgesic effect through the gating mechanism by stimulation of the A delta neurons and a pain-modulating effect through activation of the descending systems. Exercise of enough intensity has been known to increase circulating β-endorphin levels, but exercise-induced β-endorphin alterations are related to the type of exercise and special populations tested and may differ in individuals with health problems.[163,164]

It is important to include exercise in all pain management programs. Patients should be taught the appropriate exercises beginning with the first treatment session and encouraged to perform the exercises consistently when not at therapy. The ultimate end product of movement intervention is to empower the patient to modulate and control all functional activities, enabling that individual to participate in life.

Operant Conditioning

Coping strategies are learned. Individuals with chronic pain express their pain with behaviors that provide them with consistent positive rewards. For example, wincing might result in attention from a family member, or limping might allow the individual to avoid performing a particular task. Over time, the individual with pain becomes conditioned to perform certain behaviors for the behavior's rewards rather than as a reaction to the pain. Similarly, individuals with chronic pain also can condition their nervous systems through learning. If an individual expects to experience pain as the result of a particular level of activity, the individual will always experience pain at that level of activity.

Operant conditioning addresses the learned (or conditioned) aspects of pain.[165] Operant conditioning involves unlearning or separating the behavior and the response from the pain experience. If the goal of treatment is to lessen social reinforcement of the patient's pain behaviors (and thus extinguish those behaviors), the patient and the family or other involved individuals are shown how their behaviors and responses provide social reinforcement for the patient's reaction to pain. The involved individuals are provided with specific new responses to the patient's behavior. Family members might be instructed to ignore wincing, groaning, or the verbal report of pain. They might be told not to perform activities that are the patient's responsibility just because the patient reports pain. In time, the patient will become conditioned to the new response, and pain in those situations will diminish.

If the goal of treatment is to increase the patient's pain-free activity level, operant conditioning can be used to condition the nervous system to a higher level of activity before responding with pain. If the patient's usual pattern is to remain active until the onset of pain (negative reinforcement for activity) and then rest (positive reinforcement for pain), the patient is instructed to remain active to just below the pain threshold and then rest (positive reinforcement for activity). In this way the nervous system unlearns the connection between activity and pain, and the patient's activity level increases.

Hypnosis

Hypnosis is a state in which the body and conscious mind are deeply relaxed while the subconscious mind remains alert, focused, and open to suggestion.[153] This has been demonstrated physiologically by electroencephalography (EEG), which shows an increase in the number of theta waves, which are associated with enhanced attention.[166] When a hypnotized individual is given a suggestion that is in alignment with his or her existing belief system, it is accepted by the subconscious mind as reality. The suggestion is not filtered through the conscious mind, which is critical and judgmental. Hypnosis allows the individual to bypass her or his critical beliefs.[167] For example, if the individual believes that a certain activity will cause pain (critical belief), that activity is sure to cause pain. If, however, during hypnosis, the individual accepts the suggestion that the activity does not cause pain, the pain may decrease and even disappear.

When hypnosis is used for pain management, a patient is first assisted to achieve complete relaxation, then given suggestions that reinterpret the pain experience. For example, a patient might be guided to reframe the pain into a messenger and then be encouraged to listen to its message to gain understanding of the meaning behind the pain. Or a patient might be guided to view the pain as an indication to stop a particular activity to avoid being injured. Or a patient might be instructed to feel less pain. Finally, where harmless activities have become painful through learning, the patient can be guided to disconnect the activity from his or her pain.

Biofeedback

Biofeedback is a training process in which the patient becomes aware of and learns to selectively change physiological processes with the aid of an external monitor. A monitoring instrument is placed on the appropriate area of the body. The machine provides an initial readout. The patient is instructed how to change the monitored process, and as change occurs, the machine "feeds back" that information. By mentally changing a biological function, the patient learns to gain control over it. In time, the patient learns to control the process without needing an assist from the instrument.

Muscle tension, pulse rate, blood pressure, skin temperature, and electromyography (EMG) and EEG readings are some of the physiological processes that can be consciously modified with biofeedback.[150]

Biofeedback is proving to be an effective pain management tool for headaches, muscle spasms, and other physical dysfunction that leads to or increases chronic pain (see Chapters 33 and 39).

GENERAL TREATMENT GUIDELINES

As noted earlier, chronic pain management using the medical model has not been found effective. Treatment limited to correcting pathology promotes dependence on the therapist, as well as making full resolution of symptoms the measure of success.

The ICF model addresses the functional losses associated with impairments. Therapeutic interventions are not focused on pathology, but they are directed at improving the individual's function and preventing or improving disability. This does not mean that the impairment is ignored, however. Most times, addressing the individual's functional losses involves treating the impairments that caused them.

For example, patients with chronic pain frequently become sedentary, leading to the impairments of limited ROM, muscle weakness, and deconditioning. These factors can then, of themselves, cause pain, creating a cycle that spirals upward until the individual becomes disabled. During therapy, interventions are directed at the impairments with the goal of restoring function. Therapeutic interventions are selected based on their ability to improve functional outcome.

Impairments that do not affect function do not become the focus of therapy; therapeutic interventions that do not address functional deficits are not used.

The development of an appropriate treatment plan may seem overwhelming when the therapist is confronted with a patient who has chronic pain that has not responded to previous interventions or who has a chronic condition that has pain as one of its characteristics. The key is to identify the patient's functional deficits and then develop a treatment plan that addresses the causes of those deficits. In some cases, this may mean not treating the pain itself but rather its causative factors.

For example, if the patient has chronic pain because of joint hypomobility, the treatment plan includes interventions to increase joint mobility. Conversely, if the patient's pain is caused by joint hypermobility, the treatment plan includes interventions to increase support around the hypermobile joints. Merely addressing the joint pain by applying modalities will do little to resolve the pain because it does nothing to correct the precipitating cause.

When a patient has pain because of a chronic disease and the treatment plan will include instruction in pain-relieving interventions, it is important for the therapist to understand the specific causes of the pain to select the appropriate intervention. For example, pain from rheumatoid arthritis most commonly is the result of either joint inflammation or biomechanical stress on unstable joints. A patient would be instructed in pain-relieving modalities for the former and instructed to wear splints to support the joints for the latter. One intervention would not be appropriate for both causes.

CASE STUDIES

Case Studies 30.1 to 30.3 demonstrate a problem-solving approach to the treatment of patients with chronic pain.

CASE STUDY 30.1   Fibromyalgia

K. E. is a 35-year-old computer programmer with a diagnosis of fibromyalgia. She reports a 6-month history of generalized muscular pain and fatigue that increase when she performs repetitive motions or holds a position for a prolonged period. K. E. is currently unable to work because she is no longer able to perform data entry without increased neck and shoulder pain. She states she awakens from pain and leg cramps several times during the night. She awakens each morning with a headache and low back pain; she does not get much relief from pain medication. K. E. states she has not been out with friends in several months. She states she is "nervous, unable to concentrate, and depressed." She has been evaluated by several physicians. All medical test results are negative.

K. E.'s objective examination reveals pain on digital palpation of distinct points in the muscles of her neck and shoulder girdles, over both lateral epicondyles and greater trochanters, in her gluteal muscles, and just above the medial joint lines of the knees. Pain is referred from the tender points distally. K. E. sits and stands with a forward head and elevated protracted shoulders, and her cervical ROM is restricted slightly at end range because of her posture and muscle guarding. Muscle strength is 4/5 throughout. All other musculoskeletal and neurological test findings are normal.

K. E. demonstrates the impairments of pain, poor posture, decreased cervical and shoulder ROM, and decreased endurance, resulting in the activity limitations of interrupted sleep and decreased tolerance for activity and participation restrictions of inability to work at her profession.

The long-term goals of treatment for K. E. are independence with self-management of pain, normalization of posture, restoration of normal sleep, independence with a home exercise program, and return to work and appropriate social activities. The short-term goals include decreasing K. E.'s pain, helping her to achieve proper sleep positioning, correcting her postural abnormalities, improving her limited endurance, and assessing and correcting the ergonomics of her workstation. K. E. also needs intervention to address the emotional and cognitive aspects of her condition.

The lowered pain threshold and magnified pain perception seen with fibromyalgia result from a complex combination of muscle tissue microtrauma, neuroendocrine abnormalities, and changes in the levels of CNS neurotransmitters. The muscles of individuals with fibromyalgia show abnormal energy metabolism, poor tissue oxygenation, and localized hypoxia. Their blood shows decreased levels of the inhibitory neurotransmitter serotonin and increased levels of the facilitatory neurotransmitter substance P. This combination, which is unique to fibromyalgia, is thought to cause changes in the dorsal horn neurons and eventually in the areas of the brain responsible for the sensory-discriminative and affective-motivational aspects of pain.[52]

Fibromyalgia pain has been shown to respond favorably to interventions that work through the gating mechanism. These include sensory-level TENS, light massage, muscle warming, and gentle stretching. K. E. can be taught to apply localized heat or to take a warm bath before gentle stretching of her tight muscles. She should be cautioned to stretch slowly to the point of resistance and to hold the stretch for 60 seconds to allow the Golgi tendon organs time to signal the muscle fibers to relax. Quick stretching to the point of pain will cause increased tightness and pain through the pain-spasm cycle. It is important for K. E. to understand that these measures address the pain of fibromyalgia but do not have any long-term effect on the course of her condition.

Individuals with fibromyalgia, and most individuals with chronic pain, experience a variety of emotions, including depression, anger, fear, withdrawal, and anxiety.[168] These individuals have been helped with hypnosis, biofeedback, and cognitive restructuring.[52,168] In addition to giving them a sense of control over their pain, these interventions are known to bring about an increase in the individual's level of endogenous opiates, thereby activating one of the descending pain modulation systems. K. E. can be taught to perform these techniques independently.

K. E. should be asked to demonstrate her sleeping posture. Because the muscles of individuals with fibromyalgia do not relax easily, K. E. should be shown how to use pillows to support her neck and back so that they are encouraged to relax while she sleeps. This will help to decrease the frequency of morning headaches and back pain and help her to sleep through the night. She might also benefit from a warm bath before going to bed.

K. E.'s therapist can use gentle MFR to help correct the biomechanical imbalances causing her poor posture. K. E. can then be taught to selectively stretch the shortened muscles of her neck and shoulder girdles using the technique already described and to selectively strengthen their weakened antagonists using light resistance. To counter deconditioning, K. E. should be placed on a nonimpact aerobic program (walking, pool exercises, or stationary bicycle) with a goal of 30 minutes three to four times a week at 70% maximum heart rate (220 minus her age). If she is unable to tolerate 30 minutes of exercise at one time, she can be started at 3 to 5 minutes twice or three times daily and gradually progressed to three sessions of 10 minutes, then two sessions of 15 minutes, and finally one session of 30 minutes. K. E. may require a significant amount of coaxing and education to motivate her to participate in exercise; many individuals with fibromyalgia do not wish to move because movement initially increases their pain.

Before she returns to work, K. E. should be assisted with the ergonomics of her workstation. Research[169] has shown that individuals who work at computers need to vary their positions throughout the day even if their sitting posture is appropriate. Further research[87,170,171] has shown that correct mouse placement is important to minimize stress to the arms and shoulders.

CASE STUDY 30.2 Phantom Limb Pain

A. R. is a 60-year-old carpenter who underwent below-knee amputation of his right leg 4 weeks ago after a motor vehicle accident. He now reports a constant burning, piercing, throbbing sensation in the distal portion of his missing limb. He states that immediately after the amputation, he was aware of an itching or tickling in the missing portion of the leg, but the sensation gradually changed to pain. He notes that the leg feels as if it is shortening, as if the missing foot is moving closer and closer to his hip. A. R. has been fitted with a shrinker but does not wear it because of fear of increasing the pain. He does not believe he will be able to wear a prosthesis and is concerned because his employer will be unable to find work for him if he is wheelchair-bound.

A. R.'s objective examination reveals a healing surgical incision and a poorly shaped stump. Right lower-extremity hip and knee strength are 3/5 and 2+/5, respectively. Sensation to light touch is diminished in the area of the incision. All other musculoskeletal and neurological test findings are normal. A. R. ambulates short distances using a walker but relies on a wheelchair for locomotion outside his home.

A. R. has the diagnosis of a below-knee amputation and demonstrates the impairments of phantom limb pain and decreased strength in the right lower extremity, resulting in the functional limitations of inability to prepare his leg for a prosthesis, inability to ambulate, and inability to work in his profession.

The long-term goals of treatment for A. R. are independent use of a prosthesis and return to work with modified job tasks. The short-term goals include resolution of his phantom limb pain, preparation of his stump for a prosthesis, at least 4/5 right hip and knee strength, and, when appropriate, gait and balance training with the prosthesis.

There are two theories of the cause for phantom limb pain. At one time it was thought that it occurred as the result of the formation of a terminal neuroma at the site of the amputation[21]; however, this theory did not explain phantom phenomena in individuals with congenital amputations or individuals with complete spinal cord injuries who also experience painful and nonpainful sensations in their missing or anesthetic limbs. This led researchers to look at the role of the CNS in phantom phenomena, and the latest theories suggest the previously described changes in the dorsal horn neurons and changes in the spinal cord caused by the sudden loss of afferent impulses after amputation.[172]

These theories are supported by the effectiveness of interventions that stimulate the large nerve fibers and provide inhibitory input through the gating mechanism. Phantom limb pain is relieved by stroking, vibration, TENS, ultrasound, heat applications, and the use of a prosthesis. A. R. can be taught a progressive desensitization program. He should be encouraged to wear the shrinker both to prepare his stump for a prosthesis and to decrease pain. Because phantom limb pain is adversely affected by emotional stress, exposure to cold, and local irritants, he should be taught to avoid these factors as much as possible.

A. R.'s adjustment to a changed body image, a changed lifestyle, and the use of a prosthesis can be aided with any of the cognitive strategies described previously. He might also benefit from referral to an amputee support group.

It is important for A. R. to be aware of his abilities and limitations so that he remains safe when he returns to work. If appropriate, the therapist should accompany A. R. to his job and perform a job task analysis, making suggestions for necessary modifications. If this is not possible, the therapist could discuss needed modifications with A. R. based on his descriptions of his job tasks.

CASE STUDY 30.3 Complex Regional Pain Syndrome

P. S. is a 45-year-old right-handed secretary who sustained a Colles fracture of the right wrist 6 months ago. The wrist was placed in a cast for 6 weeks, during which time P. S. avoided using the extremity. Two weeks after the cast was removed, P. S. developed pain, swelling, and stiffness in the wrist and hand. She returned to her physician who diagnosed CRPS type I. She has received four sympathetic nerve blockades. The first provided 4 weeks of pain relief. The second and third provided 2 weeks of relief each. She has just received her fourth injection along with a referral for therapy.

P. S. is wearing a sling. She has 30-degree flexion contractures of her right fingers, along with swelling and stiffness of the wrist and hand. Her right wrist, elbow, and shoulder show limited motion as well. P. S. describes constant burning pain that becomes worse with any stimulation, even air blowing over the skin. She rates her pain as 4/10 since the block, but she states that the pain had slowly been escalating toward 10/10 before the injection. Her hand and wrist are cool, and the skin appears mottled and shiny. P. S. states that she is not using her arm and needs assistance at home for activities of daily living and household chores.

P. S. demonstrates the impairments of pain, swelling, stiffness, and decreased ROM of the right wrist and hand. These impairments cause activity limitations, decreasing her ability to use the right upper extremity for any functional activities, including activities of daily living, job tasks, and homemaking activities. In addition, because she is not using the extremity and carries the arm in a sling, P. S. is at risk for developing shoulder-hand syndrome.

The long-term goal of treatment for P. S. is restoration of pain-free use of her right upper extremity. The short-term goals include quieting the SNS, decreasing P. S.'s pain and edema, and restoring normal ROM of the shoulder, elbow, wrist, and hand.

Successful treatment of CRPS involves a coordinated effort by the physician and the therapist. The treatment of choice is interruption of sympathetic activity with nerve blocks and movement therapy.[173]

Interventions included in a pain management program for CRPS should be chosen for their ability to quiet the SNS as well as accomplish the desired outcome. For example, thermotherapy is more beneficial than cryotherapy because of its ability to decrease pain without stimulating a sympathetic response.[173]

A successful rehabilitation program for CRPS cannot be limited to therapy visits. Patients need to be instructed in interventions that they then perform three, four, or even five times daily. Therefore the therapist needs to become a guide, with the responsibility for performing the pain management program given over to the patient or caregiver.

Pain reduction is the first priority. This can be accomplished through the gating mechanism or through the deployment of endogenous opiates. Thermotherapy and TENS have both been found effective for pain management with CRPS. If P. S. cannot tolerate electrode placement on the right arm, the electrodes can be placed on the opposite arm or along the spinal roots of the involved segments.[41,119] P. S. can be instructed in any of the superficial heating modalities. Stroking massage along the paravertebral muscles beginning in the cervical region and continuing to the coccyx has also been found effective in quieting the SNS.

Before P. S. can regain mobility of her wrist and fingers, the edema must be resolved. This can be accomplished with elevation, massage, lymphatic drainage, and compression. P. S. can wear a compression glove or, if she is able to tolerate it, receive intermittent compression to the arm. She should be instructed to keep the arm above heart level as much as possible.

P. S. should be advised to discontinue use of the sling and begin frequent weight bearing through her arm. Immobility increases the symptoms of CRPS. Movement of the extremity is important to increase proprioception and circulation, both of which have an inhibitory effect on the SNS.[173] Therefore P. S. should

CASE STUDY 30.3   Complex Regional Pain Syndrome—cont'd

be encouraged to begin using her hand as much as possible throughout the day. If she is reluctant to use the arm, the therapist can design a functional activity program that allows her to use the arm during simple activities, which can be progressed as her symptoms improve.

There are two forms of exercise that are beneficial in CRPS. The first is active ROM exercises, which should be performed frequently throughout the day within the pain-free range to regain motion, increase circulation, and provide non-nociceptive input. Exercise of the specific ROM should be within functional activities. The activity itself will encourage ROM while the patient is concentrating on successfully completing the activity itself. The second form of exercise is stress loading,[174] which involves active compression and traction activities without joint motion. For example, P. S. can use a coarse-bristled brush to scrub

a piece of plywood and apply as much pressure as possible without causing pain (compression activity). Or she can carry a briefcase or purse in her affected hand (traction activity). Compression and traction both provide increased proprioceptive input.

P. S. should also begin performing desensitization activities, which can be modified as she is able to tolerate more stimulation to her extremity. P. S. may benefit from biofeedback to gain control over the circulation in her arm and from relaxation activities to stimulate the relaxation response and enhance parasympathetic function.

Once P. S. becomes independent in the performance of her program, therapy can be decreased to once or twice weekly to monitor and modify her pain management regimen.

ACKNOWLEDGMENTS

We would like to acknowledge the contribution of Linda Mirabelli-Susens to the writing of this chapter in the fourth edition of the textbook.

REFERENCES

To enhance this text and add value for the reader, all references are included on the companion Evolve site that accompanies this textbook. This online service will, when available, provide a link for the reader to a Medline abstract for the article cited. There are 174 cited references and other general references for this chapter, with the majority of those articles being evidence-based citations.

31

Electrophysiological Testing and Electrical Stimulation in Neurological Rehabilitation

Alain Claudel, Arvie Vitente, Miguel Garcia, Rossniel Marinas, and Rolando T. Lazaro

OBJECTIVES

After reading this chapter the student or therapist will be able to:

1. Identify electrophysiological tests performed on patients with neurological or muscle disorders.
2. Describe the instrumentation and general procedures for electrophysiological testing.
3. Recognize normal and abnormal findings of various electrophysiological tests.
4. Recognize the differences in instrumentation, signal processing, and interpretation when performing electrophysiological testing versus kinesiological electromyographic testing.

5. Differentiate the basic mechanism underlying functional neuromuscular stimulation, electrical stimulation, and electromyographic biofeedback.
6. Describe the appropriate instrumentation, signal processing, and interpretation for kinesiological electromyographic testing.
7. Describe the indications and contraindication for the use of neuromuscular stimulation, electrical stimulation, and electromyographic biofeedback.

KEY TERMS

electromyographic feedback
electroneuromyography

functional electrical stimulation
kinesiological electromyography

nerve conduction velocity
neuromuscular electrical stimulation

The goal of this chapter is to enhance the clinician's ability to recognize indications for the most commonly used electrophysiological tests and to integrate knowledge of these test indications and findings into the management of patients with neuropathological or myopathic dysfunction. The first section presents a basic description of the electrophysiological tests, including nerve conduction studies (NCSs), electromyography (EMG), kinesiological electromyography (KEMG), and the underlying neuroanatomical structures being tested. Normal and abnormal findings are discussed, with emphasis on how knowledge of these tests can assist the therapist in patient evaluation. The second section provides an introduction to the physiology, indications, contraindications, equipment, and applications of electrical muscle stimulation (EMS), neuromuscular electrical stimulation (NMES), and electromyographic biofeedback (EMGBF). The information integrates electrotherapeutic interventions into program planning for common neurological body system problems, their subsequent functional limitations, and perceived decrease in quality of life. Published evidence examining efficacy is included to assist the therapist in making choices about the use of these tools in the clinic. The third section provides a series of four case studies that illustrate the usefulness of electromyographic testing in patients with a variety of medical diagnoses.

ELECTROPHYSIOLOGICAL TESTING

Physical therapists (PTs) are uniquely positioned to understand and perform electrophysiological testing. This is because PTs examine patients with pain, numbness, and/or weakness and also because they

have a superior knowledge of neural and muscular anatomy and physiology. Electrophysiological testing is a sensitive and specific tool designed to assist in the diagnosis and the development of treatment plans for patients with diseases of the peripheral nervous system (PNS) and of the muscle itself.[1]

An informed perspective on the application of these tests will benefit the physical therapist's interaction and communication with other members of the medical team. At the completion of the electrophysiological consultation, the clinician who performed the test generates a report. Understanding this report can guide decisions in planning and modification of intervention programs or will assist in referring to other health care practitioners. A review of components of such report follows.

Electrophysiological tests are usually performed by neurologists, physiatrists, and PTs who have education, training, and experience in these procedures. Most PTs practicing in the area of clinical electrophysiology are board certified by the American Board of Physical Therapy Specialties.[2] Some states (such as California) require additional licensing.

The general goal of electrophysiological testing is to answer the following questions:

- Is there a lesion in the PNS and/or muscles?
- Where precisely is that lesion (nerve, neuromuscular junction, muscle)?
- What is the extent of the lesion (myelin, axons or both)?

Most of the electrophysiological tests described involve the application of an external electrical stimulus to a nerve or muscle and observation and assessment of the muscle or nerve response. Other tests such as needle EMG and single-fiber electromyography (SFEMG) involve the monitoring and recording of the electrical activity produced by the muscle tissue at rest or during contraction.

The electrophysiological tests most commonly used are motor and sensory NCSs, including F-wave and H-reflex latency measurements; repetitive stimulation; somatosensory evoked potential (SSEP) tests; and needle EMG. Most often, a patient referred for electrophysiological testing will undergo at least two motor nerve conduction tests, at least two sensory conduction tests, and at least one limb needle EMG. The American Association of Neuromuscular and Electrodiagnostic Medicine (AANEM) has published evidence-based guidelines, which may be found on the AANEM website at http://www.aanem.org/Practice/Practice-Guidelines.[3] A review of the patient's history, a relevant systems review, and a physical examination guide the examiner in the selection and sequencing of appropriate tests. In other words, muscle strength and tone, sensation, range of motion (ROM), cranial nerve assessment, reflex testing, neurological signs, and cognition are crucial in selecting and administering electrophysiological tests. Most subject matter experts consider electrophysiological testing as an extension of the clinical examination.[4,5] It does not replace a careful history and physical examination of the patient. It does, however, establish the precise state of the nerves and muscles and can thus determine the location of a lesion more precisely than the clinical examination alone, particularly in cases of mild weakness or ill-defined sensory changes. In very clearly defined pathologies, electrophysiological tests are not necessary (except perhaps for medico-legal reasons). For example, in the case of a unilateral ankle dorsiflexion weakness coupled with a clearly defined L5 nerve root compression on magnetic resonance imaging (MRI) of the lumbar spine, the electrophysiological test may be of little added value. However, for a similar clinical presentation (foot drop) and no clear-cut imaging, the electrophysiological tests will differentiate between a fibular palsy, a sciatic nerve neuropathy, a lumbosacral plexopathy, or an L5 radiculopathy.

Finally, evidence-based practice recommends that the practitioner have a good understanding of the implication of the sensitivity and specificity of each test to rule it in or out for a specific condition.[6]

Anatomical Review

In order to best understand the systematic interpretation of data from the electrophysiological examination of nerves, the reader is invited to review the following foundational principles. These are explored in much greater detail elsewhere in this text.

At the Cellular Level

A nerve is composed of axons covered with a sheath of myelin. Depolarization inside the axon is an "all-or-nothing" phenomenon in which an action potential moves along the surface of the cell membrane. This action potential is an electrical wave caused by a flow of ions across the cell membrane. A local current opens a sodium channel, allowing Na^+ ions to rush inside the cell. The electrical resistance to this wave is inversely proportional to the diameter of the axon. Larger nerves conduct faster than smaller nerves. In order for efficiency as an organism to be achieved, nerve conduction must be fast. In complex organisms with billions of axons, increasing the nerve diameter is not a viable option; hence, the role of the myelin sheath. The myelin is produced by Schwann cells. These are special satellite cells that separate axons from the endoneural fluid. The myelin acts as a capacitor: the conduction "jumps" between gaps in the myelin called *nodes of Ranvier*. This saltatory conduction allows human nerves to be 50 times smaller but conduct four times faster than unmyelinated nerves.[7] Consequently, recording and analyzing the *conduction velocity* of nerves primarily reflect on the state of the myelin. The amplitude of the response (if a

supramaximal stimulation is delivered) is a reflection of the number of axons available to the stimulation.

The physiology of the nerve is such that when there is an injury to the axon, the portion of the axon distal to the injury will degenerate (Wallerian degeneration). This is important because all muscles innervated by branches of the nerve distal to the lesion will show signs of denervation approximately 11 days after the lesion. Consequently, assessing a patient too early after a lesion may lead to false-negative results.[7,8]

At the Anatomical Level

The accurate performance and interpretation of the electrophysiological test—particularly the needle EMG—is significantly contingent on knowledge of the precise innervation of each muscle. As an example, an ulnar neuropathy at the elbow (UNE) clinically may be indistinguishable from a C8 radiculopathy. However, the astute clinician will remember that the cell body of the sensory nerve lies in the dorsal root ganglion, which is typically not involved in a radiculopathy. The therapist will also know that the abductor pollicis brevis is a C8- and median nerve–innervated muscle. Consequently, an ulnar nerve neuropathy is distinguishable from a C8 radiculopathy in that the ulnar sensory test will have decreased amplitude in the UNE and the abductor pollicis brevis will be denervated in the C8 radiculopathy. As a matter of fact, the clinician will keep in mind the innervation of each muscle while conducting the test. Electrophysiological testing is hence a dynamic process during which the choice of the next nerve to test or muscle to sample is predicated on the result of the previous test.[7,8]

As a result, the electrophysiological examination is not a single, stereotyped investigation but an evolutionary one during which several tests (nerve conduction, both sensory and motor, and EMG of several muscles) can be applied to a clinical presentation.[4,9]

Nerve Conduction Tests

A general overview of NCSs is presented to provide an understanding of their application and indications. Many excellent texts are available for details of the techniques.[10–14]

Motor and sensory NCSs can provide data that are helpful in establishing the presence and location of pathological conditions in the PNS. The tests may indicate the anatomical level, such as a plexopathy, versus a localized peripheral mononeuropathy. Individual and multiple nerves may be assessed, and the findings compared with responses of the same nerves contralaterally. The site of pathology may be localized, such as median nerve compression at the wrist versus a lesion of the lateral cord of the brachial plexus.

Nerve conduction velocity is faster in myelinated fibers because of saltatory conduction. Disorders involving peripheral demyelination can thus be differentiated from impairments primarily involving axonal degeneration. A mild localized compressive disorder (neurapraxia) may be distinguished from a more severe lesion in which the axons and surrounding connective tissue have been completely disrupted (neurotmesis).[12,15] In the event that the findings of nerve conduction studies (NCS) and EMG are normal, the clinician may be able to rule out most conditions involving the PNS and look for central nervous system (CNS) or other pathology. Knowledge of the rationale for NCSs and EMG should help the therapist decide when the tests may be indicated and understand the reasoning behind reports of tests that have already been performed on patients.

Motor Nerve Conduction

In motor NCSs the peripheral nerve is stimulated at various sites and the evoked electrical response is recorded from a distal muscle supplied by the nerve (a measure of orthodromic conduction). Surface

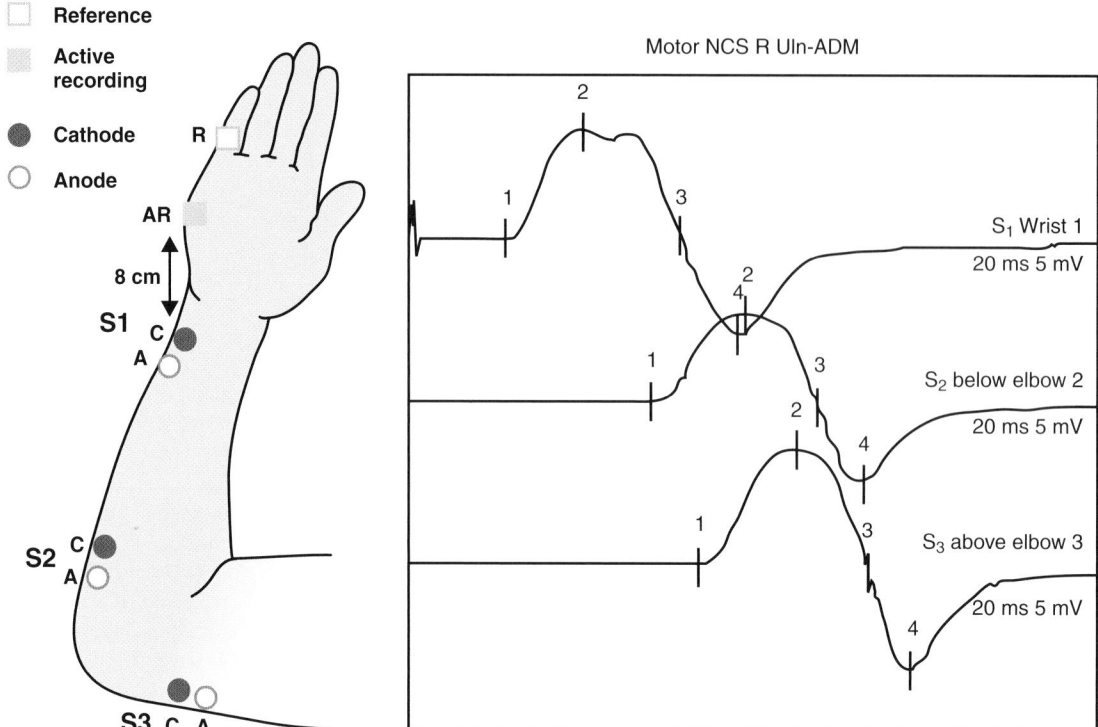

Fig. 31.1 Electrode Location for Ulnar Motor Nerve Conduction. *AR,* Active recording.

electrodes are usually used for both stimulating and recording. An example of electrode configuration for a motor NCS is shown in Fig. 31.1 (ulnar nerve study). The response represents the electrical activity of muscle fibers under the recording electrodes and is called the *compound muscle action potential* (CMAP). It is also called the *M wave* or *M response.* Measurements are taken of the latency (the time in milliseconds required for the impulse to travel from each stimulus site to the recording site) and the amplitude of the response in milli-volts (mV). The shape and duration of the response are assessed, and motor nerve conduction velocity is calculated for each segment of interest by dividing the distance between stimulus sites (in millimeters) by the difference in latency measured at each respective site.

Velocities, latencies, and the shape and amplitude of the responses (Fig. 31.2) are studied and compared with established normal values and often with values taken from tests of the uninvolved extremity (when possible). In infants and children, nerve conduction is slower than in adults and reaches adult values by age 4 years.[14] Nerve conduction velocities gradually slow after 60 years of age but generally remain within the outer limits of normal.[12,14]

Sensory Nerve Conduction

Sensory nerve conduction can be measured from many superficial sensory nerves, such as the superficial radial and sural nerves. It can also be measured from mixed motor and sensory nerves. The stimulus is applied over the nerve in question, and the recordings taken from electrodes placed over a distal sensory branch of the nerve. The recordings are called *sensory nerve action potentials* (SNAPs). An example of recording and stimulation sites is shown in Fig. 31.3. Both ortho-dromic and antidromic conduction can be assessed. Response latencies and amplitudes are measured, and sensory nerve conduction velocities are calculated for each segment by dividing the distance between two adjacent stimulus and recording sites, or two stimulus sites, by the

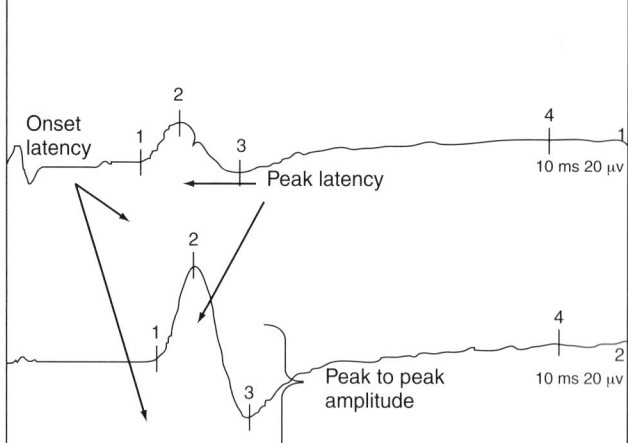

Fig. 31.2 Velocities, Latencies, and the Shape and Amplitude of the Responses.

latency (conduction time) between these same sites. Sensory nerve responses are considerably smaller than motor responses. Their ampli-tudes are generally measured in microvolts (μV). Sensory conduction velocities may be calculated with just one stimulation as, contrary to motor studies, there is no neuromuscular junction to account for in sensory nerves. Sensory recordings are more sensitive than motor recordings in cases of mixed sensory-motor neuropathies.

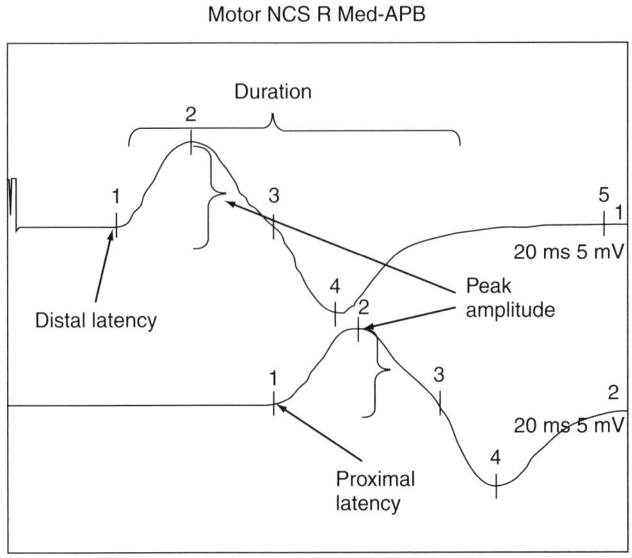

Motor NCS R Med-APB

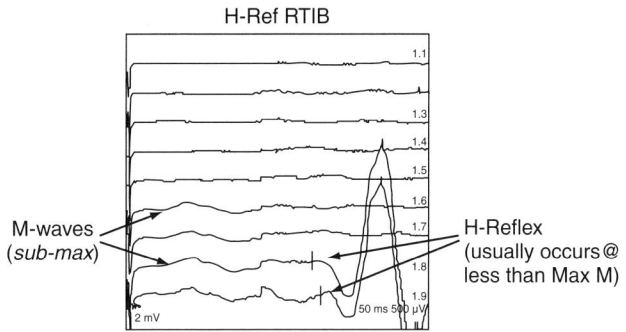

Fig. 31.3 Example of Recording and Stimulation Sites.

F-Wave Latency

When a motor nerve is stimulated in the periphery, both orthodromic (peripherally to the muscle) and antidromic (centrally toward the spinal cord) impulses are generated. A proportion of the antidromic impulses will, as it were, "bounce off" the axon hillock and return as a recurrent discharge along the same neurons to activate the muscle from which the recording is taken. This activity is termed the *F wave* (Fig. 31.4), and it is observed as a small wave occurring after the M wave.[12,14,15] No synapse is involved. Thus the F wave is not a reflex response, but rather only a measure of conduction along the motor neuron. Specific conditions of electropotential must exist at the soma-dendritic cell membrane to reactivate the efferent axon; therefore the occurrence of the F-wave response is inconsistent and variable in latency and waveform.[16]

The F-wave latency can be useful in evaluating conduction in conditions usually involving the proximal portions of the peripheral neurons (e.g., radiculopathy, Guillain-Barré syndrome, or thoracic outlet syndrome [refer to Chapter 18]). Its value, however, has been questioned by some authors because of its variability. Normal values of F-wave latency are 22 to 34 msec in the upper extremity (stimulating at the wrist) and 40 to 58 msec in the lower extremity (stimulating at

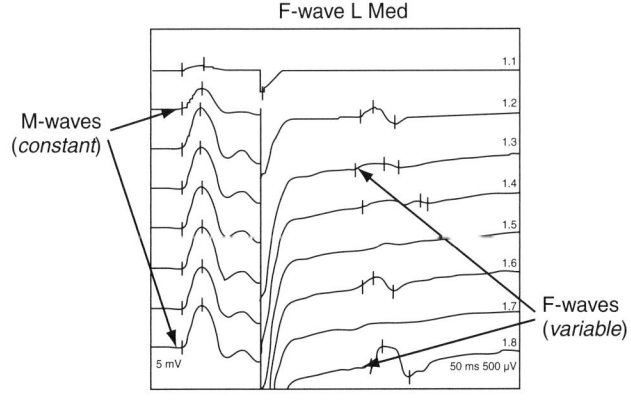

Fig. 31.4 Example of F-Wave Study.

H-Ref RTIB

Fig. 31.5 Example of H-Reflex Study.

the ankle), depending on the height of the subject, with a bilateral difference in latency of no greater than 1 msec.[17]

H-Reflex Response

The H-reflex response latency (Fig. 31.5) is a measure of the time for action potentials elicited by stimulating a nerve in the periphery to be propagated centrally over the Ia afferent (sensory) neurons to the posterior horn of the spinal cord, to be transmitted across the synapse to α in the anterior horn of the spinal cord, and then to travel distally over these neurons to activate the muscle. The response therefore measures conduction in both the afferent and efferent neurons.[12,14] It is also referred to as a "late" response (the other being the F wave).

The H reflex is constant in latency and waveform, and it occurs with a stimulus usually below the threshold level required to elicit the M-wave response (Ia afferent fibers are larger in diameter than α and thus more sensitive to electrical stimulation [ES]). This monosynaptic reflex response is most easily found by stimulating the tibial nerve at the popliteal area and recording from the soleus muscle. Braddom and Johnson[18] reported a mean latency of 29.8 msec (±2.74 msec) for the tibial nerve in normal adults, and a bilateral difference of no more than 1.2 msec. The H-reflex latency is a valuable measure of conduction over the S1 nerve root in differentiating suspected proximal plexopathy and radiculopathy from a herniated disc or foraminal impingement. Sabbahi and Khalil[19] have reported a technique for recording the H reflex from the flexor carpi radialis muscle when stimulating the median nerve. In normal human beings older than 1 year, the H reflex is usually seen only in the tibial, femoral, and median nerves. It can be elicited from several nerves in infants and in conditions of CNS dysfunction in adults.

Repetitive Stimulation Tests

The repetitive nerve stimulation (RNS) test is used to evaluate transmission at the neuromuscular junction (motor synapse) in patients with diffuse weakness. RNS tests are helpful in the differential diagnosis of disorders such as myasthenia gravis and Lambert-Eaton myasthenic syndrome (LEMS). One protocol uses a series of supramaximal electrical stimuli applied to a peripheral nerve at a distal site (e.g., median or ulnar nerve at the wrist) at a rate of three to five per second for five to seven responses. Changes in amplitude of the muscle response are assessed. Precise technical requirements are specified to prevent movement artifacts and other testing errors. Detailed descriptions of the RNS test can be found in other texts.[12,20] Under normal conditions the amplitude does not change more than 10% from that of the initial response in a series of 10 stimuli recorded before and after resistive exercise. An amplitude decrease in the fifth or sixth response of more than 10% is considered abnormal and is compatible with a physiological defect at the postsynaptic receptor site of the neuromuscular junction, as in myasthenia gravis. Because myasthenia gravis most often involves facial muscles, a muscle of choice of the RNS is the nasals muscle.

In another RNS protocol, stimuli are applied to a nerve, first at a slow rate, then at a faster rate, usually 10 to 20 per second for up to 10 seconds. Normally, the amplitude can decrease up to 40% from the initial amplitude. In some defects at the presynaptic site, the response may be lower than normal during a slow stimulation rate but show a significant amplitude increase at the higher rate. Increases in amplitude greater than 100% over the initial response are consistent with presynaptic neuromuscular junction defects such as seen in LEMS, which has a strong association with small-cell bronchogenic carcinoma, and in botulism. In 1957 Eaton and Lambert[21] reported this phenomenon as a myasthenic syndrome.

Gilchrist and Sanders[22] reported another protocol referred to as a *double-step RNS test.* This test measures amplitude before and after a temporarily induced ischemia of the extremity. They found the double-step RNS test to be slightly more sensitive than the routine RNS test, but only 60% as sensitive as the SFEMG technique. The RNS test is a good alternative test for neuromuscular transmission when the SFEMG is not available, but the examiner must meticulously adhere to technical details when conducting the test.

Blink Reflex

In some conditions (e.g., facial palsy) or to establish the presence of a widespread neuropathy, it may be necessary to assess the conduction in the cranial nerves. The stimulation of the supraorbital nerve (branch of the trigeminal nerve, cranial nerve V) elicits two separate responses of the orbicularis oculi muscles, one early and ipsilateral (R1) and one late and bilateral (R2), via the facial nerve (cranial nerve VII). The early R1 response involves a synapse in the pons, whereas the late bilateral R2 responses involve a more complex pathway involving the pons and lateral medulla. Analysis of the respective latencies of each response will help in determination of the following:

- Trigeminal neuralgia (cranial nerve V) or Guillain-Barré: all responses delayed
- Acoustic neuroma or Bell palsy (cranial nerve VII): ipsilateral responses delayed
- Pontine lesion: absence of R1
- Medullar lesion: absence of R2

Hence, the blink reflex is a nerve conduction test that assesses a portion of the CNS and has shown some utility in assisting in the diagnosis of multiple sclerosis (see Chapter 19) and Wallenberg syndrome.[8]

Clinical Evoked Potentials

Electrical potentials elicited by stimulation of nerves or sense organs in the periphery can be recorded from various sites as the impulses are transmitted centrally along the neuronal pathway and from the representative area of the brain.[12,23–25] SSEP procedures are particularly useful in assessing the integrity of afferent pathways in the CNS. They are helpful in differentiating among lesions in areas such as the plexus, spinal cord, brain stem, thalamus, and cerebral cortex. Evoked potential tests have the advantage of providing data about the integrity of both peripheral and central neuronal pathways, including transmission across axodendritic synapses.

The SSEP is valuable in assessing damage and continuity of spinal cord tracts in early spinal cord injury (SCI). For example, if an electrical stimulus is applied at the popliteal area over the tibial nerve, responses can be recorded with surface electrodes placed over the spine at the L3 and C7 spinal segments and from the lumbar representation of the contralateral sensory cortical area. Conduction time and other

parameters of the response waveforms can be measured from the recordings.

This simplified example of an SSEP illustrates how conduction over sensory peripheral nerves and afferent pathways to the cerebrum can be studied. The median nerve is usually tested to evaluate the integrity of peripheral and central pathways and their synaptic connections as the impulses travel from the upper extremity to the contralateral cortical area.

In visual evoked potential (VEP) procedures, visual stimuli such as variable light flashes of changing patterns are applied to one or both eyes under highly controlled conditions. The response is recorded from the scalp over the representative area of the cerebral cortex.[12,24,25] The term *pattern reversal evoked potentials* (PREPs), a more descriptive term for these procedures, is recommended by the American Electroencephalographic Society.[23] These tests and other VEP procedures are useful in assessing pathology of retinal photoreceptors, the optic nerve, and postchiasmal pathways. Abnormal conduction findings have been reported when VEP studies are used in demyelinating disorders such as multiple sclerosis and optic neuritis. The examiner may conclude that the patient is cortically blind because no response is recorded on the visual cortex. Although many causes for a stimulus not reaching the visual cortex are possible, the end result is considered blindness. If the cause for cortical inactivity is swelling or a neurochemical imbalance within a nuclear relay structure, once corrected, the individual may experience normal vision. A change in the reaction of the patient to the visual environment may reflect increased awareness and a change in coma scale rating. Similarly, just because an individual turns toward a light or visual stimulus does not mean an evoked potential reaches the visual cortex. Instead, the eyes as receptors and the visual tract to the brain stem may be intact even though a problem in the synaptic connections between or within the thalamus and visual cortex may exist.

Auditory evoked potential tests are used to evaluate neurological function of the cochlear division of the auditory nerve (eighth cranial nerve), central auditory pathways and synapses in the brain stem, and the receptor areas on the cerebral cortex.[12,23–25] Brain stem auditory evoked potentials are frequently referred to as BAEPs. A series of high-intensity clicks is applied to auditory receptors in the ears through headphones, and several components of the response waveforms are recorded by using surface electrodes over the representative cortical areas. The BAEP is an effective test procedure for localizing and evaluating acoustic neuromas and other space-occupying lesions in the brain stem. This test is also used for assessment of brain damage in patients who are comatose as a result of traumatic brain injury (TBI). Robinson and Rudge[26] recommend caution in using BAEP tests for this purpose because other factors, such as defective receptor organs, can cause abnormalities in BAEPs.

The evoked potential tests described in this chapter all require application of appropriate external stimuli that are rapidly repeated many times. The response is electronically averaged to sort out the desired signal from interference signals. The conduction times (latencies), waveform shape and amplitude, and sometimes conduction velocities are measured and compared with normal values. Absence of a response, increased latencies, decreased amplitudes, and slowing of conduction velocities are all abnormal findings. Normal values and details of techniques for the evoked potential tests are described elsewhere.[12,23–25]

Therapists with special interest and training administer the SSEP tests for neurological applications more frequently than other types of evoked potential tests. Because of the highly specialized techniques necessary to administer VEP tests for ophthalmological applications and BAEP tests for hearing dysfunction, they are usually performed by persons who specialize in these procedures.

Needle Electromyography

Needle EMG complements the motor and sensory NCSs; it is most sensitive in the detection of denervation.

Unlike NCSs, which use the ES of the motor nerves to elicit muscle contraction, the needle EMG is used to record and analyze muscle activity at rest and during voluntary activation. It is particularly useful in identifying pathology of the lower motor neurons and of the muscle itself. EMG can also be used to identify abnormalities of motor neuron recruitment that are associated with certain disorders of the CNS, especially when NCS findings are normal—as would be the case in radiculopathies. The primary recording studied is the insertional activity, along with activity at rest and the motor unit action potential (MUAP), which is produced by the depolarization of single motor units during voluntary or reflex activity. Spontaneous electrical activity of single muscle fibers at rest is termed *fibrillation* and is diagnostic of denervation. For recording of muscle activity, small-diameter needles are inserted within the muscles to be studied. Three electrodes are required: active (negative), reference (positive), and ground. The needles may be *monopolar,* requiring a second needle or surface electrode for reference, or *bipolar,* containing both the active and reference electrodes (usually concentric in cross section). The ground electrode is typically placed on the surface of the skin. Most commonly the needles used are disposable. The activity detected in the muscle is displayed on the video display terminal of a computer (and can be stored and printed later). It is simultaneously played through an audio amplifier. The electromyographer can often identify pathological conditions by the characteristic "sounds" of the electrical activity of the muscle. Many excellent resources are available for readers interested in details of the equipment and procedures for EMG.[10–12,27,28] Details of contraindications and special precautions are described by Currier and Nelson.[28]

In an EMG examination, four conditions are evaluated at each location: (1) activity during needle insertion (normally a brief burst [250 msec at most] of high-frequency activity that abates when the needle stops moving), (2) activity during rest (electrical silence is normal unless an electrode is placed directly over a motor endplate), (3) activity during minimal and gradually increasing voluntary contraction (biphasic or triphasic MUAPs of small amplitude composed of slow-twitch type I fibers that increase in frequency and are joined by higher-amplitude potentials as larger, predominantly fast-twitch type II motor units are recruited), and (4) activity during maximal activation (an *interference pattern* caused by the blending of potentials in which individual MUAPs cannot be identified), characterized as full (complete), reduced, or absent. Several locations in an individual muscle may be studied. The specific muscles to be studied are determined by clinical findings, and results must always be interpreted in the context of the total complex of signs and symptoms. In determining the specific location of a lesion, muscles located both proximally and distally to the suspected lesion site must be assessed. Studies may be repeated at intervals to determine if changes consistent with recovery (such as reinnervation) or exacerbation are present. EMG is typically used to help determine the presence (and extent) of the following:

- Denervation
- Reinnervation
- Myopathic or neuropathic signs
- Distribution or specific location of peripheral nerve pathology

Needle EMG is sensitive in determining the state of the axons. When axons are interrupted, there is denervation of the muscle cell. The findings in denervation and partial denervation include increased insertional activity, fibrillation potentials or positive sharp waves at rest, and a reduced or absent interference pattern. CNS dysfunction can result in no resting potentials, but if motor control was impaired, a decreased or abnormal interference pattern might be apparent because of difficulty in recruitment (Fig. 31.6). Needle EMG also informs the clinician about muscle cell disorders such as myopathies. The primary

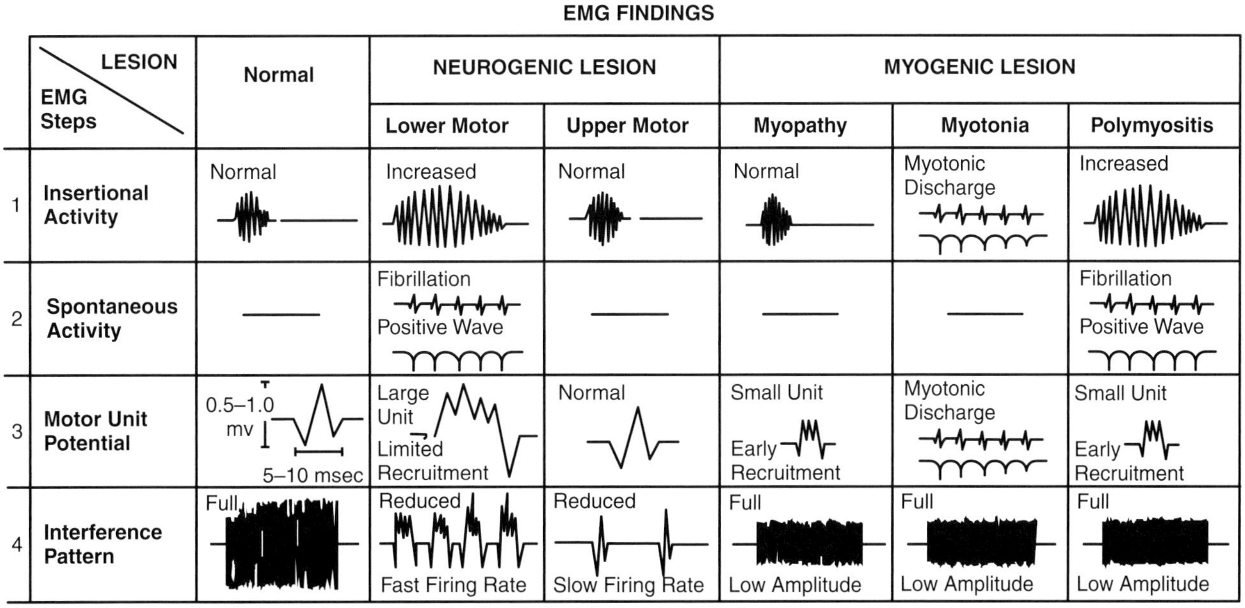

EMG FINDINGS

LESION / EMG Steps	Normal	NEUROGENIC LESION		MYOGENIC LESION		
		Lower Motor	Upper Motor	Myopathy	Myotonia	Polymyositis
1 Insertional Activity	Normal	Increased	Normal	Normal	Myotonic Discharge	Increased
2 Spontaneous Activity		Fibrillation / Positive Wave				Fibrillation / Positive Wave
3 Motor Unit Potential	0.5–1.0 mv / 5–10 msec	Large Unit / Limited Recruitment	Normal	Small Unit / Early Recruitment	Myotonic Discharge	Small Unit / Early Recruitment
4 Interference Pattern	Full	Reduced / Fast Firing Rate	Reduced / Slow Firing Rate	Full / Low Amplitude	Full / Low Amplitude	Full / Low Amplitude

Fig. 31.6 Typical findings in lower and upper motor neuron disorders and myogenic lesions. Myotonia shares many features common to myopathy in general in addition to myotonic discharges triggered by insertion of the needle or with voluntary effort to contract the muscle. Polymyositis shows combined features of myopathy and neuropathy, including (1) prolonged insertional activity, (2) abundant spontaneous discharges, (3) low-amplitude, short-duration, polyphasic motor unit potentials, and (4) early recruitment leading to a low-amplitude, full-interference pattern. *EMG,* Electromyography. (From Kimura J. *Electrodiagnosis in Diseases of Nerve and Muscle: Principles and Practice.* 3rd ed. New York; Oxford University Press; 2001.)

finding in the case of a myopathy is fibrillation potentials and small-amplitude polyphasic MUAPs.

Although patient cooperation during EMG testing is important, some aspects of muscle electrical activity can be studied in the patient who is very young (infant), who is unable to move, or who has only involuntary or reflex activity. Insertional and resting potentials can always be evaluated. MUAPs appear during the contraction of muscle fibers activated both voluntarily and involuntarily in both isotonic or isometric conditions. In normal conditions MUAPs are seen with voluntary movement; however, reflex activation of muscle also produces MUAPs with certain normal characteristics. In CNS disorders, hypertonic or spastic muscles will produce recognizable MUAPs when they are actively contracting. The electromyographer can elicit a contraction by tapping on the muscle or tendon. For example, consider a patient who is recovering from a traumatic head injury with residual spastic hemiplegia. She is unable to cooperate with the EMG exam. The patient has abnormal extensor responses in the lower extremity with the exception of the ankle and foot, which appear flaccid. An EMG of the leg and foot muscles detects abnormal resting potentials, including fibrillation and positive sharp waves in muscles innervated by the fibular nerve. Tapping on the muscles fails to elicit MUAPs. Muscles in the tibial nerve distribution have no resting potentials and respond with bursts of identifiable MUAPs when the tendon is tapped. These findings would guide the physician and therapist in looking for a possible peripheral nerve lesion in addition to the CNS dysfunction. The treatment program in this situation would differ from that for a patient without peripheral nerve pathology.

In summary, results of the needle EMG are best presented in the form of a table that indicates the following:

- Insertional activity: may be increased in acute denervation and myopathic processes
- Spontaneous activity at rest: present (positive sharp waves and fibrillation potentials) in denervation
- Fasciculations: may be present in motor neuron disorders
- Analysis of MUAPs:
  - Amplitude: Low amplitude is seen in myopathy or nascent potential; large amplitude is a sign of chronicity.
  - Phases: Normal MUAPs are biphasic or triphasic. Polyphasia is indicative of denervation-reinnervation.
  - Recruitment pattern: A less-than-full recruitment is indicative of fewer motor units discharging, as can be seen in axon loss.
  - Firing rate: If elevated, fewer motor units are contracting more often to provide the same tension in a denervated muscle.

Justification and analysis of the basic principles and results after EMG studies should assist therapists managing patients with neurological dysfunction in planning and modifying therapeutic management programs. As electrical tests are being conducted, the findings are continuously studied and used by the physician and examiner as a guide in continuing with or modifying the plan for future tests based on whether they fit the characteristics usually identified with specific pathological conditions. As previously stated, the results of the electrodiagnostic tests must be correlated with other clinical findings and data.

Summary of Clinical Electroneuromyographic and Nerve Conduction Studies

Instruments with computer-assisted analysis are now commonplace for studying electromyographic signals in great detail.[12,29–31] Parameters of the waveform, including amplitude, duration, frequency spectrum, number of turns, or phase polarity reversals and area (the integral or total voltage of the waveform), can be automatically analyzed. The data are then compared electronically with predetermined

patterns of electrical changes, which correlate with categories of neuromuscular disorders such as myelopathies and neuropathies.

The following is a summary of the more characteristic EMG and nerve conduction changes associated with selected groupings of neurological disorders. The intent is to assist in the understanding of reports of these studies and recognize changes that may be seen in sequential tests during the course of the disorders. The following is a simplified grouping of electrical changes; actual electrodiagnostic studies show considerably more detail and frequent variations of these findings.[10–12,27,28]

Electrical testing in CNS disorders typically shows normal motor and sensory nerve conduction. In the EMG, spontaneous activity is typically not seen, and individual motor units seen on muscle contraction usually have normal parameters. The recruitment pattern may show a slower-than-normal MUAP discharge frequency with an incomplete and irregular interference pattern. In the presence of tremor and other involuntary movements, bursts of MUAPs occur, consistent with the muscle contraction pattern. In cases involving the brain stem, the blink reflex may show abnormalities.[8] The tests are important in differential diagnosis between a CNS and a PNS problem, but often they are not used when clinical examinations demonstrate the problem to be definitively in the CNS.

In myelopathies, which include upper and lower motor neuron disorders (e.g., amyotrophic lateral sclerosis [ALS], poliomyelitis, cervical spondylitis, and syringomyelia), motor and sensory nerve conduction is usually normal, although mild slowing may be present.[12] Motor amplitudes may be decreased. The characteristic EMG changes, which usually appear in the more chronic stages of the disorders, are increased amplitude and duration of MUAPs because of the variable impulse conduction time in sprouting axon terminals. An increased number of polyphasic potentials with increased duration is usually found. Spontaneous activity is often seen, and on strong contraction fewer rapidly firing large MUAPs are recruited, resulting in a single-unit or partial interference pattern. Fasciculations and denervation potentials are typically found in ALS. The distribution of the EMG abnormalities determines the extent of the condition.

Peripheral neuropathies show a variety of electrical changes depending on the type and location of the pathology. In a proximal pathology (e.g., radiculopathy), motor and sensory nerve conduction generally remain normal, except F waves and H-reflex responses in specific spinal segments. If motor nerve roots are compromised, spontaneous activity and increased polyphasic potentials appear, and reduced recruitment of MUAPs results in an incomplete interference pattern. In more chronic stages MUAP amplitude and duration can be increased. As the lesion improves, spontaneous activity decreases and the recruitment patterns become more normal. If only sensory roots are injured, no EMG changes occur. Again, the distribution of the EMG abnormalities (all in one myotome) is pathognomonic, especially in the presence of denervation potentials in the corresponding paraspinal muscles.[32]

Lesions of peripheral nerves, which range from a focal mononeuropathy to plexopathy, frequently show abnormalities in motor and sensory nerve conduction, depending on which components of the nerve are involved. In the EMG, spontaneous activity, particularly fibrillation and positive sharp waves, is common. If the lesion is complete, no MUAPs are found. The presence of even a few MUAPs suggests a more optimistic prognosis. Often the location of the lesion can be identified by the distribution of the electrical changes. With regenerating axons, low-amplitude polyphasic MUAPs gradually appear. In the chronic stage, the amplitude and duration of MUAPs are often increased. Spontaneous activity decreases with reinnervation, but it may persist for several years.

Generalized, systemic peripheral polyradiculoneuropathies can be divided into primarily demyelinating, primarily axon loss, or mixed axonal-demyelinating polyneuropathies. Some involve mostly sensory nerves (e.g., hereditary sensory neuropathy types I to IV, Sjögren syndrome, Friedreich ataxia), and others mostly motor nerves (e.g., chronic inflammatory demyelinating polyneuropathy [CIDP], lead neuropathy), but most involve both sensory and motor nerves. In the primarily demyelinating type, such as Guillain-Barré syndrome, motor and sensory nerve conduction become markedly slow and F-wave latencies are delayed. EMG changes usually do not occur, except for a reduced recruitment pattern consistent with weak muscle contraction or conduction block (when the demyelination is such that the impulse does not propagate). With primarily axonal polyneuropathies, such as uremic neuropathy, isoniazid or cisplatin toxicity, and lead poisoning, motor and sensory nerve conduction is mildly slowed or may remain normal. The duration and amplitude of the response, however, decrease. During advanced stages, many polyneuropathies develop both demyelinating and axonal pathology (e.g., diabetic neuropathy, which is by far the most commonly encountered polyneuropathy). On EMG, spontaneous activity is commonly seen. These electrical changes generally become more severe with worsening of the pathology, but they also improve if the pathology is reversed. From a patient management standpoint, remyelination occurs at a much more expedient pace than reinnervation.[33–35]

Again, the scope of the NCS electromyographic test is to determine the presence and extent of a neurological dysfunction. Attributing a cause to the dysfunction (e.g., diabetes versus alcoholism) requires other tests.

With myopathic disorders, motor and sensory nerve conductions are generally normal unless neural tissue is also affected. In advanced stages, however, severely atrophied muscles can produce decreased amplitude and distorted nerve conduction responses. The characteristic findings on EMG are short-duration, low-amplitude potentials. Some spontaneous potentials, particularly fibrillations and positive sharp waves, may be found but are much more frequent in the inflammatory myopathies such as polymyositis. Specific myotonic potentials appear in certain myopathic disorders (e.g., myotonia congenita). The recruitment pattern shows many low-amplitude MUAPs, appearing in a full pattern, with little voluntary effort. This type of recruitment pattern is referred to as *early recruitment.*

Neuromuscular junction disorders involve the synapse between axons and myocytes. In LEMS, the pathology is in the presynaptic membrane (decreased release of acetylcholine [ACh]), whereas, in myasthenia gravis, the pathology involves the postsynaptic membrane. The two are differentiated by the response to RNS or jitter with single-fiber EMG (see later). In LEMS, the amplitude of the responses increases with repetitive stimulation (more quanta of ACh released), whereas, in myasthenia gravis, the responses decrease (all ACh receptors saturated). Sensory NCS findings are typically normal. Table 31.1 provides a summary of typical findings.

Single-Fiber Electromyography

Electrical activity can be recorded from two or more muscle fibers innervated by the same motor unit by using a specially designed single-fiber needle electrode. SFEMG is, at this time, the most sensitive test for evaluation of neuromuscular transmission defects such as myasthenia gravis and myasthenic syndrome. It is also used to evaluate peripheral neuropathies, motor neuron diseases, and myopathies. It is typically provided only in tertiary centers and requires a high level of patient participation.

During a carefully controlled minimal voluntary contraction, a 25 μm–diameter needle is inserted into the muscle, and several potentials from muscle fibers within the recording area are stored. Equipment with a trigger and delay line is necessary to "time lock" the tracings of the potentials. The slightly different conduction time or interpulse interval (IPI) required for impulses to be transmitted from a single motor neuron to each of its terminal endplates, cross the neuromuscular junction, and activate the muscle fiber is called *jitter.* This time difference is collected from several tracings and is converted into a mean consecutive time difference (MCD), which normally ranges from 5 to 55 msec. Values shorter or longer than this range are considered abnormal. The impulses from some axons to their muscle fibers may fail to be transmitted. This is referred to as *blocking.* Another capability of SFEMG is the measure of fiber density, that is, the average number of muscle fibers within the needle recording area. Fiber density is increased in reinnervation and also with certain myopathies because of axonal collateralization or splitting.[29]

Macroelectromyography

A variation of SFEMG uses a macroelectrode to record the majority of muscle fibers of a single motor unit as they are triggered by an initial potential, which is then time locked with all the other muscle fiber potentials recorded from a different part of the same or a nearby

TABLE 31.1	**Summary of Typical Findings**		
Disorder	**Motor Conduction**	**Sensory Conduction**	**Electromyography**
Motor neuron disease (e.g., amyotrophic lateral sclerosis [ALS])	Reduced amplitudes	Normal	Acute plus chronic neurogenic changes, fasciculations
Radiculopathies	Normal	Normal	Acute neurogenic changes in myotome
Plexopathies	Reduced amplitudes	Reduced amplitudes	Acute neurogenic changes in specific pattern
Axonal neuropathy	Reduced amplitude in affected nerve(s)	Reduced amplitude in affected nerve(s)	Acute neurogenic changes in affected nerve
Demyelinating neuropathy	Reduced conduction in affected nerve	Reduced conduction in affected nerve	Normal
Neuromuscular junction disorder	Decrement (myasthenia gravis [MG]) or increment (Lambert-Eaton myasthenic syndrome [LEMS]) with repetitive stimulation	Normal	Occasional myopathic motor unit action potentials (MUAPs)
Myopathies	Normal	Normal	Small-amplitude polyphasic MUAPs

needle.[12,30,31,36,37] Two recording channels are used. Maximal amplitude of the potentials from several muscles has been reported by Stalberg.[36] The findings are analyzed, along with findings of jitter, fiber density, and conventional EMG, to evaluate the status and prognosis of various neurological and neuromuscular disorders, such as motor neuron disease, peripheral nerve lesions, and myopathies.

In summary, the astute PT in the presence of a patient reporting weakness and/or numbness will refer that patient appropriately for electrophysiological testing based on the findings of a judicious clinical examination. In reading the report of an electrophysiological consultation, the PT will first correlate the results with the findings of the physical examination of the patient, determine whether the studies performed are complete (i.e., there are sufficient data to rule in the condition but also sufficient data to rule out other conditions), and correlate the findings with the conclusion. There is evidence that PTs performing NCSs and EMG tend to follow guidelines consistently.[38]

Kinesiological Electromyography

KEMG measures muscle activation during movement, whether it is purposeful, involuntary, dynamic, or relatively static. It is the method by which the therapist-examiner determines a muscle's (or muscle group's) onset, cessation, relative intensity, and activation sequencing during functional activities such as walking. Because normal movement depends on the CNS's ability to execute motor programs through muscle action, KEMG provides the therapist with insight, in real time, into motor function, motor control, and motor learning.

Persons with neuromuscular disorders typically exhibit control errors, including the inability to initiate, execute, or terminate movement. Selective control may be absent or abnormal with errors in muscle timing, intensity, and sequencing. Spasticity or synergistic muscle action may impede smooth execution of tasks and prevent purposeful movement. With increased emphasis on evidence-based practice, KEMG can provide objective documentation of abnormal control and intervention outcomes and provide insight into optimizing strategies for improved functional performance. Many orthopedic surgeons rely on KEMG testing to supplement clinical evaluation in planning surgical interventions (muscle transfers and releases) in children with cerebral palsy (CP),[39] in patients with TBI,[40] and in those who have had a stroke.[41]

KEMG interpretation depends on the examiner's understanding of the instrumentation chosen for testing, including electrode selection, recording techniques, signal processing, and time and intensity normalization.[42] Coupled with three-dimensional motion (infrared camera and motion capture) and force plate analysis, external moments are calculated that define internal force demands on muscles during functional activities such as walking. KEMG delineates the muscles that participate in meeting the internal force demand.

Recording Instrumentation

KEMG can be performed by using surface or fine wire electrodes (intramuscular). Controversy exists about the choice of electrodes, with the selection dependent on the clinical or research question. If the examiner is interested in "muscle groups" (e.g., dorsiflexors, quadriceps), then surface electrodes are appropriate. Fine wire electrodes are optimal if activation of individual or deep muscles is desired (e.g., posterior tibialis, iliacus). Fine wire allows for specificity of muscle action required for surgical decisions related to muscle transfers, releases, or muscle lengthening.[39,40,43]

Needle or fine wire electrodes (indwelling or intramuscular). A pair of 50-μg fine wire electrodes, also referred to as *indwelling* or *intramuscular electrodes,* are introduced through the skin and into the

muscle with a 25-gauge hypodermic needle. The 50-μg, Teflon-coated wires are threaded through the needle's core; 2 to 3 mm of the wire's distal end are stripped of insulation and, once inserted, record adjacent motor unit activity. Before insertion the electrodes are sterilized. Inserted through the skin and into the muscle of interest, the barbed end "hooks" the muscle fibers when the needle is withdrawn. Accurate placement requires that the examiner have extensive knowledge of three-dimensional anatomy and excellent palpation skills. A maximal concentric voluntary contraction is elicited to anchor the wires into the muscle fibers, preventing displacement during subsequent contraction. This ensures sampling the same motor unit pool during subsequent tasks, trials, or conditions. ES is an essential testing element to verify electrode location. Wire electrodes allow a more precise definition of muscle timing (onset and cessation) by reducing the incidence of intramuscular crosstalk.[44] Disadvantages include decreased reliability and insertional pain caused by skin penetration.[45-47] In several states, the examiner must possess specialized KEMG licensure to penetrate the skin with a needle.

Surface electrodes. When the clinical question can be answered by using surface electrodes, ES of motor points often defines optimal electrode placement over the muscle or group of muscles of interest. A maximal voluntary contraction (MVC) is elicited to confirm that optimal placement has been achieved. Standardizing electrode placement, size, interelectrode distance, and skin preparation enhances test-retest repeatability,[48] with submaximal contractions being more reliable than maximal contractions.[49] Skin displacement under the recording site may introduce movement artifact, which can be minimized by securing the electrodes to the skin with tape. To improve interday reliability, electrode placement should be marked (with ink) and standardized electrodes used. When both recording electrodes are contained in the same housing, interelectrode distance is standardized and movement artifact attenuated. Advantages of using surface electrodes include improved reliability and the ease with which they can be applied without causing patient discomfort.[45-47] Specialized licensure is not required.

Instrumentation for Kinesiological Electromyography Acquisition

KEMG signal acquisition requires either a telemetry unit (FM modulation) or a hard-wired system that relies on a "cable" tethered to the subject to transmit signals from the electrode site to the receiver. The subject's performance and nature of movement strategies performed may be altered by the cabling. Telemetry allows the subject unrestricted movement; KEMG signals are transmitted through the air from a small unit worn around the subject's waist. The optimal characteristics of the receiver include a bandwidth frequency of 40 to 1000 Hz and an overall gain of 1000 Hz.[42]

Signal processing. KEMG processing has become highly automated with the advent of high-speed computers and customized software. Once the signal has been acquired, it is stored digitally and processed by various computer programs. The "raw" signal is full wave rectified (all the negative values become positive), and a linear envelope is generated within a designated time interval. The area under the curve is mathematically integrated, and an average EMG profile is generated. Muscle-specific onset, cessation, and relative intensity are defined with a variety of software. According to a recent study, KEMG timing (onset and cessation) is optimally identified by using the intensity-filtered average (IFA) and packet analysis (PAC) when compared with ensemble average (EAV).[50] Despite a smaller recording volume with wires, Bogey and colleagues[50] demonstrated no significant difference in signal amplitude when multiple insertion sites within the same muscle were compared.

Normalization. Any acquired "raw" EMG signal needs to be referenced to a standard value. This is accomplished by dividing the raw EMG during a functional task such as walking by a reference value. The MVC serves this purpose. Subjects exert a maximal voluntary effort for each muscle that determines the maximal EMG activity possible. All subsequent efforts are compared with this maximal effort and expressed as a percentage of maximum (%MVC). In patients with neurological dysfunction who lack selective motor control, a maximal effort can be elicited in either an extensor or flexor synergy by using the upright motor control (UMC) test developed at Rancho Los Amigos National Rehabilitation Center, grading the effort as "weak," "moderate," or "strong" in synergy.[51] Maximal efforts are elicited for 3 to 5 seconds, and the software determines the maximal activity for a 1-second interval. The muscles' activation during a functional activity is subsequently expressed as a percentage of MVC.

Interpretation of Kinesiological Electromyography

Kinesiological electromyography and strength. KEMG testing does not directly measure muscle strength, and the examiner should resist equating raw EMG signal amplitude directly with muscle force or torque output. Grading the strength (manual muscle testing [MMT] or UMC test) of each maximal effort must accompany the interpretation of the muscle participation during a functional task.[52] For example, patients with postpolio syndrome (refer to Chapter 35) produce large-amplitude KEMG signals that often reflect the maximal exertion of a "weak" muscle (e.g., "MMT—Poor" or ⅖). Large-amplitude EMG signals represent activation of large motor units typical of reinnervation, not force output. Despite large-amplitude signals, the muscle is functionally weak. In other words, a 100% MVC normalized KEMG record for a muscle may represent the maximal effort of a "poor" or ⅖ muscle.

Muscle tone versus spasticity. Therapists should resist making inferences about *tone* from KEMG testing. As previously stated, KEMG reflects the contractile activity of motor units. Muscle tone refers to the amount of *resting* tension in a muscle because of its viscoelastic properties. Because tone is not a function of motor unit activity, it cannot be measured with KEMG.[42] In contrast, spasticity, defined as a hyperactive quick stretch response, can be recorded by KEMG because it reflects prolonged muscle activation (Ôºû0.1 second). Clonus has a distinct frequency characterized by a prolonged 5- to 8-Hz signal. Using signal duration in response to quick stretch, Cahan and colleagues[53] identified significant decreases in spasticity in selected lower-extremity muscles in children with CP after selective dorsal rhizotomy. In these children, spasticity interfered with agonist activation during walking.

In conclusion, KEMG is useful for delineating patterns of muscle activation in motor performance, reflecting the integrity of the neuromuscular control mechanism. The examiner's interpretation should also consider additional factors, such as the type of contraction; speed of movement; joint acceleration; and a host of physiological, biomechanical, anatomical, and neurological elements beyond the scope of this chapter.

ELECTRICAL STIMULATION AND ELECTROMYOGRAPHIC BIOFEEDBACK

NMES and EMGBF are often used as tools in the management of neurological dysfunction. EMGBF can be used both alone and in conjunction with stimulation. The primary goal of use is improvement of function by improving voluntary motor control. To that end, strengthening and alteration of abnormal tone are also common goals of treatment. EMGBF is discussed later in this chapter. More detailed explication of treatment protocols is included in a variety of published work.[54–65]

Electrical stimulators used in physical rehabilitation practice may be either small, portable, battery-operated units or larger line-powered clinical instruments. The clinical units often will offer a variety of stimulus forms and options for modulation of currents. Portable units provide the ability for patients and caregivers to carry out prescribed stimulation at home. Clinical units allow the therapist to customize programs to optimize treatment outcomes.

Neuromuscular Electrical Stimulation

NMES is often used as a tool in the management of neurological dysfunction. In NMES, muscle contraction is elicited by depolarization of the motor neurons. Electrodes may be placed over the muscle to be stimulated or over the motor nerve that controls the muscle. In NMES, muscle contraction is elicited by depolarization of the motor neurons. Electrodes may be placed over the muscle to be stimulated or over the motor nerve that controls the muscle. Firing order of neurons is a result of neuronal size, proximity of the electrical stimulus, and the intensity of stimulation.[66] Muscle recruitment patterns triggered by ES differ from those observed in normal muscle activation. In a voluntary muscle contraction, motor units fire asynchronously, with a larger proportion of type I, fatigue-resistant muscle fibers of the smaller motor units being recruited first. The order of muscle fiber firing occurs as a result of motor neuron size and the anatomy of synaptic connections.[67] Conversely, an electrically stimulated muscle contraction elicits initial responses from larger motor units, which contain a greater number of fatigable, type II muscle fibers. The type II fibers are innervated by larger-diameter neurons that have a lower threshold for ES than smaller neurons.[68] A study of healthy subjects demonstrated recruitment of these higher-threshold motor units at relatively low NMES training levels. In voluntary exercise a much greater exercise intensity is required for activation of these larger motor units.[68]

Synchronous recruitment of muscle fibers is obtained with ES. This does not occur with volitional activation. During a sustained volitional contraction, motor units periodically "drop out" and then "drop in" to reduce fatigue. With NMES, once recruited the motor units will continue to fire until the stimulus is ended. This, coupled with the early recruitment of fatigable motor units, accounts for fatigue being a major problem in the use of NMES. It also is one reason functional activities performed under control by stimulation are much less smooth and balanced than when they are performed volitionally. At the same time, relatively low levels of NMES can recruit motor units that volitionally would be recruited only with maximal effort. This provides support for observed increases in strength with low NMES training intensities.[69] Numerous potential benefits have been identified for NMES, such as improvement in ROM, edema reduction, treatment of disuse atrophy, and improvement of muscle recruitment for muscle reeducation.[57]

Parameters of Stimulation

With any ES used for patients with neuromuscular dysfunction, three parameters must be considered within the waveform: pulse (or phase) duration, pulse frequency, and pulse amplitude. Depending on the intent of the ES, instruments are available that allow all of these to be independently adjusted.

Waveform

NMES units use alternating currents. The waveform of the stimulus produced by most NMES units is either a symmetrical or an asymmetrical biphasic pulse. The two phases of each pulse continually alternate in direction between positive and negative polarity. Although an ideal waveform has not been identified, most studies have shown the symmetrical biphasic waveform to be more comfortable than either the asymmetrical biphasic or the monophasic waveform.[54,70,71]

Duration

Phase or pulse duration (also called *pulse width*) refers to the amount of time of a single pulse or phase. Stimulators with a pulse duration of 1 to 300 μs (0.3 ms) can be used to activate muscles with intact innervation. Waveforms of shorter durations require a greater current amplitude to produce a muscle contraction (because the current is on for a shorter period of time). They may be more comfortable but may not possess enough charge for good contraction levels. Longer-phase durations may be used but are less comfortable. In NMES units, pulse durations may be started at 100 μs, then increased to 200 to 300 μs if well tolerated by the patient.[72,73] Denervated muscles require significantly longer phase durations (20 to 100 msec) because of the longer chronaxy of muscle cells compared with motor neurons.

Frequency

Pulse frequency (or *pulse rate*) refers to the number of electrical pulses applied per unit time. In applications seeking to provide muscle contraction, the stimulus rate should be 35 to 50 pps. This is a typical critical frequency at which a muscle will respond with a smooth contraction (also called a *tetanic frequency*). Higher frequencies than this can result in early onset of fatigue. NMES used for spasm reduction may use a higher frequency, with the intent of fatiguing the muscle and decreasing spasm, which will result in decreased pain levels.

Amplitude

The amplitude (intensity) of the stimulus should be sufficient to achieve the desired strength of contraction. Battery-operated units usually indicate the amplitude only in a relative way (nonquantitatively) because the output of the battery declines over time. Depending on the impedance of the electrodes, coupling agent, skin, and soft tissue, the amount of current required at one location could be quite different than at another to produce the same degree of muscle contraction. This is why the amplitude of the stimulus is usually described according to the strength of the sensation felt by the patient. *Mild, moderate,* or *maximum sensory* refers to the intensity of the stimulation as felt by the patient, without eliciting a motor contraction. Similarly, *mild, moderate,* and *maximum motor* describe the amplitude of the stimulus needed to produce those visible muscular contractions using ES. If the intent is to strengthen the muscle or increase endurance, the patient is usually asked to participate by

voluntarily contracting the muscle being stimulated when the stimulation is on. The amplitude of stimulation should be graded based on the response of the patient, aiming at production of the clinically desired force output.

Additional Parameters: Ramp Time and On-Off Time Ratio

On time and off time. NMES for facilitation of muscle contraction should be used to supplement exercise, and goals for stimulation should be consistent with the goals of the exercise program. To simulate isotonic or isometric muscle contractions, as in voluntary movement for exercise, the stimulator must have the capability of setting cycles of on and off times. Each period of muscle contraction is followed by a period of relaxation (Fig. 31.7).[3,57] In most cases a shorter on time than off time is desirable to avoid fatigue. For example, a 10-second on time may be followed by a 50-second off time in a cycle, resulting in an on-off ratio of 1:5. Packman-Braun[74] investigated ratios of stimulation to rest time with NMES for wrist extension in a group of hemiplegic patients. Results supported the on-off time of 1:5 as being the most beneficial in training programs of 20 to 30 minutes because of the deleterious effects of fatigue with lower ratios (1:1, 1:2, 1:3, 1:4). If the goal is to reduce edema by providing a muscle pumping action, a ratio of 1:1 or 1:2 may be preferred,[74] as the intent is to decrease the edema by continuous muscle pumping action. Lower ratios may be used when the goal is neuromuscular reeducation or endurance training.

Ramping. Ramping is another modulation that can be set by the therapist. Ramp-up is the time taken by each train of pulses to increase amplitude or intensity sequentially from zero to maximum. Ramp-off is the period set at the end of the train of maximal intensity pulses to decrease sequentially from maximum to zero amplitude (see Fig. 31.7). Ramp time can be adjusted so that the stimulation more nearly resembles a pattern of gradually contracting and relaxing muscles. For patients with hypertonicity or spasticity and a goal of facilitation and strengthening the antagonist muscle, a longer ramp-up time may avoid or minimize activation of the stretch reflex in the hyperactive agonist muscle.

Duty cycle. The term *duty cycle* is sometimes confused with the on-off time ratio. Duty cycle is the percentage of time a series or train of pulses is on out of the total on and off time in a cycle.[3,54] For example, if the train of pulses is on 10 seconds and off 30 seconds, the total cycle time is 40 seconds. The duty cycle would be 25% (10 seconds of the total 40-second cycle). The actual on time and off time of the pulses in a cycle is a more informative description than either the duty cycle or the on-off ratio.

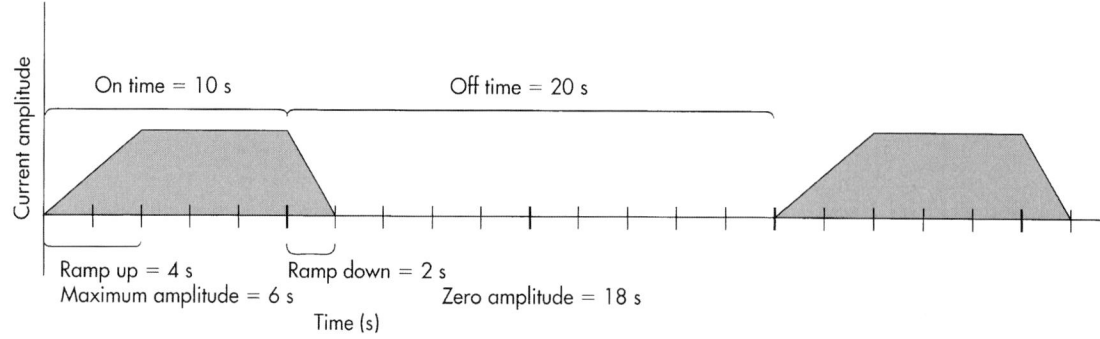

Fig. 31.7 Example of the relation between ramp times and on/off times. Each division on the horizontal axis equals 2 s. Note that the ramp-up time is considered part of the on time, whereas the ramp-down time is considered part of the off time. (Reprinted from DeVahl J. NMES in rehabilitation. In: Gersh MR, ed. *Electrotherapy in Rehabilitation*. Philadelphia: FA Davis; 1992.)

Muscle Reeducation

After an insult or injury affecting the CNS, problems with motor control frequently manifest. One of the common goals of therapy is to facilitate movement in the areas where control is lacking. If active movement is not present, NMES allows movement to occur by stimulation, which may be followed by resumption of active movement, possibly triggered by the sensory (visual and proprioceptive, among others) experience that accompanies the stimulation. When active movement is present but is weak or not well controlled, the therapist may choose to use NMES to supplement and strengthen the muscular contraction already present. Some evidence exists that NMES can increase activity in the somatosensory cortex and that the cortical activity is correlated with improvement in functional tasks.[75] In the presence of hypertonicity, the muscles serving as antagonists to the spastic muscle may be targeted for NMES, not only to strengthen the antagonist but to inhibit the spastic muscle by reciprocal inhibition.

Functional Electrical Stimulation

The term *functional electrical stimulation* (FES) has been used casually to describe various applications of NMES. However, FES is defined by the Electrotherapy Standards Committee of the Section on Clinical Electrophysiology of the American Physical Therapy Association as the use of NMES (on innervated muscles) for orthotic substitution.[3] Baker and Parker[76] use the term to describe external control of innervated, paretic, or paralytic muscles "to achieve functional and purposeful movements." Although NMES is generally considered to have therapeutic applications, such as increasing ROM, facilitation of muscle activation, and muscle strengthening, the key to application of FES is to enhance or facilitate functional control. It is used with patients with SCI, TBI, cerebrovascular accident (CVA), and other CNS dysfunction who have intact peripheral innervation.

An example of FES application is the ES of the fibular nerve to enhance ankle dorsiflexion during gait in patients with hemiplegia.[77] Two of the more common applications of FES on the market include the WalkAide system (Innovative Neurotronics, Austin, Texas) and Bioness (Bioness, Valencia, California). The L300 Go of Bioness (Bioness, Valencia, California) offers several features designed to optimize neurorehabilitation. This device uses a FES system with a three-dimensional motion detector of events in the gait cycle. Specifically, this device has a learning algorithm that analyzes the affected lower-extremity movement and induces ES directly to the phase of the gait cycle where it is required. Users of the earlier version (Legacy L300) have the tendency to be dependent on foot sensors or remote controls. This device has an adaptive motion detection feature and onboard controls to address this issue of dependency on foot sensors or remote controls. L300 Go also has a multichannel stimulation, which enables clinicians to adjust dorsiflexion and inversion/eversion with a novel new electrode options. To promote functional gains at home, a new mobile iOS application (myBioness) was developed to facilitate goal setting and tracking rehabilitation progress.[78] In terms of neurological dysfunctions, research has been published that indicates efficacy of these devices and FES in general in improving functional performance in people with CVA,[79-82] multiple sclerosis, TBI, SCI,[83,84] and CP.[85] Moreover, numerous other uses of FES have been described, ranging from isolated motor control activities, such as decreasing shoulder subluxation and reducing scoliosis, to highly technical computerized gait and bicycling capabilities, sometimes referred to as *computerized FES* (CFES).[86-94] The trigger that activates muscle contraction in synchrony with the functional activity can be manually initiated by the patient, set within the stimulator to automatically trigger on and off cycles, or programmed into a complex computer system for bicycling or gait.

Stimulation is generally applied in short-duration pulses with a frequency sufficient to provide smooth, tetanizing muscle contractions and adjusted to cycle on and off, with adequate ramp functions, as indicated by the speed and time needed to synchronize the stimulation with the functional activity. The length of the intervention depends on the purpose and may vary from a few contractions during the functional activity, building to multiple 30-minute sessions working up to several hours, repeated daily or three to five times per week. With the more complex computerized systems used for patients with complete spinal cord lesions, electrically activated functional movements are the mechanism to achieve physiological and psychological benefits. In some situations, assisted function is also an important goal, although functional community ambulation is not yet a reality.[90,92,95-102] Hooker and co-workers[96] evaluated the physiological effects of use of FES-assisted leg cycling in SCI. Compared with resting levels, significant increases were found in cardiac output, heart rate, stroke volume, respiratory exchange rate, pulmonary ventilation, and other physiological phenomena. CFES for cycle ergometry and ambulation has also been shown to increase muscle mass, electrically induce muscle strength and endurance,[91,103,104] increase circulation and aerobic capacity, decrease edema, and have a beneficial impact on self-image.[92,104,105] Jacobs and colleagues[102] compared the metabolic stress of FES-assisted standing versus frame-supported standing. Cardiorespiratory stress was significantly higher with FES, and the authors concluded that FES-assisted standing alone may provide a stress sufficient to meet minimal requirements for exercise conditioning.

The demonstrated benefits of FES clearly indicate that it is a valuable tool for supplementing functional activities. The practicality and cost of applications of the more complex computerized systems need further study, especially in terms of function in community activities. (Refer to Chapter 38 for additional discussion.)

Electromyographic Biofeedback

Biofeedback is a general term used to describe the use of visual or auditory representation of physiological processes to allow an individual to modify those processes. EMGBF makes available to the patient information regarding the electrical activity of muscle. EMGBF has several well-documented applications, including alteration of physiological responses such as heart rate, temperature, and muscle tension.[55] These applications may prove beneficial for patients with neurological dysfunction. An example would be relaxation to modify pain perception. The focus of this review is the use of EMGBF for improvement of active movement, which may include reduction of hypertonicity in addition to muscle reeducation. EMGBF units range from basic single-channel portable models to clinical units with multiple channels and multiple options for provision of feedback.

EMGBF may be used to assist a patient in attaining greater levels of muscle activation in paretic muscle, decrease levels of muscle activation in spastic muscle, or attain a balance between agonist and antagonist muscle pairs.[106] For most practicing clinicians, EMG levels are monitored through the use of surface electrodes. Monitoring of activation of deep muscles is often not feasible. Attention to size and specific electrode placement is critical to ensure feedback that will be useful. Smaller electrodes allow specific placement, although higher impedance will be encountered. Skin must be carefully prepared to take this into account.[107] Because the EMG information recorded represents the sum of action potentials from motor units between the electrodes, large interelectrode distance will increase the area of muscle recorded. This may be desirable for large muscle groups or when minimal activity is present.

Smaller interelectrode distances are preferable if interference from "crosstalk" or "volume conduction" from muscles or motor units not part of the target group is a risk. Basmajian and Blumenstein[107] provide an excellent review of electrode placements.

Reduction of Hypertonicity

DeBacher[108] described a progression of intervention with EMGBF designed to reduce spasticity. The program uses three stages of intervention: (1) relaxation of spastic muscles at rest even in the presence of distraction, mental effort, or use of muscles not targeted for EMGBF training; (2) inhibition of muscle activity during passive static and dynamic stretch of the spastic muscle, beginning with static stretch at the extremes of motion, then progressing to passive movement speed at a speed of 15 degrees per second; and (3) isometric contractions of the antagonist to the spastic muscle, with relaxation of the spastic muscle, progressing to prompt muscle contraction and relaxation of the spastic muscle, and grading of muscle contractions with movement for various force output requirements. Use of the technique in a small sample of young adults with CP demonstrated improvement in resting levels of involuntary muscle activity.[109] Improvements in function, however, were not demonstrated.

Inhibition of a spastic muscle alone may not be enough to improve function. Often the spastic muscle itself, once hypertonicity has diminished, is weak or has low functional tone. Weak antagonists to the affected muscle may contribute to the functional limitation. EMGBF to reinforce activity in the weak muscle may be done concurrently with its use to modify the tone in the agonist.[110] EMGBF can be useful in helping a patient decrease abnormal muscle activation, but persistence of control problems may be related to lack of force production, deficits in speed of muscle activation, and lack of reciprocal interaction of muscle groups.[111]

Muscle Reeducation

Therapists may opt to use biofeedback to provide information about the quality of the muscle contraction directly to the patient. The patient can then attempt to alter the contraction in accordance with guidelines provided by the therapist, whether the focus is to facilitate stronger contraction, decrease apparent hyperactivity, or modulate a balance of muscle activity during a functional task.

Concurrent assessment of muscle activity (CAMA) is an application of EMGBF in which the therapist uses biofeedback as an adjunct in evaluation of patient response to therapeutic exercise.[112] In this procedure the therapist decides which muscle group(s) are desired for activation and adjusts the position of the patient or the therapist intervention accordingly to get the correct responses. CAMA allows for the judgment of the effectiveness of a particular activity based on actual EMG responses rather than presumptions of what the intervention should cause. In a placebo-controlled study of hemiplegic patients, the addition of EMGBF to hand exercises based on the Brunnstrom approach resulted in significant improvement in active ROM in those using biofeedback compared with sham.[113]

Several authors suggest the use of biofeedback signals from homologous extremity muscles as a model for what the hemiplegic patient needs to alter muscle activity in a particular function.[114,115] This has been described as a "motor copy" and was compared with a more targeted training procedure. Indications showed that the motor copy resulted in better carryover in function than the comparison therapy in follow-up evaluations. A similar training study showed indications of benefits of the procedure, but the results were not statistically significant because of the small group size.[114] At least two studies support patterning or copying EMG from other muscles as a potentially useful tool for individuals with C4 to 7 SCI.[116,117] A meta-analysis that compared EMGBF with conventional physical therapy for upper-extremity function in individuals after stroke reviewed

only six studies and concluded that neither approach was superior to the other.[118]

Feedback Considerations

EMGBF has the benefit of being provided simultaneously with the patient's movement, consisting of accurate and objective information about muscle activity (given careful electrode application), and not requiring the same level of therapist skill as verbal feedback provision. EMGBF therefore may be beneficial for patients with deficient sensory feedback systems. The frequency of feedback provision, however, may require close scrutiny by the therapist.

Experiments examining feedback frequency in the learning of motor tasks support the use of less than 100% relative frequency for the subject to learn the task. Feedback provided on every trial may improve performance but degrades learning in normal subjects.[119] In a study of stroke patients attempting a pursuit tracking task, biofeedback was used for the experimental group (electrodes over the spastic biceps), whereas the control group performed the task without feedback.[120] Posttests revealed that the use of continuous feedback had a negative transfer effect on learning of the movement task, suggesting that the experimental learners became dependent on the external feedback in performance of the task. The clinician must therefore carefully structure the use of external feedback so the patient begins to develop a sense of muscle activation or relaxation that is present without the EMGBF apparatus. This may be accomplished by turning the screen away from the patient and turning off the auditory signal as the patient progresses.

Integrating Neuromuscular Electrical Stimulation and Electromyographic Biofeedback

The use of EMG-triggered NMES, in which NMES is initiated once the patient has achieved a predetermined level of EMG activity in the targeted muscles, is an application that has been shown to have merit,[121,122] although a more recent systematic review showed no statistically significant differences between EMG-NMES and usual care in improving upper-extremity function of the affected extremity in people who had had a stroke.[123] Threshold levels of EMG activity could gradually be increased as the patient gains the ability to activate muscles independently, with eventual discontinuance of the NMES as strength and active control allow. The success of this application has been shown in patients with hemiplegia in terms of increasing EMG activity and subsequent improvement in ROM and function in the involved arm and leg.[121] In another study, patients who had had a stroke more than 1 year previously significantly improved wrist and finger extension strength and function after treatment with EMG-triggered stimulation compared with controls.[122]

A variation of this application is NMES triggered by positional feedback, such that NMES is initiated once the patient actively moves through a portion of the available ROM at a joint.[124] The therapist may set the threshold angle in accordance with the patient's goals and abilities. This method has been shown to be effective in improving wrist motion after stroke, although it was not as effective in altering control of the knee in a similar patient group.[125]

Although discussions of EMGBF, NMES, and FES are often presented separately, the use of these modalities can be intertwined to achieve desired muscle control. NMES or FES may be initiated in the absence of active control (although lower levels of muscle activation may be discovered and facilitated with EMGBF). Once return of active control begins, EMGBF may be used to refine the control. An increase in muscle EMG should not be assumed to translate automatically to an improvement in functional use of that muscle in daily activities. Consequently, NMES and EMGBF need to be integrated into daily functional activities so that appropriate muscle activity is elicited and used in its appropriate functional context.

Applications

The application of the common principles of EMGBF and NMES to different patient populations emphasizes the role of the therapist in tailoring intervention to meet specific patient needs.

Many investigators have evaluated the use of NMES and EMGBF in patients who have had a stroke.[110,126–128] FES has been used extensively with patients with SCI. Other populations that demonstrate neuromuscular impairment or dysfunction have not been as thoroughly studied. This may be because the heterogeneity of these groups may create difficulty in research design.

Upper-Extremity Management

Electromyographic Biofeedback

EMGBF has been extensively studied, but success of the treatment is mixed, with difficulty in interpretation. A reduction in co-contraction has been observed,[129] as well as improvement in several neuromuscular variables[126,130,131]; however, a lack of significant improvement in functional skill was noted. Given the challenge of improving upper-extremity functional ability after stroke, Wolf and Binder-Macleod[131] suggested consideration of several key factors in predicting which patients may benefit from EMGBF: "Those patients who achieve the most substantial improvement in manipulative abilities initially possess voluntary finger extension; comparatively greater active ROM about the shoulder, elbow, and wrist; and comparatively less hyperactivity in muscles usually considered as major contributors to the typical flexor synergy." Attention to the chronicity of motor dysfunction also appears critical in anticipating success with EMGBF, as patients 2 to 3 months after stroke demonstrated stronger functional gains after intervention with biofeedback compared with patients 4 to 5 months after stroke. A placebo-controlled study of EMGBF showed statistically significant improvement in active ROM of the hand in patients who received EMGBF in addition to exercise.[113] A study by Doğan-Aslan[132] and colleagues found improvements in the Ashworth scale, Brunnstrom stage, upper-extremity function test, wrist extension ROM, and surface EMG potentials in their subjects who were treated with EMGBF in conjunction with neurodevelopmental therapy (NDT) and conventional treatment in a population of subjects with hemiplegia secondary to stroke.

Neuromuscular Electrical Stimulation

Common upper-extremity applications of NMES for the patient with a stroke include reduction of shoulder subluxation (FES) and facilitation of elbow, wrist, and finger extension and motor control.

FES for shoulder subluxation reduction appears beneficial for prevention of pain and subluxation, especially if used during the early stages of recovery. In 2018, Arya and his colleagues conducted a systematic review about rehabilitation methods for reducing shoulder subluxation in post-stroke hemiparesis. The researchers have reviewed 14 RCTs or controlled trials and 8 pre- and post-single group studies. In this study, researchers have indicated that FES is effective in reducing subluxation in acute stage and that shoulder support or orthosis may reduce the subluxation temporarily while in place.[133] The functional benefits over the long term are not always clear, and cost-benefit ratios need to be considered. Baker and Parker,[76] Faghri and colleagues,[87] and Chantraine and colleagues[134] have reported success in management of shoulder subluxation after stroke by using gradually increasing stimulation times that ultimately reached 6 to 7 hours per day. On-off ratios were typically 1:3.

Use of NMES after stroke to facilitate motor control and function has been studied, but many studies lack controls. The extensors of the fingers and wrist are typically the targeted muscle groups. de Kroon and colleagues[62] reported a systematic review of literature that included six randomized controlled trials. A variety of stimulation parameters were used. Three studies tested subjects with acute conditions, and three tested subjects with chronic conditions. Outcome measures for motor control included the Fugl-Meyer Motor Assessment (four studies) and strength (two studies). Functional outcomes were reported by two studies, one using the Action Research Arm test and one using the Box and Block test. The authors concluded that there was a positive effect of stimulation on motor control. Only two studies reported functional outcomes, but both were positive. Of significance is the fact that only six studies met the criteria for review in terms of rigor.[121, 122,124,135–137]

FES has also been investigated as an upper-extremity orthosis after hemiplegia, using movement of the uninvolved shoulder to trigger stimulation of elbow extension and hand opening.[138] After an extensive training period, patients were able to demonstrate functional use of the involved hand for basic reach and grasp.

Systems with more than two channels of stimulation have proved difficult for patients to use.[139] Popovic and colleagues[140] reported two studies in which they used NMES to treat patients after stroke. They termed the intervention *functional electrical therapy* (FET). The stimulation was used during an exercise program composed of voluntary arm movements and opening and closing, holding and releasing objects with the stimulation serving as an electric prosthesis. Treatment was 30 minutes daily for 3 weeks in one study[140] and 6 months in the other.[141] Outcomes were reported as better than controls. Initially higher-functioning subjects benefited more than those who were rated as low functioning. Unfortunately, outcome measures in these studies were not standardized.

A study of use of daily NMES in the form of neuroprosthetic FES (NESS Handmaster) stimulation of hand and finger extensors in patients with subacute strokes (6 to 12 months after onset) was reported by Ring and Rosenthal.[142] All subjects were receiving physical and occupational therapy three times a week. The stimulator was used at home. Those receiving stimulation had significantly greater improvements in spasticity, active ROM, and functional hand test scores compared with control subjects. The authors concluded that supplementation of outpatient rehabilitation with NMES improves upper-limb outcomes.[142]

Three-month interventions with EMG-triggered NMES, low-intensity NMES, proprioceptive neuromuscular facilitation (PNF) exercise, or no treatment were compared in a group of chronic stroke patients.[143] At 3 and 9 months after treatment, Fugl-Meyer scores improved 18% for the PNF group, 25% for the patients receiving low-intensity NMES, and 42% for the group receiving EMG-triggered NMES. The control group did not change.

These findings lend support to the use of NMES and EMGBF and NMES alone as adjuncts to physical therapy. Typically, higher-functioning patients have shown the greatest impact. Results have tended to show greater effect in patients with acute or subacute conditions, but longer-term patients sometimes benefited as well.

With the advent of the use of technology in neurological rehabilitation (see Chapter 38), an increasing number of investigations have been done to incorporate new technology with ES to improve functional performance. Sayenko and colleagues[144] described the use of a video game–based training system combined with NMES in a person with chronic SCI. Results indicated improvement in the strength and endurance of the paralyzed lower extremities of the individual after the intervention.

Lower-Extremity Management
Electromyographic Biofeedback

Several studies evaluating EMGBF for retraining lower-extremity control after stroke have focused on improvement of tibialis anterior control and reduction of gastrocnemius muscle activity. Results support increases in strength and ROM in ankle dorsiflexion with carryover into ambulation and maintenance of this improvement on follow-up evaluation.[145–147]

Wolf and Binder-Macleod[126] examined a number of variables at the hip, knee, and ankle in a controlled group study of the effects of EMGBF. Subjects were assigned to one of four groups: lower-extremity EMGBF, upper-extremity EMGBF, general relaxation training, and no treatment. No significant changes were observed between experimental and control groups for EMG levels and ROM at the hip, but improvements were noted in knee and ankle active motion for the experimental group. Although subjects in the experimental group increased their gait speed, these changes were not significantly different from findings in the comparison groups.

Use of EMGBF with the intent of improving ambulation may require use of feedback during the task of ambulation instead of during static activity, as demonstrated by this study. Positional biofeedback regarding ankle position and traditional EMGBF were compared in a group of hemiplegic subjects.[148] A computerized system provided audiovisual feedback during ambulation for both groups. Pretreatment and posttreatment measures of ankle motion, gait, and perceived exertion were conducted for the two treatment groups and a control group. The group receiving positional feedback increased walking speeds relative to the other groups, with improvements maintained at follow-up intervals of up to 3 months. The consideration of integrating feedback into functional ambulation bears further investigation.

Neuromuscular Electrical Stimulation

Fibular nerve stimulation has been documented as an assistance for patients with hemiplegia to improve ambulation.[77,149–151] Long-term stimulation with implanted electrodes has proved effective in improving gait patterns, but difficulties in achieving balanced dorsiflexion, infection, and equipment maintenance were drawbacks.[151,152]

Shorter-term use of fibular nerve stimulation as an adjunct to traditional physical therapy may be considered. In a controlled study examining the use of 20 minutes of fibular nerve stimulation six times per week for 4 weeks, the stimulated group demonstrated dorsiflexion recovery three times greater than the control group, as measured by an average of 10 maximal dorsiflexion contractions. These improvements were regardless of site of lesion, age, or time since lesion.[149] Surface electrode stimulation is effective, and gait parameters can be improved with its use.[153,154] If, however, a foot drop is the only major impediment to ambulation, lightweight plastic orthoses are a functional and much less expensive choice of intervention.

Multichannel ES has been used in the management of ambulation in patients who have had a stroke.[143,155–158] Although more effective than traditional gait training in some cases in terms of gait velocity and stride length, at follow-up evaluations 8 to 9 months after therapy the difference between groups had faded. However, the expense and availability of such systems make their use unlikely at this time.

NMES used for ankle dorsiflexion triggered by heel switch during gait and biofeedback to improve active recruitment of ankle dorsiflexors or relaxation of ankle plantar flexors has been studied in hemiplegic patients.[159] Patients who received a combination of these interventions demonstrated significantly improved knee and ankle range parameters more rapidly than those using a single modality. This

improvement was maintained over a 1-month period. Although all groups improved in gait cycle times, results in the combined intervention group were better. This may be attributable to the synergy of biofeedback and stimulation.[52] Granat and colleagues[160] also studied fibular muscle stimulation effects on gait parameters after stroke. After intervention the subjects showed significant control of eversion on all surfaces. The Barthel Index score also improved after intervention. However, no improvement occurred when the patients were not using the stimulator.

Evidence-Based Practice

Much of the literature evaluating the use of EMGBF and NMES involves patients with CVA. Although these studies have shown many significant results, interpretation of these findings in relation to what is recommended for clinical intervention is not as clear-cut. Improvements in generation of EMG activity and active movement are well documented, but the functional implications of these gains are not as well established. Clearly, in the current practice environment much of the focus is on function, so these techniques to improve muscle activation patterns must be put to functional use in the context of therapy. The therapist must consider the relevant factors that may predict success and critically evaluate outcomes during trial use of these modalities. Cost-benefit analyses must accompany any intervention using technology with the goal of regaining movement as quickly as possible and eliminating the use of equipment when practical.

Stroke

A number of studies have been published discussing the muscle recruitment problems observed after CVA.[110,127,128] Knowledge of these problems is a prerequisite for determination of the appropriate application of NMES. Delayed recruitment of the agonist and antagonist is a relatively consistent finding. Other findings include delayed termination of muscle activity once initiated,[161] presence of co-contraction of agonist and antagonist muscles,[127,128] lack of co-contraction,[110] and maintenance of agonist muscle contractions.[127]

Sander and colleagues[162] found that NMES application to the tibialis anterior muscle for 30 minutes three times a week for 4 weeks was effective in improving strength of the affected lower extremity.

Howlett and colleagues investigated the effect of FES in improving activity after stroke, and whether FES is more effective than training alone in a systematic review with meta-analysis. Following predetermined search and selection criteria, researchers included randomized and controlled trials up to June 22, 2014. Eighteen trials (19 comparisons) were eligible for inclusion in the review. Results of the study showed that FES had a moderate effect on activity compared with no or placebo intervention. Furthermore, researchers also noted that FES had a large effect on upper-limb activity and a small effect on walking speed compared with control groups, and appeared to have a moderate improvement in activity compared with both no intervention and training alone. In the study, researchers suggested that FES should be used in stroke rehabilitation to improve the ability to perform activities.[163]

Most recently, Biasiucci and colleagues demonstrated that brain-computer interfaces (BCI) coupled with FES can elicit significant lasting arm motor recovery in patients with chronic stroke. BCI translate brain signals into planned movements in patients with limb paralysis. BCI alone has an unclear efficacy and mechanisms as to motor recovery after stroke. In this study, patients who received brain-actuated functional electrical stimulation (BCI–FES) exhibit a significant arm functional recovery post intervention. The recovery lasted for 6 to 12 months after the termination of therapy. The results of the study demonstrated a promising BCI–FES combination therapy to facilitate functional neuroplasticity leading to a significant arm functional recovery patients with chronic stroke.[164]

Lee, Lee, and colleagues compared virtual reality (VR) combined with FES with cyclic FES for improving upper extremity function and health-related quality of life in patients with chronic stroke in a pilot, randomized, single-blind, controlled trial. In the study, participants were patients 3 months post-stroke. A VR-based wearable rehabilitation device was used in combination with FES. This device was used during the virtual activity-based training for the intervention group while the control group received cyclic FES only. Both groups received 20 sessions over a 4-week period. Results of the study have shown that FES with VR-based rehabilitation may be more effective than cyclic FES in improving distal upper extremity gross motor performance post-stroke.[165]

In a study done by Kuznetsov and colleagues, a tilt-table with stepping features combined with FES was applied to patients with hemiparetic ischemic stroke 3 to 6 days post-stroke. Rehabilitation may be more effective if started early; however, early training is frequently limited because of orthostatic reactions. The researchers' goal is to prevent these adverse reactions through robotic tilt-table training plus FES (ROBO-FES). The researchers compared the safety and feasibility of ROBO-FES and robotic tilt-table training (ROBO) against the control, tilt-table training alone. There were no serious adverse events occurred during the study. They concluded that robotic tilt-table exercise with or without FES is safe and more effective in improving leg strength and cerebral blood flow than tilt table alone in this patient population.[166] Hocoma has produced a device with a tilt table with a stepping movement functionality with (ErigoPro®) or without FES (Erigo®) (see Fig. 31.8).

Page and colleagues conducted a study to assess the capacity to demonstrate cortical change in individuals with stroke utilizing an ES neuroprosthesis to facilitate repetitive task specific training (RTP). Eight chronic stroke patients (mean = 46.5 months post-stroke) received RTP five times per week for 8 weeks with each session being 30 minutes long. The sessions required the use of the neuroprosthesis (Bioness H200) during functional activities. The individuals demonstrated functional improvements in the involved upper limb as indicated by results of the Action Research Arm Test and Fugl Meyer Assessment. Functional MRI results also indicated increased cortical activation. The researchers concluded that the use of a neuroprosthesis (Bioness H200) (see Fig. 31.9) appears to increase affected arm use in a functional matter post chronic stroke.[167]

Springer and colleagues conducted a study to assess the effects of a dual channel FES unit (NESS L300Plus) (see Fig. 31.10) on the stance phase of gait in patients with hemiparesis. Sixteen individuals (mean

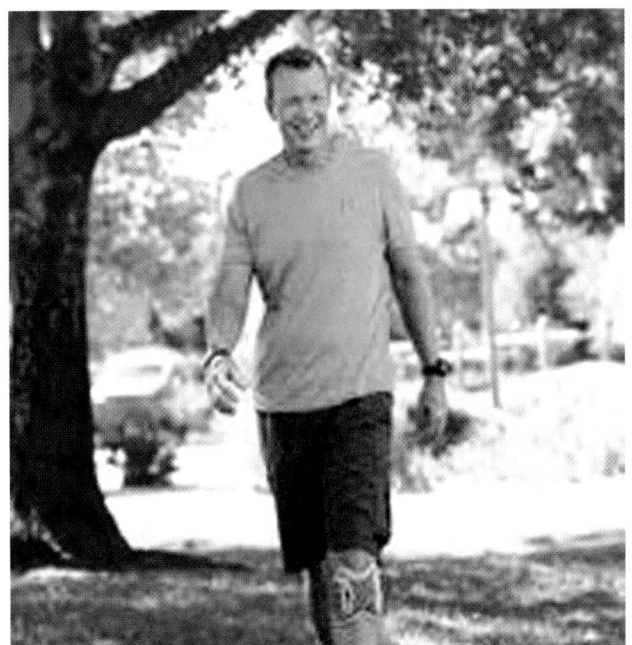

Fig. 31.9 Bioness H200.

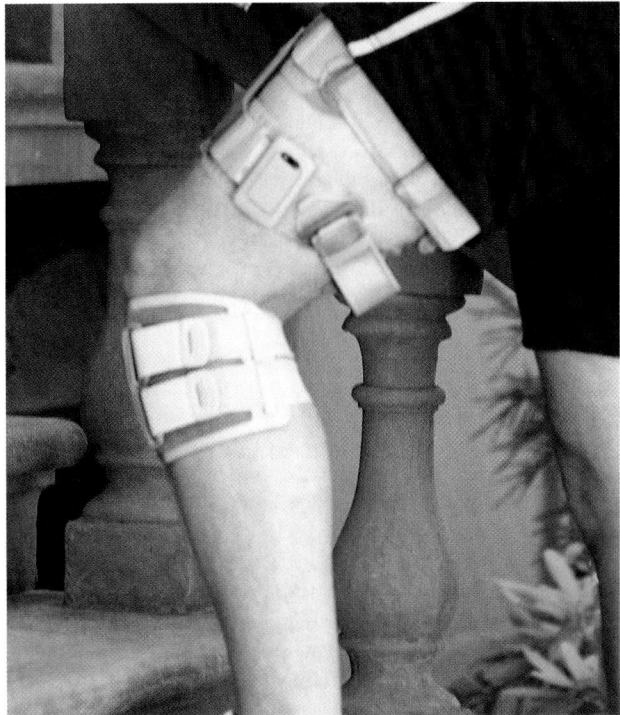

Fig. 31.10 NESS L300. Courtesy of Bioness, Inc.

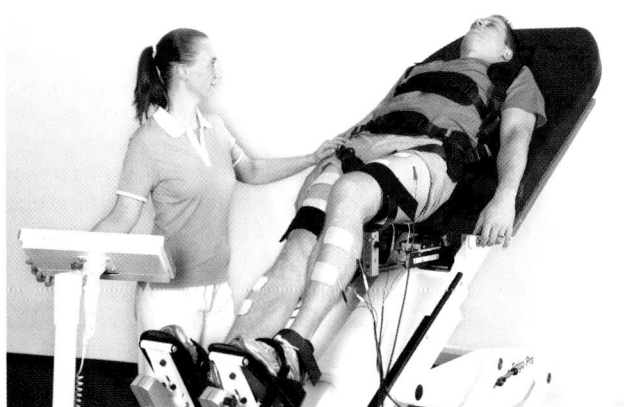

Fig. 31.8 Erigo Pro. (From: Hocoma, Switzerland.)

age = 54.2) with hemiparesis resulting in a drop foot and weak hamstrings were selected for the study and properly fitted for use of the apparatus. Gait assessments with and without the unit were completed after a 6-week conditioning program with the unit. The goal of the conditional program was to have the patients using the device the entire day by the fourth week. Dual channel FES was found to potentially have a larger effect on the functionality of the ankle dorsiflexors and hamstrings as compared to FES to solely the fibular nerve. Step length was increased in all participants.[168]

Wolf and Binder-Macleod[126] examined patient characteristics that are critical to success with biofeedback training for upper- and lower-extremity control after stroke. In a group of 52 patients with stroke, no significant relations between outcome and age, sex, number of EMGBF treatments, or side of hemiparesis were found. Lower-extremity treatment was associated with a greater probability of success, and this success did not seem related to chronicity of stroke sequelae. In contrast, success of upper-extremity treatment did appear to be related to length of time since onset of stroke, and poorer outcomes were noted if patients had received therapy to the involved arm for more than 1 year before EMGBF training. Improvements in elbow and shoulder function were obtained in this group of patients, but improvement in functional use of the hand was limited. Aphasia imposed a slight limitation to achieving improvement, but proprioceptive deficits were more significant in restricting functional gains. The role of patient motivation in success with EMGBF training was emphasized. On follow-up over a 12-month period, the improvements made in the initial intervention were maintained in 33 of 34 patients evaluated.

A number of studies have been published discussing the muscle recruitment problems observed after CVA.[110,127,128] Knowledge of these problems is a prerequisite for determination of the appropriate application of EMGBF and NMES. Delayed recruitment of the agonist and antagonist is a relatively consistent finding. Other findings include delayed termination of muscle activity once initiated,[161] presence of co-contraction of agonist and antagonist muscles,[127,128] lack of co-contraction,[110] and maintenance of agonist muscle contractions.[127] These reports emphasize the potential value of EMGBF in determining the best mode of intervention.

Jonsdottir and colleagues[169] found that the application of EMGBF in a task-oriented manner, incorporating motor learning principles, resulted in improvements in gait velocity, stride length, and peak ankle power in a population of individuals with hemiparesis. Sander and colleagues[162] found that NMES application to the tibialis anterior muscle for 30 minutes three times a week for 4 weeks was effective in improving strength of the affected lower extremity.

Lourencao and colleagues[170] studied the effects of biofeedback with FES and occupational therapy on upper-extremity function of individuals with hemiplegia. Results indicated significant improvements in upper-extremity ROM and functional recovery with the addition of biofeedback in the treatment regimen.

Lastly, a systematic review was conducted by Woodford and Price[171] on the use of EMGBF for recovery of motor function in individuals with stroke. The authors found evidence from a number of small studies that indicate that EMGBF resulted in improvement in gait, function, and muscle power compared with the usual physiotherapy interventions. The authors emphasized limitations in the results because of the small amount of evidence and problems with methodological designs and differing outcome measures.

Traumatic Spinal Cord Injury

NMES has a variety of applications for patients who have sustained SCI. Muscle strengthening may occur for muscles innervated by segments just above a complete SCI, or a variety of strengthening applications may be appropriate in the case of incomplete SCI. EMGBF may be used to identify muscle activity in weak musculature, as a tool to judge improvement in muscle activation, and as a method of facilitating increased strength.[172] Applications of EMGBF for individuals with SCI also include facilitation of unassisted ventilation in high-level quadriplegia[173] and use of biofeedback for muscle reeducation with incomplete SCI in the acute stages when immobilization may be required.[174]

The use of NMES, EMGBF, and other physical therapy was examined in a group of patients with incomplete cervical SCIs over a total treatment period of 16 weeks. Patients were randomly assigned to one of four groups receiving physical exercise, NMES, or EMGBF. Group 1 received EMGBF followed by physical exercise, group 2 received EMGBF followed by NMES, group 3 received NMES followed by physical exercise, and group 4 received 16 weeks of exercise only. Measurements of muscle strength, self-care ratings, mobility scores, and voluntary EMG were conducted at baseline, treatment midpoint, and conclusion of all interventions. All groups demonstrated improvement across the treatment period on all measures except voluntary EMG; however, no significant differences were seen among the four groups.[175] At least one other study compared conventional intervention, EMGBF, ES, and combined stimulation with biofeedback over a 6-week period in individuals with quadriplegia. An examiner who was blinded to the intervention protocol evaluated 45 subjects in the four treatment groups. All groups improved in the parameters evaluated, and no significant difference among groups was noted.[176] These results again emphasize the need to carefully consider cost as well as time and effort for setup and equipment operation in intervention planning.

A study by Carvalho and colleagues[177] studied the use of treadmill gait training with NMES to improve bone mass in people with SCI. Their research study included 21 males with chronic quadriplegia between C4 to C8, randomly assigned to a control and treatment groups. Those in the treatment group received treadmill training with NMES, unweighting the body of 30% to 50% of body weight. The training was done for 20 minutes, twice a week for 6 months. Results showed that gait training with NMES, even with 30% to 50% unweighting, resulted in the improvement of bone mass in the subjects with chronic quadriplegia. In another study also by Carvalho and colleagues,[178] NMES with partial body weight support resulted in hypertrophy of the quadriceps femoris muscle also in a population of subjects with quadriplegia. In both studies, NMES was helpful in producing stimulation that allowed for the subjects to advance their lower extremities while walking with body weight supported on the treadmill.

In a few studies, the application of NMES appears to be beneficial in improving impairments associated with SCI. Bittar and Cliquet[179] found that the use of NMES on the quadriceps and anterior tibialis of individuals with SCI was beneficial in that it allowed the feet and ankles to be placed in a better biomechanical position for ambulation. In addition, a study by de Abreu and colleagues[180] found improvements in the cross-sectional area of the quadriceps after NMES to these muscles.

In a study by De Biase and colleagues[181] EMGBF training was noted to have resulted in increased EMG response of the rectus femoris muscle in 20 subjects with chronic SCI.

A study by Street and Singleton looked to assess the overall effect in walking speed using FES for motor-incomplete SCI. 35 participants (mean age = 53) with foot drop and motor-incomplete SCI (T 12 or higher, ASIA impairment scale C or D) and who could ambulate 10 m with the use of an aide were selected. The participants underwent FES to the fibular nerve, glutei, and hamstrings over 6 months while in the community. The results of the study demonstrated initial orthotic effect, total orthotic effect, and training effect and the use of daily FES may result in improved walking speeds in individuals with motor-incomplete SCI.[182]

Craven and colleagues conducted a study to assess the efficacy of ES therapy assisted walking after chronic motor incomplete SCI on bone biomarkers and bone strength. Thirty-four individuals with chronic (≥18 months) motor-incomplete SCI (C2 to T12, ASIA impairment scale C or D) were randomized into either a treatment or conventional group. Treatment was performed three times per week,

45 minutes each for 4 months. Results of the study showed that the individuals with the FES treatment demonstrated improvements in bone turnover as compared to conventional therapy, however no significant difference in overall bone strength.[183]

Galea and colleague conducted a study to assess the efficacy and safety of FES-Assisted Cycling and Passive Cycling initiated early after SCI. The researchers randomized patients into a 12-week treatment group of either assisted cycling or passive cycling with each group undergoing treatment four times per week, 1 hour maximum, over 12 weeks. The researchers used cross sectional area measurements of the thigh and calf muscles using MRI as a primary assessment tool as well as body composition measurements. Conclusions by the researchers were that both types of modalities were shown to be safe and well tolerated after SCI.[184]

Chen and colleagues conducted a case report about the use of reciprocating gait orthosis (RGO) in combination with FES. This ambulation study of a woman with paraplegia using a RGO with FES was compared with the use of a long leg brace (LLB). The researchers concluded that RGO can help a patient with paraplegia achieve a faster and more independent ambulation. However, the combination of RGO and FES can increase the effectiveness of RGO as to locomotion. The researchers have concluded that the combination of RGO and FES is better than traditional LLB.[185]

In 2012, a systematic review was conducted by Lam and colleagues about the evidence for the efficacy of different rehabilitation strategies on functional ambulation following SCI. They have included in their systematic review pre-test/post-test or post-test only studies about the use of FES in this condition. They have concluded that FES may augment functional ambulation in sub-acute/chronic SCI.[186]

Ha and colleagues investigated on the utilization of cooperative control of FES with a powered exoskeleton. This research described this as a hybrid system that combines a powered lower limb exoskeleton with FES for gait restoration in persons with paraplegia. The general control structure consists of two control loops: a motor control loop and a muscle control loop. The motor control loop utilizes joint angle feedback to control the output of the joint motor to track the desired joint trajectories. On the other hand, the muscle control loop utilizes joint torque profiles from previous steps to shape the muscle stimulation profile for the subsequent step to minimize the motor torque contribution required for joint angle trajectory tracking. This system involves stimulation of the hamstrings and quadriceps muscles. The hip joints are actuated by the combination of hip motors and the hamstrings, and the knee joints are actuated by the combination of knee motors and the quadriceps. This study was implemented on three paraplegic subjects with motor complete SCI ranging from levels T6 to T10. Results suggested that the hybrid system provided consistent and repeatable gait motions. The researcher also noted a reduction in the torque and power output required from the hip and knee motors of the exoskeleton compared to walking without FES.[187]

Upper-Extremity Management

The use of electrically stimulated hand orthotic systems for patients with C6 or higher level SCI have been refined to allow greater functional independence for a select group of patients.[89,98,99,117,188–190] Because hand function does not occur in a cyclical pattern, the onset and termination of stimulation must be controlled by the patient in some manner, with a myoelectric or contact closing switch.[98] Multichannel stimulation is then applied with intramuscular electrodes for the flexors and extensors of the fingers and thumb, with computer-configured interplay between the different muscles to achieve a functional grasp. A chest-mounted position transducer (operated by shoulder elevation or depression and protraction or retraction) allows the user to initiate

stimulation and lock the stimulation to maintain a grasp as well as unlock it for release. A toggle switch mounted on the chest allows a choice between electronically stimulated lateral or palmar grasp patterns.[89,99] Some investigators have used contralateral shoulder slings as well as elbow accelerometers to trigger the needed stimulation.[191,192] Multiple authors have described successful implantation and use, with a few drawbacks, of upper-extremity FES prostheses.[193–196] Use of this type of system may allow patients with SCI at the C5 level to operate at the same level of independence (or even a higher level) as those with C6 quadriplegia with tenodesis, gaining the ability to perform more activities of daily living (ADLs) without an attendant. Patients with SCI at the C6 level may be able to manipulate a greater variety of objects without special adaptations.

Lower-Extremity Management

Standing. In an excellent review of the use of FES for the purpose of standing patients with SCI, Gardner and Baker[197] described the easiest approach to stimulating the quadriceps femoris to allow paraplegic patients to stand. More complex systems may incorporate stimulation of the gluteus maximus, gluteus medius, hamstring, adductor magnus, gastrocnemius, and soleus muscles for longer-duration and better-quality standing performance. Multichannel surface and implantable systems have been and continue to be developed for assistance in sit-stand and transfer activities.[198–200] Surgical procedures, patient selection, and technology are also factors cited in successful interventions. Despite these efforts, the duration of standing with electrically stimulated systems ranges from a few minutes to several hours. The patient with SCI may be able to use this technology to perform functional activities that require standing. The use of these systems depends on the functions unavailable to a patient without use of the technology, and the ease with which a system can be used and maintained. Peripheral to, but no less important, are the reactions of joints to these interventions. Two studies[201,202] have reported positive benefits to the structure and functions of lower-extremity joints of adolescents with SCI after participating in FES programs. A recent study has also identified that the physiological responses to standing in SCI may provide a cardiorespiratory stress sufficient to meet minimal requirements for exercise conditioning.[102]

Cycling. The use of systems to stimulate reciprocal lower limb motions electrically has increased for stationary cycling. The benefits of these interventions for the patient with SCI may relate to prevention of cardiovascular disease in the wheelchair-dependent patient. Physiological changes noted with electrically stimulated cycling include improvement of peripheral muscular and cardiovascular fitness, as demonstrated by increased power output after training with leg cycle ergometry.[87,96,97,103,104] Combining FES and lower-extremity cycling with upper-extremity ergometry induced a higher level of cardiovascular fitness than lower-extremity ergometry alone.[203] Exercise session frequency as little as two times a week induced positive changes in cardiovascular fitness.[204] When testing of patients with paraplegia or quadriplegia is conducted with arm crank ergometry after a training program with electrically stimulated leg cycle ergometry, patients do not demonstrate differences in pretest and posttest measures of hemodynamic and pulmonary responses. These findings may relate to the specificity of the leg exercise training or the presence of a peripheral rather than a central circulatory response to the training procedure.[97] As previously noted, many cardiovascular factors can be improved and the improvements retained for at least 8 weeks after a program of FES ergometry. In the study conducted by Sadowsky and colleagues, the effect of long-term lower extremity FES cycling on the physical integrity and functional recovery in people with chronic SCI was examined. This retrospective cohort study has a mean follow-up of 29 months, and a cross-sectional evaluation. There were 25 participants with chronic SCI that received lower-extremity FES during cycling as part of an activity-based restorative treatment regimen. Results of the study showed that FES was associated with more improvement in motor, sensory, and combined motor-sensory scores assessed using the American Spinal Injury Association Impairment scale as compared to control. Results also showed that the quadriceps muscle mass was higher and intra/inter-muscular fat was lower in the FES group. The researchers also noted that the hamstring and quadriceps muscle strength, quality of life, and daily function measures were greater in the FES group.[205]

Ambulation. As technology continues to progress, the use of electrically stimulated systems for ambulation may become more practical and useful for the patient with SCI.[100,206,207] Acceptance and use of the systems by patients outside the clinic have been mixed, but the systems have been shown to have positive effects on characteristics of ambulation.[152,208] Improvements in functional applications and use will also take place as the ability to select appropriate candidates improves.[209,210] Benefits of these systems may include increased muscle bulk, a reduced risk of pressure sores and osteoporosis, and psychological benefit. Generally, improvements in functional ability are expected to produce positive psychological factors. Addressing these factors directly, Bradley,[211] in a study measuring the effects of participation in an FES program on the affect of 37 individuals with SCI, demonstrated that positive affect was not significantly altered. Significant changes in negative affect occurred, however, with particular items of hostility and depression evident in those individuals in the treatment group who had unrealistic expectations. The author noted that these individuals need to be identified and monitored through the course of rehabilitation. Other drawbacks relate to the expense of the equipment and personnel and the lack of long-term efficacy studies. The speed with which a patient with a complete SCI is able to walk with electrically stimulated systems remains relatively low (2 to 54 m/min) compared with normal rates of 78 to 90 m/min.[212,213] Many of the published reports do not provide information on the maximal distance patients are able to walk with these systems, but reported distances range from 100 to 400 m.

Some patients may perceive the technology of electrically stimulated standing and walking as moving them toward a cure for their paralysis. With a complete injury, however, the stimulation occurs passively, without expectation that voluntary control will return.[211] In cases of incomplete injury, electrically stimulated ambulation may assist the patient in using and bolstering active control so that movement without the stimulation is more feasible. In considering use of electrically stimulated cycling and ambulation, discussion of the goals of treatment and the costs of the procedure must be conducted openly with the patient to allow an educated choice to be made about the use of this expensive technology.

Traumatic Brain Injury

NMES may be a useful tool with patients having sustained brain injury, with potential benefits of managing contractures by increasing ROM, facilitating active control, and reducing spasticity by strengthening the antagonist of a spastic muscle.[214] In cases in which an understanding of the purpose and principles of NMES is not feasible for a patient, the comfort of the stimulation may be critical in ensuring its continued use. Comfort may be enhanced by increasing the ramp-on time and selecting waveforms that allow stimulation at lower amplitudes yet still obtain the desired contraction.[37] The use of NMES with a patient at Rancho Level IV and below is not appropriate because the patient may not be able to understand the purpose and meaning of the stimulus and, hence, may perceive the stimulus as noxious.

EMGBF applications for patients with brain injury can be similar to those used with stroke, given similar motor presentations.[215]

Therapists must consider residual cognitive deficits after brain injury in determining the appropriateness of EMGBF.

Guillain-Barré Syndrome

EMGBF in patients with Guillain-Barré syndrome demonstrated improvements in muscle strength in upper and lower extremities, although inconsistent improvement in functional use of the upper extremities was noted.[216,217] Treatment regimens consisted of EMGBF for 10 trials per muscle conducted in 45-minute treatment sessions twice a week, in one case for 78 weeks and in the other case for 46 weeks.[217]

Multiple Sclerosis

In a case series, Wahls and colleagues[218] found improvements in ambulation of patients with primary or secondary progressive multiple sclerosis. The authors cited the possible positive effects of NMES application on muscle spasm, muscle pain, and disuse atrophy as possible reasons behind the improvements in ambulatory function in their subjects. Street & Singleton conducted a study to assess the long-term effects of FES on individuals with MS. One hundred and forty-five individuals with foot drop (19 bilateral, 60 left lower extremity, 63 right lower extremity, and 3 not documented) and MS were assessed with a mean age of 52 (range 28 to 74). Exclusion criteria included the capacity to walk 10 m without the use of an aide. Overall, there was a significant difference noted in the individuals who walked with FES versus those who did not. The treatment group was found to have an orthotic effect when using FES, and there was also decreased complaint of pain after 5 years.[219]

Pediatric Applications

Special considerations for pediatric patients need to be understood when addressing the use of electricity. Although contraindications and precautions are the same as for adults, acceptance and tolerance of these devices are not. Fear and apprehension of electricity, for both child and parent, must be addressed. The clinician must take extra care in explanation and demonstration, perhaps on themselves and possibly the parent, before placing the device on the child. Allowing the child as much control as possible in device operation may assist with acceptance. Of course, the attention span of the child must also be addressed.

Cerebral Palsy

The use of NMES with children with CP has been addressed to some degree, with several case study reports.[220–222] Carmick[220,221] described a variety of applications with children at 1.6, 6.7, and 10 years of age, integrating NMES into a treatment regimen that focused on a "task-oriented model of motor learning." Improvements were noted in upper- and lower-extremity movement and functional use across a variety of tasks appropriate to the age and the movement dysfunction each child demonstrated. In a study by Nunes and colleagues,[223] the once-a-week application of NMES on the tibialis anterior muscle of 10 children with spastic hemiplegia resulted in improvements in gross motor function, passive ROM of ankle dorsiflexion, and muscle strength.

Ozer and colleagues[224] studied the effect of using NMES in combination with dynamic bracing and found the dual intervention to be more effective than either alone in reducing upper-extremity spasticity in their sample of children with spastic hemiplegic CP. A similar study by Postans and colleagues[225] found that NMES combined with dynamic splinting reduced upper-limb contractures in children with CP. In another study,[226] the application of NMES to the gluteus medius improved gait parameters in children with spastic diplegia.

Advancements in technology have allowed the use of EMGBF in increasing contexts, such as the computer-assisted feedback (CAF) system, which can be used to provide feedback about muscle activity during ambulation.[227] Data examining use of this system to provide feedback about the level of triceps surae activity during gait of children with CP suggest potential improvements in gait symmetry, velocity, and appropriate muscle activation patterns as a result of this intervention. The use of this modality as an adjunct to physical therapy may prove beneficial.

When reviewing the literature, one notices controversial or lack of evidence supporting electrical modalities for the treatment of children with neurological conditions. Evidence supports the implementation of electrical modalities such as NMES and FES to treat impairments secondary to CP, however.

Arya and colleagues (2012)[228] assessed the effectiveness of electric muscular stimulation (EMS) in children with spastic CP. The current treatment for spasticity in the lower extremities include muscle strengthening, flexibility, and balance exercises. Other treatment approaches include orthotics, botulinum toxin injection, and surgical interventions. Electrical muscular stimulation is effective in improving ROM, strength, gait parameters and energy efficiency, and decreasing spasticity (Arya, et al., 2012).[228]

In their study, Arya and colleagues (2012)[228] aimed to test the effectiveness of ES in the improvement of gait parameters. This study focused on the lower extremities using surface electrodes of quadriceps and tibialis anterior in conjunction with occupational therapy and physical therapy services. The control group consisted of children with CP, who received occupational and physical therapy services, but no electrical modalities. The participants were children with spastic diplegic and spastic hemiplegic type of CP. The age groups ranged from 7 to 14 years of age (Arya, et al., 2012).[228]

This treatment approach focused on measuring the following outcomes:

- Gait: cadence (number of steps per minute), step length, and speed
- Gross motor function classification system expanded and revised (GMFCS) classification level
- Physiological Cost Index (PCI)
- Muscle power (using modified Ashworth Scale)
- Functional improvement using Gross Motor Function Measurement (GMFM) 88 scores
- MUAP Score using EMG
- Minimum strength of current needed for contraction
- Maximum tolerated current for different pulse width (100 μs to 300 μs)[228]

The parameters of the ES on the quadriceps and Tibialis Anterior consisted of EMS mode, 200 μs, 20 Hz for the quadriceps and 40 Hz for Tibialis Anterior, Biphasic rectangular pulses, for 20 to 30 minutes daily for four to five times a week. The tolerance of each child to the ES dictated the output current.[228] In this study, ES improved gait cadence, speed, and energy consumption. ES also improved functional outcome as shown by GMFM score.

A literature review indicated that ES using surface stimulation. Surface stimulation is associated with difficulty in obtaining repeatable stimulated responses, inability to stimulate deeper muscles, stimulation of unintended muscles, decreased skin tolerance with prolonged use, and stimulation of cutaneous nociceptors in patients with CP.[229] Disadvantages of surface ES are as follows:

- High levels of charge (e.g., 100 | mA for 0.2 msec), which may result in pain as cutaneous nociceptors are collaterally stimulated
- Relatively nonselective, which may stimulate untargeted muscles
- It may not stimulate deep muscles
- Donning and doffing of the equipment may be challenging for some children requiring physical assistance

- Accuracy placing electrodes over motor points to achieve repeatable motor responses[229]

The study author highlighted the importance of implanted neurostimulation devices to mitigate many of the disadvantages of surface stimulation listed above. These implanted devices provide substantially less charge (0.5 to 3 mA for 0.2 msec) and facilitate selective stimulation when the metal electrodes are implanted close to either motor nerves or the motor points where muscle is innervated.[229] This literature review concluded that ES holds promise for therapeutic value for the treatment of impairments secondary to CP. Most studies assessed the benefits of ES using surface stimulation, which suffers from nonselectivity and the potential inability to use proper dosing because of collateral stimulation of pain receptors. Consequently, the author suggests the use of long-term implantable stimulation devices such as the Radio Frequency Microstimulator (RFM) as this device mitigates adverse effects of both percutaneous and fully implanted leaded systems.[229]

Cauraugh and colleagues (2010) conducted a systematic review and meta-analysis on the effects of ES on gait in children with CP. Two hundred and thirty eight participants experienced ES treatments. Two hundred and twenty four received no stimulation and served as the control group. Common outcome measures associated with impairment and activity limitations were submitted to separate random effects models meta-analyses. The primary outcome measures for impairments consisted of ROM, torque/moment, and strength/force. For the activity limitations, the outcome measures consisted of gross motor functions, gait parameters, hopping on one foot, videotaped 6-m walk, Leg Ability Index 23, and Gillette gait index 57. Moderator variable analyses validated the positive treatment effects of ES on children with CP from both functional and neuromuscular stimulation. The systematic review and meta-analyses determined medium effect sizes for ES on gait impairment and activity limitations of children with CP.[230]

Prosser and colleagues[231] conducted a study with children with CP assessing the acceptability and clinical effectiveness of the WalkAide, a novel device that delivers FES to stimulate ankle dorsiflexion. There were 21 participants with a mean age of 13 years and 2 months. The Gross Motor Function Classification System (GMFCS) levels were I and II. The experiment group was provided with FES during gait training. The control did not receive FES treatment during gait training. The experiment lasted 4 months. Ankle kinematics and spatiotemporal variables were measured. Improved dorsiflexion was observed during the swing (mean and peak) and at initial contact subphases of the gait cycle. Gait speed was unchanged. The authors concluded the WalkAide is an effective modality to address foot drop in those with mild gait impairments secondary to CP.

Galen and colleagues[232] investigated the effects of FES combined with Botulinum Toxin A (BTXA) therapy in treating dynamic equines in children with spastic CP. This study also assessed the feasibility of this combination therapy. There were eight children: six males, two females; with ages ranging from 7 to 11 years of age. The qualifying diagnosis was CP either hemiplegic or diplegic spastic type. The ankle angle at the end of the swing phase was the primary outcome measure. All subjects participated in the study for 20 weeks, which consisted of the following periods: baseline (1 week), BTXA phase (3 weeks), first FES phase (4 weeks), first control phase (4 weeks), second FES phase (4 weeks), and second control phase (4 weeks). Each participant was assessed at the end of each phase. Results indicated that there was an increase in ankle angle at the end of swing phase in most subjects and were able to sustain the positive outcome after FES was withdrawn during the control phase. The positive results lasted longer when combining BTXA and FES. The authors concluded that combining BTXA therapy with FES is an effective treatment approach in the management of dynamic equines of children with CP.[232]

Danino and colleagues[233] evaluated the effectiveness of FES Neuroprosthesis in addressing gait deviations in children with CP hemiplegic-type. The device was the NESS_ L300TM, delivered ES to the common fibular nerve during the swing phase of the gait cycle. These stimuli facilitated the ankle to dorsiflex preventing foot drop. The participants consisted of four adolescents (mean age 16.5 years) with hemiplegic CP and one with diffuse pontine glioma. Results indicate an improvement in the Gait Profile Score (GPS), Gait Deviation Index (GDI), and Gillette Gait Index (GGI) with participants expressing high satisfaction and continuing to use the device at 1-year follow-up.[233] Danino and colleagues (2013)[233] concluded that FES targeting the dorsiflexors improves gait deviations in patients with hemiplegia (Danino et al., 2013).[233]

Spina Bifida

There is limited evidence of the effects of ES on children with myelomeningocele. Walker and colleagues[234] studied the effect of ES at night on strength and function in children with myelomeningocele. There were 15 participants, but only seven completed the treatment with ES for 9 months. ES was provided on areas of muscle weakness during sleep six nights per week. This treatment resulted in small gains in muscle strength, gait, and bowel continence, but there were no changes in physical function.

In the study by Karmel-Ross and colleagues[235] five subjects with spina bifida (aged 5 to 21 years) were treated with daily NMES over an 8-week period to strengthen the quadriceps femoris muscles. Increases in maximal quadriceps torque production were observed in two of the five subjects in the treated limb. Improvements in functional activity speeds were noted for all of the subjects. Lack of improvement in torque production by three subjects was speculated to be related to lack of adherence to the exercise regimen and the heterogeneity of the subject sample.[235]

Spinal Muscular Atrophy

Fehlings and colleagues (2002)[236] evaluated the effect of low-intensity night-time therapeutic electrical stimulation (TES) to the deltoids and biceps on upper extremity strength and function in children with intermediate type spinal muscular atrophy (SMA). After 6 to 12 months of stimulation no statistically significant differences were noted between experimental and placebo-control arms in strength, muscle mass, or function.[236]

Scoliosis

Axelgaard and Brown[86] demonstrated in the 1970s that surface NMES could reduce idiopathic scoliosis. Criteria for this treatment required curves measuring 20 to 45 degrees by the Cobb method, at least 1 year of growth remaining, idiopathic and progressive nature of the curve, cooperative and psychologically stable and compliant patient, and tolerance of the stimulation. Electrodes were placed laterally over the midaxillary line on the convex side. A paraspinous location on the convex side was sometimes used. Settings included a pulse duration of 220 μs, frequency of 25 pps, and an on-off ratio of 6 seconds on and 6 seconds off. The treatment time was gradually increased to 8 hours of stimulation per day (the stimulation was typically done at night if tolerated). High success and low dropout rates were reported.[237] Others, however, reported much lower success rates.[238] Intolerance of the treatment resulting in low compliance may be the cause of these differences. This disorder is much more common in adolescent girls. When NMES was first introduced for scoliosis, the uncomfortable and cosmetically undesirable Milwaukee brace was still the norm for treatment. With more advanced materials and orthotic management that is much more acceptable cosmetically, the use of NMES in scoliosis management has significantly declined.

Kim & Yoo[239] investigated the effect of manual therapy with FES on scoliosis in children with CP and their quality of life. Two children with CP participated in the study, which consisted of 30 minutes of manual therapy and 30 minutes of FES. These modalities were provided three times a week for 3 months. The Cobb's angle and the Pediatric Quality of Life Inventory (PedsQL) were assessed before and after the intervention to determine the effect of combing these two modalities. The authors concluded that manual therapy with FES was effective for improving the scoliosis curve and quality of life of children with CP and scoliosis.

Ko and colleagues[240] studied the effects of lateral electrical surface stimulation (LESS) on scoliosis and trunk balance in children with severe CP. The participants were children with severe CP (GMFCS level IV or V). The scoliosis was either stationary or progressive. The frequency of treatment consisted two sessions of LESS per day, 1-hour session, for 3 months at home. The intensity was set at 40 to 80 mA, pulse width at 200 μs, the frequency at 25 Hz, on for 6 seconds and then off for 6 seconds on the convex side of the spine. The following measurements were conducted at 3 months before, just before, 1 month after, and 3 months after LESS: Radiologic (Cobb's, kyphotic, and sacral angles) and functional GMFM-88 sitting score, and trunk control measurement scale (TCMS). The results revealed a median Cobb's angle of 25 degrees. There were significant improvements after 1 and 3 months of LESS treatment. The authors concluded that LESS is effective in treating scoliosis in children with severe CP and indicated that it might improve trunk balance.

Contraindications and Precautions

Any ES application is contraindicated for patients who have epilepsy or demand-type pacemakers. In addition, contraindications exist to applications over the transthoracic area or the uterus in pregnancy as well as in a cancerous area and the carotid sinus. Other factors require precaution but are not strict contraindications, such as sensory deficits, skin problems (sensitivity to stimulation, electrodes, or gel; edema; open wounds), tolerance of stimulation intensity sufficient to elicit muscle contraction, patient's capability to participate in the training process, and financial considerations.[57–59,241]

Matthews and colleagues[242] reported changes in blood pressure and heart rate suggestive of autonomic hyperreflexia when ES was applied in seven subjects with SCI above the T6 level. FES to the quadriceps produced the noted changes as stimulation intensity was increased. The mechanism for this reaction is unclear. Clinicians should monitor vital signs in patients with SCI (and possibly all patients), at least during the initial application of ES.

The use of stimulation modalities by patients outside clinical therapy sessions requires a degree of cooperation and motivation to take care of the stimulation unit, use it as instructed, and observe precautions. Long-term use of NMES (e.g., FES) may not be feasible for patients who do not have the financial resources (insurance or otherwise) to rent or purchase a unit or do not have reasonable access to support for equipment maintenance.

EMGBF does not require as many precautions because the procedure only monitors muscle activity. This form of feedback by the patient requires a basic level of attention and cognitive skill to understand the meaning of, as well as act on, the feedback to change muscle performance. Patient motivation and interest in use of this modality are also required because the patient must be able to develop sensitivity to the degree of muscle activation independently so that feedback is no longer required. EMGBF may be used in some instances that do not require the cognitive skills of the patient to use this information, such as an evaluative tool for the therapist to gather information about muscle activation to plan intervention strategies.

SUMMARY

The concepts, descriptions, and applications of electrodiagnosis presented in this chapter are intended to enrich the therapist's comprehension of these studies as applied to patients with neurological conditions. Integration of the results of these tests in differential diagnosis and in subsequent planning of intervention is invaluable.

Clearly, the use of NMES and EMGBF has numerous possibilities with patients of all ages who have sustained neurological insult or injury. Improvement of motor control has been supported in some applications, although well controlled group research in populations other than stroke and adult SCI is lacking. This underscores the need for further investigation to support the evidence for these modalities. As the therapy environment continues to change

in response to time and funding constraints, therapists must carefully evaluate the benefits of a variety of available tools to assist their patients in regaining motor control and functional ability. A benefit of FES or EMGBF is the ability of the patient to work autonomously (i.e., at home) after becoming familiar with the treatment regimen, with the therapist periodically updating a home program. This protocol allows physical and occupational therapy time to be used for direct intervention. NMES and EMGBF may efficiently assist in attaining improvement in control and may also be used in the context of functional activities, but these tools alone will not create functional changes. The case studies that follow further integrate these concepts in actual cases.

CASE STUDIES

Part 1: Electrodiagnosis

The following are cases studies from patients seen in the electrophysiology lab. The reader will receive the full benefit of studying the cases by first reading the evaluation and establishing a set of differential

possible diagnoses and dysfunctions of the nervous system. The reader can then progress through the report, test by test, and challenge the differential diagnoses. The conclusion of the study is provided. NOTE: Please refer to Appendix 31.A for a key to all the abbreviations found in the figures and tables used in the Case Studies.

CASE STUDY 31.1

The patient is a right-handed 55-year-old general contractor. He reports that 3 months prior, he purchased an exercise cycle that he started using quite vehemently. Following this bout of exercise, he started noticing muscle soreness in his hamstrings and right calf. He now reports fatigue and twitching of the muscles in both shoulders and right leg. He also has an achy back in the middle of his thoracic spine. There is no numbness. He does not have any particular stressors except for the decrease in business brought about by the change in the economy. He never lost control of his sphincters. His thinking is clear.

Prior medical history is significant only for skin cancers, which were excised from his back last year and a meniscal tear. He has no known allergies and is lactose intolerant. On questioning, the patient does report hunting and eating the game he kills but has no other exposure to heavy metals.

Physical examination shows that walks unassisted but has a slight foot drop on the right side. From an orthopedic standpoint there is some crepitus with mobilization of the left shoulder; otherwise, range of motion is full, including in the cervical spine. There is no Lhermitte sign. Inspection shows significant fasciculations in the right quadriceps and both upper arms; a mild facial asymmetry from a previously fractured upper maxilla on the left side; easily palpated dorsalis pedis pulse on both sides; and mild atrophy of the right calf, which is 1.5 cm smaller than that of the left side. Grip strength is 80 lb on the right side and 60 lb on the left side. Manual muscle testing reveals a decrease in the strength of the extensor and flexor hallucis longus on the right side, 3+/5 (⅘ on the left side); right tibialis anterior, ⅗ (⅘ on the left side); right to gastrocnemius, 3−/5; right quadriceps, 4−/5; and intrinsic muscles, ⅘ on both sides. The patient fully detects the 3.61 Semmes-Weinstein monofilament in the lower extremities and the 2.83 monofilament in the upper extremities, which is normal. Muscle stretch reflexes are 2+ in the upper extremities and 1+ in the lower extremities; there is no Hoffmann sign in either hand; plantar cutaneous reflex is equivocal; cranial nerve scan is normal including extraocular movements. Speech is normal.

Summary of Nerve Conduction Findings
Motor distal latencies are normal in all nerves tested. Conduction velocities in all segments are normal. Amplitudes of the responses are slightly decreased or at the lower limit of normal. Sensory distal latencies, amplitudes, and conduction velocities are all within normal limits.

F-wave latencies are slightly delayed in the right fibular and tibial nerves and normal in the left fibular and right median nerves.

H-reflex latencies are delayed on both sides.

Summary of Electromyographic Findings
Insertional activity was increased in the right vastus medialis, tibialis anterior, gastrocnemius, extensor feature brevis, and left tibialis anterior. Fasciculations were found in the right deltoid, triceps, first dorsal interosseous, vastus medialis, and extensor digitorum brevis, as well as in the left gastrocnemius and thoracic paraspinals. Denervation potentials were found in every muscle sampled (including the tongue) except the right biceps. Analysis of the motor unit action potentials showed them to be polyphasic in the first dorsal interosseous of the right hand, right tibialis anterior, right gastrocnemius, left extensor digitorum brevis, and left tibialis anterior. Recruitment pattern was reduced in the right biceps and in the tibialis anterior, gastrocnemius, and extensor digitorum brevis on both sides. Firing rate of the MUAPs was fast in the extensor digitorum brevis on both sides as well as in the right gastrocnemius and tibialis anterior. Refer to Tables 31.2 to 31.6, and Fig. 31.11 for a summary of various nerve conduction studies performed on this patient.

Conclusions
The results of this study are abnormal. Findings include normal sensory distal latencies, nerve conduction, and amplitudes; normal motor distal latencies and nerve conduction, slightly reduced amplitudes; widespread denervation potentials in three limbs, paraspinals, and the tongue; fasciculations. This is consistent with an acquired motor neuron disorder.

Based on this study, laboratory tests, and the physical examination, the referring neurologist diagnosed patient 1 with amyotrophic lateral sclerosis.

Prognosis
Poor.

Interventions
The patient was issued ankle-foot orthoses, first on the right side, then the left. He later required a walker, then a powered wheelchair and continuous positive airway pressure (CPAP) machine. He died 12 months after this study.

TABLE 31.2 **Motor Nerve Conduction Study**

NERVE/ SITES	REC SITE	LAT msec	AMP 1-2 MV	DISTANCE CM	VEL M/S	TEMP °C	AMP %
R Med—APB							
Wrist	APB	3.80	4.7	8		30.9	100
Elbow		7.80	4.1	23	57.5	30.8	87.1
Axilla		9.30	3.4	10	66.7	30.9	71.9
L COMM FIBULAR—EDB							
Ankle	EDB	4.55	2.6	8		31.1	100
Fib Head		11.35	1.7	31	45.6	30.9	64.4
Knee		13.30	1.6	9	46.2	30.8	60.8
R COMM FIBULAR—EDB							
Ankle	EDB	5.40	2.8	8		31.3	100
Fib Head		12.35	2.4	29	41.7	31	85.3
Knee		14.65	2.7	10	43.5	30.9	95.4
R Tibial (Knee)—FHB							
Bel. Ankle	FHB	5.85	1.8	8		30.5	100
Ab. Ankle		8.25	1.9	10	41.7	30.5	106
Knee		17.55	1.3	38	40.9	30.4	73.9

TABLE 31.3 **Sensory Nerve Conduction Study**

NERVE/ SITES	REC SITE	LAT 2 msec	AMP PK-PK MV	VEL PK M/S	DISTANCE CM	TEMP °C
R Radial—vs. Med—Thumb						
Forearm (Radial)	Thumb	2.70	6.8	44.4	12	32.3
Wrist (Med)	Thumb	3.40	14.7	35.3	12	32.4
L Sural—LAT MALLEOLUS						
Calf	LAT MALLEOLUS	3.20	2.9	37.5	12	30.5
Calf	LAT MALLEOLUS	3.35	0.42	35.8	12	30.5
R Sural—LAT MALLEOLUS						
Calf	LAT MALLEOLUS	3.60	0.29	33.3	12	31.1
Calf	LAT MALLEOLUS	3.70	0.17	32.4	12	31.1

TABLE 31.4 **F-Wave Study**

NERVE	MIN F LAT msec	MAX F LAT msec	MIN F AMP MV	MAX F AMP MV	MIN F-M msec	MAX F-M msec
L COMM FIBULAR—EDB	52.05	56.85	0.10	0.17	46.30	51.15
R COMM FIBULAR—EDB	54.50	56.55	0.16	0.27	48.60	50.70
R Tibial (Knee)—FHB	58.10	64.90	0.00	0.04	50.10	56.85
R Med—APB	27.65	61.65	0.05	0.15	23.75	57.70

TABLE 31.5 H-Reflex Study

NERVE	RESP. No MAX M	RESP. No MAX H	H LAT msec	H AMP MV	H/M AMPL %
L Tibial—GASTROCN	11	9	34.20	0.3	3.54
R Tibial—GASTROCN	21	22	35.30	0.4	9.94

TABLE 31.6 Electromyography Summary Table

	SPONTANEOUS			MUAP				RECRUITMENT	
	IA	FIB	PSW	FASC	AMP	DUR	POLYPH	PATTERN	FIRE RATE
R. Tongue	N	2+	None	None	N	N	N	N	N
R. Deltoid	N	1+	None	1+	N	N	N	N	N
R. Biceps	N	None	None	None	N	N	N	Reduced	N
R. Triceps	N	1+	1+	1+	N	N	N	N	N
R. EXT DIG COMM	N	2+	1+	None	N	N	N	N	N
R. FIRST D INTEROSS	N	1+	2+	1+	1+	N	1+	N	N
R. VAST MED	1+	1+	2+	1+	N	N	N	N	N
R. TIB ANTERIOR	2+	2+	2+	None	N	N	1+	Discrete	Fast
R. GASTROCN (Med)	2+	1+	3+	None	N	N	2+	Reduced	Fast
R. EXT DIG BREVIS	1+	2+	2+	1+	N	N	N	Reduced	Fast
L. EXT DIG BREVIS	N	2+	None	None	2+	N	2+	Reduced	Fast
L. GASTROCN (Med)	N	1+	2+	1+	N	N	N	Reduced	N
L. TIB ANTERIOR	2+	2+	2+	None	N	N	3+	Reduced	N
L. VAST Med	N	1+	1+	None	N	N	N	N	N
R. THOR PSP (Med)	N	1+	1+	1+	N	N	N	N	N
R. LUMB PSP (Med)	N	1+	None	None	N	N	N	N	N

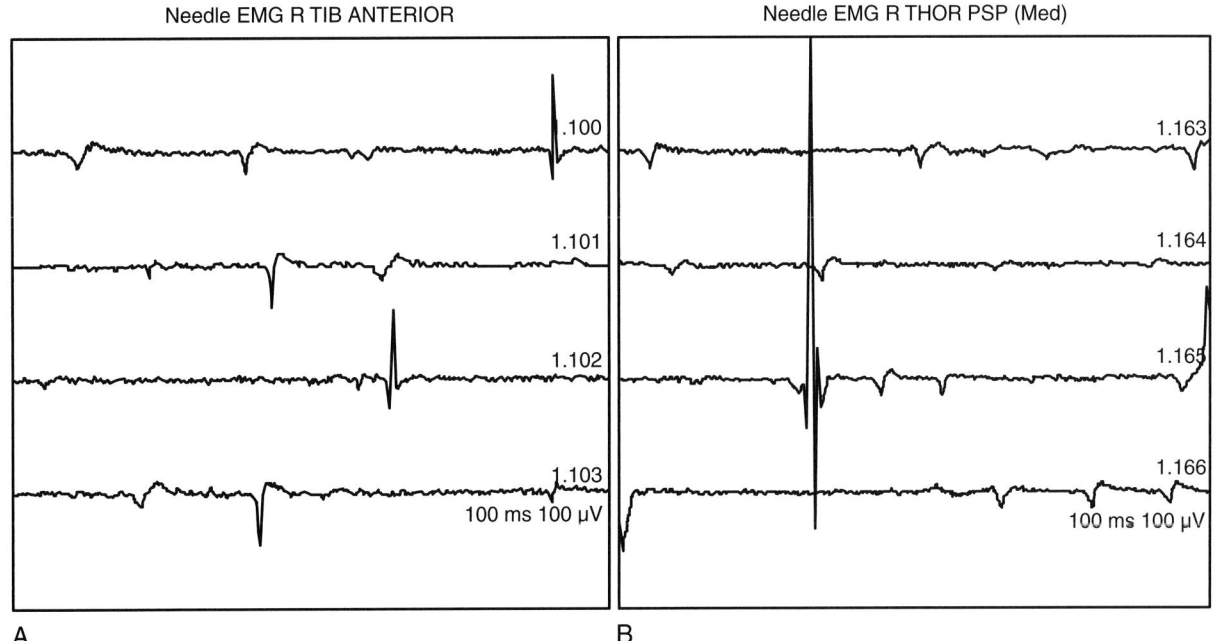

Fig. 31.11 Needle Electromyography *(EMG)*. **(A)** Positive sharp waves and fibrillation potentials. **(B)** One fasciculation and positive sharp waves.

CASE STUDY 31.2

The patient is a right-handed, 49-year-old administrative assistant. She reports a 1-year history of numbness in the right hand. Initially, this numbness was present only intermittently. The numbness involves mostly the thumb and index and long fingers. Recently the numbness has been present every morning. This impairs her ability to sleep. The patient also reports difficulty with writing. She has a positive flick sign. Finally, she reports that ibuprofen has been of some help in the sense that she no longer wakes up in the middle of the night. She has no numbness in her toes. There are no complaints regarding her cervical spine.

Prior medical history is essentially unremarkable and includes only uterine fibroids. The patient has had a hysterectomy. There are no known allergies.

Physical examination shows that the patient walks unassisted with a normal gait pattern. Inspection shows slight arthritic changes at the base of the right thumb but no noticeable muscle atrophy in the intrinsic muscles or thenar eminence. Grip strength is 45 lb on the left side and 55 lb on the right side. Sensation is slightly decreased: the patient detects the 3.61 Semmes-Weinstein monofilament at the tip of the fingers of the right hand. Result of the Phalen test is positive, and the reverse Phalen test causes wrist pain; the Finkelstein test also causes wrist pain. "Okay" sign is normal. Cervical range of motion is full in all directions; result of the Spurling test is negative. Muscle stretch reflexes are 2+ and symmetrical. Cranial nerve scan is normal.

Based on this physical examination, what is your clinical impression?

Summary of Nerve Conduction Findings

The median motor distal latency is prolonged compared with the ipsilateral ulnar motor distal latency (2.05 ms difference). Amplitudes of the median motor responses are decreased. The ulnar motor distal latency, amplitudes, and conduction velocities are within normal limits.

The median sensory distal latencies are significantly delayed. Radial and ulnar sensory distal latencies are normal. The combined sensory index (CSI) is 7.1 (cutoff value for normal conduction for the CSI is 1.3).

Median F-wave latencies are at the upper limit of normal for a patient this height. Ulnar F-wave latencies are normal.

Summary of Electromyographic Findings

Insertional activity was normal in all muscles sampled. A few denervation potentials were found at rest in the abductor pollicis brevis (fibrillation potentials). Analysis of the motor unit action potentials showed them to be of normal configuration, phases, and recruitment in all muscles tested except in the abductor pollicis brevis. In this muscle, motor units were slightly polyphasic. Refer to Fig. 31.12, and to Tables 31.7 to 31.10 for a summary of various nerve conduction studies performed on this patient.

Conclusions

This study is abnormal. Findings are consistent with a moderate to severe mononeuropathic process involving the right median nerve at or distal to the wrist. This is shown by delayed median motor and sensory distal latencies, decreased amplitudes of the median motor responses, and abnormal electromyographic findings in the abductor pollicis brevis only.

Because the ipsilateral ulnar motor and ulnar and radial sensory nerve conduction study findings are normal and because the needle electromyography findings are limited to the abductor pollicis brevis, a polyneuropathic, plexopathic, or a radiculopathic process is unlikely in the right upper extremity.

Prognosis

Excellent. The patient and her surgeon elected to go ahead with a carpal tunnel release.

Interventions

The patient started rehabilitation after surgery and went on to a full recovery in 2 months.

Sensory NCS R Uln - vs Med Palm

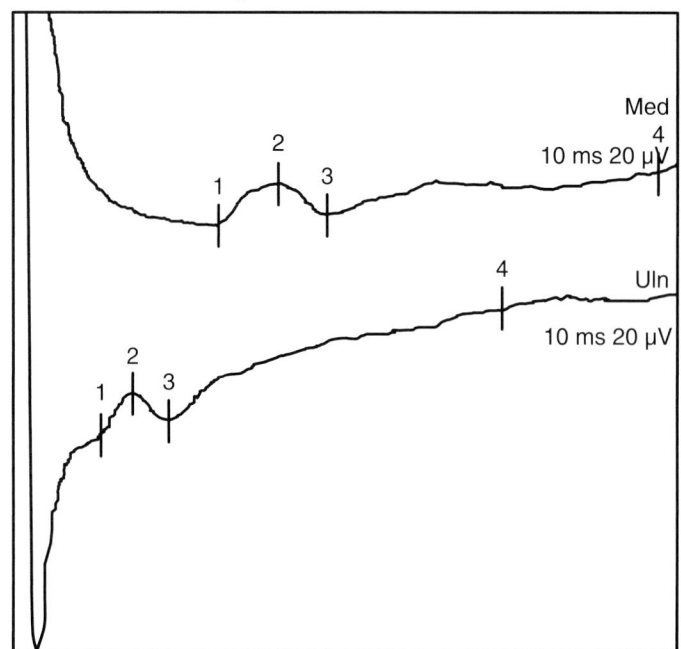

Fig. 31.12 Sensory nerve action potential difference: median *(above)* and ulnar *(below)*.

TABLE 31.7 Motor Nerve Conduction Study

NERVE/ SITES	REC SITE	LAT msec	AMP 1-2 MV	DISTANCE CM	VEL M/S	TEMP °C	AMP %
R Med—APB							
Wrist	APB	5.55	3.9	8		32.8	100
Elbow		9.60	3.8	21	51.9	32.7	97.4
Axilla		11.00	4.6	9	64.3	32.7	117
R Uln—ADM							
Wrist	ADM	2.50	9.1	8		32.3	100
bel. Elbow		6.15	8.0	21	57.5	32.3	88
ab. Elbow		7.80	7.7	9	54.5	32.3	84.9

TABLE 31.8 Sensory Nerve Conduction Study

NERVE/ SITES	REC SITE	LAT 2 msec	AMP PK-PK MV	VEL PK M/S	DISTANCE CM	TEMP °C
R Radial—vs. Med—Thumb						
Forearm (Radial)	Thumb	2.85	8.3	42.1	12	33.6
Wrist (Med)	Thumb	4.75	15.3	25.3	12	33.8
R Uln—vs. Med DIG IV						
Med	IV	6.10	8.5	23.0	14	33.6
Uln	IV	3.05	13.6	45.9	14	33.6
R Uln—vs. Med Palm						
Med Palm	Wrist	4.10	10.4	19.5	8	33.2
Uln Palm	Wrist	1.90	8.7	42.1	8	33.2

TABLE 31.9 F-Wave Study

NERVE	MIN F LAT msec	MAX F LAT msec	MIN F AMP MV	MAX F AMP MV	MIN F-M msec	MAX F-M msec
R Med—APB	28.95	32.25	0.00	0.15	23.55	26.75
R Uln—ADM	25.10	27.65	0.07	0.29	22.50	25.05

TABLE 31.10 Electromyography Summary Table

	SPONTANEOUS				MUAP			RECRUITMENT	
	IA	FIB	PSW	FASC	AMP	DUR	POLYPH	PATTERN	FIRE RATE
R. Deltoid	N	None	None	None	N	N	N	N	N
R. Tricops	N	None	None	None	N	N	N	N	N
R. EXT DIG COMM	N	None	None	None	N	N	N	N	N
R. FLEX CARPI RAD	N	None	None	None	N	N	N	N	N
R. 1st D INTEROSS	N	None	None	None	N	N	N	N	N
R. ABD POLL BREVIS	N	1+	None	None	N	N	1+	N	N
R. CERV PSP (L)	N	None	None	None	N	N	N	N	N

CASE STUDY 31.3

The patient is a right-handed, 86-year-old retired internist. He consults today for assessment of the strength in his lower extremities and numbness in his right hand. He reports having difficulty going up the 13 steps he has at home and states that his right thumb and index and middle fingers feel like "Band-Aids are on too tight at the tip of the fingers."

Prior medical history includes Waldenström macroglobulinemia, gastrectomy for recurrent bleeding, 7+ years of taking amiodarone, hypothyroid.

Physical examination shows that the patient walks with a bilateral foot drop and increased base of support. MMT shows decrease in the strength of ankle dorsiflexors on both sides, noted 3+/5; right quadriceps, ⅘; foot intrinsic muscles, ⅗; hand intrinsic muscles, 3+/5; right triceps muscle, 3+/5. All other muscles groups have normal strength. Grip strength is 30 lb on the right side and 35 lb on the left side. Sensation is decreased to the 3.61 Semmes-Weinstein monofilament at the sole of the right foot; the patient detects the 4.31 filament. It is also decreased to the 2.83 monofilament at the palm of the right hand; the patient detects the 3.61 filament. Range of motion (ROM) of the left shoulder is impaired in abduction. Cervical ROM is within normal limits. Spurling's test is negative. Toes are down-going with the plantar cutaneous reflex; there is no Hoffmann sign in the hands. Muscle stretch reflexes are 2+ in the quadriceps and upper extremities, 1+ at the ankle. Cranial nerve scan is normal. Romberg sign is positive. Refer to Fig. 31.13, and Tables 31.11 to 31.15 for a summary of various nerve conduction studies performed on this patient.

Conclusions

The study findings are abnormal. Findings are consistent with an axonal loss, mixed sensorimotor polyneuropathic process. This is evidenced by normal motor and sensory distal latencies, absent or significantly reduced amplitudes in both motor and sensory responses, delayed F-wave and H-reflex latencies, denervation in the distal more than the proximal muscles, and no findings in the lumbar paraspinals.

Prognosis

Fair to good. Improvement expected over the next 4 to 6 months with medical management of the polyneuropathy.

Interventions

The patient started balance rehabilitation and muscle strengthening and ultimately met his goal of safely climbing up and down his stairs.

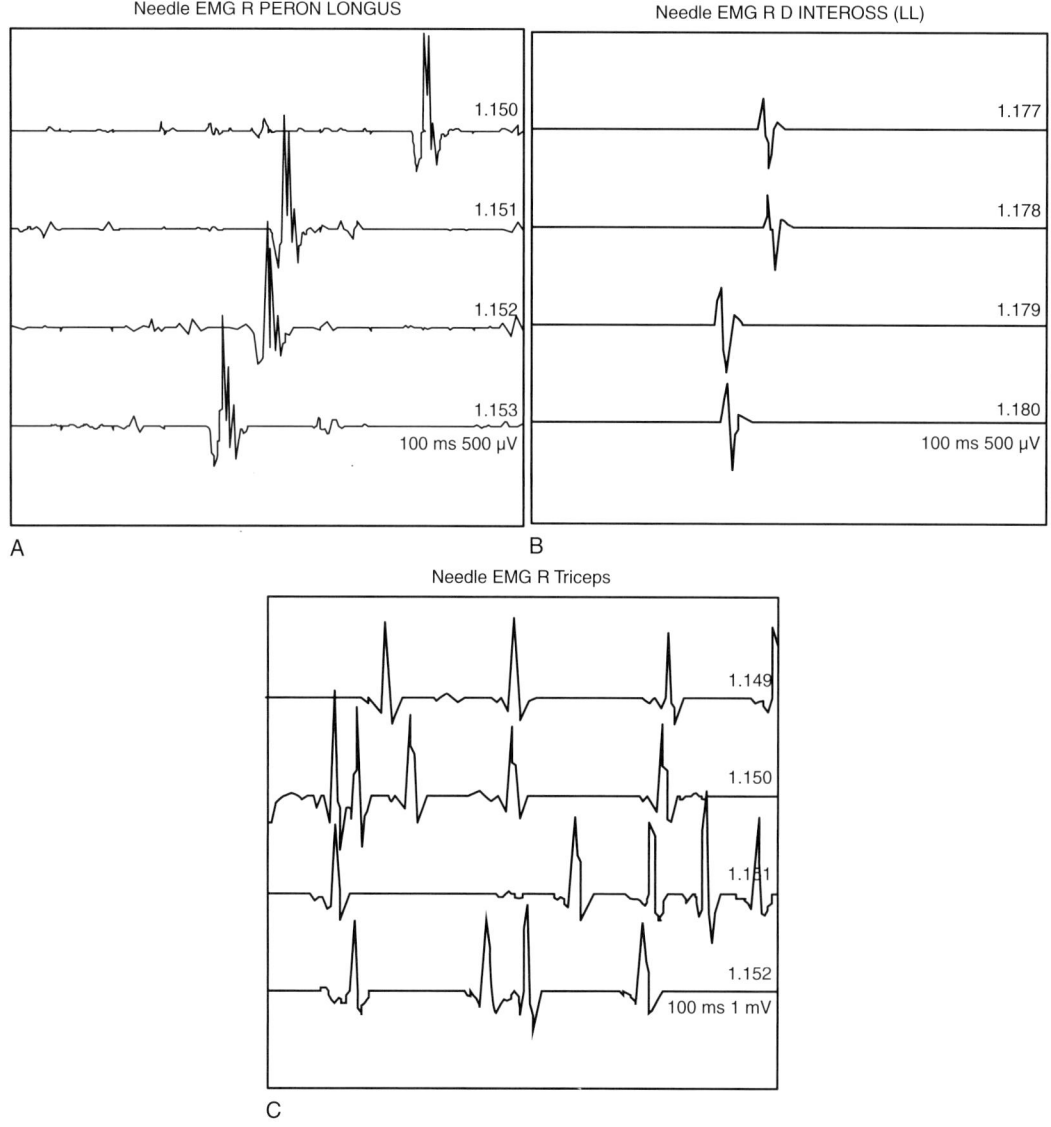

Fig. 31.13 Needle electromyography. (A) Polyphasic motor unit action potentials (MUAPs) in the right peroneus longus. **(B)** Essentially one MUAP in the foot dorsal interossei. **(C)** Fast firing MUAPs. *EMG,* Electromyography.

TABLE 31.11 Motor Nerve Conduction Study

NERVE/ SITES	RESP	REC SITE	LAT msec	AMP 1-2 MV	DISTANCE CM	VEL M/S	TEMP °C	AMP %
R Med—APB								
Wrist		APB	3.75	3.1	8		33.8	100
Elbow			8.75	1.8	25.5	51.0	34	57.7
Axilla			10.65	1.3	10	52.6	34.3	43.2
R Uln—ADM								
Wrist		ADM	3.00	6.2	8		33.9	100
bel. Elbow			7.05	6.6	20	49.4	33.5	106
ab. Elbow			9.25	5.5	10	45.5	32.4	87.9
R COMM FIBULAR—EDB								
Ankle	No	EDB	NR	NR			31.9	
R Tibial (Knee)—FHB								
bel. Ankle		FHB	5.35	0.7	8		31.1	100
ab. Ankle			7.80	0.5	10	40.8	31.1	78.4
Knee			18.20	0.5	32	30.8	31.1	66.4
R COMM FIBULAR—TIB ANT								
Fib Head		Tib Ant	2.95	0.7	8		31.3	100
Knee			5.20	0.7	10	44.4	30.9	102

TABLE 31.12 Sensory Nerve Conduction Study

NERVE/ SITES	REC SITE	LAT 2 MSEC	AMP PK-PK MV	VEL PK M/S	DISTANCE CM	TEMP °C
R Radial—vs. Med—Thumb						
Forearm (Radial)	Thumb	3.50	1.3	34.3	12	32.1
Wrist (Med)	Thumb	3.75	8.5	32.0	12	32
R Uln—vs. Med—DIG IV						
Med	IV	4.25	2.0	32.9	14	32.8
Uln	IV	5.80	2.3	24.1	14	32.5
R Sural—LAT MALLEOLUS						
Calf	LAT MALLEOLUS	3.70	0.46	32.4	12	31.6
Calf	LAT MALLEOLUS	4.05	0.79	29.6	12	31.6

TABLE 31.13 F-Wave Study

NERVE	MIN F LAT msec	MAX F LAT msec	MIN F AMP MV	MAX F AMP MV	MIN F-M msec	MAX F-M msec
R Tibial (Knee)—FHB	60.35	65.30	0.01	0.03	4.35	55.40
R Med—APB	31.25	82.10	0.04	0.26	27.30	78.10
R Uln—ADM	35.25	74.45	0.03	0.29	32.00	71.10

TABLE 31.14   H-Reflex Study

NERVE	RESP. NO MAX M	RESP. NO MAX H	H LAT msec	H AMP MV	H/M AMPL %
R Tibial—GASTROCN	13	11	33.50	1.1	102
L Tibial—GASTROCN	14	14	35.20	0.6	37.2

TABLE 31.15   Electromyography Summary Table

	SPONTANEOUS				MUAP			RECRUITMENT	
	IA	FIB	PSW	FASC	AMP	DUR	POLYPH	PATTERN	FIRE RATE
R. VAST MED	N	None	None	None	N	N	N	N	N
R. Deltoid	N	None	None	None	N	N	N	N	N
R. TIB ANTERIOR	N	None	None	None	N	N	2+	Reduced	Fast
R. PERON LONGUS	N	None	None	None	N	N	3+	Reduced	Fast
R. GASTROCN (MED)	N	None	1+	None	N	N	1+	Reduced	Fast
R. EXT DIG BREVIS	-	None	None	None	-	-	-	No activity	-
R. D INTEROSS (LL)	N	1+	None	None	N	N	N	Discrete	N
R. Triceps	N	3+	3+	None	N	N	N	Reduced	Fast
R. EXT DIG COMM	N	1+	1+	None	N	N	N	Reduced	N
R. FIRST D INTEROSS	N	1+	2+	None	N	N	N	Reduced	N
R. LUMB PSP (L)	N	None	None	None	N	N	N	N	N

Part 2: Neuromuscular Electrical Stimulation and Electromyographic Biofeedback

CASE STUDY 31.4

A 68-year-old woman is referred 3 weeks after left middle cerebral artery cerebrovascular accident with residual right hemiparesis affecting the upper extremity to a greater degree than the lower extremity. The patient's left extremities appear well controlled with at least functional strength. She exhibits a two-fingerbreadth right shoulder subluxation, with pain at shoulder flexion (150 degrees), abduction (135 degrees), and external rotation (30 degrees), and hypertonicity in a stereotypical flexor synergy pattern affecting the shoulder horizontal adductors and internal rotators and elbow, wrist, and finger flexors. She is beginning to develop upper-extremity movement with the ability to shrug her shoulder, abduct, and flex through partial range (with elbow flexed), full-range elbow flexion, partial-range elbow extension against gravity, and no wrist or finger extension. Right lower-extremity range of motion is within normal limits, although control is limited at the ankle (dorsiflexion only with hip and knee flexion, no eversion actively) and knee control is decreased (reduced eccentric quadriceps control, difficulty isolating knee flexion with hip extension). Ambulation is accomplished with the use of a quad cane and an articulating Ankle Foot Orthosis (AFO) on the right for limited distances with standby assistance. This patient lives at home with her husband, who is very supportive of her rehabilitation. Both are retired, but they have an active calendar of participation in volunteer and leisure activities.

Prognosis

Independent or isolated motor function is promising for continued improvement in the condition of the patient. Lower-extremity impairments are expected to be minimized as the return of motor control progresses. Quad cane use should continue until isolated hip and knee action improves. A need for AFO is expected for an indefinite time period.

Intervention

Interventions using neuromuscular electrical stimulation (NMES) would assist in accelerating improvement in functional control. Table 31.16 provides the various intervention options using NMES for this patient.

TABLE 31.16 Neuromuscular Electrical Stimulation/Electromyographic Biofeedback Options

Patient Problem	Goals	Modality Parameters	Measures to Determine Efficacy	Considerations
Shoulder subluxation	Decrease subluxation to 1 fingerwidth, with pain manageable within patient's daily routine.	Portable FES for home use, begin with 10:30 second on-off ratio for 15-min periods tid, amplitude to generate muscle contraction without shoulder elevation. Increase on time and treatment time as tolerated so that reduction is maintained majority of day.	Trial use for 1 month. Measure amount of palpable subluxation, pain-free ROM; if improvement is not observed, discontinue FES, with instruction to maintain shoulder flexibility, consider lapboard or arm tray when sitting, support when standing.	1. Requires rental of portable FES unit; patient/family compliance is needed for success in home program. 2. Cost of rental of FES and supplies. 3. Frequent use for reduction of subluxation requires close monitoring of skin for possible reactions to stimulation, gel, or electrodes. 4. Integrate scapular movement and stabilization exercises into program
Lack of active ankle dorsiflexion	Increase active control of ankle dorsiflexion with knee extended, allowing heel-strike without AFO for short-distance ambulation.	FES twice daily for 15-min duration; 10:20 second on-off ratio with slow ramping on-off; as active movement improves, consider EMGBF to further focus attention on balanced dorsiflexion (with eversion). Use of heelswitch requires decreased ramp time to minimum patient can tolerate. Switch should activate at heel-off to control dorsiflexion through the swing phase.	Monitor each session for increased active dorsiflexion in sitting, standing, and ambulation. Integrate use of heelswitch during ambulation without AFO. Trial use over 2–3 weeks. Discontinue if not seeing increase in voluntary control; compensate with AFO.	1. If patient rents unit for shoulder subluxation, may also use stimulator at home instead of requiring time during therapy session. 2. Similar cost, convenience issues as above. 3. Additional education necessary if stimulator settings are to be switched for dorsiflexion and shoulder subluxation interventions.
Lack of full active wrist and finger extension	Control of active wrist and finger extension to allow release in gross grasp.	NMES and/or EMGBF twice a day for 10-min sessions initially, with gradual increase in duration up to 20 min if fatigue does not alter the quality of the contractions. Other parameters as described for ankle dorsiflexion.	Trial period of 2–3 weeks; discontinue if voluntary motion is not changing significantly. Active movement in finger extensors with wrist in neutral position. Functional ability to release grasp of objects of varying shapes and sizes.	May use portable stimulator as described for ankle or shoulder interventions, with similar considerations.
Muscle imbalance, lack of right upper-extremity functional movement	Decrease hypertonicity in flexor muscle groups; increase extensor control for gross arm movements (e.g., positioning).	EMGBF to decrease flexor muscle activity (resting and with passive movement) and increase extensor activity.	Speed and control with reciprocal elbow motions, especially with extension. Use of this motion for functional activity (e.g., positioning the arm, reaching activity).	Focus on increased extensor control may prove more effective than simply decreasing flexor hyperactivity.

EMGBF, Electromyographic biofeedback; *FES*, functional electrical stimulation; *NMES*, neuromuscular electrical stimulation; *ROM*, range of motion.

REFERENCES

To enhance this text and add value for the reader, all references are included on the companion Evolve site that accompanies this textbook. This online service will, when available, provide a link for the reader to a Medline abstract for the article cited. There are 242 cited references and other general references for this chapter, with the majority of those articles being evidence-based citations.

Key to Abbreviations

The following is a key to the abbreviations used in the Case Studies in this chapter.

μV = microvolts
ABD POLL BREVIS = abductor pollicis brevis
ADM = abductor digiti minimi
Amp PK-PK = peak to peak amplitude
AMP = amplitude
APB = abductor pollicis brevis
AR = active recording
bel. = below
ab. = above
CM = centimeters
COMM FIBULAR = common fibular nerve
D INTEROSS = dorsal interosseus
EDB = extensor digitorum brevis
EMG = electromyography
EXT DIG BREV = extensor digitorum brevis
EXT DIG COMM = extensor digitorum communis
FASC = fasciculation potentials
FLEX CARPI RAD = flexor carpi radialis
FHB = flexor hallucis brevis
FIB = fibrillation potentials
Fib head = head of the fibula
FIRST D INTEROSS = first dorsal interosseus
GASTROCN = gastrocnemius
H AMP = H reflex amplitude
H LAT = H reflex latency
H/M APML = ratio between the amplitudes of the H-reflex and the M wave or motor response
IA = insertional activity

L = left
LAT MALLEOLUS = lateral malleolus
LAT = latency
LL = lower leg
LUMB PSP = lumbar paraspinals
M/S = meters per second
MAX F AMP = maximum F-wave amplitude
MAX F LAT = maximum F-wave latency
MAX F-M = Maximum difference in F-wave and M latencies
Med = median
MIN F LAT = minimum F-wave latency
MIN F-M = Minimum difference in F-wave and M latencies
msec = milliseconds
MUAP = motor unit action potentials
MV = millivolts
PERON LONGUS = peroneus longus
POLYPH = polyphasic
CERV PSP = cervical
PSW = positive sharp waves
R = right REC SITE = recording site
SNAP = sensory nerve action potential
TEMP = temperature
THOR PSP = thoracic paraspinals
TIB ANTERIOR = tibialis anterior
VAST MED = vastus medialis
VEL PK = peak velocity
VEL = velocity
vs = versus
Uln = ulnar

32

Orthotics: Evaluation, Intervention, and Prescription*

Heidi Truman and Preeti Nair

OBJECTIVES

After reading this chapter the student or therapist will be able to:

1. Identify and analyze the force systems produced by the use of an orthosis.
2. Comprehend the prescription rationale gained from an orthotic evaluation for individuals with neuromuscular dysfunctions.
3. Identify and differentiate the variables considered by the rehabilitation team to optimize outcomes during orthotic intervention.

KEY TERMS

ankle-foot orthosis (AFO)
knee-ankle-foot orthosis (KAFO)

lever arms, three-point pressure systems
thoracolumbosacral orthosis (TLSO)

OVERVIEW

An orthosis is an external device that produces a force that biomechanically affects the body to correct, support, or stabilize the trunk, the head, and/or an extremity. Orthoses are named by the sections of the body to which they are applied.[1] For example, an orthosis that controls and covers the ankle and foot is called an *ankle-foot orthosis* (AFO). The abbreviations for the device are used by professionals in clinical documentation. Orthotic use varies from temporary application to permanent use based on patient care goals. Careful evaluation is used to determine whether a prefabricated, custom-fit, or custom-made orthosis is most appropriate for the patient. A prefabricated orthosis is one that is available in "off-the-shelf" sizing and is intended for temporary use. Commonly used prefabricated items are often kept in stock by the orthotic provider. Custom-fit orthoses are customizable devices that can be modified to optimize the fit to an individual patient. These devices are intended for use on a more definitive basis and are often appropriate when the patient has adequate sensation and normal anatomy. Custom-made orthoses require very specific measurements or models of the patient to be obtained for the most specific fit and to accommodate any deformity. These devices are time and labor intensive and are worn definitively when the patient's condition is permanent or when his or her condition or anatomy does not facilitate fitting of a more basic device.[2]

Orthoses are primarily designed on three simple biomechanical concepts: pressure, force, and the lever arm principle.[3–5] The pressure principle simply means that pressure applied by the orthotic device is equal to the total force per unit area covered by the device. Because an orthosis is an external device that comes in contact with a part of the body, it has the ability to apply pressure based on the surface area it covers. If pressure is to be minimized, the surface area in contact with the device has to be maximized and vice versa. For example, a total contact orthosis will distribute pressure more evenly than a device that contacts the patient only at several points. The force principle is often used in designing orthoses that work on the three-point force system or the four-point force system. In a three-point force system, the orthosis is designed such that central components of the orthosis are able to apply force in one direction while the two terminal end parts provide a counterforce in the opposite direction, and the sum of all the three forces equals zero. For example, a knee orthosis designed to correct genu varum would consist of a central force directed medially at the lateral border of the knee joint and the terminal points of the orthosis applying laterally directed forces on the femur and tibia.[6] This way an orthosis is effectively used to permit angular change or provide control over a joint. Similarly, a four-point force system can be used to provide translational control of adjacent segments and prevent displacement of one segment over another. For example, a knee brace to prevent knee hyperextension and anterior tibial translation would consist of two parallel forces equal in magnitude and opposite in direction applied at different points on the femur to facilitate femoral flexion and two other parallel forces of equal magnitude and opposite in direction applied at different points on the tibia to facilitate tibial extension.[3,4] Finally, the lever arm principle is important in designing orthoses to determine the force at the segment of interest based on the height/length of the orthosis. As per the lever principles, the longer the orthosis, the greater the moment arm and therefore lesser will be the magnitude of force required to produce the desired effect at the joint of interest.[7,8] For example, an elbow orthosis that is just proximal and distal to the joint area will apply a greater force to immobilize the elbow, compared with an orthosis that extends to closer to the wrist and axilla. The longer orthosis will require less force to provide the same outcome of elbow immobilization.

---

*Videos for this chapter are available at studentconsult.com.

In addition to the basic biomechanical principles involved in designing an orthosis, many factors enter into the decision regarding use and type of orthosis. It is essential that the most functional, least complicated, and most cost-effective orthosis be applied to the patient. The rehabilitation team must build a priority list of desired outcomes and accept that sometimes all of the items on the list may not be achieved by either the orthosis or the patient-team combination. It is important to be aware that care may need to be attempted in stages because the patient's condition changes or if other medical concerns may arise. Effective coordination and communication between health professionals in development of patient goals are essential during the evaluation process. For instance, placing a loop closure on the side of their body that a patient cannot reach will prohibit the use of the orthotic device. A sound understanding of biomechanical and orthotic principles, as well as skilled patient management techniques, must be used to be successful with patients who require orthoses.

There are similarities in orthotic management of orthopedic and neurologically impaired patients; however, the neurological population presents additional factors that challenge prescription criteria and outcomes for the rehabilitation team. Lack of proprioception, impairments in sensation, and spasticity are some of these special considerations. Concurrent medical issues, problems with communication, and caregivers may complicate patient management.

The advancements in and access to medical technology have had a profound impact in the field of orthotics. The evolution of plastic, composite, and metals fabrication technology has dramatically improved the ability to control, support, and protect all areas of the human body. Currently, patients are fit for custom and prefabricated orthotic devices that provide a variety of functions in both a timely and cost-effective manner. These factors have led physicians to routinely prescribe orthoses for a wide range of medical conditions, whereas historically lack of availability and shortage of experienced orthotists restricted patient access and narrowed the use of orthoses.[9] Orthoses are important considerations for postoperative management, acute fracture management, and adjunct treatment in addition to more traditional uses. For many, the proliferation of the prefabricated orthosis signaled a dilution of quality orthotic care, but in reality it has had the opposite effect. These readily available, cost-effective orthoses have not taken orthoses out of the hands of the orthotist but rather have moved them into the minds of treating professionals. There has been continued growth of new and improved orthoses and expansion into other areas of treatment previously lacking in orthotic management. For example, positional and corrective orthoses can be used for premature and newborn infants, and a wide range of sizes of orthoses that previously were made only in adult sizes have become available for pediatric patients. As with any new technological advancement, there has been incorrect application and use. It is not that many of these prefabricated orthoses are difficult to apply; rather, there has been lack of a clear understanding of the indications, contraindications, and limitations these devices present to the rehabilitation team and patient caregivers.

Identifying patient functional goals and familiarity with the current state of evidence-based care for specific patient populations and diagnoses are critical in providing optimal patient care and achieving the desired clinical outcomes. In that spirit, a broad overview of the evaluation, prognosis, and intervention of orthotic devices in neurological rehabilitation is presented.

BASIC ORTHOTIC FUNCTIONS

Alignment

Anatomical and functional alignment of the extremities and spine is a common reason for an orthotic prescription. The orthosis can provide either temporary or permanent function. A thoracolumbosacral orthosis (TLSO) may be prescribed for stabilizing alignment after spinal fusion or for non-operative management off an unstable spinal cord injury (SCI; refer to Chapter 14). A supramalleolar orthosis (SMO) is commonly prescribed to hold the foot in proper alignment in multiple planes. When the goal of orthotic intervention is to correct alignment to a position well tolerated by the overlying soft tissue and/or the malalignment is a result of a muscle weakness, the new position should stabilize the joint. Clinicians need to remember that aligning one joint may result in the proximal or distal joint being placed in malalignment. An example of this is a patient with correctable genu valgum of the knee. Although this coronal plane deformity can be orthotically corrected, changes in knee alignment result in adjustments by the other joints up and down the kinetic chain. If the patient lacks inversion/eversion range of motion (ROM) at the ankle, placing the knee in a more vertical alignment will cause the patient to weight bear on the lateral border of the foot and possibly create instability at the ankle joint. Considerations such as the subtalar joint's mobility into pronation and supination must be accounted for when designing an orthosis that will provide coronal control at the knee.

Stability

Stability is often required for the patient with neurological deficits. These patients frequently lack the muscle control and strength necessary to maintain trunk balance or to ambulate. Patients with muscular dystrophy benefit from TLSOs to help maintain trunk stability, achieve sitting balance, and perform safer transfers. However, the orthotic prescription must be guided by the knowledge that maximum stability cannot compromise or restrain thoracic expansion for breathing capacity. An AFO that limits both dorsiflexion and plantarflexion can stabilize the ankle and the knee for the patient who has had a cerebrovascular accident (CVA).[10] Although this patient may require both coronal and sagittal plane ankle stabilization, controlling the lever arms at the ankle can also provide knee stability and prevent future knee impairments created by excess coronal (varus/valgus) or sagittal (hyperextension/hyperflexion) motion at the knee. The orthosis functions in the sagittal plane by maintaining ground reaction force anterior to the knee during the stance phase of gait. Most patients requiring this type of stabilization have a foot-flat gait instead of a normal initial heel-strike pattern.

Contracture Reduction

Contracture reduction is the goal for many orthotic applications in patients with neurological involvement. The increase in the use of these types of orthoses has been dramatic because even slight increases in contractures can make the difference between nonambulatory status and ambulatory community participation. Increased awareness and proactive use of prefabricated orthoses have become routine during periods of inactivity, associated surgical procedures, and "sound side" prevention. These types of orthoses can be either dynamic or static and are used in conjunction with various therapeutic modalities to reduce the contracture. Dynamic contracture-reducing orthoses use a spring-type mechanism that applies a low force to a joint over an extended period of time to gain range of motion (ROM). Static-type orthoses range from serial casts in which a manual stretch is placed over the joint for extended periods of time, to custom-made cylindrical devices designed to spread force over larger areas, to custom-fit devices with some type of quick adjustability. Dynamic-type orthoses are usually contraindicated for patients with neurological disorders that create tone and spasticity. Low-tension stretch can trigger spasticity and create skin breakdown because of the high pressure on localized skin areas. The exception for this would be individuals with lower motor neuron impairments and residual hypotonicity. Any type of tension orthosis needs to be monitored when there is sensory loss, regardless of the cause. To achieve results in contracture reduction, one must be cautiously aggressive because the amount of force required to improve ROM often threatens the soft tissue's ability to tolerate the pressure of the orthosis.[11] Experience, frequent sessions, and close communication with other members of the rehabilitation team and the family and patient are critical factors in the success of the use of orthotic devices.

EVALUATION

The examination and evaluation of the neurologically impaired patient must be comprehensive. One must not read a diagnosis and assume a total clinical picture. The diagnosis should alert the evaluator to movement patterns associated with the impairment, and these should be used to confirm potential findings. Complete patient evaluations do not end with determination of ROM, muscle test findings, assessment of proprioception, skin sensitivity evaluation, or assessment of the integrity of the affected limb or spine. The rehabilitation team must assess the total picture to determine what limitations orthotic care may impose on other important functions and activities, and patient participation in life. The evaluation must include a patient management assessment. What is the patient's or caregiver's motivation? How much equipment can the patient tolerate, and with how much can he or she function? What functional potential does the patient have once they have left the clinical or acute setting? How significant are the risks associated with orthotic intervention? As stated, the total evaluation of the patient and the patient's environment is important in developing the treatment plan, as is the communication among the physical therapist, occupational therapist, and orthotist. Whether done together or (more realistically) at separate sites, the details of the treatment plan must be discussed. The patient with neurological impairment often presents a series of complex issues: biomechanical, communication, visualization, and so on. Incomplete information or a lack of effort at communication among these professionals will not lead to a comprehensive treatment plan and ultimately optimal outcomes.

During evaluation, review of the diagnosis and gathering of patient history are extremely valuable. A complete medical diagnosis will indicate important information to the team. For example, for a patient with poliomyelitis, the orthotist is aware that it is a lower motor neuron lesion and that proprioception is intact (see Chapter 15). These patients have the benefit of skeletal balance in standing and ambulation and therefore require durable orthotic construction.[12] Compare this to a patient with T12 paraplegia with similar muscle strength. T12 level paraplegia. Assuming this is a complete lesion, patients affected at this level lack proprioception. They require other means to get feedback about standing balance and require a lightweight orthosis because they rarely use orthoses as a major means of locomotion. Although gathering patient history is a vital part of the evaluation, it is, more importantly, an opportunity to establish a productive patient management environment. Patients and family members have important information regarding the initial injury, previous medical care, reasons they sought additional care, and desired outcomes of new treatment. Most of this information can be gathered efficiently as either the therapist or the orthotist begins other professional evaluations. These are important patient and family management skills. One must hear from the patient or caregivers why they came to see the health care professional and their expectations of care. The therapist should not assume the family's goals without asking, because often patient and family goals are higher than the clinicians' expectations. Communicating at a level that is understandable is vital and

demonstrates to the patient and family that the therapist is a concerned professional, thereby engendering trust and confidence. Complete and timely documentation of these findings is vital to the evaluation and treatment plan. Whether communicating with others on the rehabilitation team, insurance carriers, or legal professionals, documentation and building medical justification are essential in treating all patients.

Evaluation of the Spine

Each area of the spinal column presents various combinations of motion and function. Beginning at the lumbar level as the base for upright position, the spinal column (1) protects vital organs, (2) serves as a supporting structure for the lungs to expand, (3) provides a base for the upper extremities to reach from, (4) acts as a scaffold for objects to be carried, (5) protects the central nervous system pathways, and (6) controls the upright position and motions of the head. The individual segments of the spine have relatively few complicated orthotic challenges. However, it is rare that only one segment is involved in the patient with neuropathic impairments. It is more common for two or more segments of the spine to be involved when there is a need for orthotic control. For example, supporting the head in a functional position is a major goal of orthotic intervention, but to accomplish this the orthosis must encompass the thoracic as well as the cervical spine to distribute the forces to minimize skin pressures.

When evaluating the cervical spine and head, one must (in addition to muscle testing) determine past what angulations the upright position of the head cannot be recovered. Limiting the head from assuming nonfunctional positions such as extreme extension is an easier orthotic function than holding the head upright. Many patients with neurological problems may have the strength to move in a 15- to 20-degree range of flexion and extension, lateral bend, and rotation but do not have the strength to recover the head from greater angles. Even the most pressure-tolerant soft tissue around the head does not tolerate long-term pressure from an orthosis; intermittent control and relief are a critical part of the design. Pressure directly on the ear is not tolerated at any time.

When the orthosis is desired to limit cervical motion due to unstable fractures or postoperative management, selecting the most appropriate design depends on how much motion is acceptable. Upper cervical motion is controlled with a Halo orthosis (Fig. 32.1) when complete immobilization is desired. If more motion is acceptable, or for lower cervical control, a collar is more acceptable to both the treating team and the patient.[13] Many types of cervical collars exist to optimize patient fit and control (Fig. 32.2).

The thoracic and lumbar spine are almost always treated concurrently with an orthosis in the patient with a neurological deficit. The major reasons for orthotic intervention in this area are to stabilize the trunk for balance, to protect surgical correction or stabilization, and to maintain respiration.[14] The pelvis is generally used as a base to prevent distal migration of the orthosis when the patient is sitting or standing. One must closely evaluate the degree of deformity, prominence of bony structure, skin sensation, and condition of soft tissue coverage. Many neurologically impaired patients also have other medical issues that need to be considered in orthotic design, such as a colostomy, gastrointestinal (GI) tubes, pressure sores, and other factors. Scoliosis and kyphosis are common biomechanical impairments within this patient group. Balance between correcting the spinal deformity to maintain respiratory function by use of a tightly fitting TLSO and the skin pressure it creates must be reached by the rehabilitation team. The evaluation of the spine and potential need for orthotic intervention would not be complete without recognizing the effect the desired orthosis may have on the extremities, whether the patient is ambulatory

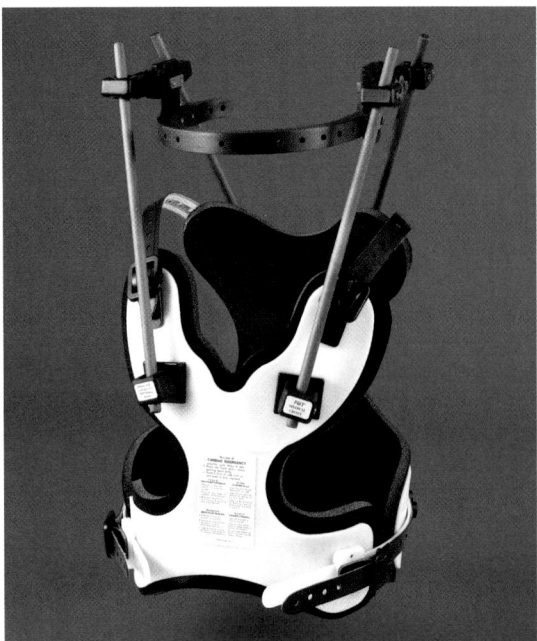

Fig. 32.1 Halo Orthosis. Courtesy PMT Corporation.

or non–weight bearing. What movements of the spine are present during ambulation, and would immobilizing the spine significantly affect the patient? Will the orthosis restrict needed shoulder elevation and arm movements? Variation in materials used for fabrication of a spinal orthosis can often significantly improve the desired outcome, increase the wear time, ease the donning process, and improve skin care. From a patient and family management standpoint, one must consider many variables in potential design of the orthosis. Can the patient or family properly don the orthosis and remove it when appropriate? Do they understand potential areas of pressure? Do they know what to do if any issues arise with fitting or skin integrity?

Evaluation of the Upper Extremities

Evaluation of the upper extremities requires multiple inputs from health care professionals, patients, family, and teachers because of the wide range of specific functions an individual performs daily. Unique to the upper extremity, multiple functions generally require multiple orthotic devices for activities of daily living (ADLs). Typical functions

of orthoses of the upper extremity include maintenance of functional wrist and hand position, reduction of contracture or tone, transfer of force available in one area to another, and support of subluxations resulting from denervation. It is common for the neurologically impaired patient to require several orthoses with different functions for use throughout the day. Strength, ROM, condition of soft tissues, and sensation are all important evaluation factors. In addition, ambulatory status, bilateral or unilateral condition, status of vision, and condition of the spine and head must be factored into the indications and contraindications in assessment of the orthotic needs of the patient. Much more critical muscle tests must be performed in the upper extremity as opposed to the lower extremity, because minor increases or decreases in strength will dramatically alter orthotic need. For example, the C5 quadriplegic has the ability to function with a wrist-hand orthosis by providing enough wrist extension to use the tenodesis effect, which can produce a three-jaw-chuck type of grip.[15] The difference between a functioning and nonfunctioning orthosis is minor, not only because there is limited muscle strength, but also because minor inefficiencies in the tenodesis splint (from friction or malalignment) could reduce function to unacceptable levels. Patients with unilateral involvement have far different needs than the bilaterally involved. The patient post-CVA with unilateral involvement may use a positional wrist-hand orthosis to prevent contracture and injury and a supportive shoulder orthosis to prevent shoulder subluxation (Fig. 32.3A–C).[16] In these cases the other extremity becomes dominant, and there is little need to fabricate complex orthoses for use by the affected extremity.

The patient with bilateral involvement presents a much different picture. Consideration for grooming, feeding, mobility, and so on must be factored into the desired expectation during evaluation. The case of the patient with neurological impairments who requires orthotic intervention is complex because this patient typically has involvement of the trunk, head, and lower extremity. These patients require specialized wheelchairs and seating systems.[17] Evaluation is most effective with all rehabilitation team members present to establish a treatment plan. Orthotic treatments maximize what limited muscle strength and ROM the patient may have. Orthoses that are used during the day to maximize function are often replaced with positional orthoses at night to preserve gains and prevent decline in ROM. The occupational therapist provides most of the functional and positional orthoses for the upper extremity. In the current rehabilitation environment, many occupational therapists work directly with orthopedic hand specialists and trauma physicians. They use low-temperature materials to mold custom devices specifically designed

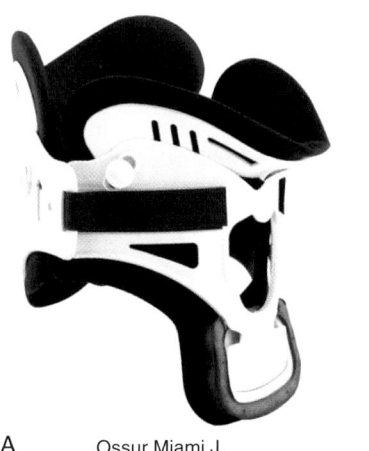

A   Ossur Miami J.

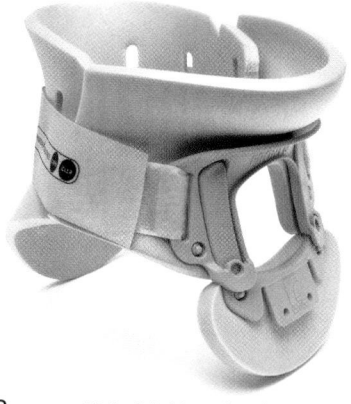

B   Philadephia orthosis.

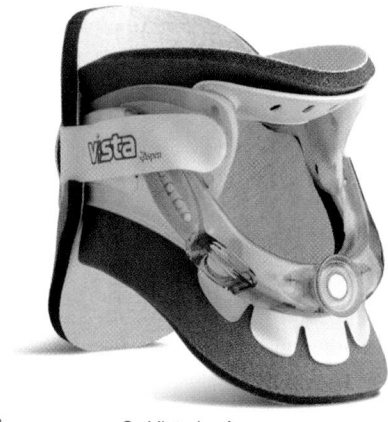

C   C. Vista by Aspen.

Fig. 32.2 Cervical Collars. **(A)** Miami J. **(B)** Philadephia collar. **(C)** Aspen Vista adjustable height collar. **(A** and **B**, Images courtesy of Össur. **C**, Photo courtesy of Aspen Medical Products, LLC.)

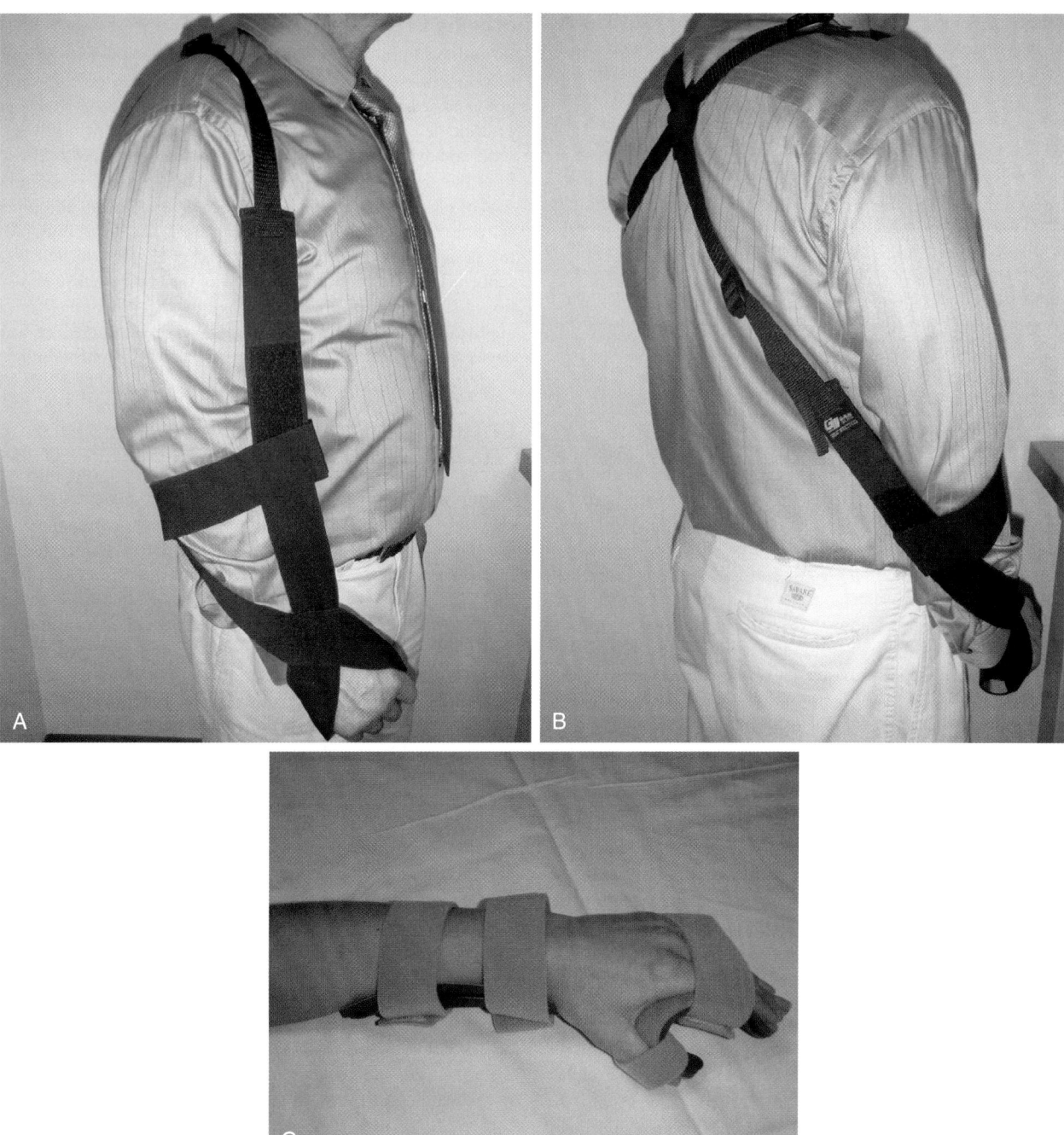

Fig. 32.3 Shoulder Sling to Support the Shoulder Against Subluxation and Pain (Givmohr Sling). **(A)** Sagittal view. **(B)** Posterior view. **(C)** Resting hand splint.

for protecting surgical reconstruction or promoting or maintaining ROM or for use as assistive devices.

Evaluation of the Lower Extremities

Evaluation of the lower extremity offers additional challenges owing to the role of ambulation and its value to independence for the patient and caregivers. ROM, strength, existing deformity, proprioception, muscle tone, soft tissue condition, and sensation must all be evaluated. Where appropriate, weight-bearing evaluation and gait analysis are completed. Patient and family assessment as it relates to the ability to comprehend and follow instructions is extremely important

because the potential for injury may outweigh the benefit of orthotic intervention to transform a patient from being non–weight bearing to having limited ambulation. Lack of ROM at the hip and knee will significantly decrease the duration of potential ambulation or may totally inhibit ambulation. Lack of ROM at the hip and knee is more critical than lack of strength. In the foot and ankle, the need for normal ROM is even more critical for efficient standing balance and ambulation. Orthoses of the lower extremity provide a combination of force lever arms acting about a joint axis at the knee, hip, or ankle. These joints are significantly compromised by the lack of ROM. Using the lever arm principles within the lower extremities substitutes for the lack of strength. For example, by blocking dorsiflexion of the ankle, the ground reaction force provides a posteriorly directed force in the sagittal plane during stance that stabilizes the knee. If the patient lacks the ability to get the ankle to a neutral alignment due to a plantarflexion contracture, this dorsiflexion limitation provides its own lever arm, which will result in a variety of undesirable forces and actions. Genu recurvatum, foot or ankle varus, a shortened stride length on the unaffected side, and the heel rising out of the shoe are common signs of this problem. These issues are further complicated when poor proprioception, spasticity, and lack of sensation are present. Lack of ROM at the ankle creates many symptoms in the lower extremity but is often overlooked during evaluation as the cause of these problems.

Genu varus and genu recurvatum are common deformities of the patient with neurological impairments. A number of factors create these problems.[18] In addition to the ankle ROM limitations, leg length differences, lack of quadriceps strength, and lack of proprioception can create deformities about the knee. The patient with a history of poliomyelitis may have both a short extremity and weak knee extensors, which lead to genu recurvatum along with coronal plane deformity. However, reducing the genu recurvatum without protecting against instability created by undesirable knee flexion would be a mistake. Patients with lower motor neuron disease have excellent proprioception, which is the reason they protect the unstable knee by hyperextending it. They may even use force from their upper extremity by pushing posteriorly on the femur with the hand to increase knee stability. Allowing some knee hyperextension in the orthotic design may be necessary to stabilize the knee during gait. Polio survivors are closely attuned to the amount of knee extension that is necessary to maintain stability, and the orthosis can be designed around this angulation.[19] A patient with upper neuron impairments, such as a patient who has had a CVA, has a similar knee alignment in gait. However, the typical cause of this patient's deformity is different. The upper motor neuron impairment often causes reduced proprioception even when there is adequate strength to stabilize the knee. Hemiplegic patients may present with knee hyperextension due to poor proprioception and reduced ankle ROM. An orthotic design for this population may need to have a heel lift to accommodate the plantarflexion contracture, and this will also help to limit knee extension in gait.[20]

Reduced strength and ROM limitations about the hip limit effective ambulation and leave a patient much more reliant on trunk stability and upper-extremity ambulatory aids. Hip flexors are more critical than hip extensors because they serve to advance the limb in reciprocal gait, whereas lack of hip extensors is compensated for by the strong hip ligaments, which tighten for stability in extension. Limited ROM to at least neutral extension about the hip creates major challenges for the patient, even if the patient has excellent upper-extremity strength. This lack of ROM will not allow stability in standing once force is removed from the upper-extremity ambulatory aids (cane or walker). The patient with a hip flexion contracture will have difficulty standing from a seated position and will stand with excess hip flexion, knee flexion, and lumbar lordosis. Once standing, they will have difficulty advancing the involved side to initiate a step as the hip flexors are already shortened and are at a mechanical disadvantage. It is difficult for the patient with a hip flexion contracture to stand without support because this alignment creates a hip and knee flexion moment that will pull them into a sitting position. Maintaining hip ROM is an important goal for the rehab team, and encouraging the patient to perform stretching exercises while supine and limiting time seated with excess hip flexion is helpful. Creating hands-free standing balance is a highly desirable outcome of orthotic intervention. The patient is then able to use both upper extremities for ADLs.

Orthotic Evaluation

In addition to the comprehensive assessment of the patient which involves assessment of the patient's ROM, muscle strength, skin condition, and spasticity, it is essential to determine appropriateness of the orthotic device being prescribed for the patient. This involves both a static and dynamic evaluation.[21] Static evaluation consists of observing fit of the orthosis on and off the patient and dynamic evaluation consists of observation of weight-bearing alignment, gait, and functional activities both with and without the orthosis and determining whether the design meets the expectations and goals for which it was prescribed. Table 32.1 summarizes some of the key aspects of this evaluation.[21] It is imperative to work closely with an orthotist for critical adjustments or modifications to optimize the fit and function of the device to best meet the goals of the patient and the rehabilitation team.

ORTHOTIC INTERVENTION

Several factors play key roles in the success of orthotic intervention. To improve function without complication or patient risk, the clinician must be sure to address the patient's major complaint. The reason the patient and family came to see the therapist or orthotist must be clearly established to ensure compliance with orthotic intervention. It is important to establish a baseline of function so that results of intervention are measurable. Validated outcome measures for certain populations are excellent tools to determine preorthosis and postorthosis function and effectiveness of orthotic management. In some situations the patient benefit is clear and immediate, whereas in others, concentrated instruction, orthotic modification, and time spend using the device are required before improved function can be observed or measured. The process of donning and doffing the orthosis as independently as possible must be well thought out by the clinician. The clinician must be conservative in setting these expectations. It is important to remember that what happens in the clinical setting may not be easily reproducible in the home situation. The orthotic interventions must be kept as simple as possible: what is the simplest orthotic intervention that will provide the expected goal? Although an obvious statement, the balance between too much and not enough can challenge the clinician's skill and experience. Patients with more impairments are more likely to use an orthotic device willingly.[22]

The use of trial orthoses can provide valuable information during the evaluation and help to guide the treatment plan. It can be helpful to maintain a small stock of presized off the shelf (OTS) devices in the orthotic clinic or therapy gym setting to give both the patient and rehab specialist an opportunity to evaluate the functional effects of an orthosis. If this fits well, it may be the patient's final device, or it can serve as justification for a more custom orthosis to be fabricated.

Various types of heat-moldable plastics have been beneficial for many individuals. Custom-made and custom-fit plastic AFOs are frequently fit because they are "more cosmetic and lighter" than AFOs made of metal and leather material. With a plastic orthosis, the user must use a shoe big enough to easily fit the orthosis. Technological advancements have led to a number of additions to the arsenal of orthotists. Prefabricated orthoses with better sizing and materials have given the clinician additional tools for evaluation and for devising permanent orthoses. Preimpregnated graphite AFOs are currently available in multiple sizes and provide toe clearance during swing phase and some knee-stabilizing forces during stance phase. Although very lightweight, these orthoses provide dynamic stance phase control. They are strong and flexible, and patients often prefer the more dynamic motion and minimal bulk of the carbon material.

TABLE 32.1 Key Aspects of Static and Dynamic Evaluation

Static Evaluation

Patient's opinion of the orthosis	Evaluate whether the patient finds the orthosis comfortable, functional, and cosmetically acceptable to promote adoption and consistent use of the device.
Donning and doffing procedures	An orthosis that is difficult to don or doff is unlikely to be used by the patient. It is essential to examine: • comfort and safety while donning and doffing the orthosis • manual dexterity while using closures and straps • effort and time required to don and doff the orthosis • consider modifications to facilitate ease of donning such as loops, tabs, Velcro, straps, etc.
Non–weight-bearing alignment	• Patient must be able to sit comfortably in a chair with the orthosis such that the hip, knees, and ankles are at approximately 90 degrees to each other. • The axis of the orthosis must lie in close proximity to the anatomical joint axis. An orthotic joint axis that is too high or too low can interfere with joint motion. • The interior surfaces and edges of the orthosis must be smooth and comfortable for the patient. A sharp edge may impinge the enclosed tissues causing skin irritation and discomfort. In the case of an insensate patient, a sharp edge can cause skin breakdown before the patient is aware of a problem • Component parts of the orthosis are comfortable and correct in size, alignment, and fit including elements such as uprights, straps, mechanical joints, inserts, and shoes. • Uprights should be aligned at midline of the leg and thigh segments and should not be too high or too low. Uprights that slide anteriorly or posteriorly can reduce the effectiveness of the forces applied by the leg and thigh bands. • Weight-bearing buildups of the orthosis should align correctly with the structures that are meant to bear weight, such as the patellar-tendon-bearing brim of an ankle-foot orthosis with the tibial tuberosity or ischial-weight-bearing brim of a knee-ankle-foot orthosis (KAFO) or a Hip Knee Ankle Foot Orthosis (HKAFO) with the ischial tuberosity. • Pressure reliefs contoured inside the orthosis for sensitive structures must be correctly aligned with those structures. For example, pressure-sensitive areas such as the fibular head and malleoli must align correctly with the pressure reliefs incorporated inside the ankle-foot orthosis.
Skin integrity	The patient's skin condition should be assessed both prior to donning the orthosis and after doffing it (and both times should be carefully documented). Prior to donning the orthosis an assessment of skin color and integrity including recording any preexisting scars or cuts should be performed. After doffing the orthosis, any color changes, skin induration, blanching, chafing, or distal edema should be noted. If these changes are present for more than 15 min, it might indicate that the orthosis is causing excess pressure, and this can lead to skin breakdown and ulceration. It is especially important to perform regular skin checks with a patient who lacks normal sensation, as they will not notice discomfort or excess pressure.

Dynamic Evaluation

Patient's opinion	During weight bearing with the orthosis, it is essential to confirm patient comfort and fit during standing and walking with the orthosis.
Weight-bearing alignment	Does the orthosis align correctly to the structures meant to bear weight? Examine if pressure reliefs contoured inside the orthosis for sensitive structures are correctly aligned to those structures.
Pregait (standing) evaluation	Assess patient's posture while standing with the device. This assessment is particularly important for patients who wear an orthosis only on one limb. The height difference when using a unilateral orthosis may need to be compensated with a heel lift on the contralateral limb to achieve balance and symmetry.
Gait evaluation	• Gait should be compared with and without the orthosis to understand if the orthosis meets the needs for which it was prescribed. If the orthosis was meant to correct excessive foot drag during walking, it can do so by either assisting dorsiflexion or controlling excessive plantarflexion. If the problem persists, the orthosis needs further modifications or adjustments. • An orthosis can correct one problem but create another one. For example, locking the knee joint during gait will stabilize the knee in stance but can prevent the knee from flexing during the swing phase and can lead to the patient using an alternate strategy to clear the limb during swing. • Assess patient effort in walking with the device. Observing how frequently the patient has to stop and start while walking with the orthosis, whether they find walking with the device tiring, and if they are able to maintain a certain speed of walking over a specific distance are important considerations of the evaluation. • Note any noise or sounds the orthosis might make while walking. Unusual sounds from the orthosis may indicate malalignment of a joint or segment. An orthosis that is misaligned might be out of phase with the limb segment and might create forces or torques that might damage the orthosis or injure the limb.

Data from Edelstein JE, Bruckner J. *Orthotics: A Comprehensive Clinical Approach.* Thorofare, NJ: Slack; 2002.

However, at times, use of a plastic or graphite AFO adds risk and complication without improvement compared with traditional AFOs fabricated with metal and leather attached to the patient's shoe. For example, if the patient requires ankle and knee stability yet lacks sensation and/or has fluctuating edema in the foot and ankle, a double-upright metal orthosis attached to the patient's shoe creates much less risk for potential skin breakdown than a rigid total contact plastic orthosis. In the case of a neuropathic foot, significant risk would be incurred by providing a total contact AFO made of plastic. A double-upright metal AFO with a well-fitting extra-depth shoe with a custom accommodative insert would fit the patient's needs and take into consideration the sensory and motor changes within the lower extremity (Table 32.2).

Introduction of biomechanical forces to the extremities may cause unwanted movements or restrictions, and careful selection of components is essential to keep the focus on the orthotic plan. For example, a patient with a CVA may need a stronger anterior lever force to provide knee stability, so one could plantar flex the orthotic ankle joint. However, this knee-stabilizing effect in stance phase may cause a toe drag during swing phase since the foot is plantarflexed. A simple fix is to provide the opposite side with a heel and sole lift for additional clearance during swing phase of the affected extremity (see Table 32.2).

Clinicians need to set realistic, manageable, patient-centered treatment goals. All too often, treatment plans are only in the minds of the clinicians and are poorly communicated with the patient and family. Often the patient and family members will expect benefits of the intervention that will far exceed what the therapist knows are possible. The time to address those gaps is prior to orthotic treatment, not when the patient and family realize that expectations regarding functional gains while using the orthosis may not be realistic. Clear and achievable goals that are clearly communicated will engender the patient's trust and guide the potential for successful future intervention. Discussing realistic achievable goals of treatment after assessing all factors, the home situation, and individual motivation with the patient and caregivers in language they understand is critical if optimal orthotic intervention is to be achieved. In the case of a patient with hemiplegia due to a CVA, orthotic goals may be to provide safe standing balance for transfers and minimal ambulation in the home. Patients and their caregivers will realize the major benefit this will have on the home situation. However, without this identified as the goal before initiating orthotic care, they may leave the therapeutic environment wondering why the patient cannot walk normally and participate in life activities that require longer distance ambulation skills.[23] This clinical error is an all too frequent patient management mistake. Integrating orthoses with physical and occupational therapy motor relearning and neuroplasticity should help to optimize functional recovery.

To provide a cost-effective orthosis in a timely manner with the current vast number of orthotic devices, the orthotist must stay abreast of the wide array of choices at his or her disposal to meet the needs of the patient. The reality of cost containment is not a recent event in the orthotic profession, because funding for these devices has always been challenged. This has necessitated the development of more cost-effective alternatives, such as prefabricated orthoses. The introduction of heat-moldable plastics into orthotics in the late 1960s and early 1970s on a custom basis replaced, to a large extent, the need to mold leather and/or metal to fabricate an orthosis (see Table 32.2). This provides total contact fit and dramatically reduced the time and skill level required for manufacturing. All orthoses produce a force field, some desirable and some undesirable. It requires an experienced clinician to make the most appropriate choices, because too often the failure of treatment is blamed on an orthosis. Usually such failure is the result of an inappropriate initial selection of orthotic components, lack of discernment between custom-made and custom-fit devices, or misidentification of the patient as candidate for a specific orthotic design. Prefabricated custom-fit orthoses are cost-effective only if they produce the desired goal over time. As a general rule, one should consider prefabricated custom-fit orthosis for patients who have an anatomically "normal" presentation and alignment at the areas the orthosis will contact and who will use the orthosis for only a short time. Custom-made orthoses for extremities or the spine are appropriately prescribed for patients who have deformity or unusual size, or who must use the device longer periods of time or indefinitely.

TABLE 32.2   Comparison of Orthotic Material Properties and Usage

Factor	Metal and Leather	Polypropylene	Lamination or Graphite	Polyethylene
Adjustability	Yes	Yes, with heat	No	Yes, with heat
Ability to change shoes	No	Yes	Yes	Yes
Weight-bearing strength	Yes	Yes	Yes	No
Skin at risk	Yes	Yes, close observation	Yes, where in contact	Yes
Best spinal use	No	Yes	No	Yes
Long-term wear	Yes	Yes, if custom	Yes	Least durable
Weight (lightest at 1)	4	3	2	1
Adjustability for functional changes (improvement or decline of patient's condition)	Yes	Limited unless initial articulation fabricated	No	No
Short-term need	Yes	Yes	Yes	Yes
Requires corrective force with good patient sensation	Fair	Good	Fair	Good
Ability of clinician to change angulation, ankle or knee	Best	Limited[a]	No	Not indicated for weight bearing
Upper-extremity orthoses	Limited	Yes	Limited	Yes

[a]Use in combination with metal joints produces best results.

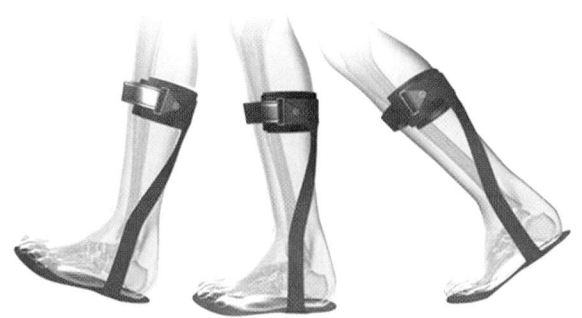

Fig. 32.4 Carbon fiber ankle-foot orthosis (AFO), preventing foot drop in swing phase of gait.

Advancements in technology have allowed the use of lighter, stronger materials in the fabrication of lower-extremity orthotics. A carbon graphite fabric with an exact amount of resin and catalyst already incorporated into the material is an example. With the fibers properly directed over a model, it can be formed with heat. Carbon graphite in other forms is used in both prosthetics and orthotics. Carbon initially had limited acceptance in orthotics because it did not significantly reduce the weight of the orthosis compared with other materials. It is difficult to modify the orthosis after the lamination process is completed. The preimpregnated graphite has a dramatically reduced weight, still maintains its strength, and gives the orthotist the opportunity to use the dynamics of loading and response during the gait cycle.[24] This allows for assistance in both the swing and stance phases of gait (Fig. 32.4). A clinical example at the end of this chapter demonstrates this material patient management.

Another significant advancement in component technology has been the introduction of stance control orthotic knee joints. The development of a lightweight, compact knee joint that allow locks to provide a patient with knee stability during stance[25] and unlocks to allow knee flexion and toe clearance during swing phase has been elusive until recently. Before this, the available knee joints for knee-ankle-foot orthoses (KAFOs) involved some type of locking mechanism that remained locked throughout the gait cycle. The joint provided stabilization of the weak quadriceps musculature during stance but kept the knee in a fully extended position, making advancement of the limb in swing more difficult for the patient. There are specific indications and contraindications for stance control KAFOs, but results are promising. This feature can potentially reduce energy output[26] and increase gait velocity[27] because it is not necessary to raise the center of gravity to clear the locked knee during swing phase. This improves patient safety when walking on uneven surfaces. Microprocessor swing and stance control knee orthosis joints also apply technology initially developed for prosthetic knee joints.[28]

New technology for externally powered orthoses has recently entered the market. These "bionic legs" are robotic aids worn during therapy sessions for gait training. They assist and augment the strength of the patient's muscle and are most typically used in rehabilitation for patients with SCI.[29] Once the patient has achieved functional improvements, the use of the orthosis can be discontinued or modified to provide only the level of assistance required.

Other advancements in orthotic technology include the development of neuroprosthetic devices. These devices act through circuitry and programming to substitute for a deficit in the neural system. External devices that provide these functions exist, and research is ongoing

regarding implantable orthotic control mechanisms and devices. Functional electrical stimulation (FES) is a method of applying low-level electrical currents to motor nerves to restore function. In the 1960s the application of FES for foot drop was demonstrated by using a simple single channel to stimulate the common peroneal nerve to activate the ankle dorsiflexors. FES has widespread applications in many other neuroprosthetic devices such as cardiac pacemakers, cochlear stimulators, bladder stimulators, and phrenic nerve stimulators. Until recently, FES devices to provide ambulation assistance were large, unreliable, complex, and restricted to use in a therapy setting. The FES used in neurological rehabilitation attempts to unmask existing voluntary control (if any) and/or initiate dormant activity of the nerves and muscles. For FES to be used, the patient must have an upper motor neuron lesion. The nerve-to-muscle pathway must be intact and the reflex arc undamaged. Goals of FES address many rehabilitative outcomes. FES can reduce spasticity, break synergy patterns, reduce swelling, and limit blood clot formation, and assist in maintaining ROM. FES used in gait can improve overall walking abilities by dorsiflexing the foot during swing to provide foot clearance, control initial contact, increase safety, decrease energy expenditure, and retrain muscles. FES has some applications in the upper extremity as well, although at this time it is purely in a therapeutic setting. Currently, there are several FES units for foot drop on the market. These devices are used by patients in their daily lives and are not limited to the rehabilitation setting. The WalkAide from Innovative Neurotronics (Fig. 32.5) and NESS L300 from Bioness (Fig. 32.6) both function to provide dorsiflexion during the swing phase by stimulating the peroneal nerve. An ideal candidate for these devices must have an upper motor neuron

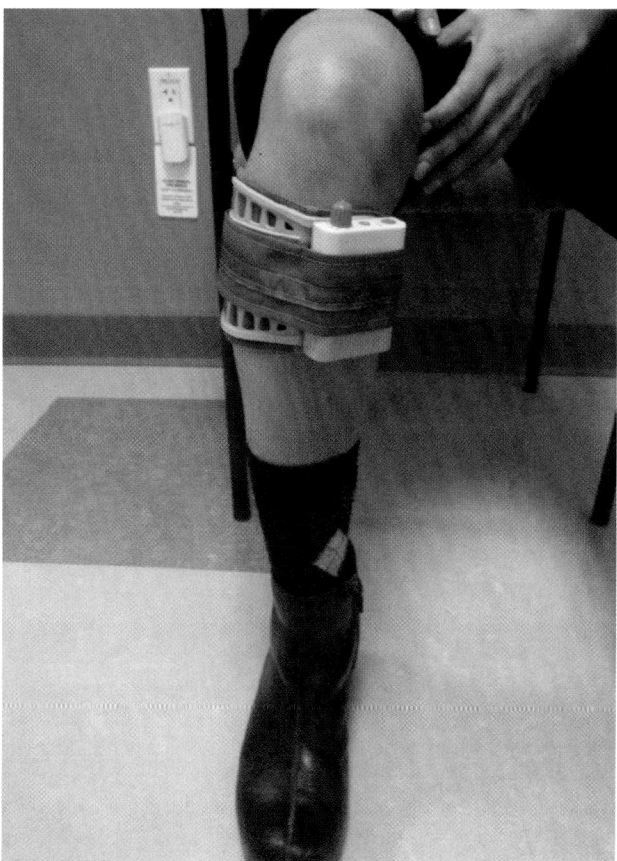

Fig. 32.5 Walk-Aide Functional Electrical Stimulation (FES) Device.

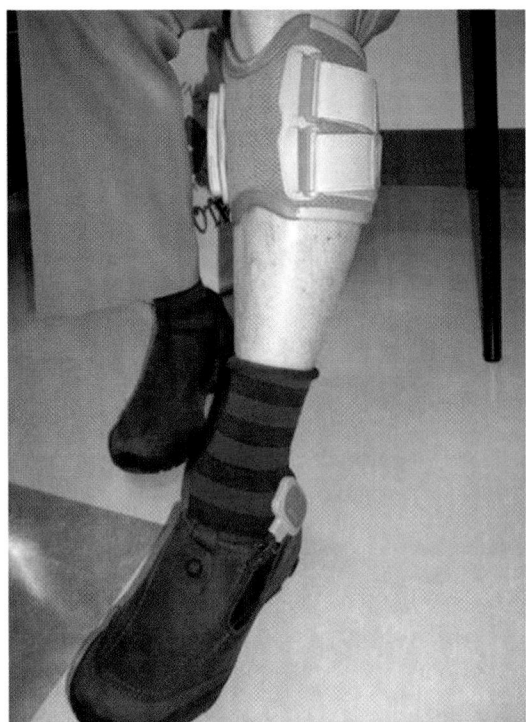

Fig. 32.6 The NESS L300 Foot Drop System.

lesion, good control of the knee joint, and drop foot. Common neurological conditions in which these devices are used are CVA, SCI, and multiple sclerosis (MS).[30–32] Both devices involve a sensor to determine when the patient is initiating swing phase and send an electrical stimulus to the nerve to dorsiflex the foot. Advantages of FES over traditional orthotic management for foot drop are that it provides activation of the muscle instead of functioning as a passive splint.[33]

Future developments in the field of orthotics will provide external power and support for patients to use in community and home settings. There are already systems that can be applied to a patient with paraplegia to allow him or her to stand and walk. "Bionic" orthoses will incorporate microchips and artificial intelligence to provide "smart," patient-specific devices. This will allow the orthosis to change its settings and parameters according to the patient's input or position during a specific task or part of the gait cycle. In more traditional types of orthoses, the materials used will continue to become lighter, stronger, and more versatile.

A common concern of both patients and the rehabilitation team is that use of an assistive device will cause muscle atrophy and increased weakness (particularly for users of AFOs). There are several ways to address this concern. Patients indicated for an orthosis already have weakness and are at risk of falls and instability.[34] If the weakness is significant enough to require orthotic management, safety outside of the therapy gym is critical. They can be provided with exercises and a program to activate the weakened musculature when in a safe environment and use the AFO when ambulating in their home and community. In addition, it has been shown that although initial muscle activation with an AFO is reduced, over time (in both healthy and paretic subjects) there is no reduction in muscle activation or electromyographic signaling.[35]

Currently orthotist and therapy teams have a multitude of devices from which to choose to meet the needs of the patient. Options range from custom-made devices using a patient mold to prefabricated custom-fit devices. A thorough understanding of the indications and contraindications for each of these devices is essential to meet patient needs. A lack of understanding of biomechanical principles, the limitations of prefabricated orthoses, and custom orthotic devices can lead to failure and increase impairment within the patient's environment.

CLINICAL EXAMPLES

Paraplegia

Lower-extremity orthotic intervention for a patient with paraplegia is generally considered for the lower extremities at the T12 level in the complete lesion.[36] Complete lesions higher in the cord leave the patient without enough trunk stability to use bilateral lower-extremity orthoses effectively. Although a thoracic extension can be added to bilateral KAFOs, this addition greatly increases the difficulty of donning the orthosis independently, and most patients will have great difficulty getting from sitting to standing.

The most appropriate orthoses for a T12 complete paraplegic are bilateral KAFOs. The patient generally uses a swing-to or swing-through gait, and successful use of orthoses requires excellent standing balance. There are three significant design requirements for these KAFOs: shallow thigh and calf bands, locking knee joints, and adjustable ankle joints. A double-adjustable ankle joint has channels on the anterior and posterior sides of the joint. This allows the orthotist to easily adjust dorsiflexion and plantarflexion position and ROM or even provide dynamic assistance via a spring added to the channel of the joint (Fig. 32.7). The shallow bands force the center of gravity forward, inducing lordosis so the patient can rest on the iliofemoral (Y ligaments) of the hip. The knee joint should lock automatically because the patient requires the upper extremities for standing. The joint will lock as the patient stands and bends over the rigid ankle joint, forcing the knee joints into extension. The lock then can catch on the back of a wheelchair seat or other chair to release and bend when the patient sits. The foot-ankle complex forms the basis for balance. A few degrees of adjustment at the double-adjustable ankle joint can make the difference between safe standing balance and limited standing balance (Fig. 32.8).

A. M. is a 21-year-old man with incomplete T12-level paraplegia secondary to a gunshot wound. A. M. has normal upper-extremity strength and ROM. He has had surgery for spinal fusion. Trunk strength is 4/5, left hip is 3/5, knee is 2/5, right hip is 1/5, and right knee is 0/5. ROM is full at hips, knees, and ankles. A. M. can transfer independently and has the goal of household ambulation, although he is aware that it "takes a lot of work." A. M. was fit with a right conventional (metal and leather) KAFO with shallow thigh bands,

drop lock knee joints, and double-adjustable ankle joints locked in 5 degrees of dorsiflexion (Fig. 32.9A and B). The left lower extremity was fitted with a conventional AFO with double-adjustable ankle joints adjusted to match the right orthosis. The distal attachment to the shoes was through a long metal stirrup with a reinforcement for stability and resistance to dorsiflexion as the pt's weight shifts forward. The patient was able to ambulate with forearm crutches.

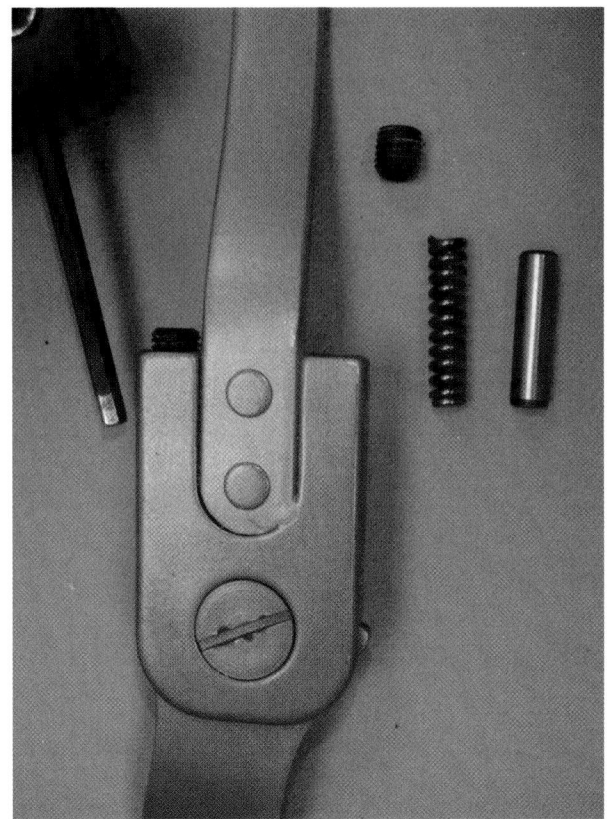

Fig. 32.7 Double-Adjustable Ankle Joint. The channels on the anterior and posterior sides allow for easy adjustment of dorsiflexion and plantarflexion range of motion. Springs can also be added to provide dynamic assistance to the movements.

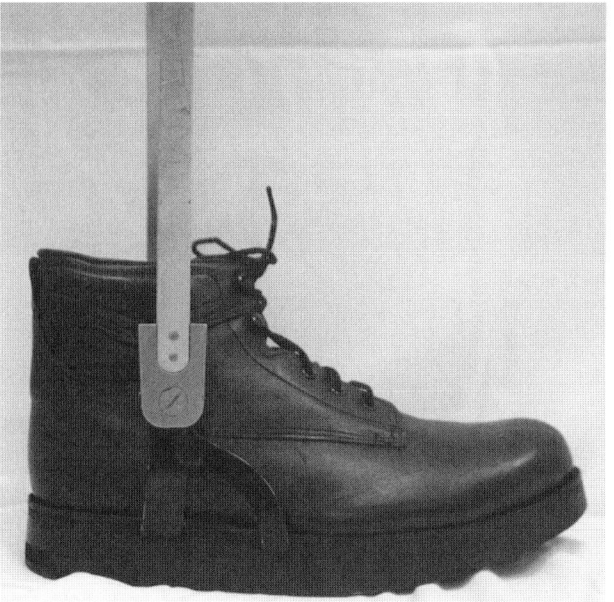

Fig. 32.8 Modifications necessary to control the ankle setting in a patient with spinal cord injury (Scott-Craig shoe or stirrup modifications).

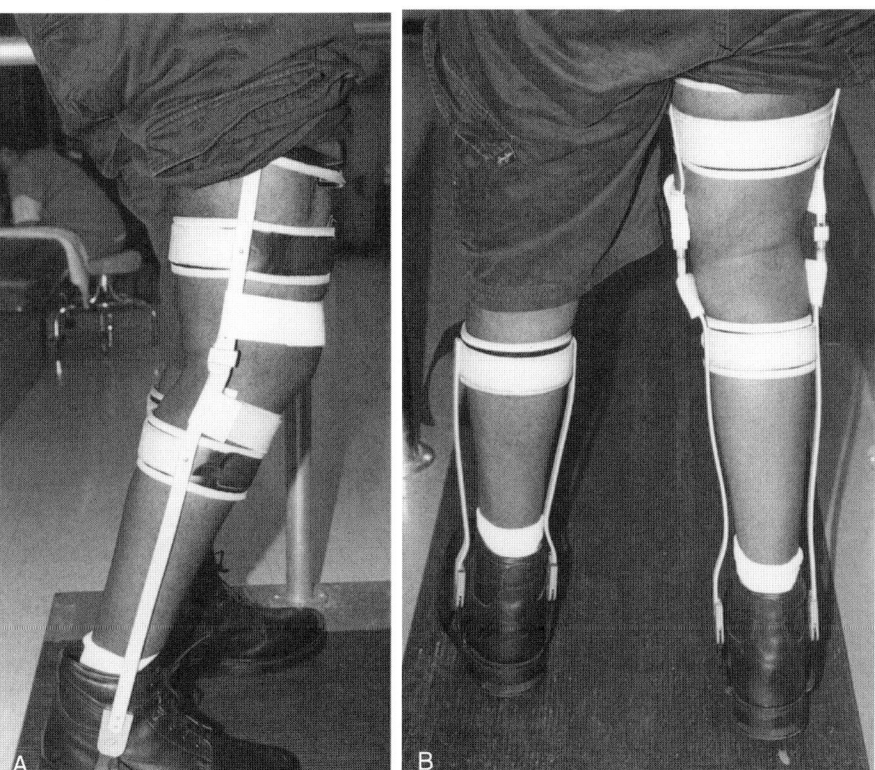

Fig. 32.9 Patient Standing Wearing a Right Knee-Ankle-Foot Orthosis. **(A)** Lateral view; **(B)** posterior view.

Hemiplegia

Patients who have had a CVA can vary widely in their need for orthotic intervention, from a simple AFO to assist toe clearance, to an AFO to stabilize both ankle and knee, to an orthosis used temporarily for training purposes. The use of a KAFO in the patient with hemiplegia is rarely indicated. Even though the more affected patient does not have knee stability, he or she rarely ambulates with a heel strike that would destabilize the knee and therefore can use an AFO with restricted ankle motion to help stabilize the knee. In addition, patients cannot don the KAFO with the use of only one upper extremity. With hip flexor weakness and knee instability on the affected side, the orthotic intervention may be to assist in transfers rather than to facilitate gait. Orthotic intervention for the patient with a CVA typically limits ankle ROM. The use of dynamic components is not effective, because they will initiate spasticity. The lack of ROM into dorsiflexion or even to neutral causes the most significant problems for these patients. An ankle that lacks dorsiflexion ROM prevents advancement of the center of gravity and produces a lever arm that induces genu recurvatum, and often the heel comes out of the shoe or the ankle rolls into varus. Because these patients lack proprioception, this constant force directed posteriorly will be significant over time. The patient may develop pain in the knee and not ambulate, the heel cord will shorten more, and the cycle will continue. Heel cords rarely gain length after the patient has been discharged from the rehabilitation setting, and one must consider the family and home situation. Heel buildups on the affected side are used to bring the tibia into 90 degrees. Buildups of 1 to 1½ inches are not uncommon. Remember to balance the opposite shoe. When selecting between different orthotic components, it is best to choose the more stable orthosis. The use of trial orthoses during evaluation is very helpful. As the patient improves, the amount of orthotic control needed will likely decrease. A three-point pressure orthosis for the knee, such as a Swedish knee cage (Fig. 32.10), is also a valuable training orthosis and, in the case of some post-CVA patients, is used daily when the degree of recurvatum exceeds the patient's ability to control the posteriorly directed force.

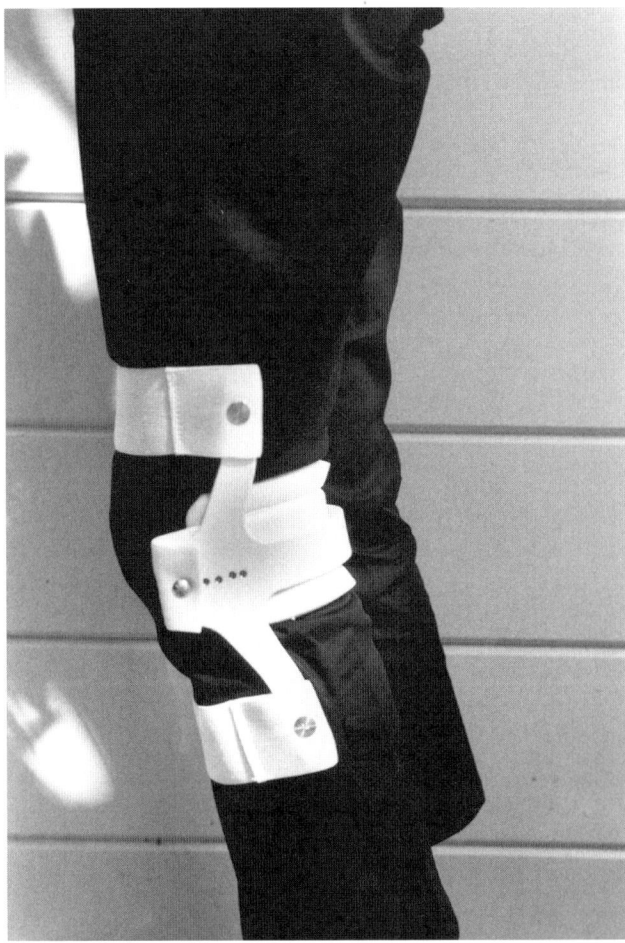

Fig. 32.10 Prefabricated three-point pressure knee orthosis (Swedish knee cage) to control genu recurvatum.

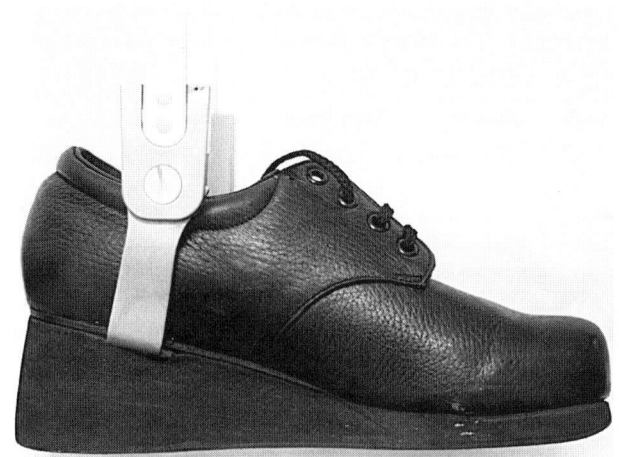

Fig. 32.11 Shoe Modification With Double-Adjustable Ankle joint.

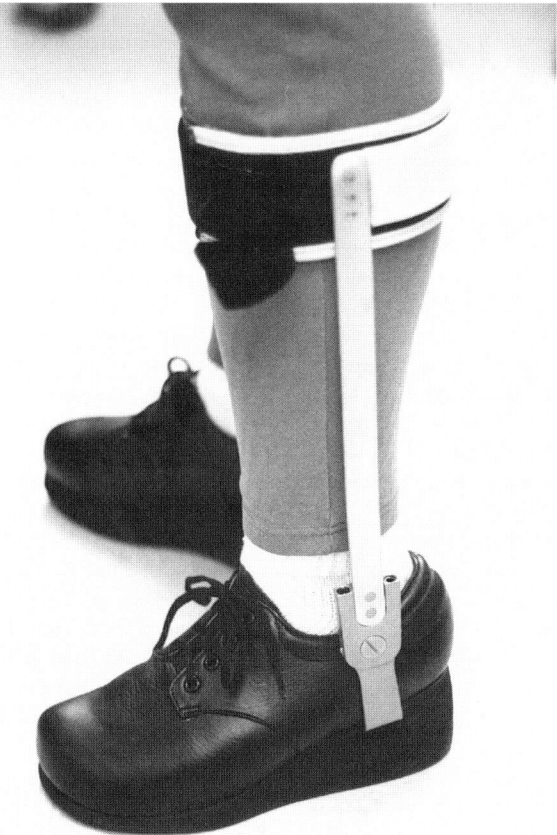

Fig. 32.12 Left conventional (metal and leather) AFO with double adjustable ankle joints and shoe build-up.

CASE STUDY 32.2   D. M.

D. M. is a 58-year-old woman who had a left CVA, resulting in a right hemiplegia, 2 years ago. She was evaluated at the request of her physician because of increased knee pain and poor standing balance. D. M. was fitted with a plastic AFO fixed at 90 degrees 14 months ago. She was wearing the orthosis, but the heel would not stay in her shoe. Evaluation showed that the patient was 15 degrees from a neutral ankle alignment (the ankle was in 15 degrees of plantarflexion), had 0/5 dorsiflexion or plantarflexion, and had fair knee extension and flexion. She also walked with the aid of a quad cane and had 10 degrees of genu recurvatum and slight genu varum at midstance. Her goal

was to walk with less pain and to be more stable. D. M. was fitted with conventional AFO with double-adjustable locked ankle joints with long tongue stirrups added to the shoe and a 1½-inch heel buildup (Fig. 32.11). The left shoe was built up 1½ inches in the heel and sole to balance the right shoe (Fig. 32.12). A Swedish knee orthosis also was used initially to help train the patient and to provide hyperextension control. A double-adjustable ankle joint gives total adjustability to change the ankle angle, or a 90-degree posterior stop also can be used in a thermoplastic type AFO. Patients who lack this much ROM provide an "anatomical" dorsiflexion stop.

CASE STUDY 32.3   M. H.

M. H. is a 59-year-old woman with a history of a CVA 1 year ago. She has left hemiplegia. She works as a facilities manager and walks through her office building several times per day. She underwent extensive therapy after the CVA and has good strength; ROM is within normal limits at her hip and knee. At her left ankle, M. H. has 3+/5 plantarflexion strength but 0/5 dorsiflexion or eversion strength, and she has extensor tone into plantarflexion and inversion. She ambulates very cautiously due to her inability to dorsiflex and evert the foot during the swing phase of gait. She has a high risk of falling because of her ankle instability and has sustained multiple inversion sprains at the ankle.

M. H. was tested using an FES device and had an appropriate response to the stimulus. The FES device consists of a cuff and control unit around her proximal calf, attached to electrodes on her skin near the fibular head. It allows her to ambulate barefoot and/or with various types of footwear because it is programmed using the angle of her leg to determine the transition from stance to swing phase in gait. The unit is inconspicuous and lightweight. Her walking velocity, safety, and stability are significantly improved with the FES unit.

Paralytic Spine

Many neuropathic diagnoses affect the spinal column. Spinal muscle atrophy, tetraplegia, myelomeningocele, and Duchenne muscular dystrophy can all require orthotic intervention. Although materials, padding versus no padding, trim lines, length of time used, and optional area openings can vary with different conditions, most spinal stabilizing orthoses are TLSOs. Orthoses used for postsurgical stabilization tend to be of more rigid material to support the healing spine. The paralytic spine that is not surgically stabilized can have either a flexible or a rigid curvature. An orthosis for a patient with a rigid curvature is used to avoid further deformity and differs from that used by the patient with a flexible curvature. If the curve is flexible, the orthosis will be used to provide of the correction. Patients with paralytic spine deformity usually undergo casting for custom orthoses, and although non–weight-bearing supine casts can greatly reduce the curve, many patients will not tolerate the pressure once in the upright sitting position. Orthotic intervention usually has one or more of the following goals: (1) improved sitting balance, (2) support of surgical stabilization, (3) prevention of further spinal deformity, (4) use as an assistive positional device for better use of head and upper extremities, and (5) improved respiratory function. Most TLSOs for these patients are total circumferential designs that use rigid materials (polypropylene) to less-rigid materials (polyethylene, foams) or a combination of padding with a rigid or semirigid frame with a heat-formable foam. The orthosis may require relief for boney prominences, g-tubes, etc. Fabrication and fitting of these orthoses require an experienced orthotist and adherence to detail. Establishing the distal and proximal trim lines of the orthosis will require a fine tuning between providing enough length to support the spine and maintaining a comfortable sitting position. Several clinic visits may be necessary to achieve the desired outcome.

Spastic Diplegic Cerebral Palsy

The goals of orthotic intervention in the patient with cerebral palsy are to control tone, prevent contractures, improve function and ambulation, and provide a secondary support after a surgical procedure.[37] As a general rule, the orthosis used to prevent contracture should be different from the orthosis used for ambulation. Some designs may incorporate modules that can key into one another or be used separately. This feature allows flexibility, assists in donning (especially in a patient with spasticity), and meets several treatment objectives. Modular articulating joints with various settings and functions used with thermoplastic orthoses greatly increase the functional and positional options to optimize orthotic management. To meet the goals of orthotic intervention stated earlier, total contact–type orthoses are generally desirable. As with any total contact orthosis and hypersensitive or hyposensitive skin, a cautious balance between correction of deformity or alignment and skin tolerance must be reached. The fitting and follow-up for these types of orthoses require experience, knowledge, and patience. Combinations of padding, wedging, straps, and heat relief methods are often necessary to enable the patient to wear the orthosis on a daily basis. A patient with spastic diplegic cerebral palsy relies heavily on her or his orthosis and wears it out faster than most other orthotic patients. In the case of a child, she or he may grow out of the orthosis before it wears out. This should be considered in the design and fabrication.

CASE STUDY 32.4 S. G.

S. G. is a 13-year-old girl with spastic quadriplegic cerebral palsy with involvement of all four extremities. She is Gross Motor Function Classification System (GMFCS) Level 5 with significant scoliosis. Her hip ROM is from −25 to 135 degrees of flexion. S. G. is fully dependent and lacks upper-extremity use.

The goal of orthotic intervention was to prevent further deformity, maintain the thoracic and lumbar column height for internal organ function, and provide trunk stability for seated balance in her wheelchair. She was fit with a custom TLSO fabricated from a cast impression (Fig. 32.13). It has ¼ inch of padding with a polypropylene outer layer, which has been modified over bony prominences for skin tolerance.

S. G. wears her TLSO while seated in her chair and also in bed. Frequent checks of the skin were made during the first few weeks of use to establish trim lines and window type modifications. She continues to be checked periodically for comfort and control as she grows, to ensure that the TLSO's fit and function are appropriate.

CASE STUDY 32.5 R. B.

R. B. is a 41-year-old woman with spastic diplegic cerebral palsy. She has tight heel cords bilaterally, with −5 degrees from neutral ROM at the ankle. Plantarflexion strength is 3+/5, and dorsiflexion strength is 3/5 bilaterally. The patient has 5–7 degrees of valgus calcaneus. The right side has pain in the midfemur and at the knee. She has a bilateral genu valgum deformity of 5–7 degrees (Fig. 32.14A). ROM at the knees is full, and strength of the quadriceps and hamstrings is good. Her hips are normal except for some internal rotation; leg lengths are equal and sensation is good.

Because the right lower extremity was painful at the knee and ankle (see Fig. 32.14B), the patient was fitted with an AFO that extended medially and proximally to the medial tibial condyle; ankle joints that had a posterior adjustment to limit plantarflexion; and a medial heel wedge and heel buildup of ⅝ inch. The ankle was fitted with a submalleolar orthosis that fit inside the AFO (see Fig. 32.14C and D). The submalleolar orthosis controls valgus of the ankle and along with the medial heel wedging exerts a varus force at the knee (see Fig. 32.14E). The heel buildup reduced the posteriorly directed force from midstance to toe off. The patient's symptoms were reduced, allowing her to be more active.

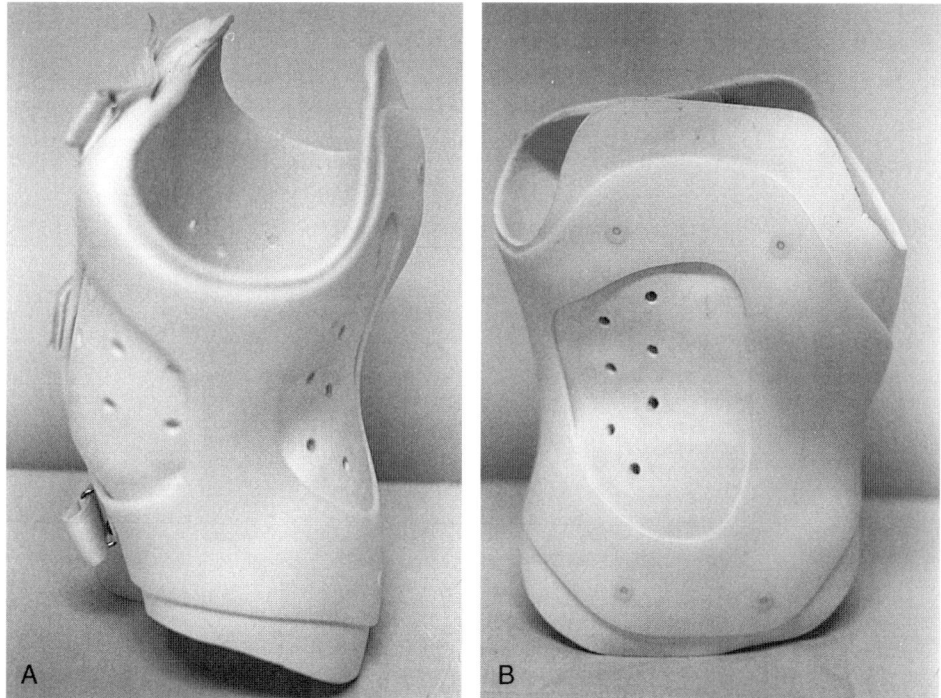

Fig. 32.13 Thoracolumbosacral Orthosis (TLSO) With Anterior Opening. **(A)** Lateral view. **(B)** Posterior view. Cutouts in rigid plastic to inner soft foam are to provide relief of deformity and expansion for breathing.

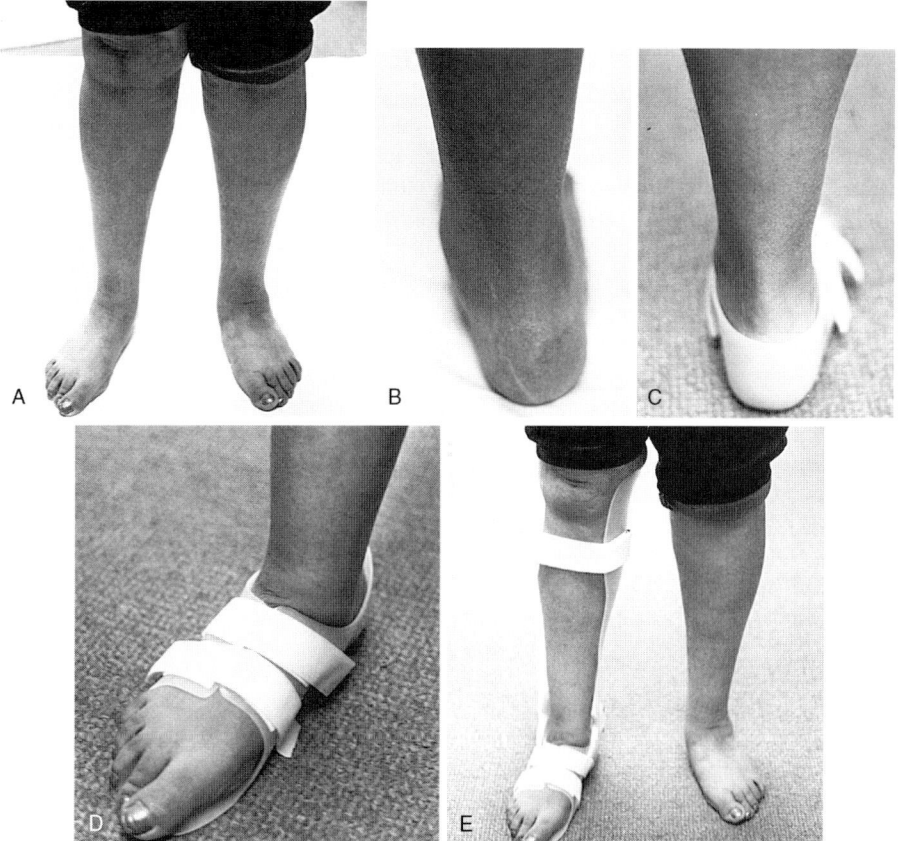

Fig. 32.14 (A) Painful right genu valgus and pronation. **(B)** Posterior view of right ankle. **(C** and **D)** Patient wearing submalleolar orthosis with pronation corrected. **(E)** Patient in AFO extended to knee to control genu valgus.

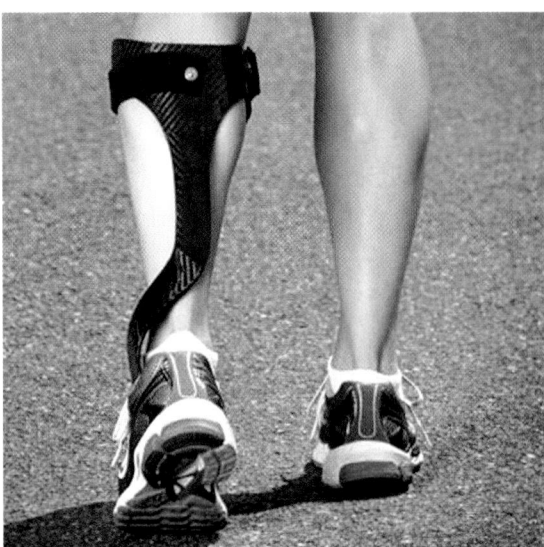

Fig. 32.15 Carbon fiber ankle-foot orthosis, which provides some stance-phase control in addition to swing-phase assistance. Image courtesy of AliMed.

Multiple Sclerosis

As MS progresses and further demyelination occurs, increased interruption of normal nerve impulses creates deficiencies in muscle control, vision, balance, sensation, and mental functions. Orthotic considerations for a patient with MS can vary as the patient's symptoms fade, recur, and change over time with the disease. Clinical presentation may vary widely over a short period of time. Fatigue plays a major role in the symptoms, and the patient's expectations and willingness to use orthotic devices changes accordingly. Typical patient reaction is reluctance to use any form of ambulatory aid or orthosis until safety is a major issue. Patients and family usually seek help when falls become more frequent. Lack of toe clearance during swing phase and poor knee stability in stance phase can benefit from orthotic intervention. The weight and simplicity of orthotic intervention must be major considerations. In many instances the evaluation will indicate the need for a KAFO, but this will be rejected by the patient because of its weight and complexity. The benefit of the KAFO for knee stability and foot and ankle control is counteracted by the patient's inability to advance the limb during swing phase. As their strength varies from day to day, they will judge their need when they are at their strongest rather than their weakest. Traditionally, plastic AFOs are used to control foot drop and provide some medial and lateral ankle control. These orthoses also can provide knee stability if the plastic is robust and if the medial and lateral trim lines are advanced anterior to the malleoli. The anterior lever arm of the AFO stops the center of gravity's forward progression at midstance. The recent development of prefabricated AFOs made of graphite has met the needs of many of these patients (Fig. 34.15). This ultralight orthosis fits inside the patient's shoe. It will provide toe clearance during swing phase and some dynamic knee stability and push off during stance phase.

CASE STUDY 32.6   D. K.

D. K. is a 38-year-old mother of three young boys and works outside the home. She was diagnosed with MS at the age of 30. Until 4 years ago she was managing the symptoms with medication and having minimal mobility problems. With the birth of her son, she had to cease use of medication, and the symptoms recurred and weakness increased. At age 36 she was limiting her activity outside the home because of safety issues—she was falling and unstable in standing and walking. She was prescribed with a right AFO because she had foot drop and knee instability and lacked the ability to recover her balance if she caught her toe. A prefabricated graphite AFO was fit to the patient (see Fig. 34.15). D. K. now has toe clearance during swing phase and dynamic knee extension during stance phase. Shortly after beginning to use the orthosis, she was able to walk safely on uneven ground and walk down stairs step over step for the first time in 3 years.

▎ SUMMARY

All orthoses create a force system. It is important to understand and integrate the appropriate force to achieve the desired outcome of intervention. A thorough initial evaluation and knowledge of the multiple orthotic options available are vital to reaching treatment goals. There has been a dramatic improvement in material technology, along with far greater access to orthotics and a much wider range of indications for orthotic intervention. This should challenge the rehabilitation team to establish measurable goals and then to develop new goals leading from the treatment interventions with the most effective outcomes. This evidence-based practice will help to provide better care and outcomes for your patients.

ACKNOWLEDGMENT

The authors would like to thank Walter Racette for his significant contributions in this chapter in the previous editions of this text.

REFERENCES

To enhance this text and add value for the reader, all references are included on the companion Evolve site that accompanies this textbook. This online service will, when available, provide a link for the reader to a Medline abstract for the article cited. There are 37 cited references and other general references for this chapter, with the majority of those articles being evidence-based citations.

33

Integrating Health Promotion and Wellness Into Neurorehabilitation*

Janet R. Bezner and Elissa C. Held Bradford

OBJECTIVES

After reading this chapter the student or therapist will be able to:

1. Define and differentiate the terms *health* and *wellness.*
2. Describe the characteristics of wellness.
3. Compare illness, prevention, and wellness paradigms.
4. Discuss theories of behavior change and their application to wellness and neurorehabilitation.
5. Determine the appropriateness of screening and standardized measures of health and wellness within the role of physical and occupational therapy.
6. Apply an evidence-based, person-centered holistic wellness approach to an individual or a population living with a chronic neurological condition.
7. Identify barriers and potential strategies to overcoming barriers to wellness for individuals living with neurological injury or disease.
8. Synthesize a wellness approach to neurorehabilitation through case examples.

KEY TERMS

health promotion	self-efficacy	wellness
perceptions	well-being	whole person
salutogenic		

In learning to cope with the often chronic nature of their conditions, individuals with neurological disease, not unlike individuals with health conditions of other systems, learn to rely on their abilities to adapt and compensate for their activity limitations and participation restrictions to regain the ability to participate in life. Although not an uncommon approach to life for any human being, the achievement of health or wellness takes on an increased focus for individuals with chronic health conditions, and it is strongly correlated with the quality of life they achieve. A casual consideration of the terms *health* and *wellness* indicates that they are similar, if not the same, in meaning, a commonly held belief among those without health conditions. This interpretation of the terms becomes problematic, however, in the presence of health conditions. Can an individual with a health condition be well? Can a person without a health condition be ill? The concepts of health and wellness and their associated meanings and measures will be explored in this chapter to provide a perspective for movement specialists that will enhance their ability to promote health and well-being in patients with neurological conditions. The evidence examining wellness approaches in patients with neurological conditions will be presented, along with common barriers and enablers to implementation. A synthesis of concepts will be promoted through case study.

DEFINITIONS AND RELATIONSHIPS AMONG TERMS

The classic understanding of the term *health* from a biomedical perspective is "absence of disease." The antonym of *health,* therefore, is

disease. The World Health Organization (WHO) contributed to the confusion between the terms *health* and *wellness* when in 1948 it defined *health* as "a state of complete physical, mental and social well-being, and not merely the absence of disease or infirmity."[1] Indeed, there are numerous illustrations of the influence of the mind and spirit on the body and thus the importance, from a public health perspective, of considering more than the physical state of the body when formulating solutions to health problems. However, there is also value in differentiating health from more global concepts such as wellness and quality of life, if for no other reason than to explain the phenomenon that an individual can be diseased and well or can experience a high quality of life while simultaneously living with a chronic disease. Considering the catastrophic nature of many neurological diseases that compromise physical health, it is even more important to distinguish between health and wellness to recognize and pursue avenues to enhance overall quality of life and well-being.

H.L. Dunn first conceptualized the term *wellness* in 1961 and offered the first definition of the term: "an integrated method of functioning which is oriented toward maximizing the potential of which the individual is capable."[2] Since Dunn's introduction of the term, numerous researchers and educators have attempted to explain wellness by proposing various models and approaches.[3–7] Although the literature is full of references to and information about wellness, including numerous definitions of the term, a universally accepted definition has failed to emerge. However, a leading wellness organization, Wellness Council of America (WELCOA), defined wellness in 2018: "Wellness is the active pursuit to understand and fulfill your individual human needs—which allows you to reach a state where you are flourishing and able to realize your full potential in all aspects of life. Every

---

*Videos for this chapter are available at studentconsult.com.

person has wellness aspirations."[8] Several conclusions can be drawn from the abundance of literature regarding wellness.

For many people, including the public, health and wellness are synonymous with physical health or physical well-being, which commonly consists of health-promoting behaviors such as physical activity, efforts to eat nutritiously, and adequate sleep. Health behaviors have been defined as "those personal attributes such as beliefs, expectations, motives, values, and other cognitive elements; personality characteristics, including affective and emotional states and traits; and overt behavior patterns, actions, and habits that relate to health maintenance and wellness, to health restoration, and to health improvement."[9] Research in the 1990s indicated that when the public was asked to rate their general health, they narrowly focused on their physical health status, choosing not to consider their emotional, social, or spiritual health.[10] This recognition has influenced researchers to ask specific questions about dimensions of health and wellness, such as physical and mental dimensions.[11] Referring to the definitions of wellness from Dunn and WELCOA, and consistent with numerous other theorists, it is clear that wellness, as it is defined, includes more than just physical behaviors or beliefs about the physical self.

The common themes that emerge from the various models and definitions of wellness suggest that wellness is multidimensional,[2,3–7,11] salutogenic or health causing,[1,12] and consistent with a systems view of persons and their environments.[2,10,12–15] Each of these characteristics will be explored.

First, as a multidimensional construct, wellness is more than simply physical health, as the more common understanding of the term might suggest. Among the dimensions included in various wellness models are physical, spiritual, intellectual, psychological, social, emotional, occupational or vocational, financial, and community or environmental.[16–18] Adams and colleagues[16] in 1997, toward the aim of devising a wellness measurement tool, proposed six dimensions of wellness on the basis of the strength and quality of the theoretical support in the literature. The six dimensions and their corresponding definitions are shown in Table 33.1.

The second characteristic of wellness is that it has a salutogenic or health-causing focus, in contrast to a pathogenic focus in an illness model. Emphasizing the factors that promote health (e.g., salutogenic) supports Dunn's[2] original definition, which implied that wellness involves "maximizing the potential of which the individual is capable." In other words, wellness is not just preventing illness or injury or maintaining the status quo; rather, it involves choices and behaviors

that emphasize optimal health and well-being beyond the status quo. Thus an individual who may or may not be *well* even though there is no physical pathology, may similarly be *well* during an acute episode, or chronic pathology or health condition whether that chronic problem results in static activity limitations or even progressive participation restrictions.

Third, wellness is consistent with a systems perspective. In systems theory, each element of a system is independent and contains its own subelements, in addition to being a subelement of a larger system.[10,13–15] Furthermore, the elements in a system are reciprocally interrelated, indicating that a disruption of homeostasis at any level of the system affects the entire system and all its subelements.[13,15] Therefore overall wellness is a reflection of the state of being within each dimension and a result of the interaction among and between the dimensions of wellness. Fig. 33.1 illustrates a model of wellness reflecting this concept. Vertical movement in the model occurs between the wellness and illness poles as the magnitude of wellness in each dimension changes. The top of the model represents wellness because it is expanded maximally, whereas the bottom of the model represents illness. Bidirectional horizontal movement occurs within each dimension along the lines extending from the inner circle. As per systems theory, movement in every dimension influences and is influenced by movement in the other dimensions.[16] As an example, an individual who has a complete T6 spinal cord injury will experience at least a short-term decrease and likely long-term challenges in physical wellness. Applying systems theory and according to the model, this individual may also have a decrease in other dimensions such as emotional or social wellness. The overall effect of these changes in these dimensions will be a decrease in overall wellness initially following the injury, and increased risk of reduced wellness through the individual's life-span.

Systems theory has been used recently to define the identity of the physical therapist. The American Physical Therapy Association (APTA) has identified the movement system, the collection of systems (cardiovascular, pulmonary, endocrine, integumentary, nervous, and

TABLE 33.1 Definitions of the Dimensions of Wellness

Emotional	The possession of a secure sense of self-identity and a positive sense of self-regard
Intellectual	The perception that one is internally energized by the appropriate amount of intellectually stimulating activity
Physical	Positive perceptions and expectancies of physical health
Psychological	A general perception that one will experience positive outcomes to the events and circumstances of life
Social	The perception that family or friends are available in times of need, and the perception that one is a valued support provider
Spiritual	A positive sense of meaning and purpose in life

From Adams T, Bezner J, Steinhardt M. The conceptualization and measurement of perceived wellness: integrating balance across and within dimensions. *Am J Health Promot.* 1997;11(3):208–218.

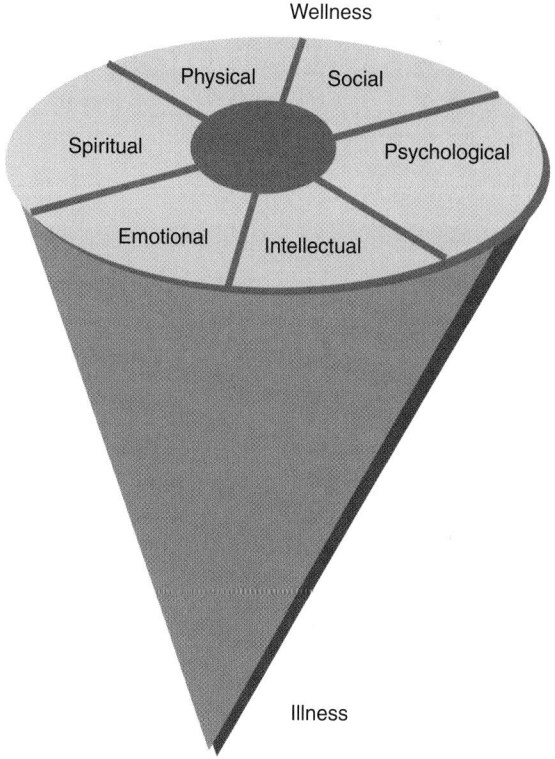

Fig. 33.1 The Wellness Model.

musculoskeletal) that interact to move the body or its component parts, to describe succinctly what physical therapists do and address with patients/patients.[19] Physical therapists address movement system issues with patients/patients along the spectrum of wellness to illness. Indeed, the majority of interventions for those with neurological disease focus on restoring or enhancing movement. The movement system typifies a systems approach as described previously, and physical therapists "maximize an individual's ability to engage with and respond to his or her environment using movement-related interventions to optimize functional capacity and performance."[19] When rehabilitation is conducted with a biopsychosocial approach, movement, health, and well-being are optimized.

A term related to wellness, *quality of life,* is also used to indicate the subjective experience of an individual in a larger context beyond just physical health. Quality of life has been defined as "an individual's perception of their position in life in the context of the culture and value systems in which they live and in relation to their goals, expectations, standards, and concerns. It is a broad ranging concept affected in a complex way by the person's physical health, psychological state, level of independence, social relationships, and their relationship to salient features of their environment."[20] Parallel to the issues related to the concept of wellness, there is lack of agreement on the definition of quality of life and its theoretical components,[21] as well as variation in the use of subjective or objective quality-of-life indicators. Implied by the WHO definition, and supported by several other authors, quality of life is best conceptualized as a subjective construct that is measured through an examination of a patient's perceptions. In other words, quality of life, like wellness, is the subjective experience of health, illness, activity and participation, the environment, social support, and so forth, and it is best measured through an assessment of patient perceptions.

A final concept important to define is the social determinants of health (SDoH)—conditions in the environments in which people are born, live, learn, work, play, worship, and age.[22] A number of social determinants have been found to relate to health and health outcomes, including access to health services, features of the built environment,

economic stability, education, and the social environment. Within the International Classification of Functioning, Disability and Health (ICF) framework, disability and functioning are the result of interactions between health conditions and contextual factors, including factors relative to the environment and those relative to the person. SDoH can be found within both the environmental (built environment, social environment) and personal (education, income) contextual factors of the ICF model.

Numerous efforts are ongoing to address SDoH across the country, for example, addressing food deserts through the establishment of farmer's markets and community gardens, public mandates to ensure all children have access to early intervention programs and preschool, and consideration for human transportation in the design and build of cities and towns.[23,24] To the extent that physical and occupational therapists recognize the contributions of SDoH to the health and wellness of the patients they treat, and they consider SDoH in the development of plans of care, more targeted and effective plans of care will be developed and there will be a higher likelihood of adherence and better outcomes.

A PARADIGM SHIFT TO WELLNESS

The importance of gaining an understanding of health and wellness is to be able to apply it and use this lens when interacting with patients/patients. The ultimate goal is thus to improve the health and well-being of the patient, as the therapist helps the patient improve movement and participation. This is critical to further the paradigm shift from a reactive illness-focused sick care system to a proactive wellness-focused health care system.[25,26] Numerous facilitators and markers of this paradigm shift exist, ranging from the Healthy People 10-year national health objectives[27] to health care reform with Triple Aim,[28] focus on value-based care[29] and the US Department of Health and Human Services' National Prevention Strategy released in 2011.[30] To learn more about these initiatives see Table 33.2 for a listing of health and wellness resources. In 2017, the National Study of Excellence and

TABLE 33.2 Health Promotion and Wellness Resources

Source	Link	Content
Council on Prevention, Health Promotion, and Wellness, APTA	http://www.apta.org/PHPW/	Links to national website resources Access to Community Hub
Academy of Neurologic Physical Therapy, APTA	http://www.neuropt.org/professional-resources/health-promotion-and-wellness	Links to national website resources Updates on health promotion and wellness initiatives in neurological physical therapy practice
National Center on Health, Physical Activity and Disability (NCHPAD)	https://www.nchpad.org/	Includes accessible fitness resources for persons with disabilities and information for health providers
Office of Disease Prevention and Health Promotion	https://health.gov	Includes Healthy People initiative and nutrition and physical activity guidelines
Academy of Geriatric Physical Therapy, APTA	https://geriatricspt.org/	Resources for healthy aging Updates on health promotion and wellness initiatives and resources through the health promotion and wellness special interest group
Exercise is Medicine, ACSM	http://www.exerciseismedicine.org/	Provides numerous resources for health care providers and exercise professionals to promote physical activity
American Occupational Therapy Association (AOTA)	https://ajot.aota.org/article.aspx?articleid=1853063	Statement from AOTA describing role of occupational therapy in health promotion and prevention
Preventive Cardiovascular Nurses Association (PCNA)	http://pcna.net http://pcna.net/clinical-tools/tools-for-healthcare-providers	Provides downloadable online forms for promoting healthy behaviors such as nutrition, smoking cessation, stress management, behavior change

Note, resources accessibility may change. Current as of July 5, 2018.
ACSM, American College of Sports Medicine; *APTA,* American Physical Therapy Association.

TABLE 33.3 The Wellness Matrix

	Illness	Prevention	Wellness
View of human systems	Independent	Interactive	Integrative
Program orientation	Pathogenic	Normogenic	Salutogenic
Dependent variables	Clinical	Behavioral	Perceptual
Patient status	Patient	Person at risk	Whole person
Intervention focus	Symptoms	Risk factors	Dispositions
Intervention method	Prescription	Lifestyle modification	Values clarification

Innovation in Physical Therapist Education stated "Individual therapists and the profession must fully commit to eliminate health disparities, address the SDoH, and improve the health care, health, and well-being of our communities and promote the health of populations."[31] To help conceptualize the implications of this paradigm shift, a comparison of the traditional "illness" paradigm with both "prevention" and "wellness" paradigms will identify ways in which a physical or occupational therapist can incorporate a wellness paradigm into the treatment of a patient with a neurological condition in the context of rehabilitation. The three approaches, or paradigms, are contrasted in Table 33.3 on six parameters, including the view of human systems, program orientation, dependent variables, patient status, intervention focus, and intervention method.

As stated previously, in a wellness paradigm each dimension or part of the system affects and is affected by every other part, resulting in an integrative view of the human body and the human movement system. In contrast, in a traditional illness or medical model, the systems are independent. There are specialties in medicine by body system (e.g., neurology, orthopedics, gynecology), and in many physical and occupational therapy education programs courses are arranged by body system (e.g., neurology, orthopedics, cardiopulmonary, physical dysfunction, psychosocial) as indicators of the independence of the systems. In a prevention approach, there is recognition that the systems interact, or influence one another, but not in the reciprocal fashion characteristic of wellness.

The program orientation of an illness paradigm is the pathology or disease-causing issue, whereas the orientation of a prevention paradigm is normogenic, meaning efforts are aimed at maintaining a normal state or condition (e.g., normal muscle length, tone). Shifting to a wellness paradigm requires a salutogenic or health-causing approach, with a focus on how to achieve greater well-being, health, or quality of life. This shift emphasizes the capabilities and abilities of the individual rather than the limitations and deficits.

The variables of interest in an illness paradigm are clinical variables, such as blood tests, VO₂max (maximum volume of oxygen use), and tests of muscle strength. Changes in these variables result in labeling the patient more or less ill. In a prevention paradigm, the variables measured are behavioral, for example whether the individual smokes, exercises, or wears a helmet. Positive improvement in a prevention approach typically results in a change in an individual's behavior. In contrast, the variables measured in a wellness paradigm are perceptual, indicating what the patient/client thinks and feels about herself or himself. Although clinical, physiological, and behavioral variables are useful and important indicators of bodily wellness and are commonly used to plan individual and community interventions, their utility as wellness measures falls short.[32] Clinical and physiological measures assess the status of a single system, most commonly the systems within the physical domain of wellness. It can be argued that behavioral measures are a better reflection of multiple systems because

of the importance and influence of motivation and self-efficacy on the adoption of behaviors, but they do not describe the wellness of the mind. On the other hand, perceptual measures, capable of assessing all systems and having been shown to predict effectively a variety of health outcomes,[16,33,34] can complement the information provided by body-centered measures insofar as they are valid, congruent with wellness conceptualizations, and empirically supportable.[32]

The influence of perceptions on health and wellness has been demonstrated repeatedly in the literature with a multiplicity of patient/client populations and in a variety of settings. Mossey and Shapiro[33] demonstrated more than 35 years ago that self-rated health was the second strongest predictor of mortality in the elderly, after age. Numerous other researchers have replicated these findings in other populations, lending support to the value of perceptions in understanding health and wellness and indicating that how well you *think* you are may be more important than how well you are as measured by clinical tests and measures or the judgment of a health professional.

Shifting to patient status in each of the three paradigms, the subject receiving treatment in an illness paradigm is called the *patient*, whereas in a prevention paradigm the subject is a *person-at-risk* because of the focus on risk factors and the maintenance of a state of normalcy. In a wellness paradigm, the patient is considered a whole person, to emphasize the multiple systems interacting to produce a state of well-being, and, more importantly, that a high-functioning or intact physical dimension, although important, is not necessary to achieve a state of well-being or a high quality of life. This concept of whole person is reflected in the ICF framework built on a biopsychosocial approach.

Consistent with the patient status elements, the focus of intervention in an illness paradigm is on symptoms, and in a prevention approach on risk factors. Consistent with a whole-person focus in a wellness approach, the intervention focuses on dispositions. Defined as a prevailing tendency, mood, or inclination or the tendency to act in a certain manner under given circumstances, dispositions produce perceptions, which can be measured to indicate a global or psychosocial assessment of the whole person, given input from all of the systems. Combined with symptom and risk factor assessment, perceptions of the individual provide valuable additional information about a patient that can enhance the therapists' ability to intervene and the success of the interventions selected. Table 33.4 lists a few measurement tools that assess patient perceptions.

The intervention method used in an illness paradigm is prescriptive. The prescriptive meaning is based on the system affected and symptoms reported. An intervention in an illness paradigm is prescribed to correct or improve the illness. Given that risk factors are the focus in a prevention paradigm and the aim is to maintain or return the person-at-risk to a normal state, the intervention method that is most appropriate is lifestyle modification in an attempt to change the behavior that is producing the identified risk. The intervention method in a wellness approach is called *values clarification*, and it is consistent with the focus on dispositions and measurement of perceptions. The

TABLE 33.4   Sample Items From Perceptual Measurement Tools

Instrument	Perceptual Construct	Sample Items (Responses)
Short Form 36[60]	General health perceptions	"In general, would you say your health is _____?" (excellent, very good, good, fair, or poor)
		"Compared with 1 year ago, how would you rate your health in general now?" (much better than 1 year ago, somewhat better, about the same, somewhat worse, much worse)
Satisfaction With Life Scale[70]	Life satisfaction	"In most ways my life is close to my ideal"
		"I am satisfied with my life" (7-point Likert scale from strongly disagree [1] to strongly agree [7])
Perceived Wellness Survey[16]	Perceived wellness	"I am always optimistic about my future"
		"I avoid activities that require me to concentrate" (6-point Likert scale from very strongly disagree [1] to very strongly agree [6])
NCHS General Well-Being Schedule[62]	General well-being	"How have you been feeling in general?" (in excellent spirits; in very good spirits; in good spirits mostly; up and down in spirits a lot; in low spirits mostly; in very low spirits)
		"Has your daily life been full of things that were interesting to you?" (all the time, most of the time, a good bit of the time, some of the time, a little of the time, none of the time)
Philadelphia Geriatric Center Morale Scale[66,67]	Morale	"Things keep getting worse as I get older"
		"I am as happy now as when I was younger" (yes, no)
Memorial University of Newfoundland Scale of Happiness[69]	Happiness	"In the past months have you been feeling on top of the world?"
		"As I look back on my life, I am fairly well satisfied" (yes, no, don't know)

aim of values clarification is to enhance self-understanding by surfacing the person's perceptions of the situation and its impact on his or her life. When values clarification can precede intervention prescription and lifestyle modification, wellness will be enhanced because the intervention will be more targeted and truly person-first or whole-person–based, rather than focused on the health condition.

THEORIES OF BEHAVIOR CHANGE

A shift to a wellness paradigm from an illness paradigm will not yield positive outcomes without consideration given to factors beyond the individual (behaviors, cognitive and physical state, experience, etc.), including the physical and social environments.[35,36] A social-ecological approach describes the multiple levels of influence on health and wellness, including individual factors, family and friends, communities and employers, policies, and social norms. Factors beyond the individual

include the SDoH and other features of the environment that impact access to and use of health and wellness enhancing resources. This approach recognizes that behavior is affected by and affects multiple levels of influence,[37] and it is necessary to do more than educate and motivate people to engage in health-promoting behaviors. Social and physical environments must support the healthy choice as the easy choice for positive health behaviors to become consistent and sustainable. There are numerous examples of the impact of health-promoting programs designed to address multiple levels of influence, but perhaps the success that has been achieved in reducing rates of cigarette smoking provides the best example, in which environmental changes occurred at multiple levels simultaneously to curb the incidence of smoking (e.g., social norms [while it was once cool to smoke, nonsmoking became cooler]), policy (cigarette taxes were increased), organizations (non-smoking sections of restaurants, airplanes, and places of employment were created). Fig. 33.2 illustrates the social-ecological model.

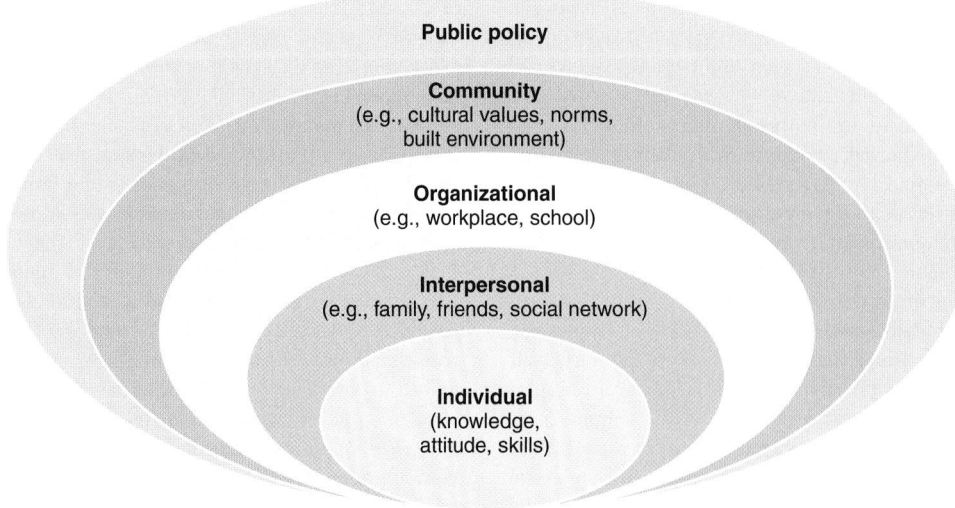

Fig. 33.2 Social-Ecological Model.

As illustrated by the social-ecological model, frameworks are useful to guide intervention programs. Theories of behavior change are frameworks that have been used for decades to explain, interpret, guide, and predict behavior in a specified context. Theories, or systematic explanations for naturally occurring phenomena, explain behavior and provide insight into ways to modify it.[38] Consistent with a wellness paradigm, the use of theories creates a more holistic approach in the provision of physical or occupational therapy because they address the cognitive and emotional factors related to readiness and motivation to behave that so frequently derail intervention programs (attitude, motivation, negative emotions, etc.). Understanding and applying theories of behavior change will enable the therapist to create more targeted intervention programs, enhance patient participation in and adherence to intervention programs, and improve outcomes. Several key health behavior change theories will be discussed in the following section, starting with interpersonal theories (social cognitive theory [SCT], resilience theory) that include environmental influences on individual behavior, and moving to individual theories (the transtheoretical model [TTM], self-determination theory [SDT]) in which variables within the person are the focus.

Social Cognitive Theory

One of the most widely used and robust health behavior change theories, SCT emerged from social learning theory, which identified that people learn from their own experiences and by observing the experiences of others.[37] There are three major constructs in SCT that interact to influence behavior: personal factors (age, cognitions, previous experience with the behavior, etc.), environmental factors (access to resources, safety, support from family/friends, etc.), and aspects of the behavior itself (vigor of the behavior, outcomes achieved as a result of practicing the behavior, competence with the behavior, etc.). Successful efforts to change behavior depend on identification of the positive supports and the detractors in each of the three constructs. For example, if a therapist is managing the physical or occupational therapy services of a patient who has multiple sclerosis and this patient is motivated to be physically active yet does not have a safe place to walk or be physically active near home, the patient will likely not be able to consistently perform physical activity. If the same patient works for an employer who provides an onsite gym, the patient could negotiate with her supervisor to utilize the gym to be physically active a few days a week.

Of the multiple additional constructs in SCT, several are worth mentioning. Albert Bandura, the author of SCT, identified self-efficacy, the confidence a person has in his or her ability to perform a behavior, as having a significant influence on behavior change.[39–41] Self-efficacy has been shown to predict the amount of effort an individual will expend to learn and practice a behavior, the persistence demonstrated in the process, and the effort expended to overcome barriers.[42,43] Self-efficacy is behavior specific. Therapists are familiar with the importance of self-efficacy in neurological rehabilitation as patients learn and relearn movement strategies after neurological insults and the way in which repetition, small steps, verbal persuasion, and observational learning build confidence and thus competence in the movement. These same strategies enhance self-efficacy for behavior change related to enhancing wellness, and self-efficacy is key to the development of sustainable health habits.

Goal setting and social support are two additional useful constructs in SCT that fall into the broad category of self-regulation, an important skill to develop when adopting new health behaviors.[41] The setting and achievement of goals can have a profound positive impact on learning new health behaviors, like the positive role goals play in physical and occupational therapy plans of care, with the additive effect of enhancing self-efficacy when goals are both challenging and achievable. When goals are not adequately challenging, they can decrease self-efficacy. Social support involves identifying others who will provide encouragement in the form of moral support, participation in the behavior, and accountability. For certain populations, social support has been shown to be significantly related to physical and mental health, pain, coping, adjustment, and life satisfaction.[44]

In summary, the application of the SCT can identify both barriers and facilitators to behavior change that can become the target of interventions that support the development of health and wellness enhancing behaviors. Attending to the self-efficacy of the patient as he or she develops a new behavior and intentionally implementing an approach that enhances self-efficacy will lead to more positive results. The use of goal setting and social support within the plan of care have been shown to support positive behavior change.

Resilience Theory

The concept of resilience arose from the science related to both the physiological aspects of stress and neuroplasticity and psychological aspects of coping.[45] Resilience, as defined by the American Psychological Association, is "the process of adapting well in the face of adversity, trauma, tragedy, threats or even significant sources of stress."[46] Resilience is thus a complex construct representing a process of adaptation to a life disturbance based on the interaction of the individual and the environment. Resilience has also been viewed as a trait or outcome.[45] As a trait, resilience is considered a protective factor. On an intrapersonal and cognitive level, resilience traits include optimism, intelligence, humor, locus of control, and a belief in purpose in life.[45,47] On an environmental level, perceived social support has been associated with higher levels of resilience. Resilience is demonstrated behaviorally through successful coping strategies, social skills, and educational abilities.[45]

Resiliency as a model or theory may be first credited to Richardson and colleagues in 1990, although the concept of resilience can be found in prior work. In the Resiliency Model, Richardson and colleagues[48] describe the characteristics of a resilient individual as protective against distress and disease. The authors describe resilience as a process of psychological reintegration with four possible levels where adversity can promote growth. In the highest level of true psychological reintegration, the individual learns new skills and strengthens characteristics of resilience from a disruptive experience ultimately reframing his or her perspective in a way that is enabling and not disabling. In 1998, Carver and colleagues[49] depicted an individual's level of functioning after an adverse event as having four possible courses similar to Richardson's levels of psychological integration: (1) succumbing, (2) survival with impairment, (3) resilience (or recovery), and (4) thriving, seen as bouncing back and *above* the stressful life event, true psychological reintegration.

Resilience has been studied across a wide range of conditions including environmental stressors such as war, developmental life stressors such as adolescence, and also health stressors such as chronic and neurological illness. Based on this work, resilience may be best conceptualized within individual domains as resiliency in one area does not necessarily equate to resilience in another, similar to the concept of self-efficacy. Given the disruption of a life-changing event such as a traumatic brain injury or a spinal cord injury, or the uncertainty and stressors associated with neurodegenerative diseases such as multiple sclerosis or Huntington disease, the study of resilience and of resilience promotion programs has grown in recent years.[50,51] In a small randomized control pilot study of the program "Everyday Matters" developed by the National Multiple Sclerosis Society, Alschuler and colleagues[51] found persons with multiple sclerosis improved their resilience and satisfaction with social roles. Trends were seen towards improvement in positive affect and well-being, and reduction in depressive symptoms. The 6-week program was delivered by teleconference and included readings, videos, and online group participation focused on improving resilience through development of optimism and happiness, and building upon opportunities for forward movement and positive outcomes.

Physical and occupational therapists can use the concept of resilience to empower choice and opportunity for patients to grow (thrive or psychological reintegration), versus simply recover or perhaps succumb[47] when faced with living with a neurological condition. By incorporating components of optimism and humor, as well as positive appraisals and reframing into therapeutic encounters, therapists can build resilience as a powerful tool to promote health and wellness. Therapists can also connect patients with existing community-based programs that build resilience for the life-long pursuit of wellness.

Transtheoretical Model

An individual theory, the TTM has four main constructs—stages of change, decisional balance, self-efficacy, and processes of change. James Prochaska, who with colleagues first described the TTM, hypothesized that individuals cycle through the stages as they adopt a specific behavior, from precontemplation (not thinking about changing the behavior), to maintenance (having performed the behavior consistently for at least 6 months).[52,53] Together with the other three stages (contemplation—feeling ambivalent about the behavior; preparation—committed to changing the behavior but hasn't started yet; action—engaged in performing the behavior), the five stages describe varying degrees of readiness to engage in a specific behavior. The processes of change can be used as interventions to move an individual from one stage to another and include cognitive (thinking about the influence of the behavior on self and others) and behavioral (cues and rewards) activities. Decisional balance, weighing the pros and cons of the behavior, influences movement from one stage to another, as does self-efficacy. The higher the list of pros for performing the behavior, the closer to the action stage the individual will move, and the higher an individual's self-efficacy, the more likely the person is to be performing the behavior. It is important to note that the stages are not meant to be linear, but cyclical, in that individuals don't progress from one stage to the next necessarily. For example, individuals who stop smoking "cold turkey" can move from contemplation to action without spending time in the preparation stage.

Identifying the stage of change an individual is in allows targeted interventions to be developed that both respect the individual's readiness to change and resonate with the person's thoughts and feelings about the change. For example, if a patient is in the contemplation stage for performing his home exercise program daily, it would be appropriate to discuss the pros and cons of the behavior and identify strategies to overcome the cons or barriers and ways to increase the pros or benefits. This approach will ideally move the individual to the preparation or action stage where performing the home program can be achieved. Geertz and colleagues[54] used TTM constructs in a study with 40 subjects with multiple sclerosis aged 35 to 65 with moderate disability. Subjects in the experimental group participated in 16 to 24 standardized exercise sessions in 8 to 12 weeks individually tailored to each participant based on baseline stage of change, self-efficacy, barriers to exercising, and social support. Following the intervention, subjects in the experimental group reported a higher stage of change compared to the control group; self-efficacy stayed the same compared to the control group in which it decreased over time, and perception of barriers changed to a less restricting view in experimental group subjects.[54]

The TTM can be useful to identify a patient's readiness to change a behavior, to identify cognitive and behavioral interventions that will

create greater readiness, and, like the SCT, to note when self-efficacy is low and to intentionally apply strategies to improve it.

Self-Determination Theory

Recognizing that human behavior is the largest single source of variance in health outcomes, that the effectiveness of most interventions is highly dependent on the patient's ability to adhere to recommendations, and that adherence is generally poor, Edward Deci and Richard Ryan created the SDT to explain how humans can successfully change their behavior.[55,56] Constructs in the SDT include three innate psychological needs of humans: autonomy, competence, and relatedness to others. Autonomy refers to the process by which behaviors become regulated over time. The authors describe motivation or regulation on a continuum, including amotivated/nonregulated, extrinsically motivated/regulated, and intrinsically motivated/regulated. When people behave to gain a reward (fit into a size 8 dress for a wedding) or avoid a negative consequence (spouse nagging, feeling guilty), they are motivated by extrinsic factors, which generally do not sustain behavior long term. Intrinsic motivation includes behaving a certain way because it is consistent with a person's deeply held values or goals, for example, to be a better parent or student or employee. Intrinsic motivation is consistent with being self-determined and can sustain behavior and health habits as lifestyle choices.[57] Competence is the degree to which individuals feel able to change and achieve goals and outcomes and is supported by the provision of skills and tools for change and effective feedback from health care providers.[58] The theory authors state that autonomy facilitates competence because when individuals choose to engage in a behavior they are more likely to take risks, learn, and apply new strategies.[58] The third construct, relatedness, refers to the degree to which individuals feel connected to others in a warm, supportive way.[56] When individuals feel respected and supported, especially by health care providers in a patient-provider relationship, they are more likely to achieve intrinsic motivation and experience success sustaining health behaviors over time.

Physical and occupational therapists can apply the SDT by providing meaningful rationale for why a behavior is recommended, acknowledging feelings and perspectives so patients feel understood, and integrating choice wherever possible in plans of care to minimize external control and pressure from the provider.[56] Numerous studies have been published illustrating the value of guiding patients toward autonomous motivation so that they can adhere to health behaviors and improve their quality of life and health outcomes.[59]

MEASUREMENT OF WELLNESS

As a result of the varied ways that wellness has been defined and understood, a variety of wellness measures exist. Consistent with the characteristics of wellness described, a wellness measure should reflect the multidimensionality and systems orientation of the concept and have a salutogenic focus. In the literature, as well as in daily practice, clinical, physiological, behavioral, and perceptual indicators are all touted as wellness measures. Clinical measures include serum cholesterol level and blood pressure, physiological indicators include skinfold measurements and maximum oxygen uptake, behavioral measures include smoking status and physical activity frequency, and perceptual measures include patient/client self-assessment tools such as global indicators of health status ("Compared with other people your age, would you say your health is excellent, good, fair, or poor?")[11] and the Short Form 36 (SF-36) Health Status Questionnaire (see Table 33.4).[60]

Although some perceptual measures assess only single system status (e.g., psychological well-being, mental well-being), numerous multidimensional perceptual measures exist that can serve as wellness measures. Perceptual constructs that have been used as wellness measures include general health status,[60] subjective well-being,[60,61] general well-being,[62] morale,[63–67] happiness,[68,69] life satisfaction,[70–72] hardiness,[73,74] resilience,[75–77] and perceived wellness[16,78] (see Table 33.4). Refer to Fig. 33.3 for the "Perceived Wellness Survey" used by professionals to help conceptualize the patient's perception of her or his wellness. This survey was first published in the *American Journal of Health Promotion* in 1997.[16] Physical therapists assess perceptions as a part of the patient/client history, as recommended in the "Guide to Physical Therapist Practice."[79] Occupational therapists assess perceptions as part of their focus on human performance and occupation. Some of the kinds of perceptions that can be assessed include perceptions of general health status, social support systems, role and social functioning, self-efficacy, and functional status in self-care and home management activities and work, community, and leisure activities. Although a few of these categories are included in overall wellness, such as general health status and social and role functioning, measuring wellness perceptions specifically can provide additional and more complete information about the patient that both the physical and occupational therapist can use to formulate a plan that can be insightful to the patient/client. Therefore perceptual tools should be used when measuring wellness.

MERGING WELLNESS INTO REHABILITATION—THE ROLE OF PHYSICAL AND OCCUPATIONAL THERAPISTS IN HEALTH PROMOTION AND WELLNESS

Incorporating wellness into rehabilitation requires that the therapist modify the traditional approach used in rehabilitation. This change

Perceived Wellness Survey

The following statements are designed to provide information about your wellness perceptions. Please carefully and thoughtfully consider each statement, then select the one response option with which you most agree.

	Very Strongly Disagree				Very Strongly Agree
1. I am always optimistic about my future.	1	2	3	4	5	6
2. There have been times when I felt inferior to most of the people I knew.	1	2	3	4	5	6
3. Members of my family come to me for support.	1	2	3	4	5	6
4. My physical health has restricted me in the past.	1	2	3	4	5	6
5. I believe there is a real purpose for my life.	1	2	3	4	5	6
6. I will always seek out activities that challenge me to think and reason.	1	2	3	4	5	6
7. I rarely count on good things happening to me.	1	2	3	4	5	6
8. In general, I feel confident about my abilities.	1	2	3	4	5	6
9. Sometimes I wonder if my family will really be there for me when I am in need.	1	2	3	4	5	6
10. My body seems to resist physical illness very well.	1	2	3	4	5	6
11. Life does not hold much future promise for me.	1	2	3	4	5	6
12. I avoid activities which require me to concentrate.	1	2	3	4	5	6
13. I always look on the bright side of things.	1	2	3	4	5	6
14. I sometimes think I am a worthless individual.	1	2	3	4	5	6
15. My friends know they can always confide in me and ask me for advice.	1	2	3	4	5	6
16. My physical health is excellent.	1	2	3	4	5	6
17. Sometimes I don't understand what life is all about.	1	2	3	4	5	6
18. Generally, I feel pleased with the amount of intellectual stimulation I receive in my daily life.	1	2	3	4	5	6
19. In the past, I have expected the best.	1	2	3	4	5	6
20. I am uncertain about my ability to do things well in the future.	1	2	3	4	5	6
21. My family has been available to support me in the past.	1	2	3	4	5	6
22. Compared to people I know, my past physical health has been excellent.	1	2	3	4	5	6
23. I feel a sense of mission about my future.	1	2	3	4	5	6
24. The amount of information that I process in a typical day is just about right for me (i.e., not too much and not too little).	1	2	3	4	5	6
25. In the past, I hardly ever expected things to go my way.	1	2	3	4	5	6
26. I will always be secure with who I am.	1	2	3	4	5	6
27. In the past, I have not always had friends with whom I could share my joys and sorrows.	1	2	3	4	5	6
28. I expect to always be physically healthy.	1	2	3	4	5	6
29. I have felt in the past that my life was meaningless.	1	2	3	4	5	6
30. In the past, I have generally found intellectual challenges to be vital to my overall well-being.	1	2	3	4	5	6
31. Things will not work out the way I want them to in the future.	1	2	3	4	5	6
32. In the past, I have felt sure of myself among strangers.	1	2	3	4	5	6
33. My friends will be there for me when I need help.	1	2	3	4	5	6
34. I expect my physical health to get worse.	1	2	3	4	5	6
35. It seems that my life has always had purpose.	1	2	3	4	5	6
36. My life has often seemed void of positive mental stimulation.	1	2	3	4	5	6

Fig. 33.3 The Perceived Wellness Survey. (From Adams T, Bezner J, Steinhardt M. The conceptualization and measurement of perceived wellness: integrating balance across and within dimensions. *Am J Health Promot.* 1997;11[3]:208–218.)

involves multiple steps, including shifting the focus from illness to wellness, being a role model of wellness, promoting active living,[80,81] incorporating behavioral[82,83] and perceptual wellness measures into the examination, and ensuring that the therapist is addressing the whole person within his or her system including values, preferences, and social context. Within the scope of rehabilitation this approach may include screenings, consultation, referral, education, resource identification, individual health behavior management, and advocacy for individual and population health.[80,83] Establishing a wellness approach also requires that the therapist assume the role of a facilitator or partner rather than that of an authority figure.[84] This shift involves utilization of practices consistent with evidence-based communication and counseling methods based on principles of shared decision making[85,86] such as the 5 A's/5 R's[87,88] motivational interviewing[89–91] and health coaching.[92,93] In this section, current recommendations for incorporating health promotion and wellness practices into rehabilitation will be shared.

There are numerous resources available to assist the therapist in facilitating health promotion and wellness into his or her practice (see Table 33.2). At minimum, the APTA recommends[94]: (1) identify patient/client health risks during the history and physical via the systems review, (2) take vital signs of every patient during each visit, (3) collaborate with the patient to develop and implement a plan to address health risks, (4) determine readiness for behavioral change, (5) identify available resources in the community to assist in achievement of the plan, (6) identify the secondary and tertiary effects of the disability, (7) demonstrate healthy behaviors, and (8) promote health and wellness in the community. This minimum skill set for the promotion of health, wellness, and prevention in physical therapist practice was developed in 2004 and updated in 2009. Since that time, work has been done at the national and global levels to clarify the role of the therapist in screening and promotion of healthy behaviors and behavior change.[25,82,83,95–97] This work has focused largely on the importance of addressing and preventing the rising prevalence of lifestyle-related noncommunicable diseases (NCDs)

(e.g., heart disease, stroke, type 2 diabetes mellitus, obesity) in developing countries across the world.[82] Based on this work, the following health behavioral domains and health behaviors have been proposed for minimum assessment in rehabilitation practice in physical therapy[25,97] (Table 33.5): physical activity (including sedentarism, lifestyle physical activity, structured exercise), nutrition, sleep, stress (representative of mental health, including depression, anxiety and stress), and smoking. Table 33.5 includes a synthesis of published work highlighting the behavioral domain, the behavioral competency or goal, and assessment and intervention recommendations.

Recently, Lein and colleagues[26] proposed a health-focused physical therapy model for incorporating health promotion and wellness into standard of care practice. The key components of this model include a needs assessment of the population served; a needs assessment of the individual for lifestyle behavior change; collaboration with the patient to classify lifestyle behavior change needs into one of three categories: does not need change, needs change but not ready to change, needs change and ready to change; and finally providing lifestyle behavior change interventions. While this model demonstrated good content validity for application to the lifestyle behaviors of physical activity and smoking cessation,[39] further research is needed to determine its validity for sleep, nutrition, and stress management, as well as its effectiveness in guiding clinical practice across diverse populations and settings, including persons living with chronic neurological conditions.

It may be most instructive to consider first how a wellness approach could be adopted with patients who are seemingly healthy or without pathology. As experts in movement problems associated with the causes and consequences of pathological conditions, physical and occupational therapists should play a significant role in primary and secondary prevention. Indeed, intervention programs designed by therapists for patients/clients with pathology generally include instruction in preventive behaviors and activities (secondary prevention). Although appropriate and worthwhile, these efforts do not produce the significant outcomes that primary prevention programs

TABLE 33.5   Lifestyle Behaviors for Assessment and Intervention

Domain	Core Competency/Goal	Assessment[a]	Intervention[b]
Physical activity	Reduction of sitting/sedentary behavior Promotion of lifestyle physical activity Promotion of structured exercise	Sedentarism (hours/day) Physical activity (e.g., GLT, PADS-R, pedometer) Structured exercise (FITT; guidelines:150 min/week moderate intensity, resistance training 2 days/week)	Advice and intervention (e.g., sedentarism and physical activity guidelines; individualized structured exercise prescription; counseling for behavior change and self-management)
Nutrition	Healthy nutrition/diet (may include weight loss)	Brief nutritional assessment BMI Waist-to-hip ratio	Potential recommendation (basic nutritional information, e.g., ChooseMyPlate.gov) or referral to other health professional
Sleep	Healthy sleep	Sleep habits (hours/night, quality; guidelines: 7–9 h)	Potential recommendation or referral to other health professional
Stress	Stress, anxiety, and depression management	Mental health (e.g., psychological stress measure, depression screen)	Potential recommendation or referral to other health professional
Smoking	Smoking cessation	Smoking history Quit attempts	Potential recommendation or referral to other health professional

[a]Patient values, priorities, and readiness to change should be assessed within each competency.
[b]Minimum intervention approach includes 5 R's if patient is in precontemplative stage of behavior change and 5 A's if in contemplative or higher stage of behavior change for each competency; additionally, follow-up, reevaluation, and progression as needed is recommended.
BMI, Body mass index; FITT, frequency, intensity, timing, type; GLT, Godin leisure-time exercise questionnaire; PADS-R, physical activity and disability survey—revised for persons with chronic neurological conditions.
See references 25, 26, 82, 83, 95–97.

might because they are applied after the onset of risk, illness, or injury. Contemporary practice includes a role for the physical and occupational therapist in primary prevention, that is, interacting with patients to promote health and improve wellness *before* they become patients.

Because individuals without overt disease are typically unmotivated to seek professional assistance, consideration must be given to how a provider recruits those without disease. Competence in communication is imperative to ensure that providers do not offend individuals or generate defensiveness when exploring opportunities for health enhancement. Strategies related to effective communication are presented later in this section. A focus on wellness and health-causing activities is a powerful solution to this dilemma. In a sports or athletic context, this approach would be considered "performance enhancing" and would be marketed to individuals who have goals and ambitions related to improving athletic performance in a specific context (e.g., improving 10K time, increasing cycling distance or speed). In a general wellness context, an appropriate marketing message might be to improve quality of life or productivity, or any subjective measure that a patient deems important. The same knowledge and skills therapists use when intervening to prevent injury, delay or prevent the progression of disease, or enhance quality of movement are useful in a primary prevention context in which the goal is to improve quality of life, well-being, and productivity. The difference is the context in which the knowledge and skills are applied. Adopting a wellness paradigm and a patient-centered perspective or focus creates an environment surrounding the patient-provider relationship that both empowers the patient to make meaningful changes and establishes a partnership that is most conducive to change and improvement. The improvement of quality of life or wellness requires a consideration of the patient as a whole person, by definition, as discussed previously in this chapter. Using a patient-centered, whole-person approach to the design of an intervention program requires a considerably different approach than the traditional, biomedical approach of measuring clinical and behavioral variables to identify impairments and functional loss and creating an intervention aimed at ameliorating the impairment.[98,99] Suddenly patients are more than their diseases, which sends a much different message and creates a much different relationship between the provider and the patient. This approach also broadens the intervention focus beyond the physical domain, opening the door to issues related to the nonphysical domains of wellness, such as emotional, spiritual, social, and psychological wellness, which at any given time could be the most important challenge to high quality of life or wellness. In this case, the therapist may refer to other providers who may be better suited to guide the patient in these domains.

COMMUNICATION STRATEGIES TO IMPLEMENT BEHAVIOR CHANGE THEORY

The way in which a physical or occupational therapist begins a conversation with a patient about a health behavior or about something more sensitive, like meaningful participation, emotional well-being, or spiritual pursuits, should be consistent with the partnership relationship discussed previously in this chapter, rather than consistent with an expert role. Patients may have limited previous experience with these types of conversations with a health care provider, so they may be surprised or caught off guard when the therapist raises these issues. Previous conversations may have been based on a paternalistic approach versus an autonomy supporting approach and weren't effective at promoting change and may have even resulted in feelings of shame or guilt in the patient. A low pressure, casual approach to beginning conversations about wellness is suggested, wherein the therapist gauges the patient's interest in discussing a topic in more depth and asks

TABLE 33.6 **The 5 A's Model for Behavior Change**

A	Definition
Ask	Ask permission to discuss behavior
Advise	Provide information about the behavior and the associated risks and provide treatment options
Assess	Assess readiness to change; assess biometric and psychosocial variables
Assist	Explore barriers and benefits; refer to another provider
Arrange/agree	Make arrangements to follow up; agree on SMART goals and intervention approach

Agency for Healthcare Research and Quality. *Five Major Steps to Intervention (The "5 A's")*. Rockville, MD: Agency for Healthcare Research and Quality; 2012. www.ahrq.gov/professionals/clinicians-providers/guidelines-recommendations/tobacco/5steps.html. Accessed August 19, 2018.

permission to discuss a topic further. The following examples serve to illustrate the type of statements that may result in patient agreement to discuss an issue in greater depth.

- I noticed that you weren't regularly physically active prior to your injury/disease; is physical activity something we could discuss? I think I can help you become more physically active if you are interested.
- Are you familiar with the relationship between smoking and risk for neurological diseases such as multiple sclerosis and stroke? If yes, "Would you be interested in discussing your smoking habit? I would like to understand more about your choice to smoke and explore ways you can successfully quit." If no, "Would it be okay if I shared some information with you about the relationship?"
- I'm concerned because you've seemed down lately. Is there something you would like to talk about with me or with another provider?
- You don't seem as committed to your home program as you were when we first started working together. Can we talk about your home program? I would like to support you to find a way to make it a consistent priority.

Another approach to entering a conversation with a patient is to use the 5 A's schemata, developed from work in tobacco cessation (Table 33.6).[87,100] The first A is to ask the patient about the behavior, similar to the approach discussed above in this section. The second A, advise, involves the provision of advice about the behavior, which should be done cautiously so as not to elicit defensiveness in the patient, and not at all if the patient is not open to discussion about the behavior. The third A, assess, means determining readiness to change, discussed next in this section. The fourth A, assist, refers to the role the provider can serve to help the patient set goals and take the next steps toward change. The final A, arrange, refers to follow-up at some point in the future to discover how the patient is progressing with the behavior change.

Once patient interest has been assessed, the therapist should determine readiness to change or stage of change from the TTM. A 5-response question assessing readiness to change the behavior of interest can be utilized, as illustrated in Table 33.7. Or a verbal 1 to 10 scale can be used to assess readiness. The therapist can ask, "On a scale from 1 to 10, with 1 being not ready to change at all and 10 being this is the most important thing I can do for myself right now, how ready are you to change?" Patient responses above 6/7 indicate readiness to change, whereas responses in the range of 3 to 5 may indicate contemplation and 1 to 2 precontemplation. For patients who appear ready to change,

TABLE 33.7 Stages of Change Question for Physical Activity

Instructions: Physical activity is defined as 150 min/week of moderate or 75 min/week of vigorous physical activity or a combination of both. Please read the statements below and select the statement that most closely describes your physical activity level.

Stage	Question
Precontemplation	I have no intention of taking action to become more physically active.
Contemplation	I intend to become more physically active within the next 6 months.
Preparation	I have taken a few steps to become more physically active and intend to start in the next 30 days, or I am active but am not meeting the current guidelines.
Action	I am currently engaged in physical activity and have been for less than 6 months.
Maintenance	I am physically active and have been for more than 6 months.

From Prochaska J, Redding C, Evers K. The transtheoretical model and stages of change. In: Glanz K, Rimer BK, Viswanath K, eds. *Health Behavior: Theory, Research, and Practice.* 5th ed. San Francisco, CA: Jossey-Bass; 2015:125–148.

the therapist can proceed to inquire about the patient's past success with the behavior, if any, and goal setting to begin to develop the behavior. Small, measurable, challenging yet achievable goals can be set to build self-efficacy and determine how the patient can successfully adopt a regular habit of the behavior of interest.[92] If goals are set too hard or too easy, the result will be decreased self-efficacy, thus the importance of determining challenging yet achievable steps toward the behavior. Patients who are in the preparation stage of change may do best to start with "thinking goals" or cognitive steps (planning) to build confidence, like finding healthy recipes, or discovering different types of physical activity of interest, or talking to family members about supporting the patient's efforts, prior to creating goals involving participation in the actual behavior. Success with cognitive goals will move the patient toward the action stage and build readiness and confidence to engage in the actual behavior of interest.[50] Behavior change goals can be set and achieved similar to therapy goals, making sure the goals are S.M.A.R.T. (specific, measurable, achievable, realistic, and time-referenced), are constructed by the patient (with assistance from the therapist), and the therapist ensures the patient has the resources and self-efficacy to achieve them. The therapist should routinely inquire about confidence in achieving a goal after setting a goal. If confidence on a 1 to 10 scale (1 = no confidence at all, 10 = I will definitely achieve the goal) is not at least a 6 or 7 for a specific goal, the therapist should consider revising the goal because it may be too difficult, or it may be unrealistic and therefore not achievable. It is suggested that therapists assess self-efficacy in this manner for each goal written, each time a goal is set to enhance the ability of patients to achieve goals and to increase self-efficacy, ensuring goals are set appropriately challenging and realistic.[84,90] Patients who are in the contemplation stage of the TTM, indicating that they are likely ambivalent about adopting a healthy behavior, or patients who are not intending to change in the near future (precontemplation), may benefit from motivational interviewing, a conversational tool used to facilitate discussion about behavior change. The goal of a motivational interview is to

identify intrinsic motivation to adopt a healthy behavior and facilitate movement to an action stage and thus readiness to change.[89] Adopting a collaborative versus a coercive approach, therapists using motivational interviewing recognize that the motivation to change comes from within the patient, rather than from the therapist (Table 33.8). The process of motivational interviewing is designed to elicit the intrinsic motivation necessary to create sustainable behavior change.[84]

Recognizing that a patient may benefit from motivational interviewing, the therapist expresses empathy for the current behavior, inquiries about the patient's history with the behavior (previous successful performance of the behavior), solicits benefits of the healthy behavior from the patient, and asks the patient to identify barriers to performing the healthy behavior. Throughout the conversation, the therapist looks for opportunities to identify discrepancy between the patient's current values and goals, and the behavior of interest and supports autonomy and self-efficacy using the four primary skills.[84,89] While motivational interviewing requires practice and feedback to learn and apply, it's use by health care providers for a variety of medical conditions has demonstrated that it is a useful adjunct to traditional approaches to behavior change.[101]

An approach parallel to the 5 A's, called the 5 R's, has been developed to discover and enhance motivation to change and is shown in Table 33.9.[88] A helpful acronym for the clinician, the 5 R's are a pneumonic that guides the therapist through the steps of decisional balance and developing discrepancy that can support the patient to develop greater readiness to change.

TABLE 33.8 Four Primary Stages Required to Conduct a Motivational Interview

- Ask open-ended questions (vs. closed-ended yes/no questions) to provide the opportunity for the patient to guide the conversation and to respect patient autonomy.
- Affirm and support the patient to prevent judgment and reflect back what the patient is saying to more easily identify discrepancy between the patient's deeply held values and current behaviors.
- Reflective listening, or mirroring what the patient says, allows the therapist to maintain a focus on the patient, avoids interjecting one's own experience, enables a deep dive into the patient's experience, and ensures the patient feels understood.
- Summarize what the patient tells the therapist periodically throughout the conversation to transition between topics, support and highlight the patient's motivations to change and progress made, and to ensure understanding.[89]

TABLE 33.9 The 5 R's of Motivation

R	Definition
Relevance	Ask the patient why the behavior is personally relevant
Risks	Ask the patient about the risks of continuing with the unhealthy behavior
Rewards	Ask the patient to discuss the benefits of adopting the healthy behavior
Roadblocks	Ask the patient about the barriers to performing the healthy behavior
Repetition	Repeat the conversation at each visit until the patient adopts the behavior

From Agency for Healthcare Research and Quality. *Patients Not Ready to Make a Quit Attempt Now (The "5 R's").* Rockville, MD: Agency for Healthcare Research and Quality; 2012. www.ahrq.gov/professionals/clinicians-providers/guidelines-recommendations/tobacco/5rs.html. Accessed August 19, 2018.

The development of intrinsic motivation is an imperative step in the process of building autonomy for sustainable behavior change and is a component of a more comprehensive communication approach to addressing health behaviors called health coaching or health counseling.[92] Health coaching "is a partnership with patients in a thought-provoking and creative process that inspires and supports them to maximize their personal and professional potential."[92] Health coaching is consistent with a wellness approach, requiring the following practitioner competencies:

- The application of a patient-centered approach,
- The ability to assist patients in identifying their goals and motives for change,
- The use of patient self-discovery to explore intervention strategies that are realistic and achievable and engage the patient in active learning,
- The ability to help the patient hold himself or herself accountable and create self-monitoring practices, and
- The attainment of health knowledge to support health behavior change.[84,102]

Therapists will likely discover that adopting more of a health coaching communication approach versus an expert approach will result in a patient-therapist partnership that will support the development of autonomy, self-efficacy, and growth and enhance both the patient's success and the therapist's satisfaction. Applying the recommendations and approach in this section is a good first step toward this shift to a health coaching communication approach and will be illustrated in the case studies that appear later in this chapter.

APPLICATION TO INDIVIDUALS WITH NEUROLOGICAL CONDITIONS

A health and wellness approach has many specific indications and benefits for those living with, and for those at risk for, neurological disease or injury. While examples have been given throughout this chapter, this section will focus exclusively on application to neurological conditions. A case study example highlighting these concepts in multiple sclerosis is available at the end of this chapter.

Benefits begin with primary prevention for those at risk but have not yet developed signs and symptoms of a neurological condition. The clearest example is stroke prevention. Strong evidence exists for the modifiable cardiovascular risk factors of physical inactivity, poor nutrition, and smoking, such that the American Heart Association in 2018 published a scientific statement calling for routine assessment and promotion of physical activity in health care settings for all adults.[103] Additionally, evidence exists for the power of healthy lifestyle behaviors and subjective well-being to potentially delay onset or prevent development of many neurodegenerative diseases.[104,105] For example, smoking has been identified as a risk factor for the onset of multiple sclerosis in individuals with a genetic predisposition.[106] Therefore screening and advocacy for not smoking and engagement in other healthy lifestyle behaviors across the dimensions of wellness may delay the onset of multiple sclerosis. Inadequate physical activity has been linked to dementia in Alzheimer disease and Parkinson disease.[104,105] Thus screening and advocacy for meeting minimum health guidelines for physical activity (150 minutes of moderate intensity physical activity or 75 minutes of intense physical activity a week)[107] may reduce overall disease incidence. While greater research is needed, the time is now for routine screening and advocacy for healthy lifestyle behaviors[82,83,97] by physical and occupational therapists within individual scope of practice.

In addition to primary prevention, healthy lifestyle behaviors including adequate physical activity, sleep, nutrition, stress management,

and not smoking may modulate and slow disease progression in neurodegenerative disorders and prevent secondary and tertiary complications of neurological injury such as stroke or spinal cord injury. Growing literature supports the benefits of exercise to enhance cardiorespiratory fitness, muscle strength, and cognition, and reduce depression in the general population[108] and in those poststroke, with spinal cord injury, and those living with multiple sclerosis, Parkinson disease, and Huntington disease.[109] Physical activity and exercise at the right dose has the potential to be neuroprotective and neuromodulatory, inducing synaptogenesis, neurogenesis, and neurotransmitter synthesis.[109–111] Determining and achieving the proper dose of lifestyle physical activity and structured exercise for individuals living with neurological conditions can be difficult. Broad guidelines include the general population physical activity health recommendations inclusive of persons with disabilities,[107] although individual disease-specific populations may differ and more research is needed. For example, for those individuals living with mild to moderate multiple sclerosis, the minimum physical activity guidelines set to demonstrate improvement in aerobic capacity and muscular strength are moderate intensity aerobic physical activity two times per week for a total of 60 minutes and moderate strength training of major muscle groups two times per week.[112] Physical activity at this level may additionally induce improvements in mobility, fatigue, and health-related quality of life, although research is insufficient to support a full claim of these benefits at this time.[112]

The physical or occupational therapist who strives for a health-focused wellness approach in neurorehabilitation must remember to look fully within and also to look beyond the physical domain to address the whole person. Within the physical domain, this includes ensuring sedentary behavior and lifestyle physical activity are addressed in addition to structured exercise during therapy encounters. Evidence demonstrates sedentarism independent of meeting the minimum guidelines of 150 minutes of aerobic activity is associated with poorer health outcomes.[113] Beyond the physical domain, a health-focused wellness approach includes addressing at minimum the emotional and psychological domains through screening assessment of stress and mental health. Additional considerations in line with the social-ecological and ICF frameworks could include the role of social support in the patient's path to recovery, identifying intellectually stimulating activities in the absence of adequate intellectual pursuits in the patient's life, supporting the patient to reframe a pessimistic attitude to a more optimistic attitude, and encouraging the patient to find meaning and purpose in life when appropriate. Incorporating perceptual and behavioral standardized measures of wellness into the systems review and examination will provide the therapist with strong evidence for decision making and tracking of outcomes and impact. As the evidence continues to grow for the system-wide benefits, including the potential neuromodulator benefits, of healthy lifestyle behaviors[114,115] and subjective well-being in various neurological conditions, routine screening and intervention will hopefully become the standard of practice. The reader is referred to Table 33.5 discussed previously for details on assessment and intervention recommendations.

For successful implementation of a health-focused wellness approach, anticipating and addressing barriers is needed. Many barriers to habitual engagement in healthy behaviors exist. In the neurological population these barriers to physical activity commonly fall across the ICF domains from impairments in body structure and function (fatigue, presence of secondary conditions) to participation restrictions (embarrassment) and to barriers in environmental and personal contextual features (lack of access to accessible equipment and facilities and decreased self-efficacy).[116] Based on a recent review of qualitative studies,[117] the most commonly reported impairments and activity and participation restriction barriers include fluctuating fatigue, lack of walking balance, muscle weakness, pain, stiffness, bladder and bowel problems, depression, thermoregulation, and fear of injury. The most common environmental barriers are accessibility, costs, transport, and insufficient information and knowledge from health professionals. The most frequent personal barriers reported are lack of motivation, feelings of self-consciousness and embarrassment in public, anxiety, frustration, and anger. Barriers may also include impaired cognition and communication skills, which can make patient-therapist interactions difficult. On the opposing end, facilitators, or motivators, commonly reported in this diverse population include maintaining independence, function, and weight; the prevention of secondary conditions; having sufficient social support; goal setting; achieving enjoyment, feeling good, and feeling "normal,"; motivation and optimism, redefining self, and escapism from everyday boundaries.[117] While it is important for the therapist to understand common barriers and facilitators to guide overall clinical reasoning and the promotion of health and wellness at a population health level, it is also crucial for the therapist to uncover and support the individual in reducing barriers and enhancing facilitators at the individual level. This approach requires strong communication and time management skills by the therapist and is where training in motivational interviewing and health coaching can be very valuable tools in the neurorehabilitation therapist's toolbox.

CONCLUSION

Individuals living with a neurological injury or disease are at increased risk for having lower levels of perceived wellness, health-related quality of life,[7] and physical activity, as well as a greater number and severity of barriers to wellness. Thus there is strong need for a wellness approach in neurorehabilitation. A wellness approach in neurorehabilitation should include the minimum skills set recommended by the APTA, the assessment of the seven lifestyle behavioral competencies recommended by Dean, education on the interrelationship between lifestyle behaviors and rehabilitation and wellness goals, direct evidence-based theory-driven interventions within scope of practice, and referral to qualified and accessible providers as appropriate to ensure a comprehensive whole person approach. Utilizing Lein's health-focused physical therapy model may assist the neurorehabilitation therapist in structuring his or her wellness approach to incorporate these components into practice. A wellness approach in neurorehabilitation may ultimately resemble the dental model with annual or biannual evaluations and intermittent episodes of care to best help the individual meet his or her health and wellness needs. This approach may include assisting the patient in the transition to community-based programs and providing skilled maintenance therapy services as appropriate. Individuals living with a chronic neurological condition can be well. Rehabilitation therapists, for both the benefit of the individual and for society, need to make a wellness approach standard practice.

CASE STUDY 33.1 Exploring Exercise and Physical Activity Motivation After Stroke: Case Script and Video Example

The patient is a 70-year-old post-stroke (cerebrovascular accident [CVA]) woman who lives with her husband, and both are retired from working, she as a librarian. The patient is very sedentary, preferring to sit and read during the day, and the physical therapist has been encouraging her to be more physically active and to do her home exercise program regularly. Recognizing that the patient lacks motivation to perform her home exercise program or to be physically active, the physical therapist decides to use health coaching communication strategies to explore the patient's motivation. The initial conversation may follow the outline below.

PT: Mrs. X, would it be okay if we talked about your physical activity?

Mrs. X: Yes, I think so.

PT: I would like to learn about another time in your life when you were physically active.

Mrs. X: I've never been physically active, always very sedentary.

PT: So, you don't really have any previous positive experiences with physical activity. How important is it right now for you to be more physically active on a scale from 1 (not important at all) to 10 (the most important thing in the world right now)?

Mrs. X: I would say a 6.

PT: Why didn't you answer a 2 or 3?

Mrs. X: Because I know it's important and I think it would make me feel better and sleep better if I did it.

PT: So, you understand the value of being physically active and you think it could enhance your sleep and make you feel better. What would it take for physical activity to be an 8 or 9 in importance?

Mrs. X: I would have to have a reminder to do it regularly, and I would have to put my reading away.

PT: So, you think you would be more physically active if you had something to remind you, how so?

Mrs. X: Yes, I just get carried away reading a book, and I don't think about it.

PT: Okay, we can talk about setting a reminder. How confident are you that you could be physically active at home on the same scale, 1 to 10?

Mrs. X: I think about a 4.

PT: Why didn't you answer a 1 or 2?

Mrs. X: Because I do the exercise when I'm in physical therapy and I know how to do it. Also, I can walk with my husband who would help me.

PT: You have exercises you can do at home, and you can go walking with your husband. What would it take to be a 7 in confidence?

Mrs. X: I think my health would have to depend on it or require me to be physically active. I can do the things I need to do right now, and there is nothing I can't really do with a little help.

PT: Let me see if I can summarize what I've learned so far from our conversation. You have never really been physically active, so it's not an automatic behavior you have like brushing your teeth. You understand and can articulate why it's important for you to be physically active, but you don't think about being active during the day. You see benefits from being physically active, and you think it would be helpful to have a reminder to be physically active, and you know how to do your exercises, and you can walk with your husband. Is all of this information accurate?

Mrs. X: Yes.

PT: What would you think about setting a goal to set a reminder to do your exercises to find out if this approach will work for you?

Mrs. X: I think that would be okay.

PT: What kind of reminder do you have in mind?

Mrs. X: I could ask my husband to remind me.

PT: That's one option, but what if he forgets or isn't around on that day? Can you think of another reminder that would not depend on your husband or another person?

Mrs. X: I could set an alarm on my iPad, which is usually with me because I read on it.

PT: Great idea. What time of day would you like to do some exercise?

CASE STUDY 33.1 Exploring Exercise and Physical Activity Motivation After Stroke: Case Script and Video Example—cont'd

Mrs. X: How about 2:30? That's a time when we are usually sitting around reading, and it would be good to get up and move around in the middle of the afternoon.

PT: Sounds reasonable. Let's say the goal will be to set an alarm on your iPad for 2:30 on Tuesday and Thursday this week to get up and exercise. How long do you want to exercise on those days?

Mrs. X: We can start with 15 minutes I guess.

PT: Okay, the goal will read, "I will set an alarm on my iPad to go off at 2:30 on Tuesday and Thursday, and I will get up and exercise for 15 minutes each time." Can you repeat the goal back to me to make sure you've got it?

Mrs. X: Yes, I will set an alarm on my iPad to go off at 2:30 on Tuesday and Thursday, and I will do 15 minutes of exercise each day.

PT: You've got it. How confident are you on a scale of 1 to 10 that you will accomplish this goal?

Mrs. X: I would say a 5.

PT: What's in the way of feeling like a 7 or 8 in confidence?

Mrs. X: Well, I might just ignore the alarm when it goes off, especially if the book I'm reading is really interesting.

PT: How can we change the goal to make you more confident that you can achieve it?

Mrs. X: I could find out if I can download a program that would turn off my iPad so I would have to stop reading and get up so I wouldn't have the option of ignoring it and continuing to read.

PT: How does that plan sound to you?

Mrs. X: I think that would be a good idea.

PT: Okay, let's write two goals. The second goal can be "I will download an app that disables my iPad at the time I set it." When can you work on finding the app?

Mrs. X: I can do that tonight.

PT: Let's revise the goal to read, "I will download an app tonight that I can set to alarm and disable my iPad for 15 minutes." How confident are you that you'll accomplish this goal?

Mrs. X: I'm an 8/10.

PT: Now, how confident are you that you'll get up and exercise for 15 minutes when the alarm goes off?

Mrs. X: I'm a 7.

PT: Sounds like you have realistic but challenging goals to work on this week. I'm confident that you will learn something from this approach.

Questions to Assess Learning

1. What was the therapist attempting to elicit by asking the question, "Why isn't your importance level a lower number?"
2. What was the therapist attempting to elicit by asking the question, "What would it take for your level of importance to be a higher number?"
3. Identify examples of motivational interviewing skills the therapist used in this role play.
4. What stage of change was the patient in for physical activity at the beginning of the conversation?
5. What stage of change was the patient in for physical activity at the end of the conversation? Answer: Action, based on the fact that she set an action-oriented goal.
6. How could the therapist debrief the patient's experience with her goals when the patient returns to therapy for the next visit?

Answers to Case Study 33.1

1. This question elicits the patient to describe the benefits she sees from physical activity. When the patient describes the benefits (rather than the therapist), it builds motivation, autonomy, and self-efficacy.
2. This question elicits the barriers that may be in the way of performing the behavior. If the patient describes barriers, a discussion about how to overcome the barriers can ensue, which will move the patient to a higher stage of change and build self-efficacy and autonomy.
3. Open-ended questions: What kind of reminder do you have in mind? How can we change the goal to make you more confident that you can achieve it? Affirm and support the patient: Sounds like you have realistic but challenging goals to work on this week. I'm confident that you will learn something from this approach. Reflective listening: So, you understand the value of being physically active, and you think it could enhance your sleep and make you feel better. Summarize: Let me see if I can summarize what I've learned so far from our conversation. You have never really been physically active, so it's not an automatic behavior you have like brushing your teeth. You understand and can articulate why it's important for you to be physically active, but you don't think about being active during the day. You see benefits from being

physically active, and you think it would be helpful to have a reminder to be physically active, and you know how to do your exercises, and you can walk with your husband. Is all of this information accurate?

4. Probably contemplation based on the fact that she was a 6/10 in importance to change and that her barriers and benefits were competing.
5. Action, based on the fact that she set an action-oriented goal.
6. The therapist should start by asking the patient if it would be okay to debrief about her experience with the goals. If the patient replies affirmatively, the therapist can ask about one of the goals by stating "Which goal would you like to discuss first?" Once the patient selects the goal to discuss, the therapist can start by asking, "Tell me about your overall positive experience with this goal." Soliciting the positive experience helps build self-efficacy, autonomy, and learning. The therapist can also ask the patient to describe what she learned from the goal and what was her best experience with the goal. Finally, the therapist can ask the patient to assess her level of success with the goal on a 1–100 scale (e.g., 75%). This method of debriefing can be applied to assess all of the patient's goals and is an important aspect of health coaching to build autonomy and self-efficacy.

CASE STUDY 33.2 Health Promotion and Wellness Strategies Applied to Neurorehabilitation in Multiple Sclerosis

The patient is a 32-year-old woman living with multiple sclerosis who is in an outpatient neurorehabilitation setting recovering from an exacerbation of her multiple sclerosis 3 weeks ago.

History and Interview

During the initial examination, the patient expresses despair and worry over her ability to care for her two small children at home, now that she needs a cane to walk and her left hand is weak. She reports prior to the exacerbation she was

barely managing and now this is just too much. The therapist notes the patient has checked difficulty sleeping and changes in her diet on the initial intake form. She reports she does not smoke, nor does she have a history of smoking.

Review of Systems

During her review of symptoms, the therapist explores her mental health asking several open-ended questions about her prior and current levels of stress. The therapist screens for depression using the 2-item depression screen for multiple

Continued

CASE STUDY 33.2   Health Promotion and Wellness Strategies Applied to Neurorehabilitation in Multiple Sclerosis—cont'd

sclerosis[118]; it is positive. The therapist also follows up on the intake form to explore current and past sleep habits regarding sleep quantity and quality as well as dietary habits and any changes in weight. The therapist explores the patient's values and how they fit or do not fit with her current behaviors and goals.

Systems Review and Tests and Measures

During the systems review as part of the therapist's standard examination, the therapist records heart rate, blood pressure, respiration, and weight. The therapist utilizes several standardized outcome measures to assess movement and abilities within reported limited activities and participation. This information guides targeted collection of tests and measures of hypothesized underlying impairments in body structure and function.

Evaluation, Diagnosis, Prognosis, Intervention

At the end of the examination, the therapist engages in shared decision making with the patient on mutual realistic goals using the goal attainment scale.[119] The therapist provides brief counsel to the patient on the role of mental health, sleep, and nutrition in her rehabilitation recovery and her long-term well-being. The therapist inquires into the patient's social support network and asks if the patient's referring physician is aware of her mood, perceived stress levels, and changes in weight. The patient reports her physician is aware. Her physician has recommended counseling, but the patient is reluctant to go because she doesn't want to appear weak. The therapist expresses empathy and encourages the patient to consider her values and goals, what it will take to accomplish them, and how her psychological and emotional health will either facilitate or be a barrier to her goals. The therapist expresses that the role of rehabilitation is to maximize her abilities as a whole person in order to achieve her movement-based wellness goals for engagement in

meaningful activities and life roles. The session ends with a preliminary action plan that includes establishing a sleep schedule to help with energy management and stress reduction, increasing lifestyle physical activity by 10 min each day over the next week while self-monitoring and adjusting for her daily fatigue levels, and following up with her physician regarding the counseling recommendation. They agree to discuss adding structured exercises at her next therapy session.

Note: The therapist-patient discussion on goals, values clarification, and action planning occurs while the patient is engaging in a submaximal exercise test on a recumbent elliptical. The therapist is providing skilled intervention through assessment and monitoring of physical activity and cardiopulmonary response and providing education.

Questions to Assess Learning:

1. To incorporate a health-focused wellness approach to practice, how did the therapist incorporate screening and assessment of the five behavioral domains of healthy lifestyle behaviors identified in Table 33.5?
2. How might the therapist's health-focused wellness approach maximize the patient's rehabilitation prognosis to achieve personal goals? Hint: There are many right answers.
3. Provide two examples of how the therapist attempted to develop a strong therapist-patient alliance.
4. Did the therapist utilize a standardized perceptual measure of wellness? If so, what was it and when was it utilized? If not, what tool could have been used and when would be the best time to do so?
5. Is this patient appropriate for application of the "dental model" of rehabilitation? Why or why not?

Answers to Case Study 33.2

1. An intake form was used for an initial screening on sleep, nutrition, and smoking. Stress was noted in the interview and the therapist followed up with open-ended questions related to stress and mental health and utilized the 2-item depression screening tool. Physical activity was assessed through standardized outcomes of movement and abilities, and a submaximal exercise test.
2. Option one: By addressing the whole person the therapist enhances the therapist-patient alliance, which has been shown to enhance rehabilitation outcomes. Option two: Through screening and identification of several at-risk lifestyle behaviors including a positive screen for depression, the therapist is able to develop a comprehensive plan that will enhance the patient's physical and mental potential and reduce barriers to goal achievement and wellness. For example, depression is a significant barrier to rehabilitation participation and is strongly linked to fatigue in multiple sclerosis. Helping the patient connect and utilize appropriate resources to help her manage her symptoms of depression will enhance the patient's potential to engage in rehabilitation for her exacerbation and her sense of well-being during and after discharge.

3. Examples may include: One, the therapist expressed *empathy* with the patient's worry of appearing weak if she sees a counselor. Two, the therapist took time to explore the *patient's values*. Three, the therapist engaged in *shared decision making* to develop mutually agreeable goals.
4. No, the therapist did not utilize a standardized perceptual measure of wellness. The therapist could have utilized the Short Form-36 or the Perceived Wellness Survey (see Table 33.4). Either of these tools could have been utilized as part of the initial pre-screening process along with the intake form, or given to the patient at the end of the session to complete prior to her next visit. These options maximize time management for both the patient and therapist and ensure a comprehensive wellness approach.
5. This patient is appropriate for several reasons. One, she presents with a chronic progressive neurological condition that will likely result in changes in functionally and across the dimensions of wellness throughout her lifespan. Two, she presents with multiple barriers and challenges across the dimensions of wellness that may require ongoing intermittent services, time, and multiple resources to best meet her needs.

REFERENCES

To enhance this text and add value for the reader, all references are included on the companion Evolve site that accompanies this textbook. This online service will, when available, provide a link for the reader to a Medline abstract for the article cited. There are 119 cited references and other general references for this chapter, with the majority of those articles being evidence-based citations.

34

Human Immunodeficiency Virus Infection: Living With a Chronic Illness*

Kerri Sowers, Mary Lou Galantino, and David M. Kietrys

OBJECTIVES

After reading this chapter the student or therapist will be able to:

1. Understand how the involvement of various systems (immune, integumentary, musculoskeletal, cardiopulmonary, and neurological) may lead to episodic disability and affect function in individuals living with HIV disease.
2. Discuss the neuropathological features of HIV infection and understand potential neurocognitive and neuropsychological alterations that may occur.

3. Incorporate psychoneuroimmunology, pain management, and movement strategies for HIV rehabilitation management.
4. Establish safe exercise parameters in the HIV-positive population.

KEY TERMS

acquired immunodeficiency syndrome (AIDS)
episodic disability
HIV disease

human immunodeficiency virus (HIV)
interprofessional rehabilitation

IDENTIFICATION OF THE CLINICAL PROBLEM

Initially recognized in 1983, human immunodeficiency virus (HIV) infection was one of the leading causes of death among young adults, peaking in 2005.[1] Since then, HIV-related deaths have declined by 48%,[1] emphasizing the metamorphosis of the diagnosis from a death sentence to a chronic medical condition. Even with significant advancements in the medical management of the disease, there continues to be a devastating impact in the developing world, where access to appropriate pharmaceutical intervention and public health initiatives remains limited.[2,3] The course of HIV disease in industrialized nations, including the United States, has changed dramatically as a result of advancements in medications used to treat the disease, as well as increased public awareness and the expansion of public health programs in poverty-stricken areas.

The long-term prognosis for those diagnosed with HIV or with acquired immunodeficiency syndrome (AIDS) has drastically changed in most industrialized countries. In the United States, HIV is no longer found in the 10 leading causes of death for the entire adult population. In fact, there has been a dramatic decline, from 10.2 (1990) to 1.9 (2015), for the age-adjusted death rate per 100,000 population[4]; consider this value in comparison to the number of deaths due to malignant neoplasms (99.0 per 100,000) or heart disease (86.5 per 100,000) in 2015.[4] HIV remains on the list of leading causes of death for those aged 25 to 44 in the United States, although it has dropped to the ninth position.[5] It is no longer found in the top 10 causes of death for other age groups. Globally, there continues to be a slow increase in

the number of people living with HIV (PLHIV); for 2016, this number totaled 36.7 million (30.8 to 42.9 million).[1] The number of new global infections continues to decline, from 3.0 million in 2000 to 1.8 million in 2016.[1] HIV-related deaths have also continued to decline globally, from 1.5 million in 2000 to 1.0 million in 2016.[1] Much of this decline can be contributed to improved global access to antiretroviral therapy (ART); an estimated 685,000 PLHIV received treatment in 2000, as compared with 20.9 million who received treatment in June 2017.[1] With only 53% (39% to 65%) of PLHIV having access to treatment in 2016, it is clear there is still room for improvement.[1]

Most epidemiologists and clinicians attribute improved life expectancy to the impact of highly effective ART and community health education and prevention practices. Implementation of these medications has resulted in a decline in HIV deaths nationally.[6,7] ART regimens have fostered longevity for many, resulting in the evolution of HIV infection into a chronic disease. Individuals previously disabled by the disease currently have the potential to return to work and functional activities and often can expect to live a normal life expectancy. However, PLHIV may experience disability that is episodic in nature, characterized by periods of wellness and illness.[8,9] Qualitative research found four phenotypes of episodic disability over time: decreasing, increasing, stable, or significant fluctuations.[8,9] Understanding a person's episodic trajectory may help to tailor interventions to promote stability, mitigate an upward trajectory of increasing disability, and increase the time between episodes of illness.[10] Therefore HIV disease, related comorbidities, and the side effects of medications used to treat the disease have a great impact on rehabilitative medicine because of the multisystem involvement. The advancements in medications that have led to increased life

---

*Videos for this chapter are available at studentconsult.com.

expectancies and improved functional capabilities have also led to a greater demand for rehabilitative services.

ART has slowed and prevented the progression from HIV infection to AIDS and from AIDS to death.[11] In communities with access to antiretroviral medications, the incidence of perinatally acquired AIDS has declined significantly because of administration of ART during pregnancy.[12] Perinatal transmission of the virus in developing nations continues to be a concern, despite a 47% decline since 2010.[1]

The clinical and pathological information about this disease is constantly increasing. Certainly, our understanding of the disease process and advances in drug regimens will change between the writing and the publication of this book. Changes in terminology reflect this evolution of clinical knowledge. The definitions used throughout this chapter reflect current usage.

The virus thought to be responsible for the transmission of HIV was first identified in 1983; it was named *human immunodeficiency virus* in 1986 at the International Conference on AIDS in Paris. A second virus, HIV-2, was identified soon after in western Africa, and the original strain was renamed HIV-1. Infection caused by HIV-2, less widely distributed, has since been established in Europe and in South, Central, and North America. Both HIV-1 and HIV-2 have resulted in AIDS, but evidence suggests that HIV-2 may be less virulent than HIV-1. In addition to these subtypes, several strains or mutated forms of HIV-1 have been identified. Different strains reflect variations in cellular affinities and resistance to medications. The context of discussion, for this chapter, will be regarding the HIV-1 strain, herein discussed as *HIV*. HIV infection is identified via a positive HIV antibody screening test (rapid diagnostic test [RDT] or enzyme immunoassay [EIA]) and confirmation with a supplemental HIV antibody test (Western blot), and/or a positive result from an HIV virological test (nucleic acid detection test, p24 antigen test, or viral culture).

The Centers for Disease Control and Prevention (CDC) recognizes three stages of HIV infection.[13] Stage 1 represents acute HIV infection. This stage is characterized by a high viral load, where acutely infected individuals are highly contagious. Some individuals may notice flulike symptoms 2 to 4 weeks following the initial infection, part of the body's natural response to an infection. Stage 2 represents a period of clinical latency and is referred to as the asymptomatic stage. HIV remains active, but there is a reduced viral load as compared with the spike after initial infection. The goal of ART during this period is to reduce the viral load to nondetectable levels. Those who do not have access to ART may eventually begin to experience symptoms and will eventually progress to stage 3, representing advanced HIV disease (AIDS). This stage is when viral replication leads to increasingly high viral loads. It is recognized when the CD4 count is less than 200 cells/µL, and/or when opportunistic illnesses are present, and/or when there is evidence of HIV-related wasting or dementia. The entire spectrum of illness from initial diagnosis to AIDS can be covered by the term *HIV disease*. In addition, the terms *acute HIV infection, asymptomatic HIV disease, symptomatic HIV disease,* and *advanced HIV disease (AIDS)* are used throughout this chapter. In general, acute HIV infection corresponds with stage 1, asymptomatic HIV disease (or symptomatic HIV disease but not yet classified as AIDS) with stage 2, and advanced HIV disease (AIDS) with stage 3. Table 34.1 presents the various modifiers of quality of life (QOL) throughout the various stages of HIV disease.

Epidemiology

It is estimated that more than 36.7 million people[1] are infected with HIV globally. In the United States the CDC estimated that 1,122,900 adults and adolescents were living with HIV at the end of 2015.[14] Because of complex social and economic factors, African Americans and Hispanics/Latinos are disproportionally affected, with approximately 44% of HIV diagnoses in 2016 being African American and 25% being Hispanic/Latino.[14] There is a higher geographical distribution of HIV diagnosis in US southern states, with 16.8 per 100,000 people in 2016.[14] Alarmingly, it is estimated that approximately 51% of young individuals (aged 13 to 24) in the United States infected with HIV are unaware of the infection.[14]

TABLE 34.1	Quality-of-Life Issues for Human Immunodeficiency Virus Disease Stages		
Stage	**Moderators of Quality of Life**		**General Quality-of-Life Issues**
Stage 1 Acute HIV Infection	**Appraisals** Anticipatory grieving, catastrophizing, and other cognitive distortions Changed expectations of future Identity and self-esteem issues	**Coping** Dealing with present and future uncertainties At risk for denial, disengagement, substance abuse, risky sex, suicide Issues of eliciting social support	**Emotional Functioning** Anxiety, anger, often increasing at diagnosis and diminishing and recycling as individual confronts realities of living with HIV disease **Role Functioning** Often able to work Possible decrements in job mobility and career opportunities Job loss **Social Functioning** Fear, isolation, issues of trust in relationships Stigmatization Changes in social support networks because of deaths Relationship and sexual changes Isolation, withdrawal **Physical Functioning** Normal but may be altered because of depression or anxiety May have hypervigilance regarding all physical symptoms **Spiritual Functioning** Opportunity to direct attention inward, thus yielding to contemplation of life's meaning, reassessment of spiritual and existential issues

TABLE 34.1 Quality-of-Life Issues for Human Immunodeficiency Virus Disease Stages—cont'd

Stage	Moderators of Quality of Life		General Quality-of-Life Issues
Stage 2 Clinical Latency	**Appraisals** Anticipatory grieving, catastrophizing, and other cognitive distortions Changed expectations of future Identity and self-esteem issues related to threats to occupational and functional abilities	**Coping** Dealing with present and future uncertainties At risk for denial, disengagement, substance abuse, and risky sex	**Emotional Functioning** Anxiety, anger, often increasing on emergence of symptoms and then fluctuating with challenges and threats to present and future functioning **Role Functioning** Often able to work May take on new roles as part of HIV support network **Social Functioning** Changes in social support networks resulting from deaths, isolation, withdrawal, relationship and sexual changes, and stigmatization **Physical Functioning** May have reduced energy levels Moderate symptomatology Possible cognitive deficits Pain **Spiritual Functioning** Anticipatory grieving, sense of relatedness to something greater than the self, unavoidable confrontation with one's own mortality
Stage 3 Advanced HIV	**Appraisals** Facing chronic illness and death Grieving about current and anticipated losses; catastrophizing and other cognitive distortions Reassessment of spiritual and existential issues	**Coping** Coping strategies may be overwhelmed in dealing with current difficulties such as financial losses, medical costs, treatment and side effects, housing May lose some traditional coping strategies such as recreational outlets	**Emotional Functioning** Anxiety and anger may cycle according to fluctuations in disease status and appraisals Relief from uncertainty **Role Functioning** Diminished capacity for work Role changes—often need care instead of being a caretaker **Social Functioning** May have diminished social networks because of lack of mobility, illness, and deaths among friends **Physical Functioning** Self-care difficulties Fatigue Wasting Much time spent in medical care Debilitation from infection and treatments Possible cognitive deficits **Spiritual Functioning** Essential worth is to provide a framework from which to pose and seek responses to metaphysical questions generated by presence of life-threatening disease Integration and transcending of biological and psychosocial nature, which gives access to nonphysical realms as prophecy, love, artistic inspiration, completion, and healing actions

HIV, Human immunodeficiency virus.

In 2017 the World Health Organization (WHO) estimated that 940,000 people died from HIV-related causes globally.[15] Worldwide, in 2017, of the 36.9 million people (all ages) living with HIV, 35.1 million are adults, 18.2 million are women, and 1.8 million are children (<15 years).[16] New HIV infections in 2017 totaled 1.8 million, with 1.6 million in adults and 180,000 in children (<15 years).[16] Global AIDS deaths have continued to decline, totaling 940,000 in 2017; adult deaths were 830,000, whereas children (<15 years) totaled 110,000.[16] For the United States, in 2015, 6465 people died from HIV disease, with 53% living in the southern United States.[17] For 2016, in the United States, there were 39,782 new infections (with approximately

50% in the southern states); 26,570 were gay and bisexual men, 9578 were heterosexuals, and 3425 were individuals who inject drugs.[14] Of those new infections, 14,740 were for ages 20 to 29, 9943 for ages 30 to 39, 6490 for ages 40 to 49, 4882 for ages 50 to 59, 1930 for ages 60 and older, and 1675 for ages 13 to 19.[14]

Normal Immunity

The immune system is complex and dynamic, comprising a multitude of components and subsystems, all of which interact continuously. The normal immune system has two main components, or lines of defense, against illness (Fig. 34.1). The first is the innate, or inborn, immune

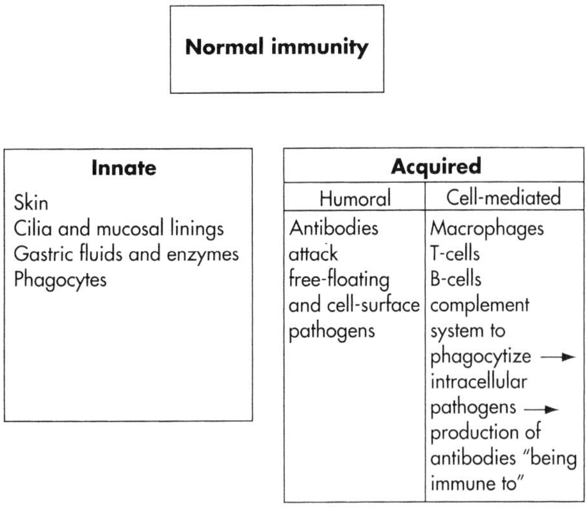

Normal immunity

Innate
Skin
Cilia and mucosal linings
Gastric fluids and enzymes
Phagocytes

Acquired	
Humoral	Cell-mediated
Antibodies attack free-floating and cell-surface pathogens	Macrophages T-cells B-cells complement system to phagocytize → intracellular pathogens → production of antibodies "being immune to"

Fig. 34.1 Main components of immunity.

system, which includes aspects such as the skin, the cilia and mucosal linings of the respiratory and digestive systems, the gastric fluids and enzymes of the stomach, natural killer cells, phagocyte cells, and the complement system. This innate component of the immune system keeps pathogens out of the body by creating barriers against them, by ejecting them, or by enveloping them and eliminating them. The second, the acquired component of the immune system, develops defenses against specific pathogens; it begins in utero and continues throughout life. It is the acquired (or antibody-based) immunity that is most pertinent to understanding HIV infection and its progression.

Acquired Immunity

Acquired immunity is divided into humoral and cell-mediated responses. Humoral immunity depends on the production of antibodies. This response is effective for disposing of free-floating or cell-surface pathogens. The cell-mediated response is required to destroy infected cells, those with intracellular pathogens. Cell-mediated immunity is essential for destroying pathogens responsible for the opportunistic infections and neoplasms that are associated with HIV infection.[18,19]

For the study of HIV pathology, it is important to consider three types of immune system cells: macrophages, T-lymphocytes (T-cells), and B-lymphocytes (B-cells). Macrophages originate in the bone marrow and then migrate to the organs in the lymphatic system. Macrophages recognize and then phagocytize antigens (substances deemed foreign to the body). All but a fragment of the antigen is digested by the macrophage. This remaining fragment protrudes from the cellular surface, where it is then recognized by T- and B-cells, allowing those cells to develop an appropriate immune response.[20]

Both types of lymphocytes (T- and B-cells) originate in the bone marrow. Their differentiation into T- and B-cells depends on where they develop immunocompetence. Immunocompetence is the ability of the immune system to mobilize in response to an antigen; it can be weakened secondary to age-related changes, radiation therapy, chemotherapy, or viral infections. T-cells migrate to the thymus to develop this ability, whereas B-cells develop it before leaving the bone marrow. T-cells travel to lymph nodes, the spleen, and connective tissues, where they wait to phagocytize the antigens in the manner previously described. B-cells function in the same way against free-floating blood-borne pathogens.[20]

There are at least eight types of T-cells with various functions. Two relevant types when considering HIV infection are helper T-cells

(CD4) and suppressor T-cells (CD8). The CD4 cells enhance the immune response, whereas CD8 cells regulate the immune response. HIV primarily attacks these two types of T-cells, impairing the body's immune response. On recognition of an antigen, CD4 cells chemically stimulate production and activation of other lymphocytes to destroy the foreign material. When the action of the T- and B-cells elicits a sufficient immune response, the CD8 cells will halt the action, thus preventing the destruction of normal (uninfected) cells. HIV causes the destruction of the CD4 cells. Declining CD4 cell counts occur in untreated disease; in healthy (uninfected) individuals, CD4 counts should be 500 to 1600 cells/μL. However, because T-cell counts fluctuate somewhat under normal circumstances, the ratio of CD4 to CD8 cells is considered a valuable laboratory value in tracking the progression of the disease (a normal ratio is approximately 2.0, whereas a ratio close to 1.0 is associated with advanced HIV infection).

In the process of identifying and destroying antigens, the normal acquired immune system retains a memory of the antigen. This allows the immune system to respond more rapidly and effectively to the pathogen if it is reintroduced into the body. Herein lies the pertinence of vaccination and the phenomenon of being immune to an illness.[20]

PATHOGENESIS OF HUMAN IMMUNODEFICIENCY VIRUS DISEASE

HIV belongs to a class of viruses known as *retroviruses,* which carry their genetic material in the form of ribonucleic acid (RNA) rather than deoxyribonucleic acid (DNA). HIV primarily infects the mononuclear cells, especially CD4 and macrophages, but B-cells are also infected.[21] HIV binds to the receptor sites on the surface of the CD4 lymphocytes, eventually fusing with and then entering the cells. Reverse transcriptase released from the HIV allows a DNA copy of the virus to be made within the host cell, which then becomes integrated into the host cell genome. Other enzymes, such as integrase and protease, turn the lymphocyte into a "virus factory," and replicated virions bud out of the cell to infect others.

Within days of acute HIV infection, lymph nodes become sites of rampant viral replication, and viral loads in the blood are high. During the stage of acute HIV infection, the individual may remain asymptomatic or may experience nonspecific and self-limited flulike symptoms including fever, diarrhea, myalgias, and fatigue; these symptoms may last for a period of 2 to 12 weeks. In the weeks after an acute infection, the body gradually produces an antibody response. The point at which antibodies can be detected with a blood test is known as *seroconversion.* Typically, seroconversion occurs within 3 to 4 weeks after the time of infection, but it can take as long as 12 months. Thus there is a period, after HIV infection, when the outcome of an HIV antibody test will present as negative, due to the delay in seroconversion. Tests for viral load can detect HIV in the bloodstream at time points earlier than antibody tests. It is important to remember that antibody testing can be unreliable in individuals with primary or secondary immunodeficiency disease.

In stage 2 of HIV disease, individuals will typically have a positive antibody test result. This stage of clinical latency may last from 1 to 20 years and is often dependent on the compliance with ART treatment. Although generally asymptomatic, individuals in this stage may express periods of generalized lymphadenopathy. Laboratory tests may reveal slowly declining immune dysfunction, as evidenced by an abnormally low CD4 cell count and an abnormal CD4/CD8 ratio. The viral load is typically at a "set point" during most of the asymptomatic stage of HIV disease. This set point is typically much lower than the viral load occurring during the period of acute infection.

In an untreated individual, the viral load will escalate as the disease progresses. In an individual successfully treated with ART, the goal is to achieve an undetectable viral load.

In an individual who is not treated with ART, the disease will progress over time. If the CD4 cell count drops to less than 200 cells/μL, and/or an opportunistic infection occurs, and/or an individual presents with HIV-related wasting or dementia, the individual has entered stage 3, advanced HIV disease (AIDS). It is possible for patients in this stage to demonstrate remarkable recovery in terms of both laboratory values and function with an appropriate ART regimen. Individuals who do not have access to ART or individuals in whom ART has failed will eventually die because of the effects of opportunistic infections that inevitably occur.

In patients with advanced HIV disease (stage 3), there may be an array of symptoms such as weight loss, weight gain, fatigue, night sweats, fever, thrush, yeast infections, prolonged recovery from other illnesses, or neurological complications. Increased rates of osteoporosis, chronic liver disease, and, in particular, cardiovascular disease (CVD) have been reported among PLHIV. With the aging HIV-infected population, the burden of these comorbid illnesses may continue to accrue over time.[22] Due to the changing nature of HIV infection to a chronic medical condition, individuals are developing a plethora of comorbid conditions and symptoms, even with the progression to advanced HIV disease (stage 3), that present new challenges in treatment and rehabilitation.

MEDICAL MANAGEMENT

CD4 Cell Counts

Medical management of HIV infection is most often guided by the CD4 cell count and viral load. For the healthy HIV-negative adult, the average CD4 cell count may fluctuate between 500 and 1600 cells/μL.[23] Typically, ART is initiated soon after an individual learns that they are HIV-positive; ideally, this is before there is a detrimental decline in CD4 cells.

Exercise, stress, seasons of the year, serum cortisol level, and the presence of acute or chronic illness and infection have all been reported to affect CD4 cell counts.[24,25] The initial CD4 count should be confirmed by repeat testing, and caution should be exercised to avoid overinterpretation of small changes in CD4 test results. The overall trend of CD4 counts is more significant than any single value. In addition to CD4 cell counts, CD4/CD8 ratios are used to evaluate the status of the immune system. In 2012 the Department of Health and Human Services and the WHO began recommending that ART be initiated for HIV-positive individuals, regardless of the CD4 count.[26] In an individual who has not been successfully treated with ART, a CD4 cell count of 200 cells/μL marks a critical point during HIV infection, often indicating that the stage of advanced HIV disease, or AIDS, has been reached. Serious opportunistic infections are likely to occur once this level of immune depletion has been attained in an individual who has not been successfully treated with ART.[27–29] Table 34.2 is a summary of common ARTs. A complete listing of pharmacological interventions to combat the opportunistic infections associated with HIV infection are beyond the scope of this chapter.

Viral Load Measurement

Testing for HIV in plasma by measuring viral RNA (copies of HIV per milliliter) has become a standard component of the management of HIV infected patients. In 2013 the WHO began recommending viral load testing as the preferred method for diagnosing and confirming ART treatment failure.[26] There are important prognostic implications for viral load in persons with HIV disease.[30] In patients with higher viral loads, disease progression is more rapid, both immunologically, in terms of the rate of CD4 cell count decline, and clinically, in terms of development of AIDS-defining illness. In addition, the plasma levels in HIV-positive pregnant women directly correlate with the risk of perinatal transmission.[31] Viral load is an important useful marker for judging the effectiveness of various antiretroviral drug interventions.[32,33] The guidelines established by the WHO recommend routine viral load monitoring at 6 and 12 months, then every 12 months after if the HIV-positive individual is stable on ART.[26] The goal of ART is to have an undetectable viral load in the bloodstream.

The WHO has concerns about the increase in HIV drug resistance, both pretreatment drug resistance and developed resistance to first-line ART.[34] There are several assays available for testing HIV for resistance to antiretroviral agents. Genotype or phenotype testing is used to determine whether the virus has mutated. The results of genotype or phenotype testing provide important information about resistance to specific antiretroviral drugs. If a mutant form is resistant to an antiretroviral drug, the ART regimen may be altered so that the potential for viral suppression is maximized. Changes in the drug combinations used for ART to respond to viral resistance are referred to as *salvage therapy*. Like genotypic testing, phenotypic testing may not detect small subpopulations of resistant HIV.[35]

Until a functional cure and/or vaccine is discovered, advances will continue to be made in ART. The primary goal of ART is to achieve prolonged suppression of HIV replication.[36,37] At this time, there are five classes of ART drugs. Entry inhibitors, such as CCR5 antagonists and fusion inhibitors, work to prevent HIV from successfully entering the cell. The CCR5 antagonist currently in use is maraviro (Selzentry); this drug works by blocking the CCR5 coreceptors on an immune cell surface, thereby preventing HIV from entering the cell.

Other classes of drugs work within the cell by interfering with one of three enzymes that are involved with the replication process: reverse transcriptase, integrase, and protease. These classes include nucleoside reverse transcriptase inhibitors (NRTIs), nonnucleoside reverse transcriptase inhibitors (NNRTIs), integrase inhibitors (INIs), and protease inhibitors (PIs). In 1987, zidovudine (AZT, brand name: Retrovir), an NRTI, was first approved by the US Food and Drug Administration (FDA). Since that time, several more NRTI drugs have been approved.[38] NNRTIs, such as nevirapine (NVP, brand name: Viramune) and efavirenz (EFV, brand name: Sustiva), also inhibit the reverse transcriptase enzyme, but they are not nucleoside analogs.[39] The NNRTIs bind to the enzymatic binding pocket of the reverse transcriptase gene and block binding by the nucleosides.[39,40] Like reverse transcriptase, integrase is an enzyme that is active in the early stages of the replication process, and INIs can be used to interrupt its function by preventing the integration of the virus in the host cell's DNA.[39] INIs include drugs such as dolutegravir (DTG, brand name: Tivicay) or raltegravir (RAL, brand name: Isentress).[39] Another drug target for anti-HIV agents is the protease enzyme, an enzyme necessary for HIV to replicate.[39] The PI drugs are structurally different from other drugs and include agents such as atazanavir (ATV, brand name: Reyataz), darunavir (DRV, brand name: Prezista), and fosamprenavir (FPV, brand name: Lexiva).[39] Pharmacokinetic enhancers, such as cobicistat (Tybost), are used to increase the effectiveness of another drug included in ART.[39]

Triple combination therapy (three different drugs from at least two different classes) has been the mainstay of ART since 1995. ART may be NNRTI or PI based (e.g., NNRTI and PI drugs are used in combination with an NRTI). The current recommendation from the Department of Health and Human Services, for a treatment-naïve patient, is two NRTIs in combination with a third drug (either an INI, an NNRTI, or a PI with a pharmacokinetic enhancer).[41] Because of the

TABLE 34.2 Human Immunodeficiency Virus Drugs, by Class, Used in Antiretroviral Therapy

Brand Name	Generic Name	Brand Name	Generic Name
Entry Inhibitors		**Protease Inhibitors**	
Fuzeon	enfuvirtide	Aptivus	tipranavir
Selzentry	maraviroc	Crixivan	indinavir
Nucleoside Reverse Transcriptase Inhibitors (NRTIs)		Evotaz	atazanavir + cobicistat
Cimduo	lamivudine + tenofovir + disoproxil	Invirase	saquinavir
Combivir	zidovudine + lamivudine	Kaletra	lopinavir + ritonavir
Descovy	tenofovir alafenamide + emtricitabine	Lexiva	fosamprenavir
Emtriva	emtricitabine	Norvir	ritonavir
Epivir	lamivudine	Prezcobix	darunavir + cobicistat
Epzicom	abacavir + lamivudine	Prezista	darunavir
Retrovir	zidovudine	Reyataz	atazanavir
Trizivir	abacavir + zidovudine + lamivudine	Viracept	nelfinavir
Truvada	tenofovir disoproxil + emtricitabine	**Single Tablet Regimens (Combination ART)**	
Videx EC	didanosine	Atripla	efavirenz + tenofovir disoproxil + emtricitabine
Viread	tenofovir disoproxil	Biktarvy	bictegravir + emtricitabine +tenofovir alafenamide
Zerit	stavudine	Complera	rilpivirine + tenofovir disoproxil + emtricitabine
Ziagen	abacavir	Genvoya	elvitegravir + cobicistat + tenofovir alafenamide + emtricitabine
Nonnucleoside Reverse Transcriptase Inhibitors (NNRTIs)		Juluca	dolutegravir + rilpivirine
Edurant	rilpivirine	Odefsey	rilpivirine + tenofovir + alafenamide + emtricitabine
Intelence	etravirine	Stribild	elvitegravir + cobicistat + tenofovir disoproxil + emtricitabine
Rescriptor	delavirdine	Symfi / Symfi Lo	efavirenz + lamivudine + tenofovir disoproxil
Sustiva	efavirenz	Triumeq	dolutegravir + abacavir + lamivudine
Viramune	nevirapine		
Integrase Inhibitors			
Isentress	raltegravir		
Tivicay	dolutegravir		

Note: Triple combination therapy, the mainstay of antiretroviral therapy (ART), involves three different drugs from at least two different classes.
Single tablet regimens (combination ART) incorporate drugs from two or more different classes.
Tybost (cobicistat) may be used to boost certain drugs used in ART.
Drugs used in ART may cause side effects that range from mild to serious or life threatening.
Side effects range from transient and manageable symptoms such as headache or nausea to severe problems that may affect neurological, musculoskeletal, cardiovascular, gastrointestinal, and/or multiorgan systems.
The US Department of Health and Human Services provides listings of side effects at http://aidsinfo.nih.gov/drugs/.

rapidly evolving nature of ART drugs, the reader is advised to consult with the CDC and WHO for the most current clinical practice guidelines. There has been a gradual evolution of pharmacology that has allowed for multiple drugs to be combined into one pill. This results in a more manageable ART dosing, which is more convenient and encourages improved patient compliance.

Side effects and toxicities are common with drugs used to treat HIV disease. Purported side effects of NRTIs include peripheral neuropathy, myopathy, anemia, gastrointestinal (GI) disturbances, hepatomegaly, and pancreatitis. NNRTIs may cause rash, liver dysfunction, cognitive problems, and lactic acidosis. PIs may cause lipodystrophy, peripheral neuropathy, GI intolerance, hyperlipidemia, hyperglycemia, and liver toxicity. This list of side effects is cursory, and the full impact of these and other HIV drugs on the various systems of the body is a

continually emerging area. Occasionally an individual's ART regimen is modified to mitigate the side effects that may occur with specific drugs.

Although ART can reduce serum viral loads to undetectable levels, it is not a cure because HIV continues to exist within the lymphoid tissue and the central nervous system (CNS).[42] Another challenge with ART is resistance to one drug in a class of agents, which may induce partial or complete resistance with other agents, depending on the specific mutations involved.[35,43] In a field that is rapidly changing, specific recommendations for ART are best made by an infectious disease specialist with experience in the management of patients with HIV disease. The major therapeutic decisions include (1) when to initiate therapy, (2) what drugs to prescribe, (3) when to modify therapy, and (4) which drugs to change to. The mortality rate of

PLHIV and the incidence of opportunistic infections decreased markedly since 1995 due to triple combination ART becoming available at that time.[7] The role of drugs with immunomodulating activity in combination with ART is also undergoing extensive research.[44,45] Drug regimens for HIV disease are dynamic, and clinical practice guidelines are consistently updated; many changes in the approach to drug interventions can be expected as HIV infection continues to be a chronic disease.[46] There remains concern regarding the occurrence of noncommunicable diseases among individuals aging with HIV, but few studies have described whether disparities between demographic subgroups are present among individuals on ART with access to care. Racial disparities in the occurrence of diabetes, chronic kidney disease, and hypertension emphasize the need for prevention and treatment options for these HIV populations receiving care in North America.[47]

Vaccines for Other Antigens

HIV-positive individuals with impaired immune systems respond less well than do uninfected persons to most vaccines for other (non-HIV) antigens. The degree of immunodeficiency present at the time of vaccination has an impact on the response to hepatitis A or B, pneumococcal, and influenza A and B vaccines.[48] Patients with a CD4 count of more than 200 cells/μL have a more successful response to the vaccine. Patients should be informed that the extent and duration of the protective efficacy of these vaccines are still uncertain.

Vaccines and Functional Cures for Human Immunodeficiency Virus

Vaccination for HIV has the potential to prevent or control disease progression, but a successful vaccine has not yet been found. The development of an effective preventative vaccine for HIV is an area of continuing research. A true cure for HIV would require complete eradication of the virus from body, which might not be feasible. Thus several routes to "functional cures" are currently being studied. This includes exploration of use of therapeutic vaccines, antibody therapy, and gene therapy.

Prevention

Transmission routes of HIV have been well known since the late 1980s. Because the two most common routes of HIV infection are unsafe sex and sharing of needles and/or syringes among IV drug users, the keys to prevention are linked to safer sex practices and, for IV drug users, use of sterile syringes. For decades, use of latex condoms was the mainstay of HIV prevention during sexual activity. More recently, using preexposure prophylaxis (PrEP), in the form of Truvada, has been shown markedly reduce the risk of HIV transmission during sex.[49,50]

Nutrition

Involuntary loss of more than 10% of baseline body weight in a 12-month period or a 5% loss in baseline body weight in a 6-month period with chronic diarrhea or unexplained weakness and fever constitute HIV wasting syndrome.[51] Early retrospective demographic research in the United States found that 17.8% of individuals with AIDS had wasting syndrome.[52,53] The ensuing malnutrition contributes to further immunosuppression.[54] With the widespread use of ART, HIV wasting syndrome has declined significantly.[55] Those PLHIV with delayed initiation of ART or poor compliance may still experience weight loss or wasting through the loss of fat mass and lean body mass; this may contribute to muscle fatigue and weakness.[55] Nutritional consultation is critical for those patients experiencing wasting syndrome and as a preventative measure for those who newly diagnosed. Studies have been done investigating the effects of nutritional counseling and other measures such as medications, hormone supplementation, and exercise on lean body mass in patients with HIV wasting syndrome. It has been shown that nutritional counseling, medications to inhibit tumor necrosis factor, androgen supplementation, growth hormone administration, and resistance strength training have all been effective in improving lean body mass. Increased caloric intake alone increases lean body mass but primarily through fat stores. Resistance strength training may prove to be the most beneficial in increasing lean body mass with minimal side effects and minimal cost.[56]

There are new nutritional concerns that have developed since the prolonged use of ART in PLHIV. The development of changes in body fat distribution, dyslipidemia, insulin resistance, lipodystrophy syndrome, sarcopenia, and frailty are currently primary concerns when considering nutritional interventions.[57] Weight loss or reduction in lean body mass may also be a problem for some patients using ART. Comprehensive nutritional intervention is advocated during the early stages of HIV infection to maintain nutritional status. ART compromises nutrition in HIV patients because of complicated drug and nutrient interactions, adverse side effects including diarrhea and nausea, and, in some cases, excessive pill loads that must be consumed. Furthermore, ART has been directly linked to HIV-associated lipodystrophy. This syndrome is marked by various combinations of insulin resistance, hyperlipidemia, visceral adiposity, loss of peripheral fat stores, and dorsocervical fat accrual.[58] Lipodystrophy is a syndrome that makes the nutritional management of HIV more difficult and may necessitate exercise, pharmacological intervention, and diet modifications.[59] Insulin resistance has been observed in approximately 50% of ART users taking a PI, compared with approximately 25% of ART users who are taking an NRTI; this can result in eventual symptomatic atherosclerosis.[57] Dietary modification has only a modest effect on serum lipid concentrations; the use of statins and ART modification may be a more effective treatment.

Diet modification and resistance exercise training have been shown to help reduce total-body and regional fat mass. In addition, the FDA approved a growth hormone–releasing factor to treat visceral fat accumulation in PLHIV diagnosed with HIV lipodystrophy.[57]

Many patients who take antiretroviral drugs also take alternative therapies, including dietary supplements. Some drug-herb-supplement combinations may result in clinically meaningful interactions. Twenty-eight pharmacokinetic studies and case-series/case reports were selected for inclusion in a recent systematic review. Calcium carbonate, ferrous fumarate, some forms of ginkgo, some forms of garlic, some forms of milk thistle, St. John's wort, vitamin C, zinc sulfate, and multivitamins were all found to significantly decrease the levels of selected antiretrovirals and should be avoided in patients taking these antiretrovirals. Cat's claw and evening primrose oil were found to significantly increase the levels of antiretrovirals. PLHIV should be monitored for adverse effects while taking these dietary supplements with antiretrovirals. This evidence shows the importance of screening all PLHIV for dietary supplement use to prevent treatment failure or adverse effects related to an interaction.[60]

SYSTEMIC MANIFESTATIONS

Integumentary System and Neoplasms

Cutaneous disorders develop as many as 90% of all PLHIV.[61] Most HIV-induced skin findings develop only when the CD4 count falls to less than 500 cells/μL. As the CD4 cell count decreases further, multiple cutaneous disorders may develop.[62] Skin conditions may be defined as infectious, neoplastic, or inflammatory; a large percentage of PLHIV will also develop primary pruritus.[61] Chronic itch may be cutaneous, systemic, or psychiatric in nature and can directly impact

QOL for PLHIV. Treatment for inflammatory skin conditions may include ART modification, oral antihistamines, topical corticosteroids, topical antipruritic agents, skin moisturizers, psychiatric interventions, or phototherapy.[61]

There are three malignancies common in advanced HIV or AIDS: Kaposi sarcoma (KS), non-Hodgkin lymphoma (NHL), and cervical cancer. KS was the first neoplastic condition to be related to HIV infection, and it remains the most common in PLHIV who have limited access or poor compliance with ART. The incidence of KS has continued to diminish because of the use of more powerful ART and maintenance of immune status.[62,63] KS can involve almost every part of the body, but the most common site of initial KS presentations is the skin or mucous membranes.[64] The disorder manifests as cutaneous purple nodular lesions or as rife visceral lesions. AIDS-KS has been intimately associated with the lymphatic system, specifically deficient lymphatic transport, nodal dysfunction, and tumors, which contribute to lymphedema.[65]

In KS there is a broad therapeutic spectrum from cryotherapy to systemic chemotherapy.[66] ART plus chemotherapy is more effective than ART alone in patients diagnosed with severe or progression KS.[63] In NHL, early therapeutic intervention is necessary because of the fast progression of the tumor.[67] A systematic review,[68] conducted in 2015, found that the prevalence of nondiffuse large B-cell lymphoma has declined significantly since the introduction of combination ART, yet the prevalence of Burkitt or Burkitt-like lymphoma has not shown the same reduction; there remains a poor prognosis for those with Burkitt or Burkitt-like lymphoma.[68] The cervical cancer in HIV-positive women seems to be more aggressive than in HIV-negative women and requires early therapeutic intervention.[69] The cancer incidence in patients with HIV is reported to be higher among nonblack patients.[70] The incidence is seven times higher in HIV-positive women, as is the prevalence of a positive HPV viral DNA test, when compared with HIV-negative women.[71]

Several other tumors occur in people with HIV infection: anorectal cancer, lung cancer, malignant testicular tumor, Hodgkin lymphoma, basal cell carcinoma, and malignant melanoma.[67,72] It is beyond the scope of this chapter to detail all aspects of integumentary and neoplastic concerns; however, the therapist needs to be aware of the importance of differential diagnosis because the skin is the first line of defense of the immune system and further work-up may be warranted. See Table 34.3 for integumentary conditions associated with HIV.

Musculoskeletal System

Musculoskeletal symptoms are common in PLHIV. Knowledge of abnormalities that may occur in the musculoskeletal system is crucial as it influences morbidity and mortality. PLHIV develop inflammatory rheumatic diseases, which require screening, assessment, and management.[73] Arthritis in HIV disease has a wide spectrum of presentations ranging from mild arthralgia to severe joint disability.[74] Arthritides seen in this population has been classified into five groups on the basis of clinical presentation: (1) painful articular syndrome, (2) acute symmetrical polyarthritis, (3) spondyloarthropathic arthritis (Reiter syndrome, psoriatic arthritis), (4) HIV-associated arthritis, and (5) septic arthritis.[75] Standardized diagnostic tests and treatments are the same for PLHIV with musculoskeletal impairments.

Primary abnormalities include osseous and soft tissue infections, polymyositis, myopathy, and arthritis. Spinal infections such as pyogenic discitis, osteomyelitis, spinal tuberculosis, and epidural abscesses can occur with avascular necrosis (AVN) and osteoporosis as common comorbidities of HIV.[73,76] Secondary musculoskeletal complications are often a result of the various compensatory patterns of gait secondary to HIV-related peripheral neuropathy syndrome or the change in biomechanics of the foot and ankle.[77] These lead to potential spinal changes and back pain. PLHIV should be evaluated from a

TABLE 34.3   Human Immunodeficiency Virus and Integumentary Conditions

Viral Infections	Acute morbilliform rash
	Herpes simplex
	Varicella zoster
	Molluscum contagiosum
	Human papillomavirus
	Oral hairy leukoplakia
Fungal Infections	Tinea
	Blastomycosis
	Candidiasis
	Cryptococcosis
	Histoplasmosis
	Pityrosorum folliculitis
	Pityriasis versicolor
	Systemic mycoses
	Pneumocystosis
Bacterial Infections	Cellulitis
	Ecthyma
	Impetigo
	Folliculitis
	Bacillary angiomatosis
Arthropod Infections	Insect bites
	Scabies
	Demodicosis
Inflammatory Conditions	Seborrheic dermatitis
	Eosinophilic folliculitis
	Psoriasis
	Eczema
	Pruritic popular eruption
Malignancies	Kaposi sarcoma
	Cutaneous B-cell lymphoma
	Cutaneous T-cell lymphoma
	Skin cancer (melanoma, squamous cell carcinoma, basal cell carcinoma, and anal carcinoma)
Other	Medication side effects
	Xerosis
	Lipoatrophy
	Postinflammatory hyperpigmentation

Many skin conditions listed in this table are seen in the general population but may be more severe or more difficult to treat in human immunodeficiency virus-infected patients.

systems perspective to underscore the primary driver of movement dysfunction.

In PLHIV, acute myopathy manifests as proximal muscle weakness and elevated creatine phosphokinase levels.[78] Patients may have initial symptoms of difficulty with basic activities of daily living (ADLs), such as rising from a chair or climbing stairs. If myopathy is in an acute inflammatory stage, resisted exercise is contraindicated.

AVN, a pathological process that is associated with a variety of medical conditions or pharmacological interventions, has been linked to prolonged use of ART. A systematic review and meta-analysis, published in 2014, found there was a statistically significant increased odds of AVN in PLHIV who were exposed to PI therapy (odds ratio 2.09, 95% confidence interval [CI] 1.01 to 4.31; $P = .05$).[79] In addition to the higher prevalence of AVN since the widespread use of ART, there is also a notable increase in the incidence of osteoporosis, especially in young men diagnosed with HIV; the higher prevalence of osteoporosis associated with ART becomes further complicated by the increased life-spans and development of frailty as PLHIV progress through the natural course of aging.[80]

Chronic pain is highly prevalent in PLHIV; it has been associated with mental health disorders and is frequently reported with other symptoms.[81–83] This is discussed in more detail in a later section of the chapter.

Patient reports of musculoskeletal symptoms may indicate possible underlying inflammation, which has been implicated as a key predictor in HIV disease progression, early aging, and non–HIV-related morbidity and mortality.[84,85] A key difference to consider is the effect of ART medications when side effects of ART may evoke symptoms that may complicate the differential diagnosis. ART drugs may limit pharmaceutical treatment options for musculoskeletal conditions, namely immunosuppressant medications. See Table 34.4 for musculoskeletal conditions associated with HIV. PLHIV continue to have high musculoskeletal symptom burden despite viral suppression and decreased side effect profiles.[86] These symptoms experienced may have underlying pathophysiology due to inflammation, even in the context of viral suppression. Clinicians should proactively ask patients about

symptoms that contribute to pain and distress, assist PLHIV with coping mechanisms, and improved QOL.

Cardiopulmonary System

Pulmonary diseases continue to be important causes of illness and death in PLHIV, but changes in therapy and demographics alter their manifestations. The risk for development of specific disorders is related to the degree of immunosuppression, HIV risk group, area of residence, and use of prophylactic therapies.[87] Sinusitis and bronchitis occur frequently in the HIV-positive population, more so than in the general public. The increasing population of HIV-positive drug users is reflected in the increasing incidence of tuberculosis (TB) and bacterial pneumonia.

Anti-*Pneumocystis* prophylaxis has reduced the incidence of and mortality from Pneumocystis carinii pneumonia (PCP). The PCP-causing organism is usually acquired in childhood, and 65% to 85% of healthy adults possess PCP antibodies. Reactivation of latent infection is responsible for the recurrent fever, dyspnea, and hypoxia that characterize PCP.[88,89] Adjunctive corticosteroid therapy has improved the outlook for respiratory failure.[87] Multiple studies have shown that the use of corticosteroids in PLHIV in acute respiratory failure did not increase the risk for the development of opportunistic infections.[90]

TABLE 34.4 Human Immunodeficiency Virus and Musculoskeletal Conditions

Condition	Symptoms and Presentation	Interventions
Acute Symmetrical Polyarthritis	Exclusive to HIV-infected patients Resembles rheumatoid arthritis Develops in the small joints of the hand Characterized by ulnar deviation of the digits and swan neck deformities Acute onset Negative rheumatoid factor test result (helps differentiate from rheumatoid arthritis) Radiographical results mimic rheumatoid arthritis (periarticular osteopenia, joint-space narrowing, and marginal erosions)	Gold therapy ROM activities
Avascular Necrosis or Osteonecrosis	Results from direct or indirect damage to the vascular supply of the affected bone (leading to in situ death of subchondral bone) Most common sites are the femoral head followed by the humeral head May occur in other locations including the wrist (scaphoid [Preiser disease] or lunate [Kienböck disease]), knee, and ankle Deep, throbbing, intermittent pain that may be insidious or sudden onset In later stages, a loss of range of motion	Early treatment by minimizing the forces across the joint (avoiding lower-extremity weight-bearing activity or by greatly limiting upper-extremity lifting and carrying activities) Advanced stages require surgical intervention to improve/restore vascularity, provide stabilization, or replace the joint ROM activities
Diffuse Infiltrative Lymphocytosis Syndrome (DLS)	Massive parotid enlargement, xerostomia, and lymphocytic hepatitis caused by CD8 lymphocytic infiltration of the liver Xerophthalmia (dry eyes), xerostomia (dry mouth), salivary gland enlargement, and arthralgias Extraglandular features may be pulmonary, neurological, gastrointestinal, renal, or musculoskeletal	Symptomatic treatment with artificial saliva and tears Antibiotics to address recurrent sinus, middle ear, and oral cavity infections Immunosuppressive therapy should be used only in life-threatening situations (pulmonary insufficiency or renal disease) Corticosteroids can be used for extraglandular features Radiotherapy to reduce the enlarged parotid gland
HIV-associated Arthralgia	Asymmetrical, oligoarticular arthritis exclusive to HIV-infected persons Occurs predominantly in the late stages Acute onset of severe pain and disability (predominantly large joints such as the knees or ankles) Self-limiting, lasts a few weeks to 6 months Mild to moderate severity Synovial fluid commonly contains only 50–2600 white blood cells/μL Radiography may show diffuse osteopenia but without erosive changes Serum is negative for human leukocyte antigen-B27 and rheumatoid factor Synovial biopsy reveals a chronic mononuclear cell infiltrate	Symptomatic relief with NSAIDs Intraarticular corticosteroid injections ROM activities

Continued

TABLE 34.4   Human Immunodeficiency Virus and Musculoskeletal Conditions—cont'd

Condition	Symptoms and Presentation	Interventions
Hypertrophic Osteoarthropathy	Systemic disorder affecting bones, joints, and soft tissues Often develops in patients with PCP Severe pain in the lower extremity, digital clubbing, arthralgias, nonpitting edema, periarticular soft tissue involvement of the ankle, knees, and elbows Skin over the affected areas is glistening, edematous, and warm Chronic erythema, paresthesias, and hyperhidrosis may be noted in the hands and feet Radiography reveals extensive periosteal reaction and subperiosteal proliferative changes in the long bones of the lower extremity Bone scan demonstrates increased uptake along the cortical surfaces	Treatment of PCP usually alleviates this condition Surgical or chemical vagotomy or radiation therapy may be necessary in refractory cases
Idiopathic Polymyositis	Bilateral proximal muscle weakness Elevated serum CK levels Often occurs early in infection Exact mechanism is still undetermined	Discontinue medication that causes inflammation or irritation of the muscle Antiinflammatory medications Corticosteroid medications
Psoriatic Arthritis	Cutaneous manifestations (macropapules on the knees, elbows, scalp and trunk), nail changes, arthritic changes or deformities, soft tissue swelling, juxtaarticular erosions, osteopenia, osteolysis Five types: asymmetrical oligoarthritis, symmetrical polyarthritis, dominant desquamative interstitial pneumonia, arthritis mutilans, and sacroiliitis or spondylitis without peripheral involvement Synovial fluid usually contains 7000–15,000 white blood cells/μL	NSAIDs Second-line agents (gold, methotrexate, and azathioprine) Intraarticular steroid injection (every 4–6 months) ROM activities
Pyomyositis	Solitary or multiple muscle abscesses that are not formed by local extension from superficial subcutaneous tissue Acute, severe muscle pain with or without erythema, fever, edema Elevated ESR and CK levels Pathogen is most often *Staphylococcus aureus* Differential diagnosis includes muscle strain, contusion, hematoma, cellulitis, deep venous thrombosis, osteomyelitis, septic arthritis, and neoplasm	Without treatment, septic shock and death can result in 3 weeks Open drainage or débridement of the site Antibiotic therapy
Reactive Arthritis Septic Arthritis Bursitis	Asymmetrical oligoarthritis or monoarticular arthritis, dactylitis, enthesopathy, joint effusion Most common in the foot and ankle May range from mild to severe Inflammation of synovial fluid, often gram negative	Surgical débridement Aspiration of fluid from the joint Antibiotics ROM activities
Reiter Syndrome	Urethritis, conjunctivitis, and arthritis Nail involvement with subungual hyperkeratosis, circinate balanitis, keratoderma hemorrhagica, oral ulcers, uveitis, AIDS foot, weight loss, malaise, lymphadenopathy, and diarrhea Severe course of persistent and erosive polyarthritis, fevers, and enthesopathies (responds poorly to treatment or has a mild and self-limited course) Common enthesopathies include Achilles tendinitis, lateral or medial epicondylitis, rotator cuff tendinitis, and de Quervain tenosynovitis Axial skeleton involvement is rare Broad-based gait and stiff ankles with weight bearing through the lateral margins of the feet because of the painful heel May become severely disabled and require use of a wheelchair	NSAIDs Second-line agents (gold, methotrexate, and azathioprine) Relief after 5–7 days of therapy Intraarticular steroid injection (every 4–6 months) Methotrexate, other immunosuppressive agents, and phototherapy should be used with extreme caution Early physical therapy and splinting of affected joints as needed to prevent atrophy and contractures
Zidovudine-associated Myopathy	Causes mitochondrial toxicity Gradual myalgias, muscle tenderness, proximal muscle weakness Elevated CK levels	Discontinue AZT therapy CK levels return to normal within 4 weeks (after discontinuing AZT) Weakness resolves in 8 weeks

AZT, Zidovudine; *CK,* creatine kinase; *ESR,* erythrocyte sedimentation rate; *HIV,* human immunodeficiency virus; *NSAIDs,* nonsteroidal antiinflammatory drugs; *PCP, Pneumocystis carinii* pneumonia; *ROM,* range of motion.

Mycobacterial infections in PLHIV usually manifest as either Mycobacterium avium complex (MAC) infection or TB.[7] Steadily increasing incidence of infection by *Mycobacterium tuberculosis* is likely the result of two factors: better medical management of HIV and the development of multidrug-resistant strains of mycobacteria. MAC infection tends to appear late during HIV infection, with the initial infection affecting the GI and pulmonary tracts; this eventually disseminates throughout the body. This disorder is probably not caused by latent reactivation of the organism but rather by primary infection by ingestion or inhalation.[91] Signs and symptoms of MAC infection include pneumonia, fever, weight loss, malaise, sweats, anorexia, abdominal pain, and diarrhea.

As in many other infections, initial signs and symptoms of TB include fever, weight loss, malaise, cough, lymph node tenderness, and night sweats. Pulmonary involvement accounts for 75% to 100% of cases of TB infection in PLHIV, but extrapulmonary infection, especially in lymph nodes and bone marrow, occurs in up to 60% of these individuals as well.[88,91–93] Less common areas of infection include the CNS, cardiac, and mucosal tissues. TB is communicable, preventable, and treatable. Tuberculin skin testing with follow-up chest radiographs when appropriate should be available and routinely offered to individuals at HIV testing sites. Individuals at highest risk for concomitant HIV and TB infections include the homeless, intravenous drug users, and prison inmates.[88,93] The risk of infection in health care personnel and in the public is a concern. Isolation rooms that provide negative-pressure, nonrecirculated ventilation, specific air filters, and higher air exchange rates offer the best protection to health care providers exposed to TB-infected individuals. Properly fitted face masks that filter droplet nuclei should be worn. Monitoring of personnel who work with these populations will identify the need for necessary preventive therapy.[88] The majority of health care facilities require personnel to have yearly screenings and have established guidelines to prevent the spread of TB in their patient population and within their workforce.

Cytomegalovirus (CMV) can affect the GI and respiratory tracts but primarily targets optic structures and the CNS; 40% to 100% of healthy adults possess CMV antibodies.[94] However, an individual who is immunosuppressed becomes more vulnerable to symptoms of infection with CMV. Predominant consequences of HIV-CMV coinfection are unilateral or bilateral deficits in visual acuity, visual field cuts, and blindness. PLHIV are more likely than the general population to have subclinical bursts of CMV replication at mucosal sites. Production of antigens can activate the immune system and stimulate HIV replication, and it could contribute to the pathogenesis of adverse outcomes of aging, such as CVD or neurocognitive impairment.[95]

Since the introduction of ART, the QOL and longevity for PLHIV have significantly improved. However, given the impact and negative effects of the virus and prolonged intervention with ART, the effects of aging from CVDs have emerged as one of the most common causes of death.[96] This accounts for up to 15% of total deaths in high-income countries.[97] As ART availability expands to low-income countries, the burden of CVD mortality will rise. Over the next decade, HIV-CVD disease burden is expected to increase globally.[97] Factors that contribute to the atherosclerotic process and its role in the development of acute coronary syndrome in the setting of infection requires close monitoring in rehabilitation settings.

Clinical CVD tends to appear approximately 10 years before in infected individuals, when compared with the general population. The pathogenesis behind the cardiovascular, HIV-associated complications is complex, involving traditional CVD risk factors, as well as factors associated with the virus itself including chronic inflammation and resultant immune activation, along with metabolic disorders related to ART regimens.[98] Determining the cardiovascular risk among HIV-infected patients, as well as targeting and treating conditions that

predispose to CVD, are currently emerging concerns among health care professionals. CVD, especially coronary artery disease, are among the leading causes of death in this population.[99]

Pericardial effusion and myocarditis are among the most commonly reported cardiac abnormalities. Cardiomyopathy, endocarditis, and coronary vasculopathy have also been reported. HIV infection, the medical management of HIV disease, and secondary opportunistic infections can all affect the myocardium, pericardium, endocardium, and blood vessels.[94,100] Cardiovascular risk in PLHIV depends on several factors: direct and indirect vascular effects of chronic exposure to the virus, metabolic effects from prolonged ART, the normal aging process (important to consider given the increased life expectancy of PLHIV), and other cardiovascular risk factors (such as diet and genetics).[101]

Body fat changes and lipid abnormalities,[102] known as *lipodystrophy* or *fat redistribution syndrome,* have been connected to PI use.[103] These body fat changes may have strong implications for patients undergoing rehabilitation interventions. Signs and symptoms of the syndrome vary, and not all need to be present in any patient. However, in both men and women, three main components of the syndrome have emerged. These include changes in body shape, hyperlipidemia, and insulin resistance. Clinically, distinct body shape changes are apparent. The most prevalent include increased abdominal growth, dorsocervical fat pad, benign symmetrical lipomatosis, lipodystrophy, and breast hypertrophy in women.[104,105] The increased abdominal growth is characterized by a redistribution and accumulation of fat in the central visceral areas of the body.[105,106] Corresponding symptoms include GI discomfort, bloating, distention, and fullness.[106] In addition to visible signs and symptoms, adverse changes in lipid, glucose, and insulin levels have been reported.[107] Several studies have revealed hyperlipidemia to be present in PLHIV, many of whom, but not all, were undergoing PI therapy.[108]

Prevention of CVD risk remains the first and essential step in a medical intervention. Lifestyle modification, including weight reduction, exercise, smoking cessation, and education on healthy dietary practices, are key target areas. Statins are the primary medication used to treat hypercholesterolemia. They have been shown to slow the progression or promote reduction of coronary plaque and could also exert an antiinflammatory and immunomodulatory effect.[109] Current ARTs are less toxic and more effective than regimens used in the early years. Lipodystrophy and dyslipidemia are the main causes of long-term toxicities. PIs may cause dyslipidemia and lipodystrophy, whereas INIs have a minimal impact on lipids profile and no evidence of lipodystrophy.[109]

Metabolic syndrome, which is a cluster of risk factors for type 2 diabetes and CVD, has become an important public health problem.[110] In HIV, new evidence suggests that the use of optimal waist cut-off points specific for the various ethnic populations is recommended.[111] Although metabolic disorders have been associated indirectly with ART, in the aging HIV population and newer, less metabolically toxic antiretroviral drugs are available. Lipotoxicity and adipokines have been key issues to explain this metabolic syndrome. Prevention strategies and therapeutic options for all metabolic syndrome and CVD need to be addressed in the light of the recent Adult Treatment Panel IV recommendations and the new antiretroviral drugs.[111]

Therapists need to be apprised of various changes in laboratory results and signs and symptoms of metabolic syndrome and cardiac disease when designing an exercise program and facilitating the return to functional activities. Screening guidelines[112,113] (from the Infectious Diseases Society of America HIV Medicine Association [IDSA HIVMA]) include the following:

- Monitor fasting lipid levels before beginning highly active antiretroviral therapy (HAART) and during the first 4 to 6 weeks of treatment

TABLE 34.5   Effects of Human Immunodeficiency Virus Treatment on Cardiovascular Factors

Cardiovascular Factor	Incidence	Effects
Lipid Metabolism HDL-C	Decreases in early infection Will increase modestly with viral suppression (not to premorbid levels)	Greater increases seen with NNRTI medications Increased visceral adipose tissue and upper trunk fat associated with low HDL-C
Lipid Metabolism LDL-C	Decreases later in infection Will increase modestly with viral suppression	No evidence of direct medication effects on LDL-C
Lipid Metabolism Triglycerides	Increases in late infection with viral suppression Decreased in early studies of AZT use	No change (primarily with PIs) with ART medications Increased visceral adipose tissue and upper trunk fat associated with elevated triglyceride levels
Glucose Metabolism Insulin Sensitivity	Decrease if untreated Trend toward decreased insulin sensitivity with viral suppression (regardless of medications)	Some PIs and NRTIs may decrease insulin sensitivity Increased visceral adipose tissue and upper trunk fat associated with insulin resistance
Glucose Metabolism Insulin Secretion	No evidence of effect if untreated No evidence of effect with viral suppression	Some PIs may decrease insulin secretion
Glucose Metabolism Fasting Glucose	No evidence of any effect if untreated No evidence of effect with viral suppression	Some PIs may increase glucose production
Glucose Metabolism Glucose Tolerance	No evidence of any effect if untreated No evidence of effect with viral suppression	May be higher rates of impaired glucose tolerance with ART
Glucose Metabolism Diabetes	No evidence of differences in prevalence or incidence rates if untreated May be a higher prevalence of diabetes with viral suppression	Higher prevalence of type 2 diabetes associated with certain PIs and NRTIs
Body Composition Lean Body Mass	Decreases disproportionately with severe wasting, if untreated Increases modestly with the initiation of effective ART	No consistent evidence of direct medication effects
Body Composition Peripheral Fat	Decreases proportionately with wasting, if untreated Will initially increase with the start of effective ART	Subsequent depletion of subcutaneous fat in the face, arms, legs, and buttocks is associated with some NRTIs
Body Composition Visceral fat	Decreased minimally when untreated Increases with effective ART	Preserved or increased visceral fat in some patients on ART
Renal Function Renal Disease	HIV-associated nephropathy, proteinuria, microalbuminuria and elevated cystatin C if untreated Decreased HIV-associated nephropathy (may still have microalbuminuria and elevated cystatin C with viral suppression)	Some ART may cause impaired renal function

ART, Antiretroviral therapies; *AZT,* Zidovudine; *HDL-C,* high-density lipoprotein cholesterol; *LDL-C,* low-density lipoprotein cholesterol; *NNRTI,* nonnucleoside reverse transcriptase inhibitor; *NRTI,* nucleoside reverse transcriptase inhibitor; *PI,* protease inhibitor.

- Monitor fasting glucose levels before and during HAART
- Monitor body weight and body shape changes on a routine basis

See Table 34.5 for effects of HIV treatment on cardiovascular factors and Table 34.6 for cardiovascular risk factors associated with HIV.

Neurological System

The neurological manifestations of HIV disease are numerous and involve the autonomic nervous system (ANS), CNS, and peripheral nervous system (PNS).[114,115] Over the course of the disease, up to 70% of patients have some form of neurological symptom.[116] Significant progress in understanding and treating the neurologically involved HIV-positive patient has been made over the past decade. However, HIV continues to affect every division of the human nervous system. HIV-positive infants show early, catastrophic encephalopathy, loss of brain growth, motor deficits, and cognitive dysfunction.[117] This static or progressive HIV-encephalopathy is characterized by acquired microcephaly, delay or loss of developmental milestones (motor, mental, and language), and pyramidal tract motor deficits.[118] Unfortunately, neurobehavioral dysfunction in early pediatric AIDS remains unchanged after therapy. Dementia develops in some adult patients despite the use of combination ART drugs, whereas other patients have subtle

neurobehavioral changes that diminish the quality of their prolonged lives. HIV infection of the CNS remains an important clinical concern.

A variety of host and viral factors are associated with an increased risk of developing HIV-associated neurocognitive disorders (HANDs). HAND is associated with a decreased survival time and is characterized by an insidious onset and slow progression of cognitive decline. In the early stages, individuals may report reduced concentration, poor memory, and impaired executive functioning.[119] As the condition progresses, the individual's affect may change, with psychomotor slowing and reduction in motor skills.[119] Approximately 18% to 50% of PLHIV who are on ART have some degree of HAND.[120,121] As PLHIV are living much longer life-spans, it is critical to differentiate HAND from the more commonly diagnosed dementias. Studies are demonstrating similarities between factors that predispose PLHIV to HANDs and the risk factors of Alzheimer dementia, suggesting the potential for a common pathological mechanism.[122] Evidence has shown that HIV-infected monocytes are carried across the blood-brain barrier and infect the macrophages and microglia in the CNS.[123,124] HIV enters the CNS early, yet HANDs may not occur until advanced stages of HIV infection. Hypotheses for the development of HANDs in the advanced stages include the loss of immune control with disease progression,

TABLE 34.6 Cardiovascular Risk Factors and Human Immunodeficiency Virus

Risk Factor	Intervention	Result
Cigarette smoking	Interpersonal counseling Medical or pharmaceutical treatment Behavioral modification	Increased rates for quitting
HTN	Dietary and physical activity counseling Calcium channel blockers Other antihypertensive agents	Reduced blood pressure Drug interactions between calcium channel blockers and PIs
Dyslipidemia	Dietary and physical activity counseling Statins, fibrates, fish oil, niacin	Modest improvements in lipids Statins improve endothelial function Multiple drug interactions with ART
Disordered Glucose Metabolism	Dietary and physical activity counseling Metformin and thiazolidinediones	Improvement in glycemia Metformin reduces insulin resistance and visceral adipose tissue Thiazolidinediones may improve subcutaneous adipose tissue
Use of ART	Modification of initial ART based on metabolic profile and CVD risk Switching ART to reduce metabolic side effects	Modest effects on lipids and insulin resistance Statins and fibrates may be more effective

ART, Antiretroviral therapies; *CVD,* cardiovascular disease; *HTN,* hypertension; *PI,* protease inhibitor.

heightened immune activation, increased transfer of infected monocytes into the CNS, and variations or mutations in the virus. Because many ART medications have reduced CNS penetration, HANDs continue to pose significant challenges for advanced HIV/AIDS patients.[125] See Table 34.7 for neurological conditions associated with HIV.

Autonomic Nervous System

Dysfunction of the ANS has been associated with HIV infection. This has implications for overall function and the design of a rehabilitation program for PLHIV disease. In one study, individuals with the greatest ANS involvement had dementia, myelopathy, and sensory peripheral neuropathy. Additional symptoms of autonomic neuropathy include orthostatic dizziness, postprandial nausea, urinary incontinence, and dysfunction in thermoregulation.[126] Variations in heart rate, including resting tachycardia, were common. Abnormal blood pressure readings were identified in response to isometric exercise and positional changes (sit-to-stand and tilting).[127] Opportunistic infections, such as CMV and varicella zoster virus, have been shown to contribute to autonomic dysfunction.[126] Individuals with suspected autonomic neuropathy should be carefully evaluated to rule out other sources, such as polypharmacy, end-organ disease, or comorbid conditions.

Central Nervous System

HIV enters the CNS during the early stages of the disease and is hypothesized to traverse the blood-brain barrier during the initial acute primary infection stage. Although the initial CNS invasion by HIV is asymptomatic in most individuals, affective and cognitive deficits may develop.[128] It is not possible in this context to discuss the neuropathological features of each of the many secondary infections and neoplasms of HIV illness. However, it is important to realize that the clinical manifestations of these pathological processes overlap with one another and with the signs and symptoms of primary HIV infection of the CNS; lesions of the CNS can be the site of more than one opportunistic disease process simultaneously. A wide variety of organisms or conditions are responsible for the neurological manifestations associated with HIV infection. These include primary and secondary viral, protozoan, fungal, and *Mycobacterium* infections, as well as neoplasms and iatrogenic conditions. Infectious processes may cause large lesions in the brain and lead to meningitis, encephalitis, or both. Such infections cause neurocognitive impairments that develop as

dementia, amnesia, or delirium.[128] Thirty percent to 40% of healthy adults have contracted toxoplasmosis, caused by *Toxoplasma gondii.*[42,129] Unchecked by the immune system, toxoplasmosis results in CNS dysfunction: altered cognition, headache, focal neurological deficits, encephalitis, and seizures. Cerebellar disorders associated with HIV infection are typically the result of discrete cerebellar lesions[130] resulting from opportunistic infections such as toxoplasmosis and progressive multifocal leukoencephalopathy or primary CNS lymphoma.[131] CNS lymphoma results in cognitive dysfunction and presentation of fever, focal neurological impairments, headache, seizures, and motor deficits.[128]

Evidence supports that the neurotoxic effect of HIV is more likely to affect the basal ganglia, the frontal neocortex, the white matter tracts connecting the regions (such as the fronto-striato-thalamocortical loops), the temporal cortices (including the hippocampus), and the parietal cortices.[132] A relationship between cerebrovascular disease and AIDS has been reported.[133,134] There are estimates of a 20% to 80% increase in ischemic or hemorrhagic stroke risk (after adjustment for established stroke risk factors) in PLHIV.[135] The most common cause of cerebral infarction in both clinical and autopsy series was nonbacterial thrombotic endocarditis. Intracerebral hemorrhages were usually associated with thrombocytopenia, primary CNS lymphoma, and metastatic KS.

HIV-related conditions in the spinal cord include not only HIV myelitis, opportunistic infections, and lymphomas, but also vacuolar myelopathy, which affects predominantly the dorsolateral white matter tracts. The cause of vacuolar myelopathy is not understood, and it has not been unequivocally linked with HIV infection.[136] Vacuolar myelopathy may affect up to 30% of untreated adults with advanced HIV/AIDS, and the incidence may be even higher in children infected with HIV.[137] Unless it is treated with effective ART, vacuolar myelopathy of the spinal cord associated with moderate clinical disability develops in many patients with AIDS.[138]

Treatment for CNS impairments includes an eclectic blend of rehabilitation strategies. Neuromuscular disturbances may first appear as movement disorders. Subtleties of altered movement can be detected early and during subsequent treatment phases. A neurological examination can be performed to determine a diagnosis and prognosis. This may include the level of the lesion, neuromuscular deficits, need for assistive devices, ability to perform ADLs, and functional abilities. Various QOL assessments used with this population can be found in Table 34.8.

TABLE 34.7 Human Immunodeficiency Virus and Neurological Conditions

Condition	Symptoms and Presentation	Prognosis and Treatment
CNS Lymphomas	Cancerous tumors (begin in the brain or result from a cancer that has spread from another site in the body) Almost always associated with the Epstein-Barr virus (EBV) Symptoms: headache, seizures, vision problems, dizziness, speech disturbance, paralysis, and mental deterioration May develop one or more CNS lymphomas	Prognosis is poor owing to advanced and increasing immunodeficiency
Cerebrovascular Accident (CVA): Ischemia or Hemorrhage	Causes include hypertension, blood vessel abnormalities (aneurysms, vein or artery malformations), hypotension, coagulopathies, thrombotic thrombocytopenic purpura, elevated lipids, viral infections of the heart muscle, herpes zoster, hepatitis C, and cocaine or heroin use Characterized by the abrupt onset of weakness, language problems, or sensory loss Symptoms often occur on only one side of the body Imaging studies help to differentiate stroke, hemorrhage, infection, and tumors	Treatment parallels the HIV-negative population CVA diagnosed <3 h after onset may be a candidate for tissue plasminogen activator (tPA); tPA is contraindicated in cases of brain hemorrhage Lipid-lowering drugs (statins), blood thinners such as warfarin (Coumadin), or antiplatelet agents such as aspirin or clopidogrel (Plavix) are indicated Specific causes of stroke may require other forms of treatment Brain hemorrhages may require surgery Prognosis depends on size and location; recovery is greatest during the initial few weeks, but improvement often continues for months Inpatient and outpatient rehabilitation is often helpful Preventive treatment parallels the HIV-negative population; includes antiplatelet agents or blood-thinning drugs, removal of plaque from the walls of carotid arteries, and newer techniques of endovascular stenting
Cryptococcal Meningitis	Manifests as meningitis, a space-occupying lesion, or meningoencephalitis The fungus first invades the lungs and spreads to the covering of the brain and spinal cord, causing the inflammation Symptoms: fatigue, fever, headache, nausea, memory loss, confusion, photophobia, stiff neck, altered vision, drowsiness, and vomiting Develops when CD4 cell counts fall to less than 100 cells/μL	If untreated, may lapse into a coma and die Treatment relies on amphotericin B (Fungizone), which may be combined with flucytosine (Ancobon) Alternative for less severe cases is fluconazole (Diflucan), which is also the drug of choice for long-term prophylaxis (preventive therapy) Amphotericin B is an alternative maintenance therapy for those who relapse on fluconazole or do not tolerate it Hydrocephalus can occur; requires a ventriculoperitoneal shunt Visual loss can be addressed by optic nerve surgery
Cytomegalovirus (CMV) Infections	Herpesvirus that causes infection of the brain, spinal cord, meninges, or nerve roots Lead to neurological problems such as encephalitis, myelitis, retinitis, polyradiculitis, peripheral neuropathy, or mononeuritis multiplex Infection of the spinal cord and nerves can result in weakness in the lower limbs and paralysis, severe lower back pain, and loss of bladder function Findings include low-to-normal glucose, normal-to-high protein, and increased numbers of white blood cells	Untreated CMV encephalitis is almost always fatal and causes death within days to weeks Anti-CMV drugs must be started immediately, often based on a suspected rather than proven diagnosis Treatment relies on ganciclovir (Cytovene) and foscarnet (Foscavir), used alone or in combination when monotherapy fails Lifelong maintenance treatment is often necessary
Distal Sensory Polyneuropathy	Damage to sensory nerves in the extremities Most common type of HIV-associated neuropathy Nerves may be injured directly by HIV or by HIV-induced macrophages that secrete neurotoxic substances May also be caused by nutritional and vitamin imbalances or drug toxicity (especially use of d4T [stavudine, Zerit], ddI [didanosine, Videx], or ddC [zalcitabine, Hivid]) Occurs at any stage of HIV disease	Treatment of symptoms may include local ointments (capsaicin, Aspercreme), antidepressant medications (amitriptyline [Elavil]), or antiepileptic medications (gabapentin [Neurontin], lamotrigine [Lamictal], carbamazepine [Tegretol]) Duloxetine (Cymbalta; an SSRI antidepressant) is FDA approved for painful diabetic polyneuropathy Pregabalin (Lyrica; antiepileptic drug) Drugs should be chosen that are unlikely to interact with or influence the effectiveness of ART Lidoderm patches may provide partial pain relief without any systemic side effects and can be combined with oral drugs.

TABLE 34.7   Human Immunodeficiency Virus and Neurological Conditions—cont'd

Condition	Symptoms and Presentation	Prognosis and Treatment
Herpesvirus Infections	Herpes zoster virus can infect the brain and produce encephalitis or myelitis Signs of shingles include painful blisters, itching, tingling, and nerve pain	Anti-herpes drugs: standard treatment for shingles is acyclovir; other medications include famciclovir and valacyclovir Nerve blocks: anesthetic drugs and/or steroids injected into peripheral nerves or into the spinal column Drugs normally used to treat depression, epilepsy, or severe pain are sometimes used for the pain of shingles; nortriptyline (antidepressant) is frequently used for shingles pain; pregabalin is an epilepsy medicine used for pain after shingles Skin treatments: creams, gels, and sprays may provide temporary relief from pain; capsaicin has shown good preliminary results; the patch form of the anesthetic lidocaine provides pain relief for some people with shingles
HIV-dementia Complex (HIV-associated Encephalopathy)	Occurs primarily in persons with advanced HIV infection Mild cognitive impairment may occur in earlier stages Symptoms: encephalitis, behavioral changes, and a gradual decline in cognitive function (decreased concentration, memory, and attention) May develop severe global dementia with memory loss and language impairment Progressive slowing of motor function (decreased balance, weakness, decreased coordination) and loss of dexterity and coordination	Can be fatal if left untreated If HIV-dementia develops during treatment with ART, additional or alternative agents should be tried Neuroprotective therapies or global memory-enhancing agents such as memantine (Namenda) or donepezil (Aricept) may be useful Polypharmacy can affect thinking and memory and make symptoms worse
Inflammatory Demyelinating Polyneuropathy (IDP)	Inflammation of the myelin sheath that surrounds the spinal and peripheral nerves Acute form of IDP (AIDP), also known as *Guillain-Barré syndrome* (GBS) Characterized by rapid onset and progression over hours to weeks Chronic form (CIDP) has slower onset and progression over weeks to months, sometimes with a relapsing course Both forms are autoimmune conditions in which the immune system attacks nerves Causes varying degrees of weakness and sensory loss, which can develop in the limbs Nerves around the head may be affected and cause symptoms of facial weakness and double vision. Other symptoms may include pain and diminished reflex responses May have difficulty with urination and bowel movements, respiratory paralysis, irregular heartbeat, and dangerously high or low blood pressure	Treatment and response rates are similar to the HIV-negative population Intravenous immunoglobulin (IVIG), a highly concentrated antibody infusion from many pooled blood donations, is the primary treatment Plasmapheresis (removal of antibodies from the blood) may be helpful CIDP may also necessitate use of corticosteroids such as prednisone
Meningitis	Inflammation of the meninges, the membranes surrounding the brain and spinal cord Signs and symptoms are malaise, fever, stiff neck, photophobia, and headache; less common are cranial neuropathies (one-sided facial weakness or double vision), confusion, drowsiness, and personality changes HIV invades the brain early and may cause meningitis within days to weeks after infection Chronic meningitis, or episodes of idiopathic acute (rapid onset) meningitis can occur anytime during the course of HIV disease	Treatment and prognosis vary by the specific cause of meningitis, severity at presentation, delay from symptom onset to treatment, and status of immunosuppression

Continued

TABLE 34.7   Human Immunodeficiency Virus and Neurological Conditions—cont'd

Condition	Symptoms and Presentation	Prognosis and Treatment
Mononeuritis Multiplex	Painful condition involving isolated nerves over the arms, legs, or trunk Nerves are affected asymmetrically Involvement of >2 nerves is generally seen in advanced HIV Burning or shooting pain down an arm or leg, then (even if resolving) another burning pain emerges over another nerve pathway in a different arm or leg Weakness in the distribution of specific nerves is common Nerves can be affected in the head and the body	Occurring early in HIV infection May resolve with ART IVIG or plasmapheresis should be considered in early or late HIV stages Advanced HIV disease may require anti-CMV medications (ganciclovir, foscarnet)
Myopathy	May be due to drug toxicity (statins, ddI, or AZT), bacterial, viral, or other infections Polymyositis is caused by an abnormal immune response HIV wasting syndrome may result from HIV infection itself. Progressive muscle weakness is the typical presentation; the speed of progression depends on the cause	If due to drug toxicity, discontinue or replaced medication Muscle infections treated with drugs specific to the responsible bacterium, virus, or other infectious agent Inflammation from an overactive immune system can be treated with corticosteroids
Neurosyphilis	Sexually transmitted infection caused by the spiral-shaped *Treponema pallidum* bacterium *T. pallidum* gains access to the body through tiny abrasions of the skin or mucous membranes; this organism may invade the CNS a few months after initial infection May proceed rapidly from the primary stage (skin chancres, or lesions, appearing about 21 days after infection) to secondary syphilis (skin rash) and tertiary syphilis (infection of different organs, including the brain) as early as 2 months after exposure Tertiary syphilis may cause hearing loss, dizziness or vertigo, headache, failing vision, cognitive impairment, personality changes, peripheral polyneuropathy, gait imbalance, seizures, or CVA	Antibiotic use depends on the stage of syphilis and follows general guidelines Most common are different forms of penicillin Although HIV-infected patients with neurosyphilis respond to antibiotics, they are less likely to have serological improvement (compared with HIV-negative individuals) HIV-associated neurosyphilis may be more difficult to treat and more aggressive
Polyradiculopathy	Damage to the nerve roots where the nerves exit the spinal cord to form peripheral nerves May be caused by CMV, or lymphoma (less likely); may be idiopathic Rapidly progressive ascending numbness, pain, and weakness affecting the legs, and later occasionally the arms, is characteristic of the CMV form Early bowel and bladder control problems may suggest the syndrome More benign, slower clinical progression characterizes the idiopathic form	CMV polyradiculopathy is rapidly fatal without therapy Treatment with foscarnet or ganciclovir may improve or stabilize the condition ART may be useful Idiopathic form may improve spontaneously, without treatment
Primary Central Nervous System Lymphoma	Characterized by the growth of abnormal lymphocytes, or white blood cells (B- and T-cells) Occurs in the brain, rarely in the spinal cord; causes brain lesions and changes in mental functioning In almost all cases, EBV is found in the lymphoma-related lesions or the CSF Often associated with CD4 cell counts less than 100 cells/μL Symptoms: impaired cognition, aphasia, hemiparesis, and seizures Onset is often subtle and progression slower	Prognosis is generally poor Whole brain radiation therapy (radiotherapy) has been the mainstay of treatment; provides for a median survival of 2–5 months Steroids are required for at least 48 h before radiotherapy to minimize swelling; steroids should be continued throughout the course of treatment High-dose methotrexate has been used with some success, given as frequently as every week for five cycles; combining methotrexate and radiotherapy can achieve survival of 1–2 years Experimental chemotherapy agents include thiotepa (Thioplex) and procarbazine (Matulane) ART should be continued

TABLE 34.7 Human Immunodeficiency Virus and Neurological Conditions—cont'd

Condition	Symptoms and Presentation	Prognosis and Treatment
Progressive Multifocal Leukoencephalopathy (PML)	Characterized by widespread demyelinating lesions (around nerves in the brain and spinal cord) and caused by the JC papovavirus Symptoms: mental deterioration, vision loss, speech disturbances, ataxia, paralysis, brain lesions, and coma Some may have compromised memory and cognition Seizures may occur when CD4 cell counts fall below 200 cells/µL Onset is usually weeks to months	Relentlessly progressive; death usually occurs within 6 months of initial symptoms Typically progresses to severe dementia and death over several months Whether ART improves survival remains controversial Survival correlates with suppression of plasma HIV viral load and higher CD4+ cell counts Death may result not from PML, but from end-stage immunodeficiency Some positive response has been reported with use of cidofovir (Vistide)
Psychological and Neuro-psychiatric Disorders	Occurs in different phases of the HIV infection; may take on various and complex forms Some illnesses are caused directly by HIV infection of the brain, whereas other conditions may be triggered by the drugs used to combat the infection Symptoms include anxiety disorder, depressive disorders, increased thoughts of suicide, paranoia, dementia, delirium, cognitive impairment, confusion, hallucinations, behavioral abnormalities, malaise, and acute mania	Treatment options include antidepressants and anticonvulsants Psychostimulants may also improve depressive symptoms and combat lethargy Antidementia drugs may relieve confusion and slow mental decline Benzodiazepines may be prescribed to treat anxiety Psychotherapy may help
Toxoplasmosis	Caused by the parasite *Toxoplasma gondii* Symptoms include encephalitis, fever, severe headache that does not respond to treatment, weakness on one side of the body, seizures, lethargy, increased confusion, vision problems, dizziness, problems with speaking and walking, vomiting, and personality changes Onset is over days to weeks	Condition is treatable, most improve by day 14 of therapy Generally responsive to intravenous antibiotics, and response to therapy is often rapid Agents of choice are sulfadiazine combined with pyrimethamine and folinic acid; for people with sulfa intolerance, clindamycin is an alternative Steroids may be used to reduce associated swelling in the brain After the initial regimen is completed, oral maintenance treatment, usually TMP-SMX (Bactrim, Septra), is continued indefinitely to suppress reactivation of the parasite Prognosis is linked to parallel treatment with ART to raise CD4 cell count
Tuberculosis Meningitis	Bacterial disease caused by *Mycobacterium tuberculosis* (can be suspended in tiny droplets in the air and transmitted person to person by inhalation) May cause persistent headache, fever, confusion, hemiparesis, seizures, stiff neck, double vision, or hearing loss Hydrocephalus associated with tuberculosis may lead to drowsiness or stupor and, later, coma Spinal cord damage can occur if the vertebrae are infiltrated by TB (Pott disease) or from abscesses inside or outside the spinal cord	Triple antibiotic therapy: isoniazid, rifampin (Rifadin), and pyrazinamide, for 12–24 months is required In cases of drug-resistant TB, a fourth drug, ethionamide (Trecator), should be administered ART should be continued Significant interactions can occur between rifampin and PIs, so an alternative anti-TB drug may be necessary
Vacuolar Myelopathy	Causes the protective myelin sheath to pull away from nerve cells of the spinal cord, forming small holes called *vacuoles* in nerve fibers Symptoms include weak and stiff legs and unsteadiness when walking; walking becomes more difficult as the disease progresses, may necessitate use of a wheelchair	Prognosis is poor, options are limited, and care is primarily supportive May improve after starting ART to stabilize spinal cord damage; maximally potent ART is required l-Methionine (also known as *SAMe,* a common dietary supplement) is an experimental treatment

ART, Antiretroviral therapies; *AZT,* Zidovudine; *CMV,* Cytomegalovirus; *CNS,* central nervous system; *CSF,* cerebrospinal fluid; *FDA,* US Food and Drug Administration; *PI,* protease inhibitor; *PML,* progressive multifocal leukoencephalopathy; *SSRI,* selective serotonin reuptake inhibitor; *TB,* tuberculosis; *TMP-SMX,* trimethoprim-sulfamethoxazole.

TABLE 34.8 Quality-of-Life Assessments in Human Immunodeficiency Virus (HIV) Disease

Outcome Measure	Dimensions	Length and Administration
AIDS Health Assessment Questionnaire (AIDS-HAQ)	Physical function, mental health, cognitive function, social health, energy, and fatigue	30 items Self-administered (5 min)
AIDS Specific Functional Assessment (ASFA)	Evaluates usefulness of functional assessment	Varies Self-administered, care provider
Functional Assessment of Chronic Illness Therapy—Spiritual Well-Being (FACIT-Sp-12)	Faith, meaning, and peace	12 items Self-administered
Functional Multidimensional Evaluation of People with HIV (VFM/HIV)	Self-sufficiency with ADL, economic resources, social resources, physical health, mental health	12 items Self-administered
HIV/AIDS-Targeted Quality of Life (HAT-QOL) Instrument	Overall function, sexual function, disclosure worries, health worries, financial worries, HIV mastery, life satisfaction, medication concerns, provider trust	42 items Self-administered (15 min)
HIV Assessment Tool (HAT)	Physical symptoms related to HIV disease, social and role functioning, psychological well-being, and personal attitudes related to well-being	34 items Self-administered
HIV Disability Questionnaire	Describes the presence, severity and episodic nature of disability experienced by adults living with HIV using six domains of disability	69 items Self-administered (14 min)
HIV Quality Audit Marker (HIV-QAM)	Captures nurse data collector's judgment of status of patient based on observations, interviews, and recorded interviews	Varies based on duration of interview Nurse
HIV-Related Quality-of-Life Questions (HIV-QOL)	Mental health, energy and fatigue, fever, limitations of basic ADL and intermediate ADL, disability days, all symptoms, sleep symptoms, neurological symptoms, memory symptoms, pain	30 items Self-administered (5 min)
HIV Overview of Problems Evaluation System (HOPES)	Global, physical, psychosocial, medical interaction, significant others, sexual components	139 items Self-administered (15 min)
HIV Patient-Assessed Report of Status and Experience (HIV-PARSE)	Physical health, mental health, general health	38 items Self-administered (5 min)
HIV Visual Analog Scale	Rates HIV-related symptom severity and general well-being	Varies Nurse or self-administered
Idiographic Functional Status Assessment (IFSA)	Patient-generated activities associated with pursuit of following goal types: achievement; problem-solving; avoidance-prevention; maintenance; disengagement	75 items Self-administered
Medical Outcomes Study HIV Health Survey (MOS-HIV)	General health perceptions, role functioning, mental health, QOL, pain, social functioning, health distress, physical functioning, energy and fatigue, cognitive function, and health transition	35 items Self-administered or interview (5–10 min)
Multidimensional Quality of Life Questionnaire for Persons with HIV (MQOL-HIV)	Mental health, physical health, physical functioning, social functioning, social support, cognitive functioning, financial status, partner intimacy, sexual functioning, medical care	40 items Self-administered (10 min)
Neuropsychiatric AIDS Rating Scale (NARS)	Assesses patient's orientation, memory, motor ability, behavioral changes, problem-solving ability, and ADL	Varies Health care provider
The Self-Efficacy for Managing Chronic Disease 6-Item Scale	Covers several domains that are common across many chronic diseases: symptom control, role function, emotional functioning, and communicating with physicians; less subject burden than other surveys	6 items Self-administered
World Health Organization-Quality of Life HIV Instrument (WHOQOL-HIV)	Physical, psychological, level of independence, social, environmental, spiritual, general QOL and health, symptoms of HIV, social inclusion, death and dying, forgiveness and fear of death	115 items Self-administered

ADLs, Activities of daily living; *AIDS,* acquired immunodeficiency syndrome.

Peripheral Nervous System

Possible neurological complications associated with HIV disease that may affect the PNS include meningitis, ataxia, myelopathy, and encephalitis. PNS diseases have been reported in up to 50% of HIV-infected individuals, resulting in distal polyneuropathy, Guillain-Barré syndrome, and mononeuropathy.[139]

Distal symmetrical polyneuropathy (DSP) is the most common form of neuropathy in HIV infection, impacting 30% to 60% of PLHIV.[126] The most frequent complaints in DSP are numbness, burning, tightness, allodynia, and paresthesias in the feet. These symptoms are typically symmetrical and often so severe that patients have contact hypersensitivity and gait disturbances. Involvement of the upper extremities and distal weakness may occur later during DSP. Neurological examination shows sensory loss or hyperalgesia to pain and/or temperature in a stocking-glove distribution, decreased vibratory thresholds, and diminished ankle reflexes compared with knee reflexes; proprioception is often spared.[126,140,141] The development of DSP correlates with increased age, increased height, exposure to ART, substance use, diabetes, hypertriglyceridemia, and metabolic syndrome. Predictors for elevated levels of pain are older age, female sex, current and past ART use, lack of virological suppression, lifetime history of opioid use, and depression.[126] The pain associated with DSP typically improves if the individual is started on ART.

The incidence of DSP increases with advancing immunosuppression, in parallel with decreased CD4 counts.[142] Thirty-five percent of patients with advanced HIV may have electrophysiological or clinical abnormalities.[143] Furthermore, pathological evidence of DSP is present in almost all patients who die of AIDS.[144] Various theories regarding the mechanism of DSP have been proposed. It was formerly thought that direct HIV invasion of the nervous system caused DSP[129]; however, most investigators currently believe that this is not the sole cause.[142] A "dying-back" neuropathy affecting all fiber types, with prominent macrophage infiltration of the peripheral nerve, has been described.[144] Additional theories include ART drug toxicity, neurotoxic effects of cytokines, toxicity of HIV proteins, and mitochondrial damage.[145] Cytokines, tumor necrosis factor, and interleukin-1 have been identified in the peripheral nerves of patients with AIDS.[146]

Oral gabapentin and cutaneous lidocaine patches are often prescribed to manage pain associated with peripheral neuropathy. Evidence for physical therapy interventions for DSP is very limited. One randomized controlled trial (RCT) found decreases in pain with use of night splints.[147] Soft tissue massage, joint mobilization, stretching exercise, yoga and low-voltage electroacupuncture,[148] and electrical stimulation have also been proposed, but more research is needed to determine their effectiveness.[149,150]

Certain ART drugs may also contribute to dysfunction of the PNS. Several NRTIs are suspected to contribute directly to peripheral neuropathy through mitochondrial toxicity (especially noted when didanosine and stavudine are used concurrently).[126] The drug stavudine has been linked to HIV-associated neuromuscular weakness syndrome.[126] This syndrome presents with acute, progressive ascending weakness (similar to acute inflammatory demyelinating polyneuropathy), lactic acidosis, and hepatomegaly.[126] Mitochondrial toxicity is thought to be the cause, and treatment is removal of the ART medication (symptoms may continue for 90 days after the drug is discontinued).[126]

Balance and Postural Mechanisms

Balance disturbances may be seen with HIV involvement of either the CNS or PNS. Polyneuropathy caused by AZT (AZT polyneuropathy) and CMV (a common pathogen in advanced HIV) may manifest in the form of a generalized asymmetrical demyelination and chronic denervation of muscles.[151] Demyelination and denervation of nerves that supply postural muscles may weaken such muscles and result in balance problems (e.g., distal pain, paresthesia, numbness, or core weakness). It is also possible that, apart from muscle demyelination and denervation, the pathological process, which also includes macrophage infiltration of neural structures, could spread to affect the vestibular neural complex of the inner ear, which is important in the maintenance of both static and dynamic balance. Clinical reports show that sensory changes are common in the lower limbs of neuropathic HIV/AIDS patients. The balance problems of these patients are likely to be connected to a lack of adequate proprioception from the legs during stance, and it is well known that diminished sensory information makes gait control more difficult. Refer to the discussion of balance dysfunction presented earlier in this text.

Peripheral neuropathy weakens the neuromuscular system and causes a limitation in functional activities. These effects on the neuromuscular system manifest in disturbances of postural control. An appropriate posture should be regarded as the starting position for a functional activity. However, compromise of the postural pattern is so characteristic of HIV peripheral neuropathy that it is diagnostic for HIV-1 infection.[152] The neurological abnormality resulting from peripheral neuropathy in HIV/AIDS produces postural disturbances[153] that may take various forms that worsen with the severity of the neuropathy[154] and compromise functional activity at various levels. This means that as the condition of HIV/AIDS patients deteriorates, balance deficits may increase.

According to Husstedt and colleagues,[155] peripheral neuropathy in HIV disease progresses much more rapidly than that associated with diabetes or hereditary polyneuropathies. Again, because of demyelination as the HIV infection progresses, distal symmetrical peripheral neuropathy increases, resulting in a depression of certain motor functions such as gait and manual dexterity, and a worsening of the condition is caused by demyelination.[155] There is therefore a need to treat HIV neuropathy as soon as it is diagnosed, to avoid complications that lead to impairments in functional mobility. This includes changing type of ART if necessary and evaluating fall risk, promoting pain management and fostering improvement in gait parameter.

One group[77] has identified DSP and its complications as causes of functional limitations in individuals with HIV disease. A patient who, for instance, has balance impairment resulting from peripheral neuropathy may not function effectively with ADLs. Functional impairments may impede a patient's ability to return to gainful employment. For PLHIV, peripheral neuropathy and its resulting pain may be a limiting factor in the ability to complete ADLs and IADLs. Use of the lower-extremity functional scale or the lower limb functional index may assist clinicians in identifying subtle changes over time. Our research showed significant functional differences in patients with DSP versus those without diagnosed HIV-DSP.[156] Emphasis on restoring range of motion through reduction of pain and improvement in ambulation skill can aid in the reduction of functional limitations should be incorporated into the rehabilitation plan of care.

Pain

Pain management is a critical part of the overall care of PLHIV. Pain is the second most common reason for hospitalization of patients with AIDS.[157] A study of 72 AIDS patients found that 97% had pain related to the disease process.[158] Newshan and Wainapel,[158] who surveyed 100 patients who had pain associated with AIDS, showed that the two reported pain types were abdominal and neuropathic pain. In a longitudinal study of HIV-positive men, painful peripheral neuropathy was one of the most common types of pain.[159]

Chronic pain is one of the most prominent and distressing symptoms for PLHIV, and it has a significant effect on QOL and psychological state. Pain may affect patients at any stage of the disease process; however, it is more frequent during the advanced stages. A systematic review in 2014 found the occurrence of moderate to severe pain for PLHIV varies from 54% to 83%[160]; this review also noted that there was less than adequate treatment of pain in the reported studies. Pain is the result of a complex process that involves psychological and neurophysiological mechanisms, and therefore it should be assessed with use of sensitive tools that examine its multi-dimensional nature. One model that evaluates the evaluative, affective, and sensory aspects of pain is the McGill Pain Questionnaire. This assessment tool is useful in evaluating HIV disease-related pain because different causes and nonsensorial factors related to the disease often make clinical assessment of pain difficult.[161]

Chronic pain in PLHIV may be attributable to a specific condition but is often multifactorial; it can be related to direct effects of HIV infection, chronic inflammation and immune activation, side effects of ART drugs or other drugs, neurological mechanisms, comorbidities/multimorbidity, opportunistic infections, aging, psychosocial influences, prescription opioid misuse and heroin use, and/or gender and ethnic differences in perception and expression of pain.[162–164] The most common characteristics of chronic pain in PLHIV are spinal pain, arthralgia, and neuropathic pain.[165] Pain in PLHIV has been shown to greatly increase the odds of impairments in mobility, self-care, and usual activities.[166]

Most PLHIV require various pain treatment interventions. Common options for pain management include nonopioid-based pharmacological therapy (acetaminophen, nonsteroidal antiinflammatory drugs, anticonvulsants, antidepressants, and topical agents), opioid therapy (which is no longer supported as the choice intervention for chronic pain), and nonpharmacological approaches (including cognitive-behavioral therapy, acupuncture, and physical therapy); recent findings are supporting that these nonpharmacological approaches to chronic pain are the most effective.[164,167] A 2016 review found that of 11 studies of pharmacological and nonpharmacological treatments for chronic pain in PLHIV, only capsaicin and cannabis have positive results.[167] There is a paucity of published research regarding physical therapy and other nonpharmaceutical interventions to manage chronic pain in PLHIV, although there some evidence to suggest a favorable role for exercise, self-management programs, and patient education.[168–170]

As discussed previously, distal symmetrical peripheral neuropathy has been shown to be the most common peripheral neuropathy complaint in patients with HIV-1 infection.[171–173] Peripheral neuropathy is one of the most common types of pain in HIV-positive men,[159] and peripheral neuropathies occur in as many as 40% to 60% of PLHIV. Peripheral neuropathy is the most prevalent neurological complication associated with HIV. CNS or PNS involvement has been found in 30% to 63% of patients across the arena of HIV and is often related to ART.[174] When neuropathy results in distal painful paresthesia, imbalance in stance and gait may result from compensatory measures aimed at relieving pain in dynamic standing activities. Postural compensations may further exacerbate musculoskeletal, cervical, thoracic, or lumbosacral back pain. DSP results in painful paresthesias that are challenging to treat with pharmacological interventions. Refer to the earlier section on the Peripheral Nervous System for more about management of pain associated with DSP.

Psychopathology

Medical and neuropsychiatric sequelae of HIV infection present a spectrum of diagnostic and treatment challenges to health care practitioners. Both HIV infection and the various opportunistic infections that manifest in patients as the result of an immunocompromised state

can affect the CNS. Epidemiological studies indicate that greater than 60% of PLHIV will experience at least one major psychiatric disorder during their infection. Depression is the most common disorder, closely followed by anxiety and substance abuse disorders.[175] It is estimated that between 18% and 81% of PLHIV will experience depression[176]; this may be further impacted by ART side effects. A 2017 systematic review attempted to determine the prevalence of anxiety in PLHIV. The study found a median value for anxiety disorders to be 22.85% (nearly 5% higher than the general population); this can be divided into panic disorders at 10.26% (7% higher than the general population), generalized anxiety disorder 5.6% (2% higher than the general population), and social anxiety disorder 9.1% (3% higher than the general population).[177] Studies have found that high levels of anxiety are related to lower QOL, poor medication compliance, and higher frequency of substance abuse.[177] Therefore therapists need to be familiar with the diagnosis and management of HIV infection–related medical and psychiatric disorders. These disorders have a great impact on the outcomes of rehabilitation.

Careful consideration of psychological function is warranted during clinical encounters with PLHIV. HIV-related psychopathologies mimic many previously described consequences of primary HIV infection, opportunistic infections, and drug side effects. These psychiatric complications can be affective or organic. Indicators include disturbances in sleep and appetite patterns, diminished memory and energy, psychomotor retardation, withdrawal, apathy, and emotional liability. Anxiety disorders (particularly posttraumatic stress disorder), adjustment reactions, reactive and endogenous depressions, and obsessive disorders frequently result.[178–180]

With use of the American Psychiatric Association's *Diagnostic and Statistical Manual of Mental Disorders,* Fourth Edition, Text Revision, one study found axis I disorders (excluding substance abuse) in 61.9% of the subjects.[181] Indeed, the virus's affinity with subcortical structures of the CNS that regulate affect and mood supports research indicating a prevalence of manic episodes that is 10 times higher than in the general population.[182] Manic episodes have been identified at all stages of the disease process and may also occur in response to AZT therapy.[21,52,183] When associated with HIV infection, mania appears to be secondary to structural CNS changes.[184,185] Described manic episodes generally respond well to psychiatric medications and may not recur.[52,186–188]

Analyses of new-onset psychosis among PLHIV yielded the following information. Psychotic episodes are preceded by a period (days to months) of affective and behavioral changes.[189] Admitting diagnoses to psychiatric units included "undifferentiated schizophrenia, schizophreniform disorder, "reactive psychosis," atypical psychosis, depression with psychotic features and mania."[189] Some psychiatric diagnoses were revised during the course of hospitalization to "AIDS encephalitis, cryptococcal meningitis, or 'organic psychosis.'"[190] Eighty-seven percent of the subjects in one study displayed delusions that were usually persecutory, grandiose, or somatic. Affective disturbances were present in 81% of the subjects. Hallucinations and thought process disorders were each prominent in 61% of patients. Several subjects received the diagnosis of AIDS during their psychiatric hospitalization.[190]

Remarkable progress has been made in recent years in the therapeutics of HIV-associated dementia. Viral replication in and outside the CNS has been greatly reduced by ART. This has resulted in partial repair of cellular immune function with improvement in, and prevention of, neurological deficits associated with HIV disease.[191] Extensive use of PIs is associated with dramatic declines in overall mortality and morbidity, including HIV-associated dementia.[44,192]

Neuropathological abnormalities seen in the brain tissue of patients with HIV-associated dementia are usually diffuse and predominantly localized to the white and deep gray matter regions. Myelin pallor and inflammatory infiltrates composed of macrophages and multinucleated giant cells are the hallmarks of this disease process, although a spectrum of lesions has been identified from encephalitis to leukoencephalopathy.[193,194] The characteristic clinical feature of HIV-associated dementia is disabling cognitive impairment, often accompanied by behavioral changes, motor dysfunction, or both.[194] Degrees of impairment have been recorded, and a five-part staging system was subsequently developed.[195–197] Motoric manifestations of HIV dementia complex include gait disturbances, intention tremor, and abnormal release of reflexes.

Differentiation between psychiatric and physiological manifestations is complicated. Psychiatric and organic disorders are initially indistinguishable based on behavior and may exist concurrently. Furthermore, other primary disease processes and drug reactions imitate psychopathological conditions. Differentiation is nonetheless essential because many disorders respond well to established therapies, both psychological and pharmacological, once differential diagnoses have been established. Research is supporting the use of psychosocial interventions, such as cognitive-behavioral therapy, over the previously preferred pharmacological interventions.[198] Awareness of the intricate interplay of all factors is essential for competent rehabilitative efforts for PLHIV.

PEDIATRIC HUMAN IMMUNODEFICIENCY VIRUS INFECTION

Pediatric HIV infection differs from that most commonly seen in adults. Symptoms develop much earlier in pediatric patients compared with adults. Children infected with HIV may be classified as "rapid progressors" or "slow progressors." Rapid progressors are children infected with HIV who manifest symptoms within the first 12 to 24 months of life. These children progress quickly to AIDS-defining conditions and have a rapid decline in CD4 count. Children who are slow progressors have a more gradual progression of symptoms and are likely to show evidence of immune system compromise by 7 to 8 years of age. A small percentage of children remain healthy and have only nominal or no symptoms of the disease and a normal to slightly decreased CD4 count through 9 to 10 years of age.[199]

An accurate understanding of the timing of HIV transmission from mother to fetus is important for the design of intervention strategies. The AIDS Clinical Trial Group (ACTG) study 076, which included treatment from the 14th week of gestation in women with CD4 counts of more than 200/μL, prompts other considerations.[200] Onset of HIV-1 infection in children has a wide spectrum of clinical manifestations.[201] Thus prevention of transmission from mother to fetus via ART is a critical component of managing this worldwide epidemic. The WHO recommends that all HIV-positive women who are pregnant or breastfeeding should receive ART regardless of clinical stage or CD4 count.[202] Without ART intervention, transmission rates from HIV positive mother to child range from 15% to 45%; with effective treatment, the transmission rate is less than 5%.[202] In 2016, clinical guidelines recommended starting ART in all pediatric HIV cases, regardless of age or immunological status.[203] Support for this recommendation resulted from the findings of the South African Children with HIV Early Antiretroviral Therapy (CHER) randomized trial; this study showed a reduction in mortality by 76% among infants randomized to immediate ART, compared with those who were given deferred ART.[203]

Pediatric HIV is neurotrophic in nature in that the virus most often initially affects the CNS rather than the PNS. As the virus spreads, pediatric HIV patients can have CNS disorders that include encephalopathy, pyramidal tract signs, receptive and expressive language difficulties, cognitive deficits, psychomotor impairments, and upper respiratory infections.[199] Neuroimaging shows HIV has an influence on neurological function in the basal ganglia, frontal cortex, and other connecting structures in the CNS. Studies also support that there is an environmental component that contributes to developmental and behavioral issues in HIV-positive children.[204]

In the first year of life, severe immunodeficiency develops in 15% to 20% of pediatric patients with serious recurrent infections or neurological dysfunction, whereas in school-age children the disease progresses more slowly and the risk for development of HIV-related encephalopathy becomes less.[205] Some infants have features of severe immunodeficiency, whereas others have nonspecific findings, such as hepatosplenomegaly, failure to thrive, unexplained fever, parotitis, and recurrent gastroenteritis. Adenopathy is common, and salivary gland enlargement occurs more frequently than in adults. Otitis media and measles, despite immunization, are also more frequent complications in children.[67,107] Cardiac involvement in children with HIV infection is a well-known entity and occurs clinically more often in patients with advanced disease.[206]

Studies have shown that children diagnosed with HIV demonstrate behaviors often associated with attention-deficit/hyperactivity disorder (ADHD), including impulsivity, hyperactivity, difficulty attending, and decreased ability to focus on stimuli. In one study, the most common behavioral issues were psychosomatic disorders (28%), learning disorders (25%), hyperactivity (20%), impulsive-hyperactive disorder (19%), conduct problems (16%), and anxiety (8%); standardized intelligence scores were lower compared with established population norms. Hyperactivity was more common in children with a Wechsler IQ less than 90, anxiety issues were more common in children older than 9 years, and conduct disorders were more often seen in children with CD4 counts less than 660 cells/μL.[204] HIV-positive children are noted to have lower cognitive and motor development scores on standardized testing, as compared with healthy, unexposed children.[207] In one study, HIV-positive children who had exposure to ART scored worse than HIV-positive children who were untreated.[207] This result should be interpreted cautiously; it does not indicate that children should not be treated, but it does provoke concerns about the impact of potentially neurotoxic medications in the developing brain.

Children are also susceptible to disorders seen in adults, especially opportunistic infections such as herpesvirus, pneumonia, toxoplasmosis, meningitis, and encephalitis. HIV encephalopathy is noted to have the most serious side effects because of its progressive deteriorating pattern and associated CNS abnormalities,[23] although static encephalopathy can be characterized by severely delayed cognitive functioning and neuromotor skills without deterioration.[208] Manifestations in children include cerebral atrophy, ataxia, rigidity, hyperreflexia, and the inability to achieve or sustain developmental milestones. Although the HIV neurodevelopmental involvement causes a prognostic worsening, most studies of pediatric cases of advanced HIV with neurological involvement demonstrate that an early diagnosis followed by adequate antiretroviral therapeutic regimens can lead to significant, even if temporary, improvement.[205]

Rehabilitation of the pediatric patient requires a multidisciplinary approach to meet the medical, emotional, and psychosocial needs of these children and their families. Children are encouraged to give form to their psychological experiences through play, writing or telling stories, and creating works of art.[209]

REHABILITATION INTERVENTIONS

The examination procedures for HIV illness are broadly outlined in the following paragraphs. Of course, each case brings about its

BOX 34.1 Evaluation Procedures for Human Immunodeficiency Virus Disease

Baseline Data (Premorbid Functional Level)
Accustomed life roles
Medical comorbidities

Stage in Disease Process
Psychosocial Issues
Coping mechanisms
Social support system
Financial resources

Cognitive/Perceptual Status
Reality orientation
Memory
Organizational skills
Visual perception
Motor planning
Safety awareness
Judgment

Communication
Oral language
Written language
Language comprehension

Sensorimotor Status
Strength
Reflexes
Muscle tone
Gait
Balance
Coordination
Kinesthesia
Proprioception
Sensation and pain

Activities of Daily Living (ADLs)
Bathing
Feeding
Dressing
Housework
Grooming and hygiene
Activity tolerance
Avocational interests
Community management
Other self-care regimens (e.g., medications)

What is the relationship of the PLHIV to the environment, both at present and in the future? The rehabilitation therapist should keep this question in mind throughout the examination process. In this context the term *environment* is meant to include not only the physical aspects of surroundings but also the psychological and emotional climate in which the individual functions (see Table 34.1).

The examination process has a different focus for different stages of the disease. If the patient is in the early stages of the disease, the therapist should determine whether she or he is still managing in accustomed life roles. Important issues may include new or adapted vocational and leisure skills. During the advanced stage, the focus may change to more basic daily functional concerns and ADLs. However, the therapist must remember that the patient may place more importance on participation in avocational interests than on independent self-care. This choice is valid and must be respected and supported by health care professionals. If the patient is evaluated in an inpatient setting, another crucial determination to be made is whether the person is to be discharged to home or some other supervised setting. It is critical to determine what kind of community-based support networks are available to the individual. Case managers or social workers are often adept at identifying home and community resources available and will assist in setting up these resources before the patient's discharge. Rehabilitation professionals need to collaborate with a variety of health care providers to achieve optimal outcomes for PLHIV. This includes physicians, nurses, social workers, case managers, recreational therapists, physical therapists, occupational therapists, speech-language pathologists, occupational health and safety officials, psychologists, and any other professions that may play a role in assisting the patient maximize their physical and emotional well-being.

Astute evaluative questions about the psychosocial status of the patient include the following:
- Does the patient's perception of his or her status and prognosis agree with that of the treatment team?
- What is the patient's predominant coping style?
- Who are the patient's caregivers?
- What is the social support system?
- What is the patient's home environment?
- What is the patient's prior level of function?

The support system can be a critical issue for many PLHIV, especially those who are part of the high-risk groups, such as homosexual and bisexual men and intravenous drug users.[210] Many of these people have traditional networks of family, spouse, and friends; a significant number have equally strong nontraditional support systems. Some will be lacking in the kinds of support needed to cope with the devastating physical and emotional effects of the disease and the need for chronic medical interventions.

It is possible to use models developed for oncology and progressive neurological disorders for HIV involvement of the CNS and PNS. An orthopedic approach may be taken when pain is a presenting factor or biomechanical alterations are a result of other disease processes. Functional fluctuations that characterize HIV infection and secondary infections must be understood; the therapist must appreciate the effects that HIV infection has on various body systems and the resultant secondary complications.

The examination of an individual who has HIV disease should include standard cognitive, perceptual, and sensory and motor function evaluative tools. The idiosyncratic nature of the disease may necessitate more detailed evaluation of these specific areas. It is recommended that cognitive and perceptual evaluations are both formal and observational. Safety, judgment, functional mobility, ADL management, community management skills, and independent financial management skills need to be assessed. Evaluation of the systemic

own unique challenges, and the evaluation process is individualized according to the specific needs of the patient (Box 34.1). Due to the widespread use of ART and improved health education program, HIV is currently considered a chronic disease, characterized by episodic disability, rather than the progressive decline to AIDS. PLHIV who are on a successful ART regimen are able to live normal life-spans and be more productive in their own lives and in their communities. Rehabilitation professionals are seeing a different HIV patient as compared with when the epidemic first began. A condition once characterized by opportunistic infections and wasting syndrome is currently characterized by obesity, lipodystrophy, and CVD; this requires rehabilitation professionals to take a more holistic approach to patient care and will require interprofessional collaboration to achieve optimal patient outcomes.

complications of HIV infection is necessary for optimal rehabilitative planning and treatment team efficacy.

The ADL evaluation is best made within the context of the immediate and projected life roles of the individual. Maximal independent functioning is the goal of rehabilitation, whatever the stage of illness. If the person is at home or is being discharged to home, a crucial component of the ADL examination is the assessment of community management skills; consider the individual's access to transportation, socialization opportunities, shopping, and banking. The ability to negotiate health care and insurance systems and participate in community activities is critical to returning to independence. Many PLHIV and their caregivers have minimal experience with disability because of their age or social status. This, combined with the stressors of a chronic illness, can create unrealistic expectations and unnecessary frustrations.

Rehabilitation Process

The neuromuscular rehabilitation intervention procedures for HIV infection and an overview of treatment techniques for opportunistic infections are presented in Box 34.2.

Cognitive deficits in attention, concentration, and memory necessitate consistency, structure, and environmental cues to minimize

---

BOX 34.2 Neuromuscular Rehabilitation Intervention Procedures for Human Immunodeficiency Virus Disease

Psychosocial Intervention
Facilitation of the expression of grief
Validation and education of caregivers

Cognitive and Perceptual Intervention
Rehabilitation
Maintenance
Compensation (including communication)

Sensory and Motor Intervention
Sensory stimulation
Tone normalization
Balance and coordination activities
Maintenance of strength, range of motion, and endurance
Functional mobility (including assistive devices and adaptive equipment)

Pain Control
Psychological modalities
Behavioral modalities
Physical modalities

Training in Activities of Daily Living (ADLs)
Energy conservation
Transfer training
Self-care retraining
Work simplification
Community management skills
Leisure or avocational skill development
Recommendations for adaptive equipment

Continuity of Care
Discharge planning and follow-up care
Community linkages
Social support services

---

confusion. Safety and judgment deficits can be countered by environmental adaptations. Lethargic patients benefit from sensory enhancement. Maintenance of endurance, strength, and passive and active range of motion are important components of any motor function treatment plan. Neuromuscular facilitation and inhibition, positioning, and splinting are feasible modalities to normalize tone as needed. Gait training, the use of assistive devices, training in motor planning, balance activities, and endurance exercises may be appropriate.

In addition to techniques and modalities, active listening, empathy, and unconditional positive regard are important aspects of the therapeutic process. The clinician must set aside personal biases and beliefs to accurately hear the perspective of the individual patient. The use of expressive modalities facilitates the development of coping skills while providing appropriate exploration and release of powerful emotions. Human touch can counter the powerful and isolating effect of fear of contagion. Rehabilitation therapists can demonstrate and educate caregivers about the safety and benefit of therapeutic touch.

Motoric manifestations of HAND and HIV infection–related dementia include gait disturbances, intention tremor, and abnormal release of reflexes. Rehabilitation and progression of independent functional mobility become more complex in these patients secondary to the cognitive involvement.

Pain management is best approached through a biopsychosocial lens. Pain reduction is achieved through training in cognitive-behavioral therapy, meditation, breathing techniques, visualization, progressive muscle relaxation, autogenics, music, meditation, and engagement in meaningful activities. Various forms of electrotherapy such as electroacupuncture, thermal agents, and manual therapy are useful therapeutic tools.

The impact of HIV infection can be evident in cerebral, emotional, psychosocial, and other physical domains, affecting the PLHIV and those around her or him. The prognosis and psychological and physical consequences of HIV infection are associated with significant emotional distress and clinical syndromes, such as adjustment disorders, depression, and anxiety in some patients.[211] Increasing focus is being placed on the potential impact of HIV infection–related stress on the course of infection because of the observed and postulated relationship between psychosocial stress, neuropsychological functioning, and immune status.[212] Minimizing stressful events throughout the management of chronic HIV infection can be approached in various ways, such as meditation, cognitive-behavioral therapy, relaxation, and various forms of exercise.

Exercise

Exercise is an intervention commonly used by movement specialists to address a multitude of impairment and functional limitations. Thus understanding of the implications of the HIV disease process on exercise prescription is important. A review of published studies[213] on the effects of exercise on individuals with HIV disease revealed the following: (1) although intense bouts of exercise may result in transient immunosuppression, there is no evidence that regular exercise by individuals with HIV disease results in a detrimental effect on the immune system over time, (2) some studies have shown actual improvement in immune system function in response to regular exercise, (3) improved cardiovascular function has been observed in response to aerobic exercise, and (4) resisted exercise may be effective in counteracting the effects of wasting syndrome and improving strength and lean body mass. A systematic review of progressive resistive exercise (PRE) showed that PRE or a combination of PRE and aerobic exercises lead to statistically significant increases in weight, arm girth, and thigh girth. Trends were also found supporting an improvement in submaximal heart rate and exercise time. In addition, PRE was found to contribute to improved strength and psychological status and to be safe and beneficial for medically stable HIV-positive adults.[214]

From a psychoneuroimmunological perspective, psychological stress has been implicated among the cofactors that contribute to the immunological decline in HIV disease. Good evidence supports the stress management role of exercise training to explain a buffering of these suppressive stressor effects, thereby facilitating a return of the CD4 cells. Early intervention with exercise, in compliance with guidelines, is most prudent to stave off opportunistic infections throughout the spectrum of HIV disease.

Precautions and Concerns During Exercise

It is important to address any orthopedic or neurological concerns before embarking on an exercise or movement therapy program. If musculoskeletal problems exist or other pain symptoms are present, a concerted effort to modulate pain is necessary for the successful completion of an exercise regimen.[215] If HIV-related peripheral neuropathy exists, it is important to implement proper foot care and supportive shoes when weight-bearing activities are performed.[77,216] In addition, appropriate safety measures, such as guarding during balance activities, should take place when working on exercise programs with patients who have decreased balance and postural stability.

There is some concern about aerobic exercise increasing the body's metabolic rate and thus increasing additional muscle loss. However, with a balanced diet and incorporation of a sound nutritional program, this should not pose a problem for the asymptomatic PLHIV. If wasting is present, the cause needs to be addressed and treatment rendered.[53] One study determined the contribution of total energy expenditure to weight changes in individuals with HIV infection–related wasting. The researchers observed a significant positive relation between total energy expenditure and the rate of weight change. During rapid weight loss, total energy expenditure fell from an average 2750 kcal/day to 2189 kcal/day. The key determinant of weight loss in HIV infection–related wasting, they concluded, was reduced energy intake, not increased energy expenditure.[217]

If fatigue is present as a symptom, a differential diagnosis for anemia, low albumin, low testosterone levels, and/or specific vitamin deficiencies must be made before any exercise regimen is begun. Proper caloric intake must be adequate to meet the energy expenditure required for the activity. Seeking the advice of a nutritionist is recommended for proper guidance. Education about sleep hygiene may also be beneficial if restorative sleep is not being achieved.

Evidence of autonomic neuropathy (a peripheral neuropathy that affects involuntary body functions including heart rate, blood pressure, perspiration, and digestive functions) on provocative testing is common in HIV infection, with estimates of incidence ranging from 30% to 60%.[218,219] Underlying cardiac parasympathetic dysfunction may need to be assessed throughout the course of HIV disease. One method described by Mallet and coworkers[220] is the use of the 4-second exercise test, which consists of pedaling an uploaded ergometer at maximal individual speed from the fourth to the eighth second of a 12-second maximal inspiratory apnea. From an electrocardiogram, vagal activity is estimated through a ratio. In that study, subjects were subjected to respiratory sinus arrhythmia, which is a valid method to detect vagal dysfunction. The researchers found that there was a tendency for lower values of the vagal function test in HIV-positive subjects. Vital sign monitoring is prudent throughout any exercise regimen. Exercise can help control long-term side effects, including altered body composition; elevated cholesterol, triglyceride, and blood glucose levels; and elevated blood pressure.[221] Certain comorbidities associated with HIV disease, such as inflammatory myopathy, acute infectious arthritis, or compromised cardiac status, may result in restrictions on exercise prescription.[213]

A supervised training program should be consistent with recommendations of the American College of Sports Medicine. Guidelines have been established for the spectrum of the stages of HIV disease.[221] During the stage of asymptomatic HIV disease, there are no limitations on maximum graded exercise testing. Exercise should consist of resistance training, cardiovascular training, flexibility training, balance training, and mind-body training.[221] In this stage, all metabolic parameters are within normal limits for most individuals. Thus unrestricted activity is generally encouraged. Most sports do not pose a significant risk of HIV transmission. However, sports such as boxing, in which there is a risk of open wounds and contamination with infected blood, should be viewed with great caution.[213]

Exercise is safe and beneficial for most individuals with HIV disease; however, caution is warranted with symptomatic HIV disease and advanced HIV disease. In individuals with symptomatic HIV disease, there may be reduced exercise capacity, Vo_{2max}, and oxygen (O_2) pulse max. There may also be other cardiovascular and pulmonary problems, anemia, and peripheral muscle abnormalities. Pain, side effects of medications, psychosocial issues, and unplanned events may also create obstacles to exercise for individuals in the symptomatic or advanced stage of HIV disease. For individuals with cardiac myopathy or hyperlipidemia, submaximal aerobic capacity testing should be followed with a staged cardiac rehabilitation program[91] because of the risk of cardiac failure in patients with compromised cardiac status.[222]

Patients with AIDS have dramatically reduced exercise capacity, vital capacity, Vo_{2max}, and O_2 pulse max. Elevated heart rate and breathing reserve persist in this stage. Neurological dysfunction, opportunistic infections, and progressive disability indicate a need for careful monitoring of the exercise program during this stage of the disease. In general, individuals with advanced HIV disease should remain physically active and exercise on a symptom-limited basis. Precautions related to comorbidities should be implemented. Individuals in this stage of the disease are at greater risk for exercise-induced injuries as a result of chronic tissue changes in both muscle and peripheral nerve. For individuals with severe morbidity and extensive disability, treatment should emphasize enhancement of basic functional tasks, ADLs, and energy conservation.[213]

As the number of older adults with HIV increases, it is important to analyze increased risk for frailty. Frailty indices have been used to establish diagnostic criteria. However, it is generally recognized as an accumulation of deficits in functional capacity and ability to perform ADLs. Using the Fried phenotype, PLHIV can be evaluated for (1) unintentional weight loss; (2) reduced walking speed; (3) weakness as measured by a grip dynamometer; (4) exhaustion by responses to a depression scale; and (5) low physical activity determined by assessing caloric expenditure.[223] Frailty may be present in up to half of older adults living with HIV and is associated with significant morbidity and mortality risk in this group.[224] Frailty in HIV can either be transient, and linked to the status of HIV-infection, or resemble a more typical gradual decline in functional capacity. Several tools have been developed and adapted to assess different domains of frailty, yet medical treatment of this condition can be complex and should include interprofessional management with appropriate medication, nutrition services, and exercise interventions. However, few concrete strategies have been developed to prevent, or treat, frailty in the context of HIV infection.[224]

Psychoneuroimmunology: Prevention and Wellness in Human Immunodeficiency Virus Infection

Psychoneuroimmunology-based interventions are used to attenuate disease progression and/or side effects of pharmacological treatment. It is the field that investigates the interrelationships among psychological constructs (e.g., stressors and mood states) of the neuroendocrine and immune systems. Psychoneuroimmunology offers a useful framework for our understanding of how stressors play a role in immunomodulation. The progression of HIV disease can be modulated by psychosocial factors and by factors such as the viral strain, genetic characteristics of the host immune system, coinfections with other pathogenic organisms, and health maintenance habits (diet, exercise, medical treatments).[225] These factors may have a profound influence on the occurrence and progression of ill health in chronic diseases such as HIV infection.

Findings of studies related to psychoneuroimmunology suggest that it is useful to evaluate the influence of behavioral factors on immune functioning and disease progression in PLHIV.[226–228] The stress response is physiologically mediated by certain immune parameters (catecholamines and glucocorticoid hormones). A study by Leserman and colleagues[229] in 2002 concluded that "stressful life events, dysphoric mood, and limited social support" are correlated to the increased rate of progression from initial HIV infection to AIDS.[229] Behavioral interventions with immunomodulatory capabilities may help to restore competence and thereby slow the progression of HIV disease, especially at the earliest stages of the infectious continuum.

A growing body of literature indicates that many different stressors have deleterious effects on the immune system.[230] It has been well documented in healthy individuals that changes in immune function and disease susceptibility are correlated with times of "psychic distress."[225] These stressors in the case of PLHIV infection may be attenuated by an exercise training program. Research indicates that continued aerobic exercise training may result in increased CD4 cell counts, heightened immune surveillance, and a potential for a slowing of disease progression.[228] Other researchers have demonstrated similar benefits of exercise for PLHIV who are at more advanced stages of disease. However, these are studies conducted on traditional modes of exercise and do not investigate alternative activities such as yoga or tai chi.

A recent systematic review evaluated the different therapeutic and/or clinical psychoneuroimmunology-based interventions associated to both psychological, neuroendocrine, and immunological variables. Decreased levels of epinephrine, norepinephrine, and cortisol were associated to interventions including tai chi, yoga, meditation, acupuncture, mindfulness, religious/spiritual practices, cognitive behavior therapy, coping, and physical exercises. From a biophysical perspective, those interventions were also associated with reduced inflammatory processes and proinflammatory cytokines in cancer, HIV, depression, anxiety, wound healing, sleep disorder, CVD, and fibromyalgia.[231] A holistic rehabilitation approach to PLHIV is key to successful outcomes.

Complementary and Integrative Therapies in Human Immunodeficiency Virus Infection

There is substantial evidence to suggest that traditional, aerobic, and progressive resistance exercises can provide notable physiological and psychological benefits for most individuals, especially those with chronic diseases. However, the mode, duration, and intensity of many traditional standardized exercise programs may not always be entirely appropriate during episodic illness. The stage of disease and the type of illness itself may preclude more strenuous exercise activities at various times. During such times, less strenuous movement therapies may prove to be more appropriate and efficacious. In fact, movement therapy includes several similar constructs used in physical therapy and can be quite complementary to an individual's program of more traditional exercise.[232,233] Refer to Chapter 39 for additional information.

The US National Center for Complementary and Integrative Health (NCCIH), formerly National Center for Complementary and Integrative Medicine (NCCIM), established five medical system categories: whole medical systems, mind-body medicine, biologically based practices, manipulative and body-based practices, and energy therapies. Whole medical systems include homeopathy, naturopathy, traditional Chinese medicine and Ayurveda. Mind-body medicine includes meditation, prayer, mental healing, tai chi, yoga, art therapy, music therapy, and dance therapy. Biologically based practices include dietary and herbal supplements. Manipulative and body-based practices include massage and spinal manipulation. Energy-based therapies include qi gong, reiki, therapeutic touch, healing touch, and electromagnetic therapy. The NCCIM, the Alternative Medicine's Strategic Plan, and the Healthy People 2020 envision a society in which all people live long, healthy lives.[234,235]

Research findings indicate that the use of complementary and integrative medicine (CIM) is often greater among people living with a chronic or life-threatening illness compared with the general population. For example, chronic pain occurs in as many as 85% of individuals with HIV and is associated with substantial functional impairment, and many PLHIV seek integrative therapies for relief.[167] Little guidance is available for HIV providers seeking to address their patients' chronic pain, especially in the current opioid epidemic in the United States. A recent systematic review found seven studies examined pharmacological interventions (gabapentin, pregabalin, capsaicin, analgesics including opioids) and four examined nonpharmacological interventions (cognitive behavioral therapy, self-hypnosis, smoked cannabis). The only controlled studies with positive results were of capsaicin and cannabis and had short-term follow-up ($\leq$12 weeks).[167]

Recent investigators evaluated the experiences and perceptions of people using integrative therapies considering the prevalence of CIM use within this population. In the United States and Canada, the rate of CIM use among HIV-positive persons is approximately 50% to 70%, whereas in Africa, rates of CIM use range from 36% to 68%. Popular forms of CIM among PLHIV include herbal or nutritional supplements, mind and body practices, and spiritual or religious healing. Worldwide, only a small percentage of persons who have access to ART refuse to take them and use CIM exclusively to treat their HIV infection.[236]

PLHIV with HIV often report using CIM because of side effects of medication, and they believe these therapies will improve their overall health and well-being. Furthermore, it provides an opportunity to take some responsibility in managing their personal health. Understanding CIM use is essential so that health professionals will have the most accurate information about which integrative therapies may or may not be helpful for PLHIV.[236] The Institute of Medicine report entitled *Integrative Medicine and Patient Centered Care* encourages health professionals to find innovative ways of obtaining evidence and expanding knowledge about diverse interpretations of health and healing.[237]

The HIV epidemic has resulted in an increase use of integrative therapies, some more traditional than others.[222] Estimates show that 53% of PLHIV in the United States report the use of at least one CIM therapy.[238] Approximately one-third of HIV patients in a recent cross-sectional study used CIM, but virtually none informed their health care provider. Medicinal herbs were the most common type of CIM, followed by spiritual therapy and vitamins, and a patient's decision to use CIM was influenced for the most part by the mass media and nonhospital health care personnel.[239] This is concerning because drug-herb interactions may render ineffective ART for viral suppression. Given people's diverse health-seeking practices, biomedical providers need to recognize the cultural importance of traditional health practices and routinely initiate respectful discussion of traditional medicine use with individuals from various cultural contexts.[240]

The impact of yoga has shown promise for PLHIV. A significant improvement in QOL scores was observed for three health-related QOL domains through Sudarshan Kriya yoga, with improvements in physical and psychological states of PLHIV.[241] A pilot study incorporating yoga and meditation showed a high level of feasibility and acceptability and modest effects on measures of QOL among PLHIV who use crack cocaine.[242] Yoga is a safe and inexpensive format to improve QOL in a population that has many medical difficulties and extenuating stressors.[242] Research has shown yoga has impact on HIV-related neuropathy with improvements in flexibility, balance, and gait speed.[150] Further yoga-based research is needed to explore the many complex dimensions of chronic HIV disease. Overall, use of integrative therapies can have preventative and additive impact on holistic treatment of PLHIV.

Social Interactions and the Association With Disease Management

The process of grieving is often mistakenly associated solely with the death of another. It is a natural reaction to loss, including the loss of one's own health and diminished independence. Loss of abstract human qualities, such as perceived attractiveness and productivity, results in grief. Such emotions are often difficult for a patient to articulate. It is the therapist's responsibility to be sensitive to the patient's individualized grief pattern (see Chapter 5).

Placement issues accompany discharge planning from acute health care facilities. The rehabilitation professional is often called on to make recommendations regarding the level of assistance the patient will need. All the previously discussed areas of cognitive-perceptual, sensorimotor, and ADL management, combined with available psychosocial and practical support, influence these recommendations. Options include a return to independent living and work, assisted independent living with help from a loved one, home with supportive services (often supplied by community-based AIDS organizations), home with hospital-based home care, hospice, assisted living facility, level I (inpatient acute) rehabilitation, level II (subacute) rehabilitation, or an extended care facility.

Literature on long-term survivors with advanced HIV is replete with anecdotal evidence linking survival to one or more of the following: (1) holding a positive attitude toward the illness, (2) participating in health-promoting behaviors, (3) engaging in spiritual activities, and (4) taking part in advocacy activities related to the HIV community.[195,243,244] Positive relationships have been demonstrated between hardiness and perception of physical, emotional, and spiritual health, participation in exercise, and the use of special diets.[245–247]

Research provides support for the hypothesis that interpersonal relationships influence patterns of physiological functions. Data from experimental studies have shown that social contact can serve to reduce physiological stress responses.[248,249] Community-based studies have also shown negative associations between reported levels of support and physiological parameters such as serum cholesterol, uric acid, and urinary epinephrine levels.[249] Studies of immune function have demonstrated that social relationships have both positive and negative impacts on immune function. Loss of a partner to cancer or HIV, family caregiving for patients with Alzheimer disease, and divorce or poor marital quality all show negative associations with immune function, whereas more supportive relationships are associated with better immune function.[230]

Exercise and movement therapy in a group context may provide the socialization necessary to foster these physiological changes and adherence to an exercise regimen. Another area of potential socialization is the workplace. The QOL issues for PLHIV are becoming more complicated as more people with the disease achieve higher CD4 counts and lower viral load levels. Improvement in health status is directly related to the improved effectiveness of newer treatment regimens, and many individuals are improving enough to either continue working or reenter the work force. Exercise and movement therapy may augment the stress and fatigue that may be associated with the adjustment to the workplace.

▍ SUMMARY

Research and resultant treatments are extending lives so that more people require rehabilitative services that maximize function and QOL. Medical management has focused on the treatment of reducing viral load, preventing secondary illnesses, and improving the immunological status of those with chronic HIV disease. Examination of the neuromusculoskeletal system and interventions for PLHIV disease are similar to those for other progressive neuromusculoskeletal disorders. HIV disease should be addressed like other life-altering diseases such as cancer, but with an emphasis on cognitive and perceptual function. Rehabilitation interventions should focus on specific impairments, disabilities, and psychosocial ramifications of the disease. Adaptive compensations, mobility, ADL retraining, pain control, and community management skills constitute a well-developed treatment plan.

The HIV epidemic is a major challenge on both a personal and professional level because of the continued natural fear of contagion. The illness originally appeared in subcultures that are often disenfranchised. Social, racial, economic status, and controversial behaviors contribute to prejudice, fear, and limited access to health care. Rehabilitation professionals have responded significantly to this challenge. Continued advocacy and compassion combined with professional enlightenment will, in a small way, alter the course of the disease.

Future Directions for Research

Although the primary focus of most research into HIV is focused on the eradication of the disease through potential vaccine development and expanding the development of effective pharmaceutical interventions that eliminate disease progression, transmission, and HIV drug resistance, novel treatments based on immunotherapy, which has been showing great promise in cancer research and clinical treatments, may prove to be an approach to treating and preventing HIV disease.

Research also needs to focus on optimal management of the comorbid conditions now associated with chronic HIV disease. The issue of HIV disability warrants a careful investigation into our current health care system. Many long-term survivors with chronic HIV, who formerly received a disability ranking, are potentially able to return to work. However, their grave concern about the long absence from work, reflected in the resume, and fears about potential opportunistic infections while on the job require specific strategies. Vocational rehabilitation and on-the-job counseling are necessary for optimal return to work. The systemic issues of acquisition of disability and the loss of all benefits when one relinquishes disability are quite complicated and overwhelming. The diagnosis of advanced HIV disease is a determining factor for disability, and many PLHIV with CD4 counts less than 200/μL have experienced considerable improvement in their immunological status with a concomitant drop in viral load. Prognosis for these individuals has great variability. Promoting QOL may be greatly enhanced using complementary therapies. An integral aspect of self-perception is often the role played in society. The workplace affords individuals a sense of identity and a self-sustaining purposefulness.

Therefore our health and governmental systems need to conduct further research on return-to-work outcomes, with ease of transition and on-the-job accommodations when necessary. Future directions in the HIV epidemic as we see people living longer will be the full return to function in all domains of ADLs and return to productive work.

CASE STUDIES

Three case studies are presented to help the reader understand and identify various stages of this clinical problem and how each stage may require a different therapeutic focus.

CASE STUDY 34.1 Asymptomatic HIV Disease Versus Symptomatic HIV Disease: Mario

Examination
History

Mario is a 58-year-old male chemistry teacher who tested positive for HIV 5 years ago. He was not experiencing any symptoms related to HIV at the time, and his CD4+ nadir was 325 cell/μL. He began antiretroviral therapy (ART; Stribild) shortly thereafter and has continued with it since, rarely missing a dose. Currently, his CD4+ count is 550 cells/μL, and his HIV viral load is nondetectable (<20 copies/mL). Mario runs 5 miles three times per week for exercise. Recently he began to experience pain and tingling in the soles of his feet that is most noticeable after running. His weight has been stable. He has noticed that he has become somewhat forgetful over the past 2 years, which he attributes to being middle aged. He is otherwise healthy and denies other symptoms. His wife and 28-year-old son serve as his primary emotional support system. The rest of his family lives in Italy. He attends church regularly. Current medications include aspirin as needed after running.

Tests and Measurements
Lower-extremity sensation testing with Semmes-Weinstein monofilaments[250] reveals normal light touch sensation in the feet bilaterally. Lower-limb neural tension test (straight leg raise with dorsiflexion) and Tinel test over the tarsal tunnel reproduce symptoms results when performed on either side. Screening of the lumbar spine, hips, and knees is negative. Foot and ankle range of motion and strength are normal. Pain is not provoked with passive stretching of the plantar fascia. Lower-extremity reflexes are normal, and no abnormal reflexes are present. Excessive pronation is noted during the gait cycle; gait is otherwise normal. In standing, an excessive calcaneal valgus angle is noted; normal medial arches are observed in non–weight bearing. Foot pain on a visual analog scale is 0/10 at rest and 5/10 after running.

Evaluation and Diagnosis
A differential diagnosis that should be considered is distal sensory polyneuropathy (DSP). DSP is the most common neurological complication in people living with HIV. DSP is a potential side effect of certain ART drugs and may also be related to chronic HIV infection itself. Sensory dysfunction with DSP involves multiple peripheral nerves and occurs first in the most distal distribution. Decreased Achilles deep tendon reflexes (DTRs) are another clinical sign of DSP.

However, Mario's toes have no sensory impairment, and his DTRs are normal. Furthermore, his symptoms are provoked by repetitive stress (running). Myelopathy should be considered in patients with chronic HIV disease who appear to have peripheral neurological symptoms, but Mario does not demonstrate any signs that would suggest myelopathy as the cause of his foot symptoms. Mario does present with signs and symptoms of flexible pes planus and tarsal tunnel syndrome bilaterally. His gait pattern of excessive pronation is likely contributing to compression and/or adverse tension on the tibial nerve within the tarsal tunnel when he runs.

Prognosis, Goals, and Outcomes
Mario is expected to have full recovery with interventions directed at reducing biomechanical stress on the tarsal tunnel during running. Mario's goal is to run for 5 miles without any symptoms within the next 3 weeks. Outcomes will be measured with the Global Rating of Change (GROC) scale and the visual analog scale for pain associated with running. Reexamination will determine changes in clinical signs (lower-extremity neural tension test and Tinel test).

Intervention Plan and Recommendations
Mario will receive low-dye taping[251] to decrease his pronation and provide temporary relief of symptoms. Orthotics will be fabricated to reduce pronation and adverse stress on the tarsal tunnel. Mario will replace running with aerobic training on a stationary bike until his orthotics are adequately broken in, after which he can slowly resume running. He will receive instruction in general lower-extremity and plantar fascia flexibility exercises. If his foot symptoms are related to running and biomechanics and his memory loss is deemed to be normal (age-related), then he will remain classified in the asymptomatic HIV disease stage. If foot symptoms are recalcitrant to biomechanically based interventions, further consultation with Mario's HIV specialist will be warranted to rule out possible tibial nerve mononeuropathy related to his HIV disease. If Mario's foot symptoms are determined to be related to his HIV disease, he will be restaged to symptomatic HIV disease. The therapist will encourage Mario to discuss his complaints of memory loss with his physician or a mental health professional. The HIV Dementia Scale[252] or other instruments may be used to assess the patient's cognitive function and rule out the possibility of HIV dementia.

CASE STUDY 34.2 Advanced HIV Disease (AIDS) and a Plan for the Future: Ruby

Examination
History

Ruby is a left hand–dominant 23-year-old woman of African-American and Hispanic descent. She has history of intravenous drug abuse and has bipolar disorder. Five years ago, she learned she was HIV positive during a hospitalization due to *Pneumocystis carinii* pneumonia and oral thrush. At that time, her CD4+ count was 15 cells/μL and her HIV viral load was 750,000 copies/mL. Her low CD4+ count and opportunistic infections classified her as having advanced HIV disease (AIDS). Her opportunistic infections were successfully treated with

antibiotics, and antiretroviral therapy (ART) was initiated prior to leaving the hospital. Within a few months, her viral load was undetectable and her absolute CD4+ level climbed to 400 cells/μL. Since then, she has had intermittent periods of homelessness. She is currently residing with a friend. She stopped adhering to her ART regimen approximately 9 months ago, during a period of depression. Recently Ruby has been working as a prostitute to earn money for crack cocaine, which she uses daily. Ruby was admitted to the hospital 12 days ago with complaints of abdominal bloating and severe left shoulder pain. Her behavior was clearly agitated. Her psychiatric consultation confirmed she was experiencing a manic episode. Her CD4+ count was 175 cells/µL and HIV viral load was 200,000 copies/mL. A large abscess was present over the left deltoid. Medical work-up revealed that Ruby had a staphylococcal infection in the left anterior deltoid and infectious arthritis of the left glenohumeral joint. Magnetic resonance imaging (MRI) of the shoulder region was negative for osteomyelitis. It was determined that she was 4 months pregnant. Ruby's abscess was incised and drained. The shoulder infection was treated with intravenous methicillin. She was placed on psychotropic medication for mood stabilization. Because during the prior months she had not been adherent to ART, her blood was genotype tested to determine if she had developed any HIV mutations that might be resistant to certain medications used in ART. Fortunately, there were no HIV mutations, and thus she was prescribed Truvada and Isentress. (HIV-positive pregnant women are placed on ART with the goal of achieving undetectable viral loads by the time of birth to minimize the risk of perinatal transmission). Consultation with nutrition services was ordered to ensure adequate nutrition during the remainder of her pregnancy. Medical clearance for examination and interventions for the shoulder was obtained from her infectious disease physician. Ruby has disclosed that her arm infection was probably caused by injecting drugs. She has agreed to see an addiction counselor and the social worker.

Tests and Measurements

Ruby has a wound over the left anterior deltoid region that was 1.5 cm × 1.1 cm with a depth of 0.5 cm. The wound appears to be clean with 100% granulation tissue, and the most recent laboratory report is negative for *Staphylococcus*. Ruby reports that the swelling and redness in her left shoulder have resolved, and no swelling or redness is observed during the examination. Left shoulder strength is 3/5 (fair) for abduction, internal rotation, and external rotation and 4/5 (good) for other motions. Passive range of motion (PROM) of the left side is limited as follows: external rotation 70 degrees, abduction 160 degrees, and internal rotation 45 degrees. Her score on the Disabilities of the Arm, Shoulder and Hand questionnaire (DASH)[253] is 85/100 for the left upper extremity. Screening examination of the cervical spine is clear; however, hypertonicity is noted in the elbow and wrist and the finger flexors on the left side. PROM of the elbow, wrist, and hand is within normal limits; however, slight resistance is noted with quick passive stretching of flexor muscles. Ruby has weakness in grasp and demonstrates a mild flexor synergy pattern with attempts to elevate the left arm. She reports her arm and hand have been "feeling this way" for a few months.

Evaluation and Diagnosis

As a result of abnormal neurological signs found during the examination, neurology is immediately consulted and brain MRI is performed. The MRI reveals a mild right cerebrovascular accident (CVA) involving the middle cerebral artery. Physical and occupational therapy will be initiated to address the following findings: impaired integumentary integrity associated with partial-thickness skin involvement over the left anterior deltoid region; impaired glenohumeral joint mobility, muscle performance, and range of motion limitations associated capsular tightness (as sequela of infectious arthritis); and impaired motor function (spasticity and weakness in the left upper extremity) associated with the right CVA.

Prognosis, Goals, and Outcomes

Ruby's outcomes will be strongly influenced by her complex psychosocial status. She states that she is highly motivated to have a healthy baby and learn how to become a stable provider, which may help her adherence to ART and drug rehabilitation. Continuing communication among all team members (infectious disease, obstetrics-gynecology, social work, addictions counseling, nutrition, physical therapy, and occupational therapy) will be critical to optimize her care. Because of multisystem involvement and multiple impairments, it is expected that Ruby will require 6–8 weeks of outpatient therapy upon discharge from the hospital. Goals specific to physical therapy include the following: facilitate wound healing and prevent reoccurrence of infection, restore full PROM to the left shoulder, improve strength and function throughout the left upper extremity, achieve independence in performance of ADLs with the left upper extremity, improve the DASH score,[253] and minimal functional limitation as per the Barthel Index score.[254] Outcomes will be measured with continuing assessment of wound characteristics, the DASH score,[253] the Barthel Index score,[254] shoulder PROM measurements, and strength assessment of upper-extremity musculature.

Intervention Plan

Wound healing will be facilitated with dressing changes and use of topical agents as prescribed by her physician. Glenohumeral impairments will be addressed with joint mobilization, therapeutic exercises, and functional retraining. Upper-extremity impairments involving tone and weakness will be addressed with motor learning techniques, functional activities, and strengthening exercises. Ruby will receive daily physical and occupational therapy until she is discharged from the hospital. Social work will facilitate discharge to a structured group home for women because Ruby's current roommate is using drugs and working as a prostitute. On discharge from the hospital, Ruby will return for outpatient therapy at a frequency of three times per week. She will continue to follow up with the social worker regarding vocational counseling.

Examination

History

Walter is a 78-year-old man who was diagnosed with AIDS in 1986. He lost his life partner to the same disease in 1988. He has no living relatives. At the time of his diagnosis, Walter had cerebral toxoplasmosis, Kaposi sarcoma, AIDS wasting syndrome, and anemia. He was one of the first patients to receive zidovudine (AZT), which, along with other medications used to treat the opportunistic infections, proved to be lifesaving. In 1995, when new classes of drugs became available, his antiretroviral therapy (ART) regimen was updated to include triple combination therapy. In subsequent years, Walter's lab values were good (nondetectable viral loads and CD4 cell counts in the 300–400 cells/µL range).

Walter lives alone in a modest studio apartment. He employs a daily home health aide to assist with food preparation and personal hygiene. Walter had been ambulating short distances in his apartment using a walker because of fatigue and unsteadiness. Walter's gait became increasingly ataxic over the past month. Currently, Walter is experiencing multiple side effects and complications of long-term HIV survival, including peripheral neuropathy in the hands and feet, fibromyalgia, myelopathy, chronic pain in his back and legs, liver toxicity, hypertension, hyperlipidemia, and severe lipodystrophy. Over the past decade, Walter's Medical Outcomes Study HIV Health Survey[255] scores have indicated worsening QOL. Walter has been hopeless and depressed about his physical appearance and level of function. Approximately 1 year ago, Walter stopped taking ART and most other medications for multimorbid conditions. His current CD4 count is 65 cells/µL, and his HIV viral load of 200,000 copies/mL. Last week, he had a seizure that resulted in the current admission to the hospital. Testing revealed progressive multifocal leukoencephalopathy (PML). Walter's physician expects that this brain infection, combined with his immunosuppression, will lead to death within a few months. Walter has refused antibiotics to treat his PML and does not wish to resume ART or other medications that

CASE STUDY 34.3   Advanced HIV Disease (AIDS) at the End Stage of Life: Walter Examination—cont'd

had been previously used for his comorbidities. Walter wishes to explore hospice placement. Current medication: OxyContin.

Tests and Measurements

Inspection of the integumentary system reveals redness over the sacrum; otherwise the skin is intact. Diminished light touch sensation is noted in a stocking-glove distribution over the hands and feet. A Hoffman reflex, consistent with his myelopathy, is present in the upper extremities. Walter rates his pain at rest as ranging from 4/10 to 7/10. His pain drawing indicates low back, bilateral leg, and foot pain. Pulse oximetry reveals 96% oxygen saturation. Vital signs sitting: heart rate 70 beats/min, blood pressure 130/70 mm Hg, and respiratory rate 16 breaths/min with no apparent distress. Pitting edema (+1) is noted in the ankles and feet.

Walter is independent with all bed mobility but moves slowly due to pain. Sitting balance is good. Standing balance is fair. Contact guard is required for sit-stand transfer and for ambulation a distance of 10 feet with a rolling walker. Vital signs after ambulating 10 feet: heart rate 110 beats/min, blood pressure 150/70 mm Hg, respiratory rate 24 breaths/min, and oxygen saturation 96%. His Borg scale rating of perceived exertion (RPE) was 15/20 ("hard") during the 10-foot walk. He demonstrates erratic foot placement and a wide base of support during gait. His Functional Independence Measure (FIM)[256] score is 4. Because of fatigue and pain, strength and range-of-motion assessments are abbreviated. The following strength data are obtained (all measured bilaterally): shoulder abduction 3/5 (fair), elbow extension 4/5 (good), knee extension 3/5 (fair), and dorsiflexion and plantarflexion 4/5 (good). Passive range of motion data (bilateral): dorsiflexion 5 degrees; knee flexion 125 degrees (full knee extension not available, 10-degree flexion contracture noted); hip flexion 120 degrees; hip extension 10 degrees; shoulder flexion and abduction 140 degrees; and elbow, wrist, hand within normal limits.

Evaluation and Diagnosis

Walter exhibits multiple impairments related to his advanced HIV disease, multimorbidity, and a current opportunistic infection (PML), including pain, impaired integumentary integrity associated with superficial skin involvement, impaired sensory integrity, impaired joint mobility and range of motion (knees, shoulders), impaired muscle performance, impaired gait, impaired balance, and impaired endurance.

Prognosis, Goals, and Outcomes

Walter's prognosis for survival is poor. It is likely that he will deteriorate slowly over the upcoming months. Goals and outcomes will thus focus on optimizing QOL during Walter's remaining days. Specifically, goals are to reduce pain, prevent adverse sequelae of immobility that would further reduce his QOL (such as pressure wounds, pneumonia, deep venous thrombosis, or joint contracture), and promote safety. Depending on Walter's energy and participation, another goal is independent ambulation with a wheeled walker up to 15 feet.

Intervention Plan

During the current hospital admission, physical therapy will first be provided at bedside. If the patient wishes, treatment may be provided in the physical therapy department. Interventions will include relaxation techniques, passive range of motion and grade I joint mobilization (knees and shoulders), gait training with a wheeled walker, balance activities, and gentle strengthening and endurance exercises as tolerated. Occupational therapy will be consulted to address bed mobility and self-care tasks. Walter's vital signs will be closely monitored during therapy because it is possible that his autonomic nervous system dysfunction may become evolved as a result of the central nervous system infection. Walter's physician will be contacted regarding Walter's pain ratings. It is likely that increased dosage of pain medication is warranted as a result of reports of moderate pain at the current dosage. Walter will be seen by a dietician. The social worker will plan for transfer to a hospice setting. In hospice care, physical therapy will focus on basic functional activities, such as transfers, gait, and endurance. Palliative interventions (moist heat, gentle massage) will be provided as needed for pain control. Caregiver education will be provided regarding prevention of the effects of immobility and safe functional mobility. The same universal precautions used in providing care to any patient apply to Walter. Staff should be cognizant of protecting all hospice patients from seasonal cold or flu contagion. In the hospice setting, Walter will have the opportunity to work with a spiritual counselor. Walter has expressed an interest in exploring Eastern medicine for pain control. Therefore a consultation with an acupuncturist will be arranged.

REFERENCES

To enhance this text and add value for the reader, all references are included on the companion Evolve site that accompanies this textbook. This online service will, when available, provide a link for the reader to a Medline abstract for the article cited. There are 256 cited references and other general references for this chapter, with the majority of those articles being evidence-based citations.

35

Aging With Chronic Nervous System Conditions and Impairments

Myla U. Quiben

OBJECTIVES

After reading this chapter the student or therapist will be able to:

1. Analyze how the aging process may affect people with lifelong functional limitations and challenges in life participation.
2. Analyze the unique challenges faced by people with chronic motor impairments such as those associated with cerebral palsy, developmental disabilities, postpolio syndrome, spinal cord injury, and traumatic or acquired head injury during the aging process.
3. Evaluate this population of patients/clients with sensitivity and skill, incorporating precautions and effectiveness of interventions.
4. Provide a framework for the examination process for individuals with chronic conditions.
5. Present holistic intervention considerations for individuals with chronic motor impairments.
6. Identify gaps in knowledge and research in the management of aging individuals with chronic neuromuscular conditions.
7. Appreciate the complexity of examination, evaluation, and management of the aging patient with chronic motor impairments.

KEY TERMS

adaptation

aging

chronic disease

developmental disability

fatigue

health disparities

health promotion

postpolio syndrome

Improvements in health care delivery, research, medicine, nutrition, and knowledge of health and physical activity have resulted in a new challenge for health care professionals—a growing population of individuals who have sustained an initial injury to the central nervous system (CNS) with resulting secondary impairments and functional limitations and who are now experiencing the added effects of aging.

The aging process typically leads to gradual physiological changes in muscle strength, flexibility, and joint mobility, and changes in balance and endurance. Physical activity and a healthy lifestyle have been shown to address age-related changes by delaying the decline and deterioration; however, age-related changes such as osteoarthritis and vascular changes are still likely to occur to varying degrees despite a healthy lifestyle. Healthy but sedentary older individuals report more problems in activities of daily living (ADLs) than do those who continue to be physically active and who previously had an active lifestyle.[1-3]

To compound the aging process, chronic diseases (multimorbidity or comorbidity), disability, and frailty are common issues that are on forefront of health prevention and rehabilitation. While multimorbidity, disability, and frailty have considerable similarities and have been used interchangeably at times, these terms are conceptually distinct.[4]

Broadly, the presence of a number of health conditions is common among many of the definitions of multimorbidity, but the cut-off point, or the minimal number of conditions, is inconsistent. No consensus on the definition of multimorbidity currently exists.

Broadly, multimorbidity has been defined with the coexistence of two or more chronic diseases,[5-7] while others have specified a number of chronic diseases that constitute multimorbidity. Frailty, a clinically recognizable geriatric syndrome of increased vulnerability from age-associated declines in function and reserve across multiple systems, results an increased risk of physical decline with aging and or further health stressors.[8,9] The overlap among frailty, multimorbidity, and disability is conceivably seen in the initial description of the frailty phenotype by Fried and colleagues.[4,8,10] Since then, evidence has shown that these entities are interrelated but are distinct from each other.[4,11,12]

In an otherwise relatively healthy aging adult, the development of multimorbidities or frailty, coupled with decreased physical activity, may lead to limitations on activity and community participation. Consider that in an individual with a preexisting chronic nervous system condition and functional limitations, the aging process may present new or *additional* losses of components of functional activities and participation in an already taxed body—a new challenge to the individual who may have had the opportunity to successfully participate in life activities after the CNS injury. Individuals with existing disabilities undergo a similar aging process; however, the typical changes associated with aging are superimposed on the body system problems and functional limitations caused by the initial CNS injury.

In the realm of chronic problems in life participation, individuals who had polio in their younger years give clinicians an enlightening example of the chronic interaction among neurological impairments, recovery, activity limitations and participation restrictions, effects of aging, and health care. As a chronic condition, individuals who dealt with polio can teach therapists to reconsider and reevaluate their approach to individuals who are now aging and likely experiencing new activity limitations, impairments, and ineffective postures and movement. The challenges of aging with chronic body system impairments are encountered by individuals who acquired CNS insult at birth (developmental conditions such as cerebral palsy [CP; see Chapter 10]) and those who acquired injury through disease or trauma sometime in the life-span development process (those who have post-polio syndrome [PPS], traumatic brain injury [TBI], multiple sclerosis [MS], and spinal cord injury). This chapter focuses on aging with chronic CNS conditions in the latter classification.

The discussion of aging with chronic disease brings several questions to the forefront:

- What is the course of age-related medical conditions common in individuals with chronic impairments?
- Do age-related conditions vary among the developmental/genetic diseases or among conditions occurring at one point during the life-span?
- What is the prevalence and/or incidence of secondary medical conditions in individuals with chronic impairments?
- Have specific treatment protocols for health provision for this population been identified?
- What is the state of dissemination of information related to aging and health to people affected by these conditions?
- How has the effect of aging with chronic body system problems changed the ability of these individuals to participate in life, as well as their perceived quality of life?

As an emerging population, individuals with chronic impairments have not been on the receiving end of much research. Much of what is known about nervous system disorders is in the pediatric realm and in the initial stages of care immediately after the initial injury or diagnosis. Only recently have studies begun to look at the health care implications of aging with chronic conditions. Therefore definitive answers to the questions posed previously are still nonexistent or in the early stages of conception. Based on a review of existing literature, the consensus appears to be that there is a dearth of definitive information on the health status and effect of age-related processes among individuals with chronic conditions from developmental or genetic disorders, or from disease or injury sustained at one point in the life-span, such as TBI or MS. Moreover, there is agreement that further evidence-based research is needed in this emerging population.

This chapter aims to provide a holistic view of the management of the chronic problems of individuals with nervous system impairments, with consideration given to the effects of aging and compensation over time. Movement emerges from the interaction among the individual, task, and environment,[13] with several variables and degrees of freedom. Therefore physical therapists (PTs) and occupational therapists (OTs) need to examine and address multisystem impairments and contributions to movement, while appreciating the changing dynamics of a highly complex movement system influenced by aging superimposed on the body system impairments and functional limitations from an existing CNS dysfunction.

DIAGNOSES WITH UNDERLYING CHRONIC CONSEQUENCES

Developmental Conditions

With increasing life expectancy, mainly as a result of innovations in health care, a unique group of individuals with chronic conditions are subject to age-related changes. Individuals with developmental disabilities constitute a growing segment of the aging society. This is a broad topic, in part because of the many conditions that are categorized as developmental disability. According to the Developmental Disabilities and Bill of Rights Act of 2000[14] developmental disabilities are severe, chronic functional limitations attributable to mental or physical impairments or a combination of both, that manifest before age 22 years and that are likely to continue indefinitely. These result in substantial limitations in three or more of the following areas: self-care, receptive and expressive language, learning, mobility, self-direction, capacity for independent living, and economic self-sufficiency. These individuals also have a continuous need for individually planned and coordinated services.[15] The definition envelops a wide range of conditions leading to significant and lifelong disabilities. This group includes those with genetic and neurological conditions, which includes CP.

The question of whether unexpected changes among people with neurodevelopmental disabilities occur as they age and how these changes compromise functioning with progressive aging is of massive importance with the emergence of a population of individuals with developmental disabilities with increased life expectancy and concurrent increase in age-related diseases. According to Heller[16] the number of adults with intellectual and developmental disabilities aged 60 years and older is projected to nearly double from 641,860 in 2000 to 1.2 million by 2030 owing to increasing life expectancy and the aging of the baby boomer generation. With the aging of adults with developmental and genetic disorders, a new societal issue looms, as individuals with developmental disabilities have a lifelong need for external support. Much is unknown about the long-term effects of aging and maturation in adults with these conditions.

Adults with several types of developmental disabilities have life expectancies similar to those of the general population, excluding adults with particular neurological conditions and with more severe cognitive deficits. Recent studies show the mean age at death ranges from the mid-50s for adults with severe disabilities to the early 70s for those with mild to moderate intellectual disabilities.[17–19]

Concurrent with an increased life-span, some evidence exists that certain individuals with developmental disabilities have experienced an increase in age-related diseases. Of the limited information available, research has shown that aging affects certain genetic and neurologically based intellectual and developmental disabilities that may increase the risk of age-related pathologies and lead to an increased occurrence of coincident conditions.[20] Among several developmental conditions, Down syndrome (DS) has been the subject of a substantial body of research. DS is known for resulting in advanced aging, which includes a higher risk for Alzheimer's disease and select organ dysfunctions.[20–22]

CP is considered a life-span disability, and evidence exists that adults with CP lose functional abilities earlier than individuals who are able-bodied.[23] In addition, evidence is also increasingly pointing to specific age-related outcomes such as the effects of deconditioning, limitations with performance reserve, and possibly a shorter life-span.[20] In adults with CP, secondary conditions commonly described in research primarily are related to the long-term effects on the musculoskeletal system, such as pain, degenerative joint disease, and osteoporosis.[20,24,25] Secondary impairments in CP can progress subtly and may not appear until late adolescence or adulthood.[24] Age-related health conditions are also seen in other genetic and neurological disorders as the affected individuals age. However, the nature of these risks lacks extensive substantiation in the literature.

Overall, knowledge of adult health issues for adults with developmental disabilities is limited.[16] Several reasons contribute to the lack of knowledge. Limited health care programs exist for this population, likely because this is an emerging population. Most of the existing literature deals with pediatric domain issues rather than dealing with age-related issues. Although these individuals were likely seen by therapists for various functional limitations throughout their lives, the professional training that health care providers have received regarding the care of these individuals has focused on early childhood and school-aged children. As a result, many adolescents and adults with developmental disabilities have difficulty accessing appropriate health care information regarding secondary conditions resulting from their specific disabilities. Moreover, in general, older individuals with developmental disabilities have more difficulty in finding, accessing, and paying for high-quality health care.[16] Communication difficulties also limit the understanding of the experiences of aging adults with developmental disabilities. Evidence exists, however, showing that obesity and inactivity are more common in individuals with developmental disabilities than in the general population.[26] Bazzano and colleagues[26] identified several reasons for this health discrepancy, including individual and community factors, physical challenges, segregation from the community, lack of accessible fitness facilities and developmentally appropriate community programs, and cognitive deficits.

Given trends of increasing survival and longevity observed among individuals with developmental disabilities, it is sensible to consider a more in-depth look at the aging process among a variety of neurodevelopmental conditions and the need for a holistic approach. Although some literature exists regarding life-span changes with these disorders, particularly DS and CP, there is lack of confirming evidence for most of these conditions. Horsman and colleagues[23] advocate for research on the expectations regarding aging for adults with CP, including preventive measures to lessen the effects of secondary impairments. This recommendation applies to developmental life-span conditions and other chronic conditions that are subject to age-related changes that may be magnified or made worse by existing impairments and limitations. Evidence-based research is necessary to better understand the long-term effects of aging on adults with developmental and chronic conditions. The challenge then is to provide a holistic examination that involves a multisystem approach and to provide appropriate referrals as necessary to address the multiple needs of individuals with developmental disabilities.

Acquired Neurological Conditions: Spinal Cord Injury, Traumatic Brain Injury, Postpolio Syndrome

In the realm of management of chronic movement dysfunction, PPS—the late effects of polio—becomes a model case for other chronic neuromuscular conditions. There is much to learn from the complex nature of the late effects of polio and the effects of aging on an already stressed system. The cause must be briefly discussed to further understand the possible effects of aging. PPS can affect polio survivors years after recovery from the initial polio infection and is characterized by multifaceted symptoms that lead to decline in physical functioning.[27] PPS manifests with progressive or new muscle weakness or decreased muscle endurance in muscles that were initially affected by the polio infection and in muscles that were seemingly unaffected; generalized fatigue; and pain.[27] The exact cause of PPS remains unknown on the basis of review of the literature. Although it is not clear what exactly causes the new symptoms, there appears to be a consensus that insufficient evidence implicates the reactivation of the previous poliovirus.[28] Underlying causes have been proposed in a variety of hypotheses from several authors, with aging playing a key role.[29-33]

The suggestion that aging contributes to PPS is supported in the literature.[30,34,35] By the fifth decade of life, loss of anterior horn cells

begins, and by age 60 years the loss of neurons may be as high as 50%.[36] Age-related changes superimposed on the already limited motor neuron pool after polio appear to be important factors in the development of PPS. With the effects of the normal aging process, the remaining anterior horn cells are further reduced to a point at which the deficits caused by the initial insult cannot be overcome. The loss of even a few neurons from a greatly exhausted neuronal pool potentially results in a disproportionate loss of muscle function.[29,37] The loss of motor neurons from aging alone may not be a considerable factor in PPS because studies[29] have failed to link chronological age and the onset of new symptoms. Rather, it is the length of the interval between the onset of polio and the appearance of new symptoms that seems to be more critical.

Another plausible hypothesis alludes to overuse and fatigue of the already weakened muscles as a factor in the development of new muscle weakness.[28,38,39] A study by Trojan and colleagues[39] provides support to this hypothesis. Their results suggest that length of time since acute polio, joint and muscle pain, physical activity, and weight gain are factors associated with PPS. Years of overuse after recovery from polio causes a metabolic failure leading to an inability to regenerate new axon sprouts. The exact cause of degeneration of axon sprouts is not known. Evidence to support this hypothesis can be inferred from muscle biopsies, electrodiagnostic tests, and clinical response to exercise.[29] McComas and colleagues[40] suggested that neurons that demonstrated histological recovery from the initial virus were possibly not physiologically normal and were potentially vulnerable to premature aging and failure.

Other proposed hypotheses include the persistence of dormant poliovirus that was reactivated by unknown mechanisms, an immune-mediated response, hormone deficiencies, and environmental contaminants.[29] Another hypothesis points to the loss of anterior horn cells during the initial polio as a factor.[28,30] Findings from Trojan and colleagues[39] support the hypothesis that the severity of the initial motor unit involvement, seen as weakness in acute polio, is critical in predicting PPS. Individuals at greatest risk for PPS had severe attacks of paralytic polio, although individuals with milder cases also had symptoms.[29] These hypotheses have not been completely examined, and currently the evidence is not strong enough to support any one possible cause. Clinically it is difficult to assume that only one factor causes symptoms. The chronicity of the disease lends weight to the possibility that more than one factor contributes to the individual's symptoms.

Medical practitioners must consider the effects of existing comorbidities and aging in the examination and management of PPS. The complexity and nonspecificity of symptoms warrant consideration of all possible contributors to the symptoms of PPS. Based on the recent literature, there appears to be some confusion regarding terminology pertaining to PPS. Compounding the general symptoms are the common problems in aging: decreasing muscle strength and endurance, joint problems, and a myriad health deficits leading to functional losses. Physiological aging, overuse, and comorbidities play contributory roles in disrupting the state of stability after the initial infection.

McNaughton and McPherson[41] state that the simple descriptive labels "late problems after polio" and "of late deterioration after polio" are less limiting and do not imply a direct link with the previous polio diagnosis. Post-Polio Health International[42] uses the terminology "late effects of polio and polio sequelae" as the most inclusive category. *Late effects of polio* and *polio sequelae* pertain to health problems that are a result of chronic impairments from polio and may include degenerative arthritis from overuse, bursitis, or tendinitis. A subcategory under this heading is "PPS leading to decreased endurance and decreased function."

Currently no definitive test exists in the literature to diagnose the late effects of polio or PPS. It remains a diagnosis of exclusion, and as such, the diagnostic process for PPS is challenging and may be long. Halstead and Gawne[43] identified cardinal symptoms of PPS as new or increased muscle weakness, fatigue, and muscle and joint pain with neuropathic electromyographic changes in an individual with a definite diagnosis of polio. Diagnostic electromyography (EMG) may be required or used when the muscle pattern or history is atypical.

The criteria most commonly used for establishing a medical diagnosis of PPS were developed by Halstead[44] and is recommended by the European Federation of Neurological Societies (EFNS)[45,46]:

1. A confirmed history of paralytic polio in childhood or adolescence
2. Partial to complete muscle strength and functional recovery after the acute paralytic poliomyelitis
3. A period of at least 15 years of neurological and functional stability
4. Gradual or sudden onset of two or more new health problems: muscle weakness or abnormal muscle fatigability with or without generalized fatigue, muscle atrophy, weakness in the limb(s), or muscle and joint pain.
5. Symptoms persist for at least 1 year
6. No other medical conditions to explain these new health problems

Dalakas[47] identified additional inclusion criteria in the diagnosis: residual asymmetrical muscle atrophy, with weakness, areflexia, and normal sensation in at least one limb and normal sphincteric function and deterioration of function after a period of functional stability unexplained by primary or secondary condition.

Several individuals who recovered from polio during the early epidemics were encouraged to exercise for years and to use heroic compensatory methods for function. An exhaustive regimen of daily stretching and strengthening, demanding compliance from individuals and their support systems, was strongly encouraged. Orthotics and assistive devices were promoted as a means toward independent mobility. The outcomes of rigorous training were individuals who adapted and compensated with their remaining capabilities. Compensations include use of muscles at high levels of their capacity, substitution of stronger muscles with increased energy expenditure for the task, use of ligaments for stability with resulting hypermobility, and malalignment of the trunk and limbs. With the late effects of polio or a diagnosis of PPS, many of these individuals may have extreme difficulty dealing with these new problems because of the attitude of "working hard" to reeducate weakened muscles and compensate for loss of function after the initial diagnosis.[48–51] The new symptoms of PPS, which limits their motor function and likely impairs established personal and societal roles, require that they not work hard or overexert themselves. These two approaches are contradictory and can leave an individual frustrated and confused over therapeutic recommendations.

Spinal Cord Injury and Traumatic Brain Injury

For people with SCI and TBI, a trend is seen toward increasing awareness on the effects of aging on the functional status of this group. Owing to medical advances, patients are now living 20 to 50 years past their time of injury. Numerous studies have been done describing quality-of-life issues for people with TBI; however, those studies seldom look specifically at changes in functional levels or what can be done to ameliorate the declines.[52–54]

Signs of "premature aging" in multiple organ systems in people with SCI have been supported in literature.[55] In a review of 92 studies by Jensen and colleagues,[55] the findings indicated several salient points about the aging adult with SCI: many secondary health conditions occur with aging, many at higher rate compared to the typical population; pain, bowel and bladder impairments, muscle spasms, fatigue,

esophageal symptoms, and osteoporosis are the most common conditions reported; and several chronic health conditions, including cardiovascular disease, diabetes, bone mineral density loss, fatigue, and respiratory complications or infections, occur with higher frequency in older individuals or those with longer SCI duration compared with younger individuals or those with shorter SCI duration.

McColl and colleagues,[56] studying the impact of aging on people after SCI, echo the major categories of problems related to aging, such as musculoskeletal problems and joint, sensory, and connective tissue changes; chronic urinary tract infections; heart, respiratory, and other chronic diseases; secondary complications of the initial lesions, such as syringomyelia; and problems related to social and cultural acceptance and access or barriers. Evidence on specific age-related changes is presented in the section on examination.

Decreases in perceived health status and in functional abilities with increases in additional assistance for ADLs have been documented for aging individuals with SCI.[57–61] In a study of 150 people aging with an SCI, nearly 25% reported decreases in the ability to perform functional activities that they had been able to handle after the acute rehabilitation phase. The subjects who reported decreases in functional ability were generally older (45 years compared with 36 years) and had longer postinjury periods (18 vs. 11 years). The most common symptoms reported by the individuals with decreases in functional status were related to fatigue, pain, and muscle weakness. The ADLs reported to be more difficult were transfers, bathing, and dressing. To maintain their functional levels, those with declines in functional ability reported needing additional equipment.[57]

The need for further assistance with ADLs was echoed in a study by Gerhart and colleagues of individuals with SCI 20 years after the initial injury.[58] The study showed that 22% of the subjects reported an increased need for support with ADLs. Compared with a general group of nondisabled men and women aged 75 to 84 years in which 78% of the men and 64% of women did not need help with ADLs, the population of people with SCI needed increasing support to remain independent, and the need for help occurred at a younger age. On average, those with quadriplegia required more help with ADLs around the age of 49 years, whereas those with paraplegia were able to maintain their functional level until age 54 years. The groups showing functional decreases reported greater fatigue, increased muscle weakness, pain, stiffness, and weight gain.[58] Other studies support the findings that 5, 10, and 15 years after the initial SCI, an association with the need for additional help with increasing age existed.[59]

Liem and colleagues,[60] referencing an international data set of people with SCI, investigated a subset of 352 people at least 20 years after their injury. Increased help with transfers and housework were needed by 32% of the subjects, compared with their functional abilities at acute hospital discharge. With increasing age, women had a higher incidence of reported musculoskeletal impairments, which may have been related to biomechanical differences between men and women (e.g., 40% lower upper body strength).

In addition to the need for ADL support, neurogenic bowel and bladder symptoms also worsen with age in some people with SCIs. With changes in general health status, polypharmacy, decreased activity, and poor nutritional patterns, bowel problems (particularly constipation) become more of an issue. Although constipation seems like a minor issue relative to paralysis, those with SCIs report significant abdominal distention and pain, an increased incidence of perineal and sacral skin breakdown, and in some cases autonomic dysreflexia. In addition to the discomfort of chronic bowel dysfunctions, the required bowel care programs may take more time, which can lead to increased psychosocial issues associated with anxiety about bowel accidents in social and work situations. Additionally, these programs may take time away from social activities for both the person with an SCI and the caregiver. For those with continuing bowel problems that interfere with life and work activities, a colostomy may be an option that increases independence from caregiver support during the bowel program.[62] Another complicating factor related to bowel dysfunction is the typical treatment for pain complaints. Because the origin of pain is often illusive, the most common treatment involves oral medications rather than referrals for therapeutic interventions. Pain medications, especially opioids, increase gastrointestinal difficulties in nondisabled populations,[63] and the problem for patients with SCI is compounded.

Charlifue and colleagues,[64] drawing on the National Spinal Cord Injury Database of 7981 individuals with SCIs that occurred from 1973 to 1998, found a slight decrease in perceived health status the longer one lived after SCI. Evidence was also found that those injured later in life had a higher number of rehospitalizations after injury than those injured at a younger age. Despite palpable problems with the statistical issues within the sample, the study clearly indicated that the best predictor of a complication is a previous history of that complication. On the basis of their results, Charlifue and colleagues[64] suggest that prevention of complications is the best approach to improve quality of health and quality of life for people aging with SCI.

In addition to many multisystem impairments that occur in this population, a recent study[65] confirmed a high occurrence of cardiovascular risk factors among older adults with long-term SCI. In 123 older adults (mean age: 63 years) with SCI with a mean time of 24 years since injury, the median number of risk factors was 3. The presence of these risk factors in individuals with existing disabilities can pose additional consequences to their health and must be addressed.

Across the literature, a call for further research and a need for longitudinal studies is a consistent recommendation. Research is needed to help understand when problems are most likely to emerge in the aging process, to identify modifiable factors can be targeted in this population, what prevention strategies may be efficacious, and to develop and test the efficacy of interventions to address and potentially prevent secondary health conditions.

Individuals with TBI are often neglected by professional health care and insurance providers after the acute rehabilitation period. According to Levin,[66] before 1980, individuals with brain injuries were considered "dead on arrival." People who would have died from the TBI several decades ago are now living into old age and are coping with the changes caused by the aging process superimposed on their physical limitations and cognitive problems. Of great concern is the possible relationship between a history of brain injury and increased cognitive changes along the dementia continuum.[67–69] Cognitive decline in the nondisabled population is a problem, but the additive effect for a person with a previous TBI may seriously impair the person's coping mechanisms when dealing with his or her own health and self-care needs.[70] TBI was found to be an independent significant risk factor in developing dementia even in mild TBI.[68] A meta-analysis in 2017[69] of 32 studies showed that head injury was associated with increased risks of dementia and Alzheimer's disease. Further, recent TBI with loss of consciousness acquired in older adulthood has been associated with an increased risk for mortality.[71]

Extensive work has been done on rehabilitation programs and quality-of-life issues related to head injury and, to a lesser extent, cerebral vascular accidents.[72] Unfortunately, the focus of rehabilitation after a TBI has been on the acute and rehabilitation stages of treatment and not the chronic problems that follow this group of patients into their older years. As with other chronic conditions, few patients see a therapist after they are discharged from rehabilitation unless they

have new acute events such as musculoskeletal problems or a medical condition that causes a change in functional status.

Although TBI is a lifetime disability, little attention has been paid to the needs of aging people with a TBI who may have recurring needs for physical and cognitive rehabilitation and retraining over the lifespan. Individuals who sustain a TBI later in life years will likely have different needs from those injured at a younger age. In a study on the effect of age on functional outcome in mild TBI, Mosenthal and colleagues[73] found that those injured later in life (after age 60) had longer inpatient rehabilitation periods and lagged behind younger patients in functional status at the point of discharge; however, similar to the younger individuals who sustained a head injury, the over-60 individuals showed measurable improvement during the 6-month study period. Therefore aggressive management of older patients with TBI is recommended, and older patients may require continuing management owing to the overlying issues of the aging process.[73] This is echoed in the National Institutes of Health (NIH) consensus document on the treatment of people with TBI, which suggests that specialized interdisciplinary treatment programs need to be put in place to deal with the medical, rehabilitation, family, and social needs of people with TBIs who are over the age of 65 years. The document also concludes that access to and funding for long-term rehabilitation is necessary to meet long-term needs; however, it recognizes that changes in payment methods by private insurance and public programs may jeopardize the recommendations.[74]

Although the authors of the NIH document recognize the need to deal with the aging processes associated with TBI, there continues to be a lack of services and trained professionals available, especially at the community level.[75] As with the SCI population, work is now being done to investigate the relationships among TBI, aging, and health. Breed and colleagues[76] found that older individuals with TBI were more likely than their age-matched nondisabled peers to report metabolic, endocrine, sleep, pain, muscular, or neurological and psychiatric problems. Their findings support those of Hibbard and colleagues[77] and Beetar and colleagues,[78] which suggest that medical personnel need to be prepared to treat a broad range of health issues in the aging TBI population. Fewer of the studies on long-term outcomes and issues in TBI extend to the 10- and 15-year postinjury periods that have been examined for patients with SCIs. In studies 5 years after the initial TBI, improvements in physical and social functions were noted in most areas for at least the first 2 years after injury, with the exception that those with a history of alcohol or drug abuse did less well. One could assume that continued abuse of alcohol or drugs would bode ill for individuals aging with a TBI.[79] In one study of 946 children and adolescents who sustained a TBI, Strauss and colleagues[80] found that patients with severe and permanent mobility and feeding deficits had higher mortality rates, with a 66% chance of surviving to age 50 years. In contrast, survivors with fair or good mobility had a life expectancy only 3 years shorter than that of the general population. However, because both severely and mildly injured individuals with a TBI can live well into and beyond their 50s, the impact of aging on the physical and cognitive deficits must be dealt with assertively to prevent superimposed disability.

Because aging individuals with an SCI or a TBI may have health problems similar to those of any aging population, primary impairments in muscle strength and endurance may be magnified. Therefore individuals with these chronic conditions who make repeat visits regarding medical problems such as musculoskeletal, cardiac, respiratory, and renal diseases should be referred for a comprehensive therapy examination and program that focuses on education, lifestyle changes, and health and wellness promotion interventions.

EXAMINATION OF INDIVIDUALS WITH CHRONIC IMPAIRMENTS

The National Council on Aging (NCOA) approximates 80% of older adults have at least one chronic disease and 77% have at least two.[81] The statistics on chronic disease continue to grow with a current estimate of approximately 45% or 133 million of all Americans having at least one chronic disease.[82] Conditions are diverse and may be related to trauma or chronic conditions such as MS.[83] Trends of increasing survival and longevity are now being observed among individuals with chronic conditions as they experience aging processes. Given the huge financial, human resource, and health costs of chronic disease, it is timely to consider how to manage individuals with chronic impairments.

Examination of individuals with chronic impairments and disabilities is challenging to say the least. Not only are the impairments and activity limitations diverse, but the combinations of these impairments and limitations are many and unique to each individual owing to societal, personal health, environmental, and psychological considerations. Moreover, the effects of aging will likely affect individuals differently depending on existing impairments, functional limitations, current health status, and each individual's attitude toward health and maintaining their functional status and lifestyle. This entails a more thorough, methodical, multisystem examination with a meticulous health interview and wellness model.

EXAMINATION: SYSTEMS MODEL

Aging with existing neuromuscular disorders, be it from a late-onset pathology or from a developmental condition, is a challenge for both the individual and the health care professional. There is a small body of literature on the later-life complications of early-onset acquired disabilities. Several problems may result from complex interactions among physical, medical, environmental, behavioral, and psychosocial factors.

Aging may confound late-onset symptoms or magnify the deficits from the initial CNS insult. With the trend of increasing longevity and survival rates from improvements in health care, it is necessary to look at how the health care provider approaches the examination of individuals with chronic impairments and activity limitations. As individuals with chronic neuromusculoskeletal impairments age, there will be an increasing number of comorbidities, and sorting out the cause of each new symptom will be increasingly complicated.

Bottomley[84] identifies essential components of a comprehensive geriatric assessment as psychosocial, functional, mental, and social health elements. These components are applicable to individuals with chronic neuromuscular impairments, who with aging are experiencing new symptoms or a magnification of preexisting impairments. Box 35.1 shows a sample examination template for this population.

Challenges of Examination of Individuals With Chronic Conditions

Assessment of individuals with chronic nervous system conditions is challenging because of the diversity of impairments, the nonspecific nature of symptoms, and the complex interaction of several factors, including the heterogeneous effects of aging. Depending on their underlying health conditions, individuals with chronic conditions may have higher risks than others of developing preventable health problems.[83] In comparing nondisabled individuals with people with disabilities, Iezzoni and O'Day[85] found that the latter group is much more likely to have higher obesity and overweight rates and higher

---

BOX 35.1   Examination Profile for Chronic Neuromuscular Impairments

Examination: Systems Model
- Examination guidelines, include nutritional and sleep screen
- Movement observation
- Health history
- Systems review
- Tests and measures
  - Musculoskeletal: strength, range of motion, power, and muscle length
  - Balance and coordination
  - Pain
  - Tone
  - Cardiovascular and pulmonary function
  - Integumentary
  - Cognition and mental function
  - Mobility
  - Posture
  - Sensory deficits
  - Sleep
  - Temperature intolerance
  - Psychosocial considerations
  - Functional assessment

---

rates of depression, anxiety, and stress. Of adults with major physical and sensory impairments, 27% are obese, compared with 19% of those without major impairments.[85] Of individuals with major difficulties in walking, 34% reported frequent depression or anxiety, compared with 3% among those without disabilities.[85] Information on predisposition to conditions such as these is important for the health care provider during the health interview and examination process.

The examination of individuals with chronic impairments presents a different challenge than examining patients or patients with acute diagnoses. For both cohorts, the task of the health care provider is to determine the effect of the active pathology on the varied systems and function. However, for the individual with chronic impairments, an added challenge exists: the impact of the active pathology can be seen with the underlying preexisting deficits in function and/or impairments that may leave the individual with a narrow margin for health.

Individuals with developmental and genetic disabilities and with conditions acquired through diseases or trauma sometime in the life-span have activity limitations and participation restrictions that are diverse and unique to each individual. Therefore some individuals may have higher risks than others of developing certain preventable health problems or may be more susceptible to developing secondary conditions owing to the long-term effects of the primary impairments from the original health condition.

The absence of specific medical diagnostic tests adds to the dilemma, as does the continuing uncertainty of the underlying cause and the lack of curative intervention. Health care professionals' limitations in knowledge of age-related medical disorders that are common in people with these conditions, including the prevalence and incidence of medical conditions with neurodevelopment disabilities also add to the complexity. Box 35.2 provides several important pointers for examining this population of patients and patients.

The individual with chronic impairments who is currently facing an active pathology likely has adapted to his or her existing system impairments and activity limitations. Depending on their underlying health conditions, some individuals with chronic conditions may have higher risks than others of developing preventable health problems.[83]

BOX 35.2 Examination Pointers

- Comprehensive: A systems approach to address the number, complexity, and diversity of the deficits is a must. Essential components are physical, functional, mental, and social health.
- Interdisciplinary: Consideration for the functional, medical, vocational, and psychosocial issues warrants a coordinated evaluation of a team versed in addressing the unique needs of individuals with chronic neuromusculoskeletal conditions and disabilities.
- Patient/client-centered: Factors that influence performance, such as fatigue, must be considered during the examination. Recognition of the individual's and family's values and goals is essential.
- Thorough: Assessment may take several hours and extend for two to four visits[86,87] to better integrate the evaluation process and allow the patient to fully participate, contend with the recommendations, and engage in long-term management.

BOX 35.3 Components of Patient/Client History

- Demographics, include body mass index
- Growth and developmental history (particularly in those diagnosed with developmental disabilities and those with acquired diagnoses such as polio in childhood or spinal cord injury as an adolescent)
- Past medical-surgical history: Include information on interventions and outcomes from initial diagnosis
- Family medical history: Critical in ruling out possible contributors to symptoms such as pain from rheumatoid arthritis; critical for possible genetic contributor to original diagnoses
- Social and vocational history: Include work status, modifications to work or home environment, and support system
- Living environment: Include adaptive equipment, modifications done or necessary to home
- General current health status: Include nutritional and sleep information
- Current functional status, activity level, and perceived quality of life

---

Thus from an examination viewpoint, the critical task of the health care provider is determining what new changes to the individual's current abilities and disabilities have been brought on by the active pathology. These changes will likely affect the current functional abilities (e.g., mobility, ADLs), as will preexisting system impairments such as deficits in strength and endurance, pain, and so on. Regardless of the level of deficit, these individuals have some prior knowledge of deficits that affect function, which may help or may hinder their willingness to participate.

On the other hand, for the patient/client who has been otherwise healthy and functional and now has an acute diagnosis, active pathology may bring on impairments and limitations that are "new" experiences to the individual. The level of education should thus be adapted to the individual, and education performed on a case-by-case basis.

Moreover, the psychosocial aspect of a new pathology and its effect on function may be very different in an individual who has dealt with chronic impairments and limitations versus one who has been active up until the disease process. As with the level of education, the health care provider's approach to a patient/client should always be professional and respectful, with open lines of communication and active listening.

PTs may develop diagnostic focuses based on movement dysfunction, activity limitations, and impairments, different from those by OTs. These variances depend on the functional activity limitations identified by the patient and the professional.[88,89]

It is critical for the clinician to examine all possible contributors to symptoms reported by the individual with chronic impairments. A thorough review of systems may identify symptoms that are related to the primary medical diagnoses, but equally important, it may identify symptoms that are associated with one or more existing comorbidities that have developed over time since the initial nervous system insult.

Health History

Therapists typically collect health history information as part of a comprehensive examination. The history information along with the symptom investigation and review of systems and physical examination will provide guidance in the differential diagnosis process and in the choice of examination and intervention techniques.

The information from the history will be useful in determining the possible cause of current difficulties or symptoms for which the patient/client is now seeking intervention (Box 35.3). Fatigue or pain may be present from unnecessary and inefficient movement strategies or from high levels of activity. Information on the habitual sleeping, sitting, standing, and walking postures along with ineffective use of devices may alert the clinician to possible factors contributing to the patient's current symptoms or difficulties.

Systems Review

A systems approach to the examination is essential because individuals with chronic conditions have a multitude of possible impairments with superimposed age-related conditions. This situation is best illustrated when examining individuals with PPS. The patient presentation in this condition is a complex interaction of all systems along with the effects of aging, previous interventions, and environmental, psychosocial, and medical aspects of care. The initial diagnosis of polio, which is critical in the diagnostic criteria, will need to be established. This may be difficult because approximately 10% to 15% of individuals who were believed to have or were diagnosed with polio did not have it, and some individuals with mild weakness were diagnosed as having nonparalytic polio.[44,90]

Chapter 7 of this text discusses the review of systems as a vital component in the PT's role in medical screening and differential diagnosis. OTs are responsible for this same vital component. Possible multisystem involvement warrants review of all systems to determine if current problems are associated with existing comorbid conditions or occult disease or are indeed late manifestations of the initial disease process, as in the case of polio.

Providing further substantiation for the need for a methodical and multisystem approach are findings of high rates of secondary conditions related to obesity and inactivity common in individuals with developmental disabilities. These secondary conditions include type 2 diabetes, cardiovascular disease, and metabolic syndrome, diagnoses that affect multiple systems.[26] Individuals with developmental disabilities also have four to six times the preventable mortality of the general population.[18,92] As therapists are entering into the decade of becoming primary care providers, anyone with a preexisting functional problem may walk into a PT or OT clinic searching for help. The importance of medical screening cannot be overemphasized.

The nonspecificity of symptoms seen in individuals with chronic movement dysfunction lends credibility to the need for review of all body systems. Fatigue, for example, a symptom frequently seen in individuals with chronic conditions such as MS and PPS, among others, is associated with several systems, such as endocrine, nervous, psychological, and cardiopulmonary.

Tests and Measures

Through system assessment by the PT and/or OT, each individual with chronic movement problems should have an opportunity to participate in development of a unique clinical profile. This profile should reflect the strengths and limitations of that individual. Simultaneously these data should aid both the patient and the therapist in identifying realistic treatment goals and selecting the most appropriate intervention strategies. The choice of outcome measures will depend on the individual's current functional skills, the medical status, and the desires and expectations of the individual. Because the severity of symptoms is variable and nonspecific, the clinician is strongly urged to perform a thorough examination and take into consideration factors that may influence performance specific to that individual's functional impairment problems, such as fatigue and pain.

Critical to the examination process is the determination of secondary conditions. Secondary conditions have been defined as injuries, body system impairments, functional limitations, or disabilities that occur as a result of a primary condition or pathology[24,93–97] as well as physical problems that were caused by small insults to one of the body systems not related to the primary condition. Musculoskeletal problems account for many of these secondary conditions; thus the musculoskeletal examination is of critical importance in individuals with developmental disabilities. Gajdosik and Cicerello[96] outlined numerous conditions that may affect the adult with CP; some can lead to significant loss in function and pain from complications such as fractures and osteoporosis. Other musculoskeletal conditions, including scoliosis, subluxations, dislocations, patella alta, foot deformities, pelvic obliquities, and contractures, further complicate the life progression of an adult with developmental disabilities.[96] Frequently these chronic conditions may have their origins in childhood, but because of the lack of sensory awareness may go undetected until later adolescence, adulthood, or well into advancing age when the body no longer has the ability to compensate for these abnormal biomechanical forces. Furthermore, as the aging process progresses, less regeneration of damaged tissue occurs, leading to greater cumulative trauma in joints and other load-sensitive structures.[97] Again, these conditions need to be closely monitored over time to ensure appropriate intervention, optimizing an individual's function and minimizing damage to various tissues.

Fatigue

Fatigue is one of the most common symptoms reported by individuals with chronic conditions such as PPS[98] and MS.[99] Movement and performance of daily activities are more energy-consuming for individuals with disabilities and may cause greater fatigue.[100] Evidence also points to individuals with disabilities aging faster than those without disabilities; cardiovascular data from individuals with SCI indicate that people with SCI may age faster than those without SCI.[101,102] Cook and colleagues[100] identified the lack of age-specific general population norms as an obstacle in the understanding and estimation of the influence of aging on the fatigue of individuals with neuromuscular conditions.

It is likely that an earlier increase in fatigue with age might be observed in other chronic neuromuscular conditions; however, the effects of chronological age on fatigue in individuals with disabilities are not entirely clear.[100] In a recent study, Cook and colleagues[100] assessed fatigue and age in four clinical populations of individuals with PPS, SCI, MS, and muscular dystrophy (MD), comparing self-reported fatigue experience in different age cohorts with age-matched, US population norms. A total of 1836 surveys were used in data analysis.

The authors concluded that individuals with disabilities reported higher levels of fatigue than the general US population, regardless of age or disability type.[100] Interestingly, the authors noted that the causes of fatigue likely vary by disability type—that is, MS, PPS, and MD are more likely to cause fatigue through a combination of central neurological processes, the effect of sleep disorders such as periodic limb movements (PLMs),[103] or increased physical effort, whereas in SCI fatigue may be a side effect of medications or result from sleep disorders.[100]

Results revealed not only that individuals with disabilities have a higher risk of experiencing fatigue than those without disabilities, but also that the risk for increased fatigue, compared with normative values, increases with age.[100] The reported mean fatigue levels were the highest observed in older PPS age cohorts among the disability samples. In the MS group, fatigue was higher than in any other clinical group except PPS. The highest fatigue reported in the MS sample was in the 35- to 44-year-old age cohort, with lower fatigue in older cohorts except for those 75 years of age and older, but the older group had a small sample size. In the SCI group, peak reported fatigue was in the 55- to 64-year-old age cohort. The results for the SCI group younger than 55 years old were very similar to those for the general population.[100]

In the general population, very little change in fatigue levels for most adults was found moving from young (65 years) to middle (75 years) old age, whereas in the disability samples the authors saw a slight but consistent increase toward greater fatigue at this point in the life-span.[100] This increase in fatigue could be associated with current physical decline associated with disease progression.[100] The authors concluded that more research is needed to determine the specific effects of fatigue on the functioning of people aging with disabilities and to further explore interventions that may shield against or reduce any negative effects that occur.[100]

Bruno and colleagues[98] state that fatigue has been identified as the most commonly reported, most debilitating, and least studied symptom in the postpolio sequelae. Generalized fatigue is typically described as overwhelming exhaustion or flulike aching accompanied by marked changes in level of energy, endurance, and mental alertness.[29] The lack of energy with minimal activity is often described as "hitting a wall," thus the term "polio wall." Polio survivors differentiated between the fatigue associated with weakness and a "central fatigue" that leads to attention and cognitive problems.[98] Severe fatigue affects not only physical function but mental function as well—hence the controversial suggestion that the fatigue associated with postpolio is caused by impaired brain function rather than the diffuse degeneration of motor units and motor junctions.[98]

Descriptors for fatigue associated with PPS are significantly different.[104] The fatigue of PPS may not appear at the time of the activity, and recovery does not occur with typical rest periods. It has also been described as a sudden and total wipeout. In a few instances headaches and sweating appear, suggestive of autonomic nervous system overload.[105] Fatigue commonly occurs in the late afternoon or early evening. Fatigue that tends to last all day is atypical in PPS[44] and should alert the therapist to consider other possible diagnoses.

Similar to the fatigue of PPS, MS fatigue profoundly disrupts multiple aspects of general well-being.[99] Krupp[106] reported that 67% of individuals with MS reported fatigue as a major limiting factor in their social and occupational responsibilities compared with no reports in healthy adults. The fatigue of MS is unique in that it is exacerbated by heat, as are many MS symptoms. Fatigue may be acute, chronic, or intermittent or persistent, whether related to a specific diagnosis such as MS, CP, or polio or having no relation to the initial medical diagnosis. It is necessary to consider the role of other symptoms related to the specific medical diagnosis during the examination of fatigue.

The evaluation of fatigue includes the various factors that can induce or worsen fatigue. The history and examination also are used to assess for new medical diagnoses or the possibility of infection, an impending relapse, heat exposure (in the case of MS), and side effects from medications.

Differential diagnoses for fatigue are extensive and may include disorders of several systems, including psychological, cardiopulmonary, neurological, and endocrine disorders, and medication use. Specific conditions that may cause fatigue include depression, myasthenia gravis, hyperparathyroidism, congestive heart failure, sleep apnea, cancer, and infections. Numerous medications commonly used in symptom management can cause fatigue, including antispasticity agents, tricyclic antidepressants, and β-blockers. The challenge is to differentiate the fatigue caused by typical activities from the fatigue of chronic conditions.

Pain

Individuals with chronic diseases often have pain as a common symptom, most likely from long-term atypical biomechanical forces on joints and muscles or from long-standing disease processes. Many developmental disabilities have a component of disordered movement, from hypomobility in the case of DS to hypermobility in the case of spastic CP. These abnormal joint stresses and strains cause long-term damage to the musculoskeletal system.[96,107,108] The natural degradation of joint structures with aging coupled with weakness and atypical ground reaction forces leads to higher incidence of musculoskeletal pain.[109–111]

Pain that occurs with chronic conditions may be muscular, joint-related, or both. The source of pain needs to be considered because pain may limit the individual's functional abilities and lead to further decline. Muscle pain is often described as a deep, aching pain similar to the pain experienced during the initial infection. The pain is frequently aggravated by physical activity, stress, and cold temperature. Pain is unusual in that it does not occur at the time of activity but rather 1 to 2 days after a precipitating event.

Joint pain in itself usually results primarily from long-term microtrauma from abnormal biomechanical forces. An example might be the overuse of the shoulder girdle muscles and joint from a lifetime of use of Lofstrand crutches to compensate for lower-extremity impairments after polio. Joint pain is frequently associated with physical activity but is rarely associated with inflammation. Interventions are complicated by the presence of osteoporosis, lack of compensatory substitutions to rest the injured part, and, often, poor response to exercise. Failing joint fusions, uneven limb size, progressive scoliosis, poor posture, and abnormal mechanics may also contribute to pain.[112]

Although pain is not a hallmark of many chronic conditions such as DS and MS, it may occur in some individuals with long-term impairments and thus should be part of a comprehensive examination. Pain frequently associated with MS is related to postural problems and inefficient use of muscles and joints to compensate for loss of function or spasticity.

More than 65% of individuals with PPS have reported neck, shoulder, and back pain radiating to the hip and leg.[113] This pain is expected because the incidence of major postural abnormalities and gait deviations is also high, as shown in Table 35.1 and Box 35.4.

Differential diagnosis for acute muscle and joint pain includes consideration of chronic musculoskeletal conditions leading to wear and tear and disorders with significant muscle or joint manifestations. The list is extensive and may include osteoarthritis, tendinitis, bursitis, fibromyalgia, rheumatoid arthritis, and polymyalgia rheumatica. The challenge is determining whether muscle or joint pain occurs from long-term wear and tear or from an acute or exacerbating occurrence.

TABLE 35.1 Major Postural Abnormalities in Sitting, Standing, and Walking in 111 Confirmed Postpolio Clinic Clients

Posture	Abnormal Deviation	No.	%
Sitting (n = 111)	Absent lumbar curve	64	54
	Forward head (loss of cervical curves)	50	45
	Uneven pelvic base[a]	29	26
	Structural scoliosis	38	34
Standing (n = 76)	Absent lumbar curve	52	68
	Uneven pelvic base[a]	40	53
	Weight bearing on stronger leg	29	38
Walking (n = 76)	Abnormal gait deviations	76	100
	Major lateral trunk oscillations	33	43
	Obvious forward lean	40	53

[a]Pelvic asymmetry was ½ inch or more.
Modified from Smith L, McDermott K. Pain in post-poliomyelitis: addressing causes versus effects. In: Halstead L, Wiechers D, eds. *Research and Clinical Aspects of the Late Effects of Poliomyelitis.* White Plains, NY: March of Dimes; 1987.

BOX 35.4 Postpolio Syndrome: Common Secondary Conditions[90,114]

- Fatigue
- Pain
- Respiratory complaints
- Sleep disorders
- Depression
- Falls
- Musculoskeletal conditions
- Cardiovascular dysfunction
- Diabetes
- Bladder dysfunction
- Integumentary impairments

Strength

Examination of strength is another critical component of the examination of individuals with chronic impairments. Long-standing weakness is an expected occurrence from decreased physical activity common in individuals with disabilities and chronic diseases. Strength deficits may result from several causes other than disuse, such as upper motor neuron weakness, fatigue, compensatory movements, pain, or spasticity. It is likely, however, that aging individuals with chronic conditions have adapted to the initial weakness associated with their diagnoses, as in the case of people with SCI or PPS who have led productive and functional lives since the initial diagnosis or acute onset.

Typical aging involves the losses of muscle strength, loss of power, and sarcopenia—processes that may intensify or build on the initial losses of strength. Delineation of weakness from age-related processes versus weakness as part of the disease process or that from lack of physical activity common in people with chronic impairments is difficult if not impractical from both research and clinical perspectives. Too many variables need to be controlled and accounted for unless specific muscle groups were examined initially and the findings well documented, which may have been the case for people with PPS. Many individuals with PPS have extreme difficulty dealing with these new problems because they were taught that hard work was the only way to correct physical problems that followed acute polio. These new problems, which also limit motor function, require that these individuals not work hard. These two concepts are contradictory and can leave an individual frustrated and confused over therapeutic recommendations.

Manual muscle testing of the entire body, although time-consuming, may be necessary to determine the muscular involvement. Muscle testing, however, may not always reveal the full extent of muscle involvement, and functional assessment may provide a better picture of individuals' potential and true difficulties. Performance and participation in daily activities will provide a better picture of a person's strengths and impairments. Therefore current functional activities are critical in determining whether current mobility difficulties are related to the aging process, represent an exacerbation of initial disease processes such as in PPS, or are signs and symptoms of new medical concerns.

Weakness and postpolio syndrome. Weakness may occur in both previously affected and clinically unaffected muscles; however, it is primarily prominent in muscles most severely affected in the initial infection.[44] It is typically asymmetrical and may be proximal, distal, or patchy.[112] Weakness is primarily observed in repetitive and stabilizing contractions rather than with single maximum efforts. The decreased ability of the muscles to recover rapidly after contracting may be a factor. Recovery of quadriceps muscle strength after fatiguing exercise was significantly less in symptomatic PPS subjects compared with asymptomatic and control subjects.[115] Overuse of muscles in relation to their limited capacity has long been associated with these new problems.[116–118] New weakness and atrophy have been attributed to metabolic overload of the giant motor units, with more pruning of muscle fibers than axon sprouting.[119,120]

New muscle involvement may also cause signs and symptoms such as muscle fasciculations, cramps, atrophy, and elevation of muscle enzymes in the blood. Yet many of these physical signs and symptoms are also present in other neuromuscular problems such as amyotrophic lateral sclerosis. Fasciculations occur at rest and during contraction and tend to persist even when muscle pain and fatigue have been resolved. Muscle cramps are common in fatigued muscles and are alleviated by decreased activity. The new weakness may or may not be accompanied by atrophy. New postpolio muscular atrophy of muscles is sometimes reported. It is very noticeable when it occurs in the gastrocnemius or the anterior tibialis owing to the effect on everyday ambulation. Elevation of muscle enzymes, indicative of muscle damage, has been found in individuals with PPS and has been related to the intensity of work.[117,121,122]

Gross muscle testing may mask the true involvement because several muscles that were initially believed to be uninvolved were truly subclinically affected by polio. The pattern of definitive manual test findings (spotty, flaccid, and asymmetrical paresis or paralysis) is also used to confirm the initial polio diagnosis.

Several polio survivors are able to function at high levels of activity with few strong muscle groups as a result of the random, diffuse nature of the motor deficits and the body's ability to compensate with uncommon muscle and joint function. This delicate balance may be maintained for years, and a disruption from late-onset weakness of a significant muscle group can lead to disproportionate functional losses.

Superimposed pathological problems have been proposed as a possible cause of the later exhibition of new signs and symptoms in postpolio survivors. Several conditions may contribute to weakness, including arthritis, fibromyalgia, deconditioning from disuse, and coronary heart disease.[123]

Range of Motion and Muscle Length

Limitations in joint motion from muscle contractures and from shortening of ligamentous joint structures are common in individuals with chronic disabilities. Likewise, hypermobile joints may also result from compensatory techniques forcing more mobility. An evaluation of the individual's activity levels and goals is vital before intervening with muscle and joint deficits. In some instances, during the convalescent stage of the initial diagnoses, as in polio or SCI, selective tightness was allowed to give some stability to joints with paralyzed muscles. In addition, the body may develop useful contractures to maintain or regain function. The presence of spasticity, particularly in severe cases, may have also contributed to the development of contractures in older adults with CP, SCI, MS, or TBI. Before making attempts to stretch contractures, therapists should carefully evaluate the functions that may be lost if gains in range of motion (ROM) are achieved. Equally important is to evaluate what functions would be gained and what the cost would be. Consider that after 20 to 40 years these contractures resist any significant elongation, and aggressive intervention may cause more harm and loss of function.

Box 35.5 lists the secondary conditions that may develop in an individual with CP. These impairments not only cause pain but also limit mobility and interfere with performance of ADLs and leisure activities. Thus a thorough evaluation of musculoskeletal status and periodic monitoring are imperative to maintaining quality of life and social participation for these individuals.

Tone

Examination of tone is a focal component of the examination of individuals with chronic neuromuscular conditions. This group of individuals may demonstrate a wide range of tone deficits from hypotonia seen with DS, to hypertonicity seen in people with TBI, SCI, MS, or CP, to a mixed type with episodes of high and low tone.

Spasticity can interfere with mobility and may coexist with weakness. It may cause pain and atypical postures, predispose the individual to contractures (particularly those with severe spasticity), and interfere with hygiene and self-care. On the opposite end of the tone spectrum, people with DS have hypotonia that may or may not limit mobility. Tone deficits in DS are not a primary limiting factor to mobility and physical activity, as the characteristic finding of marked hypotonia tends to gradually diminish with age.

Cognitive Function

Cognitive deficits may be a major disabling feature in genetic and developmental conditions such as DS and CP. Similarly, cognitive dysfunction may be a key symptom in chronic conditions such as MS, TBI, and SCI. The degree of cognitive deficits affects not only health management, but also the long-term planning for aging processes in people with chronic disabilities and conditions. The need for lifelong external support is a considerable issue for those who are unable to independently care for themselves as they age. The degree of cognitive deficits in this population may range from memory deficits to mental retardation; the degree of cognitive and perceptual deficits determines participation in functional activities and self-care, mobility, compliance, and even health status.

Standardized outcome measures exist to measure cognitive impairments; the examiner is cautioned to consider the validity and reliability of outcome measures for specific populations before use. The reader is referred to chapters discussing specific diagnoses for detailed outcome measures. Because cognition is multidimensional, examination for deficits will need to be directed at different components of cognition. Screening may be as simple as a three-item recall or short questions determining the ability to follow commands, attention, level of

Pathological Conditions
Fractures
Osteoporosis
Cardiovascular disorders
Degenerative joint disease
Spinal cord compression
Dental problems
Seizures
Pulmonary dysfunction

Impairments
Constipation
Contractures
Depression
Emaciation
Obesity
Incontinence (bowel and bladder)
Pain
Ulcers
Dysphagia
Gastrointestinal problems
Low self-esteem
Nerve entrapments
Overuse syndrome
Balance problems

Functional Limitations or Activity Restrictions
Inability to indicate toileting needs
Dependence on others for activities of daily living
Limitations in mobility
Difficulties using public transportation

Disabilities or Limitations in Life Participation
Difficulties living independently
Limited recreational opportunities
Problems with social relationships and intimacy
Social isolation
Difficulty with role as patient when medical professionals fail to make accommodations for treatment
Underemployment

Modified from Gajdosik CG, Cicerello N. Secondary conditions of the musculoskeletal system in adolescents and adults with cerebral palsy. *Phys Occup Ther Pediatr.* 2001;21:49–68.

consciousness, orientation, judgment, construction, and higher memory function.

Mobility and Posture

In individuals with chronic impairments, addressing inefficient alignments and postures is of critical importance, particularly if this area was not addressed early in their care. The dire effects of such malalignments and compensations described in the following paragraphs eventually affect functional abilities.

Asymmetrical or abnormal gait patterns, crutch walking, and propelling manual wheelchairs for several decades are frequently the major sources of the pain, weakness, and fatigue in people with chronic movement dysfunctions after a medical problem such as TBI, SCI, CP, PPS, or cerebrovascular accident (CVA). The incidence of pain

in a group of 114 patients with confirmed PPS increased from 84% in those who were ambulatory without orthotics to 100% in those who used crutches or wheelchairs for locomotion.[113] A high prevalence of osteoarthritis in patients with PPS was documented in the hand and wrist by radiography.[124] More than twice the number of subjects with PPS had osteoarthritis of the wrist or hand than would be expected in a healthy population of the same age. The risk factor was significantly increased with lower-extremity muscle paralysis and use of assistive devices.

In an electromyographic study of walking in patients with PPS, Perry[125] demonstrated overuse and substitution activity of the vastus lateralis, biceps femoris, and gluteus maximus muscles when the soleus is nonfunctional. Such substitution and overcompensation in the long term, however, lead to microtrauma of ligaments and joint structures and exhaustion of neuromuscular units.

In addition to sitting in poorly supporting chairs, sofas, auto seats, and wheelchairs, the individual with chronic impairments may have trunk muscle paresis or asymmetries of the pelvic base and may spend up to 16 h/day in the seated position. The typical posture is slumped, hanging on posterior vertebral ligaments with loss of lumbar and cervical curves. Neck, shoulder, and back pain are therefore commonly reported.

Levels and types of mobility will be diverse in individuals with chronic neuromuscular impairments. Mobility may range from independent ambulation to gait with an assistive device all the way to wheelchair dependency, depending on existing impairments and cognitive function. Thorough examination should determine the current mobility levels and possible modification needs depending on new impairments or functional limitations. It may be necessary to include a seating examination in people who are wheelchair dependent or sit for the majority of the awake hours.

Balance and Coordination

Deficits in balance and coordination in individuals with chronic conditions predispose these people to falls and limit safe mobility. As individuals with these conditions age, typical age-related changes in balance may add to the existing deficits and magnify functional limitations and impairments. Coordination and balance deficits need to be examined under functional conditions and in the context of the individual's daily activities. Standardized outcome measures are also available to objectively measure impairments; however, the reliability and validity of such measures in specific populations may be deficient. The use of outcome measures may provide a multidimensional look into deficits and provide objective baseline measures to track progress with intervention as well as progression of the movement dysfunction.

Environmental Temperature Intolerance

Consideration for the effects of heat and/or cold may be necessary when working with individuals with chronic diseases, and the examination must include a component of temperature intolerance. Two specific diagnoses embody this phenomenon: PPS for cold intolerance and MS for the negative effects of environmental heat.

Regulation of body temperature is often a problem for individuals with MS (see Chapter 17). Earlier, it was noted that a feature of fatigue unique to MS is that the fatigue is exacerbated by heat. Other MS symptoms may also be aggravated by heat. The Uthoff phenomenon[126] is an adverse response to external heat, causing fatigue or deterioration of symptoms; it often occurs with exercise. Specific recommendations for cooling during exercise intervention may be necessary to counteract the deleterious effects of heat. It is important that the examiner meticulously determine during the health interview the symptomatic effects, if any, of increased temperature in the aging individual with MS.

Sensory deficits per se are not hallmark features of polio; however, cold intolerance is a commonly reported late-onset symptom. Involved extremities in individuals with PPS are frequently abnormally cold as a result of sympathetic nerve cell involvement leading to decreased vasoconstriction and venoconstriction with heat loss to the environment.[127] The impairment may become worse with PPS. Environmental adaptation can create an easy solution to this problem as long as the individual with PPS is aware first of the problem and second of the adaptations necessary to avoid thermoinstability within the extremities. Preventing versus responding to the inadequate vasoresponse to cold empowers the individual to develop environmental control.

Sleep Disturbances

It is common knowledge that older individuals report and manifest sleep disorders.[128,129] Thus this impairment certainly can be associated with aging individuals with chronic movement dysfunction. Disturbances in sleep are a common symptom in people with chronic neuromuscular diseases. Sleep deprivation is a contributing factor to fatigue in individuals with MS. Similarly, more than 50% of individuals with PPS have been found to have sleep disturbances.[130] These disturbances may be caused by pain, stress, hypoventilation, or obstructive apnea.[131-133] Bruno[134] proposed a high incidence of abnormal movements in sleep in nearly two thirds of polio survivors, with 52% reporting sleep disturbance caused by these movements. All seven of subjects with PPS in the study demonstrated abnormal movements in sleep. The author points to the importance of eliminating sleep disorders as a cause of fatigue before the diagnosis of postpolio sequelae is made, particularly because it remains a diagnosis of exclusion.[134]

In addition to the typical symptoms of muscular weakness, pain, and fatigue associated with PPS, some individuals also develop sleep disorders such as PLMs.[103] PLMs in sleep are repetitive episodes of muscular contractions with durations of 0.5 to 5 seconds; frequencies of five or more per sleep hour are deemed pathological. The association of PLMs with insomnia or daily sleepiness suggests the diagnosis of PLM disorder.[103] Whereas PLM has been related to the pathophysiology of PPS,[134] the occurrence of PLM in PPS is not well known.[103] In a recent retrospective study of 99 patients with PPS, researchers assessed the frequency of PLMs during sleep, including other sleep-quality variables such as total sleep time, efficiency of sleep, apnea-hypopnea index, and awaking index.[103] Sixteen patients showed a PLM index that was considered pathological. The authors concluded that a close relationship between PLM and PPS exists; however, the prevalence of PPS with or without PLM and its combination with apnea-hypopnea is not clearly established, a finding in agreement with the conclusions of Jubelt and colleagues.[103,135]

A thorough history and review of systems including a sleep history may reveal the potential causes and guide the therapist in the clinical decision making process for referral and consultation. Sleep apnea, which occurs frequently in polio survivors, and other sleep disorders, including abnormal movements in sleep, may be revealed with specific questioning, triggering the referral process. The therapist plays a role when the sleep disorder is associated with the area of pain management.

Life-Threatening Conditions

Limited knowledge exists of adult health issues for older individuals with developmental disabilities. Secondary medical conditions warrant further examination, particularly in aging adults with chronic conditions. Acute onset of new symptoms may suggest exacerbation of disease or decreased functional reserves or may arise from long-standing effects of impairments from the initial disease process.

In the case of PPS, bulbar muscle dysfunction[112] may also result from the new weakness. Life-threatening conditions such as hypoventilation, dysphagia, sleep apnea,[136] and cardiopulmonary insufficiency require management by medical specialists.[131,137,138] These problems occur in people with previous bulbar poliomyelitis who may or may not be using ventilatory assistance and in those with severe kyphosis or scoliosis. Respiratory failure may occur primarily in individuals with residual respiratory insufficiency and minimal reserves.[135]

Functional Assessment

Performance in functional activities often provides a better picture of the losses stemming from chronic impairments. Decreases in strength are not usually revealed in a single-effort maximum contraction such as required in the manual muscle test. Resistive force during testing is a necessary element for two grades, 5 (normal, "N") and 4 (good, "G"), whereas the other four grades are nonresistive and mostly nonfunctional, and few examiners are now tested for reliability.[139] In a 1-year follow-up using quantitative muscle force testing, no differences were found in muscle strength, work capacity, endurance capacity, or recovery from fatigue of the quadriceps in either asymptomatic or symptomatic groups with PPS.[140] Nevertheless, there is at best a slow decline in functional ability, which patients may describe as loss of muscle strength. Clinically, individuals seeking therapy report functional loss or limitation more easily than a specific loss of muscle strength.

Functional assessment of individuals with chronic movement limitations provides a more practical and clearer picture of the abilities and limitations related to the initial condition or stemming from new impairments. Functional activities are visible and reportable performances of relevant tasks in the context of the individual's culture.[141] Functional tasks imply a specific goal and can range from simple to complex activities. In functional motor performance, the specific task and environmental context is as important as the individual functional movement (refer to Chapter 8). Consideration for these factors is necessary during examination. Detailed functional assessment is outlined by Howle[142] and Zabel.[143]

Functional limitations are difficulties in performing specific tasks. Difficulty in performing daily tasks including mobility and transfers may stem from overuse of muscles and joints that are already performing beyond their typical use, pain, fatigue, muscle weakness, weight gain, cognitive impairments, and decreases in functional endurance, among others. It can be logically inferred that individuals living with chronic movement impairments will reach a tipping point at which the performance of current activities will be hindered, or the way activities are performed will require modification.

Decreases in functional activities over time for varied chronic conditions[44,57-61,144] have been documented in the literature. As early as 5 years and up to 20 years after the initial SCI, individuals have reported decreases in functional activities and increased need for assistance with ADLs.[57-60] An association with the need for increasing support with advancing age in individuals with SCI is seen in the literature.[57-59]

According to Agre and Rodriguez,[145] postpolio survivors with significant weakness perform daily activities at a different level of effort than other individuals; muscles of polio survivors may have to work near maximal effort during activities that individuals without polio can execute at relatively lower levels of effort. Individuals with PPS commonly report difficulty in walking, stair climbing,[44] and dressing. Westbrook[144] described a 5-year follow-up study examining physical and functional abilities and health status of 176 individuals with PPS. During the course of the study, most subjects reported increases in muscle weakness, muscle and joint pain, and changes in walking. Notably, the participants reported more difficulty in four of the eight daily living activities (stair climbing, walking on level surfaces, transfers in and out of bed, and meeting the demands of home or work). Most of the participants (87%) also reported problems in meeting the demands of their job and completing household tasks. Clearly, the ability to perform motor tasks essential to completing one's goals and desires is multifactorial. Therefore functional limitations are usually related to a combination of systems impairments.

In people with PPS, to determine whether the cause of the new weakness is overuse or possibly disuse, a detailed assessment is required of home, work, recreational, and community activities.[146] This paradigm of multidimensional assessment is applicable to all individuals with chronic movement problems. If the patient is merely asked what his or her activity level is, the response may lead to assumptions that weakness is from disuse. With specific questioning, one usually finds that the patient is doing an extraordinary amount of physical activity. It is vital to establish a total picture of the patient's activities in sitting, standing, walking, lifting, carrying, climbing stairs, using a telephone or a computer, and performing daily activities such as self-care and home management.

PSYCHOSOCIAL CONSIDERATIONS

The challenges of chronic diseases are ongoing as the individual ages. Despite new pharmacological interventions, several genetic, developmental, and neuromuscular conditions remain incurable with uncertain courses as the person ages. Although individuals and their families cope effectively with the initial disease process, the incidence of depression is common in the presence of chronic disease and impairments. The impact of chronic conditions on family, marital life, and socioeconomic and financial functions is persistent. The clinician's attitudes, beliefs, support, and understanding will play a major role in the management of individuals with chronic impairments.

Most individuals living with chronic impairments and functional limitations have learned to adapt not only with their movement strategies, but also with the psychological and socioeconomic impact of the initial diagnoses. Not only have these individuals learned to live with the challenges of their initial diagnosis and its movement-related, functional, financial, and psychosocial impact, but their families and caregivers have likewise done so. It may not be surprising, then, that changes to once-established routines, either from acute medical conditions or from gradual but significant changes from the aging process, are resisted and negatively viewed. These individuals will possibly need more assistance, move slower, and need to cut back from activities once engaged in; the consequent changes in philosophy and lifestyle will not likely be welcomed by most individuals and their support systems.

Over the past years, several authors have addressed the prevalence of PPS, its causes, and the effects of aging on the development of PPS.[a] Some literature addresses the effects of aging on developmental and genetic disabilities, yet information on how aging affects individuals with existing impairments is still not conclusive. Because the population of people who are aging with chronic disabilities is increasing owing to improvements in health care delivery and nutrition, evidence concerning the consequences of the aging process remains uncertain. Similarly, the psychological effects are not widely addressed in the literature. Not much is known about the quality of life for older adults

with congenital or childhood-acquired disabilities. Psychological adjustment is difficult with any disease with an unpredictable course and differentiating organic psychological problems from adjustment issues may complicate the management of individuals with chronic diseases.

As a chronic disease, PPS provides an informative example of the interaction among neurological and functional impairments, recovery, effects of aging, and health care. Much has been written about the psychological and psychosocial issues with PPS that is applicable to other chronic disabilities as well. A brief synopsis of the psychosocial considerations of PPS follows.

Postpolio Syndrome

Although the physical manifestations of and interventions for PPS are recognized, psychological symptoms become evident in polio survivors. Bruno and Frick[48] described psychological symptoms such as chronic stress, depression, anxiety, compulsiveness, and type A behavior in polio survivors; these symptoms not only cause distress but limit these individuals in making lifestyle changes to manage late-onset symptoms. Currie and colleagues[123] generalized about adults with childhood-onset or congenital disabilities spanning a range of disability types. Understanding the background of individuals with PPS and a few of the myths that helped to shape their lives is beneficial in their care. Fear of the disease was rampant during the early epidemics. Despite safety measures, children and adolescents contracted polio. Part of the coping strategy was encouraging the child to high levels of physical achievement; approval and rewards were gained by walking farther or faster and keeping up with or exceeding the performance of other children. The best treatment available for all polio victims at that time was from the March of Dimes, which entailed hospitalization for months at a time away from the individuals' families and communities. The situation led to feelings of abandonment, anxiety, and total dependence on strangers. The "polio patient" was expected to be a "good patient" and to "work hard." Indeed, these patients did work hard to reeducate weakened muscles and compensate for lost function.[48–51] Courage, determination, and cheerfulness were attributes to be prized, self-pity was viewed unfavorably, and talking about the functional loss was not encouraged. Later in the recovery process, parents made decisions to have their children undergo multiple surgical procedures to allow removal of heavy braces so that they would "look normal" and "fit in." One can understand why patients react so negatively to the suggestion of orthotics.

Coping Strategies

The psychosocial issues confronting people with PPS often are more disruptive than the physical problems.[31,32,90,152–154] An increasing population of polio survivors is experiencing, with aging, an unanticipated late onset of new symptoms. Associated with loss of physical function and independence are social and psychological problems stemming from the inability to perform personal and societal roles. Previous research suggests that well-established, often compulsive behavior patterns may impair the ability to deal effectively with the new threats to functional independence. Bruno and Frick[33] confirmed the presence of psychological stress in survivors, noting that type A behavior and stress could precipitate or exacerbate postpolio sequelae. In a later study in 1991[48] the same researchers suggested that the acute experience conditioned survivors into lifelong patterns of compulsive type A behavior, a behavior pattern that impairs the ability to cope with new late postpolio symptoms. Kuehn and Winters[155] also noted that symptom distress and intensity were less in individuals with greater coping resources. In this study[155] in Sweden of 113 patients with postpolio sequelae, results revealed that the prevalence of distress

---

[a]References 28, 30, 34, 35, 40, 41, 44, 47, 90, 98, 112, 124, 147–151.

was highest in the physical dimensions of physical mobility, pain, and energy and lowest in social isolation. The high scores for the triad of dimensions were similar to the findings of previous studies.[136]

Individuals with PPS developed several styles to cope with their disability. Maynard and Roller[156] described coping styles according to severity of muscular involvement. Survivors with little or no obvious physical involvement were able to hide atrophy with clothing and avoided activities that revealed the weakness. Many individuals invested much energy in projecting normality and were so adept at denial that they disconnected themselves from the polio experience; often spouses do not know of the history of polio. This group can develop the most severe cases of PPS. The denial renders them detached from other individuals with PPS and thus difficult to assist.

Polio survivors with obvious physical involvement such as a limp or an atrophied extremity or who use an assistive device have usually pushed themselves to function at normal or supernormal levels. These individuals will tolerate high levels of pain before acknowledging the late effects of polio. The third group, the most severely impaired of the individuals with PPS, may have respiratory involvement or more mobility deficits. Several use or have used wheelchairs for mobility and required great effort and persistence to gain independence in self-care activities. The members of this group integrated their functional problems into their self-image and have led active, productive lives.

In a 5-year study of 176 individuals with PPS, it was unexpectedly found that participants' stress levels decreased over time.[144] The author hypothesized that eventually, lifestyle modifications and treatment contributed to the coping process. Kuehn and Winters[155] in their study found that more than half of their subjects of working age had gainful employment. Moreover, no difference in employment rate as a result of distribution of polio involvement was found, implying that this was not a deciding factor. The authors hypothesize that people with severe polio involvement were either forced to choose or encouraged to take up an appropriate profession early in life, whereas those with less involvement had not needed such planning. Nevertheless, vocational issues encompassing satisfactory accessibility and equipment are an important part of management.

Response to new diagnosis. The response to the diagnosis of PPS can range from relief to despair. Relief comes to polio survivors who have been told their symptoms were psychosomatic. Despair occurs when survivors are given a program of lifestyle changes and management suggestions that are opposed to the adage they followed during the initial infection. The proposed philosophy shift from "no pain, no gain" to energy conservation and rest may be viewed unfavorably or with disdain. Polio survivors who have led active lives may have significant difficulty adjusting their lifestyle to new symptoms and decreasing abilities, and psychological support may be indicated.[157]

The stresses of the diagnostic process also add to the challenges. Most health care professionals have limited understanding of the initial polio experience and the late effects of polio, and therefore the diagnostic process of PPS may take time and involve a series of physician consultations.[48,49,158–160] Publicity from support groups has helped refer patients to PPS clinics or to specialists with knowledge of PPS.[160]

Fear of the threat to independence, inadequate knowledge about the physiological changes, and the expectation of functional loss may contribute to the anxiety of polio survivors. Individuals with PPS will feel anxious about the prospects of changing roles with their families, friends, and co-workers.[49,156,159] Defenses and coping strategies that have been successfully used for years have broken down, and the individual experiences overwhelming anxieties and conflicts.[159]

Compliance. The patient-clinician relationship is an important determinant of compliance. Several authors[33,48,161] have identified compliance as a significant problem in type A polio survivors. Although a few individuals with PPS readily accept suggestions for lifestyle changes, a few immediately make changes, and a few refuse to consider any changes at all, most will eventually make changes but will require support, patience, and time to process. Compliance is an issue encountered not only in individuals with PPS but in many individuals with chronic conditions. Clinicians' sensitivity, support, and respect will play a major role in the response of the patient/client to management suggestions. Acknowledging the individual's current activities, values, and goals is an important step in establishing a relationship with the patient/client. Allowing patients to express feelings about the new challenges, their prior high levels of physical achievement, and previous treatment is equally important.

A health care provider perceived to be knowledgeable, interested, and concerned significantly increases compliance with recommendations.[162] Adherence of the patient/client with PPS may be improved by the therapist's ability to suggest management strategies that are accepted as conventional and the ability to alleviate pain in the initial examination. Conservative management should be attempted first before more aggressive or life-changing interventions such as orthoses, mobility changes, or motorized carts, which they may have used in the past and eventually discarded. Therapists can also be a source of information about support groups.[160] Support groups offer information about multiple facets of living with chronic impairments, and these members may be positive role models to help the newly diagnosed individual in the transition process as well as the aging individual with chronic disease and impairments in dealing with issues in terms of maturation and advancing age.

HEALTH-RELATED DISPARITIES IN AGING ADULTS WITH CHRONIC DISABILITIES

Individuals aging with chronic impairments and conditions are exposed to the effects of aging and maturation differently than the general population. People with disabilities often start at the lower end of the health continuum owing to secondary conditions that overlap with the primary disability.[163] Few will argue that despite medical advances and public health initiatives, the reality is that health disparities, including decreased access to high-quality health care, health promotion, disease prevention, and health literacy, are still present and reflect areas that need to be addressed. Outlined here are some health disparities facing adults with chronic disabilities and conditions.

- Compared with the general population, higher rates of disability and obesity are seen among adults with developmental delay.[83,164,165] Of adults with major physical and sensory impairments, 27% are obese, compared with 19% of those without major disability.[85]
- Cardiovascular disease is one of the most common causes of death among aging adults with developmental delay.[26,166,167]
- Evidence supports the earlier appearance of age-related health conditions in individuals with developmental delay. Conditions include cognitive decline, incontinence, and sensory losses.[168] Examples of health conditions that may be influenced by aging in people with developmental delay were discussed earlier regarding individuals with CP[169] (who may have increased issues with musculoskeletal deformities, progressive cervical spine degeneration, dental problems, bladder or bowel dysfunction, or osteoporosis) and individuals with DS (who have a higher prevalence of early-onset Alzheimer's disease compared with the general public).[22,170]
- Generally, individuals with intellectual and developmental disabilities have poorer health and more difficulty in finding, accessing, and paying for higher-quality health care.[16]

- Adults with developmental disabilities also have limited access to medical care, which may result in lack of obesity screening, counseling, and management.[171]
- Higher rates of depression, anxiety, and strong fears and stress are seen in people with chronic disabilities. Iezzoni and O'Day[85] found that 34% of adults with major impairments in walking reported frequent depression or anxiety, compared with 3% in those without disabilities.

MANAGEMENT OF CHRONIC IMPAIRMENTS

Aging With Chronic Impairments

The management of individuals with chronic impairments is challenging, not only because of the possibility of multisystem involvement warranting a holistic approach, but also because much is unknown about effects of the aging process on chronic neuromuscular impairments.

Aging adults with chronic conditions may be more vulnerable to conditions that will make their old age potentially more difficult with an increased possibility for infirmity and dependence.[16] Individuals with chronic and disabling impairments are often at an increased risk for the development of secondary conditions and further disability that can lead to further decline in independence and functional status and to mobility deficits. It has been suggested that people with chronic conditions, such as living with developmental delay, may age differently based on the nature and severity of their disability, other coexisting health problems, and secondary chronic conditions. With increased life expectancy, health care professions will likely see an increase in the care of those aging with chronic impairments. There is then a unique challenge for health care professionals to develop and implement programs for the management of aging adults with chronic impairments to effect optimal health status.

The heterogeneity of aging adults with chronic neuromuscular impairments lends to the need for individualized management programs. The aging process is unique for each individual, as is the recovery process in people with chronic conditions and the overall manifestation of late-onset or secondary symptoms. Therefore intervention will be dependent on the individual's current symptoms, functional needs, level of activity limitations, and values or goals.

Although evidence exists regarding interventions for individuals with chronic disease, overall, there is a dearth of information on specific treatment strategies if one considers the magnitude of associated diseases and the increasing population of individuals aging with chronic functional limitations and impairments. The reason for this is multifactorial; it may stem from the mismatch between the increase in number of individuals with chronic diseases that is resulting from longer life expectancies because of advancements in medicine and the gaps in our knowledge about the effects of aging in this population. The limitation on specific knowledge about interventions is echoed by Marks and colleagues, who state that there is a lack of framework for assessing health-related interventions for individuals aging with developmental delay.[172]

A finite number of research and treatment centers have been established to deal with comprehensive care issues for individuals with disabilities.[173] The statement by Kailes[174] regarding the lack of helpful information related to exercising for those aging with a disability is troubling yet accurate. Considering the extensive evidence showing that many of the physical limitations that occur as part of aging in nondisabled people can be prevented or delayed by changing health habits, Kailes[174] suggests that individuals with disabilities need (1) appropriate fitness assessment measures that can be used with various types of disabilities, (2) exercise guidelines that are appropriate for age and types of limitations, (3) exercise facilities that are accessible, integrated, and not separate from those of nondisabled populations, and (4) exercise equipment that incorporates universal design features.

Unfortunately, in today's health care environment, many individuals with PPS, SCI, TBI, or developmental disabilities do not have access to specialists, including PTs, who understand their complex movement limitation–related needs and how these limitations affect participation in life. Care is fragmented, and physicians and therapists, if involved in the care at all, seldom have a comprehensive picture of the person's needs. Although one might assume that the managed-care system would provide coordination of care within the provider system, the reality is that there may be more restrictions in care, particularly for disability-related care that may require a period of continuing rehabilitation treatment and retraining. Even providers within the group seldom communicate because the group is composed of practitioners who accept the insurance contract rather than practitioners working together to improve health. In my experience, hardly any individuals aging with neurological conditions such as TBI, CVA, or SCI seek therapy past their initial episode of care in the acute phase of the condition. This reality is confirmed in the literature; today people with SCI or TBI are followed in comprehensive specialty centers or clinics as they age.[175,176]

Multisystem Approach

Individuals with chronic neuromuscular conditions have multidimensional impairments across multiple systems. Chronicity of impairments in one system likely and eventually affects other systems. For example, an individual with limited physical mobility because of impairments in the neuromuscular system likely has decreased levels of physical activity, which in turn are correlated with lower muscle strength, which is associated with a greater degree of disability. Although the initial impairments may be in the neuromuscular system, over time the condition will affect the cardiovascular system because of inactivity and potentially the integumentary system. An increased likelihood of multisystem effects in an individual with chronic impairments is a reality. Therefore a multisystem, holistic approach to management is warranted.

The rehabilitation clinician is in a unique position to provide holistic care to the patient with chronic impairments. In the realm of management of chronic movement dysfunction, PPS becomes a model case for other chronic neuromuscular conditions—there is much to learn from the complex nature of the late effects of polio. Designing an intervention program may be as challenging as the evaluation because of the interactions of the systems and the influences of the environment, medical treatment, and aging. Before beginning physical or occupational therapy, it is necessary for the team to first identify and treat other medical and neurological conditions that may produce the reported symptoms.[177]

The individual's values and goals are the most significant variables to take into consideration in designing the interventions. Improvement will largely depend on the patient's commitment and thus compliance. Relatively simple interventions may result in distinctive positive changes. Conservative management should be attempted first before major life-changing interventions. Psychological considerations play a major role in designing an acceptable and appropriate management plan that will encourage compliance. Lifestyle modifications may not be favorably viewed by some individuals who have "conquered" the disease and pushed themselves to be independent, as in the case of those with PPS or SCI in their younger years. Prescription of interventions that are perceived to be "radical" should be done with sensitivity and caution. The rationale for interventions should be carefully considered in light of the patient's current functional status and goals. Introduction of orthoses, assistive devices, and mobility modifications is often difficult for the individual with chronic impairments to accept, given the long, arduous effort expended over years to avoid such devices and the movement adaptation achieved without such devices.

The long-term goals for individuals with chronic conditions center primarily on self-management of home exercise programs and appropriate lifestyle changes to reduce physical demands. No definitive, curative intervention currently exists for chronic neuromuscular conditions ranging from developmental delay (CP) to those acquired through trauma or disease sometime in the life-span (SCI, TBI, PPS); therefore symptom management is a key element in both the short and long terms. Short-term goals focus on the symptoms present and may address the following areas:

- Modified strengthening and conditioning
- Postural correction
- Energy conservation
- Lifestyle modifications
- Mobility and locomotion
- Balance during functional activities
- Walking aids, mobility devices, orthoses
- Pain reduction
- Improved functional endurance
- Ability to transfer
- Respiratory care
- Weight control

The information is presented with an evidence-based approach and will specifically address the management of adults with PPS, SCI, and TBI. When possible, the intervention approaches first offered should focus on several problems at one time (Table 35.2). The importance of individualized programs that address the variability of symptoms cannot be overemphasized. The reader is referred to specific references for further details on management prescriptions.[83,172]

Before discussion of specific intervention strategies, a shift in the philosophy of management of chronic disease and disability is presented. Within the past decade, in an effort to affect the trajectory of further decline from chronic conditions, there appears to have been a shift toward the promotion of health rather than the control of the disease itself.

HEALTH PROMOTION

Health Promotion With Chronic Conditions

Emerging in the public health arena is a call for attention to the growing population of aging adults with chronic disabilities and for reducing health disparities involving this aging population. There is consensus on a need to address issues related to the health and care of aging individuals with developmental and intellectual disabilities related to primary care, health promotion, health literacy, and health care providers.[83,172]

Decreasing health disparities affecting aging adults with chronic impairments is an increasing area of focus, as evidenced by its inclusion in the national health goals for individuals with disabilities outlined in several documents such as the Healthy People 2020 initiative,[178] the New Freedom Initiative,[179] the US Department of Health and Human Services document *Closing the Gap: A National Blueprint to Improve the Health of Persons with Mental Retardation*,[180] and the US Surgeon General's Call to Action to Improve the Health and Wellness of Persons with Disabilities.[181] Healthy People 2010 cautioned that people with disabilities would be expected to experience disadvantages

TABLE 35.2 Evidence-Based Approach to the Management of Post-Polio Syndrome

Generalized weakness	Lifestyle changes Therapeutic nonfatiguing strengthening exercises Aerobic exercise Orthoses Assistive devices Avoidance of overuse Weight loss
Pain	Therapeutic heating modalities[a] Cryotherapy[a] Activity reduction and lifestyle changes Pacing of activities Stretching Weight loss Assistive devices Orthoses Motorized mobility devices Nonsteroidal antiinflammatory drugs[b]
Dysphagia	Dietary changes or restrictions Breathing techniques Swallowing techniques Monitoring fatigue and timing eating when not fatigued
Fatigue	Lifestyle changes Energy conservation techniques Nonfatiguing exercise programs Lightweight orthoses and assistive devices Pacing of activities Frequent rest breaks Naps during the day Motorized mobility devices
Cardiopulmonary conditioning	Aquatic exercise training Endurance training Cycle or arm exercises
Psychosocial concerns	Postpolio support groups Interdisciplinary approach Counseling from psychologists, psychiatrists Vocational counseling Behavior modification
Pulmonary dysfunction	Preventive measures Noninvasive ventilatory assistance Pulmonary therapy Breathing exercises: glossopharyngeal breathing

[a]Effectiveness of heat and cold modalities are patient specific and must be used with caution.
[b]Antiinflammatory drugs have been shown to be effective in pain management in medical treatment of postpolio syndrome. The specific drug and dosage must be prescribed by the physician.
Modified from Trojan D, Finch L. Management of post-polio syndrome. *NeuroRehabilitation*. 1997;8:93–105; and Jubelt B, Agre J. Management of post-polio syndrome. *JAMA*. 2000;284:412–414.

in health compared with the general population. Five years after the release of the US Surgeon General's Call to Action, it was reported that some individuals with disabilities still lacked equal access to health care, and health promotion has been outlined as a goal to be achieved by people with disabilities.[181]

Health promotion is defined by Pender and colleagues[182] as activities motivated by the desire to increase well-being and actualize human potential. It includes self-initiated behaviors and stresses the need to enhance the responsibility and commitment of each person to achieve a healthy lifestyle. Health promotion was reflected in Healthy People 2010. Healthy People 2020 includes individuals with disabilities in all health promotion efforts as an emerging area in disability and health, reflecting a continuation of the initiative's prior goals for the well-being of people with disabilities.[178]

Shift to Health Promotion

In 1997, Patrick[183] found that research on health promotion for individuals with health disabilities was almost nonexistent. Fast-forward to 2011: a shift from disability prevention to health promotion has emerged, and literature on health promotion efforts for people with a variety of chronic diseases is emerging.

In contrast to health protection or disease-management behaviors, which are motivated by the desire to avoid illness or its effects, health promotion is not disease- or injury-specific.[182] Whereas both wellness and disease-management interventions may focus on improving similar health behaviors, a critical difference between these approaches has been proposed by Stuifbergen and colleagues.[184] They assert that the significant difference is in how the individual is viewed with regard to the interaction between his or her chronic disability and the purpose or intention of the change in behavior—that is, control and management of disease versus maximizing quality of life and health. Furthermore, whereas wellness interventions have wellness or health in the forefront and the disease in the background,[185] wellness and health promotion interventions allow the individual to choose behaviors that improve and/or sustain the quality of life within the perspective of living with chronic conditions.[186]

Part of the national initiative to improve the health of aging adults with developmental disabilities, the US Surgeon General's Call to Action to Improve the Health and Wellness of Persons with Disabilities[181] stated that people with disabilities can promote their own health through developing or maintaining healthy lifestyles. Embedded in this statement is the responsibility of the individual for his or her own health trajectory. This responsibility is shared with health care providers and support persons. A need to develop skills to improve health literacy related to health care issues is paramount to this responsibility[172] and to encouragement of active participation. Health literacy is defined by Selden[187] as the degree to which individuals have the capacity to obtain, process, and understand basic health information and services necessary to make apt health decisions.

Early education combined with opportunities for lifelong learning can help individuals develop the skills and confidence needed to improve or manage healthy lifestyles with aging.[172] Similarly, health care professionals need to improve, maintain, and use clear communication.

Health promotion and disease prevention activities should consist of specific health education programs and preventive or screening programs.[172] In the paradigm shift to health promotion, some interventions have focused on a single behavior such as exercise or nutrition or a combination of interventions for a more inclusive lifestyle approach.[184,186,188]

Community-Based Programs

With approximately 35% of Americans aged 65 and older with a disability[189] targeted by public health initiatives, assistive technology advancements, and cultural changes, many barriers still exist to access community-based programs.[179] Community-based interventions for health promotion are ideal for those with developmental disabilities

because they address social inclusion, self-efficacy, and sustainability.[190] However, few community-based lifestyle interventions targeting those with developmental disabilities exist.[26] Developing and implementing accessible programs in the community setting for adults with long-term disabilities remain challenging.[172]

Today, adults with chronic movement dysfunction have more of an opportunity to participate in sporting events and recreational activities. Therapists need to be involved in the process to ensure optimum benefit of these activities for patients to be not only successful but also safe. As research supports fitness training for people with chronic disabilities and impairments, more effort will be needed to maximize the availability of community-based facilities to meet the demand. Again, therapists can be instrumental not only in the design of equipment but also in advocacy efforts by educating governmental officials and third-party payers regarding the needs of those aging with chronic conditions. Therapists not only possess the knowledge of the physiological effects of exercise but also understand biomechanical principles critical to ensuring safety in fitness and recreational activities. Therapists can work with these individuals on maximizing strength, flexibility, body mass indices, and cardiorespiratory reserves. This focus will not only increase functional capacity and social participation of the adult with functional limitations but will lower the risk of medical comorbidities associated with the effects of physical inactivity.

Health Promotion Interventions: Evidence and Challenges

Iezzoni[83] identified several barriers faced by people with disability to accessing health care and public health interventions. Physical access, communication, financial barriers, and discriminatory and stigmatizing attitudes were identified as externally imposed barriers.

Although there has been a shift in philosophy and growing interest in health promotion in individuals with chronic impairments, the supporting evidence on the effectiveness of these interventions has not been examined in depth. Although there are published studies on health promotion in people with chronic diseases, several challenges arise. Studies often involve varied chronic diseases such as cancer, heart failure, arthritis, or human immunodeficiency virus (HIV) infection, with few studies examining individuals with chronic neuromuscular conditions. The studies often involve small experimental interventional strategies, use small population samples, and have varied intervention delivery from individual, group, or community-based programs. Moreover, Stuifbergen and colleagues[184] found that despite the benefits of health promotion for improving or maintaining function and independence in older adults, very few studies had samples of older subjects. Iezzoni[83] asserts that improving access to health promotion and disease prevention should be a national public health priority.

A mounting body of evidence regarding the positive impact of health promotion and wellness interventions on individuals with chronic conditions is seen in the literature.[184] Although these studies report significant effects and used multiple outcome measures, they had small population samples that encompassed varied chronic conditions not specific to those with neuromuscular impairments alone. Moreover, types, lengths, and delivery of interventions varied greatly from community-based to independent settings. Therefore, generalization and comparison across studies are difficult to say the least. It is noteworthy that a review of the literature supports the benefits and positive effects of health promotion and wellness interventions; however, in agreement with the findings of Stuifbergen and colleagues,[184] minimal information exists about the long-term effects or efficacy of interventions.

INTERVENTION STRATEGIES

A paucity of evidence specifically addresses precise exercise or intervention plans in individuals with chronic impairments. This lack of data is evident in specific neurological populations: SCI TBI and PPS, to name a few. Although no published studies were found on exercise plans and aging in SCI, the interest in promoting exercise and lifestyle changes to prevent secondary medical problems has been identified. Similarly, most studies are conducted in the early years after TBI, and although TBI is a lifetime disability, little attention has been paid to the needs of aging people after a TBI who may have recurring needs for physical and cognitive rehabilitation and retraining over the life-span. The information presented is directed more toward PPS, for which a body of evidence supports specific intervention strategies. There is still a marked lack of longitudinal research examining the natural course of health conditions, much less targeted interventions for aging adults with PPS. In a recent review on the treatment of PPS through the Cochrane Collaboration, Koopman and colleagues[27] found inadequate evidence from randomized controlled studies pointing to definitive conclusions on the effectiveness of different treatment options for individuals with PPS. Their results indicate that pharmacological intervention, specifically drugs such as lamotrigine and intravenous immunoglobulin (IVIG), and nonpharmacological interventions, specifically muscle strengthening and static magnetic fields, may be beneficial but need further research.[27]

As with other chronic neuromuscular conditions, there currently exists no curative treatment for PPS,[27] and therefore rehabilitation management is regarded as the key intervention. The succeeding discussion presents strategies for the rehabilitation of chronic neuromuscular dysfunction with the goals of improving and/or maintaining functional capacities and decreasing secondary impairments magnified by aging or the chronicity of the condition.

Although primarily directed at PPS, most of, if not all, the intervention strategies are applicable to people with other chronic impairments; there are commonalities to all chronic neuromuscular conditions that need to be identified and analyzed from a long-term quality-of-life perspective. Individuals who are aging with these chronic functional limitations should be allowed to age with the dignity given to any other individual. The challenge to therapists will be to step out of the model of regaining functional skill through repetitive practice and into the model of maintaining function, energy conservation, and empowerment of that function to the individual needing service. The patient/client is and should be the individual who determines what aspect of functional activities are critical to quality of life and what compensations are acceptable and unacceptable as part of an adult life expectation. From that information and the analytical understanding of what is happening to the CNS of these individuals, patients and therapists together can establish realistic goals and intervention strategies that will optimize and maintain the potential motor function of those individuals.

Therapeutic Exercise
Strengthening and Conditioning

Evidence suggests that both physical activity and strength are significant factors in severity of disability.[191] It has been shown that muscle strength has a significant role in a spiraling model of decline. Specifically, lower muscle strength is correlated with a greater degree of disability. In terms of function, difficulties in motor activities are reported by those with poor strength. It is logical, then, that the management of chronic disabilities involves a strengthening program.

A mounting body of evidence supports strengthening exercises for individuals with PPS,[112,192–196] contrary to the initial approach of no exercise because of fear of overuse or symptom exacerbation. Generally, individuals with PPS who exercised and avoided overuse demonstrated positive results without detrimental effects. Several types of nonfatiguing strengthening exercises, aerobic exercise, and the evidence supporting them have been examined. Willen and colleagues[197] suggest that water exercise may be beneficial because it decreases the biomechanical stresses on the muscles and joints. Specific exercise prescription is dependent on several factors such as the current level of function, other presenting symptoms, and the patient's interests.

Jubelt and Agre[112] note that the most important advance in the treatment of weakness in PPS involves the findings of several studies that mild to moderate weakness can be improved with nonfatiguing exercises. The benefits of nonfatiguing exercises using both submaximal and maximal contraction with limited number of repetitions are documented in the literature.[112,192]

Isokinetic and isometric dynamometers have been used to record maximum muscle forces (or torques) in PPS subjects before and after resistive exercise programs designed to increase muscle strength. Two of the studies were of single cases,[198,199] and two had 12 and 17 subjects.[193,194] Both of the multisubject studies tested the quadriceps femoris. Einarsson[193] investigated the effects of a standardized, 6-week, maximal effort and isometric strength training program on the quadriceps muscles of 12 individuals with post-polio muscles, nine of whom met the criteria for PPS. Einarsson[193] reports an average gain of 29% in isometric strength and 24% in isokinetic strength over a period of 6 weeks; muscle biopsy specimens revealed no muscle damage. In addition to the feeling of well-being in most of the subjects during and after the training program, 10 of 12 subjects stated a feeling of increased strength in the trained muscle. In subsequent follow-ups 6 to 12 months after intervention, gains in strength did not decrease, and several subjects reported better performance in daily activities such as climbing stairs, walking, and standing from a chair.[193]

Fillyaw and colleagues[194] reported a strength gain of 8% over a 2-year period. An isometric contraction was used for testing, and concentric-eccentric contractions were used for the exercise. These results do not compare with the strength gains of 100% and higher made by healthy subjects undergoing training but rather compare with serial testing when no exercise was done.[195,196] For example, Munin and colleagues[195] measured the affected and unaffected quadriceps muscle every 6 months over 3 years to document muscle weakness in people with PPS. They reported increases in muscle strength up to 25%. In older people without polio, test performance gains of the quadriceps increased an average of 174% in 90-year-old subjects[200] and 107% in 60- to 72-year-old men.[201] In these two studies, thigh muscle area (as documented by computed tomography) increased by 9% and 11%, respectively, indicating an increase in muscle bulk.

The effects of nonfatiguing resistance exercises are well documented in the literature. Fillyaw and colleagues[194] in a study of 17 subjects with PPS concluded that muscle strength may be increased in individuals with PPS and suggested supervision of exercise programs by PTs and quantitative muscle testing every 3 months to guard against overuse weakness. Agre and Rodriguez[202] suggested that a supervised exercise program could safely increase strength in subjects with PPS with at least a grade 3+ strength. Their program of a supervised 12-week nonfatiguing quadriceps strengthening program with rest intervals revealed no detrimental effects. Most of the participants reported improvements in quadriceps strength, endurance, and work capacity, and half noted increased strength recovery with rest periods after activity, walking, and stair climbing. A nonfatiguing weight lifting program used for at least 24 weeks was examined in six subjects with PPS by Feldman and Soskolne.[203] The results showed increased strength in 14 of the 32 muscle groups with maintained strength in 17 muscles.

Alternate-day, low-intensity, muscle-strengthening quadriceps exercises showed no adverse effects, with reported findings of increased endurance, strength, and work capacity. As a result of the low-intensity program, no increased muscle strength was found, although half of the participants sensed increased strength recovery after exercise.[204] The same protocol, but with a more vigorous program of 4 days per week, revealed improvements in muscular work performance and endurance without unfavorable effects noted.[204]

Because there are neural adaptations specific to the type of muscle contraction used for measurement and training, it is difficult to determine the differences in true increases in strength from the ability to improve performance on a specific test. Another term for this phenomenon or improvement in performance is *motor learning* (see Chapter 4). The theory states that the subject learns to perform the measurement or the exercise better without true gains in strength. This happens even with an apparently simple weekly maximum isometric contraction.[205] Evidence of this phenomenon can be seen when improvements are made in the opposite untrained muscle group (transfer of training), when the apparent strength gains are maintained for months after cessation of the training, and when there are no increases in the size of the muscle. The greatest improvements in test performance occur when the muscle contraction is the same for both the test and the training. Smaller increases are seen when the measurement and training muscle contractions are different and when measures to decrease the effect of motor learning have been used.

The neural adaptation specific to the type of measurement or training is illustrated in the following study on older men.[201] Multiple tests to assess strength were performed. The training program required lifting and lowering 80% of the weight of one repetition maximum (1 RM), which was assessed weekly. After 12 weeks, there were average increases in quadriceps muscle strength of 104% for the 1 RM, 7% for maximum isometric, 8% for maximum isokinetic at 60 degrees per second, and 10% for isokinetic at 240 degrees per second. In addition, there was an increase in cross-sectional area of the quadriceps of 10%, and muscle biopsy showed approximately a 30% increase in muscle fiber size.[206] This study illustrates some of the complexities of designing or evaluating studies that attempt to measure changes in muscle strength.

In chronic movement dysfunction, high tone is a symptom that may be considered a deterrent to exercise. As therapeutic procedures became based on motor control, motor learning, and neuroplasticity theories, strengthening of spastic muscles may still be underused.[207,208] In the past, placing resistance on a spastic muscle was thought to increase the spasticity. This tenet was interpreted to preclude anyone from advocating strength training in these individuals.[207,209] Interestingly, the literature identified that one of the major problems of CP is weakness. Clinicians during the 1960s and 1970s believed that the answer to this weakness underlying spasticity was to increase proprioceptive and tactile stimulation.[207,209] Current research would say that true strengthening would not occur through feedback alone and that resistance on muscle tissue is a necessary variable for strength training.[109,210,211] Damiano and colleagues[110,212–214] have shown that resistance training does not affect spasticity negatively and in fact improves many functional measures of gait. On the basis of these findings, clinicians should evaluate individual patients to determine whether the level of weakness is affecting functional performance or the attainment of personal goals. If indeed the individual's weakness is found to be clinically significant, then strength training is indicated. Strength training within functional patterns should lead to the greatest carryover.

Physical Activity

The literature clearly documents the benefits of physical activity, and in polio survivors with PPS, activity that falls within a safe range is

---

BOX 35.6 Functional Exercise: Key Points

1. Consult with a health care team before starting an exercise program. A physical and occupational therapist can provide valuable insight and recommendations on activity type and intensity.
2. Avoid overuse of muscle groups.
3. Judicious exercise programs of low to high intensity can result in positive results. Include warm-up and cool-down periods.
4. Short periods of activity are encouraged.
5. Allow for adequate rest between bouts of activity.
6. Alternate days may be necessary for full recovery (depending on activity type).
7. Individualized therapy program to address unique needs is critical.
8. Use energy conservation and joint protection techniques in regular routines.
9. Incorporate breathing, relaxation, mental imagery, and meditation exercises into daily activities.
10. Be cognizant of the body's alignment during exercise and functional activities.
11. Incorporate postural exercises and correction to address malalignments and unnecessary use of muscles and joints.
12. Compliance with clinical recommendations can significantly reduce symptoms and prevent further decline.
13. Listen to your body—pain is typically your body's way of alerting you to slow down or to stop.

---

beneficial to overall functional performance (Box 35.6). In a study involving women with disabilities in the Women's Health and Aging Study,[191] the authors found an inverse relationship between disability and physical activity, with the most disabled women being more inactive. In addition to diseases and musculoskeletal pain being directly associated with motor disability, lower levels of physical activity associated with poorer muscle strength contributed to a greater degree of motor disability.

Physical inactivity and obesity have been shown to be more common in individuals with developmental disabilities than in the general population.[26,165] Specifically, Rimmer and Wang[215] in a study of 306 individuals with physical and mental disabilities found that the rate of obesity in those with intellectual disabilities was twice as high as in the general population. More alarming was the finding that the rate of extreme obesity (body mass index [BMI] equal to or greater than 40 kg/m^2) was approximately four times higher among individuals with disabilities than in the general population. Moreover, individuals experience high rates of secondary conditions associated with obesity and inactivity, such as type 2 diabetes, cardiovascular disease, and metabolic syndrome.[166]

Although few studies have been done on the impact of exercise or the best type of exercise for people aging with a TBI, Gordon and colleagues[216] studied 240 people living in the community with a TBI. They compared exercisers and nonexercisers with a TBI and exercisers and nonexercisers without a TBI. Typical exercise activities were swimming, jogging, biking, or sports that increased heart rate for more than 30 minutes at least three times per week for a six-month period. Their findings suggest that although exercise did not decrease functional impairments related to the TBI, people who exercised reported fewer physical, emotional (less depression), or cognitive complaints (sleep problems, irritability, memory problems, and disorganization). Of interest was that the exercisers in the group with a TBI had more severe brain injuries than those who did not exercise. In their online TBI consumer report, Gordon and colleagues[216] recommend aerobic and nonaerobic exercises as beneficial. They also suggest that individuals with TBIs check out local exercise centers, independent living centers, or adult education classes and seek out videotapes that might provide encouragement or support for engaging in exercise. There is no mention of referrals to PTs or OTs for guidance in setting up exercise or lifestyle change programs or locating resources within the community.[217]

Cardiopulmonary Conditioning

Because cardiovascular disease is one of the most common causes of death among aging adults with developmental delay,[26,166,167] and physical inactivity and obesity occur at higher rates in this population, cardiovascular conditioning is a critical part of the management of individuals with chronic impairments. The following information pertains to interventions for individuals with PPS, as the evidence is strong for this population. Although limited information exists for those with SCI or TBI, one can logically infer that some benefits are likely to occur with aerobic activities in these groups.

Aerobic testing using modified protocols to reduce fatigue has been used on the treadmill,[218] bicycle ergometer,[219] and arm ergometer[220] in individuals with PPS. There were no cardiorespiratory training effects in the first study, probably owing to the low intensity of the exercise, but the duration and distance of walking increased.[195] The two ergometry studies showed an increase in maximum oxygen consumption of 15% and 19%, which is a training effect comparable to normal values for age. There were, however, no changes in blood pressure or heart rate, particularly the expected decrease in resting heart rate that occurs with aerobic training. Although the intensity of the exercise protocols had to be reduced for some of the subjects, none had to terminate the exercise because of overuse symptoms, nor did these symptoms occur at the end of the studies. A problem in evaluating these studies is that it is not always clear whether the study subjects with PPS were asymptomatic, symptomatic (PPS), or mixed.

An endurance training program in subjects with PPS demonstrated beneficial cardiovascular and strength effects without adverse consequences.[221] Aerobic exercise such as using a bicycle ergometer, walking, or swimming may be useful, but the patient must be interested in the activity to increase compliance.[177] Willen and colleagues[197] in a study of 28 individuals with late effects of polio found that a program of nonswimming dynamic exercise in warm water twice weekly resulted in decreased heart rate at submaximal work level, less pain, and positive functional impact. As with the previous studies on exercises, no adverse effects were noted. Their general fitness training, however, did not result in changes in muscle strength or endurance. Previous studies documenting improvements in muscle function and aerobic capacity were designed for three or more times per week; the authors hypothesize that a twice-a-week program was not enough to show improvements in the subjects' aerobic capacities or muscle strength.

The literature indicates that exercise within constraints can lead to several beneficial physiological and psychological adaptations in individuals with PPS.[177,192] It appears that therapeutic exercise is beneficial when performed without causing undue pain and fatigue. As with any intervention, a comprehensive examination will assist in developing a well-rounded and individualized program tailored to the specific needs of the individual with PPS.

Pulmonary Status

Older individuals with neuromuscular diseases may have increased vulnerability to respiratory complications.[123] Respiratory insufficiency and sleep apnea may mandate intermittent or constant use of ventilatory devices. Nighttime noninvasive positive pressure ventilation may be beneficial.[222] Pulmonary therapy and breathing exercises may help some individuals avoid tracheostomy.[123] In individuals with PPS who have respiratory impairments, respiratory muscle training may be beneficial in improving respiratory muscle endurance and general well-being.[223]

The role of the therapist is to modify activities and teach glossopharyngeal breathing, manually assisted coughing, or bronchial drainage as indicated.[224,225] If trunk supports are considered, vital capacity should be checked with and without an abdominal binder to determine the effect on breathing. The therapist's attention should also be directed toward prevention of problems that may occur from bed rest and maintaining as much function as can be permitted.

Fatigue Management

Use of muscles at high levels for extended periods will result in muscle overload. To perform the same activity with weak muscles, the muscles need to contract at a higher percentage of their capacity than is normally required. For example, in walking, individuals with PPS contract their muscles at both higher intensities and for prolonged or even continuous periods in the gait cycle.[118] Energy expenditure for the task is increased, and the prolonged contractions keep the capillaries compressed, limiting needed muscle nutrition. Patients with PPS are often observed using nearly maximum voluntary contractions to perform a daily activity. The muscles of individuals with PPS cannot maintain these high levels of activity indefinitely.

A general program addressing fatigue may include nonfatiguing daily activities and energy conservation techniques. Relaxation, breathing, and meditation exercises may also be useful. Lifestyle changes that incorporate methods to decrease physical demands and prevent further decline in function are the most efficacious way to target fatigue impairments. In a study by Agre and Rodriguez,[140] symptomatic subjects with PPS demonstrated the ability to perceive muscular exertion. This is indicative of a mechanism to monitor local muscle fatigue that may be used to avoid exhaustion. Their study of pacing, defined as interspersed activity with rest, revealed less local fatigue and significantly greater strength recovery in subjects who paced their activities than when they worked at a constant rate to exhaustion. The Borg Rating of Perceived Exertion (BRPE) is an outcome measure that may be used to judge effort. Finch and colleagues[226] in a study of individuals with PPS found that after one training session subjects reliably used the RPE in an exercise test to monitor their effort and complete the test. Finch and colleagues[227] have gone on to establish reliability and construct validity on an effort-limited treadmill test for individuals with PPS.

Peach and Olejnik[228] found that compliance with recommendations affected fatigue. Fatigue was resolved or improved in a group of individuals who complied with recommendations and was unchanged or increased in the group of individuals who did not.[228]

Sleep Disturbance

Sleep disturbance is a significant age-related change, with an estimated 50% of older adults reporting difficulty initiating or maintaining sleep.[128,129] Several factors may contribute to reports of sleep disturbance, ranging from relatively apparent reasons to more medically complex reasons such as sleep apnea. Habitual sleeping patterns may provide important information. Sleep disturbances from medical or psychiatric conditions (e.g., chronic pain, dementia), or a primary sleep disorder that may be age-related, or a combination of these, may further produce changes in sleep that may be reflective of typical normal developmental processes.[128] Loss of sleep with aging is often a result of the decreased ability to sleep in older adults.[129] According to Neikrug and Ancoli-Israel,[129] this diminished ability is less a function of age and more a function of other age-related factors such as medical and psychiatric diagnoses, increased medication use, and a higher frequency of specific sleep disorders.

A history of pain or numbness that is worse at night or on rising points to sleeping surfaces that are too firm or sleeping with joints in close-packed positions (usually the neck and shoulders). These problems are correctable with foam mattress covers or air pressure mattresses, cervical pillows, and modification of sleeping postures.

Given the frequency and significant number of older adults with sleep problems, health care professionals need to be more aware of sleep disturbances.[129] Changes in sleep quality and quantity in later life influence quality of life and level of function;[128] thus it is critical to distinguish typical age-related changes in sleep from pathology-related sleep disturbances. More complex reasons for sleep disturbance such as sleep apnea may necessitate referral to specialists. Sleep disturbances have been identified as common secondary conditions that develop in aging adults with chronic CNS dysfunction.[114,229]

Decreasing the Workload of Muscles

Energy Conservation Techniques

Energy conservation techniques provide the easiest way to decrease the work of muscles without loss of function. Analysis of all activities by type, time, distance, and intensity is valuable in designing interventions. Such an inventory forms the basis for setting priorities and determining where and how individuals wish to use their limited neuromuscular capacity.[146]

Questions addressed include the following:

1. Can one trip do for two or three?
2. Can the activity be performed in a less strenuous way, such as by sitting or using a rolling basket?
3. Can the activity be broken up into parts with change of activity or rest?
4. Are there easier ways to perform the activity with modern comforts and technology, including motorization and electronics?
5. Can someone else perform some of the physical aspects of the activity?

Particular attention should focus on activities that produce fatigue and pain. Specific suggestions may address breaking tasks into subtasks, making environmental adaptations such as to work height and locations, taking frequent rest breaks during activities, and using adaptive or ergonomic equipment.

Orthotics and Assistive Devices

Reduction of muscular overuse and fatigue may be accomplished with lightweight splints and braces, adaptive equipment, walkers, or crutches.[112,123] The use of orthotics and/or assistive devices is individualized and specific to the patient, whose goals, along with the therapist's expertise, will ultimately determine the use of devices. For example, unlike most individuals with chronic mobility impairments, individuals with PPS may have strong and usually negative feelings about orthotics. The use of orthotics or assistive devices may be challenging for the individual newly diagnosed with PPS and facing a relatively "new disability." Polio survivors may have previously relied on devices or may have refused such devices earlier in life, and consenting to use them again may symbolize defeat and acceptance of losses.

As with every intervention, a thorough explanation of the specific rationale and goals for the intervention not only will be helpful in gaining the patient's/client's trust but will also improve compliance. Rationale for orthotic use includes preventing falls and potential fractures, limiting joint motion and preventing pain, restoring weight bearing on the weaker extremity to decrease the work of the less affected leg in locomotion, improving posture and decreasing back pain, and decreasing energy expenditure.

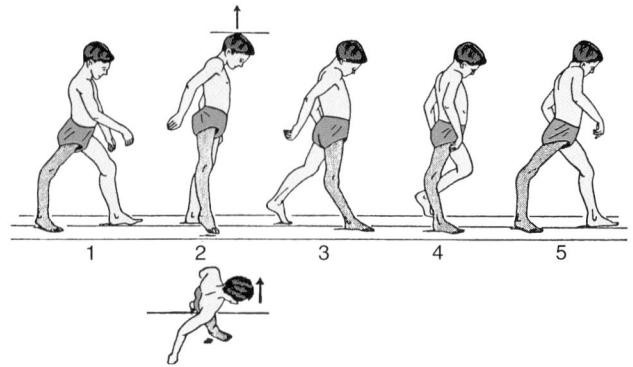

Fig. 35.1 The functional compensations of a boy with paralysis of the right lower extremity show increased energy expenditure and progressive ligamentous laxity. (Adapted from Ducroquet R, Darroquet J, Darroquet P. *Walking and Limping—A Study of Normal and Pathological Walking.* Philadelphia: JB Lippincott; 1968.)

Thoughtful consideration for the appropriateness of orthoses or assistive devices is critical; such devices should not be haphazardly prescribed or given as the only intervention of choice. They should be prescribed cautiously. Ineffective and inappropriate use of such devices will lead to malalignments, ineffective movement strategies, and postures that will cause more harm. Therapists should carefully evaluate the functions that may be lost or gained and the emotional and physical cost of the use of these devices.

Most individuals have long discarded braces and assistive devices and have relied on compensatory techniques for walking (Fig. 35.1). If an orthosis has been used and is essential for walking, it often becomes a part of the individual's body image; thus the patient/client may be resistant to changes in braces or devices. For other individuals, prior attempts to use plastic orthoses may have been painful or resulted in no functional use, and thus these patients may previously have rejected the potential of such devices. Thus it may be difficult to persuade the long-term user to consider orthoses or an orthotic change. When given the appropriate orthosis or prescription, however, polio survivors may benefit significantly enough to improve their current symptoms. A retrospective study of lower-extremity orthotic management for ambulation in 104 postpolio clinic patients by Waring and colleagues[230] revealed that 78% of patients noted that the appropriate orthotic prescription improved the ability to ambulate, increased apparent walking safety, and decreased pain.

In instances in which both the talocrural and subtalar ankle joints were fused surgically, the increased stresses on the posterior structures of the knee or the transverse tarsal joint for ambulation eventually lead to hypermobility and pain in these areas. Rocker-bottom shoes may assist with restoring motion for walking. An ankle-foot orthosis (AFO) may address pain in the transverse tarsal joint, whereas a knee-ankle-foot orthosis (KAFO) may help with knee pain.

AFOs are recommended for dorsiflexor weakness resulting in dropfoot or slapfoot, for plantarflexor weakness with absent heel rise, and for mediolateral instability. Individuals with PPS have difficulty with solid AFOs because of the structural design; they are typically made with 5 to 10 degrees of dorsiflexion and are then placed in a shoe with a slight positive heel, thus increasing the angle of the posterior shell to the floor. In standing and walking, this causes a knee flexion torque, with potential buckling of the knee if the quadriceps muscle is weak. Patients/clients may attempt to straighten the knee by pushing back against the posterior shell of the AFO, potentially causing pain. In such instances, AFOs should be made in slight plantarflexion so that the tibia is perpendicular to the floor in the usual shoes worn. This is the normal position of the ankle for toe and heel clearance.[231] In cases of plantarflexion contracture, more plantarflexion is required in the AFO. Most jointed AFOs are of limited value because of their bulk and weight. Moreover, they require a larger shoe and do not provide much control for the ankle. Jointed AFOs allow adjustment to find the best angle in function.

A floor reaction AFO prohibits all ankle motion and can place forces to control the knee.[232–234] The orthosis prevents dropfoot, promotes heel rise, provides an extension torque on the proximal tibia to supplement weak quadriceps muscles, and can limit hyperextension of the knee. It requires precision in fabrication for the knee extension torque to occur only when the tibia is perpendicular to the floor during gait. When used with rocker-bottom shoes, the patient with a flail foot can walk with a more typical gait pattern. Subjects with ligamentous laxity of the knee, excessive tibial torsion, or paralysis of the quadriceps muscles are poor candidates for this type of AFO.

Shoe inserts, heel lifts, and molded foot orthoses can provide a number of inconspicuous corrections. Positive heel shoes with a broad base, such as cowboy boots, stacked or Cuban heels, or the Swedish clog,[235] decrease the amount of dorsiflexion and plantarflexion motion and the work needed for ambulation. Rocker-bottom soles, which provide mechanical heel rise to assist the calf muscles, can be added to shoes and are commercially available. Work boots, dress boots, or basketball shoes may provide needed ankle stability.

Asymmetrical standing is typical in individuals with unilateral lower-extremity paralysis or pain. Standing is accomplished with more weight on the stronger limb, which must perform continuous, high-level isometric contractions (Fig. 35.2). Unloading the stronger leg requires restoration of weight bearing on the more involved leg using a KAFO or in some instances an AFO that prevents advancement of the tibia in the stance phase (Fig. 35.3).[113,232–234]

An obvious forward-leaning posture is seen in some ambulatory individuals with PPS. This posture requires continuous contraction of the erector spinae muscles and leads to back pain, often radiating to

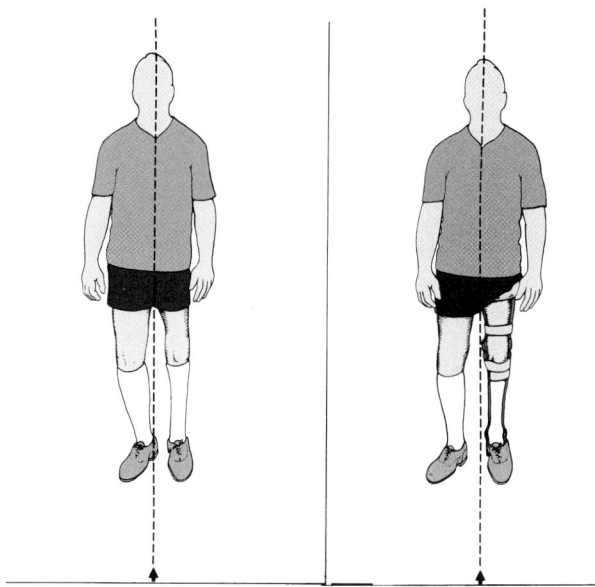

Fig. 35.3 This man has paralysis of the left lower extremity with severe fatigue, low back pain, pain and weakness in the right lower extremity, and decreased function. He can be seen to bear weight and stand on the right leg. Application of a left knee-ankle-foot orthosis with a free knee joint (with a drop lock for use in prolonged standing and walking on rough terrain) and a limited-motion ankle joint unloaded his right leg and permitted him to walk in an erect posture. His pain disappeared, and he has regained function at work and in social activities.

the hip and leg. The forward-leaning posture is found in people with quadriceps muscle paresis and in those with ankle weakness. Those with quadriceps weakness must move the center of gravity of the body anterior to the knee axis to lock the knee and prevent knee flexion in stance. This posterior force also produces ligamentous instability and genu recurvatum (see Fig. 35.1). In some instances, lightweight athletic knee braces allowing 10 to 15 degrees of hyperextension provide adequate control. More often, a KAFO with an offset knee joint allowing necessary hyperextension is required.[236–238] People with dorsiflexor muscle paralysis or ankle instabilities walk in the forward-leaning posture to watch the floor and foot placement to avoid tripping and falling. Athletic ankle supports or boots may be sufficient to control some ankle instabilities. Molded and posted plastic AFOs with or without ankle joints are needed for more control. Flexible plastic AFOs and the dynamic spring dorsiflexion assists can correct simple dropfoot.[113] Once the forward-leaning posture is addressed, the individual can walk upright and back pain will lessen and may disappear within days.

Walking with lateral trunk shift in the stance phase (gluteus medius gait) produces abnormal forces and joint dysfunction from the spine to the foot. In addition to a strengthening program, these forces may be reduced with use of a forearm crutch or a cane (see Fig. 35.2).

Long-term crutch walkers with or without orthoses and those with slow, precarious, or labored gait should be evaluated for appropriateness for use of motorized vehicles as their primary form of locomotion, whereas orthotic corrections or applications may be indicated to assist with transfers and short-distance walking.

Changes in Locomotion

In individuals with chronic neuromuscular impairments, the extent of impairment is influenced by the degree of neurological deficit in motor control, tone, and strength. This scenario illustrates the challenges

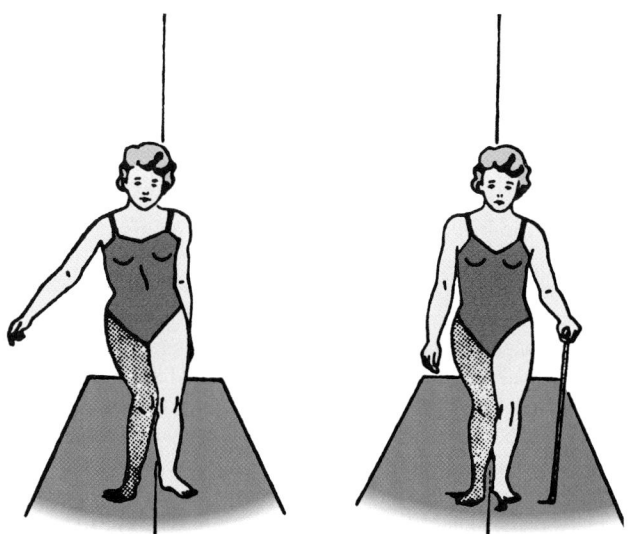

Fig. 35.2 Lateral trunk shift in a postpolio individual to illustrate abnormal forces occurring in the back, knee, and ankle with resulting joint dysfunction and pain. Prevention of these abnormal forces and some correction can be provided by use of a cane or forearm crutch. (Adapted from Ducroquet R, Darroquet J, Darroquet P. *Walking and Limping—A Study of Normal and Pathological Walking.* Philadelphia: JB Lippincott; 1968.)

associated with aging with chronic impairments and may very well be reflected in other neuromuscular diagnoses.

In a recent study that investigated the rate of decline of mobility and the potential predictors for the rate of decline in walking capacity in 48 individuals with PPS, investigators found the rate of decline could not be predicted from baseline capacities of strength, walking/mobility, or demographics.[239] Individual variations existed on substantial loss of walking capacity (27% decline) and self-reported physical mobility (38% decline).[239] Despite severe difficulties with locomotion from overuse, asymmetrical gait patterns and movement, or ineffective use of assistive devices, changes or modifications are hard for many people with chronic mobility problems, such as many polio survivors, to consider. Average walking capacity and self-reported physical mobility has been shown to decline by 6% and 14%, respectively, over 10 years.[239] As locomotion becomes more arduous or painful, many begin to limit outside activities rather than modify individual methods of locomotion. Resistance to lifestyle changes is common in the PPS population and leads to needless suffering and functional decline.[228]

Prevention of this spiraling disability and restoration of lost function require a marked decrease in the amount of walking or propelling a chair and a change to methods of locomotion that do not cause pain, weakness, and fatigue. Independent ambulators or those with inadequate assistance may need to use a cane, forearm crutches, trunk support, shoe corrections, or new orthoses. Clients who have been walking for years with crutches with or without orthoses develop shoulder, elbow, and wrist injuries, as well as new muscle weakness, muscle pain, and fatigue. Use of personal mobility vehicles (motorized carts) for distance locomotion or as the primary form of locomotion may need to be explored, with walking reserved for transfers and short distances only. Lightweight manual wheelchairs only perpetuate the problems and eventually create new ones; use may lead to development of repetitive stress injuries of the shoulder, elbow, wrist, and hand. The use of motorized mobility devices will need to be explored to prevent fatigue, muscle overuse, and further damage to joints.

The use of motorized vehicles for locomotion should be considered and explored with sensitivity and caution. Specific rationales should be thoroughly understood by a seemingly resistant patient, and perceptions regarding the use of such vehicles should be addressed. Changes in methods of locomotion may be justified to increase safety and prevent costly falls, reduce energy expenditure and decrease fatigue, prevent further repetitive injury and pain, and, most important, increase function and quality of life. Those who do make these difficult changes in their methods of locomotion seem to undergo a metamorphosis from pain and dysfunction to renewed activity and increased function.

Management of Postural Deviations

Altered biomechanics from atypical postures or faulty physiological neuromuscular processes over time may lead to deviations that may cause pain and further functional limitations. In polio survivors, common biomechanical deficits abound, including genu recurvatum, genu valgum, inadequate dorsiflexion in swing, mediolateral ankle instability, and dorsiflexion collapse during stance, as described by Clark and colleagues.[236] These deviations are very likely to be seen in people with other neuromuscular diagnoses. Strengthening exercises may be used to correct these impairments initially, with orthoses as an alternative management.

Postural exercises incorporated with breathing and stretching exercises are a way to address ineffective postures identified in all positions. Mental imagery, which may avoid impairments from fatigue, may be used early in addressing postural correction. Mechanical

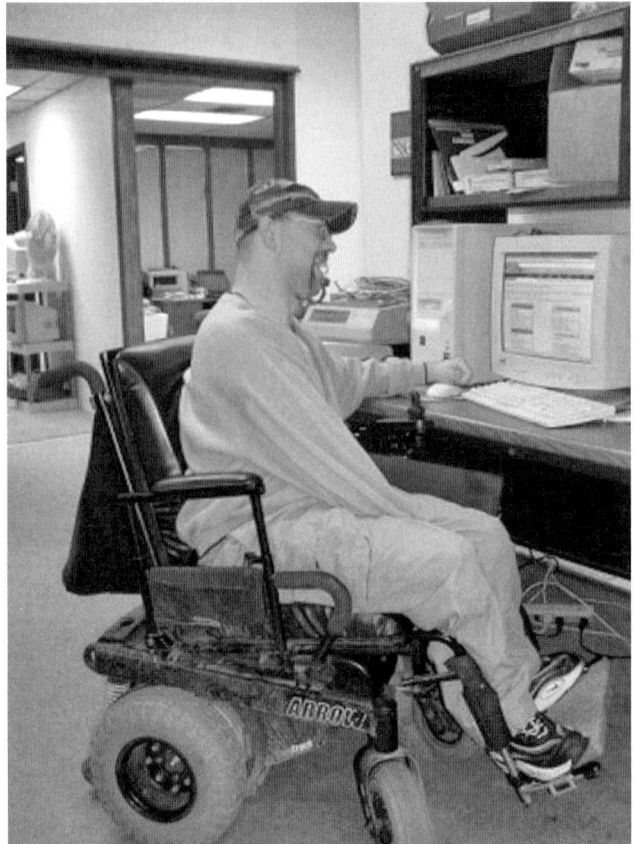

Fig. 35.4 Man with athetoid cerebral palsy working at his computer. His power chair has been modified with a back support and a seat cushion for proper positioning.

restoration of the lumbar curve in all seating and all settings and activities can address the problem if contractures do not limit motion. Properly fitted clerical chairs, ergonometric chairs, anterior tilt seats, gluteal pads, and several types of lumbar rolls, back supports, and seating systems may be beneficial (Fig. 35.4).

Individuals with abdominal muscle paralysis may benefit from custom-made thoracolumbar corsets, in which the posterior rigid stays bent to produce a normal standing lumbar curve. Paretic or paralyzed neck muscles can be rested and supported by soft foam collars or supportive microcellular neck collars. People with severe trunk muscle paralysis or scoliosis with or without spinal fusion often support the trunk or relieve pain by pushing down with their hands or elbows on chairs, on tables, and on their hips. In time, such self-traction results in pain and weakness in their arms. Chair inserts and fixed supports as well as custom-made corsets, back braces, and molded body jackets should be considered. The rigid trunk supports, however, take away mobility used for function. Usually such supports can be worn for part of the day in activities in which trunk mobility is not essential.

For people with abnormal biomechanical alignment resulting from spasticity, orthopedic deformation, or severe muscle imbalance, care must be taken to maintain proper alignment throughout the exercise. Additional positioning equipment may be required to assist the person in exercising independently. For example, people with lower-extremity spasticity frequently exhibit medial rotation of their femurs and bilateral pronation. Combined with asymmetrical patterns of weakness and tightness, a squatting motion produces an excessive valgus angle at the knee. Ensuring satisfactory alignment throughout the arc of motion improves the efficacy of the exercise. Conversely, without this attention to biomechanical alignment, these imbalances and deformities can be exacerbated.

Limitations in Range of Motion

A thorough evaluation of muscle length and ROM is critical in the overall management of life activities in individuals with chronic mobility impairments. The clinician should consider that not all tightness or limitation in motion is detrimental. Selective tightness may have provided some stability to otherwise unstable joints with paralyzed muscles, and useful contractures may have been developed by the body to achieve function. An excellent example can be seen in individuals who contracted polio as children. Muscle involvement was primarily in one lower extremity with a decrease in growth of that extremity as a result of diminished weight-bearing forces. If the individual has at least a G− (4−) manual muscle test grade in the plantarflexors, the person will walk on the toes (in some plantarflexion) to decrease large drops in the center of gravity, resulting in increased energy expenditure for walking. Over the years, a plantarflexion contracture develops that can provide up to 3 to 4 inches for weight bearing on the shortened extremity. With a custom-made shoe, gait is similar to walking in a high-heeled shoe. This can be far more energy efficient than if motion were permitted to have dorsiflexion ROM.

Gentle myofascial release can also be beneficial for recent secondary impairments of muscles to decrease pain and muscle spasms, increase nutrition to the area, and slightly lengthen muscles.

Weight Management

Adults with chronic impairments, particularly those with developmental disabilities, are at high risk for obesity and its sequelae. Weight reduction, when appropriate, addresses this health disparity and is an effective way to decrease the muscle workload, but it is one of the most difficult ways. Clinicians recommend a modest weight loss of 5% of body weight as an achievable and maintainable goal that may result in decreased hyperlipidemia, hypertension, and glucose intolerance.[240] Weight loss is slow without exercise, but it can be accomplished. Weight control needs to be incorporated as a permanent modification of nutritional habits rather than achieved in a short-term diet. Dietetic counseling and support groups are important components of this challenging lifestyle modification.

In a study of 431 community-dwelling individuals with developmental delay who participated in a community-based health promotion intervention, two-thirds of participants maintained or lost weight (mean of 2.6 pounds, median 7 pounds, range 2 to 24 pounds) over a 7-month, twice-weekly program.[26] The authors stated that even without the weight loss, the decreased abdominal girth achieved by participants may be predictive of a decrease in cardiovascular risk factors.[240]

Pain Management

Pain management in the patient with chronic movement dysfunction is dependent on the cause of the muscle or joint pain. As an example of how pain management contributes to secondary health problems, patients with SCI who reported pain from musculoskeletal problems and overuse were seldom referred for therapeutic interventions but were treated primarily with prescription medications to treat painful conditions. This medical management often resulted in increased problems, such as constipation, fatigue, irritability, and frustration.[241] The cause of pain must be carefully determined to establish appropriate intervention and management strategies. Typical interventions for pain include activity reduction, therapeutic heating

modalities, cryotherapy, stretching, or energy and joint conservation techniques.

If chronic overuse is the only or major underlying cause of the symptoms present, conservative measures can often slow or prevent further deterioration and may even lead to improved function. Conservative measures include reducing mechanical stress, pacing activities, supporting weak muscles, stabilizing abnormal joint movements, and improving biomechanics of the body. Interventions that address fatigue and weakness such as nonfatiguing functional activities, energy conservation,[146] more frequent rest periods, or change of activity[242] are also useful in pain management. Antiinflammatory agents have been used to supplement conservative measures.

Joint conservation techniques may include use of ergonomic devices, elevated chairs, bathtub bench or shower stool, and weight control. Recommendations for the neck and upper extremities include seating and workstation corrections, telephone headsets, rolling carts for carrying items, newspaper support for reading, ergonomic computer screens, wrist rests, and keyboards.

Successful intervention for joint pain, however, requires identification and elimination of the cause of the pain. This is frequently difficult because the person with chronic movement dysfunction may not have the strength in other parts of the body to compensate and carry out an essential function, or the person may be unable or unwilling to make necessary lifestyle changes. Intervention techniques may include inhibiting muscle spasm, stretching fascia and muscles, decreasing edema and increasing nutrition in joint structures, and mobilizing or stabilizing joints.[243] At some point, relaxation, meditation, modified tai chi (see Chapter 33), aquatic therapeutic exercise, or body awareness techniques such as Feldenkrais[205] may be beneficial.

Local pain and dysfunction can be treated as athletic injuries from overuse, but they require major modifications and careful monitoring of performance, pain, and fatigue. Many joint pain problems can be relieved and controlled by home program interventions such as rest for the injured part, mechanical postural corrections, cold packs, nonsteroidal antiinflammatory drugs, orthotics, and pain-free ROM exercises.

With regard to McConnell taping, although no radiological evidence shows changes in actual alignment of bone, individuals without neurological diagnoses have experienced a 50% to 78% reduction in patellofemoral pain during activities.[243,244] In the Post-polio Clinic of the Institute for Rehabilitation and Research in Houston, Texas, these taping techniques relieved anterior knee pain for several months at a time in all individuals with PPS who were selected to receive the taping. Relief occurred, although the ability to strengthen surrounding muscles was limited or impossible. The therapy program should also include assisting the patient in carrying out the home program and lifestyle changes, along with the development of a continuing program of appropriate exercises.

As with the management of fatigue, compliance of the individual with chronic impairments with suggested recommendations plays a significant role in pain management. In those with PPS, Peach and Olejnik[228] found that muscle pain was resolved in 28% and improved in 72% of people who complied with recommendations. In those who were noncompliant, muscle pain was improved in 14%, unchanged in 57%, and increased in 29%.

Alternative Pain Management

Pain sensitivity must be acknowledged by clinicians when providing therapy that may be perceived as painful, such as stretching, and in the treatment of acute pain.[245] People with chronic movement dysfunction have undergone extensive orthopedic surgery in attempts to overcome their initial deficits, as in the case of some polio survivors, and some have pain or hypersensitivities at the surgical sites. Desensitization exercises may decrease the hypersensitivities if the patient is willing to devote the necessary time. The most frequent old surgical sites of pain are in the trunk from surgery for scoliosis, the ankle near a subtalar arthrodesis, and the foot with hypermobility of the transverse tarsal joint. In most instances of foot pain, stabilization of the ankle and foot in a custom-made AFO and use of a rocker-bottom shoe has relieved the pain and permitted weight bearing and walking.[235] Custom-made corsets and trunk supports in chairs may help with the pain at previous surgical sites in the trunk. Transcutaneous electrical nerve stimulation may be helpful for pain control (see Chapter 31). Most individuals, however, stop using these devices because masking the pain permits them to physically overdo, leading to further injury to their bodies.

Static magnetic fields have become a familiar alternative approach in the treatment of athletic injuries as well as in people with PPS who have localized pain. In a double-blind randomized clinical trial, Vallbona and colleagues[246] applied active (300 to 500 Gauss) and placebo magnets in a group of 50 subjects with PPS and chronic pain. The magnets were applied to the palpable pain pressure point for 45 minutes. There was a significant ($P > .0001$) and prompt decrease in pain in the group receiving the active magnets compared with those who received the placebo.[246]

Cold and Heat Intolerance

Strumse and colleagues[247] investigated the effect of climate on the outcomes of individuals with PPS. In a randomized controlled trial of 88 individuals diagnosed with PPS, subjects received one of three interventions: (1) warm climate rehabilitation (dry and sunny, temperature around 25°C or 77°F) consisting of individual and group therapy with daily treatment in a swimming pool, physical therapy, and an individually adapted training program for 4 weeks, (2) cold climate rehabilitation consisting of indoor treatment as described for the first intervention in a rehabilitation center in Norway with rainy or snowy weather with temperatures around 0°C or 32°F, or (3) the usual health care program (control). This study was included in the review by the Cochrane Collaboration, and the authors concluded that there is low-quality evidence of no beneficial effect of rehabilitation in warm and cold climates 3 months after intervention.[27] The reviewers suggest that a more thorough description of the components of the program and outcome assessment for the usual control group would have clarified the short-term effects on both rehabilitation groups and the results of the study. The study could not demonstrate a positive effect of rehabilitation in warm or cold climate for PPS, and further studies are warranted.[27]

Most individuals with chronic conditions who have cold intolerance have learned to control heat loss as best as they can with clothing, massage, and local heat. For interventions, however, cold intolerance can pose a potential problem with the use of cold modalities in the treatment of injuries and pain. Most people with PPS are hesitant to use local cold on any part of the body. They may typically use heating pads and hot water, which feel good at the time, but may perpetuate or increase the edema, inflammation, and pain. Local cold is often more effective and is well tolerated by most people with PPS. Successful application of cold requires more patient education about the use of cold and demonstration of the effects.

In people with MS who are sensitive to environmental heat or an increase in body temperature, specific recommendations for cooling during exercises may be necessary to counteract the deleterious effects of heat. Aquatic exercises and swimming in a cool pool with temperatures at or below 82 degrees may be beneficial for cooling. The use of cooling vests, ice packs, air conditioning, and hydration during activities is also recommended.[248–250] An example of a specific exercise recommendation is the use of a Schwinn Airdyne bicycle to help with cooling while cycling.[248]

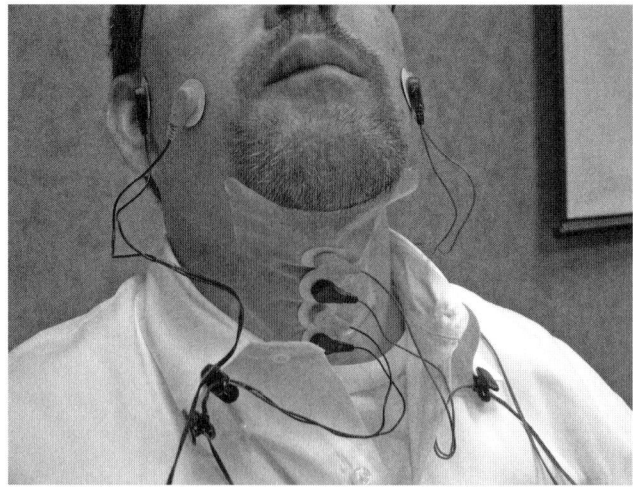

Fig. 35.5 Man with spastic cerebral palsy receiving neuromuscular electrical stimulation for facial and pharyngeal activation to improve swallowing and motor control in face.

Other Interventions

The reader is referred to specific pharmacological texts and specific chapters within this text for detailed pharmacological interventions for specific neuromuscular diagnoses. As emphasized earlier, the management of chronic conditions is individualized and dependent on the unique needs of the individual based on the interaction of multisystem involvement. Thus the pharmacological management of people with chronic conditions is also individualized and wide-ranging. Although there are classes of medications that are commonly used across varied neurological conditions (e.g., spasticity medications), the use of medication is still symptom- and patient-dependent. A literature review of pharmacological approaches for PPS revealed that controlled trials of pyridostigmine and prednisone have not been beneficial.[34,251,252] Currently, there is no specific pharmacological agent widely recommended to address the multiple symptoms of PPS.

As part of the evaluation, oral motor function is an important component in terms of sensation, speech, and swallowing. Because of their prevalence in people with developmental delay, dysphagia and aspiration potential need to be carefully explored in the history. Owing to disturbances in muscle tone, these individuals often have difficulty with feeding, which may lead to serious medical complications and potential death. In general, intervention may consist of performing breathing exercises, using swallowing techniques, monitoring fatigue levels, avoiding eating when fatigued, and initiating dietary restrictions or changes. For those with dysphagia, specific management will warrant a thorough evaluation by a speech therapist. Recent advances in treatment including deep pharyngeal neuromuscular stimulation and neuromuscular electrical stimulation, which offer people with poor motor control and weakness in pharyngeal musculature opportunities to improve safe oral feeding (Fig. 35.5).[253]

KEY POINTS

- Much individual variation exists in the aging process of individuals with chronic CNS conditions and chronic impairments. The individual variability of the development of secondary conditions and the current lack of predictive factors underscore the need for individually tailored care based on actual functional decline and restrictions in participation in society.

- Further research and longitudinal studies are consistently recommended to understand the effects of aging with a disability from a chronic CNS condition, to determine when problems are most likely to occur, and to develop and examine the efficacy of targeted interventions to prevent and/or address secondary health conditions and their negative impact on health, function, and quality of life.

REFERENCES

To enhance this text and add value for the reader, all references are included on the companion Evolve site that accompanies this textbook. This online service will, when available, provide a link for the reader to a Medline abstract for the article cited. There are 253 cited references and other general references for this chapter, with the majority of those articles being evidence-based citations.

CASE STUDY 35.1   Aging With Traumatic Brain Injury

Mark was 19 years old when he was involved in a motor vehicle accident in which a drunk driver hit Mark's car while he was stopped at an intersection. He had severe injuries that included fractures of the left femur, both forearms and wrists, and right ankle; multiple internal injuries; "swelling" of the spinal cord; and increased intracranial pressure necessitating removal of part of his skull. He had sustained frontotemporal brain injury with no injuries to the spinal cord despite severe injuries from the accident. He had complicated postsurgical sequelae and was in a coma for 3 weeks. He stayed in the acute hospital for another 3 weeks and was sent to inpatient rehabilitation, where he stayed for 4 months. At discharge he was able to stand and walk short distances at home with minimal assistance, although primarily he used a power wheelchair as his main mode of mobility. Although his upper extremities were functional, he had to learn how to write and use his dominant extremity all over again. He had dysphagia and dysarthria yet was able to communicate functionally. Mark reports he had difficulty with memory and other cognitive deficits, and those were as hard to deal with as the physical impairments from his injury. He continued outpatient physical, speech, and occupational therapy services for another 3 months and worked on the physical, cognitive, and psychological effects of his injury. He stayed with his parents who at that time became his primary caregivers as he transitioned to a new lifestyle.

In the 20 years after his injury, Mark learned to live with the chronicity of his injury and its secondary effects. He learned to walk with a walker, then a cane, and eventually walked without an assistive device with a slow, ataxic gait. He learned to use public transportation and navigate his way in the community by using landmarks for spatial orientation. He was involved with support and volunteer groups for several years that provided him the socialization and support he needed, particularly in the early stages of his injury. He married in his mid-20s, and his wife assists him with daily activities as needed, although Mark says he is independent with "everything" except with instrumental ADLs, specifically balancing the checkbook, grocery shopping, and cooking. They live in a one-level home with steps at the front and side entries and have done "some modifications" with bars and a shower chair installation in the bathrooms and wider doors in the bedrooms. Mark says he has seen a PT "maybe once or twice" in the subsequent years for back pain or walking, but has not received continued care since his long episodes of therapy after the initial injury. He candidly states that he gets by with all physical abilities, although it is "hard at times" and he does not currently engage in a specific health or exercise program. He says he

has "learned to live with it" and shares some sadness at being unable to finish his education and care for his parents, who are now in their early 80s.

Now at 48 years old, Mark reports he is starting to feel more fatigued with walking and has noticed the need for more frequent rests. He continues to walk without an assistive device indoors and short distances but uses a single-tip cane for long distances in the community and outdoors. He and his wife are saving to renovate the front and side entries of the home, which currently have five steps and handrails. Although Mark is able to navigate the steps on his own, he has noticed more difficulty over the years. In the previous year, he fell once on the steps and once in the community as he stepped off a curb. He now uses a "memory" notebook more frequently. He volunteers at the local library three times a week and continues to use public transportation as his primary mode of transportation. "I'm slower, but I get there," he states. He "feels" the secondary impairments from his initial injuries—for example, contractures of the hamstrings, decreased ROM of the ankles and shoulders, postural impairments, gait deficits, and memory deficits—"more now that I'm getting old." He has more frequent bouts of back and hip pain from a combination of biomechanical changes from chronic impairments and possible contributions from aging. He has not sought physical therapy services despite the symptoms, difficulties, and changes in the past couple of years. Although he is interested in seeking physical therapy services, he has not done so, thinking that he will not qualify for services because of the chronicity of his condition. He volunteers at a local physical therapy program where he is provided pro bono services at least twice a year.

Points for discussion (suggested answers can be found online) include the following:

- What further secondary impairments and functional limitations do you anticipate?
- What recommendations regarding lifestyle changes would you give Mark?
- If he decides to seek physical therapy services, what recommendations would you give for a holistic program?
- What specific systems need to be examined and addressed in the intervention?
- What services are available for individuals with chronic conditions? Community and hospital or outpatient-based services?
- What health care and community services *should* be available to individuals with chronic conditions?

CASE STUDY 35.2   Personal Report: Post-Polio Syndrome*

Today my life is filled with optimism and hope. This was not the case long ago. I am 58 years old and have been diagnosed with PPS. I contracted polio at the age of 2 years, but for the first time in my life I feel disabled.

It is difficult for me to determine when the symptoms began. My life has been filled with caregiving, of first my mother-in-law, who was ill for the last year of her life, and then my parents, who had special needs. I had a vague

awareness that I was slowing down, not able to do some of the things that I had always done. But at that point in my life, the focus was not on me. It seems like when I was able to take a deep breath again, I was in a lot of pain.

I was able to see a doctor who specializes in PPS. She recommended a new leg brace, and she also recommended physical therapy. The new brace, while better for my body, is asking it to do different things. I basically am trying to

Continued

learn how to walk all over again. My pain stems from weakness and tight muscles in my unaffected limb. My unaffected leg has been stressed by many years of overuse. The pain I experience is mainly in my hip and occasionally in my knee. Because of the stress of this pain, my stamina is less than it once was; my balance is not good, and just the task of moving from point A to B is a challenge. I found that I needed to use crutches to help take weight off of my leg. The pain that I felt a little over a year ago became the focus of my life. It affected everything I did. My day was reduced to struggle to even shower and dress, let alone do anything else. I had to depend on my husband to do more and more.

During this period, I would allow myself, if I was having a really bad day, to just do nothing. Some days I wouldn't even get out of bed until 11:00 AM. This didn't happen too often, but if it did, I allowed myself to not feel guilty. I think that this helped with my mental state. Yes, some days I would get frustrated and impatient and other days depressed, but it never lasted for too long. I have seen, on a personal level, what positive thinking can do. My parents were told that I would never walk again. I walked.

Having had polio, I learned at an early age how to "figure things out." If I couldn't do things one way, I perhaps could another. I think that this mindset has helped with my newest challenge. After meeting with my PT, she helped to map out a plan to achieve my goals. My goals are simple; I want to walk without pain and without crutches. I want to cross my left leg over my right knee to tie my shoe. I want to build up my stamina so that I can go shopping. I want to be in the best health that I can be in. I want to remain independent.

I am learning that achieving my goals may be a long process. It has been a little over a year, and I still have a long way to go. I have gained some strength, my stamina has increased, and I am a bit more flexible, but more important, the pain level some days is just an afterthought. I am starting to regain my life.

I have learned in the past year how important it is to listen to your body. I have learned how to manage my work, rest, and exercise time. I understand that to achieve my goals it has and will take a lot of hard, sometimes painful, work. I also understand the importance of working toward my goal and achieving it. I consider myself to still be a relatively young woman who has a lot left to do in my life. Life is a gift, and that is what I want to do—live mine fully.

Points for discussion (suggested answers can be found online):
- If this individual were to seek physical therapy consultation, what history information should the therapist ask?
- What screening questions should the therapist ask?
- What specific systems should the therapist screen?
- What specific tests and measures are appropriate for this case?
- What possible interventions are possible for this individual?
- What considerations should be considered when planning for intervention?

*Orva Klopfer, as relayed to Holly Klopfer Holton, PT, DPT.

36

Impact of Drug Therapy on Patients Receiving Neurological Rehabilitation

Annie Burke-Doe and Timothy J. Smith

OBJECTIVES

After reading this chapter the student or therapist will be able to:

1. Identify how drugs may positively or negatively affect the behavior of individuals within a neurological rehabilitation setting.
2. For a given disease state, comprehend how drugs may affect that disease state and the implications on an individual's potential for neurological rehabilitation.
3. When one or more impairments are being considered, recognize the influence of drug therapy on these impairments and on an individual's potential for neurological rehabilitation.
4. Recognize the importance of a collaborative approach in resolving drug-related issues and how those issues affect an individual's potential for neurological rehabilitation.

KEY TERMS

adverse drug reactions
disease
drug interactions

drug therapy
impairment
pharmacist

pharmacogenetics
pharmacogenomics

Drug therapy is one of the most rapidly expanding therapeutic interventions in the health care system. Whereas monotherapy (the use of one drug for treatment of a single disease state) is preferred, complex pathologies and comorbid conditions usually render this goal impossible. In addition, most of the problems associated with multidrug therapy were at one time generally isolated to geriatric patients. Today, however, such problems have expanded because of more aggressive drug treatment in all age groups. Only rarely will an occupational or physical therapist manage a patient who is not receiving drug therapy for conditions either related or unrelated to the therapist's scope of practice. Drugs used for the management of a wide variety of disease states may have unintended or undesirable effects on a therapeutic plan for a patient undergoing neurological rehabilitation. Although the occupational or physical therapist may not be responsible for monitoring all aspects of a patient's therapeutic plan, the scope of drug-related complications must be recognized. A patient's pharmacist, who is acutely aware of the prescribing practices of the patient's physician or physicians, may be instrumental in resolving the drug-related impact of any medication on a therapeutic plan. The patient will benefit greatly from an effective collaboration that includes the therapist and a pharmacist. Focusing on drug effects, diseases, and impairments, this chapter addresses these interactions from three perspectives. First, the chapter discusses what the body does to a drug (pharmacokinetics), followed by what a drug does to the body (pharmacodynamics), and then pharmacogenetics (the involvement of genes in an individual's response to drugs).[1] Second, the chapter covers a disease- or pathology-driven model that focuses on the pharmacological approaches used in drug therapy of major diseases that are often concurrent with rehabilitation. Finally, the chapter presents an impairment, activity, or functional limitation–driven model that focuses on the effects of drugs on the impairment and resulting functional deficit and the impact on

the therapeutic plan. Although defining every problem associated with a class of drugs or among patients with an impairment is not possible within the scope of this chapter, it is important to highlight common difficulties.

CLINICAL PHARMACOLOGY

Medications do not affect all patients in the same way, and rehabilitation specialists should be concerned whether a drug achieves or falls short of its therapeutic response. Many situations may alter a drug's response; drug dose, drug interactions, the patient's comorbidities, and the effect on functional recovery can be positive or negative. To understand the impact of prescriptions, this chapter discusses the pharmacology of medications used by patients. Pharmacology—or the science of drug origin, nature, chemistry, effects, and uses—is commonly divided into two important areas: pharmacokinetics and pharmacodynamics.[2] *Pharmacokinetics* refers to how drugs are absorbed, distributed, biotransformed (metabolized), and eliminated from the body, whereas *pharmacodynamics* can be defined as the study of the biochemical and physiological effects of drugs and their mechanisms of action.[2] Many patients in the rehabilitation population undergo pharmacotherapy, and clinicians must understand how drugs work in the body and how they work differently in different populations to achieve their effects.

In looking at pharmacokinetics, how the drug is absorbed into the body from its site of administration must be considered. Drugs may cross many membranes before reaching their targets, and they can be affected by factors such as the size of a tablet or capsule, its physical state, and the temperature when it is dispensed.[3] The absence or presence of food in the digestive tract, characteristics of the membrane, and the drug's ability to bind to plasma proteins can also play a role in the rate of absorption and distribution. Some medications, such as Sinemet for Parkinson disease, can be absorbed more slowly with a high-protein meal, thus decreasing their availability and potentially affecting function. When a drug binds to a plasma protein such as albumin, the drug is held in the bloodstream and thus is unable to reach its target cells.[2] The term *bioavailability* is often used to describe how much of a drug will be available to produce a biological effect after its administration.

Metabolism is the next step in pharmacokinetics, involving the biochemical pathways and reactions that affect drugs, nutrients, vitamins, and minerals. The first-pass effect is an important phenomenon because many drugs absorbed across the gastrointestinal (GI) membrane are routed directly to the liver.[2] The liver is then the primary site of metabolism before the drug is distributed to target organs. Variations in drug response and metabolism may be caused by genetic factors, the presence of disease, drug interactions, age, diet, and gender.[3] Drug doses in the elderly and young are often reduced to compensate for these patients' physiological differences. Specific prescribing guidelines for the elderly, known as the Beers criteria,[4] have been developed, and guidelines for the pediatric population are currently being developed titled Pediatrics: Omission of Prescriptions and Inappropriate Prescriptions (POPI)[5] to assist healthcare professionals. Any drug or disease that affects metabolism has the potential to affect drug activity. Excretion, which removes drugs from the body, is the last step in pharmacokinetics. Most substances that enter the body are removed by urination, exhalation, defecation, and/or sweating.[2] The main organ of excretion is the kidney. *Elimination* is another term for excretion and is often measured so that dosages of drugs can be determined more accurately. The rate of elimination is helpful in determining how long a drug will remain in the bloodstream and thus indicates for how long the drug will produce its effect.

Pharmacodynamics focuses on how the body responds to drugs; it deals with the mechanism of a drug's action or how drugs exert their effects. Successful pharmacotherapy is based on the principle that to treat a disorder, a drug must interaction with specific receptors in its target tissue. Drugs activate specific receptors to produce a therapeutic response. Optimal treatment with medications will result only when the prescriber is aware of the sources of variation in responses to drugs and when the dosage regimen is designed on the basis of the best available data about the diagnosis, severity, and stage of the disease; presence of concurrent diseases or drug treatment; and predefined goals of acceptable efficacy and limits of acceptable toxicity.[2] Rehabilitation professionals are poised to assist the other members of the medical team with the data needed to assist in determining the effectiveness of a pharmacotherapeutic plan.

Pharmacogenomics is the study of how individuals differ in their responses to drug therapy and the mechanisms underlying variable drug responses by utilizing genomics, proteomics, transcriptomics, and metabolomics-based knowledge.[6] The rationale behind pharmacogenetics is to find polymorphisms in the genes encoding the proteins and enzymes involved in drug transport, metabolism, and action that can predict the usefulness of a drug, thus increasing the number of responders and decreasing the number of subjects who experience adverse drug reactions.[7] Pharmacogenetics is a growing field in neurogenetics; it can facilitate the prescription of specific therapeutics best suited for a given individual, taking into consideration both the genetic and environmental factors that influence the individual's response to therapy. This personalized approach is being applied to the management of several neurological disorders, and there are still other such disorders undergoing investigation. Examples include Alzheimer disease, Parkinson disease, multiple sclerosis (MS), traumatic brain injury, epilepsy, stroke, major depressive disorders, and attention-deficit

disorders.[8] Although genetics contributes to only a fraction of the explanations behind interindividual difference in drug metabolism, a better understanding of how genetics influences drug responses is an emerging field and will be key to the future of individualized medicine.

DISEASE PERSPECTIVE

Many diseases and their treatment regimens may be concurrently managed while a patient is in a neurological rehabilitation environment. The pharmacological interventions for these conditions and their implications from both a physiological and a disease or pathology model are addressed in this chapter. Although not a comprehensive list, these include Parkinson disease, cancer, seizure disorders (epilepsy), cardiovascular disorders, disorders of mood, autoimmune disorders, diabetes, infectious diseases, pulmonary diseases, and GI disorders.

Parkinson Disease

Parkinson disease is a degenerative disorder involving a progressive loss of dopaminergic neurons in the substantia nigra, with the appearance of intracellular inclusions know as Lewy bodies.[2] A loss of 70% to 80% of dopaminergic function accompanies symptomatic Parkinson disease, causing a resting tremor and difficulty in the control of voluntary movement. Olfaction, sleep, cardiovascular function, bowel motility, and cognitive function are all often compromised.[9] Although not directly associated with motor system pathology, the functional deficits are emotionally devastating to the patient, resulting in depression and other mood disorders. The predominant pharmacological approach in the management of Parkinson disease is the enhancement of dopaminergic function in the affected brain regions. Among the earliest successful approaches was the use of levodopa (L-dopa), a precursor of the neurotransmitter dopamine in the central nervous system (CNS). The use of this agent (and most agents to date) only enhances dopaminergic function in the remaining neurons but has no effect on the progressive loss of neurons. In addition to central conversion of L-dopa to dopamine in the substantia nigra pars compacta, a similar conversion occurs in the limbic system, a brain center associated with the regulation of behavior. Excessive dopaminergic influence in the limbic system has been associated with aberrant disease manifestations including paranoia, delusions, hallucinations, and related psychiatric disturbances, all of which may influence sleep and mood. These behavioral changes are obviously antagonistic to any therapeutic plan. In addition to L-dopa, a dopamine precursor, agents that inhibit the breakdown of dopamine, enhance the release of dopamine, or have dopaminergic agonist activity will have similar behavioral effects (Box 36.1). Dopaminergic agents may produce postural hypotension and syncope because of their ability to produce vasodilation based on CNS and peripheral actions.[10,11] If patients are unable to take their medication, an increasing danger exists (with extended therapy) that movement may become impossible and normal chest wall expansion and contraction may be compromised.

Because Parkinson disease is progressive in nature, patients may have different presentations depending on the stage of the disease and the presence of pharmacological interventions. In the early months of the disease, the motor signs may be particularly subtle, and patients may report only slowness, stiffness, and trouble with handwriting. Attention to the history of tremor, slowness of fine motor control, a hunched and slightly flexed posture, and micrographia may lead the physician to diagnose Parkinson disease in its early phases.[12] As the disease advances, patients have increasing difficulty in activities of daily living and gait as well as bradykinesia and distal tremor.

Once a definitive diagnosis has been made, the control of symptoms and the side effects of medications is balanced with the level of

BOX 36.1 Agents Facilitating Dopaminergic Activity in the Management of Parkinson Disease

Agents That Are Converted to Dopamine
L-dopa (in Sinemet, Rytary, and DUOPA)

Agents That Stimulate the Release of Dopamine
amantadine (Symmetrel)

Agents That Reduce the Breakdown of Dopamine
carbidopa (in Sinemet, Rytary, and DUOPA)
entacapone (Comtan)
rasagiline (Azilect)
selegiline (Eldepryl)
tolcapone (Tasmar)

Agents That Are Dopaminergic Agonists
apomorphine (Apokyn)
bromocriptine (Parlodel)
pergolide (Permax)
pramipexole (Mirapex)
ropinirole (Requip)

Anticholinergic Agents
benztropine (Cogentin)
diphenhydramine (Benadryl)
trihexyphenidyl (Artane)

The effects of these agents on muscle tone are complex and dose-dependent.

functional involvement. The physician and patient may discuss the option of several medications (see Box 36.1) but must determine the best approach based on the clinical presentation. One limitation is the side effect of involuntary movements (dyskinesias). These dyskinesias can be difficult to control and are different from the involuntary movements caused by the disease itself. As mentioned earlier, dopamine agonist regimens that do not cause dyskinesias can also be prescribed, but their effect on symptoms is not as potent.[13] Often physicians may begin treatment with a dopamine agonist (Ropinirole) and continue with the agonist as long as symptoms are satisfactorily controlled. Later the physician can initiate treatment with L-dopa when the disease is in the advanced stages. With the elderly patient who has cognitive deficits, combination therapy may be the initial choice. Once a medication regimen has been initiated, the patient and therapist may notice improvements in symptoms and therefore also in functional abilities. After taking a medication over time, patients may find that the effect of the medication begins to wear off before the next dose is scheduled. At this point consultation with the rehabilitation team is recommended to potentially change the timing of the medication release ability (extended release), or they may combine the treatment with other antiparkinsonian medications.

Great emphasis is placed on treating the motor features of Parkinson disease, but patients may have nonmotor manifestations, including depression, anxiety, cognitive impairment, and dementia. Often the patient does not mention these difficulties because he or she does not link them with Parkinson disease. Patients may demonstrate some of these difficulties, and the therapist should recognize the symptoms and refer the patient for further follow-up.

The major problems that patients have after 5 years of treatment for Parkinson disease are fluctuations (both motor and nonmotor), dyskinesias, and behavioral or cognitive changes.[14,15] The mechanisms behind these complications relate both to the underlying disease and the effects of medications. Motor fluctuations take several forms. Most commonly, a predictable decline in motor performance occurs near the end of each medication dose ("wearing off"). Patients change gradually from "on," with a good medication response, into an "off" period 30 minutes to 1 hour before the next medication dose is due. Often patients have involuntary movements (dyskinesias) as a peak-dose complication, and sometimes similar movements occur at the end of the dose. Sudden and severe cataclysms of motor fluctuation occur rarely, with ambulatory patients becoming immobilized over a period of seconds ("sudden on-off").[16] Because these fluctuations occur throughout the day, accurate detection requires the cooperation of the patient, who must be trained to keep and complete a diary recording function.[17] These journals generally divide the 24-hour day into 30-minute segments to detect good medication response ("on"), poor medication response ("off"), disabling dyskinesias, and sleep. Recently two new formulations of L-dopa intended to address wearing off have been approved.[2] Rytary carbidopa-levodopa extended-release capsules contain both immediate- and extended-release beads that provide reduced off time in patients with motor fluctuations.[18] DUOPA carbidopa-levodopa intestinal gel is administered through a gastrostomy tube into the jejunum using a pump and can have a dramatic effect in reducing "off" time.[19]

In general, to meet functional goals and outcomes effectively, therapists working with patients taking antiparkinsonian medication must be aware of both the positive and negative side effects of medications. Learning the difference between tremor and dyskinesia is crucial. The therapist must coordinate therapy sessions during good medication response times to facilitate optimal outcomes. In addition, patients should be monitored for postural hypotension, dizziness, and cognitive changes. Therapists have the unique opportunity to determine the best timing, frequency, and duration of the treatment; understanding the impact of a patient's drug regimen will only enhance the outcome. Therapists must also be aware that exercise increases metabolism. Increased metabolism may use up the medication faster; thus an individual who generally remains symptom-free (no off times between doses) and whose metabolism is increased will again exhibit signs of the disease (distal tremors and axial or proximal rigidity). These increases in symptoms may stem from a problem of drug dosage, not being signs of further degeneration of the basal ganglia. All changes in symptoms should be discussed with both the pharmacist and the physician.

Cancer

Cancer is a general term for disorders associated with abnormal and uncontrolled cell proliferation. Virtually any organ system can be affected, either as the primary site of disease or as a secondary site associated with metastasis. Cancer pharmacology has improved significantly during the recent past with an expanded understanding of cancer biology and newly developed drugs that target cancer vulnerabilities. Effective early treatments, adjuvant chemotherapy, and hormonal therapy can extend overall survival and prevent disease reoccurrence. In the past 5 years the ability to harness the power of the immune system in the treatment of cancer has brought about a paradigm shift whereby some of the most feared diseases—such as melanoma, lung cancer, and even late-stage metastatic disease—can be eradicated.[20] Cancer may interfere with neurological rehabilitation in various ways. Tumors within the brain may interfere with cognitive, motor and sensory function as well as autonomic and metabolic control (see Chapter 25). Peripherally tumors may interfere with nerve function and associated motor control or may produce pain. In addition, drugs that reduce cancer pain may interfere with cognitive and

Effects on motor systems are systemic or indirect.

motor function.[21] Among such drugs, morphine and related opiate derivatives (Box 36.2) are notable. A significant degree of tolerance to the CNS depressant effects will develop with long-term administration. Currently cannabinoids are being studied not only for the treatment of cancer symptoms but also for their anticancer effects. Cannabinoids are considered useful in combating anorexia, chemotherapy-induced nausea and vomiting, pain, insomnia, and depression.[22,23] Nabiximols (Sativex), a cannabinoid drug, is still under study. An oral mucosal spray made up of a whole-plant extract with tetrahydrocannabinol (THC)/cannabidiol (CBD) is available in Canada and parts of Europe to treat pain linked to cancer as well as muscle spasms and pain from MS.[24] In cancer chemotherapeutic regimens, many antiemetic agents are used. These include dopaminergic antagonists (which may produce motor deficits similar to those of Parkinson disease), dronabinol (a chemical component of marijuana, which can affect cognitive function), and nabilone (a synthetic cannabinoid) as well as high-dose corticosteroids (which affect mood). Some antitumor agents may be neurotoxic; reduced deep tendon reflexes, paresthesias, and demyelination are associated with vincristine (Oncovin) and oxaliplatin (Eloxatin).[20,25] Naturally any change in drugs involving cancer treatment (directly or indirectly) requires the approval of the patient's oncologist.

The main role of rehabilitation specialists is to help patients with cancer recover from the physical changes that accompany their illness, promote function in activities of daily living, and help provide adaptations to activities within the limits of each patient's function and the illness. Clinicians should be aware of chemotherapy side effects and the side effects of medications given to treat the toxic effects of chemotherapy. The importance of recognizing toxic effects early in the treatment regimen cannot be overstated and will help the oncologist to alter the dose or discontinue the offending medication.

A number of chemotherapeutic and nonchemotherapeutic medications are used to fight cancer. Most anticancer therapies operate on the simple principle that because cells in tumors are actively dividing, agents that kill dividing cells will kill tumor cells.[26] Tissue cells that divide rapidly are therefore at risk, including hair, mucosal linings, bone marrow, immune cells, and skin epithelial cells. Nonchemotherapy medications called *biological response modifiers* (BRMs) are naturally made by the body but in anticancer treatment are delivered in large quantities and at higher doses than those produced by the body.[27] Interferon and interleukin are two of the most commonly used medications. Monoclonal antibodies that target oncogenic pathways are also used as chemotherapy to suppress the immune system.

Chemotherapy often has side effects that affect the integumentary, GI, hematological, and neurological systems. Each type of therapy has potential side effects along with the more general side effects of the

treatment regimen. Because of their chemotherapeutic treatment of cancer, patients often have muscular weakness, neuropathy, fatigue, pain, immobility, and reduced flexibility. Often the therapist will have to be supportive and flexible with treatment plans to accommodate for changing physiological, psychological, and social factors during treatment.

GI symptoms such as nausea and vomiting may occur; medications such as Compazine and Reglan may be given to help control these episodes. Symptoms of diarrhea may be addressed through prescriptions or the use of over-the-counter (OTC) medications including milk of magnesia and magnesium citrate. The development of mucositis or esophagitis is also possible. A prescription solution of three medications (diphenhydramine [Benadryl], nystatin, and viscous lidocaine) can help to relieve pain, inflammation, and potential associated fungal infections. Bone marrow suppression from chemotherapeutic regimens may lead to an increased risk of infection, risk of bleeding, and fatigue as well as a lack of exercise capacity and musculoskeletal weakness. Patients undergoing chemotherapy may receive one or more medications to signal the bone marrow to increase its output of white blood cells (filgrastim [Neupogen]), stimulate the production of red blood cells (epoetin alfa [Epogen]), and stimulate increased production of platelets (oprelvekin [Neumega]). These therapies may be instituted to help the patient more quickly reverse suppression of bone marrow and allow the chemotherapy to continue without interruption.[28] Generalized symptoms include fever, body aches and pains, and feelings of ill health and fatigue. No specific medications are used to improve these symptoms. In general taking medications such as acetaminophen, ibuprofen, or narcotics for fever and pain may help. The use of exercise as an adjunctive therapy for cancer treatment–related symptoms has gained favor in oncology rehabilitation as a promising intervention.[29–32] Exercise is thought to help improve endurance, functional ability, and quality of life.[29,31,32] The major side effects associated with BRMs and monoclonal antibodies are generalized as well and include fever and flulike symptoms with associated arthralgia and myalgia. Other side effects include lymphedema, which is characterized by fluid retention caused by disruption of lymphatic drainage or the removal of lymph nodes. As mentioned earlier, neurological changes may occur, with the development of neurological signs as well as forgetfulness, suicidal ideation, and depression.

In treating cancers, selection of the most appropriate treatment or treatments, dose, and dose intervals as well as the management of adverse effects requires specialized knowledge and a team effort.[20] In addition, cancer treatment regimens undergo frequent updates due to findings of ongoing clinical trials. The availability of drugs with new mechanisms of action (e.g., immune checkpoint inhibitors), good target selectivity (e.g., kinase inhibitors), efficacy in specific cancers, and different adverse-effect profiles permits the use of new drug combinations and regimens.[20] The rehabilitation professional is an important team member in oncology because his or her actions potentially affect quality of life.

Seizure Disorders (Epilepsy)

Epilepsy is associated with a diverse group of neurological disorders resulting in motor, psychic, and autonomic manifestations. Many antiseizure medications may produce drowsiness, ataxia, and vertigo (Box 36.3). Some may produce cognitive disorders in children and adults.[33,34] Although these adverse effects may be exhibited throughout therapy, they are most troublesome during its initiation, the addition of a drug, and the escalation of dosage. Sudden discontinuation of antiseizure medications may result in status epilepticus, which can be fatal. Many antiseizure medications are finding successful applications outside epilepsy, especially in the area of pain management. As with cancer, clinical evidence has shown that cannabinoids such as CBD can

BOX 36.3   Anticonvulsants

acetazolamide (various brand names)	oxcarbazepine (Trileptal)
carbamazepine (Tegretol)	phenobarbital (various brand names)
clonazepam (Klonopin)	phenytoin (Dilantin)
diazepam (Valium)	pregabalin (Lyrica)
ethosuximide (Zarontin)	primidone (Mysoline)
felbamate (Felbatol)	rufinamide (Banzel)
fosphenytoin (Cerebyx)	tiagabine (Gabitril)
gabapentin (Neurontin)	topiramate (Topamax)
lacosamide (Vimpat)	valproic acid (Depakene)
lamotrigine (Lamictal)	vigabatrin (Sabril)
levetiracetam (Keppra)	zonisamide (Zonagran
lorazepam (Ativan)	

Effects on motor systems are direct and may decrease tone at higher doses. Direct effects on muscle are minimal. This list includes benzodiazepines that have antiseizure applications.

be used to reduce seizures effectively, particularly in patients with treatment-resistant epilepsy. However, many questions remain regarding the mechanism, safety, and efficacy of cannabinoids in short- and long-term use.[35]

The practicing clinician working with patients who have a history of seizure disorders must be prepared for the onset of a seizure and be aware of any adverse side effects of medications. Adverse side effects are typically determined on a clinical basis, signifying the importance of recognition by the health care provider. Many of the common side effects can also have negative implications for motor learning, especially while the patient is getting used to the medication or the dosage is being elevated or tapered.

The treatment of seizure disorders with pharmacotherapy is typically intended to control the seizure activity completely without producing unwanted side effects. Pharmacological intervention usually begins with one medication (monotherapy); if this drug is unsuccessful, a second is added while dosage of the first is tapered. Or a combination may be needed. The effects of the medications vary and may include enhancing the inhibitory effects of γ-aminobutyric acid (GABA) (benzodiazepines); reducing posttetanic potentiation, thereby reducing seizure spread (iminostilbenes); or modulating neuronal voltage-dependent sodium and calcium channels (hydantoin).[36] The overall result is a reduction in abnormal electrical impulses in the brain. The choice of antiseizure drugs primarily depends on the seizure type and, if possible, the diagnosis of a specific syndrome. If seizures are recurrent and occur during critical periods of childhood, adolescence, and early adulthood, they may result in significant impairments in function and increased disability.

Some side effects may be slow to develop and difficult to diagnose because seizures can often be mistaken for sedation or cognitive dysfunction, especially in children, who may not report drug side effects. Practitioners can also mistakenly accept reversible drug toxicity as a necessary consequence of a seizure disorder. The number of seizures occurring during physical or occupational therapy should be tracked to assist in determining appropriate pharmacotherapy.

One common antiseizure medication, valproic acid (Depakene), may cause nausea, vomiting, hair loss, tremor, tiredness, dizziness, and headache. Valproic acid has also been reported to aggravate absence seizure in patients with absence epilepsy.[37] Metabolic side effects may include an increase in glucose-stimulated pancreatic insulin secretion, which may be followed by an increase in body weight.[38] Long-term use of valproic acid is known to increase bone resorption in adult epileptic patients and can decrease the mineral density of bone.[39]

Another seizure medication, carbamazepine (Tegretol), is considered a safe drug, but it has a long list of adverse effects, most commonly ataxia and nystagmus.[40] Other systems frequently involved are the skin, the hematopoietic system, and the cardiovascular system. Gabapentin (Neurontin) is another well-tolerated antiseizure medication with proven clinical efficacy and a low incidence of adverse events in clinical trials. Common side effects include dizziness, fatigue, and headache. Phenytoin (Dilantin) has adverse effects including ataxia, nystagmus, slurred speech, confusion, dizziness, and, at high doses, peripheral neuropathy.

Benzodiazepines (e.g., diazepam) are useful in managing status epilepticus, but their effects are not long-lasting, so they are often used along with a primary anticonvulsant. The most frequent side effects are dose-related sedation, difficulty with concentration, dizziness, and difficulty walking.

Pharmacological adverse events that occur under the influence of seizure medications must be recognized by the rehabilitation specialist to participate in a team approach to patient care. Therapists can assist in determining the effectiveness of a specific treatment regimen, appropriate timing of rehabilitation interventions, and the overall progress of the patient during rehabilitation.

Stroke, Hypertension, and Related Disorders

Stroke, by virtue of its interference with blood flow and oxygenation, produces both reversible and irreversible neurological deficits. The loss of function associated with stroke has at least two major causes. The first involves loss of oxygenation to a critical brain region, followed by glutaminergic rebound and excessive calcium influx with apoptosis (programmed cell death). Current drugs and those under development are aimed at restoring blood flow and inhibiting glutaminergic hyperexcitability and intracellular apoptotic mechanisms.[41] The second pathogenic issue is related to reperfusion injury associated with oxygen free radicals and associated cellular damage. In this case, free radical scavengers have shown some promise in animal models of stroke.[42] To reduce the damage associated with thromboembolism in such cases, tissue plasminogen activator (tPA) has been recommended.[43] However, this agent is most effective when given within an hour and up to 4.5 hours after the vascular insult.[44] Currently some studies have provided strong evidence to support the efficacy of endovascular therapy with intravenous thrombolytic treatment in patients with acute ischemic strokes due to large vessel occlusions. Speed of delivery, multidisciplinary care, and access to specialized teams with endovascular capability is required to achieve results similar to those seen in these trials.[44–48]

Drugs with other mechanisms used to improve the prognosis of stroke are under development,[49,50] showing variable promise. However, drugs used for concurrent conditions (atherosclerosis and hypertension) before and after a stroke are complicating factors for optimal outcomes from rehabilitation. These drugs include β-adrenergic antagonists, which reduce heart rate and correspondingly alter exercise tolerance. Occasionally calcium channel blockers, α-adrenergic blockers, and related agents may cause similar effects, including weakness, dizziness, syncope, and cognitive disorders. Changes in serum electrolytes induced by diuretics and the angiotensin-converting enzyme inhibitors may affect the heart, the vasculature, and skeletal muscle and ultimately cause impairments in areas such as strength of contraction.[51] Box 36.4 lists many of these drugs. Many of the cholesterol synthesis inhibitors (agents used to reduce serum cholesterol) may induce muscle weakness, which may impact rehabilitation (Box 36.5), but this adverse effect is considered rare despite the increase in prescribing.[52–55] Abrupt discontinuation of antihypertensive medications may result in a hypertensive crisis, dramatically increasing the risk of stroke and related disorders.

BOX 36.4 Commonly Used Antihypertensive and Cardiovascular Drugs

β-Adrenergic Blocking Drugs
acebutolol (Sectral)
atenolol (Tenormin)
betaxolol (Kerlone)
bisoprolol (Zebeta)
carteolol (Cartrol)
esmolol (Brevibloc)
metoprolol (Lopressor)
nadolol (Corgard)
nebivolol (Bystolic)
penbutolol (Levatol)
pindolol (Visken)
propranolol (Inderal)
sotalol (Betapace)
timolol (Blocadren)

Agents That Affect α- and/or β-Adrenergic Systems
carvedilol (Coreg)
clonidine (Catapres)
doxazosin (Cardura)
guanabenz (Wytensin)
guanadrel (Hylorel)
guanfacine (Tenex)
labetalol (Trandate)
methyldopa (Aldomet)
prazosin (Minipress)
silodosin (Rapaflo)
tamsulosin (Flomax)
terazosin (Hytrin)

Calcium Channel Blocking Drugs
amlodipine (Norvasc)
bepridil (Vascor)

clevidipine (Cleviprex)
diltiazem (Cardizem)
felodipine (Plendil)
isradipine (DynaCirc)
nicardipine (Cardene)
nifedipine (Procardia)
nimodipine (Nimotop)
nisoldipine (Sular)
verapamil (Calan)

Agents That Affect the Renin-Angiotensin System
Angiotensin-Converting Enzyme Inhibitors
benazepril (Lotensin)
captopril (Capoten)
enalapril (Vasotec)
fosinopril (Monopril)
lisinopril (Zestril)
moexipril (Univasc)
perindopril (Aceon)
quinapril (Accupril)
ramipril (Altace)
trandolapril (Mavik)

Angiotensin Antagonists
candesartan (Atacand)
eprosartan (Teveten)
irbesartan (Avapro)
losartan (Cozaar)
olmesartan (Benicar)
telmisartan (Micardis)
valsartan (Diovan)

Effects on motor systems are predominantly systemic or indirect.

BOX 36.5 Hypolipidemic Drugs (HMG-CoA Reductase Inhibitors)

atorvastatin (Lipitor)	pravastatin (Pravachol)
fluvastatin (Lescol)	rosuvastatin (Crestor)
lovastatin (Mevacor)	simvastatin (Zocor)
pitavastatin (Livalo)	

These drugs may rarely produce muscle damage through a direct effect on the muscle.

Clinicians caring for patients with stroke, hypertension, and cardiac disorders will benefit from understanding the impact of any medication on the therapeutic plan. These patients may be taking any number of medications to manage the acute and subacute complications of cardiovascular impairments and their resulting sequelae. Other complications after stroke that may require pharmacological intervention include urinary tract infections, musculoskeletal pain, deep vein thrombosis, pressure sores, shoulder subluxation, and depression. All these medications have their own issues, and health care providers must be aware of adverse events and any alteration in function of the heart that may occur in relation to exercise.

Anticoagulants such as heparin, warfarin, and aspirin (so-called *blood thinners*) are used to prevent another stroke after the first one has

occurred. Side effects may include bleeding, allergic reactions, thrombocytopenia, and, in the case of aspirin, stomach irritation.[56] New oral anticoagulants have been development for stroke prevention in atrial fibrillation. These newer agents such as dabigatran (Pradaxa), rivaroxaban (Xarelto), apixaban (Eliquis), and edoxaban (Savaysa) have a predictable pharmacological profile so that international normalized ratio (INR) monitoring and dose modifications are not required.[57–60] Their main advantages, apart from their treatment efficacy, include the reduced rate of intracranial hemorrhage, the lack of need for routine coagulation monitoring, the predictable anticoagulation response, and the limited interaction with food and drugs.[61] Blood thinners make the patient more susceptible to bruising; therefore care must be taken in patient handling and choice of activity. Antiarrhythmics are used to restore the heart's normal conduction patterns. Antiarrhythmic drugs may make some patients experience lightheadedness, dizziness, or faintness when they get up after sitting or lying down (orthostatic hypotension).[62] Antiarrhythmic drugs may also cause low blood sugar or changes in thermoregulation.[63] The most common side effects are dry mouth and throat, diarrhea, and loss of appetite.[64] These problems usually go away as the body adjusts to the drug and do not require medical treatment. Therapists must be prepared for hypotensive events and the need to educate patients on positions that will reduce the effects of orthostatic hypotension.

Hypertension is a common disorder that is frequently encountered when treating patients in the rehabilitation environment. Antihypertensive medications are used to lower blood pressure (see Box 36.4) by limiting plasma volume expansion, decreasing peripheral resistance, and decreasing plasma volume. Often patients under medical management will undergo changes in dose and additions or deletions of medication, which may lead to problems during rehabilitation. Side effects of these medications may include increased frequency of urination, increased urinary excretion of potassium, orthostatic hypotension, hypotension, dehydration, tiredness, fatigue, cold hands and feet, and dizziness.[65] Health care providers working with a patient who is taking antihypertensive medications should monitor for side effects, clinical signs, and the patient's perceived exertion. Generally people on antihypertensive medications require careful cardiovascular monitoring during any physical activity.

Many patients tend to become depressed after experiencing a stroke, a cardiac event, or another neurological disorder.[66] Such changes in mood may be attributable to a natural loss of physical function or a neurochemical response to changes in brain chemistry. Patients with signs and symptoms of depression (sadness, anxiety, hopelessness, suicidal ideation) should be referred for further follow-up by the physician. Many antidepressant medications take at least 2 weeks to achieve a therapeutic level. Antidepressants may cause temporary side effects (sometimes referred to as *adverse effects*) in some people. These effects are generally mild. Any unusual reactions, side effects, or behaviors that interfere with functioning should be reported to the physician immediately. The most common side effects of tricyclic antidepressants (TCAs) are dry mouth, constipation, bladder problems, sexual problems, blurred vision, dizziness, and drowsiness.[67] The newer antidepressants have different types of side effects, including headache, nausea, nervousness, insomnia, agitation, and sexual problems.[68] Therapists working with patients who are depressed may have to delay rehabilitation until the depression is well managed.

Hyperlipidemia is considered a modifiable risk factor for heart disease and stroke. Many patients may be receiving pharmacological treatment to reduce their cardiovascular risk. Several types of drugs are available for cholesterol lowering, including statins, bile acid sequestrants, nicotinic acid, and fibric acids.[69] The statins are considered first-line drugs and are generally well tolerated, but they can produce myopathy under some circumstances.[69] An elevation of creatine kinase level is the best indicator of statin-induced myopathy and should be checked for when patients report leg pain. Bile acid sequestrants also produce moderate reductions in cholesterol. Sequestrant therapy can produce a variety of GI symptoms, including constipation, abdominal pain, bloating, fullness, nausea, and flatulence. Nicotinic acid (niacin) therapy can be accompanied by a number of side effects. Flushing of the skin is common with the crystalline form and is intolerable for some persons. However, most persons have tolerance to the flushing after more prolonged use of the drug. The fibrates have the ability to lower serum triglycerides and are generally well tolerated in most persons. GI symptoms are the most commonly reported, and fibrates appear to increase the likelihood of cholesterol gallstones.[69]

Overall, patients taking cardiovascular medications need careful monitoring for any drug impact on cardiorespiratory or metabolic responses in relation to rehabilitation activities. Thus the effects of drugs must be considered in developing the rehabilitation plan.

Anxiety and Depression

Agents used in the management of anxiety, whether from acute or chronic disease, must be carefully titrated. Among these agents are the benzodiazepines, whose anxiolytic (anxiety-reducing) dosage range immediately precedes a dose that may affect motor skills and

---

BOX 36.6 Anxiolytic Benzodiazepines

alprazolam (Xanax)
chlordiazepoxide (Librium)
clorazepate (Tranxene)
diazepam (Valium)
halazepam (Paxipam)
lorazepam (Ativan)
oxazepam (Serax)

Note that benzodiazepines indicated for sleep induction are not included in this list. The agents listed here reduce muscle tone through a direct effect on motor systems at higher doses.

---

cognitive function (Box 36.6). In subjects of all ages but especially the geriatric population, the administration of benzodiazepines may produce paradoxical excitement, confusion, and behavioral changes.[70] Geriatric subjects also have an increased incidence of injury from falls concurrent with use of benzodiazepines and other sedative-hypnotic drugs. Although benzodiazepines may have variable effects on learning and declarative memory, these effects may differ among the benzodiazepines; there may also be considerable variation in individual responses. If producing sleep alone is desired, zolpidem (Ambien) and zaleplon (Sonata) are attractive alternatives because these agents do not have anxiolytic effects. Although the anxiolytic agent buspirone (Buspar) is relatively free of benzodiazepine-like effects, the onset time for the desired anxiolytic effect is characteristically delayed.[71] Lack of compliance with anxiolytic agents may increase panic attacks and reduce effective interactions with a therapist.

The emergence of the selective serotonin reuptake inhibitors (SSRIs) has revolutionized the treatment of depression. The older agents, such as the TCAs, are just as effective in the management of several forms of depression; however, their adverse effect profile is somewhat different. TCAs often produce drowsiness and orthostatic hypotension, effects that complicate any rehabilitation regimen.[72] Although these effects may also be produced by SSRIs, their incidence is much reduced. Certain TCAs, by virtue of their ability to inhibit the reuptake of norepinephrine in adrenergic nerve terminals, may be used at lower doses for neuralgia. Although these low-dose regimens are usually not associated with the side effects previously mentioned, some patients may be more sensitive to these effects than others. This requires increased vigilance for the care team in determining iatrogenic versus pathological sources of somnolence and syncope. A partial list of antidepressants is presented in Box 36.7. Noncompliance with antidepressant therapy may result in lack of interest in any therapeutic regimen.

Patients with stroke and other neurological diagnoses often have depression, which reduces motivation and decreases compliance with

---

BOX 36.7 Antidepressants: Examples of Tricyclic Antidepressants and Selective Serotonin Reuptake Inhibitors

Tricyclic Antidepressants
amitriptyline (Elavil)
amoxapine (various trade names)
clomipramine (Anafranil)
desipramine (Norpramin)
doxepin (Adapin)
imipramine (Tofranil)
nortriptyline (Pamelor)
protriptyline (Vivactil)

Selective Serotonin Reuptake Inhibitors
citalopram (Celexa)
escitalopram (Lexapro)
fluoxetine (Prozac)
fluvoxamine (Luvox)
paroxetine (Paxil)
sertraline (Zoloft)

These agents may produce complex direct and indirect effects on motor systems with minimal effects directly on muscle.

a therapeutic regimen. Although obviously linked, the degree of functional restoration after a stroke does not always correlate with resolution of depression.

Many patients with neurological disorders are diagnosed with or experience anxiety and depression. Affective symptomatology can be the result of cognitive and emotional deficits or impairment of brain function from the existing pathology.[66] In the rehabilitation environment, many patients may show signs and symptoms of anxiety or depression that can make the process of recovery more difficult. The rehabilitation professional must recognize the manifestations of both anxiety and depression, such as fear of dying or "going crazy," heart palpitations, shortness of breath, difficulty concentrating, depressed mood, diminished interest or pleasure in activities, sleep disturbance, changes in appetite, psychomotor retardation and agitation, and suicidal ideation.[73] Anxiety and depression may limit the patient's full participation in recovery of function and are associated with poorer outcomes.[68,74]

Anxiety and depression can be managed well when treated with the medications discussed previously, but some drugs—including centrally acting hypotensives (methyldopa), lipid-soluble β-blockers (propranolol), benzodiazepines, and other CNS depressants—may cause a depressed mood.[2] Therefore in the case of a patient with depression, review of the medication regimen can be useful as it can help to determine whether one of the medications is implicated.

Pharmacological treatments for anxiety and depression should be administered at a dosage and time that ensure the best patient response during treatment. Antianxiety medications (see Box 36.6) act within a short time after ingestion, producing their effects of sedation and relaxation and thereby reducing anxiety. Higher levels may cause drowsiness, sleep, and anesthesia and are associated with falls, which may not be ideal when the aim of treatment is to promote recovery of function. Antidepressant medications (see Box 36.7) typically take weeks for therapeutic levels to be achieved in the brain and an improvement in mood to be demonstrated. Rehabilitation may be appropriate for a patient taking these medications when they have improved the patient's mood and outlook. Side effects of antidepressants can also cause some difficulties, including lightheadedness, drowsiness, short-term memory loss, disturbed sleep, clumsiness, sedation, and low blood pressure.

Some evidence has shown that recovery from brain injury may be positively influenced by antidepressants[75,76] and that antidepressants can play a role in brain plasticity.[77] These studies suggest that recovery of function after brain injury can be influenced by experience and pharmacological intervention. Rehabilitation specialists must be prepared to assess responses to pharmacotherapy, recognize adverse effects, manage minor side effects, and seek appropriate assistance for adverse events.

Arthritis and Autoimmune Disorders

Autoimmune mechanisms play an important role in the inflammatory process and progressive joint destruction of rheumatoid arthritis (RA). Because of the constant pain associated with movement, patients tend to seek nonprescription drugs (including dietary supplements) that often escape prescription drug monitoring programs in pharmacies. It is important for all health professionals to recognize this issue, particularly with RA. In the management of RA, the therapeutic approach may influence the progress of rehabilitation. Pharmacological agents that reduce RA symptoms and impede joint damage can be categorized as either nonbiological disease-modifying antirheumatic agents (DMARDs) or biological DMARDs, which include inhibitors of tumor necrosis factor (TNF)-alpha biologics or non-TNF biologics.[78] DMARDs are the key mediations that should be initiated as soon as

possible after disease onset.[79–81] Nonsteroidal antiinflammatory drugs (NSAIDs) and/or corticosteroids can be used for symptomatic improvement as they provide rapid relief of symptoms compared with DMARDs, which may take weeks to months to have an effect.

Treatment with glucocorticoids may reduce joint pain and facilitate movement, but it may also produce changes in mood and muscle wasting.[82] Although this is reversible and limited to systemic administration of high-dose corticosteroids, its impact cannot be overlooked and certainly affects the prognosis of physical or occupational therapy. Corticosteroids should not be used as monotherapy; they are valuable in controlling symptoms before DMARDs can take effect and are used in acute RA flares as burst therapy.[78] Continuous low doses of corticosteroids may be used as adjunctive therapy when DMARDs do not provide adequate disease control. Some data suggest that they have disease-modifying activity[83–85]; however, it is preferable to avoid chronic use when possible so as to avoid long-term complications. NSAIDs and DMARDs have steroid-sparing properties that permit reductions in corticosteroid dose. Prednisone and related glucocorticoids may often produce a false sense of well-being that may exceed the ability of the patients to engage safely in certain exercise regimens. From the patient's perspective, this pharmacological effect is perceived as a "cure" and does not provide the motivation to continue with exercise therapy. The same problems may exist with the use of corticosteroids in other autoimmune disorders.[86]

NSAIDs (Box 36.8) have long been used for the relief of pain due to arthritis; however, depletion of prostaglandins in the gastric mucosa produces bleeding, which has limited their usefulness.[87] NSAIDs should seldom be used as monotherapy for RA because they do not alter the course of the disease; instead, they should be viewed as adjuncts to DMARDs. The development of newer agents that are more selective for isoforms of cyclooxygenase (COX-2 inhibitors), which are involved in joint inflammation, is a major advance. An example is celecoxib. Although bleeding disorders are dramatically reduced, the incidence of ataxia with these agents may be increased.[88] Unfortunately cardiovascular toxicity risk has led to the withdrawal of most of the COX-2 inhibitors from the market. Patients with neurological diseases or pathological processes with problems requiring antiinflammatory medications may develop side effects that interact with and complicate existing motor deficits. Failure to comply with the arthritis medication regimen will likewise reduce effective movement.

Clinically, patients with the onset of RA may have a number of systemic manifestations, including fatigue, anorexia, generalized weakness, and musculoskeletal symptoms followed by synovitis. These forewarning symptoms may continue over weeks or months before

---

BOX 36.8 Commonly Used Nonsteroidal Antiinflammatory Agents and Salicylates

aspirin or acetylsalicylic acid
celecoxib (Celebrex)
diclofenac (Voltaren)
diflunisal (Dolobid)
etodolac (Lodine)
fenoprofen (Nalfon)
flurbiprofen (Ansaid)
ibuprofen (Advil, Motrin, Nuprin)
indomethacin (Indocin)
ketoprofen (Orudis KT, Oruvail)

ketorolac (Toradol)
meclofenamate (various trade names)
mefenamic acid (Ponstel)
meloxicam (Mobic)
nabumetone (Relafen)
naproxen (Aleve, Naprosyn)
oxaprozin (Daypro)
piroxicam (Feldene)
sulindac (Clinoril)
tolmetin (Tolectin)

Only at higher doses will these agents affect motor systems directly. Most problems arise through systemic or indirect effects.

more specific symptoms occur. The initial evaluation of the patient with RA should document symptoms of active disease (e.g., degree of joint pain, duration of morning stiffness, degree of fatigue), functional status, objective evidence of disease activity (e.g., synovitis, as assessed by the number of tender and swollen joints and the erythrocyte sedimentation rate), mechanical joint problems (e.g., loss of motion, crepitus, instability, malalignment, or deformity), the presence of extraarticular disease, and damage detected radiographically.[89] Neurological complications of RA may occur in the CNS (cerebral vasculitis), the peripheral nervous system (nerve compression), the neuromuscular junction (myasthenic syndrome), and muscle (myopathy).[90] Depending on the stage of involvement, the patient may be undergoing nonpharmacological modalities (education, weight loss, range-of-motion exercises) and pharmacological therapy including analgesics, NSAIDs, steroids, DMARDs, and BRMs.

The goals of pharmacological treatment of RA are to prevent or control joint damage, prevent loss of function, decrease pain, and improve joint function.[89] NSAIDs assist in analgesia and decrease inflammation and reducing stiffness, thus allowing the therapist to work on range of motion and strengthening. Because NSAIDs regulate the production of chemicals (prostaglandins) in the body that help trigger inflammation by inhibition of an enzyme (COX), they sometimes lead to the unwanted side effects discussed previously. Data suggest that although selective COX-2 inhibitors pose a significantly lower risk of serious adverse GI effects than do nonselective NSAIDs, they are no more effective than nonselective NSAIDs, are related to cardiovascular events, and may cost as much as 15 to 20 times more per month of treatment than generic NSAIDs.[91,92]

Steroids are synthetic forms of naturally occurring hormones produced by the adrenal glands and are typically administered orally or by injection. They provide a rapid and powerful reduction of pain and inflammation resulting in improved function. Recent evidence suggests that low-dose glucocorticoids slow the rate of joint damage and therefore appear to have disease-modifying potential.[93] Side effects, depending on the dosage and length of treatment, include blood sugar elevations, cataracts, hypertension, increased susceptibility to infection and bruising, osteoporosis, and weight gain. These drugs are often used at disease onset or with disease flares as a temporary aid in obtaining control. Disabling synovitis frequently recurs when glucocorticoids are discontinued, even in patients who are receiving combination therapy with one or more DMARDs. Therefore many patients with RA are functionally dependent while taking glucocorticoids and continue using them on a long-term basis.[89]

An important foundation in the treatment of RA is the use of DMARDs, which reduce signs and symptoms, reduce or prevent joint damage, and preserve the structure and function of the joints. Their use alone or in combination has been reported to allow patients to remain active and productive.[94] The most common DMARDs in current use include methotrexate, sulfasalazine, hydroxychloroquine, leflunomide, and cyclosporine. The biological agents with disease-modifying activity include the anti-TNF drugs (etanercept, infliximab, adalimumab, certolizumab, golimumab), the costimulation modulator abatacept, the IL-6 receptor antagonist tocilizumab, and rituximab, which depletes peripheral B cells. Others include gold salts, azathioprine, and D-penicillamine. Side effects may include diarrhea, eye damage, liver damage, and nausea/vomiting; these reactions depend on the DMARD taken.

Finally, BRMs are a newly developed class of medicines that restore or stimulate the immune system to fight disease. BRMs target specific parts of the immune system that destroy joints. Some do so by blocking the effects of TNF, a protein involved in RA through the inflammatory cascade, and are credited with improving signs, symptoms, and

function in patients with RA.[95] The anti-TNF and non-TNF biological agents have proven to be effective for patients who fail treatment with other DMARDs and were previously reserved for this subset particularly due to cost. However, the American College of Rheumatology[96] now endorses the use of anti-TNF biologics in patients with early disease of high activity and a poor prognosis.

Rehabilitation therapy is important in maintaining physical function in patients with RA. With combinations of medications, health care providers can reach goals of increasing or maintaining joint mobility; decreasing pain; improving functional abilities; improving cardiovascular fitness; and educating patients on the use of assistive devices, joint protection, and energy conservation.

Infectious Diseases

Both bacterial and viral diseases may produce neurological disorders (see Chapter 26). The neurological impact of treatments and prophylactic measures must be understood. Although this may be clear for drugs, vaccines have also been implicated in causing similar problems. The association of a hypotonic-hyporesponsive episode with the pertussis vaccine is such an example.[97]

In the course of treating bacterial diseases, many antibiotics and antiinfective agents may compromise sensory, motor, and cognitive function. These functions may be compromised temporarily or permanently and may be patient specific. First, in the critically ill patient, aminoglycosides (gentamicin, tobramycin, and amikacin) and vancomycin may produce ototoxicity, such as hearing loss (reversible and irreversible) and vestibular damage (dizziness, vertigo, and ataxia). Minocycline is also associated with vestibular toxicity.[98] Extra precautions may be necessary to prevent falls during and after therapeutic exercise sessions. Fall-prevention programs must be developed in these cases as well as with the use of sedative-hypnotics, as previously noted.

A wide variety of viral diseases interfere with neurological function. Polio is historically the most widely recognized. Acquired immunodeficiency syndrome (AIDS) may manifest as a wide variety of neurological disorders. Protease inhibitors, which reduce the assembly of viral particles, may dramatically reduce and possibly reverse the neurological manifestations of AIDS.[99] Although adverse effects associated with antiviral and antibiotic agents may be intolerable, noncompliance may result in increased resistance of the virus or microorganism to retreatment.

The guiding principle of chemotherapy for infection is selective toxicity, in which the agent must cause more harm to the pathogen than to the host. Problems associated with antimicrobial therapy include resistance to drugs, side effects, allergies, and suppression of normal flora. Clinicians ask patients to exercise under conditions in which they may potentially have a compromised immune response because of trauma, a pathological condition, or surgery. These conditions may make patients more susceptible to infection, slow healing, and slow recovery.[100]

An increasing number of strains of antibiotic-resistant bacteria are now emerging (*Clostridium difficile*, carbapenem-resistant Enterobacteriaceae), in large part because of the overuse and misuse of antimicrobial drugs by health care providers.[101] Overuse of antimicrobial drugs exerts a selective pressure on bacteria, encouraging the emergence of antibiotic-resistant strains by eliminating antibiotic-sensitive strains, promoting the establishment of bacteria with rare mutations of resistance, and permitting the spread of resistant strains from infected individuals.[102] One example is the use of antibiotics for upper respiratory tract infections caused by viruses. This has been shown to have no beneficial impact on the course of the disease.[103] Infection control in the rehabilitation environment is essential to stop the spread of disease. Therapists must be diligent with infection-control procedures such as handwashing, updating vaccinations, and cleaning all equipment. Educating patients to use antibiotics only when needed and complete the entire course of medication can potentially slow the proliferation.

Common adverse effects from the use of antimicrobials and antiviral drugs include nephrotoxicity and ototoxicity (aminoglycosides), GI complications (cephalosporins, clindamycin), thrombophlebitis and vertigo (tetracyclines), jaundice (erythromycin), photophobia (vidarabine), neurotoxicity (metronidazole), and allergic reactions (β-lactam antibiotics). The therapist must be aware of adverse side effects to assist with early recognition and referral to the physician.

Antibiotics kill various normal commensal bacteria in the gut, altering the balance and allowing overgrowth of pathogens.[104] This change of bacterial flora is believed to result in increased toxins from pathogens and can cause infection with resistant microbes.[104] When patients are taking drugs to fight infection or undergoing procedures or surgeries that place them at risk for infection (indwelling catheters), they can be more susceptible to infectious agents. Abscesses or contamination because of the normal flora into a normally sterile body site is often the reason for perioperative antimicrobial prophylaxis.[105] Rehabilitation specialists will most likely see many patients who are undergoing chemotherapy with antiinfective medications and play a crucial role in preventing and controlling infectious disease in the health care setting. Therapists need to update their knowledge foundation with evidence-based protocols for specific diagnoses and treatments as well as understand when infections may or may not call for antimicrobial medications. In addition, education of patients about why antimicrobial agents are not indicated in specific situations, how to alleviate symptoms, and what signs indicate further follow-up may help them to understand the growing problem of antibiotic resistance.

Diabetes

Diabetes, as a disorder of insulin production and sensitivity, has two major forms. Type 1 has an autoimmune component based on the destruction of pancreatic islet cells, but success in modulating this pathogenic feature has been limited. As a result, patients with type 1 diabetes are necessarily insulin-dependent. The pathogenic features of insulin insensitivity characteristic of type 2 are not well understood, but a wide array of therapeutic agents have been developed for managing this condition. Although the metabolic states of type 1 and 2 pathologies may differ somewhat, the chronic pathologies associated with poorly controlled hyperglycemia are remarkably similar. The development of peripheral neuropathy, which compromises sensory and motor control, is a progressive problem in patients with diabetes. In addition to long-term management of diabetes from a glucohomeostatic perspective, other agents show promise. Treatment of diabetic neuropathy with trazodone or mexiletine is an example.[106,107]

A more acute problem is swings in blood glucose level from inappropriate diet, exercise, insulin, and oral hypoglycemic drug administration. The balance of these factors is important, and monitoring of blood glucose level is essential. Swings in blood glucose level are often associated with changes in behavior and sensorium. This may pose a safety concern because cognitive and motor function may be impaired as a result. An increase in exercise will decrease the blood glucose concentration, thereby reducing insulin requirements. These factors should be carefully considered in any exercise regimen for the patient with diabetes.[108] A list of oral hypoglycemic agents is presented in Box 36.9. Lack of glucose control because of noncompliance with medications that are useful in controlling diabetes will only return the patient to an accelerated course to peripheral neuropathies and related sequelae.

In the clinical setting the health care practitioner must remember that the main goal of diabetes management is to prevent both the

---

BOX 36.9 Oral Hypoglycemic Agents

Sulfonylureas
acetohexamide (Dymelor)
chlorpropamide (Diabinese)
tolazamide (Tolinase)
tolbutamide (Orinase)
glimepiride (Amaryl)

glipizide (Glucotrol)
glyburide (Micronase)

Related Agents
repaglinide (Prandin)
nateglinide (Starlix)

These drugs may have direct and indirect effects on motor systems by producing hypoglycemia.

---

small-vessel complications (e.g., retinopathy and neuropathy) and large-vessel complications (e.g., heart disease and amputation) of the disease linked with elevated blood glucose levels. Diabetes is therefore often controlled through intensive, tailored treatment regimens of diet and physical activity, oral agents, and insulin.[109] Each of these regimens is designed to potentially reduce hyperglycemia and can result in hypoglycemia if the patient is not monitored.

Initially the physician and patient with diabetes can work together on a treatment plan to manage the disease. An important first step includes diet, physical activity, and a program to reduce body weight by 5% to 10%.[110] The effects of exercise as a cause of hypoglycemia deserve particular consideration because physical activity represents the most variable factor in the routine of many patients, especially those in rehabilitation.[111] With vigorous exercise, glucose use can increase severalfold, and this increase can persist long after the completion of the exercise, resulting in a fall in blood glucose long afterward. Although diet and activity are important cornerstones for diabetes care, oral agents and/or insulin may eventually be required to achieve glycemic control.

Several classes of oral agents are available to help or make the body use its own insulin or lower blood sugar, including sulfonylureas (chlorpropamide), meglitinides (repaglinide), biguanides (metformin), α-glucosidase inhibitors (acarbose), thiazolidinediones (rosiglitazone), dipeptidyl peptidase-4 (DPP-4) inhibitors (vildagliptin), and sodium-glucose cotransporter-2 inhibitors (canagliflozin). These classes of medications have specific regimens and may be prescribed as monotherapy or taken in combinations that may include insulin. Side effects vary from weight gain to GI symptoms to hypoglycemia. Hypoglycemia as a side effect of pharmacotherapy is of concern in the rehabilitation setting because abnormally low glucose levels can cause alterations in cognition, cardiovascular hemodynamic changes, and an increased risk of physical injury.[112] The signs and symptoms of hypoglycemia can vary from person to person and may depend on how fast the blood sugar drops. Early signs include shaking, sweating, fatigue, and weakness. Later signs may include confusion, combativeness, and exhaustion; these may inhibit eating, which may lead to loss of consciousness.

Insulin is a primary therapy in type 1 diabetes, in which the body has no ability to produce its own insulin. When oral antidiabetic agents no longer assist in maintaining glycemic targets, insulin is usually instituted in the diabetic with low production or resistance to insulin (type 2 diabetes).[113] Many forms of insulin are available, and administration is typically through subcutaneous injection or insulin pumps. Insulin can be long-acting or short-acting and is often used in combination to maintain the optimal level of glycemic control. Hypoglycemia is the primary problem associated with insulin use because of its ability to lower blood sugar.[113]

Health professionals working with patients who have diabetes should consider a number of strategies for prevention of hypoglycemia and be able to analyze the risk and benefits of exercise. Because glycemic control is individualized, each patient must be addressed uniquely, and as a member of the health care team the rehabilitation specialist can potentially assist in education of all those involved in the care of the patient. The following are lifestyle management guidelines published by the American Diabetes Association (ADA) and should be implemented in patients with known type 2 diabetes.[114–116] Preexercise evaluation of the asymptomatic patient is currently not recommended, but a careful history, assessment of cardiovascular risk factors, and caution to be aware of the atypical presentation of coronary artery disease in diabetic patients. Before exercise begins, it is important to determine the extent of involvement and complications present. Providers should assess patients for conditions that might contraindicate certain types of exercise or predispose injury, such as uncontrolled hypertension, untreated proliferative retinopathy, autonomic neuropathy, peripheral neuropathy, and a history of foot ulcers or Charcot foot. Prepare the patient for exercise by monitoring glycemic control before, during, and after exercise. Exercise is contraindicated if fasting glucose levels are above 250 mg/dL and ketosis is present; use caution if glucose levels are greater than 300 mg/dL and no ketosis is present. The patient should ingest added carbohydrate if glucose levels are less than 100 mg/dL.

Document when changes in insulin or food intake are necessary and learn the glycemic response to different exercise conditions (e.g., light, moderate, heavy). Food intake should include consumption of carbohydrates as needed to avoid hypoglycemia. Carbohydrate-based foods should be readily available during and after exercise.

Clinicians must understand what causes diabetes, the effects of medications and exercise on the regulation of blood sugar levels, signs and symptoms of hypoglycemia, and what should be done in a diabetic emergency.

Pulmonary Diseases

Many patients with neurological problems have pulmonary disease as well. The treatment of pulmonary diseases presents an unusual challenge. Many drugs used for treatment of asthma, emphysema, and chronic obstructive pulmonary disease (COPD) are intended to have direct effects on the lung, yet systemic effects are often unavoidable. Adrenergic bronchodilators, such as albuterol (Proventil), epinephrine (EpiPen), and metaproterenol (Alupent), may increase heart rate and tremor.[117] If tremor first manifests because of a neurological insult, then these drugs may exaggerate the motor impairment. Although ipratropium (Atrovent) is an anticholinergic with bronchodilating properties, the associated systemic anticholinergic effects (such as urinary retention with prostatic hypertrophy) are not well tolerated in geriatric men.[118] Prednisone (Deltasone) and related corticosteroids may dramatically reduce the degree of pulmonary hyperresponsiveness but often produce systemic effects, as previously noted. These are often reduced (but not necessarily eliminated) with the use of inhaled corticosteroids such as beclomethasone (Qvar), budesonide (Pulmicort), flunisolide (Nasalide), and triamcinolone (Aristocort). Although the use of xanthines in asthma is declining, theophylline (Uniphyl) in asthma and obstructive pulmonary diseases can, in higher doses, produce changes in cognitive function, including delusions and hallucinations. General CNS stimulation—including nervousness, insomnia, and seizures—is well recognized.[119] Tremor and nausea are often produced with theophylline, even with the commonly accepted clinical dosage regimens. Finally, the increase in diuresis caused by theophylline in patients with prostatic hypertrophy is certainly troublesome. The metabolism of this drug is often changed by other medications, which complicates therapy. These changes in drug metabolism may increase toxicity or decrease efficacy.[120] Newer classes of disease-modifying agents known as *leukotriene modifiers* (montelukast [Singulair] and zafirlukast [Accolate]) are being favored in some regimens for the management of asthma. Although cardiovascular and neurological side effects of these drugs appear to be dramatically reduced when compared with other agents, they have been implicated in several important drug interactions.[120] For severe asthma *anti-IgE antibodies* (Omalizumab [Xolair], benralizumab [Fasenra]) bind to the IgE on mast cells or target interleukins to prevent activation and release of inflammatory mediators.[121] Lack of compliance with these medications decreases pulmonary gas exchange, ultimately decreasing motor performance.

Patients may have signs and symptoms of lung dysfunction during exercise, including nonproductive cough, dyspnea, alterations in breathing rate and chest expansion, changes in skin color, as well as changes in auscultation and percussion findings. Symptomatic pharmacotherapy may be required to reduce disease-related symptoms such as shortness of breath and improve exercise tolerance.[122] The patient should begin exercise after medications to improve exercise tolerance. With chronic lung disease, exacerbations may often be caused by an infection; therefore antibiotics may be prescribed.[123] In addition, thinning and mobilization of secretions in airways with mucolytics and chest therapy may be necessary.[124] Oxygen therapy is a secondary therapy that may be necessary for hypoxemic patients.[123] This therapy reduces the hematocrit level to more normal levels, moderately improves neuropsychological factors, and ameliorates pulmonary hemodynamic abnormalities.[125] Oxygen therapy may be indicated during exercise for patients whose levels become desaturated during low-level activity.[126] An understanding of the use of pharmacological treatments for pulmonary dysfunction can help the rehabilitation professional to promote improved strength, exercise tolerance, and functional abilities in patients with pulmonary dysfunction.

Gastrointestinal Disorders[127,128]

Among the wide variety of agents used in the treatment of GI disorders, problems with agents affecting GI motility are among the most frequently encountered. Antiemetics that are dopaminergic antagonists, such as prochlorperazine (Compazine), chlorpromazine (Thorazine), and promethazine (Phenergan), are on Beers criteria[4] and may produce extrapyramidal side effects resembling Parkinson disease through the drug's actions on the basal ganglia.[129] Dronabinol (Marinol), a cannabinoid derivative from marijuana, is an effective antiemetic but may produce cognitive and sensory disturbances, including drowsiness, dizziness, ataxia, disorientation, orthostatic hypotension, and euphoria.[130] The selective serotonin antagonists dolasetron (Anzemet), granisetron (Kytril), and ondansetron (Zofran) are effective and valuable antiemetics, especially in cancer chemotherapy. The most common adverse effect is severe headache.[131] The benzodiazepine lorazepam (Ativan) is an effective adjunct for the control of emesis. Problems associated with benzodiazepines have been discussed previously. Corticosteroids such as dexamethasone (Decadron) should be included among the antiemetic agents; their adverse effects have also been discussed.

In producing normal motility, metoclopramide (Reglan), domperidone (Motilium), and cisapride (Propulsid) are often used. The adverse effects of metoclopramide are primarily through dopaminergic antagonism. Domperidone was developed to reduce these CNS effects and has been used to treat diabetic gastroparesis with some success.[132] Cisapride, a restricted-use prokinetic agent, may have a wide variety of CNS effects, including dizziness, mood disorders, vision changes, hallucinations, and amnesia, although with low incidence compared with concerns of arrhythmias induced by this drug.[133] Compliance with medications that reduce GI problems may have little direct effect on motor performance but may prove troublesome to the patient's quality of life.

In the rehabilitation setting, GI signs and symptoms are common problems for many patients. The side effects of drugs reported in formularies show that almost all oral preparations are the potential cause of some form of GI disturbance.[134] Signs and symptoms include upper GI effects such as nausea, vomiting, indigestion, gastric reflux, and stomach pain or lower GI effects such as diarrhea, constipation, colonic pain, and blood in stools. These symptoms may be caused by an underlying GI condition (gallstones and acid reflux) or side effects from medications (nausea and vomiting). Because GI problems can be prevalent and challenging, cause poor compliance, and may be a sign of a more serious condition, the causes and potential approaches used to ameliorate the symptoms must be understood.

Medications can modify GI absorption, cause dysmotility, damage the mucosal lining, or change the bioavailability and resulting effectiveness of drugs. Some drugs modify the absorption or activity of nutrients, ions, and drugs. Drugs such as metformin (Glucophage) (used in the treatment of diabetes) may reduce the absorption of vitamin B_{12}, with the potential development of megaloblastic anemia, necessitating exercise precautions.[135] Other drugs that damage the mucosal lining (methotrexate [Otrexup], allopurinol [Zyloprim], neomycin [Mycifradin], colchicine [Colcrys], methyldopa [Aldomet]) may reduce nutrient absorption, leading to deficiencies.[104] One class of agents, NSAIDs, is estimated to be regularly used by 5% to 10% of the US population, with more than 70 million prescriptions filled annually and more than 30 billion OTC tablets sold.[136,137] These drugs are implicated in patients reporting gastric dyspepsia (pain or discomfort in the upper abdomen), and concomitant administration of proton pump inhibitors (Prilosec) (which block production of stomach acid) and prostaglandin analogs (Cytotec) (which protect the stomach lining) may often reduce mucosal erosion.[104]

Drugs that cause dysmotility of the small intestine—such as TCAs (for depression), anticholinergics (for asthma), calcium channel blockers (for heart failure), and opiates (for pain)—may be commonly administered to patients within the rehabilitation population.[104] The large intestine is more likely to have reduced motility, with abdominal pain, constipation, nausea, vomiting, and abdominal distention present. Many patients require increased activity, change of dietary habits, or laxatives to improve motility.[138] Precautions must be taken because of the potential for chronic use of laxatives, fluid and electrolyte imbalance, steatorrhea, protein-losing gastroenteropathy, osteomalacia, and vitamin and mineral deficiencies.[104]

It is important to note that some supplements and fluids (e.g., grapefruit juice) taken with medications can potentially cause changes in the bioavailability of drugs. Concurrent ingestion of iron causes a marked decrease in the bioavailability of a number of drugs such as tetracycline (an antibiotic), methyldopa (an antihypertensive agent), levodopa (for Parkinson disease), and ciprofloxacin (an antimicrobial).[139] Grapefruit juice is also known to change the bioavailability of some medications, leading to an elevation of their serum concentrations; these drugs include cyclosporine (an immunosuppressive agent), calcium antagonists (for hypertension), and coenzyme A reductase inhibitors (statins).[140]

Most medications have the potential to cause some form of GI difficulties, whether taken systemically, topically applied, or given by the parenteral route.[104] Most adverse effects can be reduced with identification of the causal relation, proper administration of the drug, and administration according to all the guidelines on the label. Therapists may suggest specific timing of medication administration to relieve symptoms and increase participation in therapy. The role of physical and occupational therapists should be recognized in observing adverse drug events to warn patients of early signs of potential problems, provide education, and refer for further follow-up by the pharmacist or physician.

AN IMPAIRMENT PERSPECTIVE

Different forms of neurological impairments are discussed in this section, and appropriate drugs are identified that either reduce or increase the degree of impairment. Although not a comprehensive list, these impairments include sensory impairments, motor problems, cognitive deficits, problems with balance and coordination, cardiovascular impairments, and problems with muscle tone; a brief overview of neuroplasticity is included. Pharmacists have been educated and work closely with physicians who have been educated in a disease or pathology model. A large portion of a physician's practice is related to drug therapy for the treatment of disease and pathology. Looking at drugs from an impairment/functional activity/life participation model is not the role of either the physician or the pharmacist. Thus movement specialists, whose model for care is based on function and quality of life, must bridge the gap between these concepts because the outcome of the interactions dramatically affects the potential of the individual after any CNS dysfunction. Currently interprofessional education has been a focus in medical professional education to assist in improved communication between the professions in order to reduce improve patient satisfaction as well as the health of the global population and reduce cost and errors.

Sensory Impairment

Drugs that affect hearing, vision, and touch may influence any type of sensory, cognitive, and motor impairment. In any impairment, the processing of accurate sensory information is crucial to modify and adjust procedural programming during movement. A subject must be able—through visual, manual, or auditory cues (even through olfactory means)—to relate to or recognize the relevance of the external environment, engage the specific motor programming centers that reach consensus regarding the specific motor response, and produce the series of signals that may progress uninterrupted through spinal mechanisms and the motor endplate to a regional muscle group for an appropriate response. Any impairment or drug that affects any component within these systems, whether early or late in this sequence, will affect the motor performance. Patients with sensory integrative problems are often given medications such as those for attention-deficit disorder, anxiety, seizure, and depression.[141] As previously discussed, certain drugs may influence hearing (as previously indicated regarding infectious diseases) or produce tinnitus (e.g., aspirin), which may be distracting and thus ultimately affect motor performance.[98] Changes in the visual field (e.g., with ethambutol and anticonvulsants) are likewise important. Analgesics and topical anesthetics may dangerously affect surface heat or cold discomfort and undermine avoidance cues. However, elimination of excessive pain (peripheral and central) may enhance cognitive focus and learning as well as allow an individual to move as part of daily living, which will help maintain power, range, balance, and thus quality of life. The CNS functions with the consensus of multiple interactions. Because the branched as well as sequential nature of systems links sensory and motor functions, the peripheral effects of drugs commonly modify the function of central systems. This is a relatively unappreciated reason why drug therapy can modify rehabilitation techniques both positively and negatively. Therapists must be aware of medications when they are working with patients who have sensory impairments. Medications can increase or alleviate signs and symptoms, as well as produce unwanted side effects. Patients may benefit from alterations in the environment to limit sensory sensitivities, timing of treatment to coincide with the most effective dose of medications, and monitoring for unwanted side effects.

Cognitive and Central Motor Control Impairment

Disorders of mood (anxiety and depression) reduce initiative in the rehabilitation process. In this context, anxiolytics and antidepressants may have a positive impact. However, if the dose is not carefully titrated, drowsiness and anterograde amnesia will cloud effective response and learning. Both antidepressants and many of the benzodiazepines may cause these effects, as previously discussed. Behavioral

BOX 36.10   Examples of Antipsychotic Agents

Standard Antipsychotics	Atypical Antipsychotics
chlorpromazine (Thorazine)	aripiprazole (Abilify)
fluphenazine (Prolixin)	asenapine (Saphris)
haloperidol (Haldol)	clozapine (Clozaril)
loxapine (Loxitane)	olanzapine (Zyprexa)
molindone (Moban)	quetiapine (Seroquel)
perphenazine (Trilafon)	iloperidone (Fanapt)
pimozide (Orap)	paliperidone (Invega)
thioridazine (Mellaril)	risperidone (Risperdal)
thiothixene (Navane)	ziprasidone (Geodon)

These drugs may produce a parkinsonian-like effect through dopaminergic antagonism.

disorders, especially those associated with untreated psychoses or dementia, impede cognitive function. Although antipsychotics may correct these disorders, the dopaminergic antagonism associated with these may interfere with the function of the basal ganglia and facilitation of movement. Many newer antipsychotic agents (also known as the *atypical antipsychotics*) have, in addition to dopaminergic antagonism, serotonin antagonist activity, which may reduce the extrapyramidal side effects of the earlier agents when analyzed as movement dysfunction (Box 36.10). The therapist should be monitoring for signs of depression, which is common in patients who have had loss of function. Effective management of depression is dependent on finding an appropriate formulation and therapeutic dose, which may take weeks, and patients will need education and support. Extrapyramidal motor signs should be monitored and reported to the health care team.

Vertigo, Dizziness, Balance, and Coordination

Many agents with histamine antagonist and anticholinergic activity have been used for treatment of vertigo and dizziness. Meclizine (Dramamine) and related antihistamines are primary examples. Occasionally sinus congestion can result in impaired vestibular function and dizziness. In the absence of hypertension or related autonomic dysfunction, an indirect-acting adrenergic agonist such as ephedrine (Primatene) or pseudoephedrine (Sudafed) can reduce this congestion and improve this condition.[142] Dizziness is a common clinical problem, affecting at least a third of the population in one form or another at some point during their lives.[143] Medications should be reviewed in all patients with dizziness, as numerous medications can be associated with this effect, including alcohol and other CNS depressants, aminoglycoside antibiotics, anticonvulsants, antidepressants, antihypertensives, chemotherapeutics, loop diuretics, and salicylates.[144] Patients should be monitored for orthostatic hypotension and hyperventilation. Depending on the cause of dizziness, patients with dizziness may benefit from canalith repositioning procedures,[145] vestibular exercises,[146] instrumental rehabilitation training on a moving platform,[147] positional education (sitting at bedside before standing), use of compression garments, dietary changes (salt and fluid intake), and use of simple physical counter-maneuvers such as squatting to temporarily but rapidly raise blood pressure.[148] Symptoms of dizziness and balance dysfunction should be reported to the health care team for determination of the underlying cause and best management strategies.

Cardiovascular Impairment

In the management of hypercholesterolemia, the 3-hydroxy-3-methylglutaryl coenzyme A (HMG-CoA) reductase inhibitors (Statins) (see Box 36.5) may produce myopathies to various degrees. Overall, statin use among US adults 40 years of age and older in the general population increased 79.8% from 21.8 million individuals in 2002–2003 to 39.2 million individuals in 2012–2013[149] indicating the increased need to be aware of potential myopathy. Changes in hemodynamics caused by antihypertensive regimens must be monitored because these agents can produce syncope and lower exercise tolerance. Weakness from intermittent claudication is a challenge that can be managed in part with cilostazol (Pletal).[150] Any drug that is used to decrease spasticity as a consequence of stroke and related cerebrovascular disorders may impair motor control and thus affect motor learning. A discussion of these drugs is outlined in the next section. Cardiovascular impairments are common in the rehabilitation setting. Knowing the pharmacological management for and side effects of medications related to the cardiovascular system will assist the therapist in providing high-quality care. Patients will benefit from education on modifiable and nonmodifiable risk factors, monitoring blood pressure and heart rate, signs of heart failure, vascular effects of modalities, and responses to exercise and positional changes.

Spasticity and Muscle Tone

Muscle spasms may be controlled with centrally acting and peripherally acting agents, all of which produce drowsiness, dizziness, and muscle weakness to various degrees.[151] Commonly used agents are listed in Box 36.11. Pharmacological management of muscle tone, spasticity, and coordination of movement is of primary importance in neurological rehabilitation.

With regard to spasticity, several additional options are available. Tizanidine (Zanaflex) is an α-adrenergic agonist available to reduce spasticity, primarily through activation of descending noradrenergic inhibitory pathways.[152] Clonidine (Catapres) has similar actions. Intrathecal administration of baclofen (Lioresal) produces an antispasmodic effect through enhancement of GABAergic function, both central and spinal.[153] Likewise, enhancement of GABAergic function and reduced spasticity can be realized through the antiseizure drug gabapentin (Neurontin).[154] Selective motor neurons can be inactivated through the local injection of botulinum toxin (Botox).[155] These agents inhibit the release of acetylcholine at the neuromuscular junction. The agent 4-aminopyridine (Ampyra) has been shown to reduce spasticity in patients with Lambert-Eaton myasthenic syndrome, MS, and spinal cord injury.[156] It acts by blocking voltage-gated potassium channels, prolonging action potentials and thereby increasing neurotransmitter release at the neuromuscular junction.[157]

The involvement of serotonin in the maintenance of muscle tone and spasticity is complex and controversial. Cyproheptadine, a relatively nonselective serotonergic antagonist, can reduce spasticity and maintain muscle tone.[158,159] However, SSRIs used as antidepressants may occasionally increase spasticity,[160] and clozapine (Clozaril), a selective serotonin antagonist, may produce muscle weakness.[161]

In addition to spinal cord injuries, MS may cause spasticity as a complication. Although several interferons have been used in the management of MS, interferon β-1b has been shown to increase spasticity.[162] Therapists often work closely with patients who are undergoing

BOX 36.11   Muscle Relaxants and Antispasmodics

baclofen (Lioresal)	metaxalone (Skelaxin)
carisoprodol (Soma)	methocarbamol (Robaxin)
chlorzoxazone (Paraflex)	orphenadrine (Norflex)
cyclobenzaprine (Flexeril)	tizanidine (Zanaflex)
dantrolene (Dantrium)[a]	

[a]Direct effects on muscle to reduce tone.
Direct effects on motor systems to reduce tone.

treatment with antispasticity medications. Knowing the underlying cause of the spasticity in the patient with neurological impairments (disruptions of inhibitory control) and using concomitant rehabilitation therapy may help to decrease pain and improve range of motion and functional ability. Therapists should have an understanding of the desired effects of agents and also their adverse effects, including sedation and addictive properties.

Neuroplasticity

The effects of drugs on plasticity are highly controversial. In Alzheimer disease a loss of plasticity may occur through deficits in hippocampal and cortical function, leading to memory loss. Many anticholinesterase agents (e.g., Aricept) improve memory, which may provide evidence that they enhance neuroplasticity.[163] Agents affecting the glutaminergic system, specifically the N-methyl D-aspartate (NMDA) antagonist memantine (Namenda), are prescribed to treat symptoms of moderate to severe Alzheimer disease.[164] These agents work by blocking the toxic effects associated with excess glutamate and regulate glutamate activation.[165] Based on the putative molecular mechanisms of the pathology, inhibitors of β-amyloid formation and related modulators may hold additional promise.[166] This rapidly evolving area of research may provide interesting avenues for the treatment of Alzheimer disease. Neuroprotective agents that aim to prevent neuronal death by inhibiting one or more pathophysiological steps in the process that follows brain injury or ischemia are currently under development for neurological disorders including stroke, spinal cord injury, traumatic brain injury, and Parkinson disease. In addition, studies on enriched environments including robotics, virtual and augmented reality, and neurogaming are[167] providing knowledge related to neuronal capacity for regeneration and repair in the adult and aging brain and spinal cord.[168] The future of neuroplasticity in rehabilitation may be enriched when medications that protect or promote neurological recovery can be paired with techniques to improve function.

RESEARCH AND DEVELOPMENT PROSPECTS

It is difficult to predict which areas of pharmacological research will have the most valuable impact on the management of neurological disorders and the resulting residual impairments. Drug development is a continuous process, although this text must have a definitive end point. Many drugs with outstanding promise for treating neurological

diseases will have adverse effects that may be less acceptable than the neurological problem (or in fact may be lethal in rare cases) and may require its removal from the market. In spite of these disappointments, many reasons for optimism exist.

Among the burgeoning areas of biotechnology that will have an influence on neurology will be the discovery, characterization, and application of neuronal growth factors, related growth modifiers, and cellular implants, which may have the long-term promise of either partially or completely restoring nerve function. Among these are stem cell implants, whose function and development have been tested in a limited number of patients.[169] It is also likely that drugs will continue to play an important role as adjuncts in disorders partially treated with stem cell therapies. Although these developments are unlikely to have extensive application within the next few years, these and related developments will take root over a period of decades and revolutionize our understanding and treatment of a wide variety of neurological disorders.

The pharmacist stands as a valuable resource for physical and occupational therapists today and will continue to do so in the future. Pharmacists must participate in the management of drug therapies that may be related to each area discussed in this chapter. Therapists should consult the pharmacist about new drug developments and discuss the potential effects that these new drugs may have on neurological rehabilitation. This is especially true when new drugs not mentioned in this text are being administered. These discussions can illuminate intended and adverse effects that may influence interventions and change patient outcomes. These drugs may cause improvements as well as exacerbations in movement function. Some of those changes are disease- or pathology-related. Other changes are attributable to spontaneous return, new learning, and neuroplasticity within the CNS. Changes can also occur because of drug therapy. Those changes, as stated, can be both positive and negative. The scope of practice for occupational and physical therapists does not involve differentiating which change is caused by which process, but these professionals certainly can recognize functional changes. When changes are positive, the team must be made aware of them, and most likely everyone will take credit for the changes. When the changes take away function, families and therapists are often the first to identify those changes. The pharmacist and physician will have to determine why the system is deteriorating. The therapist is responsible for sharing reports of those negative behavioral changes with the team and monitoring for future changes when drug regimens have been altered.

SUMMARY

The vast array of drugs, along with their intended and unintended consequences, can pose significant challenges to all clinicians. An awareness of the patient's perspective in dealing with diseases and impairments can yield valuable information that may help to prevent and/or manage the potentially adverse impact of drugs on rehabilitation. One component of this perspective is the patient's desire to self-medicate in addition to undergoing clinician-prescribed therapy. The pharmacist can often provide guidance that can be effectively relayed to a patient's therapists. This

degree of vigilance can yield greater rewards for the patient in terms of effective management of multiple diseases and reduced interference with rehabilitation. A team approach is required to resolve problems problems posed by drug treatment. When drugs play a role in a patient's treatment, the patient's physician, pharmacist, therapist, nurse, and caregiver must be aware that drugs pose a certain degree of risk with every positive step. The team must work closely to investigate possible drug problems as well as opportunities for therapeutic success.

REFERENCES

To enhance this text and add value for the reader, all references are included on the companion Evolve site that accompanies this textbook. This online service will, when available, provide a link for the reader to a Medline abstract for the article cited. There are 169 cited references

37

Use of Neuroimaging in Rehabilitation

Rolando T. Lazaro, Darcy A. Umphred, and Preeti Deshpande Oza

OBJECTIVES

After reading this chapter the student or therapist will be able to:

1. Identify conventional and advanced neuroimaging techniques.
2. Classify the different neuroimaging techniques into structural and/or functional imaging techniques.
3. Describe strengths and weaknesses of different neuroimaging techniques.
4. Recognize various slices of the central nervous system; what nuclear masses are visible in that slice; how the ventricles change from one slice to another; and how sagittal, horizontal, and coronal slices present those nuclear masses and/or ventricles differently.
5. Recognize the difference in diagnostic capabilities of radiography, computed tomography (CT), magnetic resonance imaging (MRI), and nuclear medicine scans.

6. Describe images using the correct neuroradiological descriptive terminology.
7. Recognize normal and abnormal neuroanatomy on CT scans and MRI images.
8. Analyze information obtained from imaging of the central nervous system and integrate this information into the neurological clinical presentation and the patient's intervention.
9. Recognize and analyze how neuroimaging may and may not be reflected in the movement diagnosis made by a physical or occupational therapist.
10. Summarize relevance of neuroimaging to rehabilitation and patient care.

KEY TERMS

computed tomography (CT)	diffusion tensor imaging (DTI)	magnetic resonance image (MRI)
diagnostic imaging	functional imaging	radiograph

Direct access practice for physical therapists in several states of the United States has increased the role of these professionals as primary care providers engaged in value-based and patient-centered care for improving mobility outcomes. Physical therapists are now part of the emergency department, sometimes serving to triage, and manage patients with nonsurgical musculoskeletal disorders. Physical therapists serving in the military, Public Health Service, Indian Health Service, Veterans Health Administration, Bureau of Prisons, and health care organizations, such as Georgetown University Hospital, Kaiser-Permanente, Northern California, now have imaging privileges.[1-4] Expanding roles have made it particularly important for therapists to recognize the need of diagnostic imaging and analyze diagnostic imaging for improving patient care and decisions related to patient care.

As relates to patients with neurological injuries (e.g., brain injury or stroke) and dysfunction (e.g., Parkinson disease or hereditary disorders), therapists should be able to interpret images of the nervous system to better understand how the neural insult and medical procedures affect movement and function in daily life. Expert analysis of neuroimaging, using differential diagnosis skills and knowledge of neuroanatomy, is critical in order for these professionals to know when to refer a patient to another health care

practitioner, when to refer and treat, when to merely treat, and when to neither refer nor treat.

Entry-level knowledge of content such as pharmacology, radiology, and medical screening has become an accreditation requirement for doctoral education programs in physical and occupational therapy. Orthopedic radiology is now a common part of curricula; however, content on neuroradiology, more specifically the application of neuroradiology in practice, is lacking. In a study by Little and Lazaro,[5] it was found that many of the physical therapy practitioners in California use medical imaging in their practice. When inquired about the types of imaging, the majority of respondents felt comfortable using results (and radiology reports) from radiographs obtained because of a musculoskeletal problem. This study showed the lack of access to and confidence in using medical images of the central nervous system (CNS).

In certain instances, it may be easier for therapists to recognize musculoskeletal problems when viewing radiographic images because the abnormality in the structure directly correlates with the orthopedic movement problem. When images of the CNS are viewed, correlations with movement system disorders may be much more complex, requiring knowledge of neuroanatomy, such as relationship of nuclei, tract systems, and basic neurochemistry. For example,

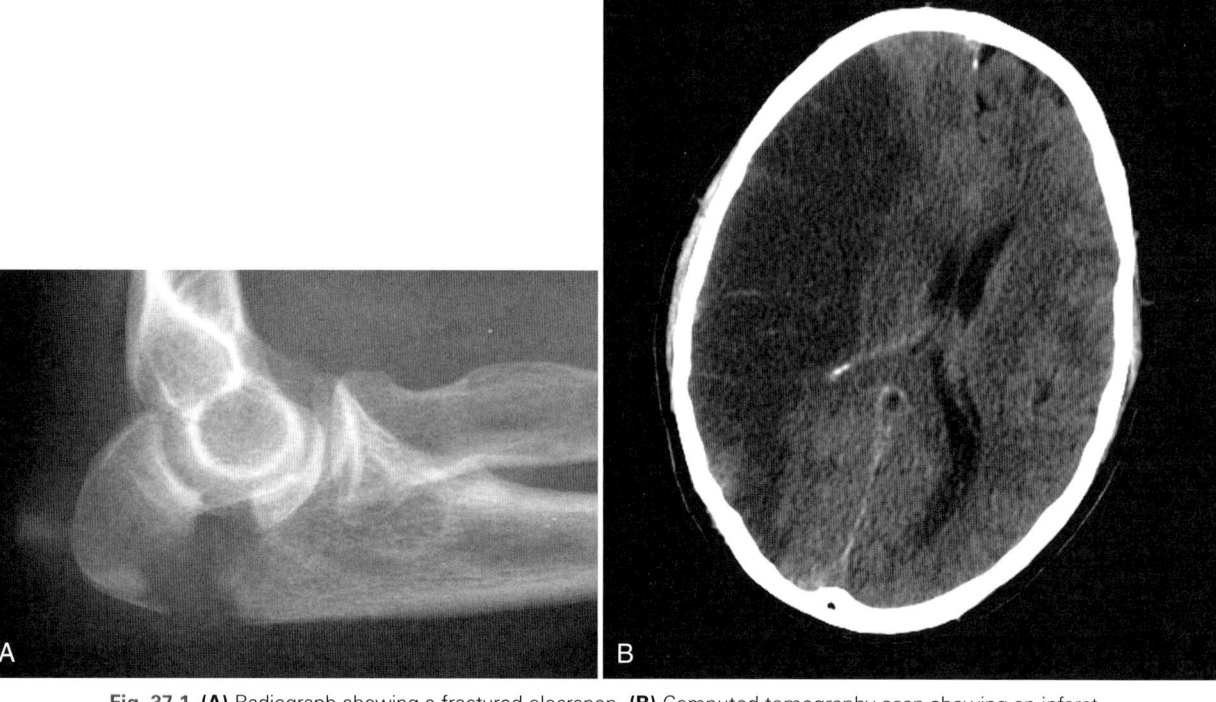

Fig. 37.1 (A) Radiograph showing a fractured olecranon. **(B)** Computed tomography scan showing an infarct of the middle cerebral artery. (B, From Wikipedia. http://en.wikipedia.org/wiki/File:INFARCT.jpg.)

when looking at a bone fracture (Fig. 37.1A) versus a vascular insult (see Fig. 37.1B), it is clear that the fracture and its effects on the bone, muscle, or skin can easily be visualized and interpreted. The second image of the CNS has many surrounding structures that must be identified in relation to the vascular insult. Good knowledge of neuroanatomy and neuroimaging is therefore essential for adopting imaging in PT practice.

In 2007, the journal *Physical Therapy* produced a special issue on neuroradiology in physical therapy practice. It is encouraging to note that this issue offered physical therapy clinicians an opportunity to understand the modalities used in the imaging of the brain and the spinal cord (for details, see the article by Kimberley and Lewis[6]). However, the rest of the article presented the application of neuroradiology in physical therapy research,[7,8] and although these articles provided valuable information for the practicing clinician, the articles did not specifically give insights as to how clinicians can use the knowledge of neuroradiology in their actual patient/client management.

It has been known for a long time that physical therapy interventions improve function by making new neural connections or by unmasking the neural networks that were previously dormant.[9] Though not a common practice in patient care, the advent of functional neuroimaging techniques has made it possible to study the benefits of the therapy and has opened more ways to guide clinical practice. Some of the benefits that therapists may have with current neuroimaging methods include being able to (1) assess the changes with therapy, (2) make treatment plans appropriate for patient by correlating clinical symptoms with neuroimaging results, (3) assess prognostic implications, (4) provide family and patient education, and (5) develop appropriate goals and accordingly develop treatment plans.

VISUALIZING THE CENTRAL NERVOUS SYSTEM

Before jumping into viewing images of the nervous system, the reader needs to be very familiar with the position and type of slices presented in those images. Fig. 37.2 illustrates the three types of slices common to the nervous system. The horizontal slices shown in Fig. 37.3 are cuts made horizontally through the brain beginning with a superior slice at the level of the beginning of the lateral ventricles. This individual would be lying supine if the brain was cut as shown. If a person were standing, the horizontal slice would be horizontal to the ground with the frontal lobes facing forward (toward the nose) and the occipital lobe in the back. The slices cut horizontally are always perpendicular to the brain stem and spinal cord or perpendicular to the upright position of the brain regardless of the position of the head in space. All right and left slices will look exactly the same as long as the nervous system has not sustained any insult. Fig. 37.4 shows the position of an upright human and what the skeleton would look like in the same position. Can you visualize what the horizontal slices would look like? The horizontal section would be perpendicular to this upright position. When viewing radiological slices in horizontal, the slices will often be on a slight angle with the lower portion slightly forward. Most of these films are taken when individuals are supine, which places the brain off vertical so a correction is made. The film usually slices horizontally through the brain as if the head were slightly tucked, similar to the image of the adult in Fig. 37.4A. Also, some radiologists want a slightly different angle to the slice because they are looking for specific orientations. When viewing these films, try to look at the radiological slice pattern (scanogram), if shown. Fig. 37.3 shows a progression of horizontal slices as if the individual were supine and the slices began anteriorly with emphasis on ventricular changes as

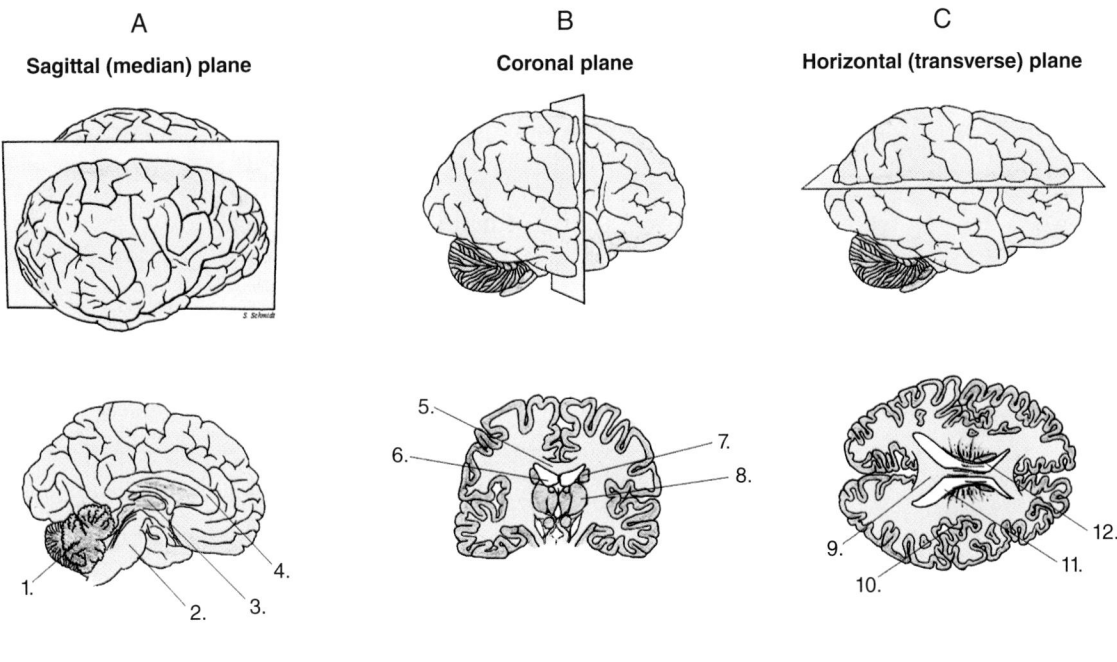

Fig. 37.2 Orientation of Brain Slices. **(A)** Sagittal. **(B)** Coronal. **(C)** Horizontal. (Courtesy Stephen Schmidt, PT, OCS, FAAOMPT.)

1. Cerebellum
2. Pons
3. Corpus callosum
4. Thalamus

5. Body of corpus callosum
6. Lateral ventricle
7. Head of caudate nucleus
8. Putamen

9. Splenium of corpus callosum
10. Insula
11. Lateral ventricle
12. Head of caudate nucleus

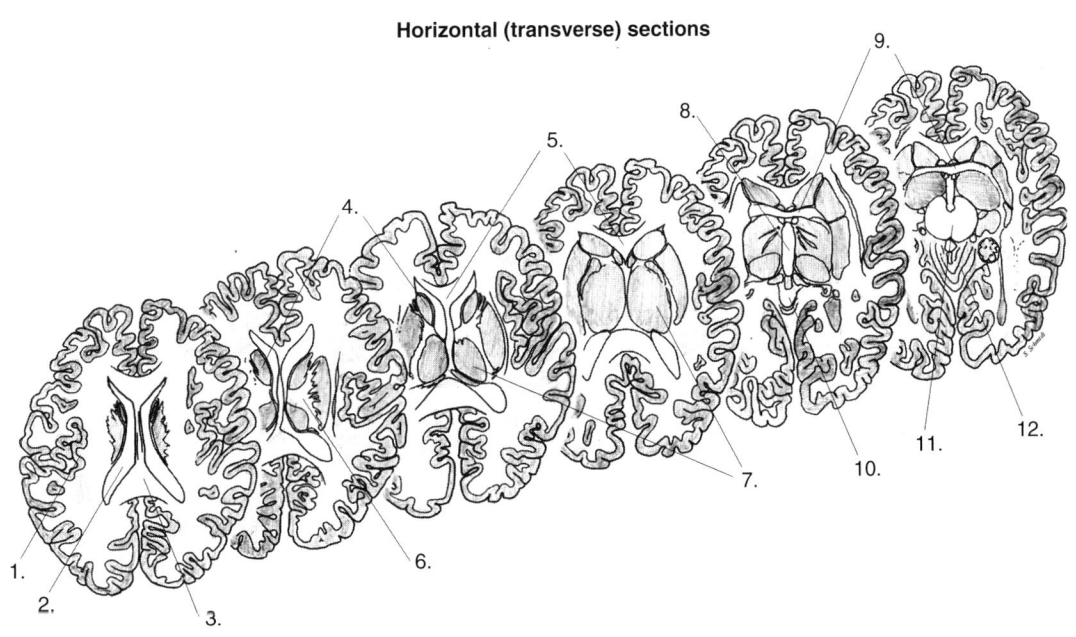

1. Insula
2. Lateral ventricle
3. Splenium of corpus callosum
4. Putamen

5. Genu of corpus callosum
6. Internal capsule
7. Thalamic nuclei
8. Third ventricle

9. Anterior commissure
10. Periaqueductal gray
11. Midbrain
12. Cerebellum

Fig. 37.3 Illustration of Horizontal Slices. (Courtesy Stephen Schmidt, PT, OCS, FAAOMPT.)

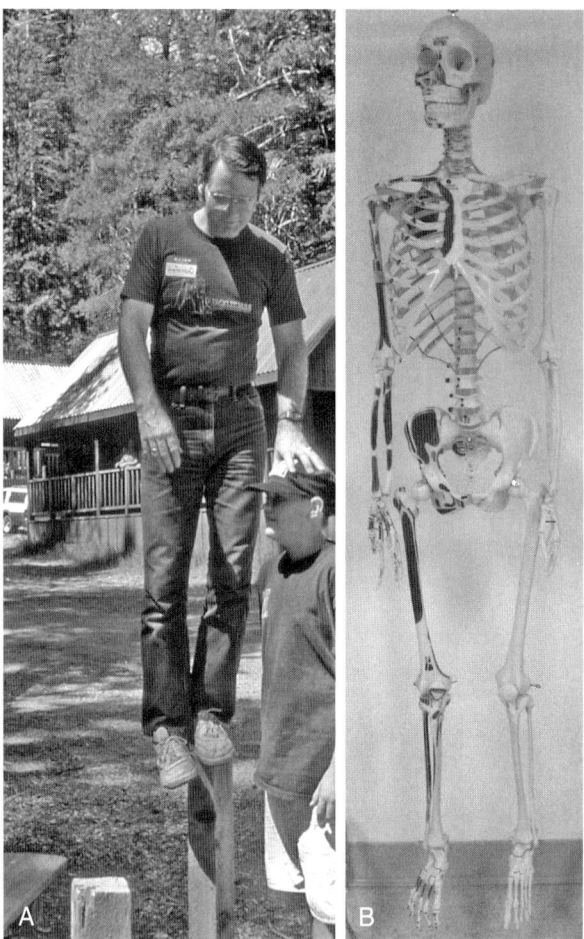

Fig. 37.4 **(A)** Photograph of a human standing. **(B)** A skeleton standing.

part of the progression. Many of the medical images of the brain are viewed as horizontal (or axial) slices or views. The person is lying supine when undergoing computed tomography (CT), magnetic resonance imaging (MRI), or positron emission tomography (PET). Therefore the imaging process cuts 90 degrees off the horizontal plane of earth in order to achieve horizontal slices of the brain. Remember to look at the scanogram, if available, to identify the position of the head in relation to the cuts.

Coronal slices in the right hemisphere look similar to those in the left hemisphere except that the top of the slice will not look like the bottom on either side (see Fig. 37.2). The two sides will reflect each other, with the tops being alike as well as the bottoms. Depending on where the cut is made, the result will be cortex on the outside, tracts (white matter) projecting downward, and gray matter again inferior and medial within the slices as the thalamus, basal ganglia, caudate, hippocampus, and so on are viewed. These slices begin at the top and cut down through both sides of the brain, with the slice ending on the inferior section. The progression of the slides can go from front (frontal lobe) to back (occipital lobe) or back to front. If visualized in a standing subject, the slice would begin in the superior frontal area and slice downward through the brain toward the feet, thus cutting equally on both sides. These slices can proceed in the posterior (backward) direction of the brain but always cutting from the top toward the bottom with equal distribution on each side. Fig. 37.5 progresses from the front of the brain toward the back using the ventricles as a point of reference.

For sagittal cuts (see Fig. 37.2), most cuts start by slicing down through the central fissure separating both sides of the brain. This cut is called a *midsagittal section*. Each sagittal slice proceeds outward toward the lateral aspect of the brain on each side respectively, depending on which side is being sliced. Anatomically, you begin as if you were slicing down through the middle of the face and the back of the head when a person is standing. Each sagittal slice moves from the inside outward toward the ear or laterally away from the midsagittal

Coronal sections

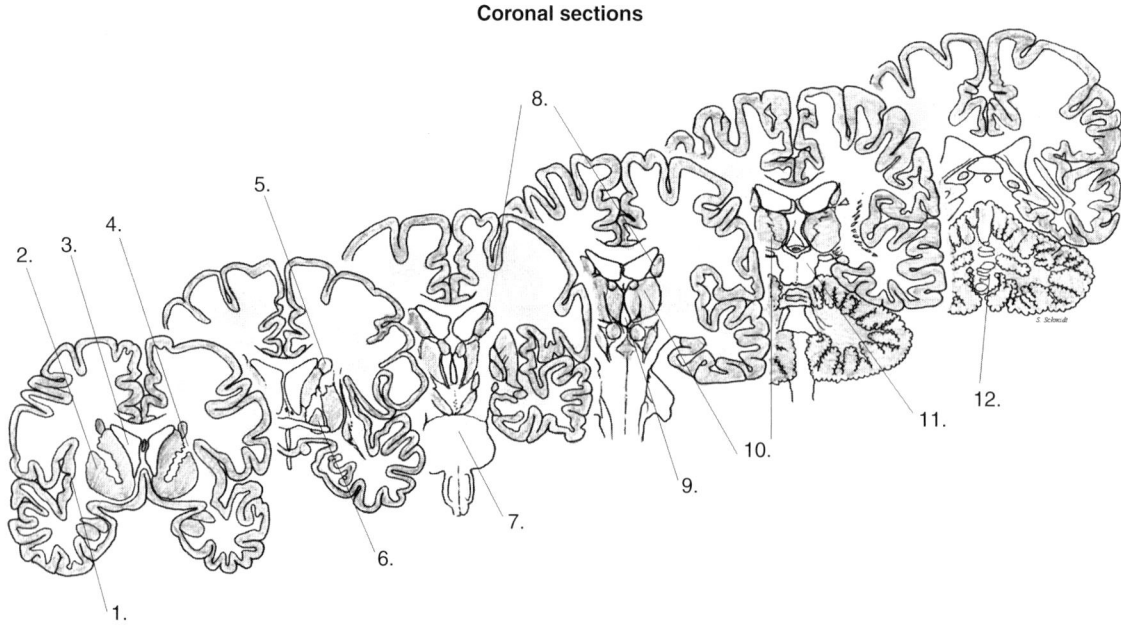

1. Insula	5. Superior long. fasciculus	9. Third ventricle
2. Putamen	6. Globus pallidus	10. Thalamic nuclei
3. Lateral ventricle	7. Base of pons	11. Colliculus
4. Internal capsule	8. Caudate nucleus	12. Cerebellum

Fig. 37.5 Illustration of Coronal Slices. (Courtesy Stephen Schmidt, PT, OCS, FAAOMPT.)

slice. Each slice cuts though the front and back of the brain from top to bottom and proceeds from medial to lateral. Sagittal images usually begin on either the right or the left side and continue slicing toward the middle to the midsagittal section separating the two sides of the brain, and then proceed toward the outside on the opposite side of the brain from the beginning slice.

Another way to conceptualize the nervous system is by visually sequencing from a view of a human in a specific position to the skeleton of a human in that position to an intact plastinated nervous system in that same position. The reader is encouraged to try to visualize what the horizontal, coronal, and sagittal slices might look like given the spatial position of the individual. Once you can easily recognize the various types of slices and where the slice was made when viewing the nervous system, you are ready to begin viewing radiological images.

IMAGING OF THE CENTRAL NERVOUS SYSTEM

It is beyond the scope of this chapter to discuss the physics behind the more common imaging modalities (see article by Kimberley and Lewis[6] for background). The purpose of this chapter is to provide the clinician a method of systematically evaluating images of the CNS and, more important, to provide examples of how clinicians can use these images to guide practice.

Neuroimaging include different techniques to directly or indirectly '"mage"' the brain and the spinal cord to understand function or physiology of the nervous system. CT and MRI remain the two most common modalities for imaging the CNS. CT scans of the brain are widely used in acute neurological injuries in which the speed of the examination is of primary importance. A common application of this is in acute traumatic brain injuries, when rapid assessment of information about hematoma formation and brain swelling is imperative to make appropriate decisions regarding medical management. Although there is less anatomical detail in CT than in MRI, the level of detail being generated by a CT is generally sufficient for the appropriate management of the patient with an acute injury. Because CT also administers the highest dose of radiation (as it is a series of x-ray exposures), it causes a higher risk of development of conditions associated with increased levels of radiation exposure.

Owing to its increasing availability, MRI can also be an ideal choice for imaging the brain and the spinal cord. MRI provides excellent resolution and can also be performed with contrast agents to enhance the detail even more. MRI, however, generally takes longer than CT to perform, and it requires the subject to avoid excessive movement while the machine is actively scanning. Also, because MRI uses powerful magnets, the use of this modality in patients with metal implants is contraindicated. With regard to cost, MRI is still more costly than CT, but this expense is rapidly coming down as more hospitals and clinics are investing in this technology.

As mentioned previously, contrast media can also be used in both CT and MRI to enhance the image, although that will increase the scanning time. There are also additional risks associated with contrast, such as possible allergic reactions to the medium being used to enhance the image.

Besides the conventional CT and MRI, advanced neuroimaging techniques such as Positron Emission Tomography (PET) scan, Functional Magnetic Resonance Imaging (fMRI), and Diffusion Tensor Imagining (DTI) may also be encountered by therapists. Whatever the technique, studying the neuro images should be made a regular practice for improved clinical decision making and prognostication.

Clinical Decisions Regarding the Need for Imaging Studies

Patients with acute neurological symptoms should be seen by a medical practitioner who will determine the type of imaging most appropriate.

For individuals with chronic neurological problems, a therapist may be in a situation to recommend the timing and type of new images. For example, when a mismatch exists between the movement diagnosis and the anatomical lesion(s) present on past images, it is the responsibility of the physical or occupational therapist to report the inconsistencies between the imaging report or medical diagnosis and the specific movement dysfunction seen and reported in the therapy situation. The objective of new images would be to render an anatomical explanation for a change in impairments and movement function. While it is outside the scope of a therapist's practice and responsibility to correct a physician's medical diagnosis, therapists should advocate for further diagnostic exploration when a patient presents with evolving clinical characteristics.

GENERAL GUIDELINES FOR REVIEWING MEDICAL IMAGES

Radiodensity

Because CT scans, like conventional radiographs, are images formed by the absorption of x-rays by the body at different densities, evaluation of CT images is the same as evaluation of conventional radiographs. Structures in the body that absorb a lot of x-ray energy are *radiopaque* and will be white on the image. Structures that absorb less x-ray energy will be different shades of gray. Air does not absorb any x-rays and will be black on the film, and is said to be *radiolucent.* Bone is an example of a radiopaque structure and will be white on the image. Because the skull is composed of bones of varying thickness, portions of this structure that have more bone will be whiter than those with less bone. Contrast media can be positive (white; heavy metals such as gadolinium) or negative (black; air, however, is not used as a contrast medium in the CNS). Brain matter and spinal cord will be varying shades of gray. The sinuses are normally filled with air and will therefore show as black, whereas the ventricles are filled with cerebrospinal fluid and will be a shade of gray on a CT image.

There are a few steps to follow when evaluating neuroradiological images. These steps are presented in the following sections.

Step 1

Gather All Pertinent Information Regarding the Patient's Neuroimaging Studies

As mentioned earlier, because of the complexity of the structure and function of the CNS, it is appropriate to have a radiologist and a neurologist or neurosurgeon to read the images first and make a report before the physical or occupational therapist reviews the images. Previous neuroimaging scans and reports will also provide additional information regarding the progression or improvement of the conditions, or the involvement of other structures that may have implications for the patient's care. Review the report thoroughly, making note of the structures that were reported to be normal as well as the ones that were reported to be pathological. This will provide insight as to the patient's potential movement disorders, as well as functions that may be normal for the patient. This review can also reveal a mismatch between the report and the presented movement diagnosis.

Step 2

Familiarize With Patient Background Information and Identify Image Type and Orientation

After reviewing the imaging report, the clinician then examines the actual images. The clinician must be familiar with the basic background information presented on the image. Normally the film will contain information such as the patient's name, age, and medical record number; the date of the scan; and the name of the hospital or facility that performed the procedure (Fig. 37.6). The date of the scan is particularly important when attempting to establish relationships between what can be seen on the image and the patient's presentation. There might be a mismatch between what is shown on the image and what the patient is doing because of either resolution of the condition or worsening of the pathology. Comparing scans taken at different intervals will also assist the clinician in arriving at some general impressions on the rate or recovery (or lack thereof) or prognoses following physical rehabilitation.

Markers may also be available. The use of markers significantly simplifies analysis by allowing the examiner to easily orient the film correctly. Common markers include *R* and *L* for right and left, respectively, and *A* and *P* for anterior and posterior.

Often a scale is provided for the clinician to relate the size of the structures on the image to actual size.

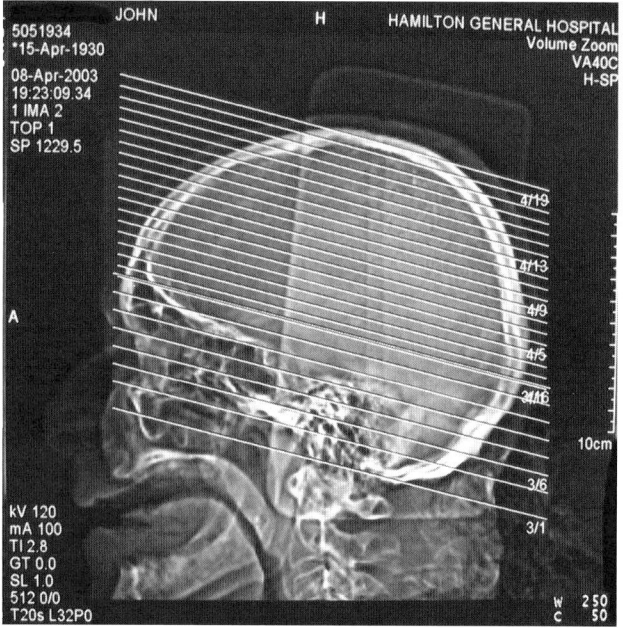

Fig. 37.6 Computed tomography scan of the brain with identifying information. (Courtesy Dr. John Wells. How to Read a CT Scan of the Brain. www.neurosurvival.ca/ComputerAssistedLearning/readingCTs/scanogram.htm.)

Next, the clinician should be familiar with some of the basic technical detail. CT and MRI can provide multiple "slices" of the brain, much like slices in a loaf of bread. Often a single large film containing all the images arranged in order can be found. Usually, the first image on the left top most corner is the "scout view" or scanogram and serves to illustrate the orientation and thickness of each slide. Depending on the suspected pathology, the slice orientation could be frontal, coronal, or sagittal, based on the specific structure in question.

Certain views of the CT image can also be produced by the radiology team by manipulating certain image parameters. These "windows" are presented in Fig. 37.7. A bone window shows bone the best and is helpful when a skull fracture is suspected. A brain window shows brain matter the best and is used when the suspected pathology is caused by or affects the brain matter (tumors, atrophy of the nuclear masses, or general atrophy of the brain itself). A subdural window is beneficial when suspecting the presence of subdural hematoma or swelling of the brain. With MRI, the images can also be "weighted" (for example, T1 vs. T2). T1-weighted images show better gray matter–white matter contrast, whereas T2-weighted images might show edema better. As mentioned previously, contrast agents may be used with either CT or MRI to improve visualization of the structures in question.

Step 3
Quick Scan Followed by Thorough Image Examination

After becoming familiar with the basic information, the clinician should then make a "quick scan" of the image, noting the pathology that quickly stands out. After doing so, a more thorough analysis of each film in the series must be done. Multiple windows and/or successive slices are often helpful in visualizing the extent of the pathology. The clinician mentally constructs a three-dimensional image of the brain from the two-dimensional scan. In a CT scan, knowledge of radiodensity is helpful in making this accurate representation, as is knowledge of normal structure and function of the CNS.

Several resources recommend slightly different methods of analyzing an image. The following are suggestions to make the process more organized and efficient.

1. Examine the symmetry.[10] Compare both sides of the brain as represented on the image. In orienting the images, the right side of the brain is usually shown on the left. Look for a midline shift by drawing an imaginary line from the anterior falx cerebri to the posterior falx cerebri. Identify the side of the greatest shift and measure it (in centimeters or millimeters). It would also be

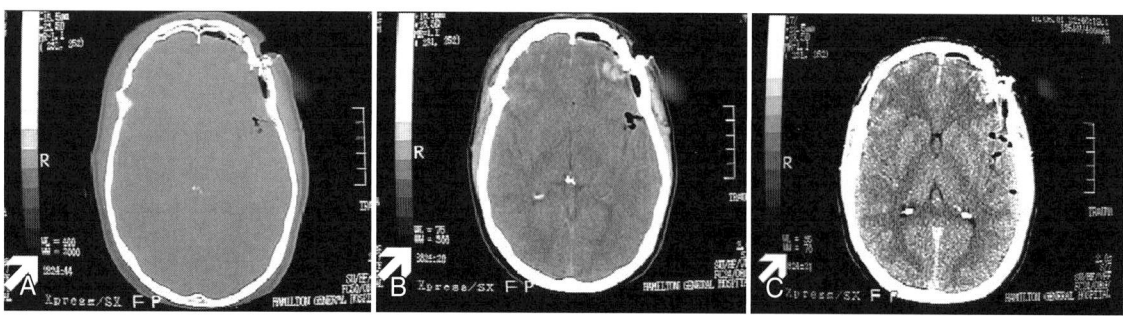

Fig. 37.7 Computed Tomography Scan of the Brain showing Three Different Windows. **(A)** Bone window. **(B)** Subdural window. **(C)** Brain window. (Images courtesy Dr. John Wells. How to Read a CT Scan of the Brain. www.neurosurvival.ca/ComputerAssistedLearning/readingCTs/windows.htm.)

helpful to look for signs of mass effect (when structures on one side are "pushed" to the other side, or a possible atrophy on the structures on one side that pushes the structures on the other side across the midline). Additional structures to inspect for symmetry include the basal ganglia, thalamus, and corpus callosum.

2. Examine the size and shape of the structures.[10] This is particularly helpful when looking at the integrity of the ventricles and cisterns. When filled with excessive fluid as in hydrocephalus, the ventricles enlarge disproportionately. This enlargement is seen in babies as a result of a variety of pathologies (see Chapter 9) and in children and adults after brain trauma (see Chapters 22 and 23). Likewise, in atrophy of the brain tissue, the ventricles may also become enlarged; this is often seen in elderly adults as the brain loses gray matter and the ventricles enlarge to fill in the extra space (see Chapter 27). Examining the size and shape of the sulci may also be beneficial when looking at atrophy of the specific structure, thereby accounting for the abnormalities of movement being observed.

3. Look for lesions in the brain. Space-occupying lesions such as brain tumors or hematoma can be visualized (Fig. 37.8). Because the brain has such a finite size to fit snugly within the cranial vault, any lesion in the brain has the potential to push brain structures to the midline or to displace the structure and create more serious pathology. Plaque formations secondary to multiple sclerosis can also be visualized as bright white spots in the gray matter (Fig. 37.9).

4. Examine densities.[10] As mentioned previously, different tissues will have different densities, and these differences are what forms the generated images. Hyperdensities may include blood, tumors, or enhancing lesions, whereas common hypodensities include air, nonenhancing tumors, and chronic hematoma.

Step 4

Establish Relationships Between the Structures Involved and the Presenting Impairments, Movement Dysfunctions, and Activity Limitations

There are two possible clinical scenarios in which the medical imaging information is reviewed. First, the therapist may be reviewing the medical imaging information before seeing the patient for the initial examination or evaluation. If this is the case, the therapist is expected to use this information in relation to other medical information in the chart (from physician's history and physical examination,

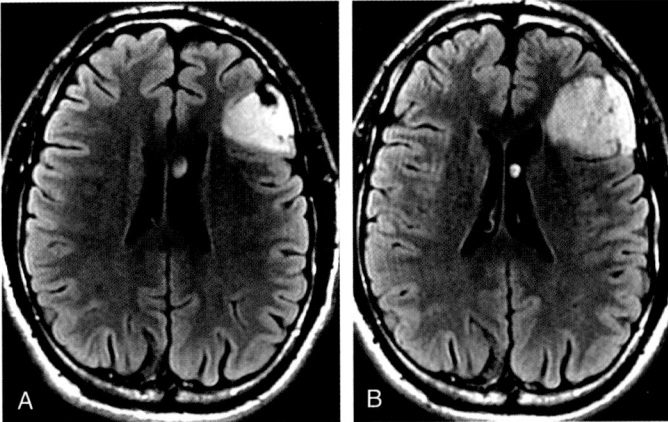

Fig. 37.8 (A) Fluid-attenuated inversion recovery magnetic resonance image showing a tumor in the in the left inferior frontal gyrus. **(B)** Follow-up imaging at 9 months shows growth of tumor. (From Brandao LA, Shiroishi MS, Law M. Brain tumors. *Magn Reson Imag Clin N Am.* 2013;21[2]:199–239.)

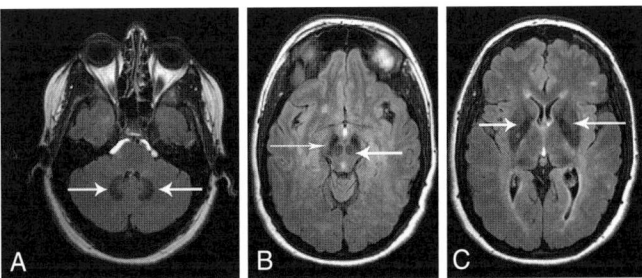

Fig. 37.9 Magnetic resonance image showing plaque formation caused by multiple sclerosis. Hypointensity noted in **(A)** dentate nucleus; **(B)** substantia nigra; **(C)** basal ganglia *(horizontal arrows)*. (From Sicotte NL. Magnetic resonance imaging in multiple sclerosis the role of conventional imaging. *Neurologic Clin.* 2011;29[2]:343–356.)

nursing notes, etc.) to get an initial sense of what the patient may be able or unable to do. This will allow the therapist to plan for the appropriate tests and measures to perform during the examination (Case Study 37.1).

CASE STUDY 37.1   A Patient With a Brain Tumor

The patient was a 71-year-old woman with history of glioblastoma multiforme, the most aggressive form of brain tumor (refer to Chapter 25). It has been reported that a second recurrence of this condition is associated with a less favorable prognosis.[11] The patient had previously undergone tumor resection, chemotherapy, and radiation. She had then been found to have another recurrence of the left frontal glioblastoma multiforme of 4 cm (Fig. 37.10), for which she had undergone a stereotactic resection (Fig. 37.11) of the tumor. After this surgery, she underwent intensive inpatient rehabilitation.

Her past medical history included history of radiation therapy, seizure disorder, diabetes mellitus, hypertension, anemia, and leukopenia. Medications include Dilantin, Lipitor, dexamethasone, fosinopril, and metformin.

The patient's primary caregiver was her husband. They were both retired, living in a single-story home with two steps to enter. She had two supportive daughters who lived nearby and were available for support as needed. Before the most recent hospitalization, the patient had been at a supervised level of assistance with ambulation outdoors and independence for household ambulation, with no assistive device required.

The medical images revealed a resected parietal lobe tumor in the left side of her brain. In the imaging report, it was noted that there was significant edema in the surrounding area and that mainly white matter tracts were affected. However, no midline shift or mass effect was noted. In addition, the tumor was reported to be located near the Broca and Wernicke areas but superficial to the ventricles.

Continued

CASE STUDY 37.1 **A Patient With a Brain Tumor—cont'd**

Based on the information provided by the imaging reports and the associated medical images, the clinician developed several initial impressions about the patient's presentation and care. First, the note about significant edema indicated more diffuse, global effects on movement and function; associated structural impairments rather than only dysfunctions specific to parietal lobe damage would be expected. The lack of midline shift or mass effect indicated a more favorable prognosis for survival for the patient. The information about the tumor being located near the speech areas indicated the possibility of deficits in expressive and receptive communication. Finally, damage to the parietal lobe indicated the potential for agraphia, aphasia, and agnosia. Because the parietal lobe is also largely important for perception and interpretation of somatosensory information, the formation of the idea of a complex purposeful motor act may also have been impaired.

The initial examination confirmed and supported all the expected movement deficits and clinical presentation of the patient. She underwent intensive occupational, physical, and speech therapy to improve her functional mobility and ambulation, self-care and activities of daily living, as well as speech, swallowing, and communication. There was a concerted effort among the rehabilitation team and the patient's family to optimize communication strategies while minimizing patient frustration. For example, more complex tasks such as transfers

were broken down into smaller components and then practiced extensively as components and as whole functions. The transfer task was broken down into three steps: (1) locking the brakes, (2) removing the leg-rests, and (3) standing and turning to sit on the destination surface. These step-by-step instructions were written on the patient's whiteboard; practiced during speech, physical, and occupational therapy; and communicated to the family and rehab team. Hand-over-hand guidance and facilitation were also included during instruction, as was use of mental rehearsal to remediate executive and visuomotor deficits to improve motor sequencing and problem solving while decreasing perseveration and frustration.[12] The rehabilitation team worked closely together to standardize treatment techniques, increase opportunity for task carryover, and decrease the patient's frustration with learning. Speech therapy started to integrate pictures and words representing tasks learned in physical and occupational therapies. In addition, therapy became more focused on repeated task training of three or four essential skills versus multiple activities, games, and skills.

This case example demonstrated how medical imaging information not only confirmed the expected presenting deficits in movement, function, communication, and learning of the patient but also included information that guided the rehabilitation team in selecting interventions that optimized function for this patient.

Case adapted from Parikh M. *The Use of Medical Imaging in Neuromuscular Physical Therapy Practice: A Case Report.* Samuel Merritt College Physical Therapy Case Report Presentations. May 2007.

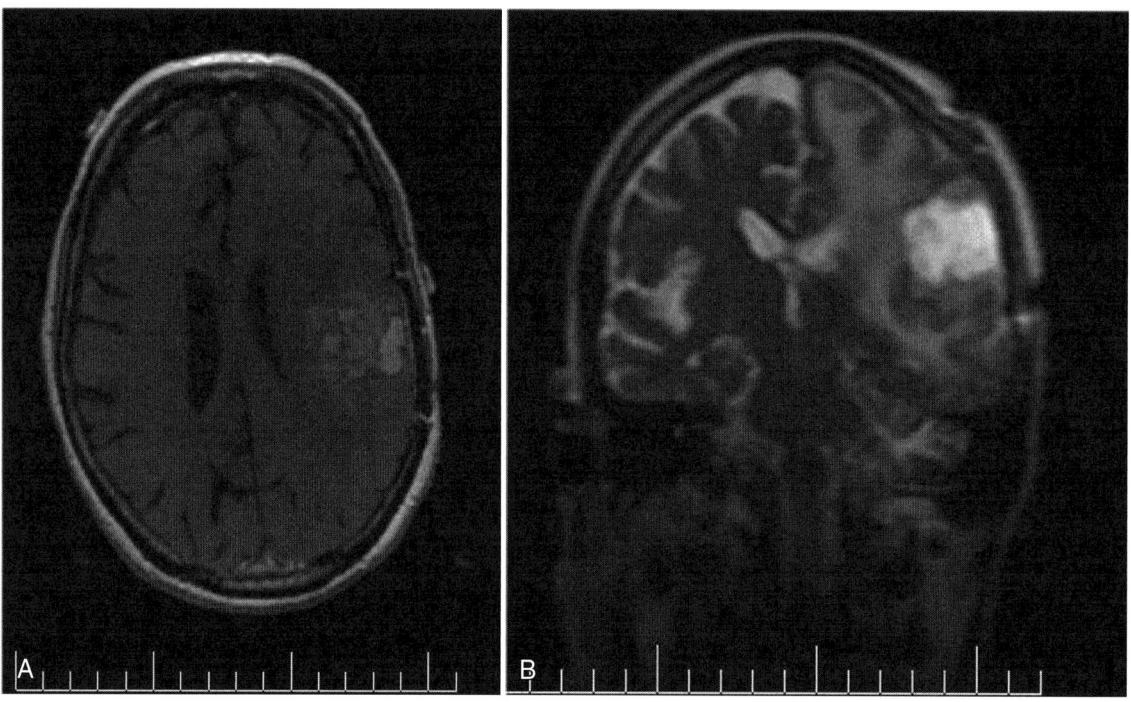

Fig. 37.10 **(A)** Axial view showing tumor. **(B)** Coronal view showing tumor.

The second clinical scenario involves the use of medical imaging information to guide clinical decisions during the actual occupational or physical therapy session. One of the major goals of this step is to make sure that the movement dysfunctions presented by the patient match the information obtained from the medical images. The therapist is expected to act accordingly and to demonstrate sound judgment, especially when the mismatch indicates a possible life-threatening situation. For example, if the imaging results indicate a small focal area involvement but the patient demonstrates

significant impairment in movement and function, the mismatch may be indicative of a worsening and potentially life-threatening condition that must be communicated to the physician and other members of the medical team.

As mentioned earlier, the complexity of the structure and function of the nervous system makes interpretation of imaging information very challenging. There may be situations in which images may not fully explain what the patient or client is able to do in terms of function and movement (as illustrated in Case Study 37.2).

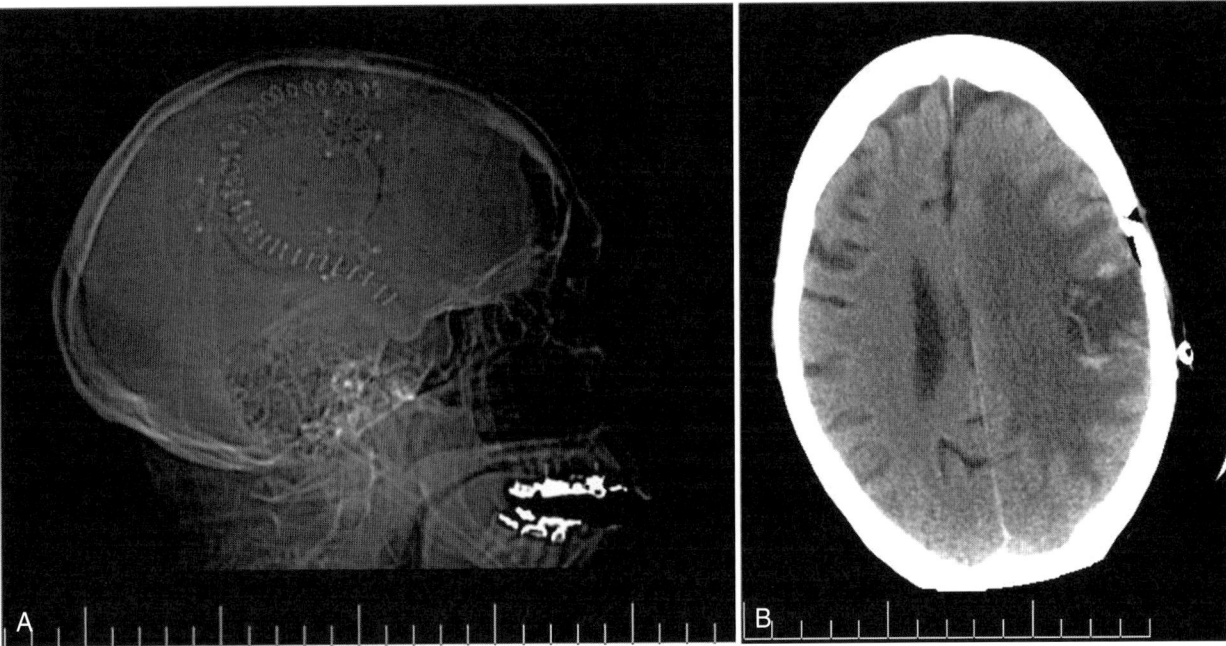

Fig. 37.11 Images After Surgery for Tumor Resection. **(A)** Lateral view. **(B)** Axial view.

CASE STUDY 37.2   A Pediatric Patient With Developmental Problems at 18 Months

An infant identified as high neurological risk based on prenatal ultrasound was eventually born full term. Prenatal findings of unusually large head were further explored after birth with computed tomography scans while the infant was in the neonatal intensive care unit (NICU). Imaging confirmed that the infant did not have closure of his lateral and third ventricles. The physicians' prognosis had been that the child would die within days after birth, and the family was encouraged to take him home and spend as much time with him as they had before his death.

Once home, the infant was evaluated by a physical therapist and asked by the child's medical team to help establish realistic expectations and treatment protocols for this child.

The child was 18 months of age at the time of this therapist's first visit. The child's motor development was very delayed owing to the large size of his head (hydrocephaly). He was also nonverbal, and the doctors had concluded that he had an extremely low level of intelligence. His loving parents played with him, fed him, bathed him, and interacted with him all day. They felt he had more ability than the pediatrician had stated.

This video case study illustrates a situation in which there is a mismatch between the medical diagnosis/medical imaging results and what the patient presents in terms of function and movement. This case will engage and guide the therapist in a clinical decision making process of analyzing the patient's movement and functional capabilities and relating those to the integrity of the specific areas of the nervous system that are responsible for the movement or behavior. It is recommended that the reader first look at and analyze the motor function of this child at 18 months and then 6 months later, looking specifically for increased motor function and potential. During the interim, the child did receive weekly therapy, but most of the practice was done at home with the parents interacting with the child. Analyze the movement from a motor learning and neuroplasticity perspective as you determine the potential for motor control. Then look at the magnetic resonance image images that lead the doctors to diagnosis the medical problem and the prognosis of death. Then ask yourself, what could be happening to cause such a mismatch between a movement and a medical diagnosis?

Note: The continuation of the case, including the video clips and imaging results, can be found on the companion website.

FUTURE OF NEUROIMAGING IN REHABILITATION

Potential use of neuroimaging to predict long-term outcomes of neuro rehabilitation and to investigate priming methods for neuroplasticity are being studied in several labs. Real time neuroimaging and neural recording for brain-computer interfaces in neuroprotheses and neuroimaging guided sensorimotor rehabilitation are some of the future possibilities.

REFERENCES

To enhance this text and add value for the reader, all references are included on the companion Evolve site that accompanies this textbook. This online service will, when available, provide a link for the reader to a Medline abstract for the article cited. There are 12 cited references and other general references for this chapter, with the majority of those articles being evidence-based citations.

38

Integrating Technology in Neurological Rehabilitation*

Jeric Uy, Sophie Lefmann, Laurie A. King, Martina Mancini, and Bradley W. Stockert

OBJECTIVES

After reading this chapter the student or therapist will be able to:
1. Summarize the need, demand, and principles for integrating advanced robotic technology in neurological rehabilitation.
2. Define common terminology used in the field of rehabilitation robotics and technology.
3. Classify the different types of advanced technology used in neurorehabilitation.
4. Apply the guidelines for integrating robotics and assistive technology into a patient's rehabilitation program.
5. Discuss the benefits of performing a cost-effectiveness analysis when considering the application of robotic technology in rehabilitation.
6. Describe the challenges of commercializing robotic devices.
7. Discuss the future of advanced technology and rehabilitation.

KEY TERMS

brain-machine interfaces
exoskeleton

human robotic interfaces
rehabilitation robotics

virtual reality training

Rehabilitation professionals face an ongoing challenge to provide clinically effective interventions that are also engaging and meaningful to the patient. The objective of rehabilitation technology is to empower clinicians and patients to take responsibility and control of the environment and facilitate physical and cognitive recovery. Technology assists patients during learning-based practice that drives neural adaptation and neural reorganization.[1] For these reasons, robotic-assisted rehabilitation technology has been embraced by allied health and rehabilitation medicine over the previous two decades. It seeks to take interventions and dosages of therapy to the "next level": a novel approach to offering high-volumes of computer/external force-guided body retraining.[2]

Timely rehabilitation maximizes people's performance of motor, speech, function, and cognition.[3] The timing and purpose of introducing rehabilitation robotics and technology into the rehabilitation process will vary greatly. The "how" and "why" of robotic rehabilitation interventions need to be just as thoughtfully targeted as any other land-based approach for function, engagement, time-efficiency, and performance optimality.

Rehabilitation approaches across disciplines consider the influence of neuroplasticity on outcomes, and also consider the relationship of intervention to the World Health Organization's International Classification of Functioning, Health and Disability (WHO-ICF). Whether the patient is an adult following a stroke or a child with cerebral palsy, the treating therapist should have a sound understanding of the principles of motor learning and neuroplasticity.

Furthermore, when reading this chapter, the clinician should reflect on the principles of experience-dependent plasticity (Table 38.1) and align how robotic rehabilitation can augment each of these components for their patient.[3]

Robotic devices come in many shapes, sizes, and price points, which must be considered in selecting the best option.[4,5] For example, is it in the patient's interest to have a wearable robotic device for everyday functional support? Is it more appropriate to access therapeutic bursts of complex, laboratory-based technology? There is no one answer, and the fine details of a patient's therapy will be individualized. However, the path pursued by therapists alongside patients should be motivated predominantly by the patient's own functional goals.

The first part of this chapter will provide an overview of the clinical utility of robotic technology in neurorehabilitation. As the field of robotic rehabilitation is dynamic, this section will not provide an exhaustive list of device options, nor will it provide explicit instructions on how to use devices. Interest in specific devices or approaches is best explored with the latest research outputs as they emerge and with the devices' manufacturers directly. Instead, the aim of this chapter is to equip the rehabilitation professional with an awareness of how robotic and rehabilitation technology can be broadly applied to patients with neurological impairments and relate it back to the overarching principles of the WHO-ICF.[6] Included in this part is the use of robotics for simulation for student education. The second part of this chapter will address other technology that is used in clinical and teaching environments, including inertia sensors, virtual reality (VR), and noninvasive brain stimulation.

TYPES OF ROBOTIC REHABILITATION AND THEIR APPLICATIONS

Robotic technology can provide service, body support, unweighting, and movement assistance that is passive, active, variable, and on-demand assistance.[7,8] Computerized and robotic technology provides the foundation for patients to practice and attend to purposeful,

---

*Videos for this chapter are available at studentconsult.com.

TABLE 38.1 Principles of Experience-Dependent Plasticity[3]

Principle	Description
1. Use it or lose it	Failure to drive specific brain functions can lead to functional degradation
2. Use it and improve it	Training that drives a specific brain function can lead to an enhancement of that function
3. Specificity	The nature of the training experience dictates the nature of the plasticity
4. Repetition matters	Induction of plasticity requires sufficient repetition
5. Intensity matters	Induction of plasticity requires sufficient training intensity
6. Time matters	Different forms of plasticity occur at different times during training
7. Salience matters	The training experience must be sufficiently salient to induce plasticity
8. Age matters	Training-induced plasticity occurs more readily in younger brains
9. Transference	Plasticity in response to one training experience can enhance the acquisition of similar behaviors
10. Interference	Plasticity in response to one experience can interfere with the acquisition of other behaviors

goal-oriented, progressive tasks spaced over time. This technology can also minimize the risk of injury during retraining. Robotic rehabilitation devices may include service robots, nonwearable assistive robotic devices, wearable assistive robotic devices, or neuromuscular stimulators. There are also vocational rehabilitation robotics, communication devices, and emotional interactive entertainment/friendly robots, which will not be investigated in depth in this chapter. Fig. 38.1 and Box 38.1 provide an overview of the classifications of robotics technology.

Service robots usually focus on task performance, movement assistance, and stability. These devices can be fixed, movable, or attached to a wheelchair.[1] Assistive robotic devices help patients perform a task with direct or indirect assistance. Some of the assistive robotics are nonwearable but assist through unweighting or movement assistance. Wearable robotic devices are specifically designed to be worn by patients to assist movements. These are designed for the upper or lower limb.[1] Vocational robotics can enhance performance at work either in terms of repetitive motions or high-force task production that would otherwise be dangerous to humans. Communication robotic devices are designed to improve communication potential for patients who cannot adequately speak or hear. Emotional support robotic devices are designed to provide emotional support for isolated individuals at home.[1]

Prosthetics for amputees, vocational robotics, communication robotics, emotional support robotics, or socially assistive devices[9-11] are not outlined in detail here as these areas are considered specialty oriented and may or may not be included in traditional neurorehabilitation programs coordinated by physical or occupational therapists.

For simplicity, we will focus on our examination on service robots, nonwearable assistive robotic devices, and wearable assistive robotic devices. It is also important to acknowledge there are a number of motorized chairs, lifts, and walkers available that can be used to transition a patient from sitting to standing, or provide unweighting

while walking, or working on balance. These devices are not usually programmable and are not classified as "rehabilitation robotics" or "advanced technology." However, these types of devices are very beneficial for helping patients maintain walking and training to improve safety and quality of gait at home and with supervision. It is important for therapists to be sure these types of assistive devices have been considered and/or integrated into a patient's rehabilitation program and at home before recommending more sophisticated technology.

SERVICE ROBOTICS

Service robots primarily assist individuals with severe disabilities. Most commonly, the robot performs everyday activities (e.g., assisting with eating, drinking, object replacing, ambulating).[12] There are three main types of schemes: desktop-mounted robots, wheelchair-mounted robots, and mobile autonomous robots. In general, these robots are used in the home, are interconnected to a variety of control systems, are programmed to the environment and consequently are not very portable.[12-14]

These types of robotic devices are often preprogrammed to perform certain tasks. There are also some autonomous robots in which the cognitive interface between the user and the robot is used to tell the robot to perform a new task or to help the patient perform the task.[15] These robotic systems are successful if the robot, the user, and the manipulated objects remain in the same initial set position every time a concrete task is performed. With the wheelchair-mounted manipulator, the relative position of the user with respect to the manipulator needs to remain the same. Although there are a variety of simple service-based robotic devices, most are complex, and setting them up at home generally requires a computer or engineering specialist.

Service robots may include smart wheelchairs[16] and smart devices in the home (e.g., The Robotic Room[10]) or wheelchair-mounted upper extremity manipulators.[17] A major consideration for patients using service robotic devices are the control options. For example, through the use of headpieces on robotic devices, information can be detected from flexion and extension, rotation, and side bending of the head to operate wheelchairs, TV sets, telephones, doors, and security systems. There are also interfaces that are sensitive to facial movements and optoelectronic detection of light-reflective head movements.[18] Other interfaces are sensitive to eye movements or use voice recognition, brain control,[19,20] and gesture recognition.[21] These interfaces not only may allow control of the robot but also may be applied to move a limb or perform a task. A more detailed discussion of robotic interfaces is included later in this section.

Service robotics is recommended when patients have achieved their maximum potential and still need assistance to live independently. A therapist may continue to work with a patient at home to maintain range of motion, minimize skin problems, and review whether the robotic technology is still providing the necessary assistance. However, an engineer will usually assume the primary responsibility for maintaining and adjusting the robotic equipment.

NONWEARABLE ASSISTIVE ROBOTIC DEVICES

This group of robotic devices primarily includes powered wheelchairs with autonomous intelligence, robots for body support, and hands-off service robotic devices. Body weight supported treadmill systems (BWSTSs) with and without robotics[22] and body weight-support mobile walking aids (BWSMWA) are also aligned to this category.[23,24] The value of BWSTSs and similar nonwearable assistive robotic devices is that patients can be supported to develop their body structures and functions (e.g., step length, weight shift abilities, balance)

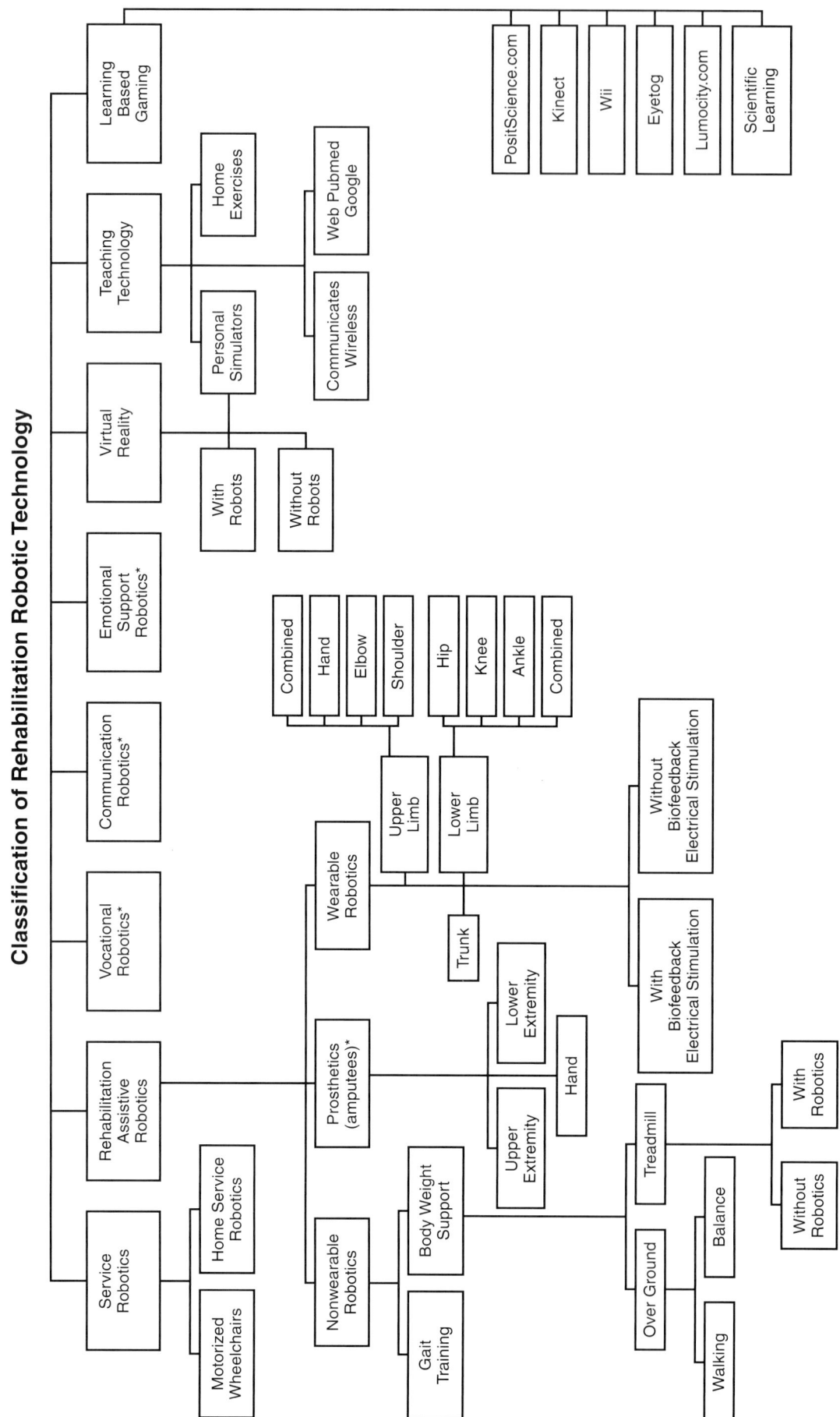

Fig. 38.1 Classification of Rehabilitation Technology.

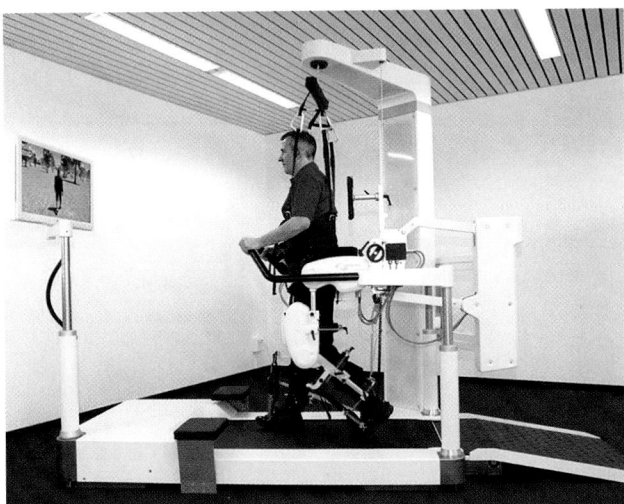

Fig. 38.2 Body weight–support trainer or body weight supported treadmill trainer: Lokomat robotic system. (Courtesy Hocoma, Volketswil, Switzerland.)

as a precursor to practicing tasks at the activity/participation level in more authentic, natural settings.[25] Body weight–supported gait training systems were initially designed to unweight the body, decrease ground reaction forces (GRFs), and protect against falling (Fig. 38.2). Under these assisted conditions, it is easier for patients to achieve intense levels of exercise such as walking, skipping, and running with less pain and less trauma to the joints.

Assistive robotic devices hold a prominent place in the rehabilitation of adults and children with neurological dysfunction.[22,26] Robotic-assisted BWSTT has been investigated for individuals with chronic spinal cord injury[27] and stroke.[28] Evidence of greatest efficacy of these robotic or electromechanical-assisted devices has been reported in the first 3 months following stroke, and of most benefit to those with very limited walking ability.[28] Furthermore, it is important to support patients to walk at community-level velocities of at least 0.8 m/s (faster than 2.0 mph).[29–33] Devices such as the Lokomat, which robotically augment joint placement and walking execution on a treadmill, have been examined in children with neurological impairments.[25] Children with cerebral palsy may experience greatest benefit when they have moderate-to-severe degrees of gait impairment (e.g., GMFCS levels II, III, and IV). The opportunity for clinically noticeable training change is greatest and more likely to achieve physiological and possibly neuroprotective benefits.[34,35]

Nonwearable assistive robotic devices can offer patients the potential for high degrees of repetitive practice by adjusting, placing, and guiding the limb through repeated movements.[2,5,36] It can help reduce the taxing physical effect and awkward positioning of rehabilitation on clinicians while offering even higher volumes of practice in a single session.[4] However, at some point, clinicians and patients must face the possibility of a ceiling effect of high-dose practice in a predictable environment. The therapeutic course should take the patient to eventually progress to task-specific training outside of assistive robotic devices, which is where conventional approaches to therapy take precedence.

WEARABLE ASSISTIVE ROBOTIC DEVICES

Assistive robotic devices are also popular in upper limb rehabilitation. The upper limb is highly complex, with a requirement for devices to be appropriately light and responsive to degrees of movement. The shoulder and hand/wrist will demand multidimensional options compared to the elbow. This becomes challenging for designers to balance aligning the device with joints, as well as incorporating motors, actuators, and cabling.[37] The clinician will therefore decide whether the patient requires an exoskeleton device (e.g., Armeo) with torque actuators that control single/multiple joints, or an end-effector-type device (e.g., InMotion 2.0), which focuses on the distal portion of the upper limb. A recent study on post-stroke intervention notes a higher degree of exploration of end-effector devices as newer exoskeleton technologies have been less commonly investigated.[38] It also notes that meaningful change, especially with earlier intervention, will be assisted with some degree of voluntary muscle initiation of wrist and fingers; timing of intervention remains an important consideration.[38]

Wearable assistive robotic devices can support patients to participate in everyday tasks with greater autonomy.[39] Structures may be exoskeleton but with rigid or soft wearable features. They may be fixed in place in a clinical training station or they may allow great portability with movement and use.[40] Examples of these include the ironHand system[41] or those that are triggered with neuromuscular stimulation, such as the Bioness upper limb or lower limb systems (see Fig. 38.3). The primary impairment that can be addressed with neuromuscular stimulation is muscle weakness, but the patient may also have neuromotor control problems or abnormal synergies of movement. These devices work only when peripheral nervous system function is preserved. The electrodes, located within the device's control unit, stimulate a peripheral nerve causing a movement effect.[42] However, in the case of patients with spinal cord injuries, multiple electrodes may need to be used to sequentially activate a series of muscle contractions to enable walking. Similar robotic devices and principles of operation are available for patients post-stroke.

Wearable assistive robotic technology extends, complements, empowers, replaces, or enhances the function or capability of the individual. For some patients, using these is an ongoing component of their rehabilitation. For others, the wearable assistive robotic device is used as it can complete the action of a task that is no longer an effective or efficient option for the patient. These robotic devices may facilitate muscle contractions in one or more directions around one joint such as the elbow, wrist, or ankle. The objectives of reducing muscular fatigue and energy conservation during task practice are met when devices are lightweight, flexible, sensitive to movement change, and easily portable.[5,41,43–45]

Upper limb and lower limb wearable robots are obviously worn by the individual, but the internal or external interface must be mapped to the anatomy, a cognitive control mechanism, or the brain. The extremities can be used to perform multiple tasks, and the redundancy of the joints and degrees of freedom (e.g., at the ankle, or the wrist) allow people to perform tasks in a variety of ways. Redundancy of the joints and degrees of freedom allow a variety of ways patients can perform a task; however, these

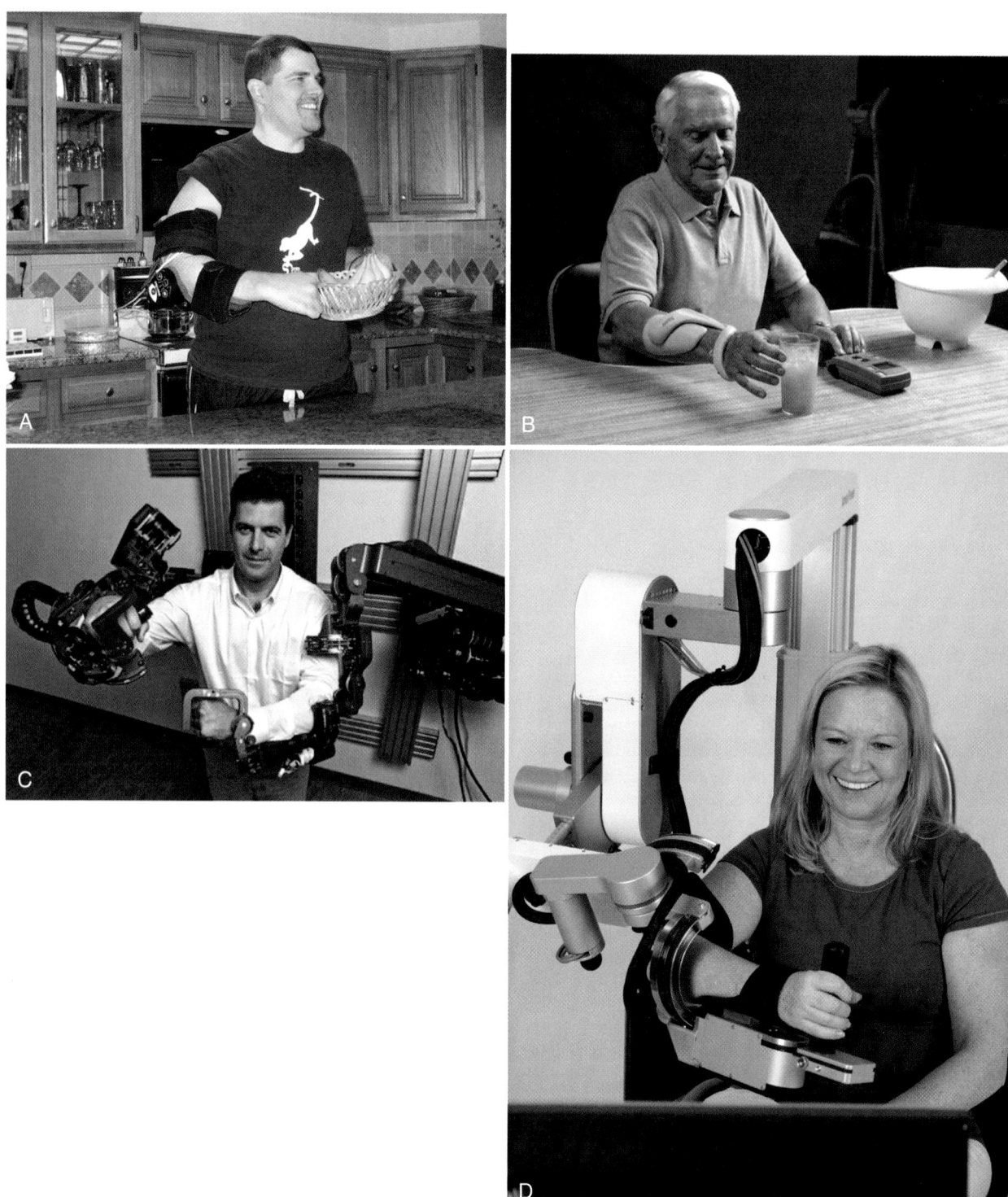

Fig. 38.3 Wearable Upper-Limb Devices and Assistive Robotic Exoskeleton Devices. **(A)** Myomo upper-limb robotic assistive device. **(B)** Bioness L200 arm and wrist trainer. **(C)** Shoulder, elbow, and wrist upper-limb assistive robotic bilateral device. **(D)** Armeo robotic arm. (**A,** Courtesy Myomo, Cambridge, MA. **B,** Courtesy Bioness, Valencia, CA. **C,** Courtesy Jacob Rosen/Jim Mackenzie, UCSC. **D,** Courtesy Hocoma, Volketswil, Switzerland.)

redundancies may be hard to control. Wearable robotic devices will vary by type of human interface system incorporated (e.g., brain neurons, cognitive, sensory [tactile, pressure], physical [movement], or breath). At a minimum, the physical interface of a wearable robot requires an actuator and a rigid structure to transmit forces to the neuromusculoskeletal system.[43]

Ideally, wearable systems use both muscle stimulation and active voluntary muscle contractions to increase functional use. Devices such as the ReWalk and the Hybrid Assistive Limb (HAL) are well known commercially, and among clinicians working in neurological rehabilitation, for their wearable design and capacity to support patients with spinal cord injuries particularly, to ambulate with relative independence.

With actuation componentry at the hip and knee, these devices facilitate gait with electromyographic triggered stimuli (HAL) or battery powered, remote-control operation mechanisms (ReWalk).[46] As with the upper limb orthoses though, wearable exoskeleton technologies guiding lower limbs have key limitations around their size, bulk, weight, and responsiveness to the external environment. There can be some limitations in transferring the device usage into more complicated, unpredictable terrains.[46] However, as a concept, wearable lower limb exoskeletons such as the ReWalk and HAL can have significant influence at the activity and participation level. If accessible to rehabilitation staff, they may be worthy of consideration for goals that align to these dimensions of the WHO-ICF. Other device examples recently cited in the literature include Ekso exoskeleton, REX Personal, and the Indego exoskeleton.[46]

ROBOTIC SYSTEM MECHANISMS FOR OPERATION

Robotic interfaces, actuators, and controllers can convert sensory, physical, and cognitive signals to:
- control robots
- permit perception of spatial relationships

- mobilize individuals in space
- assist in object manipulation
- provide emotional support
- allow individuals to call for help and communicate with others

In addition, through creative virtual training environments and gaming technology, patients can improve memory, motor skills, and movement quality.

Different robotic designs enable different performance outcomes. Understanding robotic mechanisms of operation is an important first step for a clinician as it may guide the selection of devices for patients.[47] Robotic devices in general may be active, passive, haptic, or predominantly performance feedback-oriented.[5,8] The degree of assistance offered will determine the suitability of robotic mechanical design, and vice-versa. Maciejasz and colleagues[5] best summarized different robotic systems by feature, outlined in Table 38.2.

The robotic device's mechanical design (e.g., exoskeleton) also has specific properties, which may require some understanding. These properties can help determine the degree of augmented movement available in the device,[5,49] as outlined in Table 38.3.

TABLE 38.2 Mechanical Design of Robots[5]

Term	Description
Exoskeleton devices	These use an externally-fitted framework to replicate the targeted limb/limbs' skeletal structure. The limb's joints are aligned with the framework's joints to support movement. An exoskeleton device may replicate multiple joint movements, but also can be set up to both assist and inhibit body segment use
End-effector-based devices	Usually simpler than a full exoskeleton device, end-effector designs have a single, distal point where mechanical forces are applied to the distal limb segment.[48] Note that the simplicity of the design may offer challenges when the limb position demands multiple degrees of freedom
Back-drivable devices	A feature of robotic design where the patient can move the device without robotic augmentation. Importantly, limb movement is not constrained while fitted to the device
Planar robotic devices	These devices operate in a specific plane of movement and are often associated with end effector designs
Modularity	A property of a device indicating that optional parts may adapt it to a specific condition or simply to perform additional exercises
Reconfigurability	A property of a device indicating that it mechanical structure may be modified without adding additional parts in order to adapt it to the condition of the subject or to perform other forms of training

TABLE 38.3 Glossary of Actuation Terms[5]

Term	Description
Electric actuators	Actuators powered by electric current. They are the most common because they easily provide a relatively high power and are able to store energy. There is a wide selection of commercially available electric actuators; however, some of them are heavy and/or their impedance is too high for rehabilitation settings
Hydraulic actuators	Actuators powered by hydraulic pressure (usually oil). They are able to generate high forces. Their system is relatively complex considering the maintenance of pressurized oil under pressure to prevent leakage. Commercial hydraulic actuators are also heavy; therefore only specially designed hydraulic actuators are used in rehabilitation robotics
Pneumatic actuators	Actuators powered by compressed air. They have lower impedance and weigh less than electric actuators. Special compressors or containers with compressed air are required for power
Pneumatic Artificial Muscle (PAM, McKibben type actuator)	A special type of pneumatic actuator with an internal bladder surrounded by a braided mesh shell with flexible, but nonextensible threads. Because of their specific design, an actuator under pressure shortens, similarly to the contracting muscle. It is relatively light and exerts force in a single direction. It is difficult to control because of its slow and nonlinear dynamic functions
Series Elastic Actuator (SEA)	A generic name used for a mechanism with an elastic element placed in series with an actuator. This solution is relatively often met in the design of rehabilitation robots. It decreases the inertia and intrinsic impedance of the actuator to allow a more accurate and stable force control and increase patient safety
Functional Electrical Stimulation (FES)	It is a technique that uses electrical current to activate nerves and contract their innervated muscles. It produces the movement of the limb using natural actuators of the body. However, it is difficult to achieve precise and repeatable movement using this technique, and it may be painful for the patient

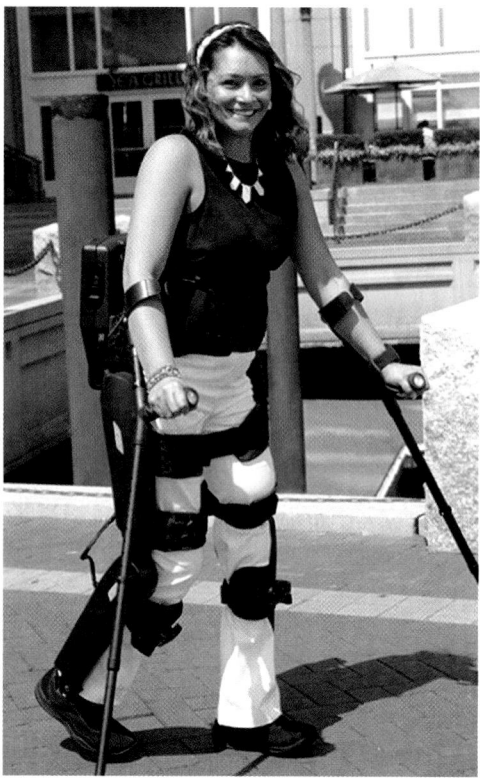

Fig. 38.4 Re-Walk Personal 6.0.

Clinical rationale for the use of robotic devices is specific to the patient and the particular device. Robotic devices can be used to improve body structure and function, activities, and participation. For example, the Lokomat (see Fig. 38.2) uses a body weight–supporting exoskeleton and provides augmented limb movement to improve the functions of weight-bearing tolerance and sagittal plane joint mobility.[8,25] Other devices, such as the ReWalk (Fig. 38.4), support the spinal cord-compromised patient to ambulate with crutches, allowing community mobility and potentially greater autonomy[50]; performance

factors that align with "participation" expectations. Patients in early rehabilitation phases may respond better to a particular type of robotic device, superseded by an alternative option as the patient's capabilities evolve or diminish. There also may be changes between genuine neurological structure recovery (e.g., CNS reactivation) and the emergence of effective compensatory strategies for movement.[47] Iosa and colleagues[8] have recently proposed the "ideal" interactional loop between the patient, the rehabilitation professional, and the robotic rehabilitation device selected (Fig. 38.5).

Aligning the device category, actuation componentry, design, and function to the patient's needs can confidently provide the clinician with a plan for robotic application. Many therapists will be limited by what their workplace has access to.

General Screening Considerations

There is a potential pitfall for patients and therapists to pursue technology for "technology's sake." A robotic device does not replace an individualized, task-specific, land-based regime and should not be a substitute for goal-oriented therapy.[47] Importantly, the patient and therapist should not become tempted to force the robotic options on offer to become a part of the patient's therapy if it does not align with functional goals. Box 38.2 summarizes the principles to support the use of technology and robotics in therapy.

The criteria used to determine which patients might benefit from rehabilitative technology will change over time. Devices will come with specific instructions and suggestions for use/contraindications to use. However, the treating therapist must also make an informed decision to use the robotic technology because it holds promise to "value-add" to the patient's performance. Before screening a patient for robotic technology, clinicians need to be certain that all standard assistive devices have already been integrated into the individual's rehabilitation program. Ultimately, guidelines should be developed to match the potential of the individual with the prognosis for independence, with and without dependable, user-friendly technology.

An objective evaluation is needed to match a patient with a commercially available robotic device. This evaluation must include a thorough assessment of anatomical, physiological, cognitive, and sensory impairments. Whenever possible, standardized tests should be used to document strength, flexibility, endurance, balance, coordination,

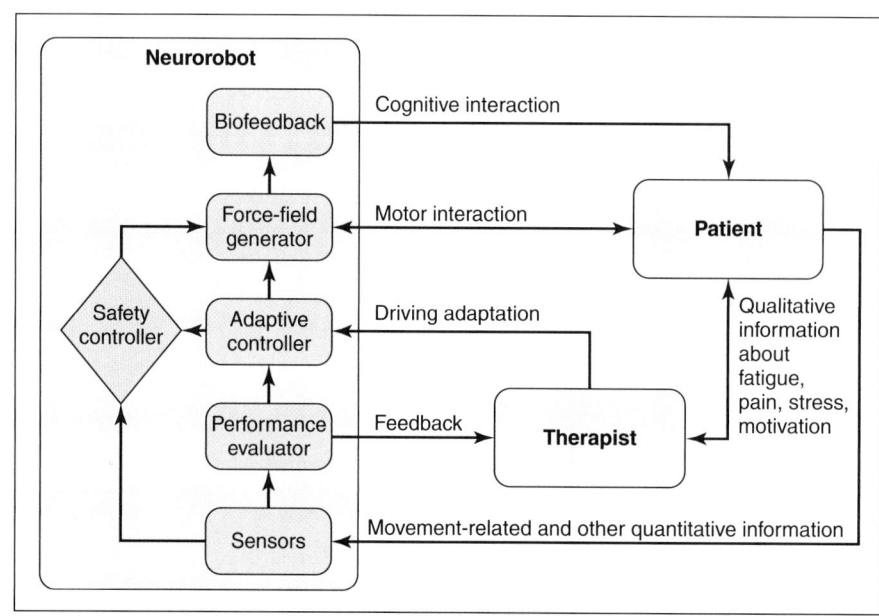

Fig. 38.5 Interactional Loop Between Robotic Device, Patient, and Therapist.[8,51(p. 8)]

BOX 38.2   Principles Supporting Advanced Technology and Rehabilitation Robotics in Neurorehabilitation

Principle I

Goals for advanced technology and rehabilitation robotics include the following:

A. *Indirectly augmenting* functional independence of individuals with impairments by:
1. performing mobility tasks for individuals at the home (e.g., using automatic motorized wheelchairs to move individuals from room to room; transitioning individuals from bed to chair and from chair to standing; moving patients who are standing; smart houses; calling for help)
2. minimizing the need for assistance from another individual
3. performing functional activities of daily living (activities of daily living; e.g., getting objects, cooking food, doing dishes, bathing, transferring)
4. helping perform difficult or repetitive tasks at work (e.g., assembly line tasks; lifting and moving heavy objects)

B. *Directly improving* human motor skill capabilities of individuals with impairments to enable them to:
1. perform functional tasks independently
2. improve voluntary control
3. perfect quality of movement
4. learn new skills

Principle II

Advanced technology and rehabilitation robotics should maximize neural adaptation and reorganization through the creation of practice opportunities that:

A. are attended, repetitive, purposeful, goal oriented, progressive, and spaced over time
B. are fun, interesting, and practical
C. are task oriented
D. provide feedback on accuracy of task completion
E. can be matched to patient abilities

Principle III

The objectives of assistive rehabilitation robotic devices need to be clearly defined in terms of:

A. unweighting a limb to reduce patient effort required for movement
B. actively canceling mechanical limitations on movement of the patient and robot arm dynamics (e.g., friction, inertia, and weight under gravity)
C. gently and progressively moving a limb to assist patient effort to perform a task
D. stabilizing a joint to enable a patient to produce a controlled movement
E. assisting the patient to improve the accuracy and quality of a movement
F. assisting the sequencing of movements
G. providing resistance to strengthen movements

Principle IV

Robotic technology must be:

A. safe for training
B. reliable in performance

C. able to reduce risks of injury (e.g., falls)
D. able to minimize injury during use

Principle V

Robotic technology should be:

A. adaptable (across patient needs, side, type of actuation)
B. able to integrate interfaces, actuators, and controllers sensitive to the ability of the individual

Principle VI

Robotic devices need to be:

A. reasonably priced and cost-effective
B. versatile
C. durable
D. repairable
E. easy to use

Principle VII

Wearable robotic devices must be:

A. lightweight
B. easy to get on and off
C. portable
D. cosmetically acceptable
E. interfaced to patient ability (sensory, motor, cognitive, brain)
F. minimally harmful to the skin
G. dynamically adaptable to performance capabilities

Principle VIII

Robotic technology for rehabilitation needs to be defined by:

A. location of the control system relative to the patient (controlled at a distance from the user [e.g., Web, Skype], controlled in proximity to the user [e.g., by a therapist or engineer], or controlled by the user [e.g., wearable device or interface])
B. environmental connection of the device and the patient (fixed to a nonmobile surface [e.g., wall], attached to a mobile platform [e.g., wheelchair], freely mobile with the patient [wearable])
C. type of control system (e.g., joystick, sensor, breath)
D. type of interface (physical, sensory, cognitive, brain)
E. type of anatomical connection (e.g., by end effector only, end effector and multiple points of attachments with serial links or temporal links)

Principle IX

Brain controlled interface rehabilitation robotics must be:

A. considered after all other alternatives have been unsuccessful
B. minimally intrusive despite surgery
C. physically accessible via remote control outside the brain
D. controlled with minimal patient risk and with safety
E. potentially controlled by cognition or the patient's mental effort
F. able to extend patient's independent task performance

---

synergistic responses, hypertonicity, gait, balance, posture, and postural righting skills. These impairments need to be integrated into functional and task-specific assessments of motor learning, motor control, activities of daily living (ADLs), work requirements, and recreational needs. Then each patient should be screened by defined objectives relative to outcomes in terms of quality of life and independence. Subjective and emotional issues such as attention, motivation, history of positive health behaviors, durability, depression,

desire for independence, and commitment to learning must also be considered. As an additional consideration for children, the parents and caregivers must confidently understand the value and purpose of including the device in a therapy regime and the therapist must feel comfortable that the child can express discomfort or displeasure with the device, to minimize adverse effects. There is evidence to suggest that with devices such as the Armeo and LokomatPro, for example, the more motivated to avatar-based games the child is, the greater the clinical effects.[2,25] Speculation is that active involvement in gaming will increase the responsiveness of body structures and functions (e.g., postural control, weight shift) to gait rather than the passivity that comes with walking on a treadmill engaging in less-interactive watching of movies on screens.[25] Indeed, recovery for patients may even be compromised if tasks are monotonous, demand less effort or focus.[5]

The patient needs to go through general and specific screenings to determine the appropriateness of integrating a nonwearable assistive robotic device into the rehabilitation program (Table 38.4). The patient who is most likely to benefit from body weight–supported gait training is the patient who has the prognosis for functional independence but needs to train to improve quality, endurance, speed, and stability of gait. Thus many patients with problems described within this text might benefit from this type of training. Those who do not have the potential for independent ambulation could still benefit from training on a BWSTS. In these cases, the training would be directed toward enhancing metabolic health, providing a sense of well-being, increasing circulation, and minimizing secondary impairments associated with excessive sitting such as decubitus ulcers and bone demineralization. These patients may need robotic, human, or harness assistance to achieve standing or stepping as well as bracing of the neck and trunk when upright. Patients with joint pain in the back or knee may also benefit from wearing supports when standing or exercising.

If a patient does not demonstrate the ability to bear weight on a single limb, then robotic control of the lower limbs may be the preferred mechanism to facilitate secondary benefits. However, when all the movements are passive, there will be minimal gains in terms of neural adaptation and reorganization. On the other hand, it may counter the secondary problems of bone demineralization and decubitus ulcers and be of value as a maintenance strategy.

In spite of advancements in rehabilitation robotic technology, some patients may still have difficulty taking advantage of this type of therapeutic assistance. In patients with challenging impairments, for safety the use of an overhead harness to access the treadmill may be required, in addition to close supervision by one or more therapists.

Specific Screening of Patients for Wearable Assistive Devices

Screening must be sensitive to the characteristics of the individual and consistent with factors in Table 38.4. After identifying the parameters of performance and the potential benefits of assistive wearable technology, the patient, the family, the therapist, and sometimes the orthotist should determine what assistive robotic devices or advanced technological equipment are available to meet the patient's needs. The team also has to assess where the devices are located, whether they are accessible, whether the device should be rented or purchased, and

TABLE 38.4 Screening Patients for Integrating Advanced Technology or Rehabilitation Robotics Into Neurorehabilitation

Screening Criteria	Service Robotic Devices	ASSISTIVE ROBOTIC DEVICES	
		Nonwearable—Mobility and Unweighting	Wearable—Mobility and Object Manipulation
Criteria for determining potential **benefit** for patient to integrate advanced or robotic technology	Patient with severe physical impairments challenged to be independent without personal assistance: 1. Has significant weakness of trunk and limbs (0, trace, poor) 2. Has minimal voluntary control of trunk and limbs 3. Cannot use a manual chair independently 4. Requires personal assistance to transfer to and from chair 5. Cannot step without maximum assistance 6. Unable to walk or stand independently 7. Unable to meet ADL needs without personal assistant 8. Is cognitively alert and aware	Patient with mobility impairments compromising safety, full independence, and quality of life: 1. Has impaired ability to walk 2. Has poor or slow balance responses 3. Demonstrates unstable single-limb support (unilateral or bilateral) 4. Is at risk of falling 5. Could benefit from fall protection when standing 6. Is weak (has poor strength) 7. Has difficulty initiating stepping 8. Lacks high-quality voluntary control for walking 9. Has involuntary synergistic movements 10. Has reduced flexibility 11. Uses an assistive mobility device 12. Needs to reduce ground reaction forces when walking or during intense exercise owing to pain, inflammation, osteoporosis, joint replacement, incoordination, and so on 13. Walks very slowly (household ambulatory but limited community ambulation) 14. Must maintain cardiopulmonary and metabolic health 15. Could benefit from stimulation of neurotransmitters and endorphins	Patient with impairments compromising mobility and/or independent task performance at home, at work, or during recreation: 1. Is unable to perform common daily tasks for independence without an assistive device or personal assistance 2. Needs assistance at one or more joints 3. Needs assistance to complete a task 4. Takes excessive time to complete task 5. Needs assistive device to ensure stability to walk 6. Has experienced a fall or an injury when performing a daily task (e.g., toileting) 7. Cannot live safely alone without personal assistance 8. Cannot cross the street in time 9. Needs more controlled forced task practice 10. Needs assistance to improve quality 11. Is not afraid of computerized or electromechanical devices 12. Is learning "abnormal" movements 13. Lives alone, but safety is in question 14. Drives but needs some assistance with transfers and/or arm or leg movements

TABLE 38.4   Screening Patients for Integrating Advanced Technology or Rehabilitation Robotics Into Neurorehabilitation—cont'd

Screening Criteria	Service Robotic Devices	ASSISTIVE ROBOTIC DEVICES	
		Nonwearable—Mobility and Unweighting	Wearable—Mobility and Object Manipulation
Screening criteria to determine if patient has the **ability** to use advanced or robotic technology	Patient has potential to achieve independent wheelchair mobility and ADLs at home with reduced human assistance: 1. Has cognitive ability to control motorized and robotic devices 2. Has the sensory, physical, and cognitive abilities to control a motorized chair (e.g., via joystick, head movement, button press, breath, piezoelectricity, voice) without human assistance 3. Can activate an automated harness system to transfer into a wheelchair 4. Can sit in a chair with or without positional assistance 5. Has sufficient understanding and ability to activate robotic service and emergency devices to be independent without human assistance (smart house designs)	Patient has the potential to improve walking quality and speed, endurance, and independence with progressive practice or training: 1. Has cognitive ability to participate in training 2. Has sufficient attention and understanding to cooperate in gait training 3. Has adequate head and trunk control to maintain postural uprightness when legs moving 4. Has sufficient strength in legs to stand up when unloaded or protected from falling 5. Has some sensation in lower limbs or can see legs 6. Has partial movement in major muscle groups in lower limb (hip, knee, ankle) 7. Has sufficient range of motion to get into standing or walking position 8. Can transfer onto the treadmill or transfer from chair to standing 9. Tone does not prevent the feet from staying on the ground or stepping when unloaded 10. Has ability to step when standing over ground or over treadmill 11. Steps after perturbation of the treadmill 12. Can swing leg through clearing floor or treadmill (with or without AFO) 13. Stepping speed can be changed with treadmill speed 14. Can tolerate training several hours a week	Patient has the sensory, physical, and cognitive ability to control a wearable device to achieve independence in mobility and/or object manipulation: 1. Has intellectual ability to understand how to use the wearable assistive orthotic device 2. Has the ability to don the wearable assistive device (or has someone at home to help) 3. Is motivated to use a wearable assistive robotic device to improve independence 4. Has basic stability of the head and trunk to move the limb(s) (even if positioning device is required) 5. Involuntary movements do not interfere with robotic assistance 6. Has adequate standing balance (with or without cane or walker) to work with a wearable assistive orthotic gait training exoskeleton 7. Has the range of motion to allow full or partial task function 8. Has adequate sensation to sense rubbing and chaffing of orthotic device 9. If inadequate sensation, has sufficient vision, audition, touch, or cognition to monitor wear and control of interface 10. Has adequate strength to lift the weight of the exoskeleton 11. Has sufficient voluntary control to assist the exoskeleton 12. Able to use the robotic assistive device several hours per day 13. Has the physical, sensory, sensorimotor, and/or cognitive skills to control the interface of the assistive robotic device 14. If unable to meet 13, may be eligible for advanced technology using a brain interface
Screening criteria to determine **temporary versus permanent need** for technology	Patient has: 1. Goals and objectives to be functionally independent without personal assistance 2. Predictable disease- or impairment-specific issues that are not going to change or may get worse 3. A support system (family or community) to check on status at home 4. Home that can be modified to accommodate robotic equipment	Patient has: 1. Goals and objectives to be functionally independent without personal assistance 2. Predictable disease- or impairment-specific issues that necessitate regular exercise to maintain independence 3. A progressive neurodegenerative condition that could be slowed with regular exercise 4. A support system (family or community) to check on status at home 5. Access to public transportation to access resources 6. The ability to drive (e.g., take driver's training or simulation; car modification) to maintain independent access to needed resources	Patient has: 1. Goals and objectives to be functionally independent without personal assistance 2. Predictable disease- or impairment-specific issues that require regular exercise to maintain and maximize independence despite injury or disease 3. Ability to maintain if not maximize independence despite injury 4. Ability to use robotic technology to improve functional recovery 5. Ability to put on and remove the assistive devices 6. Ability to slow down progression or maintain or improve function despite neurodegenerative condition that could be slowed with protected, guarded, stress-reduced intense exercise 7. A support system (family or community) to check on status at home 8. Access to public transportation to achieve community independence 9. Ability to maintain independent community driving with regular training, simulation, car modification

Continued

TABLE 38.4 **Screening Patients for Integrating Advanced Technology or Rehabilitation Robotics Into Neurorehabilitation—cont'd**			
		ASSISTIVE ROBOTIC DEVICES	
Screening Criteria	**Service Robotic Devices**	**Nonwearable—Mobility and Unweighting**	**Wearable—Mobility and Object Manipulation**
Screening criteria to determine **safety**	Patient has: 1. Ability to call for emergency help if devices do not work 2. Secondary harness systems to prevent falling with robot-assisted transfers 3. Ability to manipulate control devices to stop or encourage function of the robot 4. Ability to turn off the robot when inappropriate movements develop	Patient can: 1. Safely step on and off the treadmill 2. Tolerate the tension of the harness or unweighting system 3. Spontaneously step as triggered by the moving treadmill 4. Express concern if exercising beyond his or her limits 5. Manipulate the parameters of the treadmill 6. Tolerate the end range parameters for performance (e.g., high speed)	Patient has: 1. Adequate sensation to notice increased pressure or chaffing or skin sensitivity to electrodes 2. Ability to decrease the hypertonicity that interferes with function or causes pain 3. Sufficient cognitive awareness to recognize abnormal robotic behaviors (e.g., forced movement in abnormal directions) 4. Ability to stop excessive, abnormal movements 5. Ability to initiate self-directed movements with robotic assistance
Screening criteria to determine **accessibility** of advanced or robotic technology	Patient has: 1. Access to financial resources to afford advanced technology 2. Access to technology that is currently commercially available 3. Access to technology that is currently accessible in his or her geographical area 4. Opportunity to arrange for technical help to maintain equipment 5. Evidence available in terms of cost-effectiveness 6. Insurance that will help cover costs	Patient has: 1. Resources to purchase needed equipment for home use 2. Resources to pay to use equipment in the community 3. Equipment that is commercially available in his or her community 4. Equipment available in the community 5. Evidence on cost-effectiveness of the technology 6. Insurance that will help pay for lease or purchase	Patient has: 1. Resources to obtain assistive robotic devices 2. Access to commercially assistive robotic devices in his or her area 3. Ability to have equipment brought to his or her residence 4. Access to someone to fit, maintain, and repair the device 5. Evidence on cost-effectiveness 6. Insurance to assist with payment
Screening criteria to determine **cost-effectiveness** of advanced technology or rehabilitation robotics	There are clinical research trials reporting: 1. Objective outcomes as measured by decreased personal assistance, which can be documented in terms of hourly costs saved 2. That resource investment costs can be amortized across 5 years 3. That patients could gain 5–10 years of independent function at home 4. That the patient would be able to sustain independence at home (versus in skilled living environment) in the last few months of life	1. Objective outcomes focused on maintaining independence at home in lieu of an extended care facility 2. Patient can minimize falls and decrease risks for inpatient stay resulting from fall injuries 3. Patient able to sustain safe, independent indoor navigation without personal assistance 4. Patient able to get out of house and move in community independently or with public transportation	1. Objective outcomes focused on maintaining independence at home 2. Patient can perform ADLs and community activities safely 3. Patient uses assistive devices to minimize risk of falls 4. Patient remains committed to brain and physical fitness 5. Patient maintains safe, independent indoor and outdoor navigation without personal assistance 6. Patient able to get out of house and move in community independently or with public transportation

ADL, Activities of daily living; *AFO,* ankle-foot orthosis.

whether the insurance company will help pay for the rental or purchase of the device.

Ideally patients will use a wearable robotic assistive device to try to drive neural adaptation to recover function. Thus some patients may "train out" of the robotic device as they recover more function. Obviously, it would be better for these patients to rent rather than purchase the orthotic. Other patients would benefit from purchasing the assistive device because the robotic device improves function and independence despite ongoing impairments. Long-term use is also common when a patient has a degenerative condition, when the impairments are likely to get worse rather than better, and when with assistance independence can be prolonged.

In addition to the general and specific screening criteria, it is important to note that some assistive robotic devices may target control of one specific joint. However, given the biomechanical links, the flexibility, sensory, and motor characteristics must be assessed at each major joint above and below the primary assisted joint. The less affected side also needs to be evaluated. To maximize the benefit of a wearable assistive device, patients should ideally have some ability to voluntarily initiate movement and a grade of poor or greater strength to be able to assist in the movement.

Wearable robotics must be programmed not only to assist patient function but also to stop to avoid harm. This requires a balance between the dynamic nature of the wearable assistive device and a patient's weakness, lack of voluntary motor control, and the presence of involuntary muscle activity including hypertonicity (e.g., spasticity, dystonia, rigidity, tremor). For example, how much force would the assistive device need to provide to overcome involuntary tone? Other relevant questions must then be asked: If a robotic device is programmed to assist with flexion and the patient initiates movement into extension or abduction, will the robot have to stop assisting the limb to prevent harm? If the robot stops assisting, is there a negative effect caused by the mismatch of force between the patient and the robot? Does the patient need consistent assistance or variable assistance? How will the therapist, the robot, or the patient determine how much assistance is needed? In one case a patient may need unweighting of only a limb, and in another case, both unweighting and assistance may be needed. In theory, the amount of assistance needed should decrease with recovery of function. It is helpful if the wearable assistive device can easily be adjusted by the therapist or the patient.

Despite the advancements in rehabilitation robotics, some patients will still have difficulty wearing an assistive orthotic. For example, wearable assistive orthotic devices may not work well for patients with severe sensory impairments, severe balance problems, a fear of falling, inadequate assets to control the device or for elderly patients who are afraid of computerized technology. Sophisticated rehabilitation robotic devices (Boxes 38.3 and 38.4) also may not be recommended for patients who are disoriented, who have severe pain or neural hypersensitivity, or who cannot don the apparatus independently.

It may be appropriate and helpful for patients with severe sensory and motor impairments to train using VR technology with or without assistive technology. Patients may begin with mental imagery and practice before engaging in physical practice, without and then with the

---

BOX 38.4 Types of Nonwearable Assistive Robotic Devices

- Body weight–supported mobile walking aids
- Robotic devices for physical support (indoors, outdoors)
- Robotic devices for physical support, unweighting, and mechanical stepping in place
- Robotic devices for unweighting and controlled destabilization
- Robotic devices for unweighting and gait training
- Robotic devices for unweighting and robotic stepping on a treadmill

---

integration of wearable robotic devices. It is also possible to begin the training with the assistive technology while in a harness system to protect the patient from falling. In addition, depending on the severity of balance and voluntary abilities, it may be necessary for patients to train with technology under careful direct supervision. In cases in which balance and motor control are good but can be improved, it may be possible for patients to train at home with wireless telemetry-type supervision.

Please refer to the Evolve site for a video case illustrating the use of technology in the rehabilitation of a child with cerebral palsy.

Patient Simulator Robotics

Purpose

One area of robotics contributing to improved rehabilitative care and education of rehabilitation professionals is the development of programmable human patient simulators. This section of the chapter describes programmable human patient simulators that are currently available. Programmable human patient simulators can be used to replicate many common medical conditions. Simulation is used to train clinicians so that when those rehabilitation professionals encounter a similar clinical situation they can respond more efficiently and effectively.

Introduction

Simulation using task trainers, actors, and standardized patients is not new to the education of rehabilitation professionals. While task trainers are useful for development of specific skills (e.g., cardiopulmonary resuscitation [CPR]), immersive simulation using high-fidelity robotics can be used to simulate and practice working with a variety of medical conditions, situations, and health care personnel. In addition, these scenarios can be repeated so every student has an opportunity to deal with a variety of specific medical conditions including rare but critical events (e.g., acute myocardial infarction [MI]).

In 2011 Stockert and Brady reported that approximately 44% of entry-level physical therapist professional education programs in the United States were using some form of programmable human patient simulator.[52] In 2017 Stockert and Ohtake reported that the percentage of entry-level physical therapist professional education programs using programmable human patient simulators for immersive simulation had increased to 70% and about 40% of those programs were using the technology for interprofessional education (IPE).[53,54] Education programs reported using the technology to train health care providers from multiple disciplines for interprofessional team responses to the challenges of providing care for a patient suffering an acute MI or a patient in need of early mobility in the intensive care unit. About 90% of the programs using simulation for IPE reported including the IPE Collaborative learning objectives for interprofessional, collaborative practice.[53,55] The vast majority of these programs included interprofessional teams of de-briefers consistent with best practice patterns described in the literature.[56] The authors noted that they anticipate a

---

BOX 38.3 Types of Service Robotic Devices

- Fixed—preprogrammed task performance
- Mobile service—mechanical slaves
- Wheelchair-mounted—upper-limb manipulators
- Automatically guided wheelchairs
- "Smart houses"—designed for independence

further increase in the utilization of immersive simulation as an educational strategy for IPE in order to promote interprofessional collaborative practice and to comply with recently revised accreditation standards related to IPE in multiple health care professions.[54]

Currently available robotic patient simulators can be programmed to demonstrate clinical signs and symptoms consistent with a diverse group of clinical conditions seen by Physical Therapists and other rehabilitation professionals. The patient simulator can be programmed to present signs and symptoms that require a participant to analyze and determine the urgency of the situation, assess the "patient" status, determine an appropriate intervention, and see the consequences of their action or inaction without compromising patient safety. A wide variety of clinical conditions and situations can be presented in an effort to ensure that each participant has an opportunity to practice and receive feedback regarding their clinical performance with multiple medical conditions. Simulation experience is critical for practicing how to respond to common as well as rare but critical events (e.g., acute MI). The learner's ability to respond appropriately during a simulated event can increase the likelihood that those rehabilitation professionals are adequately prepared to respond efficiently and effectively when encountering a similar situation in the clinic.

Technology

At the beginning of 2018 there were two primary manufacturers of programmable human patient simulators. METI Learning (Medical Education Technologies, Inc.) started making patient simulators in 1996 and was acquired by CAE Healthcare in 2011 (https://caehealthcare.com/). Asmund Laerdal, with Drs. Lind and Safar, developed "Resusci Anne" for learning CPR in 1960. The Laerdal Corporation has been making a variety of patient simulators since that time (https://www.laerdal.com/us/). In this chapter on rehabilitation robotics, the properties and capacities of programmable human patient simulators are discussed based on currently available models by those two manufacturers. This analysis will hopefully help rehabilitation professionals evaluate the benefits of new robotic simulators for professional education.

Features

The number of features available on programmable human patient simulators continues to increase and raise the degree of realism (fidelity) attainable during immersive simulation. Many features, including eyes that blink and the simulated patient conversing in real-time, make the clinical scenario realistic for the participant. Several clinically relevant characteristics of human patient simulators are described on the following pages.

Size. The size of the adult human programmable patient simulator mannequins is similar to an average-sized full-grown adult, but the weight is significantly less than average (approximately 85 pounds). In addition to adult models, there are baby simulators, child simulators, and birthing simulators. Some models are wireless. This discussion focuses on the features and properties of the adult high-fidelity simulators available in 2018.

Limb and chest mobility. The upper and lower extremities of most programmable patient simulator models have very limited passive mobility with the exception of the shoulders, hips, knees, and ankles, which approach "normal" for an adult. The limited mobility of the limbs allows for some range of motion and bed exercises to be simulated. However, clinicians will note the completely passive, and somewhat awkward, nature of the movement and that the limb weight is significantly less than normal.

The chest wall moves realistically during ventilation. The excursion of the chest can be programmed to be symmetrical or asymmetrical in order to mimic specific clinical conditions. In addition, the rate and depth of ventilation can be manipulated during the course of a simulation.

Physiological features. High-fidelity programmable human patient simulators have realistic physiological features. A library of normal and abnormal breath sounds, heart tones, bowel sounds, and other sounds is available to aid in simulating a variety of clinical conditions. All of the breath sounds, heart tones, etc., can be changed during the course of a simulation to reflect a change in "patient" status during a scenario.

The simulation mannequins can be connected to multiple lines and tubes to simulate an acute care and/or critical care environment; for example, arterial line, intravenous line, nasogastric tube, electrocardiograph wires, and nasal cannula. Lines and tubes, appropriate for the simulated condition, add to the realism of the scenario. The presence of multiple lines and tubes allow the participant to practice identifying the lines and tubes, verify the patient status, and practice "clearing" the lines.

A patient monitor, similar to those found in critical care settings, is part of the setup to enhance realism. The monitor can be customized to display a number of different physiological variables including arterial blood pressure, pulmonary blood pressure, respiratory rate, cardiac rhythm, hemoglobin saturation, intracranial pressure, pH, temperature, and others. The value and number of variables shown on the monitor provide real-time patient data and can be programmed to change during the course of the simulation to simulate clinical conditions and/or a change in patient status.

Pulses are palpable in a variety of locations including the carotid, brachial, radial, femoral, popliteal, and dorsalis pedis pulses. The pulse is synchronized with the electrocardiogram (ECG), and the pulse strength can be varied during a simulation. When a simulation participant palpates the pulse, a notation is made in the computer log that specifies which pulse was palpated and at what point in time during the simulation the pulse was taken. In addition, when blood pressure is low, some pulses (e.g., the dorsalis pedis) are no longer palpable, simulating the clinical condition of systemic hypotension.

High-fidelity human patient simulators are capable of vocalizations using a variety of sounds stored in the simulation computer. However, the simulation operator is able to speak into a microphone and/or use audio files to produce sounds that appear to come from the mouth of the mannequin where a speaker is located. The capacity to converse in real-time greatly elevates the fidelity of the scenario.

Cyanosis is simulated through the use of a light contained within the mouth that makes the lips and gums appear blue. The eyes can form tears, the eyelids blink, and the pupils are reactive to light. The skin in the forehead is capable of diaphoresis. In some areas, the skin has "wound modules" that can be inserted and connected to ports that contain "blood" used to simulate bleeding from the wound site.

Cerebrovascular system features. High-fidelity human patient simulators can be programmed to display signs and symptoms consistent with an acute cerebrovascular accident (CVA) or traumatic brain injury (TBI). The simulator has the potential to display a slurred speech pattern, a drooping eyelid, asymmetrical pupils, and emotional lability. The simulator can state that their arm or leg feels heavy and that they cannot feel the limb. The patient monitor can be programmed to show a variety of changes consistent with an evolving CVA or TBI, such as changes in blood pressure, heart rate, intracranial pressure, and respiratory rate.

Cardiovascular and pulmonary system features. The onset of an acute MI is a scenario commonly used in simulation to train clinicians. The patient simulator can be programmed to complain of chest pain while simultaneously developing diaphoresis. The patient monitor can show the changes in the blood pressure, heart rate, respiratory rate, and cardiac arrhythmias consistent with an acute MI. Scenarios can be used to practice recognizing the signs and symptoms related to multiple acute medical conditions as well as to practice interdisciplinary health care team responses to acute crises. The advanced features of the cardiovascular system include the capacity to bleed from a variety of portals. The system permits health care personnel to practice advanced cardiac life support (ACLS) protocols and to practice team responses to medical emergencies. The ACLS features built into the patient simulators measure and record the rate and depth of chest compressions, as well as hand placement, during CPR. This allows "coaching" of the participants' CPR skills/technique in real-time.

The physiological response to a variety of drugs and clinical conditions is programmed into high-fidelity models. This feature allows participants to witness the response to the administration of medications as well as adverse drug reactions. The advanced clinical features for the pulmonary system include the ability to intubate (esophageal and endotracheal) and insert chest tubes into the mannequin, providing students and clinicians an opportunity to practice their clinical skills with "patients" who are intubated and/or have a chest tube. Some simulators allow the participant to practice pulmonary suctioning techniques.

A variety of cardiac arrhythmias are programmed into the patient simulators, and these can be displayed on the patient monitor, for example, atrial fibrillation and ST segment depression. This feature allows the operator to alter the ECG tracing on the patient monitor during the course of a simulation indicating a change in patient status. All of this physiological information is stored in the computer log and can be used during the debriefing session to enhance the learning experience for participants.

Programmability of Patient Simulators

In addition to the features discussed previously, high-fidelity simulators have the capacity to be defibrillated and undergo cardioversion. The physiological response to many drugs and clinical conditions is programmed into some models so that participants can witness the acute response to the administration of medications as well as adverse drug reactions and/or the physiological response to the acute onset of a clinical condition (e.g., acute MI). In addition, instructors can design custom simulations to meet specific instructional needs and learning objectives.

Costs of Establishing a Simulation Laboratory

The costs associated with establishing a simulation laboratory will vary with the type of programmable human patient simulator selected, additional equipment required and/or desired, and the amount of training needed. High-fidelity programmable human patient simulators can cost $100,000 to $200,000 for top-of-the-line models with state-of-the-art features. However, the price of the simulator(s) is only a portion of the setup costs. Establishing a simulation laboratory will also require (1) space designed for the simulation laboratory; (2) audiovisual equipment; (3) networking infrastructure; and (4) training in how to operate the system. The cost for each of these individual components can vary markedly depending on the type of equipment and infrastructure present as well as the level of sophistication desired in terms of audiovisual and networking capacity.

SUMMARY

Each new generation of programmable human patient simulators has improved our ability to teach excellence in examination, assessment, and problem solving in acute, critical care situations. Programmable patient simulators have advanced in (1) the degree of realism provided by the technology and (2) the ability of the operator to manipulate and alter the "patient" status at any point in time. Human patient simulators are now found in multidisciplinary clinical teaching centers in academic health care institutions. They have been incorporated into community-based training courses for practicing health care professionals. A high degree of realism can be provided during simulation using currently available robotics when high-fidelity simulators are placed in a realistic mock intensive care unit. The combination of a high-fidelity patient simulator and a realistic environmental setting provides an opportunity to train rehabilitation professionals to recognize and respond to changes in patient status and to practice working as members of an interprofessional health care team without compromising patient safety.

Wearable Inertial Sensors

Introduction

Assessment of mobility is complex because it includes many different neural control systems associated with balance and gait, as well as adaptive mechanisms for maintaining mobility under altered conditions.[57] Neurorehabilitation is particularly challenging since there is not one specific joint angle or measure to focus on for assessment and treatment. However, it is well accepted that balance and gait should be evaluated and monitored in patients with neurological deficits. Clinical characterization of balance and gait abnormalities can be highly dependent on examiners' expertise since subjective rating scales are typically used in the clinic.[58,59] Furthermore, there is a need for sensitive and objective documentation of deficits, either for recovery or decline, to help incrementally measure performance at all levels of disability. Although there are many performance-based, clinical tests of balance and gait, many tests suffer from ceiling effects in highly functioning or compensated individuals.[58,60] Sophisticated laboratories have been characterizing balance and gait disorders for many decades, but it has not been practical for physical therapy practitioners to routinely use information obtained in the gait laboratory for clinical decision making. In the majority of circumstance, gait laboratories and clinical spaces are entirely separate. However, these laboratory measures of balance and gait are now becoming available to physical therapists via new technologies involving small, body-worn, wearable inertial sensors. Over the past 15 years, advances in wireless technology, such as small wearable inertial sensors, have emerged as a viable tool for objective movement assessment.[61] This chapter will provide an overview of the potential uses, benefits, and obstacles of utilizing wearable sensors in the field of neuro-rehabilitation.

What Are Wearable Inertial Sensors?

Wearable inertial sensors, also called movement monitors, are small and lightweight sensors embedding usually a tri-axial accelerometer, tri-axial gyroscope, and magnetometer (for heading measures with respect to the earth magnetic field). One or more sensors placed on different parts of the body are used for mobility assessment, and synchronized data can be collected from multiple sensors, with high frequency data-sampling. Clinical user-interfaces that provide useful information and sophisticated automatic data analysis are transforming this technology for clinical use. In fact, body segment orientation and displacement in space can now be measured, replacing more expensive, time-consuming, and nonportable, motion analysis systems in laboratories.[62–64] This means that joint range of motion can be measured accurately during dynamic movements, such as gait, lunges, and stair climbing, not only in static conditions, as with goniometers. Thus gait measures, such as stride length, pitch ankle of the foot at heel strike, and foot clearance from the floor, can now be calculated from these inertial sensors.[65–67]

Some commercial systems have only one sensor, placed on the lumbar region, which allows a physical therapist to measure postural sway and, sometimes, temporal characteristics of gait, such as cadence, trunk stability, and number of steps (e.g., *McRoberts, SwayStar, BTS*). Other systems include a sensor on each foot to more fully characterize the spatial and temporal characteristics of foot motion during gait and turning (*GaitUp, APDM, and BioSensics*). Currently two systems (by *APDM and BioSensics*) allow additional synchronized sensors on the legs, trunk, and arms that allow full body characterization of balance, gait, and postural transitions, such as sit-to-stand and turning. Multiple inertial sensors can also be used to measure kinematic joint angle movements (*Xsens*), but clinically friendly systems with simple user-interfaces are needed. It is important for physical therapists to consider the quality and quantity of the validation and reliability studies of movement monitor systems as well as their ease of use, quality of reports, and supported clinical protocols, such as the Timed Up and Go (TUG) and Clinical Test of Sensory Integration for Balance (CTSIB).

Wearable inertial sensors are different from activity monitors. Activity monitors have been around for 50 years and are designed to measure the *quantity* of movement, such as how long a person is walking or running or when they are sedentary versus active. Activity monitors, such as the *StepWatch, activPAL, and Actigraph*, use only accelerometers (either uniaxial or tri-axial) to detect the number and size of acceleration spikes associated with body motion, usually to count steps or calculate time spent in different postures.[68–70] Activity monitors are popular devices for lay consumers because they can count steps per day (such as pedometers), hours of sleep (from periods of nonmoving, and horizontal posture), time spent in different postures (walking, lying down, and sitting), sedentary time, and estimates of calories burned and cadence (steps per minute). Usually, a single activity monitor is worn on the wrist or belt. They also have the advantage of a long battery life, with up to 30 days of continuous recording, and they are increasingly inexpensive. However, physical therapists should be cautioned about using widely available consumer devices, such as smart phone applications and exercise devices (e.g., *Jawbone, Basis, and NikeFuel*), in their clinical practice because they have not undergone validity testing for accuracy or reliability, especially with patient populations. Activity monitors of any type provide limited information on gross activity patterns and cannot provide physical therapists information on quality of movement, joint kinematics, or motor impairments.

Can Wearable Sensors Improve our Assessment of Balance and Gait in the Neurological Population?

Wearable inertial sensors have the potential to improve physical therapy assessments by (1) providing objective measures at the impairment level, (2) providing a greater sensitivity to detect subtle changes in balance and gait, and (3) providing data on gait and balance during regular daily function (home monitoring).

Measure Impairment

A key recommendation from the International Classification of Functioning, Disability and Health framework (ICF) is to assess a person across several levels of function and disability to include items measuring participation, activity, and impairments.[71] Many validated scales used in physical therapy measure participation (i.e., quality of life or balance confidence) and activity (i.e., Berg Balance Scale or TUG). Impairments are problems in body function and structure, such as significant deviation of symmetry, muscle weakness, or increased postural sway. An accurate impairment-level assessment of balance and gait is often difficult to obtain, but wearable inertial sensors during activity-based assessment may help. Wearable inertial sensors have recently been used to quantify aspects of mobility during the TUG test, CTSIB, and 2-minute walk.[72–83] Although each of these assessment tools fall under activity level assessment, adding inertial sensor information may provide impairment level details. These objective impairments can then be used by physical therapists to precisely target and monitor progress in their therapy (Fig. 38.6).[84–86]

Detect Subtle Deficits

Assessment tools that objectively capture deficits in the mildly impaired population are an important goal for neurorehabilitation therapists.[87–90] To make measureable treatment goals, the physical therapist must first identify objective measures of gait and balance to target. Reimbursement of physical therapy services requires evidence of the problem[91] and of gradual improvement with therapy. Many clinical balance scales and stopwatch measures are insensitive to mild impairments in high-level performers,[58,92,93] such as athletes and military populations. Even in those people with early stage disease, there is evidence to support early rehabilitation intervention for promoting neuroplasticity, emphasizing the value in early detection of balance and gait problems.

Recent research has shown added value, over traditional clinical measures, of objective measures in several neurological populations, such as multiple sclerosis (MS), Parkinson disease (PD), and mild traumatic brain injury populations (mTBI).[77–80] For example, although patients with very mild, untreated PD have normal 3m TUG performance time compared to age-matched controls, (10.8 ±_0.5 seconds

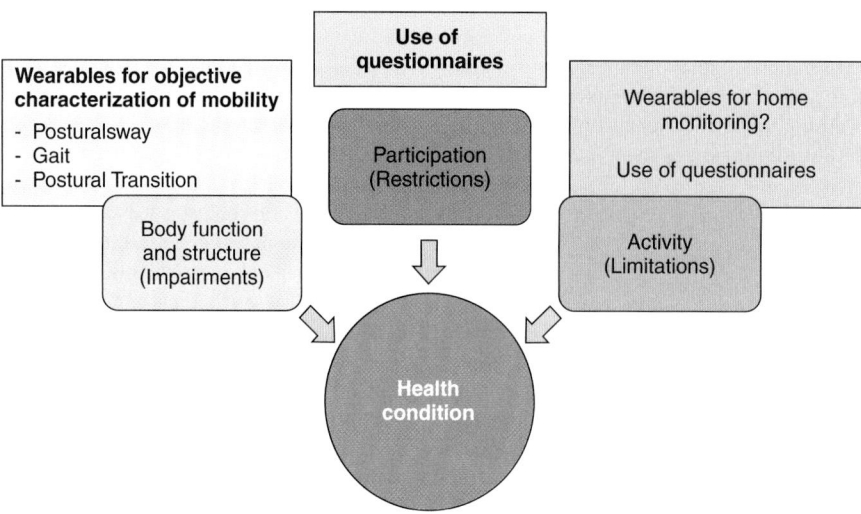

Fig. 38.6 Integrative Model of Functioning and Disability.

vs. 9.9 ± 0.3 seconds, respectively), they show other impairments in quality of walking and turning.[94] Interestingly, sometimes the same parameter can be impaired in a different neurological population but in the opposite direction (see example in new Fig. 38.7 for the trunk rotation during gait). This measure is a lower than normal value in untreated PD but is higher than normal in mild MS. These results are important since a physical therapist would address each one very differently to improve this aspect of gait.

Several studies have shown that patients with mTBI, both chronic and acutely concussed, may have normal Balance Error Scoring Systems (BESS) scores but simultaneously have abnormal postural sway profiles during the same test.[92,95] The BESS relies on the examiner to count how many errors the person makes during progressively harder stance positions, while the sensor objective details several aspects of postural sway such as amplitude, velocity, frequency, and jerkiness. Particularly, we found in a population of 76 healthy controls and 52 mTBI that the objective measures of the instrumented BESS outperformend the clinical BESS, even in the simple double stance condition (Fig. 38.8).[95]

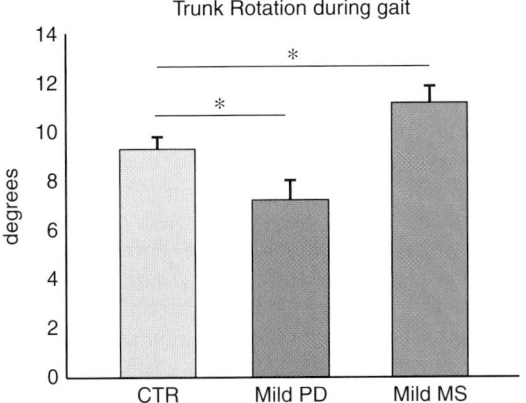

Fig. 38.7 Group mean and standard errors of trunk rotation during gait (instrumented 7 m Timed Up and Go) in healthy control, people with mild multiple sclerosis (*n* = 31), and people with mild Parkinson disease (*n* = 12).

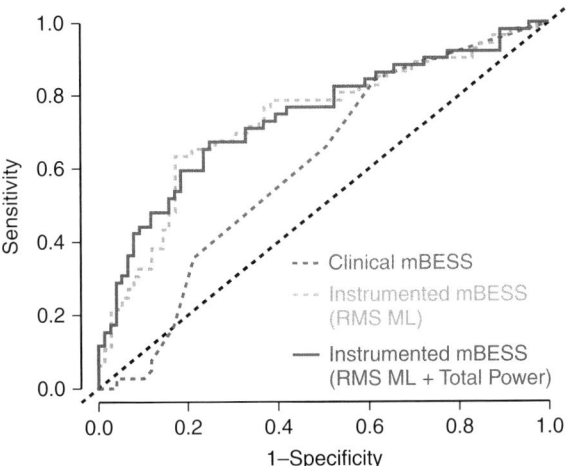

Fig. 38.8 ROC curves to discriminate among healthy controls and people with mild traumatic brain injury populations for the clinical mBESS errors count, and instrumented *mBESS* models of one or a combination of two postural sway objective measures. *mBESS*, Modified Balance Error Scoring System; *RMS ML*, root mean square medial-lateral; *ROC*, receiver operating characteristics. (Modified from King LA, Mancini M, Fino PC, et al. Sensor-based balance measures outperform modified balance error scoring system in identifying acute concussion. *Ann Biomed Eng.* 2017;45[9]:2135–2145.)

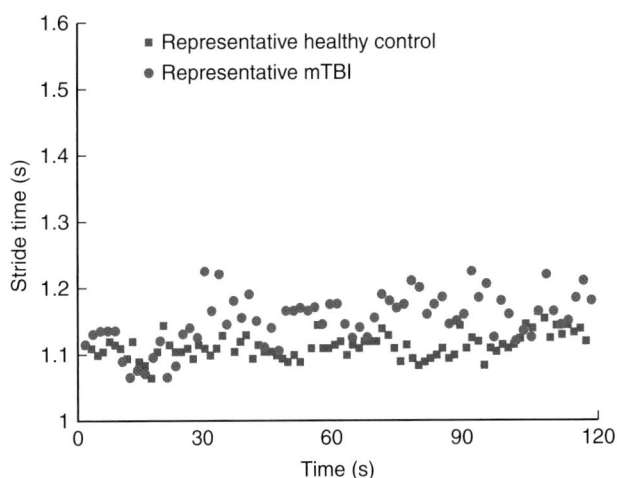

Fig. 38.9 Stride time for each gait cycle over 2 minutes of walking in a representative healthy control and mild traumatic brain injury (*mTBI*) subject. Larger spread indicates larger variability of gait. (Modified from Horak F, King L, Mancini M. Role of body-worn movement monitor technology for balance and gait rehabilitation. *Phys Ther.* 2015;95[3]: 461–470.)

This distinction may occur in gait in this population as well. For example, Fig. 38.9 compares step-by-step stride duration during a 2-minute walk in a person with mTBI and a representative control subject. Such increase in variability of stride time while walking is indicative of dynamic balance deficits during gait.[96] These relatively "high-level" mobility impairments could easily be missed by physical therapists limited to traditional balance and gait testing.

Home Monitoring

Assessment of mobility in the clinic does not always reflect mobility in daily life. It is often reported that patients walk better when they are examined in an outpatient clinic or in a research laboratory than at home. This phenomenon is known as the "white coat effect"; physical therapists who work in both the clinic and in-home health care settings may be familiar with this concept. Motor performance can be changed depending on attention, alertness, and effort to impress the examiner during testing. Therefore mobility measured during functional activities of daily life can provide further insights on function, disability, and the effect of therapies. Recent advances in better battery life and ease of use point to the possibility of continuous and/or home monitoring of specific aspects of movement. Several research groups have demonstrated feasibility including new studies that that take place in the home and community settings using wearable, lightweight inertial sensors to measure mobility for multiple days.[97,98] Novel measures of turning and gait characteristics, calculated from wearable inertial sensors, enable a detailed analysis of mobility over weeks of continuous monitoring. Previously, continuous monitoring was limited to use of activity monitors to measure the quantity of activity, but now inertial sensors allow continuous monitoring of quality of activity.[97–99] Although this approach to measurement holds promise, it is primarily limited to research studies at this point. In particular, research has been focusing on gait bouts characteristics and turning, from either a single sensor on the belt, or three sensors (two on the feet and one on the belt).[97–105] Novel measures determined from both accelerometers and gyroscopes enable a detailed analysis of variability, consistency of gait bouts and turning in both healthy and neurological populations. However, standardization or a consensus on a specific set of measures and on a definition of gait bout at home are still missing.[100]

Can Wearable Sensors Improve Treatment for Balance and Gait in the Neurological Population?

Impairment-Focused Rehabilitation

Rehabilitation focused on improving mobility may benefit from having sensitive, quantitative measures of specific impairments underlying balance and gait disorders. Performance tests of mobility, such as the Berg Balance Scale or the TUG, measure whether an individual *can* accomplish tasks, such as turn in a circle or walk a particular distance. However, inertial sensors provide objective measures of impairments documenting *how* and *why* the individual's balance and/or gait is impaired. Physical therapists can then use objective measures to guide their exercise programs to specific impairments.

Specific balance and gait impairments identified by inertial sensors are potentially modifiable when therapy is targeted to the impairments. Consider the two groups of patients with mild disability in Fig. 38.7, one with MS and the other with untreated PD. Both groups had normal gait speed, measured with a stop-watch during the Time-to-Walk 25 feet (T25FW) or the TUG. However, both groups showed abnormal balance and gait characteristics with instrumented tests. Specifically, both groups showed significant impairments in the rotation of their upper trunks while walking.[83,106] However, the patients with PD showed significantly *decreased* trunk rotation, whereas the MS patients showed significantly *increased* trunk rotation during gait, compared to healthy subjects. Therefore therapy focused for the PD group may be focused on increasing trunk rotation, such as by increasing arm swing and reducing axial rigidity, whereas therapy for the MS group may be focused on decreasing trunk instability during gait, as by increasing core strength and use of a cane. In contrast, when physical therapists are limited to measuring only the duration of the TUG, which was normal in both groups of patients, it may be more difficult to justify, focus, and measure effects of therapeutic intervention.

Therefore different impairments may reflect problems with different, independent, neural control systems.[107–109] Identification of specific types of balance problems allows for more specific rehabilitation to remediate the constraints on safe mobility.[110]

Biofeedback Rehabilitation

An important role of the physical therapist is to provide patients with accurate feedback about their performance and movement errors. Wearable inertial sensors have great potential to augment feedback (biofeedback) using more immediate and more sensitive feedback than therapists can apply without technology. Biofeedback is an approach that can use technology to provide biological information to patients in real-time that would otherwise be unknown.[111] Thus biofeedback complements normal internal feedback and acts as an additional "sixth sense" or as "sensory substitution" for patients who have lost sensory function. For example, we are currently using an audio-biofeedback approach in patients with mTBI who have excessive postural sway during quiet stance, when vision is limited.[112] In this project we will compare standard vestibular rehabilitation with the same rehabilitation program using real-time audio-biofeedback to reduce postural sway and provide feedback on body position. Audio-biofeedback is applied as a tone that increases in volume as postural sway increases, with more sound in the right ear during right direction sway and in the left ear during left direction sway. Forward and backward sway are indicated by a high-pitch tone and low-pitch tone, respectively. Since it is not possible for physical therapists to manually provide quick, accurate feedback about postural sway, biofeedback can supplement balance training (see example in Fig. 38.10).

Wearable sensors based-biofeedback is currently being developed to train dynamic tasks such as walking and turning. Preliminary data

Feet together on firm surface

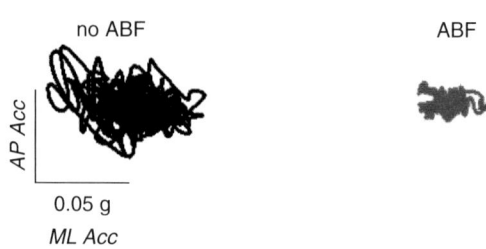

Fig. 38.10 Reduction of postural sway with audio-biofeedback from a wearable inertial sensor on the belt during stance on a firm surface with eyes closed in a patient with a mild traumatic brain injury. (Modified from Horak F, King L, Mancini M. Role of body-worn movement monitor technology for balance and gait rehabilitation. *Phys Ther.* 2015;95[3]:461–470.)

in the laboratory have demonstrated the validity and efficacy of a tactile biofeedback system to improve turning in a cohort of 43 people with PD.[113] The data collected with *a tactile biofeedback* prototype showed a significant improvement in turning mobility in the laboratory in 23 people with PD and freezing of gait (FoG) and 18 people with PD without FoG of similar age (70 ± 7 years old vs. 69 ± 7 years old), disease duration (8.2 ± 4.7years vs. 9.3 ± 6.5 years), and MDS-UPDRS III (43.6 ± 11.6 vs. 47.1 ± 10.1). Subjects turned in place for 1 minute (changing turning direction after each 360 degree turn) in a single- and dual-task (counting backward by threes) for three randomized conditions: (1) baseline (no cues); (2) turning to the beat of a metronome (open-loop); and (3) turning with phase-dependent tactile biofeedback (close-loop). All subjects who reported FoG showed mild-to-moderate freezing during the assessment. Objective measures of freezing, such as the percentage of time spent freezing and FoG ratio, were decreased when turning with both open-loop and close-loop cueing compared to baseline (Fig. 38.11A). The dual-task did not worsen FoG in freezers, but significantly slowed down turns in both groups. Both cueing conditions significantly improved turning smoothness in both groups (see Fig. 38.11B), and reduced turning velocity and number of turns compared to baseline. Interestingly, it was found that the benefit obtained with the biofeedback persisted during a turning task with a concurrent cognitive task, suggesting that these benefits could translate during everyday life. In addition, the slowing of turning with cueing has been previously reported[114–117] and could be seen as improvement considering that we previously found that larger postural instability is associated with fast turns by people with PD.[118–119]

This technology is not yet available for clinical practice, but we foresee integration of this and other systems in rehabilitation to compliment and reinforce the therapist feedback in the clinic, and ultimately, may be used to help the patient at home (Fig. 38.12).

Important Considerations in Wearable Inertial Sensors for Balance and Gait Rehabilitation

There are some important obstacles to consider when implementing wearable inertial sensors for neurorehabilitation. A major barrier to use in the clinic is the added training and time it will take for the physical therapist to add wearable inertial sensors to the evaluation (clinical utility, Fig. 38.12). Furthermore, it is unclear how billing will be handled for insurance claims.

Moreover, an ideal system based on wearable inertial sensors should be cost-effective, user friendly, and easy to use and administer (feasibility and practicality). It is of paramount importance that the

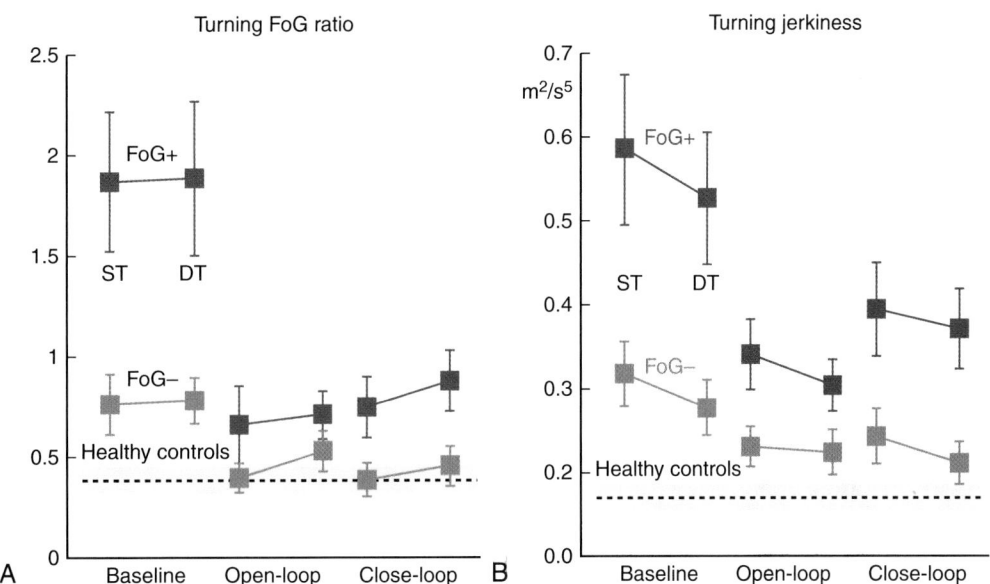

Fig. 38.11 (A) Freezing severity, measured by the FoG ratio for baseline, open-loop and closed-loop conditions in freezers (*FoG+*) and non freezers (*FoG-*) for both single-task, ST and dual-task, DT. **(B)** Turning jerkiness in the same conditions.

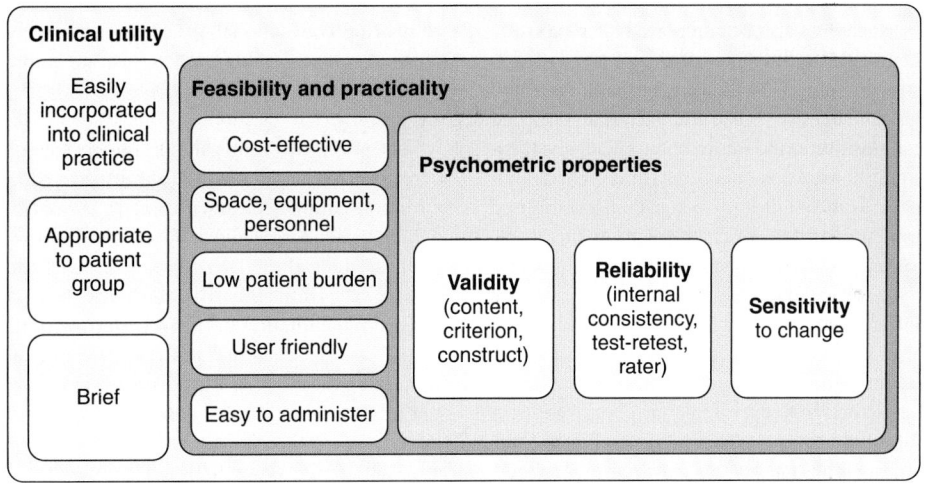

Fig. 38.12 Summary of General Requirements for Outcome Measures.

end-user of wearable inertial sensors systems understands the provided measures of mobility, and with the rapidly changing products in the market it is important to research the specific clinimetrics (validity, reliability, and sensitivity to change). As many measures extracted from wearable inertial sensors are novel, minimal detectable change and minimal important clinical difference have yet to be established.

Future Direction/Conclusions

It is an exciting time to follow the interface of technology with clinical neurorehabilitation for assessment and treatment of our patients. Ideally, the best products for use would have input during development from the end-user, the physical therapist. It is predicted that physical therapists will soon use inertial sensors to evaluate balance and gait continuously, during daily activities for more ecological and realistic understanding of patients' mobility in the real world. Physical therapists will soon be able to incorporate real-time biofeedback to improve motor learning and motor performance both during a regular training session as well as remotely. With technology becoming more and more

accessible and pervasive, physical therapists need to critically evaluate the advantages and limitations of implementing emerging technologies, such as body-worn sensors, into their clinical practice.

Virtual Reality Technology

Introduction

VR is defined as an approach to user-computer interface that involves real-time simulation of an environment, scenario, or activity that allows for user interaction via multiple sensory channels.[120] The use of VR allows for interaction between the patient and a computer-generated, three dimensional environment.[121] In VR, the user networks with an artificial world through visual, aural, and haptic interfaces. Other ways of interaction with a VR environment include a computer mouse, a joystick, or using VR goggles.[122] In some instances, the VR technology allows for customization of avatars, which provide the person another way of immersing the physical body into the VR environment.[123]

Following a neurological injury, the ability to interact with the environment can be limited by physical impairments. The availability of VR technology allows a person to interact with a realistic replica of physical space or certain situations. This has contributed to the rapidly emerging use of VR in neurological rehabilitation. This section will discuss the use and potential clinical application of VR in patients with neurological dysfunction.

The Rationale for Virtual Reality in Rehabilitation

The facilitation of neuroplasticity is what underpins neurological rehabilitation. However, not one therapy intervention is able to address the core principles of neuroplasticity.[3] As such there an impetus for therapist to find multiple, novel ways to facilitate neuroplastic change and to enhance functional recovery following a neurological injury.

Following a neurological injury, the resulting impairments often lead to activity restriction and eventually to limited participation with one's role in life and society. The use of VR has shown potential in being able to address impairment, disability, and handicap.[124] Following damage to the central nervous system, there is often an inability for a person to actively engage and interact with the environment and surroundings. This can often lead to a lack of sensorimotor stimulation and creates an impoverished environment in which one recovers.

Numerous studies in animal models have demonstrated the positive effect of environmental enrichment on the brain. Increases in brain weight[125] and cortical thickness[126] after environmental enrichment have been reported. Synaptic plasticity has also been reported after exposure to an enriched environment with studies demonstrating increased synaptogenesis,[127] synaptic strengthening,[128] neurogenesis,[129] and increased dendritic branching, length, and density.[130] The influence of an enriched environment has also been positive in the injured brain. Rats given experimental brain lesions and housed postoperatively in enriched environments were shown to perform significantly better than rats housed in impoverished environments.[131] The enriched environments comprised of opportunities to perform different activities and social interaction with other rats. The social interaction component when combined with an enriched environment was further shown to result in the best outcome.[132] The mechanism behind the beneficial effects of an enriched environment in postinjury outcome has been attributed to the increased synthesis of neurotrophic factors.[133] Neurotrophic factors are thought to be capable of promoting the neuronal survival and are likely to be involved in synaptic reorganization and alteration in receptor expression.[133,134] As neuronal changes in response to an enriched environment have been documented in the cortex, hippocampus, cerebellum, and striatum, future studies should look into its therapeutic benefits. Stimulation from an enriched environment may prove to be an important causative factor in enhancing functional plasticity following neuronal injury and damage.

Emerging experiences that bring about motor learning can also drive plastic changes in the motor cortex. The use of VR has inherent attributes that can lead to experience-dependent plastic changes and motor learning.[135] One key principle of neuroplasticity centers around the concept of practice.[3] The need for constant, intense, contextual practice is thought to be a major driver of plastic changes in the brain. With VR, clinicians are given a variety of conditions in which practice can be manipulated[135] and enable frequent and task-specific training.

Feedback is another major component in motor control and learning.[136] With VR, there are multiple sources of feedback comprising visual, auditory, and tactile.[135] This augmented feedback has been shown to have merit in terms of recovery of function in a stroke population.[137] The ability of controlling the type of feedback has added benefits in tailoring VR experiences to a particular patient's needs or goals.[138] Motivation is another key driver of motor learning.[139] Often

because of the resulting physical impairments from a neurological injury, patients are not motivated to move because of the associated difficulty and increased effort needed for movement. The visual, auditory, and tactile feedback a person receives from VR can be used easily by clinicians as an effective motivation tool.

The motor imagery that is triggered by VR can induce the activation of mirror neurons.[140,141] Mirror neurons are activated by observation and fire the same way as when one actively moves.[142] This ability to respond through perception and execution makes the activation of mirror neurons attractive in the rehabilitation and recovery of function. Practicing within a VR environment allows for observational experience and, theoretically, may enhance physical practice of a task.[143]

Clinical Application of Virtual Reality

With the potential for enhancing neuroplasticity at hand, there has been an increase in studies reporting the benefits of using VR (Fig. 38.13; a video example can be found at: www.youtube.com/watch?v=lT3Klg7_KVo) in neurological rehabilitation. Using 3D-simulated tasks practiced through a desktop computer, improvements were noted in the performance upper limb functional tasks in one of the two subjects presented in a case report.[144] In a bigger sample, enhanced feedback from VR was evaluated in terms of improving arm function in patients with stroke.[145] Following 1 hour of daily VR training in a month, improvements over baseline values in the mean scores on the Fugl-Meyer (FM) and Functional Independence Measure scales were reported. In comparing conventional therapy with one that is supported by VR, both groups were able to demonstrate improvements in FM scores with greater improvements observed in patients who had additional VR training.[146]

The effects of VR on gait parameters have also been explored. Using a treadmill mounted on a 6-degrees-of-freedom motion platform with a motion-coupled VR environment, patients with stroke were able to demonstrate increased gait speed and improved their ability to adapt to physical terrain.[147] The subjects received auditory and visual cues as a form of positive/negative feedback. In a comparison of a robot-assisted rehabilitation protocol with or without VR support, improvements in moments and powers generated in the ankle and hip of subjects in the robot-VR group were significantly greater than those in the robot-alone group.[148] A meta-analysis of 21 studies looking into the effects of VR training on balance and gait suggested that balance and gait training using a VR environment was more effective that balance and gait training without VR.[149]

The immersive nature of VR has been used in cognitive rehabilitation. A computer-simulated virtual kitchen was used to assess the ability to process and sequence information in a group of patients with

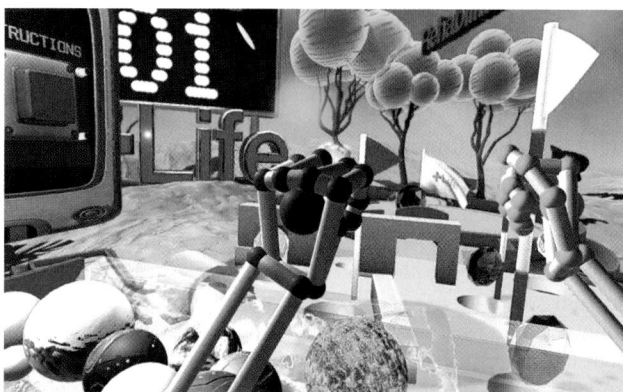

Fig. 38.13 Scene From a Virtual Reality Simulator. (Courtesy of Add-Life Technologies.)

brain injury and volunteers without brain injury.[150] Although this was not used as a therapeutic tool, the study reported the merit of using a computer-generated VR environment assessing cognitive function in persons with acquired brain injury. In a reported case study, VR was used to assess and train people with memory issues.[151] The subject was trained using a detailed computer-generated nonimmersive 3D virtual environment based on a route of an actual rehabilitation unit. Following 2 weeks' training, the subject was able to learn the route practiced in the virtual environment, but not the route practiced in the real unit, and retained her knowledge of the route in the virtual environment.

The ability of VR to provide training in a controlled and standardized setting has given it merit as a therapeutic tool in facilitating recovery following a neurological injury. Clinicians are also able to tap into the novel concept of VR to enhance neuroplasticity. The challenge there is for developers of VR technology to update the settings and scenarios to prevent adaptation and boredom with the system. The clinical effectiveness of VR in neurological rehabilitation, although increasingly being reported, lacks the statistical power to warrant recommendation as part of standard rehabilitation practice. As with most emerging technologies, further investigation into the principles, parameters, and variations of VR is needed to allow clinicians and patients to make an informed choice regarding its use in rehabilitation.

Noninvasive Brain Stimulation in Neurological Rehabilitation

Introduction

The development of noninvasive brain stimulation (NBS) techniques have enabled a quick, easy, and well-tolerated method of studying brain function in normal and pathological conditions. NBS also has been used to modulate the excitability of the cortex and enhance the functional plasticity of the brain. The clinical use of NBS has been studied in patients with stroke, PD, dementia, and other neurological conditions. Numerous studies have reported the use of NBS as a diagnostic and prognostic tool after a neurological issue as well as using NBS as a neuromodulation adjunct in rehabilitation and therapy.

The use of NBS in a therapeutic environment has primarily been aimed at modulating cortical excitability. NBS is used either to increase the excitability of the damaged motor cortex or to inhibit the activity of the intact cortical hemisphere. This neuromodulation has also been reported to balance neural activity between the two cortical hemispheres following injury. Furthermore, NBS has been reported to induce changes in synaptic efficiency, which can be used to drive motor relearning and the recovery of function.

This section will discuss two NBS techniques involving the use of transcranial magnetic stimulation (TMS) and transcranial direct current stimulation (tDCS).

Transcranial Magnetic Stimulation

TMS (Fig. 38.14) is a common technique used to activate and test propagation of impulses from the central to the peripheral nervous system. First introduced by Baker in the 1980s, TMS allows for an easy, painless and noninvasive method in obtaining information regarding the excitability of the nervous system and the functional integrity of neural structures and connections.[152] TMS also provides valuable, quantifiable measurements such as motor evoked potentials (MEP), conduction time, and cortical maps, which offer variables such as map area, map volume, and center of gravity (CoG). These variables are often used to describe and detect the subtle changes associated with neural plasticity.[153,154]

TMS works on the principle of electromagnetic induction. A high-current pulse is passed through an insulated coil, which induces a magnetic field that then passes painlessly through tissues. This magnetic field

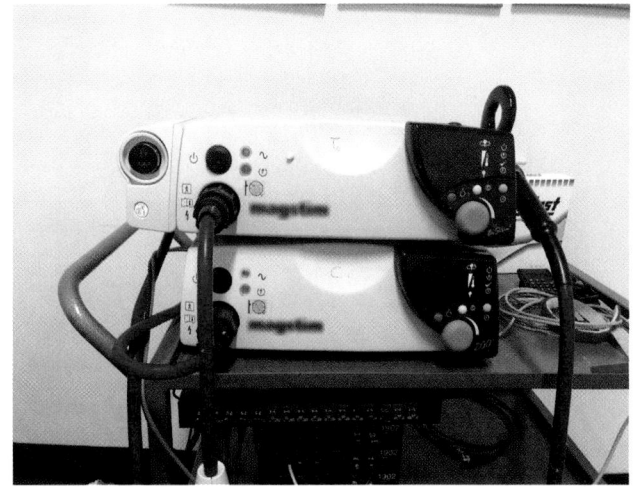

Fig. 38.14 Transcranial Magnetic Stimulator.

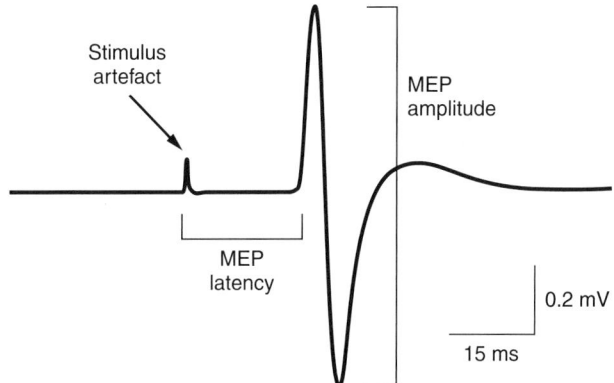

Fig. 38.15 Motor Evoked Potential *(MEP).*

runs perpendicular to the plane of the coil.[153] When the coil is held over the scalp, the skull offers very little impedance to the magnetic field produced. As the magnetic field passes through, it induces electric currents or eddy currents that flow at right angles to the magnetic field.[153,155] With the appropriate current direction, duration, and amplitude, depolarization of the motoneuron pool will occur and generate an MEP on the target muscle.[156]

The MEP (Fig. 38.15) is a common reference used to assessing corticospinal excitability in both normal individuals and those of neurological dysfunction.[157,158] The amplitude of the MEP indicates the integrity of the corticospinal tract and that there is intact propagation of impulses from the cortex to the nerve roots, down to the target muscle. In addition, the amplitude gives an indicator of the size of corticospinal projection to a given muscle as well as the excitability of the projection.[159,160]

Apart from MEP, other TMS variables reported include central conduction time[161] and motor threshold.[162] TMS is also used to produce cortical representational maps of areas of the motor cortex in normal and pathological populations.[163–166] These TMS variables provide objective and quantifiable measures to describe and detect the subtle changes associated with neural plasticity.[153]

As TMS provides focal stimulation of the motor cortex, the excitability of the cortex can theoretically be easily influenced. TMS offers differing stimulation parameters that can either induce cortical inhibition or cortical excitation.[167,168] Repetitive transcranial magnetic stimulation (rTMS) (Fig. 38.16) is a form of NBS used to drive cortical excitability and facilitate functional plasticity of the brain.

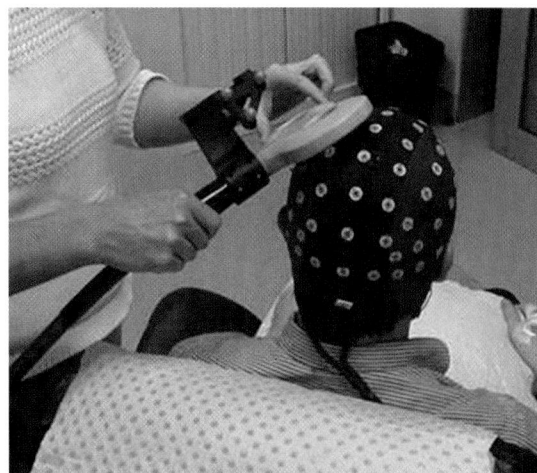

Fig. 38.16 Repetitive Transcranial Magnetic Stimulation.

Using a series of repetitive transcranial magnetic stimuli, rTMS at a low frequency (<1 Hz) has been shown to induce inhibition in the corticospinal network, while stimulation at a high frequency (>5 Hz) increases cortical excitability.[169,170]

Using high-frequency TMS bursts at 30 to 50 Hz at theta frequency has also been used to modulate cortical excitability.[171] Theta Burst Stimulation (TBS) is a form of rTMS that also leads to facilitatory and inhibitory effects on the motor cortex.[167] The desired effect of TBS works on the timing on when you apply the burst. Huang and colleagues showed that using a continuous TBS (3 stimuli at 50 Hz repeated every 200 ms) resulted in a suppression of MEPs.[167] Subsequently, using an intermittent TBS pattern (a 2-second train repeated every 10 seconds for a total duration of 190 seconds) resulted in the facilitation of MEPs.

It has been proposed that combining peripheral afferent stimulation with low-frequency transcranial brain stimulation facilitates changes in cortical excitability. Using a paired associative stimulation (PAS) paradigm, synchronously combining median nerve stimulation with low-frequency TMS over the optimal cortical activation site for hand muscles showed significantly increased resting MEP amplitude for abductor pollicis brevis.[172] The improved MEP was conditionally dependent on the timing of the arrival of the afferent stimulation and the TMS on the motor cortex. In addition, the plastic changes induced by synchronously pairing stimulation evolved rapidly, persisted, reversible, and remained topographically specific. Using a similar dual stimulation protocol, significant changes in excitability were seen together with cortical expansion of the scalp representation area for First Dorsal Interossei (FDI).[172] The expansion was accompanied by a significant movement of the CoG of the cortical map taken from FDI and the changes observed persisted for at least 2 days. The changes observed in the stimulated muscles persisted for up to 5 days without the need for further stimulation. It has been suggested that the immediate neuroplastic changes associated with a dual stimulation intervention may be analogous to mechanisms that involve fast-learning of a motor task. With repeated sessions of dual stimulation, these changes were found to be persisting and long-lasting and indicate that a process of consolidation maybe taking place.[173] The persistent and prolonged changes reported may have therapeutic value and provide another method of improving motor control and function in people with neurological injury.

Using Transcranial Magnetic Stimulation in Rehabilitation

The ability of using TMS to modulate cortical excitability has made it an attractive tool in neurological rehabilitation. Its application has been reported in patients with stroke, PD, and dementia, to name a

few. Using the ability to facilitate or inhibit cortical excitability, TMS has been shown to influence improvements of function in people with neurological issues.

The clinical application of TMS has been widely reported in stroke rehabilitation. It has been proposed that following a stroke, the inhibitory interactions between the two hemispheres are affected and can contribute to impaired function. There is a mutual transcallosal inhibition that occurs between the two hemispheres, but this is usually asymmetrical with the dominant hemisphere (usually the left) providing more inhibition to the nondominant hemisphere.[174] Following a right hemisphere stroke, the interhemispheric inhibition would be lost with the left hemisphere becoming even more dominant and providing more inhibition to the usually less dominant and now injured right hemisphere. This hyperexcitability of one hemisphere usually contributes to patients showing neglect or issues with spatial awareness on their affected side. In such situations, it is feasible to consider using TMS to decrease the excitability of the unaffected hemisphere and to modulate the balance of excitation and inhibition between hemispheres. Improved motor function of the paretic hand was demonstrated using rTMS with improved scores on with the pegboard test, and improved reaction times and force production.[175,176] Using an inhibitory rTMS protocol over the stroke-lesioned parietal cortex have demonstrated improvements in clock drawing and line bisection tests.[177–179] Significant improvements were also reported following use a continuous TBS (cTBS) protocol in outcome measure scores of the affected hand.[180–182] Although current literature is showing great potential for using rTMS to downregulate the intact hemisphere to address motor function in stroke, most of the studies have not reported any long-term follow-up and thus puts into question the possible long-term benefits of its therapeutic use. As with most approaches in physical therapy, longer, larger, and more robust trials are needed to inform rehabilitation practice.

Following a stroke, MEPs elicited by TMS have been shown to be delayed or absent[183,184] and the intensity of stimulation needed to evoke an MEP higher.[185] There is also great variability of MEP amplitude in people with chronic stroke when compared to healthy adults or the contralesional hemisphere.[186–188] The MEP response latencies were also reported to be longer in the stroke-affected side when compared to the unaffected side and was associated with impairments of the upper and lower limbs.[189,190] These parameters have been used to assist in the prognosis of motor and functional recovery following stroke.[191–193]

The ability of TMS to increase the excitability of the cortical network has been extensively reported. The use of high-frequency rTMS has been shown to assist in improving hand function across the different stages of stroke. In a group of patients in the acute stage of stroke, rTMS was shown to significantly improve disability scores following 10 days of stimulation combined with usual rehabilitation treatment.[194] Significantly larger MEP amplitudes were reported following rTMS of the affected hemisphere.[195] The increased MEP amplitude was also accompanied by improved accuracy in a sequential finger motor task. Improvements that lasted up to 1 week were also seen following rTMS in grip strength, range of movement, and pegboard scores.[196] In two groups of patients in the subacute stage of stroke who received either rTMS or sham TMS, improvements were noted for the Motoricity Index and the Box and Block test. The rTMS group showed additional improvements in motor function in the FM assessment.[197]

Changes in motor cortex excitability following rTMS targeting the lower limb areas in patients with stroke has also been reported. Applying rTMS for 20 sessions combined with physical therapy showed a significant improvement in gait velocity and TUG scores, as well as a significant reduction in physiological cost index measures.[198] This preliminary study also reported that using high-frequency rTMS at 10-second bursts at 10 Hz with 50-second intervals for 20 minutes was safe and well tolerated. Improvements in the 10 m walk test was also reported following 3 weeks of high frequency rTMS.[199] The effects persisted for 4 weeks but did not reach statistical significance owing to the small sample size. A randomized controlled trial using rTMS plus task-oriented training on people with chronic stroke showed improvements in motor control and walking ability.[200] The study used a 1-Hz stimulation frequency over the leg area of the motor cortex of the unaffected hemisphere for 10 minutes. This resulted in a reduction of interhemispheric asymmetry of MEP amplitude and increased cortical excitability as well as improved lower limb impairments. However, the subjects showed measurable MEPs from their rectus femoris, which may indicate that they may already have a higher level of function.

The use of rTMS also has been reported in the treatment of post-stroke dysphagia where the stimulus is usually applied to the pharyngeal/oropharyngeal motor cortex. This application of rTMS resulted in increased corticobulbar excitability, improved swallowing, and deglutition in both acute and chronic stroke patients.[194,201–203] Alongside conventional rehabilitation, the use of rTMS seem to provide a novel therapy in the management of swallowing issues after a stroke.

Improvements in motor function also has been reported from the application of PAS in people with stroke. In a pilot study combining TMS with a 10-Hz stimulation of the peroneal nerve, a dual stimulation paradigm was able to show an increase in neurophysiological (Fig. 38.17) and functional gait parameters in a group of patients with chronic stroke.[166] Following 4 weeks of dual stimulation, subjects showed improvements in maximal MEP amplitude and cadence, stride length, and time to heel strike. However, as it was only a small pilot study, the improvements reported were not statistically significant.

Using an inhibitory PAS paradigm applied to the contralesional motor cortex resulted in a 91% decrease in MEP amplitude of tibialis anterior (TA) in the nonaffected side and a 130% increase in the MEP amplitude of TA on the stroke-affected side.[204] The same group compared the effects of contralesional rTMS and PAS with ipsilesional anodal tDCS on walking ability post-stroke. Although the results revealed changes in cortical excitability, there was considerable variability in the responses to the protocol, and they were unable to demonstrate any significant change in lower limb muscle responses. In a single intervention of combined rTMS, peripheral nerve stimulation,

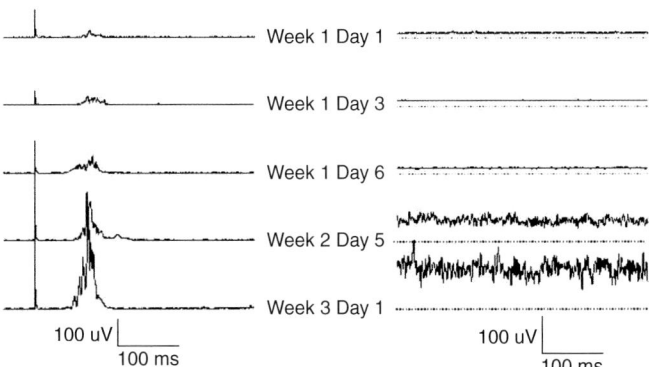

Fig. 38.17 An example of raw data traces from a subject from Uy et al.,[166] who responded positively to the dual stimulation intervention. *Left panel*: Average rectified motor evoked potentials (MEPs) in the weak peroneus longus muscle. The top trace shows that on day 1 before any dual stimulation the MEP was very small. The MEPs evoked at the same stimulus intensity increased dramatically in amplitude over successive days during the course of this intervention. *Right panel*: Mean rectified Electromyography (EMG) recorded during maximal voluntary contractions of the peroneus longus on the same days. The dotted lines are at 0 V. *EMG*, Electromuography.

and wrist and finger extension exercises, combining motor training with rTMS and neuromuscular stimulation facilitated user-dependent plasticity and improved motor function that persisted for 2 weeks.[205] A single session of rTMS applied on the ipsilesional cortex revealed improvements in index finger tapping as well as a reduced activity of the contralesional cortex as revealed by functional magnetic resonance imaging (fMRI).[206] These studies highlight the possible merit of using NBS as a method of priming and modulating the cortical excitability in stroke rehabilitation.

The effect of using TMS as a therapeutic modality of PD has also been reported. In PD, measuring the cortical silent period following TMS has been correlated to dopamine deficiency as this has been linked to cortical inhibitory circuits.[207] The cortical silent period (cSP) has also been reported to shortened when "off medication," normalizes while on medication, and is lengthened during the dyskinetic state.[208,209] The improvements reported from using TMS in PD are varied having a positive effect on gait parameters[194] or no effect at all.[210,211] The use of TMS in PD is not as widely reported as with the stroke population and with inconsistent reports on its benefits. The clinical usefulness of using TMS as an adjunct for rehabilitation in people with PD is still being questioned.

In patients with MS, the use of rTMS has been reported to have a beneficial effect on spasticity,[212] gait performance,[213] hand dexterity,[182,214] and working memory.[215] Similar to PD, the evidence to its benefits are limited and warrants further investigation to its clinical application.

Also there has been limited reports on the possible application of TMS in people with Alzheimer disease (AD). Improvements in cognitive function has been reported following rTMS, including improvements in reaction to a working memory task,[216] sentence comprehension,[217] naming performance,[218] and action naming[219] across various stages of AD. These findings again provide initial promising evidence in using rTMS as an adjunct in managing cognitive decline in AD.

Another variation of using TMS in modulating cortical excitability is TBS. This involves using high-frequency bursts of stimulation, usually around 30 to 50 Hz, delivered at theta frequency. Similarly, TBS can either have an excitatory or inhibitory effect on the cortical network. Delivering a cTBS results in a reduction of cortical excitability while intermittent bursts of TBS (iTBS) can increase the excitability of the cortical network.[167] These two protocols have been applied to patients with stroke and have resulted in increased MEP amplitude on the affected side following iTBS, and a suppression of cortical excitability in the nonaffected cortex following cTBS.[220] However, during the acute stage of stroke, both cTBS to the nonlesioned cortex and iTBS to the lesioned cortex resulted in increased excitability of the affected cortex with accompanying functional benefits.[221] Combining iTBS to the ipsilesional motor cortex with task training resulting in improvements in grip lift of the affected upper limb.[222] An interesting finding of this study was the reduction of upper limb function following cTBS of the nonlesioned hemisphere, highlighting the role of the nonlesioned hemisphere in the recovery of upper limb function following stroke. In a group of chronic stroke patients, no significant difference was found between the TBS treated and the sham group, with both groups showing clinically important improvements.[223] These conflicting reports of results from TBS puts into focus the high variability of patient response to the treatment and the need for further refinement of the parameters of TBS when applied to a lesioned brain.

Mechanism of Cortical Plasticity Following Transcranial Magnetic Stimulation

The attractiveness of using NBS in neurological rehabilitation lies in its ability to modulate cortical excitability. Various mechanisms have been proposed to explain the changes in the excitability of the cortical network. Studies using animal models, healthy human brains, and the injured cortex have provided vast evidence that the cortical changes observed following TMS are brought about by stimulation-induced neuronal activation and from changes in synaptic efficiency.[224]

The mechanism underlying the changes seen following various forms of TMS correlate to mechanisms involved in activity dependent long-term potentiation (LTP) and long-term depression (LTD).[225] LTP is defined as a sustained increase in synaptic strength brought about by high-frequency stimulation of excitatory afferents.[226,227] The process of LTP follows Hebb's postulate wherein simultaneous pre- and post-synaptic activity provide multiple inputs to a cell and results in the strengthening of synapses in the activated pathway. Another form of activity-dependent plasticity is LTD, which induces rapid, activity-dependent reduction of responses in relation to irrelevant sensory stimuli.[228,229] Heterosynaptic LTD, wherein a second pathway is activated to produce a depression in the inactive pathway, has been suggested as the possible mechanism involved in the reorganization of cortical representational maps.[230] The capacity of LTP and LTD to induce a bi-directional change in synaptic efficiency is influenced by the arrangement and organization of the stimulation arriving in the cortex, with adjustment of the strength of the synaptic connections dependent on parameters such as frequency, timing, and intensity of inputs.[231,232] The mechanisms involved in the induction of LTP and LTD in the cortex also can be influenced by the administration of drugs that interfere with glutamatergic activity. The application of N-methyl-D-aspartate (NMDA) receptor antagonists has been shown to block the inhibitory and excitatory effects of rTMS. Glutamatergic NMDA receptor activity has been linked to facilitation LTP and LTD in cortical circuits.[233,234]

The nature of the changes induced by TMS when combined with PAS also suggest a role for LTP- and LTD-like processes.[172] The process may involve the unmasking of previously silent cortico-cortical or cortico-subcortical connections. The mechanisms by which this unmasking is brought about may include both a reduction of local inhibition or changes in synaptic efficacy.[170] The significance of LTP or LTD changes is its connection to neuroplasticity. Specifically, LTP has been linked to learning and memory.[235] These attributes have given value to the use of NBS such as TMS as a substrate for functional recovery following neurological injury.

Transcranial Direct Current Stimulation

Another method of induction of cortical excitability is tDCS. This technique uses weak direct currents (DCs) to modify the excitability of cortical cells. The application of tDCS uses two surface electrodes placed over the scalp wherein a continuous electrical current of 1 to 2 mA is applied for around 10 to 20 minutes. The resulting cortical stimulation does not induce the necessary action potential and hence does not produce any visible muscle contraction. The application of tDCS in humans has been shown to be safe and without any side effects, and to date there has been no report or evidence to show that tDCS has harmful or adverse effects on humans (Fig. 38.18).[236,237]

The stimulation brought about by tDCS results in a depolarizing or hyperpolarizing effect on cortical neurons. The polarization effects result to changes in MEP amplitude and have been attributed to changes in cortical excitability.[237] Increases in cortical excitability are generally expected when using anodal tDCS, and a reduction in excitability is seen with cathodal tDCS. A reduction in TMS evoked MEP amplitude was seen following cathodal stimulation; however, TES evoked MEPs did not show any change. Similarly, no effect was found on H-reflex measurements, suggesting that tDCS influences cortical neurons and has no significant effect on spinal excitability. These induced changes were dependent on the polarity, intensity, and duration of the stimulation as well as the orientation of the electrodes.[168,238,239]

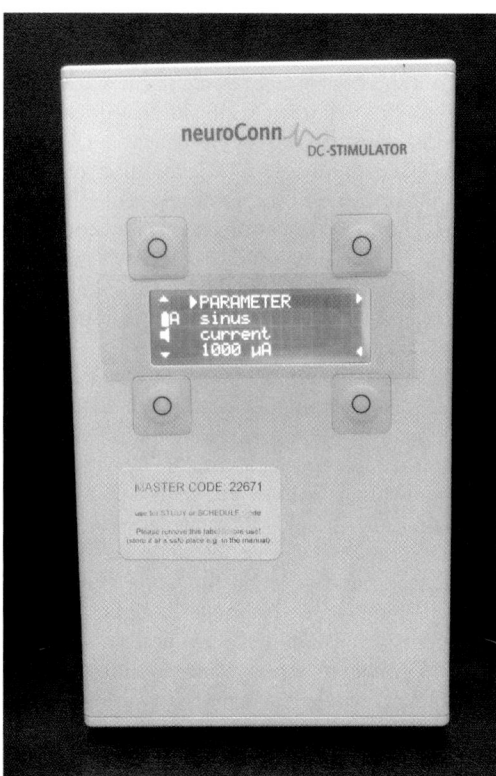

Fig. 38.18 Typical Transcranial Direct Current Stimulator.

Applying Transcranial Direct Current Stimulation in Neurorehabilitation

The use of tDCS in facilitating the recovery of function has become an emerging area of interest in rehabilitation (Fig. 38.19). The inhibitory and excitatory capacity of tDCS has been explored in people with stroke. Improvements in function was reported following anodal tDCS over the stroke affected cortex and a cathodal, tDCS on the nonaffected hemisphere,[240,241] highlighting the possible asymmetry of interhemispheric activity in stroke. The effect of using anodal and cathodal tDCS on the affected and nonaffected hemisphere also has been applied in stroke patients showing neglect. With one to two sessions of tDCS application, there were significant effects on the results of the line bisection test and the shape-unstructured cancellation test.[242,243] Using anodal tDCS over the lower limb primary cortex of the stroke affected hemisphere during motor practice of the affected ankle resulted in improvements in ankle control.[244] There was no mention of any measurement of gait parameters, and the subjects tested were either moderate to well recovered from their stroke. A meta-analysis on the use of anodal tDCS to facilitate upper limb recovery following stroke reported an overall increase in the level of upper limb motor function. There was small to moderate change in function when comparing baseline outcome scores with scores at the end of the studies analyzed.[245] Although there were encouraging results from the therapeutic use of anodal tDCS, there was still great variability in patient responses and minimal follow-up to ascertain its clinical effectiveness.

Mechanism of Change

The mechanisms underlying the effects of tDCS has been proposed to involve changes in the behavior of neuronal membranes.[246] It was suggested that tDCS manipulates ion channels or shifts electrical gradients to affect neuronal signaling and have an effect on the electrical balance of ions, involving primarily nongated and voltage-gated channels.[246]

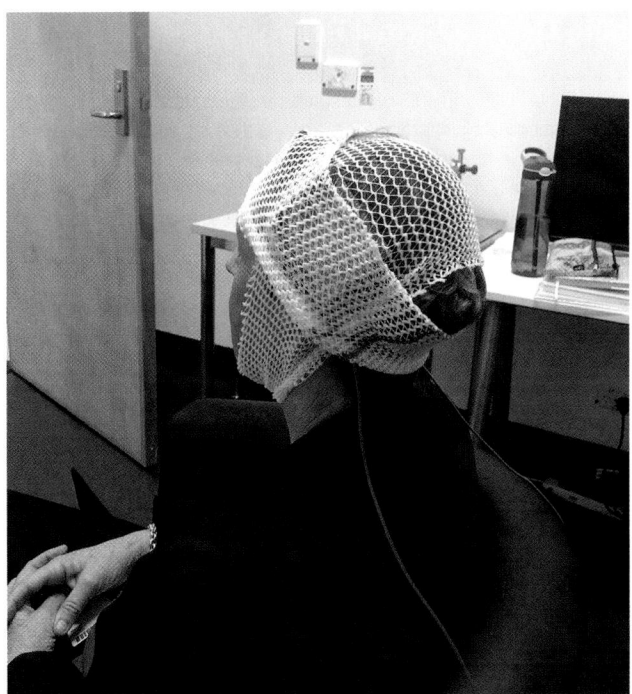

Fig. 38.19 Application of Transcranial Direct Current Stimulation on the Scalp Surface.

The application of tDCS stimulation has been shown to affect membrane depolarization. The depolarizing effect of a DC can result in the activation of voltage-sensitive events that involve presynaptic sodium channels increasing the release of excitatory neurotransmitters and postsynaptic elevation of Ca influx.[239]

The application of a Na^+ channel blocking agent carbamazepine and NMDA receptor antagonist dextromethorphan (DMO) resulted in changes in DC-stimulation-induced neuroplasticity. DMO suppressed the induced plastic change by anodal and cathodal DC stimulation in a group of healthy human subjects. Anodal stimulation has been shown to increase excitability and cathodal stimulation to reduce excitability.[239] The suppression of these effects by DMO would suggest the involvement of NMDA receptors in DC-stimulation-induced synaptic plasticity.[247] NMDA receptors in the postsynaptic neuron act as Ca channels, thus their activation will lead to an increased influx of Ca. The entry of Ca in the postsynaptic neuron activates Ca dependent

second messengers, which results in the increased availability of the glutamate receptor AMPA. This will enable the postsynaptic neuron to be more sensitive to presynaptic release of glutamate, which is necessary for maintaining LTP.

Clinical Application of Noninvasive Brain Stimulation

There is a growing interest in using NBS as a therapeutic adjunct in the rehabilitation of people with neurological issues. This is mostly from the ability of NBS to influence motor learning by priming or modulating the excitability of the cortical network (Table 38.5). The notion of being able to provide rehabilitation and training during a period of increased cortical excitability will be an attractive option for therapists.

In spite of the plausible benefits from using NBS in rehabilitation, its therapeutic effectiveness is often variable. Most of the studies available lack statistical power to warrant clinical recommendation, and with such varied protocols available, it is difficult to ascertain which one is suited for a particular type of patient. The future clinical application of NBS will be highly dependent on the development of more advanced tools of monitoring and evaluating cortical activity and the collaboration of neuroscientists and clinicians with the goal of improving the quality of life of people affected by neurological disorders.

TABLE 38.5 Summary of the Different Types of Noninvasive Brain Stimulation and Its Effects

NBS	Type	Effect
TMS	rTMS	
	Low frequency	Inhibitory
	High frequency	Excitatory
	TBS	
	Continuous	Inhibitory
	Intermittent	Excitatory
	+ PAS	Excitatory
tDCS	Anodal	Excitatory
	Cathodal	Inhibitory

NBS, Noninvasive brain stimulation; *PAS*, paired associative stimulation; *rTMS*, repetitive transcranial magnetic stimulation; *TBS*, theta burst stimulation; *tDCS,* transcranial direct current stimulation; *TMS*, transcranial magnetic stimulation.

CASE STUDY 38.1 Vestibular Rehabilitation Training Using a Virtual Reality Environment

Mrs. S. was a 52-year-old woman who came to the clinic with a diagnosis of unilateral vestibular hypofunction and the chief complaint of being unable to go into large crowds or stores or to shop without feelings of dizziness and disorientation. Clinical and laboratory findings revealed bilaterally reduced vestibular evoked myogenic potentials and a unilateral caloric weakness on the right. The patient reported onset of her symptoms 1 month ago with tinnitus and difficulty walking in crowds and in grocery stores. She was referred to physical therapy by a neuro-otologist. Mrs. S. signed informed consent to participate in a VR treatment trial. This treatment trial consisted of testing her function and symptoms pretreatment during six intervention sessions, immediately posttreatment, and at a 6-month follow-up.

PROCEDURES

The Virtual Reality Protocol

Each VR session consisted of six 4-minute exposures walking and "shopping" on the treadmill. The Balance Near Automatic Virtual Environment (BNAVE) was used as the Virtual Intervention.[248] (Fig. 38.20.)

The BNAVE consists of three walls that surround the person with a treadmill in the center. The patient was instructed to push the instrumented grocery cart (which had a force sensor on the push bar of the grocery cart) at the speed at which she wanted to ambulate through the store. The upper speed limit of the treadmill was fixed at 1.2 m/s. The specially designed treadmill was built to be wider than a normal treadmill to accommodate the turning required at the end of the grocery store aisle.

Continued

CASE STUDY 38.1 Vestibular Rehabilitation Training Using a Virtual Reality Environment—cont'd

The three rear-projected scenes were merged to form one image on the BNAVE screens with the hope that persons would be immersed and "feel" as though they were shopping in a grocery store.[248] During the 4-minute exposures to the scene, Mrs. S. was introduced first to the easiest aisle (the white paper products). There were 16 different aisles, and they were designed to be increasingly more complex either via a greater number of products on the shelves, more vibrant colors, or a greater population density of products per square inch.

Mrs. S. was asked throughout the VR experience to "find" certain products in each aisle. She reported verbally when she found the product on the shelves and then continued walking. Some patients are able to continue to "walk" and "shop" at the same time. Mrs. S. was able to fairly smoothly ambulate through the store without stopping. She would occasionally slow down significantly if she was having difficulty finding a particular product and then would continue walking in the "store."

Safety

The patient was secured to an overhead harness to prevent a fall. In addition, the therapist held a switch and could stop the treadmill if there was any indication that Mrs. S. was having a problem. The patient could also stop pushing on the grocery cart in order to stop the treadmill, plus the technician who ran the computer also had the ability to immediately stop the treadmill with a stroke of a key.

One last safety measure was incorporated into the design of the study. If the patient's leg went too far back toward the edge of the treadmill, the motor turned off the treadmill immediately in order to prevent a fall. A physical therapist stood behind and toward the side of the patient and monitored the patient's condition.

OUTCOMES

Mrs. S. tolerated the treatment well, and the sessions were never terminated because of patient intolerance of the visual surround. Mrs. S. provided subjective ratings on a visual analog scale at the beginning and end of each VR treatment session (Table 38.6[249]). The following symptoms were rated: nausea, headache, dizziness, and visual blurring. No nausea was experienced, but she did rate symptoms of headache, dizziness, and visual blurring over the six sessions. Headache was experienced during only the first VR exposure. Dizziness decreased from 1.8 (10 is the maximum score) to 0.1 at the end of the last session. Visual blurring had the highest rating at the start, at 1.9; at the end of the last session her visual blurring was self-reported to be 0.1. She appeared to be better able to tolerate the virtual experience over the six treatment sessions, and she was able to progress from the first aisle to aisle 16, the most difficult aisle, where the products were much smaller and more closely packed on the shelves.

At the beginning of physical therapy, Mrs. S. was asked to complete the Dizziness Handicap Inventory (DHI),[249] the Situational Characteristics Questionnaire parts A and B (SCQ-A and SCQ-B),[250] the Dynamic Gait Index (DGI),[251] the Functional Gait Assessment (FGA),[252] the Timed Up-and-Go Test (TUG),[253] a gait speed assessment, and the Sensory Organization Test (SOT) of computerized dynamic posturography.[254,255] Data for all of the these tests before therapy, after therapy, and at the 6-month follow-up for Mrs. S. are included in Table 38.7. Scores on all measures were better after the 6-week VR intervention program except for the TUG, and the scores remained relatively stable at 6 months. Lower scores on the DHI, SCQ-A, SCQ-B, and TUG indicate improvement, and higher scores on the DGI, the FGA, gait speed, and the SOT are "better" scores.

Mrs. S. was very satisfied, as she was able to shop again without symptoms. A clinically meaningful change on the DHI has been reported to be 18,[249] and Mrs. S. improved 34 points. The Activities-specific Balance Scale (ABC) change from 29% to 69% over the course of the VR intervention was probably meaningful, as Lajoie and colleagues[256] have reported, where scores of less than 67% are related to increased risk of falling. The patient's DGI score improved by 4, which has also been reported to be clinically meaningful.[249] Gait speed over the course of the intervention improved only by 0.07 m/s, and 0.1 m/s has been reported as a clinically meaningful change.[252] Overall, Mrs. S. made positive changes after the VR physical therapy intervention.

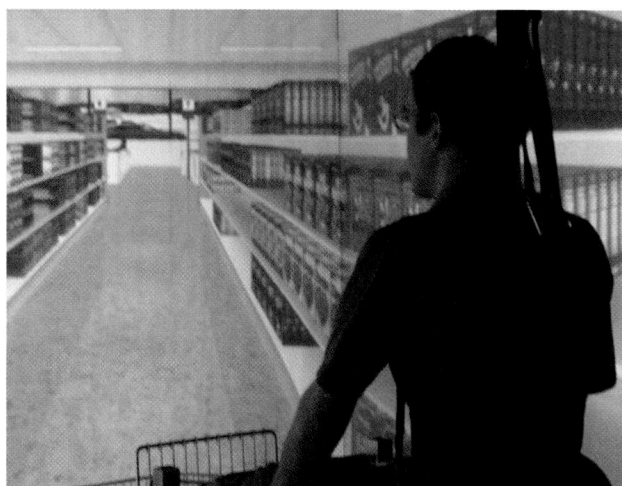

Fig. 38.20 Balance Near Automatic Virtual Environment.

TABLE 38.6 Within Session Measures: Visual Analog Scale and Simulator Sickness Questionnaire Across Six Treatment Sessions (Before and After Scores)

| | | VISIT 1 | | VISIT 2 | | VISIT 3 | | VISIT 4 | | VISIT 5 | | VISIT 6 | |
		Before	After	Before	After	Before	After	Before	After	Before	After	Before	After
VAS	Nausea	0	0	0	0	0	0	0	0	0	0	0	0
	Headache	0.5	0.3	0	0	0	0	0	0	0	0	0	0
	Dizziness	1.8	1.5	0.1	0.9	0	0.5	0	1.5	0	0.1	0	0.1
	Visual blurring	1.9	2.2	0.5	1.3	0.5	1	0	1.2	0.4	0.2	0.3	0.1
SSQ	Disorientation	6	6	3	6	3	5	1	3	3	2	3	4
	Nausea	1	1	2	2	1	3	1	1	1	3	2	1
	Oculomotor stress	6	4	4	5	4	5	4	4	4	4	4	3

SSQ, Simulator sickness questionnaire; *VAS*, visual analog scale.

TABLE 38.7 Self-Report and Performance Measures for Mrs. S. Before and After Therapy and at 6-Month Follow-Up

	ABC	DHI	SCQ-A	SCQ-B	DGI	FGA	TUG	GAIT SPEED	SOT
Before treatment	29	52	72	37	17	19	8.9	0.90	68
After treatment	69	18	18	9	21	26	9.6	0.97	81
Six-month follow-up	91	14	20	8	20	24	10.2	1.08	74

ABC, Activities-specific Balance Confidence Scale; *DGI,* Dynamic Gait Index; *DHI,* Dizziness Handicap Inventory; *FGA,* Functional Gait Assessment; *SCQ-A* and *SCQ-B,* Situational Characteristics Questionnaire Parts A and B; *SOT,* Sensory Organization Test; *TUG,* Timed Up-and-Go Test.

CASE STUDY 38.2 Noninvasive Brain Stimulation

A 68-year-old male who sustained a unilateral left pontine infarct 9 years prior to the study. He had right-sided hemiparesis with moderate spasticity of the affected side. At the time of evaluation, he had voluntary gross movement of the shoulder and minimal grasp movements of the hand. Baseline wrist extension measurement was at 31.5 cm passive and 35.5 cm active; Action Research Arm Test (ARAT) score at baseline was 16. Sensory evaluation and cranial nerve functions were both intact. Subject was ambulating independently with the use of an ankle-foot orthosis.

Hand function will be tested on three levels: impairment, activity, and participation. To test for impairment, the passive and active range of the wrist was measured. Hand disability was assessed using the ARAT. To test the level of participation limitation, a motor activity log and a general functioning questionnaire was used. Mapping of the motor cortex of both hemispheres was also performed using a Magstim 200 stimulator (Magstim Co., Dyfed, United Kingdom). Motor-evoked potential and EMG were measured from the affected wrist and finger extensors.

The patient consented to having a dual stimulation protocol for 5 days a week for 4 weeks. It involved combining TMS and peripheral electrical stimulation (ES) delivered at an inter-stimulus interval of 25 ms to allow for the afferent volley from the ES arriving at the motor cortex at approximately the same instance as the magnetic stimulus. TMS intensity was set at 15% above resting threshold. The ES consisted of a 10-Hz 500-ms train with a 1-ms pulse duration repeated every 10 seconds (McKay et al., 2002);[252a] intensity was set at the level that evoked visible twitches in the wrist and finger extensors.

Functional Test

At the end of the fourth week of treatment, the patient showed an increase in active wrist extension measures and an increase in the overall ARAT scores (Fig. 38.21). These scores were maintained on follow-up 2 weeks post-stimulation. Subjective scores also improved with the patient reporting using the affected arm twice as much prior to stimulation and found that the quality of movement improved by as much as 50%. The patient also noted that his affected upper extremity felt less stiff during the period of treatment.

Neurophysiological Measures

TMS of the affected hemisphere produced weak responses on baseline measurement. After the stimulation period, TMS responses were distinct and clear showing a 50% increase from baseline when measured during the passive state for extensor carpi ulnaris (ECU) and extensor digitorum (ED) (Fig. 38.22). EMG activity improved by 38% when compared to baseline measures. The TMS CoG measure was shown to be stable over the first two baseline measures, shifting an average of 0.5 mm. Comparison of baseline map parameters with those taken at the end of the 4-week stimulation reveals a shift in latitude. The CoG for the ECU for the subject shifted 5 mm (Fig. 38.23) and for ED shifted 2 mm.

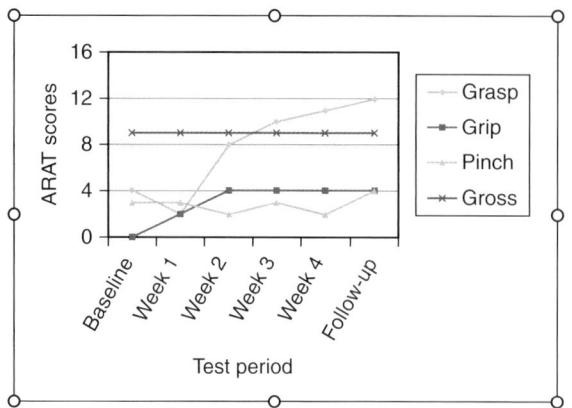

Fig. 38.21 Action Research Arm Test (ARAT) Test Results.

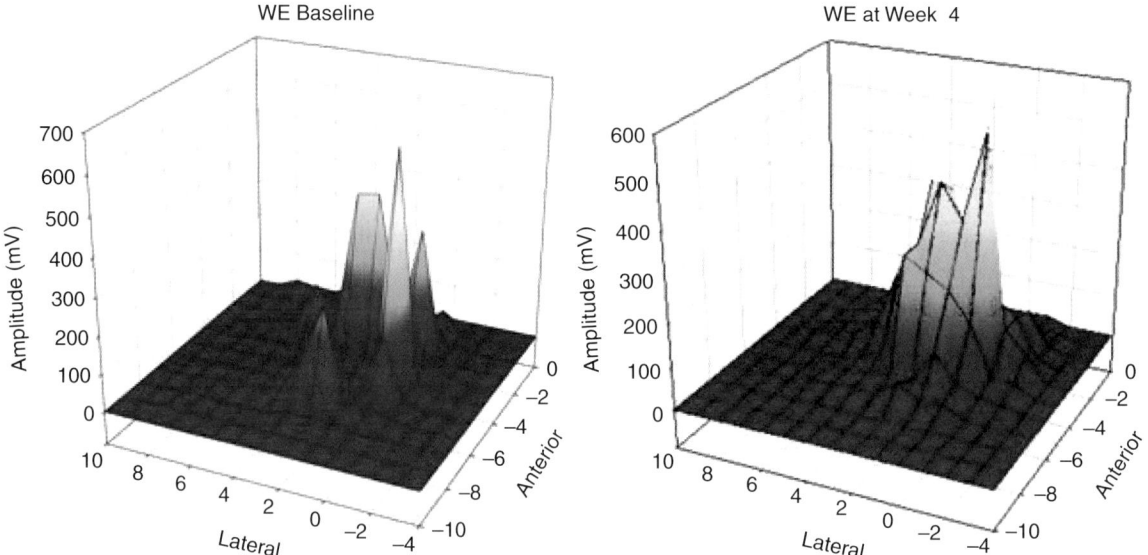

Fig. 38.22 Transcranial Magnetic Stimulation Responses.

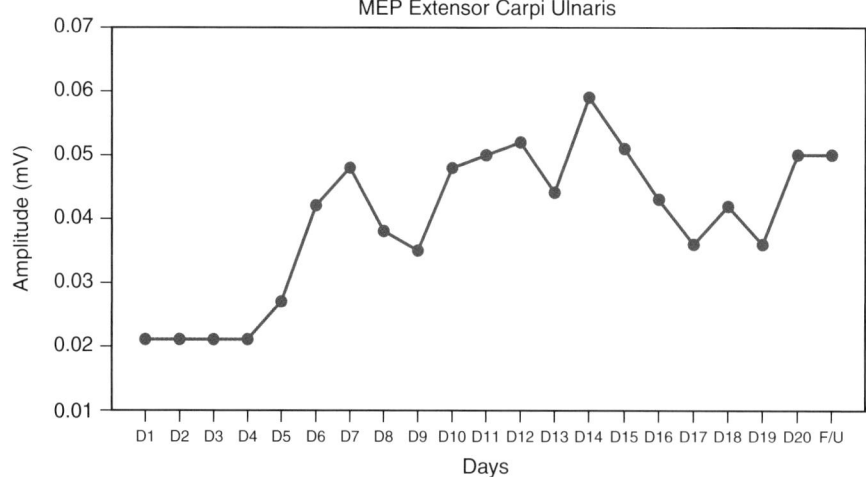

Fig. 38.23 Motor map of extensor carpi ulnaris for a subject who responded positively to the dual stimulation. Baseline and Week 4 maps show a 5-mm shift in the center of gravity. *MEP,* Motor evoked potentials.

Continued

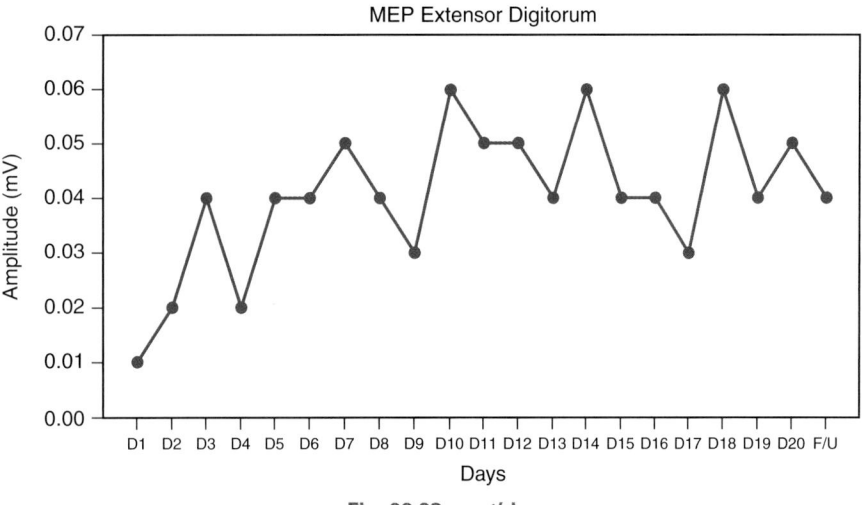

Fig. 38.23, cont'd

ACKNOWLEDGMENTS

The editors would like to thank the following for their work in this chapter in the 6th edition: Katie Byl, PhD; Nancy N. Byl, PT, MPH, PhD, FAPTA; Marten Byl, PhD; Sebastian Sovero, MS; Clayton D. Gable, PT, PhD; and Darcy A. Umphred, PT, PhD, FAPTA. The editors would also like to thank Dr. Susan L. Whitney, PT, PhD, DPT, NCS, ATC, FAPTA, for her contribution of the case study on virtual reality training for a patient with unilateral vestibular hypofunction.

Dr. Jeric Uy would like to thank Dr. Brenton Hordacre, Research Fellow, University of South Australia, for the use of the TMS and tDCS pictures. He also would like to thank Dr. Tony Aitchison of Add-Life Technologies for the picture and video used. Dr. Sophie Lefmann would like to thank her research colleagues, Associate Professor Ray Russo and Mr. Christopher Innes-Wong, from the Little Heroes Foundation's Centre for Robotics and Innovation at the Women's and Children's Hospital in Adelaide for their ongoing support in this field. She would also like to thank the patient and his family who permitted the use of video illustrating robotic rehabilitation in action.

REFERENCES

To enhance this text and add value for the reader, all references are included on the companion Evolve site that accompanies this textbook. This online service will, when available, provide a link for the reader to a Medline abstract for the article cited. There are 257 cited references and other general references for this chapter, with the majority of those articles being evidence-based citations.

39

Complementary and Integrative Therapies: Beyond Traditional Approaches to Intervention in Neurological Diseases and Movement Disorders*

Darcy A. Umphred and Mary Lou Galantino

OBJECTIVES

After reading this chapter the student or therapist will be able to:

1. Differentiate the four historical to modern worldviews of health care delivery.
2. Analyze how complementary and integrative-based health care practices overlap with allopathic traditional medical models and movement diagnoses.
3. Analyze how mind, body, and spiritual interactions have the potential to lead to health, healing, and quality of life.
4. Compare and contrast the various therapeutic models discussed and identify similarities and differences between these and the traditions of Western medicine, occupational therapy and

physical therapy practice, and the International Classification of Functioning, Disability and Health (ICF) World Health Organization (WHO) model.

5. Appreciate the role of complementary and alternative approaches in the examination and intervention of individuals with movement-based problems from neurological disorders.
6. Use evidence-based practice to measure outcomes in body system functions, functional activities, and life participation even when the science is not available to explain how and why the intervention was successful.

KEY TERMS

alternative therapies
belief-based theories
complementary models
complementary therapy interventions
energy-based theories
evidence-based practice

integrative therapies
movement diagnosis
movement-based therapies
interprofessional models
traditional concepts with new focus

The use of complementary and integrative methods or therapies (CIM/T) in the treatment of patients with neurological disorders and resultant movement problems is evolving into common practice. Clinicians and patients/clients are seeking less traditional approaches to relieve signs and symptoms of neurological diseases, syndromes, and movement disorders to attempt to alter the progression of diseases of the central nervous system (CNS) through integrative therapies and movement or manual therapeutic approaches.[1] The National Center for Complementary and Integrative Health (NCCIH), formerly known as the National Center for Complementary and Alternative Medicine (NCCAM), is the US federal government's lead agency for scientific research on the diverse medical and health care systems, practices, and products that are not generally considered part of conventional medicine. The NCCIH conducts research to help answer important scientific and public health questions about complementary health approaches and works to determine what is promising, what helps and why, what doesn't work,

and what is safe.[2] Thus the researcher, clinician, or patient can seek evidence-based information to make informed choices.

It is important that professionals working with patients with neurological problems through a traditional rehabilitation environment understand the principles and practices of complementary, alternative, and interdisciplinary approaches to the treatment of movement problems. Therapeutic approaches are proposed as options in the management of body system problems with the goal of reduction of restrictions in daily life activities and independence. The clinician needs to be cautious in the application of any treatment modalities or techniques that has paucity of research to identify the level of evidence. We do not want to accept alternative therapies as intervention solutions without significant evidenced-based research substantiating the use of these approaches, but even without evidence, some integrative approaches may be efficacious. Patients, as case studies, help us begin the path of outcome evidence, and thus it is very important to accurately measure how a patient responds to intervention. The reader must also be reminded that evidence comes from *effectiveness*, and many complementary approaches have established that result.[3]

---

*Videos for this chapter are available at studentconsult.com.

This chapter presents a sampling of integrative therapeutic models and philosophies that could potentially assist patients/clients who have movement dysfunction because of CNS pathology. Many of the techniques discussed in this chapter have been firmly established by sound research; some less–evidenced-based models are also included to widen the scope of therapeutic models with emerging evidence. Clinicians are continually being exposed to the therapeutic potential of less scientifically established theories and therefore need to be aware of their existence and impact. Creating evidence-based practice is not an all-or-none principle, nor do we suggest that models that do not have a strong research base are ineffective. We do suggest that to adopt a model because of belief or the charisma of the founder will be and should be challenged by colleagues today and in the future. Many of today's integrative health models whose theoretical constructs are based on sound rationale or that link effective-based practice across multiple areas still need to be scrutinized and approached cautiously but should not be nullified because they are considered potential complementary approaches. In time, if those models maintain their sound scientific base, more research will emerge, and efficacy may be established and become standard of care. New models may be created, and available research will develop to prove or disprove their benefit. Everything starts with a clinician using the evidence in tandem to identifying a key element that works for a specific patient, and from that strong foundation, treatment ideas develop into theories and models of practice. NOTE: A detailed historical perspective of the development of complementary and integrative therapies can be found in the online resources for this text.

ALTERNATIVE INTEGRATIVE MODELS

Darcy A. Umphred

As physical and occupational therapists, we primarily evaluate and treat movement dysfunctions that have consistencies when observed from a functional perspective and limitations in life activities. Although many of these emerging complementary approaches have not been able to show effectiveness or efficacy using a linear research model, when analyzed using social models, these approaches have been shown to create patient satisfaction and improve quality of life.[4,5] Today, models that consider patient-centered, individual's strengths can be used in conjunction with traditional therapies and will empower patients to become an active participant in his or her own health care. Many of these techniques are considered complementary or integrative therapies and are the base of most of the individual approaches presented within this chapter.[6] Personally, I have been a patient for the last three decades with interactive health issues that medical practitioners cannot explain because these medical problems fall outside of their respective evidence and always seem to overlap with other medical specialties. I have been told by more than 12 highly respected medical specialists that, when looking at their specific area of specialization, they have never seen the specific system problem that my body system presented. Thus not knowing what the causation of the specific system problem is or how it interacts with the other systems, the doctors do not know exactly how to treat the problem and each doctor reacts differently. This medical case was submitted to the National Institutes of Health (NIH) as a potential syndrome for which they might find a diagnosis. NIH returned the case, saying they do not have the finances or the ability to determine the diagnosis because it is much too complex. Obviously, there are many people with health issues that are outside current medical evidence-based practice, yet those same individuals often look to Western medicine for help. If they don't get any answers or help, they often go to practitioners outside Western medicine. Although doctors dealing with my case have had to stretch beyond their comfort zone to help and work with me in order for

my body to remain on this plane we call life, this success has led to cooperation between all individuals involved in a plan of care, with the patient playing a primary role in the key to success. Before the advent of research tools of the 21st century, doctors were constantly confronted with unknowns, and their skills in analyzing the problem and potential ways to treat it made them highly respected physician at that time. Society still refers to medicine as the "practice" of medicine, which infers that there is more to study and learn in relation to disease and pathology. This is also true for clinicians working in the area of movement science, functional recovery following any body system insult, and how an individual might regain quality of life. In contemporary medical school, the introduction and use of integrative medicine has become an intricate part of medical education and is often used by doctors if there is research to support its validity.[4,7–10]

Interprofessional practice is evolving, as are the practices of physical and occupational therapy. Future research will help validate the combination of Western and Eastern medicine along with all the theories of energy and quantum physics. OTs and PTs are movement specialists and not practitioners that evaluate and treat pathologies. Pain, a common problem among patients in our society, may be alleviated by traditional medical treatment in acute stages, but when necessary, integrative treatments may be very effective.[11,12] Movement dysfunction can be the result of pain or due to a number of system problems. As clinicians and movement specialists, we need to be able to classify movement problems and how those problems interact with function and not necessarily with the specific disease or pathology, unless that medical aspect will continue to progressively affect movement function. These problems may be specific movement functions, such as walking or reaching, or how they interact with activities, such as walking to school or reaching for a toothbrush. The patient must determine whether that activity itself has value, because if it doesn't, the patient will not practice that movement outside of therapy. Without practice, learning will not occur, as has been discussed in Chapter 3. If the patient is motivated to gain or regain specific movement function, then the probability that the motor system will regain those skills is much greater (refer to Chapter 3). Similarly, research has demonstrated the effectiveness of components of complementary approaches (refer to the list of research articles throughout this chapter for specific approaches). Additional research is needed to establish the clear reliability and validity of any methodology. In the future, some components will need to be eliminated and new creative ideas and therapeutic techniques developed. But, the true effectiveness of any integrative therapy is based on each patient's response and their ability to identify that they now can participate in activities of their choice with improved quality of life.

The models for patient management presented in this chapter have a common thread. All approaches focus on helping the patient/client maintain or regain a quality of life that cultivates their individual potential. The specific philosophy or conceptual framework embraced by any one approach may vary. As these integrative approaches are introduced in the following sections, subheadings will help the reader categorize similarities of philosophies. When we no longer need to view problems with a specific model influencing our approach, but are able to base our decisions on reliable and valid information, we will finally be able to access what is truly available to us as practitioners and give the best possible guidance and suggestions to our patients to help them regain or maintain functional control over movement as they experience life on a daily basis. In the future, there may never be a best approach but rather only options that best match the learning style of the individual and the environment and culture specific to that person. There are many ways to approach these opportunities for learning, but the clinician must remember that the patient need to learn this process, choose their path, and not be expected to just follow because he or she is being told by some practitioner that it is the best.

MOVEMENT THERAPY APPROACHES

Equine-Assisted Therapy

Kerri Sowers

Introduction to Hippotherapy and Therapeutic Riding

At the 1952 Helsinki Olympic Games, a Danish dressage rider named Liz Hartel won the silver medal and inspired a renewed interest in the field of hippotherapy and therapeutic horseback riding (THR). This master equestrian used horseback riding as a form of rehabilitation to aid her recovery from poliomyelitis, which left her lower extremities paralyzed.[13,14] The use of horses in therapy to improve physical and mental health has its founding roots in Greek culture. The term *hippotherapy* originated from the Greek word *hippos*, meaning "horse."[15,16] A renewed interest in hippotherapy and THR grew first in Europe and was especially popular throughout England.[15] In 1969, the North American Riding for the Handicapped Association (NARHA) was founded; this organization established standards for the developing THR centers in the United States.[17] The American Hippotherapy Association (AHA) was founded in 1992 and worked to establish an international protocol for hippotherapy practice.[13–16] Studies conducted in North America show that approximately 90% of children with disabilities participate in THR programs, while the remaining 10% participate in hippotherapy sessions.[18]

It is crucial to understand the differences between hippotherapy and THR, as both programs are commonly offered at the same facility and are often mistakenly thought to accomplish the same goals. According to the AHA, "term hippotherapy refers to how occupational therapy, physical therapy, and speech-language pathology professionals use evidence-based practice and clinical reasoning in the purposeful manipulation of equine movement to engage sensory, neuromotor, and cognitive systems to achieve functional outcomes. In conjunction with the affordances of the equine environment and other treatment strategies, hippotherapy is part of a patient's integrated plan of care."[19] During hippotherapy, the horse is used as a modality or treatment tool; the therapist and his or her assistants control the horse to effect a change in the patient/client. In contrast, THR teaches the patient specific riding skills that allow the rider to gain control of the horse's movement; the focus is on teaching horseback riding skills to riders with disabilities.[17] AHA attempts to clarify the difference by stating that hippotherapy "treatment takes place in a controlled environment where graded sensory input can elicit appropriate adaptive responses from the patient. Specific riding skills are not taught as in therapeutic riding, but rather a foundation is established to improve neurological function and sensory processing."[17]

Benefits, indications, and precautions. Hippotherapy and THR are perceived to be beneficial because the equine walk provides a multidirectional input, resulting in movement responses that closely mimic the movement of the pelvis during the normal human gait.[20–22] The movement is both rhythmic and repetitive, allows for variations in speed and cadence, and triggers neuromuscular responses through the stimulation of postural reflex mechanisms.[20–23] Research has demonstrated that the pelvic motion trajectories and displacement amplitudes are similar in walking and riding;[21] while there can be significant variation due to the different horses used, this variation does not cause significant alterations in the movement patterns generated. In hippotherapy, the horse is used as a dynamic base of support (BOS) to assist in improving trunk control, postural stability, core strength, and righting reactions to improve balance.[22,23] Vestibular, proprioceptive, tactile, and visual sensory inputs are incorporated during a hippotherapy session.

Hippotherapy is indicated for neuromuscular conditions. These conditions are characterized by reduced gross motor skills, decreased mobility, abnormal muscle tone, impaired balance responses, poor motor planning, decreased body awareness, impaired coordination, postural instability or asymmetry, sensory integration deficits, impaired communication, and limbic system dysfunction (impaired arousal or attention skills).[23,24]

Common conditions that may benefit from hippotherapy and THR include autism spectrum disorder, cerebral palsy (CP), developmental delay, genetic syndromes, learning disabilities, sensory integrational disorders, speech-language disorders, traumatic brain injury (TBI), and cerebral vascular accidents. There have been a multitude of suggested therapeutic benefits from hippotherapy and THR, which affect many body systems. Suggested physical benefits include improvements in endurance, symmetry, and body awareness; development of trunk and postural control; improvements in head righting and equilibrium responses; normalization of muscle tone; mobilization of the pelvis, lumbar spine, and hip joints; and improved sensory awareness.[23] Suggested cognitive, social, and emotional benefits include improvement in self-esteem, confidence, interaction with others, concentration, attention span, and communication skills.[14,25]

Contraindications for the use of hippotherapy or THR include excessive hip adductor or internal rotator tone accompanied by potential hip subluxation or dislocation. Similarly, lack of head control (in large children or adults), pressure sores, spinal instability, extreme aggressive behavior, or anxiety around animals are also contraindicated.[14,25]

Regulations. AHA offers a Clinical Specialty Certification for therapists demonstrating advanced knowledge and experience in the practice of hippotherapy. Physical therapists, occupational therapists, and speech-language pathologists must have been practicing in their profession for 3 years (6000 hours) and have had 100 hours of hippotherapy practice within the 3 years prior to application. Certification is valid for 5 years; once applicants pass a multiple-choice test, they are entitled to use the designation Hippotherapy Clinical Specialist (HPCS).[26] An entry-level certification has also been available since 2014, with the designation of American Hippotherapy Certificated Therapist (AHCB) Hippotherapy Certified Therapist; this requires 1 year of professional practice (2000 hours), completion of AHA Level I and II skills courses, and 25 hours of hippotherapy practice.[26]

American Physical Therapy Association recognizes hippotherapy as a treatment tool to address impairments and functional limitations in patients with neuromusculoskeletal dysfunction. APTA recommends that PT sessions that incorporate hippotherapy be billed as neuromuscular education, therapeutic exercise, gait training, or therapeutic activities based on the treatments completed.[27] The American Occupational Therapy Association (AOTA) also recognizes hippotherapy as an interventional tool, which can be billed as neuromuscular education, therapeutic exercise, therapeutic activities, or self-care management training.[27] The American Speech and Hearing Association (ASHA) recognizes hippotherapy as a treatment tool, which can be billed as speech-language therapy (individual or group), treatment of swallowing dysfunction and/or oral function for feeding, and therapeutic intervention for cognitive function.[27]

Evidence and clinical implications. Research and studies concerning the use of hippotherapy and THR have expanded in recent years. Research has primarily focused on children diagnosed with CP but has expanded to include conditions such as multiple sclerosis (MS), autism spectrum disorder, attention-deficit/hyperactivity disorder, psychological disorders, TBI, and stroke. In addition to the large number of articles focusing on the pediatric population, the literature has expanded to include research into the benefits of hippotherapy and THR for the adult and geriatric populations.

One systematic review investigating the use of hippotherapy and THR for children with CP found improved gross motor function;

normalization of pelvic motion; improvements in weight shifting, postural and equilibrium responses, muscle control, and joint stability; improved recovery from perturbations; and improved dynamic postural stabilization.[18] A systematic review and meta-analysis reported that short-duration hippotherapy (8 to 10 minutes of riding time) significantly reduced asymmetrical activity of the hip adductor muscles and improved postural control in children with spastic CP.[28] Another meta-analysis found that postural control and balance were improved in children with CP after hippotherapy and THR interventions.[29] A systematic review by Whalen and colleagues[30] suggests that large randomized controlled trials that utilize specific and well-defined protocols are needed to provide stronger evidence for the use of hippotherapy and THR; however, the current evidence appears to support the positive effects of these interventions on gross motor function in children with CP. Support for hippotherapy has been shown by improvements in the areas of muscle symmetry, gross motor function (as measured by valid and reliable tools), energy expenditure, and postural control.[23] Researchers suggest that hippotherapy will lead to improved head righting and equilibrium reactions and dynamic postural control, normalization of abnormal muscle tone or symmetry, improved muscle control, and better endurance.[23]

Studies have supported that hippotherapy can improve postural stability in individuals with MS and can assist in treatment of balance disorders.[31,32] A systematic review by Bronson and colleagues[33] found that hippotherapy has a positive effect on balance and enhances quality of life for individuals[20] with MS; individuals with primary progressive MS demonstrated the greatest improvement in balance, as compared with other subtypes, assessed with the Berg Balance Scale (BBS).

Hippotherapy has been shown to reduce lower-extremity spasticity in patients with spinal cord injury (SCI).[34] For individuals with hemiparetic stroke, hippotherapy, combined with conventional treatment, helped improve lower extremity motor control, independent ambulation, and gait speed and cadence; individuals treated with hippotherapy had improved normalization of gait as compared with a control group.[35]

A randomized controlled trial, conducted by de Araújo and colleagues[20], used a sample of convenience to investigate the effect of hippotherapy on functional mobility, muscle strength, and balance in a group of elderly participants. The Timed Up and Go (TUG) was used to assess functional mobility, the 30-second Chair Stand Test (30CST) was used to assess lower extremity muscle strength, and the BBS was used to assess balance.[20] After the 8-week intervention, improvements were found in muscle strength and balance in the group that participated in the hippotherapy intervention.[20] A systematic review by Hilliere and colleagues (2018)[22] investigated eight studies about hippotherapy and simulated horse riding for older adults. The results suggested that hippotherapy may lead to improvements in balance, mobility, gait ability, and muscle strength; there was also potential for hormonal and cerebral activity changes with the use of hippotherapy (Hilliere, 2018). The use of horse simulators for riding contributed only to physical fitness and muscular activity changes (Hilliere, 2018).

In addition, hippotherapy has the potential to contribute to psychosocial well-being and improved motivation by allowing interaction and acceptance with another living being and the opportunity to be mobile while astride the horse; being positioned high up on a horse gives the child the chance to be at eye level with his or her peers, and the fun of riding encourages participation and enjoyment of the therapy sessions.[36] A systematic review evaluated 33 studies involving children and adolescents with autism; hippotherapy and THR demonstrated improvements in behavior, social interaction, positive emotions, motor skills, and communication for children and adolescents diagnosed with autism.[37] A systematic review by O'Haire[38]

suggests that the research supporting the use of animal-assisted interventions, including hippotherapy and THR, for individuals with autism is promising, but further research with substantial methodological rigor is required; preliminary research suggests the potential benefits of increased social interaction and communication and reduced problem behaviors, autistic severity, and stress.

While the methodological rigor in many studies involving hippotherapy and THR is lacking, the results remain promising for a wide variety of conditions. Hippotherapy and THR are effective in the areas of gross motor function, balance, symmetry, postural control, muscle strength, gait normalization, communication, behavior, and social interaction. Continued research in hippotherapy and THR using larger, randomized controlled studies with well-defined protocols to investigate specific outcomes and account for the variations within a variety of neuromusculoskeletal conditions will be necessary to conclusively determine all potential benefits that exist.

Feldenkrais Method of Somatic Education
James Stephens
The Feldenkrais method is about learning the following:

We do not treat patients. We give lessons to help people learn about themselves. Learning comes from the experience. We tell them stories [and give them experiences of movement] because we believe learning is the most important thing for a human being. (p. 117)[39]

Development of the Feldenkrais method. Moshe Feldenkrais, a boy in Palestine, developed a method of hand-to-hand combat that was used by settlers for self-defense. Later, as a student in Paris where he trained in physics at the Sorbonne, he studied judo and became the first person in Europe to receive a black belt. When he injured his knee playing soccer, he relearned pain-free walking on his own. Later, he studied with F. M. Alexander, Elsa Gindler, and George Gurdjieff. He also studied psychology, progressive relaxation, bioenergetics, and the hypnosis methods of Milton Erickson. Also, he was familiar with the physiological concepts of his day: Sherrington, Magnus, Fulton, and Schilder. With this background, Feldenkrais developed two approaches to facilitating learning that are now known as Awareness Through Movement (ATM) and Functional Integration (FI).[40]

Feldenkrais was ultimately interested in the development of human potential. He saw that, although all people encounter trauma and difficulty in their lives, those who are most successful were able to develop new, adaptive behaviors to overcome those difficulties. He proposed that a type of learning that reconnected the brain to the control of the musculoskeletal system would be the most effective way to approach this problem of adaptation. His initial thinking in this area is set out in his first book, *Body and Mature Behavior: A Study of Anxiety, Sex, Gravitation, and Learning.*[41]

Background theory—dynamical systems theory. For Feldenkrais, learning was an organic process in which cognitive and somatic aspects were completely integrated. Presented first in 1949, this idea prefigured our current sense of dynamic systems functioning of the brain and body.[42] The learning experience should proceed at its own pace in an individualized way following the learner's intention and guided by the learner's perception that the performance of the task, movements of the body, and interaction with the environment become easier.[41] This interactive cycle of action and perception has been described well by the motor learning model proposed by Newell.[43]

Learning is a complex process with overlays from the intention of the learner, interference from environmental distraction, misperception of the task and the body, desire related to self-image, fear of injury, or incorrect performance. Thus it is possible to learn poorly, incorrectly, or in such a way as to interfere with performance and not improve it. This kind of process has been suggested by Byl and colleagues[44] as the underlying cause of focal dystonia. One of the definitions Feldenkrais gave for learning took this process into account: "Learning is the acquisition of the skill to inhibit parasitic action (components of the action unrelated to the intention behind an action but resulting from a secondary intention) and the ability to direct clear motivations as a result of self-knowledge."[43] An adult engaged in learning to walk again after a stroke with a fear-related reluctance to bear weight on the involved limb would be an example of such a secondary intention.

The process of learning proposed by Feldenkrais is one of discovery. The outcome desired is one of increased awareness. Vereijken and Whiting[45] have proposed that discovery learning, in which learners are free to explore any range of solutions in learning to perform a task in any way that they want, is as effective as or more effective than any formal approach to motor learning involving controlled schedules of practice or feedback. This process of discovery has the added dimension of allowing learners to focus on the perceptual understanding of the body/task/environment as a component of the learning process both within the human organism as well as participation within the external world. This suggests that a home exercise program should not be strictly proscribed, but patients should be encouraged to experiment with movement and be guided in that process by the therapist. In the Feldenkrais method, this discovery and perceptual learning process are explicit.

Our understanding of how experience and learning restructure almost all areas of the CNS is expanding rapidly.[46] A large focus of current thinking in rehabilitation is how to translate neuroplasticity concepts into more effective techniques for rehabilitation.[47–49] The method developed by Feldenkrais and practiced by people around the world who are trained in this method is clearly explained by these new principles, creating new approaches to rehabilitation.

Approaches to the Feldenkrais method. The two approaches to facilitating learning created by Feldenkrais, ATM and FI, are similar in terms of principle and process, although they differ in practice. They are essentially two methods for communicating a sensory experience that the patient can consider and act on. The first requirement of the process is to create an environment that is comfortable, safe, and conducive to learning, whether the learner is being moved passively or creating the movement experience voluntarily. The second requirement is that the amount of effort associated with making the movements be reduced greatly so that it is possible to make fine discriminations about the effects of forces acting on the system from inside or outside the body. The goal is to develop a rich understanding of changes throughout the system produced by small perturbations. This understanding becomes the basis for creating new solutions to movement problems as the patient progressively approaches functional movements that she or he desires to perform.[50]

In FI the practitioner will manually introduce small perturbations into the learner's system after placing the learner into a safe position closely approximating some desired activity to be learned. Here the practitioner is providing the force inputs, and the patient is asked to attend to the changes created in response to the perturbation. For example, the practitioner might press gently into the bottom of the patient's foot and ask the patient to notice where in the body movement and pressure are felt as a result. This will be repeated a number of times, and then some other forces or movements will be introduced. The guiding idea for the practitioner might be to build sensory experiences in the body that are associated with a particular movement, such as rolling. This goal is rarely explicitly expressed to the patient and is

left to emerge in the patient's understanding of the experience: "Oh, now I am rolling," or "This feels like rolling to me." Also, there is no strict expectation by the practitioner about what specific movement might emerge. Thus it is possible to create novel and unexpected outcomes of how a particular task might be best performed by this particular person at this time. This allows for a process of assessment that is continually evolving as the intervention is unfolding.[50]

In ATM the practitioner verbally provides suggestions for movements for a patient to explore and asks the patient to focus on the sensory outcomes throughout the body. Thus the patient introduces the experimental forces into his or her own system with the intention of understanding how the body as a whole responds. The underlying idea, however, is the same. In my practice, FI is used to assess body image and capacity for movement and as a form of communication when patients do not understand how a force might act on the body or when the patient is unable to produce a range of movements that we might desire to explore. An example might be in a case where spasticity prevents fine discrimination in both sensory and motor realms.

In practice with an individual patient, it is common to move back and forth between ATM and FI during the same session. The session is usually focused on the development of understanding and performing a specific function: turning, rolling, standing, stepping, a functional activity important to the patient, and so on. ATM is a verbal process in which patients perform their own movements; thus a practitioner can work with many individuals simultaneously. At the same time, individuals within the learning group are free to respond differently from one another in ways that may be appropriate only for each of them as individuals.[51] Because ATM is under the active control of the patient, this method is often a more effective tool in reestablishing voluntary control.

Note: A case study on the Feldenkrais method can be found in the online resources associated with this text.

Research

Evidence of effectiveness. In a review of studies of evidence-based studies of effectiveness up to 2004, Stephens and Miller divided[50] the literature into four different areas: pain management, postural and motor control, functional mobility, and psychological and quality-of-life impact. These categories still hold with more studies being done since in the areas of pain and posture, mobility, and balance, especially in the geriatric population. A growing amount of the literature is in the randomized, control trial format. That literature (through 2015) has been reviewed by Hillier and Worley,[52] including meta-analysis for outcomes, effect sizes, and biases.

The theory underlying the Feldenkrais method predicts that there should be changes in perception of the body or body image. Elgelid[53] reported positive changes in body perception, as evaluated by the semantic differentiation scale in a group of four subjects after a series of ATM lessons. Dunn and colleagues[54] reported that subjects who had had a unilateral sensory imagery ATM lesson perceived their experimental sides to be longer and lighter and demonstrated increased forward flexion on that side, linking the changes in perception to changes in motor control. Bitter and colleagues[55] found significant improvements in dexterity compared with a control group following a single ATM lesson. Stephens and colleagues[56] have shown that ability to image movement is improved in people post stroke after a series of ATM lessons, and furthermore that there is a high positive correlation between the Movement Imagery Questionnaire (MIQ) score and improvements in balance assessed by the BBS. In a qualitative study, Connors and colleagues[57] made a compelling argument that ATM lessons are based on principles of motor learning and therefore the general literature in an important point of reference.

Pain. The work on pain management suggests that the Feldenkrais method may be especially effective in treating pain that is biomechanical in origin. Mohan and colleagues[58] in a systematic review, conclude that there is now sufficient evidence to support the use of the Feldenkrais method for the treatment of neck and low back pain. Other examples of research on intervention that addresses pain management reach different conclusions.[59–64] A number of these papers conclude that the Feldenkrais approach to pain management is better than the traditional approaches used in comparison. Although no research has been reported that looks specifically at the Feldenkrais approach to pain management in patients with movement dysfunction from neurological insults, these treatments may help these patients, especially when the pain is caused by biomechanical malalignment. Current ongoing, not yet published, work with individuals with SCI begins to address the question of pain in this population.

Balance mobility and function. Hall and colleagues[65] found improvements in balance, mobility, functional activity, and vitality (SF-36) in a large group of elderly women compared with control subjects as a result of a 16-week ATM intervention. These results have been confirmed with other elderly subjects by a variety of researchers.[66–72]

In the areas of psychological and quality-of-life impact, Kerr and colleagues[73] have shown a decrease in state anxiety in subjects who participated in ATM lessons, and Laumer and colleagues,[74] working with young women with eating disorders, have demonstrated positive changes in self-concept, self-confidence, and behavior resulting from participation in ATM lessons.

The use of ATM with specific medical diagnoses can be found online and can be integrated with the various chapters written on the specific movement problems associated with those diseases of specific areas of the brain.

Multiple sclerosis. The initial study, done in Germany in 1994, looked qualitatively at the effects of a 30-day ATM experience on a group of people with MS. The investigators concluded that ATM improved overall well-being, resulted in greater self-reliance of the participants, and led to better self-acceptance and a more positive self-image.[75] Johnson and colleagues[76] studied the effects of FI in people with MS and reported a decrease in perceived stress in the FI compared with the massage controls. Stephens and colleagues[51] reported the cases of four individuals who participated in the same ATM classes over a period of 10 weeks. Three of four reported large improvements in their Index of Well-Being score. All individuals reported improvements in gait and balance; however, there were no measures of gait that consistently improved across the group. Instead, it was found that changes were appropriate to the participant's individual needs and resulted in a greater sense of control. In a follow-up to this study, using a randomized controlled group design, Stephens and colleagues[77] found improvements in postural control and balance confidence measures, along with a strong tendency toward an increase in self-efficacy and decreased falling. It was also found[78] that the ATM group had significant improvements in memory of recent events and perception of positive social support. It is interesting to note that they also had a decrease in pain effects.

Cerebrovascular accident. The original publication in this area is the classic work, *The Case of Nora*, in which Feldenkrais explained his work in great detail and described improvements in sensation, perception, and mobility of a woman several years after a right-sided cerebrovascular accident (CVA).[79] More recently, results from pilot studies have been reported in patients with diagnoses of CVA. Connors and Grenough[80] reported a decrease in spatial neglect as measured by line and star cancellation tests in a patient after a series of ATM lessons. Nair and colleagues[81] reported the recovery of upper-extremity function

and the return to playing golf in a 68-year-old man after an 8-week program of ATM and FI. This Feldenkrais program was begun only after a 9-month program of traditional rehabilitation had left him with a nonfunctional hand. The Feldenkrais program included mental imagery and bimanual activities. This subject was also studied before, during, and after the Feldenkrais program with functional magnetic resonance imaging. This imaging analysis showed that there was a return to higher activity in the involved contralateral primary motor cortex, with activity of the right hand compared with higher activity in the ipsilateral M1 and SMA that has been shown in other reports of CVA recovery[82] before the Feldenkrais sessions began. This finding suggests a return to more normal brain function, even after a period of 1 year after the stroke. In a small pilot study (three subjects),[83] Batson found an average 33% decrease in movement times on the Wolf Motor Function Test. In another pilot with four subjects, Batson and Deutsch[84] found significant improvements in Dynamic Gait Index ($P = .033$, 55% average) and the BBS score ($P = .034$, 11% average) and a 35% improvement on the Stroke Impact Scale (SIS). A larger study is in progress to further assess these findings. In a larger follow-up study, Stephens and colleagues[56] confirmed improvements in balance and gait and documented a strong positive correlation between improvements in balance and increased movement imagery ability.

Other Neurological Diagnoses
Cerebral Palsy

There are some preliminary findings with other neurological diagnoses. Shelhav-Silberbush[85] reported improvements in motor, sensory, kinesthetic, perceptual, and learning functions in two case studies of children with CP.

Spinal Cord Injury

The first report of a Feldenkrais method intervention with SCI was by Ginsburg in 1986.[86] He reported improvements in mobility and reductions in pain following FI and ATM classes. For several years, Allison has been writing about work with people with SCI. Her first reports documented improvements in sensory and motor function.[87] More recently, she has noted improvements in pain management.[88]

Parkinson Disease

Shenkman and colleagues[89] first reported improvements in balance, gait, and functional movement in two people with Parkinson disease (PD) as a result of interventions that were based partly on a Feldenkrais approach. This work has been supported more recently by Teixeira-Machado,[90] reporting that working with Feldenkrais method–based exercises has led to improvements in quality of life and decrease in depression scores in people with PD.

Dementia

Ann published the first case study work on people with dementia in 2006.[91] In these cases, she documented her work using FI to transform the lives of several people with dementia, not to reduce the dementia but to change the nature of their interaction with the world so that they were able to communicate better with staff and family, were less fearful, and were safer and more independent in their mobility. This study was followed by two other studies by a group in San Francisco under a guiding idea of preventing loss of independence through exercise (PLIE). This program used an integrative exercise program, combining conventional aerobic and strength exercise and complementary approaches, of which Feldenkrais played a significant part. These studies looked at function and behavior over 36 weeks in a crossover study. The first was a qualitative study by Wu and colleagues[92] which had three main findings: improved body awareness and memory for movement, more emotional comfort and positive feeling about sharing personal stories, and development of social skills leading to more positive social interactions. This study was followed up by Barnes and colleagues[93] who found clinically meaningful improvements in measures of quality of life, physical performance, and cognitive function.

Other Areas of Research

Gilman and Yaruss[94] have reported significant improvements in several young children who had problems with stuttering. Ofir[95] reported improvements in flexibility, mobility, and level of dependence in two young women who had sustained traumatic brain injuries.

Conclusion

The Feldenkrais method, in its two forms, embodies a process of somatic learning that aims to develop the perceptual capabilities of patients as it underlies the control of movement and affects function. Research literature suggests that predicted results of improved body perception and motor control are supported in work with people with neurological diagnoses, including dementia. These findings are encouraging and suggest that the Feldenkrais method makes positive contributions to our understanding and methods of rehabilitation. However, we must approach these findings with caution because many are from case studies or small pilot investigations. Research continues to substantiate these initial findings at a higher evidence-based level.

The Pilates Method

Brent Anderson

German-born Joseph H. Pilates developed his unique method of movement therapy and lifestyle in the early 1900s. As a young man, Pilates was affected by a multitude of illnesses that left him physically weak. To strengthen his frail body, Pilates studied boxing, yoga, martial arts, Zen meditation, and ancient Greek and Roman exercises. Joseph was interned in England at the Isles of Man during World War I, where he continued to develop his philosophy of health and happiness. His experiences led him to develop his own unique method of physical and mental conditioning. In 1926 Pilates brought his movement exercise program with him to New York City. Joseph Pilates's studio was soon embraced by many artists and choreographers from the dance companies of Martha Graham, George Balanchine, and Jerome Robbins. At the time, traditional allopathic medicine lacked the knowledge of how to restore injured dancers to their prior level of activity. Pilates encouraged nondestructive movement early in the rehabilitation process and worked to correct underlying biomechanical problems. This early movement intervention without pain was believed to hasten the healing process and allowed dancers and athletes to quickly return to their life activities that had meaning to them. Thus they realized that Pilates had improved their quality of life.

Almost a century later, the Pilates method has gained popularity within the rehabilitation setting because of its assistive nature in restoring functional movement. Rehabilitation practitioners are currently using the method in a variety of fields, including orthopedics,[96–104] pain management, women's health,[105] neurological rehabilitation, geriatrics, pediatrics,[102,106,107] and even acute care. Most Pilates exercises in the rehabilitation setting are performed on specifically designed apparatus: the Reformer (Fig. 39.1), the Trapeze table (Fig. 39.2), the Wunda Chair (Fig. 39.3), and the Ladder Barrel (Fig. 39.4). The apparatus regimen evolved from Joseph Pilates's original mat work, which was too difficult for many injured individuals. On the apparatus, the use of springs and manipulation of the orientation to gravity can be modified to assist an individual with movement restrictions to successfully complete movements that would otherwise be

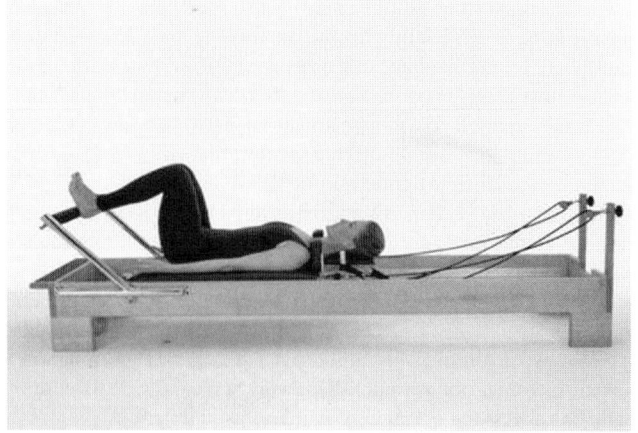

Fig. 39.1 The Reformer Apparatus Used in Pilates.

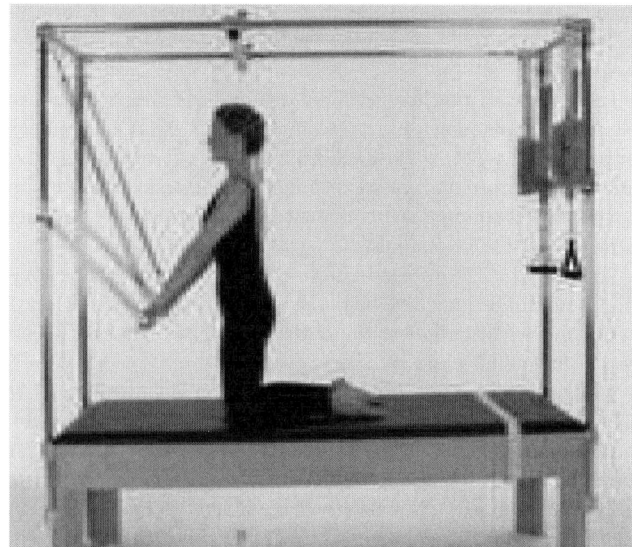

Fig. 39.2 The Cadillac Table Apparatus Used in Pilates.

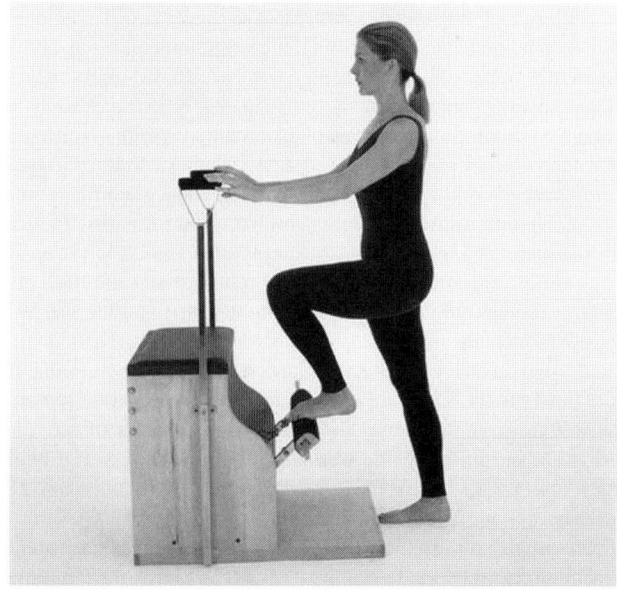

Fig. 39.3 The Wunda Chair Apparatus Used in Pilates.

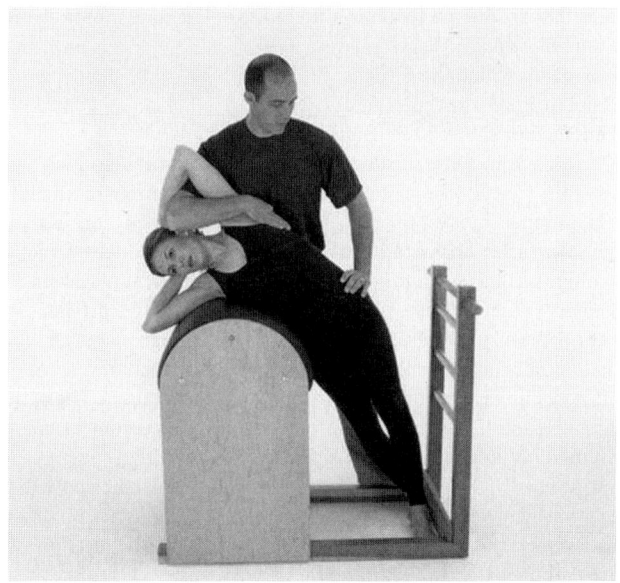

Fig. 39.4 The Ladder Barrel Apparatus Used in Pilates.

difficult. Ultimately, by altering the spring tension or increasing the challenge of gravity, an individual may progress toward functional movement safely, efficiently, and without pain.

Pilates Principles

Joseph Pilates espoused only three guiding principles according to the Pilates Method Alliance: (1) Whole Body Healthy, (2) Whole Body Commitment, and (3) Breath. A number of the first-generation Pilates practitioners known as *the Elders* expanded Pilates principles to include concentration, control, precision/coordination, isolation/integration, centering, flowing movement, breathing, and routine.[100,108] Polestar Pilates has modified the eight first-generation principles into six principles that have a greater practicality in the rehabilitation environment and stronger scientific support than the classic principles. The six Polestar Pilates principles include breathing, trunk control and axial elongation, mobility, alignment, efficiency of movement, and movement integration.*

Breathing. Faulty breath patterns can be associated with complaints of pain and movement dysfunction.[109] Pilates movements create an environment where breath facilitates improved air exchange, breath capacity, and posture. During Pilates exercise, breathing is used to facilitate stability and mobility of the spine and extremities. Because of the movement of the rib cage on the thoracic spine, inhalation can promote spinal extension while exhalation can promote spinal flexion. Breath may or may not facilitate movement based on where the breath is occurring. If accessory breath occurs while attempting spine extension, it would not have a positive movement on the spine articulating into extension. It is then important to realize that the direction of movement in the ribs facilitated by breath determines whether breath facilitates movement or not. Similarly, breath may assist with stability of the spine through the coordinated contraction of the diaphragm and the lower abdominal muscles, both of which attach to the lumbar spine and pelvis.[110,111]

Trunk control and axial elongation. Core control is the optimal recruitment of the trunk musculature required to perform a given task

in relation to the anticipated load. The transversus abdominis, internal abdominal obliques, external abdominal obliques, multifidi, erector spinae, diaphragm, and pelvic floor muscles are key organizational muscles that work together during the movement in healthy individuals.[112–114] Motor control studies indicate that the coordinated, subthreshold contraction of these local and global stabilization muscles modulate the level of spinal stability required to safely perform activities of daily living (ADLs).[115]

Axial elongation is the proper alignment of the head, spine, and pelvis that provides optimal joint spacing during movement. Correct joint spacing avoids working or resting at the end of range, which can place undue stress on the inert and contractile structures of the trunk and extremities.[116,117] Through emphasis on axial elongation of the spine and maintaining appropriate joint spacing, soft tissue surrounding the joint can move more freely, and the risk of injury can be minimized. Recent discussion has challenged the Pilates approach to trunk control and has passed through the fitness and rehabilitation fixation on core control, where the assumption is that the stronger the core muscles, the healthier the spine. Research has been leaning away from this paradigm to one of motor control and efficiency. Though Pilates uses the trunk musculature and coactivation to successfully perform the vast repertoire of exercises, the focus is on efficiency and spontaneous contractions of the trunk musculature based on the anticipated load and the amount of intraabdominal pressure required in that moment.[118]

Mobility. Spine mobility allows for the distribution of movement throughout the cervical, thoracic, and lumbar spine. This principle can also be thought of where distribution of movement equals distribution of force. It has been suggested that repetitive movement at a hypermobile spinal segment may result in microtrauma or macrotrauma.[119–121] Hypermobility is often a result of a lack of movement in a neighboring segment or joint.[122] Pilates exercise attempts to facilitate a change in movement strategy during functional tasks and distribute the forces through other motion segments. Patients are trained to distribute movement in the spine over a greater number of spinal segments, thereby decreasing potentially harmful forces at the hypermobile segment. The ability to segmentally move the spine decreases unwanted stress and shear of the spinal segments and increases the efficiency and fluidity of movement. The clinical findings of decreased low back pain because of Pilates exercise may be due to changed strategy that reduces the stress afforded to the pathological segment(s).

Efficiency of movement. Efficiency of movement is the minimization of unnecessary muscle contractions that tend to interfere with healthy movement. The excessive recruitment of antagonist muscles is obstructive and significantly increases the amount of energy required to perform a task.[123,124] This principle can be applied to functional movement skills as well as performance skills. Inefficient motor recruitment can often be recognized by the amount of tension or faulty posture in the head, face, neck, and shoulder girdle, in relation to the thoracic spine and trunk.

Alignment and weight bearing of extremities. Alignment and posture are concepts often incorporated in the field of rehabilitation. The Pilates principle of *alignment* refers to the most energy-efficient posture (static or dynamic) of the body for a given task. Proper postural organization can significantly decrease energy expenditure during daily activities by improving mechanical advantage.[125,126] Faulty alignment in the extremities and the spine can be a source of decreased range of motion, loss of joint congruency, early fatigue of muscle groups, or abnormal stresses on inert structures and may potentially cause degeneration and injury.[127,128]

Pilates provides a closed chain environment that facilitates compression and decompression forces on the axial skeleton and

---

*The six modified Pilates principles were developed by the Polestar Pilates method.

extremities through a full range of motion. Adjusting the spring resistance or patient's orientation to gravity can alter the amount of load. The ability to regulate load based on an individual's physiological limits, set by age or pathological condition, allows practitioners to more safely and effectively stress the skeletal and soft tissue systems. Theoretically, these forces can help stimulate osteoblastic activity and provide nutrition to a larger surface area of the joint and its surrounding connective tissue.[129–131]

Movement integration. Many forms of rehabilitation focus on treating limitations of anatomical structures and neglect the neuromuscular reeducation required to learn to regain the motor control necessary to perform a complex task. Pilates provides a more holistic approach by emphasizing the synthesis of mind (motor control) and body (physical strength and flexibility) to achieve fluid movement. Mobility, control, and coordination of the extremities with the trunk and the trunk with the extremities are examined and trained through motor learning and repetition of practice. In addition to the physical and mental capacity to complete a task, the environment in which a task is performed can greatly affect the success of movement organization.[132,133] Pilates provides an environment that can be modified on the basis of a patient's impairments and limitations, providing a safe, successful, and pain-free movement experience.

Clinical Application

Within the Pilates environment, faulty movement strategies are broken down into components and addressed through task-oriented interventions. By adaptation of the environmental constraints, such as gravity, assistance, and BOS, the degrees of freedom that must be controlled by the nervous system are reduced.[134] The successful manipulation of the environment can hasten the functional reeducation process and allow exercises to be safely progressed until the desired outcome is achieved. Pilates practitioners are also trained to be able to modify any exercise, so it is pain-free for the patient. It has been suggested that successful, pain-free movement, in addition to enhancing physical attributes, helps alleviate anxiety.[135,136] By decreasing anxiety levels and improving self-efficacy, the development of chronic pain and dysfunction related to the injury may be prevented.[137–139]

The potential causes of faulty movement patterns include congenital defects and abnormalities, habitual adaptations, and compensation because of injury. Motor control problems associated with the pathological condition need to be addressed before the application of therapeutic interventions that are temporary coverups for problems that have deeper roots. For example, a pathological condition at the L4/L5 segment could be a result of faulty movement patterns in the hips and other lumbar vertebrae. The lack of movement in surrounding joints might be the mechanism of the lesion; however, treatments are often focused on the site of the lesion rather than the mechanism of the lesion.

One problem often encountered in the rehabilitation setting is flawed movement progression. On a spectrum of movement progression, practitioners often jump from passive movement to resistive movement too quickly. Through facilitation of assistive movement, a pattern can be practiced without irritating the lesion. Assisted movement with the use of springs can allow for a decrease in unwanted muscle activity or guarding that is often associated with pain, weakness, or abnormal tone. As the pattern progresses and symptoms decrease, assistance decreases, and dynamic stabilization can be emphasized to challenge the newly acquired mobility or stability in a more functional and gravity-dependent position. Resistive movements are introduced only after adequate dynamic stability of the trunk is demonstrated through controlled movements that prevent excessive loading of the injured tissue. The five environmental conditions in

Pilates that are altered to allow a therapist to facilitate motor changes are the following:[132,140]
1. Narrow or widen the BOS
2. Raise or lower the center of gravity
3. Lengthen or shorten the length of the levers
4. Decrease or increase the degree of assistance (spring tension)
5. Progress from a foreign environment to a familiar environment

Traditional modes of muscle conditioning focus on isolating specific muscles and producing a maximal voluntary contraction. Although this has been found to positively alter the targeted muscle, the gains achieved have not always been shown to correlate with functional return. Pilates progresses patients through stages of motor learning via neuromuscular reeducation of functional movement patterns and emphasizes efficient recruitment of motor units. The patient is first trained to become aware of or gain a perception of current movement strategies. Then the patient must cognitively learn a new strategy. Finally, the patient must practice or act until efficient with the new strategy of movement. Task-specific interventions are progressed from a foreign to familiar environment by altering the level of assistance and the patient's orientation to gravity.

Summary

Pilates is an effective exercise system that works well in conjunction with traditional PT and OT practice.[141–143] The Pilates-evolved apparatuses allow patients to safely perform exercises that improve strength, flexibility, balance, coordination, and motor control in an environment that can be easily progressed as they advance in their rehabilitation process. In addition, Pilates is thought to address the psychosocial components of an injury that leads to chronic pain or disability by decreasing anxiety and improving self-efficacy.[137,139] Early return of functional movement after an injury helps physically and mentally empower individuals with regard to the demands of life and is crucial in the long-term success of patient outcomes. The Pilates environment is a clinical tool that can be used by practitioners to provide patients with a safe, successful, and pain-free way of restoring function and quality of life.

Tae Kwon Do

Clinton Robinson, Jr., 9th Degree, Grand Master
Darcy A. Umphred, 4th Degree

Philosophy. The overall philosophy of Tae Kwon Do (TKD) can be summed up in the student oath recited by all practitioners at the beginning of each class: *"I shall observe the tenets of Tae Kwon Do: courtesy, integrity, perseverance, self-control, and indomitable spirit."* The tenets are to be practiced outside as well as inside the training hall in all aspects of life. All aspects of these tenets reflect CNS control and neuroplasticity as well as incorporate cognitive, emotional, and motor aspects into an integrated whole. The oath continues with, *"I shall respect the instructors and seniors,"* which refers to having respect for all people—our teachers, our parents, our peers, our students, our patients—all individuals with whom the student may interact throughout a lifetime. *"I shall never misuse Tae Kwon Do."* No matter what motor skill a student develops, it is not to be used to build one's ego or to injure another unnecessarily. *"I will be a champion of freedom and justice."* Individuals are expected to develop a sense of responsibility for those less fortunate than themselves and to be active participants in the development of humanity as a whole. These tenets are basic philosophies of both occupational and physical therapy as well as in many martial arts. Empowering our students or patients to overcome their movement limitations and once again actively participate in life should be the goal of all therapeutic treatment outcomes. *"I will build a more peaceful world."* Understanding that change begins with self and developing and integrating the mind, body, and spirit while helping others do the same will set an example not only in the classroom but in our society both nationally and worldwide, so that others may improve themselves. The profession of occupational therapy has identified similar educational outcome criteria for students who graduate from an accredited educational program. Physical therapy has begun to integrate the mind, body, and spirit into outcomes, including the interactions of those three human characteristics as part of the accreditation criteria set forth by the Commission on Accreditation in Physical Therapy Education (CAPTE). There are commonalities between the practice of TKD and some of the expectations of students in educational programs in both physical and occupational therapies.

The overall goal of TKD training is the development of self-sufficiency through rigorous physical and mental practice. With this training, an inner balance or peace can be attained, thus balancing all aspects of a person's life. Students are expected to strive for their own personal excellence versus comparing that skill with another's. Thus individuals with physical challenges are always encouraged to participate.[144–146] Their challenges and expectations are different, but achieving personal excellence gives them the same respect and confidence that any other student would receive. Thus TKD as a movement science empowers participants to gain or regain a feeling of empowerment over the mind, the spirit, and the physical body. It engages all students to participation in a community of people who all begin as novices and advance only as each respective mind, body, and spirit grows as a whole unit.[147–149] At times, an individual may have physical restrictions that limit the ability to do specific techniques, but that never limits one's ability to grow and advance as a human being and continue to learn as a student of TKD.[150]

Philosophy of training.
Training in TKD consists of three primary components: forms, breaking of solid objects, and sparring. Other martial arts focus on some of the same components. The practice of tai chi focuses on the first component: forms. But with practice, a TKD student not only will have the skill to perform a sequential pattern or combinations of simple and complex movements (forms), but also will overcome a perceived obstacle (board) and interact with another person using quick movement techniques with control (sparring).

Poomsee.
Poomsee is a prearranged dance of defensive and offensive techniques against an imaginary opponent. The practice of poomsee increases the practitioner's memory, coordination, balance, and body awareness. All poomsee components have predetermined patterns of movements with a proper beginning and ending point that include various stances, along with hand and kicking techniques. The complexity and difficulty of these forms increase as the student progresses. Simple movements and combinations of patterns challenge beginners, and appropriate levels of complex patterns challenge the highest-ranking black belts. Thus all individuals studying TKD are challenged to be in a state of growth and learning.[151]

Kyukpa.
Kyukpa is breaking of solid objects such as boards, concrete, and bricks using a body part as a weapon. Kyukpa represents overcoming limitations and obstacles and facing fear. It requires tremendous concentration and belief in one's abilities. In addition, it allows participants to demonstrate the power they have attained, thereby increasing self-confidence. Self-confidence is the primary attribute in conflict resolution skills and leads to the understanding that there are few situations in life in which physical confrontation is necessary. Board breaking helps teach the student that an object, such as a board, is only an obstacle if you, the student, empower that object to have that role. Once the board is broken and the limb has passed through the obstacle, it no longer is an obstacle. This philosophy reflects life and plays a role in the establishment of values and motivation

by teaching practitioners to go beyond the known and through the obstacles that life poses. Facing the unknown is always a part of life. Some of us run from that challenge and some just keep hitting the obstacle over and over without any resolution, which causes pain and frustration. Others going beyond the obstacle allow the mind to realize that it is now in the past and no longer needs to expend energy worrying about the challenge. Kyukpa allows any student of TKD whether a child, adolescent, adult, or senior citizen to face and go beyond those perceived obstacles.

Kyorugi.
Kyorugi is actual sparring between two people using both defensive and offensive techniques learned through fundamental TKD practice. Kyorugi can be further broken down into two types. (1) In *one-step sparring*, practitioners take turns initiating a prearranged attack—one person attacks while the other defends. This allows the practitioners to engage each other without risk of injury to either party. It also allows them to practice proper distancing, execution of the techniques, and timing of that execution. This develops confidence in the ability to use the techniques properly if the need arises. (2) In *free sparring*, neither opponent knows what the other is going to do. Although free sparring may appear dangerous to one untrained in TKD, it is a relatively safe activity. Free sparring requires respect for your partner and absolutely controlled motions at all times. It is an exercise in which the aim is for all involved to increase their skill level.[152] It develops the practitioner's quick motor responses, confidence in his or her abilities, and overall awareness, as well as a cooperative learning environment.

Although both offensive and defensive techniques are viewed as equally important, all training is begun with blocking techniques to indicate that TKD never allows any initial offensive attack in its technique. Blocking techniques are practiced diligently so that they may function equally as offensive techniques. This way one can defeat an opponent, whether in the classroom or in real life, without either suffering or inflicting serious injuries. This builds self-confidence and replaces a perception of the "role of a victim."[153] Defensive techniques are not only power against power but truly reflect power of the attacker and deflection by the opposition. This deflection can stop the attacker, redirect the power back onto the attacker, or incapacitate the attacker in order for the opposition to get away. The skill in redirecting the force and intent of an attacker is not too different from redirecting a patient's motor pattern into a direction that would be functional as a motor program. The TKD practitioner and the therapist are working with the pattern of movement presented to them. The intent of the TKD student would be to disempower the attacker by redirecting energy, and the intent of the therapist would be to empower the patient with the same energy.[154–156] In Tai Chi, this would be considered the Ying and Yang of life and movement.

In TKD training, all students begin in the same place. There is no concern for one's status in life. The white belt is used to denote the beginning student. With all students beginning at that level, it allows another aspect of training that is critical to all students and individualized. Training encompasses setting and achieving goals or empowering oneself toward excellence and to one's own quality of life. In TKD, there is a belt ranking system, and the object is to progress through the various levels of proficiency, culminating in attainment of the black belt. Everyone, regardless of social status or physical skill, has the same opportunity to advance in TKD. Students who persevere and obtain a first-degree black belt soon learn that they have only begun their circle of growth and learning. With additional years of training, students may advance in black belt ranks that should reflect a greater understanding and acceptance of those initial tenets. The circle of growth will always lead to further integration of mind, body, and spirit and an inner peace and balance.[157] The balance of mind, body, and spirit is the core of other complementary therapy paradigms and ultimately seems to be an element linked to health and healing.[158]

Tae Kwon Do and complementary therapy[157–163] Although TKD is a martial arts style whose original intent was not to heal a body system condition or to allow one to regain a functional movement activity lost after some acute health care crisis, the concepts and procedures learned, repetitively practiced, and transformed into life behavior have established the foundation for health and healing in individuals. Most students in TKD fall within a health and wellness model of life.[164,165] *Their choice to participate is not based on a bodily system problem, as often seen in a physical or occupational therapy clinic. These individuals are looking to participate from a wellness perspective and expect that Tae Kwon Do will enhance their balance and their cardiopulmonary and musculoskeletal systems through exercise.* Yet many individuals have experienced some aspect of musculoskeletal system problems during their lives. These individuals, as a result of life activities, have forced the CNS to adapt and accommodate to prior bodily system problems such as ligament tears or *physical or emotional trauma from bullying in school.* These experiences create change whether the deficits are motor, cognitive, or affective.[166,167] Similarly, with identified chronic motor limitations that have caused functional *activity* restriction after a birth trauma, an external head trauma, or an internal insult, TKD can help maintain existing motor function, cognitive integrity, emotional balance, and a feeling of self-worth in the face of a long-term and possibly progressive neurological problem. All these components encourage an individual to participate in life and base advancement not only on the standards of TKD but also the individual goals set by each student.

As in all martial arts, TKD requires active participation by the student. When any TKD movement pattern is examined, certain motor control components are seen to be interacting. There are a variety of activities that generally occur during a class. First, there are warm-up exercises, after which the student will work on (1) her or his respective form or *poomsee* or *hyung* (dancelike patterns that may have 18 to 100 different movement sequences), depending on the level of advancement; (2) sparring, which is done either with one partner moving with an identified pattern while the other stays in one position or with both moving and learning to respond to the movements or feints of the other; or (3) learning to focus and perform specific strikes or blows that will lead to skills in board or brick breaking or defending oneself against a life-threatening attack.

When demonstrating the forms, the student will need to work on balance, postural tone, the state of the motor generator, synergistic patterns of movement, trajectory, speed, force, directionality, sequencing, reciprocal patterns, and the context within which the movement is being done. Similarly, memory of the specific pattern, movement sequences, and direction of the movements requires concentration. As the student progresses in rank, the specific patterns become more and more complex, increase in number of specific movements, and frequently change from quick movements to slow, controlled patterns. This repetition of practice and increase in difficulty leads to higher skill and cortical representation.[168,169] If other students are also practicing in class, then each individual needs to be aware of the total environment to respect the space of all other students. This unique individual experience during a group activity allows for variance during each class and thus should lead to greater motor learning and cortical representation.[169,170]

When students learn and practice either one-step sparring or free sparring, they not only work on learning combinations of movement patterns and how they interact or conflict with their partners, but they also learn how to control their emotional responses to threatening situations. Little in life is worth hurting another—a basic principle of

TKD. During sparring, the potential for injury is directly correlated with the control over the force and direction of movement of each individual. That control can be dramatically affected by emotion. Once students learn to control the emotional aspect, their skill and techniques become procedural, which allows their cognitive analytical ability to drive responses. The student is then ready to begin the study of the mind, body, emotional, and spiritual connections that need to intertwine and become harmonious if the student is to learn the true meaning of TKD. Sparring *should be* a controlled situation in which injury or damage to another person is never acceptable. Research over the last 15 years has pointed out the danger a student faces during TKD competition. Mistakes both in techniques themselves and in emotional force placed behind the techniques do create a potential danger to students.[171–177] Therefore safety gear is required at all TKD competitive events for color belt students, and mouth guards are always required no matter the student's age. During class the instructor is never to spar above the skill level of the student nor is the student to enter into a sparring match with the intent to prove power whether emotional or physical. In reality, when a student does take that emotional stance, the motor skills reflect only just how much more that student needs to learn. It is the teacher's responsibility to help redirect students' emotional stances and teach that TKD represents control, not lack thereof. Board and brick breaking are the activities in which a student can demonstrate force production as it interlocks with trajectory, speed, and position in space. If any perceptual or motor variables are incorrect, the student will not succeed. These skills are taught and practiced not to damage or destroy, but rather to learn to go beyond or through the obstacle. In reality, to be successful at these tasks, the hand, elbow, or foot that is used to go through the obstacle is only an extension of the body. Success is based on the learner's ability to tie the entire body's motor response, its rotation, its balance, its trajectory, its force, and its speed into a motor program that will project through one or more obstacles as a knife cuts butter. If the student, emotionally, believes that the obstacle will not break, it will not! The student will stop the movement before completing the task and often empower the wood or brick as a successful obstacle versus empowering herself or himself to overcome that obstacle as if it were not there. This concept is a critical element of TKD. It is also a critical component of any patient's learning of any motor program, turning the program into a functional activity, and improving one's quality of life and ability to participate in that life's adventure. If a patient's CNS is convinced that the movement is not possible, then that individual will fail. Without internal motivation by an individual to accept the possibility of success, acceptance of failure is embraced. This internal environment plays a key role in any individual's overcoming what he or she perceives as an obstacle in life.[178] It is the role of the TKD teacher and the therapist teacher to empower the student to the possibility of success while creating an external environment that will enhance the probability of that success.[151,168] Patients and TKD students need an environment that creates safety, promotes success, and empowers the individual to overcome life obstacles.

Those who respond best to TKD training to maintain motor function are individuals who are motivated to move, enjoy interactions with others, have cognitive integrity, and have some control over their motor system. When instructing a TKD club of individuals who had all had traumatic head injuries, the teacher, a TKD instructor, and physical therapist, whose focus had always been in neurological rehabilitation, found that using therapeutic skills through TKD movement patterns augmented the students' learning and helped them regain motor function through guided activities without the students ever realizing there had been any kind of therapeutic intervention. To those students, they were learning and advancing in a martial arts style, were tested and judged according to their development of skills, and felt accomplished as adults participating in an adult activity. Carryover and improvement in balance, postural integrity, reciprocal patterns of movement, and control of trajectory, force, and speed, as well as development of emotional stability and confidence, could be easily identified and evaluated by the use of standard objective measurement tools. As long as the student continued training, improvement would be expected and carry over into other life activities anticipated. These are the principles of neuroplasticity and have meaning both within the pre-disease or wellness model as seen in TKD[47,179] and after acute injury, disease, or insult to the CNS.[180–184]

Note: A case study on Tae Kwon Do can be found in the online resources associated with this text

As therapists, we desire all patients to continue with movement activities that encourage participation in life. TKD provides an excellent movement-based activity that leads to physical fitness,[185–191] and has been studied in relation to changes in vitamin and hormonal levels in elite athletes.[192–195] One systematic review studied martial arts training, looking at a variety of martial arts styles, including TKD and Tai Chi (TC). Both styles lead to an increase in health status of participating individuals.[196]

When considering the elderly population, a group frequently referred to both PT and OT for movement and balance disorders, TKD training has been shown to improve balance, walking abilities, and somatosensory organization in standing.[165,197] Looking at a martial art that encourages participants to stretch to their respective limits of stability both with fast and slow movement patterns, a valid question must be asked: "Would TKD be harmful to this population, especially if the participants had osteoporosis?" Two research studies investigated that question and determined that training in martial arts such as TKD can teach fall training, prevent hip fractures, and be safe for individuals with osteoporosis.[198,199] Accelerated patterns of the head and pelvis during upright walking can lead to falling in community-dwelling elderly people.[200] Individuals with Parkinson disease show evidence of body system problems causing impaired head and trunk control, thus increasing their risk of falling.[201] During TKD practice as a beginner or advanced student, individuals learn to use the head and hips in rotational patterns, which increases neural efficiency or reaction time while maintaining an upright posture and moving their upper extremities.[202–204] All these components should help maintain the physical capabilities of an elderly individual.[205]

Over the last decade, many research articles have been written that look at one aspect of TKD training, whether it be strength, balance, coordination, motivation, cardiac fitness, emotional self-control, or the effect on the many other bodily systems that interact during a TKD workout. The reader must understand that it is all those elements that make up a TKD student, teacher, or master. In the future, more research will identify this martial art as a potential form of physical exercise for all populations of individuals who have comorbidities after CNS injury (see the case study on Tae Kwon Do online). Physicians and therapists should consider recommending this martial art as an exercise activity for individuals who wish to maintain or regain their abilities to participate in life activities.[197] Until then, students of all ages will be welcomed into TKD studios and encouraged to reach beyond their perceived potential. The age ranges of TKD students now include the elderly population, with classes focusing on strength, balance, and core work, without the need for strenuous sparring or board breaking.[205] A TKD instructor will modify each senior's class experience to allow each individual to reach his or her potential without injury or trauma.

Tai Chi.
Howe Lui

As one of the more popular Chinese martial arts, TC was designed and developed 400 years ago. Its slow, gentle, and graceful movements in coordination with breathing in a calm, relaxed, and meditative way has made TC not only a defensive martial art, but a health-promotion exercise program as well.[206] Currently, TC has been recognized as an effective intervention for improving health, increasing social interaction, preventing falls, and enhancing posture not only for the general population, but for patients with neurological disorders.[207]

The term "Tai Chi" is the common English spelling of the martial art/exercise, but it is also spelled in the literature as "taiji," "tai ji quan," "tai chi chuan," and "t'ai chi"; the Chinese pinyin romanization is the form most often found in scholarly social science literature.[206,208] The Library of Congress and most university libraries also catalog Romanized Chinese with pinyin. The romanization Tai Chi is most popularly used because it is the spelling most familiar to both clinicians and patients and is the standard rendition of the term in PubMed.[208]

During TC practice, a practitioner holds a semisquatted posture and shifts his and her body weight from one leg to the other in slow, repetitive, and alternating movements that emphasize smooth trunk rotation and coordination among the body, extremities, and breathing.[206,209,210] The TC intensity is moderate and approximately equivalent to walking at a speed of 6 kilometers or 3.7 miles per hour.[211,212] Because of its beneficial effects on health promotion and improvement of human dysfunctions, including neurological disorders, TC has been considered one of the most promising exercise programs that people with neurological diagnoses can practice to improve their medical conditions.[207,213]

Tai Chi Styles and Forms

The term "style" refers to sequences of TC movements generally differentiated by lineage names (Chen, Yang, Wu, etc.). What is now known as Chen-style TC was the earliest TC, originating around the middle of the 16th century in China. The term TC or TC Chuan (supreme ultimate boxing) does not appear in historical documents until the late 19th century, but the "internal" or "soft" martial art styles that adopted the name can be documented as early as the late 18th century.[214] Besides Chen style, there are four other styles of TC that are popular today (Yang, Wu, Sun, and Wu/Hao) and claim their origins in Chen style, though this is a matter of some debate among Chen-style practitioners.[206] It should be noted that "Wu/Hao" TC bears no relation to "Wu"-style TC. Wu and Hao are family names, but the two Wus are represented by different Chinese characters.

Today, Yang style is the most popular style practiced by TC practitioners.[209,213] Its characteristics are slow, large, graceful, and sequential movements from one pose to the next with a semisquatted but upright posture (knees bent slightly, less than 30 degree).[208,209] Chen style[208,215] is ostensibly more "martial" in appearance. It requires a lower stance (knees bent more, around 30 to 60 degree) that may need more energy expenditure during practice.[216] Chen also intersperses quick, explosive movements and stamping with slow movements,[210,216] which may explain why Chen style was not as common as Yang style in patient populations. The Sun style features relatively fast hand and slow leg movements.[210] The Wu style set is slow, requiring internal power to maintain the trunk in a constant upright posture,[206] whereas the Wu/Hao style requires a high stance position (like Yang style) with relatively rapid execution of small movements.[210]

The term "form" refers to individual movements within those styles. The number of forms practiced by TC practitioners can range from 6 forms[209] to 108 forms.[217] In 1956, the Chinese Sports

Commission[206] adopted Yang style to develop a simplified 24-form TC for ordinary Chinese to learn and practice. The 24-form Yang style was the most frequently reported and commonly used among TC practitioners in the world. Currently, many short TC forms were adopted or modified from the 24-form Yang style.[208] The number of forms was selected on the basis of the subject's functional level. Healthy, functionally independent subjects could learn and practice 24 or more forms, whereas those with lower functional levels might learn much shorter forms.[207,208,213] For patients with neurological disorders, usually only TC movement components or short forms are taught.[207,213,218−220]

Characteristics of Tai Chi Movement

Several characteristics of TC performance may need to be highlighted, as they are often emphasized by a TC master to new learners.[207−209,213] *First*, to seek the quietness in moving, each TC movement should be full, gentle, calm, and graceful. The slow and alternative opening-out and closing-in of body parts (e.g., the upper extremities) may make the movements look like a moving light silk fabric or like a quiet, smoothly running creek. *Second*, to coordinate the body movements with deep-breathing patterns, when the arms move away from the body, it is time to breath in; while the arms move back toward the body, it is time to breath out. *Third*, to coordinate the body movements with the eyes focused, the trunk, neck, and head rotations should direct the eyes to focus on the palm. During this time, the practitioner should always target the hand with the palm facing up. *Fourth*, to maintain a meditative technique, the mind should be constantly clear, relaxed, and calm, with awareness of body parts in the external three-dimensional environment during TC movements.

Effects of Tai Chi Practice on Movement Science

It has been extensively studied and reported that through the practice of TC, an individual is able to improve bone density, cardiopulmonary function, physical abilities, risk of falls, quality of life, self-efficacy, psychological response, and even the immune system.[213,221,] In addition, effects of TC on posture, balance, strength, flexibility, and gait have also been largely studied and reported.[207,208] As a mind-body exercise, the main part of a TC movement is correct posture. Regardless of what styles or forms of TC is performed, the performer always tries to maintain an upright trunk with the lower extremities semisquatted—this is the starting point and foundation of each TC movement.[207,208,213,222]

Research has shown that TC practice improves the dynamic balance through assessments of posturography, stepping reaction time, maximal step length, Timed Up & Go, BBS, Tinetti Balance Scale, and functional reach. But such improvements seemed to be inconsistent to static balance, as tested with single leg stance and tandem stance.[208]

Effects of TC on strength are primarily on the lower extremity hip,[223] knee and ankle,[223]-225 and erector spinae in the trunk.[225] Additional evidence includes improvement of upper extremity function and range of motion,[226] but its effect on strength in the upper extremities is not clear. Its effect on grip strength was reportedly not improved.[227] From the authors' experience, while incorporating TC in patients with neurological disorders, the initial focus was aimed at correcting or regaining adequate range of motion. After the patient was able to demonstrate and practice TC movement patterns progressively, a cuff weight was added (starting from ½ pound) to the wrist with continued TC practice, thus improving upper extremity strength.

Studies showed improvement in function and gait with greater control of movement and breathing slowly.[228] These practitioners of Tai Chi and considered patients in a traditional medical environment demonstrated more timely posture correction, postural recovery from potential loss of balance, and dynamic postural control when body weight shifted between the left and right lower extremities or at gait initiation.[225,229,230] During double-support time, the mechanical loading on the TC practitioners' knee joint is reduced.[231]

Yin-Yang Philosophy in Tai Chi Theory and Practice

Tai Chi is developed based on the Chinese philosophy that everything, regardless in the macro- or the micro-world, is formed by Yin (the negative) and Yang (the positive). Yin and Yang are relative: Yin can be Yang and Yang can be Yin. For example, Earth is the Yin in relation to the Sun, but can be the Yang in relation to the Moon. Also, Yin and Yang are constantly and interactively coordinating to reach a dynamic harmony. Other environmental examples include the mountain is Yang and the river is Yin; the hot is Yang and the cold is Yin; the day is Yang and the night is Yin; the external is the Yang when the internal is Yin; and the rigid is Yang and the soft is Yin. As human beings, we live in a world where Yin and Yang are always working together to maintain the internal and external harmony.

According to *I Ching* (an ancient Chinese book of wisdom) and traditional Chinese medicine, Yin and Yang also coexist in the human body. For example, the Yang indicates the upper body and the back of the body, while the Yin indicates the opposite. Body extroversion (with extremities opened up) is the Yang, and body introversion (with extremities closed in) is the Yin. More specifically in the respiratory system, the nose is the Yang while the mouth is the Yin, as the nose is above the mouth. In terms of breathing action, words from I Ching, "Inspiration is the Yang, (Qi) flowing on the back of the body; Expiration is the Yin, (Qi) flowing on the front of the body. The alternating change of Yang (inspiration) and Yin (expiration) is the fundamental component of human life."

With these precepts, it is understandable that during TC practice, we emphasize the arm movements to coordinate with the respiration pattern. Namely, for Yang, one must take deep breaths in with the nose while the arms are opened up or away from the body in an upright relatively rigid posture. While for Yin, one must perform in an opposite pattern by deeply breathing out with the mouth while the arms are closed in or moving back toward the body in a relatively relaxed soft trunk posture. Through the Yin-Yang theory and activities, TC leads the learner to reach harmony within the body as well as between the body and the outside natural world. In other words, through TC practice, one may be able to develop more and more awareness of his and her body parts during movements in a conscious way and gradually and progressively toward a subconscious automatic process. Basically, TC practice is a mechanism that allows one to internally harmonize the connection between mind and body, or activities among the nervous, cardiorespiratory, and musculoskeletal systems, and externally harmonize the relationship between the physical body and the surrounding world. The final goal of performing TC is to achieve the status of ultimate harmony of external and internal body ("Tian-Ren-He-Yi" in Chinese).[232]

Mechanism of Tai Chi Effect

TC practice can promote general health and improve cardiopulmonary function, neuromuscular activities, mood, memory, cognition, and ultimately neural plasticity. In the last 20 years, the mechanism of TC benefits has been increasingly studied. TC may have immune enhancement benefits with impact on inflammatory factors to promote general health.[233,234] At the cellular and genetic level, Interleukin-6 (IL-6) and tumor necrosis factor (TNF) are proinflammatory biomarkers, and the nuclear factor kappa-light-chain-enhancer of activated B cells (NF-kB) is for proinflammatory gene expression. After 12-weeks of weekly TC practice in a group of 40 subjects with breast cancer,[234] it was found that subjects had marginal reduction of IL-6, significant reduction of TNF (RR5), and action of NF-kB, as well as downregulated genes for the generation of white blood cells—all indicating that the cellular inflammatory response may decrease after TC practice.

The effect of TC on the nervous system was investigated by studying BDNF (brain-derived neurotrophic factor), which is one of the growth factors for the central and peripheral nervous systems.[235] The investigators found significant increases in BDNF after a 6-month TC practice, indicating potential neural plasticity for improvement of memory and executive functions.[235] The mechanism was also noted through neural activity and neuroimaging levels.[236,237] Researchers reported that after TC practice, there was significant increase in parasympathetic activity in the heart and oxygen load in the prefrontal cortex.[236] Similarly, there was an increased volume of gray matter in the insula, medial temporal lobe, and putamen.[237] These changes significantly enhanced resting-state functional connectivity between hippocampus and the medial prefrontal cortex (mPFC),[237] known to be essential for the memory process.[237,238] These morphological changes in the brain may explain why TC is able to improve memory performance in TC practitioners.

The nervous and the muscular systems respond to TC practice.[239,240] After 12 weeks of TC practice, N-Acetylaspartate (NAA), an important biomarker used to assess neuronal health, was significantly increased in the posterior cingulate gyrus, a key area for emotion, meditation, and memory; recovery time of phosphocreatine (PCr), a substance often used to quantify mitochondrial function, was significantly improved in leg muscles. Toh and colleagues[240] analyzed the mechanism of TC's effect on Parkinson disease. TC practice may be able to (1) normalize neurotransmitter (e.g., dopamine) levels in the motor cortex-basal ganglia-motor cortex loops; (2) promote development of new neural pathways, particularly the somatosensory and neuromuscular control pathways; and (3) improve anticipatory postural adjustment and allow or elicit quick responses to postural changes. Together, these may indicate that neuroplasticity, neurotransmitter normalization, and extremity muscle oxidative capacity can all be improved effectively and significantly after TC practice.

Two recent reviews identified significant changes or improvement in cortical thickness, neural plasticity and functional connectivity, brain homogeneity, antiinflammatory action, motor function, pain perception, and metabolic profile, which may attribute to the mechanism of benefits with TC practice.[241,242]

Tai Chi for Neurological Disorders

TC appears to be a safe and cost-effective exercise program for patients with neurological disorders and has been shown to improve the condition of patients with a variety of neurological disorders. The use of TC with movement problems arising from brain areas associated with specific medical diagnoses can be found online and can be integrated with those chapters written on those specific medical diagnoses.

Stroke

TC improves ADLs, social interaction, general function, motor function, balance, gait, mood, and mental health.[213,242] TC has positive impact on social and general functioning for community-dwelling patients with stroke (2 times per week for 12 weeks), with improved reaction time and limits of stability in the affected and nonaffected side.[243] TC improves general health, sleep quality, anxiety, and depression[244] and demonstrates excellent adherence rates (92%) with TC exercise 150 minute/week for 12 weeks.[245]

In a meta-analysis, Ge and colleagues[220] and Lyu and colleagues[246] found that regardless of the various TC forms or components of TC

movement, significant improvement of upper and lower extremity and overall motor function were identified. However, the effect of TC on mood and mental health in stroke patients is inconsistent. Lyu and colleagues[246] reported that TC might be able to promote sleep quality and improve depression, anxiety, and cognition.

In terms of TC dosage parameters for patients with stroke, the most common recommendation is 30 to 60 minute/day, 5 to 7 times/week, for an average duration of 12 weeks (can be ranged from 2 to 52 weeks). Most TC studies were conducted with community-dwelling patients versus acute settings.[213,220,247] (Refer to Chapter 24 for additional information.)

Parkinson Disease

TC has been prescribed as a sensorimotor agility exercise program for patients with PD[248] to improve general function, balance, gait, quality of life, and mental health.[213] Patients with mild to moderate idiopathic PD, TC (60 to 90 minute/day, 2 to 3 days/week for 12~24 weeks) improves 50-foot speed walk,[249] Timed Up & Go,[249–251] functional reach,[249] BBS,[250] Unified Parkinson Disease Rating Scale (UPDRS),[250] tandem stance,[250] 6-minute walk,[250] backward walking,[250] maximum excursion, and directional control.[249] Patients in the TC group had better results as compared to the resistance training or stretching exercise programs in terms of functional capacity and fall reduction.[249]

From published literature, including a meta-analysis study,[219,240,252] patients with PD can benefit from TC practice in motor performance, in balance and functional mobility, in quality of life (assessed by Health-Related Quality of Life), and in stride length in gait and fall prevention. TC may have beneficial effects on mood and stress for PD patients.[253,254]

However, no significant difference was reported in gait speed and strength after practice for 12 weeks.[250] Later, in large and well-designed TC studies among patients with PD, after a longer 24-week TC practice, subjects could retain their improvements after 3 months.[251]

In terms of TC dosage parameters for PD, 30 to 60 minutes in session length, 1 to 5 times per week, and 4 to 24 weeks in duration were recommended,[219] but the most commonly used were 60-minute sessions, 2 to 3 times/week with 12 weeks in duration. Patients in mild to moderate severity or in Hoehn and Yahr stage 1 to 3 could benefit more from TC practice.[219]

Traumatic Brain Injury

Many patients with TBI demonstrate ADL, motor, and nonmotor functional deficits.[206,213] Manko and colleagues[255] added TC exercise to a self-care-skill goal-oriented program for 6 weeks for patients who aroused from a long-term coma. Patients had significant improvement in the skills assessed by the Standard Self-Care Skills.[213] Blake and Batson[256] did not find significant differences in physical functioning when compared with the control group, who received social and leisure activities. This might be due to insufficient short-term TC performance (only 60 minutes/week for 8 weeks). However, in a three-case report[257] with patients who suffered from TBI, but practiced TC for 2 to 4 years, patients had significant improvements in walking without assistance, and one individual even performed ADLs independently and returned to driving a car.[207,257] For the nonmotor functions, two studies[256,258] reported that TC practice could improve mood, happiness, stamina/energy, and self-esteem in patients with TBI.[256,258] TC may help patients with TBI improve their nonmotor symptoms and general mind-body health.[259]

TC parameters in the literature varied from 1 to 3 times a week for a duration of 6 weeks to 4 years.[213] Patients can benefit once aroused from a coma and able to perform.[255] This is achieved through long-term practice, which is consistent with concepts of motor learning and development of neuroplasticity.[257] (Refer to Chapters 3 and 22 for additional information.)

Multiple Sclerosis

Positive effects on patients with MS include balance, gait, flexibility, strength, quality of life, depression, and fatigue.[218] Balance was assessed by Modified Clinical Test of Sensory Organization and Balance (mCTISB),[260] single leg stance,[261] functional reach,[260] 14-task balance test,[218] and BBS,[262] but results on significant differences in quiet static stance were inconsistent.[218] Incremental improvement of lower extremity strength was reported by assessment of the chair-rise test.[218] Range of motion and gait velocity were improved.[263] Quality of life was enhanced in two studies.[263,264] Depression was also diminished.[261,264] TC effect on fatigue is mixed, and future research will have to answer this question more thoroughly. Postinterventional assessment using the Fatigue Scale of Motor and Cognitive Functions (FSMC) and Modified Fatigue Impact Scale (MFIS-5) showed significant decrease in fatigue, but no significant change was identified as measured with the Fatigue Severity Scale.[218]

The range of TC dosage parameters for MS varies from 30 to 60 minutes in session length, 6 to 50 sessions, and 3 to 25 weeks in duration.[218,262] The most commonly used parameters are short 6 TC forms, 30 to 60 minutes with multiple rest intervals per session, and 1 to 2 sessions each week for 12 weeks.[218,262] Patients in various stages of MS can learn to perform TC, but those living in the community seemed to benefit more from the practice,[218] which is consistent with current literature on motor function and the need to practice to maintain movement function. (Refer to Chapters 3 and 17 for additional information.)

Spinal Cord Injury

Wheelchaired TC exercises are modified for patients with SCIs.[265] Published studies indicate that seated TC is able to improve sitting balance, trunk and hand grip strength, quality of life, sense of pain, emotion, mental distraction, and physical sense of well-being.[266,267] However, no significant effect was identified on fatigue and depression among SCI patients.[266]

TC dosage parameters for this population may include 90 minutes per session, 1 time a week for 12 weeks,[266] while others choose 30 minutes, 2 times per day, 5 times a week for 6 weeks.[267] These indicate that short session length and high frequency with short duration might lead to more improvement in physical function, while the long session length, low frequency, and long duration would lead to more positive changes in emotion and mood. (Refer to Chapter 14 for additional information.)

Vestibular Dysfunction

There was a lack of literature in patients with vestibular dysfunction. McGibbon and colleagues[268] studied the neuromuscular mechanism of TC practice in patients with vestibulopathy. They found that after 10 weeks of TC practice, patients with vestibulopathy demonstrated a significant positive relationship between change of leg mechanic energy expenditure and change of trunk velocity and range during gait. This suggests that patients with vestibulopathy will have enhanced body control to avoid loss of balance after TC practice.

Summary

Although TC is one of many integrative approaches to enhancing both movement function, it has also been shown to motivate an individual's quality of life through participation. Group TC is often found within many communities throughout the world, which helps enhance life participation. Furthermore, social interactions through TC can improve quality of life among all ages, regardless of age or movement dysfunction.

Yoga Galantino

Mary Lou Galantino

Yoga is an ancient Indian mind-body practice that has been in existence for more than 2000 years.[269] It focuses on a combination of meditation, mindfulness, self-exploration, breathing control, and body movement to improve flexibility, focus, balance, and strength. The two types of yoga popular in the United States are Hatha and Iyengar. Hatha involves optimal breathing while holding the body in particular postures known as *asanas* for periods of time and controlling breathing rate and focus.[270] Iyengar yoga uses the aid of supports, props, blocks, and belts to allow better control to perform the *asanas*.[271,272] Although yoga has been accepted in other countries for centuries, the evolution in the United States has been a recent phenomenon. Research on the effect of yoga in the musculoskeletal areas is promising,[272–274] yet research in the neurological population is emerging and in need of larger randomized clinical trials. This section will present a general analysis of the benefits and efficacy of yoga for individuals with a variety of common neurological issues.

Carpal tunnel syndrome. Physical and occupational therapists treat carpal tunnel syndrome (CTS), an upper-limb neuropathy caused by compression of the median nerve. Symptoms involve numbness, tingling, and pain from repetitive movements that respond to a variety of treatments.[275,276] Two studies specifically explored the use of yoga to treat subjects with CTS. A yoga trial with 42 individuals tested the effectiveness of a yoga regimen on CTS symptoms. Those in the experimental yoga group were given 11 postures designed to stretch and strengthen the upper limbs, along with relaxation techniques, twice a week for 8 weeks at a local geriatric center. A control group was given wrist splints or no treatment at all.[277] Significant improvements in grip strength, pain reduction, and Phalen sign were noted. However, no statistically significant change was recorded in sleep improvement, Tinel sign, or median nerve conduction; however, improvements were noted in pain and function 4 weeks later.[277] A second study investigated the impact of yoga in patients with osteoarthritis. Twenty-six participants performed a 1-hour yoga session each week for 8 weeks with reported significant improvement in joint and hand pain during activity.[278] Larger randomized clinical trials could provide definitive evidence for patients with CTS.

The specific use of YOGA when dealing with movement problems caused by brain problems arising from specific medical diagnosis can be found on line and should be integrated with specific chapters dealing with those movement problems.

Stroke and hemiparesis. Strokes are the primary cause of adult disability in the United States and Europe, with 4.7 million individuals in the United States living with the sequelae of stroke. Extreme difficulties encountered while performing simple movements result in a sedentary lifestyle in this population, and resultant muscle atrophy further potentiates fall risk.[279]

A pilot study with four subjects observed the impact of yoga as a treatment for impairments post-stroke. Baseline measurements included the BBS, Timed Movement Battery (TMB), and SIS version 2.0. Three of the four participants had statistically improved BBS scores indicating improved balance, improved self-selected speed on the TMB indicating enhanced ability to perform everyday tasks, and positive changes in quality of life based on the SIS.[279]

Other factors may have affected the outcome of this pilot study, including differing adherence to the home exercise program with varying participation levels, degree of impairment, and fear of pain, which reduce participation with certain *asanas*. Those who adhered to the program witnessed more improvement than those who did not follow it as closely. Yoga appears to have some level of positive impact on function in post-stroke patients,[279] and a recent systematic review of eight clinical trials was done on the effects of yoga after a stroke for improvement of balance. Many stroke survivors have a least some degree of difficulty with balance, which can then affect all areas of daily living activities. The current research is not consistent with the duration or the type of yoga practice that should be performed, as studies varied based on the regions they were done. The exact reasons that yoga is beneficial in this population are unknown. It is hypothesized that it helps improve proprioception through posture, movement, and breathing techniques, but the protocol for treatment needs to be better defined.[280]

Multiple sclerosis. Individuals with MS can suffer from virtually any neuropathy, fatigue, ataxia, and chronic or acute pain. In addition, cognitive, digestive, visual, and speech problems may also occur. Although there is no cure for MS, patients have life expectancies similar to those unaffected by the disease, and yoga may be an option to manage the various impairments encountered through the years.[281,282] It is interesting to note that 65% of those diagnosed with MS use some CAM, with yoga being the most popular.[283] Perhaps the best study to date was a 6-month study that compared Iyengar yoga and exercise interventions. Participants underwent multiple cognitive assessment tests such as the Stroop Color and Word Test and the Cambridge Neuropsychological Test Automated Battery to test reaction times in performance of certain tasks that are difficult for individuals with MS. These tests measure attention and visual and auditory abilities to determine the impact of cognitive abilities. Alertness, mood, fatigue, and quality of life were also measured using the Profile of Mood States (POMS), the SF-36, electroencephalography, and physical activities such as a timed walk.[281] Of those who completed the study, both the exercise and yoga intervention groups had greater quality of life based on data from self-assessment forms (SF-36), a reported increase in vitality and energy, and a decrease in fatigue.[281]

Research exploring the use of yoga for MS is promising, and while the evidence for mind-body medicine in MS is limited, they are safe and may provide a nonpharmacological benefit for MS symptoms.[284,285]

Epilepsy. Yoga, as well as other mind-body practices, has shown promise in helping control seizures. One yoga meditation trial reported a 62% decrease in seizure occurrence at 3 months, 86% at 6 months, and 40% of the subjects becoming seizure free.[286,287] The patients in this study had hyperventilation-related epilepsy caused by anxiety, so the meditation and controlled breathing exercises along with the asanas may have led to a better understanding of how the subjects could control their diaphragm and experience relaxation, resulting in the high success rates. In this study, electroencephalographic data recorded a large shift in frequency from 0 to 8 Hz to 8 to 20 Hz, with an increase in A-band power and a decrease in D-band power. These results showed improvement in control and power of breathing. Yogic meditation regulates the limbic system, providing better control over endocrine secretions and lowering the chance of over-firing neurons.[287] Another investigation tested the use of yogic meditation for 1 year versus a control of no meditation in patients with drug-resistant epilepsy.[288] Data showed significant differences between the experimental and control groups, with the experimental group having significantly lower seizure activity over the observation period.[287]

Efficacy of a yoga meditation protocol (YMP) as an adjunctive treatment in patients with drug-resistant chronic epilepsy[289] was a trial based on the frequency of complex partial seizures, which was assessed after 3, 6, and 12 months. Participants sat in a relaxed position

with legs crossed *(sukhasana)* and focused on deep, slow, controlled breathing *(pranayama)* for 5 to 7 minutes, followed by silent meditation.[289] Patients were instructed to perform YMP daily for 20 minutes in the morning and evening at home and at supervised sessions.[289] Individuals with greater than or equal to a 50% reduction in the rate of monthly seizures were classified as responders, whereas patients with less than this percentage in seizure reduction were classified as nonresponders.[289] After the first 3 months, there was a reduction in the frequency of seizures in all but one patient. Fourteen patients continued the YMP for 6 months or more and were tested again. Of these, six were seizure free for a 3-month period, and three were seizure free for 6 months.[289] The authors of this study concluded that yoga was cost-effective with less adverse events with drug-resistant forms of epilepsy.

Human immunodeficiency virus. A pilot study examined the use of a yoga intervention for individuals with human immunodeficiency virus (HIV) infection who experienced pain and anxiety.[290] Results indicated a decrease in pain and anxiety symptoms and a reduction in amount of pain medication after an 8-week yoga program.

Another study examined the effect of yoga practice that included breathing, movement, and meditation techniques for 47 participants with HIV disease. Positive changes were noted in the Mental Health Index (MHI) and general physical health on the Medical Outcomes Study HIV Health Survey (MOS-HIV).[291] The Daily Stress Inventory showed a decrease in stress after the yoga program and improvements in activities of daily living were reported. Finally, the impact of Iyengar yoga for 1 month may reduce depression and improve immunity in individuals living with HIV disease.[292]

Fear of falling and insufficient balance. A 12-week yoga practice for adults aged above 65 years with fear of falling and balance problems included sessions of yoga asanas and breathing exercises in sitting and standing.[227] Fear of falling was measured using the Illinois Fear of Falling Measure, and balance was captured with the BBS before and after the yoga intervention. Results showed a 6% decrease in fear of falling, 4% increase in static balance, and 34% increase in lower-body flexibility.[293] Our chair yoga study showed a reduction of fear of falling and improvements in the Short Physical Performance Battery in seniors above the age of 65 years who received previous physical therapy interventions for a fall.[294] Another observational study explored the effect of yoga on balance, fear of falling, and quality of life in 26 postmenopausal and osteoporotic women aged 55 years and above. Results of the Quality of Life Questionnaire of the European Foundation for Osteoporosis (QUALEFFO) and a neuromuscular test battery revealed improvements in all aspects of the QUALEFFO for the yoga participants as well as improved ability to stand on one leg and improved perception of general health.[295]

There is also research that states yoga can help improve balance in patients with Parkinson disease, while also improving anxiety, depression, and overall quality of life. There were only two studies that were examined, so more research is needed in this area.[296]

Conclusion. Available data on the use of yoga as a therapeutic intervention for people with various neurological disorders are promising. Most studies have small sample sizes but do show trends toward improved function and reduced impairments. In general, yoga can assist in the establishment of the mind-body connection and awareness of self for individuals with neurological challenges. Greater self-awareness may explain why patients report improvements in quality of life, improved ability to better manage their disease, and a deeper understanding of their own bodies. Relaxation that results from yogic meditation fosters stress management and may improve the outlook on long-term management of neurological conditions. Yoga may serve as an adjunct to traditional exercise and can be adapted for elderly patients who are unable to perform strenuous exercise. Yoga may be modified to accommodate patients with almost any physical or cognitive disability, and potentially provide mental enhancement, which can create a significant relaxation effect. Further research is needed to further explore specific effects of yoga practice in neurological populations.

Energy Therapy Approaches
Reiki: Feng Shui, Chakras
Lexie Hashimoto

When reviewing holistic practices, it should be remembered that these practices came from ancient times when people were in tune with nature, their surroundings, each other, and ultimately the universal energy. Today we have made many strides in science and technology, but that also brings more distraction, more stress, the ability to "get more done," more comparison, and ultimately less connection with that universal life-force energy fueling our bodies, minds, and nature around us. The quote below from Lao Tzu, one of the greatest Chinese sages, touches the very importance of working on subtle energies when healing others.

> "In ancient times, various holistic sciences were developed by highly evolved beings to enable their own evolution and that of others.
>
> These subtle arts were created through the linking of the individual minds with the universal mind.
>
> They are still taught today by traditional teachers to those who display virtue and desire to assist others.
>
> The student who seeks out and studies these teachings furthers the evolution of mankind as well as her own spiritual unfolding.
>
> The student who ignores them hinders the development of all beings."
>
> —*The Unknown Teachings of Lao Tzu*
> *Hua Hu Ching*
> *Translated by Brian Walker*[297]

What Is Reiki?[298–307]

Reiki is a Japanese word for "universal life force energy." The system of healing was introduced to the United States from a lineage of Reiki called Usui Shiki Ryoho. Dr. Mikao Usui was a Buddhist monk in Japan with a desire to understand the nature of spontaneous healing like that of the Buddha and Jesus. Looking for that answer, he was guided to secluded meditation for 21 days. It has been said that he took the Yoga Sutras of Patanjali with him to Mt. Kurama and placed 21 stones in front of him to count the days.[308] On the last day, he experienced his awakening and claimed to have a Reiki as a form of healing that incorporates clear consciousness and uses strong intention not only as a healer but also from the patient.

The Seen and Unseen Influences of Energy Around and Within Us

When we begin to discuss ancient healing techniques, we need to recognize that the components of the bodily system go further than what the eye can see. Reiki works with the part of the person that doesn't need any language or belief system to be understood. The souls' connection through emotions, instinct, and intuition may be the universal language among not only humans, but all living things. Energy can be measured as over active, deficient, or stagnant. The chakra system is a way of measuring the unseen energy flow in the body. People tend to

suppress and/or store emotional or painful experiences instead of accepting and resolving the situation. These unseen energies will eventually manifest in the physical body in forms of disease or pathology. That becomes what is often seen by the person and where Western medicine often begins treatment. Looking for external healing sources for an internal soul disease may heal the manifest illness but won't resolve the disease. Aligning the body, mind, and spirit will access new levels of healing. Being able to connect that a headache may be from stress is the first part of identifying the disease, but being able to get the root source and cause of the stress someone feels may rid the person of recurring headaches over time. Reiki helps assist someone to access their soul so that the individual can tap into one's own suffering—by quieting the mind and reaching into those deep inner samskaras (emotional impressions and/or conditioning) and finding ways of healing the past to not impact the future.

Feng Shui: The Art of Arranging Your Outer World to Enhance Your Inner World

Another way of looking at the idea of energy is the ancient art of Feng Shui. This is where the placement of buildings and interior décor is used to enhance the flow of energy. Feng Shui means "wind and water," the unseen energy of wind along with the seen energy of water. When both wind and water are balanced, there is a harmonious and pleasant effect on the surroundings. If out of balance, just as a hurricane, it can be destructive. Again, this is a system of recognizing energy that may be stagnant, overactive, or deficient. When a person has a lot of clutter in a home, they may suffer from stagnant energy, finding it hard to gather the motivation to create change in their life. Or if they have a layout where their energy disperses quickly, they may always be on the run or always working from a never-ending to-do list. As an example, imagine painter's plastic hanging on a doorway in the back of first level of your house. When the front door opens and closes, unseen energy is moved. Eventually, the unseen energy will reach the plastic hanging in the back doorway, and you will see and hear the plastic move. If the plastic doesn't move eventually, that would be a signal to look at the energy flow. This is a visual way for recognizing unseen energy. Therefore the space someone lives in can drastically impact her and his quality of life. The practice of working with this invisible *ki/chi/prana*, life-force energy, can either enhance one's life or hinder it. Once again looking at the connection one has with their own *ki* is part of the cultivation that Reiki brings to light for people.[309] Taking accountability in how one lives in all areas is essential to self-cultivation. Feng Shui is not about simply placing or arranging items around a home in a certain way with set expectations of certain outcomes. It is the connection to one's intention and investing in overall subtle energies to enhance the quality of life. The more we begin to sense energy in the external sense, the more we can recognize the connection of our internal world's chaos or harmony, which eventually manifests our external reality.

Chakra: Internal Energy Wheels

The chakra system is a way of measuring energy fields within the body. Looking at the Hindu chakra system, there are seven main energy vortices stacking along the spine from the coccyx region or the root to the crown of the head considered the link to spiritual energy.[310] These energy wheels may correspond to locations in the physical body; however, they are indictive of the subtle energetic field we all have.[311] *"The chakras are connected to the functions of the way, all organs, tissues, and cells receive the energy for their various uses."*[311] Energy then is the vibration and frequency that either stabilizes, overstimulates, or slows down the chakra wheels, which then leads to other physical forms in the body that can be seen in the quality of health of a person. If you have a glass of water sitting on a table and if something hits the table, you will be able to see the water go from stillness to motion. The vibration travels and impacts the water without the water being touched by any physical outside force. When we begin to observe the body beyond the physical form and tap into the energetic field of someone, these subtle frequencies that may need work could be the starting point of treatment, saving more invasive or altering methods for cases that need immediate life-saving assistance.[309]

Five Reiki Principles and Self-Cultivation

With the right intention and working with the basic principles of Reiki (even if one is not attuned to Reiki energy), the healing effects on oneself can be powerful. Across any alternative or holistic practice, a consistent theme is *self-cultivation*. A practitioner can only help with assisting someone who comes to her and his clinic. The patient or patient also needs to have the intention of healing, and the practitioner can work with their intention. Should the patient or patient not have the will to either heal or assist in healing, the practitioner can certainly connect with the patient and plant a seed of insight that may sprout an interest in healing.

The cultivation of ones' internal peace is essential to understand the magnitude of healing. We study our whole lives to accomplish many things; however, one area that we don't spend much time mastering is our thoughts and minds. Our mind is the gateway to how we perceive everything. Creating healthy, accurate, and clear perceptions is integral in being able to handle the full array of emotions we all experience without getting stuck on any particular one. Reiki offers a daily practice of shaping how we exercise our thoughts and mind.

The five precepts of Reiki are as follows:
1. *Just for today, I will not worry.*
2. *Just for today, I will not have anger.*
3. *Just for today, I will work with integrity.*
4. *Just for today, I will be grateful.*
5. *Just for today, I will be kind to all living things.*

Reiki understands the demands on humans and how challenging it can be to keep up with virtuous habits. Therefore the precepts all start with "*just for today…*" Each day we can start fresh. It cannot be stressed enough that simply *knowing* these precepts is not a means to connection; it must be a cultivated practice. This means that someone who wishes to work with Reiki, or simply having a higher level of connection with others, must practice self-reflection, self-study, meditation, living with intention, and gaining clear perspective. Current research supports the use of Reiki as a potential method of reducing pain and improving one's well-being.[10,312,313]

Methods and Tools

There are different levels of Reiki, the first is self-healing and learning to feel energy in one's own body and, when comfortable, gifting healing to recipients who are open to receiving it. When attuned to Reiki First Degree, the individual learns the hand positions and commits to a 21-day period of self-practice. This is a wonderful way to learn what subtle energy is personal and experience what it is like to heal personal samskaras. Level II is where one receives sacred symbols to aid in healing and begin hands on healing for others along with distance healing. The third and final attunement is becoming a Reiki Master, where the practitioner becomes the teacher.

When initiating a Reiki healing session, the practitioner should be intent on calling in the highest form of healing energy for their patient and making a strong and clear connection with the patient. This means no "*to-do*" lists running through his and her head, not thinking of the

next person, and not allowing personal stressors to interfere. Single-point focus is a tool that takes practice, especially in our modern world of distractions and multitasking. When the patient arrives, having an open discussion to allow the chance to relax and become present in the healing space and release distracting thoughts is important to allow the patient to truly open herself and himself to healing.

Hands-on healing is used either directly on a patient or working a few inches above their physical body in their energy field. Other tools may be singing bowls, tuning forks, crystals, essential oils, etc. As mentioned previously, vibrations and frequencies are able to reset chakras and energy fields. These methods of sensory stimulation create a vibration within the body that will resonate throughout.[314] People may experience several forms of energy during a healing session, such as heat, vibration, pulsation, tingling, seeing colors, sensing smells, laughter, crying, muscle twitches, etc. After a healing session, patients may feel much lighter, so much that you need to allow them to have the chance to become grounded again.

Future of Healing and Interaction With Patients

People are searching for alternative forms of healing or help. There is a *tanha* (a Pali word meaning thirst or desire) among people for healing on a level much deeper than the physical body. The more each of us can become heart-minded (*kokoro* in Japanese) with our thoughts, actions, and connection, the more we will all be emanating a healing nature. When the practitioner is able to connect to a patient or patient on her and his level, that clinician may open a new form of communication that uses active listening (to their history or ongoing issues that create hindrances for that individual), thus engaging the patient from her and his perspective and offering ongoing expertise or input in forms that the patient will hear and receive and may stimulate healing in a way that individual has not been exposed to before. Effective communication goes much deeper than simply offering information. It connects to someone on an energetic level and uses empathy and compassion to relay information that may impact their life.

The energy that each therapist brings to the environment when meeting an individual can impact that person. If a clinician rushes into an appointment carrying the mental and emotional load of the day or the stress and anxiety he and she may feel, the patient will be exposed to that energy. Conversely, if the clinician is mindful, able to isolate and compartmentalize, and has intention and connection with her and his spirit for the highest good or healing possible, then that patient will also be exposed to the clinician's higher self.[315] Recognizing the importance of taking moments to do less, become comfortable with silence, and connect to the inner self is important in the current world we live in. Realizing that giving ourselves moments to calm our system down will bring clarity and allow us to ultimately heal more deeply. Sometimes just stopping long enough to take two or three deep cleansing breaths before greeting the next patient can center your emotions and allow you to regain equilibrium and inner harmony.

After a Reiki healing session is over, a practitioner releases her and his connection of healing that individual and gives back the responsibility of healing to the patient. Teaching patients about self-cultivation is also necessary to empower patients or patients to take part in her and his own healing journey. Life is an adventure from the moment we take our first breath to the moment we take our last. In between are those opportunities to grow, learn, and connect to the pure universal life-force energy within each of us.

For additional information on Reiki, chakras, and Feng Shui as a tool to help others regain balance and function in their daily lives, a suggested reading list has been provided online.

Therapeutic Touch

Ellen Zambo Anderson

Therapeutic Touch (TT) is a complementary health approach based on the concept of energy fields, sometimes referred to as *biofields*. TT is practiced by nurses, rehabilitation specialists, and others for the purposes of reducing pain and anxiety, accelerating the healing process, and promoting a sense of well-being.[316] Although not specifically named or described by the US NCCIH, TT is considered a mind and body practice.[317]

Assumptions. There are four assumptions that form the foundation for TT as an intervention that can facilitate healing and health. The first assumption, described by Delores Krieger, RN, PhD, the developer of TT, is that the body is an open energy system. The open system allows energy, often referred to as *subtle energy*, to flow within and through the body. This flow allows for a dynamic interface with the environment.[318] The second assumption suggests that individuals are bilaterally symmetrical, so that the right and left and front and back mirror each other. This symmetry allows for a balanced energy flow. The third assumption is that an imbalance or an irregular flow of subtle energy is associated with physiological impairments, illness, and disease. The fourth assumption is that the body can initiate and achieve a process of self-healing through manipulation of biofields and restoration of subtle energy balance and flow.[318]

The concept of internal and external subtle energies and their relationship to health and illness can be found in many whole medical systems, such as Ayurveda,[319] traditional Chinese medicine,[320] and Navajo medicine.[321] More specifically, the assumptions of TT described by Krieger have their roots in the ancient concepts of prana and chakras.[322,323] Prana, which is coined *chi* or *qi* in other systems of medicine, is the universal life force or energy that circulates through the universe and all living things. Chakras are the centrally aligned energy centers that are able to receive, transform, and send prana throughout the body. A blockage, interruption, void, or imbalance of prana is thought to exist when there is pathology or disease. Restoration of an individual's energy flow and balance is important for self-healing and health.[324]

Krieger, along with her colleague Dora Kunz, investigated the phenomenon and characteristics of people known as "healers" and concluded that healers possess a heightened sensitivity to their patients' states of health and being and are able to effect change through intention and energy. Through her description of sensing and effecting change in an individual's energy or biofield, Krieger has elucidated a four-step process that defines TT as a distinct therapeutic intervention different from other energy-based therapies such as Reiki and Healing Touch.

Procedure. TT is often performed with the patient or patient fully dressed and sitting. Despite the name, TT can be administered without actually touching the patient because TT practitioners are able to sense and manipulate the patient's subtle energies from a distance of 2 or more inches away from the patient's body. The first step in the TT process is called *centering*. During centering, practitioners center their consciousness so that a state of integration and quiet can be achieved. From the state of centeredness, practitioners initiate the assessment step by placing their hands 2 to 3 inches from the patient's head and slowly moving their hands down the patient's body, noting the patient's biofield. Practitioners may perceive the patient's energy as hot or cold, or sense that a patient's energy is blocked in a particular area. Perceived disturbances in a biofield suggest that the practitioner should return to that area later in the process.

Krieger has described the next step in the TT process as "unruffling the field."[318] To unruffle the field, TT practitioners sweep away bound up or congested energy, which allows the patient's energy field to become open and unrestricted. Opening the energy field sets the stage for the final step of the TT process. During the final step, TT practitioners direct and modulate the transfer and flow of energy so that the patient's energy fields can achieve balance and symmetry and healing can occur. Krieger points out that TT does not "cure" people of their diseases. Rather, she suggests that TT can have positive effects on energy fields and the flow of energy, and that these effects create an environment in which the patient's own self-healing processes can be optimized.[317,318] Sessions usually take 20 to 30 minutes, but TT practitioners have reported that frail patients and children can benefit from as little as 5 to 8 minutes of TT; other patients may require 60 minutes of TT to achieve a state of relative energy balance.

Scientific literature. The application of TT for people with neurological diseases and disorders has not been widely investigated in the scientific literature. Researchers have, however, investigated the efficacy of TT for the reduction of anxiety and pain in a variety of patient populations and disruptive behaviors in people with dementia and Alzheimer disease (AD).

Anxiety. Anxiety is a general term associated with nervousness, fear, apprehension, and worrying. An anxiety disorder differs from feelings of anxiety associated with a specific event and is characterized by an irrational dread of everyday situations or excessive and long-standing anxiousness regarding nonspecific events and objects.

Robinson and colleagues[325] performed a systematic review of the effect of TT on symptoms related to anxiety disorders but were unable to identify any studies in which subjects met the definition of anxiety disorder as defined by the *Diagnostic and Statistical Manual of Mental Disorders* (DSM-IV) or the International Classification of Diseases (ICD-10). In all of the studies of TT and anxiety included in the review, Robinson and colleagues[325] noted that pretest anxiety was measured in all subjects, but these subjects did not have "anxiety disorder" as their primary diagnosis. This systematic review helps show that individuals with neurological disorders and other medical diagnoses may not be diagnosed with an anxiety disorder but may experience some anxiety as they face the challenges of their condition.

Several researchers have investigated the effect of TT in different patient populations, such as those with severe burns,[326] cardiovascular diagnoses,[327,328] and breast cancer.[329,330] Turner and colleagues[326] found that for hospitalized patients with severe burns, TT was associated with a reduction in anxiety with no adverse effects. Quinn[327] and Heidt[328] investigated the application of TT in people with cardiovascular conditions and determined that compared with sham TT, subjects who received TT reported significant reductions in anxiety on the State-Trait Anxiety Inventory (STAI). Women with breast cancer were studied by Samarel and colleagues[329] and Frank and colleagues.[330] Samarel and colleagues[329] found that women who received 10 minutes of TT and 20 minutes of dialogue before surgery reported significantly lower preoperative anxiety than women who received quiet sitting and dialogue, but no differences in anxiety were observed postoperatively. Frank and colleagues[330] found that TT was helpful for reducing restlessness, fear, and nervousness in women who were scheduled to undergo a stereotactic core biopsy (SCB) but that the results were similar between the TT group and the sham TT group.

The application of TT with older adults has been reported by Simington and Laing[331] and Lin and Taylor.[332] Both research studies found that older subjects who received TT had significant postintervention reductions of anxiety as measured by the STAI. In the study by Simington and Laing, TT was paired with a backrub in the experimental group. The control group received just a backrub.[331] In the study by Lin, TT was compared with sham TT.[332] For inpatients with psychiatric diagnoses, TT was compared with sham TT and relaxation therapy.[333]

The researchers found that TT was more effective than sham TT but not more effective than relaxation therapy for reducing anxiety in this population.

A review of the TT literature and anxiety suggests that TT's efficacy for reducing anxiety is inconclusive. Several researchers have reported benefits of TT, yet others have found no effects when comparing use of TT with a control group or with use in patients with another condition. Reasons for the inconclusive results may be differences in the criteria for anxiety and variability in the measurement instruments. Other reasons may include research design issues such as assignment methods, blinding, and the frequency and duration of the TT intervention and comparison conditions.

Pain. Pain is strongly linked to anxiety and is associated with depression, anger, and fear. Pain also has physiological effects, including increased heart and respiration rates, and, when chronic, can result in structural changes in the brain. Pain can interfere with the ability to participate in physical rehabilitation and impair ability to function efficiently and effectively. Nonpharmacological methods for managing pain have the potential for assisting patients in their rehabilitation and achievement of functional independence without adverse effects. Investigations of TT for pain associated with neurological conditions are extremely limited. In a case report of a subject with long-standing phantom limb pain, Leskowitz[334] found that TT was effective in reducing the subject's pain from an 8 to 10 out of 10 on a visual analog scale (VAS) to a 0 in one session. Self-administered TT was then able to maintain pain at a 0 to 1 on a VAS, in which 10 is the maximum intensity. Before TT, medication, stress management, hypnosis, transcutaneous electrical nerve stimulation (TENS), and ultrasound had been successful in temporarily reducing the subject's pain to 6 to 8, but long-term pain management with these approaches was inadequate.

TT was investigated in subjects with chronic pain associated with fibromyalgia syndrome[335] and CTS.[336] Denison[335] found no significant improvement on the Short-Form McGill Pain Questionnaire (SF-MPQ), VAS, or Fibromyalgia Health Assessment Questionnaire (FHAQ) after subjects received 6 weekly sessions of TT. TT and sham TT groups both demonstrated immediate significant improvement in median motor nerve distal latencies, pain scores, and relaxation scores; however, there were no significant differences between the two groups on any of the outcome measures.

Other researchers have investigated the use of TT for pain management with older adults[332,337] and people with cancer,[329,330,338,339] osteoarthritis,[340,341] headache,[342] postoperative pain,[343,344] burns,[326] and various chronic pain complaints.[332]

In older adults, pain from a range of sources was reduced by 38% with TT,[337] and chronic musculoskeletal pain was significantly reduced following three 20 minute sessions of TT compared with sham TT and usual control groups, although no long-term measurement of pain reduction was conducted.[332] Musculoskeletal pain due to osteoarthritis was also significantly reduced with 6 weekly sessions of TT.[340,341]

Giasson and Bouchard[339] found that after each session of TT, people with terminal cancer reported improved well-being, which included a reduction in pain, compared with individuals in the control group. In a randomly controlled trial (RCT), including 90 patients with cancer undergoing chemotherapy, Aghabati and colleagues[338] found that five 30 minutes of TT significantly helped reduce pain and fatigue immediately following the session compared with those who received either standard care or sham TT. However, in a study of women with breast cancer, a session of TT had no effect on reducing their pain or anxiety when undergoing a stereotactic core breast biopsy.[330]

When utilized postsurgically, TT has been demonstrated to be effective in reducing pain when compared with a usual care group in two studies.[344,345] However, in a study that compared TT with sham TT and the standard intervention of narcotic analgesic, there were no significant differences in reports of pain. Nevertheless, TT may have decreased the patients' need for analgesic medication.[343]

The results of studies that have included TT and measures of pain suggest that TT may be helpful in managing pain that arises from many different conditions. There are, however, inconsistencies across the studies that raise questions about both significant and insignificant findings. Inclusion of a control group, use of sham TT, sample size, measurement instruments, and the duration and frequency of TT are factors related to the studies' validity that limit the ability to draw firm conclusions about the efficacy of TT for reducing pain. There is also a scarcity of information about the long-term effects of TT.

Disruptive behaviors. TT has been investigated for its effect on disruptive behaviors in people with AD and dementia. Although most patients with neurological conditions do not typically manifest AD, alterations in cognitive functioning and behavior are often observed. Studies using a within-subject design and the Brief Agitation Rating Scale (BARS) have found that TT provided twice a day for 5 to 7 minutes was beneficial for reducing overall agitation and behaviors of vocalization, pacing, and restlessness in people with dementia.[346,347] When applied in the same way in a RCT, TT was found to be helpful for significantly decreasing overall behavioral symptoms of dementia, including restlessness and vocalizations, when compared with usual care and sham TT groups.[346] In people with AD, results of an RCT that compared TT to sham TT and usual care suggest that 30 to 40 minutes TT over 5 days can be helpful in reducing physical nonaggressive behaviors but had no effect on physically aggressive and verbally agitated behaviors.[348]

Studies[332,333,349] have provided some preliminary evidence for TT's potential use for modifying at least some forms of disruptive behaviors. Additional studies need to be conducted to determine the effect of frequency and dose of TT on the duration of quelling undesirable behaviors. Application of TT to people with post-TBI or other conditions who exhibit agitated behaviors needs to be investigated.

Conclusion. As a noninvasive, nonpharmacological intervention, TT may be helpful to patients with AD or dementia who demonstrate disruptive behaviors and people with pain or anxiety. Research that investigates the mechanism by which TT may alleviate pain and the physiological changes that may occur with TT will advance the acceptance of TT as a useful modality and suggest patient diagnoses that might benefit from the incorporation of TT into a rehabilitation plan of care.

Physical Body Systems Approaches
Craniosacral Therapy
John Upledger and Mary Lou Galantino

Craniosacral therapy (CST) is a gentle, noninvasive yet powerful and effective treatment approach that relies primarily on hands-on evaluation and treatment. It focuses on the normalization of bodily functions that are either part of or related to a semiclosed hydraulic physiological system, which has been named the *craniosacral system.*

Structure of the craniosacral system. The anatomy of the craniosacral system includes a water-tight compartment formed by the dura mater, the cerebrospinal fluid (CSF) within this compartment, the inflow and outflow systems that regulate the quantity and pressure of the bones to which the dura mater attaches, the joints or sutures that interconnect these bones, and other bones not anatomically connected to the dura mater. The bones of the cranium and the second and third cervical vertebrae, the sacrum, and the coccyx are also included in the structures of the craniosacral system.[350,351] In combination with the message sent to the patient through the intentional touch of the therapist is the corrective work that is done on a basic physiological level by gentle hands-on manipulations applied both directly and indirectly to the craniosacral system. The semiclosed hydraulic system includes the dural sleeves, which invest the spinal nerve roots outside the vertebral canal as far as the intervertebral foramina, and the caudal end of the dural tube, which ultimately becomes the cauda equina and blends with the coccygeal periosteum. The fluid within the semiclosed hydraulic system is CSF. The inflow and outflow of CSF are regulated by the choroid plexuses within the brain's ventricular system and arachnoid granulation bodies, respectively. CSF outflow is not rhythmically interrupted, but its rate may be adjusted by intracranial membrane tension patterns, which are broadcast primarily by the falx cerebri and tentorium cerebelli to the anterior end of the straight venous sinus, where an aggregation of arachnoid granulation bodies is located. This concentration of arachnoid granulation bodies is known to affect venous backpressure, which has an effect on the rate of reabsorption of CSF into the blood-vascular system.[352–354]

Technique. The therapist, after mobilization of bony restrictions, focuses on the correction of abnormal dural membrane restrictions, perceived CSF activities, and energy patterns and fluctuations as they relate to the craniosacral system. It is during this time that the patient often moves from a phase of being corrected and having obstacles removed to a phase of self-healing, with the therapist serving as a facilitator of the process. The tenets of CST include the concept that the dura mater within the vertebral canal (dural tube) has the freedom to glide up and down within that canal for a range of 0.5 to 2.0 cm. This movement is allowed by the slackness and directionality of the dural sleeves as they depart the dural tube and attach to the intertransverse foramina of the spinal column.[350]

A basic assumption in CST, as it has evolved, is that the patient's body contains the necessary information for the discovery of the cause of any health problem. The treatment relies primarily on hands-on evaluation and treatment. The hands-on contact is tender and supportive. It is accompanied by a sincere intention to assist the patient in any way that is possible. In short, the therapist serves primarily as a facilitator of the patient's own healing processes. The rapport that develops during the patient-therapist interaction lends itself powerfully to the positive therapeutic effect that many patients experience.

Western medicine imparts a therapeutic modality for curative measures, whereas CST fosters facilitation, wherein the patient directs the treatment session. The inherent participation of the patient through CST promotes a holistic approach to healing. Conventional medical diagnosis will usually be more closely related to what the therapist views as the result rather than the cause. For example, the therapist would search for a cause of strabismus within the intracranial membrane system and the motor control system of the eyes, rather than considering the strabismus as a diagnosed condition to be corrected by surgery. The cause of strabismus can be found as an abnormal tension pattern in the tentorium cerebelli. The therapist then searches for the cause of the abnormal tentorial tension pattern. Quite often, these tension patterns are referred from the occiput or from the low back or the pelvis. If this is the case, the CST "diagnosis" would be intracranial membranous strain of the tentorium cerebelli as a result of occipital or low back or pelvic dysfunction, individually or severally, resulting in secondary motor dysfunction of the eyes (strabismus). The therapist would focus on the sacrum, the pelvis, the occiput, and then the tentorium cerebelli. Correct evaluation and treatment would be signified by a "spontaneous correction" of the strabismus.

Somatoemotional release is a technique that involves the bodily, and usually conscious, reexperiencing of episodes, the energies for which have been stored in the totality of body tissues. A powerful

emotional content is typically connected with this technique, and it has proved to be extremely effective in cases of severe posttraumatic stress disorder. It was tested through qualitative research with a group of six Vietnam veterans in 1993. It proved to be successful in all six of these patients.[350,351,355,356]

Outcomes. Objective responses to CST are based on the removal of obstructions to smooth and easy physiological motions of the patient's body, the absence of energy cysts, the free movement of the dural tube in the spinal or vertebral canal and the rate and quality of the craniosacral rhythm, the absence of pressing responses during the somatoemotional release process, and statements from the deeper levels of consciousness through dialogue with various images encountered in the session that "all is well."[350,351,355]

Subjectively, patients report an increased sense of well-being, improved sleep patterns, reduced manifestation of stress, reduction in or disappearance of pain, increased energy levels, and fewer episodes of transitory illness. How long it takes to achieve these results is extremely variable and dependent on the complexity of the layers of adaptation, the defense mechanism, and the level of spiritual evolution of the patient.

Use in treatment intervention. CST is useful as a primary treatment modality and as an adjunct to a wide variety of visceral dysfunctions. It works well to balance autonomic function, specifically reducing sympathetic nervous tonus. It has proved beneficial in chronic headache problems, temporomandibular joint problems,[357] whiplash sequelae, and chronic pain syndromes. We have used it as an intensive treatment for people rehabilitating from head injuries, craniotomies, spinal cord injuries, post-stroke syndromes, transient ischemic attacks, seizure disorders, and a wide variety of rare brain and spinal cord dysfunctions.[358–361] Little positive effect has been reported in people with amyotrophic lateral sclerosis. However, some remarkable success has been seen in patients with MS.[360]

CST has been used extensively and effectively in a great number of children with spastic CP, seizure disorders, Down syndrome, and a wide variety of motor system disorders, including problems with the oculomotor system, learning disabilities, attention deficit disorder, speech problems, childhood allergies, and autonomic dysfunction.[362–364] CST seems to be safe in preterm infants[365] and has cost-effective outcomes.[366] We have used CST for people living with HIV disease who have peripheral neuropathy and other chronic musculoskeletal and neurological problems. Pain management techniques can be used by the therapist and also taught to the family members to implement for a home program.[367] Future studies addressing the interaction of the immune system with the craniosacral system would be helpful in elucidating the neuroendocrine response to this technique.

Clinical experiences also suggest that CST is a powerful evaluative and treatment modality for patients with vertigo who have not responded well to or have not found relief from traditional medical treatments. CST has been found to be an effective means for treating lower urinary tract symptoms and improving quality of life in patients with MS.[368] Osseous, dural membrane, and fascial restrictions leading to asymmetrical temporal bone movement and, hence, vertigo are some of the dysfunctions of the craniosacral system. More clinical trials are necessary to verify that CST is an effective treatment as well as to determine the full range of symptoms for which CST is beneficial.

Recent studies have found an impact of CST on chronic pain pain,[369] including fibromyalgia.[370] CST improved quality of life in this population, reducing the perception of pain and fatigue and improving night rest and mood with an increase in physical function.[371]

CST along with other osteopathic techniques to treat chronic lateral epicondylitis as opposed to treating it with traditional orthopedic techniques revealed increased strength and decreased pain for both osteopathic and orthopedic groups. The assumption is that osteopathic techniques such as CST can be successful in treating chronic lateral epicondylitis;[372] however, future studies will need to isolate CST to ultimately reveal its efficacy in treatment for this problem.

To date, there have been several studies refuting the value of CST. One example is in *The Scientific Review of Alternative Medicine.* According to this group of researchers, interexaminer reliability among CST practitioners is zero.[373] Other studies suggest that the sutures that CST practitioners are attempting to mobilize are fused in the adult population; therefore the techniques are ineffective.[374–378] Future studies are necessary for CST to achieve recognition as a valid and reliable treatment option.

Training. The prerequisites for training in CST by the Upledger Institute are quite simple. It is believed that any kind of therapist who has a license to see and treat patients/clients might find CST, in its more basic form, a useful adjunct to practice.

There are six levels of training within the series that are required before one can enroll in the advanced-level workshops. The workshops are all 4 or 5 days in length and are about evenly divided between academic work and hands-on supervised practice. The training program is designed to develop the sense of touch, motion, and energy perception slightly before the academic material is presented.

A certification process was established in 1995, along with an International Association of Healthcare Practitioners, of which the American CST Association is a subdivision. The American CST Association, a nonprofit organization, was founded by a group of therapists and concerned laypersons in 1994, and the stated objectives are to bring CST into public awareness, to enhance networking among practitioners who use CST, and develop a certification program that will result in the recognition of CST as a specialty for people who are licensed as health care practitioners in other fields.

Myofascial Release (Barnes Method)
Richard Harty and Carol M. Davis
Myofascial release has become a significant method of treatment for many therapeutic professionals, with some specializing in its application. This approach can stand by itself as treatment or can be used in conjunction with other therapeutic approaches. Due to the nature of the fascial system, changes to the fascial system can have a significant influence on every system in the body. Understanding what the fascial system is anatomically, energetically, and structurally is essential to understanding myofascial release and the profound effects it can have on physical movement, pain relief, the transmission of information, the flow of nutrients, and restoration of function.[379]

The technique of myofascial release (Barnes method) discussed here encompasses both art and science, which requires the practitioner to learn how to feel the quality and direction of restriction within the fascial system with the tactile and proprioceptive senses within their hands and body, as well as understand the physical reactions to different types of force and energy being directed toward the body. Fully understanding the art of myofascial release requires one to be treated by a skilled therapist as well as apply the techniques to others.

The rationale behind this is based on the observation of the anatomical nature of the fascial system and how it responds to injury and strain. No two people are going to present the same pattern of restriction. Restrictions don't follow anatomical structures exactly, because fascia surrounds everything in the body down to the cellular level and restrictions are governed more by the patterns of damaging force placed on the fascia (or body) and how those forces move through the body. They present complex three-dimensional distortions that go in many directions. A skilled therapist should be able to map these through skilled sensory awareness.

These facts prevent myofascial release from being quantified in the same manner as when measuring range of motion, muscle strength, balance, or a functional activity. Trying to quantify the application of specific directional holds on living individuals and then looking at specific outcome measurements ignore the unique nature of every patient and assume the skill of the therapist as an artist is not a factor. This approach to measurement would assume the specific hold has the same effect on every person, which is not true. Myofascial release is a dynamic process that treats living beings whom are continually changing. Quantitative measurements only see one aspect of a single moment in time. The variables and feedback mechanisms are too complex for a simplistic double-blind study to give us any understanding of how myofascial release works or accurately predict specific outcomes. That does not mean myofascial clinicians don't have any curiosity around why it works. Myofascial practitioners can do specific studies on the tissue itself.

Dr. Paul Standley has been able to quantify the effects of sustained strain on small sections of engineered fascia and has determined that fascia produces interleukins, a crystalline protein or cytokine.[380] Interleukins (IL) play a large part in the immune system of the body. Standley demonstrated the increase in IL1b, IL3, and IL8 with the application of myofascial release. IL1b is a mediator of inflammatory response and is involved with long-term memory dependent on the function of the hippocampus. IL3 regulates hematopoiesis by controlling the production, differentiation, and function of granulocytes and macrophages. IL8 induces chemotaxis in target cells, primarily neutrophils, but also other granulocytes, causing them to migrate toward the site of infection. IL-8 also stimulates phagocytosis once they have arrived. It also stimulates the reformation of blood vessels. The increase in interleukins was more pronounced after 5 minutes of myofascial release with decreased production with holds less than 3 minutes. He also noted that tension greater than 9% of the original length caused the effect to start to fall off from the peak at 9%.

This study focuses upon only one aspect of the fascial system that interacts with a large number of components, such as the cytoskeletal microtubular network, the immune system, the lymphatic system, the circulatory system, the nervous system, the muscular system, and others, all with complex feedback mechanisms. These aspects of the fascial system present, within the living person, something far greater than the sum of its parts. So, as we explore the details of individual aspects of the fascial system, which surrounds and infuses every other system in the body, remember, the order of complexity is multiplied when these aspects are combined, not only with themselves, but when combined with each bodily system, the fascia infuses.

Fascial tissue is intimately involved in the moment-to-moment function of all of our cells and is intricately involved with central, peripheral, and autonomic nervous system tissue. It is no longer useful to view the body or the fascial system as a mechanical system alone. Nonlinear system dynamics are at work as we now understand the involvement of fascia with the neuroendocrine system, the brain, and the neurological plexus in the lining of organs, such as the stomach and gut. Fascia must not be viewed by practitioners and/or patients as static, but as innervated, alive, functional, fluid, and self-regulatory. Involving the patient or patient in the process of manipulation of fascia and its embedded tissue enhances the response of the tissue and the patient.[381]

Central to the complete understanding of the effectiveness of energy-based myofascial release for the relief of pain and the facilitation of healing are the following points:
- There are 12 different fasciae or connective tissues in the body, each with varying concentrations of collagen, elastin, and ground substance.[382]

- "Our richest and largest sensory organ is not the eyes, ears, skin, or vestibular system, but is in fact our muscles with their related fascia. Our CNS receives its greatest amount of sensory nerves from our myofascial tissue."[381]
- "The presence of smooth muscle cells within fascia, along with the widespread presence of myelinated and unmyelinated sensory and motor nerve fibers and capillaries, has led to a hypothesis that fascia is an actively adapting organ with functional importance, rather than a passive structural organ alone. This may be the root of myofascial pain syndromes."[381]
- There are 9 or 10 sensory nerve endings in the fascia for every one sensory nerve ending in the muscle. Thus fascia plays a major role in helping us to sense where we are in space and sense our inner tissue in ways not fully appreciated previously.[166]
- Fascia contains myofibroblasts that can tense or release in fascial sheets.[383]
- Fascia has been hypothesized to play a role as the seat of consciousness in the body-mind system.[384] As one example, there are 10 times as many connective tissue cells as nerve cells in the brain. Previously thought only to provide support and nutritional pathways to nerve, the latest brain scan research indicates glial cells "light up" during certain brain states, particularly emotional states. Also, they have been shown to play a role in regulating neuropeptides and neurotransmitters, thereby regulating mood.[385]
- Fascia plays a role in the maturation of stem cells. The fascia that surrounds all cells as the cell wall, and the fascia of the extracellular matrix, which is the environment of all cells in the body, determine the pressures sustained on developing stem cells into their mature forms.[386]
- Three specialized stretch receptor nerve endings in fascial structures help us sense what is happening in our tissue moment to moment as well as when receiving manual therapy. Golgi tendon organs in both tendons and in aponeuroses give feedback about the straightening of the fibers in the tendon. Paciniform endings in the myotendinous junction, joint capsules, and ligaments report vibration and rapidly changing pressures in the fascial net. Ruffini endings respond to deep and sustained pressure.[381]
- Fascia is piezoelectric tissue. Myofascial release that emphasizes sustained pressure and tension over fascial restrictions generates a flow of electrical activity, or information, throughout the fascial system. Electrical impulses are generated in the collagen by compressive and distraction forces within the musculoskeletal system. These impulses trigger a cascade of cellular, biomechanical, neural, and extracellular events as the body adapts to external stress. In response to internal stress, components of the extracellular fluid change in polarity and charge, affecting fascial motion.[387] This response is thought to be involved with the phenomenon of unwinding, an involuntary movement, and repositioning of the body to facilitate the release of emotions, holding patterns, and other reactions based on past experiences still held in the body.
- With myofascial release, the extracellular matrix softens from "gel" to "sol," allowing the fascial restriction to melt and release pressure on pain-sensitive tissue and to rehydrate to allow for conduction of flow of photons and vibration.[388] It is hypothesized that this action facilitates the cell-to-cell communication required in homeostasis and self-regulation and thus facilitates the body-mind's ability to heal itself.[389] This rehydration, combined with the gel-like water formed within the microtubular network of the fascial system as described by Dr. Gerald Pollack, provides the possibility of super conduction, because in crystal form the molecules of water line up, clearing an unobstructed path for photons and electrons to travel through the body.[390]

There are a couple of areas of research that hold great promise in helping practitioners understand why there are such powerful movements in the tissue along with shifts in consciousness reported by many patients. Patients will often express a general feeling of lightness and observe they no longer are triggered by emotions and life experiences that caused them to react in the past. They will describe being able to feel where their body is in space and being able to stand with good posture without trying to force their body into position(s). There is often a sense of peace and contentment after treatment, as if something "heavy" has been removed. While these are subjective experiences, they are desirable outcomes in regard to the quality of life experience. And these are only a few common descriptions heard from patients after treatment.

It is very possible the fascia is a major communication and computation network. It may also be involved in photosynthesis and the conversion of light energy into the flow of water down to the cellular level. This has to do with the microtubular structure of fascia, the water content in fascia, and holoenzymes on the surface of these microtubules.

The first area of research is the work by Dr. Gerald Pollack at of the University of Washington.[390] He has done extensive research on the fourth phase of water.[390] We commonly understand water to have three phases: solid, gas, and liquid. Water forms a fourth gel-like phase when it resides against a hydrophilic (water-loving) surface such as fascia. Water can build millions of molecular layers of a crystalline gel from the exposure to light energy when it is next to a hydrophilic surface such as fascia. The infrared spectrum of light is significantly more powerful than other frequencies of light in driving the formation of these crystalline layers. Infrared light is electromagnetic radiation released during the production of heat. It has longer wavelengths than the human eye can see, and it behaves both like a wave and like its quantum particle, the photon. During myofascial release, there are a number of sources of infrared spectrum light that naturally comes from living beings who naturally produce heat. The release of infrared light is also increased by the application of pressure, which is a significant aspect of myofascial release, because pressure or force creates heat through the mechanisms of compression and the piezoelectric effect.

When water forms these crystallized gel layers, the molecules of water remove impurities and form, which is called an exclusion zone or EZ water. When hydrophilic material such as fascia is in the form of a tube, the water in the center of the tube will begin to flow as an EZ layer forms on the inside of the tube. In addition to the mechanical flow of water being stimulated, there is a conversion of light energy into electrical charge as the EZ water forms an electrical differential between the non-EZ water and the EZ water forming on the hydrophilic surface. Pollack noted that this effect continued to rapidly increase up to 5 minutes and then continued to increase at a slower rate.[390]

Fascia forms microtubules in its many forms, including the cytoskeleton of the cell. Researchers have recently been able to observe fluid-filled spaces between cells with the work of Petros C. Benias and Rebecca G. Wells at Mount Sinai Beth Israel Medical Center, Icahn School of Medicine at Mount Sinai in New York, NY.[391] They describe how they discovered this new organ that they call *interstitium*: "Confocal laser endomicroscopy (pCLE) provides real-time histologic imaging of human tissues at a depth of 60 to 70‚Äâμm during endoscopy. pCLE of the extrahepatic bile duct after fluorescein injection demonstrated a reticular pattern within fluorescein-filled sinuses that had no known anatomical correlate."[391]

These researchers "propose here a revision of the anatomical concepts of the submucosa, dermis, fascia, and vascular adventitia, suggesting that, rather than being densely-packed barrier-like walls of collagen, they are fluid-filled interstitial spaces."[391] While there are many areas of this research that have to be studied in more detail, what they have shown provides a clearer view of the interstitial pathways formed by fascia that have powerful influences on the flow of nutrients and energy throughout every system in the body.

The final area of research related to fascia is the possibility that it may be involved with communication and intelligence at a much more significant level than scientists have suspected in the past. Hammeroff and Penrose have collaborated together to show how the microtubules within the connective tissue of the brain may in fact be the primary source of consciousness and the awareness of self.[392] Hammeroff, an anesthesiologist, noted that neuronal activity did not cease in patients under anesthesia. He began to question if consciousness was driven by neuronal activity as neural activity did not cease while patients were unconscious. He did studies to see what areas of the brain ceased to function while under anesthesia. He determined that anesthetics altered the quantum channels in brain microtubules to prevent consciousness.[393] It was at this point Hammeroff brought in Penrose, a quantum physicist, to determine if these microtubules within the cytoskeleton of the neuron were capable of quantum states from a physics perspective. They have since developed a theory of consciousness based on a very sophisticated mathematics based on the structures that compose the cytoskeleton of the cell called the Orch OR theory.[394]

Neuroscientist Charles Sherrington in 1940 broadly observed that the cytoskeleton was the nervous system of the cell.[395] There is precedent for this because we can observe the single celled animal called the paramecium hunt, run from predators, demonstrate awareness of its surroundings, and navigate. It can do all of this without any neurons. It does have a microtubular cytoskeleton. This suggests that the microtubules within cells might act as information carriers.[396]

Hammeroff and Penrose noted that neurons had highly organized microtubular networks within their cytoskeleton. They also noted holoenzymes on the surfaces of these microtubules and noted they had characteristics of sophisticated computational systems. The holoenzymes could alter the spiral path of energy waves traveling up the microtubules by structurally changing the molecules that formed the microtubule. Cytoskeletons exist in all cells and appear to be connected by an equally sophisticated intercellular microtubular network.[397] This suggests a much finer scale of intelligence processing. They determined that there were microscopic anatomical features present, which could produce quantum states needed to produce consciousness.[392] This might suggest that the restoration of this fascial communication and computational network might provide a global effect on many levels of well-being or peacefulness or a feeling of safety reported by patients. The simple use of touch through sustained, gentle, myofascial release, accurately directed at areas of restriction by a skilled therapist, has been reported by patients to provide significant improvement to the quality of life.

There is a saying that states, "We don't even know what we don't know." As we look at the complexity of the human body and more specifically the microscopic features of the fascial system, any claim to know how it works in total is ridiculously premature. There is a sense of wonder as we contemplate the deep complexity of what it means to be human. As myofascial therapists, we do have the art of this work and the ability to respond to feedback from our patients as we navigate these complex systems through our equally complex ability to feel and respond to our environment. Also, we see empirical results from the application of myofascial release, even though we may not understand how it works.

Researchers in science are often working at a microscopic level, while as clinicians, we are working with the entire human being. It will

take many years before the two are totally connected, but that does not mean the patients are not improving in function and back engaging in activities that they value. Thus until we can make those links, therapists need to remain keen observers through their hands, their eyes, and the emotional bond made in therapy. There is an art to myofascial release that requires specific abilities from a therapist to be applied effectively. Some therapists automatically feel and begin to change those restrictions in patients, but most need to get additional training and education before they accurately apply these techniques. For that reason, there are sequences and levels of training that can be taken to become a qualified myofascial practitioner. Training can help sharpen the focus, but to master this technique, one needs to put in the hours to hone the skills required by any art.

As an illustration of the relationship between knowledge and skill, one can be completely wrong about how the internal combustion engine of a car works and yet still be able to drive. The skill of driving depends on the ability to react to the surroundings and sense the connection between moving the controls of the car and the change in movement of the vehicle and not on the specific knowledge of how the engine processes fuel into forward motion. In fact, if you are focused on the specifics of the car's theory of locomotion and operation while driving, you won't be able to focus your attention effectively on driving itself.

A typical myofascial release technique (Barnes Method) will be applied by gently allowing one hand to sink into the skin and then, without sliding and using the skin as a handle, direct force in the direction of greatest resistance. A therapist may place the other hand in another area of the body and direct a counter force related to what they feel with the first hand. This is modified dynamically as the tissue changes and is held at least 5 minutes—many times longer. In this way, a skilled therapist, with cooperation and feedback from the patient, will map and treat restrictions in the fascial system using their proprioceptive, tactile, thermal, and energetic senses.

In regard to the fascial system, we have barely scratched the surface of understanding how it works, but experiencing myofascial release as a human being is really the best way to appreciate, feel, and comprehend what this approach can do to relieve pain, reduce tension, and restore functional movement.

Models of Health Care Belief Systems
American Indian Healing Traditions of North and South America
Richard W. Voss

Bob Prue, Member of the Rosebud Sioux Tribe

American Indians are understandably wary of the written word. Some may criticize the inclusion of this section in this chapter. This criticism is understandable, because the written word objectifies understandings out of the cultural context and can be manipulated outside the relationship in which the understanding was shared. However, not to include a discussion of American Indian views about medicine and health care is also a concern because it perpetuates the invisibility of American Indian people. The purpose here is to honor the continuing journey of understanding between medical science practitioners and traditional American Indian medicine practitioners to see how these two medicine paths can help restore health to the people and bring about increased understanding—*wo 'wableza*—among people.

Contemporary American Indian Health Care and Traditional Healing: North and South American Indian or indigenous perspectives. In a report to NIH, *Alternative Medicine: Expanding Medical Horizons,*[398] the Lakota (a Sioux people) were cited for the use of healing ceremonies by specialists who are essentially shamanic in their approach to treatment. To understand American Indian medicine ways, one cannot rely solely on written accounts. Although written ethnographical studies may provide a wealth of descriptive data, it is best to talk to authoritative sources personally. Professionals interested in learning more about traditional approaches to help and heal should contact any one of the federally recognized tribal headquarters and the tribally sponsored American Indian colleges and universities for more specific information. Many colleges conduct summer courses on Lakota culture and philosophy that are open to non–American Indians as well as American Indians interested in learning the culture. Readers wanting to know more about the cultural and linguistic revitalization with the Lakota and Dakota people are urged to visit the website for the Lakota Language Consortium.[399]

Today, many of the old American Indian healing traditions are experiencing a renaissance and are beginning to be viewed with a renewed sense of respect and credibility as an alternative and complement to more invasive or secular Western medical models of treatment.[399–405] For example, on the Cheyenne River Sioux Reservation at Eagle Butte, South Dakota, the tribe has incorporated traditional methods and approaches to a variety of social service programs, including services for at-risk youth and care for people with alcoholism, which is viewed as a problem with social, emotional, physical, and spiritual dimensions.[401,402,404,405] A survey of Urban Indian Health Organizations revealed that 100% of the responding program utilized some kind of traditional healing in their behavioral health services.[406] American Indian veterans utilize traditional healing methods to relieve the symptoms of posttraumatic stress disorder.[407] These traditional methods include the *inipi*, or purification ceremony (popularly called the "sweat lodge"), the *hanblecaya*, or pipe fast (often called the "vision quest"), and the *wiwang wacipi*, or the Sundance. The inclusion of these ceremonies within the treatment process has collectively been called the "Red Road approach."[401,402,405]

A number of medical facilities on various reservations include medicine men as consultants on a formal and informal basis,[405,408–410] and the use of traditional ceremonies in health care settings is encouraged and respected.[411] Where the ceremonial burning of sage (a common medicinal herb burned for purification) had been discouraged in the past, hospital staff report increased acceptance of this practice and now arrange appropriate space for traditional ceremonial practices both within the health care facility and outside on hospital grounds.[410,411] One Lakota friend commented on his recent hospitalization at an allopathic hospital. He was visited by a medicine man that placed a bundle of sage under his pillow. This made him feel better and showed how simple cooperation among allopathic medicine, health care practices, and alternative, complementary health care practices can be.

A Lakota centric perspective on health.
A traditional American Indian perspective on health care and medicine begins with the spiritual reality of the human being who is part of all creation and dependent on creation. Traditional understanding views human beings as intimately related to plants and all other creations in the natural world that sustain life. Reality is not linear; it is circular. Everything is connected to everything else. Good and bad, sickness and health, and physician and patient are not separate processes, they are all related aspects and part of the whole. For the Lakotas and other traditional American Indian people, there is no split or dualism in reality or creation. This traditional view challenges the intervention model and offers a prevention model as the starting place for social health and assistance. The emphasis from a Lakota-centric view is on building up the immune system and seeing the important role of the community in promoting good health care and well-being, a cultural emphasis often overlooked in conventional health care practices.

Traditional Lakota values of health and well-being emphasize the participation of the family in the healing process, including the extended family and the larger kinship community, to bring about good health to the individual. The health of the individual is connected to the health of the community, so there is an important tribal dimension to this understanding. For traditional Lakota people, the health and healing process are not impersonal but highly personalized and individualized around specific needs. The roles of medicine practitioners are multidimensional and include those of healer, counselor, politician, and priest.

Another important contribution of the Native American perspective on health is that it provides a rich topology of spirit. The human creation, like all creations, is a spirit being composed of multilayered aspects of spirit. "Spirit" here is not some supernatural reality outside the human being but an intrinsic dimension of everything that is, including the human creation (person). To speak of human beings is to speak of spiritual reality. For traditional American Indians, medical treatment or any kind of social, human, or mental health service is first and foremost a spiritual endeavor.

Ayahuasca: a spiritual pathway to consciousness and healing.
Traditional Indian people of South America have similar and yet distinctive traditions of health and healing where the rain forest provides the pharmacopoeia of medicinal plants, bark, herbs, and vines. Of course, the forest itself is viewed as a powerful source of spiritual healing. In 2004, a study in the Tambopata River area of the southeastern Peruvian Amazon (through the Amazon Center for Environmental Education and Research), Voss had an opportunity to meet with various shamans, their patients, and public health care representatives at a local community center where the regional public school and health care station are located. It is interesting to note that all members of the health care staff rotate, making visits to the area community members, including both indigenous traditional people, who mainly live dispersed through the forest (Amazon), and mestizo or mixed-blood settlers, many of whose families have lived in the river settlements since the mid-1970s.[410] Both indigenous natives and mestizo settlers seek assistance from the shaman, the curanderos, and the health station outpost, staffed by nurses and a visiting physician. The South American indigenous community Prue who visited the Tambopata River region of the southeast Peruvian Amazon used both herbal remedies and spirit-calling ceremonies, often incorporating the use of forest tobacco and other vegetation gathered from the forest as a means of purification. The use of ayahuasca, a concoction or tea made from various plants, tree bark, and vines gathered from the forest, is administered to both patient and shaman and is a common shamanic practice throughout Amazonia, according to the shamans I interviewed.[410] A detailed description of an ayahuasca ceremony is reported by Salak,[412] providing a fascinating participant observer's experience of an ayahuasca ceremony. A brief audio-video capture of the beginning of an ayahuasca ceremony may be viewed at www.nationalgeographic.com/adventure.[413] Clinical applications of ayahuasca are being studied by Jacques Mabit, Director del Centro de Rehabilitacion de Toxicomanos (Rehabilitation and Detoxification Center) at the Takiwasi Center, Peru. Mabit combines the traditional use of ayahuasca and psychotherapy techniques and holistic methods (consciousness expansion methods such as fasting, hyperventilation, and nonaddictive plants) mainly for the treatment of coca paste addictions. The center is funded by the French government. Conventional allopathic medicines are not used, except in unusual circumstances.

Riba and colleagues[414] published their neuropsychobiology study on the effects of ayahuasca. Hence traditional medicine has captured both the imagination and the attention of medical science.

Physical detoxification is accomplished through the use of medicinal plants. Conventional Peruvian approaches to addiction treatment are based on prison or military models, which have raised human rights concerns among health care workers. All studies on the clinical use of ayahuasca have European or South American sponsorship, and most have been published in Spanish.[415]

Health risks associated with ayahuasca. Religious groups in the United States have obtained a First Amendment exemption to use ayahuasca in their ceremonies. Despite the US government's opposition to the use of dimethyltryptamine (DMT), which is the main chemical substance found in ayahuasca, the government could not meet the burden of showing that ayahuasca posed a serious health risk to church members who use it in their ceremonies.[416] Gable reports that there have been no deaths caused by hoasca or any other traditional DMT/β-carboline ayahuasca brews.[416] Furthermore, he writes, "The probability of a toxic overdose of ayahuasca is seemingly minimized by serotonin's stimulation of the vagus nerve, which, in turn, induces emesis near the level of an effective ayahuasca dose. The risk of overdose appears to be related primarily to the concurrent or prior use of an additional serotonergic substance. People who have an abnormal metabolism or a compromised health status are obviously at greater risk than the normal population and might prudently avoid the use of ayahuasca preparations" (p. 29).[416] A systematic review of the scientific literature "suggests that acute ayahuasca administration to healthy volunteers is relatively safe. The literature also gives support to the idea that long-term ritual ayahuasca consumption by adults and adolescents does not appear to be seriously toxic or harmful" (p. 73).[417]

Although there is generally no known harm to ingesting ayahuasca in a ceremonial context, common sense about nonceremonial use is imperative. Using watchers to sit with the person while using ayahuasca and of course not allowing driving or use of heavy machinery is common sense. Therefore a harm reduction approach is necessary. That said, the pharmacology of ayahuasca is such that "selective serotonin reuptake inhibitors can have potentially harmful interactions with MAO inhibitors, so people taking these kinds of medications are advised to avoid ayahuasca" (p. 301).[418] This is consistent with Gable's findings. There are no significant associations between the typical dosage of ayahuasca in ceremonial usage and long-term psychosis. Gable reports that "Many or most of UDV [União do Vegetal] psychiatric episodes were transient in nature and resolved spontaneously" (p. 30).[416]

Gable notes, "The ritual context in which ayahuasca is ingested provides some control of dosage and subsequent psychological effects. Because the natural sources used in preparation of the tea do not allow UDV members to standardize their hoasca brew with respect to DMT or β-carbolines, the person conducting the ceremony drinks the brew before administering it to UDV members as a means of testing for potency. Different amounts of the brew are initially offered to individual participants, and, depending on reactions, a participant may be offered a second cup at his or her request" (p. 26).[416]

Another area of concern is risk of dependency on ayahuasca. There is no convincing evidence that ayahuasca leads to physiological dependence. Of course, this is an area worth careful attention in continuing research, although Gable notes that the general psychopharmacological profile of huasca "suggests that it lacks the abuse potential of amphetamines, cocaine, opiates, or other widely abused substances." Elsewhere, Gable notes that "tryptamine derivatives such as DMT (found in ayahuasca) result in erratic patterns of self-administration indicating that 'these compounds have weak reinforcing effects, or alternatively, mixed reinforcing and aversive effects.'" (p. 31).[416] Gable notes, "The unpredictable occurrence of frightening images and thoughts, along with predictable nausea and diarrhea, makes it a very

unlikely candidate for a 'club drug'" (p. 32).[416] On the other hand, Grob reported that "all of the 15 UDV subjects claimed that their experience with ritual use of hoasca as a psychoactive ritual sacrament had had a profound [positive] impact on the course of their lives." Most of the UDV members had a "history of moderate to severe alcohol use prior to joining the UDV" (p. 30).[416] Most therapies for alcohol or drug abuse involve a thorough and sometimes unpleasant examination of the self. Providing a psychological support system around the patient in shamanic healing is a profound aspect of the healing process in the peyote using Native American Church.[419,420] The safety in clinical settings of similar psychedelic substances (psilocybin and LSD) to treat addictions is well established.[421]

Shamanic Mythology in Palliative Care: New Frontiers

There is expanding international interest in the use of indigenous methods, and mythology and psychological processes in palliative care[422] using structured interviews and shamanic interventions studied the effect of shamanic narrative and mythology on a patient receiving palliative care. These authors noted, "[that] facing the end of life, death, evoked by serious diseases... is not only a question of techno-scientific medicine, of medical treatment, but also a therapeutic work on our narrative identity."[423] Here, both the therapist and patient enter into the shared shamanic experience and each tells their story discovered in the encounter. Santarpia and colleagues[422] state, "The shamanic tradition insists on the idea that disease is a message for the patient's soul; it marks the need for a change and a new existential meaning."[424] Elsewhere, Santarpia and colleagues note that "the patient's experience of healing does not necessarily connote a 'cure,' but it denotes instead the renewal of the person's ability to reconnect with his or her self. This relationship... extends beyond the parameters of the individual's ego and also embraces a connection with the entire universe or 'spiritual world.'"[422]

Shamanic mythology, narrative, and methods have a place in medical knowledge, care, and practice, with a long tradition dating back 30,000 and 40,000 years, with archeological evidence in discoveries of ancient cave paintings depicting shamanic activities such as dance, drumming, and use of animal skins and totems.[425-428] Shamanic practice, mythology, and methods represent both the ancient and future trajectories of medical and health sciences particularly relevant in palliative and end-of-life care.

Traditional Acupuncture

Jeffrey Kauffman and Darcy Umphred

This section has been edited by Umphred to include new references on evidence-based practice to support Dr. Kauffman's previous materials, which was based on the Laws of Five Elements. His wisdom, understanding, and appreciation of the human body and how to integrate various philosophies of health care practices were amazing. When one met him, he presented himself as another human being just trying to find ways to help others with their health care issues.

History. Acupuncture as it is practiced in the United States is a huge conglomerate of different styles of acupuncture coming from China, Japan, Korea, Thailand, Vietnam, and Western Europe. The styles differ radically depending on who is doing the acupuncture, where he or she learned it, and how much individuality has been instilled into the practice. Within this discussion, the similarities among practices are described, followed by an in-depth analysis of the style that Kauffman used.

Acupuncture is one of the five categories that make up Chinese medicine. The other four are herbal medicine, diet and nutrition, exercise, and massage. Acupuncture is a healing method that tunes a human being. Just as a piano tuner tunes a piano or one tunes a guitar or an auto mechanic does a tune-up on a car, it is possible to tune a human being. After this process, or intervention, is done, the body-mind functions more efficiently in a balanced, harmonious fashion. As a result, the aches and pains often are eliminated and illnesses and diseases reversed. Acupuncture can be used by itself and, even better, in combination with other holistic and traditional Western medical methods.

Methods. Acupuncture involves the use of tiny needles made of stainless steel, their diameter two or three times the width of a human hair, sharpened by a diamond. These needles are put into particular points on the surface of the body. There are at least a thousand of these points all over the human body.[429,430] They have a lower electrical potential compared with the surrounding skin, as is evidenced by a galvanometer. These points are also known as *acupuncture points*, *acupressure points*, *trigger points*, and perhaps by other names as well. These points are about 1 mm in diameter and are located pretty much in the same place for everyone, according to bony landmarks, skin landmarks, and anatomical structures such as nipples, umbilicus, fingernails and toenails, eyes, ears, nose and mouth, and so on. The points can be found with practice by the trained finger of the practitioner. There are electrical instruments that can help locate these points, but their reliability has not been established. Needles are put into these acupuncture points, and after being inserted, the needles are turned either clockwise or counterclockwise one revolution. They are either taken out immediately or left in for a period of time, depending on the individual patient's imbalance and illness.

Examination and evaluation. Deciding where to insert the needles is really the key and the most difficult and important part of acupuncture diagnosis. This is where styles of acupuncture come into play. There is a spectrum of acupuncture styles or methods that ranges from completely symptomatic to perfectly holistic, just as there is in traditional Western medicine. The symptomatic methods involve simply putting needles into acupuncture points at anatomical sites that are specifically related to symptoms. For example, for shoulder pain, or arthritis or bursitis, an acupuncturist using a symptomatic method would select acupuncture points that are in or around the shoulder area. Headache would be treated with needles in the head area.[431,432] Constipation would be treated with needles in the belly area. Hemorrhoids would be treated with needles around the anus and coccygeal area. This method pays little attention to where the constitutional imbalance exists within each person. An opposite philosophy, which is called *holistic acupuncture*, treats the underlying constitutional imbalance within the person. Described earlier, such imbalances are considered the vulnerable, or weak, links in the chain in each human being—the part that always gives out first because it is not as strong or disease resistant as the rest of the body-mind. The type of acupuncture Kauffman used is a holistic form. Specifically, it is called *five-element acupuncture*. It is based on the Law of Five Elements, which is a law of nature that comes from Chinese philosophy and is one of the basic foundations of Chinese medicine. It is sometimes known as the *Five Phases* and is considered the most holistic form of acupuncture available.

The law of five elements. The Law of Five Elements states that there are five elements in nature (fire, earth, metal, water, and wood) and that these elements all relate to one another in a particular fashion (Fig. 39.5). The diagram in Fig. 39.5 shows an outer creative cycle (known as *Shen*) that goes in a clockwise fashion and demonstrates that fire creates earth, earth creates metal, metal creates water, water creates wood, and wood creates fire again. Also, a star-shaped control, or destructive, cycle (known as *K'o*) shows that fire destroys or controls metal, metal does the same to wood, wood to earth, earth to water, and water to fire. These two cycles, the creative and destructive cycles, are necessary to keep balance in nature. These five elements are also found in human beings because the body is composed of elements that come from nature and return to nature when the body dies. The emotions and feelings in our personality align themselves with these same elements (Fig. 39.6).

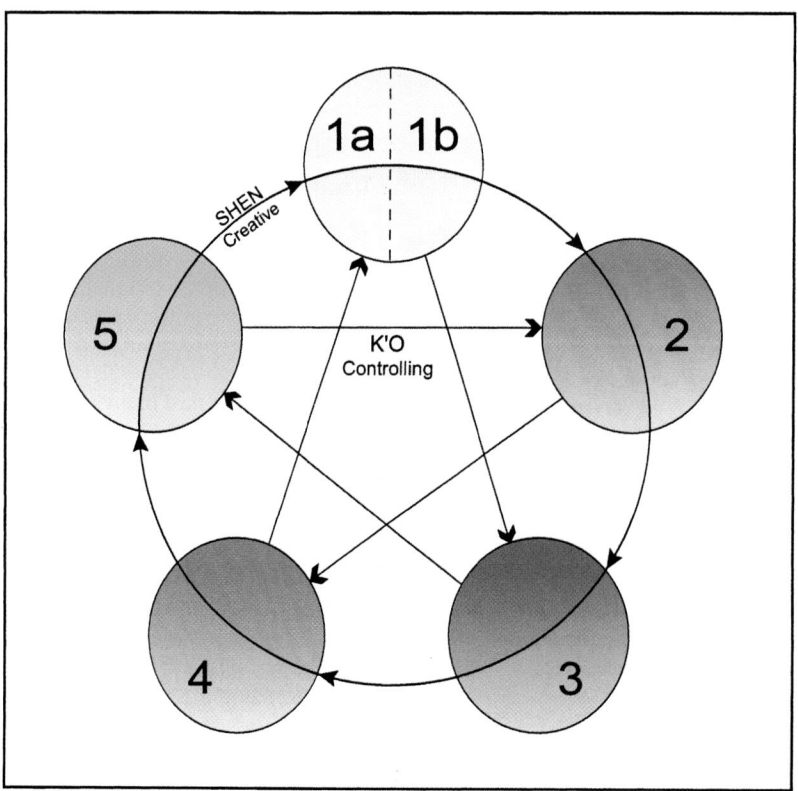

Fig. 39.5 Law of Five Elements: Demonstrating the Shen (Creative) and K'O (Controlling) Cycles.

	1a	1b	2	3	4	5
Element	Fire		Earth	Metal	Water	Wood
Meridian	Small Intestine	Three Heater	Stomach	Colon	Bladder	Gall Bladder
Organ	Heart	Heart Protector	Spleen	Lung	Kidney	Liver
Color	Red		Yellow	White	Blue	Green
Emotion	Joy		Sympathy	Grief	Fear	Anger
Odor	Scorched		Fragrant	Rotten	Putrid	Rancid
Sound	Laughing		Singing	Weeping	Groaning	Shouting

Copyright © 1999, Jeffrey D. Kauffman, M.D., M.Ac.

Fig. 39.6 Law of Five Elements Linking Fire, Earth, Metal, Water, and Wood With Interlocking Variables.

People in Western society have not been taught to think of their bodies in elemental forms, but nevertheless these elements are there. The concept of fire is present in each and every cell. The cells burn glucose to survive, and this is referred to as "burning calories." It is this burning that causes our body temperature to remain at 98.6°F throughout most of our lives. It is not difficult to picture each cell of the body having a little bonfire in the center with mitochondria sitting around roasting pieces of glucose on a stick. Obviously, water is present in our bodies. Students in grammar school are taught that our bodies are 98% water with all the tears and urine and lymph and blood. Similarly, metal can be found in the body in the form of calcium in the bones and iron in the blood, in our teeth, and so on. The concept of wood is most easily seen in the fingernails and toenails, which are similar to the bark of a tree. Also, the ligaments and tendons are much like a strong fiber. The concept of earth is best seen in the gastrointestinal tract. Picture taking a microscopic journey down the gastrointestinal tract starts from the mouth, going down the esophagus into the stomach and the intestines; the further down you get, the more the material seems earthlike, until it is excreted into the outside world.

Each of the elements has a particular color that emanates from the face, a particular emotion that comes from the personality, a particular odor that comes from the body, and a particular sound that comes from the voice, as well as a particular taste, season, climate, secretion, and body part or system that it fortifies.

Every human being has a constitutional imbalance in one of these elements. The explanation for how this happens lies in spiritual law. Suffice it to say that this imbalance is well engrained sometime during the first 5 years of life. Diagnosing this constitutional imbalance is both an art and a science and is done primarily by determining the color, emotion, odor, and sound belonging to each human being. The reader probably has noticed these colors, emotions, odors, and sounds previously with friends or even with strangers. Yet the realization that these are diagnostic clues that reveal a person's constitutional imbalance may not be as self-evident. The person who is always angry, no matter what, is displaying the emotion that goes with the wood element. The person who is always happy, joyful, bubbling over (or the opposite, more commonly seen—very sad and depressed) goes with the element of fire. The person who is always sympathetic and loves to take care of you or is always caring for children is displaying the emotion of sympathy, and that goes with earth. The person who is always grieving, who has tremendous loss and cannot seem to get over it, goes with the element of metal. The person who is always fearful, paranoid, and afraid of life fits into the water element. People have different sounds to their voice.

People who laugh excessively and are always humorous go with the fire element. People who shout a lot, their voices very powerful and strong, and knocking you over go with the wood element. People who have a singsong quality to their voice go with the earth element; groaning goes with the water element; and a weeping sound of the voice, although the person is not crying, goes with the metal element. You have probably smelled people who have a strong body odor and wondered why they did not bathe or use deodorant. There are five different odors, and each one belongs to one of these elements. And perhaps you have seen a person who is green with envy or ash white, white as a sheet, or has pallor in the face. Each one of these colors goes with an element as described in the diagram (see Fig. 39.6).

Each element also has organs relevant to it, with energetic pathways, called *meridians*, which are housed by that element.[433] These pathways, or meridians, are just under the surface of the skin, throughout the body, and serve as channels for an electrical form of energy that flows in all human beings. This energy is the life force. In Chinese it is called *chi*. In the East Indian culture it is known as *prana*. This life force is always circulating round and round the body-mind along these pathways. And the acupuncturist can get in touch with this energy at certain points on these meridians, which are the acupuncture points.

Intervention. Once the examination is complete and the diagnosis is made, paying close attention to the color, emotion, odor, and sound, and the elemental constitutional imbalance determined, it is simply a matter of treating the points along the meridians that are housed by that element on a week-to-week basis. Generally, this tunes the human being and everything starts to function more efficiently and more harmoniously, enhancing the person's quality of life.

There are 12 major meridians, two in each element, except for fire, which has four. Each of these meridians is named after the organ to which it is connected, which is also described in the diagram. Each meridian has 9 to 67 points on it. Each point has a name described by the Chinese that has been translated into English. It is the names and the functions of the different points that allow the acupuncturist to decide which points are to be used on which day and time and treatment. For example, the point Kidney-24 is actually named *spirit burial ground* and can be used to help a person suffering from grief, having lost a loved one. Taking the history at each visit and determining blockage of the chi energy flowing in the meridians are used to select the points used in treatment.

As patients get better, not only do their symptoms decrease in intensity and dissolve and often totally disappear with time, their emotional and feeling states also change for the better. People tend to become happier and peaceful and calm and more capable of handling stress. They often will say, "I feel better in myself." The reason for this is that the patient is not just having her or his symptoms treated. This form of acupuncture, the five-element style, treats the body, the mind, and the spirit and integrates these three spheres of the human being. The point names are particularly revealing. There are names connected to nature and physical objects such as *small sea, greater mountain stream, blazing valley, sea of chi*, and *skull breathing*. There are also point names that have to do with emotions and feelings, such as *palace of weariness, gate of hope, rushing the frontier gate, intermediary, little merchant*, and *abdominal sorrow*. And then there are the points that relate to the spiritual qualities of life, such as *spirit burial ground, heavenly ancestor, heavenly pond, heavenly window, gate of destiny, inner frontier gate, soul door*, and *spirit deficiency*. When these spirit points are used, the person's spirit is buoyed up—it turns back on.

Each treatment lasts 15 to 60 minutes, depending on the individual practitioner. The practitioner can also include any of the following in the treatment sessions: conversation, history taking, massage, joint adjustments, instructions on diet and nutrition, psychosocial counseling,[434] exercise recommendations, and so on. The initial visit takes longer because a history and physical examination are done and sometimes the initial treatment as well. This depends on the technique and abilities of the practitioner. In general, the treatments are done twice a week for the first two to four visits and then once a week as the patient starts to get better. The interval continues to lengthen to every 2 to 4 weeks, and as the patient improves, the optimal interval is once every 3 months—once every season, the patient comes in for a tune-up for maintenance and prevention. In general, a series of 10 treatments is a good way to start this type of therapy. Improvement in the patient's condition may be noticed as soon as the first treatment is done. It may take 5 or 10 treatments before it is noticed by the patient. Depending on the ability of the practitioner, improvement in the patient's condition generally occurs in 80% to 90% of patients. This, of course, also depends on the severity of the patient's imbalance and illness.

When acupuncture treatment is combined with psychosocial counseling, nutritional advice, exercise instruction, massage, or other forms of body work, in which the person is touched with warmth, peace, and love by another human being, great healing can take place. Acupuncture has been shown to be beneficial as part of the treatment of various medical conditions such as stroke rehabilitation,[435-438] treatment of Parkinson syndrome,[439,440] acupuncture for cardiovascular disease,[441] treatment for various clinical problems following cancer diagnosis such as anorexia,[442] pain management due to cancer,[443-448] pain due to back problem,[449,450] or patients with restless leg syndrome.[451] There are many places in the literature where the reader can find additional information on the use of acupuncture with various medical conditions.

Benefits of intervention. Five-element acupuncture can be used for all sorts of clinical problems: physical, mental, emotional, and spiritual. Any and every type of person can and does respond. There are always exceptions to this, but the general rule is one of success. This includes acute problems and chronic problems in outpatients and hospitalized patients. In China, all patients with stroke are automatically treated with acupuncture as well as the more traditional Western methods. It works on babies, toddlers, adolescents, and the elderly. It can be used as a primary form of therapy to which other therapies are added, or it can be an adjunct to surgery,[452,453] radiation, and medication or to other holistic therapies. How much all these positive outcomes stem from the individual's belief that acupuncture will be beneficial is not known. But, as Kauffman stresses, acupuncture interlinks with the mind, body, and the spirit, so possibly the one thing a clinician needs to recognize is that the patient has gotten better in daily function; pain, whether physical or emotional, had been reduced, and

the individual's quality of life is reported to have been enhanced.[454,455] Today's research continues to help all practitioners evaluate the effects of acupuncture on the human organism in relation to our understanding of the physical body.[456] Many colleagues are embracing the use of dry needling for relief of pain.[457,458] Much research is still needed regarding the efficacy of this type of intervention,[459,460] but similar to acupuncture with wet needles, dry needling seems to affect the body, mind, and spirit, and thus confuses Western researchers trying to use a linear, one variable model for research efficacy.

Future treatments. The amount of time it takes for a person to heal depends on how long the person has been ill. A rule of thumb is that for every year a person has had a particular physical or mental problem, it is going to take about a month's worth of treatment, with each session done weekly. So, if a person has had arthritis for 20 years, 20 months of treatment should be expected.

On the other hand, if symptoms have been present for only a month or two, it is possible that they could go away with one or two treatments unless they are the result of some kind of serious illness, such as the sudden onset of cancer or heart disease or something that has been present for 1 or 2 years but has been subclinical. The general average is 10 treatments over a 4- to 8-week period, with a good possibility of illness being relieved partially or almost completely during that period, depending on the severity.

Summary. In summary, acupuncture is a healing therapy that is both an art and a science that comes from the Orient, specifically starting in China approximately 4,500 years ago. Recently, they have found signs that acupuncture may have been used in the Copper Age, with the discovery of the Tyrolean Iceman as the world's oldest glacier mummy.[461] There are many styles of acupuncture, and the most holistic style is known as *five-element acupuncture*. It truly helps integrate the body, mind, and spirit. When acupuncture is combined with teaching the patient how to live a healthier lifestyle, including eating a healthy diet, reducing stress, making healthy choices, thinking healthy thoughts, and including fun and relaxation, true healing can occur. Because of the chronic and degenerative nature of many illnesses in the United States, it is possible that total healing cannot occur. Nevertheless, this type of therapy, along with the adjuncts mentioned earlier, should definitely help create a healthier human being.

Allopathic Links to Models of Health Care Belief Systems

Aquatic Therapy: A Link Between Traditional Therapy and the Community

Darcy Umphred, Matthew Baudendistel, and Arthur Baudendistel

The use of water and body immersion has been a part of physical therapy practice and intervention since the very beginning of the profession, but the clinical focus has generally been on musculoskeletal impairments and functional limitations.[462,463] In the past, these interventions have not been as frequently cited as a common therapeutic approach to assist patients with movement impairment that developed from neurological disorders. Today, research has shown the beneficial effect of aquatic therapy for both pediatric and adult patients with certain neurological disorders. Individuals with medical diagnoses of CP,[464,465] CVA,[466-470] MS,[471-474] PD,[475-477] and SCI[478] have been able to improve aspects of movement function when aquatic therapy was part of their intervention protocol. Specific benefits of aquatic therapy in patients with these disorders include evidence for improving mobility factors such as dynamic balance and gait speed, with the goal being to achieve an optimal level of quality of life.[479]

With the use of water as a medium or base for movement therapy, there are additional attributes that therapists need to consider. First, the viscosity or resistance of the water can add resistance to movement, giving the patient additional feedback, as well as slowing down movement if control is needed. Second, the water adds buoyancy or support of the body, which allows freedom of movement without the same demand for gravity when on dry land, as well as reduces the fear of falling. Lastly, the thermodynamic of water allows heat to be transferred into the water at a much higher rate than when moving against air.[473] All of these components can contribute to the patient feeling less anxious, more capable, and having greater willingness to participate in the activity.

With the development of underwater equipment such as bikes and treadmills, therapists can begin to teach movement activities that lead to strength, endurance,[480,481] cardiovascular fitness, and balance. Individuals with various movement disorders following neurological insult have benefited from aquatic therapy and improved their functional abilities.[467,478,482,483] Although different types of exercises have been introduced within the water environment without one standing out as superior, the consistent outcomes for intervention are that aquatic therapy helps patients regain functional skills and improves their quality of life.[474,482,484,485] Aquatic therapy has a beneficial effect on the cardiovascular system by reducing its demands and cardiac workload.[470] This is due to the redistribution of blood from the dependent limbs to the thoracic cavity that occurs with head-out water immersion. This is an important benefit particularly for anyone who is at risk for stroke or recurrent CVA, as it enables the patient to reap the benefits of exercise and movement while reducing cardiac workload and blood pressure, thereby minimizing the risk for stroke. This is evident by the reduction in systolic, diastolic, and mean blood pressures. In addition, the rate pressure was significantly reduced with underwater treadmill training compared with land treadmill training.[470] This is an important finding, as it allows the chronic stroke population to become more physically active through aquatic exercise while keeping their risk for recurrent insult at a minimum and preventing the deleterious effects of physical inactivity.[470] Although future research needs to be done to correlate this study with other populations of individuals with movement problems associated with neurological insult, the potential bridge is certainly present.

Individuals with neurological movement disorders may have their core postural muscle system compromised, which leads to less stability within the trunk and axial musculature and limits movement, with potential for fall risk. This risk by gravity can be reduced or eliminated within the aquatic environment. These same movement limitations and fears often lead to inactivity, which has been shown to cause additional health problems.[486,487] Thus it is critical to motivate individuals to move in a safe environment, which encourages freedom of movement in aquatic therapy.

One additional attribute of aquatic therapy is within the area of pain management. Research linking aquatic therapy with patients who have both motor impairments and back pain has demonstrated positive outcomes.[488–490] Back pain may develop prior to the neurological insult due to lifestyle choices, poor posture, and inactivity; as a result of a neurological insult and trauma; or as a secondary problem due to the postural instability of the trunk and abnormal movement patterns. The original causation of the pain is a medical problem, but the movement impairments pain causes limits function. Regardless of the etiology, back pain often causes impairments in functional mobility, strength, and self-reported disability and can increase fall risk. Patients arrive to therapy to relieve pain, regain function, and improve quality of life.[491–493] If exercise in the water reduces pain and the fear of additional pain during movement, an environment that optimizes learning

can be created and participation in activities within the aquatic environment more motivating. Aquatic therapy offers the opportunity to take away the force of gravity due to buoyancy and support the trunk through water pressure, and flotation tools can support any body part, thus reducing pain. Water can help reduce anxiety and fear of additional pain, in addition to creating a social environment where patients can interact and participate in water activities. Although no study has been done that links back pain specifically with neurological movement disorders, the obvious association can be drawn by watching individuals within this population move during any functional activity and by listening to their complaints.

Although all of these concepts when linked with pain management and musculoskeletal impairments are familiar to therapists, oftentimes the carryover to aquatic therapy's overall benefit to function in patients with neurological challenges is limited. Similarly, patients with movement limitations often never regain the total function that may have been lost following their specific insult or disease progression. For both reasons, these individuals need to maintain and/or continue to practice the movements that will lead to functional recovery or participation in life as defined by the individual. Once individuals leave a traditional therapeutic environment, such as acute, rehabilitation, or outpatient therapy, what was learned needs to become a life activity, where movements are practiced and environments challenged to facilitate nervous system learning and potential neuroplasticity. Aquatic therapy is an important link between clinic-based intervention and community-based activities. Aquatic movement exercises can become a life activity once the individual completes clinical therapeutic interventions. There is evidence that aquatic therapy can help maintain functional skills and life participation and continue to engage individuals in group activities that create a social and motivating environment.[494–500]

Note: A case study on Aquatic Therapy can be found in the online resources associated with this text.

Electroacupuncture and Dry Needling
Mary Lou Galantino

Acupuncture, a part of traditional Chinese medicine, has been used for more than 4,500 years. Mapping of 12 meridian points, which are named primarily after the visceral organs they transverse, incorporates 361 regular points. There are also "Ashi points," which are typically tender points used for treatment of pain syndromes.[501] The acupuncturist must decide which acupuncture points to stimulate on the basis of a specific diagnosis. The goal is to balance chi, which is considered vital energy. If there is an imbalance caused by disease, the altered flow of chi can be detected and subsequently treated through needles or electrical stimulation over specific acupuncture points.

Training for acupuncture varies throughout the United States (refer to the section on traditional acupuncture). Because needling is considered an invasive technique, physical therapists are prohibited from incorporating acupuncture in clinical practice. Therefore an alternative to needle acupuncture is noninvasive electroacupuncture (EA) or electrical neurostimulation. Concerning the effects of electrical neurostimulation, there are various interpretations of the methods and underlying physiological mechanisms. One mechanism is neural.[502] Another study has indicated that electrical stimulation applied to acupuncture points may activate both neurological and endocrine functions that control pain.[502] Anderson and Lundeberg's study supported the release of β-endorphin and oxytocin, which are important for the control of pain and the regulation of blood pressure and body temperature.[502]

Therapeutic effects of electroacupuncture. The use of acupuncture is gaining popularity in most Western countries,[503] and the effectiveness of EA as a modality for the treatment of pain has significantly decreased VAS scores.[504] With the increasing acceptance of acupuncture as an effective modality for pain relief, the scope of research on this modality has widened considerably to include other health care conditions. The intensive research efforts on other therapeutic effects of acupuncture have produced encouraging results.[505–507] These results point to a reduction in pain, improvement in motor function, better balance, and improved gait; the results therefore have a neurophysiological interpretation.

The conditions most commonly treated with EA include musculoskeletal, neurological, obstetric, and gastrointestinal, along with intraoperative and postoperative analgesia. EA studies, particularly with low frequency stimulation, are more likely to support the role of endogenous opioid mechanisms than manual acupuncture studies, and opioid release is more likely in the CNS than the circulation. EA is used in clinical and especially experimental research, particularly for nonpain conditions. Acupuncture does release endogenous opioids, but this probably depends on "dosage," with the evidence more consistent and convincing for EA than for manual acupuncture. Different frequencies of EA appear to activate different endogenous opioid mechanisms.[508]

The effect of spasticity has been explored by researchers for multiple diagnoses such as SCI and stroke. EA has been found to have more of an effect on spasticity the earlier the treatment is implemented, ideally within 3 weeks of injury. Findings reveal positive short- and long-term effects;[509–511] however, future research needs to include frequency of treatment and specific points of stimulation for a more comprehensive understanding.[512] Some of the possible mechanisms by which acupuncture may affect motor function include the following:

1. Stimulation of the release of endogenous opioids.[513]
2. Changing of the amplitude of end plate potential, thus facilitating the events at the neuromuscular junctions. It has been suggested that peripheral factors contributing to the potentiation of a reflex (e.g., the H reflex) may affect the afferents and the neuromuscular junction.[514]
3. Stimulation of the sensory system, which will result in integrative actions at the spinal cord level, where acupuncture may facilitate the stretch reflex arc through both the γ and α motor neurons. Facilitation may depend on the intensity and timing of the stimuli used to activate muscle afferents.[515]
4. Revealed on neuroimaging of acupuncture in patients with chronic pain, changes in cerebral blood flow associated with pain and acupuncture analgesia that correspond to areas of the brain involved in such phenomena.[515]

EA combined with conventional rehabilitation care has the potential of reducing spasticity in the upper and lower limbs and improving overall and lower extremity motor function and activities of daily living for patients with spasticity, within 180 days post-stroke.[516]

Further studies of high methodological and reporting quality are needed to confirm the effects and safety of EA and to explore the adequate and optimal protocol of EA for post-stroke spasticity, which incorporates comprehensive outcome measures with different populations. Eighteen systematic reviews were evaluated for evidence in a range of nonpharmacological interventions currently used in managing spasticity in various neurological conditions. There is "moderate" evidence for electroneuromuscular stimulation and acupuncture as an adjunct therapy to conventional routine care (pharmacological and rehabilitation) in people following stroke.[517] Electrical sensory input can contribute to routine rehabilitation to improve early post-stroke lower-extremity impairment and late motor function, with no change in spasticity. Prolonged periods of sensory stimulation, such as TENS,

combined with activity can have beneficial effects on impairment and function after stroke.

Research

Acupuncture is beneficial in some peripheral neuropathies, but more rigorously designed studies using sham-acupuncture control groups are needed to characterize its effect and optimal use.[518] Research on the effects of EA on HIV-related neuropathy found significant reduction in pain, which suggests an excitatory effect on the neuromuscular system. Such an effect may be on membrane potential (possibly through influencing ionic transport) and improvement in body fluid circulation.[519] The effect on the sympathetic system is often reduced, and the same explanation is proposed for the action of electrical stimulation on pain,[520,521] with some effects on pain-mediating neurotransmitters at the level of the spinal cord and an endogenous modulation from the brain stem.[522] All reviewed trials of acupuncture for neuropathy and neuropathic pain use acupuncture points that are closely associated with the peripheral nerves treated. Local needling is crucial for successful treatment of peripheral neuropathy.[523]

In patients after cardiac surgery, relief of pain through EA was shown to reduce the use of opioids such as fentanyl.[524] One case report showed excellent results in chronic pain reduction over a 2-year period in a patient with a pacemaker. In answer to the initial question regarding safety, EA was shown to be an excellent alternative for individuals with pacemakers.[525]

Studies have shown that EA may enhance the effect of strength training on motor function. One study compared upper-limb motor functional improvement in chronic stroke survivors who received a combination of EA and strength training with that of subjects who received strength training alone. After the combined treatment, the quantitative spastic level, active wrist extension range of motion, and Fugl-Meyer upper-limb motor score changed significantly. No significant changes were noted in isometric wrist strength. The strength training alone resulted in no significant changes to any measured variable. These results indicate that the combined acupuncture and strength training treatment reduced muscle spasticity and may have improved motor function for chronic stroke survivors with moderate or severe muscle spasticity.[526]

Although two mechanisms underlying the physiological mechanisms of EA were presented previously, it would be prudent for physical therapists to consider maximizing the benefits of electrical modalities in various musculoskeletal and neurological disorders.[527] One prospective study[528] investigated the physiological effects of stimulation of acupuncture points ST36 and ST39 of the stomach meridian with Dynatron 200 microcurrent. Hemodynamic functions and skin temperature were monitored, with no significant differences found. However, further research is necessary to elucidate the nature of physiological effects of specific surface electrodes and various types of stimulation to determine the efficacy of EA treatment.

Research applying EA on the PC6 acupoint found reduction in postsurgical nausea and vomiting. A review of 5 trails that included 426 patients studied nausea rates from 0 to 24 hours after surgery in which PC6 electroacupuncture was used to reduce nausea rates from 54.50% to 26.51%. The same studies were used to assess the use of PC6 electroacupuncture to reduce vomiting postoperatively from 0 to 24 hours; rates were reduced from 35.07% to 17.67%. When compared with PC6 acupressure and PC6 acupuncture, PC6 electroacupuncture was found to be the most effective in reducing postoperative vomiting between 0 and 24 hours after surgery and had the lowest RR rates. In addition to lowering the rate of nausea and vomiting postoperatively, electroacupuncture also has a pain-relieving effect. More research is needed to see if combining electroacupuncture of the PC6 acupoint with others would have a great effect.[528,529]

A review of different types of acupuncture used for the treatment of fibromyalgia found that electroacupuncture was the best for improving pain, overall well-being, sleep, stiffness, and fatigue. The most effective treatment sessions were found to have occurred for 25 minutes twice a week for 4 weeks with the use of 2 to 5 Hz of electrical stimulation on the acupuncture points of ST36 and L14. More research is needed in the areas of needle depth, other acupoints, and choice of needles in the treatment of fibromyalgia.[530,531]

As mentioned in the acupuncture section, dry needle therapy (DN) is used by physical therapists to reduce pain and musculoskeletal movement problems. Dry needle therapy is a method of needling the trigger points using a syringe needle without the use of a drug and is commonly used for pain at the shoulder, neck, waist, and back. The available literature shows mixed results from DN, but it is becoming an accepted treatment for pain.[457−459,460,532−537] In an RCT for patients post-stroke,[538] the inclusion of deep DN into a treatment session following rehabilitation strategies was effective at decreasing spasticity and improving balance, range of motion, and the accuracy of maintaining stability.[539,540] Specific to upper extremity fine motor skills, DN reduced wrist flexors spasticity and α motor neuron excitability in patients with stroke, and improvements persisted for 1 hour after DN.[541] This research is growing significantly as DN becomes common practice in rehabilitation settings. Thus noninvasive EA and DN may have positive impact on spasticity and result in improvements in quality of life.

Lymphedema Management for Patients With Neurological Movement Disorders

Jennifer Brooks and Arlette Godges

Edema management is a skill that belongs in every clinician's toolbox and may begin with basic elements, including elevation, rest, and other strategies taught in entry-level clinical education. Manual lymphatic drainage (MLD) and complete decongestive therapy (CDT) is an approach considered traditional physical therapy in many European countries (but not in the United States) and is often primarily associated with postsurgical cancer patients. Yet most patients with swelling problems could benefit from approaches used in this therapeutic intervention. This is often referred to as *lymphedema management* or complete or complex decongestive therapy.[542]

In the United States, there are various training and certifications available, with differing schools of thoughts regarding the approach. All forms of decongestive therapy include the same basic components: MLD, skin care, exercises to improve lymphovenous drainage, compression in some form, and patient education. The use of pneumatic compression pumps, kinesiology tape, garments, and multilayered compression bandages or alternatives are used to enhance the experience and effectiveness of treatments[543] based on an individual's need and preference.

As a bundled intervention,[544] MLD/CDT has been found to be effective in lymphedema management; however, continued compliance with self-care is of utmost importance. The intent of this section is to remind therapists that a consultation with a trained lymphedema specialist may be particularly helpful for optimal and comprehensive patient care for a patient with chronic swelling issues, with the end goal of training patients, family members, and friends to use this modality to improve function, decrease pain, and decrease the burden of comorbidities limiting functional activities. Edema may collect for many reasons, such as after trauma or injury, with infection, when a limb is left in a dependent position, or other more concerning "red flag"

causes, such as congestive heart failure, kidney dysfunction, cancer-based lymphatic obstruction, or deep vein thrombosis (DVT).[545] In the current environment of direct access practice and autonomous practice, any new swelling or edema should be viewed from a differential diagnostic perspective, and may require referral to physician for further testing, particularly in our most vulnerable populations. Swelling can be found in both healthy and unhealthy tissues, or as a result of another disease or injury process, but lymphedema is a specific condition involving abnormal accumulation of high protein lymphatic fluids as a result of lymphatic dysfunction or compromise[546] that requires physician diagnosis. It is important to embrace opportunities for a collaborative care model, including referral to physiatry or other medical specialty for proper diagnosis, followed by referral to a lymphedema specialist, for optimal and comprehensive patient care.

Integrating Lymphedema Therapy in Neurorehabilitation

Although the most common medical condition where CDT is used is in cancer survivors with lymphedema, comprehensive edema management interventions can be a bridge to a more effective and successful course in neurorehabilitation.[547] It is a concept often missed in busy practices and settings outside of oncology. Any patient will logically have better outcomes, with less swelling and collection of fluids in their tissues. Although the literature supports the use of lymphatic drainage in orthopedic injuries,[548] MLD/CDT has a place in the treatment of all individuals with diagnosed lymphatic dysfunction, no matter the underlying medical or referral diagnosis.[543] Properly implemented treatments to decrease swelling after injury or trauma will lead to a faster rehabilitation toward optimal function.

Our neurology patients can greatly benefit from this different perspective. Patients with neurological impairments, such as CVA or SCI, can develop swelling of upper and lower extremities due to low motor function and general immobility, possibly triggering a secondary lymphedema. While there is little research on these populations, one retrospective study found CDT approach to be safe and well-tolerated by patients with SCI. The intervention was associated with decreased edema, was feasible for use in a clinical setting, and recommended CDT approach for management of edema in individuals with SCI, while remaining vigilant about skin inspection.[549]

With lymphatic therapy, a body's natural pathways are utilized to return the lymph into the circulatory system and eliminate it effectively from the body without excessive strain. Many clinicians need to be reminded that MLD techniques and lymphedema management services are becoming more widely available as trained lymphedema specialists are more prevalent. Decreased swelling in extremities may lead to decreased pain and earlier ability to weight bear on extremities for functional tasks. The ability to incorporate the breath and perform active movement may enhance further healing as it increases a muscle pump, efficiently increasing lymph flow and restoring tissue homeostasis.[550] Working with diaphragmatic breathing and treatment in the abdominal region[551] may improve the patient's overall wellbeing and create opportunity for improved mobility via core awareness. A secondary benefit is increased oxygenation throughout, including imperative brain areas responsible for mood and motivation.

It is important to consider precautions and relative contraindication to consider when using MLD/CDT principles. For the diagnoses listed as follows, treatment of diagnosed lymphedema may still be indicated in individual cases and may require additional monitoring or oversight:

General: acute infections, uncontrolled asthma or COPD, cardiac edema, history of or suspicion of malignancy, acute bronchitis, renal insufficiency and/or bladder dysfunction, and hypertension.

Head and neck: cardiac arrhythmia, age >60 (possible sclerosis of vessels), thyroid disorders, and sensitivity of carotid sinus.

Abdominal treatment: pregnancy, menstrual cycle (relative), recent abdominal surgery, radiation therapy related complications, chronic inflammatory conditions (e.g., ulcerative colitis, Crohn disease, diverticulitis, etc.), undiagnosed abdominal pain of any kind, aortic aneurysm or suspicious symptoms, and diabetes (relative).

Lower extremity: acute DVT, phlebitis, thrombophlebitis, arterial disease, and acute infections.

Special considerations should be given and close multidisciplinary coordination will be required for modified or full MLD/CDT for the following populations: those with hypertension, paralysis, or paresis, sensory loss or changes, diabetes, asthma, malignant lymphedema, or pulmonale/congestive heart failure.[552]

In conclusion, the most powerful component of MLD/CDT is patient and family education. Family members and patients can be trained in edema management to the best of their ability, whether temporary or more chronic and long-lasting. There is evidence to support the adoption of remedial exercises in the management of lymphedema and for a greater emphasis on self-treatment practice. Empowerment care for themselves with access to supportive professional assistance has the capacity to optimize self-management practices and improve outcomes from limited health resources. Family members[553] and patients can be assisted with simple diagrams of the system and arrows pointing the direction of optimal flow. It is important to create a safe and encouraging environment. This can be established with informing patients and caregiver that even if their techniques are not textbook perfect, any mobility and any movement of the fluid helps. It may be less effective, or less permanent, but it still is of no harm and may provide some relief from the discomfort of the swelling via comforting touch. Explanation of why this is an effective way to help the family member and why a sedentary life is harmful and increases the risk of more fluid accumulation is also important.

The use of decongestive modalities in the care of our patients with neurological movement limitations is underutilized. Untreated swelling, lymphedema or not, becomes a cycle of pain and disuse, leading to immobility and breakdown of normal tissue. Joining lymphedema and edema management to other rehabilitative offerings and complemental care, such as yoga, Pilates, aquatic therapy, and meditative breathing, will enhance outcomes and quality of life for our patients.[554] For this reason, decongestive therapy can be considered an integrative therapy approach. It can easily be combined with other interventions along with traditional therapy services. The end result is empowering the individual back to optimal function and enhancing quality of life.

Music Therapy

Concetta M. Tomaino and Therese Marie West

Music therapy is the clinical and evidence-based use of music interventions to accomplish individualized goals within a therapeutic relationship by a credentialed professional who has completed an approved music therapy program.[555]

Although music is not a "universal language" in the sense that a particular piece of music would have the same meaning and effect for any person anywhere, music *is* a universal human phenomenon. Most people today could describe ways in which music might be used to enhance health or well-being, and we find evidence of the use of music as part of healing practices throughout history.[556,557] Within a first worldview perspective, magical or mystical powers were attributed to music, and healing occurred within a context of social structures and shared beliefs. Music was often a part of rituals conducted by a shaman or healer who served as a spiritual intercessor or guide in a process

designed to reestablish balance and harmony for the individual. Music, sometimes with dance, served as a gateway to altered states of consciousness and entry to deep altered states of consciousness, where creative experiences manifested multiple sources of information not available through observation alone. This process supported insights about the causes of and remedies for physical, emotional, social, and spiritual imbalance. Where patient, healer, family, and community members participated together in healing rituals involving the use of music, treatment occurred within the natural environment and social fabric of everyday life. Examples of music healing within a first worldview perspective can still be found within indigenous cultural groups to this day.

The rise of the second worldview brought new values that emphasized logical and rational approaches to the use of music to address health issues. During this phase in history, we see the first examples of published work asserting the theory that music could influence emotions and mood states, thereby improving physical or mental health.[556] Anecdotal evidence and case reports were used to support emerging theories and practices into the early 20th century. In the latter part of the 20th century, we began to see the scientific method applied systematically to the study of music in relation to single variable changes in (1) disease and pathological states or (2) functional activities and willingness to participate in rehabilitation treatment settings. Researchers continue to explore possible mechanisms through which music may contribute to improved physical or mental health via its influence on various factors such as emotional responses, mood states, relaxation, activation, or motivation.

History of music therapy. In the United States, music therapy began to develop as a profession after World War II, when it was found that music could facilitate both physical rehabilitation and recovery from emotional trauma in veterans returned from the war. Although early music therapists were often musician volunteers, music educators, or musician-physicians, it had become clear that specific education and training were needed, and music therapy curricula and academic programs were developed beginning in the mid-1940s. The first professional music therapy organization (the National Association for Music Therapy [NAMT]) was formed in 1950. A second professional organization, the American Association for Music Therapy (AAMT), formed in 1971. The NAMT and AAMT merged in 1998 to form the American Music Therapy Association (AMTA). The AMTA sets standards for education and clinical training in music therapy programs accredited at more than 70 colleges and universities in the United States and Canada. The Certification Board for Music Therapists (CBMT) was accredited in 1986 by the National Commission for Certifying Agencies and certifies music therapists to practice throughout the United States. Certification is via competency-based certification process that includes specialized coursework, 1,200 hours of supervised clinical training, and a certification board examination. There are currently more than 7,900 music therapists maintaining the MT-BC (Music Therapist, Board Certified) credential and participating in at least 100 hours of continuing education for recertification every 5 years to maintain and increase competencies for practice in this rapidly evolving field.[558] Music therapists may also need to obtain a state license. The development of music therapy in the United States parallels the stages of health care development as discussed earlier (see the discussion of historical perspective in this chapter). The profession has advanced in clinical research providing evidence-based models to advance the practice of music therapy. Therapists observe that patients who are unable to speak as a result of stroke or AD are often able to sing coherently when presented with familiar music. How is it that the gait of a patient with PD improves markedly in the presence of a rhythmic auditory stimulus?[559] How does music-evoked imagery (such as experienced with the Bonny Method of Guided Imagery and Music) alter physiological and psychological indicators of stress?[560,561] In recent years, advances in neuroscience have provided new understanding of how and why music and the components of music are effective in clinical interventions. In the United States, music therapy is recognized as "an established health profession in which music is used within a therapeutic relationship to address physical, emotional, cognitive, and social needs of individuals. After assessing the strengths and needs of each patient, the qualified music therapist provides the indicated treatment including creating, singing, moving to, and/or listening to music. Through musical involvement in the therapeutic context, patients' abilities are strengthened and transferred to other areas of their lives."[562]

Specialization. Music therapists develop specialized areas of practice, treating across the life-span from perinatal to palliative care, in schools, hospitals, skilled nursing, rehabilitation, outpatient, or community settings. Goals addressed support progress in developmental tasks, rehabilitation of physical and cognitive functioning, adaptation and coping, pain management, recovery from trauma, and quality of life. Music therapists work in private practice, as members of interdisciplinary teams, and as consultants and collaborators. There are many music therapists, including the authors, who work in rehabilitation settings in cotreatment, consultation, or collaboration with speech-language pathologists, physical therapists, and occupational therapists, as well as with a wide range of practitioners from other professions in medicine and mental health arenas. During early clinical collaborations in rehabilitation settings from the mid-1980s to the early 1990s, the authors found little research to support an understanding of observed phenomena in the rehabilitation clinic setting and had to depend largely on basic skills of music therapy assessment, careful documentation, and evaluation of treatment outcomes and effectiveness. In recent years, the music therapy profession has focused on increasing the quality and scope of research to support empirically validated best practice with reliable outcomes for a number of specific populations of interest to professionals in rehabilitation settings. Rehabilitation music therapists now have the benefit of empirically supported treatment protocols and continuing research regarding effectiveness and safety of music therapy methods. NIH is supporting music therapy research through the National Center on Complementary and Integrative Health (NCCIH),[563] with funding sources now available.

Music therapy in neurological rehabilitation. Music therapists have been working in neurological rehabilitation settings in the United States for more than 25 years. Tomaino[564] describes her long professional collaboration (from 1980 to 2015) with the neurologist Dr. Oliver Sacks and shares insights developed through extensive clinical application of music in the individualized assessment and treatment of various neurological diseases and injuries. Music can access intact neurological functions and is used to facilitate relaxation, increase attention and motivation, improve the readiness for (priming) and timing of motor activities, and enhance communication and emotional expression while providing supports for coping and adaptation. Tomaino[565–569] describes the music therapy process from assessment and treatment planning through treatment and evaluation of outcomes, focusing not only on physical and behavioral changes but also on the engagement of the whole person through a trust-based therapeutic relationship. Familiar music can provide the patient a sense of safety, with predictable elements of rhythm, melody (prosody), words and lyrics, and structure across time within socially and culturally relevant contexts. Musical elements are systematically applied to support functioning in cognition and memory, speech and communication, gait, and upper-extremity activities.

Music therapy has been used in many rehabilitation settings to support cognitive functioning in areas such as attention, sensory filtering and focusing, memory, sequencing, and executive functioning. Ongoing development of theoretical foundations for clinical uses of music in the cognitive treatment of those with brain insult or injury is supported by brain imaging and in vivo functional studies providing evidence of shared mechanisms among musical and nonmusical perceptual and cognitive brain functions[570] and effects of music on electroencephalographic activities in cortical networks.[571]

West has observed the phenomenon commonly reported in rehabilitation music therapy, where people with various aphasias are able to sing, but not able to speak fluently. The patient is often able to sing clearly in time with the singing of the music therapist, who adapts the tempo and other elements as needed. There appears to be an entrainment process, not only rhythmically, but also in elements of prosody and articulation. The mechanisms are not yet fully understood, but at least one study suggests that singing in synchrony with an auditory model (choral singing) may be more effective than choral speech in improving word intelligibility because choral singing may entrain more than one auditory-vocal interface.[572] Kim and Tomaino[573] have developed and pilot tested a music therapy treatment protocol for people with nonfluent aphasia, integrating extensive clinical experience with recent findings from experimental studies using cognitive-behavioral, electrophysiological, and brain imaging techniques. Whereas specific brain structures have been well established for speech and language and were thought to be distinct from music processing areas, it now appears that music and language may share some aspects of neurological processing in bilateral hemispheric activities.[573] The evolving brain research may help us better understand our clinical observations and will most certainly support increasingly effective treatment protocols for expressive aphasia.

One particularly valuable discovery in music therapy for neurological rehabilitation is the fact that rhythmic elements of music can influence the timing and execution of motor sequences in both gross motor and fine motor activities. A neuroscience approach to understanding potential effects of rhythmic auditory stimulation (RAS) and motor-rhythm synchronization phenomena in neurological rehabilitation is supported by a well-developed body of basic research and clinical studies with a number of rehabilitation populations.[574–576]

The use of music therapy with movement problems arising from brain areas associated with specific medical diagnoses can be found online and can be integrated with chapters that address specific medical diagnoses.

Music therapy as a complementary modality. Music therapy continues to play an important role in holistic care, even while some phenomena yet elude our scientific methods. West was asked to assess two different teenage boys, hospitalized and in comatose states after head injuries. The treating neurologist was preparing to recommend longer-term follow-up disposition for these young patients, and while considering all the medical evidence at his disposal, this physician also wanted to see what music therapy might discover in terms of responsiveness to stimuli. Although one patient showed no response of any kind to any auditory or tactile stimuli, the second patient proved to be a most interesting example of the mysterious recovery. His neurological tests indicated that his prognosis would be very poor; "persistent vegetative state" was the expectation. In the absence of any evidence that he could benefit from more intensive rehabilitation services, he would be sent to a facility where he would receive long-term custodial care but no therapies. During the music therapy assessment, this young man began to show signs of responsiveness to musical stimuli. A professional skeptic, West was reluctant to consider his eye gaze changes, head movement, and smiling to be meaningful responses to the music without additional testing. These could be random events coincident with the stimuli. West presented music in a popular style familiar to the patient (according to family sources) and gently applied tactile rhythmic stimulation to his hands, arms, legs, and feet in time with the music. The patient began to move his own extremities in rhythmic time to the music and continued to do so when the therapist removed her hands. The therapist carefully documented the procedures and patient responses and returned a report to the referring physician. Over the next few days, the patient's responsiveness increased dramatically. The neurologist had this young man placed in a rehabilitation treatment setting. A month later, he had begun to walk and showed promise of significant recovery of functions in a number of areas, including speech. This patient was initially medically evaluated as having little potential for recovery, yet after music therapy, he was interactive and a participant in life. This case is a good example of how music can access and bring forward what is yet intact (whole) within a person whose body has been damaged by illness or injury. More recent research by Magee illustrates the evidence for music therapy assessment and treatment for those with acquired brain injuries.[577]

Although basic and clinical research activities are increasing an understanding of "how" and "for what, when, and for whom," music therapy can be of specific benefit in neurological rehabilitation and medicine, music therapists are also facing the new challenges and opportunities of new worldviews. Music therapy is among the complementary modalities provided as part of a response to increasing demand for holistic and patient- and family-centered health care. With the increase in evidence-based practice and well as increased opportunities for collaborations between clinical and basic science researchers, the NIH has identified a new initiative to explore music and the mind.[578] Because music interacts with every domain of human experience (physical, cognitive, emotional, social, and spiritual), it has the potential to influence multiple needs simultaneously, in a unified way that respects both the uniqueness of the individual and the deep common ground of the person within the whole.

A case study presented in Box 39.1 and another case located in the online resources of this text illustrate how integrative therapy approaches can improve individuals' quality of life.

BOX 39.1   Integration of Philosophies—An Author's Experience

Darcy A. Umphred

This case study is being shared so colleagues can realize that there are many more unknowns in life than knowns. There may be clinical experiences that just do not match the available research or evidence within our profession or even in other professions or areas of science that might explain a treatment outcome.

This case began the day before I (Umphred) arrived at a Board of Directors' (BOD) spring meeting for a National Association. Each Board member was a health care provider and certainly based their practice on evidence at that time. One elected Board member had fallen on the way back to the hotel from dinner the night before. The streets were dark, the pavement uneven, and she stumbled and fell forward onto her chest and face. She went to the ED, and it was determined that she broke her nose and rib and was in a lot of discomfort/pain.[579] The next morning, I and other professional members representing various special interest groups had been invited and were present to join the meeting. During the morning, it was obvious that the BOD member that had fallen had hit her face very hard due to the swelling and distortion of her nose and the two black eyes she presented.

At the end of the day, I had planned to have dinner with that individual, who was a very cherished friend. We went to her suite to just talk and decide where to go for dinner. We began to talk, time went quickly, and we did not realize it was then 10 PM. We both decided it was too late to go for dinner. I turned to my friend and said, "Let me treat you and help reduce your pain and discomfort." I recommended that she get ready for bed, take whatever meds she needed, and then lay down on the bed, because I knew she would fall asleep during treatment if the treatment was effective in pain reduction and relaxation.

I asked her lay crosswise on the bed so I had access to her head and neck from the side of the bed. I pulled up a chair to sit and reduce the postural demand of my body. With me being relaxed, she could also relax during the treatment. I began by holding the sides of her head in my hands with my two index fingers across the occiput and C1. Her cranium rested in the palms of my hands totally supporting her head. Her ears were not covered to avoid any changes in sound. I then started doing slow gentle oscillation up and down the spine from the head region. As she began to relax, one could see that the oscillations or slight movement were beginning to flow from the head, first down into her cervical region and then down her entire spine and finally all the way to the feet.[580] Once relaxation was established, I did an occiput release to allow for full extension of the neck and increase range of motion and circulation to the head. Once released, I began to move her head slowly in a pure plane with slight flexion of the chin

(a small tucking moving) toward upper cervical flexion and then back toward extension. Then I slowly rocked the head into diagonal motions with flexion and extension. All movements were slow, and initially the range was small. I would feel the movement in the upper cervical region and then slowly increase the range as she relaxed and gave into the movement. As I moved her head, she showed no sign of resistance to the movement. As I began to increase the range of motion in all these diagonal movement, her CNS took over control and she began to move her head/neck from one position to another automatically. I did not resist any of her movement, just letting her continue in the direction and force as her nervous system directed and redirected. I just stayed connected to make sure she did not hurt herself. I am not a certified myofascial release therapist, but if one reads that literature, the term "Unwinding" can be found.[581,582] This response is often explained as a release of the memories of prior trauma to the muscles, fascia, the entire body, or the brain. Whether these memories are held in deep gray matter nuclei within the CNS or in the muscles or the fascia or the energy pattern around the person is truly theoretical, and the science not totally understood. A few years earlier, my friend had a brain tumor, which was successfully removed. I have no idea the emotional and spiritual memories or trauma that this experience may have caused my friend, and again it is not relevant. She continued to unwind and at times violently for at least 40 minutes. Finally, the movements slowed down and finally stopped. At that time, she was sound asleep and deep in relaxation.

I had just finished a level one Reiki course, which is explained earlier in a section of this chapter and as an approach is based in the philosophy of the use of energy. I knew I could not hurt my friend by trying Reiki, so I stood up in order that I could place my hands about 3 inches above the top of her head and body to feel my friend's energy field. Then I began to scan beginning above her forehead with my hands open and palms flat. As I approached the area over her eyes, the sensation I felt was a dipping toward the eyes or a valley as I approached and came over the eye sockets. So, I just held my hands over her eyes and visualized filling in the energy field under my hands until the dip was gone, and the energy felt as if it came back into balance. How exactly that thought process interacts with the energy around the person is dependent upon what you believe or have been taught. But once the process seemed complete, it gave me, a practitioner, the feeling or sensation of balance similar to having your hands on a solid surface, which is a smooth structure around the person. I continued to move off her eyes toward her nose. Again, there was a deep dip in what I felt as

BOX 39.1 Integration of Philosophies—An Author's Experience—cont'd

Darcy A. Umphred

the total energy field around my friend's nose. I used the same thought process used for the eyes until the nose area felt back in homeostasis or symmetrical. Then I continued down the body, and when I reached her ribs, especially on the right side again, it dipped. My intent was once again to pull the energy back up or to fill in the gap with energy that I perceived was coming through me and my palms into her energy field. At the time, I truly had no neuroscience research to substantiate either rationale but could not deny the sensations I felt in my hands and palms, which suggested that the energy gaps were gone. Once the gaps were no longer present, it felt as if I was pushing on a very calm, smooth surface. After I finished scanning the entire body, I turned off the light in the hallway and went down to my own room to sleep. I had been treating my friend in very little light, so I could not physically observe if any change had occurred, but my friend was very relaxed and in a deep sleep, which was my initial intent. Today, there is research to[313] substantiate the Reiki intervention I provided, but at the time I simply responded to her body and what it was telling me. (Please refer to the section on Reiki within this chapter for additional research.)

The next morning, I arrived before my friend and was sitting in my seat. When my friend walked into the room, her eyes were no longer black, her nose straight, and the swelling was reduced tremendously. I was surprised to say the least, but was pleased to see my friend out of all that discomfort. The president of the Board looked shocked and asked her: "What happened between when you left the meeting yesterday and this morning?!" She said in a relaxed voice that I had treated her and that her rib pain was also gone. So, the entire Board turned to me at one time and the President asked: "What have

you done!!??" I told him "physical therapy" because I did not know what else to say. Although today, the research may give us a better indication as to potential variables that affected the outcome of the previous evening,[313,579-583] I was as shocked as the BODs. In reality, I had not even known she had broken a rib. I just felt that dip the previous evening around her ribs and visualized bringing the energy back into balance. All I can now say is: "I did my usual approach to relaxing the body and getting rid of pain, letting her body unwind previous memories, and then treated her using Reiki." Some colleagues would say I also did craniosacral from the head, as well as Feldenkrais using gentle oscillation. It could be any if not all of these integrated techniques that helped my friend regain function and reduce the pain. The one fact that was obvious was something significantly happened that evening to change her quality of life. Whether what happened was her self-healing, the energy around her fostering recovery, some of the various techniques employed playing a role in what happened, or all of them together as an integrative whole, again does not matter. What is important to realize is that all these techniques can fall under integrative approaches to treatment. None of those present that day at the meeting would deny significant healing or change had occurred in those 12 hours. Similarly, we would have all agreed that those changes were far beyond our evidence-based research, even today when considering the evidence and environment as a whole. This case study illustrates there is much more going on in the learning environment between individuals than research can substantiate, especially when people are empowered to regain function and take hold of the quality of life they desire.

CONCLUSION

Darcy A. Umphred and Mary Lou Galantino

Before the clinician embraces any complementary or integrative approach, the individual needs to identify which philosophy or paradigm matches her or his own belief system and aligns with her or his own emotional safety issues. Tethering an understanding of any integrative approach or concepts to an established evidence-base professional model will allow clinicians to stretch beyond their comfortable paradigms. When treating patients, clinicians are not recommended to jump from one theory to another or from one intervention strategy to another without clinically reasoning why those choices have been made or without using outcome measures to illustrate clinically meaningful changes. Therapists, during their professional education, are taught to use an evidence-based model developed from current research and the most current scientific understanding of what leads to functional movement and participation in life. This quality of life is based on choices of the patients and not what functional activities professionals believe the patient should accept as important. Similarly, the student and clinician are taught to develop the ability to evaluate and analyze both normal and abnormal movement and synthesize what components within and outside the human body will influence those movements. Emphasis is placed on movements that lead to the functional skill that allow individuals to interact in daily living and work environments and those movements that the patient considers critical for quality of life. The last category encompasses valued functional movements such as golf, gold panning, fly fishing, birdwatching, hiking in the mountains, scuba diving, playing cards, social sports, leisure interactions, or any other functional activities of importance identified by the patient. Therapeutic variables that might influence the quality of movement may or may not be a result of the disease or pathology commonly considered the reason for medical management

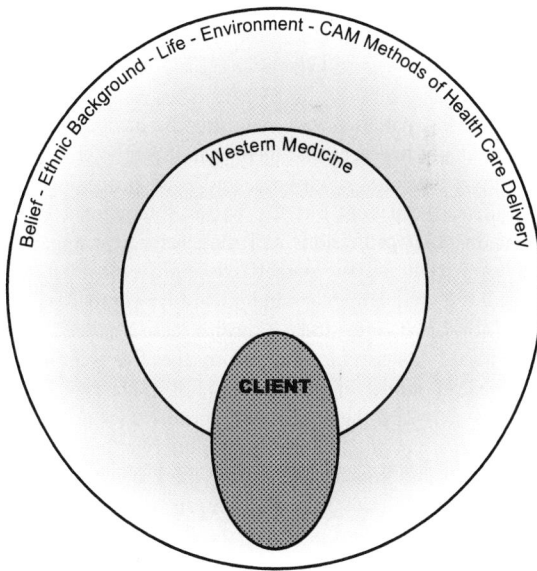

Fig. 39.7 Patient enters Western medicine owing to disease or pathological condition or with functional limitations that prevent participation in life. *CAM*, Complementary and alternative methods.

(Fig. 39.7). No one who studies and works with individuals who have had a CNS injury would imply that the medical management of that injury or disease is not critical to the outcome of the patient's motor recovery and/or quality of life. Simultaneously, clinicians in the past 20 years and today's clinicians have an in-depth scientific knowledge of motor control, motor learning, and neuroplasticity. These therapists observe, analyze, and influence motor, emotional, and

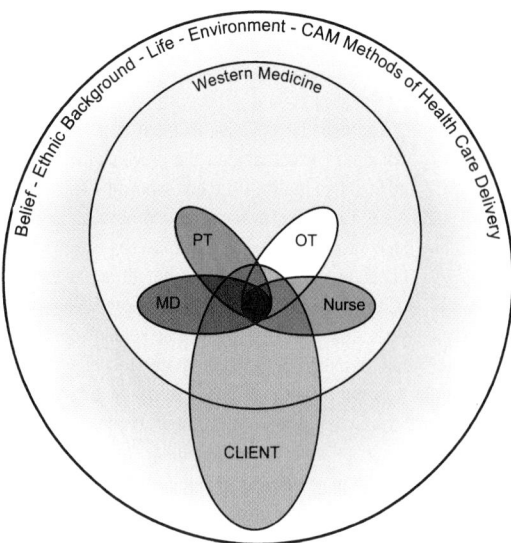

Fig. 39.8 Transdisciplinary Interactions Within Western Medical Model. *CAM,* Complementary and alternative methods; *OT,* occupational therapist; *PT,* physical therapist.

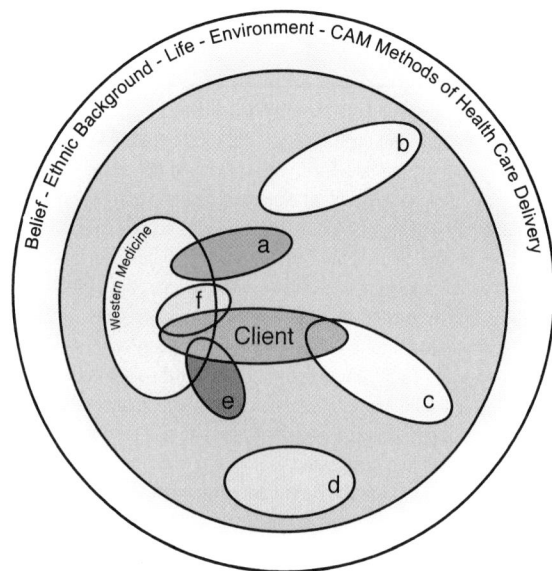

Fig. 39.9 Complementary and alternative methods *(CAMs)* of health care delivery. Some CAMs interact with Western medicine: *a, f, e;* Some alternative models do not interact with Western medicine: *b, c, d;* Some alternative models meet needs of the patient: *c, e, f;* Some alternative models do not meet the needs of the patient: *a, b, d.*

cognitive recovery in patients through movement interactions that physicians might have prognosed impossible. Physicians never want to imply false hope, but what therapists have learned about movement is that taking away hope for functional recovery can simultaneously take away motivation to drive the CNS to regain that function, which is critical for any potential recovery. (Refer to Chapters 3 and 4 regarding motor learning, neuroplasticity, and the limbic systems drive over motor function.) How an individual regains that functional control is often initially based on how the motor system easily learns to control those movements. (Refer to Chapter 2 on movement analysis across the life-span.)

When treating patients with neurological insults of any kind, students are taught to accept that there is an interdisciplinary interaction among professional disciplines, and each profession not only uniquely affects the patient but also has an interactive effect that is dependent on other professions and their respective impact on the patient's health, wellness, and potential to attain a maximal quality of life (Fig. 39.8). If complementary and integrative approaches to health care are introduced into today's health care models, then our colleagues need to determine which approaches link with the current Western medical model and which do not (Fig. 39.9). Why one approach interacts with the patient and another does not is based on the *patient's beliefs, needs, and responses* to intervention as well as the clinician's beliefs and knowledge. Because the professions of occupational and physical therapy have always been rooted and tethered to Western medicine, therapists need to critically analyze the interactions of those approaches that clearly overlap with our existing paradigm (Fig. 39.10). Disease and pathology link to medical practice and the use of surgery and medications, while PT and OT are linked to functional movement and movement analysis, which may or may not be tied closely to disease and pathology. As therapists we must realize that the CNS often learns in spite of disease and pathology, and functional outcomes are based on CNS learning and an individual's desire to learn and regain that function. Those components of integrative approaches that obviously overlap with acceptable practice and result in functional recovery following CNS trauma or change need to be identified and their effectiveness established and measured (Fig. 39.11). Evidence-based practice is considered the norm today and not just a gold standard. Yet clinicians must appreciate that evidence is often

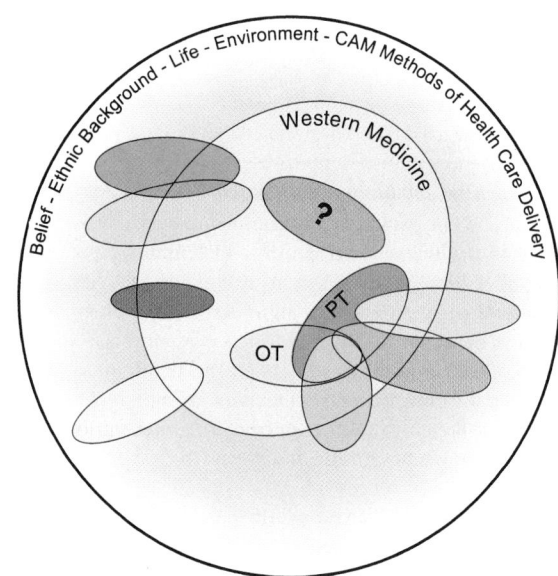

Fig. 39.10 Complementary and alternative methods *(CAMs)* interacting with Western medicine. Some models interact to a large extent with Western medicine and some to a small extent. Some models interact with both Western medicine and other complementary models. The extent of complementary interactions with either physical or occupational therapy or both reflect which models fall within respective scopes of practice and thus become part of the professional's treatment tools. *OT,* Occupational therapist; *PT,* physical therapist.

based on comparison of one variable against another and that our research tools cannot look at all variables simultaneously as seen when observing and interacting with a patient. Thus clinicians need to be constantly vigilant in analyzing the variables that affect recovery of functional movement. Accepting that a treatment will create change because the evidence suggests so does not guarantee that the specific patient will benefit optimally from the intervention. Thus when considering

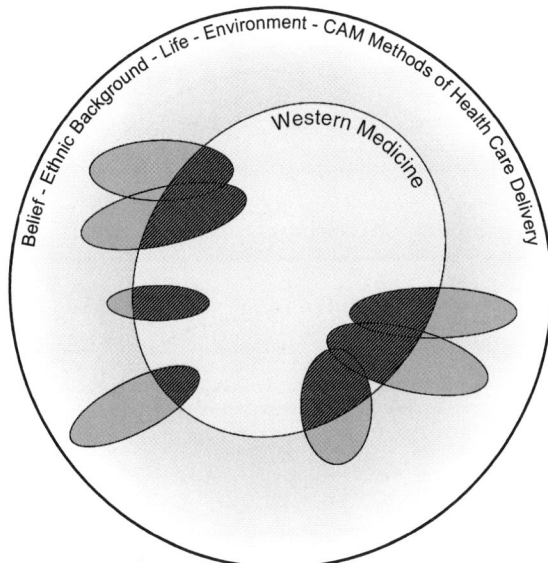

Fig. 39.11 The portion of each alternative or complementary model that overlaps with allopathic medicine and traditional occupational and physical therapy has been the focus of this chapter. As efficacy is established for those components that interlock, therapists will more readily accept these approaches as part of their practice. *CAM*, Complementary and alternative methods.

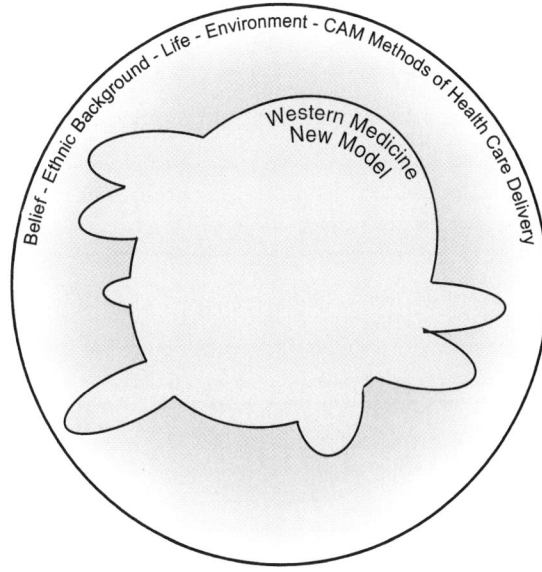

Fig. 39.12 New Model of Western Health Care Delivery Beyond Complementary Therapies. As the overlapping components of each alternative model are accepted as part of existing Western health care delivery practice, the barriers to the remaining aspects of these models become transparent. With barriers disappearing, a new model with a different shape and different alternative becomes what will be known as traditional medicine in the future. *CAM*, Complementary and alternative methods.

using a "complementary or integrative treatment approach," therapists need to remain critical in their analytical skill to determine if the patient experiences clinically meaningful change and is *actually improving*. With the establishment of those clear clinical correlations (those that match Western science models and those that show improvement in the patient), the remaining components of identified complementary paradigms seem naturally to become part of the established delivery system. As a result, a new model for Western health care practice as identified by PT and OT is formed. This new more integrative model allows the therapist to be grounded in current evidence-based interventions while enlarging a professional comfort zone to encapsulate integrative models by objectively measuring individual patient outcomes to intervention. A clinician with a neuroscience background and these individual case study measurements can conceptually establish a new model (Fig. 39.12). A clinician must always be cognizant of the fact that despite the method, philosophy, or intervention he or she selects to help a patient reach a desired functional outcome, there is no way to eliminate the fact that other aspects of human system processing will be interacting and impacting the outcome. For a century, master clinicians have been observed treating patients. Often colleagues comment that, although therapists seem to use the same methods or treatment tools, they get different outcomes. The question is are those more successful therapists using other interventions without those techniques ever being brought to consciousness? That is, if as a therapist I am aware that I use myofascial techniques along with traditional intervention, could I also be affecting craniosacral rhythm or affecting chakras and energy fields even though I don't recognize that fact? Could I be setting the stage for the nervous system to learn by optimal augmentation without knowing the literature? Could that allow the patient's nervous system to select better options for motor responses and the learning of movement function? If so, what truly is leading to somatosensory retraining, motor learning, neuroplasticity, and eventual improved motor control

and function? It may be that master clinicians use *all* these integrative approaches along with traditional treatments but only verbalize the paradigm with which they are most comfortable and that they are most capable of verbally explaining. The adventure is a process of learning, enlarging one's skill to provide the best service to patients, and differentiating what **is** effective within the clinical setting from what **is believed** to be effective. Not all evidence-based treatment approaches will be as effective for all clinicians, nor will all patients respond exactly the same way, even though their medical diagnosis may be similar. Learning to differentiate true behavioral responses on a patient-by-patient basis from what one is taught should happen may attribute to the effectiveness of master clinicians. *Best practice is constantly evolving and changing.* As movement specialists, we have the responsibility to evolve as well. That change needs to come flexibly tethered to current knowledge and models of the human CNS and analysis of how humans learn or relearn functional control over movement. This leads to many options being available for enhancement of learning, emotional openness, and freedom to venture beyond a comfort zone while objectively measuring positive change in the functional abilities of our patients and improving quality of life as defined by the patient.

Additonal material regarding this chapter, including an in-depth discussion on the history of complementary and integrative therapies and sample cases, can be found on the accompanying Evolve site.

REFERENCES

To enhance this text and add value for the reader, all references are included on the companion Evolve site that accompanies this textbook. This online service will, when available, provide a link for the reader to a Medline abstract for the article cited. There are 583 cited references and other general references for this chapter, with the majority of those articles being evidence-based citations.

INDEX

A

AAMT. *See* American Association for Music Therapy
AANEM. *See* American Association of Neuromuscular and Electrodiagnostic Medicine
AAP. *See* American Academy of Pediatrics
Abbreviations
  in cardiovascular and pulmonary problems and their effect on function, 868
  in electrophysiological testing and electrical stimulation in neurological rehabilitation, 920
ABC Scale. *See* Activities-specific Balance Confidence (ABC) Scale
Abdominal binder, for early mobilization in spinal cord injury, 420–421, 421f
Aberrant movements
  in hemiplegia from stroke, 741–742
  underlying causes of, 741–742
Abscess, brain, 778–779
Absorption, of drugs, 1020
Abstract thinking, in dementia, 802
Abuse, substance, limbic system and, 105–106
Academy of Neurologic Physical Therapy Outcome Measures Recommendation, for traumatic brain injury, 648, 648t, 649t
Acceleration, causing traumatic brain injury, 641
Accelerometer, wearable, 590f
Accessory muscles of respiration
  effects of amyotrophic lateral sclerosis on, 460t
  training of, in spinal cord injury, 418, 418f, 419f
Accommodation
  in Piaget's theory of cognitive development, 23
  visual, 826, 826f, 830
    inconsistent, 833–834t
    interventions for dysfunction of, 841
    in traumatic brain injury, 653
Accuracy, 456
ACE inhibitors. *See* Angiotensin-converting enzyme (ACE) inhibitors
Acetic acid, in iontophoresis, 883
Acetylcholine (ACh)
  in basal nuclei, 537, 538
  in learning and memory, 85–86, 85f
Acetylcholine (ACh) antagonists, 538
ACh. *See* Acetylcholine
Acid-base imbalance, in traumatic brain injury, 642
Acoustic neuroma, 638, 765

Acoustic streaming, 880
Acquired immunity, HIV infection and, 956, 956f
Acquired immunodeficiency syndrome. *See* Human immunodeficiency virus (HIV) infection
Action potential, 891
  compound muscle, 891–892
  motor unit, 895
  sensory nerve, 892
Action tremor, cerebellar, 566
Active movement patterns, in hemiplegia, 737
Active standing, in balance assessment, 588–589, 588t, 590–591, 591f, 592f
Active stepping, in balance testing, 594–595, 595f
Activities of daily living (ADLs)
  in elderly with dementia, 814, 816–817
  in Parkinson disease, 548–549
  performed by toddler, 34
  physiological fitness reserve and, 856–857
  in spinal cord injury, 406–411t, 421–428, 422t
    bathing, 424, 425f
    bladder management, 424–426, 426f
    bowel management, 426–427, 426f, 427b
    dressing, 424, 425f
    effects of aging on, 985
    feeding, 422–423, 423f, 424f
    grooming, 423–424, 424f, 425f
    home management, 428
    sexual health, 427–428, 427t
  in traumatic brain injury, 649–650
Activities Scale for Kids, 310t
Activities-specific Balance Confidence (ABC) Scale
  in balance assessment, 598–599
  in multiple sclerosis, 524
Activity
  assessment and limitations of
    in balance dysfunction, 587
    in cerebellar dysfunction, 572
    functional training for, 177–179
    in hemiplegia from stroke, 730–731, 731b
    in multiple sclerosis, 523–525
    in traumatic brain injury, 649–650
  defined, 647
  effects of aerobic training on, 862
  focus, in genetic disorders intervention, 316, 318t
  functional performance and, tests of, for differential diagnosis, 157
  goal setting in spinal cord injury, 403–405, 406–411t

Activity limitations
  in amyotrophic lateral sclerosis, 459
  defined, 647
Activity log, for amyotrophic lateral sclerosis patient, 467, 468f
Activity monitors, 1046
Actuation terms, glossary of, 1037t
Acupressure, for pain, 884
Acupressure points, 1086
Acupuncture, 1085–1088, 1086f, 1087f
  benefits of, 1088
  electro-, 1089–1090
  examination and evaluation for, 1086
  five elements, 1086–1087, 1086f, 1087f
  in future treatments, 1088
  history of, 1085–1086
  in intervention, 1087–1088
  methods of, 1086
Acupuncture-like transcutaneous electrical nerve stimulation (TENS), 882
Acute bacterial meningitis, 779–780
Acute concussion
  evaluation of, 680–682
  evidence for physical and cognitive activity in, 687
  examination of, 679–682, 679t
  neurocognitive assessment of, 680
  oculomotor assessment of, 680
  recognition of, 679–680
  removal of, 680
  vestibular/ocular motor screening for, 681, 681t
Acute HIV infection, 954, 954–955t
Acute lymphocytic leukemia (ALL), 292, 300t
Acute pain, 869
Acute symmetrical polyarthritis, in HIV infection, 961–962t
Adams closed-looped theory, of motor learning, 340
Adaptation
  cerebellar learning and, 568–569, 569f
  in motor control, 53t
  neural. *See* Neuroplasticity
  in postural control and movement, 54
  in psychological adjustment, 116–117, 118
    cultural aspects of, 118
  in vestibular dysfunction, 625–634
Adaptation/gaze stability, exercises, 716t
Adaptive devices. *See also* Assistive technology devices
  for Guillain-Barré syndrome, 498
ADED. *See* Association for Driver Rehabilitation Specialists
Adeli suit, for cerebral palsy, 276
Adenoma, pituitary, 765

Page numbers followed by "f" indicate figures, "t" indicate tables, and "b" indicate boxes.

1099

Neurotransmitters
   of basal nuclei, 537–538, 537f
   in learning and memory, 85–86
   limbic system and, 82
Neurovascular entrapment syndromes, 502
   case study, 512, 514f
   classification of, 503–504, 504t
   common signs of, 511
   examination and treatment of, 506–512,
      507t, 509f, 510f, 511f
   interventions of, 511–512, 511f
   pain associated with, 505–506
   pathogenesis of, 504–505
   symptom patterns characteristic of,
      510–511
Neutral warmth, as exteroceptive input
      technique, 187t, 194
New normal, psychological adjustment and,
      118–120
Newborn behavioral observations (NBO)
      system, 219
Nicotinic acid, effects on rehabilitation,
      1015
NICU. See Neonatal intensive care unit
NIDCAP. See Neonatal Individualized
      Developmental Care and Assessment
      Program
NJCLD. See National Joint Committee on
      Learning Disabilities
NMES. See Neuromuscular electrical
      stimulation
No Child Left Behind Act, 323
Nociceptive pain, in multiple sclerosis, 527
Nociceptors, 870
   polymodal, 870
Nodes of Ranvier, 891
Non-sports-related concussion in adults,
      690–692
Noncardiac embolism, cerebrovascular
      accident and, 726–727t
Noncomitant strabismus, 832b
Noninvasive, positive-pressure ventilation
      (NIV), 465–466
Noninvasive brain stimulation, 1051–1057
   case study on, 1057b, 1058f
   clinical application of, 1055–1057, 1055t
   transcranial direct current, 1054, 1054f,
      1055f
   transcranial magnetic, 1051–1052, 1051f,
      1052f, 1053f
Nonlinear dynamics
   of cognitive development, 24
   general systems theory and, 17
   of motor development, 28, 30f
Nonlinear learning, in elderly, 816
Nonoptical vision aids, 836
Nonsteroidal antiinflammatory drugs
      (NSAIDs)
   commonly used, 1016
   effects on rehabilitation, 1016b
Nonverbal learning disabilities (NVLDs),
      326

Nonwearable assistive devices, 1033–1035,
      1035f
   screening for, 1040–1042t
   types of, 1043b
Normalization, kinesiological
      electromyography and, 899
Northwestern University Special Therapeutic
      Exercise Project (NUSTEP), 63–64, 176
Novice stage of motor learning, 60
NPC testing. See Near point of convergence
      (NPC) testing
NSAIDs. See Nonsteroidal antiinflammatory
      drugs
Nuchal rigidity, in bacterial meningitis, 780
Nuchal thickness (NT), with genetic
      disorders, 306
NUSTEP. See Northwestern University
      Special Therapeutic Exercise Project
Nutrition
   in amyotrophic lateral sclerosis, 465
   in cerebral palsy, 260
   in spina bifida, 362
NVLDs. See Nonverbal learning disabilities
Nystagmography, video, 625
Nystagmus, 618–619
   gaze-evoked, 619–620
   geriatric supine, 636b
   spontaneous, 624
Nystatin, in cancer treatment, 1012

O

Obesity
   in developmental coordination disorder,
      336
   effects on maximum oxygen
      consumption, 858
   in individuals with developmental
      disabilities, 1000
   in spina bifida, 362, 389–390
Object agnosia, 845, 846–847
Objective outcome measures, in hemiplegia
      from stroke, 736
Obligatory movement patterns, 57
Obstacle Course Assessment of Wheelchair
      User Performance in spinal cord injury,
      405t
Occipital lobe, brain tumor in, 766, 767f
Occupational therapy (OT)
   history of, 175–176
   therapeutic models for, 2
Ocrelizumab, 520t
Ocular motor assessment, of persistent
      postconcussion symptoms, 700
Ocular motor impairment, 699–700
Oculocutaneous albinism, 291
Oculomotor assessment, in cerebellar
      dysfunction, 570–571b
Oculomotor deficits, with cerebellar damage,
      567
Oculomotor dysfunction, 832–833
Oculomotor nerve lesion, 833–834t
Oculomotor training, exercises, 716t

Older persons. See also Aging
   chronic impairments in, 982, 996.
      See also Aging
   definition of terms associated with
      801–802, 801t, 802t
   framework for clinical problem solving,
      800–803
   motor development in, 39–41, 40f
   starting point in physical or occupational
      therapy and, 799–800
   Tae Kwon Do training for, 1071
   transplantation shock in, 810–811
   vision problems in, 835
Olfactory system
   in augmented therapy techniques, 191b
   limbic involvement in, 78
Oligodendroglioma, 765
OLSTs. See One-legged stance tests
On time and off time, in neuromuscular
      electrical stimulation, 900, 900f
Ondansetron, effects on rehabilitation, 1019
One-handed adaptations, resources for, 760
One-legged stance tests (OLSTs), in balance
      assessment, 589
One-step sparring, in Tae Kwon Do, 1069–1070
Open-angle glaucoma, 835
Open environment, in motor learning, 62–63
Open-loop theory, of motor learning, 340
Openness, limbic system and, 97–98
Operant conditioning, in pain management,
      886
Opioids, prenatal exposure to, 215–216
Optic and labyrinthine righting of head, 46
Optic nerve, 829f
Optic neuritis, in multiple sclerosis, 527
Optic tract, 828, 829f
Optometrist/ophthalmologist, referral to,
      837, 837b, 839–841, 840b
Oral hypoglycemic agents, effects on
      rehabilitation, 1018, 1018b
Oral-motor coordination, in Guillain-Barré
      syndrome, 493
Oral-motor therapy, 193–194
   for neonates, 234–235, 235f
Orgasm, spinal cord injury and, 427
ORLAU. See Orthotic Research and
      Locomotion Assessment Unit
Orofacial dyskinesia, 554
Orthopedic deformities, in spina bifida, 357,
      360–361
Orthopedic management, of spina bifida,
      366–370, 366f, 367f
Orthosis
   carbon fiber, 754
   in Guillain-Barré syndrome, 498–500
Orthostatic hypotension
   in Parkinson disease, 541
   in spinal cord injury, 412–414t
Orthostatic intolerance, 636b
Orthotic Research and Locomotion
      Assessment Unit (ORLAU), for
      spina bifida, 382